MW01349734

BOARDS READY™ STEPS 1, 2, 3

1st Edition

Comprehensive Review for the USMLE Board Exams
Step 1
Step 2
Step 3 CK, CS

Tricia A. Derges, MD

Boards Ready™ Steps 1, 2 3, First Edition

ISBN 978-0-9991720-0-1
UPC 720260683217

For information on book purchases for medical schools, residency programs, bookstores or distribution, please contact us at info@boardsready.com or at Boards Ready, 3259 E. Sunshine St., Suite AA, Springfield, MO 65804

Notice

The author has compiled sources and information believed to be reliable in efforts to provide information that is complete and in accord with medical standards that were current at the time of publication. Thousands of pages of medical notes, multiple medical textbooks, and reliable websites were used to crosscheck and verify facts. However, because medicine continually evolves, the author and/or publisher do not assume any responsibility, to the fullest extent of the law, for any errors, omissions, or injury out of or related to the use of material contained within this medical textbook. This textbook is not meant to provide medical or legal advice. This advice should only be sought from a professional in their respective field. It is always important to confirm the information contained within this book with other reliable medical sources. This is particularly true in the case of pharmacology. Drugs are taken off and added to the market daily.

The author has tried to give credit to the authors of each and every image or illustration in this medical textbook. Many hours were put into reaching out to all authors/sources. In the event that an author was unable to be located, images were used which were found in various places throughout the Internet and therefore believed to be within public domain. Public domain images used are believed to be within the US Copyright Fair Use Act (title 17, US Code). If you are the owner of any of these images and feel that it infringes your copyright, please contact us and we will be very happy to credit your work or remove the image on the next edition of this book. This textbook is solely used for the education of medical students and residents; therefore we would like to extend a *sincere appreciation to all of the authors and sources that have allowed us to use their work* in order to provide excellent medical education to our future and current doctors.

Image and Error Submission

I believe you will find Boards Ready to be a fresh, new way to learn and retain the medical information you will need for your Boards, as well as for use in future practice. I have worked hard to be as accurate as possible, but being human and the fact that medicine literally changes on a day-to-day basis, I am sure there will be errors. If you find any errors, new medical information, misspellings, new drugs, or any other important information that needs to be added, I would greatly appreciate if you could email those corrections or additions to me so that I can fix them in the next edition. **For corrections: Please include your source of information.**

If you would like to submit an image (illustration or photograph) for consideration of publication in the next edition or email regarding changes, corrections, additions, etc., **please email info@boardsready.com. Please put "BOOK INFO" in the subject line so that we can easily identify it. Thank you!**

Dedications

I am so grateful to my Heavenly Father for setting forth the path of this medical journey and for allowing me to lean on Him the entire way. To complete this path would have been impossible without Him by my side every step of the way. I am thankful to be able to serve Him now by serving others.

To my amazing husband, *Dan*. Thank you for supporting me throughout this long, difficult journey and not allowing me to quit. I am sure that saying goodbye to your wife for several long years of medical school wasn't something you had planned on when we married 30 years ago. You never complained once and even became a fabulous cook by making my dinners so I could study! You were a huge part of my success. I love you so much!

To my entire family! All 8 children and 18 grandchildren (19 coming in a few months!) and my brother, *Tommy*. You were always there to pick me up and support me when I questioned what I was doing. You never once thought I was crazy, and if you did, were kind enough to never let me know! I loved all your sweet phone calls, notes and emails, they always seemed to come when I needed them the most. *Families are Forever!* You were a huge part of my success. I love you all!
Jaime, Brandi, Justin, Callie, Emily, Derick, Amy, Rachel, Chris, Jim, Rachael, David, Jim, Garrett, Hailey, Chase, Logan, Reece, Nathan, Brody, Bennett, Jameson, Tyson, Brayden, Natalie, Sydney, Lyndon, Hunter, Cambria.

To my mom and dad, *Tom and Pat Ashton*, who have cheered me on from heaven. I can never forget or repay you for your examples of hard work, integrity and determination. You always believed in me and taught me that I could do anything I wanted if I put my mind to it and worked hard enough. I heard your voices of support many times through this difficult path. I love and miss you more than you can know. It will be so great to be able to talk to you about all of this one day!

To my 4.5 lb medical school companion, Rosie, my little Yorkie. She made every flight, slept in my arms every hour of the thousands of hours I studied, went on every evening walk to chase lizards and most importantly protected me from scorpions, centipedes, fire ants and monkeys! She even weathered a hurricane! There is no doubt, she was probably the greatest medical school companion in history! Thank you Dr. Rosie! You are the greatest little doctor dog in the world!

To the greatest doctors in the world! My training was second to none because of you. Each of you are amazing! You went out of your way to insure that I received only the best in training. Thank you for believing in me and supporting me every step of the way – and you still do to this day. I will always be eternally grateful to you for your training, your integrity and your examples. You are truly not just the top physicians and surgeons in Springfield, Missouri, but the country. It was such a blessing to be able to be trained at my own hometown hospital so I could stay close to my family.
Thank you: *Dr. Michael Galindo, Dr. Timothy Woods, Dr. William Moore, Dr. Anthony Richmond, Dr. Michael Hanks, Dr. James Gibson, Dr. Edgar Galinanes, Dr. Jamie Jones, Dr. Arthur Trask and Dr. Rebecca Farinas (Jacksonville, FL).*

My last dedication is to 2 doctors in a residency program and the CEO of their hospital. Their examples are a constant reminder of what kind of a person and doctor that *I never want to be like.* Unlike them, I will always treat those with "life experience" with respect and appreciate the value of what they have to offer, instead of choosing to humiliate and hurt them. I hope that I never see the day that I would ever tell anyone, in particularly a "mature" person to go somewhere else where they would "fit in". My personal message to these men: "I pray that no one ever treats your mother's as you have treated me".

A note to all residency programs: Nontraditional students have so much to give – please give them a chance. They have excellent communication skills, are dependable, ethical, understand real empathy and compassion, aren't afraid of hard work and love to learn! Patients desperately want more doctors like this today. I can personally guarantee that you will find that these "mature" individuals have much to offer and would be a valuable asset to your team!

TABLE of CONTENTS

About the Author

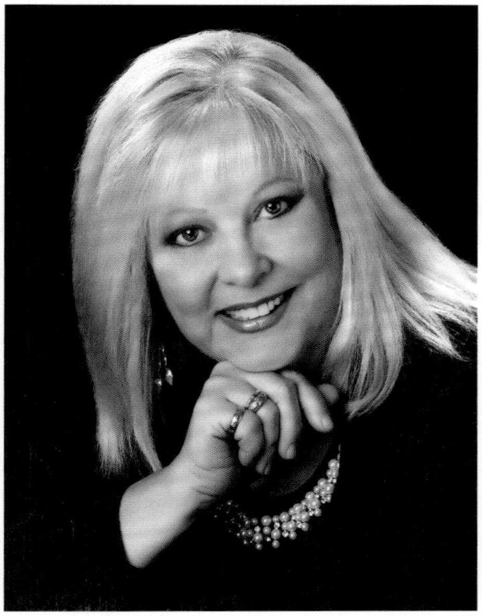

After operating as the CEO and founder of a manufacturing company for over 25 years and raising 8 children, I made the decision to go to medical school at the age of 52. This was extremely difficult. Most of the difficulty was due to the complicated medical terms and professors that seemed to think it was their responsibility to make things as difficult as possible. It was the old saying "it was hard on me, so it's going to be hard on you" mentality. I almost quit medical school because of this foolish mentality.
I am not one to quit, so I spent hundreds of hours breaking down the "complicated" terms and concepts of medicine to lay meanings, in order to better understand them. In doing so, I found out that most of these "complicated" things weren't so complicated after all. I quickly learned hat each medical term, fact, or process actually served as a parable to things I already understood in my day-to-day life. By shifting how I learned into a more visual and commonplace method, I was able to succeed; in fact, I graduated Summa Cum Laude of my medical school class. Along my journey I have seen hundreds of students fall victim to similar difficulties I faced, causing them to quit, tragically losing their dreams and thousands of dollars in tuition. So I made it a priority to try and simplify medicine so that this tragedy would stop. I founded Boards Ready in 2014, a USMLE® Step 1 and 2 review program, in which I teach "my unique method" of learning medicine.
Students from all over the world have come to me for guidance in earning the exam scores needed for the residency of their choice.

In addition to teaching Boards Ready, I have several medical clinics that students are able to take advantage of and receive core and elective rotation credits for their clinical training. These include a mission clinic, a rural clinic, and a pain management clinic. The mission clinic is named "Lift Up Springfield". During my clinical training, one of my very first patients went home to pull his own tooth with pliers because he had no money for care. I made a promise at that moment that once I became a doctor, that I would do something for those in need. In January of 2016 I founded "Lift Up Springfield", a medical and dental mission clinic. The clinic provides free medical, dental, and mental health services for the homeless, Veterans, poor, and uninsured. The clinic operates solely by volunteers and donations. As of July of 2017, the clinic has served over 8000 people. In June of 2017 I was awarded the National Jefferson Award for Missouri and the elite Jacqueline Kennedy Onassis Award for my work with the underserved at the mission clinic. Only 5 Jacqueline Kennedy Onassis Awards are awarded annually in the country. This award is considered the Nobel Peace Prize on the Community Level. I credit the awards I received to the amazing volunteers and their huge hearts that work continually to help those that are in need!

Introduction

I have spent the last 2 1/2 years compiling thousands of pages of medical school notes, verifying them with dozens of medical books and websites to bring you what I consider to be the most comprehensive USMLE® Board review book available. I wrote it from the perspective of asking myself: "If I could start all over, what is the one thing that would help me the most". My answer: "One organized book". Just one book that would cover most everything needed from day one of medical school through Step 3. Boards Ready is the only book that accomplishes this. In fact, doctors can continue to refer to it during practice. There is no longer a need to purchase multiple books. Boards Ready is written in a very simple, organized manner that provides everything you need for Steps 1, 2, and 3 all on one page. This unique arrangement allows Step 1 students to become familiar with the Step 2 and Step 3 management of pathologies. For the resident, it allows for a complete review of materials all the way from Step 1.

Information throughout the book is color-coded so that it corresponds to each Step's information: Step 1, 2 and 3, pharmacology, extremely high yield information, high yield information and general information. Important charts are repeated in each appropriate chapter to aid in seamlessly assimilating all the information needed. Every pathology in the book has its own separate subsection instead of being merged together. For example: S. aureus causes multiple pathologies. Instead of just listing the pathologies, symptoms, and their virulence factors all-together, each pathology (TSS, Impetigo, food poisoning, cellulitis, etc.) has its own individual section. This insures that you are connecting the correct facts together.

I have also provided many other tools to help you learn and retain material:

- Tips – not mnemonics, to help you recall important facts.
- Quick fact tables at the beginning of multiple chapters to help you test yourself.
- New illustrations and charts that are more visual in nature, eliminating a lot of unnecessary information.
- A visual approach to biostat equations. A huge plus for those that don't do math!
- Easy reference charts.

The book is organized very much like the way I teach my Boards Ready course. Explaining things from the perspective of activities that you have done on a day-to-day basis for years, in other words, you already understand these things. You don't have to memorize something you already understand. Then I correlate medicine to these same activities so the entire process makes sense and easily retained. Past medical students that have studied this book and taken their USMLE® Boards will all tell you that this book: (in their own words) "IS DEAD ON". Their scores have certainly reflected this. I believe that you will find that your scores will be higher too. To maximize your scores, I encourage you to combine both the Boards Ready Book with attendance at my Boards Ready Course. You can find information on my Boards Ready Review Course on the inside back cover of this book and on our website at www.boardsready.com.

The USMLE® Exam – What To Know

Step 1 has a total of approximately 280 questions divided into seven 60-minute blocks during an 8-hour testing period. There is an average of 40 questions per block.

Step 2 CK has a total of approximately 318 questions divided into eight 60-minutes blocks during a 9-hour testing period. There is an average of 40 questions per block.

The exams are testing **far more** than just your medical knowledge. They want to be assured that you are qualified to be a doctor in all aspects. Their goal is to find your faults – and they will.
They are testing:

Attention to detail. Pay close attention to:

- Similarly spelled drugs (example: Chlordiazepoxide, Chlorpromazine, Chlorpheniramine, Chloramphenicol, etc.).
- Organisms with the same first name and what specific pathology they are assocated with (example: Schistosoma haematobium, Schistosoma mansoni, Schistosoma japonicum)

Endurance and Stamina. Why are some of the most difficult questions in the final blocks? It is to find out if you are able to make critical decisions when you are exhausted. Can you push your mind and body when necessary?

Concentration and Analyzation. Can you identify the relevant signs and symptoms that will lead you to the correct differentials? The USMLE is quite gifted at turning a single question into 4 or more questions. This means in order to get to the correct answer you must have known each of the preceding parts of the question. If you are incorrect on any previous part of the question, you will not select the correct answer. The question will have led you down an incorrect path (aka: distractor).

Must Knows: Do not go into these exams without this knowledge

- The USMLE® will generally stay out of the "middle" range because "normal" or "abnormal" labs, signs/symptom ranges may vary from patient to patient. Therefore, answers will generally stay out of these middle ranges. They will almost always use the upper and lower ends of any range. There are a handful of areas that DO require exact knowledge.

- **Key Labs**. Labs are one of the key factors that can quickly lead you to the most relevant differentials. See the laboratory section to see the labs I strongly recommend knowing before going into the exams. If you have to waste time opening up the "lab" tab during your actual exam, you will be in trouble on time.

- **One of the most critical keys of the USMLE**, in particularly Step 1, is that you **MUST** know ALL of the "languages" it speaks. This means you MUST know ALL of the "AKA"'s ("Also Known As"). These AKA's are not taught in any review course or given in medical textbooks – until now. I have provided AKA's throughout my book. Medical books and classroom lectures only teach the name by which a disease, an organism, or a sign/symptom is called. However, Step 1 seldom uses those given names – they like to make up their own. If you go into Step 1 without knowing the AKA's, it may result in a lower score and could potentially cause you to fail the exam. You will read the question, know absolutely everything about the subject matter of the question but when you go to the answer choices you will not recognize anything. The sad and unfair thing is that this is what the Board's are using to determine whether or not you are qualified to be a doctor despite the fact that very few of these AKA's have ever been taught in medical school nor found in the medical textbooks. Yet, somewhere along your medical path you are somehow magically supposed to have learned these AKA words and phrases, none of which you will ever use again, especially in practice.
  So pay CLOSE attention to every AKA I have listed throughout the book.

- One of the goals of this book is to provide as many of these AKA's as possible in hopes to save excellent future doctors from being "weeded out" because they get hurt in this twisted game of words. In a time that our country is experiencing such a severe shortage of doctors, it makes far more sense to return to the methods and standards that we have used for decades to test and produce excellent doctors. This means straightforward medicine. Not word games designed around irrelevant facts designed to weed out people. The Board's should be weeding people out because of lack of knowledge, attention to detail, and endurance, but not useless words that have never been taught nor will ever used in everyday medicine! These word games come at a very high cost to medical students. Medical students at this halfway point in their studies have invested over $150,000.

  I have an entire chapter devoted to this subject in my book "Medical Swamp, Time To Drain". "Medical Swamp" covers many problem areas in the field of medicine: massive waste, residency shortages, Veterans needs, unnecessary procedures and many things that are happening which can only be considered as criminal. Its purpose is to bring to the attention of the American people and politicians things that must change. I have provided many good, common sense solutions to many of our medical problems. All easily implemented if we can get rid of the red tape that has our health industry strapped.

- **They also test: "Can You Get Back Into the Game".** There are questions that appear on the exam but do not count. They are supposedly questions that are being "tested" out. They have been doing this exam for years, they don't need to "test" any question. In my opinion, these random questions are used for two purposes:
1) The test writers know that when you get hit with one of these questions it is going to "throw you". You will beat yourself up trying to figure out why you don't know anything about the question. The purpose for this is to see if you are able to let something go, move on and immediately "get back into the game" by answering the next question correctly. Or, do you sit and waste time, beating yourself up while allowing the clock to continue to tick down and allowing it to affect your performance on the next, usually easier, question. What they are testing here is that when something goes wrong with a patient can you immediately get your mind back where it needs to be in order to treat the next patient.
2) If you are faced with something "unknown", are you able to use common sense and your knowledge in order to try and deduct the correct answer.

- According to the USMLE, they are **increasing the number of biostatistics and epidemiology** questions on all exams. In the majority of real day-to-day practice there is very little biostatistics ever used. Physicians are mostly interested in the sensitivity of a test, stats on the performance of a new drug, prevalence, incidence, NNT, NNH and p-value. It is no secret that the majority of medical students are not math experts. Yet, these exams are again basing part of their decisions on which our future doctors will be based on their ability to calculate intricate statistical formulas, which they will never use. I personally would be far more interested in my doctor knowing about prevention, disease processes, diagnosis and proper treatment rather than if they know how to calculate the attributable risk reduction. I have tried to simplify a lot of the biostatistics section in the book by making things more visual. Again, I did this with the goal of trying to keep excellent future doctors from being "weeded out" over things that they will seldom use in practice. I also recommend doing the biostatistics questions available on the USMLE® World website. The block is inexpensive and is very helpful. I also recommend the book "High Yield for Biostatistics and Epidemiology". The key in biostatistics is practice, practice, and practice. If you practice enough, eventually it will sink in.
Step 2 and 3 expand into the pharmacology advertisement area of biostatistics, most of which are 3 part questions. What I recommend on these drug questions is to save them for the very end. The advertisement will require you to scroll down as much as 3 pages. It will eat away at your time and gain you nothing. If required, pick your best guess for the first part and move to the second and third parts. Those questions are generally basic biostatistics questions from Step 1. This way you get at least 2 of the 3 parts correct. Don't waste time!

- **Step 1 now contains management questions and Step 2 and 3 contain Step 1 questions.** The days of "throwing out" Step 1 knowledge after you finish with the exam are over. This is one of the main reasons I designed this book as I did. You are able to review everything needed for Step 1, 2 and 3 for each subject all in one place, regardless of which Step you are taking. This will become especially helpful for Step 3 residents because they will not have seen Step 1 material in over 3 years. It makes review fast, easy, and convenient.

- **Knowing the wrong answer** is just as important as knowing the correct answer. This allows you to eliminate incorrect answers when you run into a question that you are not certain about. Many times these eliminations leave you with the correct answer, despite the fact that you may have no idea what is being asked. This is an area where knowing the "AKA" names are tremendously helpful.

- **Know the exceptions (the "zebra")**. Many questions focus on mechanism's of action, muscles, enzymes, drugs, ions, 2nd messengers, etc., that are exceptions to the normal rule or normal family.

- Be SURE to know what **all abbreviations stand for** because the exam will usually use the full name versus the initials that you are accustomed to using! If you forget this and look to the answers for the initials and do not see them, don't panic. Look at the first letter of each word in the long answer, you will find the initials you are accustomed too!
Example: p-anca = **p**erinuclear **a**nti-**n**eutrophil **c**ytoplasmic **a**ntibodies

- Be SURE to know the **last names** of any of the microorganisms that have the same first names and know what each does. Again, they are testing your attention to detail.
Example: Schistosoma haematobium (bladder) Schistosoma mansoni (liver)
Schistosoma japonicum (gut, hepatosplenic)

- Beware! **Do not expect** the USMLE® to use the **typical (normal)** patient profiles in the vignettes. They want to be sure you recognize the disease in an atypical situation. You MUST think outside of the box at all times!
Examples: Diverticulitis is normally seen in patients over 50, but don't be surprised to see the presentation in a 37 year old. Sarcoidosis is typically seen in African American females in the 30 to 40 year old range. Don't be surprised to see the presentation in a Caucasian, middle age male.

"My Rules" For Maximum Benefit of Boards Ready 1 - 2 - 3

The following are important guidelines and rules that I teach to help you achieve your full potential. I am an "old fashioned" teacher. I believe that we learn and retain maximum information through the repetition of reading, writing, and verbalizing. In my classes, these three skills are used extensively everyday. I credit this with being one of the most critical keys of the success of the Boards Ready Review Program (www.boardsready.com). Every single day in class, I instill each of these rules into every aspect of your thinking!

If you are a **US medical student** this book will be totally sufficient for all your boards. If you are a US student that is struggling with your boards, the Boards Ready program will get you ready!
I do recommend the Boards Ready Review program for your Step 2 CS. There are many important tips that insure that you perform at your best and more importantly insure you get everything charted within the short allotted time. Boards Ready provides a one-week intensive class for the purpose of teaching you these critical skills. One-week is generally all that is necessary.

If you are a **Caribbean or Foreign medical student** and your school does not have a 5th semester Step 1 review program, and you are having difficulty passing your school's required "NBME®" (which is NOT a standard NBME®), or you are having difficulty passing your boards, then I can't stress the **importance of coming to the Boards Ready Step 1 review program**. **Do not make the fatal error of staying home trying to study on your own**. Those that stay home and try to prepare for their Board's on their own have an 85% chance that they will never finish and quit medicine. It is critical that you have direction and focus. Another fatal and very expensive error for most students is to believe they can take a short 6-week review program and be ready to sit for their exam. This rarely works! Most students are no better off at the end of the 6-week course than when they began because they become so overwhelmed they just give up. 6-week programs lecture 8 plus hours per day on top of nighttime class and tutoring requirements, leaving no time for study.
Understand: Step 1 preparation is a huge investment of time and money, so make the right choice the first time. Do not skimp on the most important part of your medical education. ***Step 1 determines your life - your residency chances, period!*** There is NO easy way to get around this test, no magical answers. This test is designed to fail you! It does not want anyone that shouldn't be a doctor to get past this exam! So don't forget, this exam is testing FAR more than just your knowledge - and you probably didn't even realize this. It is testing your attention to detail, common sense, endurance, logic, critical thinking and your ability to move forward in case of an error. If you can't do all of these things, you probably should consider another career. Trust me, this test will be able to determine each of these factors.

For Step 1, 2 and 3 Qbanks: you must follow my rules for maximum success.

- I am very specific on how I want the Qbank done. During my course, this bank will become your best friend. In class, I will go over every one of my rules and why I want these instructions followed exactly. My unique method has proven to be extremely successful in producing higher scores. I always say: "if you are going to run the Boston Marathon, you better train for it, and that doesn't mean jogging around the track a couple of times".

Keep quick study notes with you at all times.

- It is amazing if you add up the time you spend waiting for various things. So be prepared. I recommend taking any of these quick study books with you:
  USLME® Step 1 Secrets or Deja Review. They are small and easy to carry. This continues to reinforce the critical need for repetition.
  This exam "owns" you 24/7. So be prepared to use every waking moment preparing for it.

Sleep

- You MUST get your sleep. *Minimum* of 7 hours a night. No burning the midnight oil! You must allow REM sleep in order for your brain to properly categorize the information you learned that day. Do not skimp on your sleep. This is another fatal error. Those that think they can continually study until the wee hours of the morning are only setting themselves up for lower scores and potentially failure.

Exercise

- This does not have to be a set gym "work out". That is not realistic for most people. If you can work out that is great, do it! If you are not an avid exerciser, then be sure you get out and take 30 minutes to walk, do a few dance steps, anything to get your blood moving.

Take a full day off each week!

- If you take a day off you are not going to miss out on learning more things that will help your exam! Your brain must have a breather. One day a week. Take off. Go to the movies, go shop, anything! Do not think about medicine. Let your brain take a break! You will be amazed at how much better you remember and perform if you do this!

Stop and Learn!

- When you come across a word you are not familiar with, **STOP NOW, and look it up**! Don't fall for the trick used by your brain that convinces you that you will remember to look it up later. Learn it **now**. You will be amazed how many things will suddenly connect when you learn that definition right then and there!

How to Answer QBank Questions

This is an area that we study and practice, heavily, every day during my course. You WILL get your question answering skills down during the course. These skills are critical to your success to focus on what the test writer wants so that you don't get taken down the "deception" road!

- Do NOT look at the answer choices first. If you do, you WILL see many phrases, words, drugs, etc., that you recognize. And trust me, every answer will have a "lost leader" within the question stem that will lead you right to that answer – the wrong one.
- Read the question (last line) FIRST. This will allow you to know EXACTLY what the question writer is specifically asking. **STAY FOCUSED ON THIS**!
- Read through the question stem, staying focused on the exact item you are looking for. Then go down to the answer choices with THAT target answer in mind. LOOK for that target answer written *in any other creative way*. Creative thinking ability on this exam is a positive. (Example: They describe erythema nodosum from Sarcoidosis. You know you would like to see the term "erythema nodosum" but of course, they aren't going to use that term; it won't be that straight forward. It will be there, but it could be written like any one of these options: Swollen raised areas, inflamed subcutaneous fat or adipose, diffuse patchy erythema, inflamed patches of tissue, etc.
- The USMLE wants you to recognize a disease and understand that anyone that walks into your office can present with any disease, it does not have to present "textbook". So be very careful of getting specific diseases associated with specific age rages, male vs female, African American vs Caucasian, etc. You can be rest assured that your exam questions will NOT be what you are expecting. Example: You could have a 30-year-old Caucasian male present with Sarcoidosis or a 35-year-old patient present with diverticulitis. So keep you mind open and focus on the disease. Creativity is your friend! We practice this during class!
- Read the last line (the line that gives the actual question) very carefully. Many times you do not even need to read the vignette. The question may be just a straightforward question. This saves you very valuable time. Anytime the question involves a drug side effect or a mechanism of action (MOA), stop, don't read the entire vignette, just go find the drug or MOA they want and select your answer. Be absolutely sure of what this question is asking, they can be very tricky! Beware of questions that ask about the "most common cause of", they can be very tricky! (Example: If the question simply ask what is the most common cause of death, then it wants the most common cause of death – which is: Heart disease. The person in the vignette will have some other fatal disease (usually cancer) that will lead you to automatically jump to the cancer the person had. Caution: the question did NOT ask about the person in the vignette, it just asked what the most common cause of death was. If they want the cause of what was described in the vignette, they will ask what is the most common cause of *THIS* patient's issue. If they ask about "this" patient, then you must read the vignette.
- Sometimes it is difficult to know what they want in the vignette: drug, treatment, MOA, side effect, etc. This is the ONLY time I suggest taking a quick look at the overall "subject matter" in the answers. Do not read the answers; simply squint your eyes in order to blur the words enough so that you don't see the detailed words. Glance quickly at the entire group. In this quick look you can quickly determine the category of the subject matter of the answer they are wanting: ie: drugs, side effects, MOA's, etc.
- If you read through the question and you simply have no idea, then and only then start reading each answer individually. Immediately cross out the answers you know for a fact are not correct. This is when it becomes extremely important to know what the incorrect answers mean as well. This is an area that is critical you know the AKA's. By knowing these AKA's, it gives you a tremendous advantage. It's like playing a video game. If you know exactly what brick to look behind for the golden key – then you win! This secret key lets you know what organ or disease the answer is talking about. If you know the question stem is asking about cardio, and the AKA is really saying renal, you can immediately cross that out. This will assure you can always narrow down the answers to 2 choices.
- Rules for guessing. When you just simply have **no idea** what to choose:
  1) Never select the answer choice "A" unless you KNOW for a FACT it is the correct answer.
  2) Before you begin your exam choose "high" or "low" and stick to this decision throughout the entire exam. This means that when you have narrowed down your answer choices and have no clue what to choose, you will choose either the "highest" letter choice (but NEVER A) in those final options or the "lowest" letter choice in those final options. (Example: Before your exam you decide to select "low". After you have narrowed the final answer options down to B and D, you will automatically select D (it is the lowest of your 2 choices). This helps to insure that you will get at least 50% of your guesses correct.
  3) In many cases, look for the really long answer; this tends to be the correct choice.
  4) If you are unable to narrow the answer down and you simply have no ideas: you should already have a "favorite" letter (B – E: NOT A). Just choose your favorite letter and MOVE ON! Do not beat yourself up over this: First: it is probably one of the questions that do not count and second: if it is not, if you don't know it, you don't know it. Do not allow this to affect your next question!
- **DO NOT CHANGE YOUR ANSWER unless you are willing to die for it**. You must learn to trust your brain. If you have followed everything I teach: question study requirements, sleep, exercise, etc., then your brain DOES have the information filed away, whether you can consciously remember it or not. It WILL recognize what it needs to whether you do or not. So trust this! ONLY if you absolutely know for a FACT that you have selected the wrong answer should you ever change an answer!
- Biostatistics questions: The USMLE® knows that there is only 1 minute available for each question so there are seldom any equations that will be in-depth, there simply isn't time. If you get to a question or any equation that you are not familiar with or upon reading it become totally lost – LET IT GO!! Simply pick your favorite answer number and move on to the next question! **Always be SURE to choose an answer before moving on. Never leave a question blank. If it's left blank: it is a 100% wrong answer.**
- Marking questions. Be careful with this one. There is usually barely enough time to finish a block as it is. In the case where you do have a TINY bit of extra time to go back and check a question- you only want to have 1 or 2 questions marked. That is all you will have time for! If you have marked numerous questions, it will be futile. ONLY mark the questions that you really feel a second look would be good if there is time or for equations (biostatistics, formulas, etc.). If you have an extra minute it may allow you the time to actually make the calculation and select the correct answer.

Hands on Practice:
Throughout the course, we will cover multiple other test taking skills as well as study EKG, graphs, imaging and murmurs: as all of these are on the exam. You must be confident on these important skills. We also spend a tremendous amount of time discussing cases and questions so that you learn to think "outside the box". There is nothing in medicine that comes in a perfectly packaged box! You must learn to take clues from many sources to determine the diagnosis. We spend hours correlating every physiology so that you see and understand how every body system connects to and affect each other. There is not a day in my course that I do not see "light bulbs" come on. We make sense of medicine! This makes all the difference on your exam and in how you will practice one day.

The "USMLE®" Boards Ready Clock Face©: This is a specialized "clock" that I designed to enable my students to be fully prepared for their exam. It really takes the guesswork out of the majority of the questions that will be on the exam. We use the "CLOCK" regularly throughout my course so that this "thinking method" becomes instilled as second nature!

What to do when you are ready to take the exam is just as important as the time you spent studying for it:
In my course I will outline exactly what you will do: 2 weeks before, 1 week before, the day before, the morning of and during the actual exam: down to when you will take your breaks, what you will do and what you will eat.
During my course I cover exactly what schedule you must keep during these specific periods.
These instructions can make a tremendous difference in your score!

A Word About Exam Scores and Confidentiality

I am telling you this because very few students are ever told about this "unwritten" rule and end up finding out about it the hard way.
ALL exam scores and attempts are highly private and personal. NEVER ask anyone: another student, an instructor or preceptor what their exam scores were, whether they passed or failed or how many attempts. Even those that make really high scores never speak of their scores. *It is none of your business!* It is your business if you want to share your own scores, but you should never ask others to do so, even if it's your best friend. If they want to share it, they will.
It is also important to *never judge someone on his or her score or number of attempts*! Excellent people fail these exams every day and it is not for lack of knowledge. Unforeseen situations cause people to fail: maybe they were sick that day, they had a fight with their spouse the evening before or were up with a sick child all night. Many people are poor test takers and certainly there are those that simply weren't prepared. You might be surprised to know that Abraham Lincoln, Martin Luther King Jr., and Albert Einstein were very poor test takers. Thankfully they weren't judged in the same way people are judged by their USMLE® exam or no one would have ever heard of these great men! It is not your place to make any judgments. Remember the profession of a physician is considered one of the most respected and ethical professions in the world – *live up to it!*

Step 2 CS

Step 2 CS cases will be the same as the Step 3 CS cases. The only difference being that Step 2 CS uses real "patients" and Step 3 CS uses a computerized virtual patient. Both CS exams require that you do a focused exam, good H & P, identify differentials, be proficient in labs and imaging orders and treatments. It is critical to become proficient with the USMLE® software with both Step 2 and Step 3 CS. This means practice – practice – practice! I strongly recommend that you use ***First Aid Step 2 CS*** as a guide in your actual "patient practice", it is an excellent book especially when combined with attending a one week Boards Ready Step 2 CS Course. Our Step 2 CS Course will prepare you for patient encounters, provide critical tips that expedite a focused exam and assure through, timely EMR charting and train you on the numerous things to avoid which could hurt your score or worse, cause you to fail the exam. It is important to not take the CS exams lightly. Please see the Step 3 CS chapter to review the most common CS cases.

Correlations Needed for Boards Ready 1 - 2 - 3

I have found that most students tend to be visual learners, achieving maximum learning when the subject matter is related to something they already know and understand, with material that is short and to the point. So I have tried to keep the main focus of Boards Ready 1, 2, and 3 on these facts.
Below are a few of the general key "**CONCEPT**" terms that **I will routinely refer to throughout the book and my course, so please become familiar with them**. These concepts will help you understand the basics of many processes and pathologies in the body.

1**) "BALANCE" CONCEPT. Most everything is like a teeter-totter.**
Everything in the body uses a system of checks and balances to keep homeostasis. It is like a teeter-totter. In order to keep the teeter-totter level, weights on both ends must be the same. When either of these two weights changes: decrease or increase, the other process reacts by doing the opposite.
Example 1: There is a balance between the parasympathetic and sympathetic nervous systems. At anytime if parasympathetic decreases, it allows the sympathetic to be more prominent.
Example 2: Your pH is balanced at 7.4. Meaning acid (paCO2) and Base (HCO3) are equal. If your body becomes more acidic (holding more acid/paCO2) your base (HCO3) will increase in order to compensate and bring things back into balance.

2) **"EMPLOYEE or SECURITY GUARD" CONCEPT**
Every process has an "Employee or Security Guard". The only job of this person (thing), throughout its entire life is to monitor responsibilities for that specific process. The only reason that person "goes to work" is if the process it is in charge of overseeing is not right. As long as the process is behaving properly it stays on vacation. But if something goes wrong: (levels change) this person goes to work. So it is critical to know the specific job for every "employee or security guards" in the body!
Example: Every interstate has a Highway Patrol officer that monitors it. You never see him as long as everyone is driving legally as they should. However, once someone breaks the rules, the highway patrol officer goes to work and you see him.

3) "**PATHWAY" CONCEPT©. One of the most important key concepts I use throughout my course.**
Pathway's are not just for biochemistry, but for almost all processes in the body. This requires that **YOU MUST KNOW NORMAL** before you can identify abnormal/pathologies. In all processes or product formation you must know these 3 things:
1) the normal beginning factors/enzymes
2) the normal occurring merging factors/enzymes
3) the normal end product/process
Anything that affects any one of these 3 areas can cause pathologies.
At the point where the abnormal or absent process/enzyme occurs will determine its effects:

1) Pathology can happen at this specific point
2) Processes/products/enzymes BELOW this specific point will be decreased or not produced
3) Processes/products/enzymes ABOVE this specific point will be increased and/or backed up

To make my "Pathway Concept"© visual, I will use my candle manufacturing company.
UPS delivers the wax to the door. The wax is put into the wax storeroom. The wax is then put into vats and melted at 140 degrees. Dyes and fragrances are then added. The melted wax is poured into jars. The wick is inserted. The candle is labeled. The candle is put on the finished product shelf. The candle is put into a box. UPS picks up the box and delivers it to the customer. The customer receives the box and puts the candle on the shelf. You buy the candle. A perfect process: all goes well.

If there is ANY problem at any point in this path, every process before and after that point is affected.
Example:
If the wax is never delivered = no candle (product) can be made.
If the storeroom runs out of wax = no candle (product) can be made.
If the 140 degree heat can't be generated = no wax will melt = no candle (product) can be made.
If the dye or fragrance is incorrectly measured = poor quality product.
If there are no wicks or labels, the candles will be okay up to this point, but they will now be forced to be backed up because there are no wicks or labels to allow them to continue on to the next step, so the amount of finished product will be decreased or be non-existent.
Any problem with a pathway in the body means pathology: it could be minor or major.
In biochemistry, if an enzyme is missing from a pathway, the product is reduced or not made at all. In cardiology, if a valve is stenosed, less blood will be ejected and more blood will back up behind the valve, increasing pressure.

4) **"CEO" CONCEPT**
Know the Board of Directors and the CEO, particularly in endocrine. These guys are the bosses. Every process has a CEO/Board of Directors. The workers SHOULD do what they are told by the CEO as long as the workers are normal and the boss is giving out normal instructions.
Example: If a normal TSH (CEO in the Pituitary) is telling the T3 and T4 (workers in the thyroid) that they need to work harder (increase) then the CEO will be increased and the T3 and T4 should then do as instructed and increase.
However, if the normal TSH (CEO) is decreased, therefore telling the T3 and T4 (workers) to decrease also, but instead the workers do what they want and increase, then the problem lies with the T3 and T4 (workers).

5) **"HOUSE" CONCEPT©**. This is one of the most important concepts that I use throughout my course.
Every organ is like a house. Houses have many rooms, each room has its own purpose and each room contributes to the whole. If there is anything that affects the "house" (organ) then it can affect any given room or all rooms in that house.
Example: The liver ("House") has many rooms: Clotting factor room, Alpha 1-antitrypsin room, glycolysis room, gluconeogenesis room, glycogenolysis room, albumin room, P-450 room, urea cycle room, cholesterol and bile room, bilirubin conjugation room, etc. If the liver develops cirrhosis, then every room or just some of the rooms can be affected. Know the rooms of each "house" (organ) so that you can recognize signs of problems when they occur with your patients.

6) **Do not memorize double**. This means that for any situation that has an opposite (hypo verses hyper, etc.) learn ONLY one. If you learn both, you will invariably turn them around during exam time. By only learning one you are less likely to get them confused.

7) **Memory triggers should be quick and easy!** There are 1000's of facts to learn in medicine, therefore, it is impossible to think you are going to learn about a subject and then have time to come back to create some way to remember it. You must learn now to **correlate something to trigger your memory as you go – right THEN**! This is difficult at first, but with practice, it becomes automatic. It's like those that play the piano. They are able to read treble clef and base clef simultaneously. This will save you tremendous amounts of time and insure that when you see the word on the exam that the correct correlation will always be there for you.
This could be as simple as a word or a visual to remind you. If you already have something in your mind that has worked well to remind you, NEVER try to change this correlation to another one that you might hear someone else use. If this word or visual reminds you of a specific thing, it always will. I don't care what you visual or thought you use to make a correlation is, USE IT!

8**)** ***NO, NO, NO*** **Mnemonics**. I am not a big fan of mnemonics; there are a few that are helpful, the rest are a waste of time. If you think you will have time to run down mnemonics on your exam, in front of your preceptor during clinicals or in front of your patients, you are sadly mistaken. You really just need to **learn these things**. It will make you far more successful.

9) **Memorize.** There are some things you simply must memorize; there are no shortcuts or tricks. The best way to do this is to get yourself a dry erase board and write down the facts: erase, write again, erase, write again, erase.........and do this process until you can write down the information without ANY errors. Then over the next few days, make yourself rewrite the material from memory. If you can do this, you will recognize the material on the exam. Do a reasonable amount of information at a time so you are not overwhelmed.

10) The best way to learn and remember is: **repetition, repetition, and repetition**! This is how we can remember movies or songs, in detail, from when we were children. I don't like electronic books or power points; I prefer old-fashioned note taking. This requires the use of multiple areas of your brain simultaneously: visual, motor, speech, and executive thinking. The more parts of your brain you can engage in the learning process, the more you will retain. If you want to strengthen this even further, say the notes out loud as you write or study them.

11) **LAYERING**. This is how the USMLE® turns 300 questions into 1000. Very seldom is there just a simple, straightforward question on the exam. The questions are designed in layers, kind of like how video games are designed. Many questions are 3 and 4 levels deep. This means that you must know the answer to one level before you can proceed to the next. In order to get to the correct answer you must have gotten all prior levels correct.
Example: You are given a vignette that describes a patient's symptoms, then told you prescribed "a drug" and then you are given a side effect. Then the actual question will ask is what is the receptor or MOA of the drug. So in this question, you will have had to properly identify the pathology, then know the drug you would have prescribed, as well as the drugs side effects in order to get to the correct answer. If you start off with the wrong pathology, you will not ever get the correct answer, but you will never know because they will have an answer choice that matches the pathology you got incorrect.

12) **KNOW DEFINITIONS and suffixes and prefixes!** If you are studying or doing Q banks and come across a word that you are not familiar with, STOP RIGHT THERE and look it up! Do not think you are going remember to come back and look it up later! This will be worth valuable points to you, not to mention may make important clarifications for you!

13) **Charts and Graphs**. We practice graphs and charts very heavily in my course. It is critical as this can cost you substantial points. The majority of the charts and graphs on the USMLE® are usually nothing like you have seen or studied before. The USMLE® KNOWS what you are accustomed to using – so why would you expect them to make it easy on you now? They make up new charts and graphs so that they can determine IF you actually know and understand the concept being presented. So when you see a new chart or graph on your exam, stay calm, take a deep breath, and see what concept they are asking for. **DO NOT** focus on the entire graph or chart in its entirety as this is overwhelming and unnecessary. Make the question into a two-part question. **ONLY look at half of the chart or graph, solve it first.** Start with the half that you know best. This will allow you to easily identify and cross off incorrect answers. Now, look at the last half of the graph and solve that part. This will automatically leave only one answer left...the correct one!

14) **Imaging and Murmurs.** I cover all imaging (X-rays, CT's, MRI's and Ultrasound) during my course. These are all on the exams and you must know them! We will also cover murmurs in both written description and sounds. These are guaranteed to be on the exam.

15) **TEAMS.** Know your teams! I teach "teams" very heavily in my course. Think of it this way: Every part of the body has "teams", meaning groups of things (ions, hormones, actions, etc.) that all work together to make their part work – and most importantly remember there is another team that is the counterpart to this work. Understand that ANY team player is fair game to the USMLE®. If you know what team members belong together and know their actions and the results of those actions, you can't be tricked. Once you identify the actions or see the results in a vignette, you can easily identify the team in charge. The answer has to come from one aspect of the team in charge, be it the ions, hormones, etc. This also helps you eliminate a lot of the wrong answers, as all the wrong answer will belong to the other team.

16) **Look at the WORD**. Don't get frustrated when you are hit with a word you do not know. Many times you can figure out the "category" that the word belongs to just by taking the word apart. This is especially true with anatomy.

17) **Answer choices that mean the SAME.** There can only be ONE right answer. So if you identify 2 or more answer choices that actually mean the same thing (regardless of how creative they have been presented) you can take them out, they are the wrong answers. Many times this leaves only one answer left, the right one. Again, another reason to know your AKA's.

How Boards Ready 1, 2, and 3 is Designed and Color Coded

My book is unlike any other USMLE® review textbook on the market. It is designed to be the only guide you need from the first day of medical school through Step 3 in residency. **It is the only book you will need.** All of my past students that were taught directly from this book will tell you: **"The book is dead on".** My book provides you with the necessary HIGH YIELD information for Step 1, Step 2 CK and Step 3 CK and CS. This allows the "whole picture" to be seen for all three Steps in one book and on one page. If those taking Step 1 are provided the "whole picture", they have a much better understanding of the pathology, physiology and pharmacology all the way through Step 3, which allows them to score much higher. It's the old "hind site is 20/20" routine. If you can work from Step 3 backwards, you will make far less mistakes on Step 1.
You will also find that I repeat a lot of information throughout the book. I prefer to have everything you need to study in one spot instead of having to continually flip throughout the book to find important information. This way, when you want to review a specific subject, everything will be conveniently located in that chapter. For example, you will find CSF charts in microbiology, cardiology and general pathology because they are needed in each of these areas.

The book is color coded to help you focus on what is needed for your specific exam. If you read the other information associated with your subject matter on that same page – it will only help you score higher!

COLOR CODING

BOLD GREEN: Areas that are EXTREMELY HIGH YIELD, THESE ARE HEAVILY TESTED! KNOW EVERYTHING ABOUT THIS SUBJECT! The chances of this information being on your exam are extremely high! Do NOT go into the exams without this information.

BOLD BLACK: Areas that are high yield. There is a good chance that this information will be on your exam. I would not recommend taking the exams without knowing this information.... solid.

Regular print: areas that give even more information about the subject. This is great extra reading for those going for the higher scores.

"Pharmacology" is noted in orange.
I have tried to <u>underline</u> <u>the specific drugs used mostly with Step 1</u> so that those studying for Step 1 do not get bogged down by multiple other drugs for future Steps.
Italicized Pharmacology drugs: These are strictly for Step 3. These are the brand names of that specific drug and are listed directly under that specific drug's chemical name. They are not needed for Step 1 or Step 2, but it's a good idea to start recognizing them now so that when you graduate you will be familiar with them – because these are the names that everyone actually uses.

BOLD BLUE: This information is for Step 2 and Step 3. I strongly recommend those studying for Step 1 to at least read through this information at least once because there are management questions now appearing on Step 1. It is also important to know that I also teach Step 2 along with Step 1 during my course. It is only a few lines more of information; this insures you are solid for any management questions that might appear on your Step 1. It also prepares you for Step 2, so **you are actually getting two courses in one when you take my Step 1 review.**

ABBREVIATIONS

I have written most words in long form throughout the book and included any abbreviations next to them for convenience sake. I believe it's a good idea to become familiar with the words and abbreviations at the same time verses having to stop and look them up separately. Remember that on your exam do not anticipate seeing abbreviations. When you see a long group of words in the answers, don't panic, stop, and look at the first letter of each word and you will find the abbreviation that you are accustomed to using.

A-a	Alveolar-arterial Gradient
AAA	Abdominal Aortic Aneurysm
Ab	Antibody
ABG	Arterial Blood Gas
ABP	Antigen Binding Protein
ABPA	Allergic Bronchopulmonary Aspergillosis
ABX	Antibiotics
ACA	Anterior Cerebral Artery
ACE	Angiotensin-converting enzyme
ACh	Acetylcholine
AChE	Acetylcholinesterase
ACL	Anterior Cruciate Ligament
ACom	Anterior Communicating Artery
ACTH	Adrenocorticotropic Hormone
AD	Autosomal Dominant
ADH	Antidiuretic Hormone
ADHD	Attention-deficit Hyperactivity Disorder
ADP	Adenosine Diphosphate
AF	A-fib
AFP	alpha-fetoprotein
AICA	Anterior Inferior Cerebellar Artery
AIDS	Acquired Immunodeficiency Syndrome
AIP	Acute Intermittent Porphyria
AKA	Also Known As
AL	Amyloid Light Chain
ALL	Acute Lymphoblastic Leukemia
ALP	Alkaline Phosphatase
ALS	Amyotrophic Lateral Sclerosis
ALT	Alanine Transaminase
AMA	anti-mitochondrial Antibody, Against Medical Advice
AML	Acute Myelogenous Leukemia
AMP	Adenosine Monophosphate
ANA	Antinuclear Antibody
ANCA	Antineutrophil Cytoplasmic Antibody
ANOVA	Analysis of Variance
ANP	Atrial natriuretic peptide
ANS	Autonomic Nervous System
A/O	Alert and Oriented
A-P	Anteroposterior
AP	Action Potential, Ante Partum
APC	Antigen Presenting Cell
Apo	Apolipoprotein
AR	Aortic Regurgitation, Attributable Risk, Autosomal Recessive
ARB	Angiotensin Receptor Blocker
ARDS	Acute Respiratory Distress Syndrome
AROM	Artificial Rupture of Membranes
AS	Aortic Stenosis
ASA	Anterior Spinal Artery, Acetylsalicylic Acid (aspirin)
ASD	Atrial Septal Defect
ASO	Anti-streptolysin O
AST	Aspartate Transaminase
ATN	Acute Tubular Necrosis
ATP	Adenosine Triphosphate
AR	Autosomal Recessive
AV	Atrioventricular
BBB	Blood Brain Barrier
B/C	Because
BCC	Basal Cell Carcinoma
BCG	Bacille Calmette-Guérin
BH4	Tetrahydrobiopterin
Bid	2 Times per Day
BIT	**Best Initial Test**
BLS	Basic Life Support
BM	Bowel Movement
BMI	Body Mass Index
BMR	Basal Metabolic Rate
BMT	Bone Marrow Transplant
BNF	British National Formulary
BNP	Brain Natriuretic Peptide
BPH	Benign Prostatic Hyperplasia
bpm	Beats Per Minute
BR	Bed Rest
BRP	Bath Room Privileges
BT	Bleeding Time
B/T	Between
BUN	Blood Urea Nitrogen
Ca	Calcium, Cancer
CABG	Coronary Artery By-pass Graft
CAD	Coronary Artery Disease
cAMP	Cyclic Adenosine Monophosphate
CBC	Complete Blood Count
CC	Chief Complaint
CCA	Common Carotid Artery
CCK	Cholecystokinin
CCP	Citrullinated peptide Antibody
CDC	Center for Disease Control
CEA	Carcinoembryonic Antigen
CF	Cystic Fibrosis
CFTR	Cystic Fibrosis Transmembrane Conductance Regulator
CFX	Circumflex Artery
cGMP	Cyclic Guanosine Monophosphate
CHF	Congestive Heart Failure
CHO	Carbohydrate
CI	Confidence Interval
Cl	Chloride
CIN	Carcinoma in situ, Cervical Intraepithelial Neoplasia
circ	Circumcision
CK	Creatinine Kinase
CK-MB	Creatine Kinase
CL	Clearance
CLL	Chronic Lymphocytic Leukemia

CML	Chronic Myelogenous Leukemia
CMP	Complete Metabolic Panel
CN	Cranial Nerve, Cyanide
CO	Carbon Monoxide, Cardiac Output
CO2	Carbon Dioxide
CoA	Coenzyme A
CoQ	Coenzyme Q
COOH	Carboxyl Group
COPD	Chronic Obstructive Pulmonary Disease
CPAP	Continuous Positive Airway Pressure
CPK	Creatine Phosphokinase
CPR	Cardiopulmonary Resuscitation
CRH	Corticotropin-releasing Hormone
CRP	C Reactive Protein
CS	Causes
C & S	Culture and Sensitivity
CSF	Cerebral Spinal Fluid
CMV	Cytomegalovirus
CRC	Colorectal Cancer
CXR	Chest X-Ray
CT	Computed Tomography
CVA	Cerebrovascular Accident
CXR	Chest X-Ray
DAF	Decay-accelerating Factor
DAG	Diacylglycerol
d/c	Discontinue
DCM	Dilated Cardiomyopathy
DCT	Distal Convoluted Tubule
DDAVP	Desmopressin Acetate (Vasopressin)
DES	Diethylstilbestrol
DEXA	Dual Energy –Ray Absorptiometry
DHEA	Dehydroepiandrosterone
DHF	Dihydrofolic Acid
DHT	Dihydrotestosterone
DI	Diabetes Insipidus
DIC	Disseminated Intravascular Coagulation
DIP	Distal Interphalangeal joint
DKA	Diabetic ketoacidosis
DM	Diabetes Mellitus
DMARD	Disease-modifying Antirheumatic Drug
DNA	Deoxyribonucleic Acid
DNR	Do Not Resuscitate
DOB	Date of Birth
DPA	Dead on Arrival
DPT	Diphtheria, pertussis, Tetanus
dsDNA	Double Stranded DNA
dsRNA	Double Stranded RNA
DTR	Deep Tendon Reflex
DT's	Delirium Tremens
DVT	Deep Venous Thrombosis
DX	Diagnosis
EBL	Estimated Blood Loss
EBV	Ebstein Barr Virus
ECF	Extracellular Fluid
ECG, EKG	Electrocardiogram
ECT	Electroconvulsive Therapy
EDTA	Ethylenediamine Tetra-acetic Acid
EDV	End Diastolic Volume
EEG	Electroencephalogram
EF	Ejection Fraction
EGF	Epidermal Growth Factor
EHEC	Enterohemorrhagic E. coli
ELISA	Enzyme-linked Immunosorbent Assay
EM	Electron Microscope
EMT	Emergency Medical Technician
ENT	Ear, Nose, Throat
Epi	Epinephrine
EPO	Erythropoietin
EPS	Extrapyramidal System
ER	Endoplasmic Reticulum, Emergency Room
ERCP	Endoscopic Retrograde Cholangiopancreatography
ERP	Effective Refractory Period
ERT	Estrogen Replacement Therapy
ERV	Expiratory Reserve Volume
ESR	Erythrocyte Sedimentation Rate
ESRD	End Stage Renal Disease
ESV	End Systolic Volume
ETA	Estimated Time of Arrival
ETEC	Enterotoxigenic E. coli
EtOH	Ethyl Alcohol
F	Bioavailability
FA	Fatty Acid
Fab	Fragment Antigen-binding
FAD	Flavin Adenine Dinucleotide
FADH	Reduced Flavin Adenine Dinucleotide
FACP	Fellow of American College of Physicians
FACS	Fellow of American College of Surgeons
FBC	Full Blood Count
Fc	Fragment – Crystallizable
FDA	Food and Drug Administration
FE+2	Ferrous Ion
FE+3	Ferric Ion
FEV1	Forced Expiratory Volume in 1 second
FF	Filtration Fraction
FFA	Free Fatty Acid
FGF	Fibroblast Growth Factor
FH	Family History
FHS	Fetal Heart Sounds
FN	False Negative
FISH	Fluorescence in situ Hybridization
FP	False Positive
FRC	Functional Residual Capacity
FSH	Follicle Stimulating Hormone
FTA-ABS	Fluorescent Treponemal Antibody Absorption
FVC	Forced Vital Capacity
FVC1	Forced Expiratory Volume-1 Second
Fx	Fracture
GABA	y-aminobutyric Acid
GAG	Glycosaminoglycan
GB	Gallbladder
GBM	Glomerular Basement Membrane
G-CSF	Granulocyte Colony-stimulating Factor
GERD	Gastroesophageal Reflux Disease
GFR	Glomerular Filtration Rate
GFAP	Glial Fibrillary Acid Protein
GFR	Glomerular Filtration Rate
GGT	y-glutamyl Transpeptidase
GH	Growth Hormone
GHRH	Growth Hormone Releasing Hormone
GI	Gastrointestinal

GIP	Gastric Inhibitory Peptide
GLUT	Glucose Transporter
GMP	Guanosine Monophosphate
G3P	Glucose-3-phosphate
G6P	Glucose-6-phosphate
GPe	Globus Pallidus Externa
GPi	Globus Pallidus Interna
GRP	Gastrin Releasing Peptide
Gs	G Protein, S Polypeptide
GTP	Guanosine Triphosphate
GTPase	Guanosine Triphosphatase
GU	Genitourinary
GYN	Gynecology
H/A	Headache
H2S	Hydrogen Sulfide
HAART	Highly Active Antiretroviral Therapy
HAV	Hepatitis A
Hb	Hemoglobin
HbA	Adult Hemoglobin
HbA1c	Glycated Hemoglobin
HbF	Fetal Hemoglobin
HBV	Hepatitis B
HCC	Hepatocellular Carcinoma
hCG	Human Chorionic Gonadotropin
HCO3	Bicarbonate
Hct	Hematocrit
HCTZ	Hydrochlorothiazide
HCV	Hepatitis C
HDL	High Density Lipoprotein
HDV	Hepatitis D
H&E	Hematoxylin and Eosin (stain)
HEENT	Head, Ears, Eyes, Nose, Throat
HEV	Hepatitis E
HIDA	Hepatobiliary Scintigraphy Scan
HIPAA	Health Insurance Portability & Accountability Act
HIV	Human Immunodeficiency Virus
HLA	Human Leukocyte Antigen
H&P	History and Physical
HPI	History of Present Illness
HPL	Human Placental Lactogen
HMP	Hexose Monophosphate
HOB	Head of Bed
HR	Heart Rate
H2O	Water
H2O2	Hydrogen Peroxide
HSV	Herpes Simplex Virus
ht	Height
HTN	Hypertension
HUS	Hemolytic-uremic Syndrome
HVA	Homovanillic Acid
Hx	History
IBD	Inflammatory Bowel Disease
IBS	Irritable Bowel Syndrome
IC	Inspiratory Capacity, Immune Complex
ICA	Internal Carotid Artery
ICAM	Intracellular Adhesion Molecule
ICD	Implantable Cardioverter Defibrillator
ICF	Intracellular Fluid
ICP	Intracranial Pressure
ICS	Intercostal Space
ICU	Intensive Care Unit
I & D	Incision and Drainage
I & O	Intake and output
IFN	Interferon
Ig	Immunoglobulin
IGF	Insulin-like Growth Factor
IL	Interleukin
IM	Intramuscular
IMA	Inferior Mesenteric Artery
IMP	Inosine Monophosphate
INR	International Normalized Ratio
IO	Inferior Oblique, Intraosseous
IOP	Intraocular Pressure
IP3	Inositol Triphosphate
IR	Inferior Rectus
IRV	Inspiratory Reserve Volume
ITP	Idiopathic Thrombocytopenic Purpura
IUD	Intrauterine Device
IUGR	Intrauterine Growth Restriction
IV	Intravenous
IVC	Inferior Vena Cava
IVIG	Intravenous Immunoglobulin
JGA	Juxtaglomerular Apparatus
JVD	Jugular Venous Distention
JVP	Jugular Venous Pulse
K	Potassium
Km	Michaelis-Menten Constant
KOH	Potassium Hydroxide (fungal test)
LAC	Laceration
LAD	Left Anterior Descending Coronary Artery
LAP	Leukocyte Alkaline Phosphatase
LBBB	Left Bundle Branch Block
LCA	Left Coronary Artery
LCAT	Lecithin-cholesterol Acyltransferase
LCL	Left Collateral Ligament
LCX	Left Circumflex Coronary Artery
LD	Loading Dose
L & D	Labor and Delivery
LD50	Lethal Dose
LDH	Lactate Dehydrogenase
LDL	Low-Density Lipoprotein
LEEP	Loop Electrosurgical Excision Procedure
LGN	Lateral Geniculate Nucleus
LES	Lower Esophageal Sphincter
LFT	Liver Function Test
LH	Luteinizing Hormone
LLQ	Left Lower Quadrant (pain)
LM	Light Microscopy
LMN	Lower Motor Neuron
LOC	Level of Consciousness
LP	Lumbar Puncture
LPL	Lipoprotein Lipase
LPS	Lipopolysaccharide
LR	Lateral Rectus, Lactated Ringers
LSD	Lysergic Acid Diethylamide
LUQ	Left Upper Quadrant (pain)
LVF	Left Ventricular Failure
LVH	Left Ventricular Hypertrophy
MA	Macrophage
MAC	Membrane Attack Complex, Minimal Alveolar Concentration

MALT	Mucosa-associated Lymphoid Tissue
MAO	Monoamine Oxidase
MAP	Mean Arterial Pressure, Morning After Pill
MAT	**Most Accurate Test**
MCA	Middle Cerebral Artery
MC/MCC	Most Common/Most Common Cause
MCH	Mean Corpuscular Hemoglobin
MCHC	Mean Corpuscular Hemoglobin Concentration
MCL	Middle Collateral Ligament
MCP	Metacarpophalangeal Joint
M-CSF	Macrophage Colony-stimulating Factor
MCV	Mean Corpuscular Volume
MD	Maintenance Dose
MEN	Multiple Endocrine Neoplasia
Mg	Magnesium
MGN	Medial Geniculate Nucleus
MgSo4	Magnesium Sulfate
MHC	Major Histocompatibility Complex
ml	Milliliter
MI	Myocardial Infarction
MIF	Mullerian Inhibitory Factor
MLCK	Myosin Light-chain Kinase
MLF	Medial Longitudinal Fasciculus
mm	Millimeter
MMC	Migrating Motor Complex
MMR	Measles, Mumps, Rubella Vaccine
MOA	Mode of Action
MOM	Milk of Magnesia
MPO	Myeloperoxidase
MR	Mitral Regurgitation
MRI	Magnetic Resonance Imagine
mRNA	Messenger Ribonucleic Acid
miRNA	Microribonucleic Acid
MS	Multiple Sclerosis, Mitral Stenosis
MSH	Melanocyte Stimulating Hormone
MRSA	Methicillin-Resistant S. aureus
MSO4	Morphine Sulfate
MVA	Motor Vehicle Accident
MVP	Mitral Valve Prolapse
Na	Sodium
NaCl	Sodium Chloride
NAD	Nicotinamide Adenine Dinucleotide
NADH	Reduced Nicotinamide Adenine Dinucleotide
NE	Norepinephrine
NGT	Nasogastric Tube
NH3	Ammonia
NH4	Ammonium
NICU	Neonatal Intensive Care Unit
NK	Natural Killer Cells
NKA	No Known Allergies
NKDA	No Known Drug Allergies
NL	Normal
NMJ	Neuro Muscular Junction
NMS	Neuroleptic Malignant Syndrome
NNH	Number Needed to Harm
NNT	Number Needed to Treat
NPH	Normal Pressure Hydrocephalus
NPO	Nothing by Mouth
NPV	Negative Predictive Value
NO	Nitric Oxide
N2O	Nitrous Oxide
NS	Normal Saline
NSAID	Nonsteroidal Anti-inflammatory Drug
NSR	Normal Sinus Rhythm
NSTEMI	Non ST Elevation Myocardial Infarction
NVD	Nausea, Vomiting, Diarrhea
O2	Oxygen
OAA	Oxaloacetic Acid
OB/GYN	Obstetrics and Gynecology
OCD	Obsessive Compulsive Disorder
OCP	Oral Contraceptive Pill
OH	Hydroxy
OMT	Osteopathic Manipulative Technique
O&P	Ova & Parasite (stool test)
OR	Odds Ratio, Operating Room
OSHA	Occupational Safety and Health Administration
OTC	Ornithine Transcarbamoylase
PA	Posteroanterior, Pulmonary Artery
PaCO2	Arterial PCO2
PACO2	Alveolar PCo2
PaO2	Partial Pressure of Oxygen in Arterial Blood
PAO2	Partial Pressure of Oxygen in Alveolar Blood
PAP	Papanicolaou (PAP Smear)
PAS	Periodic Acid-Schiff
PBP	Penicillin Binding Protein
PCA	Posterior Cerebral Artery
PCL	Posterior Cruciate Ligament
PCOS	Polycystic Ovarian Syndrome
PCP	Primary Care Physician, Pneumocystis jiroveci
PCR	Polymerase Chain Reaction
PCT	Proximal Convoluted Tubule
PDA	Patent Ductus Arteriosis, Posterior Descending Artery
PDE	Phosphodiesterase
PDGF	Platelet-derived Growth Factor
PE	Pulmonary Embolism, Physical Exam
PEA	Pulseless Electrical Activity
PEEP	Positive End-expiratory Pressure
PEP	Phosphoenolpyruvate
PERL	Pupils Equal and Reactive to Light
PET	Positron Emission Tomography
PF4	Platelet Factor 4
PFK	Phosphofructokinase
PFT	Pulmonary Function Test
PGE	Prostaglandin E
PGI	Prostacyclin
PICA	Posterior Inferior Cerebellar Artery
PID	Pelvic Inflammatory Disease
PIP	Proximal Interphalangeal Joint
PK	Pyruvate Kinase
PKD	Polycystic Kidney Disease
PKU	Phenylketonuria
PMN	Polymorphonuclear Leukocyte (neutrophil)
PMS	Premenstrual Syndrome
PND	Paroxysmal Nocturnal Dyspnea
PNET	Primitive Neuroectodermal Tumor
PNS	Peripheral Nervous System
po	By Mouth
post op	Postoperative

PO4	Phosphate
PPD	Purified protein Derivative
PPI	Proton Pump Inhibitor
PPV	Positive Predictive Value
preop	Before Surgery
PRL	Prolactin
PRN	As Needed
PrP	Prion Protein
PSA	Prostate-specific Antigen
PT	Prothrombin Time, Patient, Physical Therapy
PTH	Parathyroid Hormone
PTHrp	Parathyroid Hormone –related protein
PTT	Partial Prothrombin Time
PVC	Polyvinyl Chloride
PVR	Pulmonary Vascular Resistance
PWCP	Pulmonary Wedge Capillary Pressure
q	Every
qd	Every Day
qh	Every Hour
qid	4 times a day
RAAS	Renin-angiotensin-aldosterone System
RANK-L	Receptor Activator Nuclear Factor-k B ligand
RBBB	Right Bundle Branch Block
RBC	Red Blood Cell
RBF	Renal Blood Flow
RCA	Right Coronary Artery
RDS	Respiratory Distress Syndrome
REM	Rapid Eye Movement
RER	Rough Endoplasmic Reticulum
RES	Reticuloendothelial System
Rh	Rhesus Antigen
RLQ	Right Lower Quadrant (pain)
RNA	Ribonucleic Acid
RNP	Ribonucleoprotein
r/o	Rule Out
ROS	Reactive Oxygen Species
ROM	Range of Motion, Rupture of Membranes
RPF	Renal Plasma Flow
RPR	Rapid Plasma Reagin
RR	Relative Risk
RRR	Relative Risk Reduction
rRNA	Ribosomal Ribonucleic Acid
RSV	Respiratory Syncytial Virus
RUQ	Right Upper Quadrant Pain (pain)
RVH	Right Ventricular Hypertrophy
Rx	Prescription
SA	Sinoatrial
SAM	S-adenosylmethionine
SARS	Severe Acute Respiratory Syndrome
SC	Subcutaneous
SCD	Sudden Cardiac Death
SCID	Severe Combined Immunodeficiency
SCJ	Squamocolumnar Junctions
SCM	Sternocleidomastoid Muscle
SE	Side Effects
SER	Smooth Endoplasmic Reticulum
SERM	Selective Estrogen Receptor Modulator
SIAHD	Syndrome Inappropriate Antidiuretic Hormone
SIDS	Sudden Infant Death Syndrome
SLE	Systemic Lupus Erythematosus
SMA	Superior Mesenteric artery
SMX	Sulfamethoxazole
SNc	Substantia Nigra Pars Compacta
SNr	Substantia Nigra Pans Reticulata
SNARE	Soluble NSF Attachment Protein Receptor
SNRI	Serotonin – Norepinephrine Receptor Inhibitor
snRNP	Small Nuclear Ribonucleoprotein
SO	Superior Oblique
SOAP	Subjective, Objective, Assessment, Plan
SOB	Short of Breath
SS	Single Stranded, Septic Shock
SSRI	Selective Serotonin Reuptake Inhibitor
STAT	Immediately
STD	Sexually Transmitted Disease
STEMI	ST Elevation Myocardial Infarction
STN	Subthalamic Nucleus
SV	Stroke Volume
SVC	Superior Vena Cava
SVD	Spontaneous Vaginal Delivery
SVT	Supraventricular Tachycardia
SX:	Signs/Symptoms
T & A	Tonsillectomy and Adenoidectomy
tachy	Tachycardic
TB	Tuberculosis
TBG	Thyroxine-binding Globulin
TCA	Tricyclic Antidepressant
Tc Cell	Cytotoxic T Cell
TCR	T Cell Receptor
TE	Tracheoesophageal
TEN	Toxic Epidermal Necrolysis
T/F	Therefore
TFT	Thyroid Function Test
TG	Triglyceride
Th cell	T Helper Cell
THF	Tetrahydrofolic Acid
TIA	Transient Ischemic Attack
TIBC	Total Iron Binding Capacity
Tid	3 Times per Day
TKO	To Keep Open
TKR	Total Knee Replacement
TLC	Total Lung Capacity
TMJ	Temporomandibular Joint
TMP	Trimethoprim
TN	True Negative
TNF	Tumor Necrosis Factor
TNM	Tumor, Node, Metastasis (tumor staging)
TP	True Positive
tPA	Tissue Plasminogen Activator
TPN	Total Parenteral Nutrition
TPO	Thyroid Peroxidase
TPP	Thiamine Pyrophosphate
TPR	Total peripheral Resistance
TR	Tricuspid Regurgitation
trach	Tracheotomy
TRAP	Tartrate-resistant Acid Phosphatase
TRH	Thyrotropin-releasing Hormone
tRNA	Transfer Ribonucleic Acid
TSH	Thyroid-Stimulating Hormone
TSS	Toxic Shock Syndrome
TT	Tetanus Toxoid

		ADD YOUR OWN ABBREVIATIONS HERE
TTP	Thrombotic Thrombocytopenic Purpura'	
TURP	Transurethral Resection of Prostate	
TV	Tidal Volume	
TVH	Total Vaginal Hysterectomy	
TX	Treatment	
TXA2	Thromboxane A2	
UA	Urinalysis	
UC	Ulcerative Colitis	
UDP	Uridine Diphosphate	
UMN	Upper Motor Neuron	
UMP	Uridine Monophosphate	
URI	Upper Respiratory Infection	
US	Ultrasound	
UTI	Urinary Tract Infection	
UTP	Uridine Triphosphate	
UV	Ultraviolet (light)	
vag	Vaginal	
VC	Vital Capacity	
Vd	Volume of Distribution	
VDRL	Venereal Disease Research laboratory	
VEGF	Vascular Endothelial Growth Factor	
V-Fib	Ventricular Fibrillation	
VIP	Vaso Intestinal peptide	
VLDL	Very Low Density Lipoprotein	
VMA	Vanillylmandelic Acid	
Vmax	Maximum Velocity	
vo	Verbal Order	
VPL	Ventral Posterior Nucleus, lateral	
VPM	Ventral Posterior Nucleus, medial	
V/Q	Ventilation/Perfusion ratio	
V/S	Vital Signs	
VSD	Ventricular Septal Defect	
V-tach	Ventricular Tachycardia	
vWF	von Willebrand Factor	
VZV	Varicella-zoster Virus	
WBC	White Blood Cell	
WHO	World Health Organization	
WNL	Within Normal Limits	
wt	Weight	
w/o	Without	
WPW	Wolff-Parkinson-White Syndrome	
XL	X-Linked	
XX	Female Sex Chromosomes	
XY	Male Sex Chromosomes	
y/o	Year (s) old	
ZDV	Zidovudine (AZT)	

CELLULAR ORGANELLES

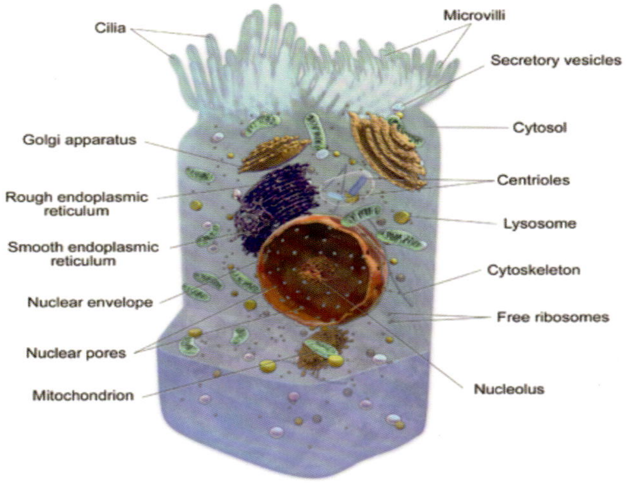

Anatomy of a Cell

PROKARYOTIC CELL	EUKARYOTIC CELLS
▪ Bacteria and Achaea ▪ Cell wall over plasma membrane* (***exception**: Mycoplasma) ▪ Cell wall is peptidoglycan ▪ Some bacteria are encapsulated ▪ DNA located in cytoplasm ▪ DNA is circular, single chromosome* (***exception** Borrelia burgdorferi) ▪ DNA condensed in a nucleus ▪ Plasmids: extra chromosomal DNA ▪ Can have flagella and pili ▪ 70S Ribosome Unit	▪ Plants, animals, fungi, protozoa, algae, slime molds ▪ Plasma membrane* (*Plasma membrane surrounded by a Cell wall in plants and prokaryotes) ▪ Cell walls may/may not be present ▪ DNA located in cell nucleus ▪ DNA is linear in form of chromosomes ▪ Can have cilia or flagella ▪ All cells contain DNA (*except **RBC b/c no nucleus**) ▪ 80S Ribosome Unit

CELL/PLASMA MEMBRANE

- Regulates what moves in and out of the cell
- Maintains electrical potential of the cell
- Protects cell from surrounding environment
- **Lipid bilayer** that is amphiphilic: Phospholipid bilayer (double layer): hydrophobic (nonpolar tail) and hydrophilic (polar head).
- Lipid bilayer provides **FLUIDITY** for diffusion. Fluidity increased by increase of temperature and degree of unsaturation of the fatty acid tails. Fluidity decreased by increases in cholesterol content
- Outer layer: phosphatidylcholine and sphingomyelin
- Inner layer: phosphatidylethanolamine and phosphatidylserine
- Allows ions and molecules to move in and out through channels or pumps
- Contains receptors
- Contains: Cholesterol, phospholipids, proteins, sphingolipid, glycolipids
- Fungal membrane contains **ergosterol**

CYTOSKELETON

- Maintains the cell's shape, anchors organelles, aids in endocytosis, "subway" system for transport inside cell
- Composed of: microtubules, intermediate filaments, microfilaments
- Microtubules made of tubulin protein
- Microfilaments made of actin protein
- **Intermediate filaments**

Intermediate Filament	Tissues	Stain
Keratin	Epithelial cells, Epithelial tumors, skin, hair, nails, bladder	Cytokeratin (AKA: Keratin)
Lamin	Fibrous: Inner membrane of nuclear envelope	Lamin
Vimentin	Mesenchymal cells: Endothelial cells, leukocytes, vascular smooth muscle, fibroblast, chondroblasts, macrophages, mesenchymal tumors	Vimentin
Neurofilament (Neurons, Neuronal tumors)	Glial Fibrillar Acidic Protein (AKA: **GFAP**) Astrocytes, oligodendrocytes, microglia, Schwann cells, ependymal cells, pituicyte cell (glial cells of the posterior pituitary, Gliomatous tumors	**GFAP**
Desmin	Muscle cells: skeletal muscle, nonvascular smooth muscle, muscle tumors	Desmin

CELL NUCLEUS

- Houses cell's genetic material: DNA (uses **histones** to form chromosomes)
- Transcription occurs: DNA replication and mRNA (AKA: RNA Pol 2) synthesis
- **Nucleolus assembles ribosomes (rRNA)** (AKA: RNA Pol 1) and exports to nucleus to make mRNA
- Nuclear envelope surrounds nucleus with double membrane
- Nuclear pores allow molecules to cross nuclear envelope

MITOCHONDRIA

- **Oxidative phosphorylation to generate ATP**
- **Location of** Krebs Cycle, Electron Transport Chain **(ECT),** Beta Oxidation, ketogenesis, 1st and last part of urea cycle

GOLGI APPARATUS

- Sorts proteins **from RER** and sends to proper locations via vesicles
- Processing and packaging the proteins and lipids made by the cell
- **O-linked glycosylation** (adds O-oligosaccharides on serine and threonine) (**tip**: think g**O**lgi for **O** link)
- **COP II** brings proteins **from RER to the Golgi** (**tip**: **2 cops** always leave the r**ER**)
- Adds **mannose-6-phosphate tag** to proteins for **trafficking (transport)** to lysosomes **(I-cell disease)**
- Proteins transported via vesicles. Endocytosis by **clathrin** coated vesicles

LYSOSOME

- Contain acid hydrolases (digestive enzymes) to digest engulfed viruses and bacteria and to digest food particles or worn organelles of the cell.
- Cathepsins (proteases that break down proteins) are found in the **lysosome and are activated by the low pHβ**. They play a roll in cell invasion (cancer) and inhibit the function of dendritic cells.
  NOTE: Cathepsin K is an exception. It is the most potent collagenase (protease). It is secreted by osteoclasts (extracellularly) so that they can break down collagen (the main component of the non-mineral protein matrix of the bone) in bone resorption. This plays a major role in osteoporosis.

PEROXISOME

- Enzymes that rid cell of toxic peroxides (hydrogen peroxide)
- Beta-oxidation of **VLCFA: Very long chain fatty acids, branched chain fatty acids and reduction of hydrogen peroxide (In the ROS: Reactive Oxygen Species). (Associated with: Zellweger Syndrome and Refsum Disease)**
  Note: Reduction: the gain of electrons or a decrease in oxidation by an atom, molecule or ion.
  Oxidation: the loss of electrons or an increase in oxidation by an atom, molecule or ion.

PROTEASOME

- Enzymes that rid cell of toxic peroxides (hydrogen peroxide)
- β oxidation of **VLCFA: Very long chain fatty acids**
- **Responsible for ubiquitin tag to cause ubiquitination (apoptosis).**
  Ubiquitination: post-translational modification (always involves the N terminal) where a ubiquitin protein (contains **76 amino acids**) is attached (tagged) to intracellular proteins for degradation by ubiquitin ligases (enzymes).
- **Misfolded proteins causing such diseases as Alzheimer's or Cystic Fibrosis are caused because the protein was not tagged with the ubiquitin tag (ubiquitin ligases).**
- Degrades viral proteins for MHC-1 and T lymphocytes
- **Ubiquitination does not exist in prokaryotes, only eukaryotes**

ROUGH ENDOPLASMIC RETICULUM

- Contains ribosomes on surface that **synthesis proteins**
- Glycosylation: process in which sugar is covalently attached to a protein
- **N-linked glycosylation** (N-linked glycan's attached to a nitrogen)
- **Cop I brings proteins back to RER from Golgi, Cop II takes proteins to Golgi**
- High in goblet cells of small intestine and plasma cells
- **Nissl Bodies** is the RER in **neurons** that make neurotransmitters for secretion

SMOOTH ENDOPLASMIC RETICULUM

- Synthesizes **steroids, lipids and phospholipids**
- High in testes, ovaries and sebaceous glands (hepatocytes and adrenal cortex)
- Metabolizes carbohydrates
- **Drug detoxification**
- Regulates calcium ion concentration in muscle cells
- Connected to the nuclear envelope
- Contains glucose-6-phosphatase (convers G-6-P to glucose in gluconeogenesis)

RIBOSOME

- Can be free floating or attached to the RER
- Free floating ribosome's synthesize cytosolic and organelle proteins
- Composed of RNA and protein molecules
- Consist of two subunits that synthesis proteins from amino acids
- Prokaryotic = 70S ribosome
  50S = (AKA: **23S** and 5S rRNA (34 proteins)
  30S = 16S tRNA (21 proteins)
- **E**ukaryotic = 80S ribosome (tip: **E** for **E**VEN numbers)
  60S = (AKA: 28S, 5S rRNA (45 proteins)
  40S = 18S rRNA (30 proteins)

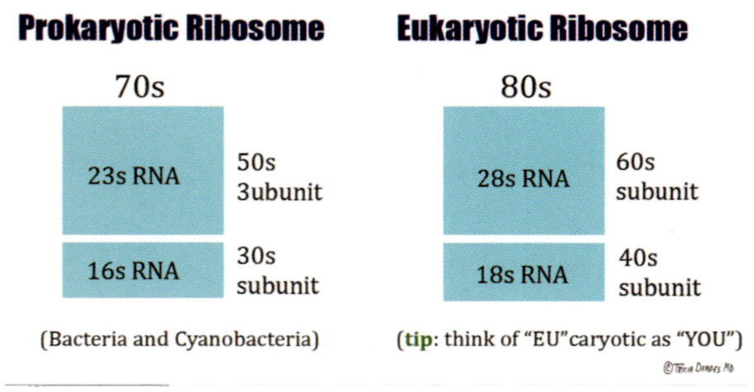

CENTROSOME

- Produces the microtubules of the cell and help form mitotic spindle

CELL WALL

- Protects cell and cell membrane from its environment
- Bacteria cell walls made of peptidoglycan
- Fungal cell walls made of chitin
- Plant cell walls made of pectin

CAPSULE

- Capsule is outside some bacterial cell walls and cell membranes
- Capsule is a virulence factor: **prevents phagocytosis**
- Can't be detected by normal staining, requires India ink or methyl blue
- **Positive Quellung** reaction: testing with serum causing a swelling appearance
- **Polysaccharide** Capsule: pneumococci and meningococci
- **Polypeptide** Capsule: Bacillus anthrax (D-glutamic acid) and streptococci
- Gram Negative Capsules: E coli (some strains), **Neisseria meningitides**, Klebsiella pneumoniae, **Haemophilus influenza**, Pseudomonas aeruginosa, Salmonella
- Gram Positive Capsules: Bacillus megaterium, Streptococcus pyogenes (hyaluronic acid and M protein), **Streptococcus pneumonia**, Streptococcus agalactiae (sialic acid), Staphylococcus epidermidis
- Yeast: Cryptococcus neoformans
- **Encapsulated organisms heavily tested!**
- **MOST IMPORTANT ENCAPSULTED: SHiN Vaccinate against these!**

FIMBRIAE aka PILI

- Filaments (hair like) make of pili protein which is antigenic
- Virulence factor: **ADHERENCE** to surfaces to cause infection (ie: UTI, gonorrhea)
- Sex pili involved in conjugation in bacteria

FLAGELLA

- Allow for cellular mobility

CILIA

- Motile and non-motile
- Motile cilia aka flagella
- Non-motile cilia are sensory organelles on cell's surface, moving in coordinated waves ie: Trachea to move mucus and dirt out of lungs; Fallopian tubes moves ovum to uterus; Sperm movement; ears
- Cilia can be damaged by 2nd hand smoke. Ie: recurrent ear infections in children
- Microtubule cytoskeleton made up of arrangement of **9 + 2 axonemal dynein**
- **Kartagener Syndrome**: Immotile cilia b/c **9:2 dynein arm defect.**
  SX: Infertility, high risk of ectopic pregnancy, recurrent sinusitis, **Situs inversus** (organs reversed to opposite side).
  Recurrent sinusitis is due to dysfunction of the **ciliated columnar epithelia cells**.
  Photo: Dextrocardia (heart on the opposite side of the chest). Described as the cardiac apex on the right.

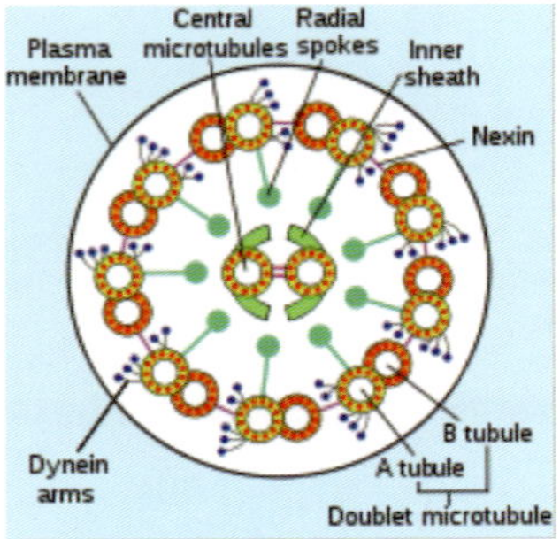

9:2 Dynein Arm (Cilia)

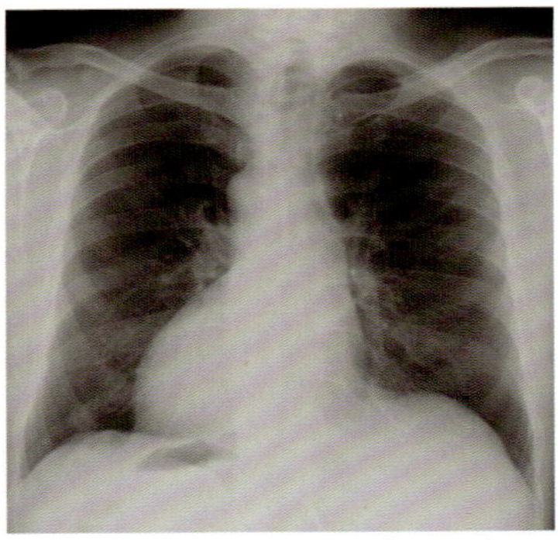
Dextrocardia, Kartagener's Syndrome

MICROTUBULES

- Composed of alpha and beta tubulin
- Component of the cytoskeleton located throughout the cytoplasm
- Makes up the internal structure of the cilia and flagella
- Major component of **mitotic spindles** that pull apart chromosomes
- Provides intracellular transport and axoplasmic transport in neurons
- Retrograde transport from + to – end of microtubule: **Dynein**
- Anterograde transport from – to + end of microtubule: **Kinesin**
- (**tip**: think "M's" = **M**icrotubules = **M** phase = **M**itotic spindle)

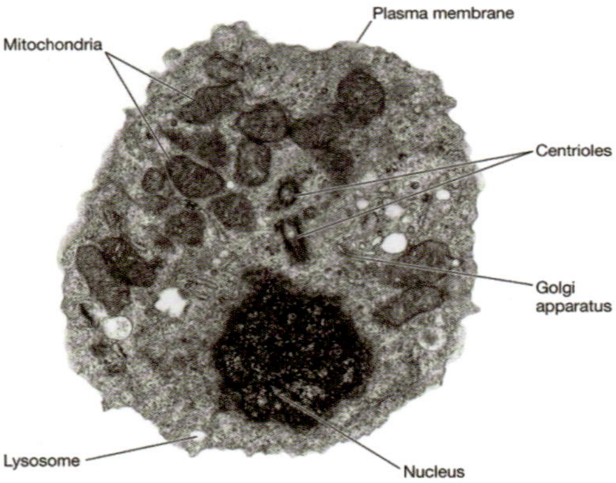

EM of a Cell

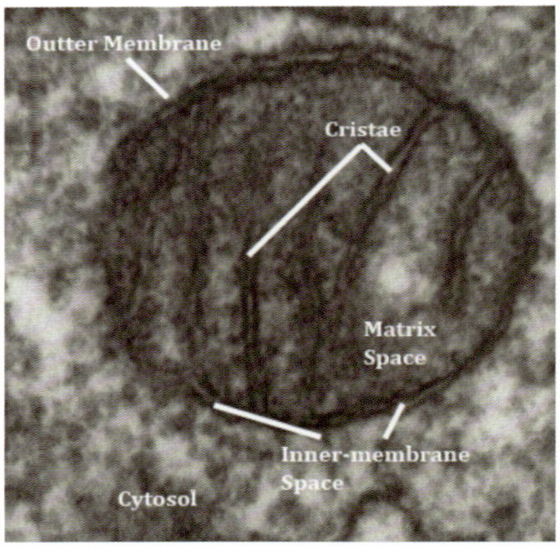

EM of the Mitochondria

HISTOLOGY

TISSUE TYPES
Epithelial, Connective, Muscle, Nervous

MACROPHAGES

- Antigen-presenting cells
- **Class II MHC** (major histocompatibility complex), **CD4, Helper T cells** and TCR (T cell receptor)
- Activated by interferon-y (gamma) and LPS (lipopolysaccharides from gram negative bacteria
- **Secrete: IL-1 (fever and mitosis of T lymphocytes); IL-6 (stimulates B lymphocytes into plasma cells, pyrogens (fever), tumor necrosis factor – a (alpha); granulocyte=macrophage colony stimulating factor.**
- **Secrete: IL-8 if the chemotaxis of PMN's are needed.**

MACROPHAGE	ORGAN
Monocytes	Blood and Bone Marrow
Kupffer	Liver
Dust Cells/Alveolar Macrophage	Lungs
Microglia	Brain (CNS)
Hofbauer	Placenta
Sinusoidal or RES (reticuloendothelial system)	Spleen
Sinus Histocytes	Lymph Nodes
Giant Cell, Histocyte	Connective Tissues
Langerhans	Skin and Mucosa
Osteoclast	Bone
Granulomas	Epithelioid
Mesangial	Kidneys

Cell Types

Cell Type	Location	Function	Cell Type	Location	Cell Type
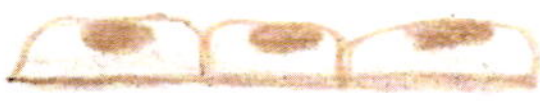 Simple Squamous Epithelium	Lines **blood and lymphatic vessels, alveoli** and lining of the heart.	Allows diffusion and filtration	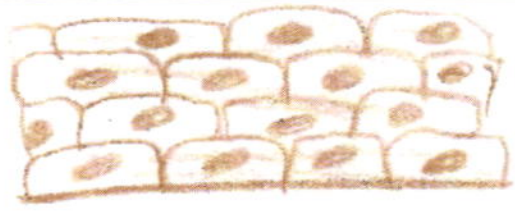 Stratified Squamous Epithelium	Lines **vagina, mouth, esophagus**.	Protects against abrasion.
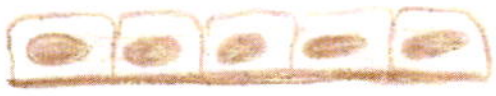 Simple Cuboidal Epithelium	Ducts in small secretory **glands, kidney tubules**.	Secretes and absorbs	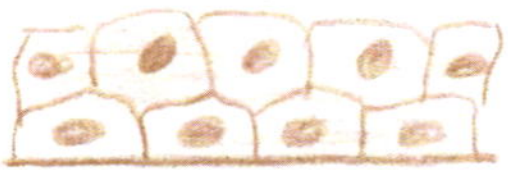 Stratified Cuboidal Epithelium	**Glands**: sweat, salivary, mammary.	Protective tissue.
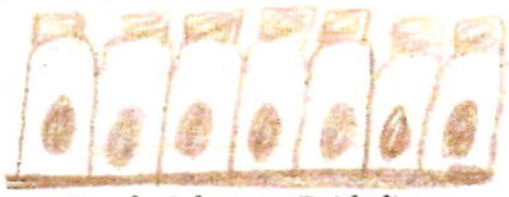 Simple Columnar Epithelium	**Ciliated tissues**: bronchi, Fallopian tubes, uterus. Non-ciliated tissues: Bladder, stomach, digestive tract	Absorption. Secretes mucus (goblet cells), enzymes.	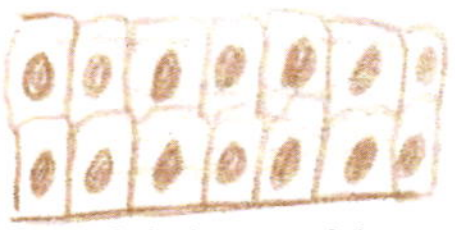 Stratified Columnar Epithelium	Male **urethra**	Secretes and protects
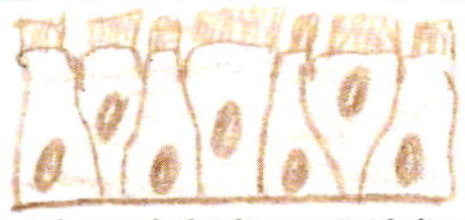 Pseudostratified Columnar Epithelium © T. Derges MD	**Ciliated tissues**: trachea, Upper respiratory tract.	Secretes mucus, moves mucus.	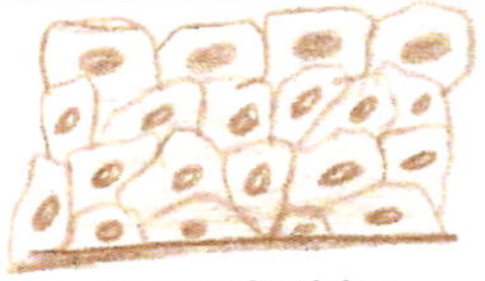 Transitional Epithelium	Lines the **bladder, ureters and urethra**	Allows expansion and stretch

HISTOLOGICAL CLASSIFICATION OF TISSUES

- Stem Cells: ability to develop into different cells types
- Neurons: conducting cells of the nervous system
- Blood Cells: red and white blood cells
- Epithelium: lines skin, bowel, glands, liver, kidney and lung
- Endothelium: lines blood and lymphatic vessels
- Mesothelium: lines pleural and pericardial spaces
- Mesenchyme: cells between organs, fat, bone, cartilage and muscle
- Germ Cells: reproductive: oocytes in women and spermatozoa in men

SIMPLE SQUAMOUS EPITHELIUM

- Function as mediators of **filtration and diffusion** allowing easy transmembrane movement for small molecules
- Kidney: lines parietal layer of Bowman's capsule and glomerulus
- **Type I Pneumocyte** in the alveoli in the lungs allows for rapid gas exchange
- Lines mesothelium of body cavities: peritoneal, pleural and pericardial
- **Endothelium** of blood and lymph vessels

STRATIFIED SQUAMOUS EPITHELIUM (Non keratinizing, moist)

- Provides protection against **friction/abrasion** and chemical damage
- **Lining upper 2/3 of esophagus** protects against stomach acid
- Cell layers of the alveoli to protect against air-born pathogens and/or toxic gases
- Lining mucosa of **oral cavity and internal lips, vagina, anal canal (below the anal valves), esophagus**

STRATIFIED SQUAMOUS EPITHELIUM (Keratinizing)

- Covers the body to withstand abrasion, is waterproof and prevents rapid desiccation
- Keratinocytes filled with keratin (a tough intermediate filament protein) that provides greater strength against abrasive forces than non keratinizing epithelium.
- Apical layer are dead keratinocytes filled with keratin, have no nucleus or cytoplasm
- Palms of hands, soles of feet

SIMPLE CUBOIDAL EPITHELIUM

- Lines **ducts of glands and organs**
- Lines the surface of renal tubules, nephrons, ovaries, parts of the thyroid and eye
- Central nucleus surrounded by cuboidal cells attached to the basal surface of the cell
- Performs secretion and absorption
- Lines respiratory bronchioles, thyroid follicular cells, lens of the eye. Pigment epithelium of retina, ependymal cells, germinal epithelium of the ovary

STRATIFIED CUBOIDAL EPITHELIUM

- Salivary glands, sweat glands and mammary glands

SIMPLE COLUMNAR EPITHELIUM

- Primary functions: protection, provide sensory input, **absorb and transport** nutrients
- **Goblet cells secret mucus** in the GI tract to coat and protect against damage. Mucins (glycoproteins/bound carbs).
- Lining of the digestive tract, stomach, colon, cornea, inner ear, nose, uterus and uterine tubes
- Nucleus located at basement membrane
- Cells connected by desmosomes and tight junctions for semipermeable membrane
- Lining of the pulmonary bronchioles
- Lining of anal canal (above the anal valves)
- Lining of large excretory ducts of glands

STRATIFIED COUMNAR EPITHELIUM

- Lining of prostate, penile inferior urethra

PSEUDO STRATIFIED COLUMNAR EPITHELIUM

- Lining of primary bronchi, trachea, epididymis, ductus deferens.
  These are the cells that are damaged with smoke inhalation.

CILIATED COLUMNAR EPITHELIUM

- Moves substances and mucus by **synchronized movements of cilia.** Cilia propels the egg forward in the **fallopian tubes.**
- Contains goblet cells that secret mucous
- Upper respiratory tract, fallopian tubes, uterus, central part of the spinal cord
  NOTE: Ciliated columnar epithelial cells are damaged in cystic fibrosis, which causes recurrent URI's.
- Viruses target cilia causing damage or death. Non movement of cilia causes build up of mucus leading to bacterial infection

NON-CILIATED COLUMNAR EPITHELIUM

- AKA: Brush boarder, Villi, Microvilli
- **Increases surface area** to allow more absorption
- Surface of small intestine
- Proximal tubule in the kidney (distal tube does NOT contain a brush boarder)

TRANSITIONAL EPITHELIUM

- Multiple layers of epithelial cells that can contract and expand to accommodate volume of fluid in an organ
- Bladder, prostate, ureters and superior urethra, renal pelvis, renal calyces

CELL POLARITY

- Apical region: area above tight junction and faces the lumen or outer surface
- Basolateral region is below tight junction, contains basolateral membrane and is in contact with the basal lamina

CELLULAR JUNCTIONS

- **TIGHT JUNCTIONS** (AKA: zona occludens): Found in apical region, closest contact b/t adjacent cells. Regulate water and solute movement **between** epithelial layers by diffusion or active transport.
  Ie: **Blood-Brain Barrier, Scrotum, Kidney**
- **DESMOSOMES**: MC in stratified epithelium. Connects plasma membrane to intermediate filaments in cytoplasm. Localized adhesive function linking 2 cells together by **cadherins.**
- **Gap Junctions**: Intercellular channels in plasma membrane (surface) of adjacent cells allowing **small molecules** to diffuse into cytoplasm of adjacent cell. Comprised of **connexins**. (ie: **Cardiac)**
- ADHERENS JUNCTIONS: Involves intercellular adhesion and interaction of the actomyosin cytoskeleton with the plasma membrane
- **HEMIDESMOSOMES**: Located on basal surface (AKA: basement membrane, basal laminae) in epidermis attaching one cell to extracellular matrix via **integrins**.
- **Desmosomes and Hemidesmosome both contain tonofilament**. (Tonofilament: fibrils (protein structures) of keratin intermediate filaments in epithelial tissues).

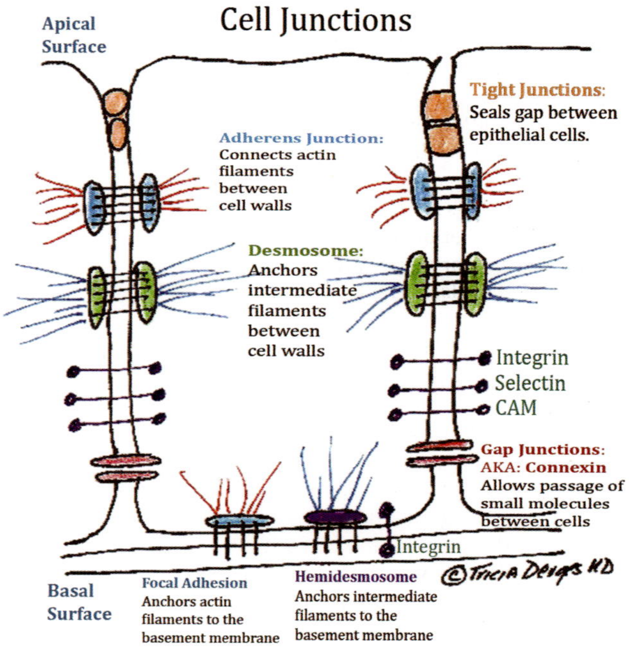

*Desmosomes and Hemidesmosomes

Desmosomes: AKA **Pemphigus vulgaris**: Antibodies attack desmoglein (Most severe form)

- **Positive Nikolsky sign**
- Sloughing, **intraepidermal** skin blisters and **MUSOCAL SORES in mouth.**
- Dx: Skin biopsy, ELISA or direct immunofluorescence for **Anti-desmoglein.**
- Linker proteins: **Cadherins** (calcium dependent cell adhesion proteins: desmoglein and desmocollin). Cadherins require **calcium** to work. Hypocalcemia can affect desmosomes.
- Attach the cell surface adhesion proteins to intracellular **keratin** cytoskeletal filaments.
  (AKA: located within **keratinocytes**)
- (**tip**: "**Demi**" needs a **pimp**, that's a bad thing because she gets ulcers in her mouth).
- (**tip**: "Ca"dherins = Ca)

Hemidesmosome: AKA Bullous pemphigoid

- **Negative Nikolsky sign**
- Bullae (blisters) formed between the **epidermis and dermis (basement).**
- Located on the inner basal **surface of the keratinocytes** in the epidermis of the skin.
- Biopsy would show the keratinocyte layer is not adherent to the basement membrane.
- Immune reaction (type II Hypersensitivity).
- IgG autoantibodies against **Dystonin.**
- Linker proteins: **Integrins**
- **(tip: HE** is a **BULL**ous and lives in the basement**)**
- (**tip**: "IN"tegrins = he is "IN" the basement)

SKIN HISTOLOGY

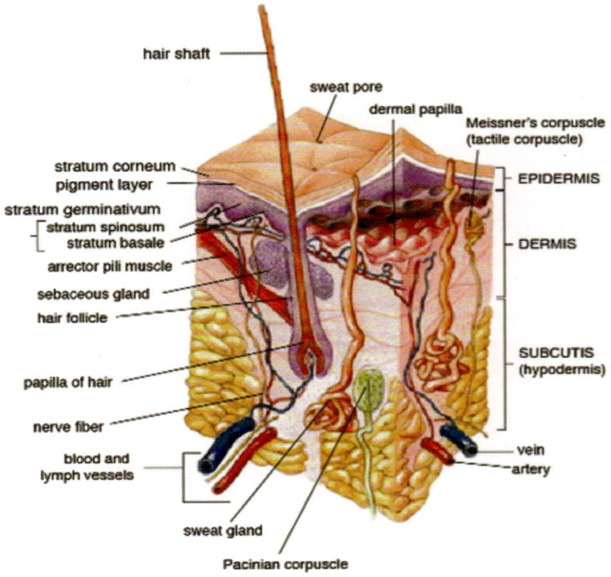

- Stratified squamous keratinized
- Epidermis is devoid of blood vessels
- **Integrins**: transmembrane receptors that bind collagen and laminin in basement membrane to maintain the integrity. (Hemidesmosome). Integrins (CD18) are defective in Leukocyte Adhesion Deficiency (diapedesis is inhibited).
- **Cadherins**: transmembrane proteins that provide cell adhesion so that cells bind together in tissues. (Desmosomes)
- **M**eissner's Corpuscles (AKA: Tactile corpuscles): Unmyelinated nerve ending responsible for **light/fine touch**. Ie: finger tips, foreskin, lips (**tip**: **M**ighty FINE tornado – looks like a tornado)
- **P**acinian Corpuscles (AKA: Lamellar corpuscles): Nerve endings responsible for **vibration and pressure**. (looks like a fingerprint). (**tip**: "P"acinan for "P"ressure)
- Merkel Cells: Cells responsible for touch of **discrimination of shapes and textures**. They are found in the stratum basale of the epidermis.
- **Basal lamina (AKA: Basement Membrane)**: **Type IV collagen.**
  Consist of 3 layers: Lamina Lucida, Lamin Densa, Lamina Fibroreticularis.
  Basal lamina is used with electron microscopy. Basement membrane is used with light microscopy.
  Stage IV Cancer: Defined when cancer has invaded through the basement membrane and metastases. The erosion/invasion through the basement membrane is via over activity of **metalloproteinases** (enzymes, **requiring zinc**).
  Don't forget: basement membrane contains: **connexins and heparin sulfate**. (**tip**: use a zinc shovel to dig)
- **Keratinocytes**: Predominant cell in the epidermis (outermost layer of skin). They form a barrier against the environment and pathogens, form cytoskeleton filaments, **desmosome** connections, provide immunity, cutaneous inflammation and tissue repair (via cytokine secretion of interleukins (IL), interferon and TNFα. They are basal-layer epidermal cells that move toward the surface while undergoing enzyme degradation to form keratin.
- **Langerhans Cells: Dendritic Cells** (AKA: **Antigen presenting cells**) of the skin and mucosa. They are found in all layers of the epidermis (MC: stratum spinosum), around the blood vessels (papillary dermis), mucosa of the mouth, vagina and foreskin. They contain **Birbeck granules**. (Cells look like tennis rackets or rods).
  MC seen in Langerhans Cell Histiocytosis: clonal proliferation of abnormal Langerhans cells that migrate to the lymph nodes.
  (**tip**: to play tennis in Burbank, CA, you have to have LONGER hands).

Layers of epidermis (deep to superficial)

- Stratum basale (deepest of the 5 layers of the epidermis). **Made up of keratinocyte stem cells: stem cells of the epidermis).**
  Cells of the Stratum Basale: Keratinocytes, Melanocytes (pigment-producing cells), Langerhans (immune cells), and Merkel Cells (touch receptors).
- Stratum spinosum (formed by migrating keratinocytes from the Stratum basale layer)
- Stratum granulosum
- Stratum lucidum (clear layer cells in the epidermis only on **palms of the hand and soles** of the feet, "the thick skin")
  Stratum corneum

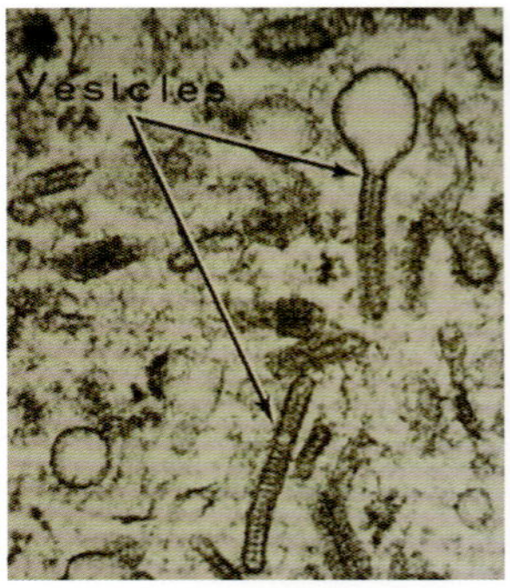

Langerhans Cells

Blood Supply to the Skin

- The epidermis does **not** have vessels.
- Blood vessels that supply the skin are located in the deep and superficial dermis

ADIPOCYTES

- Stored fat in the body
- Yellow color of fat comes from carotene
- **Synthesizes estrogen**
  One reason why "larger" women don't have as many issues with osteoporosis after menopause.
- Synthesize and store triglycerides (composed of 3 fatty acid and a glycerol backbone)
- **In WELL FED state** (increased insulin) they secrete LPL (Lipoprotein Lipase) to catalyze digestion of triglycerides into fatty acid and glycerol. Fatty acids are then stored in the adipose and the glycerol goes to the liver. (Triglycerides are carried by VLDL and chylomicrons)
- Use **Glut 4** to uptake glucose for energy (skeletal muscle also must use Glut 4 to uptake glucose)
- **In FASTING (Starvation) state** (decreased insulin and increased glucagon or epinephrine), an **increase in cAMP stimulates lipolysis, which releases hormone sensitive lipase**. Hormone-sensitive lipase cleaves the fatty acids and glycerol from the triglycerides to be used as fuel for ATP production. Fatty acids are also converted to ketone bodies in the liver and glycerol is used for gluconeogenesis in the liver.
- Secrete Leptin that decreases appetite. **Leptin is mediated in the hypothalamus in the paraventricular and arcuate nuclei.**

BONE HISTOLOGY

Osteoblast

- **Type I collagen**
- Secretes alkaline phosphatase to aid in mineralization to increase calcium and phosphate levels (lab levels monitored to assess osteogenesis and/or bone repair)
- Secretes collagen and stimulates mineralization to build bone.
- Have PTH and 1,25-dihydroxyvitamin D3 receptors
- Originates from stem cells in the periosteum

Osteoclast

- Macrophage of the bone
- Function in bone **resorption** (do not confuse resorption with reabsorption) **Resorption = break down.**
- Secrete collagenase (**breaks down Type I collagen**)
- Have calcitonin receptors
- Reside in lacunae and canaliculi
- Communicate by **gap junctions**
- Differentiated and activated by **RANK-L** (member of TNF family), **M-CSF** (Macrophage Colony Stimulating Factor)
- Regulated by PTH from the parathyroid gland, calcitonin from the thyroid gland and IL-6 (growth factor interleukin)
- PTHrP (Squamous cell lung cancer) can also stimulate bone breakdown
- IL-6 plays a major role in osteoporosis
- Osteoclast secrete cathepsin K (protease that degrades proteins) extracellularly which breaks down collagenase which directly participates in bone resorption and osteoporosis

Bone Formation

Long Bones: Endochondral ossification.

- Cartilage model of the bone made by **chondrocytes**
- Osteoclasts and osteoblasts replace this model with woven bone.
  Woven bone occurs after fractures and Paget's Disease
- Woven bone is then made into lamellar bone
- Pathology process in Achondroplasia: long bones are not developed

Flat Bones: Membranous ossification

- Woven bone is formed without cartilage
- Woven bone is then made into lamellar bone

Growth in Length of Bones: Epiphyseal plate

- Zone of proliferation: chondrocytes undergoing mitosis
- Zone of ossification: osteoblast are formed
- **Exposure to testosterone or estrogen closes the epiphyseal plate.** Precocious puberty can cause early closure of plates = short stature.
  Eligibility for growth hormones: Wrist x-ray to determine if plates are closed. If they are closed, growth hormone can be used. If they are not closed have patient recheck another x-ray in 6 months.

Growth in diameter of long bones: Diaphysis.

- Osteoblast develops within the periosteum.
- The **periosteum is the part of the bone that is active in REPAIR of bone.**

Bone Repair: Periosteum

- Hematoma – procallus – osteoblast deposit immature woven bone – mesenchymal cells form hyaline cartilage – endochondral ossification – mineralization of the bony callus – woven bone remodeled into mature lamellar bone

Hormone Action on Bones

- **PTH** acts on osteoblasts to secrete IL-I which **stimulate osteoclast to resorb bone** = increases blood level of calcium
- 1,25 (OH)2 (steroid hormone) acts on osteoblasts to secrete **IL-I** which stimulate osteoclast to resorb bone = increases blood level of calcium
- **Calcitonin** acts on osteoclasts = decrease bone resorption = lowers blood calcium levels
- Growth Hormone promotes skeletal grown and bone remodeling
- **Androgens (testosterone) and Estrogen: Closes the epiphyseal plate**
- **Precocious Puberty: growth is stunted due to premature closure of epiphyseal plate.**
  (Growth hormones should not be given to children whose growth plates have not closed. Closure of the growth plates are determined with a wrist x-ray)
- Thyroid Hormones: stimulate endochondral ossification and linear growth
- Estrogen inhibits apoptosis in osteoblasts. Induces apoptosis in osteoclast
- Estrogen deficiency (postmenopause, anorexia, surgical removal/absence of ovaries) = ↑ osteoporosis.
  ↓ Risk of osteoporosis: ↑ estrogen, African American women due to heavier bone density

Mast Cells

- **Type I hypersensitivity** reaction (immediate/anaphylactic)
- **Mediated by IgE**. The IgE **must bind (aggregate)** before mast cells can degranulate on first exposure
- Second exposure to same allergen causes mast cells to secrete:
  Heparin (anticoagulant), **Histamine** (increases vascular permeability, smooth muscle contraction of bronchi), Eosinophil Chemotactic Factor (attracts eosinophil's), Leukotrienes (increase vascular permeability, vasodilation, smooth muscle contraction of bronchi).
- Arise from stem cells in the **bone marrow**
- Degranulation (activation) of mast cells is stimulated by **tryptase**

MUSCLE HISTOLOGY

MUSCLE

- Striated (cardiac)
- Skeletal
- Smooth

ACTIN and MYOSIN

- Actins are polymers, myosin's are dimeric
- Involved in muscle contraction, cytokinesis, microvilli, adherens junctions

Fast Twitch Fibers

- **White fibers**
- **Low in mitochondria and low in myoglobin**
- **Anaerobic** glycolysis
- Larger muscles
- Weight training
- Biceps, deltoid, pectorals, latissimus

Slow Twitch Fibers

- **Red fibers**
- High in mitochondria = high in oxidative phosphorylation
- **Aerobic**
- Posture muscles: ie: paraspinal, soleus

Pain and Temperature Fibers (Spinothalamic Tract)

Type I Fibers:

- **C Fibers** = dull, aching pain and warmth. Slow Fibers. Unmyelinated

Type II Fibers:

- **A delta (δ) fibers** = sharp pain and cold. Fast fiber. Afferent.
- (**tip**: 2 legs makes you fast)

GI TRACT HISTOLOGY

- Oral cavity: squamous
- **Esophagus: Upper 2/3 = Pseudostratified squamous**
- **Esophagus: Lower 1/3 = Stratified Squamous non-keratinized**
- Cardia (where esophagus meets the stomach) = Columnar
- Stomach wall: outer mucosa, inner submucosa, muscularis externa, serosa. Simple columnar epithelium, goblet cells.
- Gastric Mucosa: epithelium and lamina propria (loose connective tissue)
- **Myenteric plexus (AKA: Auerbach's plexus)** nerves and ganglia of the GI. (Failure of **neural crest** migration)
- **Parietal Cells** (AKA: oxyntic): located in fundus. Produce gastric acid and intrinsic factor
- **Chief Cells** (AKA: zymogenic): located in fundus. Produce pepsinogen and gastric lipase
- Duodenum: Mucosa, submucosa, muscularis externa, adventitia
- **Duodenum: Intestinal Villi and microvilli**: Projections protruding from epithelial lining of the small intestinal wall. Villus has microvilli projecting from the enterocytes = brush boarder. Villi **increase the surface area** which allows for more absorption of nutrients in the intestine.
- Brunner Glands: Submucosal glands located in the duodenum (above the hepatopancreatic sphincter (AKA: Sphincter of Oddi). Produce alkaline mucus secretion (contains bicarb) to provide an alkaline environment. They also secrete urogastrone that inhibits the parietal cells and chief cells.
- Peyer Patches: In the ileum
- Paneth Cells: Cells located in the small intestine that secrete compounds to maintain the gastrointestinal barrier.
- Large intestine: Mucosa: **no villi**. Epithelium = columnar absorptive cells with **many goblet cells**, endocrine and basal stem cells.
- Large intestine: Crypts of Lieberkuhn (intestinal glands): Contained in the mucosa that contain glands and goblet cells to aid in secretion and absorption of fluids.

PANCREAS HISTOLOGY

- Islets of Langerhans: Produce the hormones of the pancreas
- **Beta Cells: Insulin and amylin**
- **Alpha Cells: Glucagon**
- **Delta Cells:** Somatostatin (AKA: **Octreotide** is analog to somatostatin)
- Gamma Cells (AKA: F Cells): Pancreatic polypeptide **(Amylin)**
- Acinus Cells: exocrine glands (found in numerous organs)

Pancreatic Cell

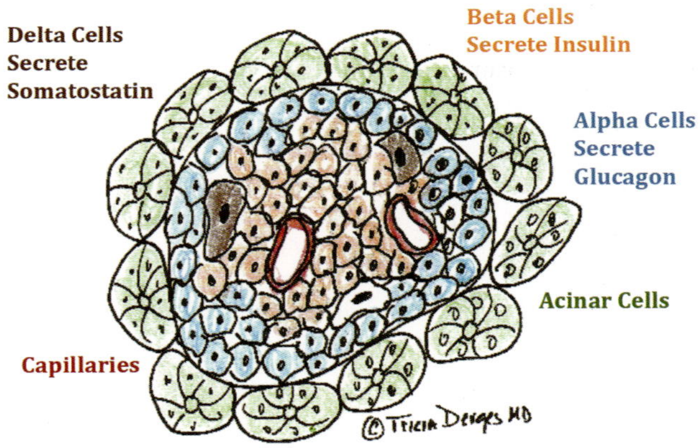

LIVER HISTOLOGY

- Hepatocytes: Parenchymal cells (bulk/functional part of an organ). **Contains abundant rough and smooth endoplasmic reticulum and Golgi bodies**. Bile originates as a secretion from the basal surface of hepatocytes.
- Sinusoids: Vascular channels lined with fenestrated endothelial cells
- **Kupffer Cells**: Macrophage of the liver
- Canaliculi: Inter hepatocytic channels for bile flow (bile flows opposite direction than blood)
- **Stellate** (AKA: Ito Cells, Perisinusoidal cells): **Stores Vitamin A**
- **B-12 is stored** in the liver. (Active form: Cyanocobalamin). **Obtained from only animal products.**

SPLEEN HISTOLOGY

- Splenic Macrophages: AKA: **Sinusoidal or RES (Reticuloendothelial System)** removes **ENCAPSULATED** organisms.
- Contains: B and T Cells, dendritic cells, RBC's, Macrophages, Natural Killer Cells.
- Tags C3 and IgG for destruction.
- Filtration system that removes damaged and old RBC's and antigens.
- **Red Pulp (non-lymphoid)**: Connective tissue (Cords of Billroth) and sinusoid (discontinuous fenestrated capillary that ↑ permeability) that filters antigens, worn out or defective red blood cells and microorganisms. Makes up approximately 75 – 80% of the spleen.
- Red Pulp consist of red blood cells, platelets, granulocytes, plasma
- **White Pulp (lymphoid):** (AKA: **Follicles** of Cortex, Malpighian bodies). White Pulp uses humoral and cell-mediated defenses.
- **B cells are found in the** follicles of the **Germinal Center. It contains adenoid tissue (lymphatic tissue). Antibodies are synthesized in the white pulp.**
- **T cells are found in the Periarteriolar lymphoid sheaths** (PALS) (AKA: **Para**cortex).
- The white and red pulp is separated by the **marginal zone**. The marginal zone contains **Antigen Presenting Cells (APC).** Taking the antigen out of circulation and presenting it to the lymphocytes in the spleen.
- After a splenectomy "Target" RBC's are noted due to the loss of Red Pulp
- In lymphoid leukemias: the red pulp atrophies and the white pulp hypertrophies.
- In myeloid leukemia, both the red and white pulp hypertrophy.
- **Peri**arteriolar lymphoid sheaths (PALS) (AKA: **Para**cortex) contain **T lymphocytes** (White blood cells)
- Lymph follicles produce IgM and IgG, **opsonization of encapsulated bacteria**
- Spleen is **extravascular** (vessels are intravascular)

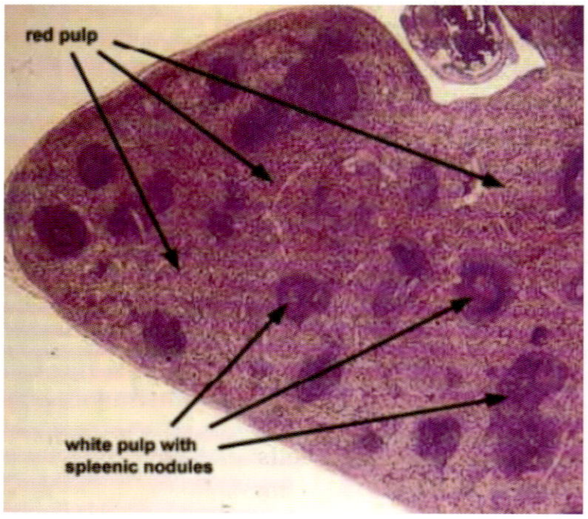

GENITOURINARY HISTOLOGY

KIDNEY HISTOLOGY

- PCT and DCT: Cuboidal
- PCT has a brush boarder to help in reabsorption

ADRENAL GLAND HISTOLOGY

- **Cortex:**
  Zona Glomerulosa (Aldosterone) (Remember: Zona Glomerulosa layer/Aldosterone is not controlled by the Pituitary/Hypothalamus hormones).
  Zona Fasciculata (ACTH, CRH, Cortisol)
  Zona Reticularis (ACTH, CRH, Sex hormones)
- **Medulla:**
  Chromaffin Cells (Catecholamines: epinephrine, norepinephrine)

CAUTION: Be careful to verify what view of the adrenal gland is shown. If it is just a section of the gland (as in the 1st slide below): then they layers go from the Zona Glomerulosa in the cortex on the top down to the medulla and chromaffin cells at the bottom. However, if they show you the entire width of the adrenal gland as shown in the 2nd slide below) , the entire outer edge (top and bottom) is the cortex (top/Zona Glomerulosa) and the center of the gland is actually the medulla.

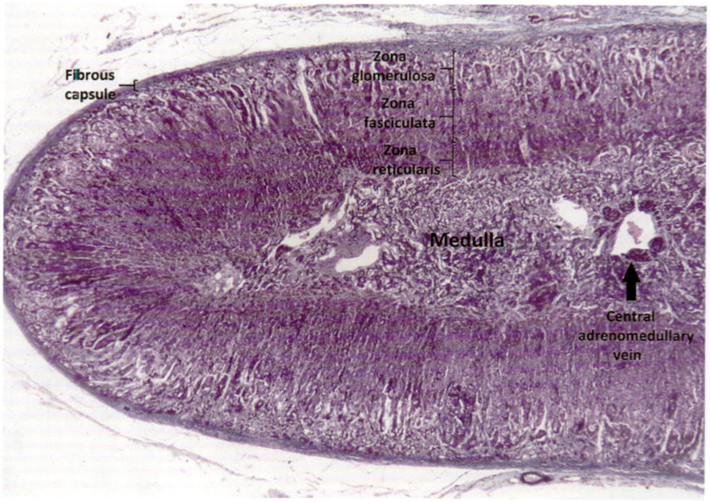

BLADDER and URETER: **Transitional** Epithelium

URETHRA

- Prostatic: Transitional Epithelium
- Penile: Stratified Epithelium

EPIDIDYMIS: Pseudostratified Epithelium with stereocilia. Stereocilia are not cilia. Their cytoskeleton is actin filaments, not microtubules.

VAS DEFERENS: Non-ciliated Pseudostratified Columnar epithelia.

OVARY: Simple Cuboidal

UTERUS: Simple Columnar

VAGINA: Stratified Squamous

FALLOPIAN TUBES: Ciliated Pseudostratified Columnar Epithelia.

BRAIN HISTOLOGY

- **Glial Cells** (AKA: Neuroglia, glia) Supportive cells in the CNS (brain and spinal cord): non-neuronal cells, form myelin, protect neurons. They do not conduct electrical impulses.
3 types of glial cells: Astrocytes, Oligodendrocytes, and Microglia.
- **Astrocytes** (AKA: foot processes) are glial cells in the brain and spinal cord. They form "feet" structures that surround brain capillaries to prevent substances from entering/exiting the capillary. This forms the **blood-brain barrier** and acts as a filter using **tight junctions**. They also help in the **repair of brain and spinal cord injuries**
- **Oligodendrocytes**: create the myelin sheath in the central nervous system (brain and spine). These are demyelinated in Multiple Sclerosis.
- **Microglia**: Macrophages in the CNS.
- **Schwann Cells**: create the **myelin sheath in the peripheral nervous system** (outside the brain and spine). Myelinating Schwann cells insulate axons of motor and sensory neurons to make the myelin sheath.
- **Nodes of Ranvier**: gaps between Schwann cells. Area that allows **influx of Na** to create the action potential
- Neuron: cell that transmits information via electrical and chemical signals (motor and sensory neurons)
Body of neuron = soma
Dendrite = receive stimulation via synapses into the neuron (action potential from other neurons)
Axon = sends impulse away from the cells body = transmits to other neurons

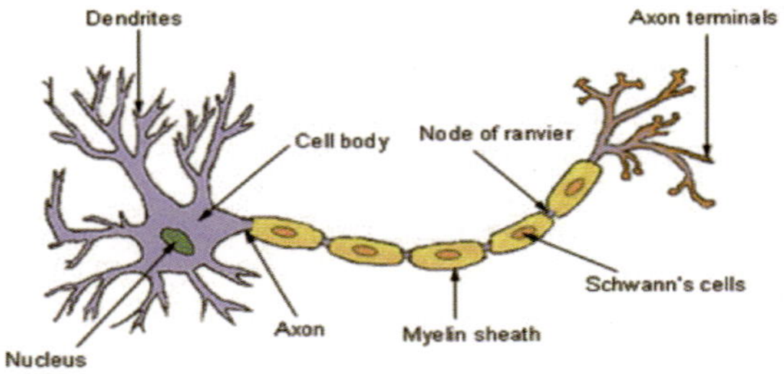

CARDIAC HISTOLOGY

- Involuntary striated muscle
- Epicardium: outer layer of the heart muscle
- Myocardium: middle layer of heart muscle
- Endocardium: inner layer of heart muscle
- **Gap junctions**: allows action potential to spread between cardiac cells
- Intercalated disc: connect cardiomyocytes to allow rapid electrical impulse transmission
- **Lines of Zahn**: In the case of an MI, if the clot shows alternating layers of platelets, fibrin and RBC. Appearance of Lines of Zahn indicates that the clot happened before death. If the clot is gelled or fatty then the clot occurred after death.

RESPIRATORY HISTOLOGY

- Nasopharynx: Respiratory epithelium
- Oropharynx: Striated squamous non-keratinized
- Trachea and upper respiratory tract: Ciliated Pseudostratified Columnar Epithelia
- Alveolar sac: Simple squamous
- **Alveoli: Type I Pneumocyte: Simple squamous (thin)**
- **Type II Pneumocyte: Cuboidal like**
- **(tip: Type I Pneumocytes are thin and long – just like the number 1 and**
Type II Pneumocytes are II (2) times the size of type I (cubed)

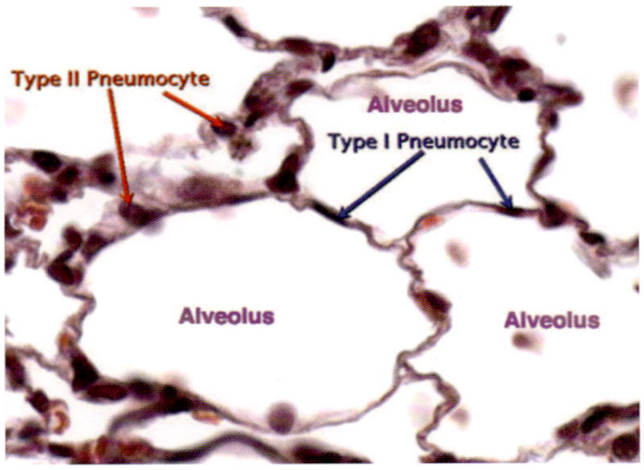

Respiratory Histology cont'd

- Trachea: (trunk of the branching tree): **ciliated** pseudostratified columnar epithelium
- Bronchi (the 2 divisions of the trachea that go into each lung): ciliated, pseudostratified epithelium
- Bronchioles: Divisions of the bronchi: ciliated, pseudostratified epithelium
- Alveoli (singular: alveolus): Bronchioles branch into the alveoli. Alveoli: simple squamous epithelium
- Intra-alveolar septum: simple squamous epithelium with capillaries in between. Each alveolus shares its wall with adjacent alveoli. Alveoli do not collapse individually, only as a group.
- Type I Pneumocyte (AKA: the squamous epithelial cells of the alveolar walls). Very thin to facilitate gas exchange.
- **Type II Pneumocyte** (AKA: the greater alveolar cells) large cuboidal type cells: Secrete **surfactant** to decrease surface tension of the alveoli. Type II Pneumocytes can change into Type I Pneumocytes to repair the lung.
- Clara Cells (AKA: Club cells) dome shaped cells with microvilli of the bronchioles: ciliated simple epithelium. Protects bronchiolar epithelium by secreting the protein Uteroglobin (similar to lung surfactant). They also detoxify the lungs and act as stem cells to regenerate bronchiolar epithelium.
- Goblet Cells: (goblet cup shape) Glandular simple columnar epithelial cells that gel-forming mucin, main component of **mucus** to protect mucus membranes. (Found in the respiratory, GI tract and conjunctiva in the upper eyelid)
- **Kerley B Lines**: Commonly seen on X-Ray in pulmonary edema, lymphomas, pneumonias, pulmonary fibrosis, Sarcoidosis.

THYMUS HISTOLOGY

- Cortex = immature T cells. Location of positive selection. T cells that are not able to recognize themselves are destroyed before moving on to the medulla for negative selection.
- Medulla = location of negative selection where mature T cells and Hassall corpuscles (concentrically arranged epithelial reticular cells (cells that contain the thymic hormones are checked to see if they recognize themselves too much. Meaning they will attack the bodies own cells. If the T cells do recognize "self" too much, then **extrinsic apoptosis (FAS/FADD via Caspase 8)** will occur.
  Failure of apoptosis = autoimmune diseases.
  (**tip**: "E"xtrensic – caspase "E"ight)
  (Remember: Intrinsic apoptosis is associate with BCL-2, Cytochrome C, BAX, BIM, BAK, and Caspase 9)

MOLECULAR CELL BIOLOGY: REPLICATION, PROTEINS, DNA, RNA

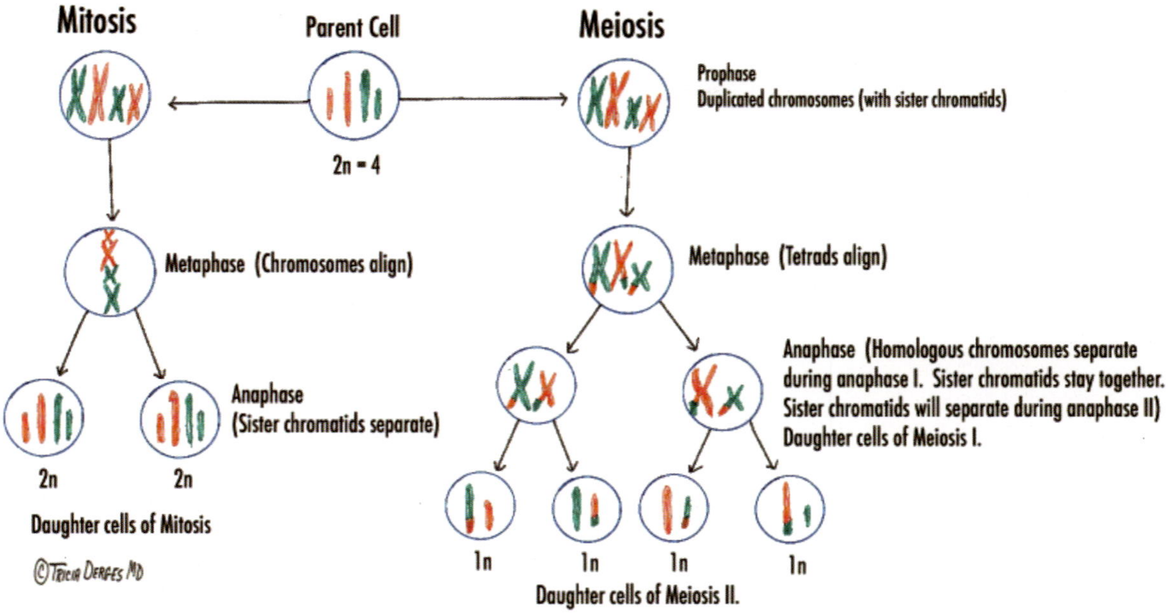

MITOSIS	MEIOSIS
• Occurs in variety of organs and tissues • **Produces diploid (46, 2N) somatic daughter cells** • Involves 1 cell division and 1 round of DNA replication • Stages: Interphase (G0, G1, S, G2), Prophase, Prometaphase, Metaphase, Anaphase, Telophase • No pairing of homologous chromosomes • Genetic recombination does not occur • Maternal and paternal homologous chromosomes are equally distributed among the daughter cells to insure genetic similarity • **Daughter cells are genetically identical**	• Occurs only in the ovaries and testes • **Produces haploid (23, 1N gametes)** • Involves 2 cell division and 1 round of DNA replication • MEIOSIS I: S Phase: DNA replication Females**: Prophase of Meiosis I last until puberty**. (**tip**: meiosis I of **P**rophase = **P**uberty) • MEIOSIS II: Identical to mitosis **Females: Meiosis II last until fertilization in metaphase.** (**tip**: a sperm MET an egg) • Pairing of homologous chromosomes • Maternal and paternal homologous chromosomes are randomly distributed among gametes to insure genetic variability • **Gametes are genetically different**

Diploid: 46, 2N = genetically identical
Haploid: 23, 1N = genetically different

Cell Cycle

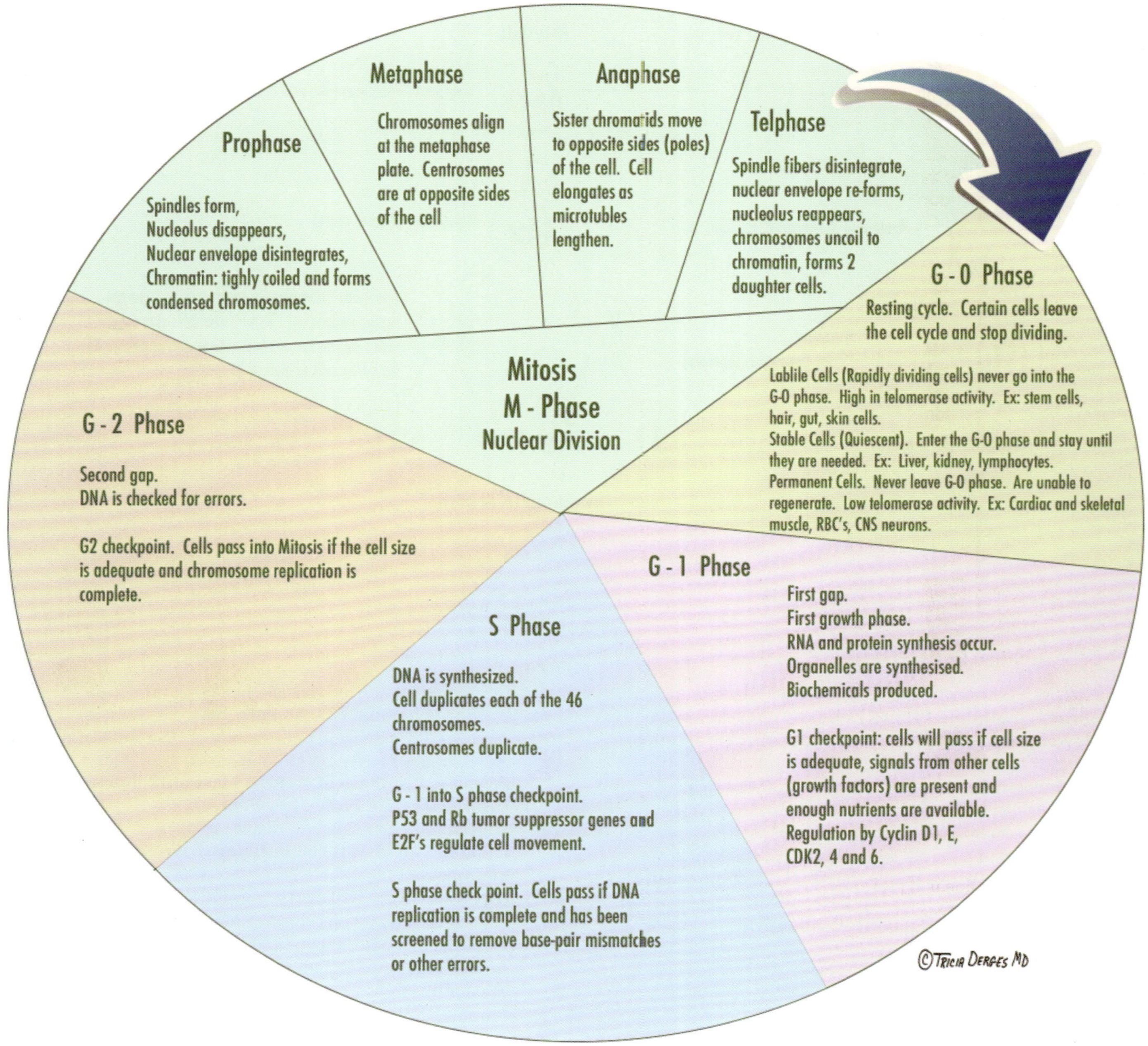
Prophase
Spindles form,
Nucleolus disappears,
Nuclear envelope disintegrates,
Chromatin: tighly coiled and forms condensed chromosomes.
Metaphase
Chromosomes align at the metaphase plate. Centrosomes are at opposite sides of the cell
Anaphase
Sister chromatids move to opposite sides (poles) of the cell. Cell elongates as microtubles lengthen.
Telphase
Spindle fibers disintegrate, nuclear envelope re-forms, nucleolus reappears, chromosomes uncoil to chromatin, forms 2 daughter cells.
Mitosis
M - Phase
Nuclear Division
G - 0 Phase
Resting cycle. Certain cells leave the cell cycle and stop dividing.
Lablile Cells (Rapidly dividing cells) never go into the G-0 phase. High in telomerase activity. Ex: stem cells, hair, gut, skin cells.
Stable Cells (Quiescent). Enter the G-0 phase and stay until they are needed. Ex: Liver, kidney, lymphocytes.
Permanent Cells. Never leave G-0 phase. Are unable to regenerate. Low telomerase activity. Ex: Cardiac and skeletal muscle, RBC's, CNS neurons.
G - 2 Phase
Second gap.
DNA is checked for errors.
G2 checkpoint. Cells pass into Mitosis if the cell size is adequate and chromosome replication is complete.
G - 1 Phase
First gap.
First growth phase.
RNA and protein synthesis occur.
Organelles are synthesised.
Biochemicals produced.
G1 checkpoint: cells will pass if cell size is adequate, signals from other cells (growth factors) are present and enough nutrients are available.
Regulation by Cyclin D1, E, CDK2, 4 and 6.
S Phase
DNA is synthesized.
Cell duplicates each of the 46 chromosomes.
Centrosomes duplicate.
G - 1 into S phase checkpoint.
P53 and Rb tumor suppressor genes and E2F's regulate cell movement.
S phase check point. Cells pass if DNA replication is complete and has been screened to remove base-pair mismatches or other errors.
©Tricia Derges MD

Cell Cycle

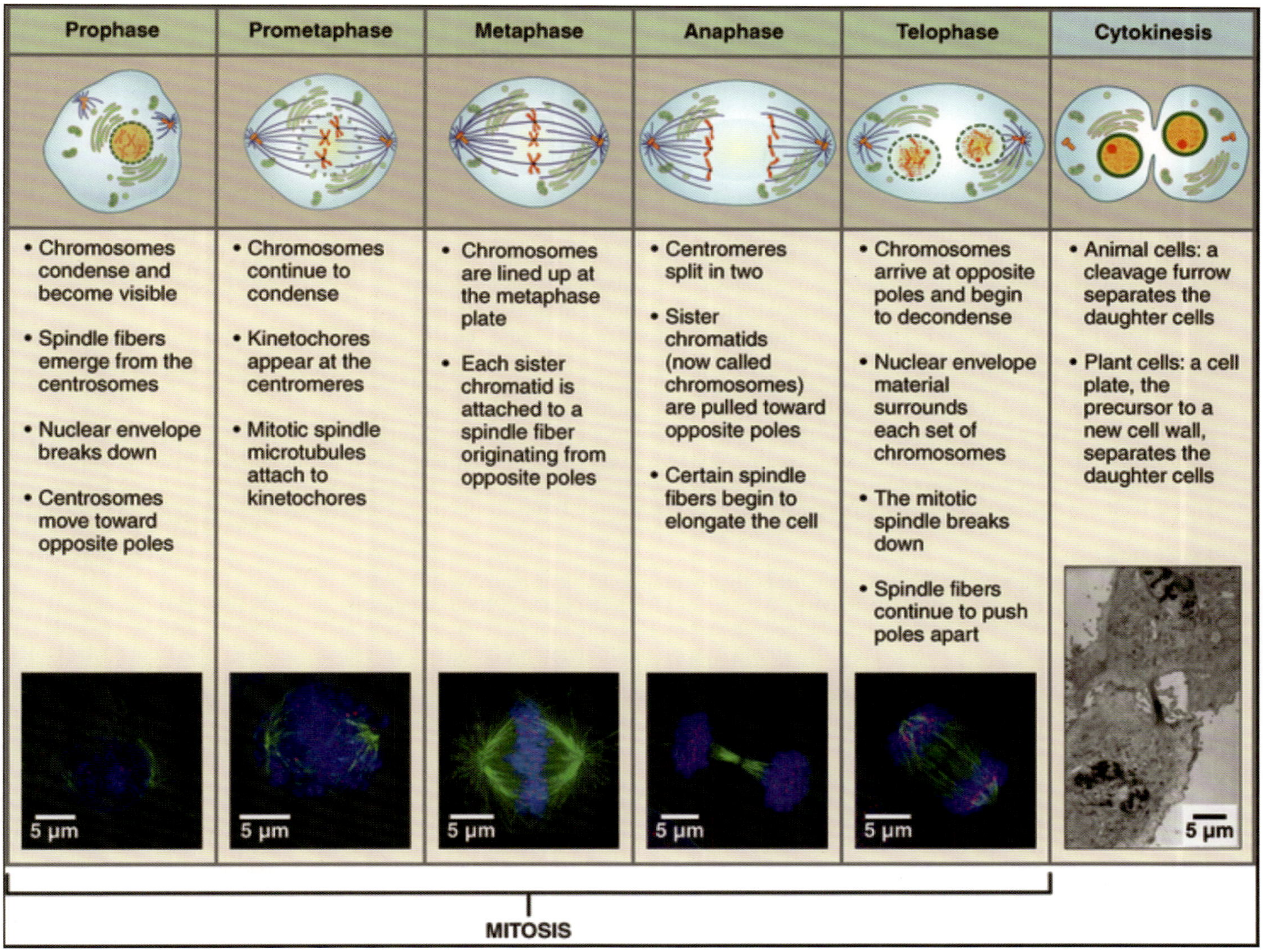

Prophase
Prometaphase
Metaphase
Anaphase
Telophase
Cytokinesis
• Chromosomes condense and become visible
• Spindle fibers emerge from the centrosomes
• Nuclear envelope breaks down
• Centrosomes move toward opposite poles
• Chromosomes continue to condense
• Kinetochores appear at the centromeres
• Mitotic spindle microtubules attach to kinetochores
• Chromosomes are lined up at the metaphase plate
• Each sister chromatid is attached to a spindle fiber originating from opposite poles
• Centromeres split in two
• Sister chromatids (now called chromosomes) are pulled toward opposite poles
• Certain spindle fibers begin to elongate the cell
• Chromosomes arrive at opposite poles and begin to decondense
• Nuclear envelope material surrounds each set of chromosomes
• The mitotic spindle breaks down
• Spindle fibers continue to push poles apart
• Animal cells: a cleavage furrow separates the daughter cells
• Plant cells: a cell plate, the precursor to a new cell wall, separates the daughter cells
5 µm
5 µm
5 µm
5 µm
5 µm
5 µm
MITOSIS

KEY DEFINITIONS

- Chromosome: linear thread of DNA associated with RNA and histones (represented by "n"
- Somatic cells contain 46 chromosomes (23 pair) including XX or XY chromosomes
- Chromatid: half of a chromosome (represented by "c"). In humans "c" is 23
- Sister Chromatid: 2 chromatids of same chromosome joined by centromere that separate in anaphase and become daughter chromosomes
- Homologous Chromosomes: One chromosome from each maternal and paternal
- Homozygous: genetically identical chromatids
- Heterozygous: NOT genetically identical due to mutations
- Diploid (2n = 46): 1 set of each homologous chromosome pairs = 2 sets of chromosomes
- Haploid (1n = 23): germ cell (sperm/egg) contains only 1 each of 23 chromosomes (or half of the diploid "2n") number of somatic cells
- Union of 2 sex cells (each only haploid) results in a diploid zygote
- Allele: One member of a pair or series of genes occupying a specific spot on a chromosome (locus) that controls the same trait.
- If both alleles are the same = homozygous
- If both alleles are different = heterozygous. If alleles are different they produce different phenotypes. (Ex: a pair of alleles that control the same trait for eye color: one codes for blue eyes and the other allele for brown eyes.
- Gene: hereditary unit of a DNA sequence in a specific location on a chromosome. It specifies the structure of a protein and is transcribed into an RNA molecule that is translated into an amino acid chain. Gene mutations occur when their DNA sequences change. Genes are responsible for physical and inheritable characteristics and phenotype.

KEY CELL CYCLE POINTS

- **Nondisjunction error**: Sister chromatids fail to separate during anaphase. One daughter cell receives BOTH sister chromatids and the other cell receives none. Causing the first cell to receive 3 copies of the chromosome: TRISOMY. The other cell is left with only one chromosome: MONOSOMY.
  TRISOMY 21 (Downs Syndrome). Due to maternal nondisjunction in meiosis 1, makes a third copy of chromosome 21.
  Turner's is due to paternal nondisjunction in meiosis 1.
  Other nondisjunction disorders: Edward's, Patau's, Klinefelter's, Cri-au-chat, Jacob's syndrome.
- Oogenesis: Primary (present at birth) **oocytes are arrested in Meiosis 1 during prophase I** until puberty (ovulation)
- Secondary oocyte arrested in Meiosis II in **metaphase II until fertilization** (When the egg **MET**s the sperm). Meiosis II is completed only if sperm penetration occurs
- G-1 Phase: Interphase. RNA and protein synthesis occur
- S Phase: **DNA is synthesized**; the cell duplicates each of the 46 chromosomes. (Many drugs work at this point to inhibit DNA. AKA: Terminate the DNA chain, intercalate DNA).
- G-2 Phase: Checking for DNA errors
- **Mitosis (M Phase)**
- Interphase (G-1 Phase): DNA doubles and chromosomes double, centrioles are copied
- Prophase: chromatin condenses into chromosomes, spindle form, nucleolus disappears
- Prometaphase: kinetochore (structure on the chromatids where the spindle fibers attach) , microtubules (centromere) assembled, nuclear envelope (membrane) disappears
- Metaphase: chromosomes align in center on metaphase plate and spindle fibers attach to chromosomes
- Anaphase: centromere (kinetochore) breaks and sister chromatids are pulled to opposite side of cell
- Telophase: nuclear envelope forms, nucleoli reappear, chromosomes unwind into chromatin
- Cytokinesis: cytoplasm divides and two daughter cells form so there is the same number of chromosomes as in the parent cell. (Myosin II and actin II cleave cell)
- **G-0 Phase:** Resting place where certain cells leave the cell cycle and stop dividing

TYPES of CELLS

- **Labile Cells:** Never go to the G-O phase. **Rapidly dividing cells**: bone marrow, gut epithelium, hair, skin.
  These cells have **low telomerase activity.** Telomerase (TERK) lengthens DNA by duplicating the ends of the chromosomes. It buffers the ends of DNA against degradation. Telomerase is high in cancer, adult germ cells and fetal tissues. Telomerase adds TTAGGG (5' to 3') to the 3' end of the DNA strand. It uses an RNA template (reverse transcriptase: making DNA from RNA: (3' to 5') AAUCCC). Telomerase protects the chromosome from degradation. Cancer cells bypass the arrest and become immortalized due to the activation of telomerase. Telomerase is rich in guanine.
- **Stable (quiescent) Cells:** Enter G-1 when needed. Kidney, liver, hepatocytes, lymphocytes
- **Permanent Cells**: Never leave G-O phase. Cardiac and skeletal muscle, RBCs, CNS neurons. Permanent cells have low telomerase activity.

CELL CYCLE REGULATION

- CYCLINS and CDKs (cyclin-dependent kinases)
- Cyclins must activate CDKs. CDKs phosphorylate to activate or inactivate target proteins to allow entry into the next cell cycle phase.
- Cyclin D phosphorylates Rb (retinoblastoma) protein which activates E2F and Cyclin E
- Cyclin E pushes cell from G-1 to S Phase
- Cyclin B breaks down nuclear envelope and initiates prophase. Deactivation of Cyclin B causes cell to exit mitosis

CELL CYCLE REGULATION: CHECKPOINTS P53 and RB

- **P53 (tumor suppressor):** Regulates cell movement from **G-1 into S Phase**. It can activate DNA repair proteins to repair DNA damage. If damage is irreparable it initiates apoptosis. It encodes proteins that bind to DNA and regulate gene expression to prevent mutations. It can initiate apoptosis (programmed cell death) if the DNA damage is not repairable. It can arrest cell growth by stopping the cell cycle from going from G1 to the S phase.
  Damage (mutations) and oncogenes activate P53 (via phosphorylation of its N-terminal) These phosphorylated sites are targets of protein kinases. (Kinases: **MAPK family, ATR, ATM**).

  Mutations in P53 (AKA: **Missense mutation** in DNA binding domain) results in uncontrolled cell division of damaged (cancerous) cells. Inactivation of P53 leads to cancer.
  (ie: Li-Fraumeni syndrome: people that only inherit one functional copy of the P53 gene).
  Causes: **HNPCC (AKA: Lynch Syndrome**, Hereditary Nonpolyposis Colorectal Cancer), **Li-Fraumeni**: Autosomal dominant: have multiple, early onset cancers (breast, brain, adrenal, etc) throughout life.

- **Rb (tumor suppressor):** Prohibits progression of damaged cell from G-1 into S Phase.
  If Rb is **inactive**/not working (**hyper**phosphorylated) it allows the **E2F proteins allow** the damaged cell to progress into S Phase.
  If Rb is **active** (**hypo**phosphorylated) it shuts off the E2F proteins and stops the damaged cell from progressing.
  (**tip:** Think: if Rb is inactive (out on vacation) then the "ELFS" are now in charge and let everything go by. If Rb is active (on the job of protection) it doesn't need the "ELFS" so they are off and the bad cells are stopped.
  Note: The Rb tumor suppressor mutation is associated with **retinoblastoma** and **osteosarcoma**.

TWO HIT HYPOTHESIS
Rb: Retinoblastoma Cancer
First Hit: (Point Mutation) To get the cancer, BOTH alleles must be knocked out. So if something mutates in one, there is still one allele remaining to stop progression of the cell cycle.
Second Hit: (Deletion) One of the two alleles is already knocked out before birth leaving only one allele left to protect against progression in the cell cycle. So any mutation at all will knock out the one remaining allele, leaving no protection for cancer cells to progress into S Phase.
"**LOSS of HETEROZYGOSITY**" is a common cause of cancer.

APOPTOSIS: PROGRAMED CELL DEATH (Apoptosis is tested heavily on the USMLE)
Apoptosis (AKA: Membrane lipid peroxidation)

- DAMAGE IN **ANY WAY** to these organelles means **IRREVERSIBLE cell damage = death.**
  Nucleus, Lysosome, Mitochondria, or Cell Membrane
- Everything else is **REVERSIBLE cell damage: bleb, cell shrinkage**
- **Pyknosis: Nuclear shrinkage**: Irreversible **condensation** of chromatin in nucleus
- **Karyorrhexis: Nuclear fragmentation**: Irreversible
- **Karyolysis: Dissolution of the chromatin** due to enzymatic degradation by endonucleases: Irreversible

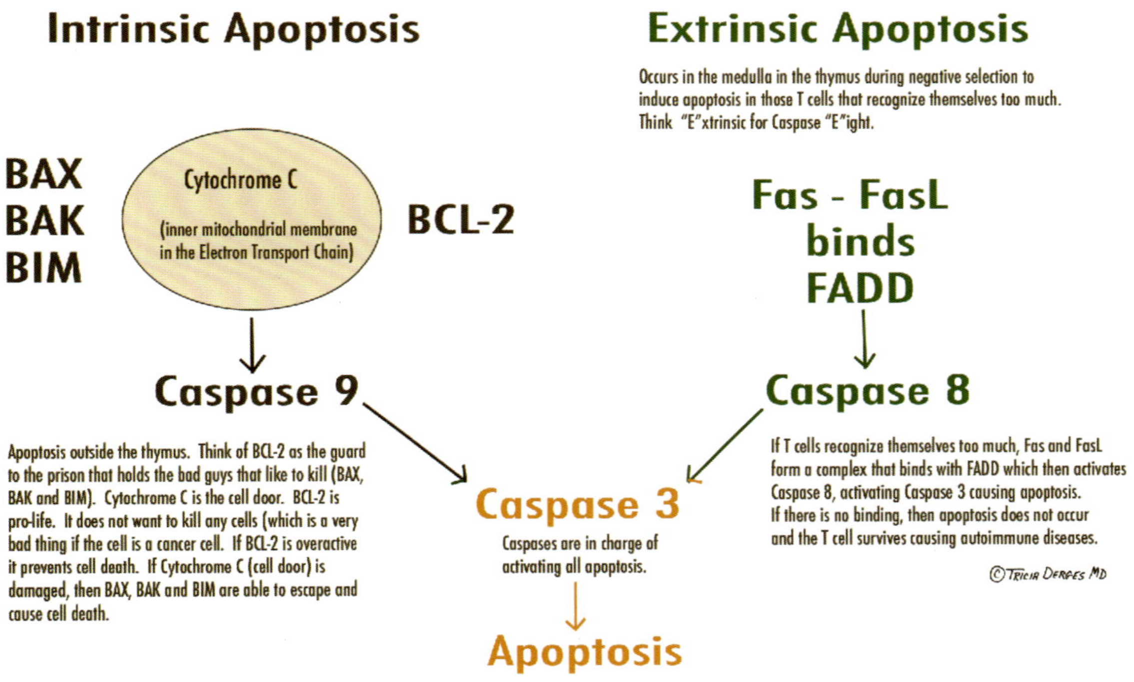

INTRINSIC APOPTOSIS PATHWAY

- **BcL2 is anti-apoptotic** and prevents release of cytochrome by **binding Apaf-1**
- Apaf-1, if free, will **activate caspase 9 and caspase 3 (tip:** Caspase 9 is "n**IN**e" for "**IN**trinisc")
- **CASPASES induce apoptosis**
- If **Cytochrome C** is released it allows **pro-apoptotic BAX , BAK and BIM out = apoptosis**
- **If BcL2 (anti-apoptotic) is overexpressed** or if Apaf-1 is overly inhibited, a cell can't be destroyed which will allow tumors/cancers to live (↓activity of caspases).
- Apoptosis is identified by **180 base pairs** (DS DNA and Histone), It is activated by endogenous endonucleases that cleave the DNA chromatin into DS NDA and Histone.

EXTRINSIC APOPTOSIS PATHWAY (2 paths) (AKA: Death receptor pathway). Occurs in the thymus.
(AKA: "T" cell education).

- **Path 1:** Occurs in the **cortex of the thymus for positive selection**. (**tip**: cor+ex = + positive). CD4 and CD8 learn to recognize MHC. If they are not able to do this, unable to recognize self then apoptosis occurs. **Fas** Ligand binds with **CD95** (Fas receptor) and activates caspases = apoptosis
- **Path 2:** Occurs in the medulla of the thymus for **negative selection**. If the T Lymphocyte cell recognizes its self too much then apoptosis will occur. Negative selection requires Fas-FasL interaction (Fas protects). For apoptosis to occur in the medulla/negative selection: Fas and FasL interact to form a complex and then bind with FADD. Once they bind, then **FADD binds caspase 8 (and caspase 3) activating them**, allowing apoptosis of the lymphocyte that recognized its self too much. If Fas is mutated, the Fas-FasL complex will not form. If this complex does not form, it is unable to bind with FADD so FADD is unable to activate caspase 8 so **no apoptosis occurs**. This allows the T cell to remain alive and be released as an autoantibody, free to attack the body and cause autoimmune disorders. The thymus is the "father of **autoimmune disorders**".
  (**Tip**: **E**xtrinsic = caspase **E**ight).
- **Simplified:** FAS + FADD = activation of caspase 8 = apoptosis
  Mutation of FAS = no binding of FADD = no activation of caspase 8 = no apoptosis.

NECROSIS IS NOT programed cell death. It is traumatic cell death that results from acute cell injury, disease or infection.

TIP: Apoptosis is heavily tested on the exams, be sure to recognize examples of apoptosis!

- Menstruation: Sloughing off of endometrial cells
- Embryo processes: spaces between digits
- Elimination of T cells that might cause an autoimmune attack
- Formation of proper synapses between neurons in the brain (requires surplus cells to be eliminated).

DNA

- Two complementary DNA strands as a double helix held together by hydrogen bonding
- DNA packaging is in the nucleosome and consist of a histone octamer of H2A, H2B, H3, H4
- Nucleosomes connected by spacer DNA to make a 10 nm chromatin fiber ("Beads on a String" on Electron Microscope)
- This 10 nm fiber is what is attacked by an endonuclease in an apoptotic cell
- Histones contain amino acids lysine and arginine. This has a positive charge so it can bind to the negative DNA (NOTE: Histones **AKA** lysine and arginine)
- **H1 histone is the only histone outside the nucleosome,** binds the 10 nm fiber to make a 30 nm chromatin fiber
- Histone **acetylation (activates)** decreases affinity between histones and DNA, allowing transcription into RNA and ultimately gene expression. Increased acetylation of histones = expression of genes.
  Note: Anytime you see the word acetylation, regardless of what other words are put with it, it means GO.
- Histone **methylation STOPS/REPRESSES** transcription and expression. **Note:** Anytime you see the word methylation, regardless of what other words are put with it, it means STOP.
- **Heterochromatin is tightly packed chromatin (H = Hard to transcribe. Inactive)**
  NOTE: The Barr Body is heterochromatin = inactive X chromosome.
- **Euchromatin is loosely packed chromatin (E = Easy to transcribe. Active)**
- Centromere = nucleotide DNA sequence that binds to the mitotic spindle in cell division
- Chromosomes have a single centromere, where sister chromatids are joined
- Kinetochores form at the centromere during prometaphase. Each sister chromatid is attached to the kinetochore.
- Centrosomes produce microtubules attach to the kinetochore to pull the sister chromatids to opposite poles during mitosis
- **KARYOTYPING:** arrest lymphocytes in metaphase or prometaphase (identification used for **Trisomy's, Klinefelter's 47XXY or XXY, Turners 45X or monosomy X**, etc).

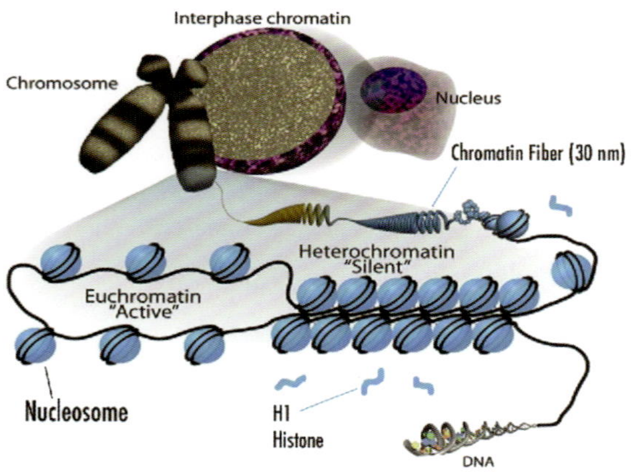

BASES: PURINES and PYRIMIDINES

- Purines: Adenine, Guanine
- Pyrimidine's: Cytosine, Thymine (DNA), Uracil (RNA)
- Thymine has a methyl
- (**TIP** for pairing bases: **A**lways **T**ouch **G**eorge **C**looney)
- G – C Bonds have 3 hydrogen bonds = Stronger than A – T bonds with 2 hydrogen's
- Nucleosides = base + sugar
- Nucleotides = base + phosphate (PRPP)
- Purine synthesis = base starts with sugar and phosphate
- Pyrimidine synthesis = base starts with an orotic acid base and adds sugar and phosphate

DNA (Chromosome) REPLICATION

- Chromosome replication occurs during **S Phase**
- Replication begins at multiple "Origin of Replication" sites = rapid DNA synthesis
- DNA **Helicase**: unwinds DNA at the "**Replication Fork**"
- **Single-Stranded Binding Proteins** stabilize the single-stranded DNA, protect it from being digested by nucleases, prevent premature annealing (binding of complementary DNA sequences) and prevent secondary structure formation
- **Topoisomerases (AKA: DNA Gyrase**) makes nicks/breaks in the coils to prevent supercoiling
  Topoisomerase I makes a single strand nick in the phosphodiester backbone and Topoisomerase II makes a double strand nick
- DNA Polymerase III goes in the 5' to 3' direction
- **Leading Strand**: **Continuous** strand, synthesized by DNA polymerase delta. Works in the **5' to 3'** direction towards the fork. Nucleotides can only be added in the 5' to 3' direction. It does not require DNA ligase. Only a single RNA primer is required.
- **Lagging Strand**: **Discontinuous** strand, synthesized by DNA Polymerase alpha. Replicates away from the replication fork in the **3' to 5' direction**.
  (Proofreading (AKA: reading, reads) goes from 3' to 5')
- RNA Primer: Several complimentary strands of RNA added to the lagging strand of DNA by RNA polymerase to begin DNA replication
- DNA Primase synthesizes RNA primers on the lagging strand that allow the DNA polymerase III to start replication
- **DNA Polymerase III replicates DNA** on leading and lagging strand.
- **DNA Polymerase III proofreads with 3' to 5' exonuclease**. It excises mismatched nucleotides (wrong base pairs).
- **DNA Polymerase I alpha removes/degrades RNA primers** from the end of the lagging strand and replaces them with DNA using Okazaki fragments. Works **3' to 5'** using exonucleases.
- **Okazaki Fragments**: short DNA fragments synthesized by DNA polymerase a (alpha). The Okazaki fragment works in the 3' to 5' direction. The start of each Okazaki fragment requires a new RNA primer. **Okazaki fragments** are 1000 to 2000 nucleotides long.
- DNA Ligase: enzyme that joins lagging strand of DNA fragments together after Okazaki fragments removed
- Proofreading is with 3' to 5' exonuclease activity. (Proofreading **AKA** "reads") Anytime the word "**reads**" is used, it **means proofreading**! They don't always use the word proofreads! (AKA: Proofreading = error-correcting process).
- **Telomerase** (AKA: Telomere Terminal Transferase, reverse transcriptase, RNA-directed DNA polymerase). Elongates the lagging strand by adding a DNA repeating sequence TTAGGG (tail) to the 3' end. Stops loss of genetic material. Telomerase stops chromosomes from losing base pair sequences at their ends (stops degradation) and stops chromosomes from fusing together. It is **high** in tumor cells, fetal tissues and adult germ cells. It is **low** in somatic (body) cells (leads to apoptosis and aging). Telomerase adds TTAGGG (5' to 3') to the 3' end of the DNA strand. It uses an RNA template (reverse transcriptase: making DNA from RNA: (3' to 5') AAUCCC). Cancer cells bypass the arrest and become immortalized due to the activation of telomerase (they are high in telomerase). **Telomerase activity protects. ↑ Telomerase = Immortal (cancer cells and anti-aging).**
  Telomere activity is controlled by either erosion or addition. Erosion occurs each time a cell divides. Addition is determined by the activity of telomerase.
- **Gene Transcription (in nucleus)**: 1st step of gene expression. Transcribes genetic information from DNA to RNA in 3 steps: 1) RNA polymerase binds DNA at the promoter region; 2) Elongation: DNA is unwound and the RNA polymerase transcribes a single strand of DNA into a single strand of mRNA (which is the template for the antisense strand); 3) Termination: RNA polymerase moves down the DNA until it reaches a terminator sequence at which time the RNA polymerase releases the mRNA polymer and detaches from the DNA. The mRNA then crosses the nuclear membrane into the cytoplasm to make proteins in the ribosome. (**Note**: rRNA comes out of the nucleolus and is called a pre-messenger RNA (pre-mRNA) and is comprised of heterogeneous nuclear RNA (hnRNA). Once the pre-mRNA has been completely processed (capping, splicing, poly-A-tail) it is then a messenger RNA (mRNA).
- **Gene Translation (in cytoplasm)**: Protein synthesis in the cellular ribosomes in four steps: 1) Initiation: mRNA and ribosome assemble and the tRNA attaches at the start codon (AUG); 2) Elongation: tRNA transfers amino acids to codons; 3) Translocation: The ribosome translocates (moves) to the next mRNA codon and the process continues in order to create a chain of amino acids; 4) Termination: Once the chain reaches a stop codon (UAA, UAG, UGA) the ribosome releases the newly formed protein (Amino acids are the building blocks of proteins).
- (**TIP**: trans**LAT**ion is the **LAT**er of the two process)
- **Repetitive DNA** contains **non-coding** sequences.
- **Non-repetitive** (unique sequence) DNA contains **functional genes**.
- Pseudo-genes: genes that are similar to another gene at a different locus but is non-functional (due to additions or deletions) that prevent normal transcription.

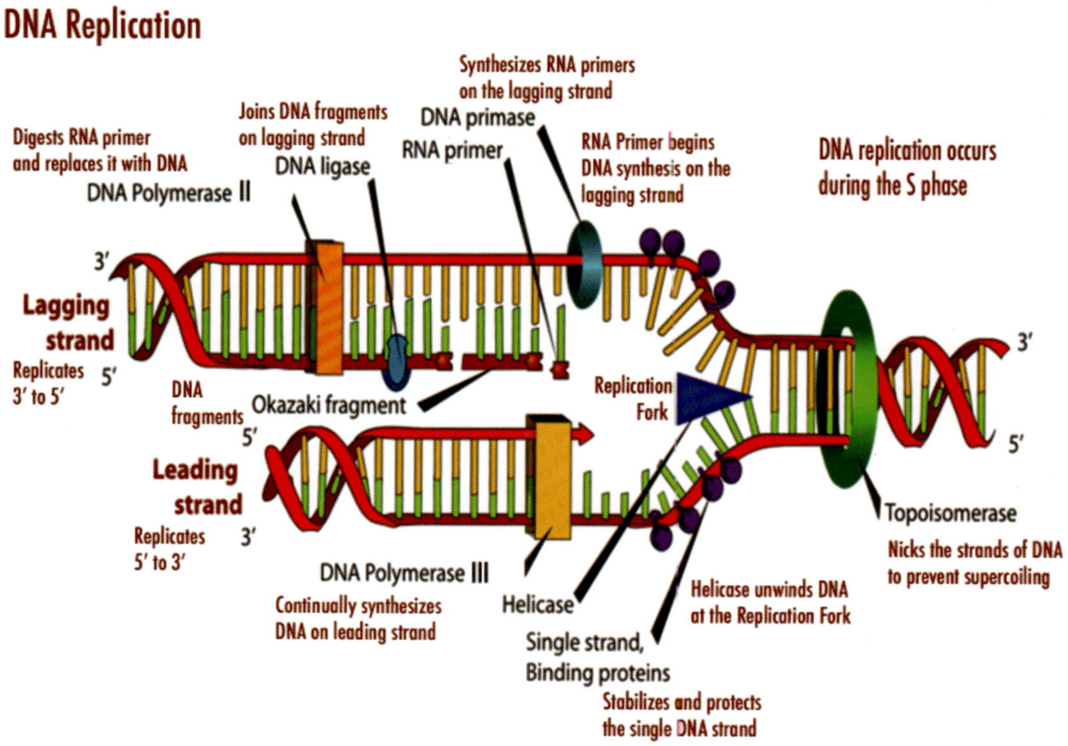

DAMAGE TO CHROMOSOMES

- Damage to chromosomes are due to breaks. Breaks caused by: ultraviolet sunlight, DNA damaging/cross-linking agents/drugs, and irradiation.
- Damaged DNA held in G1 phase for repair by DNA repair enzymes

MUTATIONS

- Silent Mutations (AKA: 3rd position **tRNA Wobble**) 1 amino acid is changed to another but there is no modification = **no change** = no pathology
- **Missense (AKA: Point Mutation, Mistake)** Puts a single base in the wrong place creating **change in the amino acids**. Proteins still stay the same size/length and are functional. This pathology presents: LATE ONSET.
  (**tip**: make a **POINT** not to make a **MIStake**)
  Example: **Sickle Cell Dz. Valine replaces Glutamic Acid at position 6. Valine is hydrophobic.**
- **Nonsense (AKA: Stops, Stop Codon)** Change results in an abnormal, **early placement of a STOP codon** creating a **shorter protein (AKA: truncated)** but still functional. (**tip**: **NO**nsense = **NO** NO means stop)
  STOP CODONS: UAA, UAG, UGA
- **Frameshift**: WORST FORM = **non-functional protein**. Deletion or insertion of nucleotides so that they are not divisible by 3. Pathology presents EARLY onset. (**tip**: **F**rameshift is worst! With **F**rameshift you are **F**.........)
  Examples: Cystic Fibrosis (CFTR Protein), Duchenne's Muscular Dystrophy XL-R, Tay Sachs)
- Transposon: Transposon alters the codon so the gene is disrupted so no protein is produced
- **Translocation**: A section of gene is moved from its original location to a different location on the same or different chromosome. Occurs due to a breakage and exchange of segments between chromosomes. Produces either no protein or a fusion protein.
  Example: **Robertsonian translocation**, Acute Promyelocytic Leukemia (APL), Chronic Myeloid Leukemia (CML)
- **Tri-Nucleotide Repeats**: Insertion of an expansion repeat sequence inside or outside the gene.
  Repeats under 50 are considered stable and have no pathology. Pathology results when there are **more than 100 repeats**.
  Examples: Fragile X Syndrome (X-link) CGG repeat; Huntington's (AD) CAG repeat

LOSS of FUNCTION

- For "Loss of Function" to be pathologic, individual must be homozygous recessive (rr)
- Heterozygotes (Rr) are normal because the individual can still remain normal by producing only 50% of the gene product.

GAIN of FUNCTION

- For "Gain of Function" to be pathologic, individual must be heterozygous (Rr) because the mutant allele (R) functions abnormally despite the presence of the normal allele (r).
  Example: a1-Antitrypsin Deficiency

DNA REPAIR

- **Base Excision Repair**: Removes a single damaged base with endonucleases.
  Order of repair process: 1) Glycosylase (removes bad base), 2) Endonuclease (cleaves sugar and phosphate/damaged nucleotide), 3) Lyase cleaves 3', 4) DNA Polymerase (replaces missing nucleotide), 5) Ligase (reconnects/seals the DNA strand).
- **Nucleotide Excision Repair: Removes a group of damaged base pairs. Repairs thymine dimers.**
  Covalent joining of pyrimidine's. Caused by UVB (ultraviolent) light.
  EXAMPLE: Xeroderma pigmentosum, AR: Excision repair is defective so no repair to thymine dimers upon exposure to ultraviolet light.
- **Mismatch Repair**: Removes a segment of the DNA strand that contains mismatched pairs.
  Mismatch is recognized by its **lack of methylation** (inability to stop).
  EXAMPLE: **HNPCC (Hereditary Nonpolyposis Colorectal Cancer),** AD, (AKA: Lynch Syndrome).
  Mismatch repair is defective so mismatched/loops nucleotides are left in.

SUN EXPOSURE

- **UVB (B=Bad) Ultraviolet radiation**
- UVA (A=Age) Causes aging
- Sun Exposure Protection:
  a) **#1 Best: Sun avoidance**
  b) Avoid mid day sun: 10 am to 4 pm (peak radiation)
  c) Apply sunscreen every 15 to 60 minutes prior to exposure (SPF 15 or higher)
- Radiation: DNA double stranded breaks = Free Radical formation (AKA: DNA breaks)
- Single strand damage is repaired by polymers
- **Sunscreens:**
  SPF 15: Filters 93% of UVB rays
  SPF 30: Filters 97% of UVB rays
  SPF 50: Filters 98% of UVB rays

Exonucleases: Remove nucleotides from the END of DNA
Endonucleases: cut DNA at a specific sequence WITHIN the DNA

PROTEINS/PEPTIDES/AMINO ACIDS

- Amino acids have an amine group and a carboxylic group. They are linked by peptide bonds (covalent chemical bond formation between two amino acid molecules).
- Peptide sequences are written N-terminus to the D0terminus (left to right). Example: a protein is translated from mRNA from N-terminus to the C-terminus and the amino acids are added to the carbonyl end.
- N-terminus (N-terminal): Start of a protein/polypeptide chain terminated by an amino acid with a free amine group (NH_2). It is the first part of the protein chain to exit the ribosome. It contains targeting signals.
- C-terminus (C-terminal): The end of a protein/polypeptide chain terminated by a carboxyl group (-COOH). It is located on the right side of the chain. It contains retention signals to enable it to sort proteins.
- C-terminal end can be modified post-translationally. (Example: additional of the GPI anchor. Defects in the GPI anchor (glycolipid) is the main cause of Paroxysmal Nocturnal Hemoglobinuria (PNH) disease).
- The amino end is what attaches to the tRNA attaches to the elongating end (carboxyl end) of the protein chain.

START CODONS in mRNA: **AUG** (always START school in **AUG**ust).
(note: most start codons code for methionine).
NOTE: A start codon can also be referred to as **ATG** from the **DNA** sequence because its complimentary 3' to 5' base pair sequence is TAC which then makes a 5' to 3' AUG of mRNA.
STOP CODONS in mRNA (**AKA**: Releasing Factors): UGA (you get A's), UAG (You Are Great), UAA (You Are Awesome).
RELEASE FACTOR recognizes stop codons = termination and the completed protein (polypeptide) is released from the ribosome.

How to Determine Anti-Codon

Example Codon: 5' **AUG**........ACGCUACCA**UUGUAA**CAAGUUAGG.........3'

1) Find STOP codon (**UAA**)
2) Going 5' to 3' find codon just prior to STOP codon (**UUG**)
3) Match the codon **U** – A **U** – A **G** – C to get the new anti-codon in the 3' to 5' direction: AAC
4) The answer choice is then written in a 5' to 3' direction. Remember to REVERSE the anti-codon: CAA

RNA POLYMERASES

- **RNA Polymerase I = rRNA, in nucleolus**
  Note: drugs that target the nucleolus, target the rRNA, the molecule in the cell which forms part of the ribosome. It is exported into the cytoplasm to help translate mRNA into protein. By stopping the rRNA, protein synthesis can be stopped.
- RNA Polymerase II = mRNA, in nucleus (largest)
  (**Note**: rRNA comes out of the nucleolus and is called a pre-messenger RNA (pre-mRNA) and is comprised of heterogeneous nuclear RNA (hnRNA). Once the pre-mRNA has been completely processed (capping, splicing, poly-A-tail) it is then a messenger RNA (mRNA).
- RNA Polymerase III = tRNA, in ribosome (**tip**: **t**RNA = **t** = RNA Pol **T**hree)
  tRNA STRUCTURE: 75 – 90 nucleotides long.
  3' CCA end is the receptor site for amino acids. (**tip**: CCA – Can Carry Amino acids)
  Anticodon end is the anti-codon loop (opposite of the 3' end).
  Aminoacyl-tRNA synthetase is responsible for accurate amino acid selection.
  tRNA wobble position (3rd position), silent mutations if incorrect amino acid in this spot.
  tRNA residues: Thymidine, Dihydrouracil, Acetylcysteine

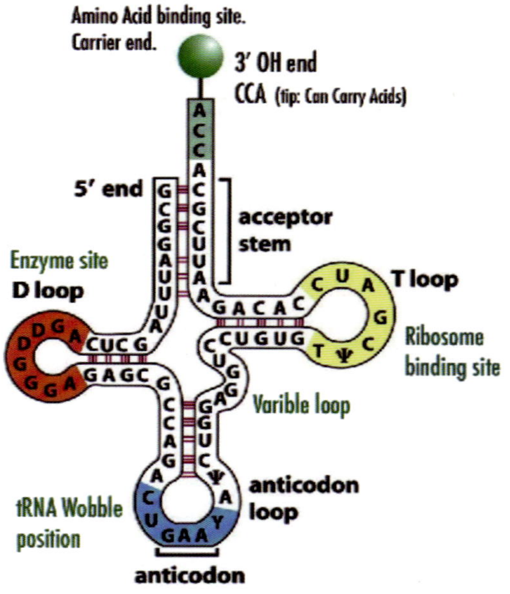

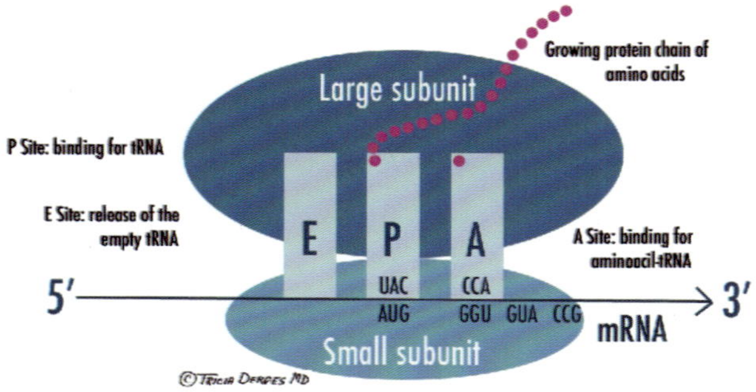

tRNA SITES and PROCESSES

- tRNA is composed of 75 nucleotides.
- **D-loop** contains dihydrouracil. It is a recognition site for the enzyme, aminoacyl-tRNA synthetase. Each aminoacyl-tRNA synthetase is very specific to each amino acid. This enzyme attaches the appropriate amino acid at the CCA site on the tRNA (5' to 3'). The tRNA is now charged.
- **T-loop** recognizes the ribosome.
- tRNA comes in to the ribosome and binds at the "A" site by matching its anti-codon with the correct mRNA codon.
- Translocation from the "A" site to the "P" site requires **GTP**.
- A 2nd charged tRNA binds at the "A" site. The amino acid at the "P" site now forms a peptide bond with the amino acid at the "A" site. This process is repeated.
- Then the tRNA at the "P" site moves to the "E" site (with GTP) and moves to the "E" site to exit.
- This translocation process continues until the stop codon at which time the finished polypeptide chain is released.
- Peptide bonds are formed between the amino acids in the direction from N (NH3) terminal to the C (COOH) terminal.

GENE EXPRESSION

- **PROMOTER**: DNA region that **Starts gene transcription**. They are located upstream.
  Process: mRNA polymerase binds to DNA UPSTREAM and promotes transcription factors
  TATA and CAAT boxes. TATA is located 25 units upstream. CAAT box located 75 units upstream
  (total between TATA and CAAT = **90 units upstream**).
  Mutation in the promoter = decreased gene transcription
- **ENHANCER**: Alters gene expression by binding transcription factors. Located **ANYWHERE** on the gene.

Gene Expression cont'd

- **SILENCER**: Site where repressors bind to switch OFF gene expression, keeps genes from being made into proteins. Located **ANYWHERE** on gene. Silencers are high in heterochromatin via histone.
- **REPRESSOR**: Binds to Silencer to repress gene transcription and binds to the operator to prevent transcription. It stops the RNA from transcribing genes. No genes = no proteins.
- **OPERATOR**: Segment of DNA that a transcription factor binds so that gene expression can be regulated. The repressor is normally the transcription factor.
- **INDUCER**: Molecule that regulates gene expression. It can bind activators or repressors. If it inhibits a repressor from binding the operator (DNA) the operon to be uninhibited.
- **OPERON**: DNA unit containing a group of genes under the control of a promoter. The group of genes is transcribed together and are either expressed together or not at all.

E. coli LAC OPERON

- LAC Genes: Z, Y, A
- In presence of **Lactose: E. Coli metabolizes** (uses/needs) Lactose. Lactose STOPS repressor. Repressor held (stopped) so operator is free to start transcription.
  (**tip**: E. coli "L"oves "L"actose) (**tip**: "L"actose will "L"ock up the repressor so the operator is free to move forward).
- In presence of **Glucose the process STOPS**: Glucose STOPS the activator so Repressor is freed so it is able to stop the operator from starting = no expression. (**tip**: **G**lucose = **G** for **G**ood that E. coli is stopped)
  Decreased cAMP = decreased adenylyl cyclase = poor binding

RNA PROCESSING

- rRNA (pre RNA) enters nucleus from nucleolus to become mRNA
- Capping of the 5' by adding 7-methylguanosine
- **SPLICING out INTRONS.**
  snRNPs form Spliceosome (loops) cut out INTRONS (AKA: cleavage of introns and non-functioning), leaving in the EXONS.
  EXONS: stay in the gene and are Expressed (functional).
  Note: Mutation of the splicing is found in Beta Thalassemia and SLE.
- **Polyadenylation of 3' end (adding a poly A tail: AATAAA/AAUAAA. Over 200 A repeats)**
  Poly A Tail is not transcribed from DNA. It is added as a POST TRANSCRIPTIONAL modification.
  It protects the mRNA from degradation in the cytoplasm after it exits the nucleus.
- mRNA exits the nucleus and meets with the P BODIES in the
- **Cytosol:** where translation, regulation and mRNA degradation occurs
- All parts of the protein (functional and non-functional) are still recognized by antibodies so can still have immune reactions

AKA's: (all are interchangeable) RNA = Protein = Gene Transcription = Gene Expression

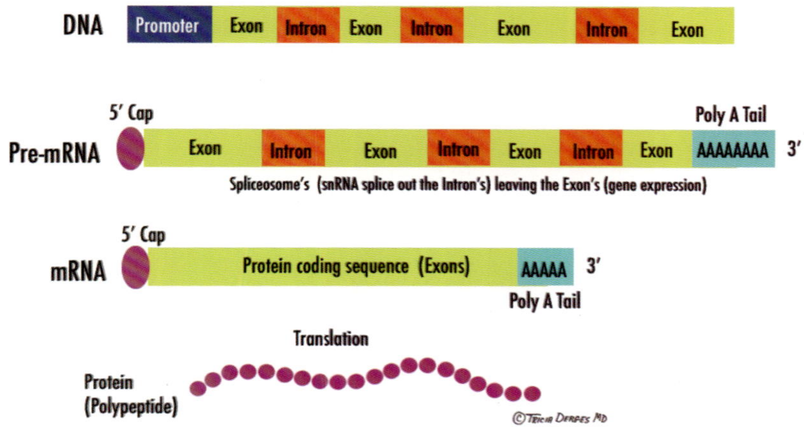

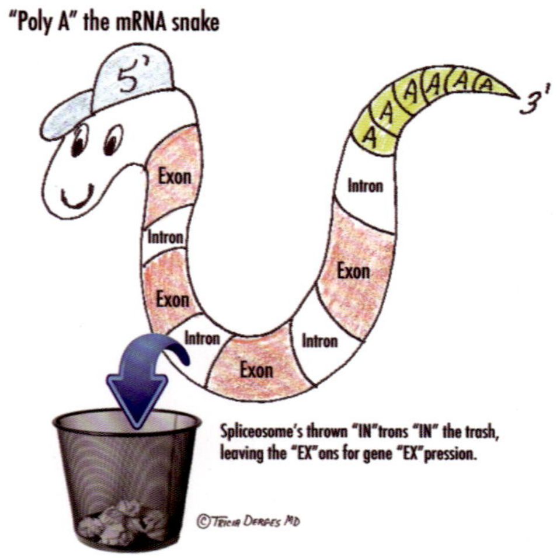

MUTATIONS in SPLICING

- Mutations in splicing leave in introns so it makes a **longer protein**
- **Antibodies to spliceosomes (snRNP) = anti-Smith Antibodies**
- **Associated with: SLE and B Thalassemia (AKA: mutates the normal splicing and makes a new 3' splice site)**
- Anti-UI RNP antibodies associated with connective tissue diseases
- Mutation seen in **Beta Thalassemia** and TTP.

INITIATION of PROTEIN SYNTHESIS

- Initiated by GTP. Ribosomal unit is assembled.
  Eukaryote Ribosome Unit: 40S + 60S = 80S (**E**ven)
  Prokaryote Ribosome Unit: 30S + 50S = 70S
- Elongation (AKA: Translocation): tRNA binds to the A site to deliver the amino acid, then translocates (moves location) to the P site and then the E site where it exits
- Termination: Release Factor recognizes the stop codon. The new protein is released.

POST TRANSLATIONAL MODIFICATIONS

- **Ubiquitination:** Tag attached to defective or **MISFOLDED proteins** to be broken down by proteases
  EXAMPLES: Alzheimer's, Parkinson's, Cystic Fibrosis
- **Removal of N or C terminal pro peptides** to make a mature protein (Example: fibrinogen to fibrin; pepsinogen to pepsin; trypsinogen to trypsin)
- Methylation, acetylation, hydroxylation, glycosylation, phosphorylation
- Chaperone Proteins: Help to fold proteins to prevent denaturing or misfolding.
  Heat Shock proteins (Hsp60) are chaperones used in yeast

LABORATORY TESTING

- **PCR (Polymerase Chain Reaction): Amplifies** a fragment of DNA by heating and cooling.
  AKA: **"Flanking"** the segment of DNA to be targeted
  Process: Denaturing **(heating, annealing to temp of 50° C**), Annealing (cooling), Elongation
- **Southwestern Blot**: Identifies **DNA** Binding Proteins with **probes** DNA Proteins: cJUN and cFOS
- **Western Blot: Identifies PROTEINS via gel electrophoresis** (**tip**: the "**P**"acific ("P"rotein) is in the WEST)
  Confirmatory test for HIV after diagnosed with ELISA
- **Southern Blot**: Identifies DNA. DNA cleaved into smaller pieces and electrophoresis
  (**tip**: good "D"inners ("D"NA) in the SOUTH)
- **Northern Blot**: Identifies mRNA
  Assesses gene expression and determines if gene is being transcribed
- ELISA: Detects the presence of an antigen (direct) or an antibody (indirect), used **HIV.** Performed on **antibodies in the blood.**
  Direct: Uses an antibody to see if an antigen is present.
  Indirect: Uses an antigen to see if an antibody is present.
- **Karyotyping**: Chromosomes are stained in metaphase. Used to diagnose **trisomy's** and sex chromosome disorders: **Klinefelter's and Turners**.
- Gene Cloning: C-Myc gene is detected by DNA probes. All signals for cloning are included in DNA
- **FISH** (Fluorescence in situ hybridization: Fluorescent DNA or RNA **probe** used to find the **location** of a specific gene on a chromosome.
- Gene Expression Modification:
  Testing on mice: Knock Out (taking gene out)/Knock In (taking gene out).
  Constitution: Random insertion of gene into mouse genome
  Conditional: Targeted insertion or deletion of gene into mouse genome
- Cre-Lox: Manipulation of genes at specific developmental points
- RNA Interference (RNAi) dsRNA synthesized that is complementary to the mRNA. When injected degrades the mRNA and stops **gene expression.**
- **Flow Cytometry**: Analysis of multiple cells in a heterogeneous population. Cell size, nucleus shape, granules, etc., are analyzed. (used a lot in **leukemia's**)
- Microarrays: Studies gene expression levels of thousands of genes simultaneously
- **Immuno*histo*chemistry:** Process of detecting antigens – antibody interactions in cells of a tissue section. Used to find abnormal cells in cancerous tumors. Test is **performed on tissues**/tumors.

Misc Genes and Transcription Factors

- **Zinc Fingers**: Mon-made molecules made of zinc and proteins. These are used to target genes and change DNA using nucleases. They can enhance or inhibit a specific gene. The zinc and protein helps to stabilize an alpha helix through cysteine and/or histidine residues that recognizes a specific DNA sequence.
- **Homeobox Gene**: DNA sequence of 180 base pairs long found within genes that regulate the formation of body structures, tissues and organs during early embryonic development. They code for transcription factors (homeodomain protein). Mutations can cause the replacement of one body part with another (aka: homeosis).
  (**tip**: The "HOME"obox gene insures that everything goes to its right "HOME").
- **Hox Gene**: Subset of the homeobox gene. The Hox gene works in the **craniocaudal direction** (head to the feet). The Hox gene is a pattern-forming gene (aka: body plan) that determines the identity of an embryonic region along the arterio-posterior axis. Example: they insure that your head is at the top of the body and the feet are at the bottom. They are **expressed below the C7 vertebra**.
- **Sonic Hedgehog (SHH Gene):** The gene that encodes hedgehog proteins that helps to pattern the structural development from the fertilized egg to the early embryo. They help in the organization of the body shape and structure: limbs, brain, spinal cord, etc.
- **Leucine Zipper:** Regulatory proteins: c-fos, c-jun, and myc family (myc, max, mdx1). These are transcription factors that help regulate normal development. Mutation or overproduction of these transcription factors can lead to cancer. They are a dimerization of the bZIP (Basic-region leucine zipper) that is 60 – 80 amino acids in length. The bZIP is in the N-terminal where it interacts with lysine and arginine. The C-terminal is an amphipathic α helix that dimerizes to form the leucine zipper.
- **c-jun and c-fos**: regulatory proteins that help in transcription. They are produced at the end of the MAPK pathway. They also play a roll in apoptosis. C-jun is anti-apoptotic. Overexpression of c-jun results in ↓ levels of P53 and P21, which cause accelerated cell proliferation.

GENETICS

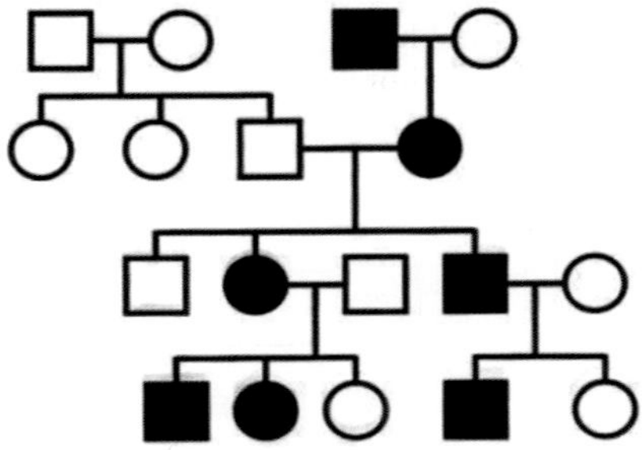

Autosomal Dominant
Vertical transmission

- Presents early on, usually due to **structural defects in the proteins**
- Affects both male and female
- **If 1 parent is affected = 50% of kids get**
- **If both parents affected = 75% of kids get**
- Family history important

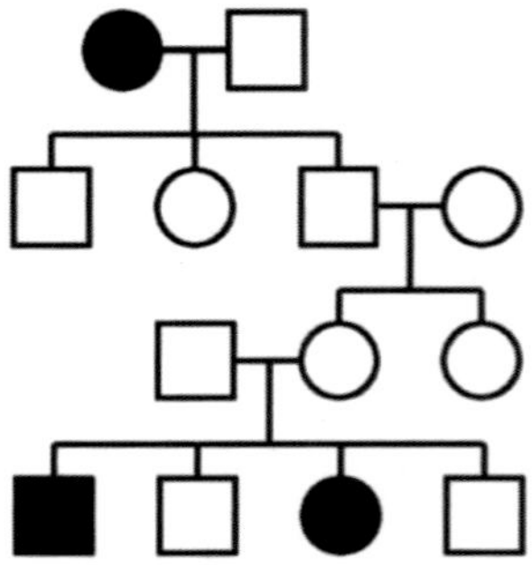

Autosomal Recessive

- **Sporadic** transmission, usually seen in 1 generation
- Presents later, usually due to **enzyme problems**
- High risk in consanguineous families
- **25% of kids will have**
- **67% of kids will be carriers**

X Link Recessive

- 50% of sons of heterozygous mothers affected
- No transmission from dads to sons
- All daughters of dad are carriers

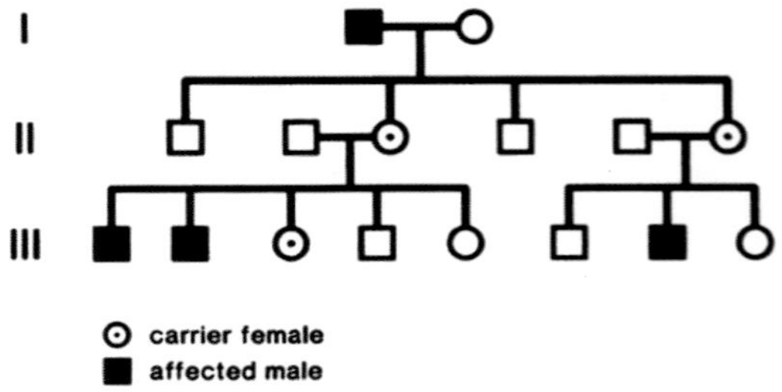

X Link Dominant

- Transmitted through both parents
- Mothers transmit to 50% of all sons and daughters
- No transmission from dads to sons
- Fathers transmit to all daughters

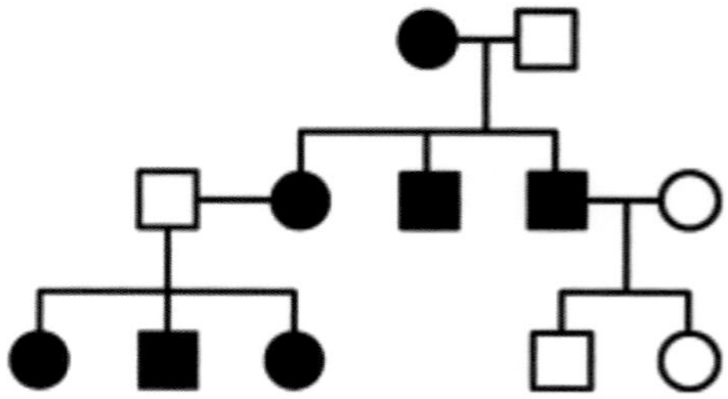

Mitochondrial (AKA: **Heteroplasmy**)

- Mother transmits to all children
- Variable expressivity due to heteroplasmy
- Mitochondrial myopathies biopsy show **"red ragged fibers"**
- Diseases: Leber's (loss of central vision)
  Myoclonic Epilepsy,
  Mitochondrial Encephalopathy

DEFINITIONS

- Hardy-Weinberg:
  Requirements: Random mating, no migration, no natural selection, no mutation occurring at the locus
  p2 + 2pq + q2 = 1
  p2 = frequency of homozygosity for allele p
  q2 = frequency of homozygosity for allele q
  2pq = frequency of heterozygosity (carrier frequency)
  Frequency X Link Recessive in males = q, females = q2

- Probability
  Probability: The likelihood that a specific event will occur. It is expressed as the ratio of the number of actual occurrences to the number of possible occurrences.
  1) Calculate sex probability and make a fraction:
  (Chances of a boy 50% = 1/2 Chances of a girl 50% = 1/2)
  2) Take what chance of the child having the disease (based on the inheritance) and multiply the two (#1 and #2) together:
  (Ex: AD = 50% of child having = 1/2)
  1/2 child x 1/2 AD chance = 1/4 = 25%

- Mendelian Inheritance: Simple genetics' rule: a gene only comes in dominant or recessive forms.

- Normal human cell contains 46 chromosomes: 44 autosomes and 2 sex chromosomes (XX in females and XY in males)

- **Variable Expressivity**: severity of the disorder can vary between individuals.
  Example: A parent with Marfan's has long fingers but his child is tall.

- Reduced or Incomplete Penetrance: Many individuals have the same disorder but do not develop symptoms, but can still transmit to their offspring.
  Example: Some women with mutations in the BRCA1 gene do not develop breast cancer but others do.

- **Pleiotropy**: When a single gene is responsible for a variety of traits. The disorder has multiple effects on the body.
  Example: Marfan's can have issues with the eye, heart and skeleton.
  (**tip**: pleio......trouble = multiple troubles).

- Polygenic Trait: A trait that is determined by genes at two or more loci. Environmental factors can also influence the trait.
  Example: Skin and hair

- Phenotype: What you physically see.

- Allele: Alternative (variations) of a gene.

- Genotype: An organism's entire genetic makeup or the alleles at a particular locus
- Heterozygous: A genotype consisting of two different alleles of a gene for a particular trait (Aa).

- Homozygous: Having the same allele at the same locus on both members of a pair of homologous chromosomes. A genotype consisting of two identical alleles of a gene for a particular trait. Homozygous recessive (aa), Homozygous Dominant (AA).

- Homologous Chromosomes: Chromosomes that are paired during meiosis. They have the same genes, but not necessarily the same alleles at the same locus.

- Uniparental Disomy: When both copies of a chromosome are inherited from the same parent.
  Isodisomy: (heterozygous) One copy is an identical copy of one homolog of a chromosome from one parent. Meiosis 1 error.
  Heterodisomy (homozygous) both homologs of a chromosome are passed from one parent. Meiosis II error.

- **Imprinting**: At one locus, one allele is active and the other is inactive because it was imprinted (**AKA: methylated**). If the one active allele is deleted the individual will develop the disease.
  Example: **Prader-Willi:** Gene passed from mom is inactive. Prader-Willi is developed once the active gene from the father is deleted.
  Angelman: Gene passed from dad is inactive. Angelman is developed once the active gene from the mother is deleted.

- **Heteroplasmy (AKA: Mitochondrial), biopsy on muscles show "red ragged fibers".**

- **Mosaicism**: Different cell lines with different genotypes in the same individual who developed from a single fertilized egg. Due to mitotic errors after fertilization.
  Somatic Mosaicism: mutation in multiple tissues and/or organs.
  Germline (Gonadal) Mosaicism: mutation is only in the egg or sperm cells.
  Example: **Robertsonian**, McCune Albright

- Aneuploidy: An extra or missing chromosome (abnormal number of chromosomes). Chromosomes do not separate properly during cell division.

- Monosomy: Having only one chromosome instead of two due to unbalanced translocations or deletions.
  Example: Turners (XO)

- Trisomy: Presence of tree copies of a chromosome instead of two.
  Examples: Downs, Edwards, Patau's

- **Non-Disjunction**: Failure of homologous chromosomes or sister chromatids to separate properly during cell division.
  Non-Disjunction results in daughter cells with abnormal chromosome numbers (aneuploidy).
  Non-Disjunction in Meiosis 1 is failure of homologous chromosomes to separate properly and in Meiosis II is failure of sister chromatids to separate properly.
  Example: **Downs is a result of non-disjunction in maternal Meiosis I.**
  Turner's is a result of non-disjunction in paternal meiosis I.

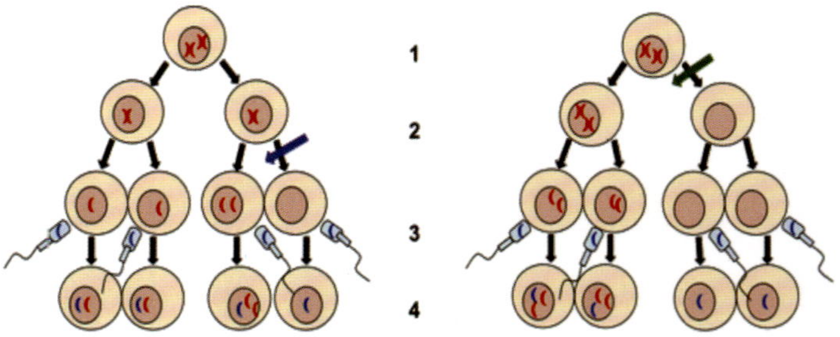

1) Meiosis I 2) Meiosis II 3) Fertilization 4) Zygote

- Co-dominance: Both alleles contribute to the phenotype.

- Translocation: Transfer of a piece of one chromosome to a non-homologous chromosome. It does not always produce abnormal development.

- Deletion: When a chromosome breaks and a portion is lost.

- **Loss of Heterozygosity:** (**AKA: Two Hit Hypothesis**) Loss of an entire gene and surrounding chromosome region. Individual inherits/mutates a tumor suppressor gene (NOT an oncogene) the other allele must be deleted/mutated before cancer can be developed.
  Example: Retinoblastoma, BRCA1, BRCA2

- Locus Heterogeneity: Single disorder, pattern or trait caused by mutations in genes at different loci. These mutations produce similar phenotypes.
  Example: Albinism, hypertrophic cardiomyopathy, osteogenesis imperfecta.

- Linkage Disequilibrium: Non-random association of alleles at different loci. In populations alleles are not equally linked, they are linked more than they should be.

- Allelic Heterogeneity: Different mutations at the same locus produce the same phenotype.
  Example: B-Thalassemia (different mutations on the B globin gene)
  Alkaptonuria, Achondroplasia, Phenylketonuria.

- **Anticipation:** Earlier onset or increased severity of symptoms of a disease in succeeding generations.
  Example: **Huntington's and ALL other trinucleotide repeat disorders.**

- Genetic Drift: Evolution or change in gene pool frequencies, resulting from random chance. Occurs most rapidly in small populations.

- **Genetic Shift (AKA: Antigenic Variation):** Two or more different strains of a virus combine to form a new subtype of virus.
  This is the **worst type** of shift.
  (**tip**: Oh SH.....ft, this is bad") Example: **Influenza virus and all other segmented viruses.**

GENETIC DISEASES*

AUTOSOMAL DOMINANT

Achondroplasia
Alport syndrome
Ehlers-Danlos syndrome
Familial adenomatous polyposis
Hereditary nonpolyposis colorectal cancer (HNPCC)
Hereditary spherocytosis
Marfan syndrome
Neurofibromatosis
Retinoblastoma
Tuberous sclerosis
Adult polycystic kidney disorder
Charcot-Marie-Tooth disorder
Epidermolysis bullosa simplex
Familial hypercholesterolemia
Porphyria cutanea tarda
Huntington disorder
Myotonic dystrophy 1 and 2
Osteogenesis imperfecta
Von Willebrand disorder
Acute Intermittent Porphyria

AUTOSOMAL RECESSIVE

a1-Antitrypsin Deficiency
Alpha thalassemia
Ataxia telangiectasia
Branched chain ketonuria
Cystic fibrosis
Dwarfism
Erythropoietic porphyria
Friedreich ataxia
Galactosemia
Pompe
Andersen
Hers
Homocystinuria
Tay Sachs
Niemann-Pick
Sandhoff
Hurler
Peroxisomal disorders
Pyruvate kinase deficiency
Sickle cell anemia
Xeroderma pigmentosa
Albinism
Alkaptonuria
Beta thalassemia
Childhood polycystic kidney disorder
Cystinuria
Ehlers-Danlos syndrome
Fanconi anemia
Fructosuria
Von Gierke
Cori
McArdle
Hemoglobin C disorder
Hypothyroidism
Gaucher
Krabbe
Metachromatic leukodystrophy
Osteogenesis imperfecta
Phenylketonuria
Retinitis pigmentosa
Tyrosinemia

X LINK DOMINANT

Hypophosphatemic rickets
Rett syndrome
Goltz syndrome

X LINK RECESSIVE

Duchenne muscular dystrophy (Dystrophin)
Fabry disorder
G6PD deficiency
Hunter syndrome
Lesch-Nyhan syndrome (HPRT1)
Ornithine transcarbamylase deficiency
Agammaglobulinemia
Alport's (COL4A5)
Ehlers-Danlos (Type IX)
Fragile X syndrome (CGG on gene FMR-1)
Hemophilia A & B (F8 and 9)
Menkes Kinky hair syndrome (ATP7A, copper efflux protein)
Wiskott-Aldrich syndrome (WASP protein)
Bruton's (BTK gene)
SCID (IL receptor mutation)

TRINUCLEOTIDE REPEATS (can show anticipation)

Fragile X	CGG
Huntington Disease	CAG
Friedreich Ataxia	GAA
Myotonic Dystrophy	CTG

TRISOMIES (AKA: aneuploidy)

Downs Syndrome, Trisomy 21
Edwards Syndrom, Trisomy 18
Patau Syndrome, Trisomy 13

MICRODELETION

Cri-du-chat Syndrome
Williams Syndrome

DELETION
DiGeorge Syndrome

IMPRINTING/MICRODELETION
Prater Willy
Angelman's

MUSCULAR DYSTROPHIES'
Myotonic Type I
Duchenne's
Becker

MONOSOMY
Turners

MOSAICISM
Robertsonian Translocation

MITOCHONDRIAL (AKA: **Heteroplasmy**)
Leber's
Myoclonic Epilepsy
Mitochondrial Encephalomyopathy

*Not a complete list of genetic diseases. Diseases listed are the most common seen on the USMLE.

GENETIC CARDIAC DEFECTS
Downs Syndrome: ASD, Endocardial Cushion, Intra Atrial Septum
Kartagener's: Situs Inversus
Tuberous Sclerosis: Cardiac rhabdomyoma, Myxoma
DiGeorge: Tetralogy of Fallot, Truncus Arteriosis
Marfan's: Necrosis of Aorta, MVP, Thoracic Aortic Aneurysm, Aortic Dissection
Fredericks Ataxia: HCM
Neonatal Lupus: Heart Block
Williams: Aortic Stenosis
Lang Neilson: Long QT Syndrome
Edwards: VSD
Congenital Rubella: PDA
Kawasaki: Coronary Artery Aneurysm
Turners: Coarctation of the Aorta, Bicuspid Aortic Valve
Infant of Diabetic Mother: Transposition of Great Arteries

Mental Retardation

- MC genetic cause of mental retardation: Trisomy 21 (Down Syndrome). It is seldom inherited.
- MC form of inherited mental retardation: **Fragile X**

GENETIC PATHOLOGIES

ANEUPLOIDIES

Trisomy 21, Downs Syndrome

- **Maternal Meiotic (Meiosis I) nondisjunction of homologous chromosomes in stage 1 and 2 of anaphase**
- Third copy of chromosome 21
- Higher risk with **increased maternal age** (over 35)
- **Increased risk of ALL and Alzheimer's**
- SX: **Hirschsprung** disease, mental retardation, single palmer simian crease, cardiac endocardial cushion defects, **ASD** (Fixed S2), **Brushfield spots** (white specs in the iris), gap between first two toes, **duodenal atresia** (AKA: double bubble), flat faces, epicanthal folds, large protruding tongue, short neck, instability of the atlantoaxial joint
- Ultrasound Fetal Findings: Increased **nuchal translucency** (thick area at back of neck)
- **Labs: Decreased: AFP, Estriol, PAPP-A**
  Increased: Inhibin A, B HCG
- **MC: Robertsonian translocation between chromosomes 13 and 21** (2 short arms of chromosome are lost).
  Can also be due to **Mosaicism** Post fertilization mitotic error
  No association with maternal age

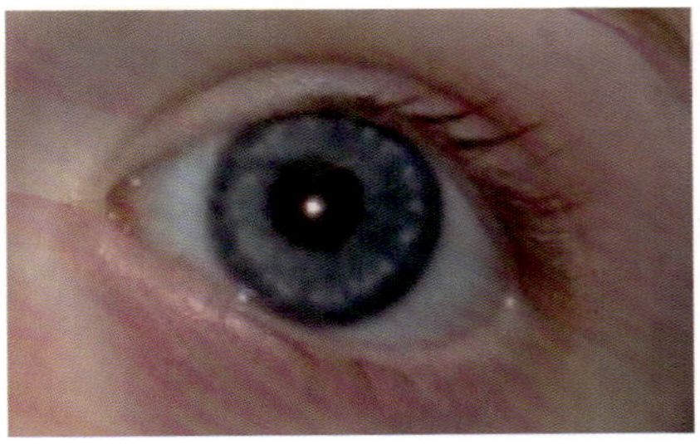

Brushfield Spots

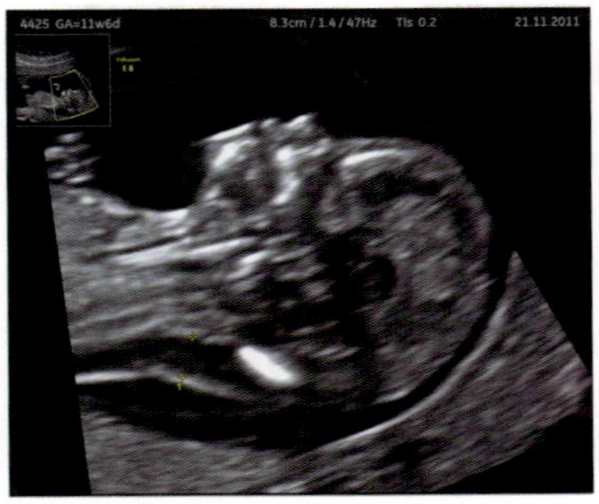

Nuchal Translucency

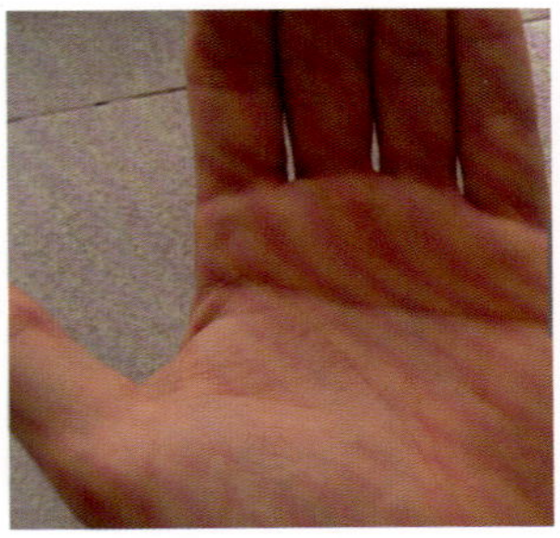

Palmar Simian Crease

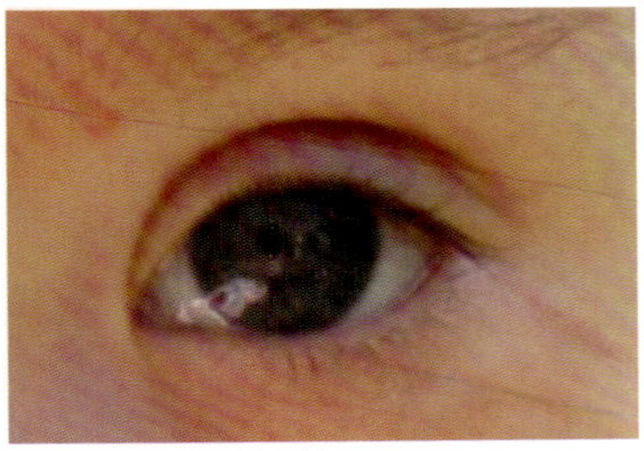

Epicanthal Folds

Trisomy 18, Edwards

- SX: **Micrognathia (small jaw), clenched hands, VSD**, prominent occiput, rocker bottom feet, mental retardation, malformed low set ears
- Labs: ALL Down: AFP, Estriol, B HCG, PAPP-A, and Normal Inhibin A

Trisomy 13, Patau's

- SX: **Cleft lip, cleft palate, polydactyl**, rocker bottom feet, microcephaly, cyclopia
- Ultrasound: increased nuchal translucency
- Labs: Decreased B-HCG, PAPP-A

Trisomy Quad Screen Labs

Trisomy	afp	estriol	β HCG	A Inhibin	PAPP
Trisomy 21, Downs Syndrome	↓	↓	↑	↑	↓
Trisomy 18, Edwards Syndrome	↓	↓	↓	Normal	↓
Trisomy 13, Patau's Syndrome			↓	↓	

(**tip**: Trisomy 21 quad screen: little vowel's (a and e) are little so they are down. The big letters β and A are up)

SEX CHROMOSOME DISORDERS

Turner Syndrome (45XO) Monosomy

- 45XO/46XX due to mosaicism
- SHOX gene
- Nondisjunction in **paternal** meiosis I
- No Barr body
- Decreased estrogen = **increased LH and FSH**
- SX: **Absent ovaries (AKA: streak ovaries)** (no menses because no estrogen, but they can still carry a fetus with in-vitro), **coarctation** of the aorta (different BP in upper body verses lower body), notched ribs, cystic **hygroma** (posterior neck swelling and extra skin at birth), **dactylitis** (swelling of hands and feet due to lymphedema due to dysgenesis of lymphatic network), low hairline, short 4th metacarpal, **horseshoe kidney (due to inferior mesenteric artery)**, nail dysplasia, discolored spots on skin (nevi), web neck, wide chest (AKA: shield chest), bicuspid valve, arched palate
- Note: There is a small percent of Turners **that do have ovaries**, therefore they will have normal cycles and are able to get pregnant. So if your vignette describes a girl who has the other signs of Turner's but has periods or was able to get pregnant, it still is Turners.

Klinefelter's Syndrome (47 XXY, or XXY)

- Inactivated Barr body (X chromosome)
- Dysgenesis of seminiferous tubules (no sperm) = **decreased inhibin = increased FSH**
- Dysfunction of Leydig cells = decreased testosterone = **increased LH = increased estrogen**
- SX: **Infertility**, testicular atrophy, long extremities, **gynecomastia,** decreased libido, impotence
- Labs: **↑ FSH, ↑** LH
- Histology: Shows many Leydig cells, few Sertoli cells and **absent germ cells.**
- XXY males can also have health problems that typically affect females: breast cancer, osteoporosis and autoimmune disorders.
- Due to a **nondisjunction during paternal or maternal meiosis I.** (Nondisjunction: when homologous chromosomes (X and Y or two X chromosomes) fail to separate).
- Error in chromosome **segregation in anaphase** during the **primary spermatocyte** stage of spermatogenesis.

True hermaphroditism (46XX/46XY, 47XXY, 46XX/47XXY)

- Individual born with both testicular and ovarian tissue
- Ambiguous external genitalia depending upon amount of testosterone produced between 8 and 16 weeks of gestation

Female Pseudohermaphrodite (XX)

- Ovaries present, external genitalia virilized
- Due to excessive exposure to androgens during early gestation
- (Girl inside, boy outside)

Male Pseudohermaphrodite (XY)

- Testes present, external genitalia are female
- Due to androgen insensitivity (testicular feminization)
- (Boy inside, girl outside)

Double Y Males (XYY)

- Phenotypically normal
- Severe acne, high risk of anti-social behavior, very tall

TRINUCLEOTIDE REPEATS

Note: Anticipation is a pattern of inheritance that can be seen in any trinucleotide repeat, however, Huntington's is the most common. Trinucleotide repeat pathologies occur when there are more than 100 repeats.

Fragile X Syndrome, XL

- **Methylation of FMR1 gene**
- Fragile sites on the long arm of the X chromosome
- Trinucleotide repeat: **CGG**
- High association with autism
- Fragile X in an X-linked dominant pattern is associated with premature ovarian failure in women (AKA: FXPOI)
- SX: **Large protruding ears**, long faces, **macroorchidism (large testes)**, hypotonia, flat feet, difficulty with social and emotional issues

Myotonic Dystrophy, AD

- CTG trinucleotide repeat expansion in DMPK gene
- SX: Can't release an object (can't let go of a door knob), muscle wasting, cataracts, frontal balding, arrhythmias, testicular atrophy

Friedreich Ataxia, AR

- **GAA** trinucleotide repeat in FXN gene
- Reduced expression of **Frataxin** protein
- Degeneration of nervous tissue in spinal cord = lose of myelin sheath
- SX: **Loss of coordination (ataxia**), vision and hearing impairment, high plantar arch, **HCM, hammer toes**

Huntington Disease, AD

- **CAG** trinucleotide repeat in the huntingtin gene on **chromosome 4**
- **Hypermethylation** of histone gene (AKA: deacetylation)
- Basal ganglia lesion
- Atrophy of **caudate nuclei**
- Neuronal death via NMBA-R binding and glutamate toxicity
- **Anticipation**
- **Decreased ACH and GABA, Increased Dopamine**
  Ach comes from Nucleus of Meynert
  GABA comes from Nucleus of Accumbens
  Dopamine comes from **Ventral tegmentum area (VTA) and SNc (midbrain).** (SNc: Substantia nigra pars compacta)
- SX: **Aggression, personality changes (frontal lobe)**, dementia, cognitive physical decline, **chorea** (random, uncontrolled movements)

MICRODELETION'S

DiGeorge Syndrome

- **Abnormal 3rd and 4th brachial pouches = no thymus (no T cells)**
- Microdeletion on chromosome **22:11**
- Recurrent infections: virus, fungus, parasites, atypical bacterial
- **Hypocalcemia (no parathyroids)**
- SX: Cleft palate, abnormal faces, **thymic aplasia** (AKA: Thymic shadow on x-ray), T cell deficient, **Truncus arteriosis**

Cri-du-chat Syndrome

- Microdeletion of short arm of chromosome 5
- SX: high pitched crying (mewing like a cat), cardiac abnormalities = VSD, microcephaly

Williams Syndrome

- Microdeletion of long arm of chromosome 7
- Deleted region includes the elastin gene
- SX: Extreme friendliness, "elf" faces, hypercalcemia, mental retardation

Prader-Willi

- Maternal Imprinting: maternal gene is imprinted (silenced – DNA methylation)
- **Paternal gene is deleted on chromosome 15**
- SX: **Hyperphagia (excessive eating), obesity**, hypotonia, mental retardation, hypogonadism, infertility, almond shaped eyes, scoliosis, excessive sleeping, strabismus (crossed eyes)

Angelman

- Paternal Imprinting: paternal gene is imprinted (silenced – DNA methylation)
- **Maternal gene is deleted on chromosome 15**
- SX: **Inappropriate laughter**, **seizures**, hand flapping, **extremely friendly**, ataxia, mental retardation, prominent mandible, microcephaly, speech impairment

Neurofibromatosis Type I (AKA: Von Recklinghausen Disease), AD

- Tumor disorder caused by **microdeletion on the NF1 gene on chromosome 17 that encodes for the protein neurofibromin**
- **MC tumor: Pilocytic astrocytomas**
- SX: **Lisch nodules** in the iris, flat pigmented skin lesions (café au lait spots), **freckling of the axillae** and/or inguinal areas, dermal neurofibromas (single/multiple firm rubbery bumps) on the skin, scoliosis, kyphosis, ADHD, **neurofibromas (derived from Schwann cells** or fibroblasts)

Neurofibromatosis Type II, AD

- Mutation of the **Merlin** gene (influences the form and movement of cells)
- **Microdeletion of the NF2 gene located at chromosome 22**
- **Bilateral acoustic neuromas (Schwannomas)**
- Schwannomas, meningioma's, ependymomas
- Symmetric, non-malignant brain tumors in the **region of cranial nerve VIII** by the internal auditory meatus
- Schwannomas are **neural crest** derivatives (S-100 marker)

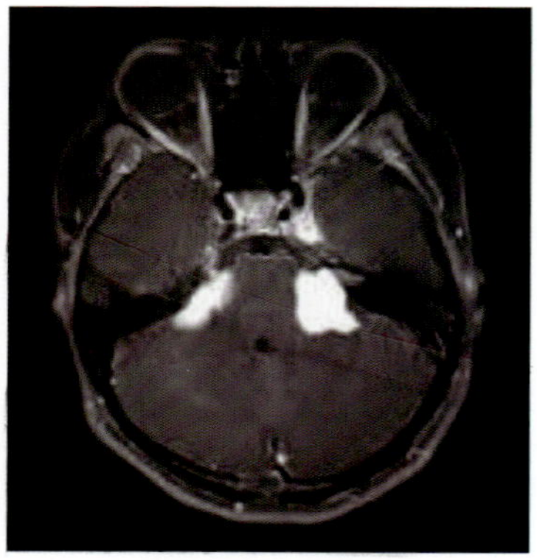

Bilateral Schwannomas

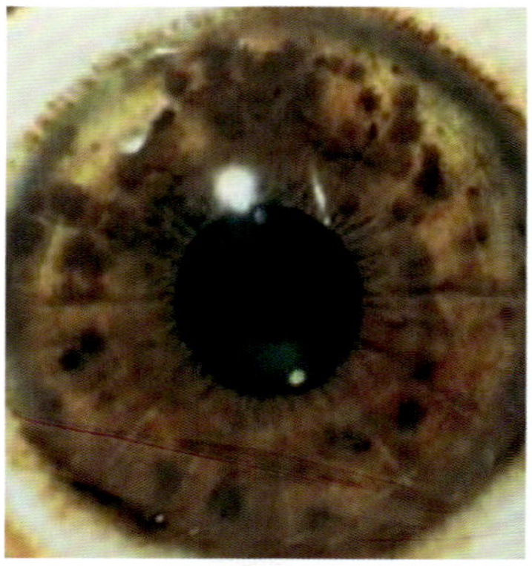

Lisch Nodules

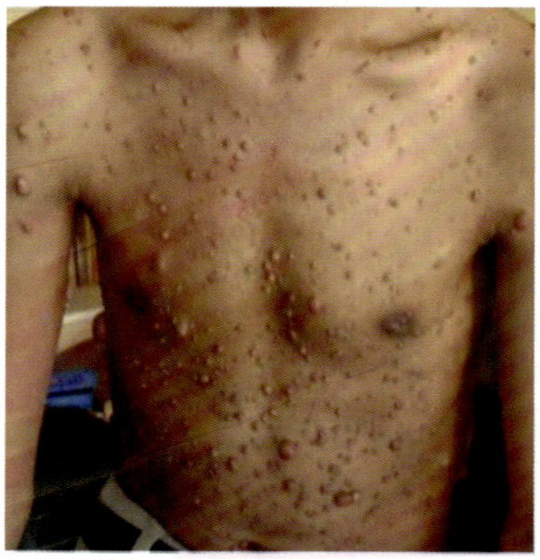

Neurofibromas

MISFOLDED PROTEINS

Cystic Fibrosis, AR

Defect in the CFTR protein that regulates sweat and mucus by the movement of water and chloride.

Normal: The CFTR protein helps produce digestive fluids, sweat and mucus. The CFTR protein is a channel for the movement of chloride in and out of cells (exocrine glands). This provides for the balance of salt and water in the body. Sweat glands secrete salt and water into the sweat ducts. Then reabsorbs the salt from the sweat back into the ducts. Sodium moves through sodium channels and chloride moves through the CFTR channel.

Abnormal: The CFTR protein channel does not work causing chloride ions to be trapped inside of the cells. Negatively charged chloride ions attract the positive charged sodium ions outside the cell. Chloride and sodium combine to produce salt, which is lost. The high concentration of chloride and sodium trapped inside the cell backs up and becomes thick mucus. It affects the pancreas, lungs, kidneys and intestines.

- **Autosomal recessive**
- Defect of **CFTR gene on chromosome 7**
- **Deletion of PHE (Phenylalanine) at position ΔF508 in CFTR protein, which keeps the protein from reaching the cell membrane surface. (ΔF508 mutation is 90% of cause).**
- **Frameshift** mutation +/- base pair (tip: If you have cystic fibrosis you are "F"..... = Frameshift)
- AKA: **Misfolded protein (was not tagged with ubiquitin for apoptosis)**
- AKA: No intracellular folding
- AKA: Defect in cellular transport of Cl
- AKA: Defective ion transport at epithelial surfaces
- AKA: Decreased Cl secretion = increased intracellular Cl = increased Na reabsorption = increased H2O reabsorption = thick mucus excreted into lungs and GI
- AKA: Increased concentration of Cl ions in sweat
- AKA: No intracellular folding
- AKA: No glycosylation of protein
- AKA: CFTR encodes an ATP gated CL channel that secretes Cl in lungs and GI and reabsorbs Cl in sweat glands.
- G551D mutation (3rd MCC Cystic Fibrosis) is a missense mutation that adds an aspartate instead of a glycine amino acid.
- Number one cause of malabsorption in Caucasians
- DX: Sweat chloride test (measures the concentration of chloride that is excreted in sweat): shows increased Cl in sweat.
- SX: **recurrent** pulmonary infections (esp. **Pseudomonas**), infertility in males (due to lack of vas deferens = no sperm), malabsorption = steatorrhea, malabsorption = deficiency of fat soluble vitamins D, E, A, K, **nasal polyps**, **meconium ileus** in newborns, chronic bronchitis, bronchiectasis, clubbing of the fingers, easily dehydration in hot weather.
- TX: **N-acetylcysteine MOA**: mucolytic – cleaves disulfide bonds
  Ivacaftor (VX-770) restores the function of the mutated CF protein by decreasing sweat chloride levels and decreasing pulmonary symptoms in CF with the G551D Mutation.
  Must also replace amylase, lipase and chymotrypsin to ↓ malabsorption (**Pancrelipase**)

Alzheimer Disease

- **Decrease in ACH (ACH synthesis is in Nucleus of Meynert)**
- **Cerebral cortex atrophy**
- Decreased glutamate with MMDA receptor
- Misfolded protein
- AKA: No intracellular folding
- Early onset for Downs Syndrome (before age 35)
- Early onset: Chromosome 21 and APP protein
- Late onset: Chromosome 19 and **Apo E4 protein** (Apo E2 is protective)
- B-amyloid core, AB (Amyloid B) made from APP protein. Plaques are formed **outside the neuron**
- Neurofibrillary **tangles** (tangles determine the degree of the disease)
- **Tau proteins** are hyperphosphorylated, which form the neurofibrillary tangles. (tau forms microtubules this leads to the collapse of the microtubule structure). They are cytosolic aggregations (**inside the neuron**).
- **SX:** First stage: Patient has subtle memory loss (progressive, not sudden), difficulty in language, apraxia (loss of ability to perform task they were once able to do: ie: pay bills)
  Second stage: Impaired judgment and personality changes
  Third stage: Psychotic features (ie: hallucinations) present LATE
  Alzheimer patients do not realize there is a problem, it is usually their family that brings them in concerned.
- TX: **Donepezil**
  MOA: Increase ACH

Alpha-1-Antitrypsin Deficiency (A1AT)

- Protease inhibitor
- Protects tissues from enzymes of **neutrophil elastase** (neutrophil elastase breaks down elastin in the lungs)
- Causes loss of recoil (rebound of lungs after inhalation). Inversely related to compliance.
- Increased compliance, increased TLC and RV
- Misfolded protein
- **Made in periportal hepatocytes in the liver**
- Liver biopsy: **PAS +** globules in periportal hepatocytes
- Patient may indicate a history of neonatal jaundice
- Results in **panacinar emphysema** and COPD (**Obstructive** lung pathologies)
  (**tip**: **O**-bstructive lung DZ can't breath **O**-ut)

Amyloidosis

- Accumulation of **misfolded proteins** (amyloids)
- Proteins are insoluble in water and deposits in organs and tissues in **Beta (B) pleated sheets** causing pathologies
- Stain: **Congo red stain showing apple green birefringence**
- Amyloids are referred to by different names depending upon where they deposited

AMYLOID	PATHOLOGY
AB	Alzheimer's (B Amyloid)
AL	Ig Light chains (Bence Jones Proteins) Multiple Myeloma
Amylin	Pancreas
AA	Rheumatoid Arthritis (Amyloid A)

Achondroplasia, AD

- Defective **fibroblast growth factor receptor 3 (FGFR3) which inhibits chondrocytes**
- **Endochondral ossification**
- Dwarfism, short limbs, normal head and trunk, normal life span, normal fertility
- Affects the long bones (longitudinal bone growth)
- **Chondrocytes**
- Higher risk with advanced **paternal age**

Duchenne Muscular Dystrophy, XL

- **Frameshift mutation**
- **Shortened (truncated) dystrophin protein (AKA: Dystrophin gene: DMD)**
- Pseudohypertrophy of calf and deltoid muscles because muscle is **replaced by fat and fibrous tissue**
- Proximal muscle weakness of legs and pelvis and loss of muscle mass, lumbar lordosis, muscle atrophy, congestive heart failure
- **Gower maneuver**
- High creatine kinase blood levels (CPK)
- Genetic errors in the Xp21 gene
- DX: muscle biopsy (or immunohistochemistry) shows absence of dystrophin
- **Early** onset, usually by 2

Becker Muscular Dystrophy, XL

- **Point mutation** (missense) in the dystrophin gene leading to instability I the structure of muscle cell membrane
- Similar symptoms, but less severe than Duchenne's
- **Later** onset, usually in adolescence

Myotonic Muscular Dystrophy, AD

- **CTG trinucleotide repeat of CTG in the DMPK gene (myotonic dystrophy protein kinase) on chromosome 19**
- Abnormal expression of myotonin protein kinase
- **Myotonia (Can't let go of an object. If you shake their hand or if they grab a door handle, they can't let go)**, muscle wasting, cataracts, testicular atrophy, problems with executive functioning, hypersomnia

MITOCHONDRIAL DISORDERS (AKA: Heteroplasmy)

Leber's Hereditary Optic Neuropathy, Mitochondrial

- Mitochondrial DNA point mutation
- Degeneration of retinal ganglion cells
- **Loss of central vision**
- Majority affected are males
- SX: Acute onset of vision loss in one eye followed by the other eye in weeks to months

Myoclonic Epilepsy, Mitochondrial

- **Myoclonus**: brief jerks of the body (majority in the limbs and facial muscles)
- Myoclonic epilepsy with **red-ragged fibers** seen on biopsy (AKA: MERRF syndrome)
- **Heteroplasmy**
- SX: Epilepsy, falls

Translocations

- 8:14 = Burkitt's Lymphoma (C-myc gene over expression)
- **9:22 = Philadelphia Chromosome**. CML. Bcr-Abl over expression. P210KD Tyrosine Kinase.
- 11:14 = Mantle Cell Lymphoma (Bcl-1 gene (AKA: Cyclin D)
- 11:22 = DiGeorge's
- 12:21 = in ALL is a better prognosis. In ALL the 9:22 translocation is the worst prognosis
- 14:18 = Follicular NHL (Bcl-2)
- **15:17 = AML M3** (Auer Rods, DIC)

Chromosome Pathology Summary

1	2	3	4	5	6
Gaucher Presenilin 2 (Alzheimer) L-myc (small cell CA)		**Von Hippel Lindau (VHL gene)**	**Huntington's CAG** Achondroplasia (FGFR3 gene)	Cri-Du-Chat APC (FAP gene)	Hemochromatosis (HFE gene)
7	**8**	**9**	**10**	**11**	**12**
Cystic Fibrosis (CFTR, 508 gene) Williams Syndrome	C-myc Burkitt's Lymphoma	Melanoma (P16 Tumor Suppressor gene Friedreich's Ataxia (Frataxin gene, GAA trinucleotide repeats)		Niemann Pick (sphingomyelinase) Beta Thalassemia (Beta Globin Chain) Cyclin D (BCL-1 gene) C-1 Esterase Inhibitor Deficiency	
13	**14**	**15**	**16**	**17**	**18**
Patau Trisomy Retinoblastoma and Osteosarcoma (RB gene) BRCA 2	Alzheimer (Presenilin 1 gene)	Tay Sachs (Hexosaminidase A) Marfan (FBN1 gene) Prader-Willi and Angelman (Imprinting)	Polycystic Kidney DZ (PCKD1, polycystin 1 Gene) Alpha Thalassemia (alpha globin chain) Tuberous Sclerosis (TSC2 gene)	**Neurofibromatosis Type 1, (NF1, Von Recklinghausen)** P 53 BRCA 1	**Edwards Trisomy** BCL 2 Colon CA (DCC gene)
19	**20**	**21**	**22**	**23**	**SEX DISEASES**
Familial Hyper Cholesterolemia (LDL receptor mutation) Myotonic Muscular Dystrophy (DMPK gene)		**Downs Trisomy** Alzheimer (B-APP Protein) Superoxide Dismutase (SOD1 gene)	**Neurofibromatosis 2 (NF2, Merlin protein)** DiGeorge Syndrome (Locus 11 deletion)		**Klinefelter's XXY (Barr Body)** **Turner's XO (SHOX gene)**

BIOCHEMISTRY

Amino Acids

Amino acids are the building blocks of all proteins. tRNA attaches the amino acid on its 3' CCA site and transports to the A site in the ribosome for protein production.

DESCRIPTION	AMINO ACIDS
Essential Amino Acids (Body can't make de novo (from scratch), it must come from the diet)	Phenylalanine, Valine, Threonine, Tryptophan, Methionine, leucine, Isoleucine, Lysine, Histidine
Smallest	Glycine
Branched Chain	Leucine, Isoleucine, Valine
Aromatic	Phenylalanine, Tyrosine, Tryptophan
Ketogenic	Leucine, Lycine
Kinky (used anywhere there are bends/turns)	Proline
Disulfide	Methionine, Cystine (**tip**: "My" "Cister")
N-Bonds	Asparagine, Glutamine
Both Ketogenic and Glucogenic	Phenylalanine, Isoleucine, Tryptophan, Threonine
The ONLY "IMINO" acid	Proline
Acidic	Aspartic Acid and Glutamic Acid (Negatively charged at body pH)
Basic	Arginine, Lysine, Histidine. Arginine is the most basic. **Histidine has no charge at body pH**

Buffers

Intracellular Buffer: Amino Acids (Histadine)
Extracellular Buffer (blood): Bicarb (**tip**: "B"lood = "B"icarb)

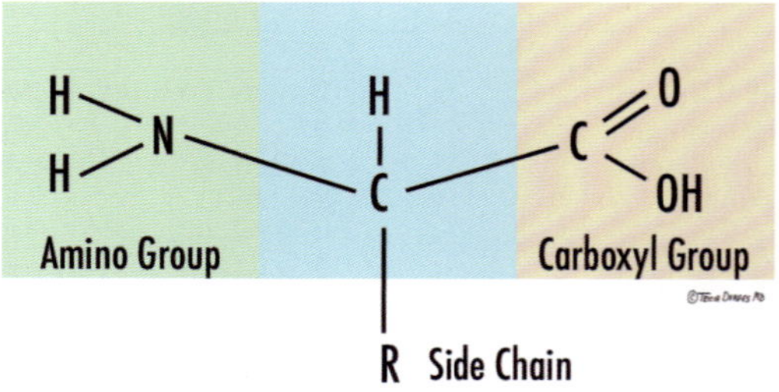

Denaturing of Proteins

Alcohol or acetone (organic solvents). Destroys the cell membrane.
Heat
Iodine
Extremes of PH
Disruption (beating of egg whites)
Chaotropic agents (disrupts the hydrogen bonding) ie: urea, guanidine
Ionic detergents

Acid and Base

- **Acid**: COOH to COO^- = **IONIZED/CHARGED** (have a charge: either positive or negative. Acid is negative, base is positive). Does **NOT cross** membranes. Gives up H+ (AKA: Protons).
  (Acid starts out neutral and becomes charged when it dissociates its hydrogen ion).
  Has high solubility and decreased bioavailability. (Tip: **C**OO = **C**harged). Acids give away their protons.
- **Base**: NH3+ to NH2 = **UNCHARGED/NEUTRAL**. Easily **crosses** membranes. Has low solubility and **high bioavailability**. (Base starts out charged and becomes neutral when it dissociates its hydrogen ion).

pH = pka when there is 50% acid and 50% base.

Restriction Enzyme Test

ENZYME	AMINO ACIDS
Trypsin	Cuts to the RIGHT of TRP and TYR
Chymotrypsin	Cuts to the RIGHT of PHE, TRP, TYR
Elastase	Cuts to the RIGHT of GLY, ALA, SER
CnBr	Cuts to the RIGHT of MET
Aminopeptidase	Cuts to the RIGHT of amino acids
Carboxypeptidase	Cuts to the LEFT of carboxy terminal
Mercaptoethanol	Breaks disulfide bonds

Titratable Amino Acids (3 PH points)

- HIS, ARG, LYS, ASP, GLUT, CYST, TYR

Co-Factors

Cofactor	Pathway/Process
Vitamin B1 (AKA: Thiamine)	**Pyruvate Dehydrogenase and a-Ketoglutarate Dehydrogenase** (TCA) **Transketolase (HMP Shunt/AKA: TPP),** Branched chain **Ketoacid Dehydrogenase**
Vitamin B2 (AKA: Riboflavin) AKA: **FAD**	**Pyruvate Dehydrogenase and a-Ketoglutarate** (TCA), Branched chain Ketoacid Dehydrogenase Goes to complex II of the ETC.
Vitamin B3 (AKA: Niacin) AKA: **NAD**	**Pyruvate Dehydrogenase and a-Ketoglutarate** (TCA), Branched chain Ketoacid Dehydrogenase Goes to complex I of the ETC.
Vitamin B5 (AKA: Pantothenate)	Coenzyme A (AKA: CoA) CoA is a cofactor for acyl transfers and fatty acid synthase
Vitamin B6 (AKA: Pyridoxine)	AA Transamination (ALT, AST), Decarboxylation, Glycogen Phosphorylase. Synthesis of: Niacin, Heme, Cystathionine, Histamine, Serotonin, Epinephrine, Norepinephrine, Dopamine, GABA (Note: must add B6 to INH treatments and do not add B6 to Parkinson's drug treatments).
Vitamin B7 (AKA: **Biotin**)	**Carboxylase** (Pyruvate, Acetyl CoA, Propionyl CoA)
Vitamin B9 (AKA: Folic Acid)	Nucleotide Synthesis of DNA, RNA, **Tetrahydrofolate** (THF) in methylation
Vitamin B12 (AKA: Cobalamin)	Homocystine Methyltransferase, **Methylmalonyl** CoA
Vitamin C (AKA: Ascorbic Acid)	**Collagen**, Hydroxylation's, Purines, Dopamine B-Hydroxylase, **Iron Absorption**
Vitamin D	1,25 Hydroxylation
Vitamin K	**Gama Carboxylation** of glutamic acid (clotting factors 2, 7, 9, 10, C & S)
Vitamin A (AKA: Retinol, Beta-Carotene)	**CSF** Production, PTH with Mg
Zinc	Taste buds, hair, **sperm**
BH4 (AKA: Tetrahydrobiopterin)	Tyrosine, Dopa, Serotonin, Nitric Oxide
Normal Flora	Folate, Vit K, Biotin, B-5 (Pantothenic Acid)
Md (Mendelevium)	Purine breakdown (Xanthine Oxidase)
Mn (Manganese)	Glycolysis
Se (Selenium)	Heart
Sn (Tin)	Hair
Mg (Magnesium)	Kinase, PTH with Vit. A
Fe (Iron)	Hemoglobin, ETC
THF	Nucleotides
Cu (Copper)	Lysyl oxidase (synthesis of elastin and collagen)

(See Vitamin/Mineral/Herb chapter for full information)

Organs that USE Ketones

Brain, heart, kidney, skeletal muscles

Organs that cannot use Ketones

RBC and Liver (hepatocytes): because **liver has no thiophorase**.

Organs that do not need insulin in order to take up glucose

(BRICKLE) Brain, RBC, Intestines, Cardiac, Kidney, Liver, Exercising Muscle

GLUT receptors

Glut Receptor	Organ
Glut 1	RBC, Fetal tissues, Brain
Glut 2	Liver, Pancreatic B Cells, Hypothalamus, basolateral membrane of small intestine and renal tubular cells
Glut 3	Brain
Glut 4	**Adipose, Striated Muscle** (Skeletal and Cardiac) by **Facilitated Diffusion (Carrier Mediated) – INSULIN DEPENDENT**
Glut 5	Intestine

Reaction/Enzyme Definitions

- **Majority** of the enzymes used in bio chem reactions are named based on the substrate and enzyme. Use this as a general rule in determining the enzyme's name:
  - The name of the substrate is the "first name" of the enzyme
    Example: Phenylalanine to Tyrosine is done by Phenylalanine Hydroxylase. (1st name: Phenylalanine)
  - What was done to the substrate in the reaction is the "second name" of the enzyme
    In the above example, the substrate was hydroxylated to form Tyrosine (2nd name: Hydroxylase)

Reaction	Definition and Notes
Carboxylation	Chemical reaction in which a carboxylic acid group is added to a substrate (COOH). Co-Factor: **Biotin.**
Decarboxylation	Chemical reaction that removes a carboxyl group (COOH) and releases carbon dioxide (CO2). Co-Factor: Decarboxylate Complex: **Complex Consist of:** **Vitamin B1 (AKA: Pyrophosphate, Thiamine, TPP- Thiamine Pyrophosphate)** **Vitamin B2 (AKA: FAD, Riboflavin)** **Vitamin B3 (AKA: NAD, Niacin)** Vitamin B5 (AKA: CoA, Pantothenate) Lipoic Acid
Methylation	Addition of a methyl group. It is an alkylation with a methyl group, replacing a hydrogen atom. Methylation **STOPS**. **Mediated by SAM** (S-adenosyl methionine). Methylation of a histone. (Post-translational modification).
Transamination	ALT/AST. Chemical reaction that replaces an amine functional group with another amine by transaminases. **Co-factor: B6 (Pyridoxine).** (NOTE: Must replace B6 when taking INH to prevent neuropathies: INH pulls B6 out of the body). (NOTE: Do not give B6 with Parkinson's drugs).
Phosphorylate	Addition of a phosphoryl group (PO3) to a molecule. This is done with phosphorylase, which makes the phosphate (Pi) available (dephosphorylation). Post-translational modification.
Dephosphorylation	A phosphorylated substrate donates a phosphate group so that ADP can gain an ATP.
Dehydrogenase	Oxidizes a substrate by a reduction reaction that transfers hydrides (H-) to an electron acceptor. Used mostly with NAD/NADP and FAD/FADH reactions.
Hydroxylase	Enzyme that oxidizes two donors by incorporating oxygen into one of them.
Kinase	Enzyme that transfers phosphate groups to substrates (AKA: Phosphorylation). The substrate gains a phosphate group and ATP molecule. Requires the use of ATP in order to phosphorylate. Co-factor: Mg.
Hydrolase	Enzyme that catalyzes the hydrolysis (addition of water) of a chemical bond.
Thiol	Required to break disulfide bonds. MC thiol 's: Mercaptoethanol, Dithiothreitol (are reductants).
Epimerase	Used for inversions: MC: Glucose to Galactose and Galactose to Glucose.
Isomerase	Used to covert a molecule from isomer to another. MC: Glucose to Fructose and Fructose to Glucose. A-B ➔ B-A
Lyase	Enzyme that catalyzes the breaking down of a chemical bond. Required to cut a carbon bond.
Mutase	Enzyme that catalyzes a functional group from one position to shift to another position in the same molecule. Required to move a side chain from one carbon to another carbon.
Synthase	Enzyme that catalyzes a synthesis process. 2 substrates used to make a product with or without use of ATP.
Synthetase	Synonymous with ligase.
Ligase	Enzyme that catalyzes the joining of two large molecules by forming a new chemical bond. Hydrolysis is usually involved. Synonymous with Synthetase. Example: Ab + C ➔ AC + b.
Enantiomer	Two stereoisomers that are non superimposable (non-identical) mirror images of each other.

PATHWAYS and CONTROLLING ENZYMES
(RLE = Rate Limiting Enzyme) (Reg = Regulators)

- **Glycolysis:** This pathway is ON when we are in well-fed state.
  RLE = PFK-1 (Phosphofructokinase)
  Reg turns ON Glycolysis (we need to make energy): AMP, Fructose 2, 6 bisphosphate
  Reg turns OFF Glycolysis (we have enough energy): ATP, Citrate

- **TCA Cycle:** This pathway is ON when glycolysis is on, sending pyruvate.
  RLE = Isocitrate dehydrogenase
  Reg turns ON TCA (we need to make ATP and NADH): ADP
  Reg turns OFF TCE (we have enough ATP and NADH): ATP, NADH

- **Gluconeogenesis (GNG):** This pathway is ON when we have used up our glucose from eating and need to make more. It is glycolysis in reverse.
  RLE = Fructose 1, 6 bisphosphate
  Reg turns ON GNG (we need to make energy): ATP, Acetyl-CoA
  Reg turns OFF GNG (glycolysis is working): AMP, Fructose 2, 6 bisphosphate

- **Glycogenesis:** This pathway is ON when we are in well fed state, we are storing.
  RLE = Glycogen Synthase
  Reg turns ON glycogenesis (we need to make energy stores): Glucose 6 Phosphate, Insulin and Cortisol
  Reg turns OFF glycogenesis (we have enough energy stored): Epinephrine, Glucagon

- **Glycogenolysis:** This pathway is ON when we are in starvation state.
  RLE = Glycogen Phosphorylase
  Reg turns ON glycogenolysis (we need energy from our stores): Epinephrine, Glucagon, AMP
  Reg turns OFF glycogenolysis (we are in fed state, making energy): Glucose 6 Phosphate, Insulin, ATP
  Allosteric activator: Acetyl CoA (first step in GNG, it increases the activity of Pyruvate carboxylase

- **HMP Shunt** (AKA: PPP Pentose Phosphate Pathway): Pathway is ON when we need NADPH
  RLE = Glucose-6-phosphate dehydrogenase (G6PD)
  Reg turns ON HMP (we need NADPH): NADP
  Reg turns OFF HMP (we have enough NADPH): NADPH

- **Fatty Acid Synthesis** (making of fatty acids)
  RLE = Acetyl CoA carboxylase (ACC)
  Reg turns ON Fatty Acid Synthesis (We need to make FA stores): Insulin, Citrate
  Reg turns OFF Fatty Acid Synthesis (We have enough FA stored): Glucagon, Palmitoyl CoA

- **Fatty Acid Oxidation** (breaking down of fatty acids for energy) (AKA: Beta Oxidation)
  RLE = Carnitine acyltransferase I
  Reg turns ON Fatty Acid Oxidation (We are in starvation and need energy): none
  Reg turns OFF Fatty Acid Oxidation (We have enough energy): Malonyl CoA

- **Cholesterol Synthesis:** This pathway is on when we are well fed.
  RLE = HMG CoA **Reductase**
  Reg turns ON Cholesterol Synthesis (We need to make cholesterol): Insulin, Thyroxine
  Reg turns OFF Cholesterol Synthesis (We have enough): Glucagon, Cholesterol, cAMP

- **Ketogenesis**: This pathway is on when we are in starvation and need ketones
  RLE = HMG CoA **Synthase**
  No Reg enzymes

- **Urea Cycle**
  RLE = Carbamoyl phosphate synthetase I
  Reg turns ON Urea Cycle: N-acetylglutamate

- **Purine Synthesis**
  RLE = PRPP (Glutamine-Phosphoribosylpyrophosphate amidotransferase)
  Reg turns OFF purine synthesis: AMP, IMP (Inosine monophosphate), GMP

- **Pyrimidine Synthesis**
  RLE = Carbamoyl phosphate synthetase II
  No reg

Pathway Metabolism Sites

Pathways that in occur in both, mitochondria and cytoplasm

- **H**eme synthesis, **U**rea cycle, **G**luconeogenesis (**tip**: takes two to HUG: both locations)

Pathways that occur in the mitochondria

- Fatty acid oxidation (AKA: Beta oxidation), Acetyl CoA production, TCA Cycle, Oxidative phosphorylation, CPS/OTC of urea, Pyruvate carboxylase, Ketogenesis

Pathways that occur in the cytoplasm

- Glycolysis, Fatty acid synthesis, HMP shunt (AKA: PPP), Protein synthesis (RER), Cholesterol synthesis, Steroid synthesis (SER)

Shuttles

From Mitochondria to Cytoplasm

- Malate Shuttle: OAA (Oxaloacetate) to Gluconeogenesis in liver
- Citrate Shuttle: Acetyl CoA to Fatty Acid Synthesis in liver
- Ornithine Shuttle: Citruline to Urea Cycle in liver

From Cytoplasm to Mitochondria

- Carnitine Shuttle: Acetyl CoA to Beta Oxidation of Fatty Acids in liver and muscles

ATP Production

Aerobic: 32 ATP via malate-aspartate shuttle in heart and liver
30 ATP via G3P shuttle in muscle
Anaerobic: 2 ATP in RBC
ATP's from Fatty Acid Oxidation: From 1 cycle of Palmitate: 129 ATP
ATP"s from Glucose to Pyruvate: 2 ATP

Well Fed State vs Fasting/Starvation State **(in a nut shell)**

You **must know** what is on and off during each of these situations and what hormones/enzymes are at work. Heavily tested.

Well Fed to Starvation State Time Line

Fed State: up to 4 hours after a meal. Fasting: more than 4 hours after a meal.
Fasting - In between meals: After 4 hours.
Starving: 3 or more days of fasting.
Sympathetic system stimulates hepatic gluconeogenesis (liver and kidney), glycogenolysis (liver) lipolysis (adipose) and decreases glucose uptake in the muscle and adipose tissue.
Parasympathetic system suppresses hepatic gluconeogenesis, glycogenolysis, and lipolysis.
Processes that produce glucose: Glycolysis, beta-oxidation, and ketolysis.

Well Fed State (within 4 hours of a meal)

Glycolysis and aerobic respiration. ATP is produced.
Insulin stimulates glycolysis and lipogenesis and suppresses gluconeogenesis.
Insulin stimulates synthesis of glycogen, lipids, and proteins.
Glycolytic products synthesize fatty acids via de novo lipogenesis.
Long chain fatty acids are made into cholesterol, triacylglycerol, and phospholipids.
Proteins are synthesized from dietary amino acids.
The brain and RBC's use glucose as a fuel (insulin has no effect on their metabolism).

Fasting (in-between meals)

Drop in blood sugar stimulates glucagon release from the alpha cells of the pancreas so that it can maintain blood glucose levels.
Fatty acids are converted to ketone bodies via ketogenesis, which is used as fuel by the brain and skeletal muscles.
Glucose generated from the liver and ketone bodies provide the metabolic fuel for extrahepatic tissues during periods of exercise and starvation.
The kidney can help maintain blood glucose levels in prolong fasting by gluconeogenesis.
The kidney helps protect against ketoacidosis caused by high levels of ketone bodies. The kidney metabolizes glutamine, which produces ammonia in the NH3 form so that it is able to pick up the extra protons (H+) and convert to NH4 in order to be excreted in the urine. By decreasing the extra H+ the body's pH will normalize.

After glycolysis (4 hours) all pathways will help maintain blood glucose.
In the early part (short term) of the fasting state glycogenolysis maintains blood glucose levels.
Glycogen stores are the main source of energy for the first 24 hours and are depleted by end of the 3rd day.
Glycogen is resynthesized from lactate (Cori cycle) and alanine (from muscle via the glucose/alanine cycle).
Gluconeogenesis is the main source of energy after the first 24 hours.

During prolonged fasting (once glycogen is depleted), gluconeogenesis is the primary source of glucose production.
Gluconeogenesis synthesizes glucose using pyruvate, glycerol, lactate, and amino acids.
Amino acids generate glucose by gluconeogenesis.
Glucagon stimulates glyconeogenesis (it counteracts insulin) so that amino acids are made into glucose.
During starvation, skeletal muscles use fatty acids as fuel so that the ketone bodies are reserved as the energy source for the brain.

Lipolysis (beta-oxidation) also occurs in adipose tissues to release fatty acids, which are converted into ketone bodies (ketogenesis) to be used for fuel by the brain and the skeletal muscles.

After day 3, Free Fatty Acids from adipose is the main source of energy for the liver, adipose tissue and skeletal muscle. The liver converts the fatty acids into ketone body which are used for energy by the brain.

Proteins (muscle wasting) are broken down as the last source of energy.

In summary:

WELL FED (high glucose/fructose)	FASTING/In-between meals
Glycolysis is working **Insulin is on** **ON: 2, 6 Bisphosphate, PFK 1** **OFF: 1, 6 Fructose,** Alanine, Glycine **OFF: cAMP** **Turns it off: Citrate and ATP** **Turns it on: AMP, Fructose 2, 6 bisphosphate**	**Glucagon (alpha cells in the pancreas), cortisol, epinephrine: are on.** **Gluconeogenesis and Glycogenolysis is working.** **OFF: 2, 6 Bisphosphate, PFK 1** **ON: 1, 6 Fructose,** Alanine, Glycine **ON: cAMP** **Turns it ON: ATP and Acetyl CoA** **Turn it OFF: AMP, Fructose 2, 6 bisphosphate** **Allosteric Activator: Acetyl CoA**

WELL FED: Food eaten within 4 hours is used to make immediate energy/ATP and to build up (anabolic) storage of ingredients in various sites in the body to make ATP for between meals and extended periods of no food. Insulin is in charge of this period.
Insulin is ON (membrane receptor tyrosine kinase)
Insulin from Pancreatic Beta Cells is required to pull glucose into adipose and muscle cells by Glut 4 receptors.
Insulin stimulates building up and storage of glycogen, lipids and proteins.
Insulin and well fed state facts:

- Glucose (eating) stimulates insulin
- Turns off glucagon (cortisol, epinephrine)
- Insulin promotes the building of amino acids, proteins, nucleic acids
- Glycolysis is turned on
- Lipogenesis is turned on
- Glycogenesis is turned on: storing glycogen for future use
- Synthesis of triglycerides, proteins, amino acids
- High K uptake (Without K INSIDE the cell, NO insulin can be released.)
- Glucose is transported into adipose tissue and skeletal muscles
- VLDL from the liver and chylomicrons from the gut are transferred into and stored as fatty acids
- RBC only fuel is glucose. There is no fuel reserve. RBC requires a continuous supply of glucose. RBC has no mitochondria so there is no Krebs cycle (TCA cycle). Lactate is released and goes to the liver for the Cori cycle.
- RBC's need the Pentose Phosphate Pathway (PPP) It produces NADPH in order to regenerate glutathione. Glutathione in turn fights free radical damage from H2O2 and peroxides so the REC membrane is not oxidized.
- RBC's produce 2,3 BPG from 1,3 BPG in glycolysis
- Brain (Glut 1 receptor) uses 20% of all oxygen. Main fuel is glucose; there is no fuel reserve. Glut 3 is used for neuronal cells.
- Cardiac muscle uses fatty acids as its energy source.
- Liver (Glut 2 receptor) builds up stores of glycogen, is responsible for gluconeogenesis, synthesizes proteins, synthesizes all blood proteins except for immunoglobulins), and is the detoxification center for the body.

BETWEEN MEALS/FASTING/STARVATION: After 4 hours the body must rely on the breakdown (catabolic) of its various stores to provide energy/ATP. Glucagon is in charge of this period (cortisol and epinephrine are counterparts to glucagon).
Glucagon/Cortisol/Epinephrine (**protects from hypoglycemia, maintains blood glucose levels**)
Glucagon stimulates:

- Glycogenolysis
- Gluconeogenesis
- Lipolysis
- Ketones
- Protein breakdown
- Growth hormones
- **Kidneys also help to maintain blood glucose levels in fasting states.** They synthesize and release glucose during fasting states through **gluconeogenesis.**
- The **brain uses glucose (Glut 2) and then ketones once glucose** is unavailable. (Glut 2).
- Cardiac muscles use fatty acids (stored fat) and ketones.
- RBC, WBC, the retina, and adrenal medulla use glucose.
- Muscles, kidney and liver use glucose, fatty acids (stored fat) and ketone bodies.
- Muscle and liver also use amino acids.
- During fasting the liver runs glycogenolysis, gluconeogenesis (lactate through the Cori cycle, amino acids from muscle protein and glycerol from adipose tissues), ketogenesis from fatty acids (adipose tissue) and amino acids (muscle), and disposes of nitrogen via the urea cycle.
- Note: glucagon does not have any affect on skeletal muscle.

Stress Response to Starvation: Hypoglycemia stimulates Growth Hormones, which decrease glucose uptake so that lipolysis occurs and raises blood sugar levels.
Glucagon has no affect on adipose or skeletal muscle.

Hexokinase verses Glucokinase (Induced by insulin)

Hexokinase and Glucokinase are the first enzymes used by the body to start the process of glycolysis.
Glucokinase is **only in the liver and Pancreas**. If there is no glucokinase = no insulin = hyperglycemia.
Hexokinase: Is used by the rest of the body and can be used as a back up when Glucokinase is not available in the pancreas or liver.
Glucokinase: FASTER enzyme it is used by the liver and pancreas so that it can quickly glycolysis and the release of insulin. **Glucokinase is the FASTER** enzyme because **it has a higher Vmax** than hexokinase.

Metabolic Fuel Use Calculation

1 gm protein	4 kcal
1 gm carbs	4 kcal
1 gm alcohol	7 kcal
1 gm fat	9 kcal

Example: A patient is given 3000 calories a day. How many grams of protein did they get? 20% of this amount was protein (20% of 3000 = 600). 600 divided by 4 = 150 gm.'s of protein.

Hyperglycemia in relation to diabetics: After the fed state, normal metabolic processes that breakdown glucose do not occur because of lack of insulin or lack of insulin signaling. This causes the body to continue to process as if it was in the fasting/starvation states. Prolonged high blood glucose can lead to: neuropathy, retinopathy, renal disease, stroke and cardiovascular disease.

Hypoglycemia: When blood sugar levels drop **below 40 mg/dL**. Hypoglycemia can cause CNS symptoms: headache, confusion, altered mental status, coma, and death. The body tries to over come hypoglycemia by: releasing epinephrine and causing tremors, anxiety and palpitations.
Types of hypoglycemia

- Postprandial: Transient hypoglycemia after a meal when too much insulin was released.
- Insulin-induced: Happens in diabetics that are on insulin treatment. Treated by intake of oral carbohydrates or glucagon injection.
- Fasting: Can be caused when there is liver damage that reduces glyconeogenesis, adrenal insufficiency, over production of insulin (pancreatic beta cell tumor), or G6PD (liver is not able to supply glycogen or perform gluconeogenesis).
- Alcohol-induced hypoglycemia: Overproduction of NADH by alcohol dehydrogenase inhibits gluconeogenesis because OAA uses malate to get rid of the excess NADH and pyruvate is shifted to lactate to get rid of the excess NADH.

BIOCHEMISTRY PATHWAYS

Common Enzymes (numbered) in Biochemistry Pathways

Enzyme	**Pathway and Notes**
1α Hydroxylase	

Enzyme	**Pathway and Notes**
1α Hydroxylase	Converts 25-hydroxyvitamin D3 to 1,25-dihydroxvitamin D3 (active form of Vitamin D: Calcitriol) in the kidneys
α 1,4 Glucanotransferase	AKA: Acid Maltase. Glycogenolysis (Glycogen storage disease. Pompe Disease)
α 1,6 Glucosidase	AKA: Debranching enzyme. Glycogenolysis (Glycogen storage disease, Cori Disease)
PFK 1 and 2,6 Bisphosphate	ON in glycolysis (insulin)
1,6 Bisphosphate	ON in gluconeogenesis (glucagon)
3β Hydroxysteroid	Synthesis of cortisol, aldosterone and sex steroids in the adrenal gland
5α Reductase	Converts testosterone to DHT in the testes
5' Deiodinase	Converts T4 to the active form T3 in the periphery
7α Hydroxylase	Rate limiting enzyme in the synthesis of bile acid from cholesterol
11β Hydroxylase	Synthesis of cholesterol, steroids and converts 11-deoxycortisol and corticosterone to cortisol in the adrenal cortex
14α Demethylase	Converts lanosterol to cholesterol (humans) and ergosterol (fungus)
17α Hydroxylase	Converts pregnenolone and progesterone to DHEA and androstenedione (sexual development in the fetus and puberty)
21α Hydroxylase	Synthesis of steroid hormones, cortisol and aldosterone. Deficiency leads to Congenital Adrenal Hyperplasia.
N^5 N^{10} N-acetyl-glutamate (aka: NAG)	Cofactor for Carbamoyl phosphate synthetase I (CPS I)

GLYCOLYSIS PATHWAY

- Glycolysis is at work in well-fed states. AMP tells us we need to make more ATP. The key of glycolysis is to get to Pyruvate, which then enters the TCA cycle to make ATP. It also makes Acetyl CoA so cholesterol and ketones can be made.
- Pathways of: Glycogen, Galactose, HMP Shunt (AKA: PPP) all require Glucose 6 Phosphate from Glycolysis
- Fructose enters into the Glycolysis pathway at G3P (Glyceraldehyde-3-P)
- Occurs in the cytoplasm
- Total of 2 ATP net are produced for each glucose molecule
- Total of 2 NADH net are produced
- RBC are only able to do Glycolysis, producing 2 ATP (Anaerobic)

Glucose – Alanine cycle

- Amino acids (amino group) from degradation in muscles are transaminated (amino group + keto acid) into glutamate
- Glutamate can transfer this amino group to pyruvate via ALT to form alanine and α-ketoglutarate
- Alanine can now be transported via the blood to the liver to participate in gluconeogenesis to make glucose to return which is then returned back to the muscle
- Glutamate enters the mitochondria and is degraded into ammonium ions via glutamate dehydrogenase which then go into the urea cycle to form urea to be excreted

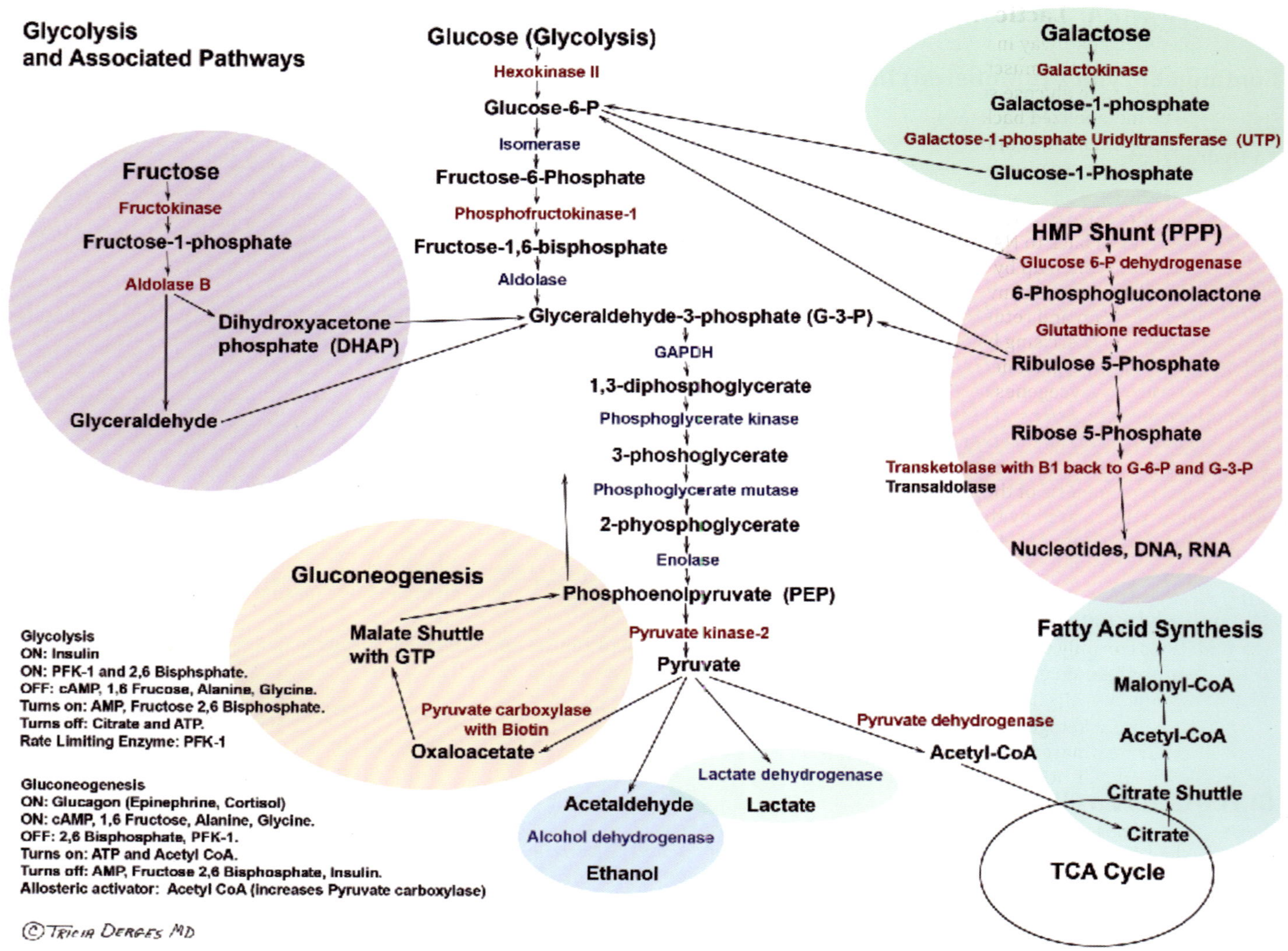

Paths of Pyruvate

1) **Pyruvate to Acetyl-CoA** by Pyruvate dehydrogenase and then into the Krebs cycle. Irreversible step.
   Deficiency of Pyruvate Dehydrogenase Complex (common in alcoholics because B1 deficiency)
   Acetyl-CoA enters the Krebs cycle (aka: TCA cycle or Citric acid cycle).
2) **Pyruvate to lactate** by lactate dehydrogenase (LDH) causing lactic acidosis. Reversible step.
   Generated in anaerobic glycolysis: Allows conversion of NADH to NAD.
   In the liver: LDH converts lactate to pyruvate for gluconeogenesis or for metabolism to acetyl-CoA by the **Cori cycle.**
   Note: Common in alcoholics because of vitamin B1 deficiency. Alcohol ➔ Pyruvate is unable to enter the TCA cycle or initiate gluconeogenesis. Because pyruvate is unable to enter the TCA cycle or gluconeogenesis, blood glucose levels cannot be maintained causing hypoglycemia.
3) Pyruvate to Ethanol. Pyruvate decarboxylase to Acetaldehyde and then to ethanol via **alcohol dehydrogenase causing an increased NADH: NAD ratio**.
4) **Pyruvate to Oxaloacetate** (OAA) by **Pyruvate carboxylase (cofactor: Biotin).** Irreversible step.
   Enters gluconeogenesis. (OAA to Malate shuttle to Phosphoenolpyruvate (PPE), using **GTP for energy**). **(GTP made from Succinyl-CoA to Succinate by Succinate by Succinyl-CoA synthetase).**
5) **Pyruvate to alanine** by Alanine transaminase (ALT). Reversible step.
   Alanine carries amino groups to the liver from muscle.
   In the liver Alanine transaminase (ALT) **converts alanine to pyruvate** for gluconeogenesis.

Cori Cycle (AKA: Lactic Acid Cycle)

- Metabolic pathway in which lactate is produced by anaerobic glycolysis in the muscles and is then moved to the liver to be converted to glucose so that it can then return back to the muscles to be metabolized back to lactate.
- During intense use of muscles, energy is released through anaerobic metabolism creating lactic acid.
  Lactic acid fermentation ➔ pyruvate ➔ lactate via lactate dehydrogenase. The fermentation oxidizes NADH (produced by glycolysis) back to NAD.
  Lactate is taken up by the liver (Cori cycle) into gluconeogenesis so that the lactate is converted back to glucose. The glucose enters the bloodstream and returns back to the muscles (during exercising states). If exercising has stopped then the glucose that was generated via gluconeogenesis is then used to build up glycogen stores via Glycogenesis.
  This process keeps the lactic acid from building up in the muscle causing lactic acidosis and to produce ATP during muscle activity.
- **NOTE: Side effect of Metformin**: lactic acidosis because it inhibits gluconeogenesis of the Cori cycle. This build up of lactate is normally cleared by the kidneys, but in patients with renal failure, the lactate is unable to be cleared causing lactic acidosis.

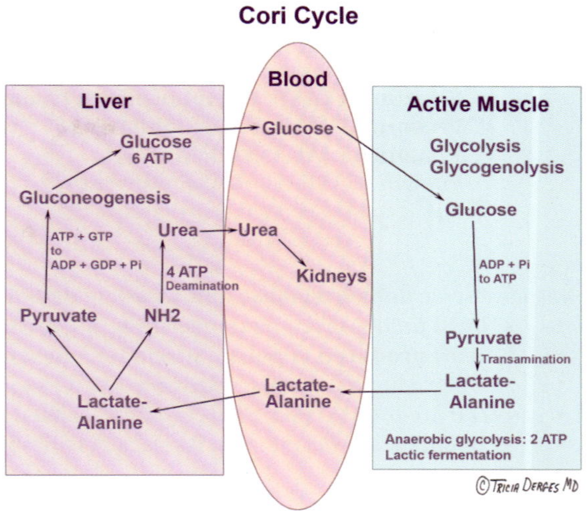

Pyruvate Kinase Deficiency (AKA: Erythrocyte Pyruvate Kinase Deficiency)

- RBC's can only use Glycolysis to manufacture ATP. They have no mitochondria.
- Causes **LACTIC ACIDOSIS**
- Common in alcoholics due to Vit B-1 deficiency
- Requires a ketogenic diet: **Leucine and Lysine**
- Pyruvate Kinase is required to make Pyruvate. Without pyruvate = no ATP
- Without ATP, RBC will shrink/deform into echinocytes (burr cells) = cell death
- Causes increase in 2,3 BPG = right shift in Oxy Hb curve
- RBC lysis leads to hemolytic anemia in the newborn = jaundice from increased bilirubin
- TX: Blood transfusion or removal of spleen

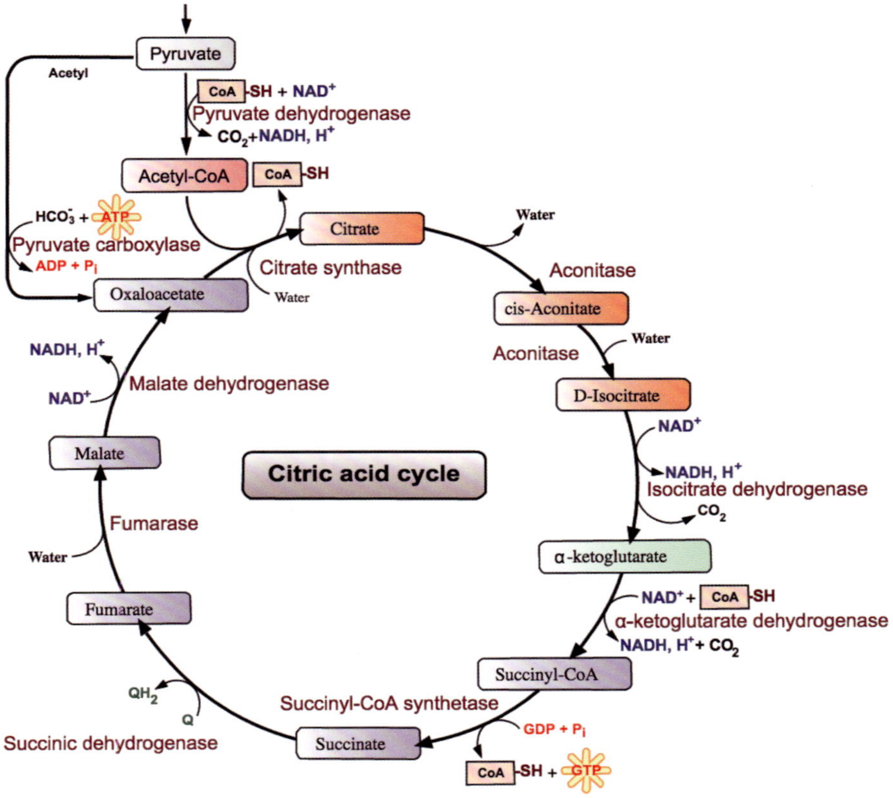

TCA Cycle (aka: Tricarboxylic Acid Cycle, Citric Acid Cycle, Krebs's Cycle)

TCA Cycle cannot work without pyruvate. Pyruvate is the end product of glycolysis.
Pyruvate can NOT enter the TCA without the **Pyruvate dehydrogenase*** **(AKA: Complex Dehydrogenase)**

Complex Consist of:
Vitamin B1 (AKA: Pyrophosphate, Thiamine, TPP)
Vitamin B2 (AKA: FAD, Riboflavin)
Vitamin B3 (AKA: NAD, Niacin)
Vitamin B5 (AKA: CoA, Pantothenate)
Lipoic Acid

***α-Ketoglutarate dehydrogenase and Ketoacid dehydrogenase requires the same complex requirements**

- 3 NADH produced at points: Isocitrate, a-Ketoglutarate, Malate an sent to Complex I of ETC
- **1 FADH produced at point: Succinate and sent to Complex II of the ETC**
- 2 CO2 produced at points: Isocitrate and a-Ketoglutarate
- **1 GTP** produced at point: Succinyl CoA. Is **used for energy by OAA** back to PEP in GNG
- Alcoholics are deficient in Vit B1 so can't enter the TCA cycle

Amino Acid Entry Points into the TCA Cycle

Acetyl CoA
Isoleucine*
Leucine*
Lysine*
Phenylalanine*
Tryptophan*
Tyrosine

Succinyl CoA
Isoleucine*
Methionine*
Valine*
Threonine*

Oxaloacetate
Asparagine
Aspartate

***Essential Amino Acids and must come from diet.**

a-Ketoglutarate
Arginine
Histidine*
Glutamate
Glutamine
Proline

Fumarate
Phenylalanine*
Tyrosine

Pyruvate
Alanine
Cysteine
Glycine
Serine
Threonine*
Tryptophan*

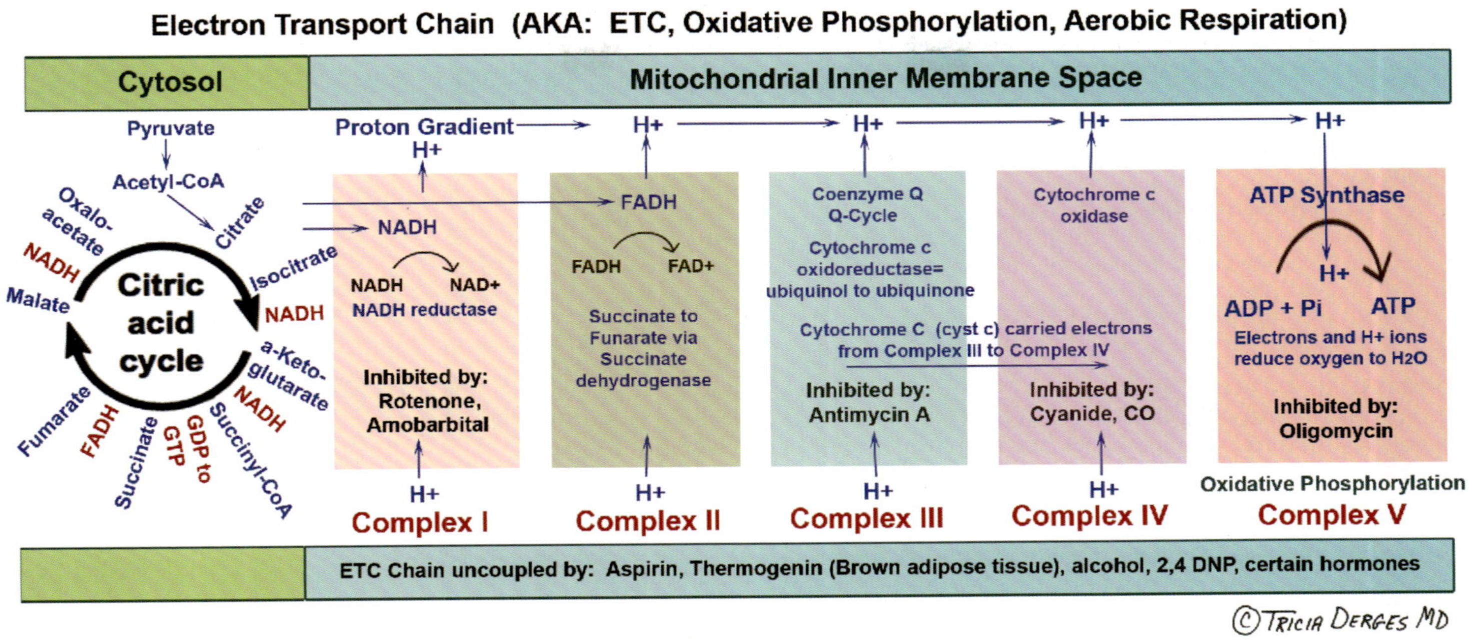

Electron Transport Chain (AKA: ETC, Oxidative Phosphorylation, Aerobic Respiration)

- Occurs in the **inner membrane of the mitochondria.**
- **Glycolysis occurs outside the mitochondria in the cytoplasm.**
- ETC is a series of redox reactions (donor to acceptor) that transfer electrons from electron donors to electron acceptors.
- Oxygen is the electron acceptor.
- The force driving the redox reactions is the Gibbs Free Energy (△G). This is the "free" energy available to do the work. **If the △G is < 0 = favors reaction (spontaneous). If △G is > 0 = disfavors reaction (nonspontaneous)**. If △G is 0 = no change either way.
- Oxygen produces the greatest Gibbs free energy and produces the most energy.
- Proton pumps pump protons (H+ ions) across the membrane to create a proton gradient. **The ↑ of H+ ions across the inner mitochondrial membrane causes an ↑ in the ratio of oxygen consumption to ATP generation.**
- Proton gradient drives ATP synthesis.
- ETC generates superoxide (highly reactive molecule that contributes to oxidative stress, AKA: Free Radicals).

Complex 1

- NADH electrons enter from glycolysis (by G3P) and TCA (by malate-aspartate shuttle)
- NADH Reductase
- NADH electrons changed to NAD and moved down the ETC by a protein gradient from H+
  The reduced product of this change is ubiquinol (QH2)
- Complex I **stopped by <u>Rotenone and Amobarbital</u>**
- **NADH (NAD AKA: NIACIN, VIT B3)**
- H+ (AKA: Proton) sent to Complex V creating a proton gradient

Complex II

- FADH enters from TCA from process of **Succinate being converted to Fumarate via the enzyme Succinate Dehydrogenase.**
- FADH electrons changed to FAD and moved down ETC by a proton gradient from H+
- **FADH (FAD AKA: RIBOFLAVIN, VIT B2)**

Complex III

- **Coenzyme Q (AKA: CoQ, ubiquinone**) is the transport that moves electrons from NADH and FADH from Complex I and II to Complex III and **Cytochrome C**
- Cytochrome Reductase
- Complex III **stopped by <u>Antimycin A</u>**
- Organs with the highest energy requirements (heart, liver and kidney) have the highest CoQ
- H+ sent to Complex V (creating a proton gradient)

Complex IV

- Complex IV **stopped by Cyanide** (almond breath) **and CO** (Carbon Monoxide = 1st sign: headache, cherry red blood)
- Cytochrome Oxidase
- H+ sent to Complex V (creating a proton gradient)
- Electrons are removed from Cytochrome C
- Electrons and Hydrogen ions (H+) reduce Oxygen to water (H2O)

Complex V

- Complex V is **stopped by Oligomycin**
- Trans membrane proton gradient is used to make ATP
- ATP Synthesis (AKA: Oxidative phosphorylation): ADP phosphorylated to ATP by ATP Synthase (adds a phosphate Pi)

Uncoupling of the ETC

Occurs when an alternative flow of protons back into the inner mitochondrial matrix. This alternative flow causes thermogenesis (creation of heat: non-shivering thermogenesis) instead of creation of ATP by bypassing ATP Synthase.
Proton gradient decreases, oxygen use increases, ATP synthesis stops, electron transport continues causing **extreme heat, rigid muscles**.

- **Thermogenin (Brown adipose tissue** in babies)
- **Aspirin** (AKA: Salicylic acid)
- 2,4 Dinitrophenol (AKA: DNP or 2,4 DNP) (in some: herbicides, diet pills, explosives)
- Uncoupling proteins are increased by: thyroid hormone, leptin, epinephrine, Nor Epi
- Alcohol
- DX: **Malignant Hyperthermia**
- **TX: Dantrolene**
  MOA: Blocks ryanodine receptors and stops release of ind from the sarcoplasmic reticulum

(**NOTE:** Shivering is the body's way of raising its temperature. It produces heat because the conversion of chemical ATP energy to kinetic energy causing heat.)

Cytochrome C

Is in the inner membrane of the mitochondria. Release of Cytochrome C results in apoptosis (cell death) by activation of **Caspase 9 (intrinsic killing).**

- **Cytochrome C is protected from release (cell death) by anti-apoptotic BCL-2.** As long as BCL-2 is in charge, it keeps the cell from dying. This is good if the cell is normal, but is NOT if the cell is cancerous. Overexpression of BCL-2 allows the cancer cells to survival.
- **If BCL-2 is not working, Cytochrome C is released.** If Cytochrome C is released then the pro-apoptotic (BAD boys) BAK, **BAX, BIM** are able to go free and kill the cell.
- In the case of the negative/positive selection process in the thyroid, **FAS** is not able to protect the cell from apoptosis, so apoptosis occurs when **Caspase 8 (extrinsic killing)** is activated.

GLUCONEOGENESIS

- Occurs mainly in the liver to maintain blood glucose levels (euglycemia) in-between meals and fasting/starvation states
- **Does NOT occur in muscle because it lacks glucose 6 phosphatase**
- Works for approximately the first 24 hours

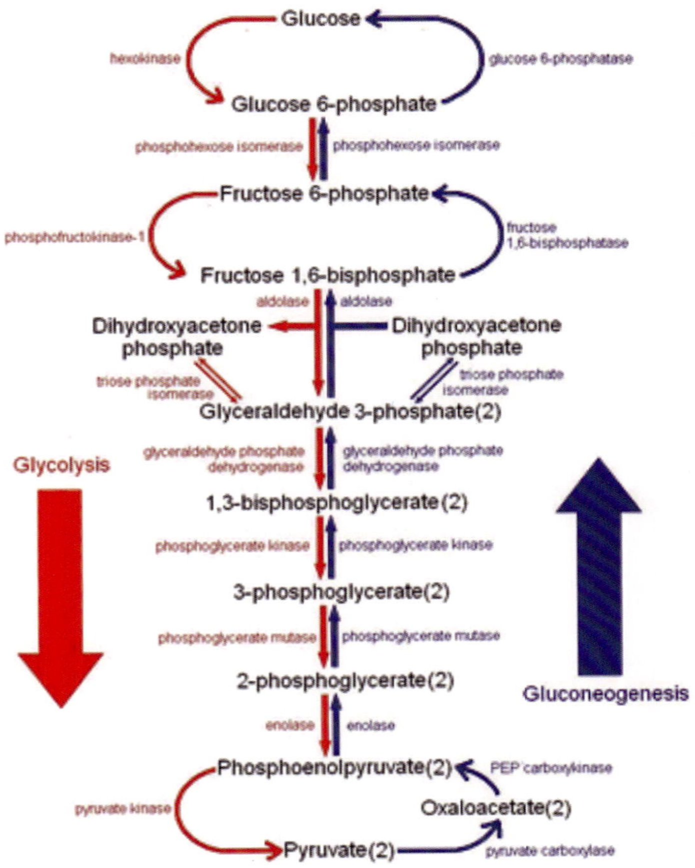

FASTING/STARVATION

Glucagon (alpha cells in the pancreas), cortisol, epinephrine: are on.
Gluconeogenesis and Glycogenolysis is working.
OFF: 2, 6 Bisphosphate, PFK 1
ON: 1, 6 Fructose, Alanine, Glycine
ON: cAMP
Turns it ON: ATP and Acetyl CoA
Turn it OFF: AMP, Fructose 2, 6 bisphosphate
Allosteric Activator: Acetyl CoA

Pathway's To Glucose Production

In Mitochondria: Pyruvate to Oxaloacetate via Pyruvate Carboxylase
Cofactor: **Biotin** (Carboxylase), Allosteric Activator: ***Acetyl CoA**, Energy: ATP.
In Cytosol: Oxaloacetate to Phosphoenolpyruvate (PEP) via Phosphoenolpyruvate carboxykinase. Energy: **GTP: made from Succinyl CoA to Succinate step in TCA cycle.**
In Cytosol: Fructose 1,6 BP to Fructose-6-P via Fructose 1,6 Bisphosphatase.
In Endoplasmic Reticulum: Glucose-6-P to Glucose via Glucose-6-Phospatase.

NOTE: Cortisol causes hyperglycemia by stimulating gluconeogenesis. Protein breakdown releases amino acids which act as precursors to gluconeogenesis to stimulate lipolysis. When lipolysis occurs, free fatty acids are released and act as the energy source for gluconeogenesis.

*Acyl-CoA dehydrogenase Deficiency

- Acetyl-CoA is the allosteric regulator of pyruvate carboxylase in gluconeogenesis.
- Without Acetyl-CoA there is decrease in glucose because there is no gluconeogenesis (=hypoglycemia), no ketones and no cholesterol.

Carbohydrates

Monosaccharides

- Glucose: monosaccharide
- Fructose (fruit sugar): monosaccharide
- Galactose (milk sugar): monosaccharide

Disaccharides

- Sucrose (sugar): Glucose and Fructose
- Lactose (breast milk): Glucose and Galactose
- Maltose (malt sugar): Glucose and Glucose

Oligosaccharide: contains 3 to 9 simple sugars (monosaccharide's) O or N linked to amino acids
Polysaccharide: polymeric carb molecules of long chains of monosaccharide's bound by covalent bonds (stable sharing of positive and negative electron pairs between atoms).

GALACTOSE PATHWAY

Galactose to Galactose -1-Phosphate via **Galactokinase***
Galactose-1-Phosphate to Glucose-1-Phosphate via **Galactose-1-Phosphate Uridyltransferase*****
Glucose-1-Phosphate to Glucose-6-Phosphate (Glycolysis Cycle)
AND
Galactose is also being converted to Galactitol (AKA: dulcitol) via **Aldose Reductase****

*** "Glycolysis and Associated Pathways" to see where the Galactose pathway enters Glycolysis.*

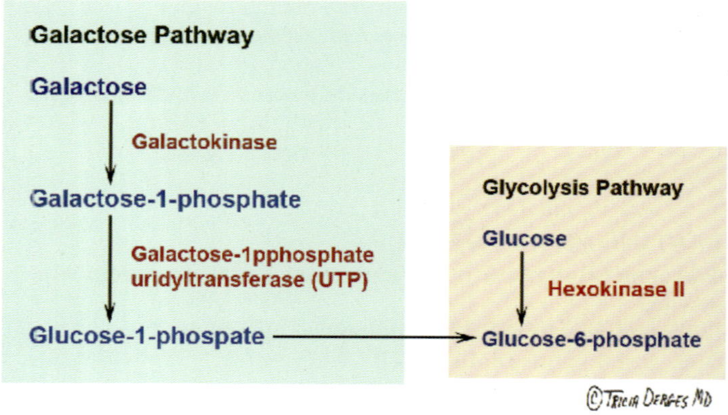

Galactose Pathway Pathologies

***Galactokinase Deficiency (mild), AR**

- Hereditary deficiency of Galactokinase
- Galactitol accumulates
- Galactosuria: Galactose seen in blood and urine
- TX: Exclude lactose from diet

****Aldose Reductase Deficiency** can result from

1) Build up of galactose in the conversion of Galactose to Galactitol via **Aldose reductase**
2) Build up of **sorbitol** in the conversion of sorbitol to fructose via **Sorbitol dehydrogenase**

BOTH CAUSE

- **Sorbitol accumulation** that causes **osmotic damage = cataracts**, retinopathies or peripheral neuropathies in diabetics with chronic hyperglycemia

*****Galactose-1-Phosphate Uridyltransferase Deficiency (UTP) AR = GALACTOSEMIA**

- **Begins soon after the start of breast feeding**
- **Accumulation of Galactose-1-P** and Galactitol in blood and eyes
- High levels of galactose in blood = **galactosemia**
- High levels of neonatal sepsis
- SX: Failure to thrive, jaundice, hepatomegaly, infantile cataracts, mental retardation
- TX: Exclude galactose and lactose (galactose, glucose) from diet

Lactase Deficiency (AKA: Lactose Intolerance)

- Inability to digest lactose (milk sugar) into galactose and glucose due to a deficiency of lactase
- Common in African, Asian and Native Americans
- Accumulation of lactose in GI
- SX: abdominal bloating, cramps, osmotic diarrhea, nausea, borborygmi (rumbling stomach), vomiting
- DX: Hydrogen Breath Test shows high H+ (bacteria ferment lactose)
  Stool Test: Low pH of <5.5 in stool = acidic. If lactose is not digested in small intestine it reaches the colon. The bacteria in the colon digest it leaving acidic stools.

FRUCTOSE PATHWAY

Fructose to Fructose-1-Phosphate via **Fructokinase***
Fructose-1-Phosphate to DHAP/Glyceraldehyde via **Aldolase B****
DHAP/Glyceraldehyde to Glyceraldehyde-3-P (G3P in Glycolysis)

*** "Glycolysis and Associated Pathways" to see where the Fructose pathway enters Glycolysis.*

Fructose has the **fastest metabolism**: it bypasses PFK-

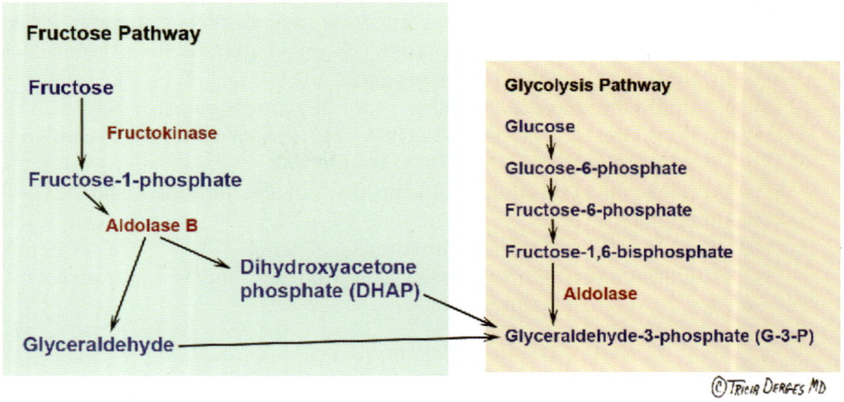

***Fructokinase Deficiency = Fructosuria (mild)**

- Benign because fructose can still be processed by using hexokinase
- Fructose appears in urine and blood = Fructosuria
- Appears in babies around 6 months old (time of introduction of fruits/fruit juice into their diet)
- TX: Discontinue any foods/beverages with fructose from the diet. **NOTE: This includes no intake of sucrose (sucrose is a disaccharide of fructose and glucose).**

****Aldolase B Deficiency (AKA: Fructose Intolerance, Hereditary fructose Intolerance)**

- Fructose-1-P accumulates which **decreases/stops production of ATP** (oxidative phosphorylation) so inhibits gluconeogenesis and glycogenolysis
- **Begins after the first introduction of fruit, juice, honey into a babies diet (about 6 months old)**
- SX: hypoglycemia, jaundice, cirrhosis, vomiting
- TX: Exclude/decrease intake of fructose and sucrose (glucose and fructose)
- (**tip**: Aldolase **B** for **B** = **Bad**. Don't mix up with Aldolase Reductase in the Galactose pathway. This leads to cataracts, not death).

HMP SHUNT PATHWAY (AKA: Pentose Phosphate Pathway: PPP)

Glucose-6-Phosphate to 6-Phosphogluconolactone via **Glucose-6-Phosphate Dehydrogenase***
Glucose-6-Phosphogluconolactone to Ribulose-5-Phosphate
Ribulose-5-Phosphate to Fructose-6-Phosphate via **Transketolase (cofactor: Thiamine Vit B1)**

HMP Shunt (AKA: Pentose Phosphate Pathway), XL

- Provides **NADPH** for: **Glutathione in RBC**, Fatty Acid Synthesis, Cholesterol Synthesis
- Provides **Ribose** for nucleotide synthesis
- Occurs in the cytoplasm
- Located in: Adrenal cortex, liver, RBC, mammary glands, fatty acid and steroid synthesis sites

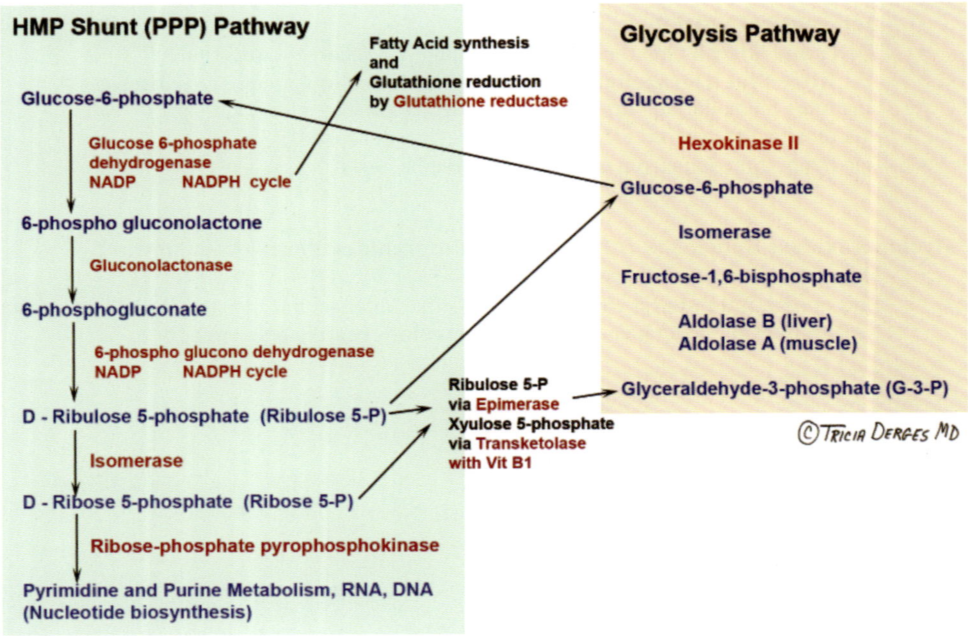

Glutathione

- **Glutathione:** Protects RBC's from free radical damage. Biosynthesized by amino acids: cysteine, glutamic acid and glycine.
- **Glutathione Reductase** converts (recycles) glutathione disulfide back to Glutathione.
- Glutathione is made from **Glutamate.**
- Glutathione is needed by the liver for detoxification processes.
- Glutathione is needed to make bile (bile is required for **digestion and the breakdown of fats**). **Without glutathione the β-oxidation pathway (Acyl CoA) is affected.**
- Glutathione is essential for the production and immune responses of IL-2 and killer cells. It is especially important in cell-mediated immunity.
- Glutathione reduces inflammation.
- Glutathione is important for oxygen transport, amino acid transport, and protection of DNA, protection of B12 inside the cells and for the removal of heavy metals.

*Glucose-6-Phosphate Dehydrogenase Deficiency (G6PD)

- Highest in Africans and Mediterranean decent
- **Protective against malaria**
- **X Linked** condition that predisposes to hemolytic anemia and jaundice in oxidative stress
- Neonatal jaundice can lead to kernicterus due to large numbers of RBC sequestered (taken out of circulation) in the spleen
- **MCC**: Fava beans (broad/flat beans, bean dip), drugs (esp. sulfa drugs, anti-malarial drugs, INH, aspirin, sulfa diuretics, dapsone), illness.

Reactive Oxygen Species (ROS) (AKA: Respiratory Burst, Oxidative Burst)

Our first line of defense: Phagocytes (neutrophils and macrophages) require **NADPH Oxidase*** to produce the respiratory burst used to kill the bacteria they ingest. NADPH produces superoxide anions (reactive oxygen species). Superoxide is then reduced and oxidized into hydrogen peroxide (H2O2) by **Superoxide Dismutase** (SOD). **Myeloperoxidase**** **(AKA: Azurophilic granules, Peroxidase enzyme)** then oxidizes hydrogen peroxide (H2O2) into hypochlorite (bleach) which kills the bacteria. (It is like a bomb that the phagocytes throw at the bacteria and blow them up).

If the CGD individual is infected with bacteria that are not catalase positive, the phagocytes can use the hydrogen peroxide from these bacteria and still make bleach and create the respiratory burst (bomb) and kill the bacteria. However, if the bacteria are **CATALASE positive**, they neutralize their own hydrogen peroxide so there is none left for the phagocytes to use in individuals with CGD. So the phagocytes are unable to create the respiratory burst. **This causes recurrent infections by catalase, gram-positive bacteria.**

CATALASE POSITIVE BACTERIA

Staph aureus, Pseudomonas, Enterobacteriaceae family (Serratia, E. coli, Citrobacter, Klebsiella, Shigella, Yersinia, Proteus, Salmonella), Aspergillus, Listeria, Corynebacterium, Nocardia, Candida, **Burkholderia**, Mycobacterium tuberculosis, Cryptococcus, Rhodococcus. (Catalase negative: Streptococcus and Enterococcus).

*Chronic Granulomatous Disease (AKA: CGD, NADPH Oxidase Deficiency)

- **Deficiency of NADPH**
- PMN's and MR can't kill the bacteria they ingest = recurrent infections
- DX: **Nitro Blue Tetrazolium (NBT) Test**. If blue color appears = NO disease (meaning an oxidative burst occurred), if NO color (or yellow) appears = Positive for Disease (meaning no oxidative burst occurred)
- Recurrent infections from **catalase positive** bacteria

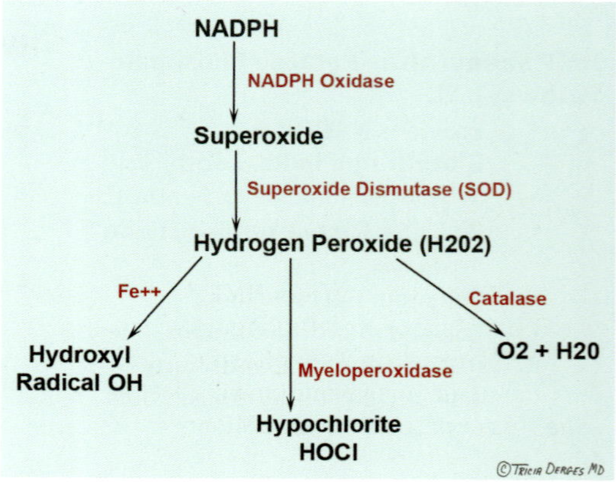

**Myeloperoxidase Deficiency (AKA: Azurophilic granules, Peroxidase enzyme)

- Most common infections by Candida
- Have a respiratory burst with a **NORMAL** nitro blue test because they have NADPH but can't form bleach because of **myeloperoxidase** deficiency

PYRIMIDINE PATHWAY

Glutamine and CO2 to Carbamoyl phosphate via **Carbamoyl phosphate synthetase II * (CPS II)**
Carbamoyl Phosphate to Orotic Acid via **Aspartate** and Dihydroorotate dehydrogenase
Orotic Acid to UMP (Orotic Aciduria)**
UMP to UDP
UDP to dUPD via Ribonucleotide reductase
dUDP to dump
dump to dTMP via Thymidylate synthase:
Cofactor: DHF (Dihydrofolate) to THF (Tetrahydrofolate) via **Dihydrofolate reductase**
THF to DHF via N5 N10 Methylene THF

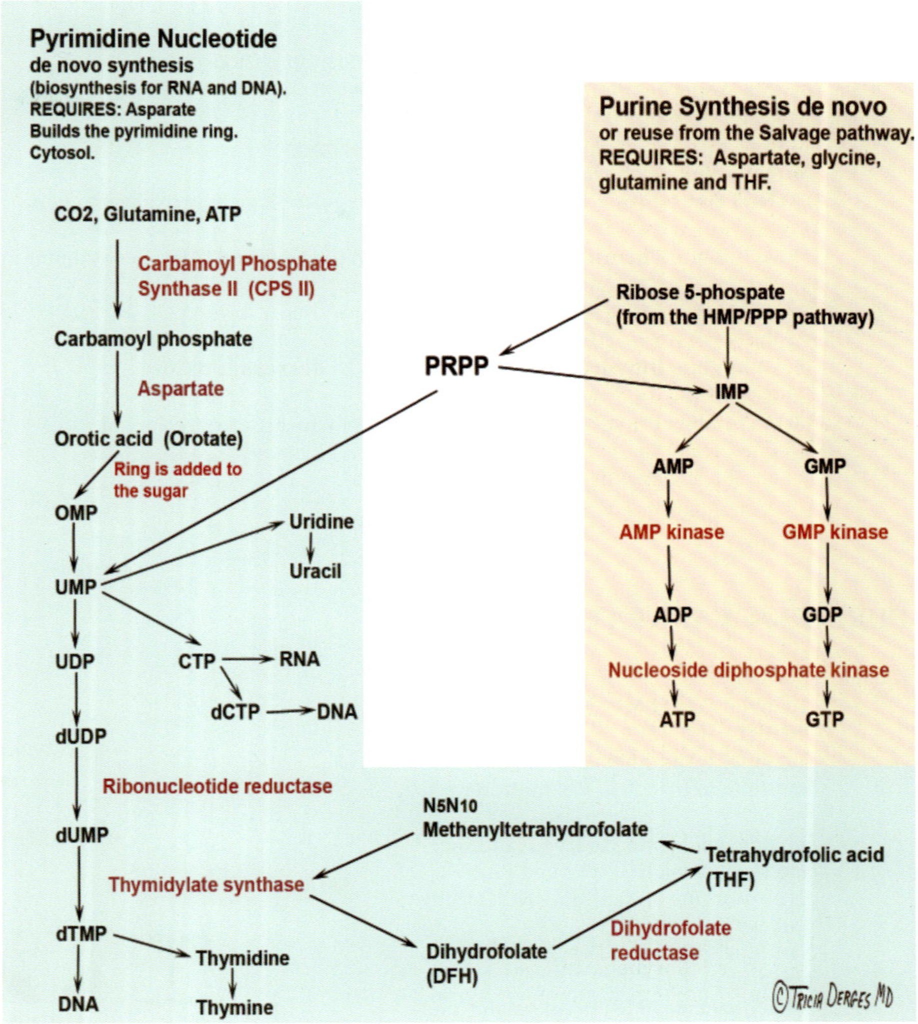

*Carbamoyl phosphate synthetase II (CPS II)**

- Occurs in the cytosol
- **No ammonia**
- **DO NOT** CONFUSE THIS WITH CPS I, which occurs in the Urea Cycle. CPS I will show HIGH ammonia – see details in the Urea Cycle section

****Orotic Aciduria**

- **Inability to convert orotic acid to UMP** (UMP synthase deficiency)
- Excretion of orotic acid in the urine
- Crystals look like white needles
- Causes megaloblastic anemia due to decreased pyrimidine synthesis which decreases erythrocyte synthesis in bone marrow
- SX: **NO AMMONIA, excessive orotic acid in urine,** megaloblastic anemia that can't be cured with administration of Vit B12 or folic acid
- TX: **Uridine**

PURINE PATHWAY

Ribose 5-Phosphate (from HMP Shunt) to **PRPP** (Phosphoribosyl pyrophosphate) via PRPP Synthetase. PRPP goes two directions:
1) to IMP (Inosine Monophosphate) which produces AMP and GMP.
2) then joins the pyrimidine pathway at UMP.
The rest of pathway from UMP on, is the same as the pyrimidine pathway (see above).

Drugs MOA with Purine and Pyrimidine Pathway

- **Hydroxyurea**
  Use: Used in **Sickle Cell to increase HBF** (increase affinity for oxygen)
  MOA: Inhibits Ribonucleotide Reductase
  SE: **Pulmonary Fibrosis**, **Pancreatitis**, Myelosuppression
- **Mycophenolate** inhibits IMP dehydrogenase
- **Ribavirin** inhibits IMP dehydrogenase
- **6-Mercaptopurine (6-MP) (AKA: Azathioprine)**
  MOA: Inhibits de novo purine synthesis
  DO **NOT** use **Allopurinol** with 6-MP. 6-MP requires Xanthine oxidase to work
- **5-Fluorouracil (5-FU)**
  MOA: Inhibits **Thymidylate Synthase which decreases dTMP** (Deoxythymidine monophosphate)
- **Methotrexate (MTX)** (Used in Eucaryotes)
  Trimethoprim (TMP) (Used in Procaryotes)
  Pyrimethamine (Used against parasites)
  MOA: Inhibits **Dihydrofolate reductase** which **decreases dTMP**
- **Leflunomide**
  MOA: Inhibits Dihydroorotate dehydrogenase which stops orotic acid

PURINE SALVAGE PATHWAY

Nucleic Acids make:

- Guanylic Acid (**GMP**) to Guanine via **HGPRT*** and PRPP
  Guanine to Xanthine
  Xanthine to Uric Acid via Xanthine oxidase
- Inosinic Acid (**IMP**) to Hypoxanthine and Inosine via **HGPRT*** and PRPP
  Hypoxanthine to Xanthine by Xanthine oxidase
  Xanthine to Uric Acid via Xanthine oxidase
- Adenylic Acid (AMP) to Adenosine and Adenine
  Adenosine to Inosine via **Adenosine deaminase* (ADA)**
  Inosine to Hypoxanthine
  Hypoxanthine to Xanthine via Xanthine oxidase
  Xanthine to Uric Acid via Xanthine oxidase

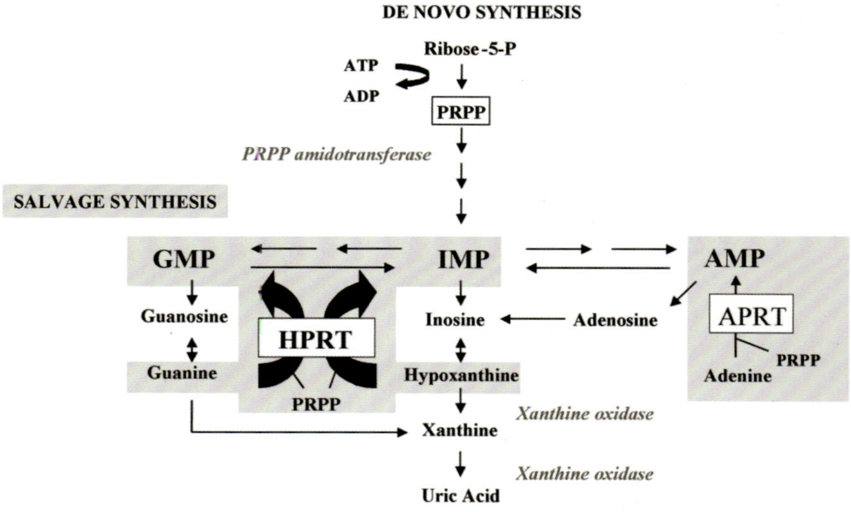

***Lesch-Nyhan Syndrome (HGPRT Deficiency), XL**

- **Deficiency of HGPRT** (Hypoxanthine-Guanine Phosphoribosyltransferase)
- **Build up of PRPP**
- SX: **Self mutilation, high uric acid levels = gout**, mental retardation, aggression, seizures
- TX: **NSAID, Colchicine (for acute gout)**
  MOA: Targets inflammation, stops chemotaxis of PMN's
- TX: **Allopurinol (for chronic gout)**
  MOA: Inhibits Xanthine Oxidase so stops production of uric acid
- TX: **Febuxostat (2nd line after Allopurinol)**
  MOA: Inhibits Xanthine Oxidase so stops production of uric acid

****SCID (Severe Combined Immunodeficiency Disease) (Adenosine Deaminase Deficiency), AR**

- AKA: Combined Immune Deficiency
- Deficiency of **Adenosine deaminase**
- Defective IL receptor mutation
- Defective antibody response to defective activation of B lymphocytes because of non-functional T-Helper cells so that both B and T and Natural Killer cell defenses are impaired **(no humoral or cell mediated defenses)**
- Ribonucleotide Reductase is inhibited preventing DNA synthesis
- Eliminates excess adenosine in cells
- "Bubble Boy" Recurrent infections: bacterial, viral, fungal, atypical bacteria, and parasites

TIP: When reading a vignette that starts listing the different specific infections an individual has had, note exactly what of each of the infections is: bacterial, viral, fungal, atypical bacteria, parasites, tumors. **Be VERY careful of the atypical bacteria!** (Mycoplasma, Chlamydia, Rickettsia, Ureaplasma, Borrelia, Treponema, Legionella, Coxiella burnetii) Atypical bacteria are fought by T cells, NOT B cells). Once you have each type of infection identified you will be able to see if the individual was deficient in B cells only, T cells only or both). On the exam, I recommend writing this down on your note page so that you keep each straight. It is not a good idea on exam day to try and keep numerous things straight in your mind. This includes ALL answers that have the up/down arrow choices or answer choices that list a specific order. Do NOT take a chance on a careless error. Write it down and mark through the incorrect answers as soon as you identify them!

UREA CYCLE

- Urea Cycle is located in the liver
- Occurs in both the mitochondria and cytoplasm
- Cycle converts dangerous ammonia in our bodies (from metabolites/cell death) to safe urea which is excreted by the kidneys
- **Most urea is absorbed in the collecting tubules in the kidney**
- Ammonia is dangerous and therefore must be "escorted" to the liver by **Alanine (in the blood)** and **Glutamate (NH3 shuttle).** Glutamate combines with pyruvate to make alanine.
- To much ammonia (too much uric acid, too much cell breakdown) can cause a build up of ammonia in the body. To much ammonia (NH4) depletes a-ketoglutarate which stops the TCA cycle
- **ANY liver failure or dysfunction** can cause the urea cycle to function poorly or not at all, which causes ammonia to build up in our blood and go to our brain – **Hepatic Encephalopathy**.
  SX: Jaundice, Asterixis (AKA: Flapping tremor, Liver Flap), confusion, somnolence (excess sleep), blurred vision, cerebral edema, coma (anything that indicates there are problems in the head)
  TX: **Lactulose** and limit protein in the diet (decreases amino acids)
  MOA: **Acidifies the GI and converts NH3 (ammonia) to NH4+ (ionized) for excretion**

Urea Pathway

CO2 + NH3 (ammonia) to Carbamoyl Phosphate via **Carbamoyl Phosphate Synthetase I (CPS I)** with **Cofactor N-acetylglutamate* (NAG)**
Carbamoyl Phosphate to Citrulline via **Ornithine transcarbamylase** (OTC)**
Citruline to Argininosuccinate via Argininosuccinate synthetase and **Aspartate adds the nitrogen.**
Argininosuccinate to Arginine via Argininosuccinase
Arginine goes two directions:
1) Ornithine via Arginase
2) Urea to the kidney to excrete

Urea Cycle

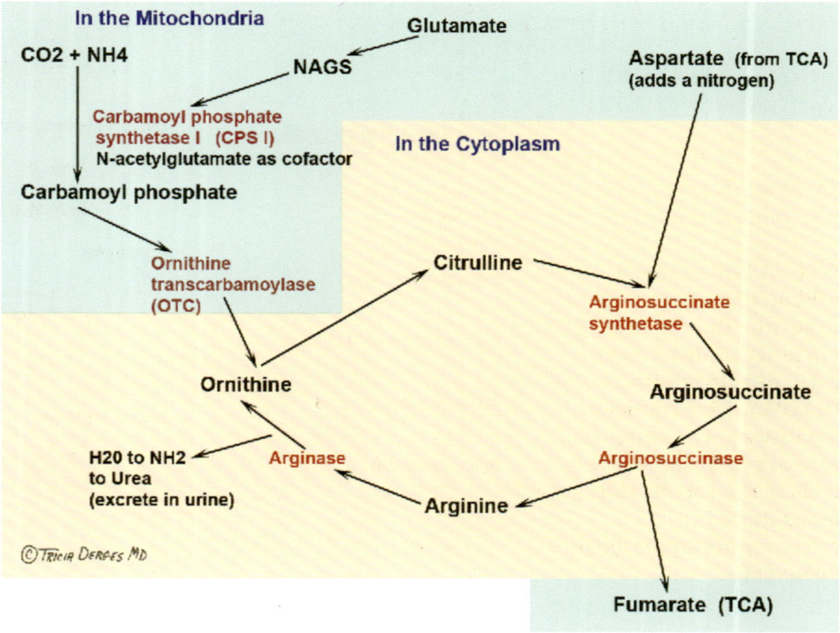

Urea Pathologies

***N-acetylglutamate (NAG) Deficiency (N⁵ N¹⁰)**

- Cofactor for Carbamoyl phosphate synthetase I (CPS I)
- Causes build up of ammonia in the blood (hyperammonemia)

****Ornithine Transcarbamylase Deficiency (OTC), XL**

- Deficiency of Ornithine transcarbamylase not allowing Carbamoyl phosphate to convert to Citruline
- Carbamoyl phosphate builds up causing excess Orotic Acid to be made in the Pyrimidine Pathway
- SX: High Orotic Acid levels in blood and urine, **Hyperammonemia**, **NO megaloblastic** anemia
- High ammonia can cause: neural damage and hepatic encephalopathy (TX: **Lactulose**)

(Don't confuse this with Orotic Aciduria in the Pyrimidine Pathway. This is due to OTC deficiency and **DOES HAVE high ammonia).**

Remember: CPS 1 is in the Urea Cycle (**tip**: you pee out of ONE hole) and **HAS** ammonia
CPS II is in the Pyrimidine Pathway and has **NO** ammonia

PHENYLALANINE (PHE) and CATECHOLAMINE PATHWAY

PHE to Tyrosine via **Phenylalanine hydroxylase*** and cofactor **BH4 (Tetrahydrobiopterin)**
Tyrosine goes three directions:
1) to Thyroxine (T4)
2) to Dopa via Tyrosine Hydroxylase and **cofactor BH4**
3) to Homogentisic Acid to Maleylacetoacetic Acid via **Homogentisate oxidase****
Maleylacetoacetic Acid to Fumarate in the TCA Cycle

Dopa (Dihydroxyphenylalanine) goes two directions:
1) to Melanin via **Tyrosinase*****
2) to Dopamine via Dopa decarboxylase and **cofactor B6**

Dopamine to Norepinephrine with **cofactor Vitamin C**

IN THE ADRENYL MEDULLA

Norepinephrine to Epinephrine by **SAM** (S-Adenosyl methionine) and PNMT (Phenylethanolamine N-methyltransferase).

Cortisol controls PNMT, if cortisol is ON, PNMT is ON

(**tip**: **SAM**, SAM the Methyl Man (**methyl = stops)**

NOTE: Anytime there is a build up of a product in the serum, the cause is a deficiency of the enzyme or its co-factor that FOLLOWS this product in its pathway. Example: If there are ↑↑ dopamine levels in the serum, this means there is a deficiency of Dopamine β-hydroxylase.

Phenylalanine (PHE) and Catecholamine Pathway

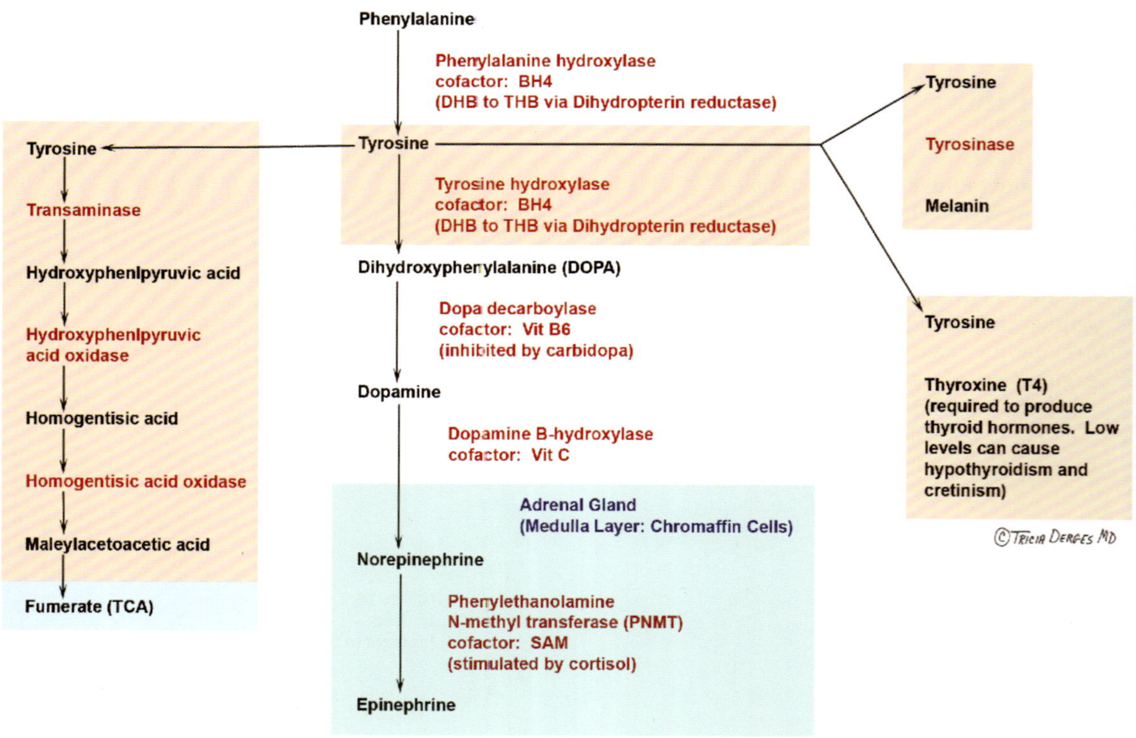

Breakdown products of catecholamines (Shows in urine)
These breakdown products are found in the urine in pheochromocytoma (MEN)

- **Norepinephrine** to Normetanephrine (NMN) to **Vanillylmandelic Acid (VMA) (urine)**
- **Epinephrine** to Metanephrine (MN) (in blood serum) to **Vanillylmandelic Acid (urine)**
- **Dopamine to Homovanillic Acid (HVA) (urine)**

Phenylalanine and Catecholamine Pathway Pathology

***Phenylketonuria, AR**

- **Decrease of Phenylalanine hydroxylase**
- **Decrease of BH4 Tetrahydrobiopterin cofactor**
- Disorder of **AROMATIC amino acid metabolism**
- Without PHE, **Tyrosine becomes essential** (needed to add into diet)
- Screened for several days after birth because PHE levels will be normal at time of birth due to mothers enzymes
- Both Tyrosine and Phenylalanine stimulate prolactin secretion
- SX: mental retardation, seizures, eczema, growth retardation, fair skin, musty body odor
- **DX: Guthrie Test**
- TX: Avoid artificial sweetener aspartame (diet drinks) that contain PHE
- **BE CAREFUL: Chediak-Higashi Syndrome** signs are very similar to albinism and to PKU. Chediak-Higashi is a defect in cellular transport of the lysosome through the microtubules to the phagosome to form a phagolysosome.

Maternal PKU

- Women with PKU must maintain low PHE levels
- PHE crosses the placenta
- Causes: Congenital heart disease, microcephaly, mental and growth retardation

****Alkaptonuria (AKA: Ochronosis), Homogentisate oxidase Deficiency, AR**

- **Deficiency of Homogentisate oxidase**
- Occurs in the pathway of **Tyrosine to Fumarate** (enters the TCA cycle)
- No metabolism of PHE
- SX: **Pigment deposits in connective tissues (AKA: blue-black tissue on the nose, ears** or cheeks), **urine turns black** upon exposure to air, arthralgia
- Homogentisic Acid is toxic to cartilage = weakens cartilage
- Benign

*****Albinism (AKA: achromia), AR, Tyrosinase Deficiency**

- **Deficiency of Tyrosinase**
- No synthesis of melanin from tyrosine (AKA: **Defective tyrosine transport**)
- Lack of migration of neural crest cells
- Complete or partial absence of pigment in the skin
- Albino is the complete **absence of melanin**
- SX: White skin, white hair, pink eyes, nystagmus, sensitivity to sun
- **BE CAREFUL**: Chediak-Higashi Syndrome signs are very similar to albinism and to PKU. Chediak-Higashi is a defect in cellular transport of the lysosome through the microtubules to the phagosome to form a phagolysosome.
- **NOTE**: Albinism is a problem with deficiency of tyrosinase. Vitiligo is an autoimmune disease that attacks the melanocytes in the skin.

TRYPTOPHAN PATHWAY

Tryptophan can go two directions:
1) Tryptophan to ***Niacin** to NAD+/NADH via cofactor B6
2) Tryptophan to Serotonin to Melatonin via Cofactors B6 and BH4

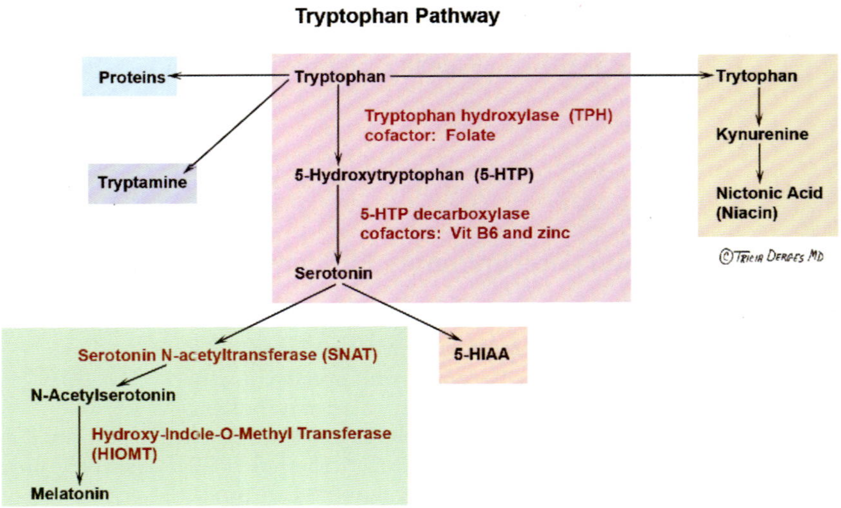

***Pellagra**

- Deficiency of **Niacin** (AKA: Vitamin B3, NAD/NADH) or **Tryptophan**
- SX: "the 3 D's": Diarrhea**, dermatitis, dementia**
  Aggression, glossitis (beefy red inflamed tongue), sensitivity to sunlight
- Associated with high diet of corn (maize) due to lack of niacin
- **Hartnup Disease** ("Pellagra Like") disorder affecting the absorption of tryptophan

Additional Amino Acid Pathways

- Histidine to Histamine via cofactor B6.
- Glutamate can go two directions: 1) to GABA via cofactor B6 OR 2) to Glutathione (RBC).
- Arginine can go three directions: 1) to Creatine; 2) to Urea OR 3) to Nitric Oxide via cofactor BH4.

ADDITIONAL AMINO ACID METABOLISM PATHOLOGIES

Cystinuria, AR

- Defect of amino acid transporters for (COLA) Cysteine, Ornithine, Lysine, Arginine in the intestine and PCT of the kidneys.
- AKA: No amino acid transport
- See high amino acids in urine
- Excess cystine in urine = cystine stones (AKA: cystine staghorn calculi)
- Cystine = 2 cystines connected by a disulfide bond
- In the urine the crystals look like envelopes
- TX: **Acetazolamide or potassium citrate** (**urinary alkalization**) and hydration
  MOA: Carbonic anhydrase inhibitor. Causes diuresis and decreases HCO3 in body.
  SE: Metabolic acidosis, sulfa allergy, not for use in DKA

Homocysteine Pathway

- Synthesized from Methionine.
- Homocysteine made from Methionine is by demethylation.
- Methionine made from homocysteine is by methylation.
- Methionine to SAM (S-adenosyl methionine) via S-adenosyl-methionine synthetase. (receives an adenosine group from ATP)
- SAM transfers the methyl group to an acceptor molecule (Ex: norepinephrine is the acceptor group during epinephrine synthesis and DNA methyltransferase is the acceptor group during DNA methylation).
- The adenosine group is then hydrolyzed to Homocysteine.
- Homocysteine can then go two different directions:
  - It can convert to cysteine or
  - It can covert back to Methionine by Tetrahydrofolate (THF)

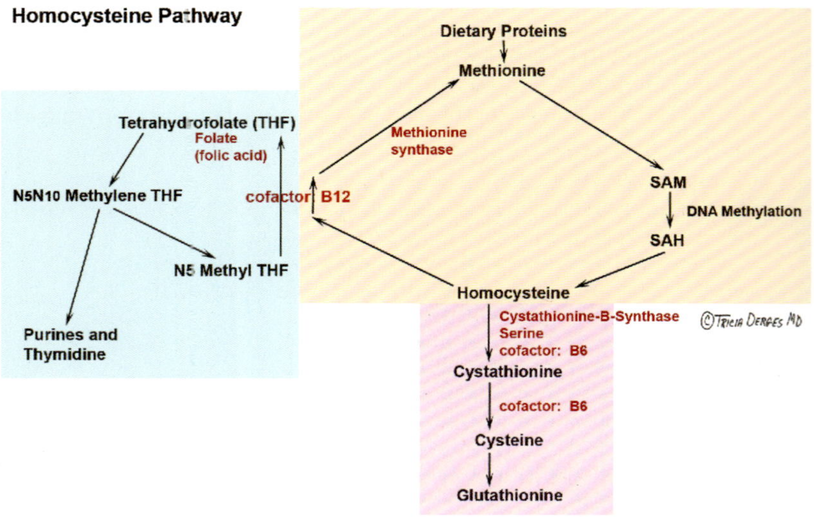

Homocysteine to Cysteine (aka: Transsulfuration pathway)

- Homocysteine combines with **Serine** to form Cystathionine via **Cystathionine-β-synthase**. Cystathionine to Cysteine via Cystathionine-γ-lyase and **cofactor B6.** Cysteine will continue on to synthesize **glutathione.**
- If there is a deficiency in this pathway: **Cysteine becomes essential** (need in diet).
- If there is a deficiency in Cystathionine-β-synthase: **Homocystinuria**
    - High homocysteine in urine.
      ↑ **Methionine levels** and ↑ Homocysteine in the serum.
      SX Marfan-like symptoms
      TX: Give B6 and cysteine in the diet

(**Tip: If question discusses homocystine and cysteine = choose B6**)

Homocystinuria, AR

- Due to **Cystathionine synthase deficiency**
- Homocysteine cannot be metabolized efficiently, and therefore backs up/accumulates in the blood.
- The accumulated homocysteine is metabolized to methionine by Homocysteine methyl-transferase (HMT) and cofactor B12.
- Mental retardation, **Marfan like features:** tall and slender with long arms, kyphosis, abnormally long, slender fingers and toes (arachnodactyly), lens subluxation (downward and inward), have high levels of homocystine = **hypercoagulability** (clotting).

Homocysteine can **convert** back to Methionine (aka: Regeneration of Methionine from Homocysteine)

- **Homocysteine methyltransferase** (HMT) methylates homocysteine to Methionine. This needs cofactors: B12 and 5-methyltetrahydrofolate (N5 MeTHF).
- Methyl group is transferred to Homocysteine to form Methionine.
- **Methionine synthase** catalyzes the final step of Homocysteine into Methionine with **cofactors B12**.
- If deficiency in **Homocysteine methyltransferase (HMT)** there is **no increase in methionine.**
- High **Methylmalonic in urine**.
- B12 Deficiency causes ↑ **Methylmalonic acid (MMA) and ↑ Homocysteine levels.**

(**Tip: If question discusses homocystine and Methionine = choose B12**)

Folate deficiency

- ↑ **homocysteine levels.**
- B12 needs a methyl group from folate so that it can pass it to homocysteine to synthesize methionine. If folate is deficient, B12 is unable to give a methyl group to Homocysteine, therefore Homocysteine builds up.
- Folate deficiency **does not cause** an increase in Methylmalonic acid or neurological symptoms.
- Folate deficiency results in: macrocytic/megaloblastic anemia, fatigue, weakness, hypersegmented neutrophils.
- MCC of elevated homocysteine levels in the USA is folate deficiency, secondary to alcoholism.

Methyl groups: Folate and B12 work together with methyl groups. If folate does not need the methyl group it gives it to B12. If B12 doesn't need the methyl group it is given to methionine. B12 is a cofactor in the recycling of methyltetrahydrofolate back into tetrahydrofolate so that DNA can be synthesized. If B12 is deficient it can cause folate to be deficient: so both B12 and folate deficiencies are similar with macrocytic/megaloblastic anemia and hypersegmented neutrophils and increased homocysteine levels. Deficiency of B12 can cause neurological symptoms, loss of vibration and proprioception, hematologic and psychiatric symptoms, dementia, depression.

Maple Syrup Urine Disease (MSUD), AR, Decreased a-ketoacid dehydrogenase

- Defect in branched chain amino acids: **Leucine, Isoleucine, Valine**
- **a-ketoacid dehydrogenase** requires **same Complex Cofactors as Pyruvate dehydrogenase** (**B-1 Thiamine/TPP**, B-2, B-3, B-5, Lipoic Acid)
- Appears in the first few days of life
- See high levels of leucine, isoleucine, valine, and ketoacids in the blood and urine
- Urine and ear wax has sweet smelling maple syrup scent
- Sotolon is compound responsible for scent.
- SX: Rigid muscles, poor feeding, seizures

Peroxisome Diseases

Peroxisome Diseases: Very Long Chain Fatty Acid Pathology (VLCFA)

- Odd # fatty acids with phytanic acid
- No alpha and beta oxidation
- **Peroxisome** is non-functional. Error in peroxisome biogenesis.
- Neuro defects, CNS myelination problems
- Peroxisomes normally degrade VLCFA (Very Long Chain) and BCFA (Branched Chain)
- Not tagged with **ubiquitin** for degradation in the proteasome

Zellweger Syndrome, AR, (AKA: Floppy Baby Syndrome, Cerebrohepatorenal Syndrome)

- Absent or reduced number of peroxisomes
- **No formation of myelin** in the CNS
- Impaired neuronal **migration**
- SX: Hypotonia, seizures, hepatomegaly, renal cyst

Refsum Disease, AR

- Deficiency in peroxidase **alpha oxidation** because of accumulation of VLCFA of phytanic acid
- Deficient **phytanic acid** catabolism
- Hypotonia, adrenal dysfunction, hepatomegaly

Neonatal Adrenoleukodystrophy, AR

GLYCOGEN PATHWAY

Occurs in hepatocytes and skeletal muscle.
Glycogenolysis helps maintains blood sugar in fasting/starvation states.
Glycogen stores run out by the 3rd day in the starvation state. Then energy stores rely on adipose tissue, followed by proteins.

PATHWAY to make Glycogen (branched chains) stores:
Glucose-6-phosphate to **Glucose-1-phosphate to UDP-glucose via UDP-glucose pyrophosphorylase,**
UDP-glucose to Glycogen via Glycogen synthase.
Activators: Glucose-6-phosphate

PATHWAY of Glycogenolysis (Breakdown of Glycogen stores):
***Glycogen phosphorylase** cleaves off Glucose-1-phophate residues until 4 remain.
****a-1,4** glucanotransferase (AKA: **Acid maltase**) cleaves of 3 of the 4 residues.
*****a-1,6** glucosidase (AKA: **debranching enzyme**) cleaves off the final residue of Glucose-1-P.
Activators: cAMP and Ca2 (muscle)
Inhibitors: Glucose, Glucos-6-phosphate, ATP

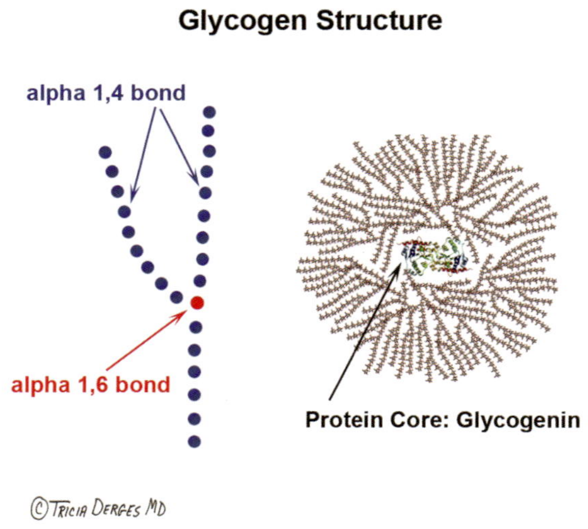

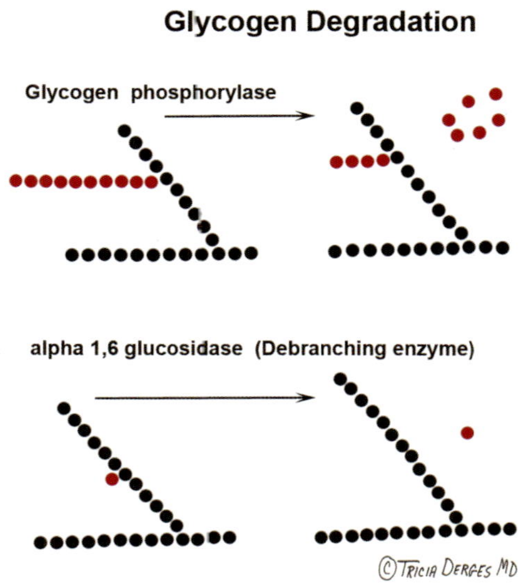

GLYCOGEN STORAGE DISEASES

Glycogen is a molecule the body uses to store carbohydrate energy.
Pathology processes involve:

- Abnormal glycogen metabolism.
- Accumulation of glycogen inside of cells.

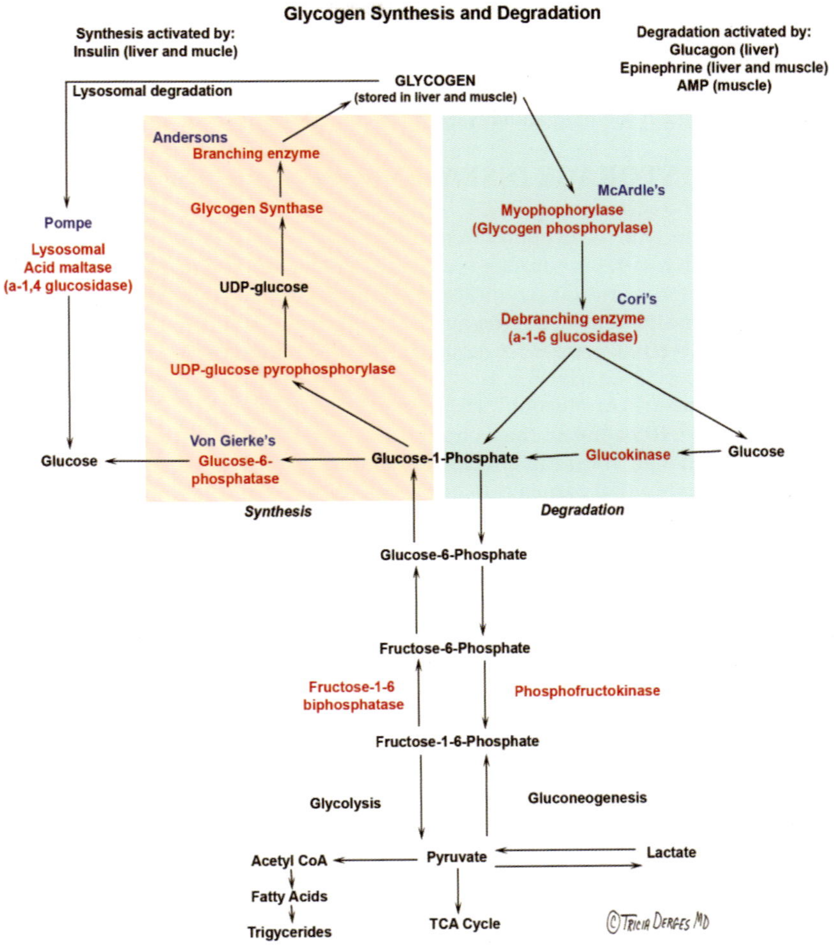

Von Gierke Disease (Type I), AR

- Deficiency: **Glucose-6-phosphatase**
- **Mutations on G6Pc gene or SLC gene**
- High **lactic acid** in blood and urine
- **Hyperuricemia**
- High glycogen in liver (glycogen can't be broken down) – hypoglycemia.
- SX: **NORMAL spleen and heart**, high urea, seizures, doll face, short, protruding abdomen, growth failure.
  3 H's: Hypoglycemia, Hepatomegaly, Hyperlipidemia
- TX: Avoid fructose and galactose

****Pompe Disease (Type II), AR**

- Deficiency: **a-1,4**, glucosidase
- Mutation on **acid maltase** gene on chromosome 17.
- Build up of glycogen in **heart**, skeletal muscles, liver and nervous system.
- SX: NO Hypoglycemia, NO hyperlipidemia, Yes: **Hepatomegaly**
- (**tip**: **PUMP**e disease. **PUMP = Heart** = Pump is **4** letters (1,4))

*****Cori Disease (Type III), AR (AKA: Forbes Disease)**

- Deficiency: **a-1,6, glucosidase** (AKA: **debranching enzyme**)
- Gluconeogenesis is working
- TX: High protein diet to induce gluconeogenesis
- **NORMAL** blood lactate levels, **"limit dextrin-like"** structures in the cytosol.
- Milder form of Von Gierke (Type I)
- SX: 3's H's: Yes: Hypoglycemia, Yes: Hepatomegaly, Yes: Hyperlipidemia

Andersons (Type IV)

- Deficiency: Glycogen branching enzyme
- Mutation on the **GBE1 gene.**
- SX: Cirrhosis. No Hypoglycemia, Yes: Hepatomegaly, No Hyperlipidemia

***McArdle Disease (Type V),** (AKA: Muscle phosphorylase – myophosphorylase deficiency), **AR**

- Deficiency: **Glycogen phosphorylase (AKA: myophosphorylase**) in skeletal muscles
- Mutations in the **PYGM gene** on chromosome 11q13.
- **Rhabdomyolysis because of strenuous exercise**: **Myoglobin** in urine (red urine but is **NOT** RBC) Myoglobin is a sign of muscle breakdown and is toxic to the kidneys = renal failure. Will see high glycogen in the muscle and cardiac cells.
- Myoglobin causes a left shift in the oxy-hb curve
- NO H's: No Hypoglycemia, No Hepatomegaly, No Hyperlipidemia

Hers Disease (Type VI), AR

- Deficiency: Liver glycogen phosphorylase
- YES H's: Yes Hypoglycemia, Yes Hepatomegaly, Yes Hyperlipidemia

Danon Disease (Type IIB), XL Dominant

- Deficiency of the lysosomal glycoprotein **LAMP2 gene** (Lysosome-associated membrane protein 2) resulting in abnormal protein structure.
- **Hypertrophic cardiomyopathy**, skeletal muscle weakness and mental retardation, Wolff-Parkinson-White, **autophagic vacuoles** in skeletal and cardiac muscle. (Autophagic vacuole contains fragments of ribosomes and/or mitochondria delivered to the lysosome).
(Can be mistaken for Pompe Disease)
- Accumulated autophagic materials in striated myocytes
- **Normal acid maltase levels**
- Earlier onset in boys, later onset in girls
- It is both a lysosomal and glycogen storage disease

LYSOSOMAL STORAGE DISEASES

Hurler Syndrome (AKA: Mucopolysaccharidosis Type 1, MPS I), AR

- Deficiency: **a-L-iduronidase** (enzyme that degrades mucopolysaccharides in lysosomes)
- Accumulated: **Heparan sulfate, Dermatan sulfate (in basement membranes)**
- **Facial malformations (gargoyle faces), cornea clouding**
- Defective **IDUA gene** on chromosome 4. (**tip**: he **HURL**'s when he sees his **face**)

Hunter Syndrome (AKA: Mucopolysaccharidosis II, MPS II), **XL-R**

- Defective **IDS gene** on the X chromosome. Deficiency: **Iduronate sulfatase**
- Accumulated: **Heparan sulfate, dermatan sulfate (in basement membranes)**
- **Clear vision** (NO cornea clouding), **aggressive** behavior
- (**tip**: a **HUNTER** is a **MAN** (XL) that must be able to **SEE WELL** (no corneal clouding)

Fabry Disease (AKA: Angiokeratoma corporis diffusum), **XL-R**

- Dysfunctional metabolism of sphingolipids
- Deficiency: **a-galactosidase A**
- Accumulated: **Ceramide trihexoside** (globotriaosylceramide)
- Accumulates in the vascular endothelium resulting in fat bodies (Maltese crosses) in the urine
- SX: **Renal trouble**, strokes: thrombotic events (clotting), decreased sweating, burning peripheral neuropathy, angiokeratomas (tiny, painless papules on the body), cardiovascular disease

Gaucher Disease, AR

- **GBA gene (beta-glucosidase)** mutation on chromosome 1. Deficiency: **Glucocerebrosidase (AKA: B-glucosidase)**
- Accumulated: **Glucocerebroside**
- Bone problems: DX: X-Ray: distal femur Erienmeyer Flask **pathological fractures**
- Gaucher Cells (AKA: **Lipid laden macrophages** (microscope: looks like crumpled tissue)
- SX: bone pain, easy bruising, anemia, thrombocytopenia, hepatosplenomegaly. Can also be seen in Ashkenazi Jews.
- (Tip: Think of Oscar the Grouch: all crumpled up inside a trash can so his bones hurt and
The 3 G network is "sweet" = Gluco: Gaucher, Gluco, Gluco)
- This is affecting the bone so you can expect to see decreased cell counts and anemia. This does **not** have a cherry red macula.

Krabbe Disease, (AKA: Globoid cell leukodystrophy), AR

- Mutation in the **GALC gene** on chromosome 14. Histology shows multinucleated globoid cells.
- Deficiency: **Galactocerebrosidase**
- Accumulation: **Galactocerebroside**
- Demyelination and accumulation of globoid cells in the CNS. Affects the myelin sheath of the nervous system.
- SX: Blindness, optic atrophy, mental retardation, seizures, no myelin, peripheral neuropathy, psychomotor retardation

Metachromatic leukodystrophy, (AKA: Arylsulfatase A Deficiency), AR

- Deficiency: **Arylsulfatase A (ARSA).** Arylsulfatase is activated by cofactor Saposin B.
- Accumulation: **Cerebroside sulfate**
- Has sulfate so it **demyelinates**
- SX: Central and peripheral demyelination, ataxia, dementia in adults

Niemann-Pick Disease, AR

- **Missense** mutation in the **SMPD1 gene**. Deficiency: **Sphingomyelinase**
- Accumulation: **Sphingomyelin**
- Accumulates in liver, spleen, **bone marrow** and brain. Involves the reticuloendothelia system.
- Histology shows: Foam cells (AKA: **cytoplasmic vacuolization**, **lipid laden macrophages, foamy histiocytes**) and **zebra bodies**.
- Ashkenazi Jews. Early death.
- SX: **Hepatosplenomegaly**, red spot on macula eye exam, **cervical lymph node swelling**, progressive weakening/regression.

Tay-Sachs Disease, AR

- Mutation of **HEXA gene** on chromosome 15. Deficiency: **Hexosaminidase A**
- Accumulates: **GM2 ganglioside** (buildup of gangliosides in the lysosomes)
- Ashkenazi Jews. Early death.
- Histology and labs: cells show **onion skinning lysosomes,** lipid droplets in cytoplasm, gangliosides deposited in CNS neurons
- SX: **NO Hepatosplenomegaly** (a **normal**, soft palpated abdomen exam), **red spot on macula** eye exam (aka: Cherry red macula), **NO cervical lymph node swelling**, mental retardation, seizures, progressive motor weakness/regression (dysphasia, clumsiness, ataxia, dysarthria), hypotonia, hearing loss.
- (**tip**: to help remember the difference between Tay-Sachs and Niemann-Pick: remember, Tay-Sachs has NO cervical lymph node swelling, NO hepatosplenomegaly, So think of a kid named "Tay" and say "NO, NO Tay").

I-Cell Disease (AKA: Inclusion Cell Disease, Mucolipidosis Type II), AR

- **Defective trafficking** of enzymes into **lysosomes**
- Deficiency of GlcNAc phosphotransferase (an enzyme in the Golgi)
- Defective proteins are not tagged for destruction with the **mannose-6-phosphate tag on the N-linked** glycoprotein in the Golgi
- High concentration of lysosomes are found in the blood
- SX: Failure to thrive, course facial features, stiff claw-shaped hands, large spleen and liver, short trunk - dwarfism (lack of growth), clouding of the cornea

Danon Disease (Type IIB), XL Dominant

- Deficiency of the lysosomal glycoprotein **LAMP2 gene** (Lysosome-associated membrane protein 2) resulting in abnormal protein structure.
- **Hypertrophic cardiomyopathy**, skeletal muscle weakness and mental retardation, Wolff-Parkinson-White, **autophagic vacuoles** in skeletal and cardiac muscle. (Autophagic vacuole contains fragments of ribosomes and/or mitochondria delivered to the lysosome).
  (Can be mistaken for Pompe Disease)
- Accumulated autophagic materials in striated myocytes
- **Normal acid maltase levels**
- Earlier onset in boys, later onset in girls
- It is both a lysosomal and glycogen storage disease

FATTY ACID SYNTHESIS – CHOLESTEROL SYNTHESIS - BETA OXIDATION – KETONE SYNTHESIS

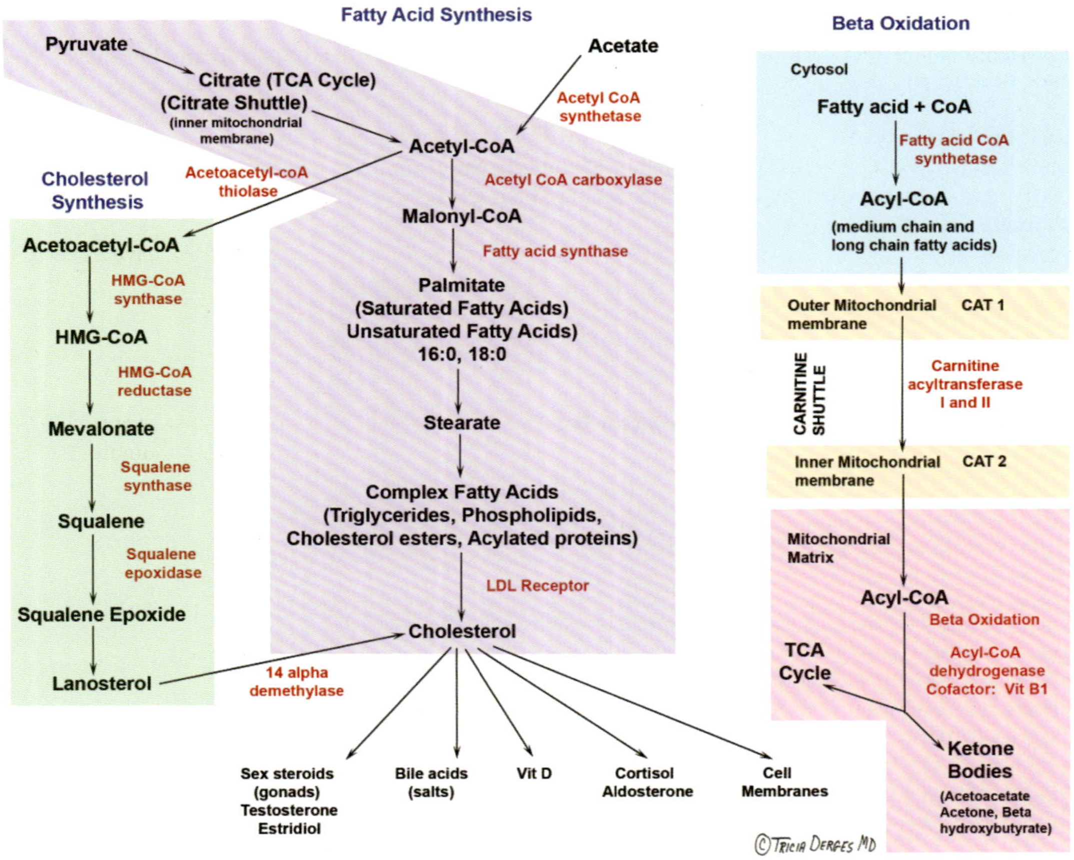

FATTY ACID SYNTHESIS (AKA: Lipogenesis)

Pathway (Cytoplasm)
Pyruvate (and Citrate from TCA via Citrate shuttle and Citrate lyase) to **Acetyl-CoA via Pyruvate Kinase**
Acetyl-CoA to Malonyl-CoA via **Acetyl-CoA carboxylase** to Fatty Acid with **cofactor Biotin.**
It is the synthesis of fatty acids from acetyl-CoA via malonyl-CoA
Malonyl-CoA inhibits the rate-limiting step in beta-oxidation (aka: fatty acid oxidation) of fatty acids. It inhibits carnitine acyltransferase (carnitine shuttle), which inhibits fatty acids from crossing over into the mitochondria and therefore inhibits beta oxidation.
Activator: Citrate acts to activate acetyl-CoA carboxylase when there are high levels of carbohydrates so that fatty acid synthesis can take place and energy can be produced in the Krebs cycle. **NOTE:** High serum insulin levels will dephosphorylate acetyl-CoA carboxylase so that fatty acid synthesis can occur. This promotes the formation of malonyl-CoA from acetyl-CoA so that carbohydrates are converted to fatty acid.
Inhibitor: Palmitoyl-CoA, **cAMP.** High levels of palmitoyl-CoA allosterically **inactivates acetyl-CoA carboxylase** to inhibit fatty acid synthesis so that fatty acids do not build up.
NOTE: Glucagon, epinephrine, cortisol (hormones released "in-between meal", starvation states and during exercise) will phosphorylate acetyl-CoA carboxylase so that fatty acid synthesis is inhibited and fatty acid oxidation (beta oxidation) occurs.

FATTY ACID METABOLISM (AKA: Beta Oxidation, Lipolysis) and KETONE BODIES SYNTHESIS

Long and medium chain fatty acids requires the Carnitine Shuttle (AKA: CAT-1) to be transported into the mitochondria to be made into ketones and acetyl-CoA (for the TCA cycle).
Remember: the KEY reason for beta-oxidation is to make **KETONES**.
Note: Remember that when calorie intake is decreased during dieting, **β oxidation is ↑** (aka: hepatic lipid oxidation)

Pathway
In Cytoplasm:
Fatty acid and Acetyl-CoA to Acyl-CoA via Fatty acid CoA synthetase
***Carnitine Shuttle** (disassembles and reassembles Acyl-CoA)
Acyl-CoA via Acyl-CoA dehydrogenase with Cofactor Vitamin B1 (aka: ****B-oxidation** (broken down) goes in to two directions:
1) Acetyl-CoA that goes into the TCA cycle
2) **Ketone bodies (AKA: Acetoacetate, Acetone, Beta hydroxybutyrate)**
Inhibitor: Malonyl-CoA

A deficiency in either carnitine or Acyl-CoA dehydrogenase will cause a ↓ in fatty acid oxidation and ketones.

***Carnitine (AKA: CAT-1) Deficiency, AR**
- Carnitine shuttle takes Acyl-CoA across plasma membrane into the mitochondria
- **Impaired fatty acid oxidation (AKA: error of fatty acid transport)**
- **No ketones made**
- High triglycerides
- Low plasma carnitine levels
- Increased urine carnitine levels
- SX: Chronic muscle weakness, myoglobin, cardiomyopathy, hypoglycemia, liver dysfunction

****Medium Chain acyl-CoA dehydrogenase (MCAD)**
- **Deficiency of Acyl-CoA Dehydrogenase with cofactor B-1**
- Mutation in the ACADM gene
- Inability to metabolize medium chain fatty acids
- No ketones made
- Build up of medium chain fatty acids in tissues, liver and brain

Ketone Bodies
- Ketone bodies used in brain, heart, kidney and skeletal muscles
- NO ketones can be used in RBC's.
- NO ketones can be used by the liver (hepatocytes) because the liver has **no thiophorase**
- No ketone bodies are made in prolonged fast because impaired Beta Oxidation = severe hypoglycemia
- Alcoholics: **excess NADH builds up acetyl-CoA** which shunts glucose and free fatty acids to make ketone bodies
- Fruity breath odor
- Ketone bodies produced during starvation/fasting and DKA
- **Ketone bodies (AKA: Acetoacetate, Acetone, Beta hydroxybutyrate)**

CHOLESTEROL

- Cholesterol is a **precursor** to: steroid hormones, bile acids, Vitamin D
- Precursor to: cortisol, aldosterone, progesterone, estrogen, testosterone
- Component of cell membrane to maintain structural integrity and **fluidity**
- Ingested cholesterol is esterified (poorly absorbed), esterified by LCAT (lecithin-cholesterol acyltransferase
- Cholesterol is recycled. Non-esterified cholesterol is excreted by the liver by vile into the digestive tract
- Assist in cell signaling by assisting in formation of lipid rafts in plasma membrane
- Myelin sheaths in neurons are rich in cholesterol to aid in nerve conduction
- Cholesterol converted to bile (bile salts) in the liver and stored in gallbladder to aid in absorption of fat molecules and fat-soluble vitamins

CHOLESTEROL SYNTHESIS

Pathway (See illustration above)
Acetyl-CoA to Acetoacetyl-CoA to HMG CoA to Mevalonate via ***HMG CoA reductase**
Mevalonate to Squalene to Lanosterol via Squalene epoxidase
Lanosterol to Cholesterol
Inhibitor: Cholesterol and cAMP

***HMG CoA reductase: MOA: Statins inhibit this enzyme.**

LIPID TRANSPORT and LIPOPROTEINS

- Dietary fat and cholesterol
- ***Apo lipoprotein B-48 = Chylomicron** (chyme) **assembly** and release. Shows in the plasma as "buffy coat" (AKA: turbid plasma). White layer on the top of plasma
- Three stages of the chylomicron:
  - Nascent Stage: (B-48) formed in the ER in small intestines (emulsified by bile and hydrolyzed by lipase), passes from intestinal lumen into enterocytes to be re-esterified into triglycerides to form nascent chylomicrons. Then released into lymphatic vessels and secreted into the bloodstream at the thoracic duct and subclavian vein.
  - Mature Chylomicron State: Circulate in the blood. HDL (High density lipoproteins) donate Apo lipoprotein C-II and Apo E to covert the nascent chylomicron to mature. CII is also the cofactor for LPL (lipoprotein lipase).
  - Chylomicron remnant: Mature chylomicrons distribute triglycerides it returns the CII back to HDL, but keeps the APO E and B-48. The APO E and B-48 allow the liver to recognize the remnant for endocytosis and breakdown.
- ***Apolipoprotein B-100 binds with the LDL receptor** to allow uptake of LDL, IDL by extrahepatic cells.
- **Apolipoprotein E mediates uptake** of chylomicrons, VLDL, IDL, HDL into the liver.
- **LPL (Lipoprotein lipase)** degrades triglycerides (TG) in chylomicrons and VLDL 's and requires cofactor **apolipoprotein C-II.**
- **LCAT (lecithin-cholesterol acyltransferase)** esterifies cholesterol activated by **apolipoprotein A-1.**
- HSL (Hormone Sensitive Lipase) Degrades triglycerides stored in adipose tissues.
- Hepatic triglyceride lipase: Degrades triglycerides remaining in LDL.
- Pancreatic lipase: Degrades triglycerides in small intestine (without lipase = mal-absorption).
- Chylomicron remnants (remaining parts of chylomicron after TG removed) go to liver and enter through Chylomicron remnant receptors.
- Chylomicron delivers triglycerides to peripheral tissues.
- Chylomicrons secreted by intestinal epithelial cells.
- Triglycerides are broken down into Free Fatty Acids and sent to adipose tissues and skeletal muscles.
- HDL mediates cholesterol delivery from tissues to liver ("good" cholesterol).
- LDL mediates cholesterol delivery from liver to tissues ("Bad" cholesterol).
- Increased Free Fatty Acids and triglycerides = insulin resistance in overweight people leading to Type II Diabetes.
- Note: Increased cholesterol production can lead to the development of cholesterol **gallstones.** Anytime there are cholesterol gallstones, there is **increased cholesterol production in the liver**.

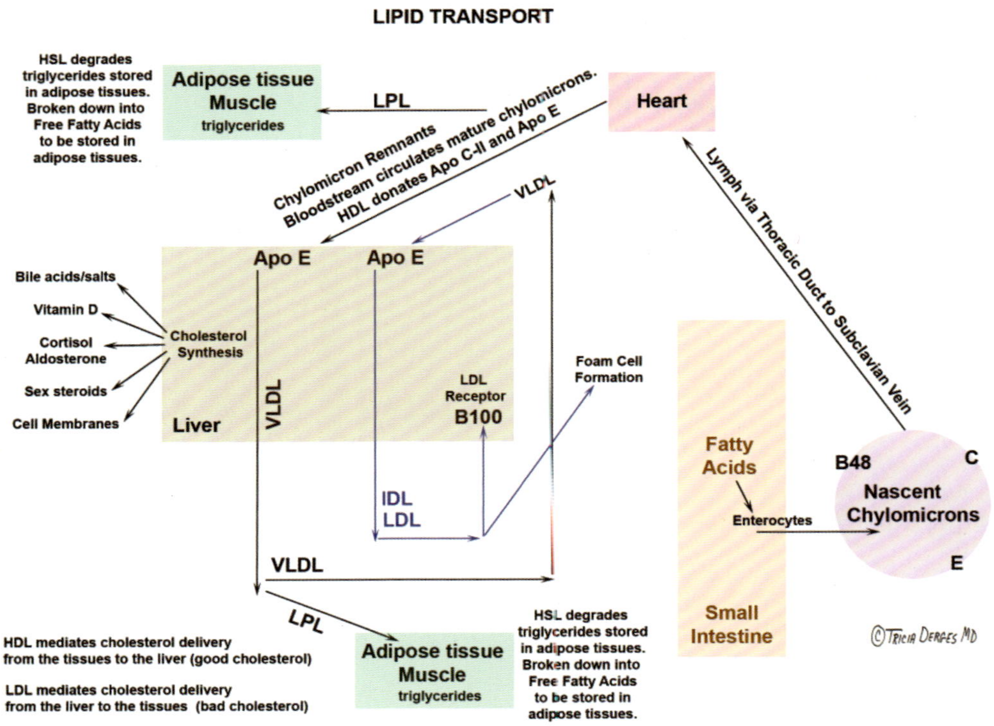

CHOLESTEROL, TRIGLYCERIDE, APOLIPOPROTEIN PATHOLOGIES

***Abetalipoproteinemia**

- Deficiency of **B-48 and B-100** apolipoproteins
- Inability to absorb chylomicrons
- See "buffy coat" on top of plasma
- **Acanthocytosis (AKA: Spur cells)** (be sure to recognize these on a slide)
- SX: Failure to thrive, night blindness, ataxia, abdominal pain

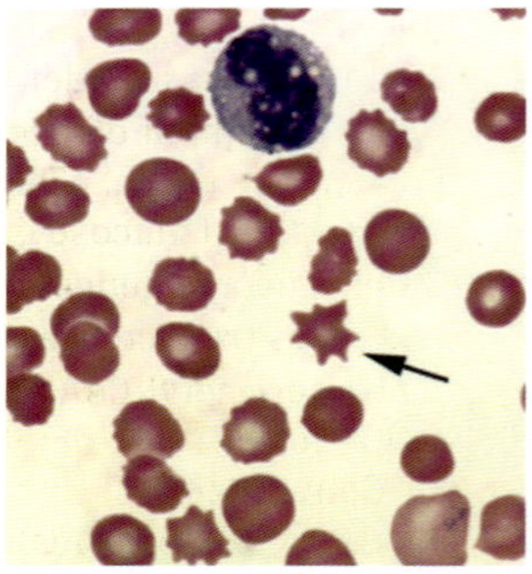

Acanthocytes "Spur Cells"

Marasmus

- **Malnutrition, lack of calories**
- Develops in months to years
- **Severe Muscle wasting**
- Loss of fat, loss of peripheral protein
- SX: Emaciated appearance, ≤80% of normal weight
- Labs: ↓ muscle mass = ↓ creatinine
- (tip: **M** = **M**uscle)

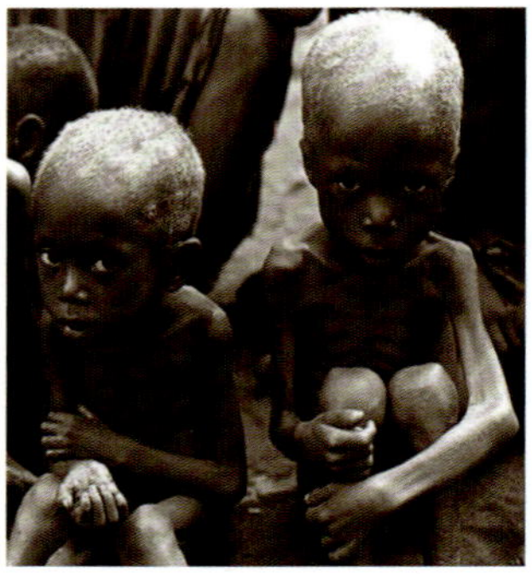

Kwashiorkor

- **Malnutrition of protein (despite overall caloric intake) or severely increased catabolic rate due to stress from a critical illness or major surgery**
- Develops in weeks
- Loss of visceral protein with increased visceral fat
- Decreased Apo lipoprotein synthesis causing fatty change
- **No LDL synthesis (Apo B100)**
- **Apo lipoprotein E**
- SX: **Swollen belly** = extreme edema (pot belly look), fatty liver, anemia, severe hypoalbuminemia, scaly skin, hypopigmented hair, poor wound healing, impaired immune functions, increased risk: pneumonia, sepsis.
- Labs: Low serum albumin (<2.8 mg/dL)
- (**tip**: "sKwash" the protein)

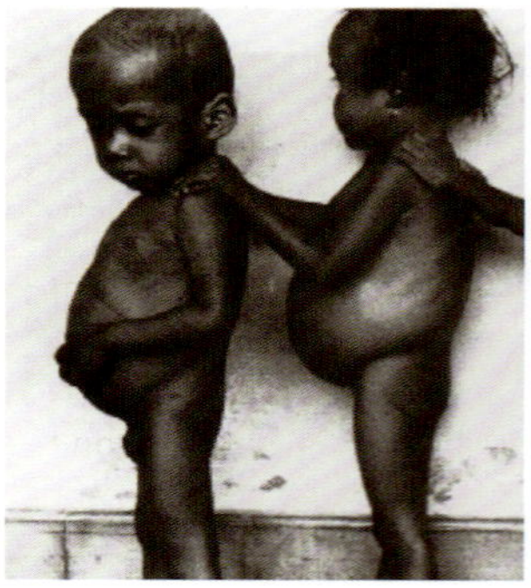

Type I Hyperchylomicronemia, AR

- **LPL (Lipoprotein lipase) deficiency** or Lipoprotein C-II deficiency
- Chylomicrons, Triglycerides
- SX: pancreatitis, xanthomas

Type IIa Familiar Hypercholesterolemia, AD

- Defective or **absent LDL Receptors**
- Accelerates atherosclerosis
- SX: **xanthomas** on Achilles tendon, cornea arcus (light ring around the edge of cornea in eyes) early age of MI

Type IV Hyper-Triglyceridemia, AD

- Hepatic overproduction of VLDL and triglycerides
- Increased triglycerides
- SX: **pancreatitis**

ETHANOL (Methanol, Ethylene Glycol)

Pathway

Ethanol to Acetaldehyde via **Alcohol dehydrogenase** (changes NAD to NADH)
Acetaldehyde to Acetate by **Acetaldehyde dehydrogenase** (changes NAD to NADH). This is what contributes to the disulfiram reaction (Disulfiram, Antabuse: **Inhibits Acetaldehyde dehydrogenase** so that "hangover" effects occur).

Ethanol metabolism: Increased NADH to NAD ratio. (Too much NADH) Causes:

- Most common deficiency: **Vitamin B-1 (Thiamine).**
  Without Vitamin B-1, the Pyruvate dehydrogenase complex can't be formed so Pyruvate is not able to proceed into the TCA cycle or initiate gluconeogenesis. It is shunted via **Pyruvate decarboxylase** to **Acetaldehyde**.
- Alcoholics are also deficient on **folate.** Without folate there is ↓ purine and pyrimidine synthesis = ↓ Thymidine synthesis.
- In the treatment of alcoholics: B-1 (Thiamine) must be given BEFORE any glucose is given. If glucose is given first before thiamine, it can cause death. (Thiamine is one of the requirements in the dehydrogenase complex that allows entry into the Krebs cycle to make ATP. If glucose is given first, it will not be able to enter the Krebs cycle).
- Stops gluconeogenesis = hypoglycemia
- Increases triglycerides = hepatosteatosis
- Increases acetyl-CoA = ketogenesis
- Depletion of NAD inhibits:
  1) Conversion of pyruvate to lactate
  2) Oxaloacetate to malate = no gluconeogenesis

Methanol - Ethanol Metabolism

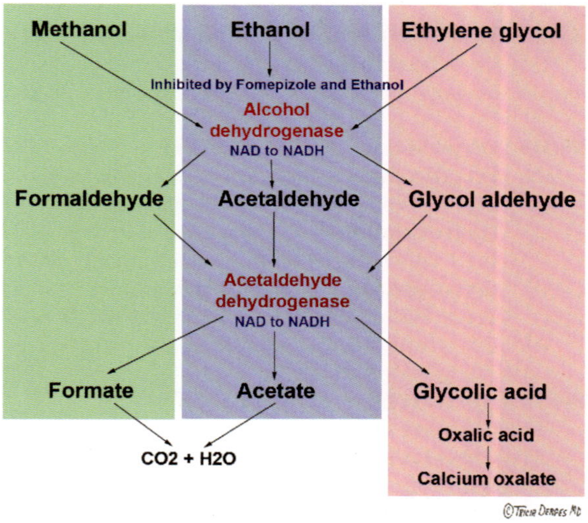

Ethanol Overdose

- Fomepizole, **Ethanol**
  MOA: inhibits **Alcohol dehydrogenase** (stops NAD conversion to NADH)
  Also treatment for: Methanol and Ethylene glycol poisoning
- **Disulfiram**
  MOA: inhibits **Acetaldehyde dehydrogenase so that Acetaldehyde builds up** causing hangover symptoms
  Drugs causing Disulfiram reaction if alcohol is used while on the drugs:
  Metronidazole, Cephalosporins, Griseofulvin

COLLAGEN

- Most abundant protein in the body
- Tensile strength
- Main component in: cartilage, tendons, ligaments, skin, blood vessels, bones, gut, intervertebral discs, corneas, dentin in teeth, fascia,
- **Fibroblast cells: most common "Collagen Factory" in the body**
- Responsibility of skin strength and elasticity
- Collagen is attached to the cell by **fibronectin and Integrin**
- Fibroblast show up on the 7th day of the healing process in the body to manufacture collagen

Aging Process

- Wrinkles due to **decrease in collagen and fibril and elastin production**
- TX: **Tretinoin** (retinoid, Vitamin A, retinol)
  SE: **Severe teratogen**

Types of Collagen

- Type I (strongest)
  Skin, **scar tissue**, cornea, bone, tendon, artery walls, fascia, **teeth** (late wound healing), Osteogenesis imperfecta
- Type II
  Hyaline cartilage, vitreous humor, nucleus pulposus (center of intervertebral disc)
- Type III
  Granulation tissue, reticular fiber, lymphatic system, **keloid**, embryonic tissue, uterus
- Type IV
  Basement membrane (basil lamina), eye lens, filtration system in capillaries and glomeruli
- Type V
  Elders-Danlos

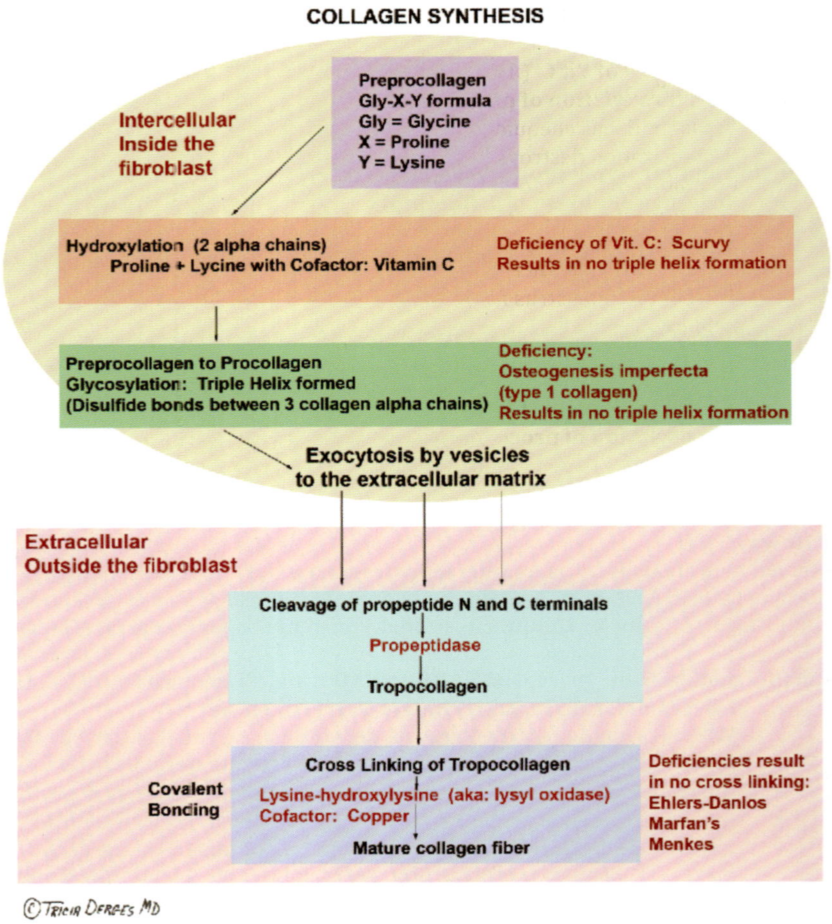

COLLAGEN SYNTHESIS (Think of fibroblast as mobile collagen factories)

NOTE: Remember: Collagen is the most common PROTEIN in the body, so beware if the vignette ask where this process is taking place and they do not show fibroblast in the choices: then look for: **rough endoplasmic reticulum**.

INSIDE (Intracellular) the FIBROBLAST in the **RER** (Rough Endoplasmic Reticulum)

1) Preprocollagen: alpha collagen chains in Gly-X-Y formula **(Gly = Glycine, X = Proline, Y = Lysine).** Glycine is one third of the collagen formula.
2) **Hydroxylation** of (2 alpha chains) Proline and Lysine with **cofactor *Vitamin C** and **iron**. Without Vit C, there is no formation of the Triple Helix (AKA: helical structure). **Scurvy**
3) **Glycosylation** of preprocollagen into procollagen to form a ****TRIPLE HELIX via collagen peptides (proteins).** Triple Helix: **disulfide bonds** between three collagen alpha chains. **Osteogenesis imperfecta (Type I collagen)**.
4) Exocytosis via vesicles in the Golgi. Procollagen triple helix is sent extracellular.

OUTSIDE (extracellular) FIBROBLAST

1) **Cleavage** of the Propeptide **N and C terminals** into **tropocollagen** via **Propeptidase**
2) **Cross Linking:** Tropocollagen to make collagen fibrils by covalent bonding of **lysine-hydroxylysine**. (AKA: **lysyl oxidase with cofactor of Copper).**
3) **Ehlers-Danlos, Marfan's, Menkes.** Elastin is made extracellularly. **Defects can lead to: poor arteries (subarachnoid hemorrhage, aortic dissection, aortic aneurysm, dilated aorta), mitral valve prolapse, spontaneous pneumothorax, ribcage deformity, elasticity in tissues (stretchy skin), scoliosis, flexible joints, flat feet, slender/tall limbs, subluxation of the lens (lens dislocation), weak tissue of dural sac encasing the spinal cord.**

NOTE: Cathepsin K is the most potent collagenase (protease). It is secreted by osteoclasts (extracellularly) so that they can break down collagen (the main component of the non-mineral protein matrix of the bone) in bone resorption. This plays a major role in osteoporosis. (All other Cathepsins are found in the **lysosome and are activated by the low pH**).

Collagen Pathologies

*Scurvy

- **Deficiency of Vit C (AKA: ascorbic acid)**, leading to defective collagen production
- **No hydroxylation of proline and lysine** occurs, so **no triple helix occurs**
- Breast milk has adequate Vit C
- Pasteurization destroys Vit C so all commercial baby formulas add Vit C
- Common among sailors: lack fruits and vegetables on long sea voyages
- Common among the **elderly on the "tea and toast" diet**
- SX: **bleeding gums** and mucous membranes, lethargy, **spots on skin** (esp. thighs/legs), **loss of teeth**, jaundice, neuropathy
- TX: **Diet** rich in citrus fruits (oranges, lemons), tomatoes, strawberries, kiwi, carrots, broccoli, potatoes, spinach, cabbage, bell peppers

** Osteogenesis imperfecta (AKA: Brittle Bone Disease), AD

- **Glycosylation of procollagen into triple helix so problem forming bone matrix**
- Deficiency of **Type I collagen**
- Often mutations of COL1A1 and COL1A2 genes
- SX: bones fracture easy, blue sclera (blue-grey color due to translucency of the connective tissue over choroidal veins), hearing loss, dental problems (lack of dentin)
- Often **confused with child abuse** (both children will have x-rays showing previously healed fractures and fractures in different stages of healing).
  Child abuse fractures: show as spiral fractures

***Ehlers-Danlos

- Problem with the structure, production or **processing of collagen (Type V Collagen)**
- **No cross linking**
- SX: **Hyper-flexible joints**, unstable joints prone to sprain and dislocation, **hyper elasticity of skin**, easy bruising, skin tears easily, **mitral valve prolapse (mid-systolic click), arterial aneurysms and/or dissections, berry aneurysms (AKA: sub arachnoid hemorrhage (SAH)**
  (**tip:** when **Elders** return from a mission they always go to **COLL**age)

***Marfan's

- **Misfolding of fibrillin-1 (glycoprotein that forms sheath around elastic fibers)**
- Mutated fibrillin binds poorly to TGF-B (Transforming growth factor, beta) = **excess TGF-B** in heart valves, lungs, aorta, eyes
- Mutation on **FBN1 gene on chromosome 15** (encodes for fibrillin-1), extracellular
- **Cross linking gives elastin its elastic properties**
- Common for **pneumothorax** (blebs bursting). (tip: be aware of the patient coming into your ED that is young, tall and short of breath)
- SX: Unusually **tall, long limbs, long thin fingers and toes (AKA: Arachnodactyly** (spiderlike), **mitral valve prolapse, arterial aneurysms and/or dissections, berry aneurysms (AKA: SAH) due to decrease of Collagen Type III, subluxation of the eye lens** (dislocation so they can't look up, identified by slit-lamp).
  (**tip:** MarFans. **F** = **Fibrillin**, but be sure and think of elastin with this.
  tip: Marfans: can't look UP to see Mars)
- Don't forget: Marfan **"like"** symptoms can appear in: **Homocystinuria, MEN 2B**

***Menkes Disease (AKA: Kinky Hair Syndrome), XL

- **Impaired copper absorption and transport**, due to decrease in copper
- **Decreased lysyl oxidase** because **copper is a cofactor in cross linking**
- Mutation in the ATP7A Copper Efflux Protein
- Decrease in copper in the system
- SX: Hair is brittle and "kinky", hypotonia, growth retardation, deterioration of the nervous system, seizures, blue sclera, subnormal body temperature
- DX: homovanillic acid/vanillylmandelic acid ratios

Alport Syndrome, XL

- Problems with their basement membrane (Type IV Collagen) in their ears (deaf), kidney glomerular basement membrane (urinary problems) and eyes (vision problems)

ELASTIN (AKA: Tropoelastin)

- Made by linking tropoelastin proteins **catalyzed by lysyl oxidase**
- Allows tissues to resume their shape after stretching or contracting (AKA: Recoil)
- Recoil (Example: recoil in the lungs is what pulls the lungs back after breathing out)
- Associated with pathologies: *Marfan's, ****Alpha 1-Antitrypsin deficiency (A1AT)**, *Menkes Disease

Elastin Pathologies

*Marfan's and Menkes **Disease:** See above

****Alpha 1 – Antitrypsin Deficiency (A1AT)**

- Protease inhibitor
- Protects tissues from enzymes of **neutrophil elastase** (neutrophil elastase breaks down elastin in the lungs)
- Misfolded protein
- **Made in periportal hepatocytes in the liver**
- Liver biopsy: **PAS +** globules in periportal hepatocytes
- Patient may indicate a history of neonatal jaundice
- Results in **panacinar emphysema** and COP

HEME PATHWAY

Pathway

Glycine and succinyl-CoA to d-aminolevulinic acid (d-ALA)
via ***d-aminolevulinic acid synthase**
(rate limiting step) with cofactor B6
d-ALA to Porphobilinogen via ****ALA dehydratase**
Porphobilinogen to Hydroxymethylbilane via
*****Porphobilinogen deaminase**
Hydroxymethylbilane to Uroporphyrinogen
Uroporphyrinogen to Coproporphyrinogen III via
******Uroporphyrinogen decarboxylase**
Coproporphyrinogen III to Protoporphyrin to Heme via
****Ferrochelatase** with cofactor Fe

Decrease in heme = increase in ALA synthase
Increase in heme = decrease in ALA synthase

(tip: To help remember the starting substances and general order of the enzymes: "Guys Suc" ALA and Poor Bill is sad, but "URO" a "Fella")

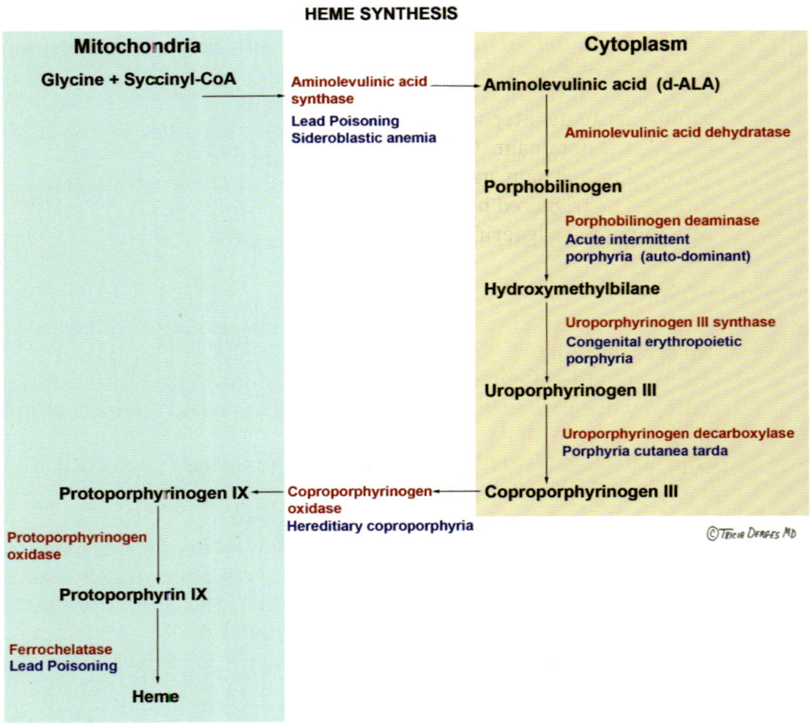

Heme Pathway Pathologies

****Lead Poisoning**

- Deficiency or absence of **ALA dehydratase and accumulation of d-ALA**; **OR**
- Deficiency of absence of **Ferrochelatase and accumulation of Protoporphyrin**
- Stops heme synthesis
- Higher rates with low socio-economic status
- Lead Exposure Risk: House paint in houses pre 1978, painted children's **toys from China**, plumbers, miners, auto mechanics (batteries), **battery** factory workers, paper hangers, hunters (lead bullets), **ammunitio**n factory workers, imported toys, crayons, or cosmetics
- PICA: eating unusual things (ie: ice, paper, dirt)
- Pregnancy: miscarriages and still births
- SX: **Spoon nails**, abdominal pain, fatigue, irritability, **basophilic stippling in RBC**, difficulty concentrating, HTN, kidney failure, headache, cognitive and behavior problems, constipation, hemolytic anemia
- DX and TX: **Dimercaprol, penicillamine, succimer, EDTA**
  X-Ray shows dense "lighter" lines in bones at the metaphyseal lines
  Blood Lead levels < 45 = remove child from house and retest in one month
  Blood Lead levels > 45 = Chelation Therapy
  Blood Lead levels 45 – 69 = DMSA
  Blood Lead levels >70 = EDTA

*****Acute intermittent porphyria (Autosomal Dominant)**

- Deficiency or absence of **Porphobilinogen deaminase** and accumulation of Porphobilinogen
- Autosomal dominant
- See Coporphobilinogen in the urine
- Precipitated by stress, drugs, alcohol, starvation
- SX: **Severe abdominal pain**, **urine turns dark**, **psychological** problems, seizures, anxiety and paranoia
- TX: Glucose and heme (IV hematin)

Congenital erythropoietic porphyria (CEP) (AKA: Gunther disease)

- Deficiency or absence of **Uroporphyrinogen III synthase** and accumulation of Coproporphyrinogen III
- Porphyrins accumulate in the teeth and bones. Increased porphyrin levels in the bone marrow, plasma, RBC's and urine.
- Causes skin to thicken and produce vesicles that can rupture and become infected
- Porphyrins accumulate in the bone and teeth causing erythrodontia (red discoloration of teeth)
- Limit or eliminate sun exposure. Sunscreens that have zinc oxide and titanium dioxide.

Hereditary coproporphyria (HCP)

- Deficiency or absence of **Coproporphyrinogen oxidase and accumulation of ALA and Porphobilinogen**
- Similar to Acute intermittent porphyria.
- Autosomal dominant. Coded by the CPOX gene.
- SX: Abdominal pain, nausea, vomiting, hypertension, seizures and cutaneous lesions (bullous lesions) upon exposure to sunlight.
- HCP can be triggered by drugs, alcohol, hormone changes, stress and diet changes.
- TX: Eliminate triggering factors. IV hemin (hematin).

******Porphyria cutanea tarda (Autosomal Dominant)**

- Deficiency or absence of **Uroporphyrinogen decarboxylase and accumulation of Uroporphyrin**
- Blistering reaction to sun exposure due to high porphyrin accumulation in the body.
- See Uroporphyrin in urine = tea color urine
- Labs: Increased 24-hour urinary uroporphyrins.
- Associated with Hepatitis C, alcoholism, liver disease (hepatitis, hemochromatosis), diabetes.
- Precipitated by estrogen and OCP 's
- **Photosensitive** (only come out at night)
- SX: **Blistering on sun-exposed skin** (painless blisters), excessive hair growth on the face (Werewolf syndrome, hypertrichosis).
- TX: No estrogen or alcohol, avoid the sun or use high SPF sunscreen, phlebotomy (or **Deferoxamine**) if due to hemochromatosis

Vitamins, Minerals, Herbs

Vitamins

Substance	Function	Deficiency Symptoms	Excessive Intake Symptoms: Overdose	Notes
Vitamin A (AKA: Beta-Carotene, Retinol, Retinoic Acid, Isotretinoin)	Antioxidant, Acne, **Measles, AML, subtype M3**, Improve skin, Differentiation of epithelial cells. **Cofactor**: in CSF production, with Mg for parathyroid production, and for Rhodopsin (rod photoreceptors).	Night blindness (AKA: nyctalopia) ↓ ability to drive at night or ↓ ability to see well in low light), dry skin, cheilitis (dry lips), **Hypoparathyroidism** (↓ Ca ↑ Phos)	Joint pain (arthralgia's), yellowing of skin, **Pseudotumor cerebri, hyperparathyroidism**, Alopecia, osteoporosis, Hepatic abnormalities. **Dry, scaly skin**. Severe teratogen.	Sources: Preformed A: meat, poultry, fish, dairy. Provitamin A: Fruits, vegetable, plant-based products. **Severe teratogen.** Vitamin A is stored in **hepatic Stellite cells.** Retinol is produced in the retina by Vitamin A. Orlistat (weight loss drug) can ↓ absorption of vitamin A.
Vitamin B1 Thiamine TPP (Thiamine pyrophosphate)	Cofactor for **Dehydrogenase enzyme Complex reactions**: Pyruvate dehydrogenase, α-ketoglutarate dehydrogenase, **Transketolase (HMP Shunt/PPP Pathway)**, Branched chain ketoacid dehydrogenase Growth, development, function of cells.	Impaired ATP production. Wernicke-Korsakoff syndrome. Wet beriberi: High output cardiac failure (dilated cardiomyopathy). Dry beriberi: diabetic gangrene, polyneuritis	Water soluble: no toxicity	Sources: Whole grains, meat, fish, pork, legumes, beans, seeds, nuts
Vitamin B2 Riboflavin	**FAD for ETC Complex II.** FAD from the TCA cycle: **Succinate to Fumarate via Succinate dehydrogenase.** FAD gives 2 ATP. Growth, development, cell function.	Angular cheilosis (dry lips: fissures at the corners of the mouth), stomatitis, glossitis (smooth, red tongue due to loss of lingual papillae), (inflammation of the mouth and lips), corneal vascularization, cataracts, reproductive and nervous system problems.	Water soluble: no toxicity	Sources: Eggs, organ meats (kidneys, livers), lean meats, green vegetables, low fat milk.

Vitamin B3 Niacin	**NAD for ETC Complex I.** Derived from Tryptophan (requires B2 and B6). Raises HDL levels. Cofactor: NAD/NADH	**Pellagra and Hartnup** disease due to ↓ **tryptophan** absorption. **Carcinoid** syndrome (↑ **tryptophan** absorption: for DX see ↑ **5-HIAA in urinalysis**), Glossitis. SX: **"4 D's"**: Dermatitis (rash), diarrhea, dementia (memory issues), death. Diets high in corn can lead to Pellagra/Hartnup Diseases.	**Flushing,** hyperglycemia, hyperuricemia. (Flushing due to prostaglandins)	Niacin vasodilates so can ↑ effects of HTN drugs so **HTN medication doses must be ↓.** Niacin causes insulin resistance so **insulin medication doses must be ↑.**
Vitamin B5 Pantothenate Acid	Acetylation. Component of coenzyme A (CoA).	Dermatitis, alopecia, adrenal insufficiency. "Burning feet" syndrome (severe burning/aching of the feet and vasomotor problems that lead to excessive sweating. Associated with lack of B5, hypothyroidism, diabetes, rheumatoid arthritis, renal failure).	Water soluble, no toxicity	Acetyl CoA is a cofactor for: Acyl transfers and fatty acid synthase. (EX: OAA to Citrate in the TCA cycle)
Vitamin B6 **Pyridoxine**	Cofactor for **transamination (ALT, AST), decarboxylation** and glycogen phosphorylase. Synthesis of neurotransmitters (Dopamine, Serotonin, Norepinephrine, Epinephrine, GABA), heme, cystathionine, niacin, histamine.	**Peripheral neuropathy,** sideroblastic anemia (defective heme synthesis and iron excess), convulsions.	Water soluble, no toxicity	**Sources: Poultry, fish, starchy vegetables (potatoes), fruit (other than citrus)** **Must supplement B6 with INH.** **Do NOT give B6 with Parkinson's drugs.**
Vitamin B7 **Biotin**	Cofactor for **Carboxylation.** (Pyruvate carboxylase in Pyruvate to Oxaloacetate, Acetyl-CoA carboxylase in Acetyl-CoA to Malonyl-CoA, Propionyl-CoA carboxylase in Propionyl-CoA to Methylmalonyl-CoA)	Causes by **excessive ingestion of raw egg whites** and antibiotics. Alopecia, dermatitis, enteritis.	Water soluble, no toxicity	**Note:** Excessive ingestion of raw egg whites, smoking seizure medications and dialysis may cause a **deficiency** in biotin. SX of deficiency: lethargy, hallucinations, hair/nail problems, loss of appetite.
Vitamin B9 **Folic Acid/Folate**	Converted to **THF** (Tetrahydrofolate). Cofactor: Nucleotide synthesis. Synthesis of nitrogenous bases in **DNA, RNA.**	**Macrocytic, megaloblastic anemia (MCV >100), hypersegmented PMNs, glossitis.** **NO neurologic symptoms (B12 has neuro symptoms)**	Water soluble, no toxicity	Sources: Green leafy vegetables, fruits, juices, nuts, beans, and grains. **Absorbed in jejunum.** **Goat's milk has no folic acid. Must supplement.** **In the Homocysteine pathway**: Folate is needed to go to cysteine. **Without folate, cysteine becomes essential.** If there is a deficiency of folate then there will only be ↑ levels of homocysteine. (verses B12, see below)

Vitamin B12 Cobalamin	Cofactor for homocysteine methyltransferase and methylmalonyl-CoA mutase.	**Macrocytic, megaloblastic anemia (>100), hypersegmented PMN's, paresthesias (neuro symptoms), degeneration of dorsal columns,** lateral corticospinal tracts, spinocerebellar tracts) Stored many years in the liver. Deficiency seen in: vegans, malabsorption, Diphyllobothrium latum, lack of intrinsic factor (associated with Pernicious anemia, gastric bypass surgery or Anti-intrinsic factor antibodies), colectomy of terminal ileum (Crohn's DZ). **NOTE**: If an a patient presents with possible **dementia** or depression. you **MUST check B12 and TSH levels first.** Deficiencies in either of these can mimic dementia.	Water soluble, no toxicity	**Source: Animal products.** Stores last in the liver 5 – 7 years. **Depleted by 5 years if person is on a vegan diet.** Must supplement B12 for these individuals. Vitamin B-12 deficiency **stops erythroid lines** in the bone marrow = ↓ erythropoiesis = anemia and ↑ indirect bilirubin **Absorbed in the ileum with intrinsic factor. Without both: Vitamin B12 and Intrinsic factor → pernicious anemia.** **In the Homocysteine pathway**: B12 is needed to go to Methylmalonic. If there is a deficiency of B12 then there will be an increase in both homocysteine and Methylmalonic levels. (verses Folate, see above) **NOTE:** Deficiency in Vitamin E can produce the same symptoms as B12 deficiency. If the problem is due to **B12 there will be megaloblastic anemia with hypersegmented PMNs and no ↑ methylmalonic acid.** Can be confused with copper deficiency. Copper deficiency is evaluated with serum copper or ceruloplasmin. B12 is evaluated with methylmalonic acid.
Vitamin C Ascorbic Acid	Cofactor for **hydroxylation** of proline and lysine in **collagen** synthesis.. Cofactor for **Dopamine β-hydroxylase**, the enzyme that converts dopamine to norepinephrine. Antioxidant to the gut. Helps in absorption of iron (reduces it to the Fe^{2} state). Used with Met Blue in treating methemoglobinemia to reduce Fe^{3} to Fe^{2}.	**Scurvy.** **Swollen gums, poor wound healing,** "corkscrew" hair, bruising, hemarthrosis, anemia, subperiosteal hemorrhages.	↑ iron absorption = iron toxicity, diarrhea, nausea, stomach cramps. Patients with hemochromatosis could worsen due to ↑ absorption of iron. Water soluble, no toxicity	Sources: Fruits and vegetables.

Vitamin D	Bone mineralization. Reabsorption of calcium and phosphate in the gut.	**Rickets in children. (Lateral bowing of the legs/femurs)** **Osteomalacia in adults.** (bone pain, muscle weakness) Factors that affect Vitamin D intake: Darker skin tones, low sun exposure, prematurity. NOTE: **Breastfed infants must be supplemented with Vitamin D.**	**Hypercalcemia,** hypercalciuria, ↓ appetite. (Polyuria and polydipsia) The more Vitamin D = more calcium is reabsorbed in the gut. NOTE: **Granulomatous diseases** have increased calcium levels. Granulomas increase activation of Vitamin D.	D3 (Cholecalciferol) D2 (Ergocalciferol) D3 and D2 ingested from diet and supplements. (Diet sources: fatty fish, beef liver, cheese, egg yolks) Skin: major source (sun) . Liver: D3 converted to 25-OH (Calcidiol). Kidney: **Calcidiol** converted to 1-25 OH (**Calcitriol**, active form). Gut: Calcitriol reabsorbs calcium and phosphate.
Vitamin E Tocopherol Tocotrienol	Antioxidant for the blood (RBC's). ↑ affects of warfarin.	Posterior, **dorsal column** demyelination, spinocerebellar tract demyelination, retinopathy, muscle weakness, acanthocytes (spur cells), instability (unstable, ataxic gait), ↓ deep tendon reflexes, ↓ coordination, loss of proprioception, fatty stools, hemolytic anemia.		Source: Vegetable oils, nuts, green vegetables. **CAUTION: Deficiency in Vitamin E can produce the same symptoms as B12 deficiency.** If the problem is **due to B12** there will be megaloblastic anemia with hypersegmented PMNs and no ↑ methylmalonic acid. **Vitamin E deficiency is not associated with megaloblastic anemia, hypersegmented PMN's or methylmalonic acid/homocystine.**
Vitamin K	Cofactor for clotting factors II, VII, IX, X, Proteins C, S. **Gamma (γ) carboxylation of glutamic acid which inhibits clotting factors II, VII, IX, X, proteins C, S**	**Bleeding due to no presence of clotting factors.** **Neonatal hemorrhage** (watch for the question that presents a baby born at home. It did not receive the Vitamin K shot so it hemorrhages because the baby has no gut flora yet so can't synthesis Vitamin K on its own)		Source: Green leafy vegetables (spinach, kale, broccoli, lettuce), blueberries, figs, meat, cheese, eggs, soybeans, vegetable oils. Note: made by gut flora. Note: Vitamin K is an **antagonist of warfarin.** Used when the warfarin's PT/INR is above therapeutic level. Newborns are given injection of Vitamin K at birth because their gut is sterile and have not produced vitamin K yet.

Minerals, Nutrients, Elements

Substance	Function	Deficiency Symptoms	Excessive Intake Symptoms	Notes
Calcium	Bones, teeth, action potentials	↑ risk osteoporosis, osteopenia, arrhythmias, convulsions, numbness, tingling	Kidney stones, constipation	Sources: dairy, dark vegetables (broccoli, kale), fish, grains
Copper	Neurological function, antioxidant, neurotransmitter synthesis, proper cellular function. **Cofactor with Lysyl Oxidase** in the synthesis of elastin and collagen (cross-linking).	Gait changes, peripheral neuropathies, paresthesias, altered vibration perception, anemia, ↓ WBC.	The body regulates copper storage through biliary excretion, so toxicity is rare unless ingestion of excessive copper or a genetic predisposition: Wilson's Disease. Excess copper deposits in the liver, causing cirrhosis and deposits in the basal ganglia in the brain causing degeneration and neurological symptoms. SX: Parkinsonian symptoms: dystonia, tremor, Kayser-Fleischer rings in the eyes.	Can be confused with B12 deficiency. Copper deficiency is evaluated with serum copper or ceruloplasmin. B12 is evaluated with methylmalonic acid. Copper deficiency associated with: ALS, Alzheimer's and Parkinson's Diseases.
Iodine	Thyroid hormone synthesis	Harm to the fetus (stunted growth, mental retardation), Goiter. Depression.	Goiter, thyroid inflammation, GI symptoms	Sources: Iodized Salt, seafood, diary products, fruits, vegetables
Iron Fe	Hemoglobin, Myoglobin, ETC	Iron Deficiency anemia Microcytic anemia (<80)	GI symptoms, constipation, abdominal pain, fainting. Large doses: coma, death.	Sources: Lean meat, seafood, poultry, beans, peas, nuts, dried fruits.
Magnesium Mg	Muscle and nerve function, blood sugar levels, blood pressure, making proteins, DNA. PTH with Vitamin A, Kinase	Fatigue, ↓ appetite, nausea, vomiting, weakness, tingling, muscle cramps, seizures, arrhythmias.	Diarrhea, nausea, abdominal cramping. High levels: arrhythmias, cardiac arrest	Source: Legumes, nuts, seeds, whole grains, green leafy vegetables, dairy.
Manganese Mn	Glycolysis			
Mendelevium Md	Purine breakdown			
Selenium Se	Heart, thyroid gland function, reproduction, DNA production, protection from free radicals.	Heart disease, male infertility, arthritis	(Brazil nuts contain high selenium): garlic breath, diarrhea, skin rashes, discolored teeth, brittle hair and nails, metallic taste, loss of hair. High doses: heart failure, tremors, kidney failure.	Sources: Seafood, meat, poultry, eggs, dairy, breads, grains
Tin Sn	Hair			
Zinc Zn	Taste buds, sperm, hair, Zinc fingers (transcription factor), Immune system, proteins, DNA, **Metalloproteinase** (Excess action by metalloproteinase is what causes the invasion by cancer leading to metastasis. Metalloproteinase requires zinc (**tip**: to invade (dig) you need a metal shovel made of zinc).	↓ adult body hair, Dysgeusia (↓ taste), ↓ sperm (anosmia), Hypogonadism, delayed wound healing.		Sources: Oysters (best source), red meat, poultry, seafood, beans, nuts, dairy.

Herbal Supplements

Herb	Function	Side Effects
Aloe	Relieve constipation (internally taken), relieve irritated skin and burns (externally)	Internally: can cause arrhythmias when taken for long periods
Black Cohosh	Relieves menopausal symptoms.	Causes lower blood pressure at high doses
Ephedra (Ma-Huang)	Obesity	↑ heart rate and blood pressure. Fatal.
Garlic	Lower cholesterol, prevent colds and certain infections	↑ risk of **excess bleeding** when taken with blood thinning drugs
Ginger	Alleviate nausea/motion sickness, lower cholesterol, decrease platelet aggregation	Interferes with blood clotting and ↑ risk of excess bleeding when taken with **blood thinning** drugs. High doses: arrhythmias and blood pressure changes.
Ginkgo	Improves memory, mental function	↑ risk of **excess bleeding** when taken with blood thinning drugs
Ginseng	Improves mental and physical capacity, increase sexual performance, boost immunity	Interferes with blood clotting and ↑ risk of excess bleeding when taken with **blood thinning** drugs
Hawthorn	Alleviate congestive heart failure and HTN	↑ risk of excess bleeding when taken with blood thinning drugs
Kava	Reduces anxiety.	Liver damage, death, nerve damage, skin changes.
Licorice Root	Cough's, stomach ulcers, cirrhosis	**Increases blood pressure** (renin effects) and arrhythmias.
Real licorice		Inhibits 11 β-hydroxysteroid
St. John's Wart	Depression	P-450 Inducer. Decreases the effectiveness of other drugs.
Supplements that should be avoided due to heart attack, arrhythmias, stroke, kidney damage, liver damage: Aconite, Bitter Orange, Chaparral, Colloidal Silver, Coltsfoot, Comfrey, Country Mallow, Germanium, Greater Celandine, Kava, Lobelia, Yohimbe. (**tip**: Note that most all of the herbs beginning with "G" all affect the blood = thinning it)		

Action Potentials, Receptors and Messengers

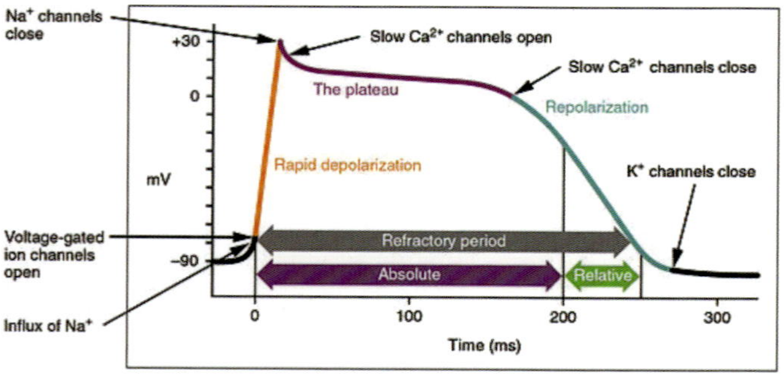

(a)

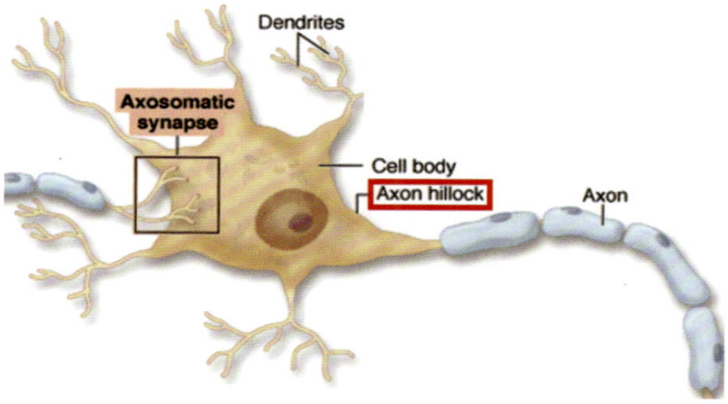

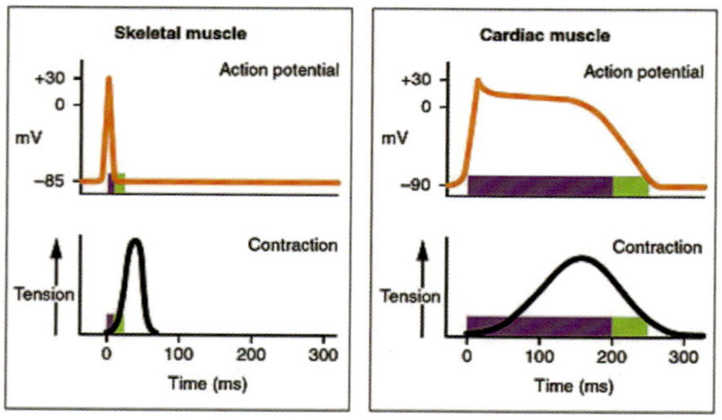

(b)

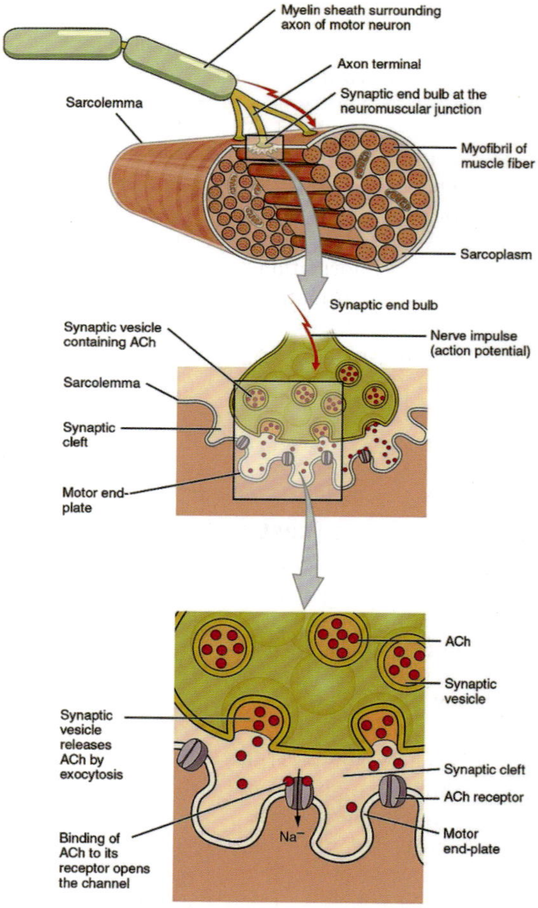

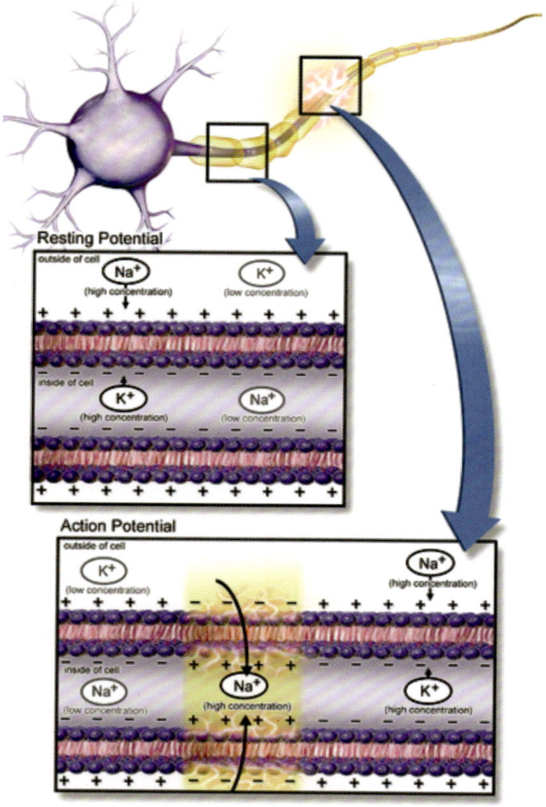

AUTONOMIC NERVOUS SYSTEM

Spinal Nerves

- Mixed nerve carrying motor, sensory and autonomic signals between the spinal cord and body
- 31 pairs of spinal nerves on each side of vertebral column
- Regions of Spine: Cervical, thoracic, lumbar, sacral, coccygeal
- Cervical Nerves: 8 pairs; thoracic nerves: 12 pairs; lumbar nerves: 5 pairs; sacral nerves: 5 pairs; coccygeal: 1 pair
- Each nerve: posterior and anterior root
- Posterior root: carries afferent sensory info to brain
  Anterior root: carries efferent motor info from brain
- Spinal nerve leaves spinal column through intervertebral foramen (between vertebra)*
- *Exception: C1 (first spinal nerve) exits between occipital bone and atlas (first vertebra)
- Cervical vertebra are numbered by the vertebra below, except spinal nerve C8 (exits below C7 and above T1). All other spinal nerves are numbered by the vertebra above.
- After leaving the vertebral column, the nerves divide into the Posterior ramus and anterior ramus.
- Posterior (Dorsal) ramus: nerves that innervate the posterior trunk carrying: visceral motor, somatic motor and somatic sensory information to and from the skin and muscles of the back (epaxial muscles).

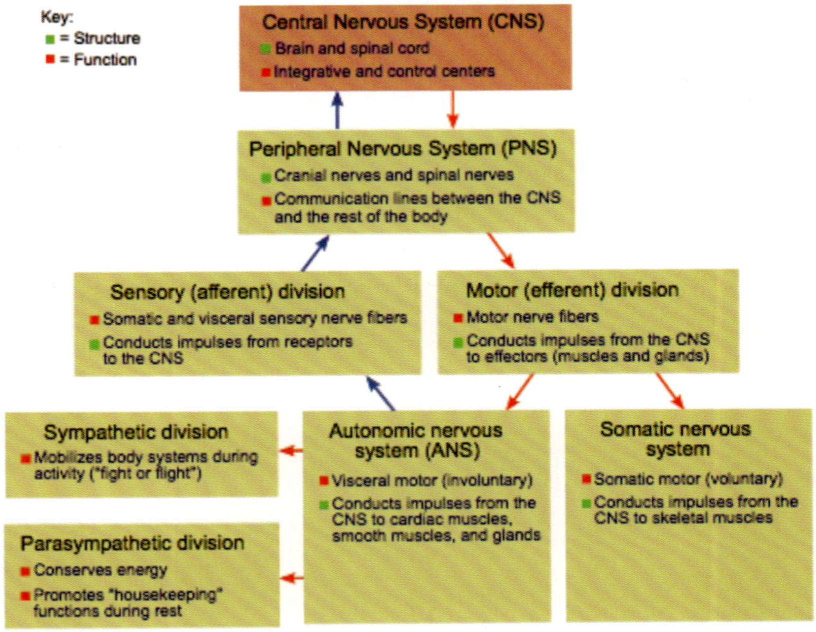

- Anterior (Ventral) ramus: nerves that innervate the anterior trunk and upper and lower limbs (hypaxial muscles) carrying visceral motor, somatic motor and sensory information.
- Sensory Information: Afferent fibers transmit sensory information from internal organs back to the CNS are not divided into parasympathetic and sympathetic. They are conducted by general visceral afferent fibers.
- General visceral afferent: unconscious sensations (reflex arcs) from hollow organs and glands. Can send pain sensations as referred pain. Pain is referred to dermatomes on the same spinal nerve level.

Parasympathetic (rest and digest, feed and breed) Overview

- Nerves arise from the CNS (Central Nervous System)
- Efferent parasympathetic nerves are carried from the CNS by two neurons. 1st Neuron = preganglionic (AKA: presynaptic) in the CNS and its axon extends to synapse with the dendrite of a postganglionic (AKA: Postsynaptic) neuron close to the target organ.
- Both synapses: preganglionic and postganglionic are cholinergic and use ACh as the neurotransmitter to activate nicotinic receptors (presynaptic) and muscarinic (postsynaptic) receptors.
- CN III, VII, IX, X
- CN III, VII, IX synapse in different nuclei in the cranial ganglia (ciliary, pterygopalatine, otic, submandibular).
- The **Edinger-Westphal nucleus (CN III)** sends preganglionic fibers to the ciliary ganglion via branches of the oculomotor nerve. **Ciliary ganglion** sends postganglionic fibers via **short ciliary nerves** that innervate the **sphincter pupillae muscle: constricts pupil (miosis) and ciliaris muscle of the lens causing contraction (making lens more convex, AKA: accommodation)**.
- *Pterygopalatine ganglion*: innervates the lacrimal glands and nasal mucosa, heating and cooling the air in the nose.
- **Superior Salivatory nucleus (CN VII)** sends preganglionic fibers to the sphenopalatine and submandibular ganglia. The **Submandibular ganglion** sends postganglionic fibers to the submandibular and sublingual salivary glands.
- **Inferior Salivatory nucleus (CN IX)** sends preganglionic fibers to the **Otic ganglion**. The Otic ganglion sends postganglionic fibers to the parotid gland for salivation.
- **The Dorsal Motor nucleus and nucleus ambiguous (X)** sends preganglionic fibers to the ganglia in the larynx, pharynx, thorax, and abdomen. These ganglia send postganglionic fibers to various glands and smooth muscle in these areas.
- **Vagus gives off** other parasympathetic nerves: **recurrent laryngeal nerve** (supplying parasympathetic innervation to the trachea and esophagus); the Cardiac nerves (forming the cardiac and pulmonary plexuses)
- **Vagus nerve provides parasympathetic presynaptic innervation** to the proximal 2/3 of the kidneys, gall bladder, transverse colon, smooth muscles and glands of the gut, pancreas, liver, and stomach.

- Spinal nerves in the sacrum S2, S3, S4 (Pelvic splanchnic nerves, innervation to hindgut)
- Pelvic splanchnic nerves reside in the lateral gray horn of the spinal cord at the T12 – L1 vertebral levels.
- Pelvic splanchnic nerves arise from the anterior rami (AKA: ventral ramus), the anterior division of a spinal nerve (S2, S3, S4) and enter the sacral plexus via parasympathetic efferent fibers. Then travel to the inferior hypogastric plexus (AKA: Pelvis plexus). Hypogastric plexus is located on sides of rectum in both males and females and on the sides of the vagina in the female. (hypogastric nerve).
- Pelvic splanchnic nerves innervate: pelvic and genital organs, emptying bladder, controlling open/close of internal urethral sphincter, motility in the rectum and erection.
- Pelvic splanchnic nerves contain both preganglionic (nerve fibers from the CNS to the ganglion). All preganglionic fibers (whether parasympathetic or sympathetic are cholinergic, using ACh as their neurotransmitter).
- Pelvic splanchnic nerves provide parasympathetic and pain sensation in the distal 1/3 transverse colon, sigmoid, rectum and cervix.
- **Sexual response**: Males: Cavernous nerves from the prostatic plexus allow blood to fill the **corpus spongiosum** to allow for erection. Females: Parasympathetic fibers innervate the fallopian tubes to promote peristaltic contractions to move the oocyte to the uterus for implantation.

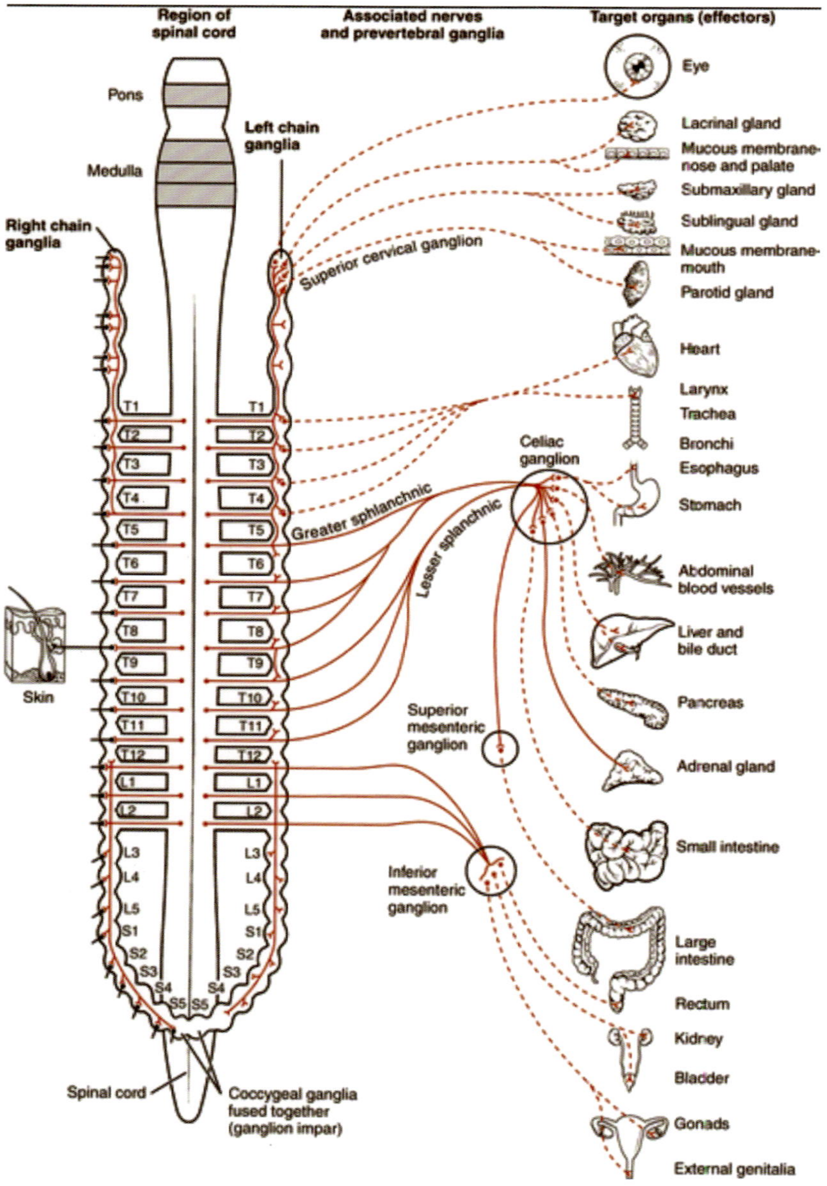

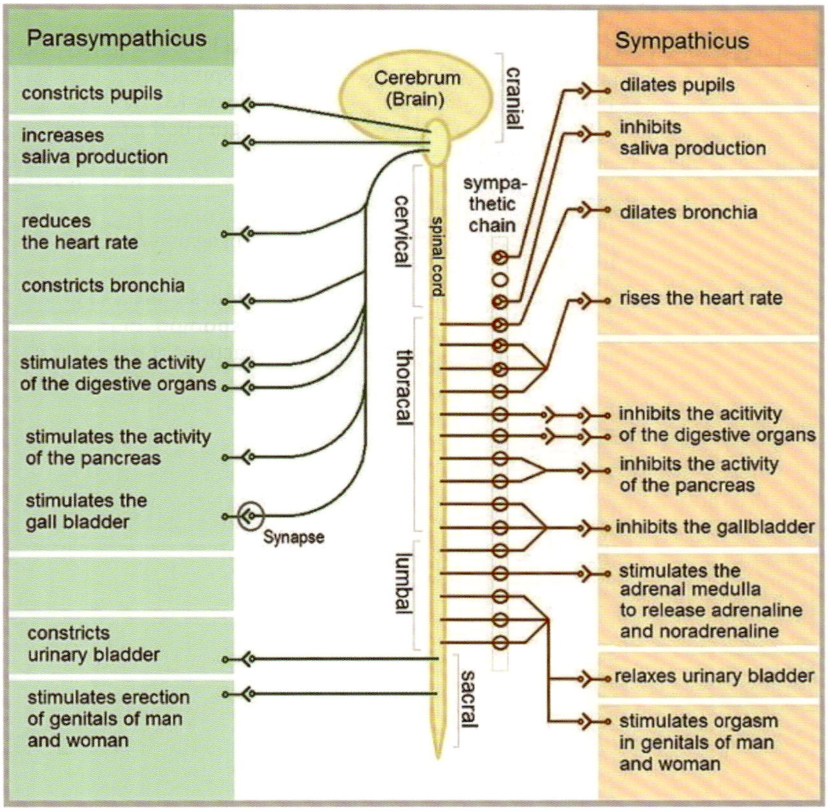
Parasympathicus
constricts pupils
increases saliva production
reduces the heart rate
constricts bronchia
stimulates the activity of the digestive organs
stimulates the activity of the pancreas
stimulates the gall bladder
Synapse
constricts urinary bladder
stimulates erection of genitals of man and woman
Cerebrum (Brain)
cranial
cervical
spinal cord
sympa-thetic chain
thoracal
lumbal
sacral
Sympathicus
dilates pupils
inhibits saliva production
dilates bronchia
rises the heart rate
inhibits the acitivity of the digestive organs
inhibits the activity of the pancreas
inhibits the gallbladder
stimulates the adrenal medulla to release adrenaline and noradrenaline
relaxes urinary bladder
stimulates orgasm in genitals of man and woman

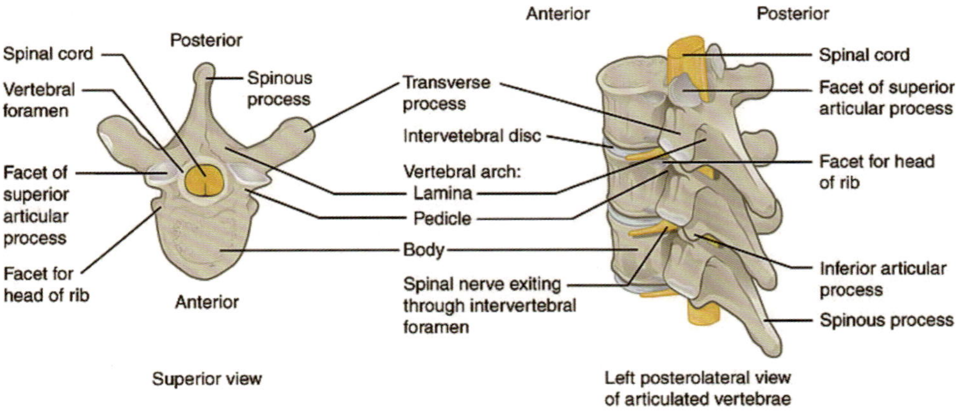
Posterior
Spinal cord
Vertebral foramen
Spinous process
Facet of superior articular process
Facet for head of rib
Anterior
Superior view
Anterior
Posterior
Transverse process
Intervetebral disc
Vertebral arch:
Lamina
Pedicle
Body
Spinal nerve exiting through intervertebral foramen
Spinal cord
Facet of superior articular process
Facet for head of rib
Inferior articular process
Spinous process
Left posterolateral view of articulated vertebrae

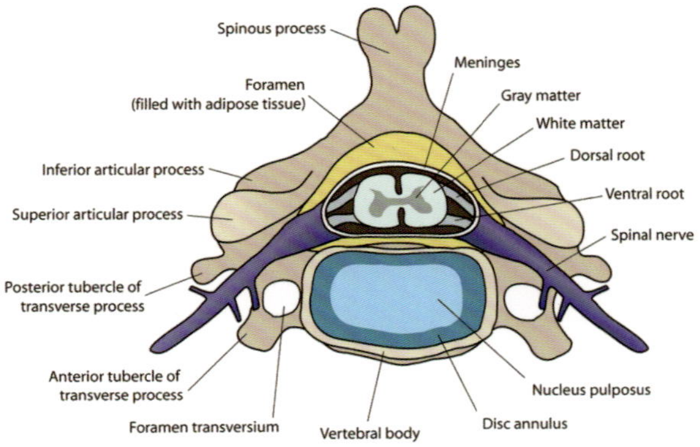
Spinous process
Foramen (filled with adipose tissue)
Meninges
Gray matter
White matter
Dorsal root
Ventral root
Spinal nerve
Inferior articular process
Superior articular process
Posterior tubercle of transverse process
Anterior tubercle of transverse process
Foramen transversium
Vertebral body
Disc annulus
Nucleus pulposus

Sympathetic (fight or flight) Overview

- Two neurons transmit signals in the sympathetic system: pre-ganglionic from the thoracolumbar region of the spinal cord (levels T1 – L2) that travel to ganglion to synapse and the post-ganglionic that travel to the organ.
- Preganglionic neurons release ACh as the neurotransmitter that activate nicotinic receptors
- Postganglionic neurons (there are 2 exceptions*) release norepinephrine that activates adrenergic receptors on the target tissue.
- *Postganglionic neurons of sweat glands and the adrenal medulla (chromaffin cells) release ACh to activate muscarinic receptors.
- Sympathetic nerves arise from the spinal cord in the intermediolateral nucleus of the lateral grey column.
- Axons of the sympathetic nerves leave the spinal cord through the anterior root and enter the anterior rami of the spinal nerves, separating through the white rami communicans (preganglionic sympathetic outflow nerve tract from the spinal cord).
- Presynaptic nerves terminate and synapse in the paravertebral or prevertebral ganglia.
- Paravertebral and prevertebral ganglia include: sympathetic trunks, cervical ganglia (superior, middle, inferior), celiac, and mesenteric ganglia.
- Superior cervical ganglia (SCG): Innervates the head and neck. Lies deep to the internal carotid artery and internal jugular vein. Part of the cervical plexus (C1 – C4).
  Gray rami communicantes to cervical nerve I - IV
- Middle cervical ganglia: Located at C5 – C6) and by the inferior thyroid artery.
  Gray rami communicantes to cervical nerve V and VI.
- Inferior cervical ganglia: Located at C-8 and first rib beside the costocervical artery.
  Gray rami communicantes to cervical nerve VII and VIII.
- Postsynaptic nerves then innervate target organ.

RECEPTORS

Ligand channel receptors: transmembrane ion channel proteins that open for ions. Allow ions: Na, K, Ca, Cl to pass through the membrane in response to the binding of chemical messenger such as neurotransmitters. It has an allosteric binding site.
Allosteric binding site: regulation of the protein by the binding of an effector molecule that regulates the gene expression, cell signaling or ↑ or ↓ of enzyme activity in that protein. MC found in synapses to covert chemical presynaptic signals into postsynaptic electrical signals. This conversion can be regulated by membrane potential, channel blockers and allosteric ligands
3 types of ligand channel receptors:

- Cys-loop: loop formed by disulfide bonds between two cysteine residues in the N terminal at the extracellular domain and conduct anionic or cationic ions.
  Example: **Nicotinic acetylcholine receptor**. Positive Na ions flow down the electrochemical gradient into the cell to depolarize the postsynaptic membrane in order to initiate an action potential.
  Nicotinic acetylcholine receptors (Sensitive to nicotine from tobacco). **Cholinergic/ionotropic receptors: they respond to nicotine, choline and the neurotransmitter, acetylcholine (Acetylcholine originates from the basal optic nucleus of Meynert). There are two types: muscle receptors and neuronal receptors. Nicotinic receptors use ion channels, the do NOT use 2nd messengers (like the metabotropic receptors do). They open to allow ions: Na, K, Ca to diffuse into or out of the cell. They transmit outgoing signals to both sympathetic and parasympathetic systems. They bind chemicals in the extracellular domain at the** N terminal. **Ion channels open to these chemical messengers so that positive ions (cations), sodium is able to move in and potassium is able to move out. So the net flow of positive ions is inward. The inward movement of these cations causes depolarization of the plasma membrane passing on the action potential.**
  The somatic nervous system (muscles) uses nicotinic receptors. Acetylcholine is released into the neuromuscular junction.
  (**tip**: "**N**"icotinic binds at the "**N**" terminal).
- Ionotropic Glutamate receptors: Tetramer that binds glutamate. Example: GABA and NMDA receptors. One of the major sites that anesthetics and alcohol have their effect.
- ATP-gated ion channel: Channels that open in response to the binding of ATP. Form dimers with two transmembrane receptors and the N and C terminal is on the intracellular side.

Metabotropic receptors: Receptors that use second messengers. Three types: Hydrophobic (non-water soluble: DAG, phosphatidylinositols), hydrophilic (water soluble: cAMP, cGMP, IP_3, Ca), and Gases (are able to diffuse across the cytosol and cell membranes: NO, CO, H_2S).

- **Second messengers:** Intracellular signaling molecules released during the intracellular signaling transduction cascade in response to a first messenger's stimulation (extracellular molecules). This causes physiological changes within the cell: apoptosis, proliferation, differentiation.
  Examples: **G protein Receptors: Gs, Gi, Gq.**
  Gq: Calcium ions: Phospholipase C = DAG (diacylglycerol), IP3 (Inositol trisphosphate).
  Gs/Gi: cAMP (Adenylate cyclase, PKA). G Proteins are guanine nucleotide-binding proteins: GDP: Guanosine diphosphate and GTP: Guanosine triphosphate: cGMP.
- **Muscarinic receptors** (Sensitive to muscarine, substance found in the Amanita muscaria mushroom). Receptors that form **G protein receptors in the cell membranes** and are stimulated by acetylcholine released by postganglionic fibers (fibers from the group of nerve cell bodies (AKA: Ganglion) to the effector organ) in the parasympathetic system. (Preganglionic fibers are from the CNS to the group of nerve cell bodies). Most effector organs are in the parasympathetic system.
  EXCEPTION: Preganglionic fibers from the sympathetic system terminate at the muscarinic cholinergic receptors at the chromaffin cells in the **adrenal medulla** (which secretes norepinephrine and epinephrine into the bloodstream) and the **sweat glands**.
  Muscarinic receptors have alpha-subunits. The receptors differ based on which G protein they are bound to. Gs, Gi, Gq.
  They rely on a second messenger. For activation of the G protein: Acetylcholine is the ligand (signaling molecule) that binds with a transmembrane receptor (Receptor that is able to take the signal across the membrane. This transmembrane receptor spans the membrane 7 times). Once the signal crosses through the receptor into the cell it binds with the metabotropic G protein receptors. Upon binding the signal cascades into the cell.
  G protein receptors have subtypes: M1, M2, M3, M4 and M5. Each responsible for a specific location and job.

	cAMP System	cGMP System	Phosphoinositol System	Arachidonic System	Tyrosine Kinase System
First Messenger: Neurotransmitters	Epinephrine: α2, β1, β2 Acetylcholine: M2	---------------	Epinephrine: α1 Acetylcholine: M1, M3	Histamine receptor	----------------------------
Frist Messenger: Hormones	ACTH, CRH, ANP, CT, LH, FSH, hCG, MSH, PTH, TSH Glucagon	ANP, Nitric oxide	GnRH, GHRH, AGT, TRH, Oxytocin	-------------------------	IGF, PDGF, INS
Signal Transducer	Gs: β1, β2 Gi: α2, M2	----------------	Gq	Unknown G protein	RTK
Primary effector	Adenylyl cyclase	Guanylate cyclase	Phospholipase C	Phospholipase A	RasGEF
Second Messenger	cAMP	cGMP	IP3, DAG, Ca2+	Arachidonic acid	RAS.GTP
Secondary effector	Protein kinase A	Protein kinase G	PKC, CaM	5-Lipoxygenase, Cyclooxygenase	MAP3K (c-Raf)

First messengers: Extracellular factors: neurotransmitters or peptide hormones (peptide hormones are hydrophilic so can't cross the phospholipid bilayer cell membrane. They must use the 2nd messengers to send their extracellular signal intracellular. Examples: Ras, MAPK). Examples of first messengers: Serotonin, epinephrine, and dopamine.

Voltage-gated ion channels: channels that open and close depending upon the membrane potential. (Cell membranes are impermeable to ions so ions must diffuse through transmembrane protein channels). Located along the axon and at the synapse. Gated channels are specific to one ion: Na, Ca, K, Cl and open/close based on the ions concentration (ie: gradient) between the outside and inside of the cell.

Stretch-activated ion channels: channels that open/close in response to the stress in the cell membrane. Used in detection of taste, smell, stretch, heat, volume, vision, sounds, vibration, and pressure.

Steroid receptors: Intracellular receptors. They are in the plasma membrane, nucleus and cytosol and initiate signal transduction for steroid hormones to affect gene expression. MC is the nuclear receptors (transcription factors). They are either in the cytosol and move into the nucleus upon activation or are in the nucleus waiting for the steroid hormone to activate them. **Heat shock proteins (HSPs)** are bound to the receptors until the steroid hormone replaces them. (HSP act as chaperones. **Chaperones** help stabilize new proteins to ensure correct **folding** or help to **refold damaged proteins**).
Examples: Cortisol (ACTH regulates cortisol by cAMP and PKA), Aldosterone (regulated by blood volume and Angiotensin II activate aldosterone by Phospholipase C to IP3 to Ca), Progesterone, Estrogen, Testosterone (GnRH regulates sex steroids by FSH and LH).
Non-steroid hormones that use steroid receptors: Vitamin D3, thyroid hormones (T3 and T4), and retinoic acid.

Parasympathetic Innervation in the Head (Eyes and Glands)

NUCLEUS/CN	PREGANGLIONIC	POSTGANGLIONIC	ACTION
Edinger-Westphal, CNIII	Ciliary Ganglion	Short ciliary nerves. Sphincter pupillae muscle. Ciliaris muscle of the lens.	Constricts pupil (miosis) Contraction, making lens more convex (AKA: accommodation)
Superior Salivatory nucleus (CN VII)	Submandibular ganglion	Submandibular glands Sublingual glands	Salivation
Inferior Salivatory nucleus (CN IX)	Otic ganglion	Parotid gland	Salivation
Dorsal Motor nucleus and nucleus ambiguous (CN X)	See table above		

Parasympathetic Innervation in the Body

PARASYMPATHETIC	1st Stop		2nd Stop		
ORGAN	**1st RECEPTOR**	**NT**	**2nd RECEPTOR**	**NT**	**ACTION**
Heart (Via Vagus)	Nicotinic	ACh (AKA: Cholinergic)	Muscarinic	ACh	Slows heart beat
Lungs (via Vagus)	Nicotinic	ACh (AKA: Cholinergic)	Muscarinic	ACh	Constricts bronchi
Stomach (via Vagus)	Nicotinic	ACh (AKA: Cholinergic)	Muscarinic	ACh	Peristalsis & secretion
Liver (via Vagus)	Nicotinic	ACh (AKA: Cholinergic)	Muscarinic	ACh	Release of bile
Bladder	Nicotinic	ACh (AKA: Cholinergic)	Muscarinic	ACh	Contracts (detrusor)

G Protein Class (color coding used in each of the tables below)

All G proteins are transmembrane spanning proteins. (AKA: 7 transmembrane domain receptors).

cAMP 2nd Messenger System:

Endocrine hormones that bind the receptor in the cAMP pathway: (**tip**: FLAT CHAMP)
FSH, LH, ACTH, TSH, CRH, hCG, ADH (V2=kidneys), MSH, PTH, GnRH, Calcitonin, Glucagon.
Endocrine hormones (ligand) binds a receptor (stimulates) either a Gs (stimulatory) or a Gi (inhibitory) protein. The receptor is bound to a trimeric transmembrane protein (7 spanning). The trimeric protein has 3 subunits: alpha, beta, and gamma. The receptor determines whether the Gs or Gi is stimulated. (Most of the receptors are Gs: stimulatory). The majority of the Gi receptors are α2. Once the G protein is stimulated it activates Adenylyl cyclase. Adenylyl causes ATP to become cyclic AMP. Cyclic AMP stimulates PKA (Protein Kinase A). Protein Kinase (takes ATP and gives AMP, taking phosphates to phosphorylates proteins and enzymes in the cytoplasm). PKA also phosphorylates the CREB protein (transcription factor). CREB diffuses across into the nucleus to bind CRE (cAMP response element), the promotor on the DNA. Once CRE is activated starts the transcription of a gene leading to a specific protein or enzyme.

- **Gs = (stimulates) = Adenylyl cyclase = ATP and cAMP = PKA (Protein Kinase A) = phosphorylates proteins.**
  1) increases Ca in the heart = ↑ heart rate, ↑ contractility
  2) stimulates myosin light chain kinase in smooth muscle = contraction
  Gs receptors: Beta 1, Beta 2, D1, H2, V2

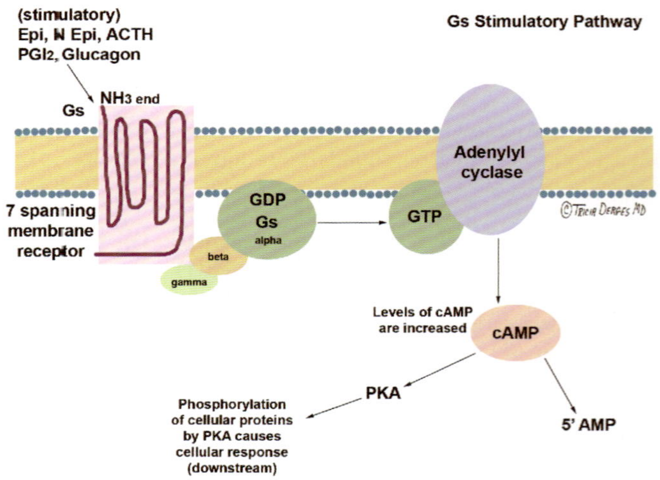

- Gi = (inhibitory) = Blocks/decreases Adenylyl cyclase activation= ↓cAMP
  1) decreases Ca, ↓ adenylyl cyclase, ↓ cAMP, ↑ K channels = decrease in the heart rate and contractility.
  2) ↓ sympathetic (adrenergic) outflow

  Gi receptors: alpha 2, M2, D2

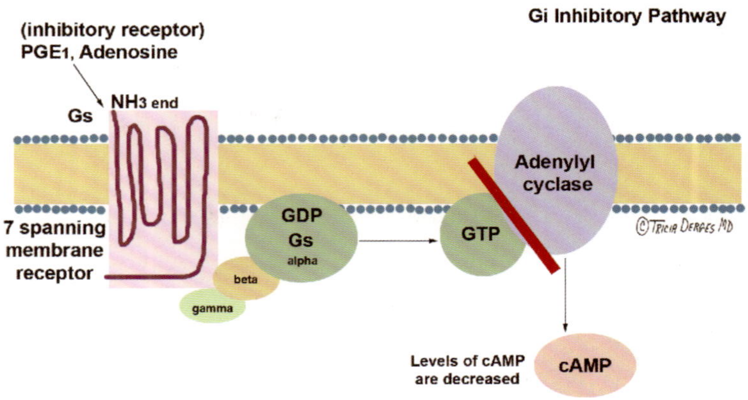

- Gq = Phospholipase C = PIP2
  PIP can go two ways:
  1) DAG to PKC (Protein Kinase C)
  2) IP3 to increase Ca to contract smooth muscle

  Gq receptors: alpha 1, M1, M3, H1, V1

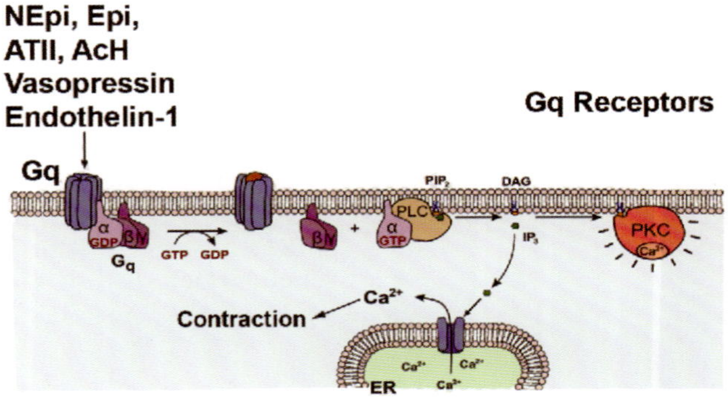

Muscarinic Receptors (AKA: Cholinergic, ACh neurotransmitter)

(see color coding above)

MUSCARINIC RECEPTOR	ORGAN	ACTION
M1, 2nd messenger, 7 transmembrane Gq protein segments	**Neural – CNS, enteric: gut.**	**Gq, IP3 and DAG cascade. ↓ K conductance. Mediates EPSP in the CNS. Enteric system in the gut. Secretions from salivary glands and stomach**
M2, 2nd messenger, 7 transmembrane Gi protein segments	**Heart.**	**Gi, Inhibits cAMP, activates K channels Slows down heart rate, ↓ contractile forces in the atrium and ↓ conduction velocity of the AV node. ↑ K conductance and ↓ Ca conductance.**
M3, 2nd messenger, 7 transmembrane Gq protein segments	**Multiple Organs**	**Gq, IP3 and DAG cascade Bronchoconstrict the lungs. Vasodilates vessels. Increases gut motility, dilates sphincters. Increases exocrine gland secretions: lacrimal, salivary, gastric acid. Contracts detrusor muscle of bladder to micturate. Increases papillary sphincter contraction = miosis. Increase ciliary muscle contraction = accommodation.**
M4, 2nd messenger, 7 transmembrane Gi protein segments	Produce inhibitory effects	Decreased cAMP in the cell.
M5, 2nd messenger, 7 transmembrane Gq protein segments	Not fully understood at this time	Gq: upregulates phospholipase C

SYMPATHETIC	1st Stop		2nd Stop		
MAIN ORGAN	**1st RECEPTOR**	**NT**	**2nd RECEPTOR**	**NT**	**ACTION**
Heart	**Nicotinic**	**ACh (AKA: Cholinergic)**	**Adrenergic, Beta 1 Gs, ↑ cAMP**	**NEpi**	**Increases heart rate Increases contractility Increase renin release Increase lipolysis Stimulates adenylyl cyclase, ↑cAMP**
Lungs	**Nicotinic**	**ACh (AKA: Cholinergic)**	**Adrenergic, Beta 2 Gs, ↑ cAMP**	**NEpi**	**Dilation bronchi Vasodilation (relaxes smooth muscle) Increase insulin release Activates glycogenolysis in liver Stop uterine contractions (↓ tone): Tocolysis Ciliary muscle relaxation Increase aqueious humor Increase heart rate Increase contractility Increase lipolysis Stimulates adenylyl cyclase, ↑cAMP**
Vessels	**Nicotinic**	**ACh (AKA: Cholinergic)**	**Adrenergic, Alpha 1 Gq, ↑ IP3**	**NEpi**	**Vasoconstriction Increase papillary dilator (mydriasis) Increased bladder sphincter contraction (bladder retention) Forms: IP3, DAG, ↑intracellular Ca**
General	**Nicotinic**	**ACh (AKA: Cholinergic)**	**Adrenergic, Alpha 2 Gi, ↓ cAMP**	**NEpi**	**Decrease sympathetic tone (makes everything MORE parasympathetic) Decreases release of NEpi Decrease insulin release Decrease lipolysis Increase platelet aggregation Inhibits adenylyl cyclase, ↓cAMP**
Adrenal Medulla	Nicotinic	ACh (AKA: Cholinergic)			Releases Epinephrine and Norepinephrine
Muscles (somatic system)	Nicotinic	ACh (AKA: Cholinergic)			
Sweat Glands	Nicotinic	ACh (AKA: Cholinergic)	Muscarinic	ACh	Sweat

NOTE THE EXCEPTION in the sympathetic system: **Adrenal medulla and sweat glands are innervated by ACh (AKA: Cholinergic fibers).**
NOTE THE EXCEPTION in the somatic system: **Muscles are only innervated by ACh at nicotinic receptors at the neuromuscular junction.**

(**Tip:** For action potential synapses for all parasympathetic and sympathetic regarding receptors and neurotransmitters. Think of it like a trip. Let's say that everyone in your class is going to take a train to a different country, but the trains that go to the individual countries are all located at the transfer station. EVERYONE in your class must FIRST stop at the same transfer station (Nicotinic – first synapse) using the exact same fuel (Ach). Once everyone arrives at the transfer station each person exits and gets on a different train that will take them to a different country (different receptors: ie: adrenergic, muscarinic, dopaminergic etc.) and they will be using a different fuel to get there (different neurotransmitters: Ach, Norepinephrine, Epinephrine, Dopamine, etc). There are 2 classmates that will not get on a second train to get to their destination. They will get off at the transfer station because their destination is at the transfer station (Nicotinic receptor using Ach as the fuel). The two destinations that are located AT the transfer station are: Skeletal muscles (AKA: somatic) and the Adrenal medulla (innermost layer, below the cortex layer) that releases its own fuel (neurotransmitters: Epinephrine and Norepinephrine). Everyone but these two classmates boards another train.

Additional Receptors

(See color coding above)

MAIN ORGAN	NT	ACTION
Kidneys	D1, Dopamine	Arteriole dilation of renal vessels Stimulates adenylyl cyclase, ↑ cAMP
Brain	D2, Dopamine	Dopamine release Inhibits adenylyl cyclase, increases potassium conductance
Lungs	H1, Histamine	Increases bronchial and nasal mucus production, Increases vascular permeability Increases constriction of bronchioles, pain, pruritus
Stomach	H2, Histamine	Increases gastric acid release
Vessels	V1	Vasoconstriction
Kidneys	V2, ADH, Vasopressin, Desmopressin, DDAVP	Increases water reabsorption in collecting tubules

Signaling Pathways of Endocrine Hormones

Signal	Hormones	Notes
cAMP	HCG, PTH, Calcitonin, Glucagon, ADH (V2 receptors), FSH, LH, ACTH, TSH, CRH, GHRH,	Adenylate cyclase
cGMP	NO, ANP	Vasodilation
IP3	ADH (V1 receptor - constrictor), Oxytocin, GnRH, TRH, Histamine (H1 receptor), Angiotensin II, Gastrin	Phospholipase C

Steroid Receptor (lipophilic) Circulate bound to globulins, which increase solubility. **Intranuclear**	**T3/T4** (thyroid hormones), Testosterone, Estrogen, Vit D, Cortisol, Aldosterone, Progesterone	These receptors are **intracytoplasmic, nuclear receptors** and go directly to gene expression. They are NOT on the cell surface. Associated with **Chaperones (heat shock proteins hsp90 and hsp 56)** Chaperones assist in folding/unfolding, assembly/disassembly of proteins. Thyroid hormones are required for growth hormone synthesis. SHBG (Steroid Hormone Binding Globulin) ↑ SHBG lowers free testosterone = gynecomastia ↓ SHBG raises free testosterone = hirsutism ↑ SHBG raises with OCP 's and Pregnancy

Tyrosine Kinase (AKA: **RTKs** = receptor tyrosine kinase) (**Cell surface** receptor for growth factors/insulin. Transmembrane receptor. Extracellular. Ligand binds and then auto-phosphorylates the tyrosine residues.	**Insulin** **Growth Factors**: IGF-1, FGF (fibroblast), PDGF, EGF	**MAP kinase pathway**. (**RAS/MAP** Kinase pathway) Triggers a **cascade** of events through phosphorylation that **transmits the extracellular signal** to the nucleus causing changes in gene expression.
Tyrosine Kinase (Intrinsic) (AKA: nRTK's = non-receptor tyrosine kinase) **Cytoplasmic**, No surface receptors, no transmembrane domains). Do not bind to a ligand. Transfers a phosphate group to tyrosine kinases.	**Cytokines**: IL-2, IL-6, IL-8, IFN, Prolactin, EPO, TCR (T cell receptors), BR (B cell receptors), **Growth Hormones**: Acidophils (organisms that thrive under acidic situations)	**JAK/STAT pathway.** Transfers a phosphate group from ATP to a tyrosine residue (phosphorylation) - **downstream**. Regulates cells growth, signal PMN's, proliferation, differentiation, adhesion, migration, apoptosis and regulate the immune system. **LACK:** extracellular ligand-binding domain, transmembrane-spanning. Regulation: Tyrosine phosphorylation

Tyrosine kinases receptors verses G protein receptors: Tyrosine kinases do not require the use of a 2nd messenger; G protein receptors do require a 2nd messenger.

Adrenergic Neurotransmitter Release

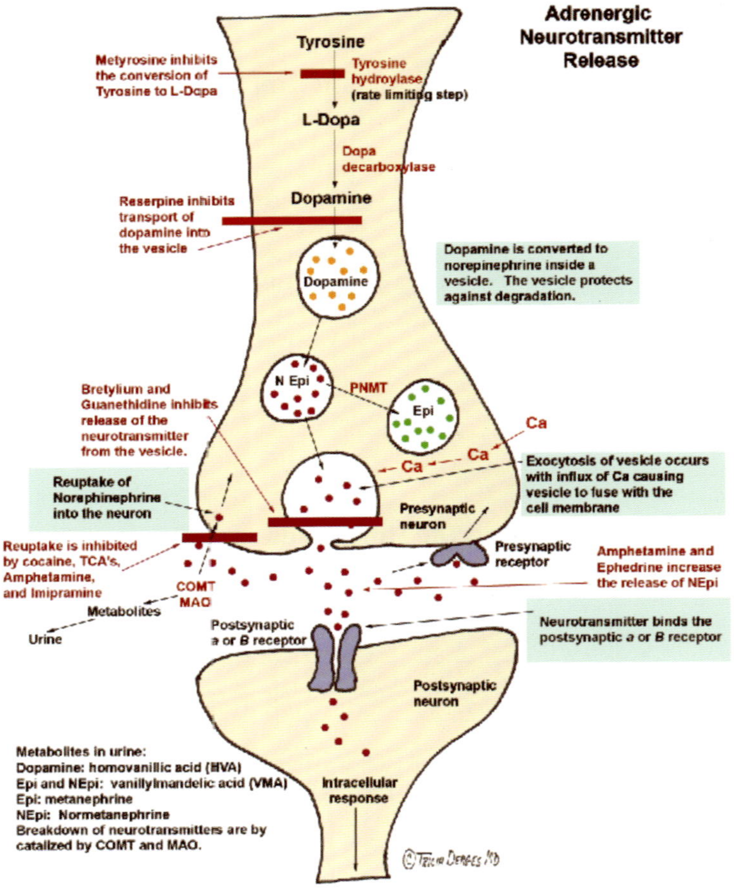

Cholinergic Neurotransmitter Release

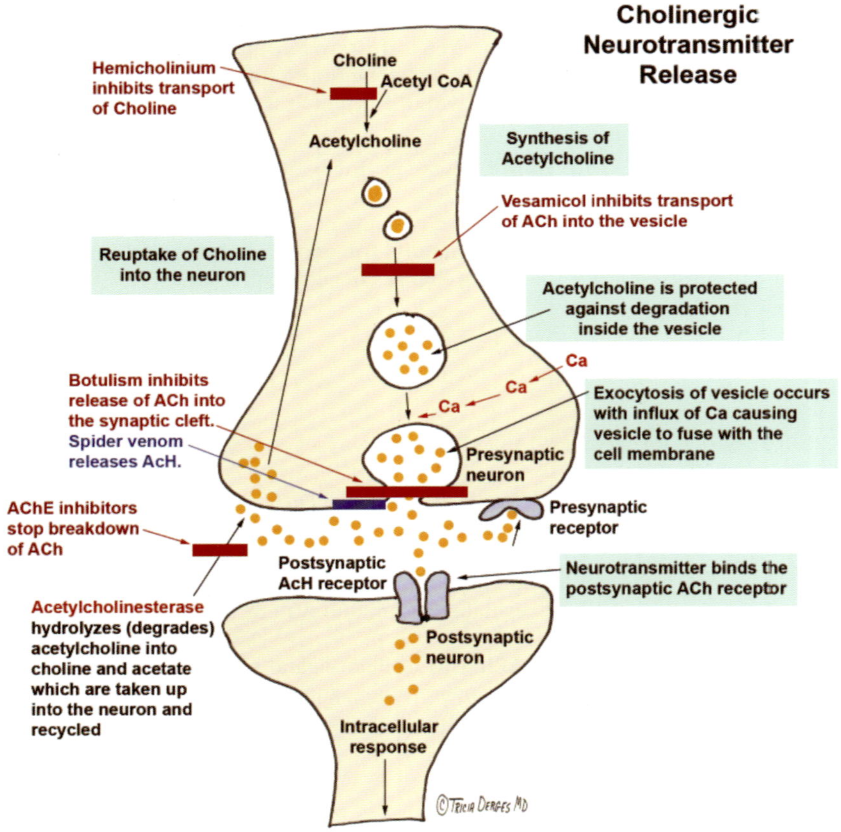

Cholinergic (Cholinomimetic)

Parasympathetic

OVERALL CAUTION: When using **Cholinergic/Parasympathetic** agents with any patients that have difficulty breathing (asthma, COPD, emphysema) because it will cause ↑pparasympathetic effects causing
↑ difficulty in breathing land lead to an exacerbation. Caution also when using with patients that have peptic ulcers. Parasympathetic agents ↑ parasympathetic effects causing
↑ release of HCL in the stomach.

Toxicity for all Cholinergic/Parasympathetic: ↑↑ parasympathetic effects: ↑ muscle tone in the GI, nausea, vomiting, cramps, diarrhea, bradycardia, heart block, hypotension, ↑ sweating, ↑ salivation,
↑ lacrimation.

DRUG GENERIC name Trade name	Clinical Use	Mechanism of Action and Resistance	Toxicity and Notes
MUSCARINIC DIRECT AGONIST: Neurotransmitter binds directly to the receptors.			
Bethanechol	**Bladder (urinary) retention,** postoperative ileus, neurogenic ileus.	Neurotransmitter binds directly to the muscarinic receptors.	Activates bladder and bowels.
Carbachol	Glaucoma	↓ intraocular pressure	(**tip**: CARBon copy of ACh)
Pilocarpine	Open and Closed glaucoma. Stimulates tears, saliva, sweat.	Open-angle glaucoma: contracts ciliary muscle. Closed-angle glaucoma: contracts pupillary sphincter.	(**tip**: drool on your PILOw)
Methacholine	Asthma challenge test. Causes an asthma attack.	Stimulates muscarinic receptors in airways (parasympathetic = bronchoconstriction = difficulty breathing).	
MUSCARINIC INDIRECT AGONIST: Anti-cholinesterase (Stops the enzyme acetylcholinesterase from breaking down ACh = enhances the action of the Neurotransmitter acetylcholine).			
Donepezil	Alzheimer Dz	↑ endogenous ACh	(**tip**: I am DONE with Alzheimer's)
Edrophonium (AKA: **Tensilon Test**)	Myasthenia Gravis Challenge test. Used to DX Myasthenia Gravis and to monitor the need to adjust dosage on medication.	↑ endogenous ACh	If there is improvement with the test (↑ amount of ACh during the test) then dosage of medicines are ↑. **Antibody test:** Anti-AChR Ab (anti-acetylcholine receptor antibody).
Neostigmine	**Reverses succinylcholine.** Postoperative ileus, neurogenic ileus, bladder (urinary) retention.	↑ endogenous ACh	(**tip**: **NO**, NO more succinylcholine)
Pyridostigmine	**Myasthenia Gravis.** NO CNS penetration.	↑ endogenous ACh	(**tip**: py**RID**ostigmine gets **RID** of MG)
Physostigmine	**Atropine overdose, Jimson weed poisoning.** (Any anticholinergic toxicity: inhibits parasympathetic effects = causing sympathetic effects) **Crosses Blood Brain Barrier)**	↑ endogenous ACh	(**tip**: **PHY**sostigmine **PHI**xes atropine)

Organophosphate Poisoning (Cholinesterase Inhibitor poisoning) Irreversibly inhibit AChE.

- Cause: Insecticides, nerve gas (farmers crop dusting, people that work with pesticides, military)
- MOA: Inhibit acetylcholinesterase. Because there is no degradation of ACh (the enzyme acetylcholinesterase is inhibited) there is a ↑↑ build up of ACh in the synaptic cleft = overstimulation of ACh = ↑↑ parasympathetic activity.
- SX: Urination, miosis, diarrhea, bronchoconstriction = bronchospasms, bradycardia, seating, salivation, tearing (lacrimation), ↑ excitation of skeletal muscle, ↑ excitation of CNS.
- TX: Requires 2 treatments. **Atropine acts on the muscarinic receptors** as a competitive inhibitor to ↓ cholinergic effects **and Pralidoxime to act on the nicotinic receptors** to ↓ muscle excitation.
- TX: Must **remove clothing** FIRST and wash down the patient. Medical personnel should be protected so they are contaminated and so that they do not spread the contaminant. The toxin is absorbed through the skin.

Muscarinic Antagonist (AKA: Anti-cholinergic/Anti-parasympathetic/Anti-muscarinic) = allows ↑ sympathetic effects.

MOA for all Muscarinic Antagonist: (AKA: Anti-cholinergic) ↓ IP3 and ↓ Ca = smooth muscle relaxation = sympathetic response.

DRUG GENERIC name Trade name	**Clinical Use**	**Mechanism of Action and Resistance**	**Toxicity and Notes**
Atropine Cyclopentolate Homatropine Tropicamide	**Mydriasis (dilation) during eye exams,** Paralysis of the ciliary muscle (AKA: cycloplegia = loss of accommodation). ↓ airway secretions, HCL secretions in stomach, GI motility, urinary urgency. **TX: Organophosphate poisoning** (at the muscarinic receptors). TX: **Digoxin overdose**. TX: **Heart Blocks/bradycardia (blocks the Vagus nerve)**		Topical application in the eye. NOTE: **Jimson weed** (Datura stramonium). Used to relieve asthma and analgesic during surgery. Narrow therapeutic index causing toxicity and death. Plant alkaloids contain high levels of atropine and scopolamine. (Atropine overdose). The question may describe someone that was working out in the yard. TX: **IV Physostigmine.** **Atropine toxicity:** SX: Dry skin, confusion/disorientation, ↑ body temperature (no sweating), tachycardia, and cycloplegia. TX: **Physostigmine.**
Benztropine	**Parkinson DZ**	Selective M1 muscarinic acetylcholine receptor antagonist. Blocks cholinergic activity and **increases dopamine by blocking its reuptake**.	(**tip**: PARK my BENZ)
Glycopyrrolate	Preoperative anesthesia medication to ↓ secretions in the airway. Hyperhidrosis. ↓ HCL secretion to TX ulcers. ↓ excess saliva.		Does not cross BBB. Causes dry mouth, constipation, headaches, difficulty with urination.
Ipratropium **Tiotropium** *Atrovent*	COPD, acute asthma.	↓ cholinergic effects on the bronchial musculature. Promotes ↓ cGMP on intracellular calcium = ↓ contractility of smooth muscle in the lung = ↓ bronchoconstriction and ↓ mucus secretion.	(**tip**: I **PRA**y I can breath with COPD)
Oxybutynin Tolterodine Darifenacin Fesoterodine Solifenacin Trospium	↓ urinary (bladder) urgency. ↓ bladder spasms (detrusor muscle).	Antispasmodic effect on smooth muscle.	Do not use in closed-angle glaucoma, GI obstruction, hiatal hernia, GERD, Myasthenia Gravis, Ulcerative colitis.

Scopolamine	Motion sickness, postoperative nausea.	Crosses BBB so can affect the CNS.	Note: Scopolamine overdose: TX: Physostigmine (crosses BBB) is antidote to treat CNS.

Drugs with anti-muscarinic side effects

- TCA's, Atropine, H-1 Antagonist (Diphenhydramine), Neuroleptics, Anti-Parkinson's drugs.

Nicotinic Receptor Drugs

DRUG GENERIC name Trade name	Clinical Use	Mechanism of Action and Resistance	Toxicity and Notes
Succinylcholine Mivacurium	Induce muscle relaxation (short term paralysis), Tracheal intubation, relaxation before anesthesia, muscle relaxant during ECT.	Depolarizing neuromuscular blocker that acts on the nicotinic receptors causing continual depolarization of the motor end plate. It is not broken down by acetylcholinesterase so the membrane potential is held above threshold so that the cell is not able to repolarize.	Reversed by **Neostigmine**. **Side effects:** malignant hyperthermia, rhabdomyolysis, hyperkalemia, bradycardia, cardiac arrest. In individuals with a **Pseudocholinesterase deficiency**, the paralyzing effects of succinylcholine will be prolonged.

α- Blockers

MOA for all α-blockers: Blocks the activities listed below:

- α-1 receptors (adrenergic) cause sympathetic effects on the vessels: vasoconstrict.
- α-2 receptors decrease the sympathetic outflow (so ↑ parasympathetic effects)

DRUG GENERIC name Trade name	Clinical Use	Mechanism of Action and Resistance	Toxicity and Notes
α-1 Blockers – Sympatholytic drug. Selective. All end in "zosin or osin"			
The "osin's" **Prazosin** **Tamsulosin** **Terazosin** **Doxazosin**	**BPH .** Prazosin: PTSD, anxiety, panic disorder. (**first line:** SSRI)		Toxicity: **First dose hypotension, syncope**, and priapism (rare). (Difficult for body to control BP without active α adrenergic receptors).
α-2 Blockers - Increases sympathetic output			
Mirtazapine	Depression, Appetite stimulant, Sleep aid, anxiety.		Toxicity: Weight gain, ↑ cholesterol. Mirtazapine is an atypical antidepressant (specific serotonergic)
Nonselective			
Phen-oxybenzamine	Given prior to pheochromocytoma surgery to prevent HTN crisis. (Men 2B)	Irreversible.	**MUST GIVE α-blocker FIRST, BEFORE the β-blocker** otherwise there is an unopposed α adrenergic effect causing hypertensive crisis.
Phentolamine	Treatment for tyramine crisis (MAO inhibitors that eat food that contain tyramine).		

β-Blockers

- ↓ **HR and contractility** = ↓ **Oxygen demand** of the heart
- ↑ **Filling time in diastole**
- ↓ **MI mortality**.
  Drugs that ↓ mortality: β-Blockers, Ace Inhibitors, Aspirin, Spironolactone
  Procedures that ↓ mortality: Implantable fibrillator, Angioplasty (balloon, stent, PCI: Percutaneous Coronary Intervention)

DRUG GENERIC name Trade name	Clinical Use	Mechanism of Action	Toxicity
The "lol's" **Acebutolol** **Atenolol** **Betaxolol** **Bisoprolol** **Carvedilol** **Esmolol *(short acting)*** **Labetalol** **Metoprolol** **Nadolol** **Nebivolol** **Pindolol** **Propranolol** **Timolol** (**Tip**: **Selective: A – M.** **Non-Selective: N – Z** **Exception:** C and L Carvedilol Labetalol: These **both** selective **and** non-selective **and** work on α and β	SVT (↓ AV conduction velocity), V-Tach, Rate control (A-fib, atrial flutter), CHF (↓ progression of chronic heart failure), ↓ HTN (↓ CO = ↓ Renin (β-1 Receptor blockade on JG cells), MI (↓ mortality), angina pectoris (↓ HR and contractility = ↓ O2 consumption) **Timolol:** Glaucoma (↓ aqueous humor) **Propranolol:** Thyrotoxicosis, Essential tremors, migraines, portal HTN, Performance anxiety Nebivolol: combines β-1 and β-2 activate nitric oxide. Used to treat HCM because it allows the heart to slow so there is more time to fill. More blood in the heart is important for HCM.	↓ cAMP and ↓ Ca currents = ↓ SA and AV nodes activity. **↓ Afterload, ↑ EDV, ↓ BP, ↓ Contractility, ↓ HR.** **↓ Phase 4 and ↓ conduction through AV node.** ↓ Conduction of AV node = ↑ **PR interval**. **(Prolongs the interval)** ↓ Ventricular rate and peripheral resistance (AKA: **Afterload**). **Inhibits release of renin** = ↓ vasoconstriction = ↓ Na and H_2O retention. Negative chronotropic effect. Negative inotropic effect. Give with Nitrates to ↓ affects of reflex tachycardia.	All: **Bradycardia, AV block**, CHF, sedation, depression, **impotence**, **mask the signs of hypoglycemia.** ↑ risk impotence in African American males. **Use CCB instead: Amlodipine**. **Do not use non-selective with ANY breathing problems** (asthma, COPD, etc.)- must use only selective. Causes exacerbation. Metoprolol = dyslipidemia (↑ Cholesterol). **DO NOT GIVE in Cocaine MI's** (users) due to unopposed α-adrenergic activity and ↑↑↑ HTN. **Give ONLY CCB.** Prior to surgery for pheochromocytoma: must **give α-Blockers before β-Blockers** or will cause unopposed α-adrenergic activity. Propanolol: exacerbate vasospasms: Do not use in: Prinzmetal angina, Raynaud's. Pindolol, Acebutolol: Contraindicated in angina because they are partial beta agonist. **TX for OD: Glucagon** (↑ cAMP)

Sympathomimetics

Stimulants. Mimic effects of agonists of the sympathetic nervous system (catecholamine's).
MOA for all sympathomimetics.

- Direct acting: α-adrenergic agonist, β-adrenergic agonists, dopaminergic agonists.
- Indirect acting: MAOI's, COMT inhibitors (reuptake inhibitors that ↑ levels of catecholamine's.

Inotropic: Force of contraction.
Chronotropic: Speed of contraction.

DRUG GENERIC name Trade name	Clinical Use	Mechanism of Action and Resistance	Toxicity and Notes
Direct Sympathomimetics			
Epinephrine (AKA: adrenaline)	**Anaphylaxis IM (Epi-pens),** hypotension (pressor), OPEN angle glaucoma.	Greatest effects on **all β receptors**, Lesser effect on α receptors. **β > α**	**Do NOT use on CLOSED angle glaucoma.**
Norepinephrine (AKA: noradrenaline)	**Hypotension.** (Pressor).	Greatest effects on **α-1 receptors**, then α-2 receptors and the least effect on β-1 receptors. Vasoconstriction = ↑ BP. **α-1 > α-2 > β-1**	↓ Renal perfusion.
Dopamine	**Hypotension.** (Pressor). Unstable bradycardia, heart failure.	Greatest effects on **D1 receptors**. **D1 = D2 > β > α**	
Isoproterenol	Evaluation of electrical currents of the heart for arrhythmias.	Greatest effects on **β-1 receptors**. **β-1 = β-2** **PURE β agonist (has no α action).**	Can worsen ischemia.
Dobutamine	Stress test. Cardiogenic shock (Cardiac failure).	Greatest effects on **β-1 receptors**. ↑ Inotropic effects. **β-1 > β-2 and α**	
Phenylephrine **Methoxamine**	Hypotension. Decongestant. Mydriasis for eye exams/procedures. Priapism.	Greatest effects on **α-1 receptors.** Vasoconstriction = ↑ BP. **α-1 > α-2** **PURE α agonist (has no β action).** Priapism: vasoconstriction of blood vessels entering penis = ↓ blood flow.	Toxicities: May cause reflex bradycardia via Baroreceptors. **Rebound nasal congestion**. ↑ BP due to vasoconstriction.
Metaproterenol	Asthma	Greatest effects on **β-2 receptors**. Bronchodilator. **β-2 > β-1** **PURE β agonist (has no α action).** ↑ cAMP = relaxation of bronchial smooth muscle and inhibits the degranulation of mast cells.	Dizziness, tachycardia, weakness, nervousness, headache.
Albuterol **Salbutamol**	Acute asthma – rescue inhaler.	Greatest effects on **β-2 receptors**. **β-2 > β-1** **PURE β agonist (has no α action).**	Tremor, anxiety, headache, dry mouth, palpitations, muscle cramps.
Salmeterol	Long-term asthma, COPD.	Greatest effects on **β-2 receptors**. **β-2 > β-1** **PURE β agonist (has no α action).**	Dizziness, migraines, ↑ BP, sinus infection.
Terbutaline	**Tocolytic**: ↓ uterine tone (stops contractions in premature labor).	Greatest effects on **β-2 receptors**. **β-2 > β-1** **PURE β agonist (has no α action).** **Relaxes uterine smooth muscle**.	Tachycardia, anxiety, tremors, headaches, hyperglycemia, hypotension, hypokalemia.

Indirect Sympathomimetics			
Amphetamines *Adderall* *Vyvanse* *Adderall XR* *Dexedrine*	**ADHD, narcolepsy,** obesity. Memory/cognitive enhancer.	CNS stimulant. Releasing agent of stored catecholamines and reuptake inhibitor of dopamine and norepinephrine.	**Hypokalemia.** TX: In addition to medical treatment of amphetamines for narcolepsy, the patient should be instructed to schedule a daytime nap. Overdose: **(see drug chapter for details)** Arrhythmias, ↑ or ↓ BP, tremor, ↑ RR, urinary retention, ↑ body temperature, confusion, agitation, rhabdomyolysis, psychosis.
Methylphenidate *Concerta*	**ADHD, narcolepsy,** obesity. Memory/cognitive enhancer.	CNS stimulant. Dopamine-norepinephrine reuptake inhibitor. Binds and blocks dopamine and norepinephrine transporters.	Appetite loss, anxiety, insomnia, dry mouth, restlessness (akathisia), lethargy, palpitations, tachycardia.
Cocaine **"Coke"**	Recreational street drug. Local anesthetic for procedures in the mouth or nose.	Reuptake inhibitor of serotonin, norepinephrine, dopamine causing increased levels. CNS stimulant.	Toxicity: **(See drug chapter for details)** Vasoconstriction. **DO NOT GIVE β-Blocker in cocaine overdose** because of unopposed α-1 effects (vasoconstriction) causing HTN crisis and **sudden cardiac death. Must use Calcium Channel Blockers.** SX: **Diffuse ST elevation on EKG.** Agitation or extreme happiness, tachycardia, sweating, mydriasis, ↑ BP, ↑ body temp, loss contact with reality. Snorted, inhaled, injected.
Ephedrine	Nasal decongestion, appetite suppressant, (↓ gastric emptying and an aid in weight loss)	Stimulant. Bronchodilator.	Tachycardia, arrhythmias, angina, HTN, vasoconstriction, difficulty in urinating (constricts the internal urethral sphincter), delusion, dyspnea, hyperglycemia.

Sympatholytics (Adrenergic antagonist)
A-2 agonists

MOA for all sympatholytics.

- Inhibits sympathetic activity.
- Inhibits epinephrine and norepinephrine

DRUG GENERIC name Trade name	**Clinical Use**	**Mechanism of Action and Resistance**	**Toxicity and Notes**
Clonidine	ADHD, High BP, anxiety, withdrawal (drugs, alcohol, smoking), migraines, hot flashes.	Stimulates α2 receptors in the brain which ↓ peripheral vascular resistance.	Orthostatic hypotension, anxiety, sedation, nausea, delusions, constipation. (Do not confuse with: Clomiphene or Clozapine)
Methyldopa	Gestational HTN. (Safe in pregnancy), HTN.	Inhibits DOPA decarboxylase (enzyme that converts DOPA to dopamine).	Depression, nightmares, anxiety, lethargy, sedation, headache, restless leg syndrome, hypotension

PHARMACOKINETICS and PHARMACODYNAMICS

Pharmacokinetics: Effects of the **body on the drug** (tip: MADE)
M=Metabolism, A=Absorption, D=Distribution, E=Excretion

Pharmacodynamics: Effects of the **drug on the body** (potency, efficacy, toxicity)

Goal: Achieve efficacy without toxicity. Plasma concentration must be within the therapeutic window

DEFINITIONS and FACTS

- **Competitive Antagonist**: Decreases potency, shifts curve to the right, and can be overcome.
- **Non-Competitive Antagonist**: Decreases efficacy, shifts curve down and **can't be overcome**.
- **Partial Agonist**: Tones down the effect of the stronger drug (if initial drug given is to strong, a partial agonist can be added to tone it down). It uses the same receptors.
- **Full Agonist**: Maximum efficacy
- **Inverse Agonist**: Binds to the same receptor as an agonist but induces a response opposite to that agonist. An agonist increases the activity of a receptor above its base level and an inverse agonist decreases the activity of a receptor below the base level.
- **Efficacy**: **Vmax.** Maximum effect a drug can produce.
- **Potency (Km).** Amount of drug needed to achieve a given effect.
- **Permissive Effect (AKA: Synergy, Potentiate, Enhance**). When the presence of a 2nd drug is required in order for the first drug to achieve its full effect.
- **Synergistic:** When the effect of both drugs together is greater than what their individual effects are. (Example: Aspirin and Clopidogrel).
- **Adjuvant therapy**: (used with chemotherapy) any treatment given after primary therapy to increase the chance of long term survival.
- **Additive**: When the total effect of two drugs used together is the same as adding the individual effect of each drug together.
- **Tachyphylactic**: The acute decrease in the response of a drug after its initial or repeated administration.
- Antagonism: Shifts curve to the right.
- The most important thing is that efficacy is achieved.

Km and Vmax

Km: AKA: Potency
Km is inversely related to affinity
Km is the "X" axis
The amount of drug needed to get the desired effect
Vmax: AKA: Efficacy
Vmax is the "Y" axis
How effective the drug is. Does not depend on the dose to achieve maximum effect.

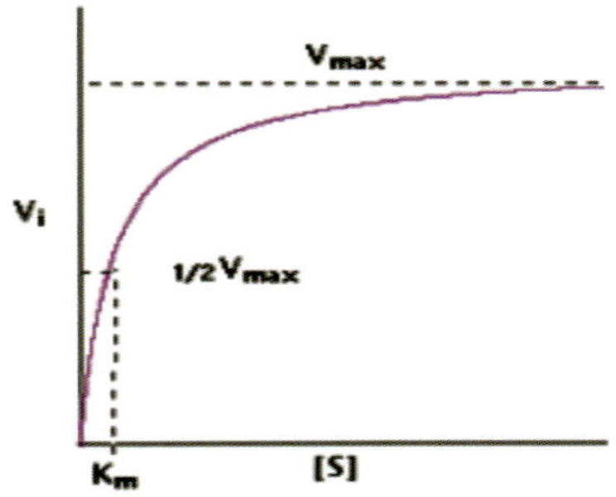

V_i = initial velocity (moles/time)
[S] = substrate concentration (molar)
V_{max} = maximum velocity
K_m = substrate concentration when V_i is one-half V_{max} (Michaelis-Menton constant)

RULES of Km and Vmax

	Competitive	Non-Comp
Km	↑	------
Vmax	-------	↓

Km and Vmax Examples

- If lines cross (not parallel), drugs work on different receptors so can't compare affinity
- If lines do not cross (are parallel), drugs work on same receptor so the affinity (potency) can be compared
- A is higher potency (Km) than B or C
- B is higher potency (Km) than C
- B is higher efficacy (Vmax) than A or C
- A and B will cross so can't compare the drugs
- A > B in potency in low doses
- B > A in potency in higher doses
- A and C are partial so have the same efficacy
- B has full efficacy
- C is less potent and has less efficacy than A or B

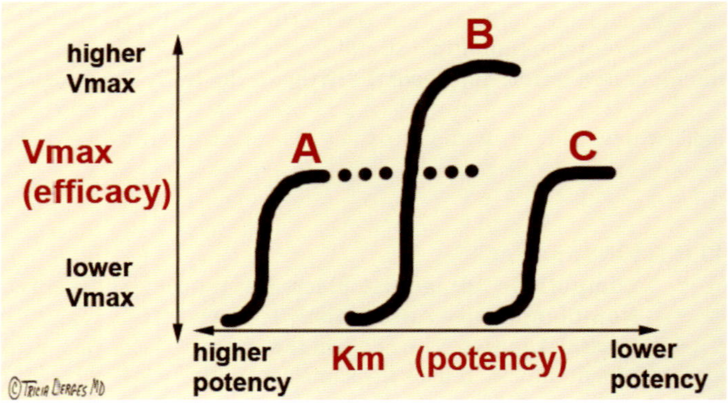

Examples of Drugs:

- High efficacy drugs: **Analgesics, antibiotics, antihistamines, anti-congestive**
- High potency drugs: **Chemo, anti-hypertensive, anti-lipids (cholesterol)**
- Non-competitive drugs: **Digoxin, allopurinol, PPI, aspirin, phenoxybenzamine**

Lineweaver-Burk Plot

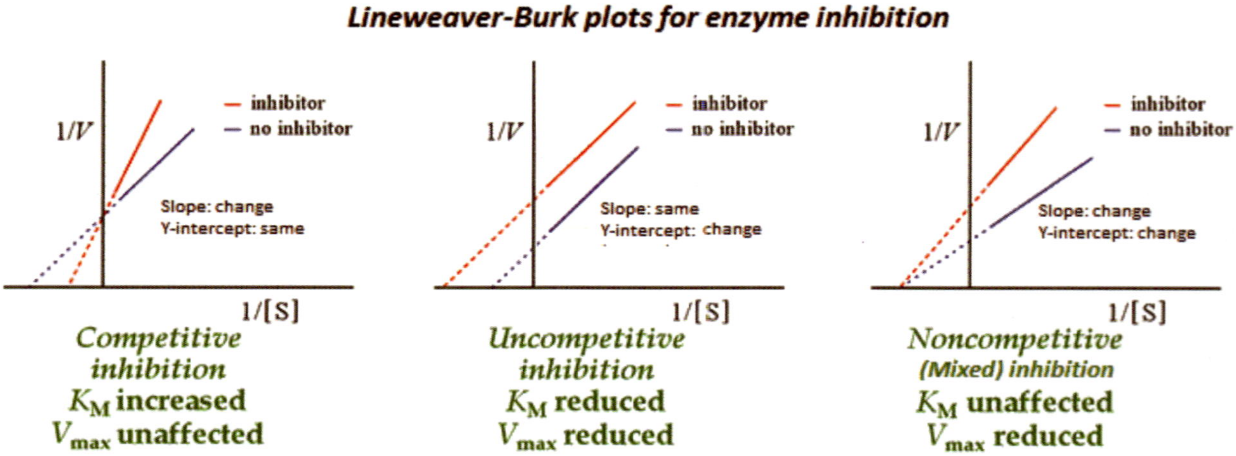

How to read this plot: **REFER TO THE CHART "RULES of Km and Vmax" at the beginning of this section.**

- Remember: the "Y" axis is Vmax, the "X" axis is Km
- Look at the 3rd image. BOTH lines (red and blue) start at the SAME location on the "X" axis (Km) therefore, **Km did NOT change**. If you look at the "RULES of Km and Vmax", find the column where Km does NOT change. You will note that this is in the NON-COMPETITIVE column. Therefore, the new red line (drug) added is a NON-COMPETITIVE drug.
- Look at the 1st image. The new red line does NOT start at the same location on the Km line. The new red line starts at a different location, therefore **Km has now CHANGED**. Look at the "RULES of Km and Vmax" and find the column where Km CHANGES. You will note that this is in the COMPETITIVE column. Therefore, the new red line is a COMPETITIVE inhibitor.
- Then for the final answer, because these are 1/v (fractions) you must remember to make your answer into a fraction, meaning put a "1" over your answer!
- Note in the center image, the lines are parallel, they do not cross. So there is no inhibitor or non-inhibitor.

Synergism and Permissiveness

- Synergism (multiple stimuli, more than additive)
- Permissiveness (needs a second hormone to get full expression)
- Antagonism (opposes. Ie: glucagon opposes insulin)

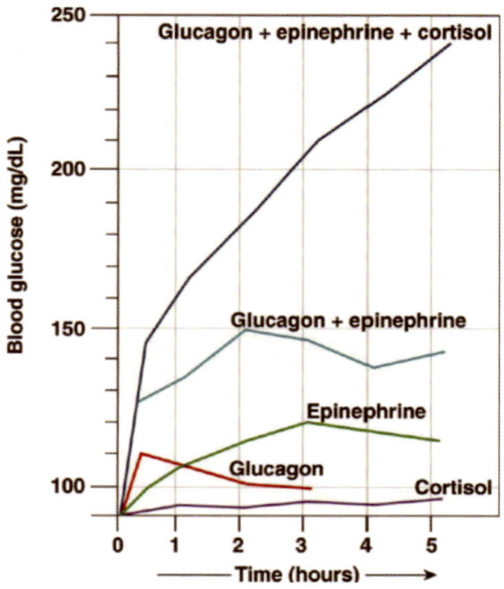

Pharmacology P-450 Interactions

- Note: anytime a question mentions that a patient has been on a drug for a while and has been properly responding, THIS is NEVER the problem. Always look for what is ADDED into the question. THIS is what will be the cause of the new side effects now presenting. If the "new" addition is a drug, check to see if it is a P-450. If a patient is on a statin and the "new" addition is red urine (myoglobin) look for a new strenuous activity the patient has begun (pushing their muscles: ie: training for a marathon, increased weight lifting – anything that is pushing muscles more and then look for the new drug added to be a P-450 inhibitor. (Usually a fibrin).
  (If someone has pushed their muscles and myoglobin is presenting, but the patient is not on any medications: remember to check for other clues that could point to McArdle's).
- It is critical to be aware of all drugs a patient is on. A P-450 inhibitor is MCC for toxicity. If a patient is on a P-450 inhibitor, all other drugs will not be cleared normally and will build up. This is especially dangerous if the patient is on a drug that has a narrow therapeutic margin (esp: **warfarin = building up = ↑ bleeding**) or a drug that had major side effects (ie: **statin** = muscle damage).
- If the drug is a P-450 inducer, it means that any other drugs the patient is on is being cleared quickly, so the original drug will not be working as well. The main drugs that this would affect would be: OCP's (patient could become pregnant), warfarin (PT/INR is ↓ so clots can be formed). Look for someone that has A-fib (irregularly irregular rate) that has been well controlled with warfarin and now present with signs of a stroke. This is due to clots being made due to ineffective warfarin. This can also be seen with other drugs. This would present as no improvement in the patient's condition despite therapy because the therapeutic drug is being cleared out of the system (therefore not being allowed to work) because of an inducer P-450 drug.

P-450 Inhibitors: **Causes other drugs to build up = toxicity.**	**P-450 Inducers:** **Clears other drugs so they do not work.**
Acute Alcohol abuse	Chronic Alcohol
Fibrates (Gemfibrozil)	Modafinil
Ciprofloxacin	St. John's wort
Isoniazid	Phenytoin
Grapefruit Juice	Phenobarbital
Quinidine	Nevirapine
Amiodarone	Rifampin
Ketoconazole	**Griseofulvin**
Erythromycin (Macrolides: except Azithromycin)	Carbamazepine
Sulfonamides	
Cimetidine	
Ritonavir	

P-450 Substrates: Warfarin, Theophylline, Birth Control (OCP's), Anti-epileptics (These drugs can become a problem with either inducers or inhibitors)

Zero Order and First Order Elimination and First Pass Metabolism

Zero Order Elimination

- A constant amount of drug is eliminated per unit of time – elimination rate is **CONSTANT.**
- Drug decreases LINEARLY with time.
- Rate of elimination is independent of the drug. Elimination rate does not increase as drug concentration increases.
- No true half-life.
- Zero Order Drugs: **Aspirin, Phenytoin, Ethanol** (tip: an APE has zero tolerance)

First Order Elimination

- A proportional amount of drug is eliminated per unit of time. Drug concentration is directly **proportional** to the dose.
- Drug decreases **EXPONENTIALLY with time**.
- Half life is constant regardless of time
- Elimination rate increases as drug concentration increases.

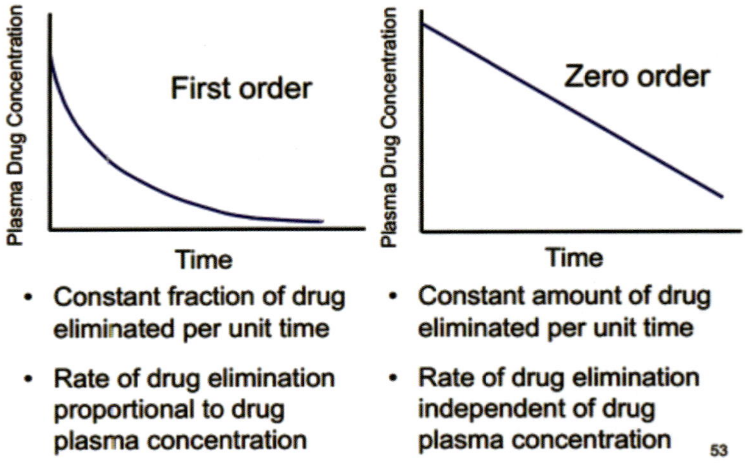
Plasma Drug Concentration
First order
Time
• Constant fraction of drug eliminated per unit time
• Rate of drug elimination proportional to drug plasma concentration
Plasma Drug Concentration
Zero order
Time
• Constant amount of drug eliminated per unit time
• Rate of drug elimination independent of drug plasma concentration
53

Zero order constantly goes straight to zero.
First order has to stop along the way.

First Order Drug Metabolism

A = First Order
B = Metabolism switches to zero order
C = Constant amount of drug is metabolized per unit of time (zero order) = steady state

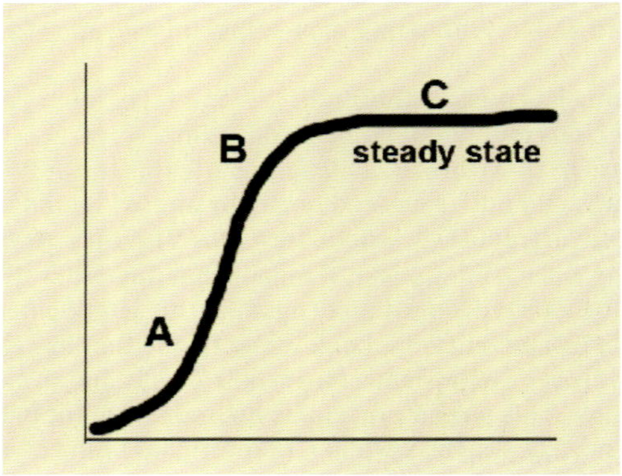
C
B
steady state
A

Drug Metabolism

Phase	Description	Notes
Phase I	Oxidation, reduction, hydrolysis via P-450 system (zone 3 of the liver).	Elderly patients lose phase I first.
Phase II	Conjugation (AKA: Methylation, Glucuronidation, Acetylation, Sulfation).	Elderly patients become **"slow acetylators"** which causes them increased risk

First Pass Metabolism

- The concentration of a drug is greatly reduced before it reaches the systemic circulation. Part of the drug lost is **due to the absorption in the liver** and gut wall, therefore the bioavailability is reduced.
- Path of the drug: Swallowed = absorbed by the digestive system = enters portal system = liver = then finally reaches the rest of the body.
- Routes of drug administration that avoid the first pass metabolism of the liver: IV, intramuscular, sublingual and suppository.

Bioavailability: Amount of drug that reaches the systemic circulation unchanged.

- IV drugs bioavailability is 100%
- Oral drugs bioavailability is dependent on first pass metabolism and amounts not absorbed.
- Oral drugs have a **decreased bioavailability due to first pass metabolism in the liver.**
- Factors that affect bioavailability: poor hepatic or renal function, interactions with other drugs or foods, if the drug was administered in the fed or fasting state, solubility of the drug, health of the GI tract.
- As the drug spreads throughout the body the plasma concentration falls

Acetylation: How quickly the drug is metabolized. CAUTION: Elderly, individuals with renal and/or liver impairment, neonates or individuals with enzyme inhibitions are SLOW ACETYLATORS (AKA: low clearance, increased volume of Distribution) so the dose of their drugs may need to be reduced!
ADDITIONAL NOTE: Deacetylation means: STOPS. This term can be used as an AKA for methylation.

DRUGS THAT DO DECREASE MORTALITY – MUST KNOW!!!!

- **Aspirin (decreases MI mortality 50%)**
- **Beta Blockers**
- **Ace Inhibitors (ARB's)**
- **Spironolactone**

Drug Absorption/Metabolism

Water Soluble drugs (AKA: hydrophilic, polar)

- Readily excretable by the kidney
- Methyl groups are added to some drugs (ie: penicillin) to increase their potency because they are excreted so quickly
- Larger molecules so penetrates membranes more slowly
- More **difficult to absorb** and are not retained in the body very long
- High plasma albumin binding capabilities
- **Ionized** (high rates of ionization)
- **Polar**
- **Charged**
- **↓ Volume of distribution**
- Polar substances will mix with polar substances but not mix with non-polar substances
- Example: Water, alcohol

Fat Soluble drugs (AKA: hydrophobic, lipophilic, non-polar).

- Hydrophobic molecules in water stick together in micelles
- Nonpolar drugs can **easily pass through cell membranes** (plasma membrane is a lipid bilayer)
- Absorbed easier and are retained in the body longer
- Low plasma albumin binding capabilities
- **Non-ionized** (low rates of ionization)
- **Non-polar**
- **Uncharged**
- **↑ Volume of distribution**
- Small molecules so that it penetrates membranes more rapidly
- Can **cross the blood-brain barrier**
- Example: Oil, most gases, hydrocarbons
- ↑ Bioavailability
- **(tip**: fat is a negative word, so notice that all words sound negative: "**non**-ionized, **non**-polar, **Un**charged")

Ionized molecules = charged = polar = water-soluble = difficult to cross membranes.

Non-Ionized molecules = uncharged = non-polar = easily crosses membranes = ↑ volume of distribution.
Non-ionized form is what is useable, the rest is excreted.

Henderson-Hesselbach

$$pH = pK_a + \log\left(\frac{[\text{base}]}{[\text{acid}]}\right)$$

$$pH = pK_a + \log(1)$$
$$pH = pK_a$$

Relates the pKa of a buffered solution to the relative amount of an acid and its conjugate base.
Acid: More acid = more drug is used to ↓ pH. (Start neutral and become charged when they dissociate)
Acids want to give away (dissociate) their H+.

- Weak acid: pH 4 – 7
- Strong acid: ph 2 – 3
- Acids like acids

Base: More basic = more drug is used to ↑ pH. (Start charged and become neutral when they dissociate)
Bases want to keep/take their H+.

- Weak base: pH 7 - 9
- Strong base: pH >10
- Bases like bases

The non-ionized form is what is usable, all else is excreted.

To determine what is ionized (excreted) and non-ionized (usable - bioavailable)

Note: that at 50% the pKa and pH are equal.

1) If you put a weak acid (pKa value given) in a more acidic environment it acts more basic so will keep its H+ = non-ionized/neutral/not charged/high volume distribution/usable (bioavailable).
(EX: Given a pKa of 5 and a pH of 3. The difference is -2, which means that 99% is usable (bioavailable) and 1% is excreted).
(EX: Given a pKa of 5 and a pH of 4. The difference is -1, which means that 90% is usable (bioavailable) and 10% is excreted).

2) If you put an acid (pKa value given) in a basic environment it acts like an acid, so it gives the H+ away (AKA: dissociates) = ionized/charged/excreted.
(EX: Given a pKa of 5 and a pH of 7. The difference is +2 which means that 99% is excreted and 1% is usable (bioavailable).
(EX: Given a pKa of 5 and a pH of 6. The difference is +1 which means that 90% is excreted and 10% is usable (bioavailable).

3) If you put a base (pKa value given) into an acidic environment it acts like a base and keeps its H+ = ionized/charged/excreted.
(EX: Given a pKa of 7 and a pH of 5. The difference is -2 which means that 1% is usable (bioavailable) and 99% is excreted).
(EX: Given a pKa of 7 and a pH of 6. The difference is -1 which means that 10% is usable (bioavailable) and 90% is excreted).

4) If you put a weak base (pKa value given) into a strong base environment it acts more acidic so the weaker base gives its H+ to the stronger base so that it keeps the H+ = it is non-ionized/neutral/not charged/high volume distribution/usable.
(EX: Given a pKa of 5 and a pH of 7. The difference is +2 which means that 99% is usable (bioavailable) and 1% is excreted).
(EX: Given a pKa of 5 and a pH of 6. The difference is a +1 which means that 90% is usable (bioavailable) and 10% is excreted).

Bottom line: To keep this simple:

If you put an acid into an acid: It is non-ionized/usable. (means it keeps the larger % and excretes the smallest % number).
If you put an acid into a base: It is ionized/excreted. (it dissociates) (means it excretes the larger % number and keeps the smallest % number).
If you put a base into an acid: It is ionized/excreted. (it dissociates) (means it excretes the larger % number and keeps the smallest % number).
If you put a base into a base: It is non-ionized/usable. (means it keeps the larger % and excretes the smallest % number).

To keep it simple: If you put a like into a like: it is non-ionized and usable.
(an acid into acid or base into a base)

Difference between pKa and pH. If the difference goes up (pKa of 5 to pH of 7 = +2) If the difference goes down (pKa of 7 to pH of 5 = -2)	**-3**	**-2**	**-1**	**0** **pKa = pH**	**1**	**2**	**3**
Result of the H+ ions. (Use the % that corresponds to the above difference. EX: If the pKa is 5 and the pH is 7 there is a +2 difference. Go to the +2 column and use the % shown in the box below, which would be 99% in this case).	**<1%**	**1%**	**10%**	**50%**	**90%**	**99%**	**>99%**

PH Levels in the Body

- **Blood** = 7.4
- Small Intestine = 8
- Stomach = 1 to 3
- **Vagina = 3.8 – 4.5**
- Semen: 7.2 – 7.8
- Urine = 6.0
- CSF = 7.5
- Pancreas secretions = 8.1
- Saliva (mouth) = 6.5 – 7.5

Protein Binding of Drugs

- Acidic drugs bind to serum albumin.
- Bound drugs are unavailable. They must be unbound from the protein to be cleared.

Drug Absorption Methods

- Passive Diffusion: Crossing a cell membrane from a region of high concentrations (ie: GI fluids) to region of low concentration (ie: blood). It is directly proportional to the gradient but depends on the molecules lipid solubility, size, degree of ionization and the area of absorptive surface. No ATP (energy) required.
- Facilitated Passive Diffusion (Carrier mediated): Carrier molecule in the membrane binds with the molecule (substrate) on the outside of the cell and the carrier/substrate complex diffuses across the membrane. The availablity of the carriers limits the process. No ATP (energy) required
- Active Transport: Requires ATP (energy). Energy allows it to transport against a concentration gradient.
- Pinocytosis: Fluids or particles are engulfed by the cell. The cell membrane invaginates and encloses the fluid or particle and moves it into the cell interior. ATP (energy) is required.

Drug Administration

- Enteral: Through or within the intestine or GI tract
- Parenteral: Not in or through the digestive system.
  IV (Intravascular): directly into blood stream.
  IM (Intramuscular): drug injected into skeletal muscle.
  Subcutaneous: Absorption of drug from the subcutaneous tissues (under the skin, beneath the epidermis and dermis).
- Inhalation: Absorption through the lungs.
- PO (Oral): Mouth
- Sublingual: Under the tongue
- Suppositories: Rectal and Vaginal
- Transdermal: Patch
- **Intraosseous: Injection directly into the marrow of the bone. This is used in PEDIATRIC EMERGENCIES when IV access cannot be obtained. It can be maintained for 24 – 48 hours until another route can be obtained.**
- **Intrathecal: Injection into the spinal canal. (ie: spinal anaesthesia, chemotherapy, pain management)**

Prescriptions

Abbreviation	Abbreviation	Abbreviation	Abbreviation
q = every (once)	**cf = with food**	tab = tablet	O.D. = in the right eye
q.h. = every hour	a.c. = before meals	nebul = spray	O.S. = in the left eye
q.d. = every day	p.c. = after meals	syr = syrup	O.U. = in both eyes
q.o.d. = every other day	**p.o. = by mouth**	ung = ointment	A.U. = in both ears
b.i.d. = twice daily	supp = suppository	susp = suspension	A.S. = in the left ear
t.i.d. = three times daily	vag = vaginally	T.P.N. = total parenteral nutrition	A.D. = in the right ear
q.i.d. = four times daily	SL = sublingually	tsp = teaspoon	T = One
q.4h = every four hours	SC = subcutaneous	tbsp = tablespoon	TT = Two
q.6h = every six hours	Rectally = rectally	qtt = drop/s	TTT = Three
q.h.s. = at bedtime	I.M. = Intramuscularly	oz = ounce	TTTT = Four
prn = as needed	I.V. = Intravenous	a.m. = morning, before noon	Y.O. = year old
w = with	top. = Topical	p.m. = evening or afternoon	X = times
w/o = without	Disp. = dispense #___ and spell out the #		d/c = discontinue/discharge

A prescription should contain: Name, address, telephone, DEA of prescriber, date, generic name of the drug, strength of the drug, dosage form and route of administration and frequency to be taken, total amount of the drug, special instructions (ie: take with food, don't take with alcohol, refrigerate, shake before taking, etc), warnings, refill number (if no refills: then write out "none" or ⊘), reason for drug (diagnosis), name, address, birthdate of patient and the signature of the prescriber.

Example: If you write a prescription for Colace 100mg and you want the patient to take 1 tablet at bedtime and you want 30 pills to be dispensed with no refills:
Write: Colace 100mg 1 tab PO qhs, Disp #30 (thirty), Refills: none or ⊘

Example: If you write a prescription for Zofran 4mg and you want it to be taken by mouth every 4 hours as needed for nausea and you want 15 tablets to be dispensed with 1 refill:
Write: Zofran 4 mg, PO q.4h prn, Disp #15 (fifteen), Refills: one

Sympathomimetic Reactions

It is common to have one of these charts on your exam. Be sure to follow the instructions in the beginning of the book where it explains how to answer charts and graphs. Only answer one section at a time.
Take the first segment and determine what happened to the body (increase/decreased heart rate or BP) and then look at all of the first drugs listed in the answer choices and determine which one(s) would cause the reaction that occurred in the first segment. Then cross off ALL of the other drugs that do NOT elicit this reaction. That will get rid of at least half of the answer choices.
Then move to the last segment of the chart and see what changed in the body (increase/decreased heart rate or BP) after the administration of the 2nd drug. Now look at the 2nd drugs listed in ONLY the answer choices that you have not marked off. You will find that only ONE of the remaining 2nd drugs listed will cause the change that occurred.

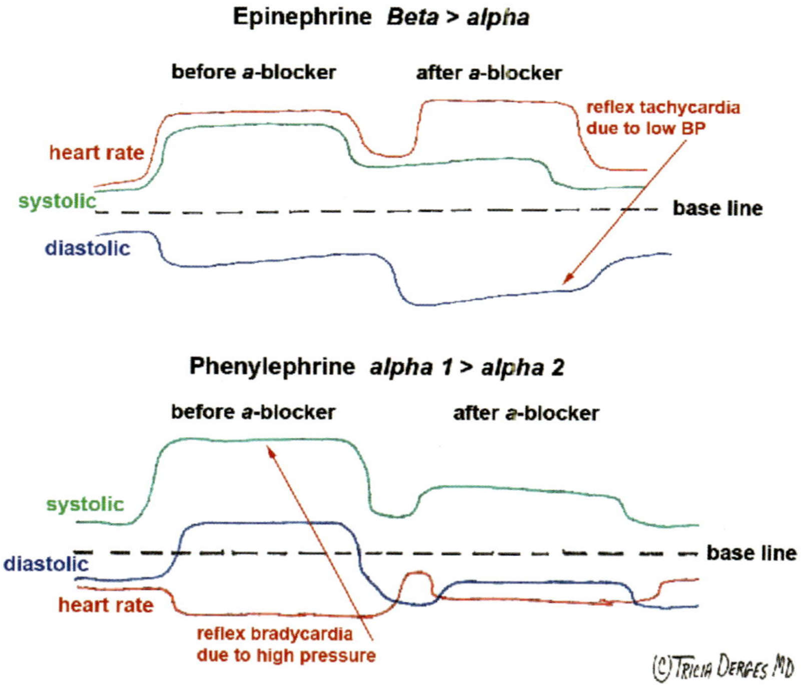

First segment:
Bodies reaction (BP and HR) to the first drug given.

Second segment:
Bodies reaction (BP and HR) to the second drug given.

Example of body response based on drug administration: (Take each drug and determine its MOA)
Given: Labetalol: will ↓ heart rate.
Given: Epinephrine: will ↑ peripheral resistance.

Pharmacology Equations

Vd = Volume of Distribution: distribution of a drug between plasma and the rest of the body after oral or parenteral dosing.
CL = Clearance: Rate at which dugs are cleared from the blood

- **Vd** = Amt of Drug in Body / Amt of Drug in Plasma

- **CL** = Rate of Elimination (AKA: Flow) / Amt of Drug in Plasma

- **Loading Dose: Desired Dose x Vd**
  Loading doses are larger than normal doses given at the beginning of treatment to rapidly increase the plasma concentration

- **Maintenance Dose: Desired Dose x CL**

- **Half Life (time to steady state) = .7 x Vd / CL**

  (Quick Method to Calculate Half Life)
  You can also multiple the half life given by 4. It takes between 4 and 5 half lives to get to steady state.
  Example: If drug has a half life of 4 hours: multiply that half life (4 hours) by 4 = 16 hours to steady state. Keep in mind, some people (test writers) may multiply the half life by 5 = 20 hours (they can use either 4 or 5). So look for the answer to be anywhere between 4 and 5 (16 and 20 hours). There will never be two answers within this range. The answer within this range is the answer.

  Half Life is directly proportional to Vd (high ½ life = high Vd)
  Half Life is inversely proportional to CL (high ½ life = low CL)

- **TI (Therapeutic Index): Lethal Dose / Effective Dose**

  Safe drugs have a higher TI
  Drugs with a low TI must be monitored closely! They can become toxic quickly.
  Drugs with a low TI: **Digoxin, warfarin (Coumadin), lithium, and theophylline.**

- **Bioavailability:** AUC po / AUC iv (AUC = **Area Under the Curve**)
  Bioavailability is the AUC po (oral). The AUC is the oral dose given which determines bioavailability. Since IV administration is always 100% there is nothing to determine. So if you are asked about bioavailability, it is the determination of the oral drug given which is represented by the curve under the IV line.

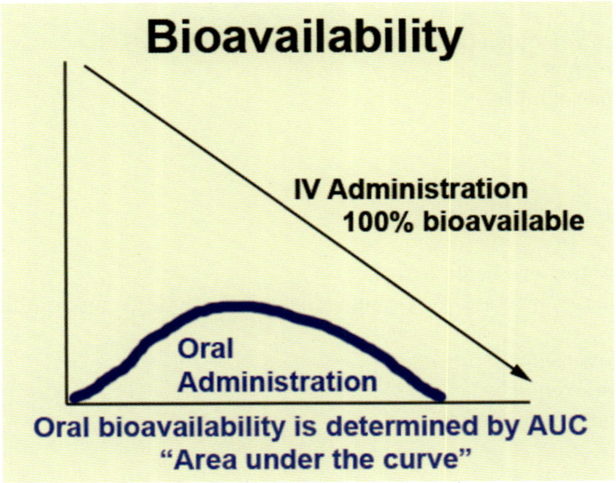

EMBRYOLOGY

Organ Morphogenesis
Malformation: Primary defect in cell that forms an organ (ie: congenital heart DZ)
Deformation: Abnormal structure due to external force (club feet, Potters, hip)
Disruption: Secondary breakdown of normal tissue (amniotic bands: amniocentesis if before 9 weeks, best at 16 wks)
Sequence: # of abnormalities from a single defect (Potters)
Syndrome: group of developmental abnormalities pathologically related (ie: Turners)
Agenesis: Absence of an organ (renal agenesis)
Hypoplasia: Incomplete organ development (lung hypoplasia)
Aplasia: Absent organ

Surfactant: Fetal Lung Maturation: L/S Ration 2:1
- **Lecithin (AKA: Phosphatidylcholine) to Sphingomyelin**
- **Fetus lungs mature after 34 weeks**
- Steroids given prior to 34 weeks to mature lungs (causes stress = release surfactant)
  Betamethasone, Dexamethasone
  Decrease Respiratory Distress Syndrome (AKA: RDS, Hyaline Membrane Disease)
- **Surfactant produced by Type II Pneumocytes in the lungs**
- **Surfactant decreases the surface tension of the lungs**

Embryogenesis

KEY PHYSIO
- Placenta: Cytotrophoblast and Syncytiotrophoblast
- Trophoblast: outer cells of the blastocyst providing nutrients to embryo: first cells to differentiate from the fertilized egg: develop into placenta
- **Syncytiotrophoblast: Synthesizes and secretes HCG. Stimulates corpus luteum to secrete progesterone during the first trimester. Lacks MHC-1 expression so there is a decreased risk of attack from the maternal immune system.**
- Cytotrophoblast: Inner layer of chorionic villi
- Decidua Basalis (from endometrium) becomes the maternal part of the placenta. Interacts with trophoblast (outer cells of the blastocyst and provides nutrition to embryo) and is under influence of progesterone
- **B-hcG produced by syncytiotrophoblast** (part of the placenta), has alpha and beta sub units. Alpha subunits are **same as** in LH, FSH and TSH. Beta subunit is used for pregnancy test (it is exclusive to pregnancy).
  B-hcG maintains the corpus luteum in the beginning of pregnancy (corpus luteum secretes progesterone in the first trimester) until the placenta takes over.
  B-hcG can be detected in the urine 2 weeks after implantation.
  B-hcG levels double every 2 days in normal pregnancy until 16 weeks. **High levels of B-HCG after 16 weeks** can mean a molar pregnancy.

Genes
- Homeobox (HOX) Gene: Organization of appendages/organs in proper location (cranial to caudal). If mutated: appendages/organs are in the wrong place.
- Hedgehog gene: produced at the base of limbs

Fetal Landmarks
- Day 0 = Fertilization (zygote)
- 1 week: B-HCG secretion begins after blastocyst implants
- 17 days: Notochord forms
- 3 weeks: Neural plate, mesoderm notochord begin to form
- 3 – 8 weeks: Neural tube formed (closes by week 4). Organogenesis, EXTREMELY susceptible to teratogens. Give folate to help prevent neural tube defects.
- 4 weeks: **Heart beats**, upper and lower limbs forming
- 8 weeks: **Fetal movement** (aka: quickening)
- 10 weeks: Genitalia have male/female characteristics

Placenta
- **Decidua basalis** (aka: maternal part of the placenta)
  - Derived from the endometrium.
  - Contains the maternal artery and maternal vein.
  - Maternal circulation provides the fetus with: Oxygen, nutrients, hormones, IgG, electrolytes and any pathologies that would come from drugs, bacteria, viruses, crossing over to the fetus.
  - Under the influence of progesterone.

Placenta cont'd

- Cytotrophoblast (fetal part of the placenta): Inner later of chorionic villi.
- Syncytiotrophoblast (fetal part of the placenta): Outer layer of the chorionic villi. **Synthesizes and secretes HCG. HCG maintains the corpus luteum during the first trimester until the placenta takes over.** Stimulates corpus luteum to secrete progesterone during the first trimester. Lacks MHC-1 expression so there is a decreased risk of attack from the maternal immune system.

Umbilical Cord

- One umbilical vein that supplies oxygenated blood to the fetus. **This is the location of the highest oxygen content in the fetal blood supply. Note: the remnant of the umbilical vein is the falciform ligament.**
- Two umbilical arteries that carry away waste products, urea, CO_2 and hormones from the baby and send back into the maternal circulation.
- Allantoic duct: duct of extra embryonic membrane that helps the embryo exchange gasses and other materials with the uterus.
- **Wharton's' jelly:** gelatinous substance in the umbilical cord (same substance is in the vitreous humor of the eye). It protects and insulates the umbilical blood vessels.

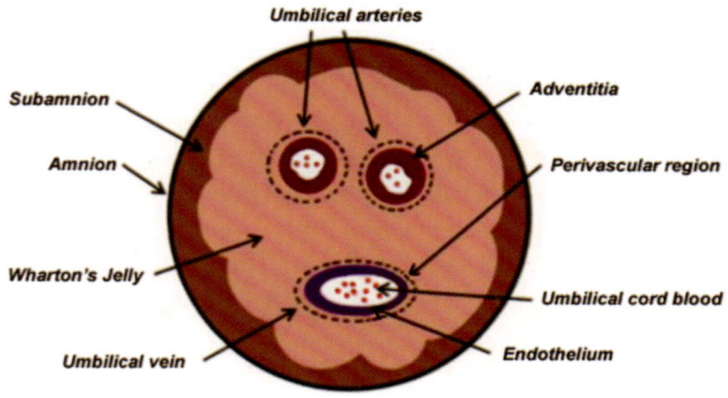

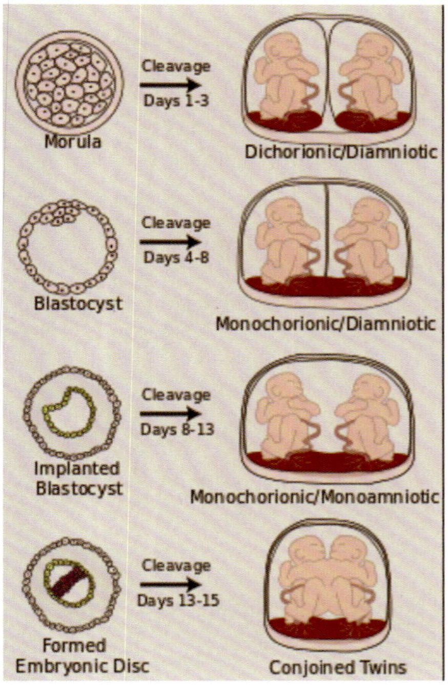

Twins

Monozygotic: 1 egg, 1 sperm

- Same Sex: Genetically IDENTICAL
- Monochromic (1 placenta) with Diamniotic (2 sacs) or monoamniotic (1 sac)

Dizygotic: 2 eggs, 2 sperms

- Can be different sexes or same, but NOT identical
- Dichromic (2 placentas) or Monochromic (1 placenta) with Diamnionic (2 sacs)

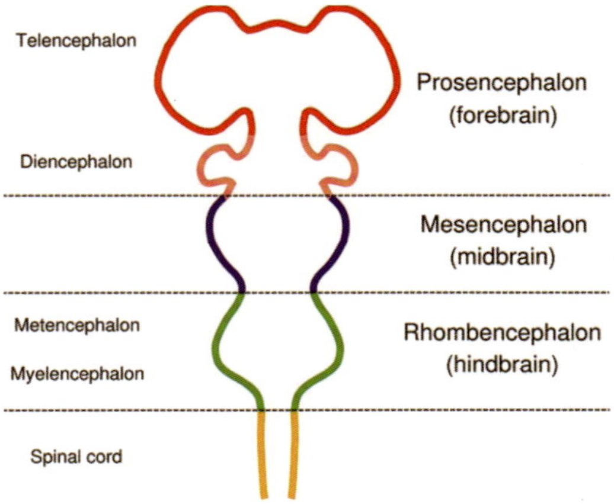

Neural Development

- Notochord differentiates into neuroectoderm and forms neural plate
- Notochord formed on day 17 of embryonic life
- Neural plate forms neural tube and neural crest
- **Notochord** becomes **nucleus pulposus** in the intervertebral disk

Fetal Layers

Endoderm layer becomes:

- Digestive system, Liver, Pancreas, Lungs (inner layers)
  (GI and tube above the pectinate line, liver, lungs, pancreas, thymus, thyroid follicular cells, parathyroid, bladder, urethra, serous linings of body cavity)

Mesoderm layer becomes:

- Circulatory system, Lungs (epithelial layers), Skeletal system, Muscular system
  (muscles, connective tissue, bone, cartilage, blood, lymph, spleen (from foregut), adrenal cortex, kidney and ureter, skin, INTERNAL genitalia: ovaries, testes, vagina)

Ectoderm layer becomes 3 Layers

- **Surface**
  Anterior Pituitary (AKA: Adenohypophysis from Rathke's Pouch). Roof of mouth.
  (NOTE: If there is pathology with the pituitary and the vignette brings it into the embryo category: this is the location: it is due to a diverticulum of the roof of the mouth in the embryonic oral cavity).
  Where **Craniopharyngioma occurs with cholesterol crystals)**, lens, sensory of smell and hearing,
  glands: sweat, mammary, salivary, anal below pectinate line, hard palate, bitemporal hemianopsia.
- **Neural Tube**
  CNS and brain, **posterior pituitary (AKA: Neurohypophysis)**, retina, CNS neurons, oligodendrocytes, astrocytes, spinal cord
- **Neural Crest**
  ANS, cranial nerves, melanocytes, chromaffin cells of adrenal medulla, parafollicular cells of the thyroid, melanocytes, larynx, Schwann cells, pia and arachnoid skull, cranial nerves, odontoblast, aorticopulmonary septum (SPIRALING): Transposition of Great Vessels, Tetralogy of Fallot, Truncus Arteriosis and Migration in Hirschsprung, S-100 markers.

Neural CREST (crown) Queen

Think of: big heart (spiraling congenital heart issues), pair of CATS, (Catecholamines of chromaffin cells in adrenals), para SWANS (Schwann cells), para FOALS (Thyroid Follicular cells), Singing (larynx), Teeth (Odontoblast), Thick skull (skull: pia, arachnoid, cranial nerves), tan (melanocytes), S-100 markers, Guts (Hirschsprung's).

The Neural Crest Queen

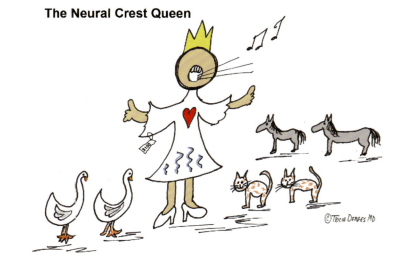

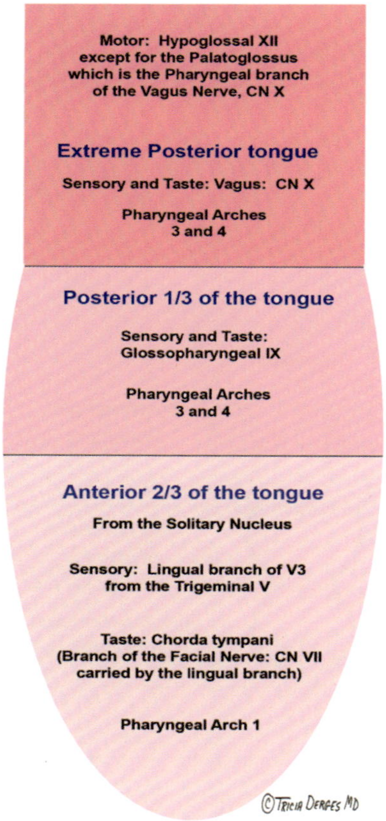

Tongue Development

- Anterior 2/3: 1st and 2nd brachial arches
- Posterior 1/3: 3rd and 4th brachial arches

Taste Development: From the **Solitary Nucleus**

- **Anterior 2/3: CN VII (AKA: Chorda tympani, Facial nerve**
- Posterior 1/3: CN IX
- Very Back (extreme posterior): CNX

Sensory Development

- Anterior 2/3: CN V3
- Posterior 1/3: CN IX
- Very Back (extreme posterior): CNX

Motor Development

- CN XII
- Muscles are from the occipital myotomes

Sweet vs Bitter

- Sweet taste receptors are controlled by CN VII on the anterior 2/3 of the tongue
- Bitter taste receptors are controlled by CN IX and X on the posterior of the tongue

(This is why there is a bitter taste in the mouth in the morning when one suffers from GERD)

CONGENITAL and NEONATAL
Embryology, Pathologies

Neural Congenital and Developmental Pathologies

Anencephaly

- Malformation of anterior neural tube = no forebrain
- High AFP
- Polyhydramnios due to absence of swallowing center of brain
- Higher risk with maternal diabetes type I
  Decrease risk by supplementing folate

Holoprosencephaly

- Failure of brain hemispheres to separate
- Mutations of hedgehog gene
- SX: Cleft lip, cleft palate or cyclopia (one eye)

Posterior Fossa Malformations
Arnold-Chiari Malformation (AKA: Chiari II)

- **Herniation** of cerebellar vermis and tonsils through foramen magnum
- Aqueduct stenosis
- Hydrocephalus
- Myelomeningocele and paralysis

Dandy Walker

- Agenesis of cerebellar vermis
- **Enlargement of 4th ventricle**
- Non communicating hydrocephalus and spina bifida
- (**tip:** have a large ventricle to WALK around in)

Neural Tube Defects:

- **#1 Cause of high AFP: DATING ERROR or multiple gestations**
- Amniocentesis shows: **↑ AFP, ↑ AChE-AF (Acetylcholinesterase)**
- **Due to failure to fuse**
- Gastroschisis (intestines NOT covered by peritoneum (**tip**: "gast"ly)
- Omphalocele (intestines covered by peritoneum)
- Spina Bifida Occulta: No herniation: failure of bony spinal canal to close (tuft of hair)
- Meningocele: Meninges herniates through spinal canal
- Meningomyelocele: Meninges and spinal cord herniated
- Anencephaly

Neural Crest Migration Failure

- **Hirschsprung**
- 12th week: **Ganglion cells do not migrate to rectum**
- No **Meissner** (sub mucosal), no **Auerbach** (bowel wall) Plexus
- Biopsy shows no ganglion cells
- Higher risk in Downs Syndrome
- Transposition of the Great Vessels: No **SPIRALING of aorticopulmonary septum (AKA: Failure of septation)**

Pituitary Pathologies
NOTE: If there is pathology with the pituitary and the vignette brings it into the embryo category: the location of the origin of this organ is in the **anterior pituitary (AKA: Adenohypophysis from Rathke's Pouch).** It is due to a **diverticulum of the roof of the mouth in the embryonic oral cavity.**

DERIVATIVES of the PHARYNGEAL ARCHES

ARCH	BRANCHIAL POUCH (Endoderm)	SKELETAL (Mesoderm and Neural Crest)	AORTIC ARCH (Mesoderm)	MUSCLES (Mesoderm)	CRANIAL NERVE (Neural Tube)	Cleft
1 Mandibular	Ear (Middle ear, Eustachian tube)	Incus, malleus, mandible, maxilla, temporal bone, sphenomandibular ligament, sphenomalleolar ligament (**Meckel's** cartilage), zygomaticum	**Maxillary branch** of the carotid artery	Jaw muscles, floor of mouth, soft palate, Muscles of the ear. **Muscles of mastication**. Tensor palatine muscles, **anterior** belly of digastric, mylohyoid, tympani	5	External acoustic meatus
2 Hyoid	Palatine Tonsil	**Stapes** bone of middle ear, **styloid process** of temporal bone, stapedius, hyoid bone of neck, (**Reichert's** cartilage)	Cortico-tympanic artery (adult), **stapedial** artery (embryo), arteries to the ear	Muscles of facial expression, jaw and upper neck muscles, stapedius, Stylohyoid, **posterior** belly of digastric muscle	7	Cervical sinus
3	Thymus, **Inferior** Parathyroids	Lower rim and greater horns of the hyoid bone	**Common carotids, Internal carotid**	Stylopharyngeus (elevates pharynx)	9	Cervical sinus
4	**Superior** Parathyroids, C Cells of Thyroid	Laryngeal cartilages	Arch of the Aorta, Right **Subclavian** Artery	Constrictors of pharynx and vocal cords, larynx, striated muscle of the esophagus	10 **Superior laryngeal** branch of Vagus nerve	Cervical sinus
6		Laryngeal cartilages	**Pulmonary Artery**, Ductus Arteriosus	Intrinsic muscles of the larynx, pharynx, striated muscle of the esophagus, Sternocleidomastoid, Trapezius	10 - XI **Recurrent laryngeal** branch of Vagus nerve, Spinal accessory	

Thyroid

- **Thyroid origin: Foramen cecum**
- **Thyroid is enclosed by the pretracheal fascia**

Heart and Circulation Development

- Truncus Arteriosus: Ascending aorta and pulmonary trunk.
- **Cardinal Veins (of heart): SVC**
- Septum secundum/septum primum: Atrial septum, Foramen Ovale.
- Endocardial cushion separates atria from ventricles (valves), affected in Downs Syndrome.
- **Fetal Erythropoiesis**
  3 – 8 weeks: Yolk Sac; 6 – 30 weeks: liver (main) and spleen (secondary);
  28 weeks to birth: bone marrow
- **Fetal Blood Hb**: 2 alpha, 2 gamma (adult: 2 alpha, 2 beta).
  Hb F = Higher affinity for O2 than mother.
  Hb F = Left shift in Oxy Hb curve.
  Hb F = ↓ 2,3 BPG (2,3 BPG loves to give oxygen away to mothers tissues).
  Hydroxyurea: given to **sickle cell patients to increase Hb F.**
  SE: Pulmonary Fibrosis and bone marrow suppression
- Blood Flow to Fetus: Umbilical Vein (one) via ductus venosus to IVC. Umbilical arteries (two) return deoxygenated blood to mother.
  Highest Oxygen content in fetus: Umbilical Vein
  Oxygenated blood reaching the heart goes through the foramen ovale and pumped out of heart to brain and body.
  Deoxygenated blood from SVC sent to pulmonary artery through Ductus arteriosus to lower body of fetus
- Umbilical Cord: 2 arteries, 1 vein
- **Foramen Ovale (AKA: Fossa Ovalis) closes after birth due to high left atrial pressure and decreased prostaglandins.**
- **Patent Foramen Ovale**: Failure of septum primum and septum secundum to fuse after birth causing ASD. ASD's allow venous emboli to enter arterial circulation. (ASD: Fixed S_2 split)

- Smooth part of the right ventricle is derived from the bulbus cordis
- Truncus arteriosis develops into the proximal pulmonary artery and ascending aorta
- Ostium Primum: Gap between the two embryonic atria
- Septum Primum: Fills the gap (Ostium Primum) between the two embryonic atria
- Endocardial cushion: Cells in the developing heart tube that give rise to the valves and septa
- ASD (Ostium Primum Type ASD): Failure of Septum Primum to fuse. (Defect in the development of the endocardial cushion)
- Failure to form the Septum Secundum results in fetal death. No hole between the atria provides no oxygenation for the fetus
- Valve of the Foramen Ovale is made up of the Septum Ostium (part that does not regress)
- Pathway of development of the Foramen Ovale: Ostium primum closed by Septum primum ➔ Ostium secundum ➔ Septum primum fuses with the endocardial cushions ➔ Septum Secundum develops
- The Septum primum fuses with the endocardial cushions (the Septum secundum does not fuse)

Cardio Pulmonary Embryo Remnants

Embryonic Tissue	Remnant
Umbilical vein	Falciform Ligament (AKA: Ligamentum teres)
Umbilical arteries	Medial umbilical ligament
Ductus arteriosus	Ligamentum arteriosum
Ductus venosus	Ligamentum venosum
Foramen ovale	Fossa ovalis
Septum secundum	Foramen ovale

Cardiac and Pulmonary Congenital and Developmental Pathologies

Congenital Heart Pathologies

Downs Syndrome: ASD, Endocardial Cushion defect of the atrioventricular canal, Intra Atrial Septum
Kartagener's: Situs Inversus
Tuberous Sclerosis: Cardiac rhabdomyoma
DiGeorge: Tetralogy of Fallot, Truncus Arteriosis
Marfan's: Necrosis of Aorta, MVP, Thoracic Aortic Aneurysm, Aortic Dissection, SAH
Fredericks Ataxia: HCM
Neonatal Lupus: Heart Block
Williams: Aortic Stenosis
Lang Neilson: Long QT Syndrome
Edwards: VSD
Congenital Rubella: PDA
Kawasaki: Coronary Artery Aneurysm
Turners: Coarctation of the Aorta, Bicuspid Aortic Valve
Infant of Diabetic Mother: Transposition of Great Arteries

Kartagener Syndrome (AKA: Primary Ciliary Dyskinesia)

- Immotile cilia b/c **dynein arm defect**.
- SX: Infertility, high risk of ectopic pregnancy, recurrent sinusitis, situs inversus (organs reversed to opposite side)

Early cyanosis ("blue babies"), right to left shunt: Must keep the PDA open.

Transposition of the Great Vessels

- Failure of the aorticopulmonary septum to **spiral – neural crest cells**
- Great arteries are reversed: Pulmonary artery leaves the left ventricle, Aorta leaves the right ventricle. Loud, single S2.
- MC in **diabetic mothers**
- **Must maintain PDA** with **Misoprostol** (PGE1) or there is no oxygenation. (So patient must keep a PDA, ASD or VSD)
- Right to left shunt
- Evident immediately after birth, early cyanosis
- TX: Surgery. Incompatible with life. Two surgeries are required, each carries a 50% mortality rate.

Truncus Arteriosus

- **Failure of truncus arteriosus to divide** into aorta and pulmonary
- **VSD**: right to left shunt
- Common in **DiGeorge's** (22:11)
- Evident immediately after birth, early cyanosis
- Right to left shunt
- Must maintain patency of **PDA (Ductus Arteriosus)** – keep PDA's open with **Misoprostol** (decreasing cAMP)

Total Anomalous Pulmonary Venous Return (TAPVR)

- Pulmonary vein drains into right heart circulation (no venous return between pulmonary veins and left atrium)
- 2 forms: with and without obstruction (angle of the veins) of the venous return.
  With obstruction: presents early: respiratory distress/severe cyanosis.
  Without obstruction: presents after 1 year old with right heart failure/tachypnea.
- Must maintain PDA
- Right to left shunt
- Evident immediately after birth, early cyanosis
- TX: Surgical repair

Tricuspid Atresia

- Absent tricuspid valve
- Hypoplastic right ventricle
- ASD and VSD to survive, early cyanosis
- Right to left shunt

Hypoplastic Left Heart Syndrome

- Left side of the heart is severely underdeveloped
- Aorta and left ventricle are underdeveloped, the aortic and mitral valves are either closed or too small to allow for sufficient flow of blood
- PDA must be kept open
- Requires multiple surgeries, carries a high mortality rate

Tetralogy of Fallot

- The most common early cyanotic heart defect in children
- **Degree of Pulmonary Stenosis determines prognosis**
- Right ventricular hypertrophy: x-ray shows **boot shaped heart**
- Overriding aorta
- **VSD** (holosystolic murmur)
  VSD 's are common in the Trisomy's: 13, 18 and 21 (Patau, Edwards, Down's)
- Right to left shunt
- Associated with **chromosome 22** deletions
- CXR show a "boot shaped" heart and decreased pulmonary vascular markings.
  CXR shows decreased pulmonary vascular markings which indicates a decrease in pulmonary blood flow.
- TX: β-Blocker, PGE1 (if there is cyanosis at birth). Surgical repair before 12 months.
- **"TET spells": child squats to improve oxygenation and decrease cyanosis. Squatting increases TPR (AKA: Systemic vascular resistance, PRELOAD) which increases blood flow to the right heart, forcing more blood to go through the stenosed pulmonary valve into the lungs which allows it to get more oxygen, instead of going through the VSD.**

Left to Right Shunts, no cyanosis at birth

Patent Ductus Arteriosus

- Ductus arteriosus: blood vessel connecting pulmonary artery to aorta to bypass the fetus's non-functioning lungs. Closes at birth to become **ligamentum arteriosum**
- PDA murmur: continuous **"machine like" murmur**
- PDA normal in fetus (right to left shunt), closes after birth
- PDA is required in congenital cyanotic heart conditions to sustain life
- Patent PDA is maintained by prostaglandins (PGE), kept open by **Misoprostol** (decreasing cAMP)
- PDA's are closed (ended) by **Indomethacin** (prostaglandin synthetase Inhibitor)

Atrial Septal Defect

- **ASD: Fixed Split S2 murmur, systolic ejection murmur. Heard on left upper sternal border.**
- **Septum secundum**
- **ASD allows venous paradoxical emboli to cross over to the arterial system = arterial clots, strokes**
- **MCC: Failure of fusion of septum primum and secundum**

Ventricle Septal Defect

- Holosystolic (pansystolic) S2 murmur heard at left lower sternal boarder
- Usually closes within 6 months of birth
- Due to a defect in the formation of the intraventricular septum that inhibits complete closure of the intraventricular foramen.
- Most self resolve, otherwise surgical repair if there is a right to left shunt, pulmonary hypertension or failure to thrive

Eisenmenger Syndrome

- Begins with left to right shunt, increasing blood to right ventricle causing right ventricular hypertrophy (RVH)
- Increases pulmonary blood flow
- RVH causes shunt to become right to left causing cyanosis
- Cyanosis leads to polycythemia and clubbing

Coarctation of the Aorta

- Infants: Aorta narrowing proximal (preductal) to ductus arteriosus (closed to heart)
- Adults: Aorta narrowing is distal (postductal) to ligamentum arteriosum
- MC originates from the left subclavian artery
- High association with **Turners Syndrome**
- **Differences in BP** in upper extremities (HTN) and lower extremities (weak)
- X-ray shows **notching of the ribs**

Acyanotic Cardiac Defects

Defect	Description and Treatment
ASD	**Fixed splitting of S2**, Systolic ejection murmur. Heard on left upper sternal border. Patent foramen ovale will allow paradoxical emboli to cross from right to left atria.
VSD	Harsh **holosystolic** (pansystolic). Loud S2, heard over left lower sternal border. Closes within 6 months of birth. Due to defect in the formation of the intraventricular septum. Surgical repair if right to left shunt, pulmonary hypertension or failure to thrive.
Pulmonary stenosis	Determining factor of **severity of Tetralogy of Fallot**. Ranges from asymptomatic to severe. TX: Prostaglandins (PGE1) at birth. Balloon valvuloplasty.
Patent Ductus Arteriosus	Harsh, **continuous "Machinery" murmur**. Wide pulse pressure. Bounding pulses. MCC: Maternal rubella infection. Connects the pulmonary artery and descending aorta in the embryo so that blood bypasses the lungs. TX: Close with Indomethacin or surgical closure.
Atrioventricular Canal	Combination of ASD, VSD and the common atrioventricular valve. TX: Surgery to prevent pulmonary hypertension.
Coarctation of the Aorta	MC location: origin of the left subclavian artery. Blood pressure is higher in the upper body. TX: Prostaglandins (PGE1) to maintain patent ductus

Pulmonary Development

- Breathing in utero: by aspiration and expulsion of amniotic fluid. This causes ↑ vascular resistance.
- Breathing at birth: Fluid is replaced by air. This ↓ vascular resistance.
- Amniotic fluid is required for lung maturation. **Oligohydramnios can cause lung hypoplasia.**

Development Stage	Development Process	Notes
Embryonic Weeks 3 – 6 weeks	Formation of **lung bud.** Differentiation into trachea and bronchi	Errors in the embryonic stage can lead to TE fistulas
Pseudoglandular (Fetal period) Weeks 7 – 17	Branching of the bronchial tree. Formation of the respiratory parenchyma. Beginning of capillaries. **Type II pneumocytes appear**.	It is not possible for the fetus to have any respiratory functions at this stage. It is incompatible with life.
Canalicular (Fetal period) Weeks 17 – 27	Formation of lung periphery and terminal bronchioles. Increased vascularization (capillaries). **Type I pneumocytes appear**. Air-blood interface formed.	Respiration is possible at 25 weeks.
Saccular (Fetal period) Weeks 27 – 36	Formation of alveolar saccules/ducts. Detectable surfactant in amniotic fluid.	
Alveolar (Birth and postnatal) Weeks 36 to 8 years	Formation of mature alveoli/terminal sacs. Proliferation and expansion.	There are 20 – 70 million alveoli at birth. There are 300 – 400 million alveoli by the time a child is 8 years old.

Pneumocytes

- **Type I Pneumocytes: Simple squamous (thin). 97% of alveolar surface). Gas exchange. (AKA: the simple squamous epithelial cells of the alveolar walls). They are very thin to facilitate gas exchange.**
- **Type II pneumocytes (AKA: the greater alveolar cells) large cuboidal type cells: Secrete surfactant (dipalmitoyl phosphatidylcholine) to decrease surface tension of the alveoli. Type II pneumocytes can change into Type I pneumocytes to repair the lung.**

Pulmonary Pathologies

Lung Hypoplasia

- Incomplete development of lungs
- **Oligohydramnios**: amniotic fluid helps to mature lungs
- Congenital Diaphragmatic Hernia. Shows loops of **bowel in the chest**. MC on left side.
  Presents as RDS and scaphoid abdomen.
  TX: Immediate intubation and surgery

Respiratory Distress Syndrome (AKA: RDS, Hyaline Membrane Disease)

- **Surfactant: Fetal Lung Maturation**: L/S Ratio 2:1
- **Lecithin (AKA: Phosphatidylcholine) to Sphingomyelin**
- **Fetus lungs mature after 34 weeks**
- **Steroids given prior to 34 weeks to mature lungs (causes stress = release surfactant)**
  Betamethasone, Dexamethasone
- **Surfactant produced by Type II Pneumocytes in the lungs**
- **Surfactant decreases the surface tension of the lungs**
- SX: Hypoxemia, **Nasal grunting, flaring**, tachypnea, intercostal retraction, hypercarbia and respiratory acidosis.
  NOTE: If hypoxia (diffusion) does not improve with oxygen, the problem is probably cardiac in nature.
- DX: CXR shows ground glass appearance, atelectasis
- **TX: Oxygen and nasal CPAP, Lucinactant (exogenous surfactant administration)**
  NOTE: RDS and pneumonia look the same on CXR (ground glass appearance): give antibiotics

Neonatal Polycythemia

- Due to hypoxic situations (ie: **RDS, respiratory distress**)
  ANY hypoxic situation will stimulate **erythropoietin** in the **peritubular capillary bed (AKA: interstitial fibroblast) in the kidney)**
- High RBC count, high Hb and Hct
- SX: Lethargic, hypotonic, apnea, hypoglycemic
- TX: Partial exchange transfusion and hydration

Bronchogenic Cysts

- Solitary cyst, formed in the 16th week due to an abnormal budding of the tracheal diverticulum.
- Composed of cartilage, smooth muscle, fibrous tissue, and mucous glands. Located in the suprasternal notch or over the manubrium (top part of the sternum).
- SX: due to compression of the cyst: dysphagia, dyspnea, cough, chest pain, chronic infections
- TX: Excision

Meconium Pulmonary Pathologies

Meconium Aspiration

- Occurs in a term or post-term neonate with hypoxia or fetal distress in utero
  (meconium can be aspirated in utero or in the first breath at birth)
- Hypoxemia
- Presents like RDS
- CXR shows: flattening of diaphragm, barrel chest, patchy infiltrates
- Prevention: Airway suction or endotracheal intubation
- TX: Nitric oxide, Positive pressure ventilation, high-frequency ventilation

Meconium Plugs obstruct the lower intestine

- Hirschsprung, maternal drug use, Cystic fibrosis, Idiopathic Onset Diabetes Mellitus (IODM)

Meconium Ileus: obstruction in the ileum

- **Cystic fibrosis**

Meconium DX: Abdominal X-ry
Meconium TX: Gastrografin enema

GI Development and Pathologies

Area of Development	Organs Included	Blood Supply - Notes
Foregut	Pharynx to duodenum. Referred pain: Epigastrium	Celiac artery **(Celiac artery also supplies spleen)**
Midgut	Duodenum to transverse colon. Referred pain: Umbilical	Superior Mesenteric Artery (SMA)
Hindgut	Distal transverse colon to rectum. Referred pain: Hypogastrium	Inferior Mesenteric Artery (IMA)
Spleen	Spleen	Derived from the embryonic dorsal mesentery
Greater Omentum (greater sac)	Greater Omentum. Any rupture of the posterior stomach will drain into the greater sac.	Derived from the embryonic dorsal mesentery
Omental bursa (Lesser sac)	Formed from an infolding of the greater omentum. The open end is the omental foramen and is next to the stomach. Any ruptures of organs around the stomach will leak into the lesser sac (omental bursa).	

	Presynaptic Sympathetics	Sympathetic Ganglion	Postsynaptic Sympathetics	Parasympathetics
Foregut	Thoracic splanchnics (T5-T12)	Celiac ganglion	Celiac plexus	Vagus (Cranial Nerve X)
Midgut	Thoracic splanchnics (T5-T12)	Superior mesenteric ganglion	Superior mesenteric plexus	Vagus (Cranial Nerve X)
Hindgut	Lumbar splanchnics (L1,L2)	Inferior mesenteric ganglion	Inferior mesenteric plexus	Pelvic Splanchnics (S2, S3, S4)
Pelvic Viscera	Lumbar splanchnics (L1,L2)	Small scattered unnamed ganglia	Superior hypogastric plexus (more details later in pelvis)	Pelvic Splanchnics (S2, S3, S4)

Retroperitoneal Organs (SAD PUCKER)

- Suprarenal (adrenal) gland
- Aorta and IVC
- Duodenum (2nd, 3rd parts)
- Pancreas (head), NOT tail
- Ureters
- Colon (ascending and descending)
- Kidneys
- Esophagus, lower 2/3
- Rectum

Vomiting

Occurs due to the stimulation of either the vomiting center in the medulla (near the respiratory center) or the chemoreceptor trigger zone in the area postrema on the floor of the fourth ventricle.

Paths:

- Vomiting due to psychological stress occurs via the cerebral cortex and limbic system to the vomiting center.
- Anticipatory vomiting occurs via the cerebral cortex and limbic system to the vomiting center.
- Vomiting due to motion sickness occurs via the vestibular/vestibulocerebellar system from the labyrinth of the inner ear to the vomiting center.
- Vomiting due to chemical (drugs, chemotherapy drugs, toxins) occurs via the chemoreceptor trigger zone in the area postrema when chemical signals are detected in the bloodstream and cerebrospinal fluid.
- Gastrointestinal distention, irritation and delayed gastric emptying stimulate the vagal and visceral nerves.

Bilious Vomiting Causes Due to anything that can obstruct the GI tract or any of its tributary's. These require immediate evaluation. • **Hirschsprung's' disease** • **Annular pancreas** • Small bowel atresia (aka: **duodenal atresia**). MC: **Down's Syndrome** (aka: double bubble sign) • Biliary atresia • Intestinal malrotation • Volvulus • Meconium ileus • Meconium plug • Colonic atresia • Intussusception • Lactobezoar (aka: Inspissated Milk Syndrome): Obstruction of the small bowel by milk curds.	**Non-Bilious Vomiting Causes** • **Pyloric stenosis** (**hypertrophy of the muscle** surrounding the opening of the pylorus: pyloric sphincter). • Foreign bodies: MCC: swallowed coins. MC places of obstruction: cricopharyngeus and the lower esophageal sphincter. • Gastroesophageal reflux (aka: GERD: poorly coordinated swallowing and delayed gastric emptying),

GI and Upper Respiratory Congenital and Developmental Pathologies

DiGeorge Syndrome

- **Abnormal 3rd and 4th brachial pouches = no thyroid gland (no T cells)**
- Microdeletion on chromosome **22:11**
- Recurrent infections: virus, fungus, parasites, atypical bacterial
- **Hypocalcemia (no parathyroids)**
- SX: Cleft palate, abnormal faces, **thymic aplasia**, T cell deficient, Truncus arteriosis

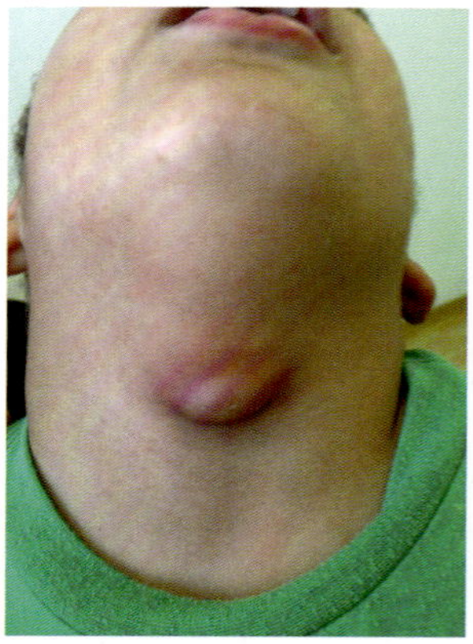

Thyroglossal Duct Cyst

- Failure to **descend/migrate**
- Most common at base of tongue
- Moves when swallowing or protruding tongue
- See Thyroglossal cyst in **midline of neck** (see a lump on the side of the throat)
- TX: surgery if causes problems in swallowing or breathing

Branchial Cleft Cyst

- Epithelial cyst caused by failure of obliteration of the second branchial cleft (AKA: failure of fusion of the second and third branchial arch)
- Mass is **lateral to the midline**
- TX: Infected cyst: antibiotics. Large cyst: surgical removal

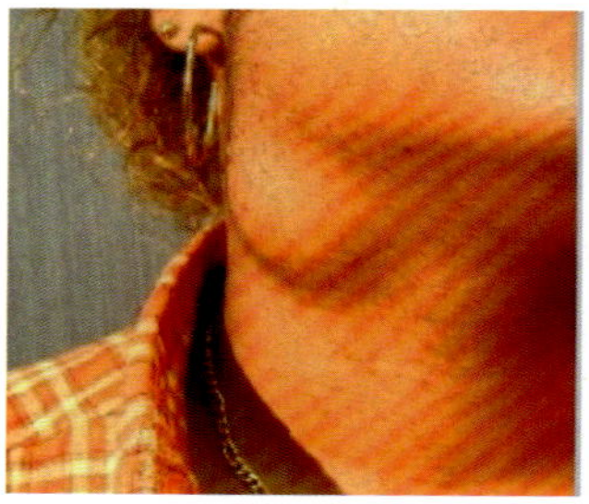

Cleft Lip and Cleft Palate

- Risk: gestational diabetes, smoking during pregnancy, medications, Patau's Syndrome.

Cleft Lip: Failure of maxillary and medial **NASAL** processes to fuse (opening in the upper lip that extends into the nose).
Cleft Palate: Failure of **palatine** process (nasal septum), which is the two plates of the hard palate of the roof of the mouth that do not fuse. (The roof of the mouth opens into the nose).

Esophageal Atresia

Esophagus does not connect to the stomach. It can end in a blind pouch or connect via a fistula with the trachea.

- DX: CXR shows esophageal and gastric air bubble, inability to pass an NG tube to the stomach
- TX: Surgical repair. Antibiotics if aspiration pneumonia has developed.

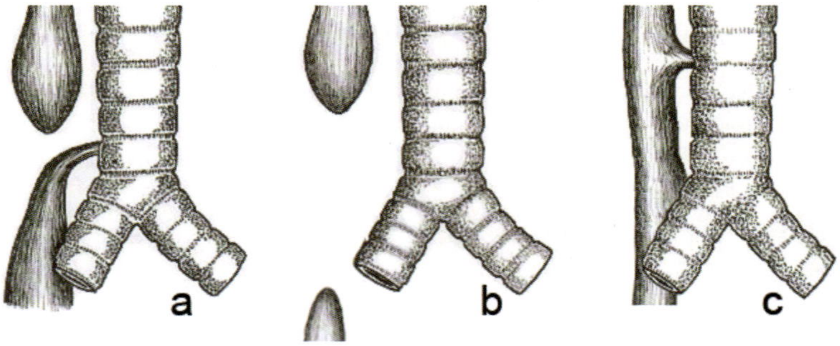

Tracheoesophageal Fistula (Most common form of esophageal atresia)

- Abnormal connection b/t **trachea and esophagus**
- Cyanosis and choking with **first feeding** (**high cause of aspiration pneumonia in a baby due to abscess formation in the respiratory system due to anaerobic infection**)
- Can not pass an NG tube to stomach
- Causes: **polyhydramnios** because fetus can't swallow amniotic fluid

Choanal Atresia

- **Bone or soft tissue mal-development** that obstructs the back of the nasal passage (choana).
  AKA: **Buccopharyngeal membrane**.
- Baby turns blue (cyanosis) with feeding (babies must breath through nose) and is relieved by crying (baby turns pink)
- Can not pass an NG tube to stomach
- DX: CT
- TX: Endoscopy and surgery to reconnect the pharynx to the nostrils
- Associated with CHARGE syndrome. (Group of congenital defects in newborns).
  C: Coloboma of the eye and CNS abnormalities
  H: Heart abnormalities
  A: Atresia of the choana
  R: Retardation of growth
  G: genital/urinary defects (hypogonadism)
  E: ear and eye abnormalities (deafness, blindness) NOTE: CHARGE syndrome is the leading cause of congenital deaf/blindness

Immature Lower Esophageal Sphincter

- Non-bilious spitting up (uncomplicated reflux)
- From 0 to 4 months, peaks 2 – 4 months, outgrows usually by 7 to 8 months
- Usually occurs right after eating or within 2 hours
- Benign

Laryngomalacia

- Collapse of the immature cartilage of the upper larynx during inhalation causing airway obstruction and inspiratory stridor
- Presents in the first few months of life and resolves by 2 years old
- SX: Chronic noise during breathing (inspiratory stridor)
- Must keep child upright for ½ hours after feedings

Pancreas Development (foregut)

Ventral Bud: Main pancreatic duct and small amount of head

Dorsal Bud: Tail, small ducts and main part of head

Tail is peritoneal, head is retroperitoneal

Annular Pancreas

- **Ventral** pancreatic BUD (AKA: **Uncinate process**) encircles the 2nd part of duodenum.
  Bilious vomiting within the first few days of life.

Pancreas division: Dorsal and ventral buds **fail to fuse.**

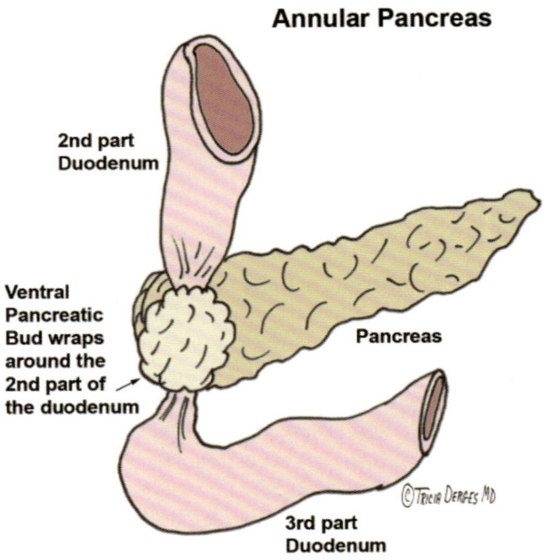

Congenital Diaphragmatic Hernia

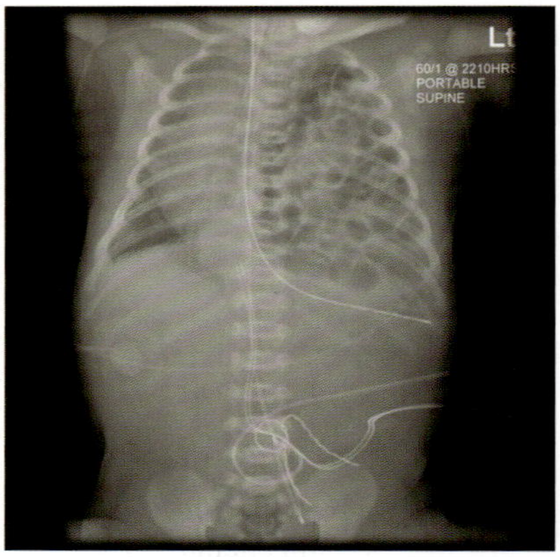

- Failure of diaphragm to close during development
- **Due to a defect in the left pleuroperitoneal membrane of the diaphragm**
- MC on left side
- Intestines herniated into chest cavity and lungs do not develop causing **pulmonary hypoplasia** and pulmonary hypertension.
  Pulmonary hypoplasia: incomplete development of lungs = decreased number of alveoli.
- X-ray shows intestines (loops of bowel) inside the thoracic cavity
- Presents as RDS and scaphoid abdomen.
- TX: Immediate intubation and surgery

Pyloric Stenosis

- **Non bilious** projectile (forceful) vomiting, beginning at 2 to 3 weeks
- **Hypertrophy** of the pylorus muscle
- Palpable "olive" mass (AKA: "Olive sign")
- Single primary developmental defect
- Most common in boys
- **Erythromycin** can cause pyloric stenosis
- SX: Projectile vomiting, dehydration, failure to thrive
- Physio/LABS: vomiting causes **metabolic alkalosis** (vomiting out H+ and CL = hypokalemia and hypochloremia), decreased volume (vomiting) activates Renin-Angio system = water retention = loss of more H+
- DX: Ultrasound
- TX: Surgery: Pyloromyotomy.
  (**NOTE: Electrolytes must be normalized BEFORE surgery is performed**)

Infant GERD

- Frequent vomiting/spit up due to incompetent esophageal sphincter tone.
- Peaks at 4 months, resolves by 12 – 24 months
- Infant's growth is fine and maintains weight
- DX: Esophageal pH monitoring
- TX: Feed thickened milk or formula, sit infant up when feeding.
  1st line: **H2 Blockers (Ranitidine), PPI**

Meckel's Diverticulum (AKA: Vitelline Duct)

- Failure of obliteration of **Omphalomesenteric** duct (AKA: **Vitelline Duct, Yolk Stalk**)
- **AKA:** Failure of vitelline duct to close
- **AKA:** Persistence of the Vitelline Duct (AKA: **Yolk Stalk, Omphalomesenteric duct**)
- **AKA**: Remnant of connection from yolk sac to the small intestine
- Omphalomesenteric Cyst: Dilation of vitelline duct
- **TRUE diverticulum** (contains all 3 layers: mucosa, submucosa, muscularis propria)
  (Other true diverticulum: Crohn's)
  (Not true diverticulum: Zenker's, Diverticulitis)
- Location: distal **ileum** by the ileocecal valve
- Contains **ectopic tissue**: gastric and pancreatic
- Can progress to an obstruction and intussusception
- SX: painless rectal bleeding (melaena), **intermittent** (AKA: wax and wane, episodic) severe abdominal pain, chronic iron deficiency anemia, positive stool for occult blood.
- **DX: technetium-99m (99mTc) pertechnetate scan** (AKA: Meckel scan)
- TX: Laparoscopic surgery

Intussusception

- Telescoping of intestine. MC in children < 2 years old.
- SX: Rectal bleeding: black "currant jelly" stool (AKA: blood and mucus from necrosis), Palpation of "sausage shaped mass" in lower quadrant, **Intermittent**, **colicky**, severe abdominal pain, fever, ↑ WBC, shock, **bilious vomiting.**
- DX: BIT: Ultrasound shows a "doughnut sign" or "target sign". Plain X-ray of abdomen to rule out obstruction (air/fluid levels show obstruction). X-ray shows a "target" shape on ultrasound (**NEVER** use a scope for ANY diagnosis in the colon except for a colonoscopy, due to risk of perforation of intestine).
- TX: **Barium or air contrast enema. Barium enema is both diagnostic and therapeutic,** NT tube to decompress bowels.
  NOTE: Do not use enema if child has signs of perforation, peritonitis or shock.

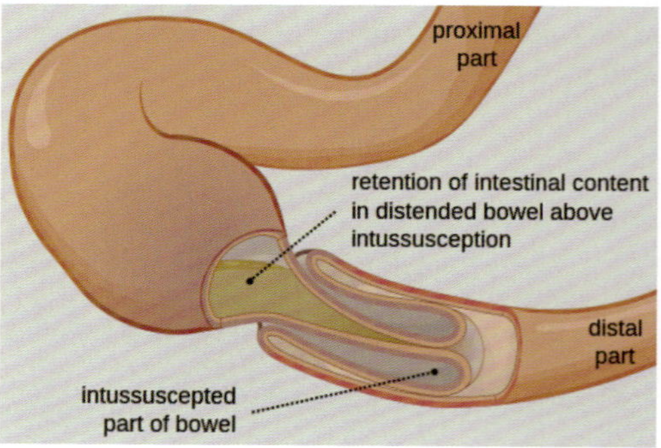

Hirschsprung

- 12th week: **Ganglion cells do not migrate to rectum**
- No **Meissner** (sub mucosal), no **Auerbach** (bowel wall) Plexus
- Biopsy shows **no ganglion cells**
- Higher risk in Downs Syndrome
- **Always involves rectum**
- Dilated colon proximal to narrowing segment produces **"string stool"**
- **Chronic constipation** early in life
- SX: Difficulty in passing meconium. Will not pass meconium for at least 48 hours or not at all.
  (**Do NOT confused Meconium Ileus in Cystic Fibrosis**), inability to pass flatus, tight rectal sphincter, bowel obstruction
- BIT: Abdominal X-ray shows distended bowel loops and no air in the rectum. Contrast enemas show retention of barium.
- DX: BIT: Rectal examination. (Digital exam causes baby to pass large amounts of stool)
  Confirmatory test: Rectal biopsy shows **absent ganglionic cells in the submucosa.**
- TX: Gastrografin enema, surgical resection

Meconium Pathologies

Meconium Plugs obstruct the lower intestine

Causes: Hirschsprung, maternal drug use, Cystic fibrosis, Idiopathic Onset Diabetes Mellitus (IODM)

- **Cystic fibrosis: Meconium Ileus: obstruction in the ileum.**
- **Hirschsprung's always involves the rectum.**

Meconium DX: Abdominal X-ry

Meconium TX: Gastrografin enema

CYSTIC FIBROSIS, AR

Defect in the CFTR protein that regulates sweat and mucus by the movement of water and chloride.

Normal: The CFTR protein helps produce digestive fluids, sweat and mucus. The CFTR protein is a channel for the movement of chloride in and out of cells (exocrine glands). This provides for the balance of salt and water in the body. Sweat glands secrete salt and water into the sweat ducts. Then reabsorbs the salt from the sweat back into the ducts. Sodium moves through sodium channels and chloride moves through the CFTR channel.

Abnormal: The CFTR protein channel does not work causing chloride ions to be trapped inside of the cells. Negatively charged chloride ions attract the positive charged sodium ions outside the cell. Chloride and sodium combine to produce salt, which is lost. The high concentration of chloride and sodium trapped inside the cell backs up and becomes thick mucus. It affects the pancreas, lungs, kidneys and intestines.

- **Autosomal recessive**
- Defect of **CFTR gene on chromosome 7**
- **Deletion of PHE (Phenylalanine) at position ΔF508 in CFTR protein, which keeps the protein from reaching the cell membrane surface. (ΔF508 mutation is 90% of cause).**
- **Frameshift** mutation +/- base pair (tip: If you have cystic fibrosis you are "F"..... = Frameshift)
- AKA: **Misfolded protein (was not tagged with ubiquitin for apoptosis)**
- DX: Sweat chloride test (measures the concentration of chloride that is excreted in sweat): shows increased Cl in sweat.
- SX: **recurrent** pulmonary infections (esp. **Pseudomonas**), infertility in males (due to lack of vas deferens = no sperm), malabsorption = steatorrhea, malabsorption = deficiency of fat soluble vitamins D, E, A, K, **nasal polyps**, **meconium ileus** in newborns, chronic bronchitis, bronchiectasis, clubbing of the fingers, easily dehydration in hot weather.
- TX: N-acetylcysteine MOA: mucolytic – cleaves disulfide bonds
  Ivacaftor (VX-770) restores the function of the mutated CF protein by decreasing sweat chloride levels and decreasing pulmonary symptoms in CF with the G551D Mutation.
  Must also replace amylase, lipase and chymotrypsin to ↓ malabsorption (**Pancrelipase**).
- TX: **Day to day: Macrolides, TMP/SMX, Ciprofloxacin.**
  Infection with Pseudomonas or S. aureus: Piperacillin plus Tobramycin or Ceftazidime.
  Resistant organisms: Inhaled Tobramycin.

Forms of Intestinal Atresia

- **Duodenal Atresia (AKA: Double Bubble, Intestinal atresia).**
  High risk: Downs Syndrome.
  SX: **Bilious vomiting within 12 hours of birth.**
  DX: Abdominal x-ray shows the "**double bubble**" sign.
  Failure to recanalize. Due to **lack of apoptosis** so the lumen of the duodenum is not recanalized.
  (NOTE: Jejunal atresia, Ileal atresia, colon atresia: due to vascular accident).
  TX: Surgical repair (duodenostomy). Must replace electrolytes prior to surgery due to vomiting (low K), NG tube to decompress the bowel.

- **Apple Peel Atresia**
  Terminal ileum spirals around the **SMA.**
  Due to **malrotation.**
  "Apple core" sign on x-ray.
- **Midgut Volvulus**
  Malrotation of gut causing bowel obstruction.
  Abdominal distension, bilious emesis, colicky abdominal pain.
  MC in babies < 1 year old.
  Ischemia to affected part of intestine.
  DX: Ultrasound or barium enema. Enema shows a "birds beak" appearance at rotation site.
  TX: Surgery

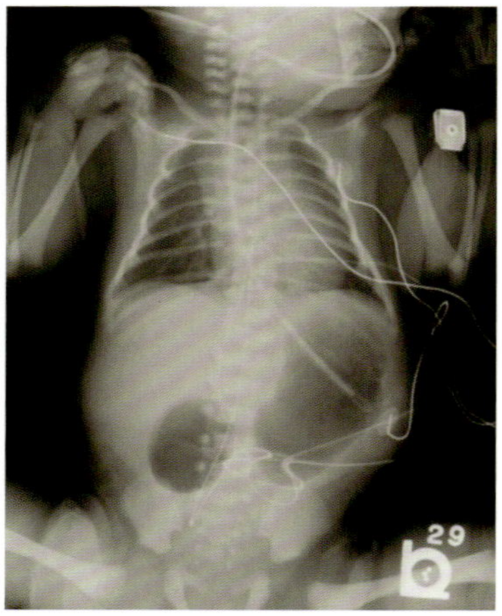

Duodenal Atresia (Double Bubble)

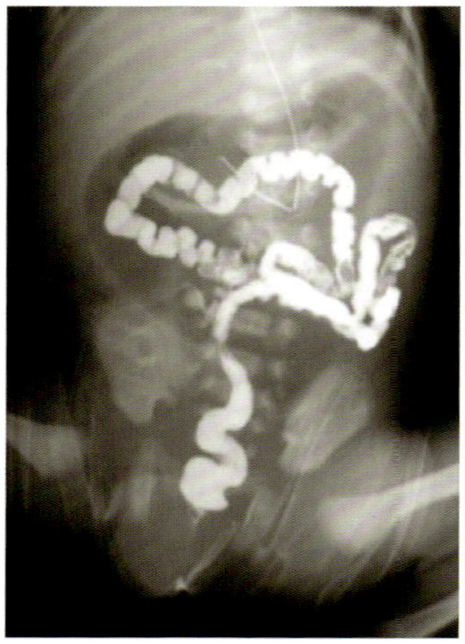

Apple Peel Atresia

Necrotizing Enterocolitis (NEC)

- Premature infant (always in the NICU).
- ↓ Apgar scores
- **Bloody stools**, apnea, lethargy, vomiting, low weight, cardiac issues, poor feeing.
- **Abdominal x-ray shows: Pneumatosis intestinalis: gas/air filled intestines = distended abdomen.**
- TX: Surgery (bowel resection), NPO, decompress gut and give broad spectrum antibiotics.

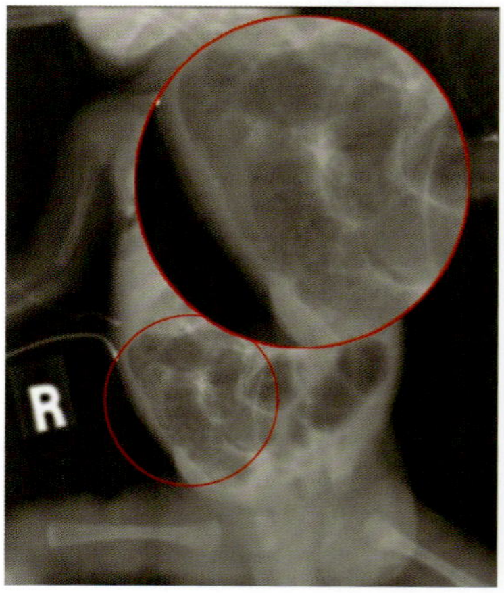

Necrotizing Enterocolitis

Imperforate Anus

- "Dimple" instead of anal opening.
- Rectum ends in a blind pouch.
- Common to see other abnormal development of rectal structures and urinary/urogenital tract defects
- SX: Extreme constipation.
- Associated with Down's syndrome.
- Associated with VACTERL syndrome (non-random co-occurrence of birth defects)
  V: Vertebral abnormalities
  A: Anal atresia
  C: Cardiovascular abnormalities
  T: Tracheoesophageal fistula
  E: Esophageal atresia
  R: Renal abnormalities
  L: Limb abnormalities

Anus formation

Upper Anus: **above pectinate line.**
Formed from hindgut.
Internal hemorrhoids (Painless).

Lower Anus: **below pectinate line.**
Invagination of surface ectoderm.
External hemorrhoids **(Painful).**

Abdominal Wall Defects
Intestines are located outside of the abdomen
Elevated levels of **AFP** and **AChE-AF** (Acetylcholinesterase)
Caused by **malrotation**

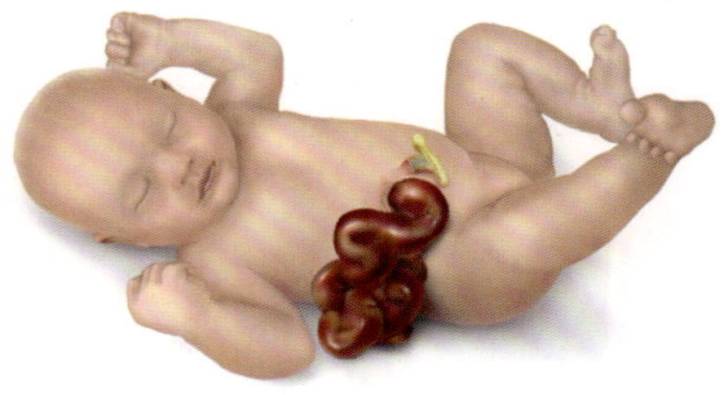

Gastroschisis

- **Gastroschisis**
  Intestines NOT covered by peritoneum. (**tip:** "gast"ly)
  Does not involve the umbilical cord and not midline
  Failure of lateral fold closure of abdominal wall
  Treatment: wrap with sterile saline dressing and cover with plastic wrap. Surgery.

- **Omphalocele**
  Intestines covered by peritoneum.
  Intestines protrude through the umbilical cord and is midline.
  Failure of lateral fold closure of abdominal wall

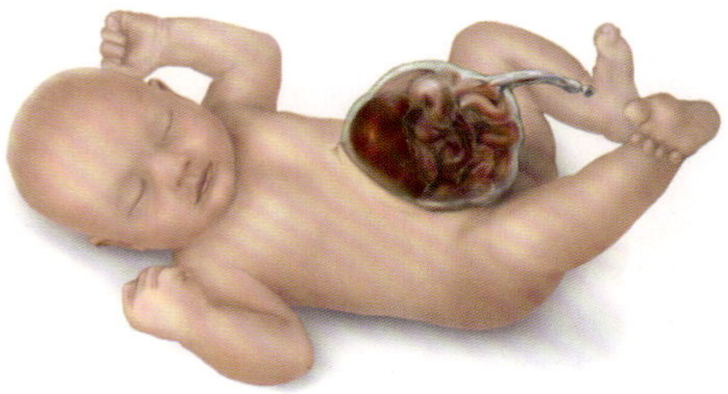

Omphalocele

Renal Development

- Pronephros degenerates at week 4
- **Mesonephros** function as kidneys for the first trimester
- Metanephros (permanent) give rise to:
- **Ureteric bud** (main kidney body): Ureter, pelvises, calyces, collecting ducts
- **Metanephric mesenchyme** (Glomeruli system): Glomerulus, PCT, Loop, DCT, collecting tubes

Renal Congenital and Developmental Pathologies

Fetal Hydronephrosis
- Back up of urine into the kidneys
- MCC: Area of obstruction: **Ureteropelvic junction**

Bladder Obstruction
- MCC in males: **Posterior Urethral Valves**
- Obstruction in bladder can cause urine to back up and cause hydronephrosis

Horseshoe Kidney
- Higher risk: Turners Syndrome (45XO)
- Caused by **Inferior Mesenteric Artery** (keeps kidney from ascending)

Potters Syndrome
- **Oligohydramnios** due to inability of fetus to urinate = decreased amniotic fluid
- Example of sequence birth defect
- Malformation of Uretic Bud
- Bilateral **Renal Agenesis**
- **Pulmonary Hypoplasia** = respiratory distress. Amniotic fluid matures lungs. If there is no fluid = hypo lungs. MCC of death in this baby = respiratory failure
- SX: Flat faces, club feet, jaw deformity
- Example of sequence and deformation

Polyhydramnios
- Increased amniotic fluid. Fetus has **decreased ability to swallow due** to: GI obstruction, esophageal obstruction, duodenal atresia, anencephaly
- Fetus is urinating too much: Increased cardiac output because anemia or twin to twin transfusion syndrome
- **Dangerous risk**: uterine enlargement, preterm labor risk

Posterior Urethral Valves

- Posterior urethral valves and renal agenesis: MCC of oligohydramnios
- Most common reason for newborn male not to urinate during first day of life
- Catheterize
- DX: Voiding cystourethrogram

Congenital Urinary Anomalies

- UTI's in young children (ie: vesicoureteral reflux)
  DX: Voiding cystourethrogram
- Hematuria from minor trauma in young children
- Little boys should not get urinary tract infections. If they do, must rule out a congenital anomaly

Abnormal Ureter Development

- Ectopic ureter: Ureter that does not connect properly to the bladder and drains somewhere outside the bladder
- Low implantation of the ureter in a girl: a low placed ureter empties into the vagina (it is below the sphincter). The girl folds normally but is constantly wet because there urine in the vagina.
- Ureteropelvic Junction Obstruction: MCC: symptoms present when person drinks a large amount of beer (beer-drinking binge) and develops colicky flank pain. DX: Ultrasound and repair.

Urine at the Umbilical Cord

- **Patent Urachus (AKA: Remnant of Allantois, Persistent Allantois Remnant)**
- Urachus connects bladder with yolk sac
- Urachus connects the apex of the bladder to the umbilicus
- Urachus runs within the umbilical cord
- Urachus goes on to form the medical umbilical ligament

Urinary Tract Infections (UTI's)

- MC in girls >2 and boys < 1 by gram negative rods
- Can progress to pyelonephritis if the UTI is not treated
- Testing: Voiding cystourethrogram (VCUG) used when:
  Children that have ≥2 febrile UTI's
  Children that have one UTI with any of the following complications: Hypertension, infection with any organism other than E. coli, family history of urological or renal problems, failure to thrive.
- BIT: urinalysis
  MAT: Urine culture
- UTI TX: **TMP/SMX, Amoxicillin** (not use in infants < 1 month old)
  Pyelonephritis TX**: IV Ceftriaxone or Ampicillin plus Gentamycin**

Vesicoureteral Reflux (VUR)

- Condition when urine flows backwards from the bladder into the ureters and kidneys
- Anatomical causes: posterior urethral valves, urethral or meatal stenosis
- Complications: pyelonephritis, scarring of the kidney and kidney failure
- DX: Voiding cystourethrogram
- TX: TMP/SMX

Genitalia Development

Female

- Paramesonephric: Internal structures: **Ovaries, Fallopian tube, uterus and upper 1/3 vagina**
  (**tip: paramesonephric** for woman = woman has a "para" ovaries).
- It is the absence of anti-mullerian hormone that keeps male internal genitalia from forming (from the Sertoli cells, which causes Mullerian apoptosis causing the Wolffian ducts to regress).
- Lower 2/3 of vagina develops from the **urogenital sinus**.

Male

- Mesonephric (AKA: Wolffian). Allows the development of the male internal genitalia (urogenital structures): trigone of the bladder, epididymis, vas deferens, seminal vesicles. In the adult, this system stores, matures sperm and provides semen.
- Wolffian ducts are exposed to testosterone via androgen receptors during embryonic development.
- SRY gene on Y chromosome = testes development
- **Sertoli Cells: Release Mullerian Inhibitory Factor (MIF) and stops paramesonephric (woman)**
- **Leydig Cells: Release androgens to make mesonephric ducts (AKA: testosterone)**
- **Mesonephric Ducts (AKA: Wolffian) forms internal structures: Seminal vesicles, epididymis, ejaculatory duct, ductus deferens, but NOT the prostate**
- **DHT (not testosterone) is responsible for development of external male genitalia**

External Genitalia Homologues

- Males: Dihydrotestosterone to develop external genitalia
- Females: Estrogen to develop external genitalia

Embryologic Tissue	**Male**	**Female**
Genital tubercle	Glans penis	Glans clitoris
Genital tubercle	Corpus cavernosum	Vestibular bulbs
Urogenital Sinus	Bulbourethral glands (AKA: Cowper)	Vestibular glands of Bartholin
Urogenital sinus	Prostate gland	Urethral/Paraurethral glands of Skene Urogenital folds
Urogenital folds	Ventral shaft of penis/penile urethra	Labia minora
Labioscrotal swelling	Scrotum	Labia majora
Processus vaginalis	**Tunica vaginalis** (Associated with a **hydrocele)**	Obliterated
Gubernaculum	**Anchors testes inside scrotum**	**Ovarian and round ligament**
Yolk Sac		**Oocytes**

Genitalia Congenital and Developmental Pathologies

No Sertoli cells or lack of anti-mullerian hormone

- Child develops both male and female internal genitalia and male external genitalia

5 alpha-reductase deficiency

- **Testosterone can't be converted to DHT**
- Child has internal genitalia (because testosterone is present) and has ambiguous external genitalia (looks female) until puberty

Hydrocele

- Remnant of **tunica vaginalis**
- Painless, fluid filled scrotum (spermatic cords). **Will transilluminate**.

Varicocele

- Dilation/swelling of the veins (like a varicose vein) in the **pampiniform plexus**. (AKA: Bag of worms)
- Usually disappears upon lying down.
- MC on the left side due to the drainage route through the left renal vein to the IVC.
- Does not transilluminate.
- DX: Ultrasound both testicles (problem is bilateral in many cases)

Bicornuate Uterus

- **Incomplete fusion of paramesonephric ducts**
- Urinary tract abnormalities and infertility

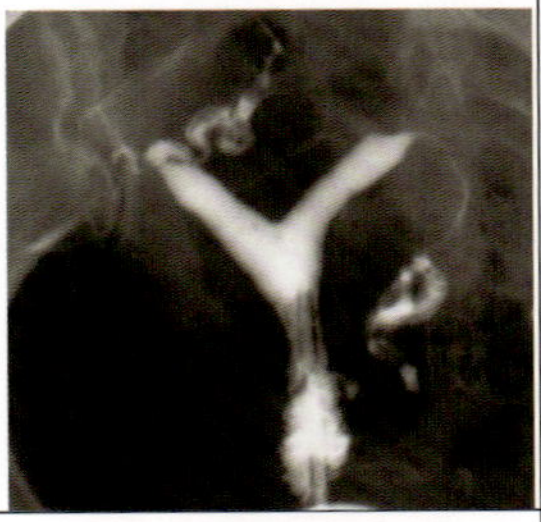

Cryptorchidism

- Absence of one testicle (testicle has not dropped into the scrotum from the inguinal canal)
- TX: Orchiopexy after 1 year
- Without repair there is an increased risk of sterility and cancer

Epispadias

- Faulty positioning of genital tubercle. Malformation in which the urethra opens on the upper (dorsal) side of the penis.
- Urethra opens on **dorsal** (superior) side of penis
- Associated with exstrophy (AKA: Ectopia vesicae) of the bladder (bladder outside of abdomen). Exstrophy of bladder: due to failure of caudal fold closure. Urinary incontinence.
- TX: Surgical correction
- (**tip**: E "**PEE**" spadias. On the side that you will **PEE** in your eye)

Hypospadias

- **No fusion of urethral folds**
- Urethra opens on ventral (inferior) side of penis
- Risk of UTI's if not repaired
- In the female, no fusion of urethral folds = vagina

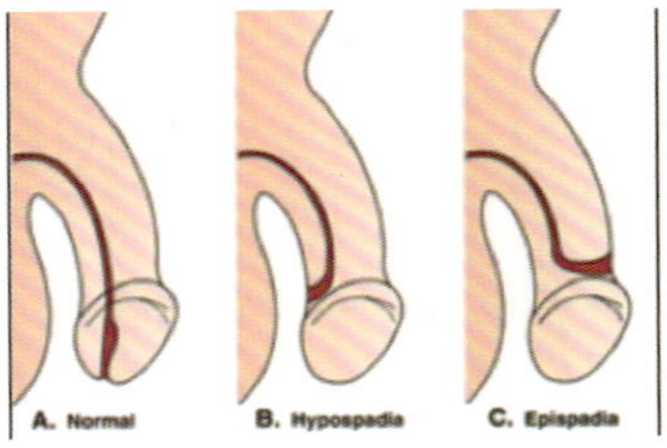

- Associated with inguinal hernias and cryptorchidism
- Do not perform circumcision, prepuce used for reconstruction
- TX: Surgical correction.

Additional NEONATAL and INFANT PATHOLOGIES

Neonatal Polycythemia
- Due to hypoxic situations (ie: **RDS, respiratory distress**)
  ANY hypoxic situation will stimulate **erythropoietin** in the **peritubular capillary bed (AKA: interstitial fibroblast) in the kidney**
- High RBC count, high Hb and Hct
- SX: Lethargic, hypotonic, apnea, hypoglycemic
- TX: Partial exchange transfusion and hydration

Congenital Hypothyroidism (AKA: Cretinism)
- **Umbilical hernia**
- Course facial features
- **Enlarged, protruding tongue**
- Low set hairline, mottled skin, hoarse cry, dry and cold extremities, mental retardation

*Bacterial Meningitis, Neonatal Sepsis
Must treat with empiric antibiotics until culture results come back. Do NOT wait to treat until culture results return.

DX: CBC, blood cultures, UA, urine culture, CSF cell count,
CSF culture (do not do lumbar puncture if there are signs of ICP: bulging fontanelles or fixed visual gazes).
Do not use Ceftriaxone (with babies under 2 months) or use Sulfonamides.

Empiric treatment:
- **Vancomycin plus Cefotaxime or Ceftriaxone*** (Do not give babies <2 months Ceftriaxone. Liver is not mature and can increase bilirubin levels causing kernicterus).

Treat for specific organisms once test results return
Babies <1 month: **Strep B, E coli, Listeria**
TX: Strep B and E coli: **IV Amp B and Gentamycin**
TX: Listeria: **Ampicillin and Cefotaxime.**

Babies >1 month: **Strep pneumo, Neisseria.**
TX: **IV Vancomycin and Ceftriaxone*, Penicillin, 3rd generation Cephalosporin.**
*SE: **Ceftriaxone: Do NOT give to babies under 2 months**. Liver is not mature and can increase bilirubin levels causing kernicterus.
Babies: HiB: **Ampicillin**

Rifampin for prophylaxis for all close contacts in cases involving HiB or N. meningitis

Gestational Diabetes Affect on the Infant
- **Macrosomia** (big baby)
  Big baby = more weight = difficulty breathing = RDS
  ↑ risk of shoulder dystocia (anterior shoulder of the infant can't be delivered without ↑ manipulation)
- Surfactant decreased
- Hypoglycemia (after birth)
- Respiratory Distress = EPO = Polycythemia
- Heart issues (ASK, VSD, truncus arteriosus)
- Hypocalcemia
- Polyhydramnios
- Physiologic jaundice (Hyperbilirubinemia)
- IUGR
- Hypocalcemia
- Hypomagnesemia
- Polycythemia
- Abdominal distension (small left colon syndrome).
- ↑ risk of childhood obesity
- ↑risk of developing diabetes
- **Caudal Regression**

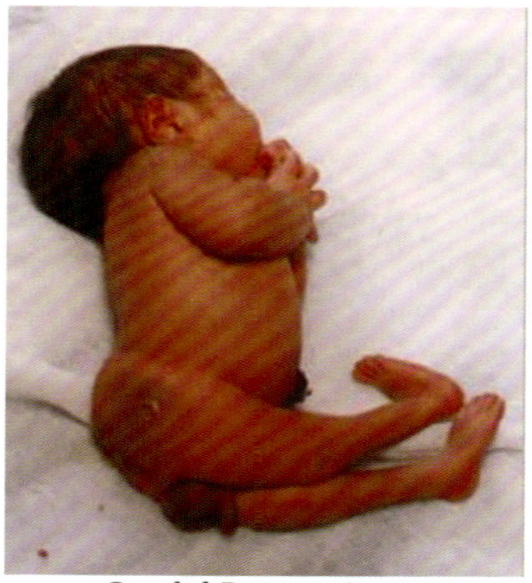
Caudal Regression

All Febrile Neonates **DX: CBC, blood cultures, UA, urine culture, CSF cell count, CSF culture (do not do lumbar puncture if there are signs of ICP: bulging fontanelles or fixed visual gazes).** **Do not use Ceftriaxone (under 2 months) or Sulfonamides.** **Do NOT wait to give empiric treatment until test results return.**	**Cerebral Palsy** • Permanent movement disorders that appear in early childhood. MC movement disorder in children. • Causes: Cerebral **anoxia**: lack of oxygen to the baby's brain, genetic causes, premature birth, infections during pregnancy (ie: toxoplasmosis, rubella). • SX: tremors, weak muscles, seizures, difficulty in swallowing, speaking, hearing and vision. Slow development of milestones. Hypotonia and increase of deep tendon reflexes. Mental retardation and disabilities.
Baby Rashes **Milium** (Milia): (AKA: Milk spot) Keratin filled cyst just under the epidermis of the nose, eyes and genitalia (look similar to whiteheads). Resolves within 2 to 4 weeks. 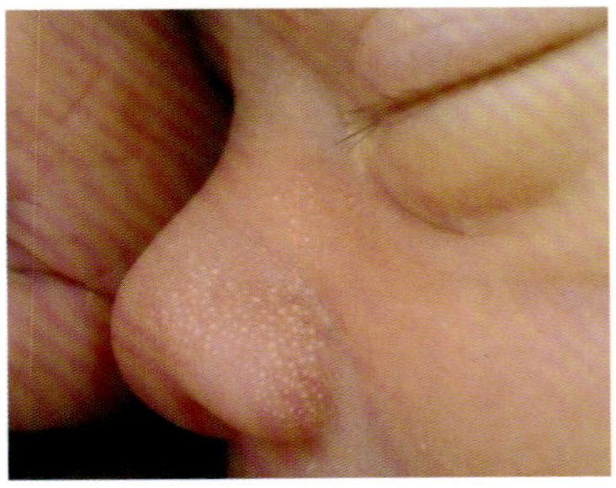	**Baby Rashes** **Erythema Toxicum:** Occurs between days 2 – 5 after birth. Blotchy red spots on the skin with overlying white or yellow pustules. Eosinophils. Resolves within first 2 weeks. 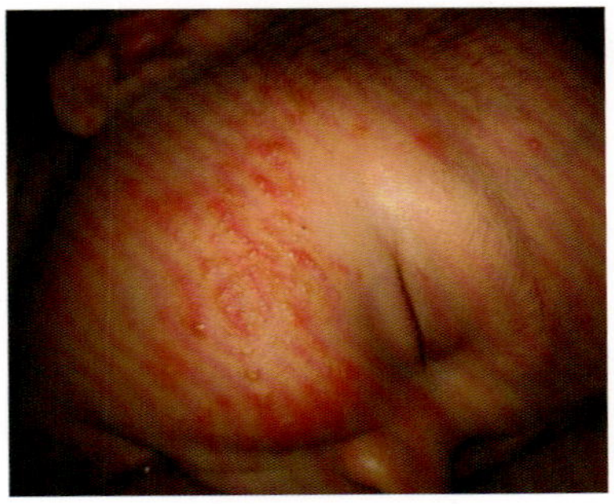
Transient Conditions of the Newborn • **Tachypnea of the Newborn** MC seen in cesarean section babies. Fluid from the lung was not removed by compression in the birth canal. Tachypnea should not persist >4 hours or it is considered pathological and must be evaluated with urine and blood cultures. • **Polycythemia of the Newborn** Hypoxia during birth stimulates erythropoietin, which causes an ↑ in RBC. This normalizes once the baby is breathing normally. • **Hyperbilirubinemia** Excess RBC breakdown (due to removal of Hgb F) sends increased bilirubin to the liver for conjugation leading to jaundice. This may also be due to lower levels of UDP in the liver due to prematurity. • **Subconjunctival Hemorrhage of the Eyes** Tiny hemorrhages in the eyes of the newborn may be seen due to the increase of intrathoracic pressure from the compression in the birth canal.	**Delivery Associated Injuries of the Newborn** • Caput succedaneum (does cross suture lines) • Cephalohematoma (does not cross suture lines) • Clavicular fracture (due to shoulder dystocia) • Facial nerve palsy (due to forceps deliver) • Brachial Plexus Injury: Klumpke Palsy (paralyzed hand with Horner's SX) Duchenne-Erb Palsy (shoulder dystocia) • Skull fractures (linear, basilar, depressed)

Pneumonias

Bacterial Pneumonia Presentation

- Acute onset, high fever, chills, cough, decreased breath sounds, pleuritic chest pain

Viral Pneumonia Presentation

- MCC: **RSV**
- Low-grade fever, tachypnea (fast breathing), URI symptoms (sore throat, headache, runny nose, cough, malaise, loss of appetite), can be wheezing

Bronchiolitis **AKA: Respiratory Syncytial Virus (RSV)** Viral family: RSV, Paramyxoviridae, Adenovirus. MCC of pneumonia in children under < 2 years old. Most severe in children 1 – 2 months. Spreads: direct contact. Remains viable for half an hour on hands and 5 hours on countertops. ↑ rate in child care centers. SX: Coughing, wheezing, upper respiratory tract infection symptoms, grunting, nasal flare, retractions (accessory muscles used in breathing), tachypnea, cough, apnea, prolonged expirations, hyperinflation of the lung because of air trapping due to the inflammation. **DX: BIT: CXR shows hyperinflation and patchy atelectasis.** **MAT: RSV antigen in nasal or pulmonary secretions.** **Complications: Acute otitis media** **TX: Supportive measures, humidified air. Inhaled bronchodilators: Albuterol or epinephrine (β-agonist nebulizers). No steroids.** **Hospitalize if severe symptoms of fever, tachypnea (> 60/min) and use of accessory muscles in breathing.**	**Chlamydia trachomatis Pneumonia** MC: Infants 1 – 3 months old. SX: Slow onset, no fever or wheezing (differentiates it from RSV), staccato cough and peripheral eosinophilia. **DX: CXR shows unilateral lower-lobe interstitial pneumonia.** **TX: Erythromycin (Macrolides)** **Pneumonia Treatments** **Mild outpatients: Amoxicillin, Cefuroxime, Amoxicillin/Clavulanic acid (*Augmentin*)** **Hospitalized patients: IV Cefuroxime, IV Vancomycin if S. aureus** **Viral: Initially give no antibiotics. If signs of worsening condition add antibiotics.** **Chlamydia and Mycoplasma: Erythromycin (Macrolides)**

IV Access on Children

- **If unable to get an IV line established must do: Intraosseous cut down.**
  Do not leave in more than 24 – 48 hours.
  (For an adult: saphenous vein cut down)

NEONATAL JAUNDICE - BILIRUBIN

Bilirubin Lab Levels
Total bilirubin levels are the total of both conjugated and unconjugated together
Indirect bilirubin levels are calculated from the Total Bilirubin minus the Direct Bilirubin

Pathologic Jaundice

- Hyperbilirubinemia appears on the first day of life
- Hyperbilirubinemia last more than 2 weeks
- Bilirubin rises more than 5 mg/dL/day
- Bilirubin rises above 19.5 mg/dL in a full term baby
- Direct bilirubin rises above 2 mg/dL anytime
- MC with conditions of hemolysis (ABO and Rh incompatibility) and Crigler-Najjar
- SX: Kernicterus (deposition of bilirubin in the basal ganglia), seizures, lethargy, hypotonia, chorea (irregular contractions), athetosis (twisting, writhing), hearing loss
- TX: Phototherapy (blue-green light) breaks down the bilirubin to allow for its excretion.
  Exchange transfusion if bilirubin rises above 20 – 25 mg/dL.

UNCONJUGATED (INDIRECT) PATHOLOGIES – Fat Soluble

Crigler-Najjar Syndrome, Type I, AR • Unconjugated • Bilirubin levels of >20 umol/l • **Absence of UDP glucuronosyltransferase**. **They are not able to conjugate.** • Extreme jaundice and high levels of serum bilirubin in first few days of life • **Kernicterus** • Treatment with phenobarbitol will not decrease levels of bilirubin • Death unless liver transplant	**Crigler-Najjar Syndrome, Type II, AR** • Unconjugated • **NO Kernicterus** • Bilirubin levels of <20 umol/l Treatment with phenobarbitol WILL decrease levels of bilirubin
Gilbert's Syndrome • Unconjugated • **Reduced** activity of UDP glucuronosyltransferase. • Patient leads normal life, basically asymptomatic • Jaundice only occurs when patient is **stressed** (ex: exams, break up, etc.), exertion, fasting or infections	**Unconjugated Bilirubin (Indirect) Complication and treatment** • **Kernicterus**: build up of unconjugated bilirubin into the brain = bilirubin encephalopathy. • Bilirubin is neurotoxic = severe brain damage or death • Labs: high levels of serum bilirubin • SX: lethargy (won't wake up to feed), decreased feeding, hypotonia, high pitched cry, spasmodic torticollis (AKA: cervical dystonia) are involuntary neck movements, opisthotonus (muscle spasms), vertical gaze palsy, fever, seizures • TX: **Exchange transfusion (AKA: Plasmapheresis)** (patients blood is removed and replaced)
Physiologic Jaundice • Unconjugated • **Appears after first day of life, during the first week.** • Due to decreased activity of UDP-glucuronosyltransferase because the liver is **immature** and is not conjugating adequately and that Fetal Hb is being broken down and replace by adult Hb. • Last about 2 weeks in term infants, and up to one month in premature and exclusively breastfed infants. • Higher risk with premature babies. • **Mildly** elevated serum bilirubin. • Higher risk with diabetic mothers, Asian and Native American infants. • TX: **Phototherapy: converts unconjugated bilirubin to water-soluble form.**	**Breast Feeding Failure** • Unconjugated due to a "mechanical" problem • Occurs **within the first week of life** (overlaps with physiologic jaundice). • Due to **inadequate breast milk volume or intake** = bowel movements to remove bilirubin from the body. • Failure to thrive. • Work with mother on longer for more frequent feedings to stimulate adequate milk production. Can also supplement with formula.

Breast Milk Failure • Unconjugated due to a "biochemical" problem • Develops **after the first week (between 1 and 2 weeks).** • Due to interaction between hormone and enzymes in breast milk affecting conjugation. • Stop breast-feeding for a few days, use formula, then restart breastfeeding. • Self-Limiting.	**Hemolytic Disease of the Newborn (ABO)** • Unconjugated • **AKA: Erythroblastosis fetalis (Parvo B19)** • **Maternal IgG antibodies** pass into the fetal circulation and cause hemolysis to the fetal RBC's. Anti-A and anti-B antibodies are usually IgM and do not pass through the placenta. • Can cause hydrops fetalis (heart failure). • **Can occur in a first-born baby** (Unlike Rh Disease which first occurs in the 2nd baby). • More common in mother's with blood type O, very seldom to mother's with A or B. • **Jaundice develops in the first day of life.** • Fetal anemia. • TX: High bilirubin levels = exchange transfusion.
Rh Disease (AKA: Rhesus, Rhesus Hemolytic Disease of the Newborn) • Unconjugated • **Mother is Rh negative, father is Rh positive and baby is Rh positive.** • **Mother's antibodies (IgG) against Rhesus D antigen on babies RBC's.** • In first birth mother is exposed to infant's blood causing development of antibodies so that all **subsequent pregnancies are in danger.** • Severe disease causes erythroblastosis fetalis (AKA: hemolytic disease of the newborn), hydrops fetalis or stillbirth. • DX: **Indirect Coombs test for IgG in the mother.** • TX: Rhesus D negative mothers given an anti-RhD IgG immunoglobulin injection (AKA: RhoGAM) **at 28 weeks gestation** Non-sensitized mothers are given RhoGAM immediately (within 72 hrs) after birth.	Other pathologies that cause unconjugated bilirubin: Spherocytosis, Arteriovenous malformations, G6PD deficiency, Pyruvate Kinase deficiency, Sickle Cell Disease, Alpha-Thalassemia, Polycythemia, Hypothyroidism, Sepsis, UTI.

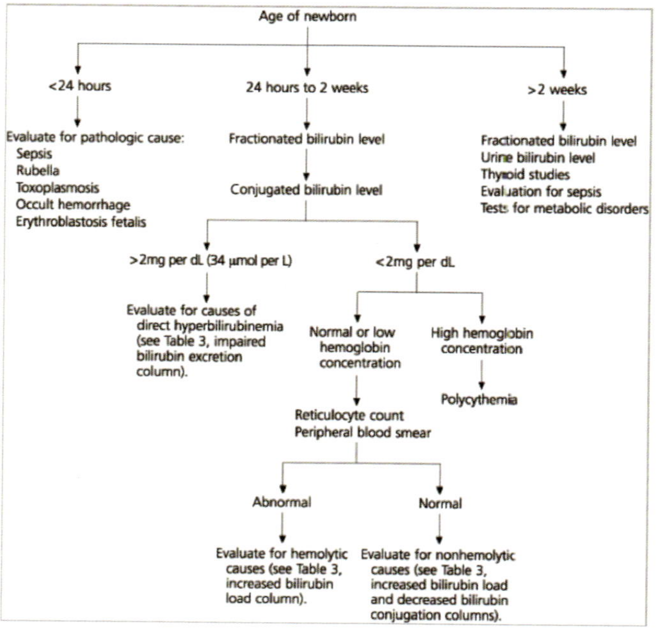

CONJUGATED (DIRECT) BILIRUBIN

Water-soluble

Biliary Atresia • Conjugated • Occurs about 2 weeks of age. • **Light stools and dark urine** (sign of conjugated bilirubin). • **Extrahepatic**: bile duct is blocked or absent • NO kernicterus • Leads to Neonatal Cholestasis • **Negative coombs test** • **↑ risk with Downs Syndrome**	**Dubin-Johnson*** • Conjugated • Problem is with **excretion** of conjugated bilirubin • **Liver is black** • Deposits of **epinephrine metabolites in hepatic lysosomes** • Normal LFTs • **Increased urinary coproporphyrin** • (**tip**: Johnson's outboard motors are black)
Rotor Syndrome* • Conjugated • Problem is with **storage** (milder form of Dubin-Johnson) • Jaundice triggered by: Stress, OCP 's, Pregnancy • **Liver is NOT black** • Deposits of epinephrine metabolites in hepatic lysosomes • Normal LFTs • Increased urinary coproporphyrin	***Excretion of conjugated bilirubin**: **Active ATP transport**. If these channels are blocked the conjugated bilirubin can not go to the biliary system but will go into the plasma (water soluble) and will increase the urinary excretion of bilirubin (**UA = increased levels of coproporphyrin**). If the active ATP transport is not working, the bilirubin can still be excreted from the liver into the plasma by **passive organic ion diffusion.** UA = normal urinalysis should never show bilirubin. If bilirubin shows in urine, urine will be dark and the bilirubin will be conjugated (water soluble). Other pathologies of conjugated bilirubin: TORCH infections, HEP A and B, Alpha-1-antitrypsin deficiency, Cystic Fibrosis, TPN (total parenteral nutrition), Bile duct obstruction, Choledochal cyst

Bilirubin Differentials

	Crigler-Najjar	**Dubin-Johnson Syndrome**	**Rotor's Syndrome**	**Gilbert Syndrome**
Pathology	No bilirubin conjugation.	Defective excretion conjugated bilirubin. Water-soluble.	Defective storage of conjugated bilirubin. Water-soluble.	Decreased bilirubin conjugation.
Liver Histology	Normal	**Black liver**	Normal	Normal
Defective Gene	UGT1A1	MRP2		UGT1A1
Prognosis	Death in infancy if not treated	Normal	Normal	Normal. May show mild signs of jaundice during stressful times
Treatment	Transplant	No estrogens	None	None

NEW BORN EVALUATION

APGAR SCORING, taken at 1 minute and 5 minutes after birth

- **1 minute reflects the effects of labor and delivery**
- **5 minute reflects the response to resuscitation**

	SIGN	0 POINTS	1 POINT	2 POINTS
A	Activity (Muscle tone)	Absent	Arms & Legs Flexed	Active Movement
P	Pulse	Absent	Below 100 bpm	Above 100 bpm
G	Grimace (Reflex, Irritability)	No response	Grimace	Sneeze, cough, pulls away
A	Appearance (skin color)	Blue-gray (dusky), pale all over	Pink body, blue-grey (dusky) extremities	Pink all over: body and extremities
R	Respiration	Absent	Slow, Irregular	Good, Crying

Scoring: 8 – 10 Excellent   5 - 7 Moderately Depressed   0 - 4 Severe Depression – Requires immediate resuscitation

General Baby Evaluation and Procedures

- APGAR
- Height and Weight (low birth weight considered <2500 gms)
- **0.5% Erythromycin eye DROPS or 1% silver nitrate eye drops**
- **1 mg Vit K injection IM**
- **SCREENING TEST: PKU, Biotinidase, Cystic Fibrosis, MSUD, Galactosemia, Homocystinuria, CAH, MCAD, Hypothyroid, Lysosomal Storage Diseases; if applicable: Sickle Cell, Thalassemia**
- **Hearing test (rules out congenital sensorineural hearing loss)**
- **First HEP B Vaccine and Ig within 12 hours of birth**
  2nd vaccine: 1 – 2 months
  3rd vaccine: 6 months
  HEP B Serology (HBsAg and Anti-HBsAg) between 9 – 15 months

Sutures and Fontanels

Sutures: separate the bones in the skull

Fontanels: where the major sutures intersect in the anterior and posterior portions of the skull

- Anterior Fontanels: closes between 4 and 26 months
- Posterior Fontanels: closes by 2 months
- Fullness of the fontanels = intracranial pressure
- Normal fontanels: flat and soft
- Full fontanels = increased ICP due to baby crying or vomiting
- Pulsations of the fontanels = peripheral pulse
- Depressed (sunken) fontanels = dehydration
- Bulging fontanels = increased ICP due to pathology

Scalp Swelling

- **Cephalohematoma**
  subperiosteal hemorrhage from birth trauma
  Localized swelling of the scalp
  Swelling does NOT cross suture lines
  Resolves by 3 weeks
- **Caput Succedaneum**
  Asymmetrical head swelling
  Swelling over the occipitoparietal region
  Capillary distention and extravasation of blood from rupture of amniotic sac
  Swelling crosses suture lines
  Resolves in 1 – 2 days
- **Craniosynostosis**
  Premature closure of sutures
  Causes: abnormal growth and shape of skull
- **Hydrocephalus**
  Bulging anterior fontanelles
  Eyes deviated downward showing upper sclera (AKA: "Setting Sun Sign")

Microcephaly

- Due to premature closure of sutures or microcephaly
- **Microcephaly** causes: congenital infections (ie: Zika virus), chromosome abnormalities, neurologic pathologies, maternal metabolic disorders

Macrocephaly (>95 percentile)

- Macrocephaly causes: hydrocephalus, brain tumor, subdural hematoma, inherited genetic issues

Failure to Thrive: Inadequate weight gain for age.

- Signs: growth <5th percentile for age
- Causes: Any serious pathology can cause failure to thrive

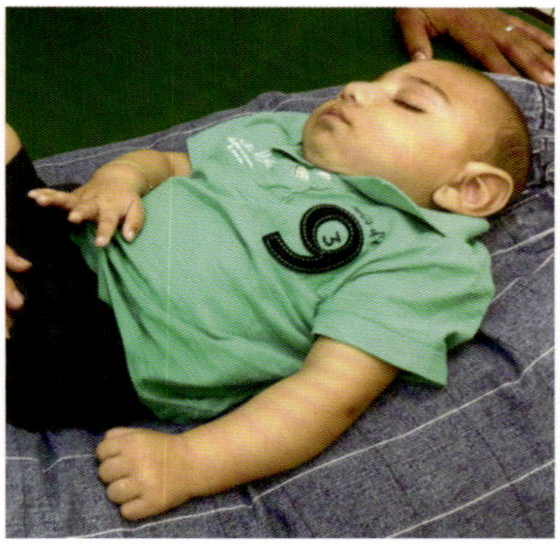

Microcephaly

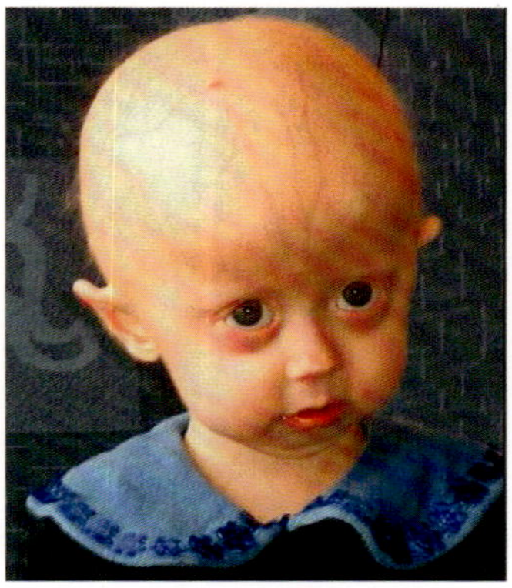

Macrocephaly

Home Delivery Newborn Complications

Vitamin K Deficiency (AKA: Hemorrhagic Disease of the Newborn)

- Baby born at home
- No Vit K prophylaxis was given at birth
- Appears from 24 hours of birth to one week
- Bleeding
- **No gut flora developed yet. Lactobacillus** (primary gut flora in breastfed babies) produces Vitamin K.
- Breast milk contains only small amounts of Vit K.
- **No Vit K = no gamma carboxylation of the clotting factors 2, 7, 9, 10, C & S = bleeding.**
- Risk Factors: Maternal anti-seizure meds (interfere with Vit K metabolism), anticoagulant's (Coumadin, aspirin, warfarin), antibiotics (cephalosporin's), breastfeeding exclusively.
- SX: **Bleeding** in the umbilicus, GI tract (melena), skin, nose, surgical sites (ie: circumcision), brain, skin bruising, mucosal bleeds.
- TX: **Vitamin K**

Neonatal Tetanus

- Baby born at home, umbilical cord cut with a **non-sterile instrument.**
- Baby has not acquired passive immunity because **mother has not been immunized.**
- Appears about one week old.
- Best way to prevent: Tetanus toxoid vaccine to women of childbearing age.
- SX: **Muscle rigidity**, irritability, **dysphagia** (foaming at mouth b/c can't swallow), facial grimacing, muscle spasms, poor sucking.

CONGENITAL DISEASES (TORCH)

Congenital Syphilis

- Treponema pallidum
- Syphilis is transmitted through the placenta so C-sections will not prevent the disease.
- **Ulcers (peeling skin)** on body, **rhinorrhea (looks like a cold, runny eyes/nose**), jaundice, crusted eyes, Osteochondritis and Periostitis (inflammation of periosteum. DX: x-ray of bones shows distorted bones)
- Later in life: Mulberry molars, Hutchinson teeth, saber shins (anterior bowing of legs), saddle nose, deafness, keratitis, and high arch palate.
- DX: BIT: VDRL screen
- DX: MAT: IgM-FTA-ABS or dark field microscopy.
- TX: **Penicillin** (If allergic, **desensitize** mother)

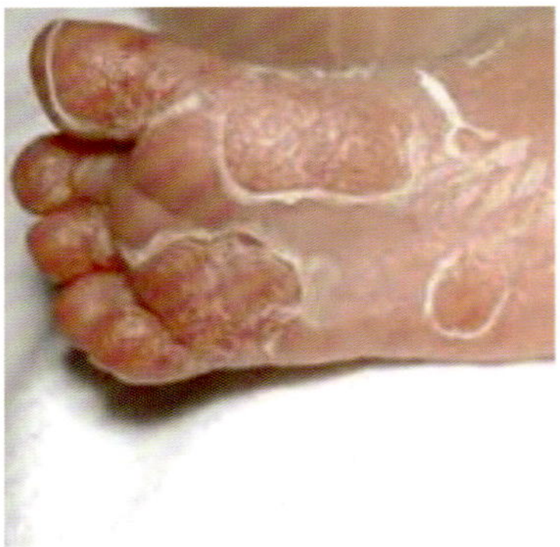

Peeling skin (desquamation)

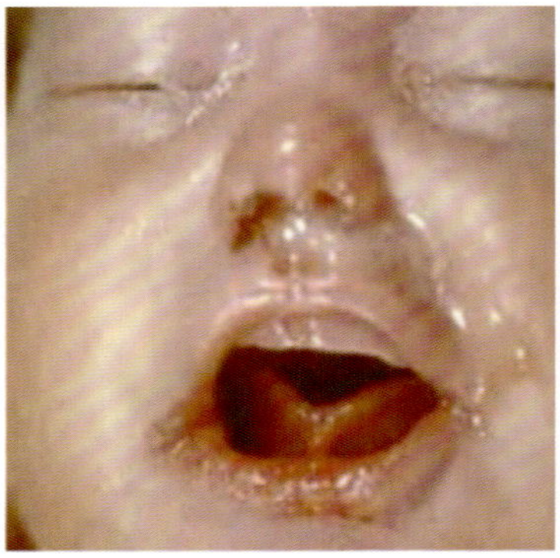

Rhinorrhea

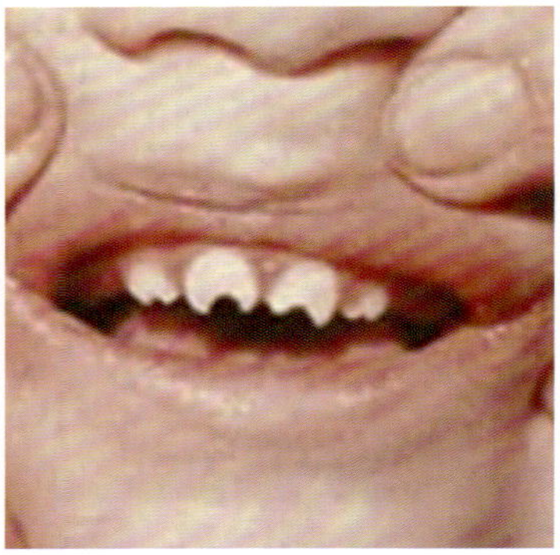

Hutchinson teeth

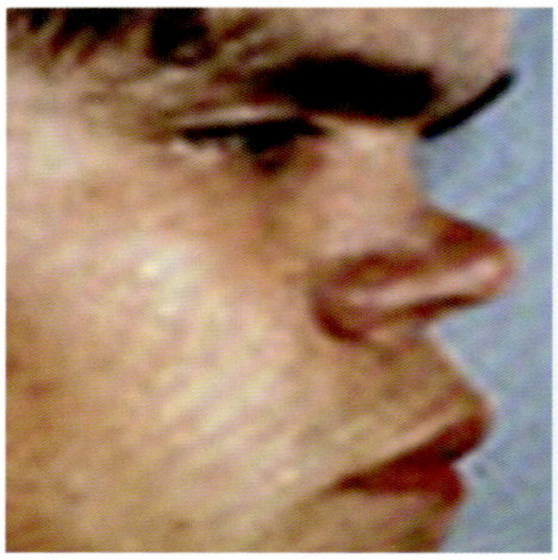

Saddle nose

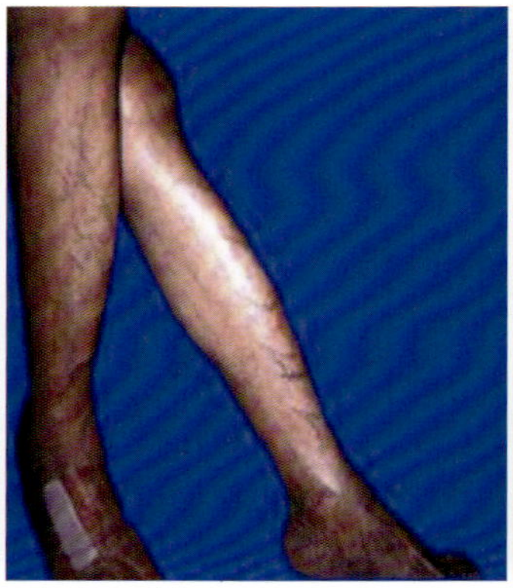

Saber shins

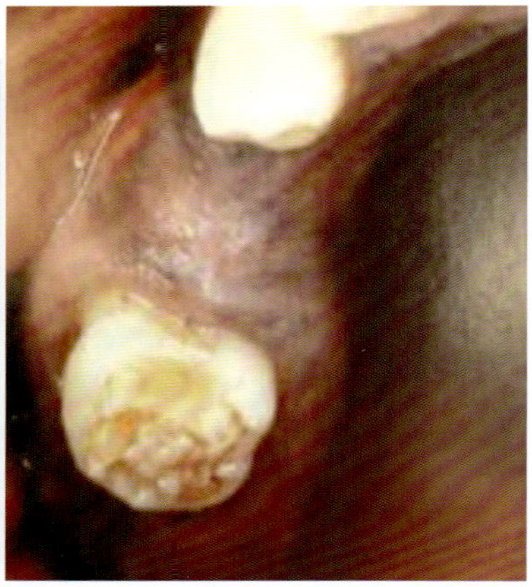

Mulberry molars

Congenital Rubella

- **Petechia** (blueberry muffin rash, thrombocytopenic, purple skin lesions), **cataracts (white eye reflex), heart problems (PDA)**, microcephaly, deafness, large liver/spleen, IUGR, hyperbilirubinemia.
- Transmission: first 4 weeks of pregnancy
- Spread: **respiratory droplets**
- DX: IgM against rubella
- TX: Supportive

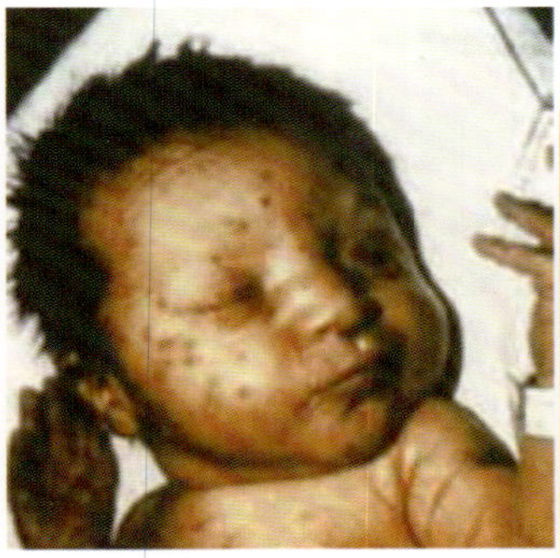
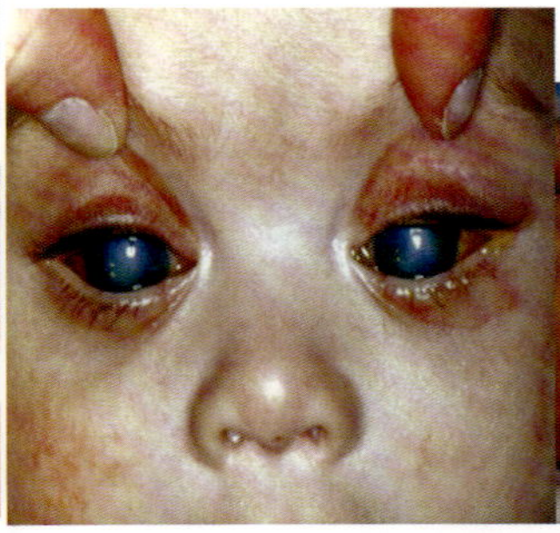
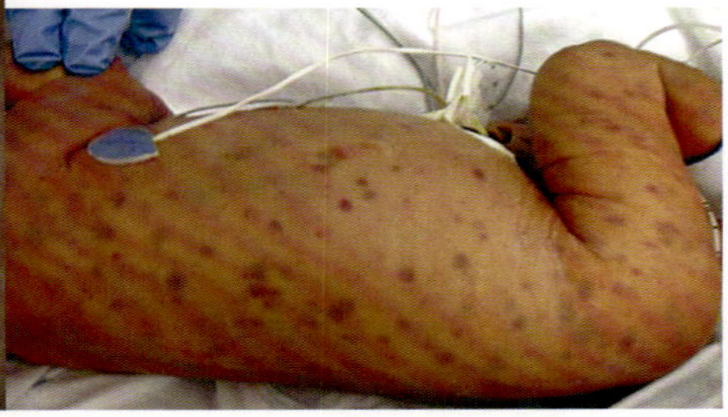

Congenital CMV

- **Petechia** (blueberry muffin rash, thrombopenic), **eye problems (red eye – chorioretinitis), periventricular calcifications**, microphthalmia (small eyes), deafness, IUGR, hepatosplenomegaly, **microcephaly**, mute, **hearing loss**.
- Spread: sexual contact
- DX: BIT: CMV IgM and urine or saliva viral titers. (Negative urine or saliva CMV excludes CMV). MAT: Urine or saliva PCR for viral DNA.
- TX: **Ganciclovir**

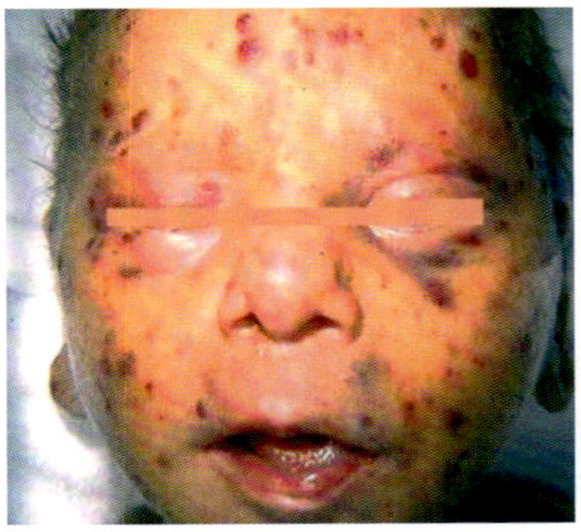
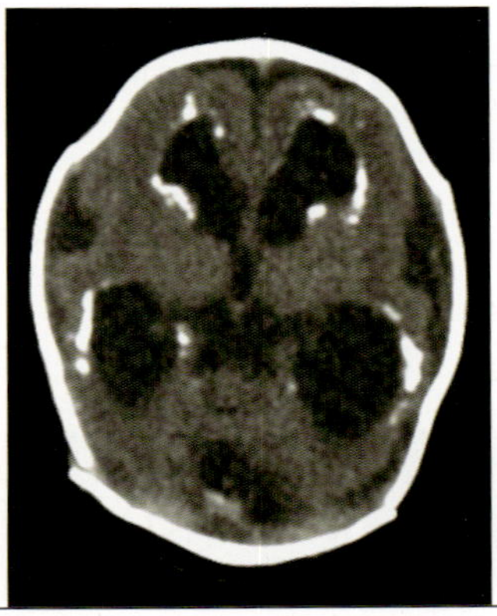

Neonatal Chlamydia – Gonorrhea

- Acquired through vaginal canal
- 1st complication in newborn (eye):
  If it shows in the **first week (2 – 5 days)**: Gonorrhea (**tip**: "**GO"norrhea** for **"GO"**es first)
  If it shows **after first week (5 – 14 days): Conjunctivitis, mucopurulent or watery discharge.**
- **Chlamydia is MCC.** Neonatal pneumonia due to Chlamydia can also be seen.
- **Gonorrhea usually has a heavier mucopurulent discharge and a cloudy cornea.**
- **TX: Erythromycin ointment**
- 2nd complication in newborn: Pneumonia: shows 4 to 12 weeks.
- **Chlamydia pneumonia SX: Staccato cough**, nasal congestion, hyperinflation on CXR, rales in lungs.
- Spread: sexual contact – vertical transmission

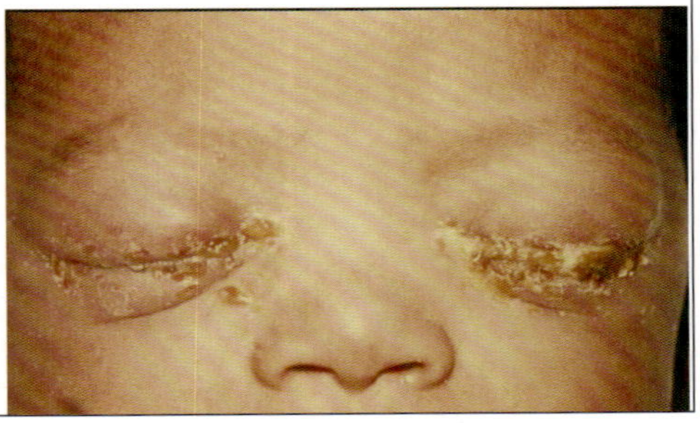

Congenital Toxoplasmosis

- **Hydrocephalus, macrocephaly, intracranial calcifications**, seizures, large spleen and liver, red eyes – retina (Chorioretinitis).
- **Source: Toxoplasma gondii from** cat feces, deli meats, undercooked meats, skins of vegetables (peel veggies).
- DX: BIT: IgM against toxoplasmosis. MAT: PCR for toxoplasmosis.
- TX: **TMP/Pyrimethamine** **(Sulfadiazine and Pyrimethamine)**

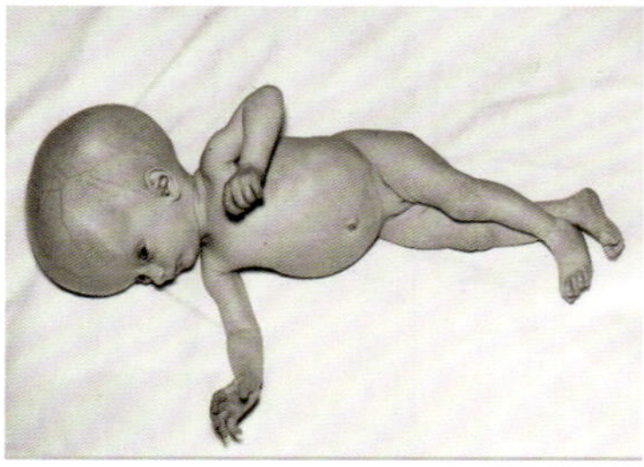
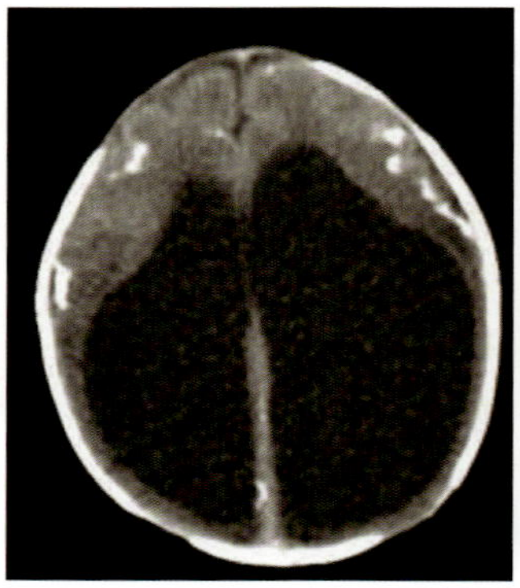
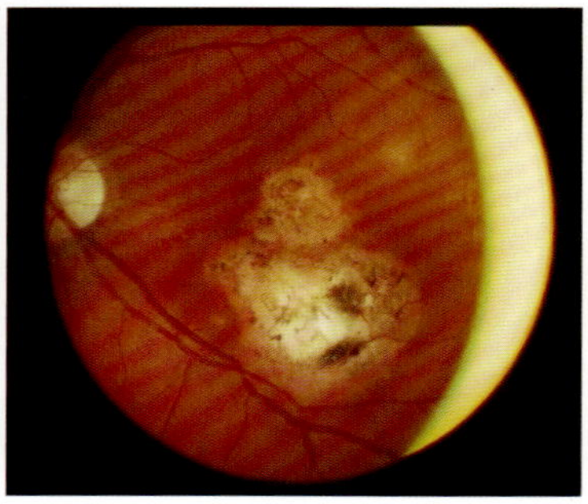

Neonatal Herpes

- Majority of cares are due to vertical transmission of herpes simplex virus from mother to newborn in the vaginal canal. Small percent is due to infections in utero and postnatal.
- **Vesicular skin lesions** (located at trauma sites from scalp electrodes, forceps, vacuum extractors, in the eyes, nose or circumcision), affects on the liver, **temporal encephalitis** (seizures, lethargy, irritability, poor feeding), **meningitis**, bulging fontanelle, sensitivity to light, unstable temperatures, sepsis, DIC.
- Mother's with active genital herpes lesions at the time of labor should be delivered by caesarean section.
- DX: BIT: Tzanck smear. MAT: HSV PCR
- TX: **Acyclovir** and supportive care.

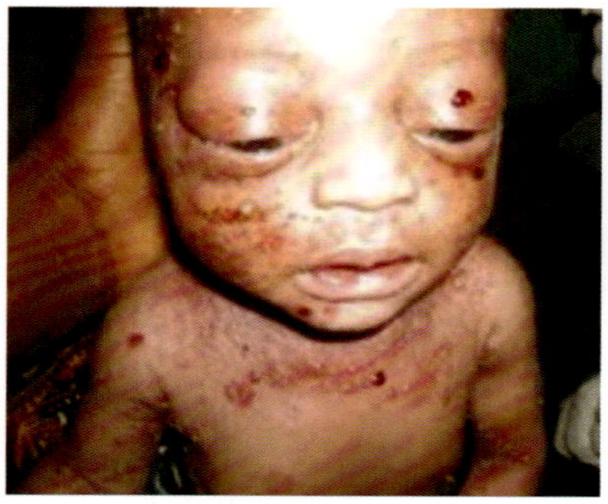
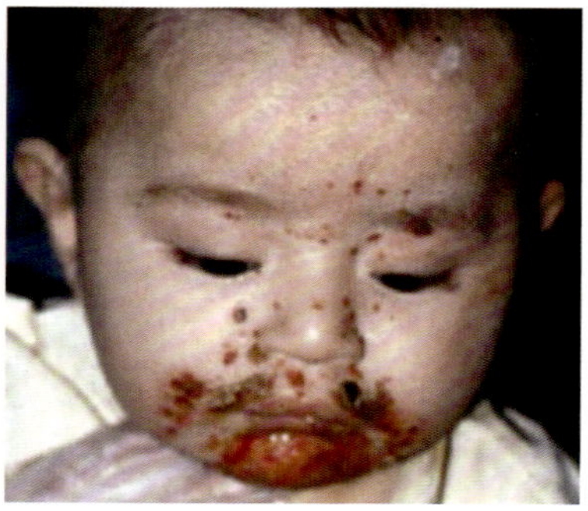

Congenital HIV

- **Oral thrush, lymphadenopathy**, eczema, large liver and spleen, recurring fevers, **irretractible diarrhea**, failure to thrive (does not gain weight), recurrent infections
- Asymptomatic at birth. Does not show until later in the first month
- Vertical transmission from mother
- C-section must be done if the mother's viral load > 1000 at the time of delivery.
- TX: **AZT IV** in labor and oral **AZT** for the **baby for 6 weeks**

Congenital Varicella – Zoster

- Due to mothers with a primary infection with **chickenpox** (maternal varicella zoster) prior to 20 weeks gestation. Condition is very rare.
- IUGR, **skin lesions** (thickened, overgrown hypertrophic scar tissue, indurated hardened and inflamed. **Skeletal** anomalies (Malformation of the arms and/or legs (hypoplastic), hypoplasia of fingers and toe)s. Cortical atrophy, dilated ventricles, mental retardation, **eye diseases** (nystagmus, cataracts), abnormalities of the nervous system and skeletal anomalies.
- DX: BIT: Serology
- DX: MAT: PCR of amniotic fluid
- TX: Varicella-zoster IVIG

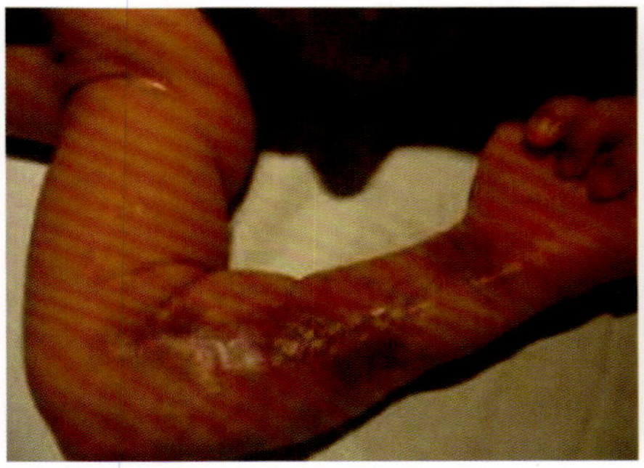
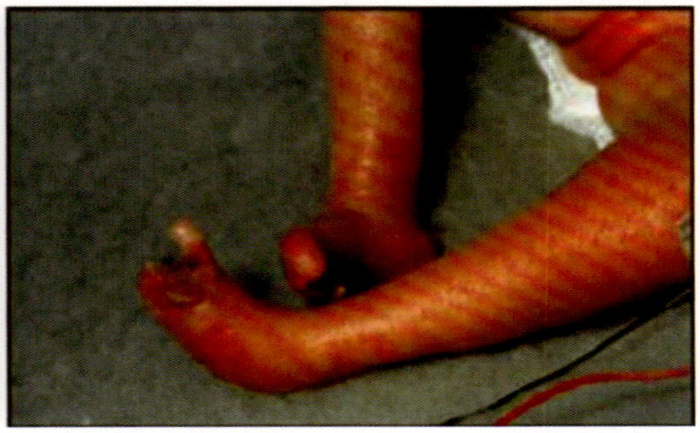

Newborn Seizures

- **SX: Repetitive movements: tongue thrusting, staring, chewing, blinking, apnea, sucking movements. Jittery movements do not improve when limb is passively moved, deviation of the eyes.**
  TX: Correct the underlying cause (ie: electrolyte abnormalities)
  TX: Acute seizures: Lorazepam, Diazepam (rectally).
  TX: Absence seizures: Ethosuximide

DRUGS DURING PREGNANCY – NEONATAL

Withdrawal (AKA: Neonatal Abstinence Syndrome)

- Withdrawal can begin within a few hours to an average of 3 days after birth, but can take as long as 5 – 10 days.
- MC Withdrawal substances: Opiates (Heroin, Codeine, Oxycodone). Amphetamines (Cocaine), Barbiturates, Marijuana, Benzodiazepines, Alcohol.

Cocaine

- Winds you up! Stimulates the CNS. **High suckling**, high and **pronounced reflexes** (startles easily), jitters, irritable, increased risk of SIDS.
- Last 8 to 10 weeks
- This is a withdrawal from the mother. Shows up 1 – 2 days after birth (once cocaine has left the babies system).
- Babies have higher chance of learning and growth disorders.
- Mothers: Risk of **abruptio placenta**, preterm labor.

Heroin (other opioids: hydrocodone, morphine, codeine)

- **Sneezing**, yawning, seizures, **Inconsolable crying**, **high-pitched cry**, difficulty sleeping, vomiting (emesis), diarrhea, tachycardia, difficulty maintaining a normal temperature, hyperactive reflexes (easily startled), poor weight gain.
- Symptoms appear between 24 – 36 hours
- Mom: High chance of premature labor or still birth
- Babies have high chance of learning disorders

SSRI

- Jitteriness, seizures, exaggerated startle reflex, weak cry, poor muscle tone, low blood sugar, increased motor activity, yellow discoloration of the skin.
- When mom takes SSRI 's in the last trimester of pregnancy.
- Symptoms appear between hours and days.

Marijuana

- Normally does not cause withdrawal symptoms.

Fetal Alcohol Syndrome

- #1 most common cause of birth defects
- Symptoms appear within 3 to 12 hours after birth.
- **Smooth philtrum; thin upper lip, microcephaly, palpebral fissures** (small eye openings), lung fistula, mental retardation, cardiac defects, hypoplastic fifth fingernails.

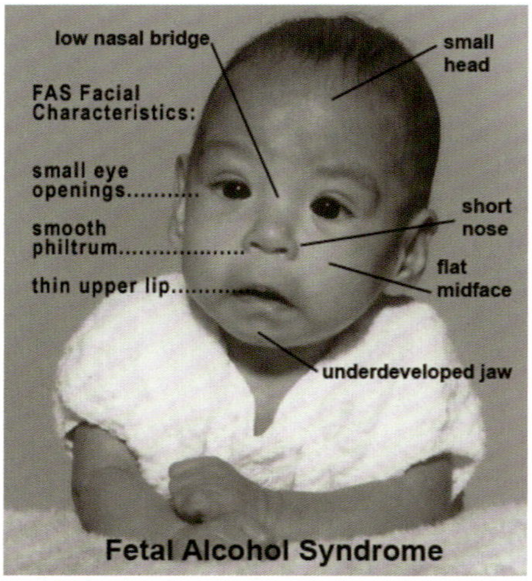

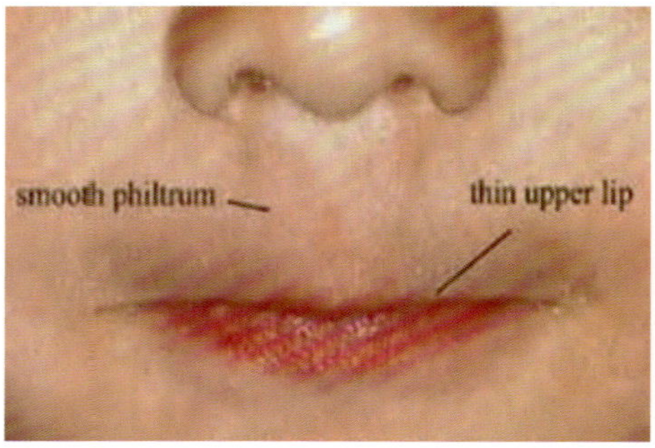

Smoking

- Mothers risk: preterm labor, placental problems
- Babies risk: **IUGR, premature**, ADHD

IUGR

Poor fetal growth. Fetal weight is estimated to be < 10th percentile of its gestational age that result in low birth weight.

Asymmetrical IUGR (most common 70%)	Symmetrical IUGR
Restriction of weight followed by length. Head grows normally but body is thin, out of proportion to head. Exam shows normal head measurement but ↓ abdominal measurements.	Overall growth restriction indicating that the fetus has grown slowly since the beginning. The head and body are proportional. Exam shows all measurements are ↓.
Causes occured > 28 weeks (MC: due to maternal causes)	Occurs occurred < 28 wks (MC: congenital causes)
HTN, smoking, hypoxia, pre-eclampsia, vascular dz, malnutrition, infarction of placenta, alcohol, drugs	TORCH infections, chromosome problems, structural anomalies, aneuploidy, anemia

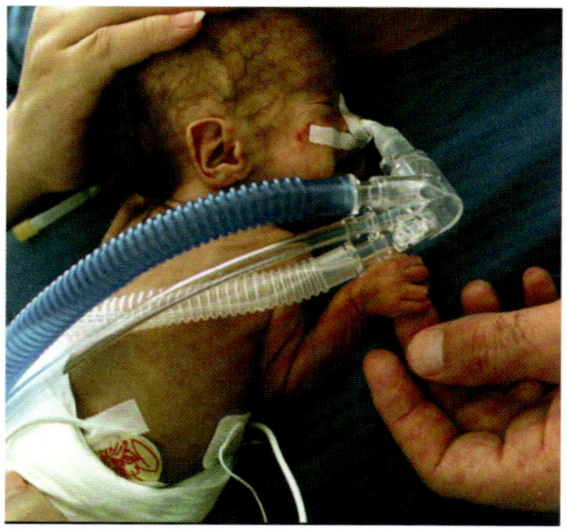

Premature

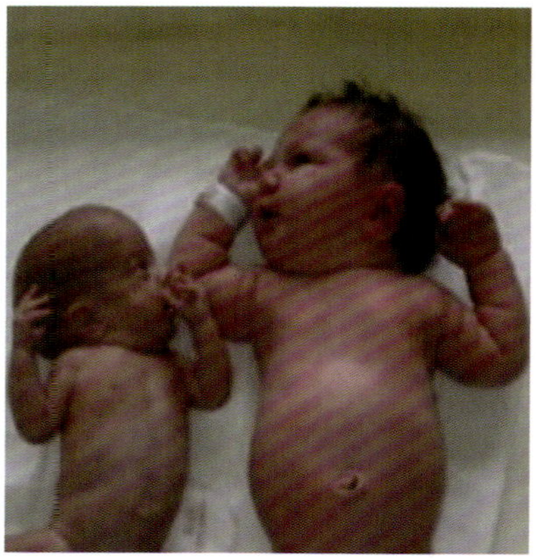

IUGR Normal

TORCHES and TERATOGEN PATHOLOGIES

Pregnancy Drug Categories

- Class A Human and animal studies done: safe
- Class B Animal studies show no fetal risk, no human studies, OR animal studies show fetal risk but human studies: likely safe
- Class C Animal studies show fetal risk, no human studies: use ONLY if potential benefit outweighs risk
- Class D Fetal Risk, Potential benefit may justify use in severe cases
- Class F Fetal Risk, Do not use in any case

Medications with High Teratogen Risk

- ACE Inhibitors: Renal problems, craniofacial abnormalities
- Aminoglycosides: Ototoxic (CN VIII)
- Anesthetics: Respiratory depression
- Barbiturates: Respiratory depression, CNS, depression
- Carbamazepine: Neural tube defects, fingernail hyperplasia, craniofacial (odd faces), IUGR (Intrauterine growth restriction).
- Chloramphenicol: Grey Baby Syndrome (UDP Glucuronyl Transferase), Aplastic Anemia (AKA: Pancytopenia).
- Clarithromycin: embryotoxic
- DES (Diethylstilbesterol): Clear Cell Vaginal CA, Adenomyosis
- Fluoroquinolones (Cipro 's): Tendonitis, tendon rupture, cartilage damage.
- Folate Antagonist: Neural tube defects
- Griseofulvin: embryotoxic
- Isotretinoin: Face and ear abnormalities, heart disease
- Lithium: Ebstein's Anomaly (Right atrium)
- Magnesium sulfate: Respiratory depression
- Metronidazole: Can take during pregnancy but must stop for a few days if breastfeeding.
- NSAIDS: Premature closure of ductus arteriosus
- Phenobarbital: Vitamin K deficiency
- Phenytoin: Microcephaly, odd faces, hypoplastic nails, cardiac problems, mental retardation.
- Ribavirin: embryotoxic
- Sulfonamides (TMP/SMX, Sulfa Drugs, Thiazides): Kernicterus (displaces bilirubin from albumin).
- Tetracyclines: Teeth discoloration and bone problems
- Thalidomide: abnormal limbs ("Flappers") Taken off the market
- Valproate: Neural tube defects, mental retardation (stops maternal folate absorption).
- Warfarin: Fetal hemorrhage, abortion, bones, eyes, chondrodysplasia, facial abnormalities (must use Heparin).

Misc Teratogens

- Iodide: Goiter, hypothyroidism
- **Maternal Diabetes**: **Caudal Regression Syndrome** (anal atresia to sirenomelia), heart defects, neural tube defects, **macrosomia**, baby is hypoglycemic after birth. (Baby is used to outputting a lot of insulin due to mother's constant high glucose levels. After birth, the mother's glucose is no longer available, but the babies insulin levels remain high, depleting the baby of glucose creating hypoglycemia)
- **Vitamin A (Retinol):** Spontaneous abortions and birth defects, cleft palate, cardiac problems
- X-Rays: Microcephaly, mental retardation

Neonatal Conjunctivitis

Non-specific signs: red conjunctiva, tearing, mucopurulent or non-purulent discharge, chemosis, edema in the eyelid (swelling).

- Chemical causes: Due to the silver nitrate drops put into the newborns eyes at birth. Usually occurs in the first 24 hours.
  SX: Mild conjunctiva, tearing, self-resolving 2 – 4 days.
- Neisseria gonorrhea
  Usually occurs between 2 and 5 days. (**tip**: "GO"norrhea "GO"es first).
  SX: Acute conjunctivitis, chemosis, severe eye lid edema, heavier mucopurulent discharge, potentially corneal involvement (clouding, edema, ulceration), superficial keratitis.
  DX: Culture on chocolate agar or Thayer-Martin media.
  TX: **Erythromycin ointment.**
- Chlamydia trachomatis
  Usually occurs 5 – 14 days after birth.
  Note: Can also see neonatal pneumonia due to Chlamydia.
  SX: Lighter mucopurulent discharge, eyelid edema, chemosis (swelling of conjunctiva), pseudomembrane formation, mild hyperemia (increase in blood flow).
  DX: Conjunctive scraping w/Gram stain and Giemsa stain.
  TX: **Erythromycin ointment**.

- HSV Neonatal Conjunctivitis
  Edema, nonpurulent discharge, moderate conjunctiva, serosanguineous discharge (watery discharge of serum and blood), possible herpetic keratitis (dendritic keratitis is seen in adults).
  DX: Exposure to maternal herpes outbreak during vaginal delivery.
  TX: **Acyclovir IV**

Perinatal Infection

- **Transcervical** (Ascending)
  Inhalation of infected amniotic fluid: pneumonia, sepsis, meningitis, high risk with PROM (premature rupture of membranes).
  Passage through infected birth canal: herpes (caesarian section with active herpes).
- **Transplacental** (hematogenous)
  Viral and parasitic: HIV (at delivery with maternal to fetal transfusion), TORCH, Parvovirus B19 (AKA: Fifth Disease, Slapped Cheek, Erythema Infectiosum).
  Bacterial: Listeria monocytogenes.

CHILD DEVELOPMENT

NORMAL Child Development Chart

Age	MOTOR	SOCIAL	VERBAL - LANGUAGE
Birth – 3 mos	Holds head up, Rooting Reflex, Moro Reflex (Reflexes disappear At 4 – 6 months)	**Social Smile**	Responds to voices
3 mos – 1 year	**Sits** alone, holds toys, crawls, cruises, Rolls over, **pulls to stand**, **thumb-finger (pincer) grasp**	**Stranger anxiety**	Plays peek-a-boo, plays ball, Responds to simple words
1 to 18 months	Walks, Climbs stairs, stacks 3 blocks, Makes lines and scribbles	Separation anxiety	Can say a few words
2 years	Feeds self, kicks/throws ball, Stacks 6 blocks, turns pages, removes clothes, goes up and down stairs jumps with 2 feet, eats with spoon, threads shoelaces.	Will leave mother for a short time	**200 words,** 2 word phrases
3 years	Rides tricycle, copies simple **lines or circles/shapes,** feeds self, helps with chores, walks downstairs with alternating feet, knows age, knows sex	Parallel/group play, gender identity	**900 words,** Complete sentences
4 years	Brushes teeth, **buttons**, zippers, **Hops on 1 foot**, draw stick figures, draws person (stick figure), jumps over objects, throws ball overhand, tells stories.	**Imaginary friends**, Cooperative play, Imitates adults	Tells stories, uses plurals and prepositions, Counts to 10

Tip: Be VERY aware of the verbal skills (number of words) given in the question. If they are decreased from the normal, **you must have their hearing tested!**

Gestational Age

- Preterm <34 weeks
- Late preterm 34 – 36 weeks
- Term 37 to 42 weeks
- Post-term >42 weeks

Neonatal: First 28 days of life
Infancy: >28 days to first year of life
Preschool: Ages 1 – 4 years
School Age: Ages >5

Mortality

Perinatal morality: deaths after 22 weeks gestation
Neonatal mortality: deaths in the first 28 days of life
Postneonatal mortality: deaths after 28 days but before one year
Child mortality: deaths within the first five years of birth

Birth Weights

Low Birth Weight: <2500 gm (<5.5 lbs) = < 10th percentile

- Causes: Prematurity, IUGR, STD's
- Complications: SIDS, impaired thermoregulation, polycythemia, infections, respiratory distress (RDS), low immunity, hypoglycemia, impaired emotional development, necrotizing enterocolitis, increased risk for developing DM II later in life, high mortality.

Normal Birth Weight: **3500 gm** (7.7 lbs) with average being 2500 to 5000 kg (5.5 – 11 lbs), 10 to 90th percentile.

Large Birth Weight: **>5000 gm** (>11 lbs), >90th percentile

- Causes: Postmature newborn (over 42 weeks), diabetic mothers
- Complications: hypoglycemia, reduced function of the placenta = decreased nutrition, respiratory distress, meconium aspiration.

Pediatric Vital Sign Normal Ranges

Age Group	Respiratory Rate/Min	Heart Rate/Min	Systolic BP	Weight Kilos	Weight lbs
Newborn	30 – 50	120 – 160	50 – 70	2 – 3	4.5 – 7
Infant (1 – 12 months)	20 – 30	80 – 140	70 – 100	4 – 10	9 – 22
Toddler (1 – 3 years)	20 – 30	80 – 130	80 – 110	10 – 14	22 – 31
Preschool (3 – 5 years)	20 – 30	80 – 120	80 – 110	14 – 18	31 – 40
School Age (6 – 12 years)	20 – 30	70 – 110	80 – 120	20 – 42	41 – 92
Adolescent (13 + years)	12 – 20	55 – 105	110 – 120	>50	>110

Fetal Growth and Maturity

Pre Term Infant	Post Term Infant
< 37 weeks gestation, < 2500 gm Few creases in the feet, they are smooth. Covered in lanugo "Peach fuzz", ↓ fat causes hypothermia, thin skin so veins are visible, ↓ cartilage in the ears, hypoglycemia, ↓ temperature stability. Risk: immature lungs, RDS, ↑ infections	> 42 weeks gestation, peeling skin, long fingernails. Risk: meconium aspiration

Newborn Procedures/Test

In delivery room at birth

- **STEPS if infant is NOT in distress: 1) Suction the mouth and nose, 2) then clamp and cut the cord, 3) dry and wrap the baby, 4) place under a warmer.**
- **2 opthalmic antibiotics: 0.5% Erythromycin or Tetracycline ophthalmic ointment to prevent ophthalmia neonatorum (infection due to N. gonorrhea or Chlamydia trachomatis). Silver nitrate drops.**
  Conjunctivitis in a newborn:
  1st day: due to irritation from silver nitrate eye ointments/drops.
  1st week (2 – 7 days): due to N. gonorrhea.
  >3 weeks due to herpes.
  After 7 days due to C. trachomatis.
  TX for N. gonorrhea or Chlamydia: Erythromycin ointment.
  TX for herpes: oral Acyclovir and topical Vidarabine.
- **1 mg Vitamin K IM (gut flora is not established yet so Vitamin K is not produced in order to cause gama-carboxylation of clotting factors II, VII, IX, X, protein C & S) Babies born at home that do not get the vitamin K shot have a higher risk of hemorrhage (hemorrhagic disease of the newborn).**
- **NOTE: Tiny hemorrhages in the infant's eyes may be seen and are normal due to the increase of intrathoracic pressure from the chest being compressed in the birth canal.**

Screening and other treatments during hospital stay (before discharge)

- **Phenylketonuria (PKU)**
- **Cystic Fibrosis (elevated sweat chloride)**
- **Congenital Adrenal Hyperplasia (CAH)**
- **Galactosemia**
- **G6PD deficiency**
- **Beta thalassemia**
- **Homocystinuria**
- **Hypothyroidism (cretinism)**
- **Biotinidase**
- **Hearing test**
- **Hepatitis B vaccine if mother is HBsAg negative.**
  If mother is HBsAg positive: administer both Hepatitis B vaccine and Hepatitis IVIG

Newborn Reflexes (additional reflexes in the Neurology Chapter)

- Suckling reflex (baby will automatically suck on any nipplelike object)
- Grasping reflex (baby will grab and hold a finger)
- Moro reflex (when startled, the babies arms will swing outward simultaneously)
- Rooting reflex (touch the babies cheek and it will turn to that side)
- Babinski reflex (sweep the bottom of the babies foot and the toes will extend/fan out)
- Stepping reflex (when the babies toes touch they ground they will make walking movements)
- Superman reflex (when the baby is held up facing the floor, the arms will go out)

Breastfeeding

NO Breastfeeding Allowed With These Pathologies

HIV	TB	**HSV** (if active breast lesions)
Malaria	Sepsis	Typhoid Fever
Eclampsia	Nephritis	**Substance Abuse** (actively on illicit drugs)
Breast Cancer	**Varicella** (active)	Chemotherapy
If baby has Galactosemia		

Breastfeeding Allowed With These Pathologies
Hepatitis B
Hepatitis C

Supplements For Infants

- Breast milk has sufficient iron for the infant. Formula fed babies should be supplemented with iron-fortified formula.
- Begin supplements of **Vitamin D** (400 IU per day) in 2-month-old infants that are strictly **breast-fed.**
- Folic acid for babies taking **goats milk.**

Breast Feeding Newborns

- **15 – 20 minutes on each breast 8 times per day**
- **4 – 6 wet diapers per day**
- **8 – 12 stools per day**

Breast milk

- Human milk protein (whey)
- Absorbs better, easier to digest, improves gastric emptying, ↓ reflux, ↓ colic

Breast or Bottle Feeding Timeline

Birth to 6 months	6 months to 12 months	12 months
If breastfed, Must add: Iron (supplement till 1 year. #1 most deficient in kids) Vitamin D (400 IU/Day. Start within 1st month)	Add pureed vegetables And fruits. Add one at a time to watch for allergies.	Introduce cow's milk

Child Normal Weight and Height Development

- Weight:
  Regains birth weight by 2 weeks
  Double the weight in 5 – 6 months
  Triple the weight in 1 year
  - Newborns can lose up to 10% of weight in the first week and retain it by 10 days
- Height:
  Growth of 50% of the original height by 1 year
  Doubles original height by age 4
  Triples original height by age 13
  - Growth spirts: Occurs from: 2 – 12 years old
    Pain: bilateral, at night, lower extremities (thighs and calves)
    TX: Massage, muscle stretch, analgesics
- Head Circumference
  0 – 2 months: 0.5 cm/week
  2 – 6 months: 0.25 cm/week

Dehydration in Children

1 kg acute weight loss = 1 L fluid loss
TX: IV Bolus of isotonic fluid. 20 mL/Kg of normal saline.

- Mild: 3 – 5 % volume.
  Cause: ↓ intake or ↑ fluid loss.
  Minimal or no symptoms.
- Moderate: 6 – 9%
  SX: ↓ skin turgor, dry mucus membranes, tachycardia, irritable, delayed capillary response (refill) of 2 – 3 seconds, ↓ urine output.
- Severe: 10 – 15%
  SX: Cool clammy skin, cracked lips, dry mucous membrane, sunken eyes, sunken fontanelle, lethargy ↓ urine output, hypotension, delayed capillary response (refill) > 3 seconds, tachycardia, shock.

High Risk Children for Cholesterol and CAD

- ↑ Risk if: parents, grandparents, aunts, uncles with ↑ blood cholesterol > 240 or premature CAD.
- For high risk children: check random cholesterol at 2 years old
  Results:
  If ↑ levels, repeat test in 1 – 2 weeks
  If levels are < 170 recheck at 5 years old
  If levels are > 200 do lipid profile

Failure to Thrive (FTT)

- Growth rate less than expected for a child
- Weight is usually affected before length
- Weight and length are affected before head circumference (usually spared in FTT)
- MCC is inorganic FTT (inadequate caloric intake due to a disturbed child/parent bond.

Cleft Palate

- Cleft Lip and Cleft Palate Repair: Rule of 10's: By 10 weeks, or 10 lbs or 10 Hb

Enuresis

- Inability to control urination.
- Nocturnal enuresis: bedwetting between 5 and 10 years old.
  Normal: More ADH is produced at night to decrease the need to urinate.
  MCC: Causes: small bladder capacity, longer sleep periods, immature signals in the brain that signal a full bladder.
  These will disappear as child matures.
- TX: Moisture alarms (wakes child when they begin to urinate)
  Desmopressin (AKA: DDAVP) (increases ADH levels), Imipramine

Encopresis

- **Voluntary or involuntary fecal passage after child has been toilet trained, usually in underwear or on floor (> 4 years)**
- **MCC: Retention due to constipation. Stood remains in the colon too long so that water is removed and the stool becomes hard and painful to expel.**
- **Other factors due to retention: stress, Hirschsprung dz, and ulcerative colitis.**
- **TX: Stool softeners and behavior therapy**
- **Factors due to non-retentive: abuse**

Normal Sexual Growth (2 – 5 years old)

- Play doctor, imitate laying on another, clothed (if having seen parents doing this), talk about their genitals, occasional masturbation, curiosity about naked bodies (theirs or others), cross dressing

Abnormal Sexual Growth

- Pre-occupation with masturbation, extensive sexual knowledge, simulating of foreplay or intercourse, excessive talk about sex, touching others genitals

Infant/Child Deprivation

Child is being deprived of a life that a normal child would live. This can be due to the living environment, malnutrition, etc. This is something that is not done on purpose, many times the parents **don't know any better**.

- Deprivation over 6 months can cause irreversible damage
- Severe deprivation can lead to death
- Deprivation can cause child to be:
  Withdrawn, underweight, no trust, poor language and social skills, illness

Child Neglect

Maltreatment of a child. Caregiver is **aware of the failure** to provide:

- Food, shelter, education, affection, supervision
- Signs: withdrawal, malnutrition, lack of hygiene, emotional or social impairment
- **MUST be reported to child protective services**

Pathologies Involving Regression of Milestones

- Rett's Syndrome
- Niemann-Pick Disease
- Subacute Sclerosing Panencephalitis (SSPE) (history of measles < 2 yrs old)

Child Abuse

- Child abuse, even if you are remotely suspicious, MUST be reported to authorities
- Physicians have no liability risk in reporting child abuse. They can't get into any trouble.
- Children most at risk
  - Stepchildren
  - ADHD/extremely active children
  - Children, 1 year (especially babies because they cry often)
  - Handicapped children (require continual, high care)
  - Premature children (require continual, high care)
- Ophthalmology exams are necessary for any infants/children that may have been abused.
- Never send a child home in cases where there may be suspicion of abuse: admit them to the hospital. If parents refuse, get an emergency court order.

Risk Factors and Signs of Child Abuse

	Sexual Abuse	Physical Abuse
Age	Peak: 9 – 12 years old	Less than 3 years old
Abuser	Usually male. Victim usually knows the abuser	Parent or guardian, esp. mother Young babysitters, young and/or low social economic parents
Signs	STDs, UTI's, Genital, oral, anal trauma	X Rays show healed fractures or fractures in different stages of healing, **spiral fractures** (see picture below), scalding burns: show a straight burn line, cigarette burns, **bruises** in multiple locations or in **different stages of healing**, belt, electrical cord or switch marks on skin, rib fractures, **retinal hemorrhages** or subdural hematomas due to **shaken baby,** unexplained injuries or inconsistent stories, delay in seeking treatment, demanding or dominant parent after delay in seeking treatment, history of repeated injuries or accidents, alcohol or drugs in the family history, repeated vaginal infections, repeated STD's, vaginal bruising or lacerations, pain in sitting, female circumcision (is considered abuse, regardless of culture).

Child Abuse

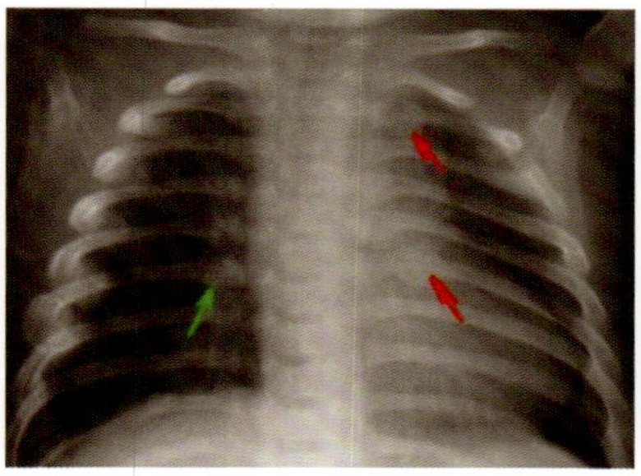

Broken ribs

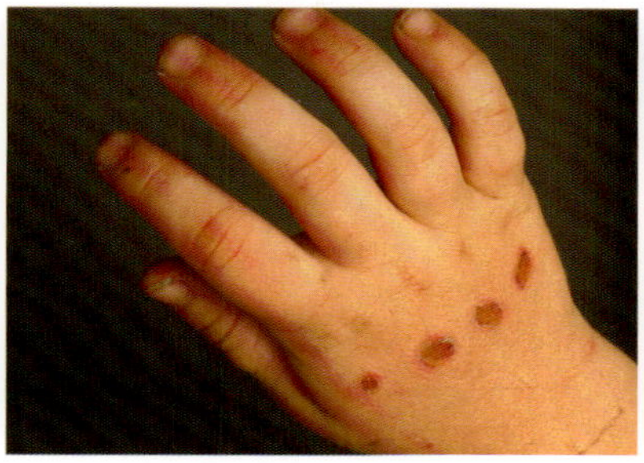

Cigarette burns

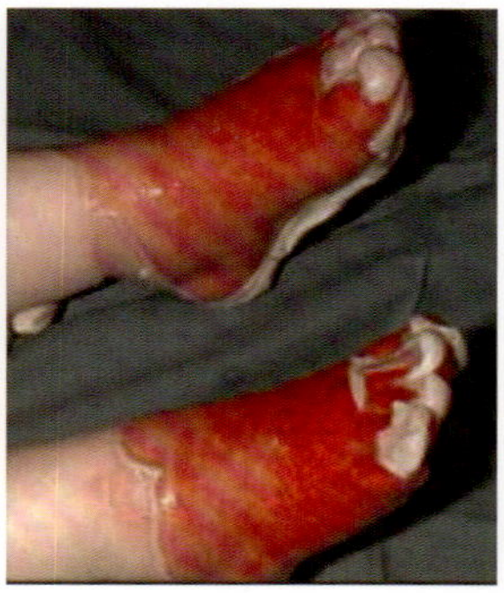

Scalding burns
Note the water lines

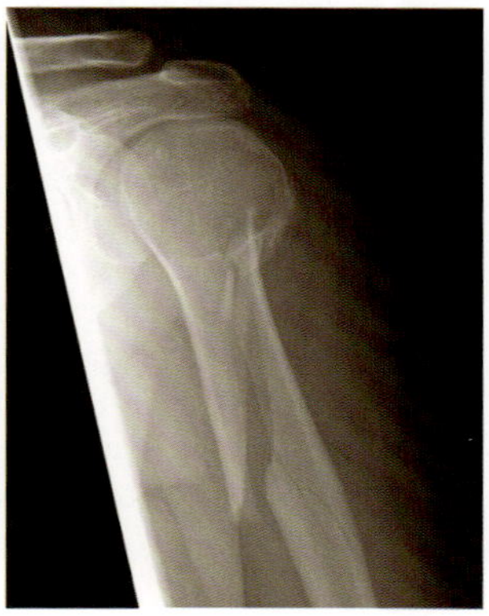

Spiral fracture

NOT FORMS of CHILD or ADULT ABUSE
Be careful **not to confuse these with child abuse**

Name of Marking	Description
Mongolian Spots	Common among Asian population 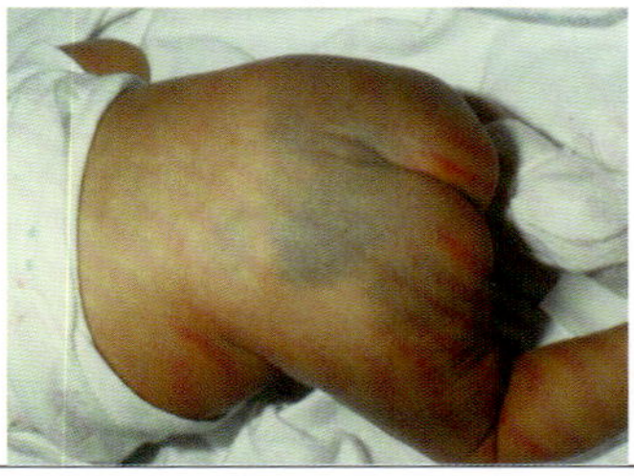
Coining AKA: Moxibustion	Chinese medicine used in acupuncture in which herbs and heat is applied to the body. Some forms can leave scars. 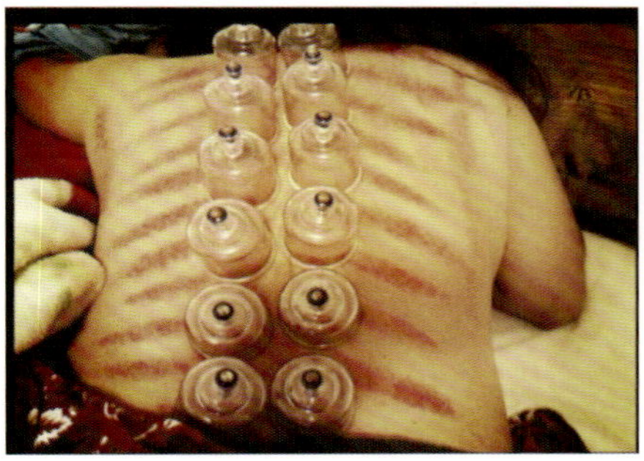 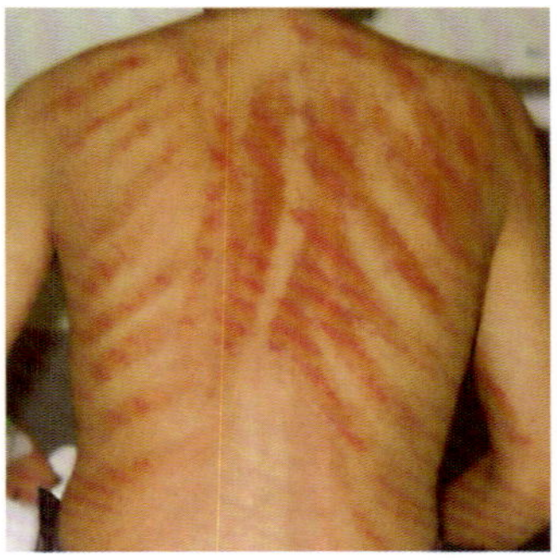
Osteogenesis imperfecta	Children present to the ER often with broken bones. X-rays will show breaks in different stages of healing. But child abuse will show "spiral" fractures. 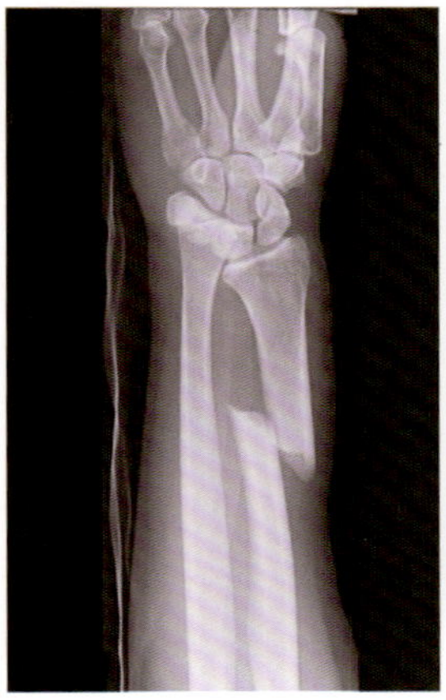 Osteogenesis fracture 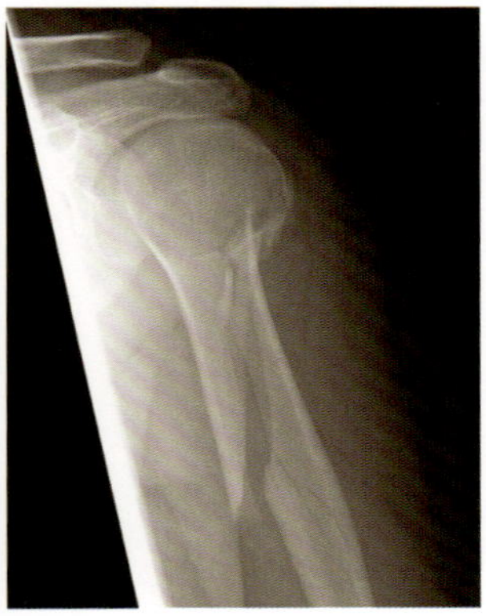 Child abuse spiral fracture

Spousal Abuse

- Can occur to both males and females
- MC occurs to females. #1 MC cause of injury to females.
- Highest risk
  - Married young
  - Dependent personality
  - When alcohol or drugs are involved
  - Last trimester of pregnancy (highest risk category)
  - History of past abuse background in the family (parents, etc.)
- It is not reportable
- Do **NOT** ever advise the victim to leave their spouse! This is for your safety and the spouse's safety.
- Provide information on how they can get help: Women's shelters, counseling.
- Be aware of children in the household. If the spouse is being abused there is a **high probability that the children are being abused.**

Elderly Abuse

- MCC is neglect
- Types of abuse: Neglect, physical, exploitation (the taking, misuse, of funds, property, assets) for someone else's benefit, emotional, abandonment, self-neglect.
- SX: Suffering is usually done in silence. Be aware of changes in personality or behavior, bruises, broken bones, abrasions, burns, depression, bruises around breast or genitals, sudden changes in financial situations, unattended medical needs, unusual weight loss, strained/tense relationships, arguments between caregiver and elderly person.
- Be aware of the individual that accompanies the patient that answers all the questions for the patient or if the patient answers the questions but will not look at you. Always ask the additional person to **leave the room** so you can speak to the patient in private.
- Caregivers are the most common to abuse.
- Risk factors of caregivers to cause abuse:
  Inability to cope with stress, depression, lack of support from other potential care givers, substance abuse, alcohol or drug involvement, view of caregiver that the elder is burdensome.

IMMUNOLOGY

Primary Organs: Thymus and Bone Marrow: Concerned with production and maturation of lymphoid cells.
Secondary Organs: Tonsils, lymph nodes, Peyer's patches, and spleen: Sites in which the lymphocytes localize and identify antigens to mount a defense.

Organs involved in immunity

- **Spleen**
  Spleen (**Extravascular**). (Note: blood vessels are intravascular).
  Filtration system that removes damaged and old RBC's and antigens.
  Tags C3 and IgG for destruction.
  Contains: B and T Cells, dendritic cells, RBC's, Macrophages, Natural Killer Cells.
  Red Pulp (non-lymphoid): Connective tissue (Cords of Billroth) and sinusoid (discontinuous fenestrated capillary that ↑ permeability) that filters the blood for antigens, worn out or defective red blood cells and microorganisms. Makes up approximately 75 – 80% of the spleen. Red Pulp consists of red blood cells, platelets, granulocytes, and plasma.
  White Pulp (lymphoid): (AKA: **Follicles** of Cortex, Malpighian bodies).
  White Pulp uses humoral and cell-mediated defenses. **B cells are found in the** follicles of the **Germinal Center. It contains adenoid tissue (lymphatic tissue). Antibodies are synthesized in the white pulp. T cells are found in the Peri**arteriolar lymphoid sheaths (PALS) (AKA: **Para**cortex).
  The **marginal zone** separates the white and red pulp. The marginal zone contains **Antigen Presenting Cells (APC)** that take antigens out of circulation and present them to the lymphocytes in the spleen.
  Splenic Macrophages: AKA: **Sinusoidal or RES (Reticuloendothelial System)** removes **ENCAPSULATED** organisms.
  Lymph follicles produce IgM and IgG, **opsonization of encapsulated bacteria**
  In lymphoid leukemias: the red pulp atrophies and the white pulp hypertrophies.
  In myeloid leukemia, both the red and white pulp hypertrophy.
  After a splenectomy "Target" RBC's are noted due to the loss of Red Pulp.
- **Thymus**
  T Cell differentiation.
  Positive Selection (Cortex), Immature T Cells.
  Negative Selection (Medulla), Mature T Cells and reticular epithelial cells (Hassall corpuscles).
- **Tonsils and Adenoids**
  Independent immune organs.
  Trap bacteria and viruses.
  Adenoids: Nasopharynx, above the uvula in the soft palate.
  Tonsils: Back of the throat.
- Appendix (AKA: Vermiform appendix).
  Located at the end of the cecum.
  Enhances intestines defense.
  Helps signal lymphocytes where to go to attack an infection.
- **Bone Marrow**
  Houses stem cells.
  Hematopoiesis: produces the stem cells of all cells of our immune system: B cells, granulocytes, immature thymocytes, RBC's, WBC's, platelets, natural killer cells.
  Stem cells separate into precursors of cells that leave the bone marrow and mature elsewhere or stay and develop into mature cells in the bone marrow.
  Fights bacteria, viruses, fungi, parasites, and tumors.
- Peyer's Patches
  Lower ileum
  Lymphatic cells
- Lymph Nodes
  Cluster of lymphatic tissue surrounded by coat of connective tissue.
  Captures bacteria and cancer cells.
  Separates out the lymphatic fluid.
- Lymphatic System

LYMPH DRAINAGE
Four main groups of lymph nodes

Sacral Nodes	Internal Iliac Nodes	External Iliac Nodes	Common Iliac Nodes
Lie in the hollow of the sacrum. Receive drainage from: pelvic, perineal and gluteal regions. Drain to the **internal iliac or common iliac nodes**.	Lie around the internal iliac artery. Receive drainage from the pelvic viscera, perineum and buttock. Drain to the **common iliac nodes.**	Lie around the external iliac artery. Receive drainage from the **superficial and deep inguinal nodes**, some of the pelvic viscera and abdominal wall below the umbilicus. Drain to the **common iliac** nodes.	Receive drainage from the **external and internal iliac nodes** and the **sacral nodes**. Drain to the lumbar nodes.

Lymph Node	Drainage
External Iliac Nodes Along the external iliac vessels and *drains into common iliac nodes.* *Receives drainage from the superficial and deep inguinal nodes.*	**Superior bladder**, upper 1/3 vagina**, anterior cervix** and lateral cervix (drains with uterine arteries and cardinal ligaments at base of broad ligament) legs, buttock, ductus deferens, superior uterus, and **ultimately drains into the Paraaortic/Aortic nodes.**
Internal Iliac Nodes Along the internal iliac vessels and *drains into the common iliac nodes.* *Receives drainage from the sacral nodes.*	**Prostate, base of the bladder,** middle 1/3 vagina**, lower uterus, posterior cervix,** lateral cervix (drains with uterine arteries), all pelvic structures**,** upper anal canal (above pectinate line), and **ultimately drains into the Paraaortic/Aortic nodes.**
External and Internal Iliac Nodes	Seminal vesicle, bladder, urethra, ureter, vagina
Deep Inguinal Lymph Nodes Between the leg and pelvis under cribriform fascia. Affected due to infections of STD's, leg and foot infections. *This drains into the external iliac nodes.*	**Penis,** scrotum, **vulva, clitoris,** perineum, gluteal region, lower abdominal wall, lower anal canal (below the pectinate line)
Superficial Inguinal Nodes Beneath inguinal ligament and **drain into the deep inguinal** lymph nodes. *This drains into the external iliac nodes.*	**Scrotum**, tunica vaginalis, **rectum**, **lower 1/3 vagina**, **vulva**, perineum, (below the hymen), lower anal canal (below the pectinate line).
Paraaortic (Lumbar)/Aortic Nodes *Receives drainage from the internal and external iliac nodes.*	Upper uterus, fallopian tubes, **ovaries, testes**, kidneys
Common Iliac Nodes *Receives drainage from the external and internal iliac nodes and the sacral nodes.*	
Lumbar Nodes (AKA: lateral aortic nodes) Between the diaphragm and pelvis along the IVC and aorta. *Common iliac drains into the Lumbar nodes and converge to become the* **THORACIC DUCT**	Intestinal trunk
Popliteal Nodes Located at back of knees in popliteal fossa of posterior leg	Lower leg and foot
Celiac Nodes	Spleen, stomach, pancreas, upper duodenum, liver
Superior Mesenteric Nodes	**Small intestine**: Lower duodenum, jejunum, ileum, ascending colon, transverse colon to the splenic flexure
Inferior Mesenteric Nodes	**Colon**: Splenic flexure, sigmoid colon to the upper/superior rectum. **Location of metastasis of cancer of the descending colon.**
Gastroepiploic Nodes	Greater curvature of the stomach
Subpyloric Nodes	Distal stomach, duodenum, pancreas
Axillary Nodes Underarm to the collar bone	**Breast**, upper chest wall, upper limbs
Hilar Nodes Lungs	**Lungs**

Supraclavicular Nodes In the cavity over the clavicle (Right and Left sides).	Lymph from the abdomen and thoracic cavity drain through here. **RIGHT NODE:** Drains mediastinum lungs, esophagus. Enlargement: It is a location of metastasis of various malignancies: gastrointestinal, lung, retroperitoneal. Location of: **Virchow's node** (left supraclavicular node with lymph drainage, especially the stomach, passing through the thoracic duct. **LEFT NODE**: Drains thorax, abdomen via thoracic duct. Enlargement: Lymphoma, thoracic or retroperitoneal cancer, bacterial or fungal infection.
Mediastinal Nodes Along the trachea, esophagus, between lungs and diaphragm	Trachea, Esophagus. Location where lymph drains into the **subclavian vein**
Cervical Nodes Over and below the Sternocleidomastoid muscle	Posterior: Scalp and neck, thorax, cervical, auxiliary nodes, thyroid gland, posterior pharynx, tonsils, head, neck. Enlargement: TB, lymphoma, head and neck malignancy.
Sub-Mandibular (AKA: Tonsilar Nodes) Beneath the mandibular angle, base of jaw	Tongue, lips, mouth, molars, submaxillary gland. Enlargement: infections of head, neck sinus, ears, eyes, scalp, pharynx.
Sub-mental Nodes Beneath chin	Lower lip and tip of tongue, floor of mouth, teeth, skin of cheek, submental salivary gland. Enlargement: CMV, Mononucleosis, EBV, Toxoplasmosis, dental periodontitis.
Postauricular Nodes Behind ears	External auditory meatus, pinna, scalp. Enlargement: local infection, **mononucleosis**
Preauricular Nodes In front of ears	Eyelids, conjunctivae, temporal region, pinna. Enlargement: External auditory canal infection, **strep throat.**
Suboccipital Nodes Between back of head and neck	Scalp and head Enlargement: Local infection

(**tip:** You have a "**Para**" testes and ovaries, **S**crotum is **S**uperficial and the penis goes **Deep**)

Lymphatic System

- Originates as plasma (fluid portion of blood)
- 2 – 3 liters of lymph is filtered per day
- Lymph (AKA: extracellular fluid: fluid that flows between cells)
- Flows in a continuous loop in one upward direction in its own system, independent of blood
- Upward movement dependent on movement of muscles and joint pumps (lymph has no pump)
- Passes through lymph nodes (afferent vessels) that filter out pathogens, waste products, cancer cells so fluid can be returned to circulatory system
- Lymphocytes (WBC) inside of the lymph node destroy these pathogens
- Damaged or destroyed lymph nodes do not regenerate
- **Thoracic duct (AKA: alimentary duct),** largest lymphatic vessel. Begins at 2nd lumbar vertebra to the neck. **Drains systemic circulation at the left subclavian vein. It drains lymph from most of the body: legs, trunk, left chest (thorax), left arm, left head and neck.**
- **Right lymphatic duct drains the right arm, right chest (thorax), right head and neck. It combines with the right subclavian vein and right internal jugular vein.**
- **Filtered lymph flows into (efferent vessels) the subclavian veins**

IMMUNITIES: Innate and Adaptive

Innate Immunity (AKA: Born With) **(tip:** is IN you when you are born or "IN"fant)	**Adaptive Immunity (AKA: Acquire/develop)**
Skin, IgA (mucus membranes protect) PMN's, macrophages, monocytes, dendritic cells, natural killer cells, compliment	B Cells, T Cells, Antibodies
Compliment, lysozyme, CRP	Immunoglobulin's
TLR (Toll Like Receptors) recognize PAMP (Pathogen associated molecular patterns. Note: **CD14 on the macrophages** act as a receptor for PAMP's), bacteria, viruses. NF-KB turns on acute response.	Memory cells. Activated B and T Cells from PREVIOUS EXPOSURE. (ie: vaccinations, get the disease or have been exposed). FASTEST immune response.

IMMUNITIES: Passive and Active

Passive Immunity ("Active" humoral immunity)	Active Immunity (Naturally acquired immunity)
Temporary, passes on, does not last	Long lasting
Borrows antibodies from someone else = "ready made antibodies", FAST onset. Antibodies are given.	Can be acquired naturally or artificially. Requires exposure to an antigen. Slow onset.
Transferred artificially or through the placenta: Antitoxin Good for travel Humanized monoclonal antibody IgA in breast milk. **IgG CROSSES placenta** (IgM does NOT cross, its too large). (**tip**: Ig**G** = **G** for **G**oes across) Babies get IgG from mom, it last 2 months (this is why babies start vaccinations at 2 months).	**Naturally**: Person is exposed to disease, develops disease and then becomes immune as a result of the primary immune response. **Artificially**: Induced by a vaccine.
Used for: After exposure to: Tetanus toxin, botulism, HBV, Rabies	Used for: Combined passive and active vaccines can be given for HEP B or Rabies exposure

VACCINATIONS

Pieces of bacteria are attached to a **hapten** that causes the body to set off an immune response.

Vaccine Failure

- The hapten falls off during vaccination so no bacteria are induced, therefore no immune response
- To verify if the vaccine is working, check the titers

Anergy Vaccine Failure

- Patient is very sick. The antibodies are to busy fighting off the illness and do not stop to respond
- Verify with an anergy panel. If bumps = response and the vaccine is working. No bumps = no immunity

Dependent Vaccines: Conjugated vaccines. Once a polysaccharide (independent) is conjugated with proteins (peptides), it becomes dependent. They need each other. (**tip**: it takes "two" to conjugate. Two: polysaccharide (T cell) and proteins/peptides).
Peptides: Need B and T cells. T cells DEPEND upon B cells to help.
NOTE: If a vaccine is "Dependent", it means that proteins have been used to conjugate the polysaccharide. **This means that the vaccine is used against polysaccharides (encapsulated organisms):**
Examples: **H. influenza and N. meningitis**.
Both H. influenza type B and N. meningitis were polysaccharides that were conjugated with proteins.

Independent Vaccines: One cell is independent = not around to help the other.
Polypeptides: Need only a B cell response.
Polysaccharides: T cell is independent and is of no help to B cells.
T cell independent vaccine is less immunogenic because it has no Ig or memory cells (no interleukin as no T cell is involved. Interleukin is required for class switching).
Once the vaccine is conjugated with protein it becomes T cell dependent and more immunogenic.

Vaccination rules for children

- It is ok to give all of the required vaccinations at once during a well child visit. Vaccinations do not need to be spaced out
- It is ok to give vaccinations to a child that is mildly ill or after a mild illness (colds, low grade fever)
- Do NOT give vaccinations to a child that is sick (high fever, not eating, etc.)
- **Premature babies**: vaccinations are given on chronologic age – meaning that the baby will start their regular vaccination schedule 2 months after the date of their birth.

Vaccination reactions to Dtap (Diphtheria, Tetanus, Pertussis)

- **Severe reaction (anaphylaxis, encephalopathy, CNS complications) = Do not give any more shots**
- **Mild reaction: Give ONLY the DT (Diphtheria and tetanus) on the next vaccination, do not give the pertussis.**
- **Pertussis is normally what children react to.**

Vaccinations and Pregnancy

- Moms can be vaccinated during pregnancy with tetanus toxoid. IgG will cross the placenta and protect baby.
- Vaccinations against Rubella should not be giving during pregnancy, however, if the mother is vaccinated and is concerned, the answer will be to just REASSURE her. The chances of any problems are extremely small.
- If the vignette asks what is the best thing that can be done to reduce congenital birth problems in developing countries, the answer is always to vaccinate the women of childbearing age against rubella.

Live Attenuated Vaccines

- **T cell response (Cell mediated)**
- Pathogen is denatured making it inactive so the body can make antibodies
- Induces lifelong immunity
- Can cause the disease: Chance of getting the disease: 1 – 3%
- **Contraindicated in pregnancy and immunocompromised conditions**
- Live Vaccines: **Polio (Sabin), Varicella (chickenpox), Measles, Mumps, MMR (rubella), Yellow fever, Influenza (nasal spray), Zoster (Shingles), BCG (TB).**

Killed/Inactivated Vaccines

- **B Cell response (Humoral)**
- Pathogen inactivated by heat or chemicals
- **Stops viral entry into cells**
- Safer than live vaccines: No chance of getting the disease
- Weaker immune response so boosters required
- **Killed Vaccines: Polio (Salk. Tip: K = Killed), HEP A, Influenza (injection), Rabies, Cholera**

Toxoid Vaccines are **bacteria exotoxins**. Toxins have been inactivated (purified inactivated toxins) by heat or chemicals while the immunologic properties are preserved. Toxins are what cause the illness (the illness is not directly caused by the bacteria, it is caused by the toxin it produces).
Vaccines against toxins. (Gram + rods)

- Diphtheria toxoid
- Tetanus toxoid from the tetanospasmin produced by Clostridium tetani (Vaccine: Dtap)
- Botulism toxoid from botulin produced by Clostridium botulinum

Recombinant Vaccines (aka: Purified protein vaccines) are purified antigens from the infectious organism. The vaccinated person produces antibodies to the protein antigen, which protects from the disease.

- HBV (antigen)
- HPV

Conjugate (aka: Subunit) are vaccines that only use pieces of the pathogens they protect against.

- HEP B, Haemophilus influenza type B, Pertussis, Pneumococcal, Meningococcal

Antigenic Variation (AKA: Antigenic Shift)

- DNA rearrangement or RNA segment reassortment
- Most common: **Influenza (AKA: VIRUS)**
- Reason why we can't make a vaccine that will cure the flu. It is constantly changing because of Antigenic Variation (Antigenic Shift)
- **Antigenic Shift is much worse (tip:** Oh "Shi.....t) than antigenic drift

Methods to decrease antigens

- Detergents (soap): **stops adhesion**, loosens and disrupts membranes.
- Disinfectants are antimicrobial (ineffective on spores).
- Alcohol/Anti-septic/disinfectant: kills 99% of antigens, **destroys membranes**, stops endotoxins by denaturing the protein and dissolving the lipid membrane.
- Hydrogen peroxide, chlorine: (oxidizing agents) oxidizes cell membrane = lysis.
- **Sterilization/Autoclave is the ONLY way to kill spores (Bacillus, Clostridium).**
  Autoclave at 121° for 15 – 20 minutes with vapor/steam/ gas/pressure.
  It also kills bacteria, viruses, and fungi.
- Autoclaving **can't kill prions** or the Archaean Geogemma barosii at 270° for 90 minutes.
- To kill prions: must denature the protein (soak in bleach and water for 30 min., caustic soda, acidic detergents, 1N NaOH).

DEFENSE CELLS

B Cells (AKA: Humoral immunity, **PLASMA CELLS**, Antibody mediated, Neutrophils)

- **Fight/kills BACTERIA (tip: B = B Cells, Bacteria, Blood, Bone), but NOT atypical bacteria (atypical bacteria: Chlamydia, Rickettsia, Mycoplasma, Legionella, Uroplasma)**
- Antigen Presenting Cells (APC)
- Differentiate into plasma cells to produce antibodies and memory
- Hyperacute organ rejection (AKA: Antibody mediated)
- **Cell markers: CD19, CD21 (EBV), CD22**
- (**TIP:** If you see high numbers/recurrent humoral infections (ie: pneumonia, sinusitis, GI) check Ig serum levels, this usually indicates the patient has no/low levels of Immunoglobulin's)
- **CR3 (Complement Receptor 3), type of integrin:** receptor located on: PMN 's, Natural Killer Cells and Macrophages. CR3 binds to foreign cells causing phagocytosis and destruction of the cell.

T Cells (AKA: Cell mediated)

- Fight/kills **VIRUSES, PARASITES, FUNGUS, ATYPICAL BACTERIA, TUMOR/CANCERS.**
  (T cells can NOT fight Candida, must use an Azole medication)
  Atypical bacteria: Chlamydia, Rickettsia, Mycoplasma, Legionella, Uroplasma
  (**Beware! Know your atypical bacteria.** The exam will give you a list of various infections that the patient has had and wants to know what cells are involved. If you do not recognize the atypical bacterial infection you will chose B cell response and you will be WRONG!)
- **Cell marker CD4**
- **CD4 and MHC II**
  (**ALWAYS think of the terms: T Cells, CD 4, MHC 1 and Macrophages TOGETHER**!)
- CD4 and T cells stimulate B cells to make antibodies and produce cytokines
- Associated with **Hypersensitivity Type IV (AKA: Delayed)**
- Cytotoxic organ rejection: acute and chronic
- Undergo positive and negative selection in the thymus
- **MHC-1 expressed by ALL host cells except non-nucleated cells (RBC's)**
- **MCC of ALL infections are viruses. Fought by T cells and macrophages (cell mediated).**
  (**Tip:** All "Penia's" are causes by viruses or drugs. Viruses love DNA so they have a high occurrence in the bone marrow)
- **NOTE:** when a vignette describes a sickness and wants to know what type of cell would be decreased: decide first what type of sickness it is. Is it one that involves T cell defense (virus, fungal, parasite, cancer, atypical bacteria) or B cell defense (bacteria), then look in the answer for ANY of the cells that are in that pathway: TH1 or TH2.

Cytotoxic T Cells (T-killer cell, CD8 + T cells, killer T cell, cytotoxic T lymphocyte)

- **Fights/kills virus, cancer and donor graft cells**
- Express **TCR's (T-cell receptors)** that recognize antigens, **CD3 markers** and B cell receptors
- Stimulates Natural Killer Cell activity by secreting **INFγ**
- Cell marker CD8
- **CD8 and MHC-1 class**
- Undergo positive and negative selection in the thymus
- Kills directly by **releasing cytotoxins: perforin, granzymes and granulysin** that triggers the caspase cascade which causes **apoptosis (programed cell death)**

Natural Killer Cells

- Cytotoxic lymphocyte (type of WBC) part of the **innate immune** system
- Mature in: bone marrow, spleen, thymus, lymph nodes, tonsils
- **DO NOT** express TCR's or CD3 or B cell receptors
- Cell Markers: **CD56 and CD16** (binds to the Fc region of the Ig for activation)
- Activated by: IL-2, IL-12, IFNα, IFNβ
- Kills cells that do not display an MHC I marker or that display the stress marker MIC-A which means the cell is invected with a virus or cancer

Helper T Cells

- CD4 and MHC II
- Differentiate into **TH1 or TH2** helper T cells

Eosinophils

- **Induced by IL-5**
- Bi-lobed nucleus with granules
- Destroys parasites (AKA: helminthes) by **MBP (Major Basic Protein).** MBP can cause damage to epithelial and endothelial cells in the bronchioles
- **High levels of eosinophil's are seen with**: Neoplasms (lymphomas), allergies, asthma, Addison's, collagen (Vascular), parasites (AKA: helminthes), drug damage to organs (esp: kidneys), esophageal eosinophilia
- **PATHOLOGY:** In asthma **NOT** induced by a pathology or exercise, sputum will show **eosinophil's** and **Charcot Leyden crystals (AKA: Crystal bodies)**
  TX: Zafirlukast, Montelukast (Leukotriene antagonist)

MHC I Class (MHC: Major Histocompatibility Complex)

- **Binds CD8 and TCR** (T Cell Receptors)
- Expressed on all nucleated cells (no RBC's)
- Located: HLA-A, HLA-B and HLA-C
- Has β2 Micro globulin and TAP peptide transporter to aid in presenting antigen on cell surface
- (**tip** for the HLA's in the MHC I class category: "I" class = 1. 1 letter behind the HLA: A, B, C)

MHC II Class

- **Binds CD4** (AKA: Naïve T Cell) **and TCR** (T cell receptor)
- Expressed only on APC (Antigen presenting cells)
- Located: HLA-DR, HLA-DP, HLA-DQ
- Utilizes an endosomes to aid in presenting antigens on cell surface
- (**tip** for the HLA's in the MHC II class category: "II" = 2. 2 letters behind the HLA: DR, DP, DQ)

Cell Types

- Leukocytes: **ALL** white blood cells (WBC): Neutrophils (PMN's), Monocytes, Granulocytes (Basophil, Eosinophil, Neutrophil: BEN), Lymphocyte
- Lymphocytes:
  B cells (Antibodies, plasma cells, memory, activate compliment),
  T cells (CD4 Helper T cells, TCR, MHC Class II on APC (Antigen presenting cells) make cytokines),
  Natural Killer Cells (kills cells that do not display an MHC I marker or that display the stress marker MIC-A which means the cell is infected with a virus or cancer),
  Macrophages (monocytes),
  Cytotoxic T cells (CD8, MHC I)
- Basophils: (AKA: Granulocytes): (**tip**: BEN) Basophils, Eosinophil's, Monocytes
  Basophils: responsible for allergic and antigen response. Releases histamine-causing vasodilation of vessels.
  Eosinophils: Responsible for parasitic infections and allergic/allergies.
  Neutrophils (AKA: Polymorphonuclear leukocyte): Most abundant WBC. Fight bacteria and fungal infections.
  Forms pus (pus is dead PMN's).
- WBC Normal Labs
  Neutrophils (PMS's): 60 – 70%
  Lymphocytes: 20 – 30%
  Monocytes: 3-7%
  Eosinophil's: 1 – 3%
  Basophils: 0 – 1%
  Note: PMN's must be monitored in patients to detect any complications due to infection, in particularly those that are immunocompromised.
  Note: IL-8 recruits PMN's.
- **Leukocytosis** (AKA: left shift): When there are more immature leukocytes than mature because of an abnormal increase in WBC. Seen with acute inflammation against Compliment (C3). (Similar to a leukemoid reaction).

Immunology Pathway

Antigen Presenting Cells (APC)
Macrophages
Dendritic Cells
B Lymphocytes

T Cell Path: TH-1

AKA: Cell mediated immunity
Location: Tissues
Kills: Virus, Fungus, Tumors
Atypical Bacteria, Tumors,
Self Antigens

B Cell Path: TH-2

AKA: Humoral immunity, Antibody mediated
Location: Blood
(tip "B"cells for "B"lood and "B"acteria)
Kills: Bacteria

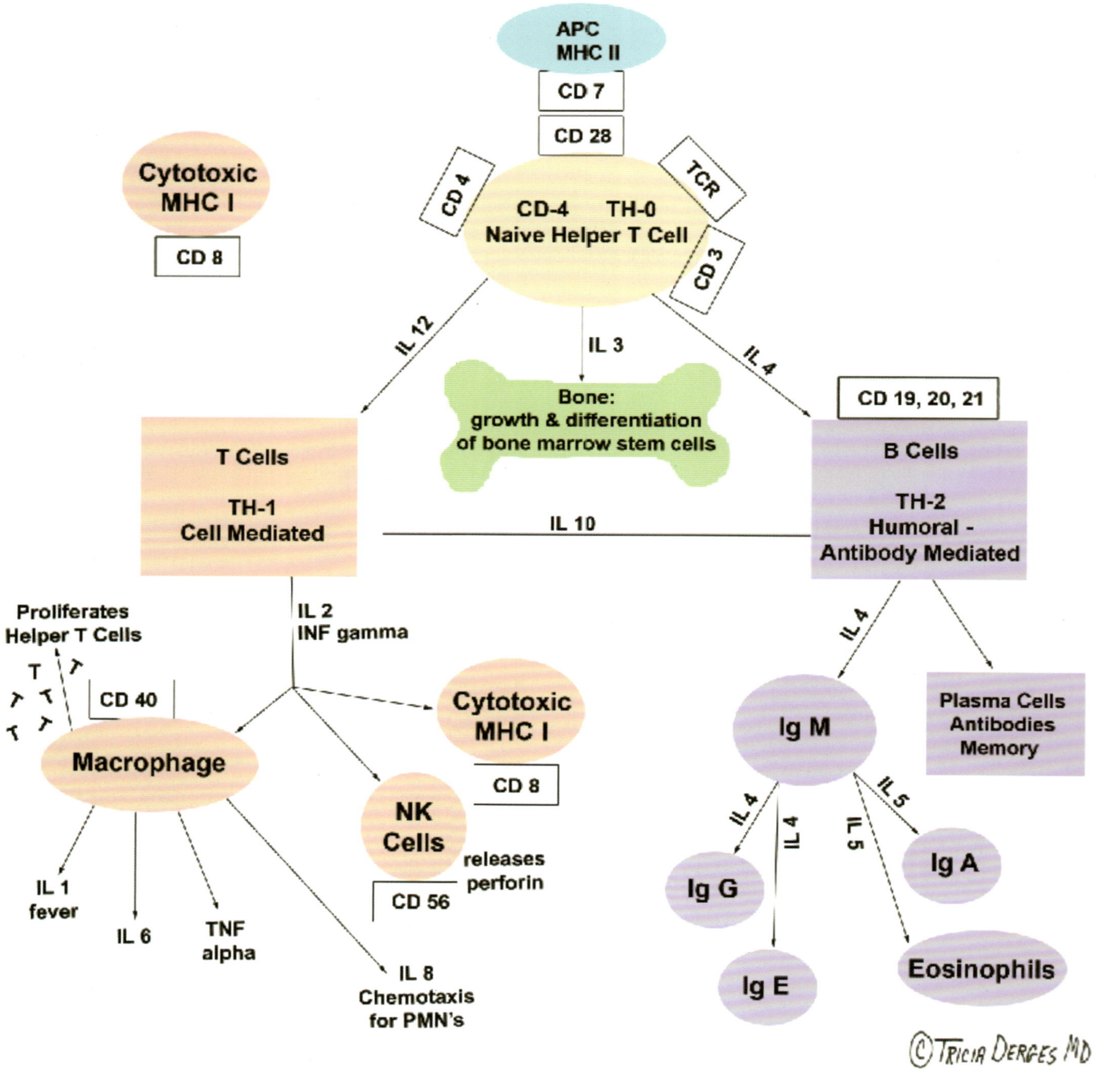

HLA (Human Leukocyte Antigen)

- Are the locations of genes that encode proteins responsible for the regulation of the immune system. HLA genes are the human versions of the MHC genes.
- **HLA Class A, B and C correspond to the MHC I class (AKA: HLA = MHC I)** . These bring the fragments of the antigen to the surface of the cell so that it can be destroyed by the Cytotoxic T Cells.
  (Association example: HLA-B27 is associated with several arthritis pathologies, such as Ankylosing Spondylitis. If the question asks what is associated with this disease or what would need to be evaluated to see if the children of the diseased would be susceptible, you must first recognize that this pathology is a HLA-B27. HLA-B27 is an **HLA Class B**, which is associated with **MHC I**).
- HLA Class DP, DM, DOA, DOB, DQ and DR correspond to the MHC II class. These bring the fragments of the antigen to the surface of the cell to be presented to the T-lymphocytes that stimulate T-helper cells and B-cells to produce antibodies.
  (Association example Celiac DZ: Any of these HLA **Class D's** would be associated with **MHC II**).

CELL SURFACE MARKERS (Proteins)

CELL	MARKERS
Macrophages	CD14 (receptor for PAMPs: Pathogen-associated molecular patterns: pathogens recognized by the innate immune system. Recognized by TLR's (Toll Like Receptors), **CD40, CD33,** CCR5 **MHC II, B7** (binds with CD28) APC (Antigen Presenting Cell) Fc and C3b (Phagocytosis)
B Cells	**CD19, CD20, CD21** (EBV), CD40 **MHC II, B7** (Binds with CD28), APC (Antigen Presenting Cell), Kills typical bacteria **(Caution: Atypical bacteria are killed by T cells)**
T Cells	**CD4, CD8** **TCR** (binds with MHC-antigen complex) **CD3** (Signals with TCR), **CD28** (Binds B7 on APC (Antigen Presenting Cell) CXCR4, CCR5 (HIV) **Kills viruses, parasites, fungus, tumors, atypical bacteria** **T Cells can NOT fight Candida, must use an Azole med)** **Atypical bacteria: Chlamydia, Rickettsia, Legionella, Mycoplasma, Uroplasma**
Helper T Cells	**CD4**, CD40L
Cytotoxic T Cells	**CD8** **MHC I** CXCR4, CCR5 (HIV)
Regulatory T Cells	CD4, CD25
NK (Natural Killer) Cells	**CD56, CD16** (binds Fc of IgG)
Hematopoietic Stem Cells	**CD34**
Dendritic Cell	CD11, CD123, CD40
Granulocyte	CD66
Erythrocyte	CD235
Platelet	CD41, CD61, CD62
Endothelial Cell	CD146
Epithelial Cell	CD326
Stem Cell Precursor	CD34
PECAM Adhesion Molecule	CD31
Lymphocyte Function Associated Antigen (LFA-3)	CD58
TNF Receptor	CD40 (CD40 is expressed on: B cells, follicular dendritic cells, dendritic cells, activated monocytes, macrophages, vascular smooth muscle cells, several tumor cell lines, endothelial cells

INTERFERONS

IFN	Function
IFNγ	Stimulates T cells and NK cells
IFNα and β	Produced by many cells in response to viral infections. Acts as a cytokine on neighbor cells so they make anti-viral proteins to stop viral mRNA so that synthesis is stopped

HLA ASSOCIATIONS WITH DISEASES

HLA	Disease Associations
HLA-A3	**Hemochromatosis**
HLA-B27	Most arthritis: Reactive arthritis (AKA: Reiter Syndrome), Psoriatic arthritis, **Ankylosing Spondylitis**
HLA-DQ2, DQ8	Celiac Disease
HLA-DR2	Goodpasture Syndrome, SLE, Multiple Sclerosis
HLA-DR3	**Graves** Disease, Diabetes Type I, SLE
HLA-DR4	**Rheumatoid Arthritis**, Diabetes Type I
HLA-DR5	**Hashimoto** Thyroiditis, Pernicious Anemia (B-12/Intrinsic Factor)

CYTOKINES (aka: Interleukins, growth factors). Use the Tyrosine Kinase Receptors (cell membrane receptor, membrane spanning)

CYTOKINE	RESPONSIBILITY
IL-1	1st cytokine to be released. FEVER, secreted by Macrophages, acute inflammation, and secretions to recruit leukocytes. Causes secretion of IgA in mucosal surfaces (where infections usually enter)
IL-2	Secreted by T cells. Stimulates: Helper T cells, Cytotoxic T Cells, regulatory T cells
IL-4	Differentiation into TH2 cells. Stimulates B cells, Class switches to IgG and IgE (tip: GE makes light bulbs 4 you)
IL-5	Class switch to IgA and eosinophil's
IL-6	Stimulates Acute Phase reactants (C-Reactive protein, complement, fibrinogen, prothrombin, factor VIII, VWF, plasminogen, ferritin, hepcidin, haptoglobin, alpha 1-antitrypsin, serum amyloid A, ceruloplasmin)
IL-8	Chemotaxis for neutrophils (PMN). (AKA: recruits PMN's)
IL-10	Inhibits TH1 and T cells (anti-inflammatory)
IL-12	Differentiates T cells into TH1, activates NK cells
TNF-α	Septic shock, increases vascular permeability
INF-γ	Activates NK cells (kills viruses, parasites, fungus, tumors, atypical bacteria)
Septic Shock	**IL-1, IL-6, TNFα** (septic shock: **must have the triad**: fever, low BP, tachycardia) MCC: e coli. Can also be caused by Staph.

Growth Factors

- Signaling molecules (cytokines or hormones) that stimulate cell growth, cell differentiation, proliferation and healing.
- Are either proteins or steroid hormones.
- Utilize the **Tyrosine kinase receptors: Membrane receptors** (aka: 7 spanning, membrane spanning).

Growth Factor (GF)	Action
Angiopoietin	Angiogenesis. Vascular growth factor
Interleukins (IL)	Cytokines (see above)
Colony-stimulating factor	m-CSF Macrophage colony-stimulating factor. Stimulates hematopoietic stem cells to differentiate into macrophages. Have paracrine effects on osteoclasts. It causes resorption of the bone, which leads to increased calcium plasma levels. **m-CSF is associated with RANK-L** in the stimulation of osteoblast for bone resorption. G-CSF Granulocyte colony-stimulating factor. Stimulates bone marrow to produce granulocytes (neutrophils, basophils, eosinophils, mast cells) and stem cells. (Pharmacology analogs of G-CSF are Filgrastim and Lenograstim).
Epidermal growth factor	EGF stimulates cell growth, proliferation, differentiation by binding EGFR receptor
Erythropoietin	EPO, Hematopoietin. Cytokine for RBC precursors in the bone marrow. In the adult, EPO is produced by **interstitial fibroblasts in the kidney** with peritubular capillary and the PCT. In the fetus, EPO is produced in the perisinusoidal cells in the **liver**.
Fibroblast growth factor	FGR Involved in angiogenesis, endocrine signaling pathways, wound healing and embryonic development. They are heparin-binding proteins associated with heparin sulfate. They use the FGFR (fibroblast growth factor receptor). FGR are more potent angiogenic factors than VEGF or PDGF.
Insulin	Peptide hormone produced by beta cells of the pancreatic islets. Metabolism of carbs, proteins and fats and absorption of glucose from the blood into adipose tissue, skeletal muscle and the liver.

Growth Factors cont'd

Insulin-like growth factors	IGF-1, IGF-2: Proteins similar to insulin. They have two cell-surface receptors (IGF1R and IGF2R) and two ligands (IGF-1 and IGF-2). **IGF-1 is produced in the liver, stimulated by GH** from the anterior pituitary. IGF-2 promotes growth during gestation.
Keratinocyte growth factor	KGF Stimulates epithelial growth and wound healing.
Placental growth factor	PGF Stimulates angiogenesis in embryogenesis. It is produced from the placental trophoblast.
Platelet-derived growth factor	PDGF Dimeric glycoprotein that helps regulates cell growth and division, angiogenesis. Helps stimulate cell growth by stimulating mitosis for fibroblast, smooth muscle cells, glial cells and mesenchymal cells. It is produced and stored by the alpha granules of platelets and is released upon activation of the platelets. It is also produced by macrophages, endothelial cells and smooth muscle cells.
T-cell growth factor	TCFG Stimulate the production and development of T-cells. Produced by the thymus.
Thrombopoietin	THPO (aka: megakaryocyte growth and development factor). Hormone produced by the liver (in sinusoidal endothelial cells and parenchymal cells) and in the kidney (in the PCT) that regulates the production of platelets. IL-6 assists in the production of THPO in the liver. Stimulates the production and differentiation of megakaryocytes, which leads to platelet production. Located on chromosome 3.
Transforming growth factor	TGFα and TGFβ TGFα is produced in macrophages, keratinocytes, brain cells and stimulates epithelial development. TGFβ helps regulate the immune system, assist in tissue regeneration and cell differentiation. They are upregulated in Marfan's syndrome.
Tumor necrosis factor	TNF (aka: cachexin) Cytokine involved in inflammation and the acute phase reaction. It regulates the immune cells and can produce fever (IL-1), cachexia, apoptosis, inflammation, inhibit tumor formation, viral replication and responds to sepsis by IL-1 and IL-6. It is produced by predominately by macrophages. It can also be produced by CD4 lymphocytes, NK cells, neutrophils, eosinophils, mast cells and neurons. **Expresses CD40** (transmembrane glycoprotein).
Vascular endothelial growth factor	**VEGF** stimulates **angiogenesis** and vasculogenesis. It creates new blood vessels in the embryo, after any form of injury (including damage to muscles due to exercise), create collateral circulation due to blocked vessels (ie: due to thrombosis), vasodilation (by nitric oxide release from endothelial cells), chemotaxis for macrophages and granulocytes, mitosis and migration of endothelial cells. Overexpression of VEGF helps cancers grow (increases metalloproteinase activity) and metastasize or create neo-vascularization in the retina (diabetics).

Thymus and T Cell Selection

- T-cell precursor goes from bone marrow to Thymus

Positive Selection

- Occurs in the **Cortex**
- Involves: CD4, CD8, TCR
- T cells that are able to bind "SELF" MHC molecules survive. (**tip:** It is POSITIVE that the cells recognize themselves).
- Cells that can't recognize themselves go through Extrinsic Apoptosis (see below).
- Cells that do recognize "SELF" go on to the Medulla to participate in negative selection.

Negative Selection

- Occurs in the **Medulla**
- T cells CD4, CD8, TCR that recognize "SELF" too much are destroyed through Extrinsic Apoptosis (see below). (**tip**: is NEGATIVE for you to want to destroy yourself).
- Cells that pass this final test "graduate" and go on into the lymph node to go to work.
  CD8 cells become **Cytotoxic T cells killing viruses, cancer/tumors and donor graft cells.**
  CD4 cells become **Helper T cells** that go on to differentiate further into TH1 and TH2.
- **Cells that recognize "SELF" too much and are not destroyed in apoptosis are the root cause of autoimmune disease.**

EXTRINSIC APOPTOSIS PATHWAY (2 paths)

- **Path 1: Fas Ligand binds with CD95** (Fas receptor) and activates caspases = apoptosis
- **Path 2:** Occurs in **negative selection in the thymus**. Negative selection requires Fas-FasL interaction. **Fas protects.** If Fas and FasL interact to form a complex they bind with FADD. **FADD binds to the inactive caspase 8 and activates them**, thereby allowing the apoptosis of lymphocytes that recognize "self" too much. If Fas is mutated, the Fas-FasL complex will not form, FADD is not able to bind caspases, so negative selection does not occur allowing lymphocytes out that recognize "self" too much to be released, which **causes autoimmune disorders**.
- (**tip: E**xtrinsic = caspase **E**ight)
  (Remember: Intrinsic Apoptosis pathway: associated with BCL-2, Cytochrome C, BAX, BAD, BIM)

Thymoma

- Tumor originating from the epithelial cells of the thymus.
- Associated with **Myasthenia Gravis.** (Can be associated with other autoimmune diseases).
- SX: Compression of surrounding organs causing: dysphagia, superior vena cava syndrome, hoarseness
- DX: CT, FNB
- TX: Surgery, chemotherapy or radiation

IMMUNOGLOBULINS (AKA: Ig)

IgM

- "M" = MAIN ONE, MAIN – 1st response
- **Primary/Immediate, first Ig to respond, ACUTE stages**
- Does **NOT cross the placenta** (too large) (**tip**: "M" for "M"assive)
- **Monomer** on B Cells
- **Pentamer** when secreted
- Found in the blood
- Fixes complement (activates classical compliment pathway)
- **Stimulated by IL-4**
- On the surface of mature B cells
- IgM = Cold agglutination (tip: "M" for "M"iserable when its cold)

IgG

- **Second antibody to respond, DELAYED, CHRONIC stages – shows up later**
- **CROSSES placenta (small), provides passive immunity to fetus.** Last 2 months after birth. This is why childrens vaccines are started at 2 months old. Their mother's immunity is gone. (**tip**: Ig"G" = "G"oes across the placenta)
- Fixes compliment, opsonizes bacteria (activates classical pathway).
- Found in the blood
- **Activated by IL-4**
- IgG = Warm agglutination (**tip**: "G" for "G"ood when its warm)

IgA

- Protects mucus membranes
- Contained in **secretions: colostrum (first breast milk), mucus, saliva, tears)**
- Does NOT fix complement
- Monomer in the blood (circulation)
- **Dimer** in secretions (Dimeric)
- **Activated by IL-5**
- Must have **"J" chain (AKA: Secretory piece)**

IgE

- Mediates **Hypersensitivity Type I (Immediate reaction: Anaphylaxis, Allergies, Asthma)**
- **Two IgE MUST cross link (AKA: Aggregate, bind) to activate mast cells can degranulate to release histamine and heparin**
- **Releases histamine and heparin,** histadine, proteases, leukotriene's, prostaglandins
- Bound to FcR1 receptors on the surface tissue of mast cells and blood basophils
- Kills parasites via antibody-dependent cytotoxicity (eosinophils with FC receptors are the cells that destroy with MBP (Major Basic Protein).
- Activates eosinophil's (**Eosinophil's are activated by IL-5**)
- **IgE is stimulated by IL-4**
- CD23 is the receptor for the Fc portion of IgE

IgD

- Found on the surface of **immature B cells**
- Co-expressed with IgM
- Monomer

Anaphylaxis
Cause: Insect stings/bites, foods, latex (gloves, condoms), medications (MC drugs: Sulfa, penicillin, quinidine, phenytoin, quinidine, rifampin)

SX: Acute: Immediate hypersensitivity. Hypotension, tachycardia, difficulty breathing, swelling of lips/tongue/face causing inspiratory stridor, urticarial.

TX: **Intramuscular epinephrine** (1:1000), Corticosteroids, Diphenhydramine, Hydroxyzine, be prepared to intubate.
MOA: Epinephrine: Works on α-1 receptors to cause vasoconstrict and works on β-2 receptors to cause dilation of the bronchi.
MOA: Steroids: Inhibits the arachidonic pathway so leukotrienes are inhibited from constricting the bronchi and also stimulate α-1 receptors to vasoconstrict.

Angioedema
Sudden **swelling of airway, tongue, face, lips, face**.

Causes: Minor trauma to hands or face (example: person hit in face with pillow or particles hitting the hands), **Hereditary C1 esterase inhibitor deficiency** (will see low levels of C2 and C4), **side effect to Ace Inhibitors**.
Admit to ICU.

SX: Stridor, abdominal pain. No urticaria or pruritus.

TX: 1st line: **Ecallantide (inhibits kallikrein which blocks bradykinin production).**
Acute occurrence: Fresh frozen plasma.
Androgens: **Danazol, Stanazol (Androgens raise levels of C1 esterase inhibitor)**
Hereditary angioedema does not respond to glucocorticoids.

Allergic Rhinitis
AKA: Hay fever.

SX: Recurrent: rhinorrhea (runny nose), sneezing, stuffiness, nasal itching, watery eyes, eye itching, **inflamed boggy nasal mucosa, nasal polyps.**

Labs: Eosinophil's increased IgE levels. (IgE dependent triggering of mast cells).

TX: Avoid allergen: Get rid of pets, use A/C and close windows to avoid pollens, cover mattress and pillows, dust filters.
For allergens that are unavoidable: Desensitization.

Drug TX: **1st line: Intranasal steroids (most effective). Antihistamines, Intranasal antihistamines (Azelastine), Cromolyn (Mast cell stabilizer), Ipratropium, Leukotriene inhibitors, nasal saline spray.**

Mast Cell Pathology

Systemic Mastocytosis:
Mass proliferation of mast cells.
Mast cells release histamine = increases HCL production in stomach on H2 receptors = hypersecretion of gastric acid = **thick rugae**

(**Note:** don't forget for mast cells to degranulate (activate) and release histamine it requires the enzyme **Tryptase**.
(**Tip**: when you go on a boat TRIP it requires a MAST).

TX: Antihistamines, Leukotriene antagonists, Mast cell stabilizers (Cromolyn), Proton pump inhibitors, Corticosteroids.

Urticaria
Sudden swelling of superficial layers of the skin due to mast cell reaction/allergy to medications, insects, cold, pressure (dermatographism: "skin writing").

TX: Antihistamines, Leukotriene Receptor Antagonists

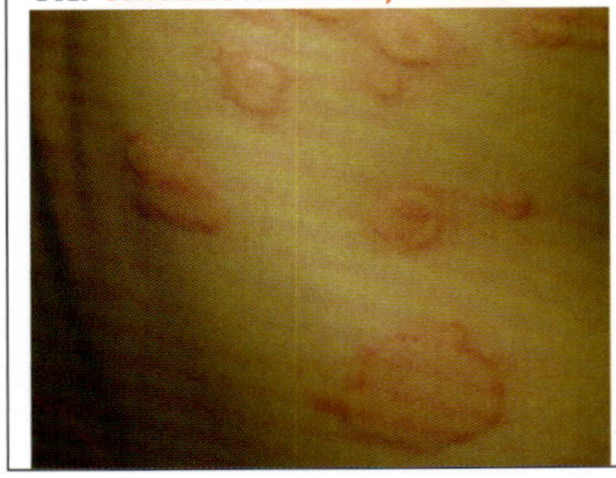

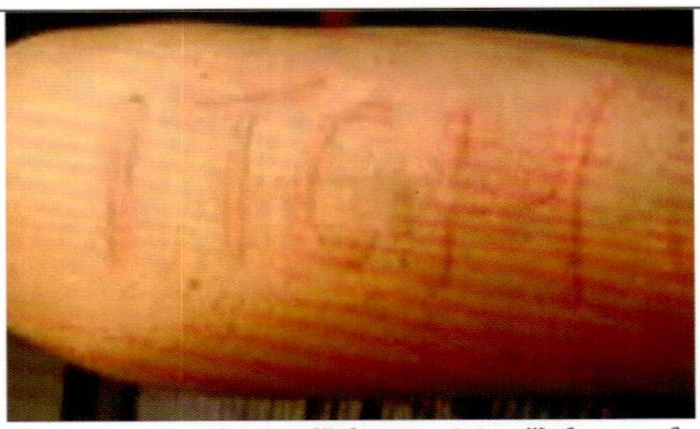

Dermatographism ("skin writing") form of urticarial

Acute Phase Reactants

- Released from the **liver** in acute and chronic inflammation.
- **Induced by IL-1, IL-6, TNFα, INFγ**
- **High ESR = indication of inflammation**

Acute Phase Reactants (APR)	**Function**
Ferrit**in** (high levels)	Sequesters iron to storage form. Keeps iron "**IN**" so that the microbes will not utilize it for their own fuel
Fibrinogen (high levels)	Fibrinogen converts to Fibrin to repair endothelial damage.
C-Reactive Protein (AKA: CRP) (high levels)	Fixes compliment and promotes phagocytosis
Hepcidin (high levels)	Prevents release of iron in storage
Amyloid A (high levels)	Chronic high levels = amyloidosis
Albumin (low levels)	Conserves amino acids
Transferrin (low levels)	Used by macrophages to sequester iron

ANTIBODIES

Antibodies Function

- Neutralization: prevents bacteria from attachment
- Opsonization: coating the bacteria to promote phagocytosis
- Complement Activation: "complements" or helps antibodies and phagocytic cells to destroy pathogens. Complement works with antibodies.
- Antibodies are made by plasma cells (aka: B cells, Humoral)

Antibody Structure

- **Fab Region** (fragment, antigen-binding)
  AKA: **Epitope** binding site
  Antigen binding (traps antigens; virus and toxin neutralization)
  Variable region
  Direct antimicrobial activity
  Composed of one constant and one variable from each heavy and light chain
- **Fc Region** (fragment, crystallizable)
  Complement binding (fixation)
  Constant region
  Binds to phagocytes
  Antibody dependent, cell mediated, Cytotoxicity
  Carboxy terminal
  Carbohydrate side chains|
  Composed of two heavy chains
  Determination of isotypes (phenotypic variations in the constant regions of the heavy and light chains)
- **Heavy Chain**: IgA, IgD, IgG, IgE, IgM
- Light Chain: K, λ (Kappa Light Chain is the most common in antibodies)
- Immunoglobulin class switching: Changes heavy chains but not the light chains
- Hinge Region: flexible stretch of amino acids in the center of the heavy chains of IgG and IgA
- Variable region determines idiotype
- Heavy Chains determine isotypes
- "J" Chain (AKA: **Secretory** piece) must be present on IgA
- IgE must crosslink (aggregate) to activate mast cells

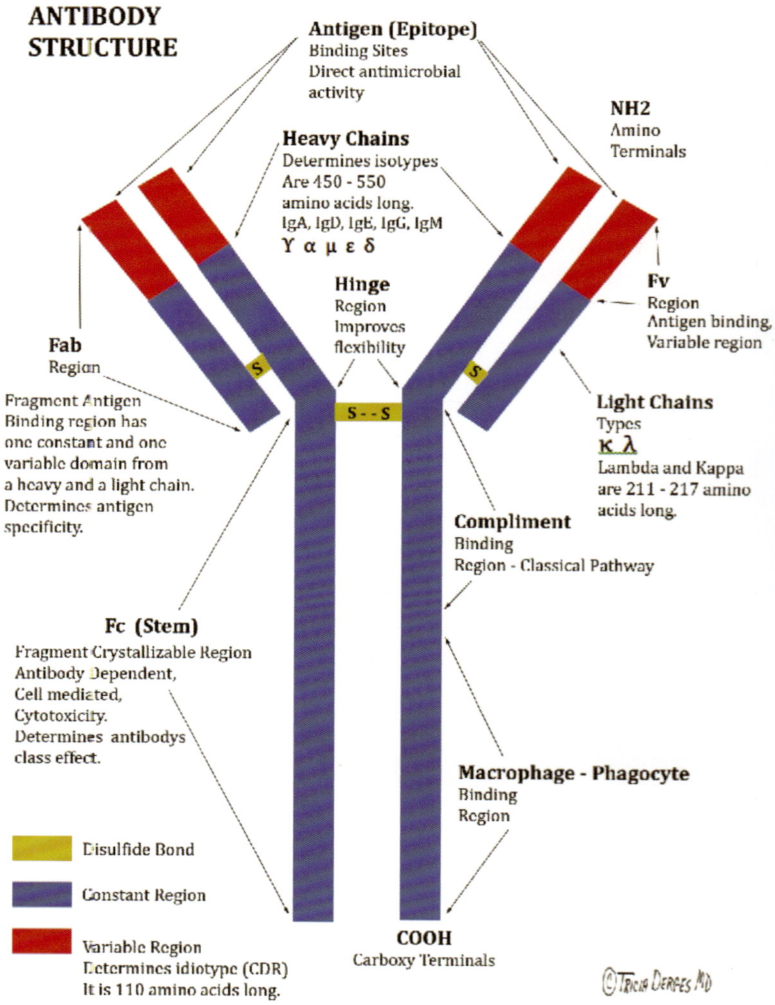

Causes for no antibodies being made

- Class switching is not working
- IL-4 is not working (IL-4 influences ALL class switching)
- CD-40 is not working
- Tyrosine Kinase (2nd messenger) is not working (seen in Bruton's Agammaglobulinemia)

AUTOANTIBODIES

Pathology	Autoantibody
Graves Disease	Anti-TSH receptor
Hashimoto Thyroiditis	Antimicrosomal Antithyroglobulin
Myasthenia Gravis	Anti-Ach receptor
Lambert Eaton Syndrome	Antibodies against voltage-gated calcium channels
Polymyositis Dermatomyositis	Anti-Jo-1 Anti-SRP (Signal-recognition particle) Anti-histidyl-tRNA synthetase Anti-aminoacyl-tRNA synthetase Anti-Mi-2
Mixed Connective Tissue Dz	Anti-U1 RNP (ribonucleoprotein)
Scleroderma, Limited (CREST)	Anticentromere
Scleroderma, Diffuse	Anti-Scl-70 Anti-DNA Topoisomerase I
SLE (Lupus) Antiphospholipid	Anti-cardiolipin Lupus anticoagulant
SLE (Lupus)	**Anti-dsDNA (specific)** Anti-Smith Antinuclear antibodies
Drug Induced Lupus	Antihistone
Rheumatoid Arthritis	**Anti citrullinated Protein Antibodies (anti-CCP) (specific)** IgM antibody against the IgG Fc region. Rheumatoid Factor (RF) (RF is NOT specific for Rheumatoid Arthritis. Several diseases are associated with RF).
Pemphigus Vulgaris	Anti-desmoglein
Bullous Pemphigoid	Anti-hemidesmosome
Sjogren Syndrome	Anti-SSA Anti-SSB anti-Ro, anti-La
Autoimmune Hepatitis	Anti-smooth muscle Antinuclear antibodies
Primary Biliary Cirrhosis	Antimitochondrial antibodies
Celiac Disease	Anti-gliadin IgA anti-tissue transglutaminase IgA antiendomysial Anti-reticulin
Wegner's Granulomatosis with polyangiitis	c-ANCA PR3-ANCA
Churg-Strauss Syndrome Microscopic Polyangiitis	p-ANCA MPO-ANCA
Goodpasture Syndrome	Anti-basement membrane
Type 1 Diabetes	Anti-glutamate decarboxylase
Primary Sclerosis Cholangitis	Anti-smooth muscle antibody
Dermatomyositis	Anti-Mi2 antibody
Primary Membranous Nephropathy	Anti phospholipase A_2 receptor

Autoimmune Diseases (most common)

Heart
- Myocarditis
- Dressler's
- Subacute bacterial endocarditis

Kidney
- Goodpasture's (Anti-Glomerular Basement Nephritis)
- Interstitial cystitis
- Lupus
- Addison's DZ

Liver
- Autoimmune hepatitis
- Primary biliary cirrhosis
- Primary sclerosing cholangitis

Skin
- Alopecia areata
- Angioedema
- Autoimmune urticaria
- Bullous pemphigoid
- Dermatitis herpetiformis
- Erythema nodosum
- Lichen planus
- Lichen sclerosus
- Pemphigus vulgaris
- Pityriasis
- Psoriasis
- Systemic scleroderma
- Vitiligo

Eyes
- Autoimmune uveitis
- Graves ophthalmopathy
- Optic neuritis
- Scleritis

Ears
- Meniere's DZ

Reproductive
- Autoimmune Oophoritis
- Endometriosis

Pancreas
- Autoimmune pancreatitis
- Diabetes mellitus Type I

Thyroid
- Autoimmune thyroiditis
- Grave's DZ
- Ord's thyroiditis

Salivary Glands
- Sjogren's

Digestive
- Celiac DZ
- Crohn's DZ
- Ulcerative colitis

Blood
- Antiphospholipid syndrome
- Aplastic anemia
- Autoimmune hemolytic anemia
- Autoimmune neutropenia
- Autoimmune thrombocytopenia
- Cold agglutinin DZ
- Essential cryoglobulinemia
- Paroxysmal nocturnal hemoglobinuria
- Pernicious anemia
- Pure red cell aplasia
- Thrombocytopenia

Muscle
- Dermatomyositis
- Fibromyalgia
- Myositis
- Myasthenia gravis
- Polymyositis

Connective Tissue
- Ankylosing spondylitis
- CREST syndrome
- Drug-induced lupus
- Eosinophilic fasciitis
- Felty syndrome
- Juvenile arthritis
- Lyme DZ (chronic)
- Mixed connective tissue DZ
- Psoriatic arthritis
- Reactive arthritis
- Rheumatic fever
- Rheumatoid arthritis
- Sarcoidosis
- Systemic Lupus

CNS
- Guillain-Barre
- Hashimoto's
- Lambert-Eaton
- Multiple sclerosis
- Sydenham chorea
- Transverse myelitis

Vascular
- C-ANCA
- Behcet's DZ
- Churg-Strauss
- Giant cell arteritis (Temporal)
- Henoch-Schonlein purpura
- Kawasaki's DZ
- Lupus vasculitis
- Rheumatoid vasculitis
- Microscopic polyangiitis
- Polyarteritis nodosa
- Polymyalgia rheumatic
- Urticarial vasculitis
- Vasculitis

COMPLEMENT

- Complements are small inactive proteins synthesized in the liver. When stimulated (activated) they result in a cascade pathway that activates MAC (Membrane Attack Complex) to kill the pathogen cells.
- Functions of complement:
  Opsonization: enhancing phagocytosis of antigens.
  Chemotaxis: attracting macrophages and PMN's (neutrophils) to produce inflammation.
  Cell Lysis: rupturing membranes of foreign cells (rupture) by MAC
  Agglutination: (AKA: Sticking) clustering and binding of pathogens together.
- Complement Pathways:
  Classical Pathway: activators are **antigen-antibody complexes (IgG and IgM).**
  Initiated by: Binding of the Fc region to C1 (**tip:** GM cars are classic).
  Alternative Pathway: Opsonize and kill pathogens.
  Initiated by: C3b binds the microbe (hydrolysis of C3).
  Lectin Pathway (AKA: **Mannose**-binding protein): Mannose binding lectin binds to mannose or glucose.

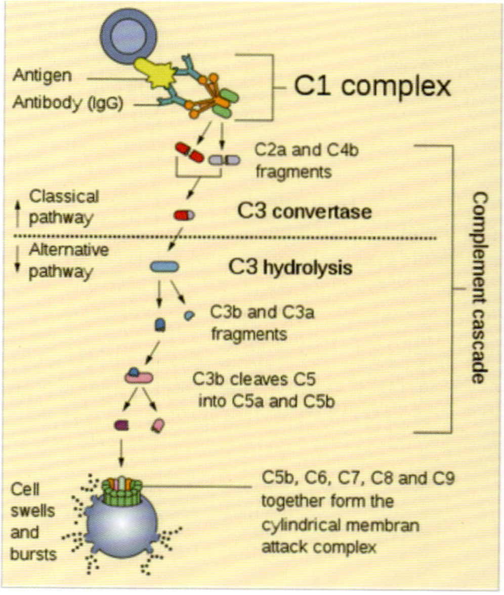

Complement cont'd

- Functions of Specific Complement
  C3b: Opsonization (**tip**: **b** = **b**acteria and **b** = **b**ite (makes it taste better so you can **b**ite it).
  C3a, C4a, C5a: Anaphylaxis (**tip**: a = anaphylaxis).
  C5a: PMN chemotaxis.
  C5 - C9 = MAC (Membrane Attack Complex). Deficiency of the MAC can cause recurrent infections by Neisseria.
- Deficiencies in compliment regulators can also cause:
  Paroxysmal Nocturnal Hemoglobinuria (PNH). Destruction of RBC due to deficiency of GPI anchors (DAF).
  Hereditary angioedema. Unregulated bradykinin due to mutation in the C1 esterase gene.

Margination/Leukocyte Extravasation Steps

STEP of Leukocyte extravasation	Process	Additional Molecules Involved
1) **Margination**	PMN's marginate to the sides of the blood vessel	**Rouleau** of RBC to the center of the vessel
2) **Rolling**	PMN's roll along vessel walls "**SELECTIN**" a spot to stop. **(E-selectin, P-selectin**)	GlyCAM-1 Sialyl-Lewis (AKA: Weibel Palade bodies/VWF), L-selectin (Sialyl-Lewis bodies are like the "glue factory" and VWF is the "glue" for adhesion.
3) **Adhesion (binding)**	PMN's adhere to the side of the blood vessel, ready to to "INTO" (**INTEGRINS**) the tissues. Without integrins: diapedesis can not occur.	**ICAM-1 (CD54)** VCAM-1 CD11-18 INTEGRINS (CD18) VLA-4 INTEGRIN
4) **Diapedesis** (AKA: extravasation, transmigration, gaps between epithelial cells, **increased vascular permeability**)	**PMN's exit** (squeeze through) the blood vessel endothelial cells. **(AKA: separation of the endothelial junction).** **This leads to swelling – edema.** **Swelling is the first sign of inflammation.**	**PECAM-1** (CD31) (**tip**: Pecan trees must grow OUTside (exit:out)
5) **Chemotaxis**	**Chemotactic signals** guide leukocytes (by "TAXI") to the site of injury/infection	Products and signals released: Signals sent to **liver** to release **Acute Phase Reactants.** Chemotactic products released: C5a (PMN's), IL8 (PMN's), LTB4 (PMN's), **Kallikrein (Bradykinin)** to vasodilate so more room is made in the vessel to bring in more leukocytes and help and increased in vascular permeability to let more leukocytes out into the tissue, platelet-activating factor (to stimulate platelets)

Demargination and Stress

- Normal state of our WBC is that half of the WBC are always in circulation. The other half stay on the wall of our blood vessels waiting for a "call" to go to work (margination).
- Infection will "call" these WBC on the blood vessel walls to work. So there is an ↑ in the WBC count (Leukocytosis) due to the Leukocyte Extravasation physiology above.
- When cortisol and/or catecholamines (norepinephrine and epinephrine) are in play, they can cause the WBC that are waiting on the side of the blood vessel walls to go into circulation without need for an infection (margination).
  Thereby causing a state of leukocytosis in states of stress.

Margination (Leukocyte Extravasation)

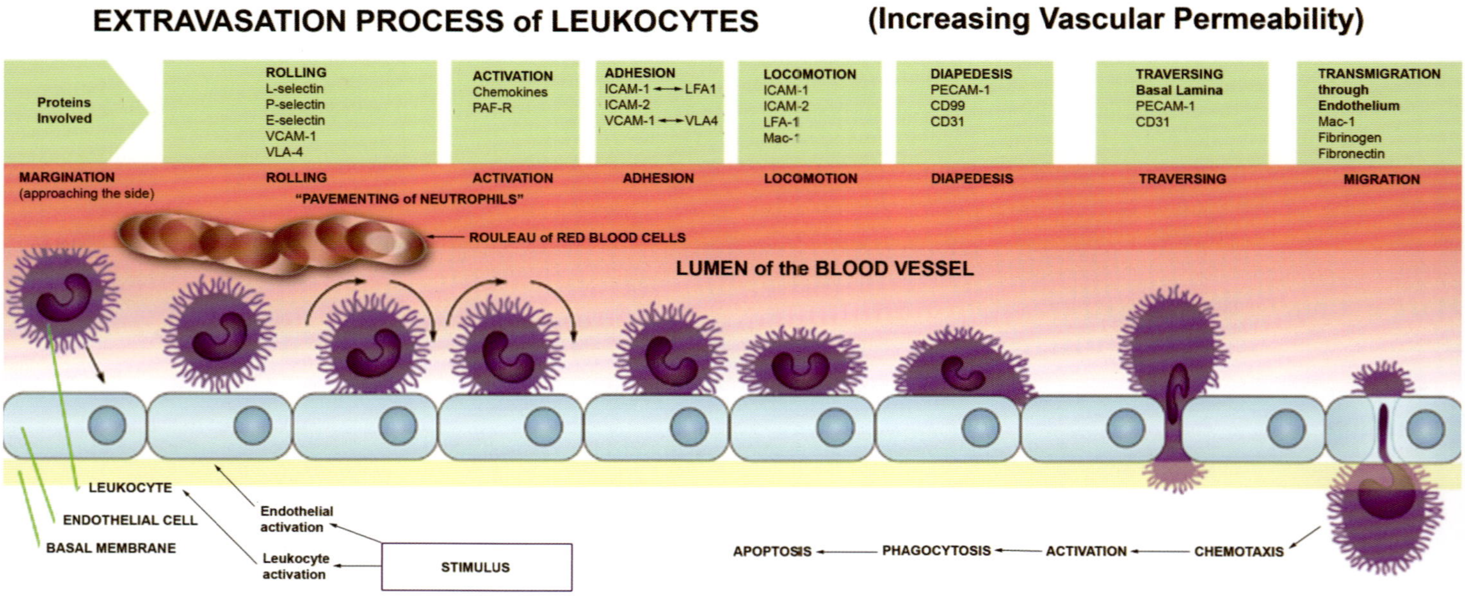

Adhesion Pathology (Integrins, I-CAM's)

Leukocyte Adhesion Deficiency, AR

- No chemotaxis of **integrins** (impaired PMN migration. Margination/Pavementing is not working)
- Defect in LFA-1 integrin (AKA: CD18), which inhibits diapedesis (AKA: extravasation, transmigration).
- Impaired wound healing, **delayed separation of umbilical cord.**
- Absence of PMN's at infection site
- No pus formation because leukocytes can't exit blood stream and get to infection (AKA: no diapedesis).

ARACHIDONIC PATHWAY

- Arachidonic acid (AKA: eicosatetraenoic acid) forms PG2 (2 double bonds, 20:4).
- Formed from polyunsaturated fatty acids (PUFA) (an omega-6 fatty acid) in the phospholipids of cell membranes.
- Highest in brain, liver and muscles, but found in most all tissues and cells.
- Arachidonic acid is cleaved from the phospholipid molecule by either **Phospholipase A2 (PLA2) or by DAG by diacylglycerol lipase.**
- Precursors in the synthesis of eicosanoids (metabolites of arachidonic acid) are: cyclooxygenase (COX-1, COX-2), lipoxygenase, P450 monooxygenase epoxygenase and anandamide. These eicosanoids are synthesized on demand and act locally where they are found.
- Modulates cell function.
- Eicosapentaenoic acid (EPA) forms PG3 (3 double bonds, 20:5) is high in fish oil and increased in individuals that consume larger amounts of fish. EPA completes with arachidonic acid. Increased EPA reduces formation of PG2.

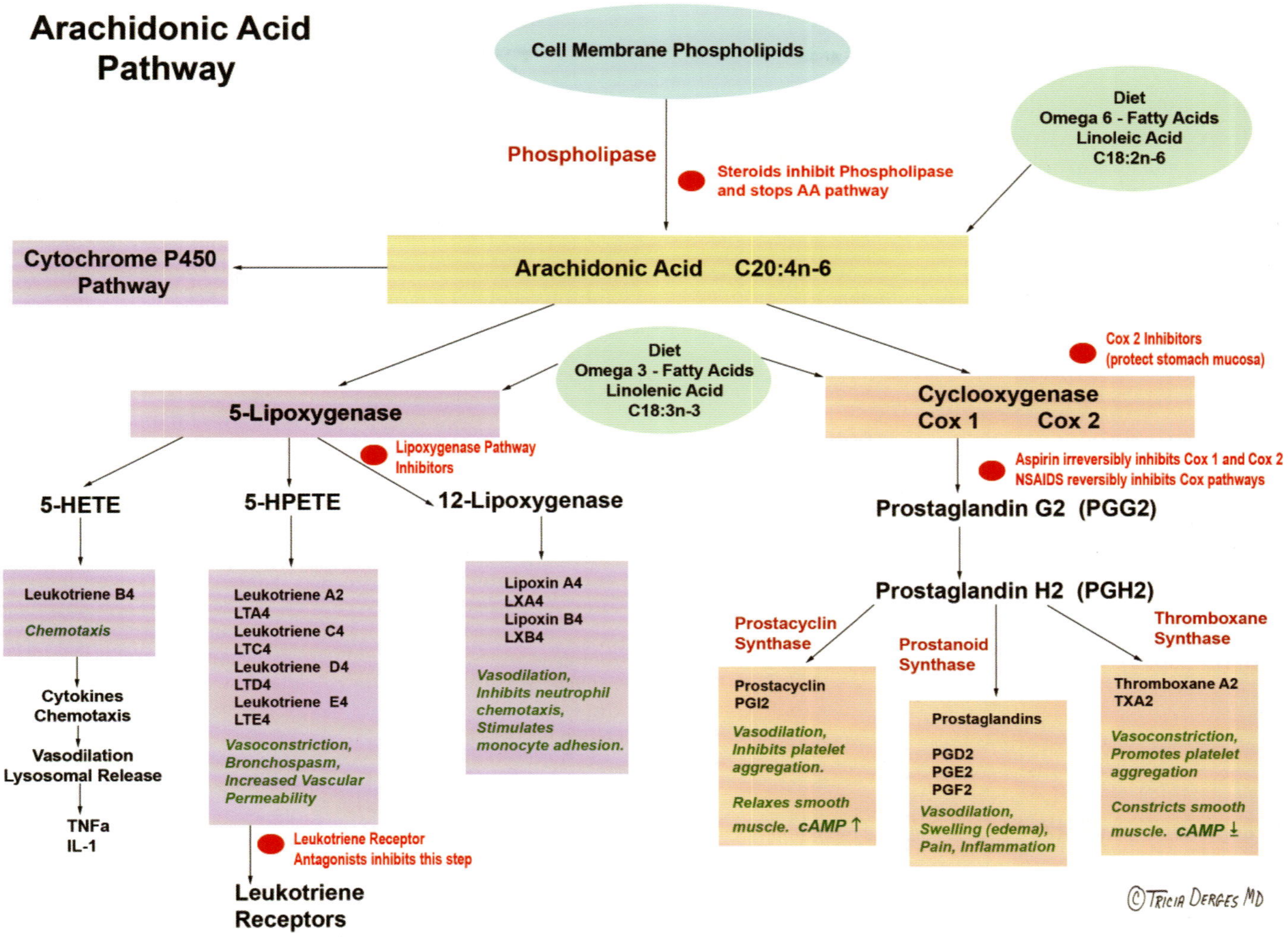

Eicosanoids

- **Increases capillary (vascular) permeability**
- Induces local vasodilation and erythema
- Promotes infiltration of inflammatory cells
- Produces tissue injuring oxygen free radicals during synthesis of PG's and LT's
- Producing inflammation pain (hyperalgesia)

Cyclooxygenase (COX-1, COX-2)

- Endoperoxides convert to PGG2, PGH2) which are then converted to PGI2, PGE2, PGF2, TXA2
- COX-1 found in most all tissues and functions to increase mucus in the stomach for protection. NSAIDS inhibit function, which causes increased risk of ulcers. It also affects kidney function (hemodynamics) and stimulates platelet thrombogenesis.
- Isoleucine at the 6th position
- COX-2 found in the brain and kidneys. It is associated with areas of inflammation and injury. It is not associated with stomach protection. It is upregulated by cytokines, growth factors, tumor promotors and bacterial lipopolysaccharides.
- Valine is substituted for Isoleucine, creating a hydrophobic side pocket

Lipoxygenase

- P-450 monooxygenase epoxygenase (LTB4, LTC4, LTD4, LTE4)
  Converts arachidonic acid to HPETE 's (hydroperoxides, hydroxyeicosatetraenoic acid) and EET's (epoxy eicosatrienoic acid).

Anandamide

- Anandamide binds marijuana receptors and causes analgesia and decreased movement

Cyclooxygenase pathway (PG = Prostaglandins (PGE), Prostacyclin (PGI2), Thromboxane (TxA2)

- Modulators of neuronal activity: increasing or decreasing release of neurotransmitters and causing changes in behavior
- Sensitize pain receptors
- **Aspirin irreversible stop this entire pathway (Cox I and Cox II)**

PGI2 (Prostacyclin)	Produced by vascular tissue (endothelium)	Relax muscles **Inhibits platelet aggregation,** **Decreases uterine tone** (stops uterine contractions), Vasodilation, **Decreases bronchial tone** (dilates), Inhibit gastric acid secretion, Increase GI mucus secretion, Renal diuresis and increase Na and K excretion	(**tip**: "I" = inhibits (down): platelets, vessel tone, bronchial, uterus) ↑ cAMP, ↓ Ca, ↑ K, ↓ TxA2, ↓ PDGF, ↓ IL-1, ↓ IL-6, ↑ IL-10, ↓ VEGF, ↓ TGFβ
PGE 2, PGF 2 (Prostaglandins)		Relax muscles, **Increases uterine tone** (causes uterine contractions), Vasodilation (decreases vascular tone), **Decreases bronchial tone** (dilates), Renal diuresis and increase Na and K excretion, Inhibit gastric acid secretion, Increase GI mucus secretion	Induction of abortion and induction of full term labor. Normal uterine production of PG's contributes to menstrual cramps (**NSAIDS** effective in relieving menstrual cramps)
Thromboxane A2 (TxA2)	Produced by platelets	Contracts muscles, Vasoconstriction (Increases vascular tone), **Induces platelets to aggregate**, Increases bronchial tone (increases airway resistance)	

Lipoxygenase pathway (Leukotrienes LT's)

LTC 4, LTD 4, LTE 4		Contracts muscles Vasoconstriction **Vasoconstriction of airway** smooth muscle Increases vascular permeability Bronchoconstriction: (increases airway resistance; increases bronchial tone) in asthma and immediate hypersensitivity	
LTB 4		**Neutrophil chemotaxis**	(**tip**: PMN's get there B-4 everyone else)

Arachidonic Pathway Pharmacology is located in the Immunosuppressant Pharmacology at the end of this chapter.

HYPERSENSITIVITIES

Type I

- **Immediate** reaction because of **PREFORMED** antibodies
- Mediated by **IgE (must crosslink/bond) before mast cells can degranulate to release histamine and heparin** that act on postcapillary venules
- For mast cells to degranulate (activate) and release histamine the enzyme **tryptase** is required.
  (**tip**: to go on a boat TRIP a MAST is required)
- **Anaphylaxis** (bee stings, drugs, foods)
- **Allergies and atopic disorders** (hay fever, hives, eczema, asthma), food allergies, allergic rhinitis.
- DX: Skin testing, assay test

Type II

- **Cytotoxic: antibody compliment mediated** by macrophages and/or Natural killer cells.
- Antibody and complement binding lead to destruction by MAC.
- **Mediated by IgM and IgG**. Must bind to lysis cells.
- Hyperacute transfusion reaction: Anti-ABO antibodies = DIC. Antibodies in recipient bind antigens on donor RBC = Ag/Ab complex.
- Hemolytic disease of the newborn = RH incompatibility
- Mostly related to autoimmune disorders: Antibodies directed against antigens cause destruction of tissues and/or cells.
  Goodpasture syndrome, Bullous pemphigoid, Pemphigus vulgaris, Hemolytic diseases of the newborn,
  Pernicious anemia, Acute transfusion reaction, Idiopathic thrombocytopenic purpura, Rheumatic fever.
  NOT: Lupus
- DX: Direct and Indirect Coombs test.

  ANTIBODY DETECTION TEST (Autoimmune)
  Direct Coombs Test: (Ex: RH factor. RH negative mother and an RH positive fetus)
  Detects antibodies that have adhered to patients RBC's
  Indirect Coombs Test: (Ex: RH positive woman for RH positive antibodies)
  Detects antibodies that can adhere to other RBC's

Type III

- **Antigen – Antibody immune complex**
- **Mediated by IgG** to activate compliment (attracts neutrophils)
- Deposits **circulating immune complexes** of antibodies – antigens that are deposited in tissues causing damage that is compliment mediated.
- Shows low compliment (C3 levels)
- MCC: treating viruses with antibiotics
- SLE, Serum sickness*, Post strep glomerulonephritis, Polyarteritis nodosa, Arthus reaction (swelling after a tetanus vaccination), rheumatoid arthritis, hypersensitivity pneumonia.
- DX: Immunofluorescent staining.
  Labs: WBC count, serum complement levels, serum C3 and C1q levels.

Type IV

- **Delayed reaction**
- Cell Mediated
- Macrophages are activated by T cells (lymphocytes), **NO ANTIBODIES INVOLVED.**
- **Mediated by TH1 cells: T Cells (Helper T Cells) and Macrophages (CD-4).** TH1 cells activate macrophages creating an inflammatory response over 12 – 72 hours.
  (Path: CD4 = IL-12 = TH1 = IL-2 and INFγ = Macrophage). The damage is from cytotoxic T lymphocytes and activated macrophages.
- MUST have been exposed to the antigen before.
- **Poison ivy, PPD test (TB), Contact dermatitis** (occurs at the site of the direct contact. TX: **corticosteroids**), most transplant rejections**, candida test (tobacco injection** under skin), granulomas (Macrophages make up granulomas), **graft vs host rejection** (bone marrow or liver), **nickel allergy (AKA: contact dermatitis (tip:** watch for a rash around the neck, finger or wrist = nickel jewelry), Multiple sclerosis, Guillain-Barre syndrome.
- DX: Patch test

BLOOD TRANSFUSION REACTIONS (Blood transfusions are the #1 MC organ transplant)

Reaction	Timeline	Pathology	Signs	Treatment	Prevention
Allergic-Urticaria	2 – 3 hrs	Donor anti-leukocyte antibodies Lung infiltrates, **IgE Mast** Cells, **Type I hypersensitivity**	Wheezing, flushing, pruritis, angioedema, pulmonary edema, fever	Antihistamines	
Anaphylactic	**Seconds** to Minutes	**Anti-IgA Antibodies**. Patient is IgA deficient (**tip**: **A**naphylactic = Ig**A**)	Dyspnea, hypotension, bronchospasm, urticaria, respiratory arrest, angioedema	1- **STOP** transfusion 2- IM Epinephrine	Wash RBC, Give blood that has no IgA
Delayed Hemolytic	2 – 10 days	+ Coombs, Hemolytic anemia antibody response	Mild Fever		
Febrile	1 – 6 hrs	**Host antibodies against donor HLA antigens** and Leukocytes. Caused by cytokine accumulation in **blood storage.** **Type II Hypersensitivity**	**Chills, fever**, flushing		**Wash RBC** and decrease WBC (Leukocyte antigen)
Hyperacute Hemolytic	Within 1 hour	**ABO group incompatibility**. **Extravascular hemolysis.** **Hemolytic Disease of the Newborn.** **Host antibodies against foreign antigen on donor RBC**. **+ Coombs**. Due to mismatched blood type. **Antigen/Antibody complex.** **Type II hypersensitivity. RH incompatible activates compliment which activates MAC = lysis of RBC.** **DIC** (Compliment mediated cell lysis)	Fever, flank pain, chills, **jaundice** = extravascular **hemolysis**, hypotension, hemoglobinemia = intravascular, tachycardia. **Urinalysis shows Hb**. Labs: ↓ haptoglobin (haptoglobin levels measure the free (unbound) globin. They only become bound when there is Hb that has been released from dead/lysed RBC's. So when more RBC die and more Hb is released: haptoglobin levels ↓ because they are binding up with the free Hb)	1- **STOP** transfusion 2- Hydrate with normal saline	Careful cross and match

Transfusions

Transfusion Product	When to Transfuse
Fresh Frozen Plasma **Note: do NOT use vitamin K in active bleeding, it is to slow.**	**Active bleeding when on warfarin (Coumadin).** Increased PT/INR
Platelets 1 unit of platelets increases the platelet count by 5000. If adequate platelets are given to bring the count to normal and then the platelets quickly drop = antibodies against the platelets.	If platelet count is < 50,000 and the patient is going to surgery or an invasive procedure or is actively bleeding. If patient is stable and not bleeding: < 10,000. If patient is stable, non-bleeding and has fever: < 20,000. Only in HIT or TTP when life-threatening hemorrhage occurs due to potential thrombosis. Sickle Cell Anemia, acute blood loss > 30% of blood volume.
Packed Red Blood Cells Note: Treats hemorrhage and ↑ oxygen delivery to the tissues.	When Hb levels are < 7 g/dL in adults or children Younger patient: When Hct is < 20,000 Elderly patient: When Hct is < 30,000
Plasma	Patients with INR > 1.6 with active bleeding. In patients on anticoagulant therapy before an invasive procedure.
Cryoprecipitate (Prepared by thawing fresh frozen plasma and collecting the precipitate. It contains high concentrations of Factor VIII and Fibrinogen.)	Used in massive hemorrhage and consumptive coagulopathy.

ORGAN TRANSPLANT REJECTION

Rejection	Timeline	Pathology	Signs
Hyperacute	Minutes	**Antibody Mediated**. **B Cells**. Host **preformed antibodies against Donor's ABO** or HLA's. Anti-HLA antibodies. **Type II hypersensitivity**	"White graft". **Ischemia or necrosis**. Graft must be removed immediately.
Acute	Weeks to Months	**T Cell Mediated.** **CD8, T cells, Macrophages, CD4.** Lymphocyte infiltrate. Host T cells against MHC graft antigens.	Vasculitis of graft vessels with interstitial **lymphocyte infiltration**
Chronic	Months to Years	**T and B Cells.** T and B MHC are seen as self. Host T cells are sensitive against MHC graft antigen. (**Non-self foreign MHC graft is seen as self MHC** but is showing a "non-self_ antigen)	**Fibrosis.** Renal: vascular obliteration. Lungs: Inflamed bronchiole airways. Fibrosis of graft and vessels. Heart: athero**sclerosis**
Graft versus host		**T cells**. **T cells in donor graft see host MHC cells as foreign.** Graft CD8 and CD4 destroy host cells. **Hypersensitivity Type IV.**	Jaundice, hepatosplenomegaly, maculopapular rash. Usually seen in **bone marrow and liver transplants.**
NO rejection		Eye lens (cataracts) Stem cells	

Transplant Match Evaluation Criteria

- 1st Choice: Siblings without any HLA mismatches
- 2nd Choice: Blood relative with ≤ 3 HLA mismatches
- 3rd Choice: Non-relative with ≤ 4 HLA mismatches
- If there are 1 – 2 HLA mismatches, it is the same as a blood relative or non-relative
- Cadavers: Must have no HLA mismatches to be better than a living donor

Transplant Ethics and Laws and Facts

- No child **under the age of 14** or adult over the age of 65 can donate an organ
- If the closest donor match for a child is an only parent that is responsible for the home/finances, another donor must be used
- Even if a patient has signed their driver's license to authorize their organs to be donated in the event of their death, **the family can override this decision**.
- Blood transfusions are the most common transplants performed

GRAFT TYPES

Graft	Source
Autograft	From self
Allograft	From non-identical individual of same species
Xenograft	From different species. MC: Pig is used for heart valves
Syngeneic	From identical twin

IMMUNOLOGY PATHOLOGIES

COMPLEMENT PATHOLOGIES

Paroxysmal Nocturnal Hemoglobinuria (PNH)

- PNH: Stem cell defect.
- Destruction of RBC by **over activation of complement**.
- **DAF** (Decay-Accelerating Factor) protects RBC's, displays cell markers: **CD55 and CD59**
- AKA: **GPI anchored** enzyme deficiency
- Mutation in the **PIG A gene (leads to absence of GPI anchors on cell membrane)**
- Without **GPI anchor** on membrane complement lyse the RBC's
- MCC death: Thrombosis (MC site: Hepatic and Mesenteric Veins)
- SX: red discoloration of the urine due to presence of Hemoglobin and hemosiderin from breakdown of RBC's, seen mostly in the morning from concentrating overnight.
- Complications: Aplastic anemia, acute leukemia, myelodysplasia.
- DX: Flow cytometry shows ↓ CD55/CD59.
  DX: positive **HAM test** (RBC become fragile when placed in mild acid). Negative Coombs test.
  (**tip**: a "PIG" gene is a HAM)
- Labs: hemolytic anemia, low Hb, increased LDH (Lactate dehydrogenase), ↑ bilirubin, ↓ haptoglobin, ↑ reticulocytes, pancytopenia, iron deficiency anemia.
- TX: **Prednisone. Eculizumab** (inactivates C3).
  Folic acid replacement.
  Transfusions if necessary.
  Cure: Allogenic bone marrow transplant.

MAC (C5 – C9) Complex Deficiency

- **Recurrent infections with Neisseria bacteria**

C1 Esterase Inhibitor Deficiency (**AKA: Hereditary Angioedema**), AD

- C1 Esterase Inhibitors suppress activation of complement
- Family history of angioedema (episodic swelling of the face, GI tract, upper airways, extremities, genitals
- Complement activates **kallikrein which causes a build up of bradykinin** which causes vasodilation which causes angioedema
  (Note: kallikrein is from the precursor: prekallikrein which is stimulated by **Factor XII**)
- Located on chromosome 11
- **Ace Inhibitors are contraindicated because of bradykinin accumulation**

C3 Deficiency

- Recurrent sinus and respiratory tract infections
- Type III Hypersensitivity reactions

Additional Complement Facts

- **The progression of SLE is monitored by complement levels**
- **Membrano Proliferative Glomerulonephritis: low C3 complement**
- **Acute Poststreptococcal Glomerulonephritis: low C3 complement**
- **Diffuse Proliferative Glomerulonephritis: (SLE) low C3 complement**

IgA Pathologies

IgA Deficiencies will cause **recurrent sinopulmonary infections**, mucosal, respiratory, GI infections. Also seen in Celiac, IBD, and diarrhea.

Henoch-Schönlein Purpura, Small Vessel Vasculitis (HSP)

- IgA Complex deposition
- **ONE WEEK** after an URI (**Post Strep** Glomerulitis is **TWO** weeks post URI).
  Common infections that can lead to HSP: Strep A, Parvo B-19, Coxsackievirus, H. pylori, rubella, adenovirus, measles, and mumps.
- TRIAD: Arthritis (joint pain) + purpura (rash, tiny hemorrhages) = abdominal pain.
  SX: Purpura (AKA: rash) on lower legs and buttocks, arthritis/joint pain, abdominal pain, melena (blood in stool), renal issues. (**tip**: you always want your hens (chicken) grade A). Many people have kidney involvement that can lead to hematuria, proteinuria.
  (**tip**: Vignettes can make Henoch sound *exactly* like Post strep, so WATCH the time line, 1 week or 2)

IgA Nephropathy (AKA: Berger's Disease) – Nephritic Syndrome

- IgA immune complex deposits in mesangium
- Normal compliment levels
- Occurs a few days after an URI or gastroenteritis
- DX: Light Microscopy: mesangial proliferation; Electron microscopy: mesangial immune complex deposits
- SX: Painless hematuria after an URI

Chronic Giardia

- **Deficiency of IgA**
- Mucosal surface of the intestines are not protected
- IgA prevents adhesion (attachment) of giardia to the intestine walls
- Chronic diarrhea that will not clear up after the standard treatment of **Metronidazole** **(Side effect: Disulfiram effect)**. (tip: patient will have visited somewhere and either **swam or drank "clear" lake or stream water.** (**Beware**: this "outside" water source could also be from the water faucets of campgrounds/latrines).
- SX: Bloating, flatulence, steatorrhea, foul smelling diarrhea

T Cell Pathologies

T Cells fight viruses, parasites, fungus, atypical bacteria and tumors/cancer. So deficiency will cause recurrent infections with these pathogens.

IL-12 Receptor Deficiency, AR

- Decreased TH1 responses
- Decreased IFNγ

Chronic Mucocutaneous Candidiasis

- Chronic infections by Candida albicans
- Infections of mucosal membranes, nails and skin.
- Assocated with chromosome 2

DiGeorge Syndrome (AKA: Thymic aplasia)

- Failure to develop **3rd and 4th pharyngeal pouches** = no thymus and no parathyroid glands (↓ Ca)
- 22q11 deletion shown on FISH test
- Deficient in: T cells, PTH
- SX: **Recurrent infections** with all pathogens that T cells fight (shown above), **hypocalcemia** due to no parathyroid glands, **truncus arteriosis**, tetralogy of Fallot, **dysmorphic facial features**
- DX: **Absent thymic shadow on CXR**

Hyper IgE Syndrome (AKA: Job Syndrome), AD or AR

- **Increased IgE** and decreased INFγ
- Decreased INF-γ prevents macrophage activation causing a greater TH2 response, leading to an increased IgE and increased histamine, which inhibits PMN chemotaxis.
- Neutrophils are impaired to respond to infection
- **STAT3** mutation due to deficiency of TH17 cells
- **Recurrent skin infections caused by Staph** and candida
- SX: Eczema (rashes), abscesses, course facial features, lung infections (lesions of pus or air), difficulty in losing their primary teeth or have two sets of teeth.
- TX: **Dicloxacillin, Cephalexin**

B Cell Pathologies

B Cells fight bacterial infections. So deficiency will cause recurrent bacterial infections, esp. from encapsulated bacteria.

Selective IgA Deficiency

- Deficient IgA, but **NORMAL IgG and IgM levels**
- Recurrent sinus and pulmonary infections
- Cannot have ANY blood transfusions from persons who have normal levels of IgA or will result in anaphylactic shock.
- Can see other autoimmune diseases in connection with this: ie: rheumatoid arthritis, vitiligo, thyroiditis.
- TX: Transfusions only from persons that are IgA-deficient or from blood that has been washed.
- (**SEE ADDITIONAL IgA pathologies above**)

Bruton Agammaglobulinemia, XL
(AKA: X-Linked Agammaglobulinemia)

- Males (**tip**: Brut's a boy)
- Low levels of **all Ig classes.** Only the IgG is found in the serum.
- Normal CD19 and B cell count, but B cells are not able to mature.
- **B cells and all Immunoglobulins are decreased or absent (🡇 B cells and 🡇 or absence of lymphoid tissues: lymph nodes, tonsils, spleen, adenoids), T cells are normal.**
- Defective **BTK gene (tyrosine kinase)** (**tip**: **BRUT**al **TYR**ant)
- Babies lose maternal IgG protection at **6 months old**, so look for **recurrent pyrogenic bacterial infections to begin around 6 months old.**
- **SX: Small or absent lymph nodes, spleen, tonsils, and adenoids.**
  Recurrent respiratory tract infections.
- **TX:** **IVIG** and add antibiotics for specific infection.

Common Variable Immunodeficiency (CVID)

- Decrease in plasma cells and all Immunoglobulin's. There normal amount of lymphoid tissues (tonsils, lymph nodes, adenoids, spleen) and B-lymphocytes but a **decrease in the quantity of B lymphocyte output**. Antibodies (immunoglobulins) are being made, just too little.
- **Total IgG levels are low**.
- B cells are not able to differentiate
- Usually occurs **after 20's** (where in **Bruton's is a baby** and does not involve plasma cells)
- High risk of autoimmune diseases in addition to recurrent bacterial infections (esp. sinus)
- SX: **Recurrent episodes of sinopulmonary infections** (bronchitis, sinusitis, pharyngitis, pneumonia), enlarged lymph nodes, adenoids, and spleen and Celiac Spruelike disorder: Malabsorption, steatorrhea, diarrhea, and Giardiasis.
- DX: IG levels are 🡇 and 🡇 **response to antigen stimulation of B cells**.
- 🡅 risk of lymphoma
- TX: **IVIG** plus antibiotics for specific infection.

T and B Cell Pathologies

Recurrent infections in all areas: bacterial, virus, fungus, parasites, and **atypical bacteria**.

Ataxia-telangiectasia

- **ATM gene defects**, DNA double strand breaks
- 🡅 AFP
- 🡇 IgA, IgG and IgE
- Defect in the 11q22-23 (codes for DNA repair) deletion leads to T cell defect
- Increased risk of lymphoma
- SX: **Ataxia** (cerebellar defects and cerebellar atrophy), skin and conjunctiva telangiectasia (angiomas), IgA deficiency, cerebellar degeneration.

SCID (Severe Combined Immunodeficiency)

- Deficiency of **Adenosine deaminase** (autosomal recessive)
- Equivalent to HIV
- Defective **IL receptor mutation** (X link)
- **Deficiency of both B and T cells**
- **No B cells = recurrent sinopulmonary infections beginning at 6 months old**
- **No T cells = recurrent infections (same infections that would be seen in HIV)**
- Defective antibody response to defective activation of B lymphocytes because of non-functional T-Helper cells so that both B and T and Natural Killer cell defenses are impaired **(no humoral or cell mediated defenses)**
- Ribonucleotide Reductase is inhibited preventing DNA synthesis
- Eliminates excess adenosine in cells
- "Bubble Boy" Continual recurrent infections: bacterial, viral, fungal, atypical bacteria, parasites
- DX: absence of thymic shadow on CXR, flow cytometry for T cells
- TX: Bone marrow transplant

Hyper IgM Syndrome, XL

- **↑levels of IgM**
- **↓ levels of IgG, IgA, IgE**
- Defective CD40L so defective class switching
- High infection risk for opportunistic infections: CMV, Pneumocystis, Cryptosporidium

Wiskott-Aldrich Syndrome, XL

- X-Link
- **Decreased IgM** and platelets
  (**tip**: remember to turn the "W" in Wiskott upside down to an "M")
- **Increased IgE and IgA**
- **Normal B and T cells**
- Mutation is WAS gene
- High risk of infections by encapsulated organisms (polysaccharide capsules)
- SX: **Thrombocytopenic purpura, eczema** (atopic dermatitis), recurrent infections.
- TX: Bone marrow transplant
- (**tip**: "**Wisk**"ers the cat has a **MITE**: "**M**", **I**nfection, **T**hrombocytopenia, **E**czema)

Phagocyte Pathologies

Infections from catalase positive and encapsulated bacteria. High risk when there is no spleen.

Chédiak-Higashi Syndrome

- **Phagosome-lysosome fusing** dysfunction (AKA: **microtubule** dysfunction)
- Abnormal lysosome inclusions
- Defect in lysosome **trafficking**, **LYST gene** (**tip**: "**list**"en to Chediak)
- SX: (Careful: Signs in vignette will **sound like PKU**): albinism, light skin, blue eye, blond hair, and neuropathies. Recurrent staph and strep infections.

Chronic Granulomatous Disease (CGD), XL

- Genetic disease.
- Defect of **NADPH oxidase (NADPH generates superoxide)** so **can't make a respiratory (oxidative) burst**
- NADPH (aka: nicotinamide adenine dinucleotide phosphate oxidase)
- SX: **Abscesses of the tissues, lymph nodes, organs, ulcers/inflammation of the nose, granulomas in GI or urinary tract (these can become obstructive)**
- DX: Negative **nitroblue tetrazolium test** (will have a yellow color), meaning that no oxidative burst occurred.
- High infections from **Catalase positive** bacteria (**S. Aureus, Pseudomonas**, Listeria, Candida, E. coli, Serratia, **Aspergillus**, **Nocardia**, **Burkholderia**)
- See additional info under CGD in the Biochemistry chapter

Leukocyte Adhesion Deficiency, AR

- No chemotaxis of **integrins** (**impaired PMN migration**. Margination/Pavementing is not working)
- Defect in LFA-1 integrin
- Impaired wound healing, **delayed separation of umbilical cord**
- Absence of PMN's at infection site
- No pus formation because leukocytes can't exit blood stream and get to infection (AKA: no diapedesis)

Phagocyte Pathologies cont'd

INF-γ Receptor Deficiency

- Defective INF-γ receptor inhibits macrophage activation which inhibits the killing of intracellular pathogens
- SX: Severe systemic mycobacterial infections

IL-12 Receptor Deficiency

- Defective IL-12 receptor inhibits the TH1 response
- SX: Severe systemic mycobacterial infections

Immunosuppressant Pharmacology

- Drugs that help decrease transplant rejection
- Block lymphocyte activation and proliferation
- Commonly combined to increase efficacy
- Suppresses cellular immunity
- MAB's (Monoclonal antibodies): antibodies must be humanized

DRUG GENERIC name Trade name	**Clinical Use**	**Mechanism of Action and Resistance**	**Toxicity and Notes**
Azathioprine 6-mercapto-purine (6-MP) 6-thioguanine (6-TG)	**Prevents organ rejection**, SLE (Azathioprine), RA, Leukemia, AML, IBD (6-MP, 6-TG). Azathioprine is a precursor of 6-mercaptopurine.	Antimetabolite. Purine analog. ↓ purine synthesis = interferes with DNA synthesis. Activated by HGPRT. Blocks nucleotide synthesis which Inhibits lymphocyte proliferation.	**Bone marrow suppression** (anemia), hepatotoxic, GI symptoms, thrombocytopenia, leukopenia, and neutropenia. Fetal Effects: IUGR, fetal myelosuppression. Do not use when breastfeeding. Azathioprine and 6-MP: require xanthine oxidase to be metabolized so **do NOT use Allopurinol** or **Febuxostat** with these drugs. You must use another chronic gout drug instead. Allopurinol inhibits xanthine oxidase so 6-MP can't be broken down and metabolized so it builds up → toxic.
Corticosteroids *Prednisone* ***SEE BELOW** FOR COMPLETE INFO (UNDER ARACHIDONIC PATHWAY DRUGS)*	**Inflammation, autoimmune diseases, decrease transplant rejection.**	Inhibits chemotaxis and expression of cytokines which inhibits T cell activation. Inhibits NF-κB (protein that controls transcription of DNA and cytokine production). Induces apoptosis of T Cells. Blocks IL-1 and IL-6.	**Osteoporosis, avascular necrosis** of the femoral head, HTN, **adrenal insufficiency**, **Cushing's** syndrome, atrophy and thinning, ecchymosis, cataracts, psychosis, acne, hyperglycemia. Fetal Effects: IUGR, cleft lip, thymic hypoplasia, adrenal insufficiency. OK to use with breastfeeding.
Cyclosporine	Rheumatoid arthritis, psoriasis, decreases risk of transplant rejection.	Calcineurin inhibitor. Binds **cyclophilin.** **Inhibits IL-2** transcription, which **inhibits activation of T cells.**	**Nephrotoxicity (kidney failure),** HTN, HUS, ↑ herpes infections, gingival hyperplasia, neurotoxicity, hyperlipidemia, hirsutism, malignancy, **hyperkalemia**, Fetal Effects: IUGR, myelosuppression. Do not use when breastfeeding. Note: used synergistically with Sirolimus.

Tacrolimus FK506	Decrease risk of transplant rejection, Eczema, Atopic dermatitis, Seborrhoeic dermatitis, Malassezia furfur	Calcineurin inhibitor. Binds **FKBP12** protein. **Inhibits IL-2** transcription, which inhibits activation of T cells.	**Nephrotoxicity**, HUS, neurotoxicity. ↑ herpes infections. Increased risk of diabetes due to hyperglycemia, hyperkalemia, hypomagnesemia, insomnia, seizures, tremors, catatonia. (note: no gingival hyperplasia or hirsutism). Fetal Effects: neonatal hyperkalemia, prematurity.
Sirolimus Rapamycin	Decreases risk of kidney transplant rejection	Inhibits **mTOR**, binds FKBP. Inhibits IL-2 transcription, which inhibits activation of T cells. It also inhibits B-cell differentiation.	Insulin resistance, hyperlipidemia, pancytopenia, thrombocytopenia, **hyperkalemia**, hypomagnesemia, hypertriglyceridemia. Fetal Effects: Low fetal weight, delayed skeletal ossification.. **Not nephrotoxic.** Note: used synergistically with cyclosporine.
Daclizumab **Basiliximab**	Decreases risk of kidney transplant rejection	MAB: Monoclonal antibodies (must be humanized). Inhibits IL-2, which inhibits activation of T cells.	HTN, headache, dyspnea, GI symptoms, insomnia, tremor, edema.
Mycophenolate	Decrease risk of transplant rejection, SLE	Prevents purine synthesis of B and T cells by reversibly inhibiting IMP dehydrogenase. (Derived from penicillin molds)	Pancytopenia, neutropenia, anemia, thrombophlebitis, thrombosis, hyperglycemia, HTN, GI symptoms, spontaneous abortion, malignancies (mc: lymphomas), pure red cell aplasia, pulmonary fibrosis. Fetal Effects: Cleft lip, cleft palate, ear malformations. Do not use when breastfeeding.
ATG (Polyclonal) OKT3 (Monoclonal)	Decrease risk of transplant rejection	Depletes T and B cells	Allergic reactions, ↑ risk of infections, cytokine-release syndrome. Monoclonal: Renal failure. Polyclonal: Pancytopenia.
CP-690 Tyrphostin AG490	Decrease risk of transplant rejection	Synthetic. Binds cytoplasmic tyrosine kinase JAK3 that inhibits cytokine signaling.	Anemia (due to effects on JAK2)

MAB Antibody Pharmacology
Autoimmune Treatments

DRUG **GENERIC name** **Trade name**	**Clinical Use**	**Target**	**Toxicity and Notes**
Infliximab Adalimumab Certolizumab	**Ulcerative colitis, Crohn's,** rheumatoid arthritis, psoriasis, ankylosing spondylitis.	TNFα	**Must do a PPD test due to risk of reactivation of TB.**
Eculizumab	Paroxysmal nocturnal hemoglobinuria	Complement C5	
Natalizumab	Multiple sclerosis, Crohn's disease	A4-intigrin	

MAB Antibody Pharmacology
Cancer Treatments

DRUG **GENERIC name** **Trade name**	**Clinical Use**	**Target**	**Toxicity and Notes**
Alemtuzumab	CLL, Multiple sclerosis	CD52	
Bevacizumab	Colon cancer, Renal cell carcinoma	VEGF	
Cetuximab	Colon cancer (stage IV), Head/neck cancer	EGFR	
Rituximab	CLL, ITP, Rheumatoid arthritis, B-cell non-Hodgkins lymphoma	CD20	
Trastuzumab	Breast Cancer	**HER2/neu**	(**tip:** "Tra"ining bra (bra = breast)

MAB Antibody Pharmacology

DRUG **GENERIC name** **Trade name**	**Clinical Use**	**Target**	**Toxicity and Notes**
Abciximab	Antiplatelet used in treatment of MI's and stents.	Platelet glycoproteins IIb/IIIa	(**tip:** Michael J's song: **A, B, C**....1, **2, 3**)
Denosumab	Osteoporosis	RANKL (inhibits osteoclast)	
Digoxin immune Fab	Antidote for digoxin toxicity	Antidote for digoxin toxicity (along with: magnesium, atropine)	
Omalizumab	Allergic asthma	IgE, prevents IgE from aggregating and binding to FcεRI	
Palivizumab	**RSV** prophylaxis	**RSV F protein**	
Ranibizumab	Macular degeneration	VEGF	

Cytokines and Recombinant Pharmacology

DRUG **GENERIC name** **Trade name**	**Clinical Use**
Aldesleukin (IL-2)	Melanoma, Renal cell carcinoma
Epoetin alfa (erythropoietin)	Replacement of EPO in renal failure
Filgrastim (G-CSF: granulocyte colony stimulating factor)	Neutropenia (stimulates bone marrow to ↑ production of neutrophils. Also used to ↑ hematopoietic stem cells in the blood before stem cell transplantation.
IFN-α	**Hepatitis B, Hepatitis C**, Kaposi, Melanoma
IFN-β	**Multiple sclerosis**
Oprelvekin (IL-11)	Thrombocytopenia
Romiplostim	Thrombocytopenia
Sargramostim (GM-CSF)	Bone marrow recovery

Arachidonic Pathway Pharmacology

NSAIDS

- NSAIDs: Aspirin, Non-selective NSAIDs and COX-2 inhibitors
- Acetaminophen is not normally considered an NSAID because it does not have anti-inflammatory effects
- **Aspirin: irreversibly**, competitively inhibits COX-1 and COX-2
- Non-selective NSAIDs and COX-2 inhibitors reversibly, competitively inhibits COX-1 and COX
- Non-selective NSAIDs: Ibuprofen, Naproxen, Indomethacin, Ketorolac (Indomethacin is used to close a PDA)
- Non-selective NSAID effects: Analgesic, anti-inflammatory, anti-pyretic, anti-platelet
- **NSAIDS** inhibit platelet aggregation = increased bleeding time
- NSAIDS alter kidney function **(constrict afferent arterioles that decreases GFR)**
  Contradicted in kidney failure or those that are dependent on renal flow.
- NSAIDS block mucus secretion, which may lead to stomach ulcers.

Celecoxib

- Only Cox 2 inhibitor (does not affect stomach)
- Selective reversible inhibitor of COX-2. Inhibits the transformation of arachidonic acid to prostaglandin precursors.
- Effects: Antipyretic, analgesic and anti-inflammatory
- By inhibiting COX-2 the drug reduces inflammation and pain while minimizing GI stomach ulcers (common with non-selective NSAIDS and aspirin).

Aspirin

- NSAID that **irreversibly**, competitively inhibits COX-1 and COX-2, decreasing formation of prostaglandins and thromboxanes. Forms covalent bonds.
- Analgesic, anti-inflammatory, anti-pyretic and anti-platelet. These effects are achieved by inhibiting the COX pathway and reducing prostaglandin production.
- Overdose: **mixed acid/base disorder** (**respiratory alkalosis and metabolic acidosis**), presents with **tinnitus and rapid breathing (Kussmaul breathing).**
- Side effects: gastric ulcers, **Reye syndrome** if used in children for viral illnesses (flu), acute renal failure, **interstitial nephritis, tinnitus.**

Acetaminophen *(Tylenol)*

- Does **not** provide any anti-inflammatory effects: **ONLY** treats fever and pain.
- MOA: Blocks COX-2 in the CNS.

Zileuton *(Zyflo):* MOA: 5-lipoxygenase **enzyme** inhibitor, stops the formation of leukotrienes.

Montelukast *(Singulair)*, **Zafirlukast** *(Accolate):* MOA: competitive leukotriene **receptor** blocker (antagonists).

Steroids (Glucocorticoids)

- **Intranuclear receptor**
- Inhibits Phospholipase A2 so that the COX and Leukotriene pathway are both inhibited shutting down the entire inflammatory axis (**shuts down the entire ACTH axis**).
- Increases PMN's, decreases lymphocytes – monocytes – basophils – eosinophil's
- Side effects: **Cushing's syndrome**, truncal obesity (**increased hip to waist ratio**), muscle wasting, **osteoporosis**, (treat with **bisphosphonates**) **avascular necrosis**, peptic ulcers, dermal (skin) atrophy and thinning (**decreases dermal collagen**), easy bruising (**ecchymosis**), telangiectasia, **atrophied adrenal gland (Remember when steroids are being used, they are taking the place of the endogenous cortisol, so the adrenal gland does not have to work. Remember: Since there is cortisol present, the ACTH from the hypothalamus/pituitary axis will not be affected).**
- **Chronic use of Steroids: individual is considered immunocompromised.**
  Adrenal insufficiency (AKA: Adrenal Crisis) if drug is abruptly stopped after chronic use. (Drug must be tapered if used for more than one week). **WATCH** for the patient that is admitted for surgery (or other inpatient procedure) and goes into adrenal insufficiency due to stress but the body is not able to supply cortisol (stress hormone) because entire ACTH axis has been shut down due to chronic steroid use. Steroids must be continued in hospitalized patients in order to avoid adrenal insufficiency.
- **NOTE: In any pathology** where systemic steroids (glucocorticoids) are being used, even as an adjunct (ie: RA, Lupus) remember that **any of the side effects or signs from steroid use can be seen** in the patient: osteoporosis, atrophied adrenal gland, avascular necrosis.
- **NOTE: Anytime steroids are being used it is not uncommon to see infertility problems because steroids suppress the gonadotropins.**

MICROBIOLOGY - BACTERIA

Bacterial Components

- Ribosome: 50S and 30S ribosomal subunits for protein synthesis
- Spores: Asexual reproduction. Allows long-term survival. Resistant to dehydration, heat and chemicals.
- Capsule: Polysaccharide (exception: Bacillus anthrax contains **D-glutamate**)
- Peptidoglycan: Protects against osmotic pressure, cellular support
- Cell wall = Gram-Positives: Lipoteichoic acid: induces TNF and IL-1
- Cell membrane = Gram Negatives: Endotoxin, lipopolysaccharide (LPS), Lipid A induces TNF and IL-1
- Cell membrane = Gram Negatives: O Polysaccharide antigen
- Glycocalyx: Allows adherence to surfaces (ie: indwelling catheters)
- Plasmid: Small, circular, double-stranded DNA molecule
- Flagellum: appendage from the cell body that allows motility
- Pilus/Fimbria (AKA: Adherence): appendage made of glycoproteins. Allows adhesion, virulence factor for E. coli and other bacteria, conjugation between bacteria

Bacterial Shapes

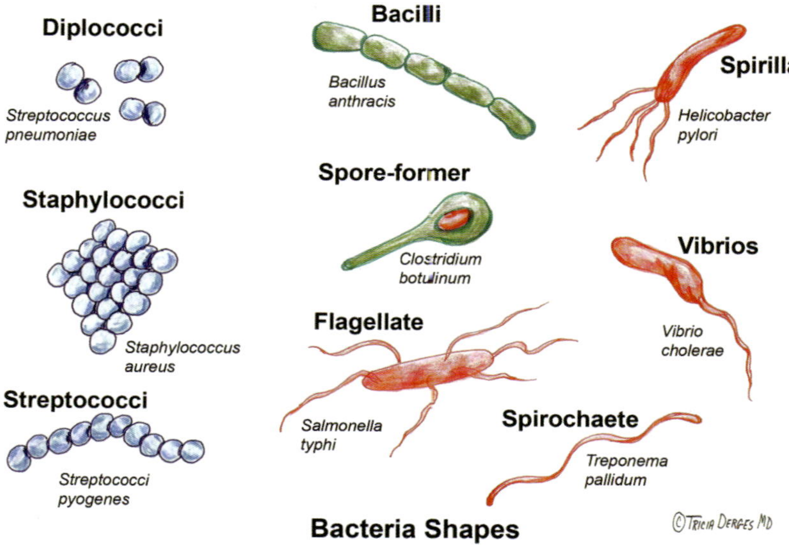

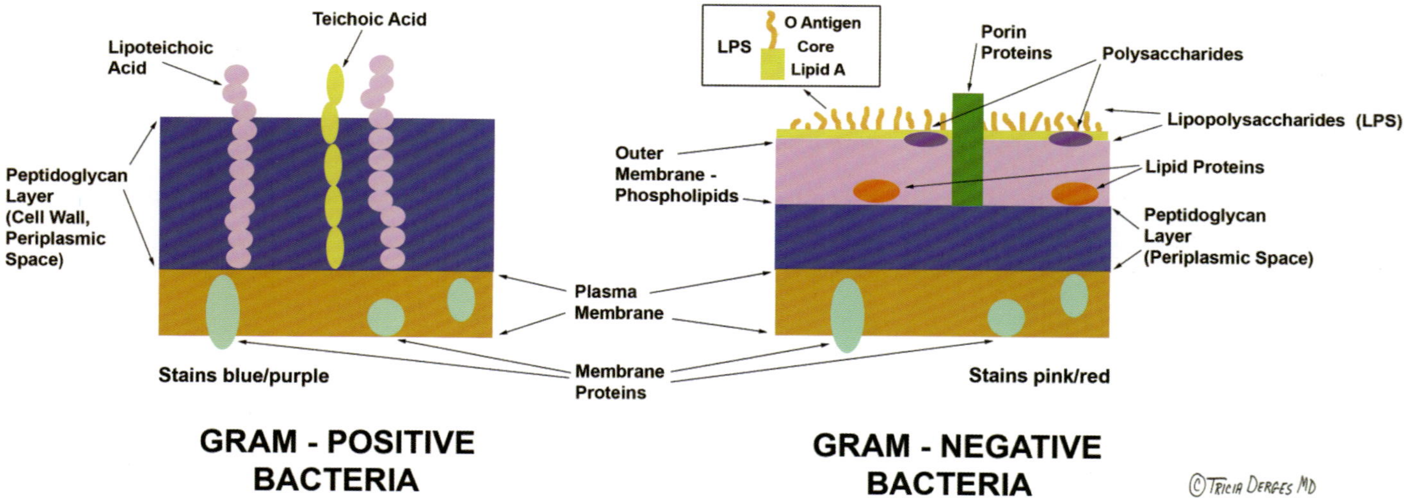

Gram-Positive Bacteria – produce EXOTOXINS (except Listeria)

Gram positive bacteria stains purple due to their thick peptidoglycan layer.

- **(tip:** eXotoxin. X looks like a +, positive)
- **Coccus shape (cocci, circular)**
  Staphylococcus (Staph): form clusters
  Staphylococcus aureus
  Staphylococcus epidermidis
  Staphylococcus saprophyticus (AKA: Honeymooners cystitis)
  Streptococcus: forms chains
  Streptococcus pneumoniae (AKA: pneumococcus)
  Streptococci pyogenes (Group A Strep, GAS)
  Enterococci (Group D Strep)
  Streptococcus agalactiae (Group B Strep, GBS)
  Streptococcus bovis
  Streptococcus Viridans Group (mouth): S. mutans, S. viridans, **S. sanguinis**, **Eikenella, Kingella**, Cardiobacterium, Aggregatibacter, Hemophilus, S. gordonii,
- **Rod shape (AKA: Bacillus) Shapes: Bacillus (one), diplobacillus (two), streptobacillus (chain)**
  Mycobacterium (Ziehl-Neelsen stain (AKA: carbol fuchsin), acid fast stain, cell wall contains mycolic acid) (Culture: Löwenstein-Jensen agar)
  Corynebacterium (Culture: Tellurite agar, Löffler)
  Listeria (**ONLY** gram-positive endotoxin)
  Bacillus
  Clostridium
  (**tip**: My Corny List is in the Back of the Closet)

Gram-Negative Bacteria – Produce ENDOTOXINS

Endotoxins: Bacteria membrane lipopolysaccharides (LPS) that consist of a toxic fatty acid: Lipid A core and a polysaccharide coat containing O antigen.

Gram negative bacteria stains red due to the thin peptidoglycan layer.

- (**tip**: eNdotoxin. N = Negative)
- (**tip**: poly**SAC**charide. Encapsulate organisms are in a **SAC**)
- **Coccus Shape (Cocci, Circular)**
  Neisseria (AKA: Diploici) (Culture: **Thayer-Martin**: Vancomycin, Polymyxin, Nystatin)
  Neisseria gonorrhea (Gonococci)
  Neisseria meningitis (Meningococcal)
- **Enterics (Rod, Bacillus shape)**
  E. coli (Pink colonies on MacConkey agar, Eosin-methylene blue agar)
  Pseudomonas (MacConkey agar)
  Helicobacter pylori (Silver stain)
  Bacteroides
  Bordetella pertussis (Bordetella medium)
  Fusobacterium
  Proteus
  Klebsiella
  Vibrio
  Shigella
  Salmonella
  Yersinia
  Coxiella
  Haemophilus influenza (AKA: coccobacillus) (Chocolate agar with **Factors V (NAD) and X (hematin)**
  Bordetella pertussis (AKA: Whooping cough) (Culture: Bordet-Gengou – potato agar)
  Tropheryma whipplei (**PAS** stain (Periodic Acid-Schiff: stains for glycogen (sugar)

Spirochetes

- Treponema (Dark Field microscope)
- Borrelia (Wright or Giemsa stains)
- Leptospira

Spores

- Bacillus
- Clostridium tetanus and anthrax
- SPORE GROWTH. **Maximum** spore growth is in stationary phase

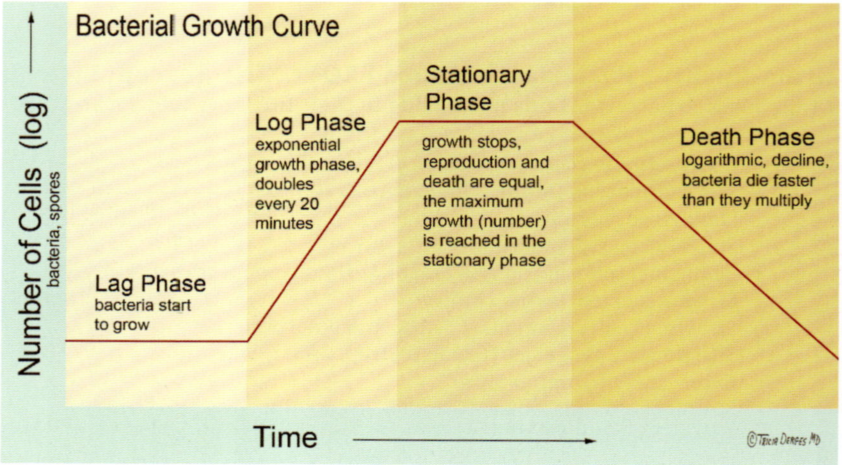

Intracellular

- Chlamydiae (Giemsa stain)
- Rickettsiae (Giemsa stain)
- Legionella (Culture: Charcoal yeast extract) (Silver stain with cysteine and iron)

Branching Filaments (gm +)

- Actinomyces
- Nocardia (Ziehl-Neelsen stain (AKA: carbol fuchsin), weak acid fast)

No Cell Wall – contains sterols

-
- Mycoplasma (does not gram stain, lacks peptidoglycans) (Culture: Eaton agar, requires cholesterol)

Exotoxins (Gram-positive) verses Endotoxins (Gram-negative)
(**tip**: e**N**dotoxins = **N**egative
e**X**otoxin = the **X** looks like a **+**)

Property	Exotoxin	Endotoxin
Bacteria	Mainly Gram-positive	Mainly Gram-negative
Toxin	**Teichoic acids (Lipoteichoic), Polypeptide**	**LPS (Lipopolysaccharide), Lipid A, O Antigen**
Toxicity	Highly toxic: fatal on few micrograms	Low toxicity: requires 100's of micrograms to be fatal
		Septic Shock: Fever, Tachycardia, Hypotension, DIC **Macrophages release: IL-1, IL-6, TNFα**
Vaccines	Vaccines made from toxoids	No vaccines
Heat Stability	Destroyed at 60°C	Stable at 100°C

VIRULENCE FACTORS

Bacteria	Virulence Factor
Staph aureus	Protein A (heat stable enterotoxin) Exotoxin (preformed enterotoxin = food poisoning) SSS (Scalded Skin): AB Toxin
Staph epidermitis	Biofilm (AKA: polysaccharide slim, extracellular polysaccharide)
Staph pneumonia	Encapsulated, IgA protease
Strep pyogenes (Strep A)	Protein M, Exotoxin A, Strep O (ASO), β hemolysis, Erythrogenic toxin
Strep agalactiae (Strep B)	CAMP
Corynebacterium	ADP-ribosylation of EF2 (elongation factor), AB Exotoxin
Clostridium botulism	Botulinum toxin. Preformed toxin (swallowed) or Inhaled spore
Clostridium perfringens	A Toxin, β Toxin, lecithinase
Clostridium difficile	Toxin A and B
Clostridium tetani	Tetanospasmin. Inhibits release of GABA and glycine
N. gonorrhea (Gonococci)	Antigenic pili (AKA: fimbria, adherence)
N. meningitis (Meningococcal)	IgA protease
Nocardia	Cord factor, catalase and superoxide dismutase (inactivates reactive oxygen species that are toxic to the bacteria)
Pseudomonas	Ribosylation of EF2, Exotoxin A, Elastase (destroys vessels), Pyocyanin (reactive O2 species), Biofilm (lungs), Phospholipase C (destroys cell membranes)
Shigella	Shiga Toxin (AKA: Verotoxin), inactivate 60S ribosome

Virulence Factors cont'd

E. coli (EHEC)	Shiga-like (Endotoxic shock)
E. coli (ETEC)	Fimbriae, Pilli Heat labile = ↑ adenylate cyclase = ↑ cAMP = ↑ Cl secretion in gut, H2O efflux Heat stabile = ↑ guanylate cyclase = ↑ cGMP = ↓ NaCl and H2O in gut
E. coli meningitis/pneumonia	K Capsule
B. pertussis	Pertussis toxin, Edema factor. ↑ adenylate cyclase = ↑ cAMP by inhibiting Gi
V. Cholera	Cholera toxin. ↑ adenylate cyclase = ↑ cAMP activating Gs = ↑ Cl secretion in gut
H. Influenza	Capsule B, IgA protease
Bacillus anthrax	Polypeptide capsule with D-Glutamate, Lethal Factor, Edema Factor = ↑ cAMP

Septic Shock

Gram-negative: **LPS Endotoxin (Lipopolysaccharide) contain Lipid A and O antigen**
Can be caused by gram positive and gram negative bacteria
Gram-positive: Exotoxin (Most common: Staph aureus: TSST-1 Toxic Shock Syndrome)
Gram-negative: Endotoxin (Most common: E. coli)
Sepsis must show the triad of: Severe hypotension, fever and tachycardia **(tachycardia is the FIRST physical sign that can be detected that indicates a falling blood pressure)**
In gram-negative sepsis: LPS toxin binds CD14 receptor on macrophages, monocytes and PMNs which signals TLR (toll-like receptors) to release cytokines: IL-1, IL-6 and TNFα to trigger the immune system. **High levels of these cytokines can cause septic shock.**

- Macrophages: release IL-1 (fever), TNF (fever and hypotension), Nitric oxide (hypotension)
- Compliment: C3a (hypotension, edema)
  Compliment: C5a (chemotaxis of PMN's)
- Tissue factor: activates the coagulation cascade causing DIC

SX: Systemic vasodilation (hypotension), decreased myocardial contractility, multiple organ failures, endothelial injury, alveolar capillary damage triggering the Tissue Factor which activates the coagulation system resulting in DIC and death.

Bacterial Reproduction

Reproduction Form	Process
Transduction	**Phage** infects bacteria = leaves his RNA behind leading to bacterial DNA. DNA transferred by bacteriophage (virus)
Transformation (Dumpster diving)	**Inpatient setting**. Due to in hospital antibiotic overuse. Taking up naked DNA from environment (hospital). Plasmin from one patient left for another patient to pick up. Combines 1 strain with another =- stronger strain
Natural Transformation	Is dependent on DNA **recombination**. DNA fragment is taken into a bacterial cell and recombination occurs between this DNA fragment and the bacterial chromosome by crossing over resulting in a double stranded DNA. The two strands of DNA are not complementary because part of one strand came from a different source. Both of the new strands now replicate so that the new DNA molecules are **genetically different**. One daughter cell is genetically the same as the original cell and the other contains a different allele from the DNA fragment that was taken up.
Conjugation	Sex pilus mediated transfer of DNA
Transposition	Transpose one segment of DNA into another. Excision of one segment and reintegration into another location

α and β Hemolytic Bacteria

Hemolysis (breakdown of RBC's).
This test is used to classify microorganisms based on their ability to cause hemolysis on blood agar.
Description:

- α Hemolytic: (aka: green hemolysis). The agar remains a dark green. There is only a small amount of destruction of RBC's. The bacteria produce hydrogen peroxide, which oxidizes the hemoglobin to green methemoglobin.
- β Hemolytic: (aka: complete hemolysis). The RBC's around the colonies of microorganisms are completely destroyed. The area is either transparent or light yellow.
- ϒ Hemolytic: Non-hemolytic. The organisms do not produce any hemolysis.

α Hemolytic	β Hemolytic	Υ Hemolytic
Strep pneumonia	**Staph aureus**	Enterococcus faecalis
Strep viridans	**Strep pyogenes (Group A): Streptolysin O (SLO), Streptolysin S (SLS)**	Staph saprophyticus
	Strep agalactiae (Group B)	Staph epidermidis
	Listeria monocytogenes	
	Clostridium perfringens	

Action of catalase: Degrades H202 into H20 and 02. Decreases killing effect of PMN's and monocytes on the bacteria.
Action of coagulase: Allows bacteria to induce blood clotting.

QUICK BACTERIAL REFERENCES, CHARTS and DEFINITIONS

Anaerobes

- Clostridia
- Bacteroides
- Actinomyces
- Fusobacterium
- Peptostreptococcus

Atypical Bacteria (fought by T cells, TH-1)

- Mycoplasma (lack peptidoglycans)
- Chlamydia (lack peptidoglycans)
- Legionella
- Coxiella
- Rickettsia
- Ureaplasma

Bioterrorism Agents

- Yersinia pestis
- Bacillus anthracis
- Ebola virus
- Francisella tularensis
- Smallpox

Black eschar lesions

- Bacillus anthrax
- Francisella tularensis
- Pseudomonas
- Mucor, Rhizopus

Bloody Diarrhea

Infectious diarrhea SX: Fever, tachycardia, hypotension, bloody diarrhea, abdominal pain, metabolic acidosis
SX: **Abdominal pain and NO fever** and bloody diarrhea

- EHEC 0157:H7 (E. coli) leading to HUS and TTP

SX: **Fever and NO abdominal pain** and bloody diarrhea

- Shigella (Daycares. HUS)
- Salmonella (puppies, poultry)
- Campylobacter (can lead to Guillain Barre)
- Yersinia enterocolitica (Thrives with iron and diseases associated with ↑ iron: blood transfusions, hemochromatosis)
- Amoeba histolytica (protozoan)
- Vibrio parahaemolyticus (Shellfish)
- Vibrio vulnificus (Shellfish)
- Clostridium difficile (antibiotics, MC: nosocomial. WBC and RBC in stool)

Non-Bloody Diarrhea

- Giardia (unfiltered fresh water, streams, lakes, camping, latrines in campsites)
- Staphylococcus (vomiting)
- Bacillus cereus (vomiting)
- Viral causes (Rotavirus)
- Cryptosporidiosis (HIV < 100 CD4 count)

Catalase Positive Bacteria (tip: PLACES SN)

Most dangerous for those deficient in NADPH or myeloperoxidase because the PMN's can't make the respiratory (oxidative) burst.
Staph aureus, Pseudomonas, Enterobacteriaceae family (Serratia, E. coli, Citrobacter, Klebsiella, Shigella, Yersinia, Proteus, Salmonella), Aspergillus, Listeria, Corynebacterium, Nocardia, Candida, **Burkholderia**, Mycobacterium tuberculosis, Cryptococcus, Rhodococcus.
(Catalase negative: Streptococcus and Enterococcus).

CSF Findings in Diseases (Lumbar punctures)

Disease	PMN's	Glucose	Lymphocytes	Protein	Pressure	RBC	Other
NORMAL	0 – 5	45 – 80		18 – 58		0	
Bacterial Meningitis	↑↑ >1000	↓ <40		> 400	↑		
Fungal Meningitis		↓	↑↑	↑	↑		
Viral Meningitis (AKA: Aseptic Meningitis)		NORMAL	↑↑ > 90%	Normal	↑		Note: there is a ↑ in WBC over the normal ratio of WBC and RBC in meningitis. In a subarachnoid hemorrhage the WBC is ↑ but the ratio is normal. **Normal ratio:** 1 WBC to every 500-1000 RBC
TB Meningitis	5 – 1000	↓↓ <10		↑↑ >400			
Lyme, Cryptococcus, Rickettsia		↓	↑↑	↑			
Guillain Barre	Normal	Normal		↑↑ 45 - 1000			
Tertiary Syphilis							Positive VDRL
Pseudo Tumor Cerebri					↑↑		
Multiple Sclerosis				↑↑			
Subarachnoid Hemorrhage (SAH)						↑	Xanthochromia Note: there is an ↑ in WBC but the WBC and RBC ratio is **normal**. In meningitis the WBC is ↑ than the normal ratio. **Normal ratio:** 1 WBC to every 500-1000 RBC.
Injury/improper stick technique						↑↑	
Herpes			↑↑ > 90%	↑	↑	↑↑	(RBC with viral profile)
HIV Toxoplasmosis							EBV DNA
Creutzfeldt-Jakob Disease				14-3-3 Protein			
Normal Pressure Hydrocephalus (NPH)				Normal			
Subacute Sclerosing Panencephalitis (SSPE)							Antibodies to the measles virus

Lumbar Puncture Rules

- **BEFORE performing an LP, a CT of the head must be obtained if the patient has ANY of these signs:**
  Papilledema (Indicates increased intracranial pressure), confusion, focal neurological abnormalities or having/had seizures
- **Do any cultures BEFORE starting antibiotics**
- **If no LP can be performed start antibiotics immediately**
- **LP (or spinal anesthesia)_ Anatomy: Landmark: Iliac crest for L3 to L4**
  Layers to penetrate (in order): Skin, fascia, supraspinous ligament, interspinous ligament, ligamentum flavum, epidural space, dura mater, subarachnoid space.
- **Normal WBC to RBC ratio in CSF: 1 WBC to every 500 – 1000 RBC.**
  Note: In SAH: there is a higher WBC's count but the ratio to RBC is still normal.
  In meningitis: there is a higher WBC count but that count is higher than the normal WBC:RBC ratio (abnormal).

Encapsulated Bacteria (SHiN are the MOST COMMON) (Strep pneumo, H. influenza, Neisseria)

Most dangerous for asplenic patients (Sickle Cell, removal of spleen due to an accident or Hereditary Spherocytosis

- **Strep pneumonia**
- **H. Influenza B**
- **Neisseria**
- Salmonella
- Group B Strep
- Klebsiella
- Pseudomonas
- Citrobacter
- Cryptococcus (yeast)
- (**tip**: Some Killers Have Some Pretty Nice Citric Crypts)

Endocarditis

- **AKA: Deposit/aggregate of fibrin and platelets**
- Due to the infection or damage of the **endocardium** (**inner lining of the heart muscle** that also covers the heart valves)
- **Endocarditis can involve the heart muscles, heart valves or the lining of the heart (not just the valves)**
- **Complications:** Blood clots and emboli, brain abscess, CHF, glomerulonephritis, neurological problems, arrhythmias, stroke, severe valve damage.
- **Fever and new murmur**
- **Splinter hemorrhages**
- Flat, painless lesions (Janeway lesions)
- Raised, painful lesions (**O**sler nodes) (**tip**: **O** for **O**uch)
- Microemboli to brain, lungs, arterial vessels, eyes, kidneys
- **Roth spots in the eyes**
- If TIA's occur, check ECHO to see if an endocarditis is the source of the micro emboli
- Always get cultures **FIRST** before treatment. After culture, IMMEDIATELY start empiric treatment, **DO NOT WAIT** until result of culture come back. Once the culture results are back the treatment can be switched to the best-recommended treatment for that organism.
  Best empiric treatment: **IV Vancomycin and Gentamicin**
- Subacute Endocarditis: occurs on pre-existing damaged valve
- Acute Endocarditis: occurs on healthy valve

Endocarditis Diagnosis

Diagnosed by Duke's Criteria (must involve 2 major symptoms, or 1 major and 3 minor symptoms or 5 minor symptoms).
Diagnostic Test: Best Initial Test: TTE (Transthoracic Echocardiogram). If TEE is negative: perform TEE (Transesophageal Echocardiogram).
TX: Empiric TX: **Vancomycin and Gentamicin** combined.

Duke's Criteria

Major Symptoms	Minor Symptoms
• **2 positive blood cultures with: S. aureus, S. bovis, S. epidermis, Candida, Viridans, Streptococci, Enterococci, gram-negative rods.** • **Abnormal echocardiogram showing: Valvular vegetation, abscess, dehiscence of prosthetic valve, mass**	• **Fever** • **IV drug use** • **Prosthetic heart valve** • **Hx of endocarditis** • **Dental procedure with bleeding** • **Structural heart DZ** • **Janeway lesions (flat, painless)** • **Splinter hemorrhages** • **Osler's nodes (raised, painful) (tip: O = Ouch)** • **Roth Spots on retina** • **Arterial emboli** • **Mycotic aneurysm** • **Pulmonary infarcts (septic)** • **Conjunctival hemorrhage** • **Glomerulonephritis** • **Positive blood cultures (not falling under major SX)**

Endocarditis Prophylaxis

The ONLY time that prophylaxis is given for endocarditis is:
(Prophylaxis: **Amoxicillin for oral/dental procedures**. **Cephalexin** *(Keflex)* for skin procedures.
If patient is allergic to penicillin: Azithromycin, Clindamycin, Clarithromycin, Vancomycin)

- Prosthetic valve
- Unrepaired cyanotic heart disease
- Previous endocarditis
- Dental work involving blood
- Cardiac transplant with valvulopathy
- Respiratory tract surgery
- Transplant patients (recipients)
- Surgery of infected skin

Otherwise: NO prophylaxis is needed for: endoscopes, OB Gyn procedures, urology, all murmurs, MVP, valve heart disease, atrial or ventricular septal defects, pacemakers, implantable defibrillators, septal defects, dental fillings, flexible scopes, cystoscopy, urinary procedures.

Endocarditis Organisms – Characteristics - Treatments

Organism	Characteristics	Treatment
Staph aureus	IV Drug use, indwelling catheter: ie: hemodialysis. (NOT central lines) Goes to healthy valves (MC: tricuspid valve) **CAUTION**: if murmur gets louder inhalation it is tricuspid if it gets louder on expiration it is the mitral.	**Nafcillin, Oxacillin, Cefazolin** **If prosthetic valve, add Rifampin**
Strep Viridans (Mutans, other mouth organisms: ie: Eikenella, Kingella, Peptostreptococcus, Fusobacterium, Bacteroides, Actinomyces, H. aphrophilus, H. parainfluenzae, Actinobacillus, Cardiobacterium)	From poor dental hygiene. Normally goes to pre-damaged valves. MC: Mitral valve.	**Ceftriaxone (4 wks)**
Staph epidermidis	From prosthetic devices (valves, joints) and from central lines	**Vancomycin**
Enterococci (Group D) E. faecalis, E. faecium	Follows GI/GU manipulation procedures (AKA: **cystoscopy**) from contaminated instruments. MC: Elderly men	**Ampicillin and gentamicin**

Endocarditis Organisms cont'd

Strep bovis (Group D) Clostridium septicum	Colonizes the gut. Indicates possible **colon cancer** or GI tuberculosis. **Next Step: Colonoscopy**	**Ampicillin and gentamicin**
Fungus		**Amphotericin** **Surgery: Valve replacement**
Culture Negative Endocarditis	MC: Coxiella, Bartonella Other culture negative: **HACEK:** H. aphrophilus, H. parainfluenzae, Actinobacillus, Cardiobacterium, Eikenella, Kingella.	**Ceftriaxone**
Non-bacterial Endocarditis (AKA: Marantic endocarditis)	Associated with terminal illness :(cancer or sepsis), SLE (Libman-Sacks), hypercoagulability, trauma. Sterile fibrin deposits. **NO bacteria**	
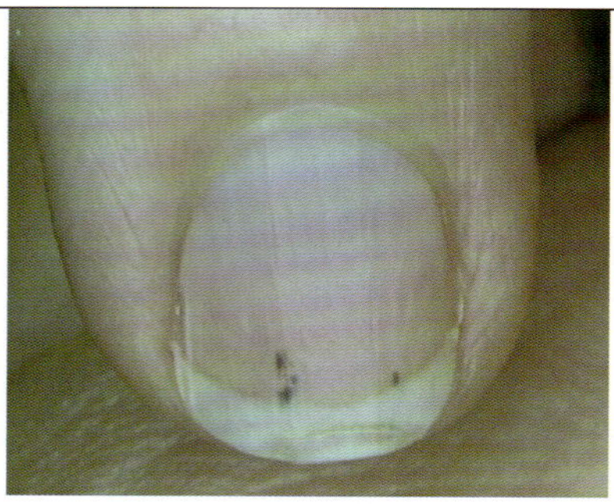 Splinter hemorrhages	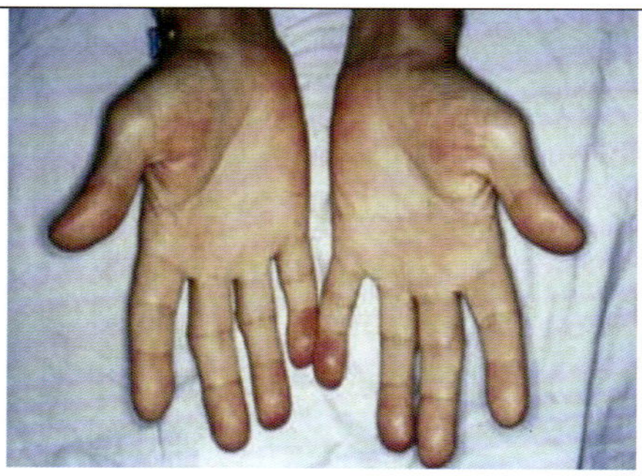 Osler's Nodes	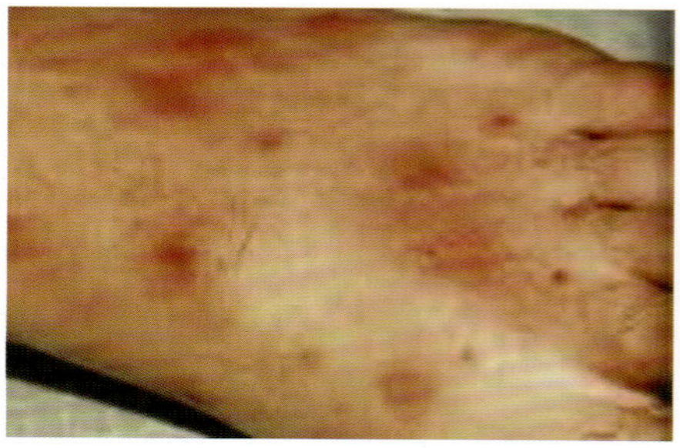 Janeway lesions

FOOD POISONING

Organism	Source of Food Poisoning	SX - MOA – TX - Notes
Bacillus cereus	Reheated rice, leftover sauces, soups and other prepared foods that have sat out too long at room temperature.	SX: Diarrheal type: Watery diarrhea and abdominal cramps. Emetic Type: Nausea and vomiting. MOA: Spores survive cooking. Enterotoxin. TX: Supportive, fluids. Duration 24 hours. Keep hot foods > 140° and keep cold foods < 40°. Store food in wide, shallow container and refrigerate as soon as possible.
Campylobacter	Raw and undercooked poultry, unpasteurized milk, contaminated water. Fecal-oral transmission, person to person contact.	SX: GI symptoms, diarrhea may be bloody, fever, cramps. TX: Mild cases: Supportive, stay hydrated. Severe: Antibiotics. Duration 2 – 10 days Campylobacter can lead to Guillain-Barré
Ciguatoxin (AKA: Ciguatera)	Reef Fish contaminated with a toxin made by dinoflagellates (marine plankton) that are on coral, algae and seaweed that the fish eat. (Barracuda, Moray Ell, Snapper)	SX: Mimic cholinergic symptoms: GI and neurological effects. Nausea, vomiting, diarrhea, paresthesia, numbness, ataxia, hallucinations, vertigo, **cold allodynia** (burning sensation when exposed to cold (AKA: hot feels cold), dyspareunia. SX can last weeks to many years. Relapses occur: alcohol, chicken, eggs, nuts, exercise. MOA: Opens Na channels ➔depolarization (stops action potential)

Food Poisoning cont'd

Clostridium botulinum	Canned food, home canned food that is spoiled (bulging cans) Food left out that spores could fall into (esp: turkey at Thanksgiving), honey, cheese sauce, bottled garlic, herb-infused oils, corn syrup.	SX: descending paralysis. 1st sign: Loss of gag reflex. Infants: Lethargy, weakness, poor feeding, constipation, poor suckling reflex, poor head control. Adults: Double or blurred vision, ptosis, slurred speech, difficulty swallowing, dry mouth, weakness. MOA: Adults: Ingestion of preformed, heat-labile toxin that inhibits ACh vesicle release at the neuromuscular junction = no action potential. Babies: Ingestion of spores (honey) or inhalation of spores (environmental "dust") TX: Emergency
Clostridium perfringens	Beef, poultry and gravy.	SX: Diarrhea, abdominal cramps (no fever or vomiting) TX: Supportive, stay hydrated. Duration of mild cases: 24 hours. Severe cases: 1 – 2 weeks. MOA: Cells that the spores grow into. Cooking kills C. perfringens cells that cause food poisoning but not the spores (spores grow into cells). Bacteria thrive between 40-140° so they grow quickly at room temp, but can't grow when refrigerated or are frozen. Thoroughly cook foods (meat, poultry). MC in foods prepared in large quantities and kept warm a long time before serving.
E. coli 0157:H7	Undercooked meat (esp. hamburger), unpasteurized mild and juice, soft cheeses, raw fruits and vegetables (sprouts), contaminated water, swimming in contaminated water. From animals (cows, sheep, goats) if hands are washed. Feces of infected people.	SX: Severe (commonly bloody), severe abdominal pain, vomiting, no fever. Can progress to HUS: Oliguria, anemia, blood in urine, and renal failure due to micro thrombi, thrombocytopenia, and schistocytes. MOA: Shiga-like toxin. Toxin causes necrosis and inflammation. TX: Supportive, stay hydrated. Duration: 6 – 8 days. (HUS would occur after 1 week)
Hepatitis A	Raw or undercooked shellfish from contaminated water, raw produce, contaminated drinking water, uncooked foods and cooked foods that are not reheated after contact with an infected food handler.	SX: Diarrhea, dark urine, jaundice, fever, headache, nausea, abdominal pain, loss of appetite, lack of desire to smoke. MOA: Virus TX: Supportive: Stay hydrated. Duration: 2 weeks – 3 months. Vaccination for all children 12 months and older, travelers to other countries, immunocompromised.
Listeria	Deli meats, hot dogs, meat spreads, unpasteurized dairy products, soft cheeses, raw sprouts, refrigerated smoked seafood.	SX: Fever, stiff neck, confusion, weakness, vomiting, diarrhea. ↑ risk: Pregnant women, immunocompromised, organ transplant patients, elderly. TX: Antibiotics Listeria grows in cold temperatures. Cooking and pasteurization kill listeria.
Norovirus Norwalk Virus	MC cause of acute gastroenteritis (infection of stomach and intestines) in the USA. (AKA: Stomach flu, viral gastroenteritis) Produce, shellfish, ready-to-eat foods touched by infected food workers (salads, sandwiches, ice, cookies, fruit)	SX: GI symptoms, watery diarrhea. Diarrhea more common in adults, vomiting more common in children. TX: Supportive, stay hydrated. Duration 1 – 3 days. Norovirus survives on surfaces that have been contaminated and can spread through contact with an infected person.

Salmonella	Poultry, eggs, meat, unpasteurized milk, juice, cheese, raw fruits, vegetables, nuts. Animals: Reptiles (snakes, turtles, lizards), frogs, baby chicks, pet food/treats	SX: GI symptoms: Diarrhea can be bloody, fever, abdominal cramps, vomiting. MOA: Endotoxin. Infectious dose is very high, requires a lot to infect. TX: Supportive. Last 4 – 7 days. Cooking and pasteurization kill salmonella. Antibiotics prolong infection.
Scombroid (Extremely fast onset) (AKA: Histamine)	Decayed fish (mahi-mahi, tuna, sardines, anchovies, bluefish, mackerel)	SX: **Fast onset**, within 30 minutes: Burning sensation in mouth, urticarial, pruritus, flushing, and tachycardia, wheezing. Possible anaphylaxis (angioedema, hypotension, bronchospasm) MOA: Bacterial toxin is histamine, which is formed as the fish decays. **Histamine** is not degraded by cooking. Bacterial histidine decarboxylase converts histidine to histamine. Histidine decarboxylase is produced by the bacteria Morganella morganii. (Store fish in the freezer). Self-limiting: last 1 – 2 days. Note: This is often mistaken as a fish allergy. TX: Antihistamines, Albuterol, Epinephrine
Shigella	Contaminated food/water or contact with infected person. MC: Salads and sandwiches that involve hand contact in preparation. Raw vegetables contaminated in the field.	SX: GI symptoms: Diarrhea that may be bloody with mucus, abdominal cramps, fever, diarrhea, nausea, vomiting. MOA: Endotoxin. Bacteria are shed from infected people in their feces. Resistant to gastric acids. Highly infective: infectious dose takes only a tiny amount of toxin. TX: Supportive, hydration. Antibiotics shorten duration.
Staph aureus	Mayonnaise based foods (potato salads, Cole slaw), custards (cream pies), Cream filled donuts.	SX: Fast onset: < 6 hours. GI symptoms: Nausea, vomiting, abdominal cramps, and diarrhea. MOA: **Preformed enterotoxin** (heat stable = not destroyed by cooking) TX: Self-supportive. Antibiotics are NOT helpful.
Tetrodotoxin	Puffer fish, Porcupine Fish, Ocean Sunfish, Triggerfish	SX: Fast onset, within 30 minutes. If dose is fatal: symptoms occur within 17 minutes of digestion. Paresthesia, nausea, loss of reflexes, hypersalivation, headache, lethargy, incoordination, dysphagia, seizures, paralysis, arrhythmias. MOA: Toxin inhibits action potential by binding fast voltage-gated Na channels in nerve and cardiac tissue, inhibiting depolarization. TX: Activated charcoal, Supportive therapy
Vibrio vulnificus Vibrio parahaemolyticus **Hepatitis A (virus)**	Ingestion of contaminated shellfish/seafood or exposure to an open wound. (Oysters, crab, clams). Affects marine or brackish waters.	SX: GI symptoms, abdominal pain, non-bloody diarrhea. Can infect bloodstream: fever, chills, hypotension, septic shock, blistering skin lesions. TX: Supportive, preventing dehydration and monitor electrolytes. Duration 2 – 8 days. Vibrio naturally occurs in waters where oysters/shellfish live.

Genital Lesions

Pathology	Ulcers on genitals	Lymph nodes	Treatment
Syphilis chancre	NOT painful, ulcerated lesions	Not painful lymphadenopathy	Penicillin G (single dose)
Haemophilus ducreyi (**tip**: "you cry")	Painful ulcers	Not painful lymphadenopathy	Azithromycin (single dose)
Klebsiella inguinale (AKA: Donovanosis, Granuloma inguinale)	NOT painful, Beefy red granulation	NO lymphadenopathy	Doxycycline, Tetracycline
Lymphogranuloma venereum	NOT painful	Painful lymphadenopathy	Doxycycline
Genital herpes	Painful ulcers	Not painful lymphadenopathy	Acyclovir, Famciclovir, Valacyclovir. (Foscarnet for acyclovir resistant)

Intestinal Biomass

- 1000's of bacteria fill the gut (good and bad: they live in a balance)
- When something affects this balance (such as antibiotics that kill off the good bacteria) then sickness occurs because of overgrowth (biomass overgrowth) of the bad bacteria. They overtake the good.

Jarisch-Herxheimer Reaction

- Reaction to endotoxin-like products released by the death of harmful organisms during antibiotic treatment.
- Occurs within a few hours of the first dose. SX: Similar to bacterial sepsis. Fever, chills, headache, hypotension, tachycardia, vasodilation, flushing, myalgia. No treatment, self-limiting.
- Most commonly associated with penicillin treatment of syphilis.
- Increase of inflammatory cytokines: IL-1, IL-6, IL-8, TNFα

Meningitis, Most Common Causes

Age	Organism
0 to 6 months	Group B Strep, E. coli, Listeria
6 months to 6 years	Strep pneumoniae, Neisseria meningitides, H. influenza B, Enteroviruses
6 years to 60 years	Strep pneumoniae, **Neisseria meningitides (#1 in teens)**, Enteroviruses, HSV
> 60 years	Strep pneumoniae, Listeria

Normal Body Flora

"Intestinal biomass" are the 1000's of bacteria that normally fill the gut. This is what keeps healthy people from becoming sick when they ingest bad bacteria. The bad bacteria are overtaken by these biomasses.

Organ	Organism
Dental plaque	Strep mutans
Oropharynx	Strep viridans, Fusobacterium
Nasopharynx	Strep pneumoniae
Nose	**Staph aureus, EBV (virus)**, Staph epidermidis
Skin	Staph epidermidis
Colon	Bacillus fragilis, E. coli
Vagina	**Lactobacillus**, E. coli, **Strep agalactiae (Group B Strep)**

Nosocomial Infections

- Infection is **not** considered to be a nosocomial cause if it is **under 48 hours** of admission.
- Pneumonia: Klebsiella (due to aspiration: strokes, seizures, alcoholics, post surgery, altered mental status, difficulty swallowing)
- Pneumonia if water source is cause: Legionella
- Ventilators: Pseudomonas
- UTI's: E. coli
- Wound infections: MRSA (Staph aureus)
- Urinary catheterization: E. coli, Proteus mirabilis
- Transplants: CMV
- Newborn nursery: RSV

Pigment Producing Bacteria

- Pseudomonas aeruginosa: blue green pigment
- Staph aureus: yellow pigment, golden
- Serratia **marc**escens: red pigment (**tip**: **mar**aschino cherries = red)
- Actinomyces israelii: yellow sulfur granules

PNEUMONIAS

- Community acquired pneumonia verses nosocomial pneumonia (hospital acquired): Pneumonia is NOT considered nosocomial unless patient develops the pneumonia **AFTER 48 hours of admission**. If the patient develops pneumonia **less than 48 hours after admission it is considered community acquired.**
- **Most common community acquired pneumonia**: **Strep pneumonia**
  TX: Ceftriaxone, Azithromycin (or doxycycline), Fluoroquinolones, Ampicillin + Sul Bactrim
- **Most common nosocomial acquired pneumonia and UTI**: **Klebsiella**. Due to **aspiration causes**: after surgery, alcoholics, after stroke, unconscious or altered mental status.
- **TX:** **Vancomycin, Ciprofloxin, Cefepime**

Pneumonia – Most Common Causes

Patient	Age	Organism
Neonates	<4 weeks	**Group B Strep**, E. coli
Children	4 wk – 18 yrs	**RSV**, Mycoplasma, Chlamydia
Young Adults	18 yrs – 40 yrs	**Mycoplasma**, Strep pneumoniae
Adults	40 yrs – 65 yrs	**Strep pneumonia**
Elderly	>65 yrs	**Strep pneumonia**, Influenza virus Secondary Bacterial Pneumonia: Pneumonia that occurs after the elderly come down with the flu, usually spread to them by grandchildren (**Strep pneumo, Staph aureus**, H. influenza)
HIV or any immunocompromised (chemo, COPD, steroids, etc.)		**>200 CD4 count: Strep pneumo** **200 CD4 count: Pneumocystis jiroveci (AKA: Pneumocystis pneumonia, PCP, PJP)** **<50 CD4 count: Mycobacterium avium** <50 CD4 count: CMV (virus) M <50 CD4 count: Aspergillus fumigatus (fungus)

Silver Stainer' s

- Legionella
- Pneumocystis
- Bartonella
- Helicobacter
- Chlamydia
- Borrelia recurrentis

Spirochetes

- Treponema (Dark Field microscope)
- Borrelia (Wright or Giemsa stains)
- Leptospira

Spores

- Clostridium tetani
- Clostridium botulinum
- Clostridium perfringens
- Bacillus cereus
- Bacillus anthracis
- Coxiella burnetii

To kill spores: pressurized steam In an autoclave for 15 minutes at 121°C.
To kill prions: Prions must be killed with bleach, caustic soda or autoclaved at 274° for 15 minutes using pressurized steam.

UTI's

Leading cause of UTI's

- **#1) E. coli** #2) S. saprophyticus #3) Klebsiella

UTI in women ("suprapubic pain") and prostatitis in men

- **E. coli is #1 cause (D-Mannose binds/adheres to the E. coli fimbria)**
- UA test: **+ Leukocyte esterase** = bacterial infection
  + Nitrate test = gram negative organisms
  + Urease test = Klebsiella, Proteus
  - Urease test = E. coli, Enterococcus

UTI - Nosocomial causes (associated with catheters)

- Klebsiella
- Pseudomonas (blue-green pigment with fruity odor)
- Serratia marcescens show red pigment. (**tip**: "maraschino" cherries are red)

UTI - stones if urine **pH is >7**, caused by urease positive organisms (alkaline urine)

- Struvite stones (AKA: Staghorn, Magnesium)
- **Protease**, Klebsiella, Morganella, Pseudomonas, Providencia, Staph, Urease

UTI if urine **pH is <7**, caused by urease negative organisms (acidic urine)

- **E. coli**, Candida, Citrobacter, Enterococci

Vaginal Infections

Organism	Inflammation	Physical Exam	Labs	Treatment
Candida vulvovaginitis – Not STD	Yes	Thick, white discharge (Cottage cheese)	Pseudohyphae **Normal pH 4.0 – 4.5**	(Fungus) **-Azoles**
Bacterial vaginosis (BV) (Gardnerella) Not STD	No	Thin white discharge, Fishy (odd) odor	Clue cells **pH >4.5**	**Metronidazole**
Trichomoniasis STD	Yes	Red, inflamed vaginal/cervix tissue, gray-green, foul smelling discharge	Motile trichomonads **pH > 4.5**	**Metronidazole** Must treat partner (**tip**: "tricky dicky")

BACTERIA - GRAM POSITIVE BACTERIA

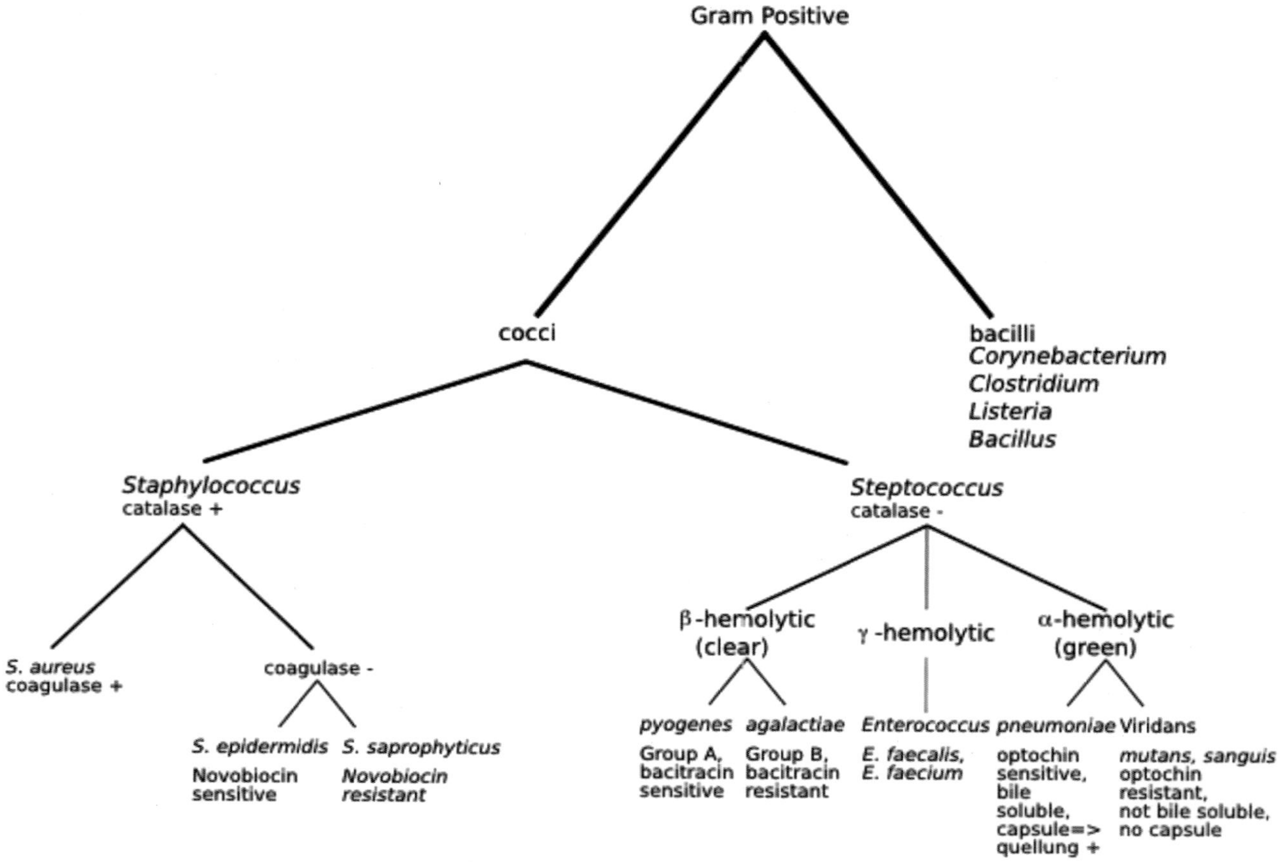

GRAM POSITIVE: COCCI BACTERIA – STAPH – CLUSTERS

Staphylococcus aureus		
Gm +, Staphylococci **Catalase positive +** **Coagulase positive+** Mannitol positive+ **B Hemolytic**	**Colonizes the Nose** (aka: Nares)	**Virulence Factors:** Protein A (Ø C3) = Heat stable enterotoxin Exotoxin (Preformed enterotoxin) = Food poisoning AB Toxin = Scalded Skin Syndrome
Food Poisoning **Preformed Enterotoxin** Heat stable Acute onset **< 6 hours** Custards, Mayonnaise base foods (potato salads, Cole slaw), cream pies, cream filled donuts. Tx: Supportive	**Endocarditis** Likes healthy valves (normally tricuspid)* **IV drug users, IV lines, hemodialysis,** Indwelling catheters. (**NOT** central lines) **(*Careful on ALL endocarditis murmurs: if murmur louder on Inhalation = tricuspid. If louder on expiration = mitral)**	**Osteomyelitis** MCC in young children (including Sickle Cell) **Periosteal reaction = pain in long bones of children.** (Sickle Cell: #1 cause in older children = **Salmonella**)

Cellulitis
From skin infections, MCC **venous stasis**

SX: Irregular, elevated boarders.
Tender, erythema, fever on the skin. Can lead to skin ulcers.

TX: **Minor: Cephalexin** *(Keflex)* **or Dicloxacillin**
Severe: IV Nafcillin, IV Oxacillin, IV Cefazolin

DO NOT DO SURGICAL DEBRIDEMENT on ULCERS– antibiotics ONLY.

Caution: Cellulitis and DVT can present the same. Rule out DVT with a Doppler.

Also caused by S. pyogenes

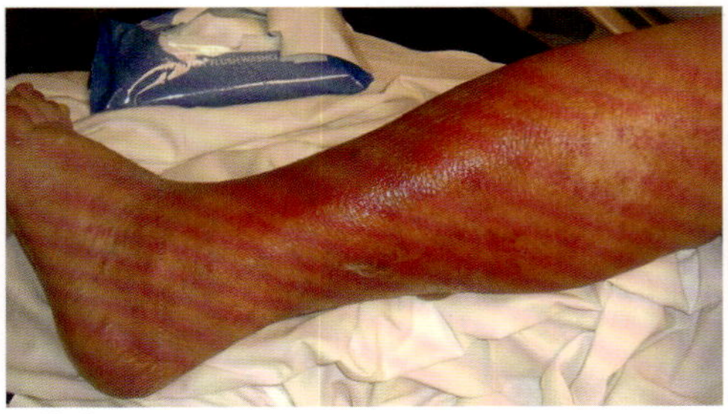
Cellulitis

Septic Arthritis (destroys joints)
(AKA: Bacterial arthritis) in **children** and **non-sexually active** adults.

SX: Usually proceeded by cellulitis.
Unilateral joint, pain, swelling, erythema, high WBC: **PMN's >50,000, ↑ ESR,** turbid synovial fluid, can't bear weight

DX: Arthrocentesis
TX: **Vancomycin**

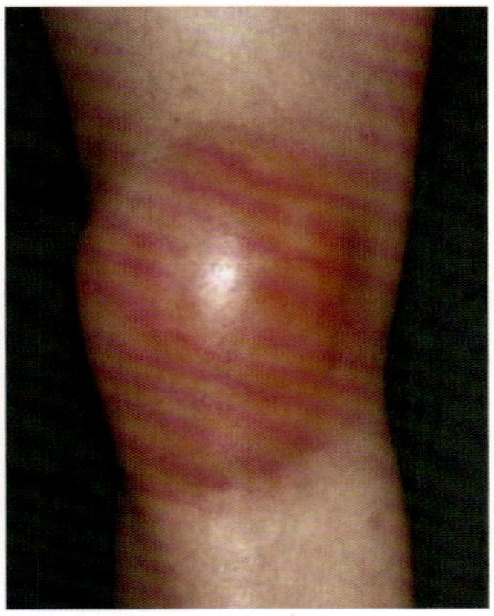
Septic Arthritis

Bacterial tracheitis
Acute respiratory infection of the trachea following a viral upper respiratory infection. Can be confused with the croup.

SX: high fever, brassy cough, respiratory distress, no dysphagia or drooling. If severe distress, may require intubation.

TX: Antistaphylococcal antibiotics

Impetigo
SX: weeping, oozing, **honey color crusted** lesions. Most commonly around mouth, but can be anywhere.
Skin infections can lead to **Post-Strep Glomerulonephritis (NOT rheumatic fever)**
TX: Topical **Mupirocin** (most effective) **or Retapamulin, Erythromycin (oral)**
TX Severe case: **Oral dicloxacillin, Cephalexin** *(Keflex)*
Also caused by S. pyogenes

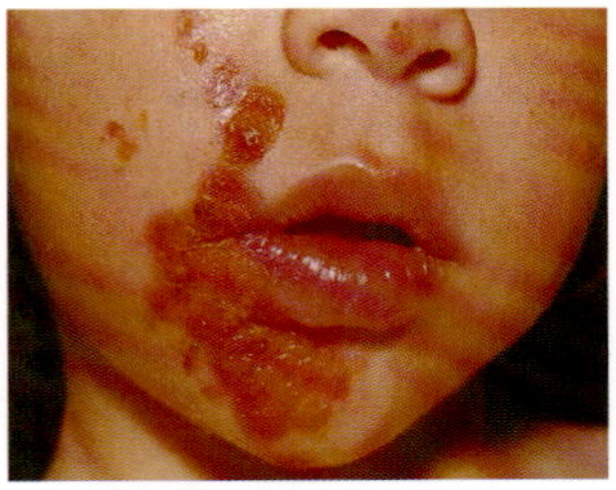
Impetigo

SSS – Scalded Skin Syndrome (SSSS)
AB Toxin
Dermatomes separate the granulosum layer.

SX: Skin rash like a sunburn (desquamation of skin). Normal BP and no involvement of other organs (as in TSS).
Splits the only the superficial layer of skin.
+ Nikolsky's sign, fever, blisters, painful skin.
Complications: cellulitis, sepsis, pneumonia.

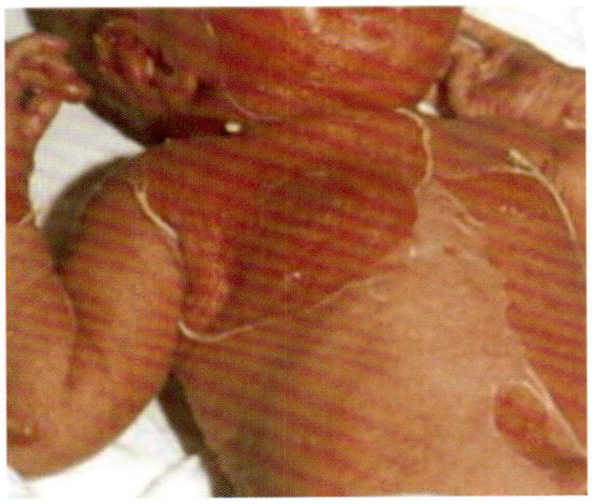
Scalded skin syndrome

TSST-1 Toxic Shock
Superantigen, binds to MHC II and T Cell receptor.

SHOCK = LPS = LIPID A = activates IL-1, IL-6, TNFα

SX: Fever, rash, shock, tachycardia, hypotension

Vaginal or nasal **tampons,** surgical material retained in the body (retained sutures).

MRSA
Methicillin Resistant Staph aureus.
Resistant to methicillin, oxacillin and nafcillin because of **altered penicillin-binding protein.**
TX: **Vancomycin or Linezolid and add a Beta Lactamase**

Secondary Bacterial Pneumonia
Common in the elderly after they acquire viral influenza.

Abscess>Boils> Carbuncles> Furuncles>Folliculitis
All are infections at the base of the hair follicle: differentials: size. (Abscess is the largest).
(Folliculitis can also be caused by pseudomonas: **hot tub folliculitis**)

Complication: Post-strep glomerulonephritis.

TX: Larger (Abscess and boils may require drainage).

TX: **Minor: Cephalexin** *(Keflex)* **or Dicloxacillin**
Severe: Nafcillin, Oxacillin, IV Cefazolin

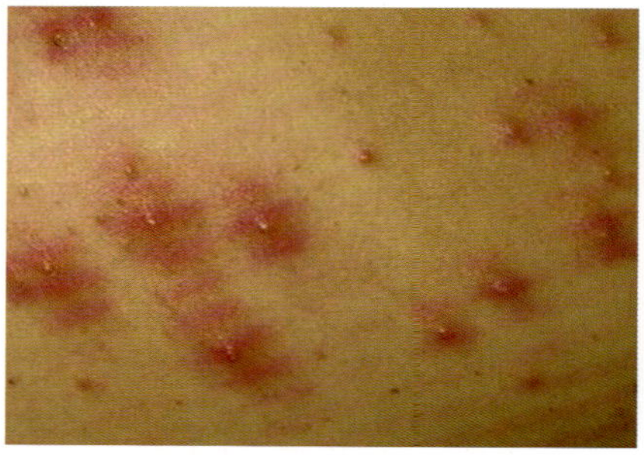

Folliculitis

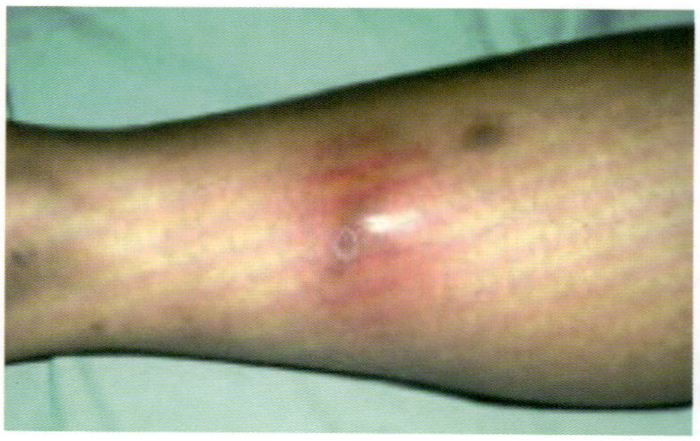

Boil

Staphylococcus epidermidis

Gm+, Staphylococci Catalase positive+ Coagulase negative – **Novobiocin sensitive**	**Virulence:** Adherent **biofilms** (**AKA**: polysaccharide slime, extracellular polysaccharide)	Infects prosthetic devices, central line catheters, stents. Anything that is indwelling inside the body. This does **not** include needles (IV's, dialysis, etc): these would be Staph aureus.
MCC **Septic arthritis** in prosthetic joints	**Endocarditis** Due to infection of central lines	TX: **Vancomycin**

Staphylococcus saprophyticus (AKA: Honeymoon cystitis)

Catalase positive + Coagulase negative – Novobiocin resistant	2nd MCC uncomplicated UTI (E. coli is MCC)	Girls 5 – 10 yrs old Little girls (putting objects up vagina) and sexually active girls.

GRAM POSITIVE – COCCI BACTERIA – STREP – CHAINS = EXOTOXINS

Streptococcus agalactiae (Group B Strep)		
Gm +, Streptococci Bacitracin resistant (**tip**: BRAS: Strep B = Resistant Strep A = Sensitive) (**tip**: Group "B" Strep is for the "B"ottom) β Hemolytic Colonizes vagina	Virulence Factor: CAMP factor (AKA: Hippurate test)	**Meningitis in babies** Onset: between 1 week of birth up to a few months. SX: Fever (rectal >100.5°F), lethargy, poor feeding, irritable, fontanels can be bulging. Spread: Spread to infant before or during delivery. Bacterial meningitis CSF profile in LP TX: Empiric: **Vancomycin and Cefotaxime (or Ceftriaxone)**
Prevention of S. agalactiae transmission during birth: 35 – 37 weeks: vaginal and rectal culture. Positive culture for GBS = **Intrapartum IV Ampicillin or Penicillin G**		

Streptococcus pneumonia (AKA: Pneumococcal, Gm Positive diplococci)

Gm +, Streptococci
Catalase negative –
α hemolytic
Diplococci (Cocci in pairs)
Optochin sensitive
Does NOT grow in bile (bile soluble)
ENCAPSULATED
LANCET shaped
Resides in the nasopharynx

Vaccine (Pneumovax) = **is against the polysaccharide capsule.**

#1 MCC Community acquired pneumonia

#1 MCC Meningitis in adults
(Teens: #1 MCC: Neisseria)
Meningitis mode of transmission: droplets from infected person inhaled through nasopharynx or kissing/sharing things coming in contact with the mouth, then Hematologically spread to the CNS.

Meningitis
(see CFS profile above)
SX: High **fever**, **nuchal rigidity** (stiff neck), irritability, **headache**, **photophobia**, vomiting.
DX: Lumbar puncture
TX: Ceftriaxone, Vancomycin and steroids

Otitis Media (children)
MC: 6 – 36 months old
Swelling of the Eustachian tube (inflamed isthmus)

SX: **Bulging**, erythematous, **non-mobile tympanic membrane**. Fever, irritable, ear drainage, fluid in middle ear, decreased hearing.
High Risk: **2° smoke** (smoke damages cilia), allergies, formula, facial deformities)
Healing: Takes up to 2 months. Tympanic membrane will continue to be swollen, but no other SX. Reassure patient.

TX: Amoxicillin or Amoxicillin plus clavonic acid (Augmentin)

(**tip**: otitis Media. M = mini (children)
Otitis Externa. E = elderly)
(other Otitis Media causal organisms: Haemophilus, Moraxella)

Pneumonia
#1 MC Community acquired
(to be considered a nosocomial pneumonia, patient must have been in the hospital 48 hours)
Lobar pneumonia
Consolidated, ↑ fremitus

Vaccine:
Vaccine is against the **polysaccharide capsule**.
Vaccine: ⊘present to T cells, **T cells independent and B cells respond**.

TX: Ceftriaxone

Prophylaxis: **Pneumococcal vaccine at age 65 or to all immunocompromised (HIV, chemo, asplenic, COPD). If given prior to age 65, must give booster at 5 yrs.**

Bacterial conjunctivitis
(AKA: Keratitis)
SX: Unilateral infection,
Purulent discharge, not itchy,
No adenopathy (swollen lymph nodes),
low level contagious
TX: topical antibiotics: Erythromycin, Gentamicin, Bacitracin

Differentials:
Viral conjunctivitis: Bilateral, watery discharge, contagious, itchy, adenopathy (swollen nodes)

Allergies: Bilateral, itchy, watery

Bacterial Sinusitis
Inflammation of the sinuses.
MCC: Viral
Other causes: infections, allergies, air pollution, and structural problems in the nose.

SX: headache, facial tenderness, poor sense of smell, sore throat, fever, tooth pain, nasal discharge.

Antibiotics indicated if: last > 10 days, > 102° fever, purulent nasal discharge (yellow/green mucus), face pain (maxillary sinus) > 3 days or if SX continue to worsen after 5 days.

Complication: Can lead to Bacterial Orbital Cellulitis (see next block)
Reoccurrence risk ↑ with **2° smoke**

TX: Amoxicillin with Clavulanic Acid *(Augmentin)*

Orbital Cellulitis

Pre-Orbital and Orbital SX:
Eyelid edema, erythema, tenderness,
Fever, leukocytosis.

Orbital Cellulitis (dangerous), caused by Bacterial Sinusitis:
Additional SX: (above Sx) **plus**:
Ophthalmoplegia (weak eye muscles), pain with ocular movement, proptosis (forward push of eyeball).
Complication: blindness, intracranial infection.

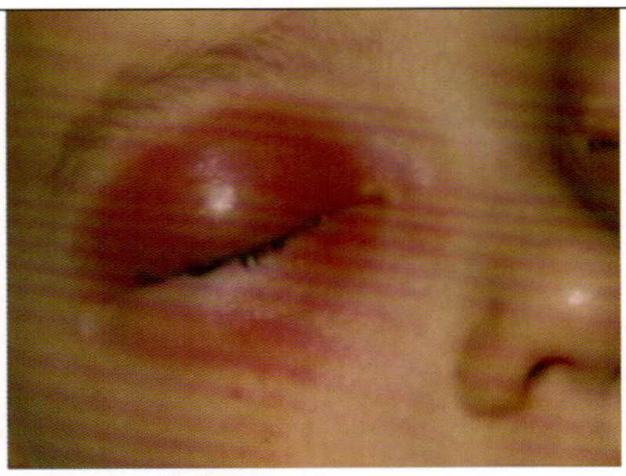
Orbital cellulitis

Streptococcus pyogenes (Group A Strep)

Gm +, Streptococci Catalase negative – β Hemolytic Exotoxin Erythrogenic toxin **Bacitracin sensitive** (**Tip**: BRAS: Strep B = Resistant Strep A = Sensitive)	**Virulence Factors:** **M Protein** **Exotoxin A** **ASO** (anti-streptolysin: antibody made against streptolysin O) **β Hemolytic** **Complications:** All Strep A skin infections can lead to Post-Strep Glomerulonephritis. All Strep A throat infections can lead to both Post-Strep Glomerulonephritis and rheumatic fever.	**Rheumatic Fever** MC: **Immigrants**, developing countries MCC: Untreated strep throat (AKA: Pharyngitis) SX: **Rash** (erythema marginatum), **chorea** (involuntary movements), **arthritis** (joint pain), cardiac. Labs: ↑ ESR **Heart:** Young patients: Mitral regurg Older patients: **Mitral stenosis**. **Mitral stenosis causes hemoptysis.** TX: Lifelong treatment of **penicillin** for prophylaxis so no reoccurrence.
Impetigo SX: weeping, oozing, **honey color crusted** lesions. Most commonly around mouth, but can be anywhere. Skin infections can lead to **Post-Strep Glomerulonephritis (NOT rheumatic fever)** TX: Topical **Mupirocin** (most effective) **or Retapamulin,** **Erythromycin (oral)** TX Severe case: **Oral dicloxacillin, Cephalexin** *(Keflex)* Also caused by S. aureus	**Pharyngitis (AKA: Strep throat)** SX: Erythema throat, fever, **anterior** lymphadenopathy**, exudate** on tonsils/throat/pharynx. **NO COUGH or HOARSENESS.** BIT: Rapid Strep Test (best initial test) MAT: Culture TX: **Amoxicillin or Penicillin** **If allergies: Azithromycin or Clarithromycin** * Can lead to Post-Strep glomerulonephritis **and** rheumatic fever. *If Amoxicillin is given and the patient returns a few days later with a rash, the patient had mononucleosis, not Strep throat.	**Scarlet Fever** SX: Erythema rash with a "**sandpaper" texture that blanches**, **red (erythema) tongue** or oral mucosa, abdominal pain. TX: **Penicillin** 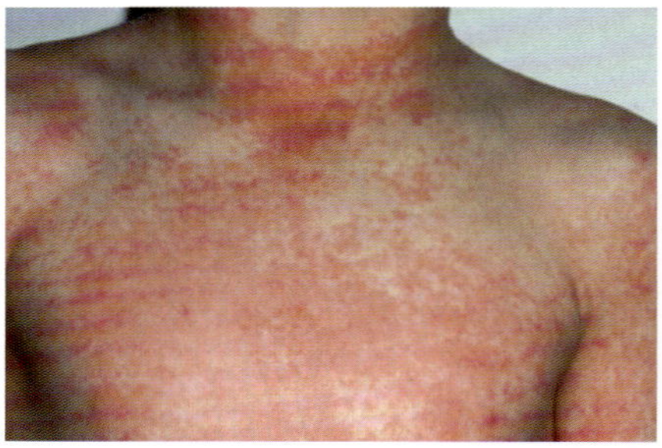 Scarlet Fever
Erysipelas SX: Shinny, erythema with swelling and heat, borders are sharply demarked and raised (clearly defined, where as cellulitis is difficult to see exact boarders), fever, chills. MC seen on face or legs. TX: **Oral Cephalexin** *(Keflex)*, **or Dicloxacillin** If blood cultures confirm Strep A: **Penicillin** 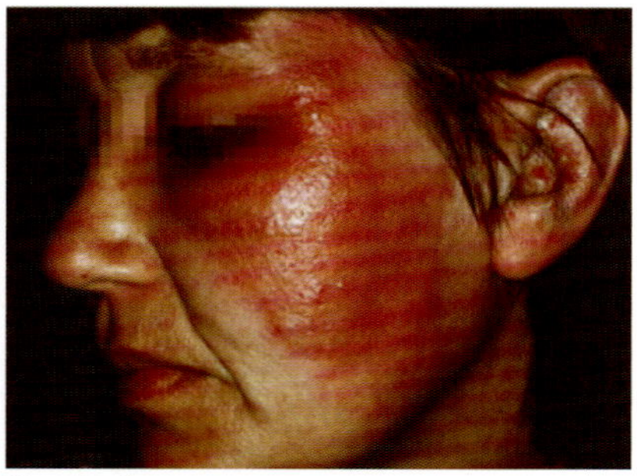 Erysipelas	**Necrotizing fasciitis** **Type II** (AKA: gas gangrene, flesh eating bacteria). Occurs in healthy persons due to injuries, IV use, and surgery. SX: **Crepitus** (gas), rapid spread, blisters, **shock**, erythema This involves the **deep fascia and muscles**. If it involves **only** the superficial tissues and fascia it is caused by C. perfringens. (AKA: necrotizing fasciitis Type I) TX: **Clindamycin** and **surgical debridement.**	

Strep Comparisons (AKA: Tonsillitis, Pharyngitis) verses No Strep verse Viral

Strep (AKA: Tonsillitis, Pharyngitis)	No Strep	Viral
Can lead to Rheumatic fever Can lead to Post Strep Glomerulonephritis **NO URI, NO COUGH** **Rapid onset**, abdominal pain, vomit **Fever**, sore throat, erythema, **exudate, anterior cervical lymphadenopathy**, TX: Rapid strep test. If negative= repeat test WITH culture. TX: Amoxicillin	Cough NO fever +/- Lymphadenopathy	Rhinorrhea Conjunctivitis

Streptococci – Viridans Group		
Gm +, Streptococci α hemolytic Optochin resistant Cause endocarditis on pre-damaged valves (MC: Mitral) Normal flora of oropharynx	Normal flora: Streptococci, Lactobacilli, Staphylococci, Corynebacteria, **Peptostreptococcus**, **Eikenella**, Neisseria, Haemophilus, Actinomyces, **Kingella**, Fusobacterium, Porphyromonas, Prevotella, Capnocytophaga, Bifidobacterium, Treponema, Veillonella, Capnocytophaga	S. mutans S. viridans Colonize the dental surface and gingiva.
S. salivarius Cold agglutinin test for EBV monospot test. Quickest to colonizes a newborn baby. S. sanguinis Makes dextrans that bind to fibrin platelet on heart valve	**Eikenella** Gram negative, oxidase positive, MC: **Fight bites** Bleach smell SX: appear in 1 week **TX: Amoxicillin**	**HACEK Organisms** Haemophilus aphrophilus Haemophilus parainfluenzae Actinobacillus Cardiobacterium **Eikenella** **Kingella** **TX: Ceftriaxone**

Streptococcus bovis (Group D Strep)

Gm +, Streptococci Endocarditis SX: See endocarditis SX above	S. bovis colonizes the gut. **Colon cancer** and GI tuberculosis can cause S. bovis endocarditis and GI pathologies. Next Step: **Colonoscopy**	**Note:** Caution: Endocarditis can also be caused by **Clostridium septicum,** an organism that can also indicate colorectal cancer.

Enterococci (Group D Strep)

Gm +, Streptococci **Grows in 6.5% NaCl and Bile** **Negative - Nitrate**	Enterococcus faecalis Enterococcus faecium	**Subacute Endocarditis** SX: See endocarditis SX above. Cause: **Contaminated instruments** in **genitourinary** manipulation or **cystoscopy**. MC in elderly men.

GRAM POSITIVE - RODS (AKA: BACILLUS) BACTERIA
Shapes: Bacillus (one), diplobacillus (two), streptobacillus (chain)

Bacillus anthracis		
Gm +, Bacillus/rod **SPORE** forming rod **ONLY** bacteria with polypeptide capsule with **D-glutamate**. "Box Car" shaped capsule (long rectangle) **Must autoclave to kill spores: steam and pressure for 15 minutes at 121°C. Will not kill prions. Prions must be killed with bleach, caustic soda or autoclaved at 274° for 15 minutes using pressurized steam.**	**Virulence Factor:** Anthrax toxin ↑ cAMP with edema factor. **Lethal Factor and Edema Factor**. ↑ cAMP causes PMN dysfunction. Polyglutamic acid allows anthrax to stop phagocytosis. Culture shows: "medusa head" colonies.	**Pulmonary anthrax** Inhalation of spores SX: Pulmonary hemorrhage, mediastinitis on chest x-ray. AKA: Widened mediastinum. (Inflammation of tissues in mid chest), shock, death. TX: **Ciprofloxacin and Doxycycline** Source: **inhaled spores** from contaminated animal wool/hair: sheep, goats, people working with animal hides, tanning hides, taxidermist. **Terrorism agent.**
Cutaneous anthrax **Black eschar** lesion Boil like lesion, necrotic	**Bacillus cereus** Food poisoning by **Cereulide: preformed toxin.** Cause: **reheated rice** and **pasta.** Quick onset: 1 to 5 hours SX: Watery, nonbloody diarrhea, GI pain TX: Supportive	**Bacillus anthracis** 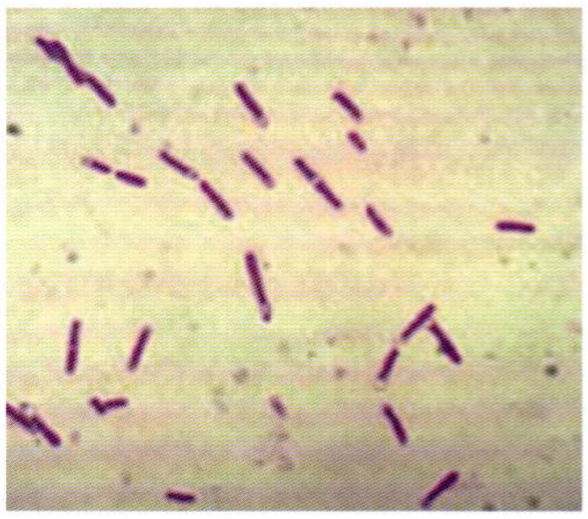

Clostridia		
Spore Gm +, Bacillus, Spore forming Spores: dipicolinic acid in their core Anaerobic bacilli **Must autoclave to kill spores: autoclave/pressure for 15 - 20 minutes at 121° C**	**Clostridium tetani** Exotoxin = **tetanospasmin** Causes paralysis: **Blocks glycine and GABA** in Renshaw cells in the spine. (Glycine is the major inhibitory neurotransmitter in the spinal cord (GABA is the major inhibitory transmitter in the brain) so tetanus toxin cleaves the snare complex at the presynaptic terminal preventing the release of the neurotransmitters. So nothing is inhibited so all muscles are contracting without any inhibitory action to stop the contractions. SX: Dysphagia (foaming at mouth), paralysis, **trismus** (lockjaw), **risus** sardonicus (spasm of facial muscles that looks like a grin).	**Neonate tetanus** Will be a baby born at home and the umbilical cord will have been cut with a contaminated (dirty) knife or scissors. 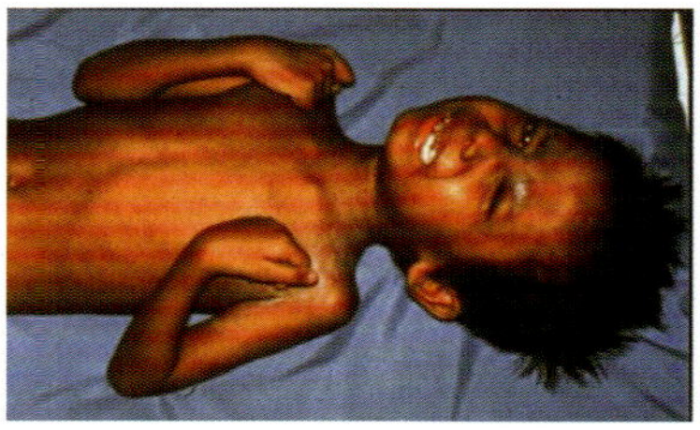 Risus 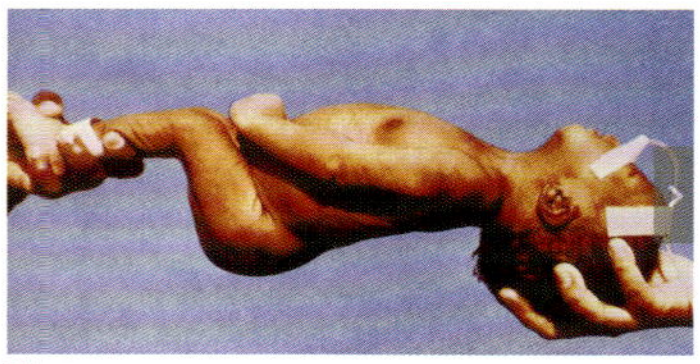 Tetanus

Clostridium botulinum	Clostridium difficile	Clostridium perfringens
Transmission: **Babies under 6 months old**: (is still on bottle) by "environmental dust". The germ grows in dust, the baby breaths it in and the toxin is produced in gut. It is **NOT** passed through breast milk. **Babies over 6 months** (eating food): ingest the preformed toxin in the spore. (MCC: ingestion of honey) **Adults**: Bad food (dented cans) SX: **DESCENDING** paralysis. First: **loss of gag reflex** (CN IX), diplopia, dysphagia, dystonia. ("Floppy baby") **BOTOX:** treatment for dystonia, spasms, migraines, and cosmetics. **MOA botulism:** Botulism inhibits the vesicle of the neurotransmitter acetylcholine to be released into the synaptic cleft (nerve terminal) DX: Check **stools for bacterial toxin**	(AKA: **Pseudomembranous colitis**) **Grey pseudomembrane** lining the gut. AKA: Overgrowth of bacteria in the colon. (Biomass) Virulence**: Toxin A and B.** **Toxin A** enterotoxin binds brush boarder in the gut **Toxin B** cytotoxin disrupts the cytoskeleton by actin depolymerization **Cause: MC due to antibiotic use** (esp: **Ampicillin, Amoxicillin and Clindamycin**) SX: **Mucosal death (necrosis)** and water in gut = diarrhea. Abdominal cramps, ↑ PMN's. DX: **Toxins in the stool.** Complication: Megacolon 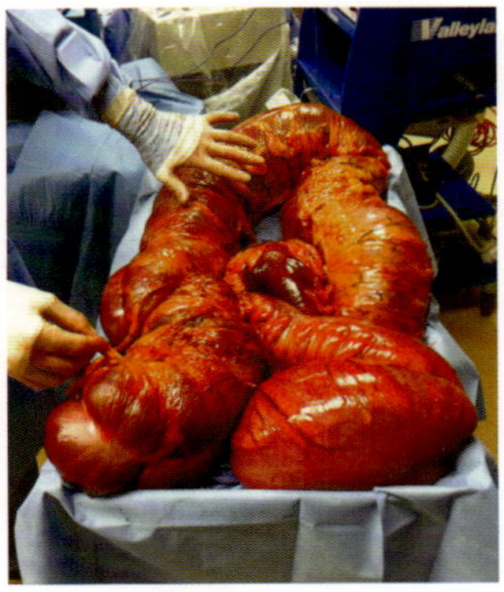 Megacolon	**(AKA: Necrotizing Fascitis Type I, flesh eating bacteria, gas gangrene)** Virulence: **α toxin** (lecithin's phospholipase) MOA: **Splits phospholipids** of cells causing gas between the layers causing necrotizing fasciitis. Occurs in previously ill (ie: Diabetes, vascular disease, etc.) SX: **crepitus** (gas gangrene) (flesh eating bacteria) of subcutaneous tissues and fascia. DX: Surgical debridement. NOTE: Perfringens does **NOT** involve the deep fascia or muscles. It involves **only** the superficial fascia layers. If it involves the deep fascia and muscles it is caused by **S. pyrogenes** (Group A Strep)

Clostridium septicum
Normal gut flora. Drumstick-like shaped, motile (flagella).
Toxin: Alpha toxin.
Causes: myonecrosis by gas gangrene. (Extensive tissue destruction, edema, thrombosis, bullae). No tissue damage is required to establish gas gangrene with C. septicum as with C. perfringens.

Associated with **colorectal cancer** and other colon pathologies.
If patient presents with SX of **endocarditis** (fever, new murmur) and cultures show C. septicum, the **next step is a colonoscopy.**
Caution: Remember, endocarditis caused by **Strep Bovis** also indicates possibility of colorectal cancer.

Tetanus Vaccinations and Prophylaxis

Vaccination Schedule (vaccine used to prevent: diphtheria, tetanus and pertussis)

- **Vaccines: Dtap, Tdap, DT and Td.**
  Dtap and DT: children <7 years old
  Tdap and Td: >7 years old and adults
- **Children <7: receive 5 doses at 2, 4, 6, 15/18 months and 4/6 years old.**
- **Adolescents and adults booster: Td every 10 years**
- **Tdap (similar to Td, but contains protection against pertussis):**
  Adolescents 11 – 18 should receive a single dose of Tdap
- **Tdap: Adults 19 and older should receive a single dose**
- **Tdap: Pregnant women should receive during each of their pregnancies in the 3rd trimester**
- **Tdap: Children 7 – 10 who have not been immunized against pertussis**

Prophylaxis after injury: cut, bite, etc.

- Patient has never received any tetanus vaccine or does not remember their last booster:
  Must receive **BOTH: Tetanus toxoid and Immunoglobulin** (Ig)
  MOA: Tetanus toxoid: Gamma-Aminobutyric Acid stops tetanus toxin. Provides humoral immunity with circulating antibodies that neutralizes bacterial toxins.
- Patient has received a Td booster between 5 and 10 years: must receive another Td booster
- Patient has received a Td booster within the past 5 years: no need to vaccinate

Corynebacterium diphtheria		
Gm +, Bacillus/rod **Tellurite** agar grows black colonies Elek test for toxin (**tip**: I'll **TELL U RIGHT** now that I better have butter on my **CORN**)	Virulence AB Exotoxin: Stops ribosome function by inhibiting protein synthesis by **ADP-ribosylation of EF-2** (elongation factor) (Note: Pseudomonas also ADP ribosylates the EF-2) (EF: Elongation Factor -2)	Diphtheria SX: Grey-white pseudomembrane in the throat – **DO NOT SCRAPE OFF = patient can bleed to death**! Lymphadenopathy, myocarditis (endocarditis), arrhythmias.
Toxoid Vaccine **Diphtheria Anti-toxin** Prevents diphtheria Provides **IgG passive immunity against exotoxin of B protein**	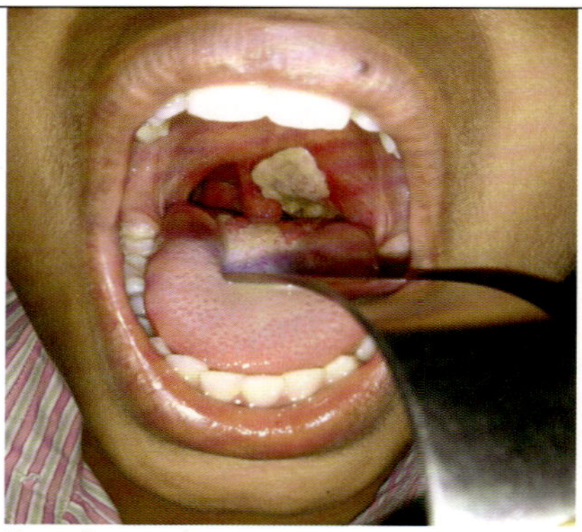 Pseudomembrane	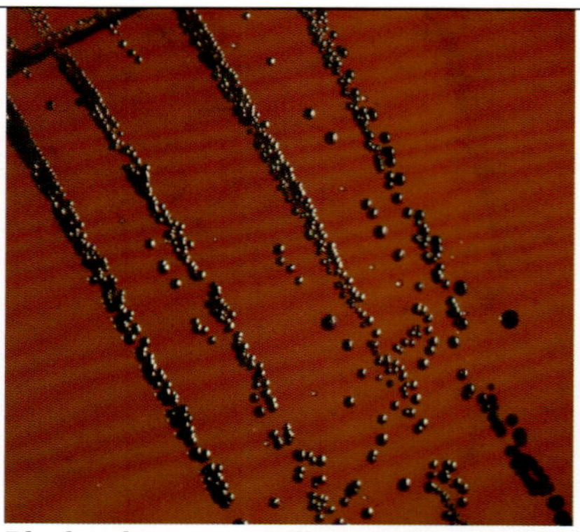 Black colonies on Tellurite agar

Listeria monocytogenes		
Only POSITIVE endotoxin (produces LPS) **Tumbling motility by actin polymerization**. (**tip**: **LISTERI**ne mouthwash **tumbles** in your mouth) ↑ Neutrophils in CSF. Likes cold temperatures: can live in the refrigerator.	Acquired by: Ingestion of **unpasteurized dairy products, deli meats**. Uncooked meats and vegetables and fruits. Skins of vegetables can be contaminated by run off water from livestock. Can also be found in soil. Animals can also be carriers. Can also be transmitted through the placenta or vaginal transmission during birth. SX: Non-invasive: Fever, chills, muscle aches, GI symptoms. SX: Invasive: CNS symptoms.	MC: Meningitis in neonates, pregnant women, immunocompromised (HIV) and elderly. Also common in HIV, asplenic, steroid use, have leukemia or lymphoma, hemochromatosis and associated with pregnancy. TX: Must use **Ampicillin**. **Ampicillin must be added to ALL medicine regimens when treating Listeria**. Causes: meningitis, spontaneous abortions, septicemia, gastroenteritis.

Mycobacterium (TB)

Gm +, Bacillus/rod Cell wall: contains **Mycolic Acid.** **Löwenstein-Jensen media** It will not gram stain because of mycolic acid, must use carbolfuchsin (aniline dye) **Sputum culture: Acid Fast Bacilli by Ziehl-Neelsen stain** **Latent TB Testing:** Test for TB: **PPD test** (Purified Protein Derivative). This test will show positive/react if patient has had a BCG vaccine. (See PPD below). Positive test requires a chest x-ray. **If negative CXR**: Must take **Isoniazid (INH) and B6 for nine (9) months** for prophylaxis. Test for latent TB: IGRA (QuantiFERON Test: Interferon gamma release assay) blood test. More specific than PPD. This test will not cross-react with BCG vaccine.	Virulence: **Cord Factor**: grows in **serpentine cords (parallel)** with cord factor. Inhibits macrophage maturation stimulates release of TNFα Spreads: **Respiratory droplets** BCG Vaccine (bacilli Calmette-Guérin): Given intradermal. If given subcutaneously it may lead to infection and spread to the regional lymph nodes. Vaccine against TB in many other countries. Vaccination will give a false-positive result for PPD test. Even if the patient has had a BCG vaccine and gets a positive result: **they must still take** the 9 months of treatment with INH and B6 for 9 months for prophylaxis.	**Mycobacterium tuberculosis** MC: **Immigrants** or developing countries. ↑ Risk: HIV, prisoners, alcoholics, Diabetes mellitus, heme malignancies, healthcare workers, exposure to someone with TB. SX: Fever, night sweats, weight loss, hemoptysis, chronic cough, sputum. DX: BIT: CXR. **Sputum stain: positive for acid-fast bacilli** (mycobacteria). Primary Infection: Mid to lower lung, **Ghon complex**. Secondary Infection*: **Upper** lobes of lung, fibrous cavity. **Caseating granulomas** (Central necrosis with multinucleated Langhans cells). Causes caseous necrosis in the lungs. **TX: Isoniazid (INH) plus B6, Rifampin, Pyrazinamide, Ethambutol.** **Treatment schedule:** **INH and Rifampin: 6 months.** **Pyrazinamide and Ethambutol: 2 months.** **Must treat > 6 months if comorbidities:** **Meningitis, Pregnancy, Miliary TB, Cavitary TB, Osteomyelitis.** ***Infliximab**: (TX: Crohn's and Ulcerative Colitis). Can **reactivate TB** so you must do a **PPD test** before starting this drug. (**tip**: I'm "**FIX**'in" crohn's and ulcerative colitis)
Extrapulmonary TB (outside lungs) Tuberculosis meningitis (CNS system) Tuberculosis pleurisy (pleura) Tuberculosis urogenital (GU system) **Pott's Disease** of the spine	**Miliary Tuberculosis** (AKA: disseminated tuberculosis) Dissemination throughout the body. MC: lungs, liver, spleen DX: Many 1-5mm lesions (spots) throughout the body, seen on x-ray	**Mycobacteria avium** Pneumonia in HIV when the CD4 count reaches **<50**. **Prophylaxis of Azithromycin should be started when CD4 counts are at 200.**

Mycobacterium leprae (AKA: Leprosy, Hansen's Disease) Infection of skin and nerves. Likes **cool temperatures**: infects nose, ears, fingers, toes (areas of cooler temps). Transmission in US: **Armadillos** 2 Forms: 1) Tuberculoid. TH1 cell mediated response. Invades Schwann cells. SX: Hypopigmentation and skin thickening and red edges 2) Lepromatous: TH2 humoral mediated response. Proliferates within the Macrophage SX: Disfigured faces ("Lion Faces"), loss of eyebrows, nasal collapse, lumpy ear lobes, bones, fingers, toes. TX: **Dapsone and Rifampin (Dapsone SE: G6PD and myositis. Rifampin SE: Orange body fluids and ↑P-450.**	**Tuberculosis luposa** (AKA: Lupus Vulgaris (Skin TB) Trauma of the skin of infected lymph node. Granulomas with necrotic centers in the dermis. SX: **Red-brown nodules**/lesions on eyelid, lips, cheeks, ears. TX: Full TB, 4 drug, treatment	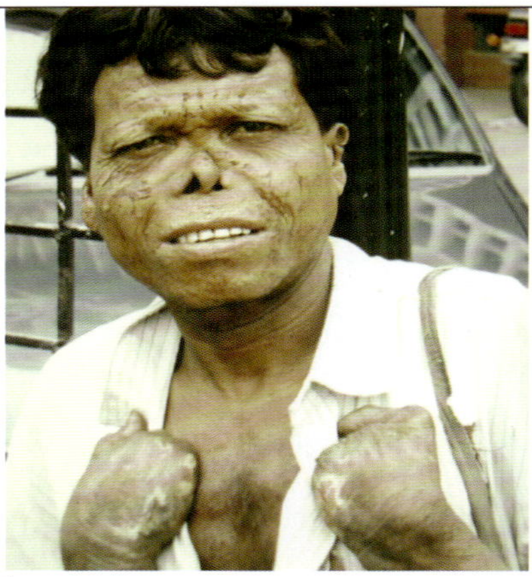 Leprosy 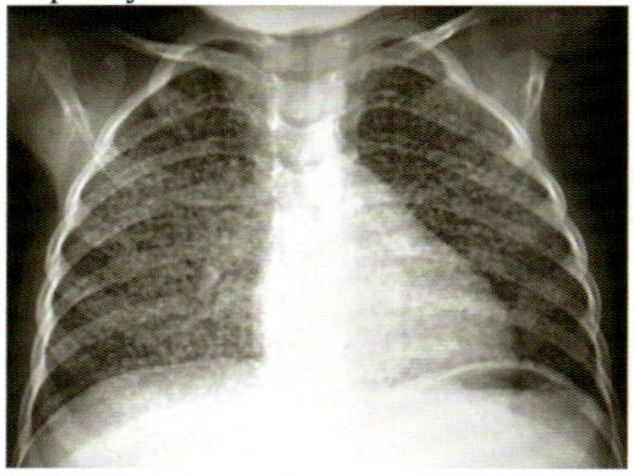 Miliary Tuberculosis

PPD Testing (Purified Protein Derivative)

PPD Results and Treatment

PPD: **Type IV Hypersensitivity involving CD4, T cells and macrophages.**

PPD: Will react (positive) if patient has previously had a BCG vaccine.

Positive PPD Results

- Positive if **>5mm** in high-risk group: immunocompromised, HIV, recent exposure, transplants, steroid users, close contacts with active TB patients, abnormal calcifications on CXR.
- Positive if **>10mm** in: IV drug users, healthcare personnel, travelers from high prevalence countries, people in close quarters (prisons, nursing homes, etc.), prisoners, alcoholics, Diabetes mellitus, heme malignancies
- Positive if **>15 mm** in persons with no known risk.

If Positive PPD Test

- If first PPD test patient has ever had and the result is negative, must give another PPD within 1 – 2 weeks (to rule out false negative). If first test is positive, no need to do another test, patient must do a chest x-ray.
- If second test is negative, patient is negative. If second test is positive, patient must go for chest x-ray.
  Note: Once a PPD is positive, the patient will always test positive in any future test so do not repeat PPD's.
- Chest X-Ray
  If negative: Must take **Isoniazid (INH) and B6 for nine (9) months** for prophylaxis.
  If positive (active case): 1st step: Sputum staining to confirm acid-fast bacteria. 2nd step on positive staining: Quarantined in hospital in a negative (-) air flow (pressure) room. (There is no return of the air back into the room).
- **High risk of false negative PPD in HIV, Sarcoidosis, Mononucleosis, Hodgkins, Immunocompromised, steroid therapy, malnutrition.**
- **False positive PPD test: BCG Vaccine (Bacillus Calmette-Guérin). Can have a false positive for years after the vaccine.**

PPD Ethics

- **If PPD test is positive with a negative chest x-ray, the individual (employee, job applicant for any job, including medical jobs) can refuse the prophylaxis treatment of INH and still be hired. It is not required to take the prophylaxis treatment.**
- **If PPD test is positive and a positive chest x-ray, it is mandatory quarantine and must be reported to the CDC. Full treatment for tuberculosis: Isoniazid plus B6, Rifampin, Pyrazinamide, Ethambutol**

GRAM POSITIVE – BRANCHING FILAMENTS

Actinomyces

Gm +, Branching filaments
Anaerobe
Normal oral flora

MC in immuno**COMPETENT** people. Occurs due to dental or facial trauma.

SX: **Gingival** ("lumpy jaw") Facial or oral abscesses that drain through tracts, usually to outside of the face. Drainage is from cysteine and forms **sulfur granules (yellow).**
Cervical: IUD use with women with PID

TX: **IV Penicillin for 6 to 12 weeks**

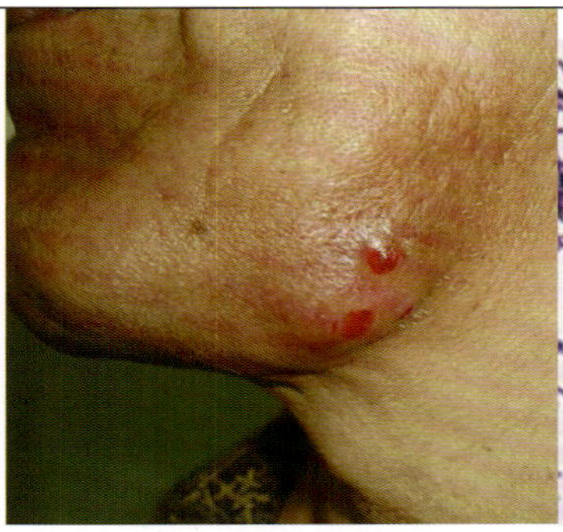
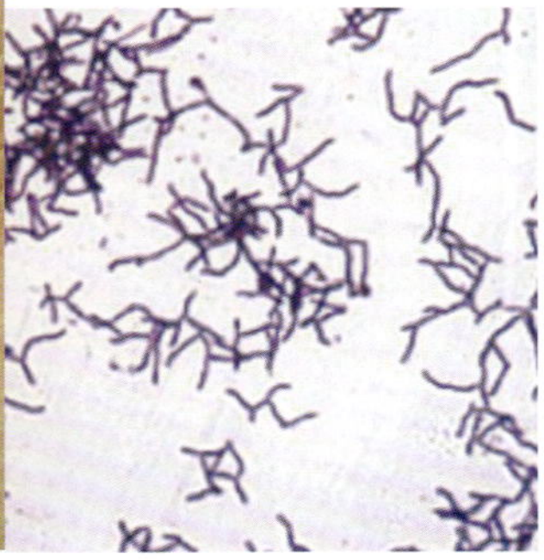

Nocardia

Gm +, Branching filaments
Aerobe
45° angle, **beaded** appearance
Catalase positive
Partially (weakly) acid fast
Virulence factor: **Cord factor**
Source: Soil

MC in immunocompromised people.

SX: Pulmonary infections in immunocompromised
Cutaneous infections after trauma in immunocompetent.

Risk of: Endocarditis, **slowly progressive pneumonia**, cough, dyspnea, fever, can spread to pleura of chest, subcutaneous abscesses.

DX: BIT: CXR
MAT: Culture.

TX: **TMP/SMX (sulfonamides)**

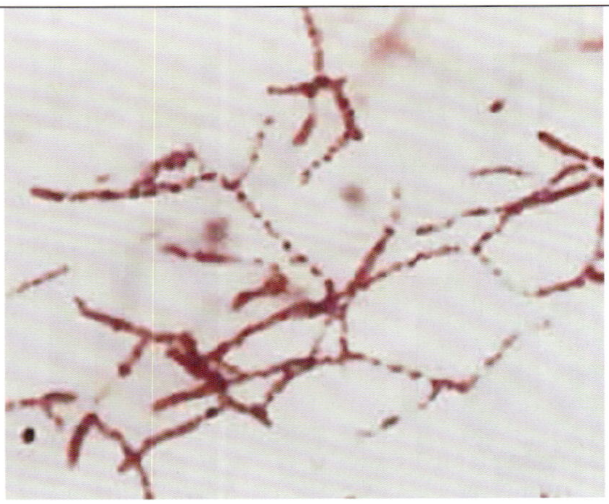

GRAM NEGATIVE BACTERIA = ENDOTOXINS (LPS)

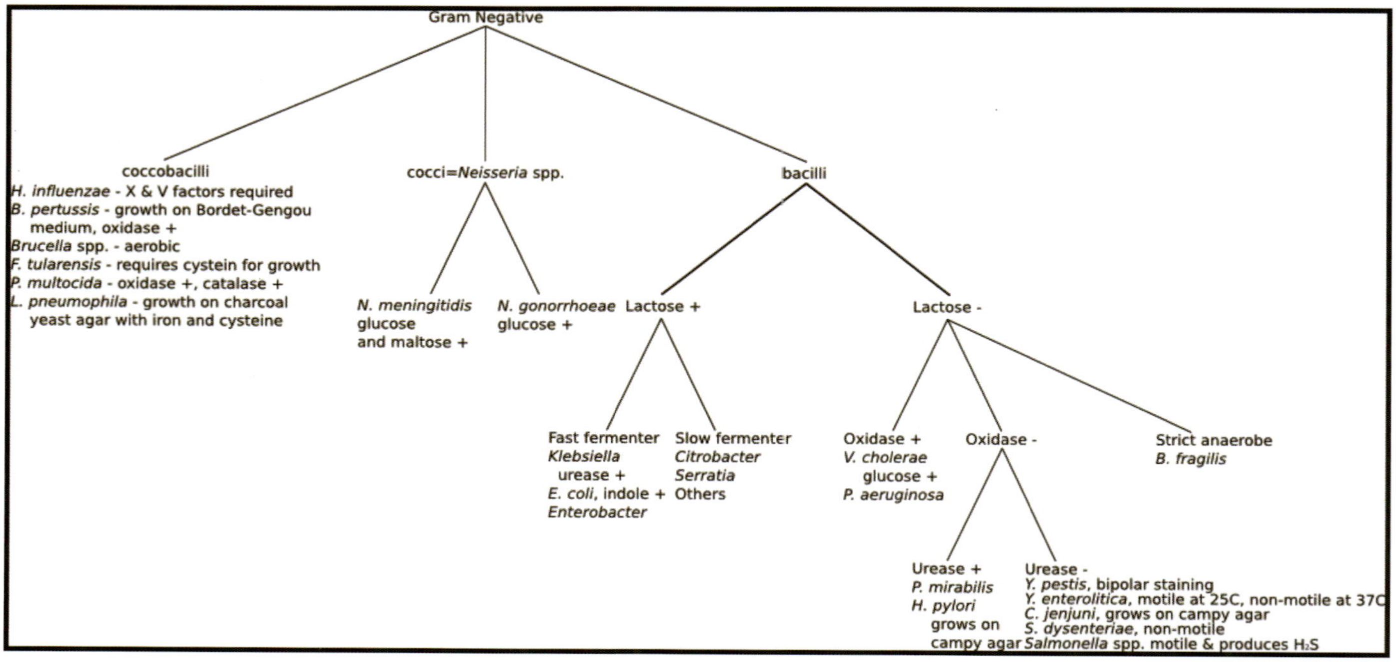

Neisseria: Neisseria gonorrhea		
Gm Negative, Diplococci **ENCAPSULATED** Ferment glucose Produce IgA proteases allow Neisseria to survive on mucosal surfaces. (AKA: attach, penetrate, pili) Media: **Thayer Martin** (AKA: Selective media). Testing for Gonorrhea and Chlamydia: Gram stain: BOTH organisms must be treated. PCR: Very specific. If this test shows only one organism, then just that one organism can be treated. NAAT (Nucleic Acid Amplification Test: DNA probe): best test for both gonorrhea and chlamydia. In men: urine. In women: vaginal swab.	**Neisseria gonococci (gonorrhea)** **STD** No polysaccharide capsule No vaccine due to antigenic variation Transmission: sexual **Virulence Factor: Pilli (Fimbriae, adherence).** SX: **Muco/Purulent discharge, cervical motion tenderness.** (Chandelier sign). BIT: NAAT (Nucleic Acid Amplification Test) for both Chlamydia and Gonorrhea. NAAT can also be done on the urine (men and women). TX: **Must treat partner and MUST treat for chlamydia also.** **Ceftriaxone IM for gonorrhea and oral Azithromycin (or Doxycycline) for Chlamydia.** (Be careful of a woman that is DX with gonorrhea that is vomiting. Remember, you must treat for both gonorrhea and chlamydia. Because the ceftriaxone is oral, you must **admit her to the hospital** to give IV treatment)	**Neisseria gonorrhea cont'd** **Additional complications: septic arthritis, PID (pelvic inflammatory disease, neonatal conjunctivitis, Fitz-Hugh-Curtis syndrome.** **Septic arthritis (Destroys joints)** SX: Red, swollen, tender joint, **mono-arthritis** DX: Arthrocentesis, **Labs: WBC > 100,000, ↑ ESR** High risk with arthritic or prosthetic joint. (Also caused by S. aureus and Strep) (**tip**: WBC count in "GOnorrhea GOes much higher) TX: **IV ceftriaxone and vancomycin** 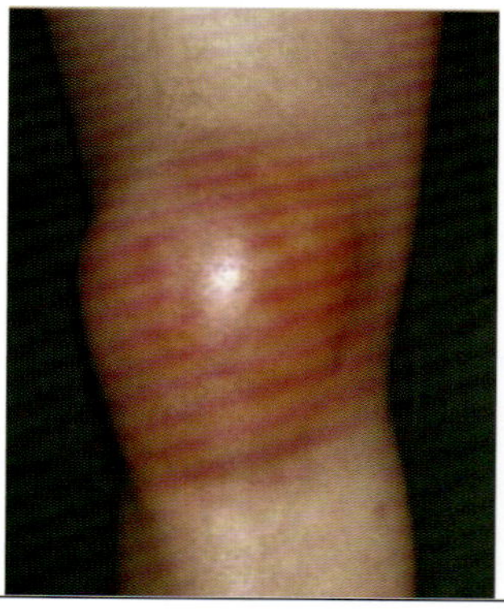

Neisseria: Gonorrhea cont'd

Pelvic Inflammatory Disease (PID)
Cause: Chlamydia trachomatis and Neisseria gonorrhea.
MC bacterial STD in the USA.
MCC of infertility in women <30 with normal periods.

SX: **Cervical motion tenderness** (Chandelier sign), **purulent (mico-purulent discharge), infertility,** endometritis, tubo-ovarian abscess, **salpingitis** (inflammation of fallopian tube), hydrosalpinx (blocked fallopian tube with serous or clear fluid), fever, leukocytosis (↑ WBC), adnexal tenderness, lower abdominal pain.

Complications:
Hugh-Curtis Syndrome: infection of liver capsule leading to adhesions (AKA: Violin string adhesions).
If no treatment: may develop abscesses, peritonitis, sepsis.

Risk Factors: Because PID causes the fallopian tubes to become scared, sperm cannot reach the eggs causing **infertility**. If they are able to get through to fertilize the eggs, the eggs can't make it through the tubes so implant in ectopic locations causing **ectopic pregnancies**. Adhesions can cause intestinal **obstruction** (air/fluid levels on abdominal x-ray).

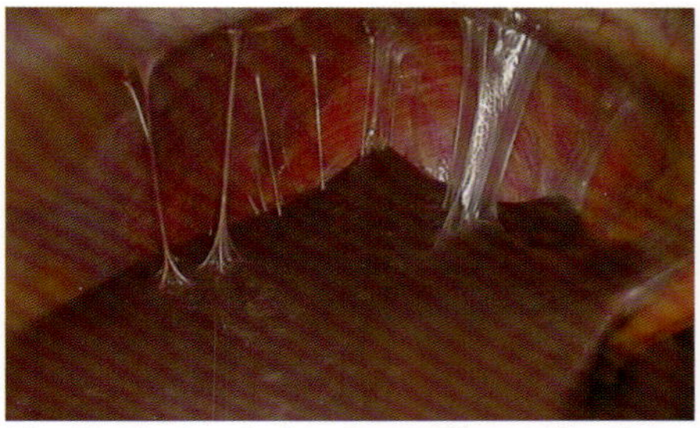

Fitz Hugh-Curtis Syndrome (complication of PID)
("violin string" adhesions can cause intestinal obstruction)

Pelvic Inflammatory Disease (cont'd)

TX: Must start TX immediately, do now wait for results of cultures.
YOU MUST TREAT FOR BOTH GONORRHEA and CHLAMYDIA.
Outpatient TX: **Oral Azithromycin (or Doxycycline) and IM Ceftriaxone**.

CAUTION: watch the vignette: if the patient has been throwing up: you must hospitalize her to use IV meds (she will not keep the oral meds down). This goes for ANY situation in which a patient must receive medication but is throwing up.
In Patient TX: IV Cefoxitin or Cefotetan and IV Azithromycin (or Doxycycline OR IV Clindamycin and IV Gentamycin.

BIT: β-hCG, cervical culture
MAT: Laparoscopy.
Be sure to rule out pregnancy in a woman with lower abdominal pain or cervical motion tenderness.

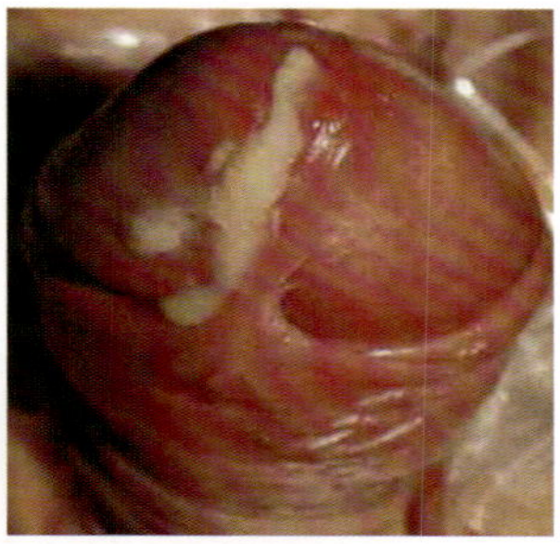

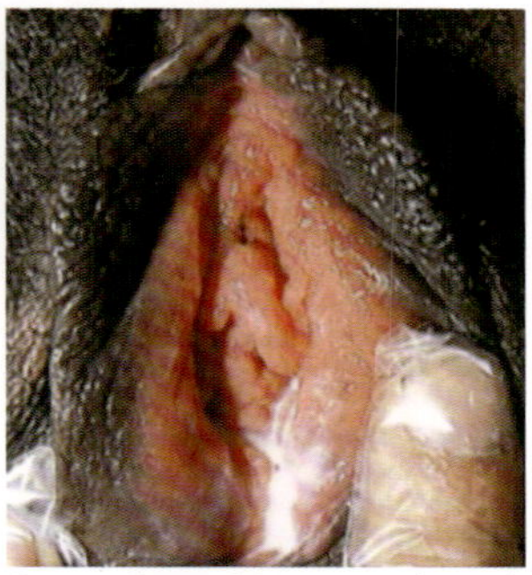

Gonorrhea: Mucopurulent discharge

Gonococcemia
(Disseminated gonorrhea)

SX: painful and swollen joints (arthritis-like), inflammation of the wrist and heel tendons (tenosynovitis), rash of pus filled bumps, chills, fever

Neonatal conjunctivitis
Occurs in the **first week** after birth.
(Chlamydia conjunctivitis occurs in the 2nd week after birth)
(**tip**: "GO"norrhea Goes first)
SX: Mucopurulent discharge from eye
TX: **Ceftriaxone**, **Erythromycin ointment**

Neisseria: Meningitis		
Neisseria meningococci **ENCAPSULATED: Polysaccharide capsule** "**Kidney Bean**" shaped nuclei **Intracellular, inside PMN's** and will show on a gram stain. Maltose fermentation **Endotoxin (LPS: Lipo-oligosaccharide)** Transmission: **Respiratory and oral** secretions. Complications: Meningitis and Meningococcemia **Meningococcal Vaccine: Targets the polysaccharide capsule**	**Neisseria meningococci** **MENINGITIS** **ROUTE of infection**: Pharynx to blood to choroid plexus to meningitis. SX: Fever, **stiff neck (nuchal rigidity), headache**, petechiae (non blanching rash), nausea, photosensitivity. MC in **close quarters**: dorms, army barracks, prisons, etc. TX: **Ceftriaxone or Penn G and respiratory isolation.** **Prophylaxis to close contacts: Rifampin** Routine contacts: school and work do not need prophylaxis. (NOTE: If vignette has a patient with Neisseria along with a variety of people that they have been around and want to know which one is the **closest contact** – or most likely to contract the disease without prophylaxis: pick the person that would be doing the intubation because they would be **directly exposed to respiratory droplets**). Other "close contact" examples that would need prophylaxis would be kissing, sharing cigarettes, household contacts and eating utensils/glassware).	**Neisseria meningococci complication:** **Waterhouse-Friderichsen Syndrome.** (AKA: Hemorrhagic adrenalitis) This is **severe bleeding in the adrenal gland** due to bacterial infection. This causes organ failure, shock and DIC. **Recurrent Neisseria infections** are due to lack of **MAC** (Membrane Attack Complex). Compliment C5 – C9. MC neurological damage due to untreated bacterial meningitis is deafness (damage to CN VIII).

GRAM NEGATIVE BACTERIA = RODS/BACILLUS = ENDOTOXINS (LPS)

Bacteroides fragilis		
Gm -, Bacillus/rod Beta lactamase producer **Makes Vitamin K for host** Inactive LPS = NO endotoxic shock Normal gut flora Anaerobe	Bacteremia due to: intraabdominal infections, peritonitis and abscesses due to rupture of an organ (**appendix**) spilling into the peritoneum, abscesses or burns near the anus	TX: **Piperacillin with Tazobactam, Metronidazole**

Bordetella pertussis (Whooping Cough)	
Bordet Medium Culture: Bordet-Gengou- potato agar Virulence Factors Pertussis Toxin **AB Toxin** **ADP Ribosylates** and stops the GI Filamentous Hemagglutinin Adhesion Factor in respiratory tract (FHA).	MOA: Extracellular **Adenyl cyclase ↑ cAMP,** PMN chemotaxis and oxidative metabolism is defective because of ↑ Adenyl cyclase. SX: **"Machine Gun" cough.** Can be severe enough to burst organs. **Many coughs on single expiration followed by a deep inspiration (whoop)** Cough with green phlegm DX: Bacterial nasopharyngeal culture or PCR TX: **Treat patient and close contacts with: Erythromycin (Macrolides)**
3 Phases of Bordetella 1) Catarrhal Phase: 1 – 2 weeks: fever, conjunctiva, cough, malaise 2) Paroxysmal Phase: 2 – 3 months: "Whoop" cough, vomiting after cough, cough can be started by yawn, laughing, yelling **3)** Convalescent 1 – 2 weeks with no cough	Vaccine: Dtap (Diptheria, Tetanus, Pertussis) Children's vaccine schedule: given at 2, 4, 6, 15-18 months and then a final one between 4 – 6 years old. Reactions to Dtap are usually due to Pertussis Sever reaction (anaphylaxis, encephalopathy, CNS complications) = Do not give any more shots Mild reaction: Give ONLY the DT (Diphtheria and tetanus) on the next vaccination, do not give the pertussis. Pertussis is normally what children react to.

Campylobacter jejuni	
Gm -, Bacillus/rod Comma shape (S shape) **Grows at 42°** Oxidase positive Zoonotic Labs: ↑ CSF protein **Major complication: Respiratory failure (diaphragm – phrenic nerve), monitor "chest expansion"** Do NOT use steroids – worsen condition TX: **Plasmapheresis, IV IG** (Guillain-Barré can also be caused by CMV and follow an URI)	**Bloody** diarrhea Fecal – oral transmission Source: **puppies**, poultry, undercooked meat, unpasteurized milk. (watch for new puppies at home). 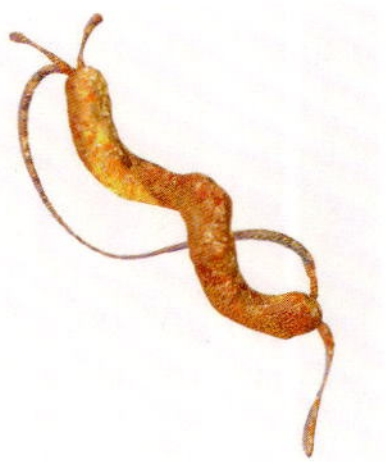 Commonly precedes **Guillain-Barré.** Demyelination of peripheral nerves (Autoimmune dz that destroys Schwann cells) = ↓ neuron firing **SYMMETRICAL ascending** paralysis starting from lower extremities or arms/hands. **NO sensory loss.**

Citrobacter
Gm -, Bacillus/rod Non-spore forming **Produce citrate** Indole negative Source: soil, water, wastewater, human intestine. Seldom source of illness

Enterobacter	
Gm -, Bacillus/rod Ferments Lactose at 37° in presence of bile salts Oxidase negative Indole negative	↑ Nosocomial Pathology: Cause opportunistic infections in immunocompromised. Ventilators, urinary and respiratory infections. TX: **Cefepime, Imipenem, Amikacin, Quinolones**

Escherichia coli (E. coli)		
Gm - Bacillus/rod McConckey Agar Eosin, Methylene Blue Green metallic sheen Hemolysis on blood agar Colonizes the GI tract Indole positive Ferments Lactose	**ETEC (Travelers diarrhea)** Heat stable and heat labile (**tip:** Heat stable = c**G**MP, stable on the **G**round. cAMP = labile) Enterotoxins Ferments sorbitol Watery diarrhea: no inflammation or invasion Promotes fluid and electrolyte secretion from intestine. Virulence: **Cholera like toxin** SX: **Mucus and epithelial cells in stool.** **↑ cAMP and ↑ cGMP**	EIEC Invasive to intestinal mucosa causing necrosis and inflammation. (Similar to Shigella) Dysentery Ferments sorbitol EPEC Virulence: M Cells MOA: Flattens villi and stops absorption. Pediatric diarrhea

EHEC 0157:H7

Virulence: **Shiga Like Toxin**

Endotoxin = Lipid A of LPS causes septic shock.
MOA: Stops production of glucuronidase.
Inactivates ribosomal units and stops protein synthesis of the 60s subunit.
Does **NOT** ferment sorbitol
Dysentery: necrosis and inflammation

HUS (Hemolytic-uremic syndrome) = triad of renal failure, anemia, thrombocytopenia)
Microthrombi form causing hemolysis of RBC causing **schistocytes** in the blood.
Labs: ↑ LDH, ↓ haptoglobin, schistocytes, anemia (↓ HB and HCT)

SX: Presents 5 – 10 days: Abdominal pain, bloody diarrhea, pallor (due to microangiopathic hemolytic anemia) oliguria and hematuria, proteinuria, DIC.

DX: Helmet cells, burr cells, schistocytes, negative combs test, thrombocytopenia.

MCC: eating contaminated food or water (esp: undercooked ground meats).
Can also be caused by Shigella, Salmonella, and Campylobacter.

EHEC TX: Supportive. Early dialysis. Do NOT give antibiotics when caused by E. coli 0157:H7 due to increased risk of developing HUS.

Escherichia coli (E. coli) cont'd

Cystitis (UTI), Pyelonephritis, Epididymitis and Prostatitis in older men. (Younger, sexually active men: Epididymitis and Prostatitis is due to gonorrhea and chlamydia).
Virulence: Fimbriae (AKA: pili, adhesions)

D-Mannose-specific adherence (fimbriae) associated with bladder infections. D-Mannose binds/adheres to the E. coli (a normal microflora of the intestinal tract). It is not a normal flora of the bladder or urinary tract. This binding leads to a UTI.

Cystitis (women or men)
MCC: E. coli
SX: **Burning and pain on urination**. "**Suprapubic pain**".

BIT: Urinalysis shows **Leukocyte esterase** positive: this indicates there are **WBC** in the urine.
If UA shows **Nitrite positive**: this indicates the cause is due to **gram-negative** bacteria.

MAT: Urine Culture

TX: **TMP/SMX** *(Bactrim)*, **Ciprofloxacin, Fosfomycin, Cefixime.**
Pregnancy: Nitrofurantoin *(Macrobid)*, **Fosfomycin**
Pregnancy is the only time an asymptomatic cystitis should be treated. Start treatment immediately.

Treatment: 3 days if an uncomplicated cystitis with TMP/SMX, Nitrofurantoin, fosfomycin.
If complicated: treat 7 days with TMP/SMX or Ciprofloxacin. (Complicated: if there is an anatomic abnormality, stone present, tumor, obstruction or patient is a male.* If there is a cystitis in a male patient: must do an ultrasound).

Pyelonephritis
Infection in the kidney due to an ascending infection from an untreated cystitis.

SX: **Flank pain or Costovertebral pain,** WBC in the urine, **fever.**

UA: **White cell cast, WBC**

TX: **Ceftriaxone, Ciprofloxacin**
Empiric until culture results:
Ampicillin and Gentamicin

Complication:
Perinephric Abscess
Pyelonephritis that will not resolve.
SX: Persistent fever for a week following treatment of pyelonephritis.
DX: CT and biopsy.
TX: Drainage of fluid, culture.
Quinolone with Oxacillin, Nafcillin or Vancomycin.

Septic Shock
(Severe infection and sepsis)
Must have **triad** for septic shock:
Severe hypotension, fever, tachycardia (the first physical sign of a falling blood pressure is tachycardia)

Endotoxin = LPS
TLR (Toll-like receptors) release cytokines: IL-1, IL-6, TNFα
(See septic shock details)

Additional complications:

Spontaneous Bacterial Peritonitis (SBP)
SX: Cirrhosis, ascites, fever, mental status change
DX: Paracentesis with PMN's >250
TX: Third generation Cephalosporin.

(Can also be caused by Klebsiella)

Prostatitis in older men.
(Chlamydia is the cause in younger men, more sexually active men)

SX: Frequency, urgency, dysuria, tender prostate on exam, perineal or sacral pain.

BIT: Urinalysis
MAT: WBC in urine after prostate massage

TX: **TMP/SMX, Ciprofloxacin**

Neonatal Meningitis
Top 3 causes of neonatal meningitis

Pneumonia
Top 3 causes of neonatal pneumonia
236

Fusobacterium

Gm -, Bacillus/rod Anaerobe Rod shaped bacilli with pointed ends Normal flora of oropharynx Virulence: Biofilm, LPS Associated with colon cancer, ulcerative colitis, periodontal disease, skin ulcers and Lemierre 's syndrome	**Lemierre 's Syndrome** Peritonsillar abscess due to progression of throat infection Thrombophlebitis of the internal jugular vein = clot formation and bacteremia (septic emboli) SX: sore throat, spiking fevers, lethargy, swollen cervical lymph nodes, painful neck, sepsis Labs: ↑ ESR and C-reactive protein and WBC TX: **Clindamycin**

Haemophilus influenza

Gm -, Bacillus/rod **ENCAPSULATED** Coccobacillary rod Quellung positive Oxidase positive Virulence Factor: **Capsular Type B** (polysaccharide, polyribosylribitol phosphate conjugate) Produces **IgA protease** Culture: **Chocolate agar** with **Factor V (NAD) and X (hematin)** (**tip:** when I get the FLU, mom gets me CHOCOLATE at the 5 and 10 store) **Vaccine:** **HiB**: Targets PRP Polyribosyl-ribitol Phosphate Capsule causing a T cell response Vaccine Schedule: HiB given at 2, 4, 6 and 12-15 months	**Epiglottitis** Swelling of the epiglottis compromising the airway. SX: **INSPIRATORY STRIDOR**, **drooling,** dysphagia, high fever, muffled voice. Patient will **lean forward** when sitting. DX: Lateral neck X-ray shows **"Thumbprint" sign.** TX: Emergency - **Send to the OR to intubate**- do NOT do this in the ER TX: Prophylaxis to household contacts: **Rifampin** (also caused by S. pneumonia, S. aureus, S. pyogenes, Mycoplasma)	**Haemophilus ducreyi** **PAINFUL** genital ulcer **Inguinal lymphadenopathy** Chocolate agar shows **satellite cells** Histo: shows **parallel chains** or "School of Fish" appearance TX: **Azithromycin, Ceftriaxone** (**tip**: this ulcer is painful so you "Do Cry") Other complications in children: Meningitis Otitis media Pneumonia

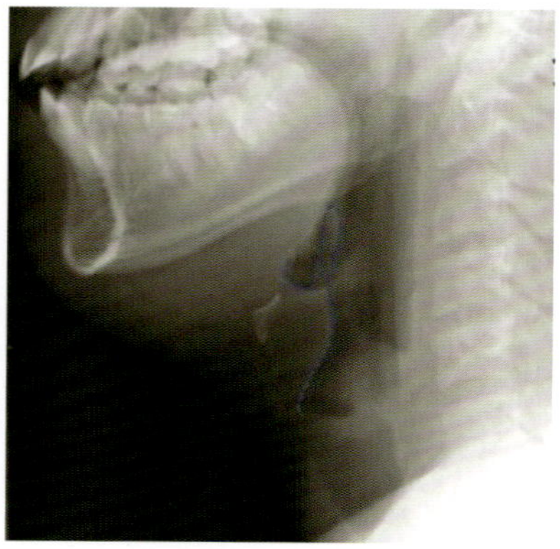

"Thumbprint Sign" Epiglottitis

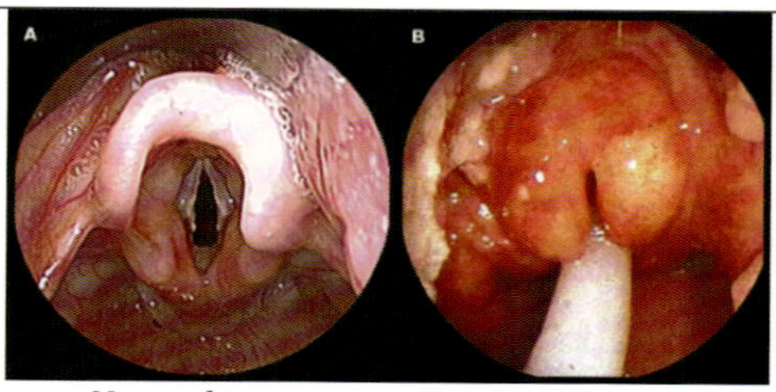

Normal Epiglottitis

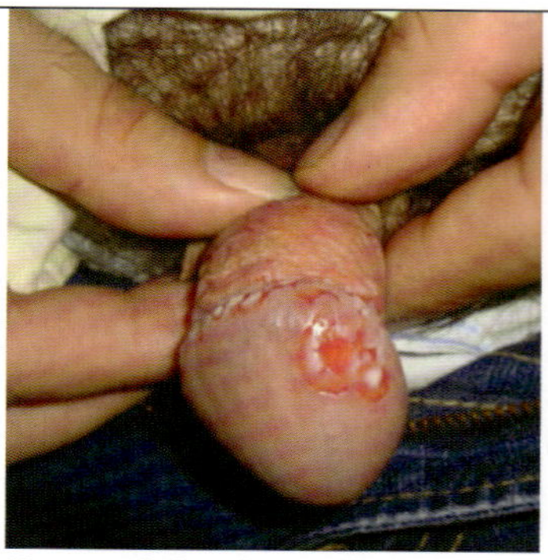

Haemophilus ducreyi

Helicobacter pylori		
Gm -, Bacillus/rod Positive Hydrogen Test **Silver staining** (**tip**: think of the **silver** blades on a helicopter) Urease positive Catalase positive Oxidase positive Likes alkaline environment 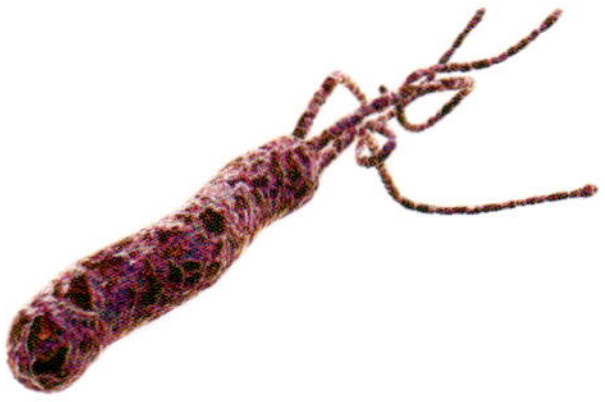	**Complications:** Gastritis Peptic Ulcer Disease due to: Gastric Ulcers or Duodenal Ulcers **Gastric Ulcers:** Usually more painful when eating, so weight loss **Duodenal Ulcers:** Usually more painful on an empty stomach, so weight gain (keeping food on stomach). Ulcers: **destruction of mucosal tissue via urease and proteases**.	DX Test: **Positive Urea breath test** **Positive Fecal antigen** TX: **Requires a PPI (Proton pump inhibitor) and 2 antibiotics.** **PPI and Clarithromycin and Amoxicillin** If treatment fails, **use PPI and metronidazole and tetracycline.** If treatment fails again: **test for Zollinger-Ellison** ***If patient is >45 years old, must do an endoscopy to rule out gastric cancer** **Also be aware:** H. pylori like alkaline environments. By taking PPI's or H2 blockers, the environment is made more alkaline, so problems persist.

Klebsiella	
Gm -, Bacillus/rod **Lactose positive** **MCC: Nosocomial UTI and Pneumonia** Can also cause staghorn calculi	**Pneumonia – Nosocomial** Right upper lobe **Due to aspiration of food particles, vomit** (alcoholics, IV drug users, post surgical patients under anesthesia, stroke victims, **COPD**, renal failure, diabetics, malignancy, altered mental status, drug overdoses, esophageal fistulas in neonates, ANY weakened immune system, Zenker's diverticulum, etc.) SX: **bloody sputum** (current jelly sputum) Cause: aspiration causes abscess in lungs TX: **3rd generation Cephalosporin**
Klebsiella granulomatis AKA: Klebsiella Inguinale AKA: Donovanosis, granuloma venereum AKA: Granuloma inguinale SX: Ulcerative genital lesions – **NOT PAINFUL** (do NOT mistake this for syphilis), **red, beefy granulation ulcer**, mucus and blood leakage, NO lymphadenopathy. DX: Wright-Giemsa stain show **intracellular inclusion bodies: Donovan Bodies** (intracytoplasmic cyst) **TX: Doxycycline or Azithromycin**	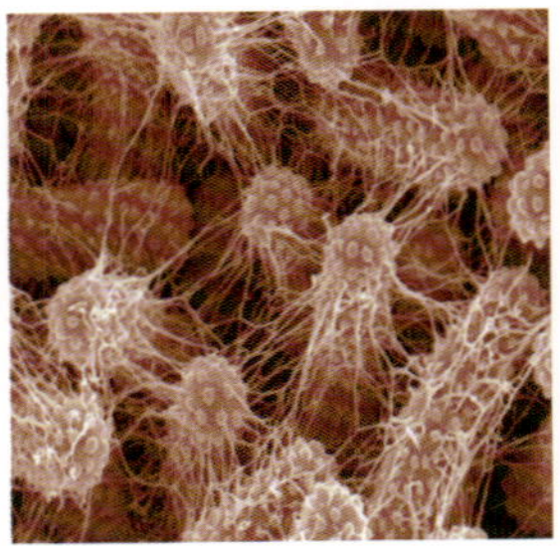 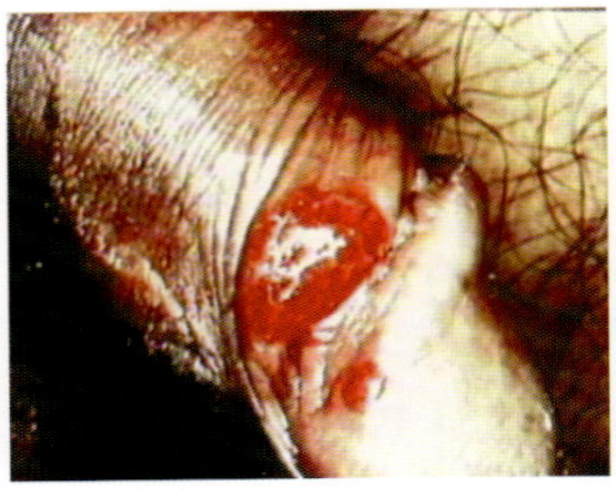 Klebsiella pneumonia Klebsiella granulomatis

Proteus mirabilis

Gm -, Bacillus/rod
Oxidase negative
Catalase positive
Nitrate positive
Flagellar H antigen
Positive urease test
Swarming pattern of movement (school of fish)
Produces H_2S (hydrogen sulfide)

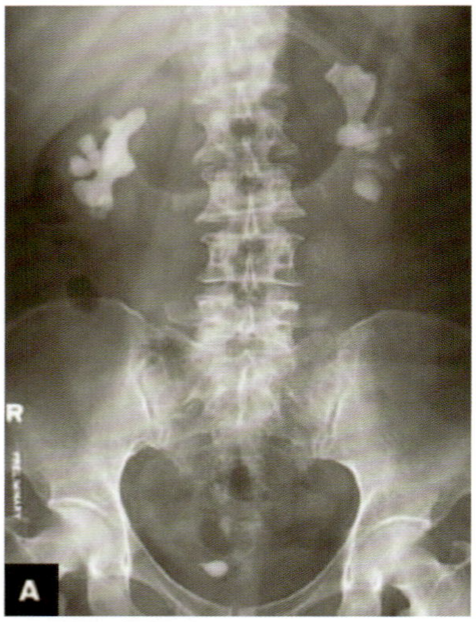

Staghorn calculi

Proteus mirabilis
AKA: **Struvite stones** (crystals)
AKA: **Staghorn calculi**
AKA: **Ammonium magnesium phosphate**
Forms in high pH
MOA: Urine is alkalized when urease enzyme splits urea into ammonia and carbon dioxide and raises pH
DX: **Radiopaque** (can be seen on X-ray), **>7.4 pH**
Cause: from waste water/sewage
SX: **Flank or costovertebral pain**. Calculi can take up a large part of the kidney
TX: Surgical removal
(can also be caused by Klebsiella and Staph)
(**tip**: "Mag"nificient STAG)

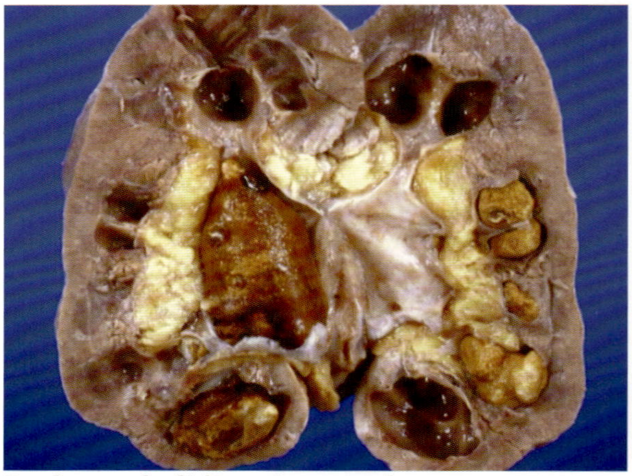
Staghorn calculi (Struvite stones)

Pseudomonas aeruginosa

Gm -, Bacillus/rod
ENCAPSULATED (**polysaccharide capsule**)
MacConkey's agar
Non-lactose fermenting
Oxidase positive
Pigment: Pyo**cyan**in (blue/green) with a sweet grape like odor
Motile with flagella

Highest Risk Patients:
Cystic Fibrosis
Burn patients
Intubated ventilator patients
(NO flowers or plants allowed in intubated inpatient rooms!)
Diabetics
Immunocompromised
Neutropenic

Virulence Factor:
Endotoxin for fever and shock
Exotoxin A (inactivate the **EF2 elongation factor stopping protein synthesis, ribosylation of EF2**)
Biofilm in lungs b/c mucus secretions
Produces **elastase** that cleaves elastase and collagen to destroy vessels
Phospholipase C = destroys cell membranes
Pyocyanin produces reactive O_2 species

Cystic Fibrosis: Pneumonia is due to the **biofilm** from pseudomonas

Pseudomonas Antibiotics
Piperacillin with Tazobactam, Ticarcillin, Cefepime, Ceftazidime, Cephoperazone, Imipenem, Meropenem, Amikacin, Tobramycin, Aminoglycosides PLUS a beta lactamase inhibitor (Clavulanic acid, Sulbactam, Tazobactam)

Folliculitis (Hot Tub Folliculitis)
Superficial infection of the hair follicles.
MC: hot tubs, therapy pools, water slides due to improper sanitation due to poor chemicals maintenance.
SX: rash that resembles a pimple at the base of each hair follicle
TX: **Topical Mupirocin**
If infection worsens from a simple folliculitis into a furuncle (collection of infected folliculitis) or into a carbuncle (abscess) you must **TX with: Dicloxacillin or Cefadroxil**

Can also be caused by S. aureus

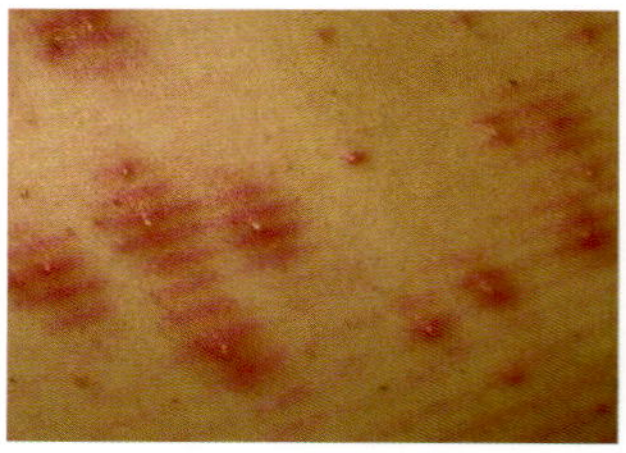

Pseudomonas aeruginosa cont'd		
Acute External Otitis Media (AKA: Otitis Externa) (AKA: **Swimmers Ear**) Infection by bacteria due to water remaining inside the ear after swimming (showers). SX: **NORMAL** tympanic membrane, **purulent drainage and itching from external auditory canal, severe pain** TX: **Topical Ciprofloxacin w/dexamethasone (steroid to ↓ swelling and itching) otic drops, Ofloxacin, Polymyxin/neomycin.** **Add acetic acid and water solution to re acidify the ear.**	**Malignant Otitis Externa** (MC in elderly adults – not connected with swimming) (Different than Otitis Media). AKA: Osteomyelitis of the skull. (**tip**: "E"lderly = "E"xternal) **Granulation tissue** (fibrous tissue) deposits inside ear canal MC: in-patient with diabetes. Complication: brain abscess, destruction of the skull. SX: **NORMAL** tympanic membrane, **purulent drainage, severe pain.** DX: MRI, bone biopsy/culture. TX: Pseudomonas antibiotics and surgical debridement.	**Osteomyelitis** MC seen with a puncture wound that penetrated the **rubber sole of a tennis shoe** TX: Surgical debridement and a Fluoroquinolones
Ecthyma gangrenosum Necrotic cutaneous lesions MC seen in neutropenic individuals Cause: invasions of blood vessels, **Exotoxin A** destroy vessels. SX: Round or oval lesion with a halo of erythema with a center **sepsis** of **black necrosis** TX: **Pseudomonas antibiotic**	**UTI** MC: inpatients with indwelling catheters	**Contact Lens Keratitis** Infection of the cornea usually caused by S. aureus or Pseudomonas. MC: contact wearers SX: Eye pain, redness, blurred vision, sensitivity to light, excessive tearing, eye discharge Cause: leaving contacts in to long (overnight), poor disinfecting, sharing contacts, storing and rinsing with water TX: Remove contacts, antibacterial eye drops. Other types: Dendritic keratitis: Herpes simplex keratitis or Herpes zoster keratitis (form of shingles). Onchocercal keratitis from the blackfly bite in Africa (AKA: River blindness).

Salmonella

Salmonella	
Gm -, Bacillus/rod Enterobacteria **Virulence factor: O antigen** and flagella H antigens. Hektoen agar: colorless colonies with black centers. **Mobile** with flagella (**tip**: salmon swim). Spreads hematogenously. **Produces H_2S (hydrogen sulfide)** on ferrous sulfate media. SX: **Bloody diarrhea**, fever, headache, and splenomegaly. **TX: <12 years old or immunocompromised: Cipro or TMP/SMX. >12 is self limiting** **Complication: Heart Block**	**Salmonella Enteritis** **Food poisoning** SX: bloody or non-bloody diarrhea, fever, abdominal cramps, nausea, vomiting, fever, chills, headache, muscle and joint pain 12 – 72 hrs after exposure Source: **Infected or undercooked poultry, fish, milk, eggs**. Unwashed hands of an infected food handler. Feces of pets with diarrhea. **Reptiles** (**turtles**, iguanas, lizards, snakes). DX: Stools show salmonella TX: Self limiting Complications: Reiter's Syndrome (AKA: Reactive arthritis) SX: Joint pain, conjunctivitis, and painful urination. Resolves in a year but can lead to chronic arthritis
Salmonella Sickle Cell Osteomyelitis MCC in older children and adults with Sickle Cell (In younger Sickle Cell patients < 6 – 8 with a normal working spleen, MCC osteomyelitis is due to S. aureus). Path: Macrophages of the RES (Reticuloendothelial system – in the spleen) normally eliminate salmonella from the body. In Sickle Cell patients, the macrophages are loaded with the breakdown products of the RBC's (sickled cells) and aren't able to ingest and kill Salmonella. Sickle Cell patients become asplenic by the ages of 6 – 8. Without a spleen, the salmonella can not be removed from the body.	**Salmonella typhi** **Typhoid Fever** Spread: Food or drinks that have been handled by an infected person, contaminated **sewage**. Once eaten spreads to the blood stream. MC seen in developing countries but is in the US. SX: flat, **Rose spots** on abdomen, fever, diarrhea, headache, **sustained high fever** of 103° to 104° DX: Stool or blood samples TX: **Fluoroquinolones, Ceftriaxone, Azithromycin**

Shigella sonnei

Shigella sonnei	
Gm -, bacillus/rod Enterotoxin **Shiga Toxin** Virulence factor: O antigen **AB Exotoxin stops the 60s Ribosome** No hematogenous spread	Bloody diarrhea **Invades M Cells (Peyer patches)** in the ileum causing mucosal ulcers. **MC in daycares and nursing homes**, one of the leading causes of diarrhea worldwide Spread: **Fecal-Oral** DX: Fecal samples SX: bloody diarrhea, fever, nausea, vomiting, abdominal pain, flatulence, large painful bowel movements TX: **Ampicillin, TMP-SMX**

<table>
<tr><th colspan="2">Vibrio cholera</th></tr>
<tr><td>Virulence factor: Cholera toxin
Oxidase positive
Comma shaped
Motile at 25°, flagellum at one cell pole
Grows at 42°
Grows on Bile and alkaline media (tip: think Vi- BILE)
TCBS agar shows flat yellow colonies</td><td>Profuse watery diarrhea (rice-water diarrhea) up to 3 Liters per day
Developing countries (so look for travel to these areas)
MOA: Enterotoxin activates Gs and ↑ cAMP
"Rice" is the mucus and intestinal epithelial cells in stool
Cause: drinking water contaminated by feces of infected person
SX: Extreme dehydration, must keep hydrated, abdominal cramps, dry mucous membranes, sunken eyes, hypotension, weak pulse, tachycardia, oliguria, coma, death
Sensitive to gastric acid (does not like acid) so condition will worsen if patient is on a PPI or H2 blocker because these drugs raise the ph.</td></tr>
<tr><td>Vibrio vulnificus
Is a relative of Vibrio cholera
Lactose fermenting
Motile, curved, rod-shaped bacillus

Its capsule protects it from phagocytosis.</td><td>Causes: Contaminated marine or brackish water that infects injured skin causing formation of blisters or ulcers. Eating raw or undercooked shellfish (seafood, oysters).

SX: Vomiting, explosive diarrhea, abdominal pain. Rapidly expanding cellulitis, septicemia (fever, chills, confusion).
It can be life threatening to the immunocompromised, especially individuals with liver disease (virulent forms adhere to the iron bound to transferrin).</td></tr>
</table>

<table>
<tr><th colspan="2">Yersinia</th></tr>
<tr><td>Yersinia enterocolitica
Gm -, rod-shaped coccobacillus
SX: Bloody diarrhea: invades colon, mesenteric adenitis that mimics an appendicitis
Source: Pet feces (esp. puppies), contaminate milk, pork</td><td>Yersinia pestis (Zoonotic)
Bubonic Plague
Infection of the lymphatic system
Bubonic F-1 antigen in macrophage
Bipolar staining (safety pin shape)
MC: SW United States
Reservoirs: Fleas, prairie dogs, rats
SX: Bloody diarrhea, black necrosis ("Black death"), buboes (lymphadenitis, infection of lymph glands), gangrene, DIC
TX: Antibiotics in first 24 hrs to prevent death. Aminoglycosides, doxycycline</td></tr>
</table>

ATYPICAL BACTERIA

Caution: T cells fight atypical bacteria.

Chlamydia		
Atypical Bacteria **Intracellular:** can't make ATP. Cell wall **lacks muramic acid** (amino sugar acid that is found in most bacterial cell walls). **No peptidoglycan in cell wall.** **Silver Staining.** **Elementary Body (Extracellular)** enters the cell via endocytosis and becomes a reticulate body. **Reticulate body (Intracellular)** replicates in the cell by fission and becomes Elementary bodies. (**tip**: **E** in elementary for **E**xtracellular and **E**nters. **R** in reticulate for **R**esident) Labs: Shows NO bacteria. Giemsa stain shows: **intracytoplasmic inclusion bodies.** The **ONLY** way it is ok to treat only for gonorrhea is if a **PCR** is done and shows no Chlamydiae infection. **Beware:** If a stain is done in the office lab and shows negative for Chlamydia, you **MUST** treat for **BOTH** because Chlamydiae will not be seen, they are intracellular.	**Chlamydia trachomatis** **STD** **Co-Infection with gonorrhea** History: High # of sex partners SX: **Mucopurulent discharge, cervical motion tenderness**, dysuria and frequency, increased urethral infections (non-gonococcal urethritis), **PID** (Pelvic Inflammatory Disease), **reactive arthritis** (Reiter syndrome: HLA-B27)). Conjunctivitis in neonates. BIT: NAAT (Nucleic Acid Amplification Test) for both Chlamydia and Gonorrhea. NAAT can also be done on the urine (men and women). TX: **MUST TREAT FOR BOTH CHLAMYDIA and GONORRHEA.** **Must treat partner.** **Chlamydia: Azithromycin IM (or Doxycycline)** **Gonorrhea: Ceftriaxone oral**	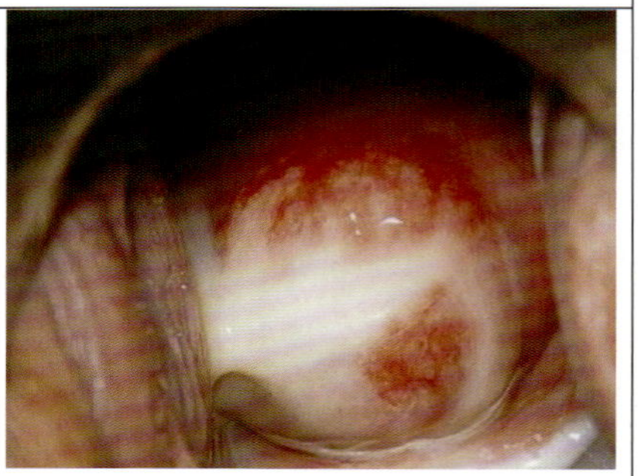 Mucopurulent discharge from cervix 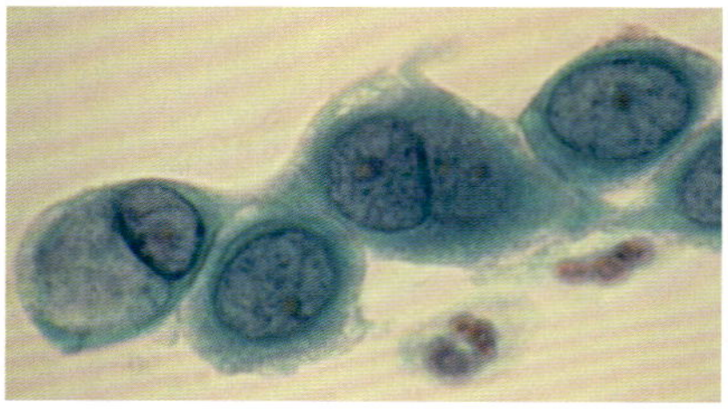 Chlamydiae - Intracellular
Chlamydia psittaci **Chlamydia atypical pneumonia** Source: **birds, chickens, pigeons.** High risk for: Veterinarians, pet shop workers, chicken farmers, zoo workers Transmission: aerosol SX: **dry cough, non-productive cough**, sore throat, fever, CXR shows **patchy** pneumonia TX: **Azithromycin IM or Doxycycline IM**	**Chlamydia Neonatal Conjunctivitis** #1 MC cause of preventable blindness in the world Occurs in the **2nd week** after birth. (Gonorrhea conjunctivitis occurs in the 1st week after birth) (**Tip**: "**GO**"norrhea **G**oes first) SX: **Mucopurulent/purulent** discharge from eye, **neo-vascularization** of cornea TX: **Erythromycin ointment**	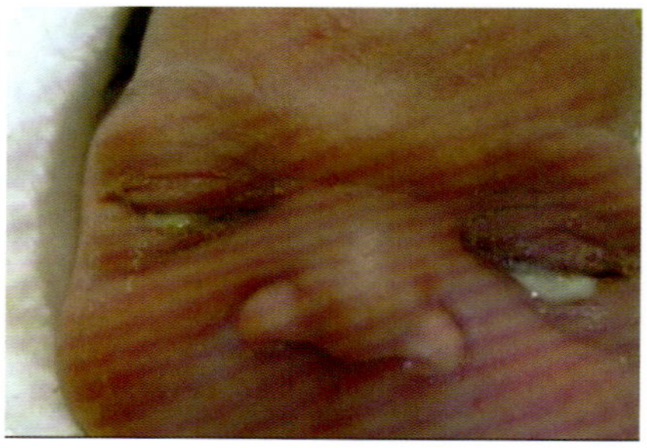 Chlamydia Neonatal Conjunctivitis

Chlamydia cont'd		
Chlamydia Lymphogranuloma Venereum **SX: Painless** genital ulcers, **painful, swollen inguinal lymph nodes that ulcerate (buboes)** **TX: Doxycycline** 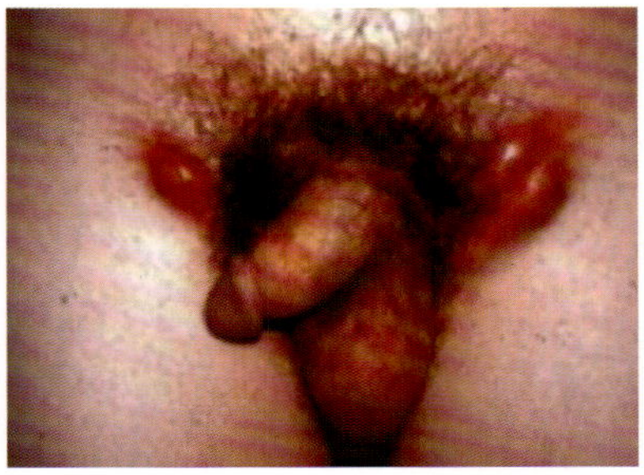	**Chlamydia Neonatal Pneumonia** **Transmission: birth canal** **SX: Staccato cough** **Fitz-Curtis Syndrome** due to PID ("Violin string" adhesions can cause **intestinal obstructions**) 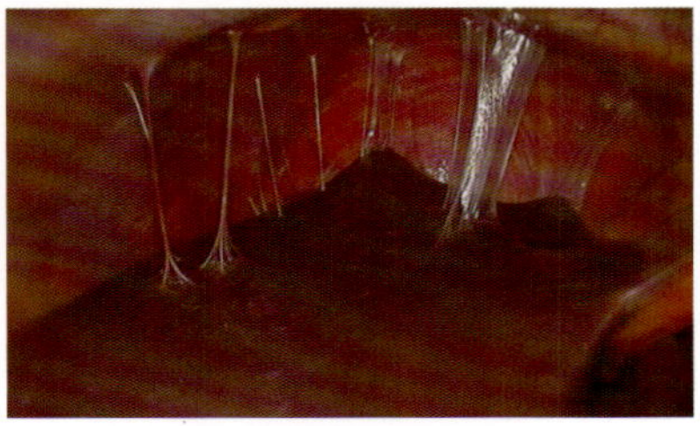	**PID (Pelvic Inflammatory Disease** Cause: Chlamydia trachomatis and Neisseria gonorrhoeae. MC bacterial STD in the USA SX: **Cervical motion tenderness** (Chandelier sign), **purulent (muco-purulent discharge), infertility,** endometritis, tubo-ovarian abscess, **salpingitis** (inflammation of fallopian tube), hydrosalpinx (blocked fallopian tube with serous or clear fluid). **Fitz Hugh-Curtis Syndrome**: infection of liver capsule leading to adhesions (AKA: Violin string adhesions). **Risk Factors**: Adhesions can cause intestinal **obstruction** (air/fluid levels on abdominal x-ray), **infertility**, **ectopic pregnancy**

Coxiella burnetii			
Atypical bacteria	**Q Fever** **Endospore** inside of cells. Atypical pneumonia, Myocarditis Negative Weil-Felix test	Pneumonia	**Amniotic** fluids, aerosols of cattle/sheep/livestock. (MC: farmers, veterinarians). Spores inhaled.

Legionella pneumophila (AKA: Legionnaires Disease) (Milder form: Pontiac Fever)		
Atypical Bacteria **Silver staining** Culture: **Charcoal yeast with iron and cysteine** DX: Antigen in urine Source: **Water source**: air conditioning, water mist in grocery stores, outdoor water cooling mist, whirlpools, fountains, ice machines, dental equipment. Aerosol transmission, no human-to-human transmission.	SX: only pneumonia with both **GI symptoms with pneumonia**. Fever, diarrhea, confusion. PMN's form abscesses. SX Pontiac Fever: milder, flu-like Labs: ↑**PMN's**, hyponatremia Infects: Alveolar macrophages High risk: older, smoking and drinking men TX: **Fluoroquinolones, Azithromycin**	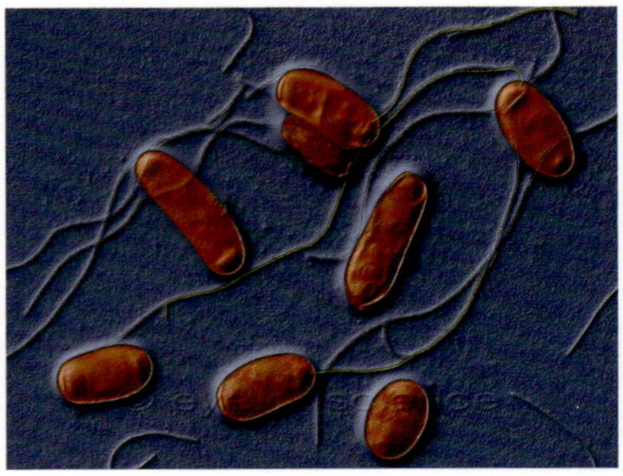

Mycoplasma pneumonia (AKA: Walking pneumonia)	
Atypical Bacteria Has no cell wall, lacks peptidoglycans Only bacteria containing **cholesterol** Bacteria membrane contains sterols Medium: **Eaton agar: requires cholesterol** to grow Labs: Cold agglutinins (IgM) **(tip:** being **COLD** is **M**iserable, being **WARM** is **G**ood**)**	SX**: Nonproductive cough**, headache. CXR shows diffuse interstitial infiltrate. **X-ray looks worse** than patient. High risk in **close quarters**: dorms, prisons, and military bases. MC under 30 years old. **TX: Macrolides, Doxycycline, Fluoroquinolones**

Rickettsia			
Rickettsia rickettsia **ATYPICAL bacteria** **Zoonotic bacteria**	Rocky Mountain Spotted Fever DX: Positive Well Felix	SX: **Rash on palms/soles**. Rash **starts on wrist** and then spreads to trunk, DIC, shock (**tip**: **R**ash starts on the **R**ist)	**Dermacentor tick**
Rickettsia typhi	Typhus	Same as prowazekii	Fleas

Ureaplasma urealyticum
Atypical Bacteria STD No cell wall Belongs to family of Mycoplasmataceae Transmission: sexual activity and vertically in birth canal Risk: PID, urethritis, infertility, stillbirth, premature birth TX**: Doxycycline, Azithromycin**

Spirochetes

Leptospira interrogans		
Spirochete **Source:** infected **animal urine** with direct contact or contaminated water. Invades through open skin. Replicates in liver and kidneys. Higher risk: farmers, sewer workers, recreational water activities (surfing), tops of cans (soda, food) due to rat/mouse urine. SX: Jaundice, flu-like symptoms, photophobia Most severe form: Weil disease	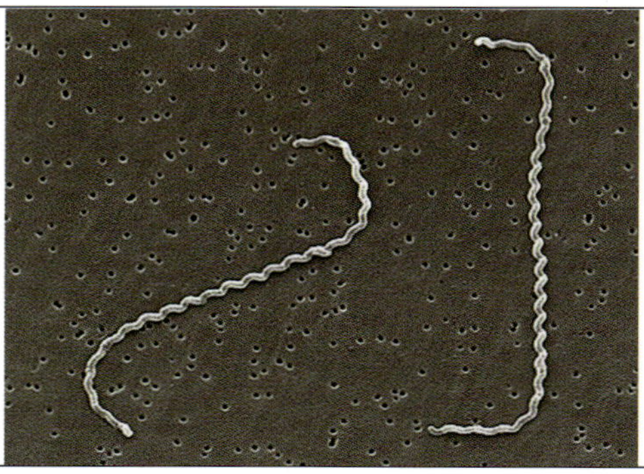	Spirochete. Looks like the old ice block tongs.

Treponema pallidum (Syphilis) – STD

(**tip**: syphilis is not my "pal")

1° Syphilis

SX: **PAINLESS** chancre appears 6 weeks after exposure. Heals spontaneously without treatment.

DX: 1° **Dark-field microscope shows spirochetes**
(**DO NOT** use VDRL/RPR testing to diagnose 1° Syphilis due to ↑ false negatives).
If dark-field is positive for spirochetes, no additional testing is necessary.

NOTE: Please see Congenital Disease chapter for Syphilis pathology in the fetus and newborns.

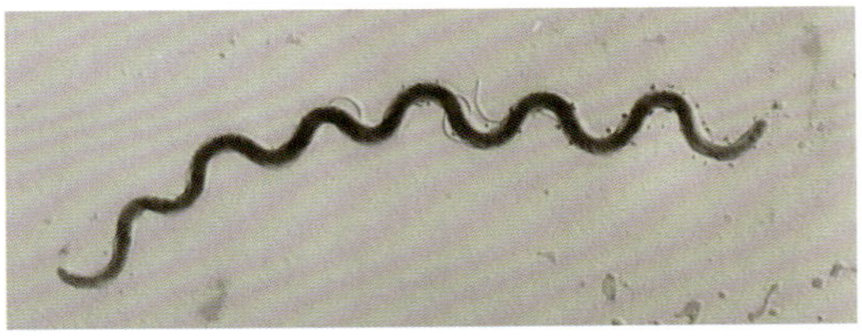

2° Syphilis

SX: **Diffuse, maculopapular rash** (bronze rash) starting on trunk and spreads to extremities (can include palms and soles of feet), alopecia areata, **condylomata lata** (wart like lesions on genitals), lymphadenopathy.

DX: **VDRL/RPR** and **confirmatory test FTA-ABS**

TX: IM Penicillin (Doxycycline if allergic)

Condylomata lata TX: Imiquimod (sloughs off the lesion without harm to surrounding tissues. **Tip**: "I" for "Ideal". Imiquimod also treats basal cell cancer and actinic keratosis), Liquid nitrogen, cryotherapy, podophyllin or trichloroacetic acid (melts away the lesions).

3° (Tertiary) Syphilis
Neurosyphilis

SX: **Gummas** (granulomas: on skin and bone), Argyll Robertson pupil (Pupils do not respond to light but constrict on accommodation), **aortitis (AKA: Vasa vasorum destruction leading to aortic aneurysm, aortic regurgitation)**, broad based ataxia, positive Romberg, meningovascular stroke (does not involve HTN, this stroke is from vasculitis), Charcot joint, **Tabes dorsalis** (loss of vibratory sense and position, incontinence), memory and personality changes.

Neurosyphilis (AKA: tabes dorsalis – dorsal columns). Takes 5 to 10 years to develop.
TX: **IV Penicillin** **(Must desensitize if allergic to penicillin)**

DX: LP shows a **positive VDRL and granulomas in the CSF.**
Neurosyphilis: excluded with a negative CSF FTA.
The most sensitive test for the CSF is the FTA.

TX: 1° and 2° Syphilis: **IM Penicillin G**
TX: Tertiary Syphilis: **IV Penicillin**
If **allergic** (even in pregnancy), patient must be **desensitized** to penicillin if the patient is pregnant or has neurosyphilis. Can't use Doxycycline.
(Can use **doxycycline** if allergic to penicillin and patient is not pregnant or suffering from neurosyphilis).

VDRL/RPR moa:
Test separates sediment from the fluid. Serum is added to **cardiolipin** and lecithin (**fats**). If test is positive **"Flocculation"** (separation) occurs.

VDRL/RPR False Positives risk in:
Viruses (mono, hepatitis), HIV, Malaria, IV drug use, Rheumatic fever, Endocarditis, Infection, Elderly, **Lupus (anti-phospholipid syndrome)**, Leprosy

Jarisch-Herxheimer Reaction
Reaction to endotoxin-like/lipoprotein products released by the death of microorganisms during an antibiotic treatment. Usually occurs a few hours after the first dose of antibiotics.
SX: fever, chills, hypotension, tachycardia, flushing myalgia, fever.
TX: Prophylaxis with an anti-inflammatory medicine. Oral aspirin or ibuprofen, oral or IV prednisone.

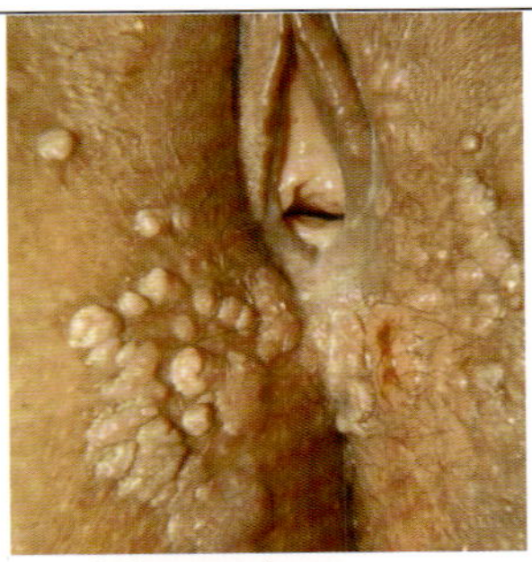

Condylomata lata

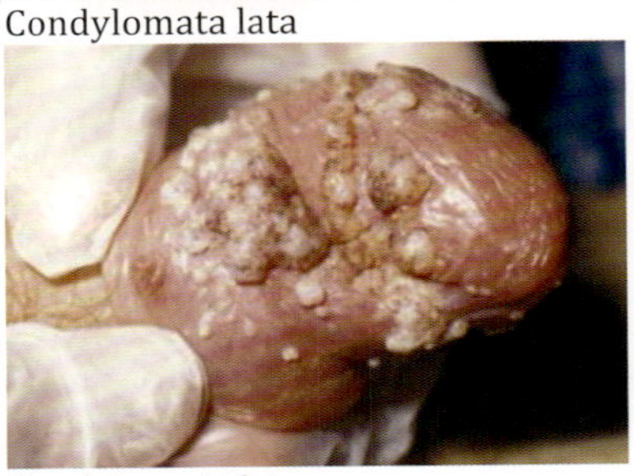

Condylomata lata

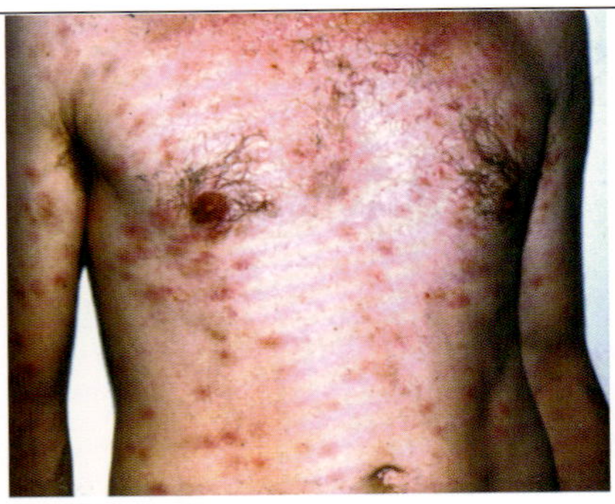

Syphilis rash

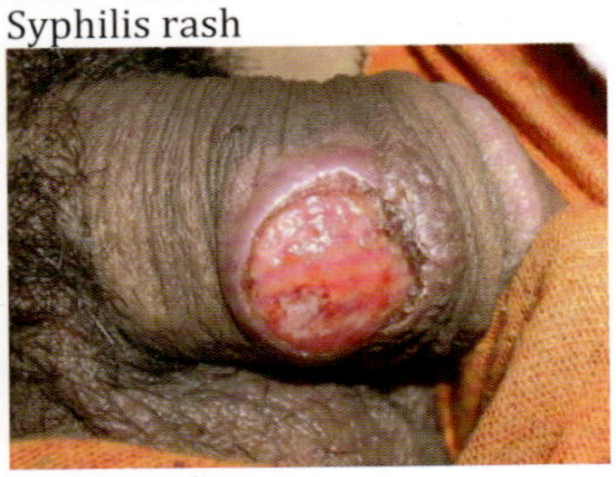

Painless chancre

Misc. Bacteria (variable staining of gm – and gm +)

Gardnerella vaginalis (Bacterial vaginosis, BV)	
Vaginosis Gm variable Is **NOT an STD** but is associated with sex SX: **Gray vaginal discharge, fishy smell**, is NOT painful, **NO redness or inflammation.** DX: **Clue cells (squamous epithelial cells covered with adherent bacteria** due to an overgrowth of anaerobic bacteria in the vagina) TX: **Metronidazole** Nursing moms: discontinue nursing while taking meds and then resume once meds have stopped	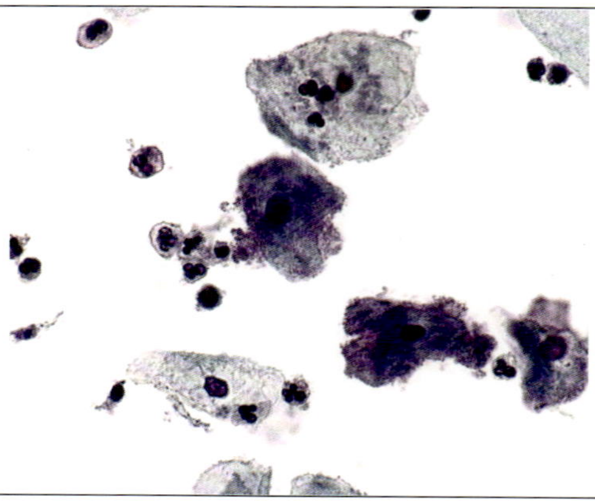

Tropheryma whipplei	
Been shown to be Gm + and Gm - **PAS stain positive** (Periodic Acid-Schiff) stains for glycogen (sugar) in the macrophages in the lamina propria Non-acid fast bacteria Actinobacteria Complications: Whipple's Disease, Endocarditis	**Whipple's Disease** Malabsorption SX: diarrhea, abdominal pain, weight loss, joint pain, wasting and enlargement of lymph nodes in the abdomen, steatorrhea, flatulence, abdominal distension, peripheral edema MC: in farmers and those exposed to soil and animals TX: **Ampicillin, Tetracycline**

Zoonotic Bacteria – Transmitted from animals to humans

Organism	Disease/DX	Symptoms/TX	Source and Transmission
Anaplasma	**Anaplasmosis** DX: Giemsa	SX: hemolytic anemia, hematuria, diarrhea, anorexia, granulocytes with morulae (berry-like inclusions) MC: tropical regions TX: **Doxycycline**	Ixodes tick (on deer, mice), Hematogenous spread
Bartonella	**Cat Scratch Disease** Bacillary Angiomatosis DX: Warthin Starry Stain	SX: Granulomas, pus, nodular **lymph nodes** TX: **Azithromycin**	**Cat scratch** (**tip**: Bart the cat)
Babesia (protozoan)	**Babesiosis** DX: **Maltese cross** on blood smear, PCR. AKA: merozoites attached together. AKA: Tetrads of intraerythrocytic rings.	SX: Similar to malaria, **hemolytic anemia**, chills, sweats, thrombocytopenia. MC in asplenic persons. Babesia infects RBC, so the spleen normally removes these infected cells. TX: **Azithromycin, Atovaquone**	**Ticks bites**

Borrelia burgdorferi* (See below zoonotic section for additional details and pictures)	**Lyme disease** DX: ELISA, Western blot, PCR, serologic testing	**SX: Erythema migrans (target lesion), unilateral or bilateral bells palsy (CN VII)**, flu-like symptoms, arthritis (knee MC joint), **and heart block. Can become systemic if not treated.** TX: **Doxycycline >8 years Pregnant and <8 years: Amoxicillin**	**Ixodes tick** (on deer, mice) MC in **NE United States**
Borrelia recurrentis	**Relapsing fever** DX: Giemsa, **Silver staining**	SX: Morulae (berry like inclusions)	Louse
Brucella	**Brucellosis** AKA: Undulant fever due to LPS virulence DX: granulomas in the macrophages	SX: Undulant fever (fluctuant). Enlargement of **lymph nodes**. MC: TX, CA, VA, FL	Unpasteurized dairy
Campylobacter	Bloody diarrhea (Can lead to Guillain Barré)	Bloody diarrhea	**Puppies,** undercooked meat, unpasteurized milk. Fecal-oral
Chlamydophila psittaci	Psittacosis **Atypical pneumonia**	Dry cough, patchy pneumonia on X-Ray, sore throat, fever. TX: Self resolving: get rid of bird/s	Birds (parrots, chickens, etc) transmitted: aerosol (MC: Pet shop workers, veterinarians, etc)
Coxiella burnetii **ATYPICAL bacteria**	**Q Fever** **Undulant fevers.** **Endospore** inside of cells. Atypical pneumonia, Myocarditis Negative Weil-Felix test	Pneumonia	Amniotic fluids, aerosols of cattle/sheep/livestock. (MC: farmers, veterinarians). Spores inhaled. (**Remember**: Atypical bacteria is fought by T cells)
Ehrlichia chaffeensis	**Ehrlichiosis.** **Anaplasma.** DX: Clumps of bacteria in leukocytes that stop protein synthesis. Kills WBC. AKA: PCR, Monocytes with **morulae** (AKA: berry like inclusions or inclusion bodies in the WBC)	SX: **NO rash** **Leukopenia** (↓ WBC) **Thrombocytopenia** ↑LFT (ALT and AST). MC: Central/Eastern USA (ie: Missouri, Arkansas) TX: **Doxycycline**	Lone Star tick.
Francisella tularensis Coccobacillus Non-spore forming Non-motile	**Tularemia** Needs cysteine for growth. (High virulence: classified as a potential bioterrorism agent)	Sx: Granulomas **Black ulcers, conjunctivitis, lymphadenopathy.** TX: **Gentamicin, Streptomycin**	**Rabbits, squirrels (AKA: furry little animals),** ticks, flies. **Hunters** can be infected (skinning animals, taxidermist, etc.)
Leptospira interrogans (Spirochetes)	**Leptospirosis** AKA: Well's Syndrome DX: "Ice tong" appearance, ELISA, PCR	SX: headaches, fevers, **kidney failure**, abdominal pain, myopathy, hemoptysis, meningitis, **jaundice** from liver failure. MC; Tropical regions, developing countries TX: **Doxycycline, Ceftriaxone, Penicillin**	Person was **exposed** to **animal urine** (food contaminated by urine). Rodents MC: Veterinarians, farmers, slaughterhouse workers, waste facility workers.
Mycobacterium leprae	**Leprosy** (2 forms) Tuberculoid (TH1) and Lepromatous (TH2)	SX: Loss eyebrows, nasal collapse, lumpy ear, loss fingers, toes DX: Acid fast bacilli on skin	Armadillo

Pasteurella multocida	**Cellulitis, Osteomyelitis** DX: oxidate positive Catalase positive. Bi-polar staining. Polysaccharide capsule. LPS, Lipid A (Lipid A anchors the LPS to the outer membrane).	SX: Musty odor of suture wounds. TX: **Amoxicillin plus Clavulanic acid (Augmentin)** **TX: Bite on hand or puncture wound: leave open to drain.** **Face and other lacerations: stich closed.**	**Animal bites** or scratches from domestic pets. Soft tissue inflammation within 24 hours, localized cellulitis. Serious cases: Osteomyelitis, endocarditis. Can cross the blood-brain barrier causing meningitis.
Rickettsia prowazekii **ATYPICAL bacteria**	**Typhus**	SX: Rash SPARES palm/soles, rash **starts on trunk** and spreads (Pictures below)	Louse, lice, flying squirrels
Rickettsia rickettsia **ATYPICAL bacteria** (see additional information and pictures at end of zoonotic section)	**Rocky Mountain Spotted Fever** DX: Positive Well Felix, DX: ELISA, Western blot, PCR, serologic testing	SX: **Rash on palms/soles**. Rash **starts on wrist** and then spreads to trunk, DIC, shock. (**tip**: **R**ash starts on the **R**ist) TX: **Doxycycline** **If pregnant or <8 yrs old: Amoxicillin**	**Dermacentor tick**
Rickettsia typhi	**Typhus**	Same as prowazekii	Fleas
Yersinia pestis	**Bubonic plague** F-1 antigen in microphages. Bipolar staining, (safety pin shape)	SX: Bloody diarrhea, DIC, **black necrosis** ("Black death")	Fleas, rats, prairie dogs MC: SW United states
Viral Tick Born Diseases			
Bourbon Virus		SX: High fever, fatigue, joint pain, maculopapular rash, SOB, joint pain, muscle aches, nausea, vomiting, diarrhea, low WBC and low platelets, loss of appetite.	Ticks Midwest USA: MO, KS, TN Orthomyxoviridae Virus
Heartland Virus		Same as Bourbon	Ticks: Lone Star Tick Midwest USA: MO Bunyaviridae Virus
Powassan Virus		SX: Flu-like symptoms. Affects the brain, causing infection and inflammation, neurological problems. (Viral encephalitis)	Ticks: Ixodes, Dermacentor North America Flavivirus

Tick Diseases and Facts

Tick Removal

- No disease and no treatment if tick has been attached <24 hrs
- Remove with **tweezers** so it can't release toxins
- Start prophylaxis with **Doxycycline (or if pregnant or under 8 years old: Amoxicillin)** if
  a) The tick is an adult tick or a deer tick
  b) The tick has been attached >24 – 48 hours – start prophylaxis within 72 hours of removal
  c) The tick is identified as Ixodes scapularis
  d) Patient is from an endemic area
  e) The tick is an engorged nymph-stage tick
- Lyme Disease: MC location: NE United States. The infection rate is 20%

Tick Paralysis

- Can occur between hours and days after tick attachment
- **Ascending paralysis**
- **Remove tick** and paralysis resolves in 24 – 48 hrs

Borrelia burgdorferi	**Rickettsia rickettsii**	**Ehrlichia chaffeensis**
Lyme Disease **Ixodes tick (Deer/Mouse tick)** Target lesion with central clearing (erythema lesion) NE United States **SX: Erythema migrans (target lesion), unilateral or bilateral bells palsy CN VII)**, flu-like symptoms, **arthritis** (knee MC joint), **heart block, dilated cardiomyopathy. Can become systemic if not treated.** TX (Rash, joints, Bells Palsy): **Doxycycline if >8 years old.** **Pregnant or <8 years old: Amoxicillin** **TX: Cardiac or neurologic symptoms:** **IV Ceftriaxone.**	**Rocky Mountain Spotted Fever** **ATYPICAL bacteria** Dermacentor tick Mid to South Eastern United States SX: **Rash on palms/soles**. Rash **starts on wrist** and then spreads to trunk, DIC, shock. (**tip**: **R**ash starts on the **R**ist) DX: Positive Well Felix TX: **Doxycycline.** **Pregnant and <8 years: Amoxicillin**	**Ehrlichiosis** Lone Star tick Central/Eastern USA (ie: Missouri, Arkansas) SX: **NO rash** Leukopenia (↓ WBC) Thrombocytopenia ↑LFT DX: Clumps of bacteria in leukocytes that stop protein synthesis. Kills WBC. AKA: Monocytes with morulae (berry like inclusions) TX: **Doxycycline.** **If pregnant or <8 yrs old: Amoxicillin**
Bourbon Virus SX: High fever, fatigue, joint pain, maculopapular rash, SOB, joint pain, muscle aches, nausea, vomiting, diarrhea, low WBC and low platelets, loss of appetite. Ticks Midwest USA: MO, KS, TN Orthomyxoviridae Virus	**Heartland Virus** SX: High fever, fatigue, joint pain, maculopapular rash, SOB, joint pain, muscle aches, nausea, vomiting, diarrhea, low WBC and low platelets, loss of appetite. Ticks: Lone Star Tick Midwest USA: MO Bunyaviridae Virus	**Powassan Virus** SX: Flu-like symptoms. Affects the brain, causing infection and inflammation, neurological problems. (Viral encephalitis). Ticks: Ixodes, Dermacentor North America Flavivirus
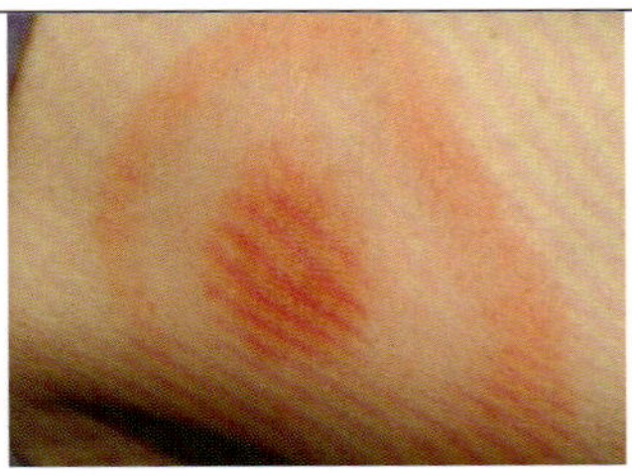 Lyme Disease Target Rash 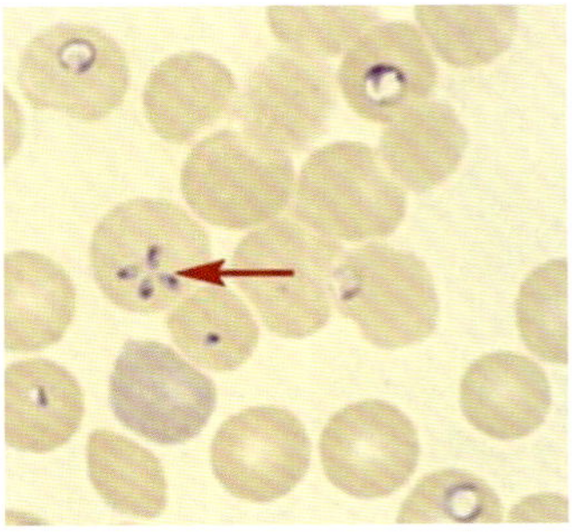 Maltese Cross in Babesiosis	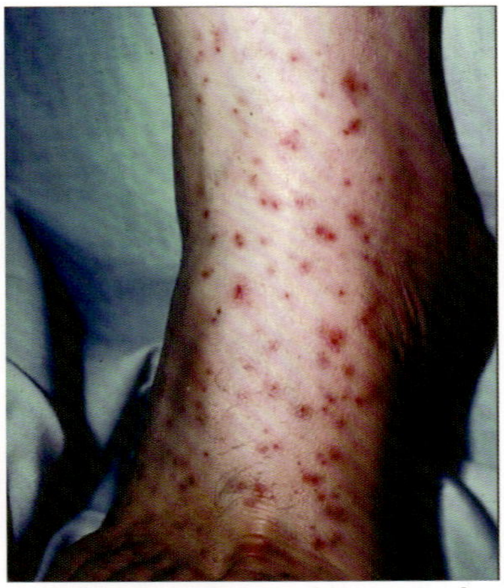 Rocky Mountain Spotted Fever Rash	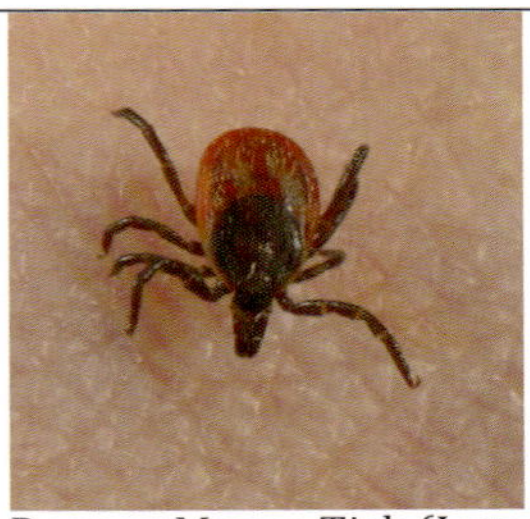 Deer or Mouse Tick (Lyme Disease) Ixodes Tick 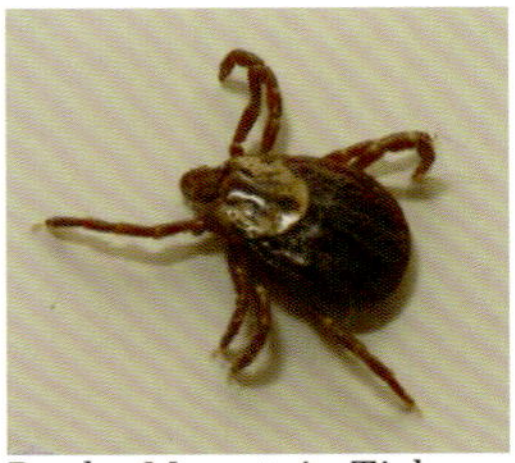 Rocky Mountain Tick Dermacentor Tick

Fleas, Lice , Scabies (Mites), Bed Bugs

Fleas Siphonaptera Located: Pets, carpets, pet bedding and upholstery. Can spread disease. SX: Raised red and swollen bump (wheal) <1 hour after bite. Small clusters of dots. Intensely itchy. Bump will have a punctured spot in the center. Bump (wheal) can become open sore or blister within 1 day. Legs and feet are most common areas. (do not appear as red as bed bug bites) TX: OTC: **Hydrocortisone cream, calamine, Benadryl** for pruritis and inflammation. Prescription: **Hydroxyzine** Prevention: Vacuum upholstery and carpets, beat rugs outside, treat pets and pet bedding with anti-flea products, spray house for fleas.	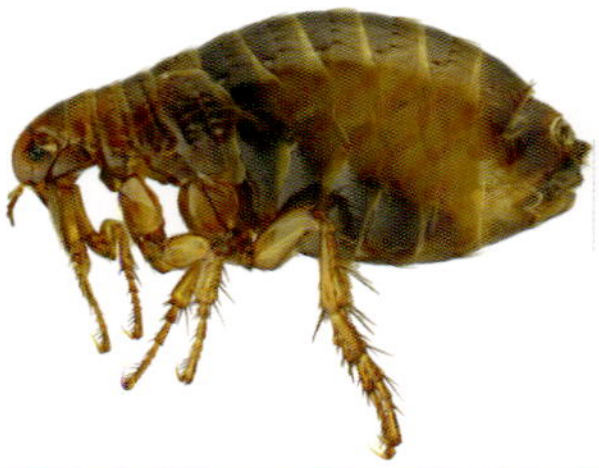 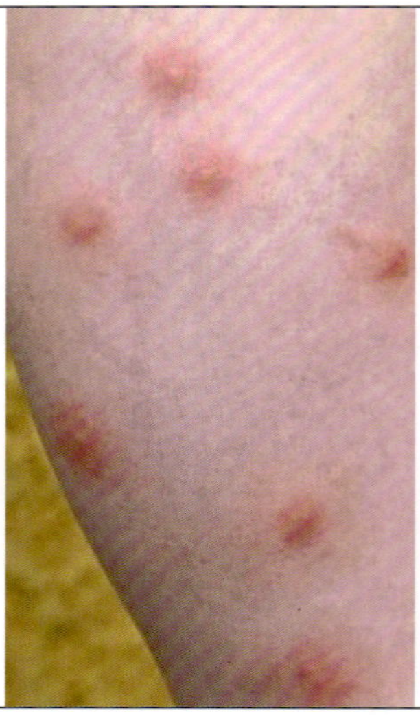
Head Louse (Lice) Pediculus humanus capitis. Live on the human **scalp** feeding on human blood Do not carry disease **Nits:** egg of the louse that attach to hair shaft Transmission: close contact: shared combs, hats, towels, clothing, beds, head to head contact TX: Launder bedding, clothing, stuffed animals, hats, towels. OTC shampoos: **Nix, Rid** or soak hair in vinegar for several minutes. Prescription: **Malathion lotion, Benzyl Alcohol, Lindane Shampoo**	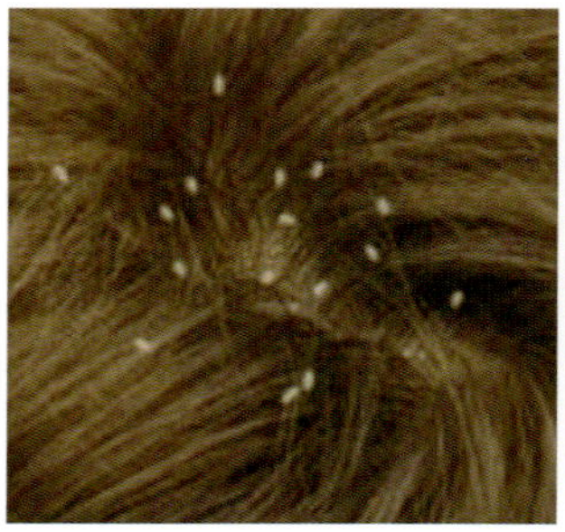 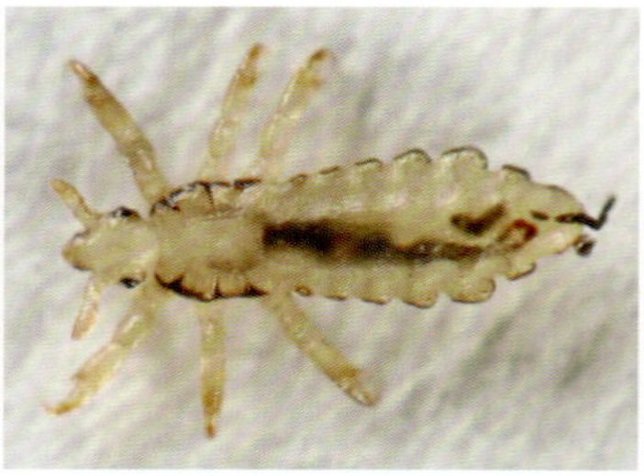
Body Louse (Lice) Pediculus humanus Same as Head Louse, but attaches to **clothing** instead of the base of hair.	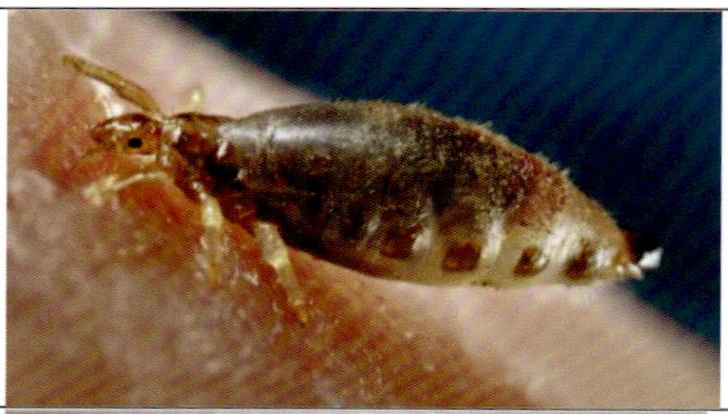
Pubic Louse (Crab Louse) Pthirus pubis, Pediculosis pubis Lives on **pubic hair** or other course hair: eyelashes. Feeds on blood Transmission: Close contact; sexual intercourse. Shared towels, clothing, beds. SX: Itching TX: **Lindane shampoo, Malathion lotion, Permethrin**	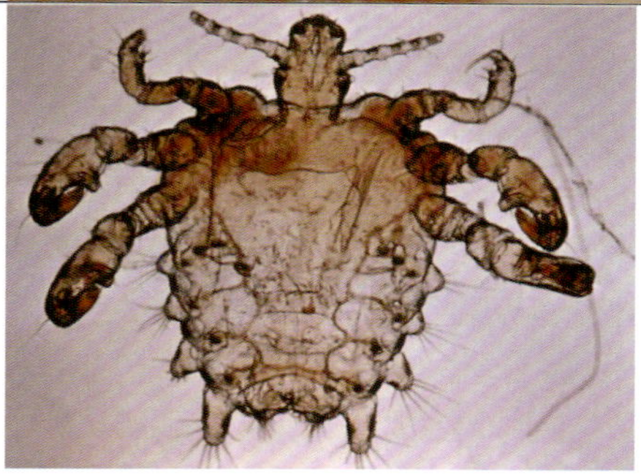

Scabies (Mites) Sarcoptes scabiei SX: Severe itchiness, pimple like rash. **Burrows** under the skin: wrists, finger webs and along waistline (under belt area). Symptoms due to allergic reaction to mites High risk of spread: close quarters: child care facilities, group homes, prisons TX: **Permethrin, Lindane creams, Crotamiton, oral Ivermectin.**	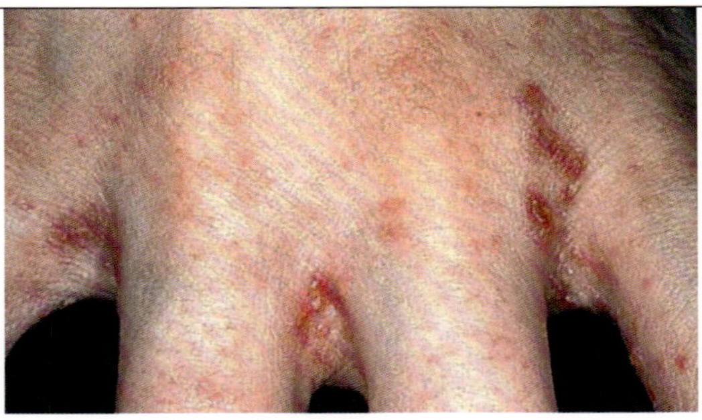
Bed Bug Cimex lectularius Does not spread disease. Located: warm houses, inside of beds and **bedding**, Mainly nocturnal, feeding on blood. Can survive up to 300 days without eating. Dark spots on bedding, rusty stains on sheets. Give off an odor of rotting raspberries. SX: Bites cause red bumps with central dark red spot, pruritus, bites are usually in linear pattern, but can be a cluster. (look hard and red like mosquito bites). Can turn into blisters. Most common on face, neck arms and hands. (Bed bug bites are more red than flea bites). No puncture spot in the central of the bite as seen in a fleabite. TX: Pesticides for the home. Topical steroid creams or oral antihistamines. Oral antibiotics if infection occurs. Prevention: Encase mattress and box spring in an impermeable mattress cover. Put infested bedding and clothing in a dryer for 20+ minutes on high heat, reduce clutter in the room, seal/caulk any holes or cracks, wear PJ's that cover as much skin as possible, tuck in sheets and blankets so no floor contact, place legs of bed into containers of paraffin oil or water to prevent bugs access to bed.	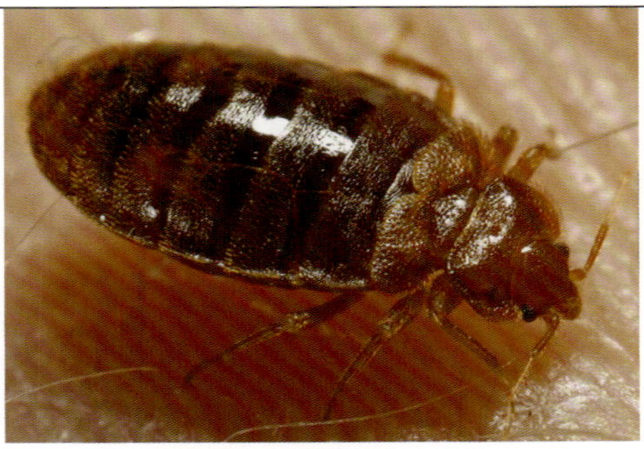 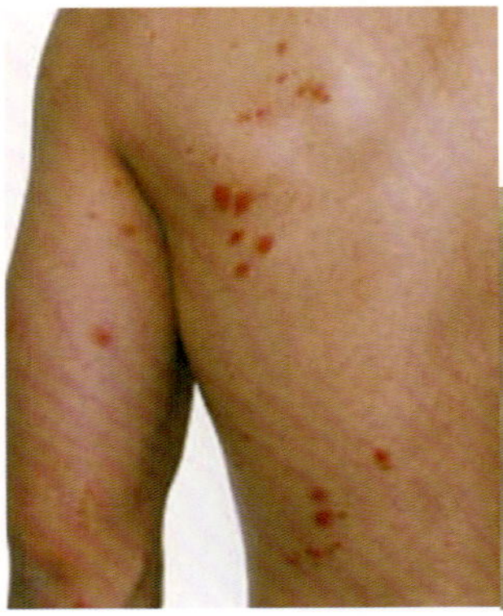 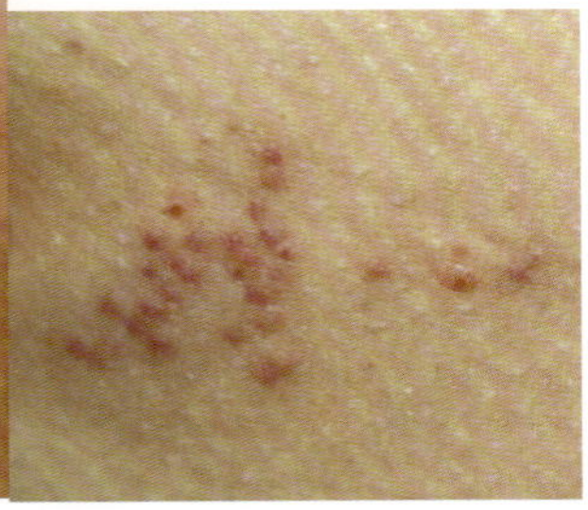

MICROBIOLOGY PHARMACOLOGY
ANTIMICROBIALS

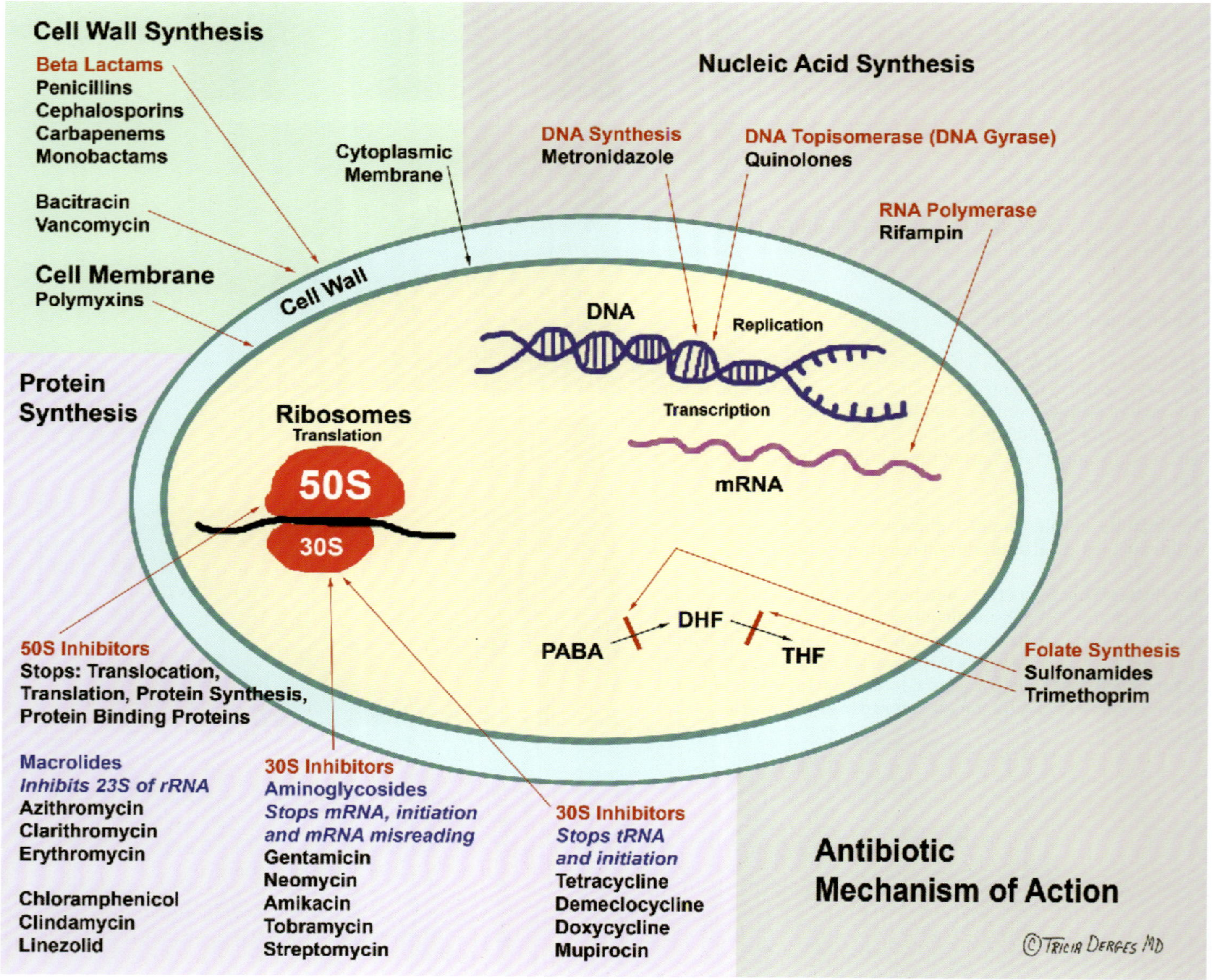

Bacteriostatic

- A biological or chemical agent that stops bacteria from reproducing. It does not kill them. It holds the bacterial "static" until the host defense system can eradicate the bacteria.

Bactericidal

- A biological or chemical agent that kills bacteria.
  Antibiotics.
  Disinfectants: chlorine, iodine, alcohol, acids.
  Antiseptics: iodine, peroxides,, alcohols

The "cillin's"
Penicillin G (IV and IM), V (oral), Ampicillin, Amoxicillin, Oxacillin, Nafcillin, Dicloxacillin, Ticarcillin, Piperacillin

- **MOA: Any of these terms may be used to describe the mechanism of action of the "cillin's"**
  Penicillin-binding proteins (PBP) (AKA: transpeptidase), Blocks transpeptidase cross-linking, blocks cross-linking of peptidoglycan, peptidoglycan cross-linking, changes structure of PBP and stops antibodies from binding.
  stops gene expression, stops initiation, misreading, ANYTHING that stops protein synthesis.
- **Penicillinase enzymes are β-lactamase that hydrolyze and inactivate penicillin**
- **Penicillinase breaks down β-lactam rings in penicillin**
- **B-Lactamase inhibitors are added to the "cillin's" to extend the use of the "cillin". It protects, it keeps the bacteria from breaking down the "cillin". (AKA: It makes the penicillin stronger. AKA: Prolongs the drug.)**
- **Best for Strep Infections: Amoxicillin, Ampicillin, Penicillin**

DRUG **GENERIC name** **Trade name**	**Clinical Use**	**Mechanism of Action and Resistance**	**Toxicity and Notes**
Penicillin G, V (β-lactam drug)	Gram positives cocci and rods, Gram negative cocci, Spirochetes, N. Meningitis, **Syphilis (T. pallidum)** **Penicillinase sensitive.**	See above. Resistance: Penicillinase (used by bacteria) to cleave β-lactam rings.	MCC: **Hypersensitivity reaction**. **Syphilis: if person is allergic to penicillin they must be desensitized and treated. Is also used to treat syphilis in pregnancy.**
Ampicillin **Amoxicillin** (Augmentin: amoxicillin and clavulanic acid)	Same as penicillin but is a wider spectrum (covers more gram negative) and enterococci. **Penicillinase sensitive.** **Ampicillin:** Listeria and intrapartum (during labor) for GBS. **ALWAYS add Ampicillin to any drug regimen when treating Listeria.** **Amoxicillin** (add clavulanic acid): Covers most infections in the "head" region: **Strep, otitis media, bites (animal or human), mouth.** MC drug used in pediatrics.	See above. Resistance: Penicillinase (used by bacteria) to cleave β-lactam rings.	**Hypersensitivity reaction, Pseudomembranous colitis** (AKA: C. difficile) (MC drugs for pseudomembranous colitis: **Clindamycin, Ampicillin, Amoxicillin**) **Jarisch Herxheimer Reaction** (rash): Rash that appears a few days after **Amoxicillin** is used to treat **Strep throat** because the patient actually had **mono**. **Add β-lactamase inhibitor to protect against penicillinase.** **(Clavulanic Acid, Sulbactam, Tazobactam)** **Lyme Disease: If child is under 8 years old or patient is pregnant, must treat Lyme DZ with Amoxicillin** and **not** Doxycycline. Bacteria covered by Ampicillin: **HELPS** (H. influenza, E. coli, Listeria, Proteus, Salmonella.
Nafcillin **Oxacillin** **Dicloxacillin** Methicillin*	**S. aureus** **(does not cover MRSA** because of altered penicillin-binding protein site) (**tip**: Naf for Staff) *Methicillin is no longer on the market. Removed due to ↑↑ interstitial nephritis.	See above. MRSA: (Methicillin Resistant Staph aureus) Resistant to all β-Lactam antibiotics and β-Lactamase resistant antibiotics because penicillin- binding proteins (PBP) are altered so they can't bind.	**Hypersensitivity reaction,** Interstitial Nephritis Nafcillin is high in Na = ↑ risk for heart arrhythmias, kidney problems and seizures. Patients with: Burns, diabetics, Cystic Fibrosis, Neutropenic, ventilators, immunocompromised must be treated with antibiotics that treat **BOTH staph and pseudomonas.**

Piperacillin, Ticarcillin **(add: Tazobactam)**	**Pseudomonas**	See above. Patients with: Burns, diabetics, Cystic Fibrosis, Neutropenic, ventilators, immunocompromised must be treated with antibiotics that treat **BOTH staph and pseudomonas.**	**Add β-lactamase inhibitor to protect against penicillinase. (Clavulanic Acid, Sulbactam, Tazobactam)**

Beta-Lactamase Inhibitors

DRUG GENERIC name Trade name	Clinical Use	Mechanism of Action and Resistance	Toxicity and Notes
Clavulanic Acid Sulbactam Tazobactam	Added to the "cillin's" (penicillin's) to **prevent** the drug from being **broken down**/destroyed by the β-lactamase (penicillinase). It **extends** the use of the drug. (AKA: Makes the drug **stronger**)		Beta-Lactamase drugs are safe in pregnancy.

Penicillin Allergies

- **Most common drug hypersensitivity**
- Only penicillin can be used to treat for syphilis. **If the patient is allergic they must be de-sensitized to penicillin and then treated.**
- Carbapenems are closely related to penicillin so may produce allergic reactions
- **Treatment for penicillin allergies:**
  Anaphylaxis reaction: Epinephrine (IM)
  Allergic reaction: Penicillinase
- **In drug allergies there will eosinophilia**
- **Penicillin Allergy Alternatives**
  - If only a rash reaction: **Cephalosporins**
  - Anaphylaxis: **Macrolides, Clindamycin**
  - For minor infections: **Macrolides, Clindamycin, TMP/SMX**
  - For major infections: **Vancomycin, Linezolid, Telavancin (Vancomycin derivative), Daptomycin**

DRUG GENERIC name Trade name	Clinical Use	Mechanism of Action and Resistance	Toxicity and Notes
Aztreonam	**Monobactam: Penicillin-allergic** patients. (No cross-reaction with penicillin). Patients that can't use aminoglycosides with renal insufficiency. Gram negatives only. Pseudomonas.	Inhibits peptidoglycan cross-linking by binding to PBP.	SX: GI
Macrolides Azithromycin, Erythromycin, Clarithromycin	Use with patients with penicillin allergies.		

Anaphylaxis Reactions

- #1 = Penicillin's
- #2 = Sulfa drugs
- #3 = Cephalosporin's

MSSA Drugs (Staph Sensitive)

- IV: Nafcillin, Oxacillin, Cefazolin (2st generation cephalosporin)
- Oral: Cephalexin (1st generation cephalosporin), Dicloxacillin

MRSA Drugs (Staph Resistant)

- Minor MRSA infections: TMP/SMX, Doxycycline, Clindamycin
- Severe MRSA infections: Vancomycin, Linezolid, Daptomycin, Tigecycline, Telavancin (Vancomycin derivative), Ceftaroline

DRUG **GENERIC name** **Trade name**	**Clinical Use**	**Mechanism of Action and Resistance**	**Toxicity and Notes**
Vancomycin	**MRSA,** Empiric TX with Gentamycin for endocarditis. Gram positives only. C. difficile.	Inhibits **cell wall** peptidoglycans by binding **D-ala D-ala**. AKA: Glycopeptide polymerization stops **cell wall** synthesis. AKA: **Punches holes** in membranes so that **ions leak** out. AKA: Binds **D-ala** on **cell wall** glycoproteins and stops **transpeptidase and PBP** from **cross linking** so that it stops protein synthesis. Resistance: Modification of D-ala D-ala to D-ala D-lac. Resistance: Plasmids encode resistances to vancomycin. **So a ↓ in plasmids lead to a ↓ in vancomycin resistance.** (Plasmids also encode resistances to erythromycin, gentamicin and streptomycin).	Ototoxic, Nephrotoxic, Thrombophlebitis. **Red Man's Syndrome**: Diffuse flushing and itching due to **too rapid** of infusion rate. **Mediated by histamine**. (Mast cells are irritated and degranulated releasing histamine). TX: pretreat with antihistamines (diphenhydramine) and reduce rate of infusion.
Linezolid	**Use when Vancomycin allergy/resistant.** In Vancomycin resistant: Isolate patient in a negative pressure room and switch to Linezolid.	Inhibits 23s subunit of the 50s ribosome and stops protein synthesis. It specifically stops the **initiation** complex.	**Bone marrow suppression** (must monitor CBC), thrombocytopenia, optic neuritis, and serotonin syndrome. (**tip**: "Line"zolid is in a line, your bones are in a line = bone marrow)
Daptomycin	**Alternative to Vancomycin**	Depolarizes cell membrane. Disrupts the cell membrane.	**Myopathies (↑ CPK),** muscle weakness. Inactivated by surfactant. (**tip**: dapto "mycin" = Mycin has to do with muscles)

Cephalosporins

Mechanism of Action

- **Inhibit cell wall synthesis.**
- **AKA: Stop transpeptidases**
  AKA: Stops binding of PCP

Toxicities

- Do not use with Aminoglycosides (↑ risk of nephrotoxicity)
- Hypoprothrombinemia and disulfiram-like reaction:
  This is because the **MTT side chain** (N-methylthiotetrazole, the make up of cephalosporin's) blocks the enzyme **Vitamin K epoxide reductase** (causing hypothrombinemia because of Vitamin K deficiency = ↑ bleeding) and blocks aldehyde dehydrogenase (causing alcohol intolerance). (AKA: They **deplete prothrombin** = ↑ risk of bleeding). This is most common with Cefoxitin and Cefotetan.
- MRSA, Listeria, Enterococcus are resistant to all forms of cephalosporin's (except Ceftaroline that covers MRSA).
- Cephalosporin's can be used as an alternative if there is a penicillin allergy (indicated by a rash) because there is <3% chance of a cross reaction. However if there is an anaphylactic reaction to penicillin then do not use a cephalosporin, use a non-beta-lactam antibiotic.

DRUG **GENERIC name** **Trade name**	**Clinical Use**	**Mechanism of Action and Resistance**	**Toxicity and Notes**
1st Generation			
Cefazolin (IV) **Cephalexin** *Keflex* Cephradine *Infexin, Intracef* Cefadroxyl (**tip**: the xins and lins)	Gram positive cocci, E. coli, Proteus, Klebsiella (narrow gram negative spectrum) **Cefazolin:** **Antibiotic administered prior to surgeries to prevent S. aureus infections.**	See above.	See above
2nd Generation			
Cefaclor Cefoxitin Cefuroxime Cefotetan Cefprozil Loracarbef (**tip**: the "F"s. it's a FACt the FOX has FUR)	Gran positive cocci, wider gram negative spectrum: 1st generation gram negatives plus: H. influenza, Enterobacter, Serratia, Neisseria. Cefoxitin, Cefotetan: cover anaerobes.	See above.	See above Note: Cefoxitin and Cefotetan are the only cephalosporins that cover anaerobes. Cefoxitin and Cefotetan may ↑ the risk of bleeding due to depletion of prothrombin (see details under toxicities of cephalosporin's above).
3rd Generation			
Ceftriaxone **Ceftazidime** Cefotaxime Cefoperazone (tip: the "**T**'s" for the **T**hird: TRI, TAZ, TAX)	Gram negatives. **Ceftriaxone: Gonorrhea, Meningitis: they penetrate the CNS.** (**tip**: ceftriaxGONE for GONEorrhea) **Ceftazidime** **Cefoperazone:** **Pseudomonas** (**tip**: the "**pime**'s and **dime**'s are for pseudomonas)	See above.	See above **Ceftriaxone**: **Do not give to babies** < 2 months because is liver is not mature (↓UDP-glucuronyl transferase = jaundice and kernicterus). Use Cefotaxime instead. **Ceftriaxone: When treating gonorrhea: MUST add Azithromycin or Doxycycline to cover Chlamydia.**

4th Generation			
Cefepime	**Pseudomonas** (nosocomial pneumonia) (**tip**: the "**pime**'s and **dime**'s are for pseudomonas)		See above
5th Generation			
Ceftaroline (**tip**: "Tar"ribly expensive!)	**C. difficile,** Gram positive, gram negative, simple anaerobes, MRSA. Does NOT cover Pseudomonas. (**very** expensive drug)		See above Ceftaroline is the only cephalosporin that covers MRSA.

Carbapenems

DRUG **GENERIC name** **Trade name**	**Clinical Use**	**Mechanism of Action and Resistance**	**Toxicity and Notes**
Imipenem Meropenem Ertapenem Doripenem (**tip**: CARBON copy of penicillin)	**Gram-positive cocci, gram-negative rods, anaerobes, pseudomonas.** Ertapenem is the only Carbapenem that **does not** cover pseudomonas.	B-Lactamase resistant	Seizures, Stevens Johnson, CNS toxicity, GI symptoms. **Imipenem** = ↑ **risk of seizures**. MUST administer **Cilastatin** with it. (Cilastatin inhibits **dehydropeptidase** – enzyme in the kidney that degrades imipenem. Cilastatin protects Imipenem from this enzyme and prolongs its antibacterial effects) **Meropenem** = has **least** risk of seizures. Do not use if patient has penicillin allergies. There is a 50% cross over of having the same reaction. Carbapenems are "carbons" to penicillin.

ANTIBIOTICS “SHORTSTOP” CHART

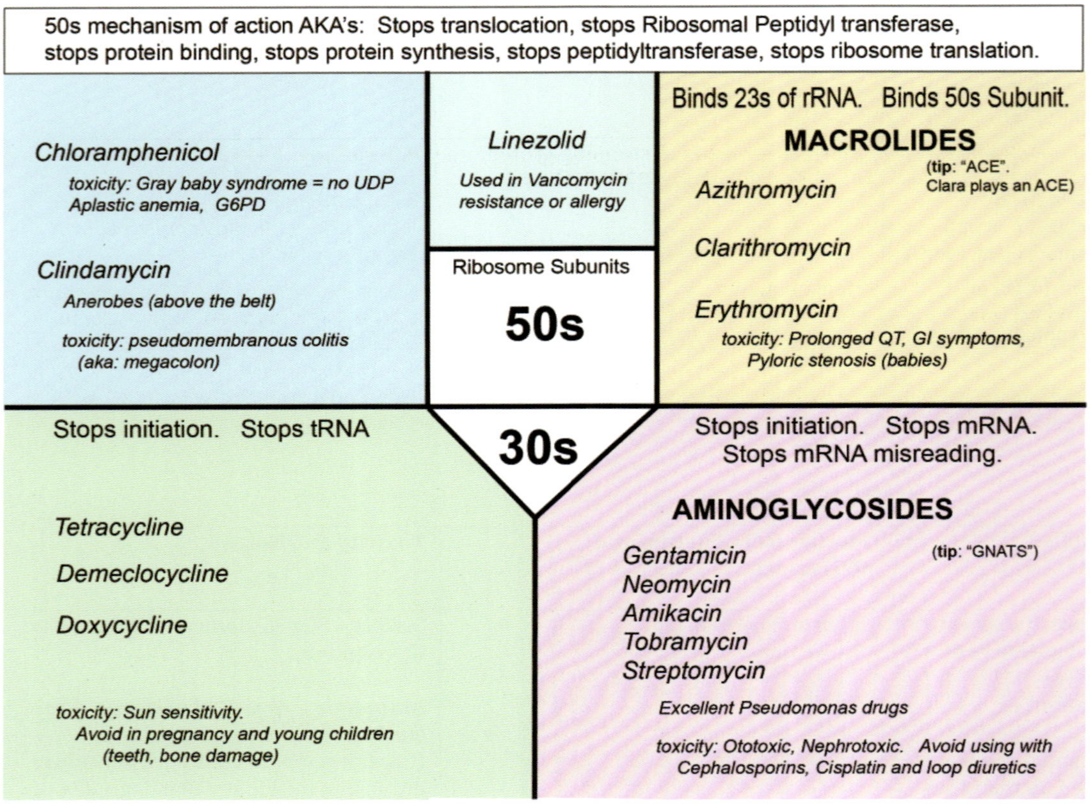

Chloramphenicol, Clindamycin

DRUG GENERIC name Trade name	Clinical Use	Mechanism of Action and Resistance	Toxicity and Notes
Chloramphenicol	Bacterial meningitis, S. Pneumo, Rocky Mountain Spotted Fever	Blocks peptidyltransferase at 50S ribosomal unit. AKA: Stops ribosome peptidyltransferase. AKA: Stops protein synthesis. Stops protein binding. Bacteriostatic. Resistance: Plasmid-encoded acetyltransferase inactivates drug.	Aplastic anemia, pancytopenia, **Gray baby syndrome** (MC: premature infants due to lack of **UDP-glucuronyl transferase**)
Clindamycin (**Tip**: Clindamycin stops anaerobes above the belt, Metronidazole stops anaerobes below the belt)	**Anaerobes.** C. perfringens, Bacteroides, aspiration pneumonia, lung abscesses, Group A Strep.	Stops translocation at 50S ribosomal unit. AKA: Stops ribosome peptidyltransferase. AKA: Stops protein synthesis. Stops protein binding.	**Pseudomembranous colitis** AKA: C. difficile. AKA: Biomass overgrowth. (MC drugs for pseudomembranous colitis: **Clindamycin, Ampicillin. Amoxicillin**)

Macrolides

DRUG GENERIC name Trade name	Clinical Use	Mechanism of Action and Resistance	Toxicity and Notes
Azithromycin **Clarithromycin** **Erythromycin** (**tip**: ACE)	Atypical pneumonias (Outpatient pneumonias), **Chlamydia,** Patients with penicillin allergies for gram-positive cocci infections. **Azithromycin:** Prophylaxis treatment for **Mycobacterium Avium.** Must start prophylaxis once CD4 count reaches 200. Avium is contracted with the CD4 count drops to 50. Erythromycin **ointment:** TX for neonatal Chlamydia or Gonorrhea conjunctivitis.	Blocks translocation stopping protein synthesis. Binds the 23S rRNA of the 50S ribosomal unit. AKA: Blocks peptidyltransferase at 50S ribosomal unit. AKA: Stops ribosome peptidyltransferase. AKA: Stops protein synthesis. Stops protein binding. Bacteriostatic.	**Macrolides: P-450 Inhibitors.** **Prolonged QT interval, GI issues** (diarrhea), cholestatic hepatitis. Note: **Azithromycin and Doxycycline** can be **interchanged**. Either can be used. Example: If you look in the answers for Azithromycin for TX of Chlamydia and do not see it, look for Doxycycline.

Aminoglycosides

DRUG GENERIC name Trade name	Clinical Use	Mechanism of Action and Resistance	Toxicity and Notes
Gentamicin **Neomycin** **Amikacin** **Tobramycin** **Streptomycin** (**tip**: GNATS can kill pseudomonas)	**Pseudomonas,** Gram negative. Synergistic with β-Lactam antibiotics. No anaerobe coverage. Synergistic with beta-lactam's for staph and enterococci infections. (Need oxygen to enter the bacteria's cell membrane). **Neomycin** used for bowel surgery. **Gentamicin**: used in empiric therapy with vancomycin in endocarditis.	Stops initiation. Misreads mRNA. Stops translocation (aka: protein synthesis intracellularly) at the 30s subunit on the ribosome. Resistance: Bacterial transferase enzymes inactivate the drug.	**Do not use with Cephalosporin's or with Loop Diuretics = ↑ risk of ototoxicity and nephrotoxicity (kidney failure).**

"Cyclines"

DRUG GENERIC name Trade name	Clinical Use	Mechanism of Action and Resistance	Toxicity and Notes
Tetracycline **Doxycycline** Minocycline	**Doxycycline:** **Lyme Disease (Borrelia burgdorferi), Rocky Mountain Spotted Fever (Rickettsia), Chlamydia, Ehrlichia, Mycoplasma, MRSA (cellulitis: skin/soft tissue)** **M. pneumonia (Walking pneumonia)** **Tetracycline: Acne**	Stops tRNA. Binds to the 30S ribosomal subunit. Resistance: **Transports pumps (ATP** generated) pumps drug out of the cell (AKA: ↑ **efflux**).	**Teratogen and in young children: Discolors teeth and inhibits bone growth.** **Photosensitivity:** blisters skin after being in sun or sunbeds. (watch for teens on tetracycline for acne). Do not take with Ca, Mg or Iron products (milk, antacids) because absorption in the gut is inhibited. **Doxycycline for Lyme DZ: If child is under 8 years old or patient is pregnant, must treat Lyme DZ with Amoxicillin.** **Expired Tetracycline: Fanconi's Syndrome** (leads to renal tubular acidosis)

Fluoroquinolones (AKA: the "Floxacin's")

DRUG GENERIC name Trade name	Clinical Use	Mechanism of Action and Resistance	Toxicity and Notes
Ciprofloxacin **Levofloxacin** Norfloxacin, Ofloxacin, Sparfloxacin Moxifloxacin Gemifloxacin Enoxacin Nalidixic Acid	Gram-negative rods, gram positives. UTI's and GI tract infections. N. meningitis, Best TX for **Community acquired pneumonia**, pseudomonas. Ciprofloxacin: cystitis, pyelonephritis. Diverticulitis (multi-drug TX): Ciprofloxacin, Levofloxacin, Gemifloxacin can be used but must be combined with Metronidazole. Diverticulitis: Single drug TX: Moxifloxacin (do not need to add Metronidazole).	**Inhibits DNA gyrase (AKA: topoisomerase).** AKA: Binds DNA gyrase. Bactericidal. Resistance: Genes encoding for DNA gyrase. Efflux pumps.	**Tendon rupture, tendonitis, cartilage damage.** Do not take in pregnancy. Prolonged QT interval, GI symptoms. **Ciprofloxacin: P-450 Inhibitor.**

Misc. Antibiotics

DRUG GENERIC name Trade name	Clinical Use	Mechanism of Action and Resistance	Toxicity and Notes
Metronidazole *Flagyl*	**Giardia, Entamoeba, Trichomonas, Bacterial Vaginitis (Gardnerella), Anaerobes (C. difficile, Bacteroides).** (Treats anaerobes below the belt, clindamycin treats anaerobes above the belt) (**tip**: GET GAP on the metro) **Used with Triple Therapy for H. pylori infection with: Clarithromycin and Omeprazole (PPI).** **Antabuse:** Disulfiram-like effect to aid in stopping drinking.	Forms free radicals that damage the DNA in the bacteria. Bactericidal.	**Disulfiram-like reaction**. ("Hangover symptoms" when alcohol is used while on this drug). Metronidazole **inhibits aldehyde dehydrogenase.** Metal taste in the mouth. Do not use in pregnancy: mutagenesis. If breastfeeding: Must stop breastfeeding for 2 – 3 days while on the drug, then resume breastfeeding.
Sulfonamides: **Sulfa-methoxazole (SMX),** **Sulfisoxazole, Sulfadiazine.**	**Sulfamethoxazole is used in combination with Trimethoprim** **TMP/SMX: used for UTI's, Pneumocystis jiroveci (PCP), MRSA (cellulitis: skin/soft tissue)**	Inhibits **folate synthesis**. **PABA** (Para-aminobenzoic acid inhibits **dihydropteroate synthase**. AKA: Stops nucleotides. Bacteriostatic. Resistance: Alters the dihydropteroate synthase to decrease uptake or increase synthesis of PABA.	**If patient is G6PD deficient will cause hemolysis, nephrotoxic (interstitial nephritis), photosensitivity, kernicterus in infants.** **Sulfonamides: P-450 Inhibitor.** **Do not use TMP/SMX in UTI's during pregnancy. Can use: DOC = Nitrofurantoin** (Macrobid), Amoxicillin, Amoxicillin + Clavulanate acid, Cephalexin.
Trimethoprim **Pyrimethamine**	**Sulfamethoxazole is used in combination with Trimethoprim** **TMP/SMX: used for UTI's, Pneumocystis jiroveci (PCP). MRSA (cellulitis: skin/soft tissue)** **TMP/Pyrimethamine: prophylaxis for toxoplasmosis.**	Inhibits Dihydrofolate Reductase. Bacteriostatic.	Megaloblastic anemia (lack of folate), supplement with folinic acid (folate). Note: When treating PCP (Pneumocystis jiroveci) you must **add steroids** in the PaO2 < 70% or the A-a gradient is > 35. It will improve their breathing.

Nitrofurantoin	**Treatment of UTI's in pregnancy.** (Other antibiotics approved for UTI's in pregnancy: Amoxicillin, Cephalexin)	Damages bacterial DNA.	Nausea, headache, flatulence, dizziness, pruritus, **pulmonary fibrosis**
Mupirocin *Bactroban, Centany* **Retapamulin** *Altabax, Altargo*	**Impetigo**, furuncles, MRSA (for short term only. Long term will develop resistance).	Reversibly binds tRNA synthetase on 50S subunit in S. aureus and Strep to inhibit protein synthesis.	Resistance may develop if used for prolong periods.
Bacitracin (triple antibiotic ointment) Neosporin	**Group A Strep** Gram positive, gram negative. (**tip**: BRAS: Strep B = Bacitracin resistant, Strep A – Bacitracin sensitive)	Stops cell wall synthesis.	
Fidaxomicin	Clostridium difficile, Gram positives.	Inhibits RNA polymerase to stop protein synthesis and cause bacterial cell death. Bactericidal.	

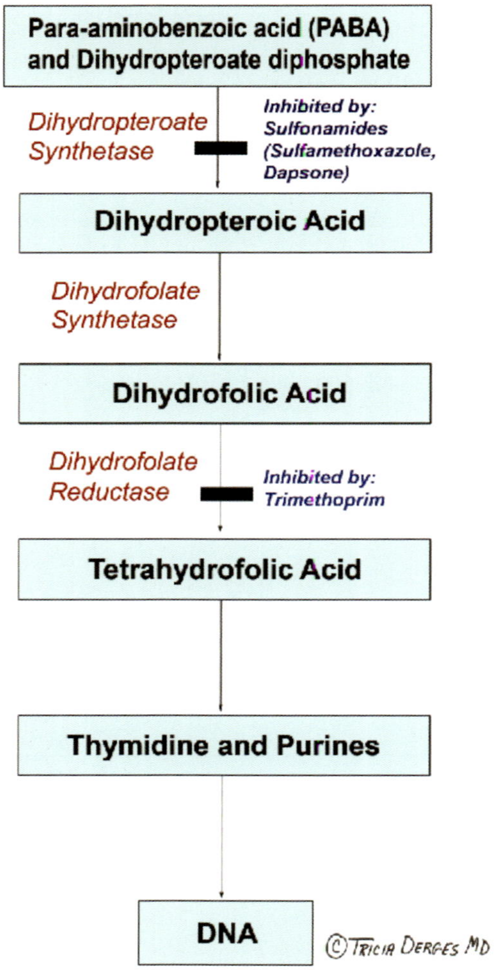

Mycobacterium Tuberculosis Treatment Regimen

- Pathway to TB: IL12 = TH-1 = INFγ = macrophages and CD8 = granulomas = inflammation and caseous necrosis = damage to lung tissue.

DRUG GENERIC name Trade name	Clinical Use	Mechanism of Action and Resistance	Toxicity and Notes
Isoniazid (INH)	Treatment and Prophylaxis for Mycobacterium Tuberculosis Prophylaxis treatment given with a positive PPD test and a negative chest x-ray. **INH and Vitamin B6 (Pyridoxine)** are **given for 9 months.**	Enzyme catalase-peroxidase (AKA: katG gene) inhibits the synthesis of mycolic acid (component of the cell wall in TB). Resistance: No expression of catalase peroxidase.	**P-450 Inhibitor.** **Hepatotoxicity.** Neurotoxicity (prevented with B6), **Drug induced SLE.** The only TB drug that can be used as a solo prophylaxis for TB (with B6).
Rifampin **Rifabutin**	Treatment regimen for TB. **Prophylaxis for:** **N. meningitis exposure and H. influenza type B.**	Inhibits DNA-dependent RNA polymerase. Resistance: Stops RNA synthesis. AKA: Altered structure of enzymes in RNA synthesis.	**P-450 Inducer** **Orange body fluids** (Benign) (Orange tears, sweat, urine) Can't be used in TB prophylaxis because of genetic mutations.
Pyrazinamide	Treatment regimen for TB. TX intracellular organisms.	Inhibits mycolic acid by stopping mycobacterial fatty acid.	**Hyperuricemia (Gout),** Hepatotoxicity
Ethambutol	Treatment regimen for TB.	Blocks **arabinosyltransferase** so ↓ carbohydrate polymerization in the cell wall.	**Color blindness** (optic neuropathy)

Pneumonia Treatments

Community Acquired

- Ceftriaxone (S. pneumo)
- Azithromycin/; Doxycycline
- Fluoroquinolones
- Ampicillin + Sulbactam

Nosocomial

- Vancomycin
- Cefepime (Pseudomonas)
- Ciprofloxacin

Bugs: Mites, Louse, Scabies

DRUG GENERIC name Trade name	Clinical Use	Mechanism of Action and Resistance	Toxicity and Notes
Permethrin	**Scabies, head lice, louse, mites**	Neurotoxin. Affects neuron membranes by ↑ Na channel activation.	Skin irritation, burning.
Ivermectin	**Scabies,** Onchocerca volvulus, Loa Loa, Onchocerciasis (river blindness)	Interferes with nervous system and muscle function by inhibiting neurotransmission.	CNS depression, ataxia.

Antibiotics General Quick Reference

Penicillin Allergy Alternatives If only a rash reaction: **Cephalosporins** If Anaphylaxis: **Macrolides (Azithromycin, Clarithromycin), Clindamycin** For minor infections: **Macrolides (Azithromycin, Clarithromycin), Clindamycin, TMP/SMX** For major infections: **Vancomycin, Linezolid, Telavancin (Vancomycin derivative), Daptomycin**	**MSSA Drugs (Staph Sensitive)** **IV: Nafcillin, Oxacillin, Cefazolin (2st generation cephalosporin).** (More effective than Vancomycin in organism is sensitive). **Oral: Cephalexin (1st generation cephalosporin), Dicloxacillin**
MRSA Drugs (Staph Resistant) **Minor MRSA infections: TMP/SMX, Doxycycline, Clindamycin, Linezolid** **Severe MRSA infections: Vancomycin, Linezolid** (thrombocytopenia), **Daptomycin** (↑ CPK, myopathy), **Tigecycline (also gm negatives), Telavancin (Vancomycin derivative), Ceftaroline**	**Pseudomonas Infections** Aminoglycosides (Amikacin), Ceftazidime, Cefepime, Quinolones (Ciprofloxacin, **Levofloxacin, Gemifloxacin, Moxifloxacin**), Piperacillin plus Tazobactam, Ticarcillin plus Tazobactam, Polymyxins, Aztreonam, Carbapenems (Imipenem, Meropenem. Note: Ertapenem **does not** cover Pseudomonas)
Strep Infections Amoxicillin, Augmentin (Amoxicillin plus beta lactam), Penicillin, Ampicillin (Both Strep and Staph: Amoxicillin, Ampicillin, Penicillin)	**Anaerobic Infections** Respiratory Infections (**Above the diaphragm**): **Clindamycin**, Penicillin G, Ampicillin, Amoxicillin. GI Infections (**Below the diaphragm**): **Metronidazole (most effective)**, Piperacillin plus Tazobactam, Piperacillin plus Tazobactam, **Carbapenems (Most effective: Strep, Staph (sensitive)**, Cefotetan, Cefoxitin. (only cephalosporin's that cover anaerobes).
Strep Infections Amoxicillin, Augmentin (Amoxicillin plus beta lactam), Penicillin, Ampicillin (Both Strep and Staph: Amoxicillin, Ampicillin, Penicillin)	**NO Anaerobic Coverage** Fluoroquinolones, Oxacillin, Nafcillin, Aminoglycosides, Aztreonam, All Cephalosporins except Cefotetan and Cefoxitin
Gram Negative Infections (Aminoglycosides) Gentamicin, Amikacin, Tobramycin, (Penicillins) Piperacillin plus Tazobactam, Piperacillin plus Tazobactam, (Quinolones) Ciprofloxacin, Levofloxacin, Moxifloxacin, Gemifloxacin, (Cephalosporins) Cefepime, Ceftazidime, (Monobactam) Aztreonam, (Carbapenems) Imipenem, Meropenem, Doripenem, Ertapenem.	**Skin Infections** Impetigo: Topical Mupirocin, Retapamulin. Cellulitis: Minor: Oral Dicloxacillin, Cephalexin (*Keflex*). Severe: IV: Oxacillin, Nafcillin, Cefazolin. Erysipelas: Oral Dicloxacillin, Cephalexin (*Keflex*). Abscess/Boils/Carbuncles/Furuncles/Folliculitis: Same TX as used in Cellulitis.
Infections of: Head, Neck, Ear, Throat, Bites Otitis Media (children): Amoxicillin plus beta lactam (Augmentin) Otitis Externa (adults): Polymyxin/Neomycin, Ofloxacin Bites (animal or human): Amoxicillin plus beta lactam (Augmentin) Pharyngitis (Strep Throat): Amoxicillin plus beta lactam (Augmentin) or Penicillin. Sinusitis: Amoxicillin plus beta lactam (Augmentin) and add inhaled steroids.	**Endocarditis** Empiric: Combination of Gentamicin and Vancomycin Prophylaxis: Amoxicillin Staph aureus: IV Nafcillin, Oxacillin, Cefazolin Staph epidermidis: Vancomycin Staph (resistant): Vancomycin Enterococci: Ampicillin and Gentamicin Fungal: Amp B and valve replacement Strep viridans: IV Ceftriaxone
STD's Gonorrhea: Ceftriaxone IM Chlamydia: Oral Azithromycin or Doxycycline In Patient: Gonorrhea: IV Cefoxitin Chlamydia: Oral Doxycycline In Pregnancy: Gonorrhea: Ceftriaxone IM Chlamydia: Oral Azithromycin 1° and 2° Syphilis: IM Penicillin Tertiary Syphilis: IV Penicillin	**Tick-Borne Diseases** Lyme: Early: Oral Doxycycline Late (CNS/Cardiac involved): IV Ceftriaxone Pregnancy or children < 8 yrs old: Amoxicillin Babesiosis: Azithromycin, Atovaquone Ehrlichia: Doxycycline

UTI's, Pyelonephritis, Prostatitis, Epididymitis	Synergistic Drugs
Uncomplicated: Oral TMP/SMX for 3 days. If resistant: Oral Ciprofloxacin, Levofloxacin Complicated: Oral TMP/SMX for 7 days or Ciprofloxacin. (Complicated: anatomic obstruction: stone, tumor) Pregnancy: Nitrofurantoin, Ampicillin, Cephalexin, Erythromycin. Prostatitis: Oral Ciprofloxacin. Epididymitis due to gonorrhea and chlamydia : Oral Azithromycin and Cefixime Epididymitis due to E. coli: Oral Ofloxacin, Levofloxacin.	**Aminoglycosides (against Staph and enterococcus)**

Antibiotics to Avoid in Pregnancy

Aminoglycosides	Ototoxicity
Chloramphenicol	UDP – Gray baby
Clarithromycin	Embryotoxic
Fluoroquinolones	Cartilage/tendon damage
Griseofulvin	Teratogenic
Ribavirin	Teratogenic
Sulfonamides	Kernicterus
Tetracyclines	Discolored teeth, inhibits bone growth

MYCOLOGY and PARASITES
MYCOLOGY

- DX: KOH prep (KOH picks up the chitin in the fungi outer wall because it does not break down)
- Cold = mold
- Heat = yeast (in the body)

Systemic Mycoses

Blastomycosis

Broad base budding **Dimorphic fungi (cold = 20° is a mold) and (heat = 37° is a yeast in the body/tissues)** Found: **NE and SE US, East of Mississippi river and Central America.** **Infection source**: soil, rotting wood. No person-to-person transmission. (**tip:** Atlantic City is in the NE United States so you think of having a BLAST in Atlantic City) 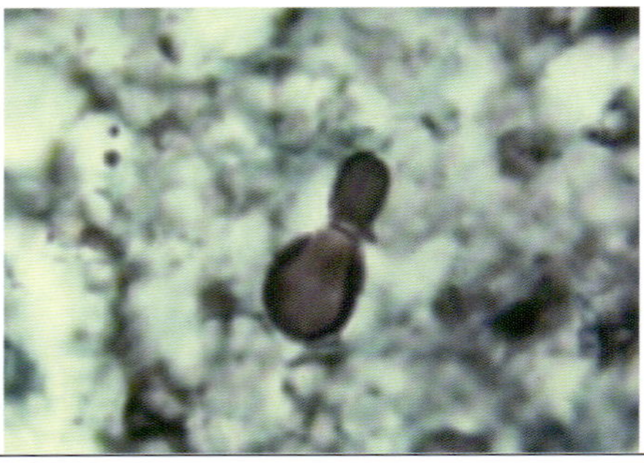	↑ Pneumonia in **immuno COMPETENT (non-sick)** CXR: lungs show **dense consolidation and granulomatous nodules** that can disseminate to skin and bone. SX: Skin, **bone lesions**, fatigue, weight loss, **prostate** problems, joint/**bone** pain, **ulcers or blisters on skin.** Heaped up lesions on skin with violet color with well-marked boarders. 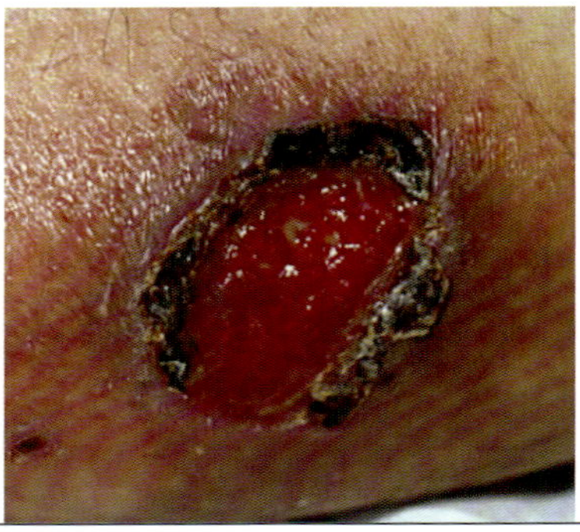	DX: check sputum with Potassium hydroxide TX: Local infections: **Fluconazole or Itraconazole** Systemic infections: **IV Amphotericin B** (**tip**: Blastomycosis: Think all "B"s: Affects the **B**alls (prostate), **B**ones, **B**oils, (ulcers on skin), **B**listers, looks like a **B**owling **B**all and is **B**road **B**ase **B**udding).

Coccidioidomycosis

Spherule filled with endospores AKA: San Joaquin Valley Fever (**tip**: they fight cocks in the SW) **Infection source**: Dry areas. Spores are in the dust and are breathed in most commonly after dust storms and earthquakes. Shows hyphae at 25° and single cells (**endospores** at 37°) Found: **Southwestern USA (CA, NM, AZ, UT).** (**tip:** Las Vegas is in the SW United States and when you think of this city you think of "coc's") 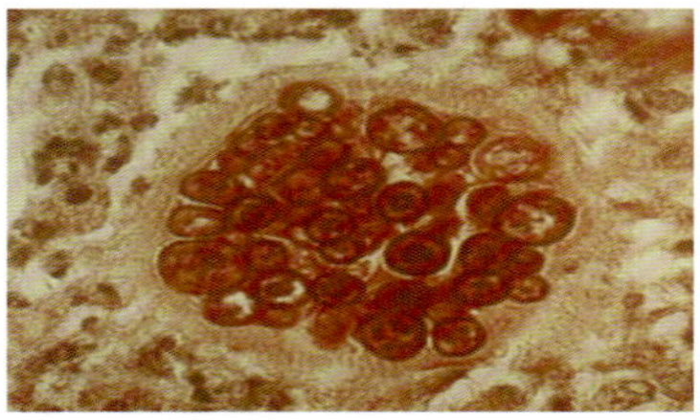 **Endospores**	Pneumonia and meningitis Usually seen in **HIV only** CXR: lungs show **pulmonary infiltrate, hilar adenopathy**, pleural **effusions**. Can disseminate to skin and bones. SX: Night sweats, fever, cough, **granulomas**, pleuritic chest pain, bone lesions, **maculopapular rash** (AKA: "desert bumps" = **erythema nodosum**), joint pain (AKA: "desert rheumatism" = **arthralgia** No person to person transmission	TX: Local infections: **Fluconazole or Itraconazole** Systemic infections: **IV Amphotericin B** 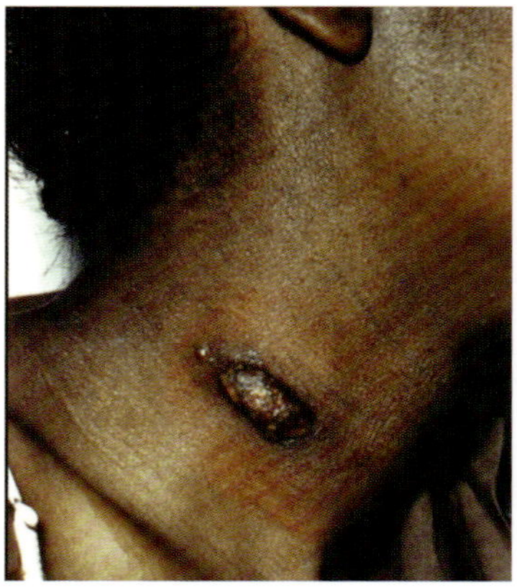

Histoplasmosis

Macrophage filled with Histoplasma Spores with budding yeast (**tip:** "**Histo hide**"s in macrophages) AKA: Intracellular **macroconidia** with spikes. AKA: **Ovoid cells** in macrophages AKA: Yeast cells with thin walls AKA: Huge hepatocytes Found: **Ohio River valley, MS, MO.** **Infection Source**: Wet/damp areas: Cave explorers due to contact with infected bat guano (AKA: spelunking), chicken farming, raccoons. No person to person transmission	**Acute** Pneumonia CXR: lungs show **reticulonodular** (**nodules**) pattern with hilar lymphadenopathy SX: Fever, weight loss, **mouth ulcers**, **palate ulcers**, hepatosplenomegaly, night sweats. Most common with HIV patients DX: BIT: **antigen in urine or sputum** **MAT: Biopsy with culture.** 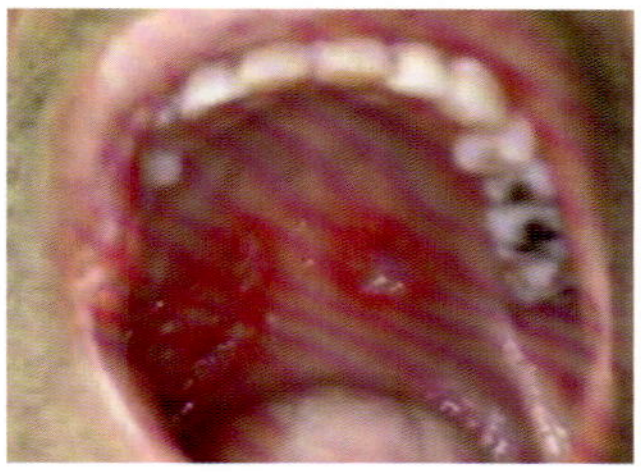	TX: Local infections: **Fluconazole or Itraconazole** Systemic infections: **IV Amphotericin B** 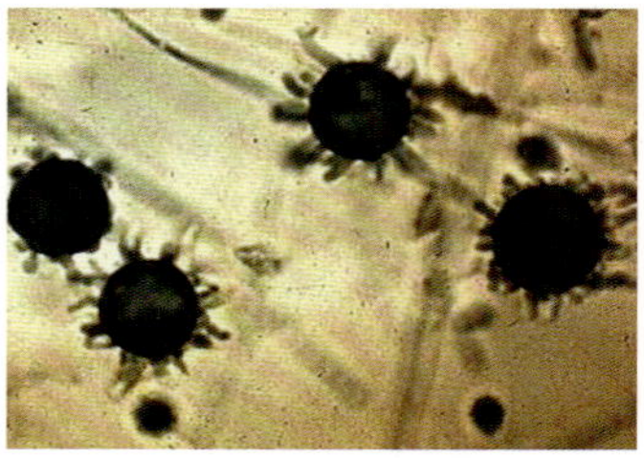 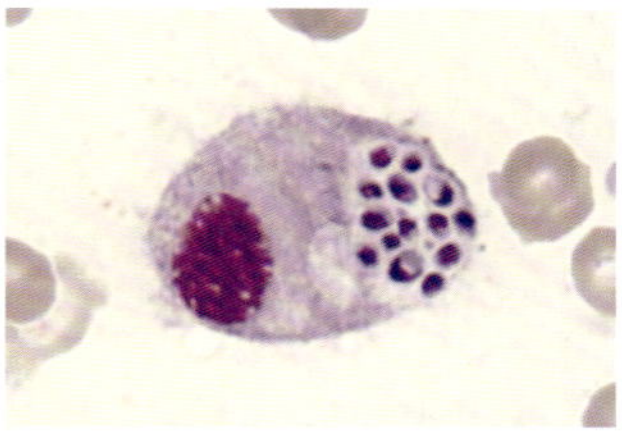 Histo hides in macrophages

Paracoccidioidomycosis
(AKA: Brazilian blastomycosis, South American blastomycosis)

Cells covered in budding **blastoconidia** Dimorphic fungus AKA: Budding yeast in a "Captains wheel" or wheel shape formation. Multiple buds differ from Coccidiomycosis Found: **Latin America** (South America, Brazil)	Can affect immunocompetent host Begins as lobar pneumonia or pleurisy. SX: **Painful lesions on lips and on oral mucosa (cutaneous ulcers),** weight loss, fever, cough	**TX:** **Sulfonamides, Itraconazole or Amphotericin B** Looks like a captains wheel of a ship. (**tip**: The ship is going south to Brazil). 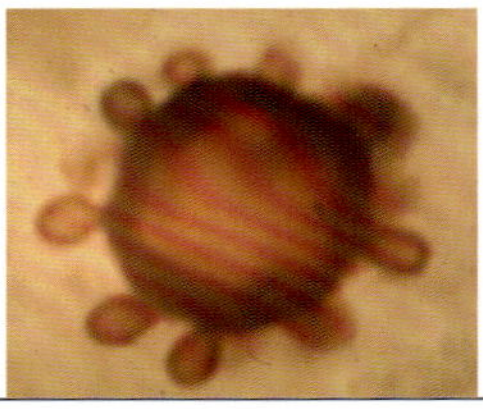

Cutaneous Mycoses

Tinea versicolor

Cause: Malassezia furfur MOA: degradation of lipids produces acids that damage melanocytes. Occurs most often (after being overheated) **after sun exposure, tanning beds, after hot shower, exercise** SX: pigmented patches (hypo or hyperpigmented) DX: microscope shows "spaghetti and meatballs" TX: **Miconazole, selenium sulfide (Selsun), Ketoconazole**	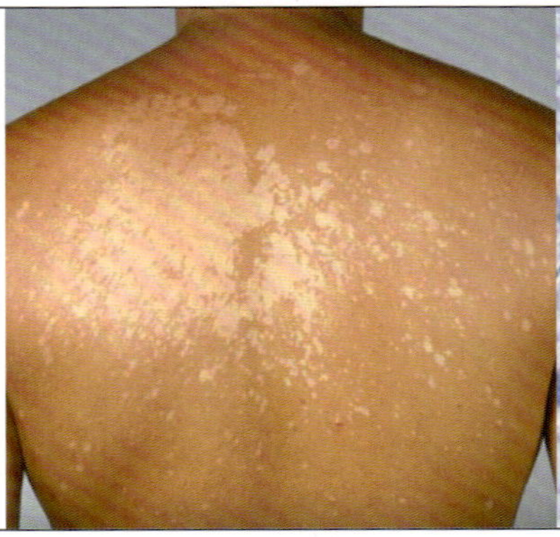 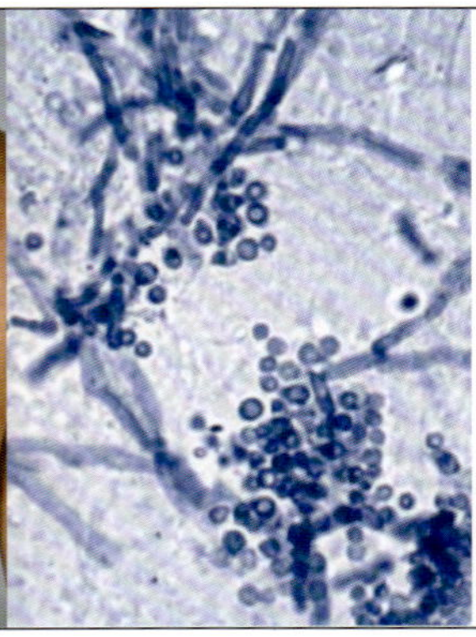

Dermatophytoses

- Keratinized epithelium (dead layer)
- For all Tinea infections:
  BIT: **KOH** (potassium hydroxide prep) (dissolves skin cells but leaves the fungi visible).
  MAT: Fungal culture.
  TX: For all tinea infections **EXCEPT** nail (tinea unguium) and hair (tinea capitis) infections: use topical antifungals.
  For nail or hair treatment: use oral medications: **Terbinafine** (check LFT's first) or **Itraconazole.**

Tinea cruris (**groin**, jock itch, eczema marginatum) Dermatophyte	Source: Tight, restrictive clothing (jockstraps) trap heat and moisture, sharing towels. SX: Inflammation of: groin, anal area, upper thigh (does not include genitals), sharp boarders, spreading with central clearing, skin is raised, red, scaly. TX: Topical antifungals: **Azoles**
Tinea pedis (foot, **athletes foot**) Dermatophyte Trichophyton rubrum (AKA: **Trichophyton epidermophyton**)	Source: warm/moist environment: barefoot in locker rooms, swimming pools, shared towels, inside of shoes. SX: Interdigital (between toes). Skin red and/or ulcerative, scaly, itchy. DX: KOH test TX: Topical antifungals: **Azoles (Miconazole)**
Tinea capitis (scalp, **hair**, head, ringworm of the **scalp**) Dermatophyte Trichophyton, Microsporum	Source: Direct contact with affected individuals (schools, close quarters, etc.) SX: Thick, scaly, boggy swelling raised rings. Itching, dandruff, bald patches. DX: Woods lamp: yellow/green fluorescence of hairs. (this differentiates it from psoriasis and seborrheic dermatitis) TX: **Oral terbinafine, griseofulvin**
Tinea corporis (ringworm on **body**, body infection) Dermatophyte	Source: Person to person, animal to human. High risk in contact sports (wrestling, soccer), tight clothing, immunocompromised, humid/wet environments. SX: Raised red rings with central clearing. Edge of rash elevated and scaly/flaky, hair loss in areas of the infection. DX: KOH skin scrapings TX: Topical antifungals: **Azoles**
Onychomycosis (infection of **fingernails or toenails**) AKA: Tinea Unguium Dermatophyte (Western countries) or Candida (tropics)	Source: Risk factors: aging due to diminished blood circulation, moist/humid environments, shoes with no ventilation, shower rooms, gyms, athletes foot, skin or nail injury, diabetes, immunocompromised. SX: Thickened, discolored nail (black, white, green), brittle nails, pain, foul smell, scaly skin. DX: Potassium hydroxide smear TX: **Terbinafine** (be sure and check LFT's first)
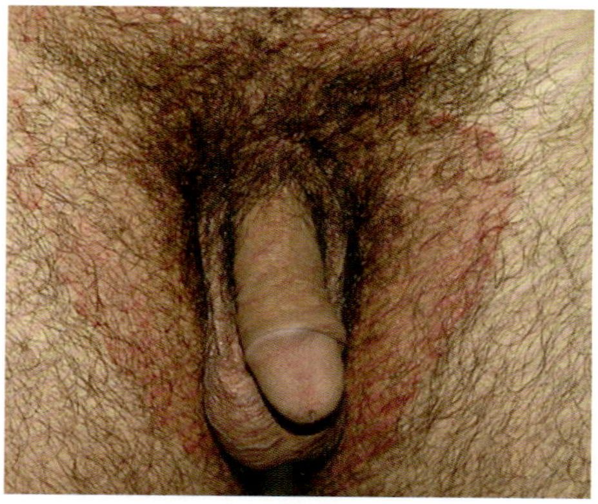 Tinea cruris - male	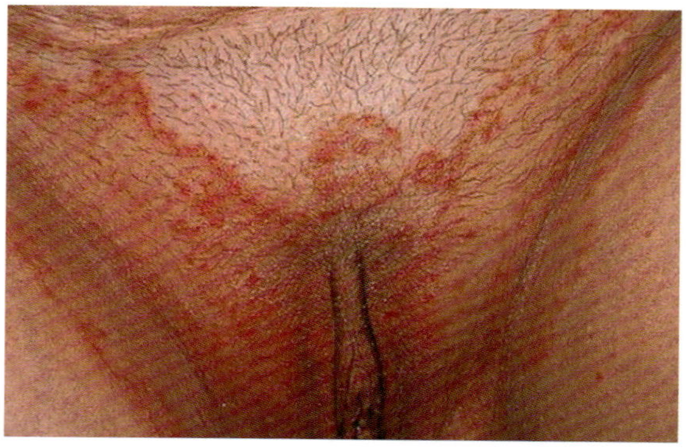 Tinea cruris - female

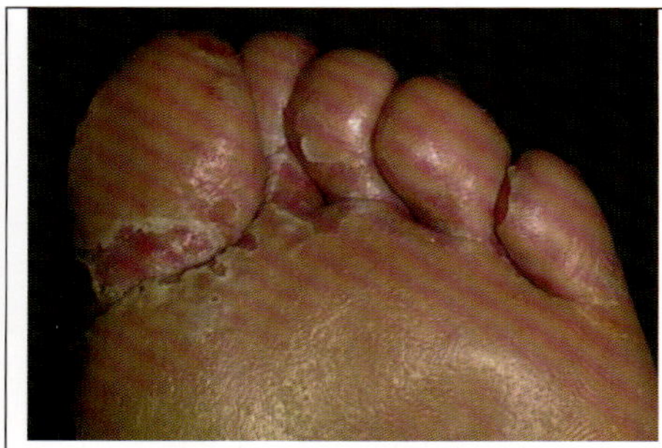 Tinea pedis	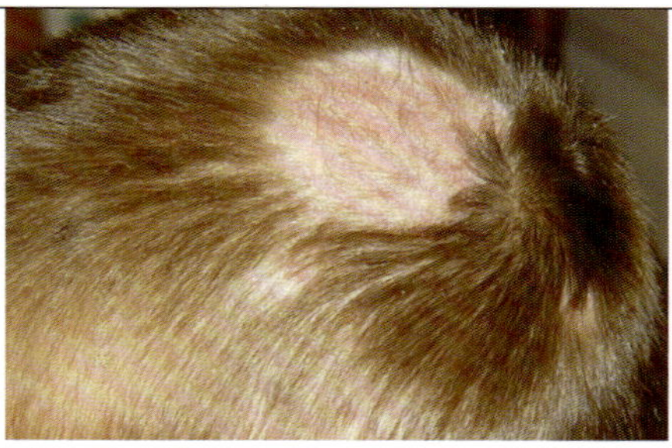 Tinea Capitis
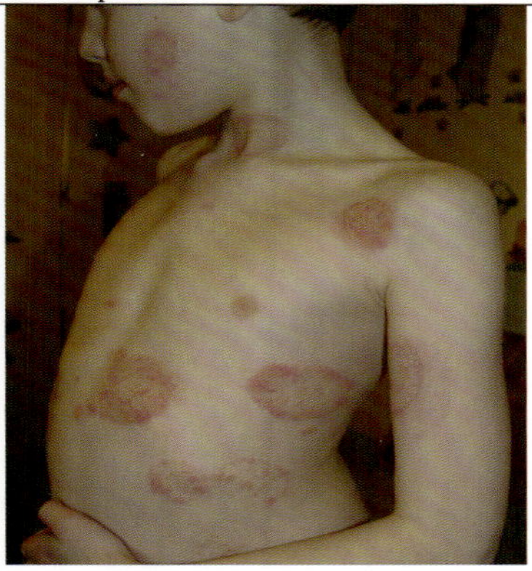 Tinea Corpus	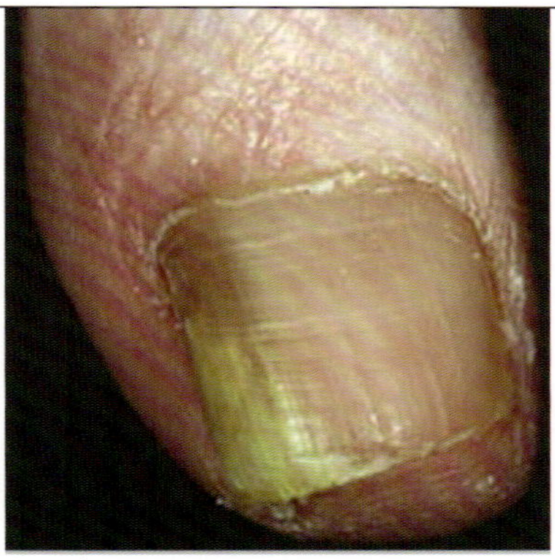 Onychomycosis

Opportunistic Fungal Infections

Aspergillus fumigatus

45 ° branching, hyphae with septae Spores (Conidiophore) with **"Chains" of spores** "Fiber balls in lungs" or "**Colonizing** in lungs" (because it takes over old cavities, esp. after TB infection) Mobile (moving ball) Can show a **crescent** shape (moon) in the ball or "halo sign" 🡅 Eosinophil's, IgE response	ABPA (Allergic bronchopulmonary aspergillosis): associated with cystic fibrosis, asthma, sinusitis. High risk: Immunocompromised, CGD **CD4 count < 50 with HIV** SX: Pulmonary **nodules, hemoptysis**, MC upper right lung, fever, cough TX: Amp B
Hepatocellular carcinoma Cause: **Aflatoxins** from Aspergillus flavus and Aspergillus parasiticus Source: decaying vegetation, hay, grains, **peanuts**, olive/peanut/sesame cooking oils MC: SE Asia	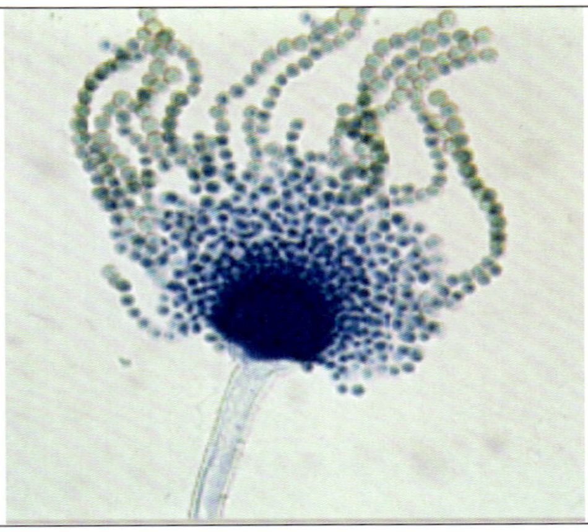

Candida albicans

Dimorphic yeast.
Pseudohyphae and budding yeast at 20° C
Germ tubes at 37°C
NO β 1-3 Glucan in the walls
↓ Glucan = osmotic instability

Vaginal Candidiasis: Not sexually transmitted (due to overgrowth of Candida, normally because of antibiotic use).

Vulvovaginitis (Vaginitis/yeast): due to antibiotic use (esp. in diabetics). Antibiotics, steroids, diabetes, OCP 's, immunocompromised allow for the **decrease in the normal flora bacteria Lactobacilli**, which allows for the **overgrowth of Candida**. (AKA: Yeast infection).
SX: White **"cottage cheese"** coating.
TX: **topical "azole" cream**

Local infections: T cells
Systemic Infections: ↑ in neutropenic patients

DX: **Germ Tube test**

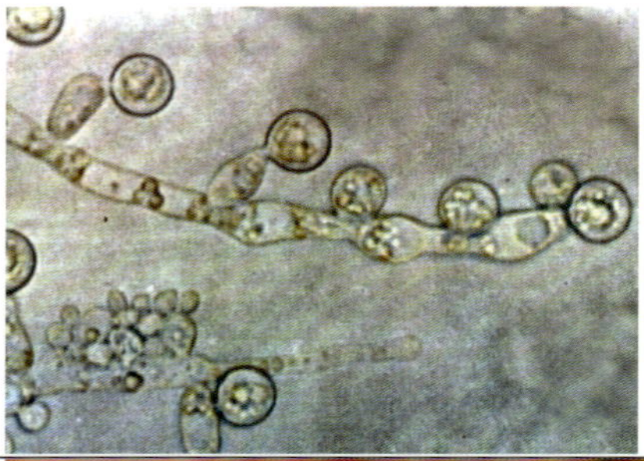

Pathologies:
Candida Esophagitis: Oral and esophageal thrush in immunocompromised (esp. HIV with <50 cd4 counts and neutropenic patients).
SX: Difficulty and pain with swallowing, white coating will scrape off.
Oral Flucytosine is BOTH diagnostic and therapeutic in Candida

Fungal Diaper rash: Candida (tip: Ca "IN" dida albicans = IN the skin fold creases). SX: Bright red, rash is inside the skin folds.
TX: **Topical azole** for fungal.

Bacterial diaper rash: NOT in the skin fold creases.
Bacterial due to staph or strep (Impetigo: blisters and pustules).
TX: **topical or oral antibiotics**.

Other diaper rash causes: Contact dermatitis (contact with urine or stool) – is not in skin folds. TX: **Zinc oxide (Desitin) or petroleum jelly (Vaseline)**.

Vulvovaginitis (Vaginitis/yeast): due to antibiotic use (esp. in diabetics). Antibiotics, steroids, diabetes, OCP 's, immunocompromised allow for the **decrease in the normal flora bacteria Lactobacilli**, which allows for the **overgrowth of Candida**.
SX: White **"cottage cheese"** coating.
TX: **topical "azole" cream**

Endocarditis in IV drug users.
Systemic Infections: **IV Amp B, Fluconazole, Caspofungin**

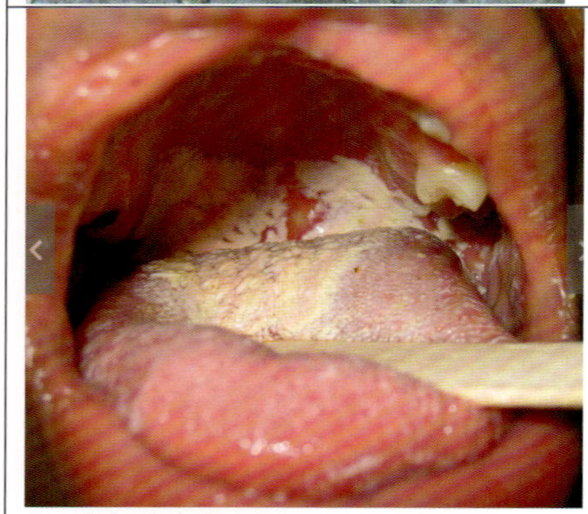

Candida Esophagitis

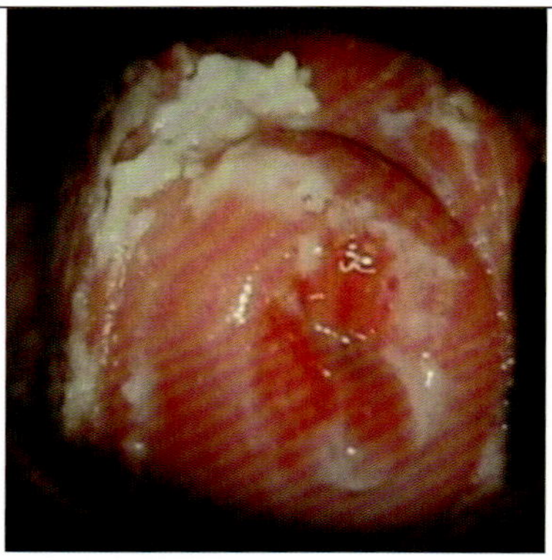

Vulvovaginitis

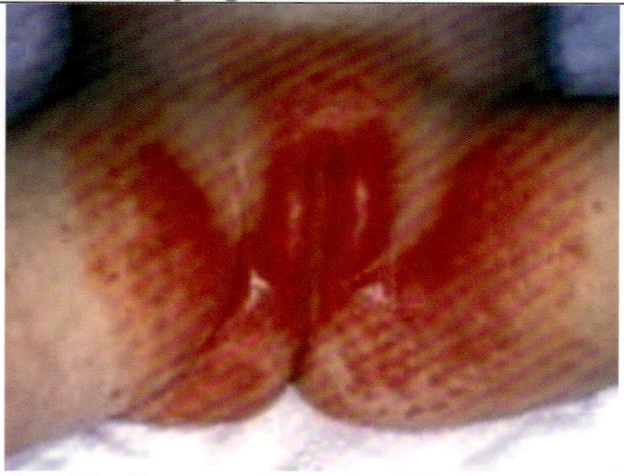

Candida diaper rash (in the folds)

Cryptococcus neoformans

Encapsulated yeast Capsule **"halos" around budding yeast** Budding yeast **ONLY fungus with a polysaccharide capsule** Source: soil, pigeon droppings DX: **Culture: Sabouraud agar** **Stains: India Ink, stains red with mucicarmine** **Capsule: Latex agglutination test against polysaccharide capsule.**	**Cryptococcus meningitis** Spread: **hematogenous** dissemination to meninges. Risk: HIV 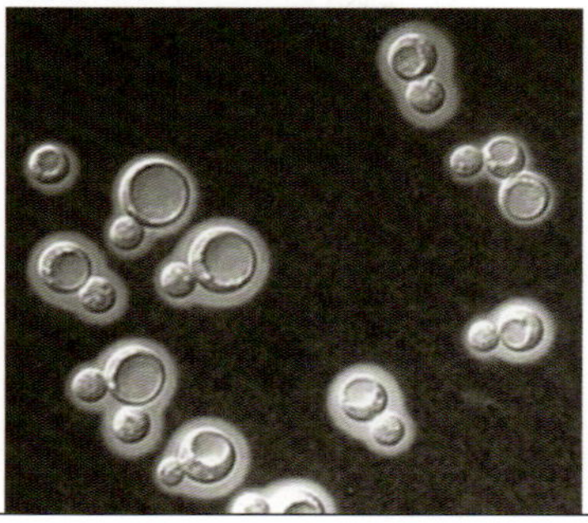

Mucor (Mucormycosis), Rhizopus (AKA: Zygomycosis, Absidia)

90° branching Highest risk: **Diabetics** (proliferates when there is excess glucose and ketones) Enters brain through **cribriform plate** to form a frontal lobe abscess. DX: Mucosal biopsy SX: Headache, facial pain, **black eschar lesion** (nose or face). ↑ exudate with surfactant and Type II pneumocytes TX: IV Amp B	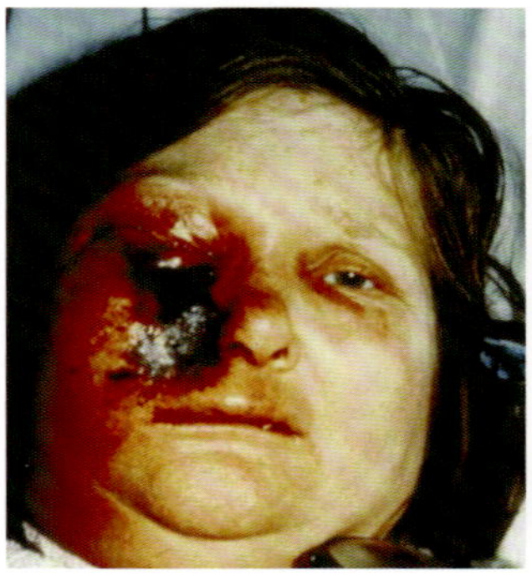 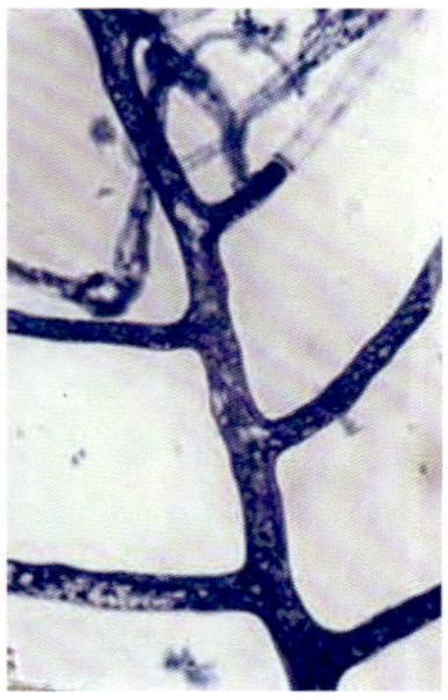

Pneumocystis jiroveci (PCP, PJP) (AKA: Pneumocystis carinii)

Yeast "Sporozoites" = Dark **oval** bodies Stain: Methenamine **silver staining** Highest Risk: **#1 AIDS defining disease. CD4 <200** (**tip:** if given ANY HIV patient with a CD4 count of **ANYTHING** over 200, the pneumonia is due to **Strep pneumonia**) ↑ pneumonia in premature infants Immunocompromised	DX: Lung biopsy SX: CXR shows: **Diffuse bilateral infiltrates** (interstitial pneumonia). Dry, **non-productive** cough. **Prophylaxis of Azithromycin for Mycobacterium avium should be started at this time.** TX: **TMP-SMX and add steroids** to aid in breathing Prophylaxis for PCP can begin at CD4 of 200 with **Atovaquone or Dapsone**.
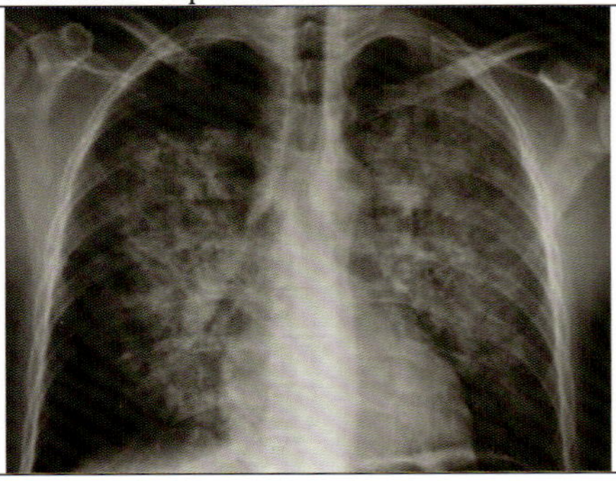	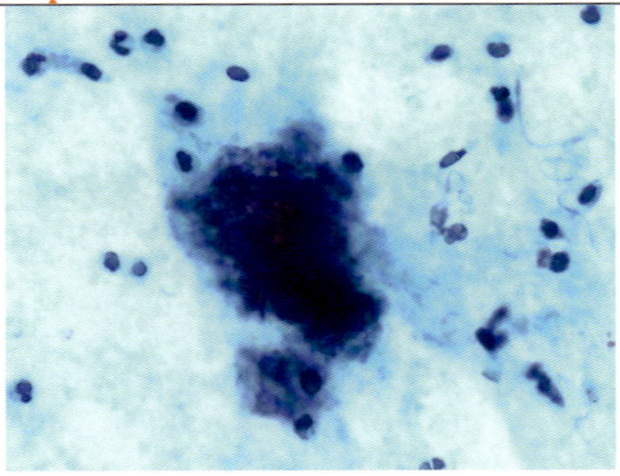

Sporothrix schenckii (AKA: Rose Gardner's Disease)

Dimorphic
Yeast at 37° C
Fungi (oval conidia) at 25°
Cigar shape budding yeast living on plants
Source: spores enter the skin through thorn prick, tree bark

SX: Subcutaneous **nodules/ulcers** along ascending **lymphatic's.**
TX: **Potassium iodide, Itraconazole**

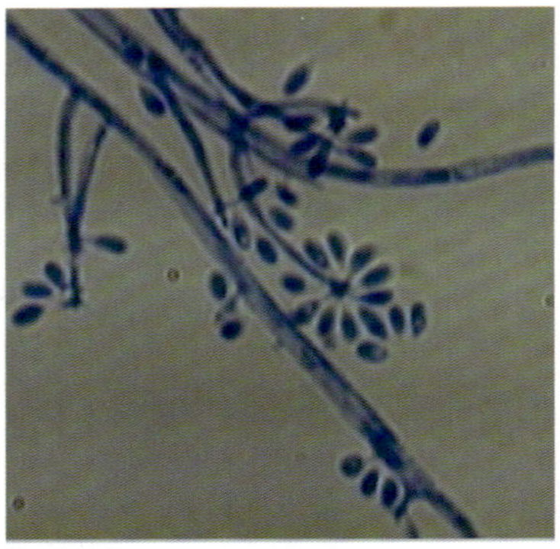

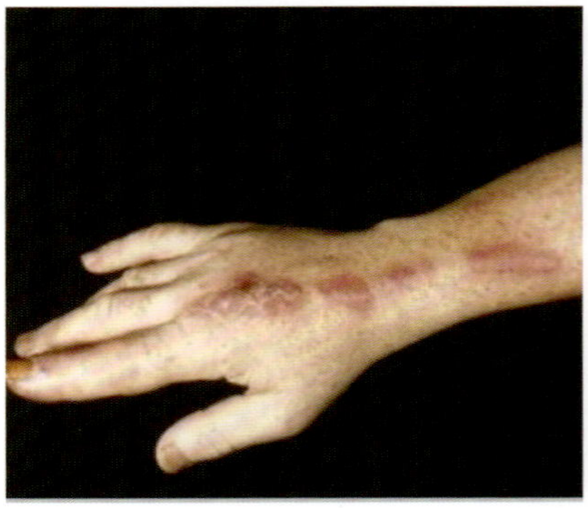

PARASITES – PROTOZOA - WORMS

Protozoan CNS Pathologies

Naegleria fowleri

Naegleriasis
Protozoan

Fatal primary amoebic meningoencephalitis
Enters brain through cribriform plate.

SX: Severe frontal headaches, vomiting, fever, stiff neck, seizures, coma, death.

Source: **Warm freshwater** ponds, lakes, rivers, hot springs, poorly chlorinated swimming pools, warm water discharges from industrial plants (is not found in salt water)

DX: Amoebas in spinal fluid
TX: **IV Amp B, Miltefosine**

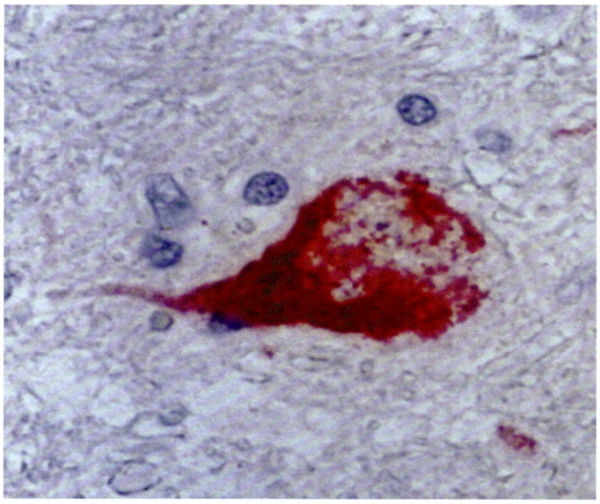

Naegleria fowleri

Toxoplasma gondii

Toxoplasmosis
Intracellular, parasitic protozoan

Source: Ingestion of oocysts (sporozoites). **Cat feces, deli meats,** skin from raw vegetables (peel vegetables).
Pregnant women must avoid these things – **oocysts cross the placenta** and infect the fetus.

Highest risk: HIV

SX: Brain CT shows **Ring Enhancing Lesions**
Triad of: Chorioretinitis (cotton like- white/yellow lesions in the eyes), hydrocephalus, **intracranial calcifications**.
(**Tip**: tOxOplasmosis: the "O"s make a RING)

DX: Blood sample showing tachyzoites

TX: **Sulfadiazine and pyrimethamine**
(If the TX of Sulfadiazine and pyrimethamine does not work then the differential DX is Primary CNS Lymphoma

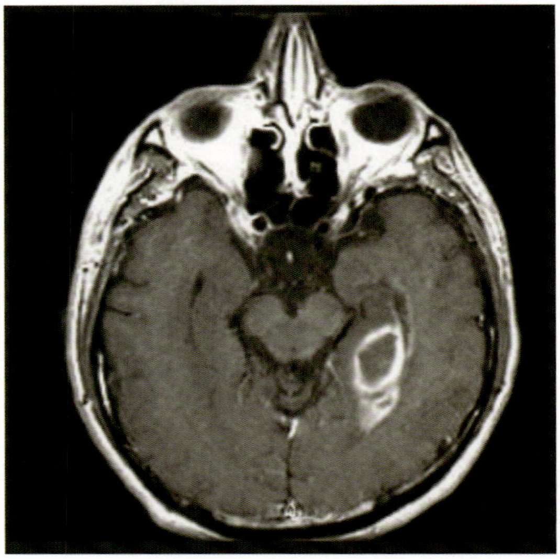

Trypanosoma brucei

African Sleeping Sickness
Protozoan
Can cross blood brain barrier
Have variable surface glycoproteins that undergo **antigenic variation,** which allow chronic infections.

Source: Tsetse fly

SX: Anemia, skin rash, **swollen lymph nodes**, **recurrent fever**, thrombocytopenia, confusion, insomnia, **somnolence**, coma

DX: Blood smear

TX: **Suramin** for blood borne infection (**tip**: I'm **SUR**e Sleepy)
Melarsoprol for CNS infection

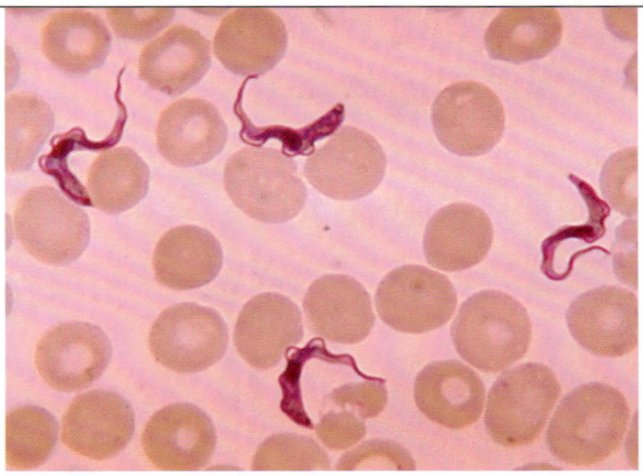

Protozoan Hematologic Pathologies

Babesia

Babesiosis
Parasite

Source: **Ixodes tick** (same tick as Lyme disease)
Location: Northeastern USA

SX: Hemolytic anemia, fever
High Risk: Asplenic patients. Spleen is responsible for removing the infected RBC's infected with Babesia.

DX: Blood smear, smear will show "Maltese Cross".
AKA: merozoites attached together.
AKA: Tetrads of intraerythrocytic rings.

TX: **Atovaquone, Azithromycin**

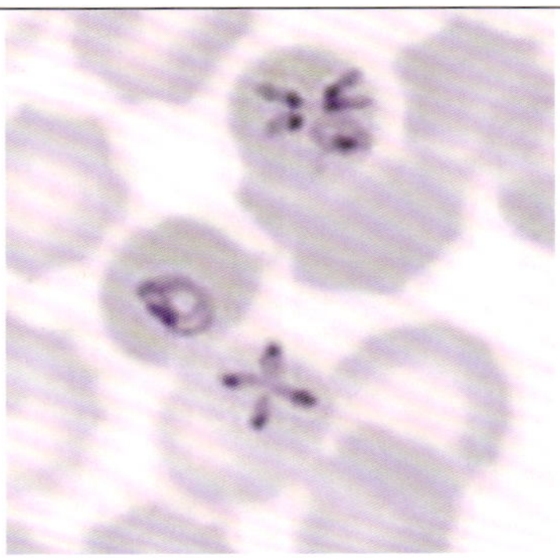
Babesiosis (maltese cross)

Plasmodium
Malaria

<table>
<tr>
<td>Malaria
RBC lysis by parasites

Anopheles mosquito

SX: Fever, headache, anemia, splenomegaly, GI symptoms.

DX: Blood smear shows trophozoites inside of RBC

Life cycles:
sporozoites (injected by saliva of mosquitoes into the host's blood and then invade the hepatocytes in the liver);
Merozoites (infect the RBC's);
Trophozoites (grow in the RBC's);
Schizonts (divide in the RBC's);
Hypnozoites (stay latent in the liver for up to 30 years: P. vivax, P. ovale (tip: "H"ypnozoites = "H" for "H"epatic)

Tissue Stages:
1) Exo-erythrocytic (liver stage: Chloroquine is not effective on this stage, requires Primaquine)
2) Erythrocytic (Blood stage. Infects the RBC's)
3) Sporogonic (Mosquito stage)</td>
<td>Mosquitos and Fevers

P. falciparum (sub-Saharan Africa)
Fever: irregular fever cycles
MCC death

P. vivax and P. ovale
48 hour fever cycles
MC malaria to reoccur b/c hypnozoites in the liver
(tip: "P" = Pair of mosquitos: Ovale and Vivax, Pair of places it goes: liver and RBC, Pair of treatments: Chloroquine and Primaquine, Pair (2 days) of fevers)

P. malariae
72 hour fever cycles

P. knowlesi (Southeast Asia)
24 hour fever cycles
Affects primates and humans</td>
<td>Tx:
<u>Chloroquine</u>
DOC for sensitive areas.

(Areas resistant to Chloroquine are:
Africa, India, Pakistan, Bangladesh = must use <u>Mefloquine</u>)

MOA: blocks Plasmodium heme polymerase.</td>
</tr>
<tr>
<td>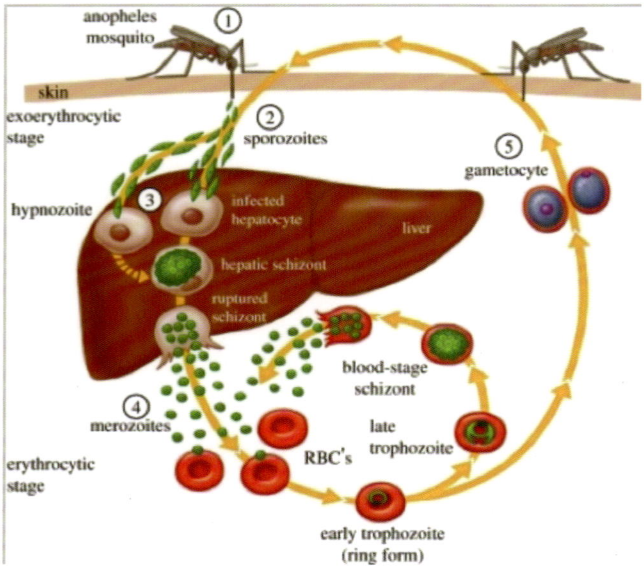
</td>
<td>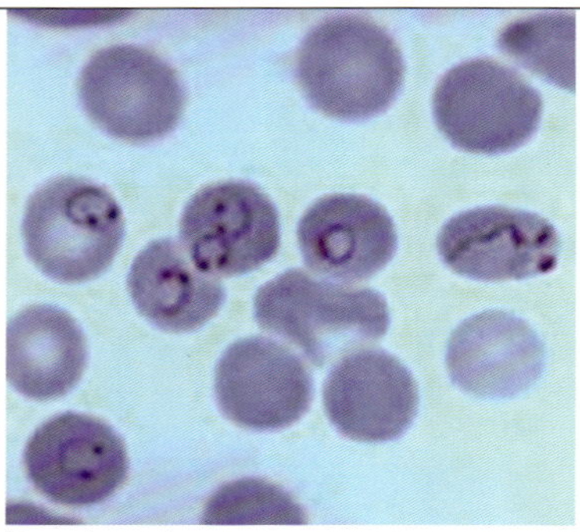
Trophozoites
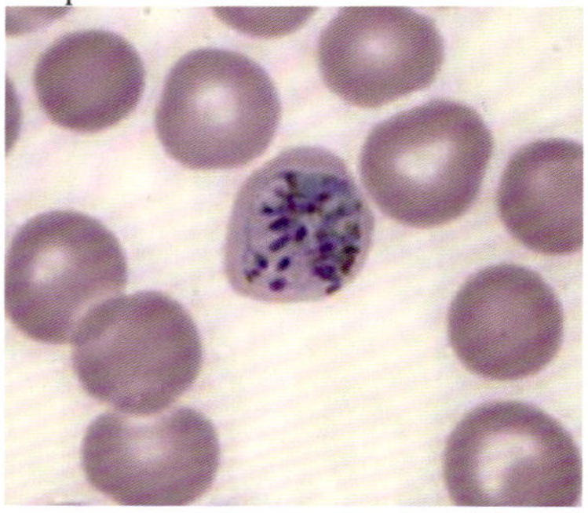
Merozoites</td>
<td>For Chloroquine resistance, use:
<u>Mefloquine, Atovaquone</u>
Proguanil
Side effect of Mefloquine:
psychedelic nightmares.

For P. vivax and P. ovale must add <u>Primaquine</u> to kill the hypnozoites in the liver.

Antimalarial Drug Side Effects:
Primaquine, pamaquine, chloroquine can cause acute hemolysis in people with G6PD</td>
</tr>
</table>

Protozoan GI Pathologies

Cryptosporidium parvum

Severe watery diarrhea in AIDS

Mild watery diarrhea in immuno**COMPETENT**
High risk of Sclerosing cholangitis

Source: Oocysts (AKA: **Red oocyst**) in poor water supplies, swimming pools.
Prevention: **Filtering water**

SX: Watery diarrhea (no blood), flatulence, bloating, increased Alk Phos.

DX: Acid fast stain shows Oocysts

TX: **Nitazoxanide** in ImmunoCOMPETENT

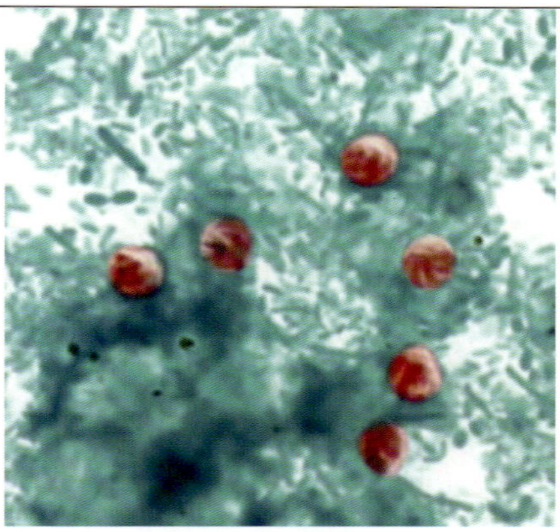

Cryptosporidium parvum

Entamoeba histolytica

Amebiasis
Anaerobic protozoan

Source: Cyst in water

SX: Dysenteric **Bloody diarrhea**, **liver abscess** (thick exudate). Ultrasound shows a hypoechoic lesion (dark area) in the liver. Weight loss, fatigue, abdominal pain, amoebae (amebic granuloma, lesions inside the bowel)

DX: Needle aspiration shows brown fluid.
Trophozoites with RBC's or Cysts with **4 nuclei** in the stool.
Cyst shows a "Cartwheel" distribution in the nucleus.
No microorganisms are seen.
DO NOT BIOPSY the LIVER or RUPTURE CYST

Tx: **Metronidazole** in the liver,
Nitroimidazole in the intestine

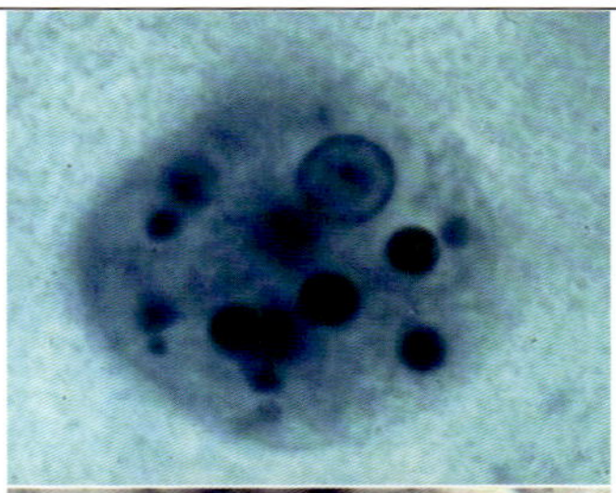

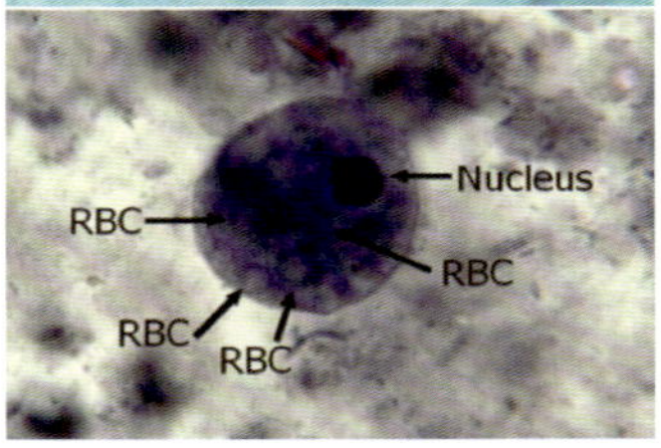

Entamoeba trophozoite

Giardia lamblia

Giardiasis
Protozoan

Source: Cysts in water. **Mountain streams,** campers/hikers

SX: **Foul-smelling stools**, fatty diarrhea, bloating, gut inflammation and **villous atrophy (no invasion), malabsorption**

DX: Trophozoites or cyst in stool

Chronic Giardia: due to IgA DEFICIENCY. Normal: IgA protects the gut wall and stops adhesion/attachment of Giardia.

Tx: **Metronidazole**

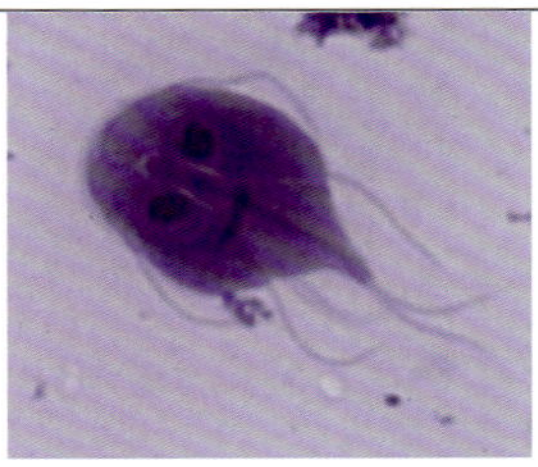

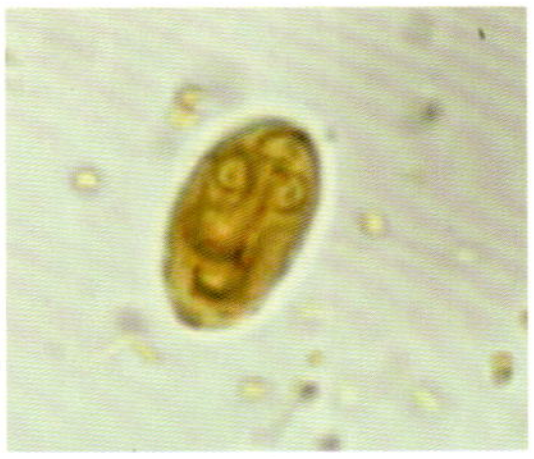

Giardia lamblia

Protozoan Misc. Pathologies

Leishmania donovani

Leishmaniasis (AKA: Black Fever)
Protozoan

Source: **Sandfly**

SX: Anemia, spiking fevers, hepatosplenomegaly, leukopenia, weight loss, pancytopenia, heavy dark skin pigmentation, and hard/course skin with warty eruptions.

DX: Macrophages with **amastigotes and external flagella**

TX: Amp B, Sodium stibogluconate

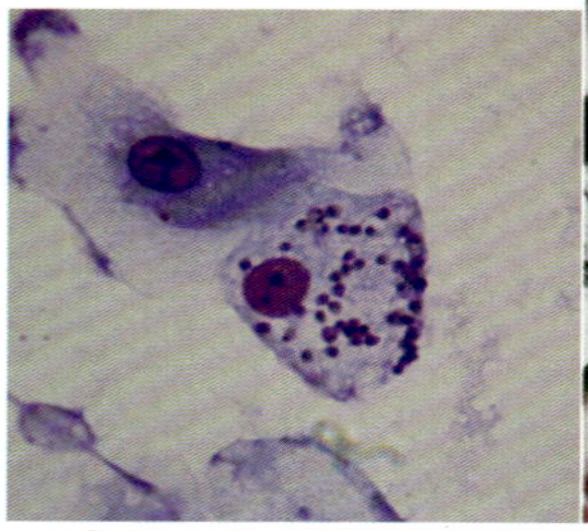
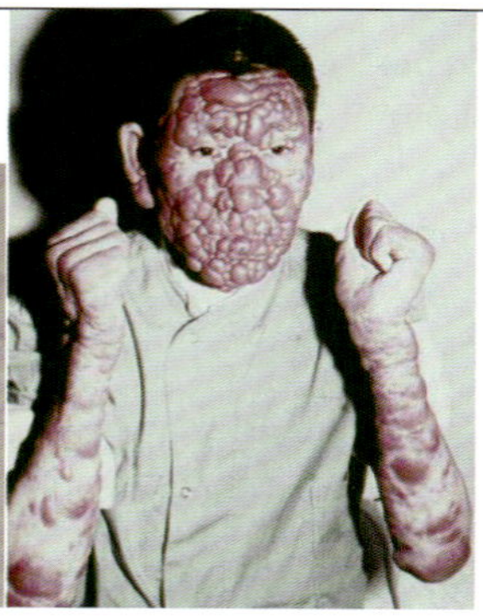

Leishmaniasis

Trichomonas vaginalis

Vaginitis
Protozoan

Source: **STD**

SX: Vaginal **pruritis and burning**. **Red vaginal mucosa** (AKA: Strawberry cervix), dyspareunia (pain with sex). Inflammation of vagina and vulva.

High risk for: preterm labor, premature rupture of membranes (ROM).

DX: Motile Trophozoites on wet mount in pear shape with flagella
Vaginal pH of >5 (alkalotic)

TX: Metronidazole
MUST treat partner also. (**tip**: "tricky dicky").
Nursing mothers: Must stop nursing for a few days while on the medicine and then resume.

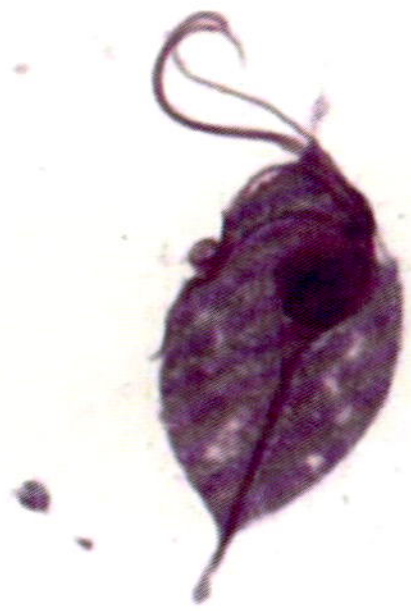
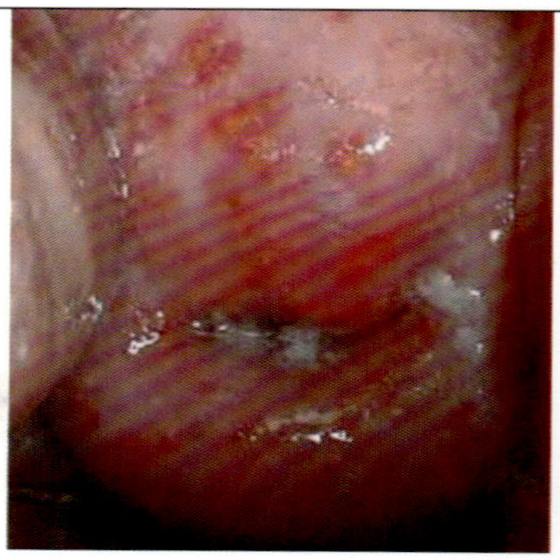

Trichomonas vaginalis

Vaginal Infections

Organism	Inflammation	Physical Exam	Labs	Treatment
Candida vulvovaginitis – Not STD	Yes	Thick, white discharge (Cottage cheese)	Pseudohyphae **Normal pH 4.0 – 4.5**	(Fungus) -Azoles
Bacterial vaginosis (BV) (Gardnerella) Not STD	No	Thin white discharge, Fishy (odd) odor	Clue cells **pH >4.5**	Metronidazole
Trichomoniasis STD	Yes	Red, inflamed vaginal/cervix tissue, gray-green, foul smelling discharge	Motile trichomonads **pH > 4.5**	Metronidazole Must treat partner (**tip**: "tricky dicky")

Trypanosoma cruzi

Chagas Disease
Protozoan

Source: **Reduvid beetle** (aka: "Kissing bug", Triatominae beetle)
Location: **South America, Brazil**

Transmission: Bite from the bug that occurs MC on the face during the nighttime. It can be transmitted from an infected person via blood transfusions or transplantation of infected organs. Can be acquired by eating undercooked meat/food that is contaminated with the parasite. Infected mother's can transmit the disease to the fetus.

Three phases of the disease:
Acute phase: **swelling and erythema** around the areas bitten, fever, swollen lymph nodes, body aches, nausea, vomiting, liver or spleen enlargement.
Intermediate phase: progression
Chronic phase: **Cardiomyopathy**, CHF, **megacolon,** megaesophagus

DX: Protozoan in blood smear

TX: **Benznidazole, Nifurtimox**

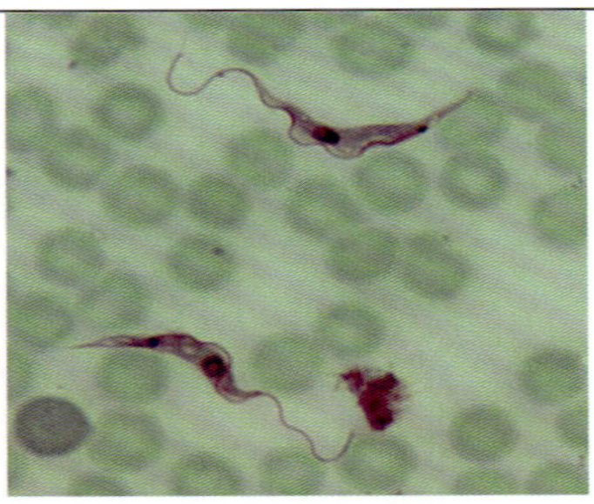

Trypanosoma cruzi (Chagas)

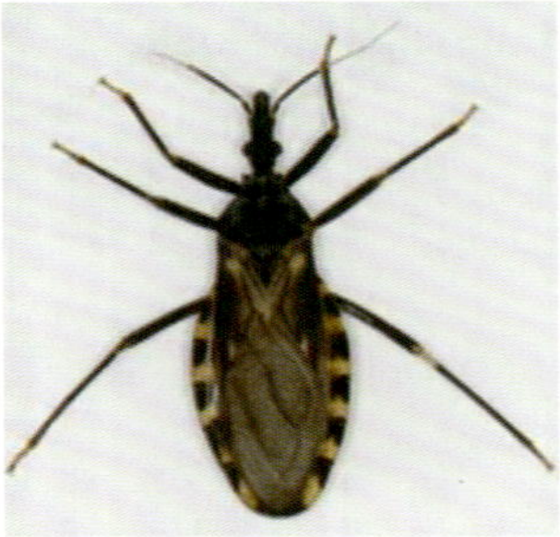

Reduvid beetle

Cestodes (Tapeworms)

Diphyllobothrium latum

Source: Ingestion of larvae from raw freshwater fish

Pathology: **Pernicious anemia** due to Vitamin B12 deficiency. D. latum completes for the **B12** so it is not available to bind with intrinsic factor in the ilium.

TX: **Praziquantel**

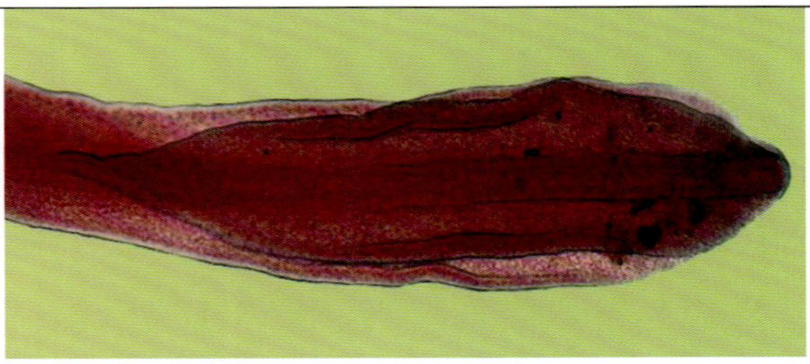

Diphyllobothrium latum

Echinococcus granulosus
(AKA: **Hydatid Cyst**)

Source: Host: Sheep and dogs with sheep. Ingestion of eggs from dog feces (fecal/oral).

SX: **Hydatid cyst in liver**, lung, kidneys and spleen with daughter cyst inside, granulosus

TX: Surgery. **DO NOT BIOPSY or CUT OPEN THE CYST, ANTIGENS WILL BE RELEASED CAUSING ANAPHYLAXIS AND DEATH**. Ethanol must be injected into the cyst to kill it before it can be removed.

TX: **Albendazole**

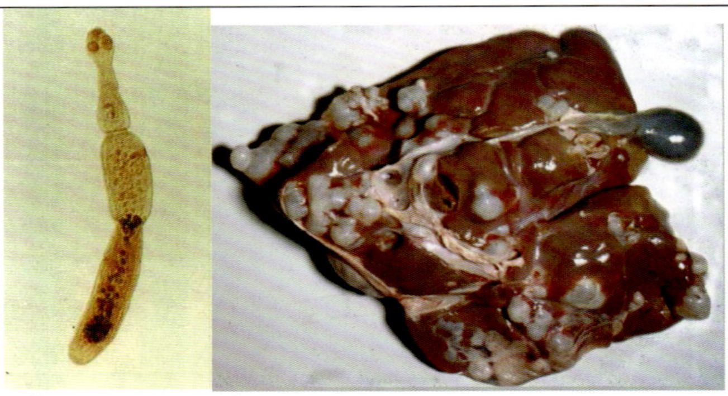

Echinococcus granulosus
(AKA: Hydatid Cyst)

Taenia solium (Pork tapeworm)
Cysticercosis

Worm lives in the intestine and infections are asymptomatic unless infection occurs during the larval stage causing **Cysticercosis or Neurocysticercosis**
(Very common in Mexico, South America, India, and Eastern Europe).

Source: Ingestion of larvae in **uncooked or undercooked pork (infected pork)**, eggs, undercooked vegetables

SX: Seizures, **Cysticercosis** (tissue infection: **calcified thin walled cyst**), **neurocysticercosis** (brain infection causing seizures)

DX: **Eosinophil's in the CSF, CT/MRI of brain shows multiple cysts that will calcify over time.**

TX: **Albendazole, Praziquantel** for Cysticercosis
Albendazole for Neurocysticercosis if uncalcified.

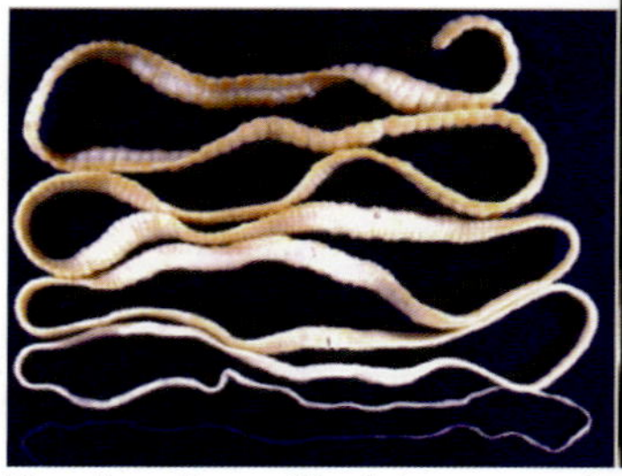
Taenia solium (Pork tapeworm)

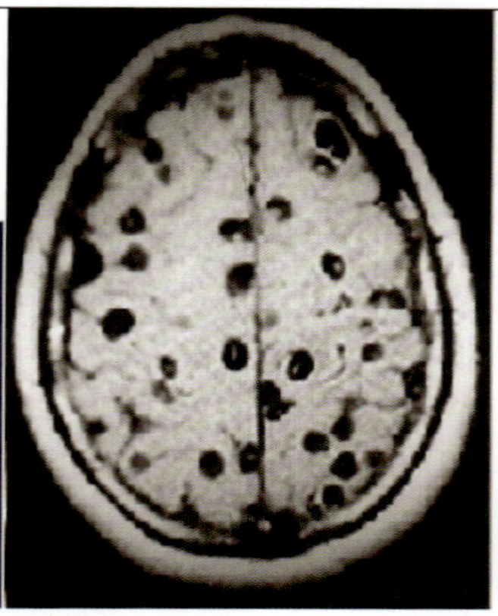
Cysticercosis

Nematodes (Roundworms)

Ancylostoma duodenale (hookworm)
Necator americanus (hookworm)

Source: Larvae in soil/sand **penetrate skin** (feet). Animal feces infect areas with sand: beach, sand box.

SX: Intestinal infection. Anemia (caused by hookworms attaching to the **intestine** and sucking blood), Itchy red papules

TX: **Bendazoles, Pyrantel Pamoate**

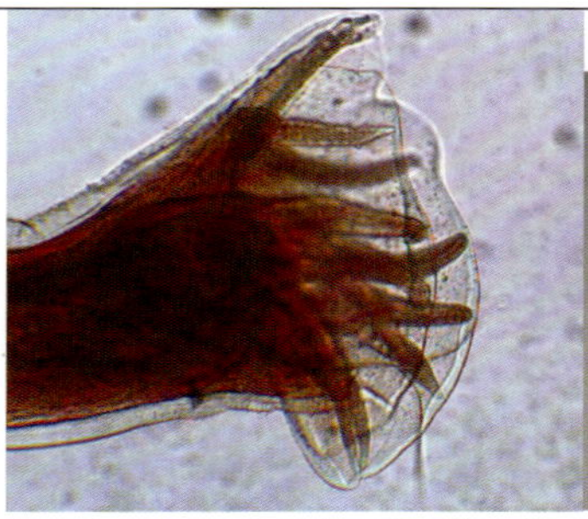
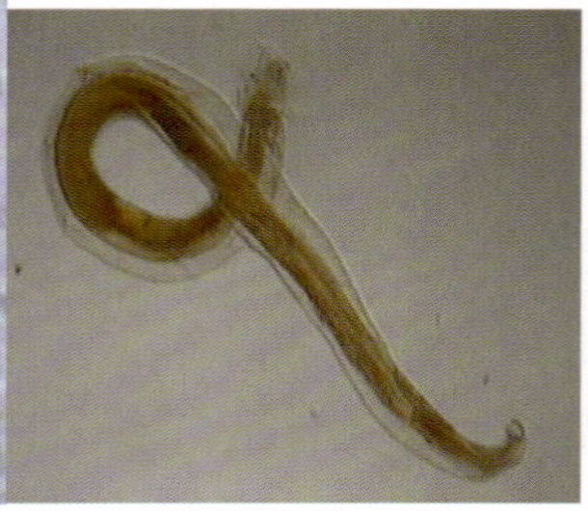
Ancylostoma duodenale (hookworm)
Necator americanus (hookworm)

Ascaris lumbricoides (Giant Roundworm)

Source: **Fecal/oral**. Eggs in feces

SX: Intestinal infection. Eosinophilia, **risk for small bowel or biliary obstruction**, GI symptoms
Lung phase: no productive cough

TX: **Bendazoles, Pyrantel Pamoate**

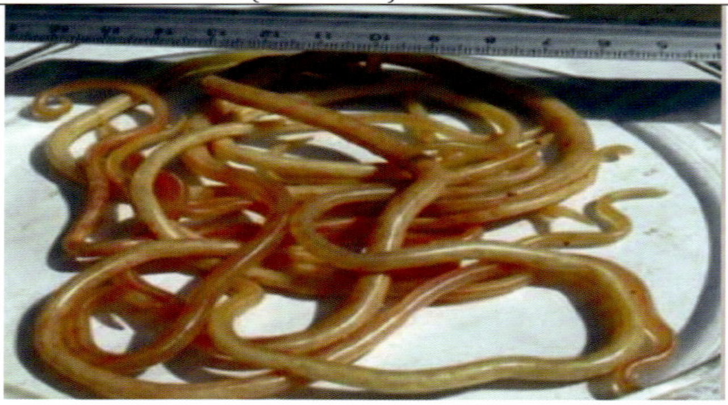
Ascaris lumbricoides (Giant Roundworm)

Enterobius vermicularis (pinworm) #1 MC helminth infection in the USA Source: Fecal/oral. SX: **Anal itching**, vulvo vaginitis, abdominal pain, nausea, vomiting (females exit anus during the night and lay eggs on the outside of the anus and then return back inside the body) DX: **Scotch tape test** TX: **Bendazoles, Pyrantel Pamoate** Do NOT use during pregnancy	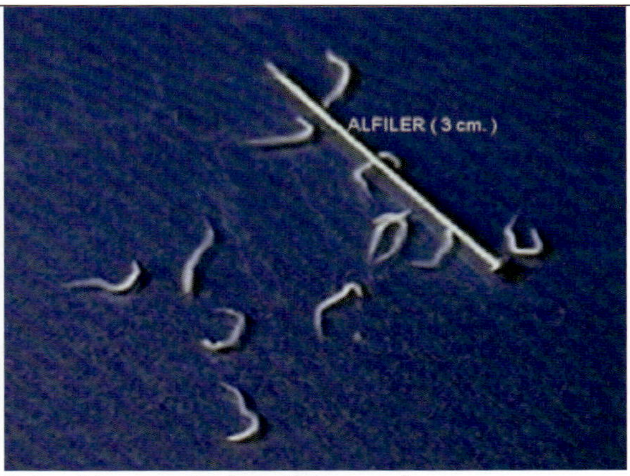 Enterobius vermicularis (pinworm)
Loa loa (Eye worm) Africa, India Source: Deer or Horse fly SX: **Worms in conjunctiva**, inflammation in skin, itching, joint pain, fatigue, death DX: **Diethylcarbamazine, Ivermectin**	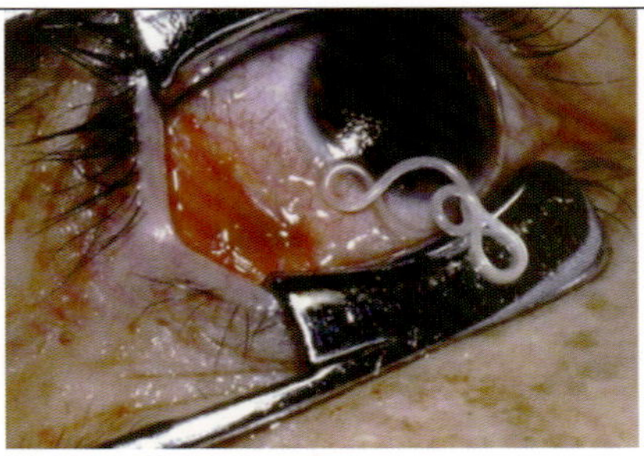 Loa loa (Eye worm)
Onchocerca volvulus Africa Source: Female blackfly SX: **River blindness** (thickening of the corneal stroma leading to blindness) TX: **Ivermectin**	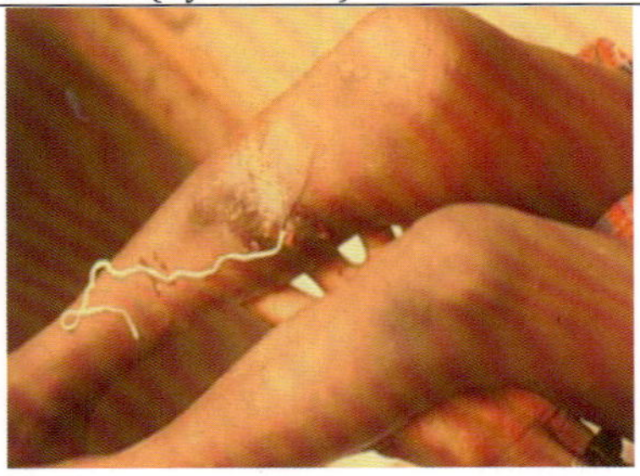 Onchocerca volvulus
Strongyloides stercoralis (roundworm) "Threadworm" Source: Larvae in soil/sand penetrate skin (feet) SX: Intestine infection: GI symptoms: diarrhea, vomiting, epigastric pain, dermatitis, swelling, itching. If lungs become infected with the worm (Löffler Syndrome: eosinophilic pneumonia): wheezing, cough, pneumonia-like symptoms, feeling of a burning chest TX: **Albendazole, Ivermectin**	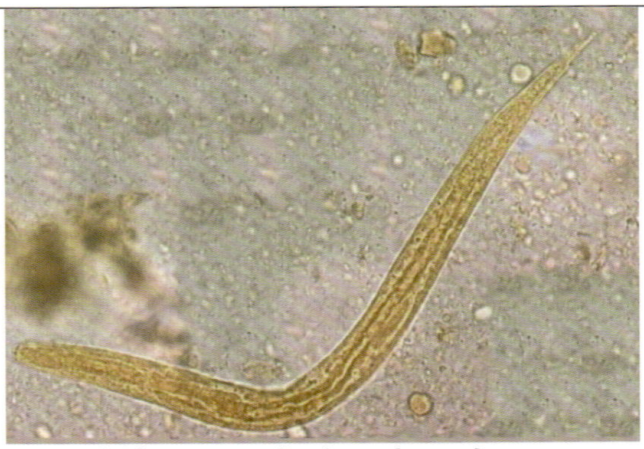 Strongyloides stercoralis (roundworm)

Toxocara canis (dog roundworm)

Source: Fecal/oral

SX: Visceral and ocularis larva migrans (Migrate through the intestine wall and travel in the blood stream to organs causing inflammation and damage)
Visceral: Heart = myocarditis, CNS = seizures and coma, liver
Ocularis: Unilateral visual problems, strabismus, eye pain

TX: **Albendazole, Mebendazole**

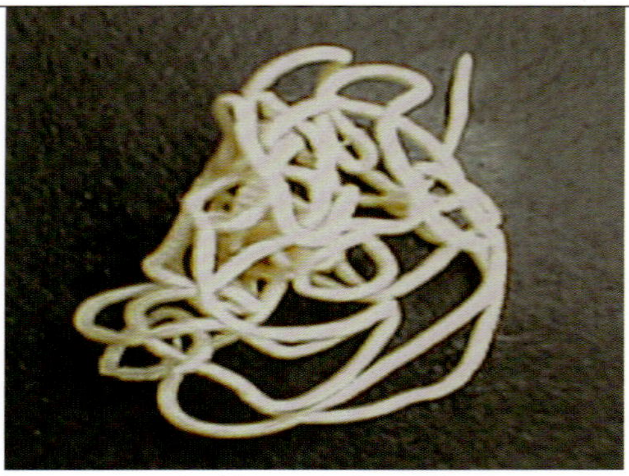

Toxocara canis (dog roundworm)

Trichinellosis (Trichinosis) (Roundworm)

Source: Trichinella larvae from **undercooked pork or wild game**

SX: High **eosinophil's** in the blood, GI issues (heartburn, dyspepsia, diarrhea, nausea), periorbital eye edema, facial edema, myositis (inflammation of muscles), swelling of conjunctive (chemosis).
Larvae migrate causing **splinter hemorrhages and retinal hemorrhage.**

TX: **Mebendazole, Albendazole**

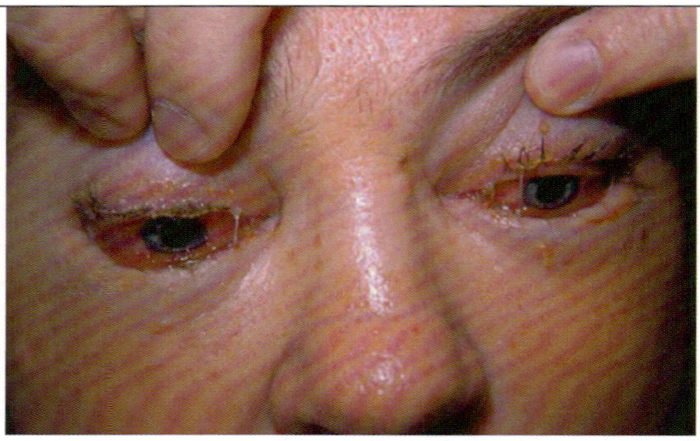

Trichinellosis (Trichinosis) (Roundworm)

Wuchereria bancrofti (Elephantiasis)
(roundworm)
Africa, South/Central America, tropical regions of Asia, southern China

Source: Female mosquito

SX: appear after 9 months from bite. Lymphatic filariasis: blocks lymphatic vessels.
Asymptomatic phase: Microfilaremia infection, no symptoms
Inflammatory (acute) phase: female adult worm's antigens cause disruption of lymph flow = lymphedema, painful lymph nodes, epididymitis (inflammation of spermatic cord)
Obstructive (chronic) phase: Lymph varices, hydrocele, lymph scrotum, and elephantiasis. In women: legs, arms and breast are affected. In men: legs, arms, scrotum affected.

TX: **Diethylcarbamazine, Ivermectin, Albendazole**

(**tip:** "Wucherria bancrofti" looks like "**water** buffalo – water buffalos are in Africa, so are **elephants** . So also think that this is a problem with "**water**" (**lymph**).

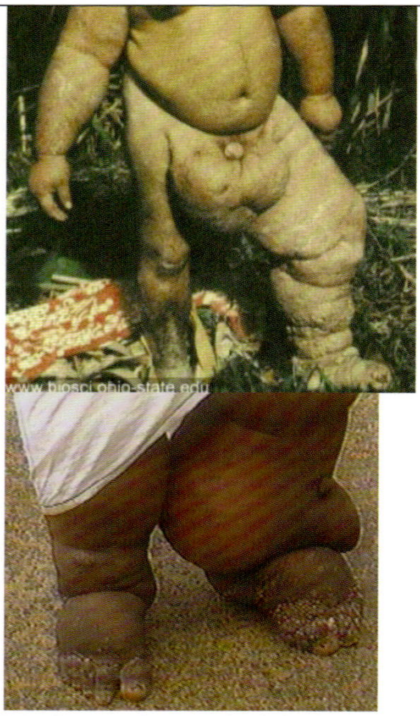

Wuchereria bancrofti (Elephantiasis)

Trematodes (Flukes)

Clonorchis sinensis Source: Undercooked fish SX: Biliary tract inflammation, pigmented gallstones. Associated with: **Cholangiocarcinoma** TX: **Praziquantel**	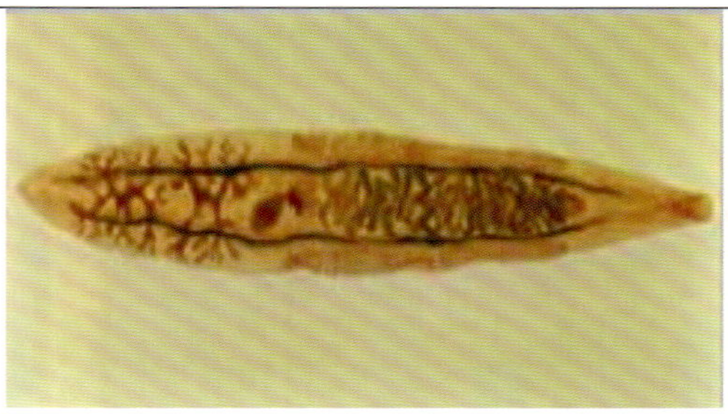 Clonorchis sinensis
Paragonimus westermani Paragonimiasis "Japanese lung fluke" Eastern Asia, South America Source: Raw or undercooked **freshwater crab meat**, freshwater crayfish SX: Lung infection: cough, **bronchitis, and hemoptysis**. Granulation tissue. If dissemination: can go to the spinal cord = paralysis or to the heart and = death. DX: Eggs in stool or sputum, CXR shows worms	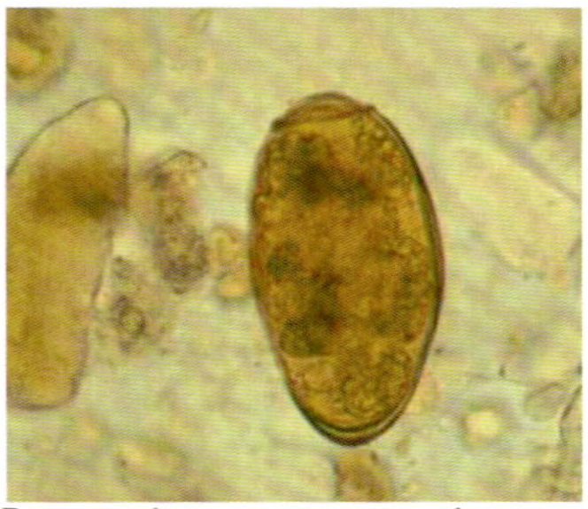 Paragonimus westermani
Schistosoma haematobium Associated: **Bladder Cancer** (painless hematuria) Africa, Middle East Source: Human waste in water supplies. Snails. Cercariae penetrate the skin SX: Hematuria and fibrosis of the bladder, hydronephrosis. Granulomas and multinucleated giant cells DX: Eggs in the urine TX: **Praziquantel**	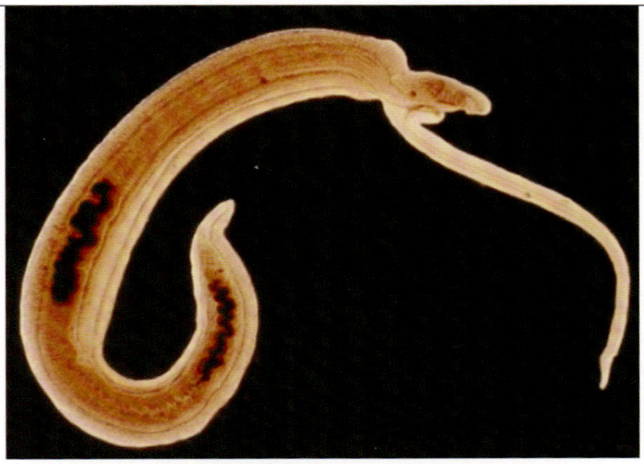 **Schistosoma haematobium**
Schistosoma japonicum China Intestinal and hepatic Schistosomiasis Source: Human waste in water supplies, fertilization of crops with human waste, snails SX: Katayama fever (fever, lethargy, urticarial rash, hepatosplenomegaly), liver fibrosis, liver cirrhosis, liver portal HTN, splenomegaly, ascites TX: **Praziquantel**	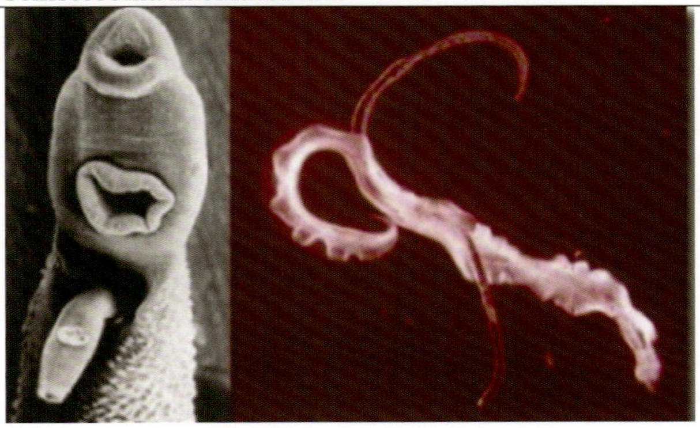 Schistosoma japonicum

Schistosoma mansoni
Intestinal and hepatic Schistosomiasis
Caribbean, Africa, South America, Middle East

Source: Freshwater snail (Biomphalaria species)

SX: Rash ("Swimmers itch"), Katayama Fever, aching, cough diarrhea, lymphadenopathy., collagen deposition and fibrosis. Granulomas impair blood flow in the liver = portal HTN and ultimately lead to cor pulmonale. Granulomas obstruct the colon and cause blood lose in the intestines.

DX: Eggs in stool

TX: **Praziquantel**

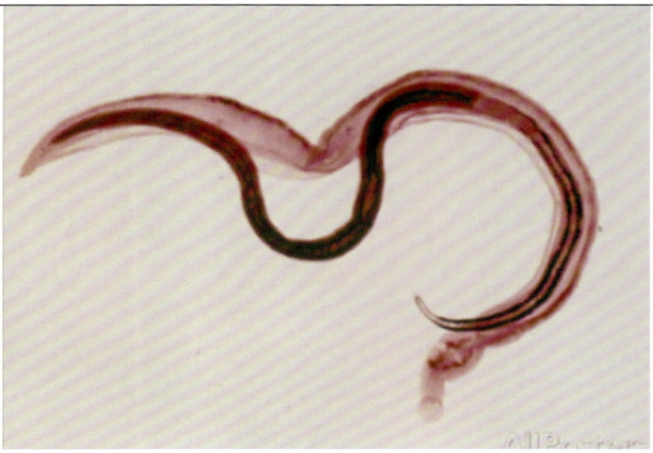

Schistosoma mansoni

MYCOLOGY and PARASITE PHARMACOLOGY

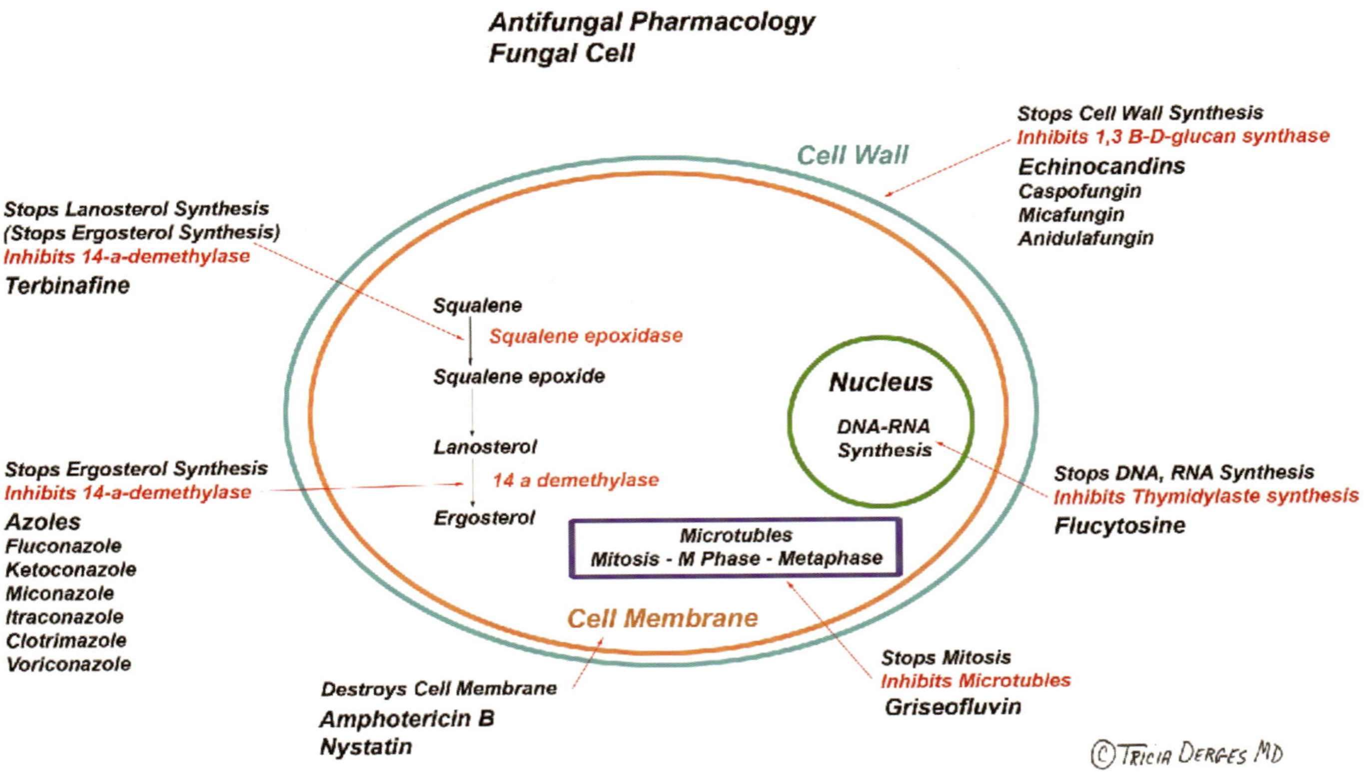

Antifungal Pharmacology

DRUG GENERIC name Trade name	Clinical Use	Mechanism of Action and Resistance	Toxicity and Notes
Amphotericin B	**All serious systemic fungal infections.** Histoplasmosis Blastomycosis Coccidioidomycosis Candida albicans Mucor/Rhizopus Fungal Meningitis Aspergillus Cryptococcus	Binds **ergosterol and cholesterol. Makes holes** in cell membrane so that **ions leak out** = cell lysis. (**tip**: Amp "**B**" = "**B**" for **BOTH** ergosterol and cholesterol and ↓ in **BOTH** K and Mg)	**Loss of K and Mg** causing **arrhythmias. Hypokalemia (U wave, inverted T wave), Metabolic acidosis, fever, chills.** It also causes **renal tubular acidosis** (RTA – nephrotoxic/↑ Creatinine) (AKA: altered permeability in DCT) because of loss of K and Mg and retention of Hydrogen ions. TX: Use liposomal amphotericin instead. **"Shake n' Bake" symptoms (fever, chills) after infusion.** **MUST supplement K and Mg.** **Flucytosine IV is given (inpatient) with Amp B. When patient goes home it is changed to Fluconazole (oral).**

Nystatin	Oral for mouth and esophagus (oral "swish and swallow") for candidiasis. (MC: HIV) Topical for Fungal infections: skin (diaper rash), vagina yeast infections.	Same as Amp B. Binds **ergosterol and cholesterol.** Makes holes in cell membrane so that **ions leak out** = cell lysis.	SX: GI, Stevens-Johnson syndrome, rash.
Flucytosine	Used IV for inpatients in combination with Amp B for serious systemic fungal infections. (Changed to Fluconazole (oral) when patient is discharged home)	**Inhibits DNA and RNA synthesis** by conversion to **5-fluorouracil** by **cytosine deaminase**.	Bone marrow suppression: AKA: anemia, agranulocytosis, pancytopenia, leukopenia, aplastic anemia. CNS SX: Photosensitivity, can affect liver and kidneys.
"Azoles" **Fluconazole** **Ketoconazole** **Itraconazole** **Miconazole** Clotrimazole Voriconazole Posaconazole	Fungal infections. **Fluconazole**: is both diagnostic and therapeutic in HIV esophagitis. **Crosses BBB.** **Best for Candida.** **Itraconazole**: Blastomycosis, Coccidioidomycosis, Histoplasmosis Miconazole, Clotrimazole**: topical** fungal infections. Posaconazole: Mucormycosis/ Mucorales/Zygomycetes /Rhizopus Voriconazole: Best for Aspergillus.	Inhibits **ergosterol synthesis** by inhibiting **14 α Demethylase** so that **lanosterol is not converted** to **ergosterol**. **Resistance:** Mutation of lanosterol C14 Demethylase active site.	**Ketoconazole: gynecomastia due to inhibition of testosterone synthesis.** **P-450 Inhibitor.**
Griseofulvin	Treats dermatophyte infections (tinea 's and ringworms)	Causes dysfunction of **microtubules, which** inhibits mitosis. (Microtubules: transport/movement) (**tip**: picture a big "grisly" bear bending a tube in half)	**P-450 Inducer.** **Teratogen,** CNS symptoms (headaches, confusion)
Echinocandins "the Fungins" **Caspofungin** **Micafungin** Anidulafungin	Aspergillosis, Candida Caspofungin: Neutropenic fever (more effective than Amp B). Echinocandins do NOT cover Cryptococcus.	Inhibits **cell wall synthesis** by inhibiting the synthesis of the polysaccharide **β-glucan**. Exhibits 45° branching. (**tip**: CASPer the friendly ghost goes through WALLS) (**tip**: CASPer AN MICA go thru walls)	Flushing (histamine release), GI Sx.
Terbinafine	Onychomycosis. Fungal infections of **fingernails, toenails, hair.** Ringworm (tinea corpus).	Inhibits lanosterol synthesis by inhibiting **squalene epoxidase**.	**Hepatoxic:** Must check LFT's before prescribing.

Antihelminthic, Anti-malarial, Antiprotozoan

Antihelminthic

DRUG GENERIC name Trade name	Clinical Use	Mechanism of Action and Resistance	Toxicity and Notes
"Bendazoles" **Mebendazole** **Albendazole**	Helminthic 's. **Pinworms**, ascariasis, hookworms, roundworms, tapeworms, Echinococcus granulosus (hydatid cyst)	↓ cell membrane **permeability to calcium** → kills the parasite.	SX: headaches, vomiting, tinnitus, GI symptoms.
Praziquantel	Flukes/Trematodes (**Schistosoma**), **Diphyllobothrium** latum, Cysticercosis (pork tapeworm), Paragonimiasis westermani.	Not currently known.	Somnolence, fatigue, vertigo. dizziness, headache, CNS affects, seizures. (**tip**: think of "Pray" to get rid of the "P"arasites. If it's a parasite, best bet, treat it with the "P" drug. Also: "Praz the flukes")
Ivermectin	Onchocerca volvulus, Loa Loa, Onchocerciasis (river blindness), **Scabies**	Interferes with nervous system and muscle function by inhibiting neurotransmission.	CNS depression, ataxia.
Pyrantel Pamoate	Hookworms, roundworms (Ascaris lumbricoides: AKA: Ascarids).	**Depolarizing neuromuscular** blocking agent causing paralysis.	If there is a heavy worm load that is destroyed it could lead to intestinal obstruction.
Diethyl-carbamazine	Filariasis (roundworms of the Filarioidea type). Wuchereria bancrofti, Loa loa, Onchocerca volvulus.	Inhibitor of arachidonic acid metabolism making the microfilariae more susceptible to innate immune attack. (Does not kill the parasites).	

Antimalarial

DRUG GENERIC name Trade name	Clinical Use	Mechanism of Action and Resistance	Toxicity and Notes
Chloroquine	Malaria: Prophylaxis and Treatment. Chloroquine: not for use against P. falciparum in Africa, Southeast Asia, South America due to resistance. Must use **Mefloquine.**	Crystallizes heme to form **hemozoin**, which collects and becomes toxic to parasite. **AKA:** Blocks plasmodium heme polymerase. Parasites that do not form hemozoin are resistant to chloroquine. Resistance: Membrane pump that ↓ intracellular concentration of drug.	Hemolysis in **G6PD patients. Sulfa** allergies, retinopathy.
Quinidine	Malaria treatment for P. falciparum malaria when there is Chloroquine resistance.	Blocks fast Na current. (Class 1a antiarrhythmic)	↑ QT interval leading to torsades de pointes (is a Class 1a antiarrhythmic drug), thrombocytopenia, myasthenia gravis. **P-450 Inhibitor.**

Quinine and Doxycycline Atovaquone and Proguanil Artemether and Lumefantrine	Treatments for P. falciparum malaria when there is Chloroquine resistance.		
Mefloquine	Malaria prophylaxis in Chloroquine resistant regions. Malaria treatment.		**Neuropsychiatric (weird) dreams with vivid colors.** Cardiac arrhythmias.
Primaquine	Treats P. vivax and P. ovale hypnozoites in the liver.		**This must be added to malaria treatments when treating for P. ovale and P. vivax parasitic infections.**

Antiprotozoan

DRUG **GENERIC name** **Trade name**	**Clinical Use**	**Mechanism of Action and Resistance**	**Toxicity and Notes**
Metronidazole Flagyl	**Giardia, Entamoeba, Trichomonas, Bacterial Vaginitis (Gardnerella), Anaerobes (C. difficile, Bacteroides).** (Treats anaerobes below the belt, clindamycin treats anaerobes above the belt) (**tip**: GET GAP on the metro)	Forms free radicals that damage the DNA in the bacteria. Bactericidal.	**Disulfiram-like reaction**. ("Hangover symptoms" when alcohol is used while on this drug). Metronidazole **inhibits aldehyde dehydrogenase.** **Metallic taste**. Do not use in pregnancy: mutagenesis. If breastfeeding: Must stop breastfeeding for 2 – 3 days while on the drug, then resume breastfeeding.
Trimethoprim Pyrimethamine	**TMP/Pyrimethamine: prophylaxis for toxoplasmosis.**	Inhibits Dihydrofolate Reductase. Bacteriostatic.	Megaloblastic anemia (lack of folate), supplement with folinic acid (folate).
Suramin	Trypanosoma brucei (sleeping sickness)		Nausea, vomiting, urticarial rash.
Nifurtimox	T. cruzi (Chagas Dz)	Creates free radicals that are toxic to T. cruzi.	Hypersensitivity reactions.
Sodium Stibogluconate	Leishmaniasis		Phlebotoxic (toxic to veins), pancreatitis.

MICROBIOLOGY – VIROLOGY

Virus structure

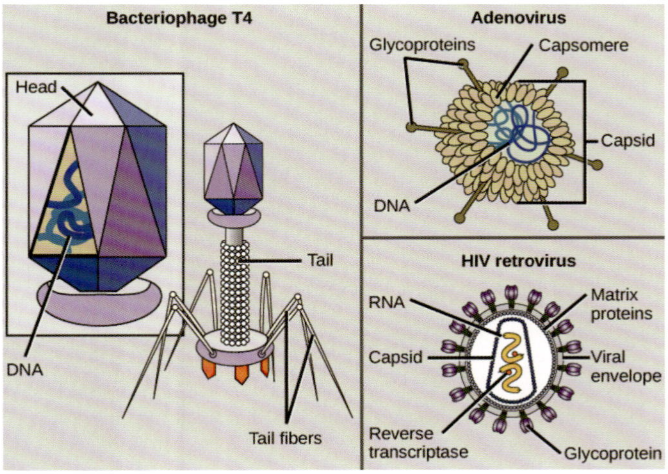

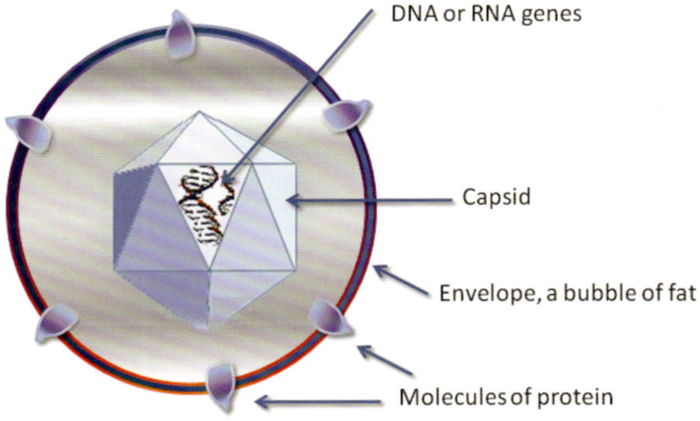

QUICK VIRAL REFERENCES, CHARTS and DEFINITIONS

Antigenic Variation (Antigenic shift, Genetic shift) (tip: "oh sh.....t, its bad)

- Cause of pandemics (infection of infectious disease that spread across large areas, multiple continents/world. (ie: flu, smallpox, tuberculosis, HIV)
- **Reassortment** of viral genome. Heavily associated with the influenza virus and other segmented viruses. (**tip**: reas"S"ortment – "S"egmented viruses).
- Reassortment allows the viruses to become **resistance** and makes **long lasting immunity difficult**, the viruses change constantly

Genetic Drift, Antigenic Drift

- Cause of epidemics (rapid spread of infectious disease to a large number of people in a population within short periods of time: 2 weeks or less. It is not required to be contagious. Ie: meningococcal infections, contaminated water or food supplies, measles).
- Changes in the virus are due to random mutations in the **hemagglutinin or neuraminidase** genes.
- Not as serious as Antigenic Shift

HEPATITIS

Virus	Classification	Transmission	Carcinoma Risk	Additional Facts
HEP A (HAV)	RNA - Picornavirus	Fecal-oral	No	Acute – self limiting Vaccine: 2 doses
HEP B (HBV)	DNA - Hepadnavirus	Sexual	Yes	Vaccine: 3 doses
HEP C (HCV)	RNA - Flavivirus	Blood	Yes	No vaccine
HEP D (HDV)	RNA – Delta Virus	Sexual, Parenteral	Yes	Must HEP B
HEP E (HEV)	RNA Herpesvirus	Fecal-oral	No	↑ mortality in **pregnant women**

(**tip**: HEP B, C, D: Sex, blood, parenteral. HEP A, E: Food and water)

MEASLES Differentials

RUBELLA (German, 3 day measles)	**Rubeola (Measles)**	**Roseola**
RNA, Togavirus	RNA, Paramyxovirus	DNA, HSV 6 (Herpes Virus)
Rash: Face to trunk	Rash: Face to trunk	Rash: AFTER fever, truck to limbs
Lymphadenopathy, Arthritis (joint pain), thrombocytopenia	NO lymphadenopathy, NO arthritis (joint pain), Koplik spots, 3 C's: cough, coryza, conjunctivitis	Very high fever then rash. Rosy, non-pruritic rash
	SSPE (Subacute sclerosing Panencephalitis)	

Segmented Viruses
- All segmented viruses are RNA
- (BOAR) Bunyaviruses, Orthomyxoviruses, Arenaviruses, Reoviruses

Viral Genetics

Complementation
- When 2 viruses infect a cell and one of the viruses is muted so produces a non-functional protein. The other normal virus makes functional proteins that provide for both viruses.

Phenotypic Mixing
- When 2 viruses infect a cell and the first virus is coated with the surface proteins of the second virus, but the progeny show only the first viruses genetic material.

Reassortment
- When **SEGMENTED** viruses exchange **segments**. Most common among influenza.
- (**tip**: rea**S**sortment = **S** for **S**egmented, or SORT the segments)

Recombination
- When viruses COMBINE and EXCHANGE **GENES** between 2 chromosomes by crossing over.

Virus Cell Receptors and Binding of Cells
- CMV: cellular integrins
- EBV: CD21 (EBV gp 350 binds with CD21)
- HIV: CD4 and CXCR4 and CCR5 (HIV gp120 binds with CD4)
- Rabies: Nicotinic (ACh receptor)
- Rhinovirus (acidic): ICAM1 (CD54)
- Parvo B-19 binds with RBC and P antigen

Viral Replication
- **DNA viruses replicate in the nucleus** (**except** for the pox virus that replicates in the cytoplasm)
- **RNA viruses replicate in the cytoplasm** (**except** for influenza, Retrovirus)
- Viruses must use eukaryote ribosomes for protein synthesis and put their genome into the mRNA

Virus Structure
- DNA viruses are all double stranded DNA (**except for Parvo**). (**tip**: "D"NA for "D"ouble stranded)
- RNA viruses are all single stranded RNA (**except for Reoviridae**)
- Viral **envelopes**: **All HSV (Herpes) Viruses get their envelope from cell host nuclear membrane**. All others get their envelope from the outer membrane of the host cell

Virus Vaccines
- **Live Vaccines**: Induce BOTH cell-mediated and humoral immunity
  Influenza (intranasal), MMR (Rubella), Zoster (Shingles), Polio (Sabin), Smallpox, Yellow Fever, Varicella (Chickenpox), BCG (TB), Rotavirus, Mumps
- **Killed Vaccines**: Induce ONLY humoral immunity
  HEP A (HAV), Influenza (injected), Salk Polio, Rabies, Cholera
- Recombinant Vaccines (Purified proteins: protein antigens that have been produced from large amounts of the pathogenic organism so that the individual produces antibodies to the protein antigen)
  HEP B (HBV, HBsAg), HPV (types 6, 11, 16, 18)

Virus Identification on RFLP (Restriction Fragment Length Polymorphisms) Polyacrylamide Gel Cultures

- Restriction enzymes are used to help differentiate between DNA and RNA viruses.
- The key is to determine from the vignette which type of virus the patient has based on the description of the signs and symptoms. Either DNA or RNA.
- If it is DNA, these viruses are not segmented, which means all culture patterns will look the same.
- If it is a segmented RNA virus, then all of the culture patterns will all be different (due to reassortment). If it is not a segmented RNA virus, then all of the culture samples will look the same.

DNA Viruses

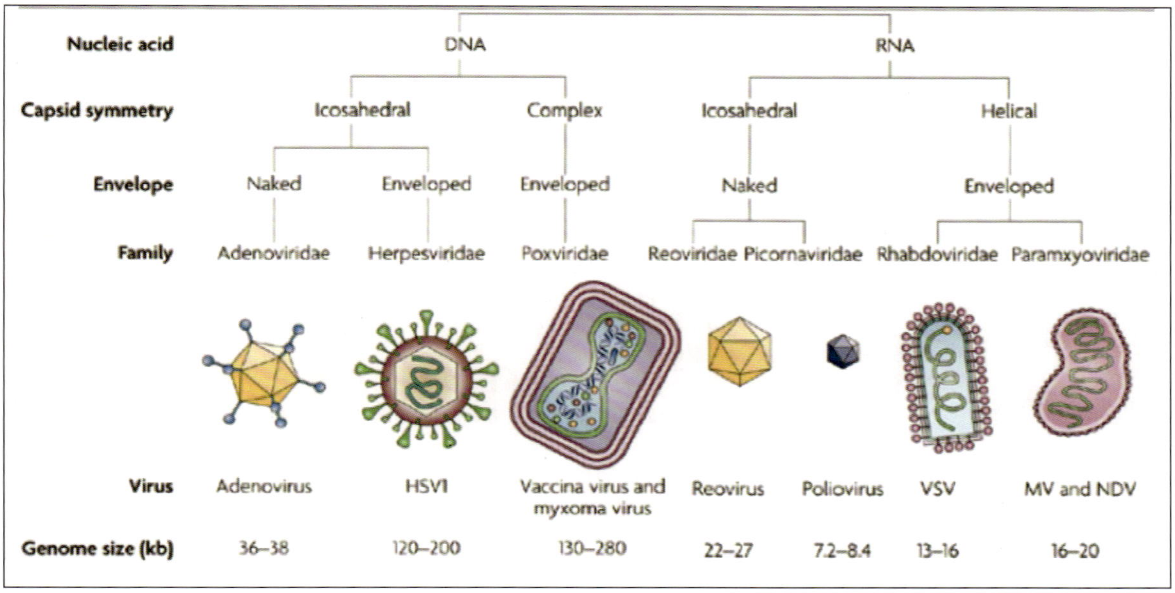

DNA VIRUS

All DNA viruses are Double Stranded *except* Parvo (Single Stranded)
All DNA viruses replicate in the nucleus *except* Pox (Cytoplasm)

ENVELOPED DNA VIRUSES

HERPES

HSV

Linear shape.
Only virus that gets its envelope from the *nuclear membrane,* all others get their envelope from the cell membrane.

HSV-1 Oral. Dormant in trigeminal ganglia.
HSV-2 Genital. Dormant in sacral ganglia.
HSV-1 and HSV-2: Test: Tanzack. Histology: Cowdry bodies, Inclusion bodies, multi-nucleated giant cells.
HSV-3 VZV, Chicken Pox, Shingles (Herpes zoster). Dormant in dorsal root ganglia.
HSV-4 Positive Monospot. Histology: Atypical lymphocytes. Burkitts, Hodgkin's
HSV-5 Negative Monospot.
HSV-6 Roseola. High fever, then rash.
HSV-8 Kaposi's. Endothelial cancer. Associated with HIV.

Hepatitis B

Circular shape.

Hepatitis B Only DNA Hepatitis. Has reverse transcriptase. Has speres and tubes.

Pox Virus

Linear, brick shape.

Pox Only DNA that replicates in the cytoplasm.
Largest DNA virus.
Mollusum contagiosum, Small Pox, Cow Pox,
If in adults is assocated with HIV.

NON - ENVELOPED DNA VIRUSES

Adeno Virus

Linear shape.

Adeno Virus: #1 UTI in daycares, pink eye, gastroenteritis, sore throat/cough.

Parvo Virus

Linear shape.

Parvo: Only single-stranded DNA. Smallest DNA.
AKA: Slapped cheek, 5th Disease, Erythema Infectiosum.
Aplastic crisis, Hydrops fetalis in pregnancy,
Pure RBC aplasia, Mimics rheumatoid arthritis (symetrical).

Papillo Virus (HPV)

Circular shape.

Papillo Virus (HPV). HPV 6, 11 Condylomata acuminata (warts),
E6 = P53, E7 = Rb, Koilocytes, Anal cancer in males.

Polyo Virus

Circular shape.

Polyo Virus. JC Virus: Aids defining, Multi-focal leukodystrophy, demyelination in the brain.
BK Virus: Kidney disease, trasplants.

Enveloped DNA Viruses

Herpes Virus (HSV)

Enveloped
Double stranded, linear

ALL Herpes viruses get their **envelope** from cell host **NUCLEAR membrane**. All other viruses get their envelope from host outer cell membrane

DX:
Genital herpes: **Tzanck test**: smear of open vesicle shows **multinucleated giant cells.**
Cowdry A inclusions in infected cells

Encephalitis: **CSF PCR shows HSV DNA**

TX for ALL forms of Herpes:
TX for neuralgia pain: Gabapentin or Amitriptyline
TX for Herpes outbreak: Acyclovir oral
TX for Herpes encephalitis: IV Acyclovir
TX for Herpes in the CSF: IV Acyclovir
Acyclovir requires thymidine kinase

HSV-1 Herpes I
Mostly oral lesions ("cold sores"), but can include genital lesions or other areas of body.
(Dangerous if in eyes)
Can be brought on by stress, sun exposure and injury (ie: permanent lip cosmetics)

Transmission: respiratory secretions, saliva (ie: kissing).
Contagious if open lesions isolate or cover until crusted over.

SX: Painful Vesicles (lesions) in the oral mucosa of the mouth, on the lips or genitals.
Herpes LOVES the **temporal lobe**:
Temporal lobe encephalitis: most common sporadic encephalitis in the USA
Keratoconjunctivitis (inflammation of cornea and conjunctiva),
gingivostomatitis (canker sores in mouth).

Latent: Lies latent in **trigeminal ganglia**

Labs: Cowdry A Inclusion bodies in infected cells. Smear of open vesicles shows: **Multi nucleated giant cells**)

TX: **Acyclovir – oral**
Requires thymidine kinase

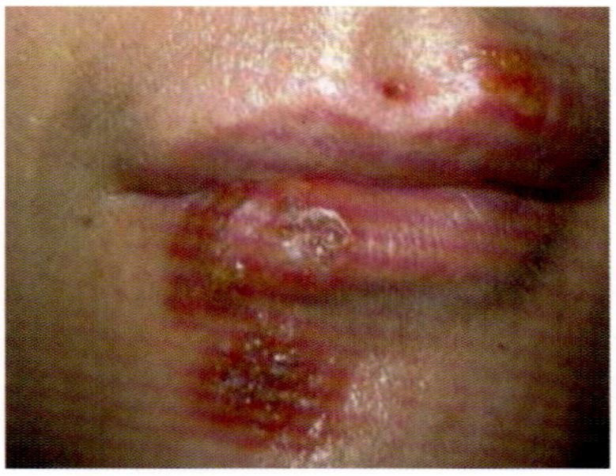

HSV-2 Herpes 2
Genital herpes.

Transmission: sexual contact

Latent: Lies latent in **sacral ganglia**

SX: Painful **vesicles** (lesions) on the genitals.

TX: **Acyclovir – oral**
Requires thymidine kinase

To reduce future outbreaks of Herpes: Treat with either Valacyclovir, Acyclovir, Famciclovir AFTER first episode

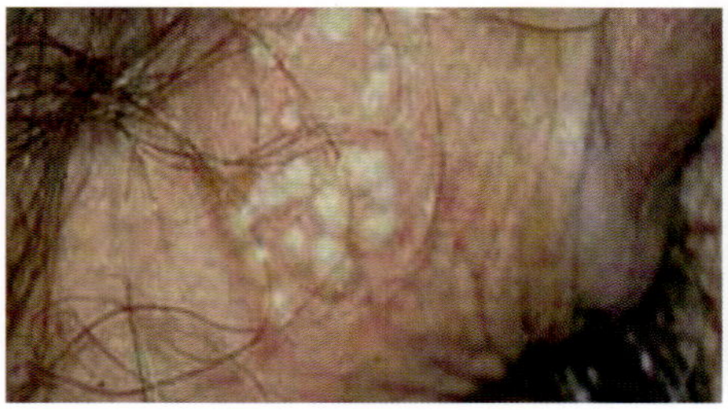

VZV Chickenpox, Shingles (HHV-3)
(AKA: Varicella, Varicella-zoster)
Transmission: respiratory secretions

Chickenpox: SX: Vesicles in **different stages of healing (papules, vesicles, pustules, crusting),** low grade fever, malaise.

Chickenpox vaccine: live
DO NOT give live vaccine to pregnant women or immunocompromised. Vaccine will help those that have already had shingles outbreaks.

Chickenpox exposure:
If patient is immunocompromised give IV Ig within 96 hours. If patient has had previous vaccine, just monitor

DX: MIT: Tzanck smear shows multinucleated giant cells.
MAT: Viral culture.
TX: Supportive treatment with topical ointments to relieve itching.

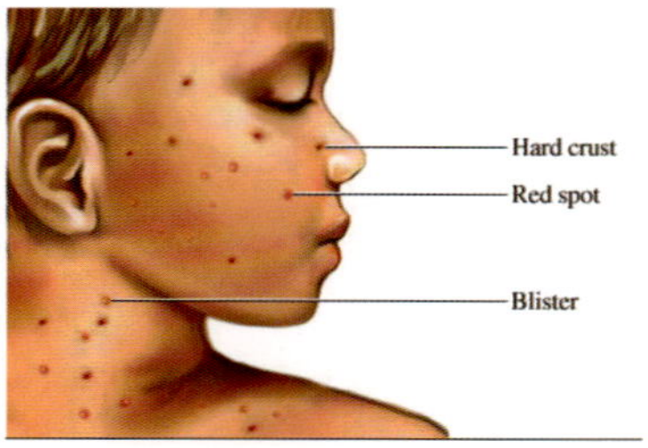

Shingles
AKA: Dermatomal Herpes Zoster.
Vesicular outbreak **along dermatomes**.
Burning and itching precedes outbreak.
Latent: Lies latent in **dorsal root ganglia**

TX: **Famciclovir** (**tip:** "Famous for shingles")
Requires Thymidine kinase.
TX: Nerve pain: **Gabapentin** (*Neurontin*), **Topical capsaicin, Pregabalin** (*Lyrica*), **Tricyclic antidepressants.**
Complications: Hepatitis, pneumonia, dissemination.

Vaccine: Varicella-zoster (Shingles) vaccine recommended to patients over 60.

Neuralgia (nerve pain) = BURNING

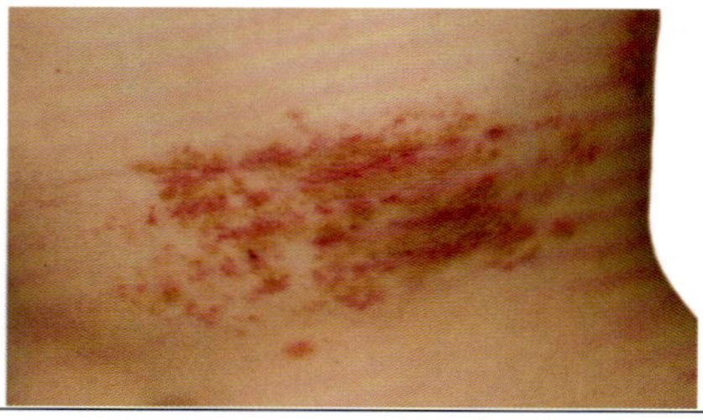

EBV (HHV-4)
Mononucleosis, Burkitt Lymphoma, Hodgkin Lymphoma, nasopharyngeal carcinoma

Mononucleosis
Transmission: **respiratory** drops and **saliva** (kissing)
MC: teenagers and young adults
B-Cell (CD 21) disease

SX: Gradual onset. (Resembles strep throat: if you treat with Amoxicillin for Strep Throat and patient returns in a few days with a rash, **they had Mono, not Strep. Strep is acute onset**)
Fever, **posterior lymphadenopathy**, pharyngitis (red, swollen throat, swollen tonsils, exudate), lethargy, mild autoimmune hemolytic **anemia***, hepatosplenomegaly.

*Autoimmune hemolytic **Anemia**: **Compliment mediated RBC destruction** (transient anemia).
Cells infected with mono look very similar to normal RBC's, so antibodies attack both, but not enough to cause major anemia. **Anemia is self-resolving.** DO NOT treat (do not give iron, this is NOT iron deficiency anemia, MCV will be normal).

DX: **Positive monospot test (AKA: Heterophile antibodies, latex agglutinin test, agglutination** of sheep or horse RBC's).
IgM Cold agglutination

Labs: ↑ PMN's, Blood smear shows host immune response of cytotoxic **CD8 and T cells against infected B lymphocytes (CD 21) resulting in atypical lymphocytes (Downey T cells).**

Risk: Spleen rupture. NO contact sports till **cleared by doctor before returning to sports** (no test or x-ray can show recovery)

TX: Self-limiting. Bed rest and fluids. If worsens to include respiratory problems, add **IV steroids**.

(See oncology section for Burkitt's, Hodgkins, nasopharyngeal carcinoma)

CMV (HHV-5)
Associated with HIV, congenital CMV, mononucleosis, CMV retinitis, pneumonia, CMV esophagitis

CMV Mononucleosis
Negative monospot test
SX: (resembles flu), ↑ lymphocytes, fever, muscle and joint aches, NO sore throat, NO lymphadenopathy,

CMV Pneumonia
High risk with bone marrow transplants

HIV CD4 counts <50 diseases:
CMV retinitis (Cotton wool spots)
CMU esophagitis (thrush) and linear ulcers

CMV with transplants
Creatine will rise with ↓ in WBC (neutropenia), fever, and intracellular inclusion bodies. (Neutropenic patients have high risk of bacterial infections)

High risk HIV and blood transfusions, sexual contact, saliva, urine, transplants

Labs: Smear shows **large "owl eye" giant inclusion bodies**

TX: **Gancyclovir**
Requires thymidine kinase

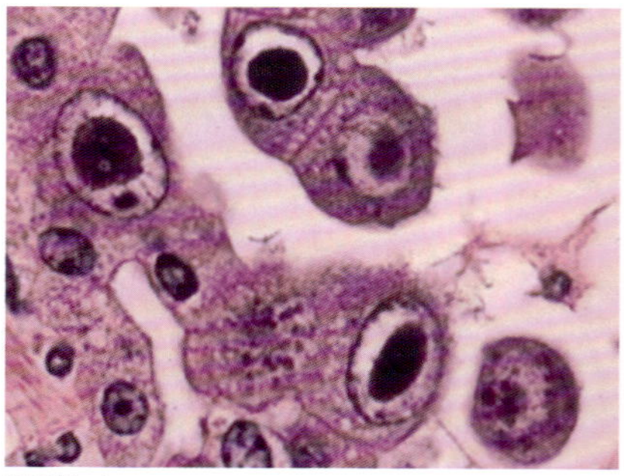
CMV virus

Roseola (HHV-6)
(AKA: Exanthem Subitum)

(HHV-7) Also causes Roseola

SX: **High fevers for 2 – 3 days and URI followed by rosy, non-pruritic rash once fever subsides.** Rash begins on trunk and spreads to legs and neck. Risk of febrile seizures with high fevers.

Transmission: saliva

TX: Supportive

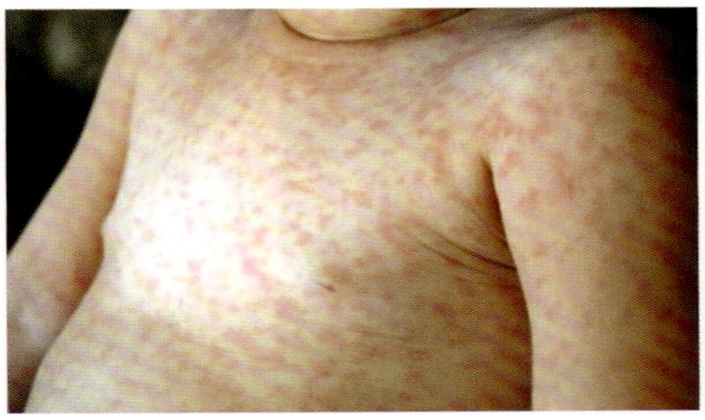

Kaposi Sarcoma (HHV-8)
Neoplasm of endothelial cells
Associated with HIV and transplant.

Caution: this is a vascular lesion, not a skin lesion. If the question asks the origin, it is **endothelial**, not epithelial.

Note: Kaposi sarcoma can also be located inside the small intestines, colon, lungs, liver, spleen, heart, bone marrow.

Transmission: Sexual contact

SX: **Dark (purple), flat and nodular/papular skin lesions.**

DX: Smear shows **spindle cells.** Biopsy.

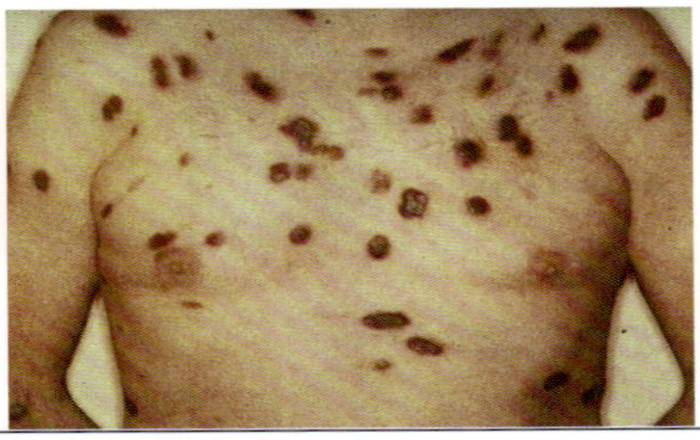

Herpes Encephalitis
#1 cause of sporadic encephalitis

Temporal lobe
Acute onset (2 – 3 days)

SX: fever, confusion, ataxia, encephalopathy. Death without treatment

DX: LP **shows viral CSF profile with RBC's.**
CSF PCR shows HSV DNA

TX: **IV Acyclovir**

Mononucleosis EBV vs CMV

EBV	**CMV**
Positive monospot test	Negative monospot test
↑ PMN's	↑ Lymphocytes
Posterior lymphadenopathy	NO lymphadenopathy
Sore throat (pharyngitis)	NO sore throat (pharyngitis)
Fever, myalgia	Fever, myalgia, joint pain

Hepadnavirus (AKA: Hepatitis B, HBV)

Enveloped with Spheres and Tubes
Double stranded, **circular**. (**tip**: write the "B" in "Hep B" using zero's "0")
Has: Reverse Transcriptase
ONLY DNA Hepatitis

Replicates DS DNA → template → progeny DS DNA

Viral hepatitis:
1st stage: Viral prodrome = fever, malaise, nausea, vomiting
2nd stage: ↑ ALT verses AST

Vaccination recommendations for HEP A: Travelers.
Vaccination recommendations for HEP B: Health care workers, diabetics/dialysis.
Vaccination recommendations for HEP A and B in adults:
IV Drug users, close contacts of people with HEP A or B, homosexual men, chronic recipients of blood transfusions, liver disease, immunocompromised.

HEP B (HBV) Serologic Markers
Acute Infection: HBsAg, **HBeAg, IgM**
Window phase: Anti-HBe, IgM
Chronic (high infectivity): HBsAg, **HBeAg, IgG**
Chronic (low infectivity): HBsAg, **Anti-HBe, IgG**
Recovery: **Anti**-HBs, **Anti**-HBe, **IgG**
Vaccination: **Anti-HBs**

Key:
s = surface antigen HBs = current infection (bad)
Anti-HBs = recovery (good)
IgM (core)= immediate/current
IgG (core)= chronic
Anti= antibody (good)
e = infectivity HBe=Active infection (bad)
Anti HBe= inactive virus, not infecting (good)
Core (marker of present or past infection: IgM, IgG)
HBV DNA: a measure of virus activity

Hepatitis B Infections	Hepatitis Prophylaxis
High risk for hepatocellular carcinoma. Show high LFT's: ↑ ALT and ↑AST. (Viral liver causes usually show a higher ALT while liver problems due to alcohol show a higher AST (**tip:** "S" = scotch) Acute hepatitis infections show ↑↑ ALT and ↑ AST with normal Alk Phos Associated with: **Polyarteritis Nodosa (PAN)**, Membranous Glomerulonephritis. Chronic TX: **INF-α, Lamivudine, Tenofovir, Telbivudine, Adefovir, and Entecavir.**	Newborns with moms of HEP B: HEP B vaccines (active immunity) and Ig (passive immunity) Needle Stick from active HEP B patient: 1st: HBV titer is checked. If high titer (have had HEP B vaccine series, showing HBsAb**) no shots** are required. If **low titer or no immunity** because no HEP B shots have ever been received: **Get BOTH, Ig and HBV** vaccines within 24 hours. If patient does not develop immunity after the first 2 of the 3 HEP B series, give the HEP B series over.

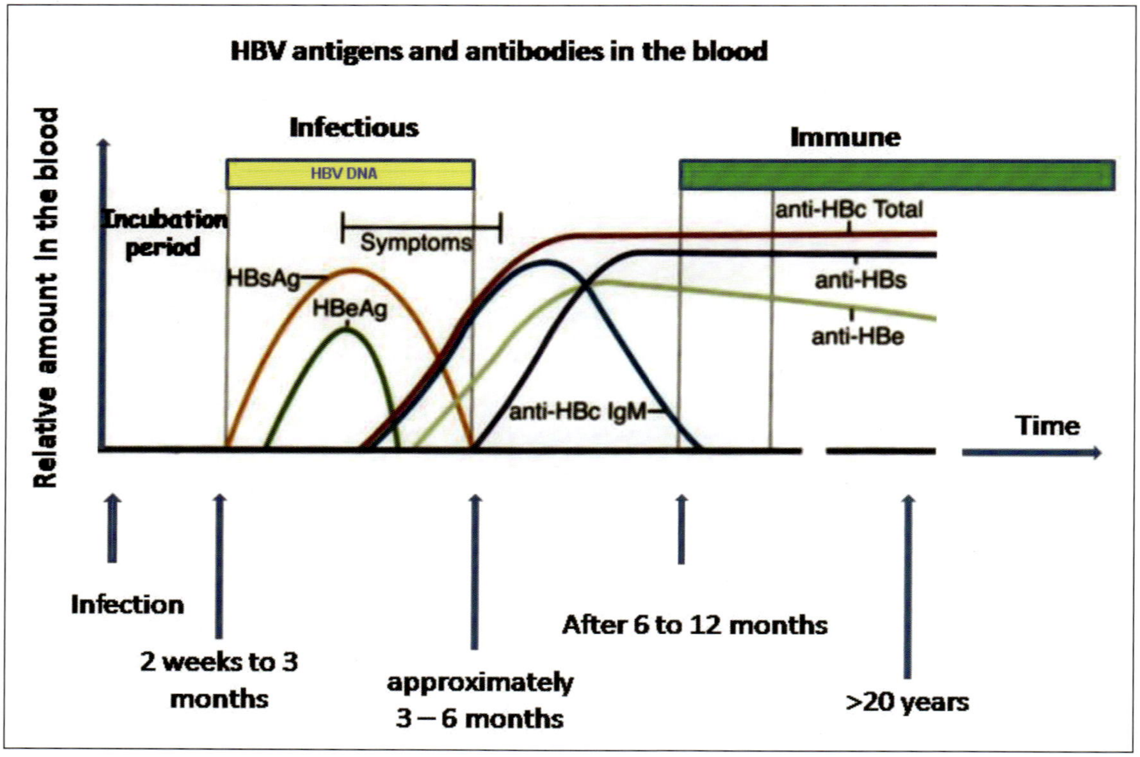

Hepatitis B Markers

	Surface Antigen	e-Antigen	IgM	Core Antibody	Surface Antibody	IgG
Acute, Infective	Positive	Positive	Positive	Positive	N	N
Window Period-recovery	N	N	Positive and then IgG will become positive	Positive	N	N
Healed-Recovered, past infection	N	N	N	Positive	Positive	Positive
Vaccinated	N	N	N	N	Positive	N
Chronic – low infectivity	Positive	N	N	Positive	N	Positive
Chronic-high infectivity	Positive	Positive	N	Positive	N	Positive

Hepatitis B Infection

- E-antigen: correlates with the active viral replication. Presence of e-antigen means high infectivity.
- E-antigen with IgG: Indicates a chronic disease with high infectivity. This condition must be treated with anti-viral meds.
- Presence of E-antigen is best indicator that an infected mother will transmit to her fetus.
- Surface antigen: Measures the active virus (viral particles). It is the first thing thing to be abnormal when person becomes infected.
- No surface antigen: indicates the person is no longer a risk for transmission.
- Chronic infection: presence of surface antigen for >6 months.

Poxvirus

Enveloped Double stranded, linear **Largest DNA virus** **Replicates in the cytoplasm**	**Cowpox** ("Milkmaid Blisters") Zoonotic with cattle. Subfamily includes: **Smallpox (Poxviridae virus)** Bioterrorism agent. SX: Maculopapular rash, raised fluid-filled blisters. Transmission: respiratory droplets, body fluids, fomites (clothing/bedding)	**Molluscum contagiosum** SX: Flesh colored, round, shinny, dome shaped lesions/bumps, pearly in appearance, umbilicated papules (central dimple). Usually 2 – 4 mm in diameter. Contagious. Common in children: self-limiting in 1 – 2 years. Adults: Associated with HIV 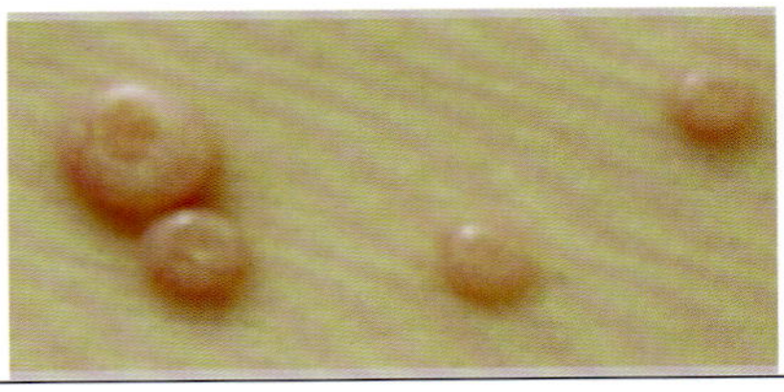

NON-ENVELOPED DNA VIRUSES

Adenovirus

No Envelope Double stranded, linear Causes: **Kids UTI's**, viral myocarditis, pneumonia, acute hemorrhagic cystitis (dysuria and hematuria), **febrile pharyngitis (sore throat),** upper respiratory infections, **Conjunctivitis (Pink Eye)** 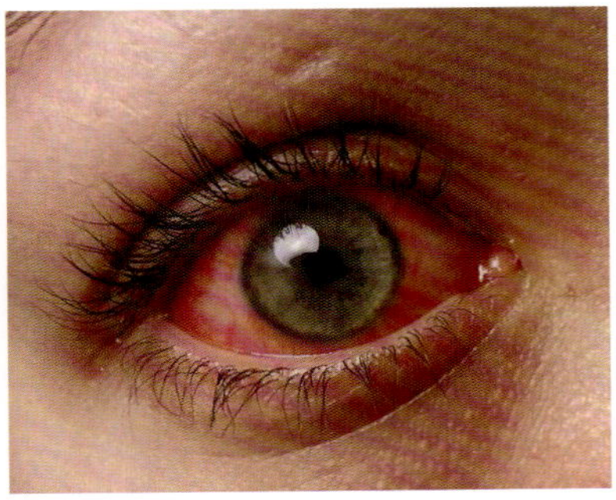 Pink Eye	High risk groups: People in close quarters. **Day care**, military, dorms, prisons **Kids UTI (MCC of children's UTI's), in daycares** **Febrile pharyngitis**: Mistaken for Strep throat. Most causes of sore throats are viral – do NOT treat with antibiotics. SX: Sore throat, **cervical lymphadenopathy** **Viral Conjunctivitis: Pink Eye** Inflammation of the conjunctiva. Highly contagious. Transmission: contact with eye discharge. SX: Eye redness, discharge of fluid from the eye/s, eye/s can be stuck shut in the morning. **Cobblestone** appearance of the conjunctiva. Associated with: URI, common cold, sore throat. Usually in one but can spread to both.

Conjunctivitis Comparisons

Viral	Bacterial	Allergies
1 or both eyes Discharge of fluid: red and crusty Assoc. with common cold, URI, sore throat 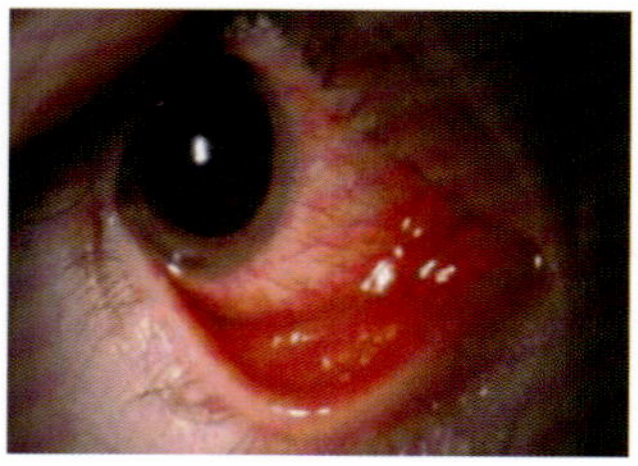	1 eye **Mucopurulent** discharge Redness, swelling of eyelid 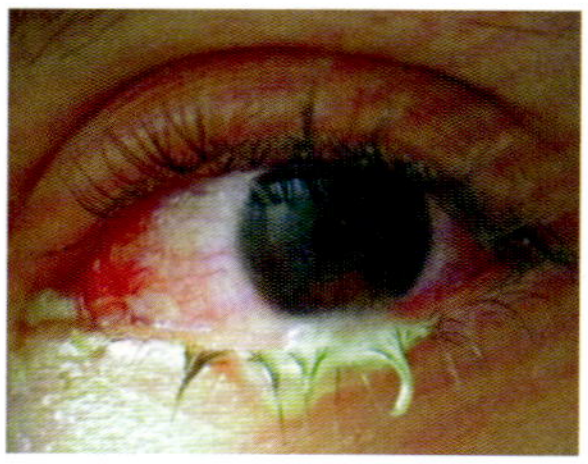	Both eyes **Bilateral itching** and redness Nasal congestion (pale, boggy mucosa) Increased tearing (lacrimation) **Cobblestone** appearance of conjunctiva SX due to histamine from mast cells 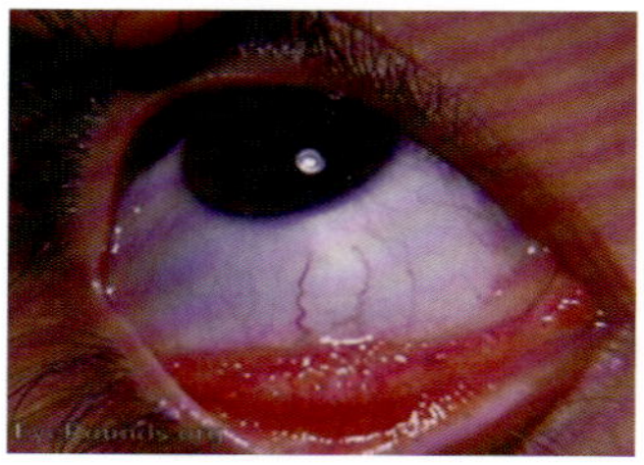

Parvovirus

(AKA: Parvo B-19, Slapped Cheek, 5th Disease, Erythema Infectiosum)

No Envelope **Only Single Stranded DNA** **Smallest DNA virus** Linear Replicates in bone marrow **P Antigen** **Causes:** Aplastic Anemia (Crisis) in **Sickle Cell**, Erythema infectiosum: "slapped cheek" rash in kids **Hydrops fetalis** in fetus Rheumatoid arthritis-like symptoms in adults, **Pure RBC aplasia** 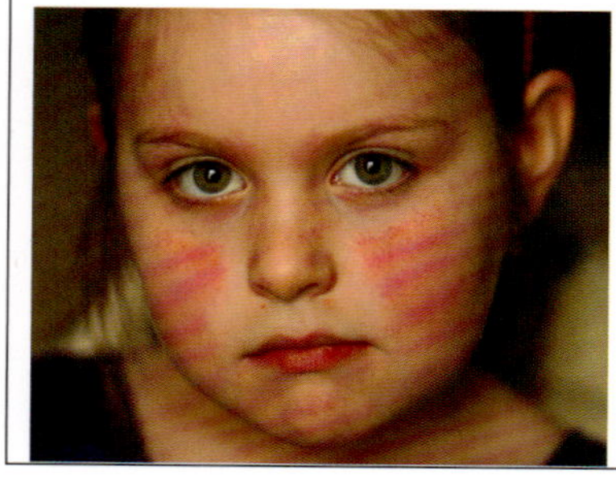	SX: "Slapped cheek" rash that is preceded by fever and URI. DX: Clinical TX: Supportive **Associated With:** **Sickle Cell: Aplastic anemia.** Parvo replicates in the bone marrow **Hydrops fetalis** in fetus: Parvo is cytotoxic to fetal blood precursors, which causes severe anemia. **Pregnant women MUST avoid contracting Parvo.** **Erythema infectiosum** (Fifth Disease, Slapped Cheek): circumoral rash around mouth/nose **Rheumatoid arthritis-like SX in adults**: This will usually be someone that works with young children (**day care, schools**) that will have contracted this from a child. Only other "arthritis" that **mimics rheumatoid arthritis** because it is **SYMMETRICAL.** Will also have fever and rash for 2 days. Self-limiting

Papillomavirus (HPV, Human Papilloma Virus)

No Envelope
Double stranded, circular

Causes:
HPV 1, 2, 6, 11, CIN (Cervical Intraepithelial Neoplasia), Cervical Cancer (HPV 16, 18, 31, 45),
Anal cancer in men, genital warts

Transmission: Sexual activity
High risk: due to higher number of sexual partners or having sex with a man who has had many other partners.
Condoms do NOT totally protect against HPV because areas around genitals and thighs are not covered.

Additional HPV Pathologies

HPV warts, associated with HPV 6, 11
Condylomata acuminata.

SX: Heaped up, white, flesh, transparent colored. (Resembles cauliflower)

TX: **Cryotherapy** with liquid nitrogen, laser removal, trichloroacetic acid, **podophyllin** (melts them away, but is potentially teratogenic, do NOT use during pregnancy), **Imiquimod** (sloughs off wart **without any damage to surrounding tissues** and causes no pain).

Anal Cancer in Males
Due to anal intercourse
Associated with HPV 6, HPV 16, HPV 18, HPV 31

Oropharyngeal or Laryngeal Cancer (throat)
Associated with HPV 6, 11
Finger shaped lesions on the vocal cords, epiglottis or larynx.
Histology: Finger shaped **fibrovascular** core lined with benign **squamous epithelium.**

CIN (Cervical Intraepithelial Neoplasia)
Cervical Cancer

Location: **"Transitional zone": squamocolumnar junction.**

CIN 1, CIN 2, CIN3 (carcinoma in situ) is the extent of the dysplasia

MCC associated with: **HPV 16, HPV 18, HPV 31, HPV 45.**
MOA: **HPV 16 and 18 produce the E6 and E7 gene** products.
E6 inhibits p53 suppressor gene. (**tip**: E**6** is next to p**5**3). **E6 promotes cell growth and malignancy by degrading P53 with ubiquitin ligase.**
E7 inhibits RB suppressor gene.

Risk: #1 Multiple sex partners, smoking, early sexual intercourse, or having sex with men who have had sex with many other partners, HIV.

Early dysplasia:
Koilocytes (squamous epithelia cells) that has undergone structural changes due to HPV. Shows **enlarged dark, wrinkled (like a raisin) nucleus** (2 – 3 x normal size) with **halo around nucleus (perinuclear halo)** and irregular nuclear membrane;.

Dysplasia on a PAP smear are preneoplastic cells: **Koilocytes** and atypical cells.
Histology: Shows neoplastic cells in the **sub-basement membrane.**

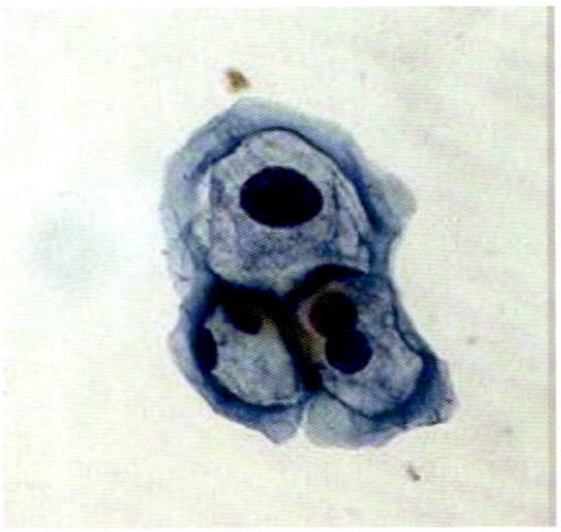

Koilocytes

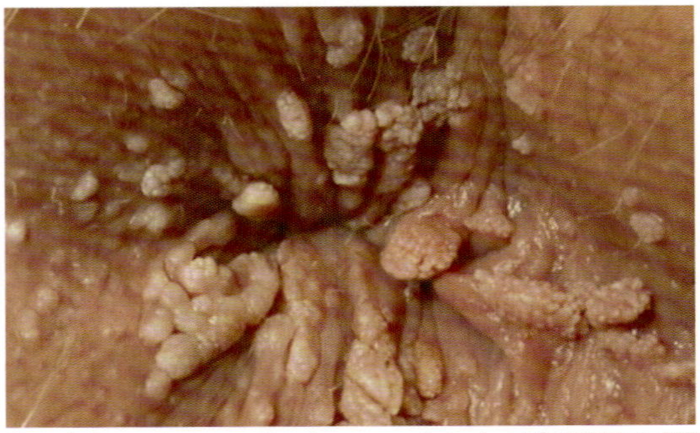

Condylomata acuminate, associated with HPV 6, HPV 11

HPV Screening Guidelines (PAP Smears)

- **Normal healthy patients: Begin PAP's at age 21 until 65 every 3 years**
- **You MUST also test for Chlamydia in sexual active women**
- **In immunocompromised patients (HIV, SLE, transplants) do PAP at time of 1st sexual activity, twice in 1st year and then every year.**
- **No screening required if no risk and no DES exposure (ie: hysterectomy with cervix removed)**
- **If cytological abnormality occurs on a PAP smear:**
  1) Colposcopy is performed. Acetic acid is applied to cervix at the squamocolumnar junction (transformation zone). Areas that turn white or have an abnormal vascular pattern are biopsied.
  2) If biopsy shows dysplasia then a LEEP (loop electrical excision procedure) procedure is done. (End of cervix is removed using a wire loop with an electric current. Future risk of LEEP is cervical incompetence during pregnancy (cervix is tied shut until term) and increased potential of spontaneous abortion.

Polyomavirus (JC Virus, BK Virus)

No Envelope Double stranded, circular	**JC Virus** (Progressive Multifocal Leukoencephalopathy, **PML in HIV**) – AIDS DEFINING Path: JC Virus crosses blood brain barrier into CNS infecting astrocytes and oligodendrocytes. (**tip**: J "C" = Cerebellum = **brain**) BK Virus Virus disseminates to **kidneys** and urinary tract (usually found in transplants). Virus is generally asymptomatic except in the immunocompromised/immunosuppressed. (**tip**: B "K", "K" = Kidneys)

RNA VIRUS

All RNA viruses are Dingle Stranded except REO (Double Stranded)
All RNA viruses replicate in the cytoplasm except the Ortho virus
Segmented Viruses: (BOAR) Bunyaviridae, Ortho, Arena, Reo

No Envelope

No Envelope
All Positive Sense +
All Icosahedral Linear

tip:
"HELP CALlie PICk REO"

HEP E: Associated with death in pregnancy

CALICI: AKA: Norwalk virus. Viral gastroenteritis. Cruise ships, hotels

PICORNA:
- POLIO: Anterior horn, Trendelenberg gait, Paralytic encephalitis
- ECHO: Aseptic menengitis
- RHINO: Common cold (tip: Rhino's long nose) Acid liable: does not colonize GI
- COXACKIE A: AKA: Hand, Foot, Mouth DZ, Pericarditis, MCC viral meningitis
- HEP A: Travelers, Oysters, Shellfish. Anti-HAV IgM = Active Disease

REO: ROTAVIRUS. *Segmented.* #1 fatal diarrhea in children

All Postivie Sense, Enveloped Linear (except Corona) Icosahedral +

RETRO: HIV. Reverse Transcription. RNA dependent DNA polymerase activity. T cell leukemia.

TOGA: RUBELLA (German Measles): Lymphadenopathy, joint pain. East, West Encephalitis

FLAVI: HEP C. No 3' to 5' proofreading. Dengue, Yellow Fever, West Nile, St Louis Encepalitis, Zika Virus, Chikungunya Fever.

CORONA: Helical Shape. SARS, common cold.

tip:
"I'm POSITIVE the guy in the RETRO TOGA wants FLAVored CORONA"

All Negative Sense Enveloped −

ORTHO: INFLUENZA. *Segmented.* Hemaglutin, Neuraminidase

PARA:
- CROUP. Parainfluenza, Barking cough.
- RSV. #1 Broncholitis in babies.
- RUBEOLA Measles. Koplik spots. Acute encephalitis.
- MUMPS. Orchitis

RHABDO: RABIES. Linear. .

FILO: EBOLA, Marberg

ARENA: *Segmented.* LASSA, LCMV. Circular.

BUNYAVIRIDAE: *Segmented.* HANTA, Congo Fever. Vector: Sandfly. Circular

DELTA: HEP D. Requires Hep B. Circular

tip:
"I'm NEGATIVE about flying DELTA to PHILLY (FILO) to see an ORTHOdontist pull a PARA teeth from a RABID BUNnY in an ARENA"

Laura A Deyer MD

RNA VIRUSES

- **All RNA viruses are single stranded except Reovirus**
- **All RNA viruses duplicate in the cytoplasm except influenza and retrovirus**
- **Positive sense viruses (5' to 3') are the most dangerous. These viruses RNA sequences may be directly translated into viral proteins and immediately be translated by the host cell.**
- **Negative sense (3' to 5') is complementary to the mRNA and must first be converted to a positive sense RNA by an RNA polymerase before it can translate.**

NON-ENVELOPED RNA VIRUSES

Calicivirus (Norovirus, Norwalk Virus)

No Envelope Single stranded, linear **Positive Sense** Icosahedral	Viral gastroenteritis. Associated with cruise ships, hotels.

Hepatitis E (HEV)

No Envelope Single stranded, linear **Positive Sense** Icosahedral	Associated with **pregnancy** Causes death (**tip**: **E** for **E**mbryo (pregnancy)

Picornaviruses

No Envelope Single stranded, linear **Positive sense** Icosahedral **Causes: "PERCH": Poliovirus, Echovirus, Rhinovirus, Coxsackievirus, HAV (HEP A)**	**Poliovirus** **Anterior horn damage** **Transmission: fecal/oral** Enterovirus SX: **Asymmetric** paralysis. Affected: **Trendelenburg gate (Superior gluteal nerve and the gluteus medias and gluteus minimus muscles)**, aseptic (viral) meningitis Risk: High in immigrants DX: LMN and meningitis **Vaccines: Salk = killed; Sabin = live**
Echovirus Enterovirus MC Infection: **Aseptic (viral) meningitis** Transmission: fecal/oral Virus uses proteases to cut up larger virus into several **Echovirus and Enterovirus: MCC Aseptic Meningitis**	**Rhinovirus ("Common Cold")** Only Picornavirus that is **not** fecal/oral transmission. **Acid labile**: destroyed by stomach acid so can't infect the GI tract. All other viruses are able to pass through the stomach, colonize and infect the GI tract. (**tip**: RHINO's have a very long NOSE (colds affect noses) Cell receptor: ICAM1 (CD 54)

<table>
<tr>
<td>

Coxsackie Virus
Enterovirus

AKA: Hand, foot, mouth disease, aseptic (viral) meningitis, **pericarditis** (leaning forward, f**riction rub, diffuse ST elevations** on EKG), **and myocarditis.**

Hand, Foot and Mouth Disease: Fever followed rash that blisters the hands, feet and oral cavity.

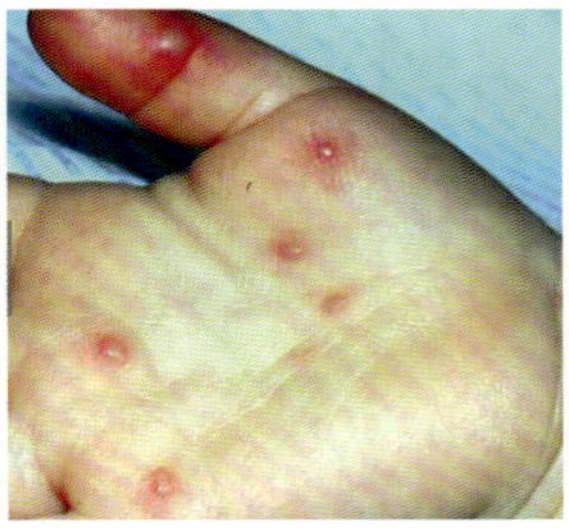
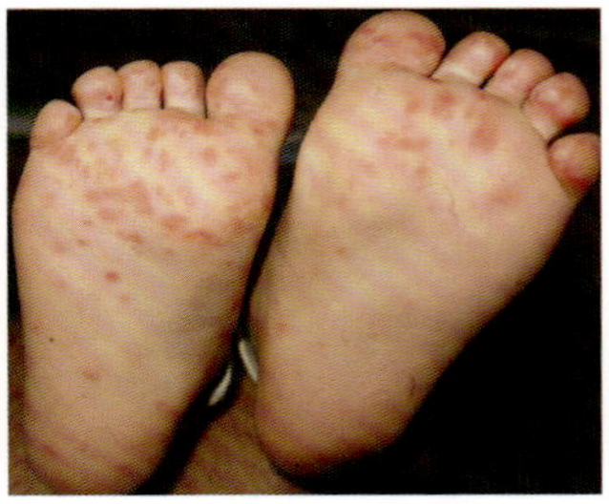
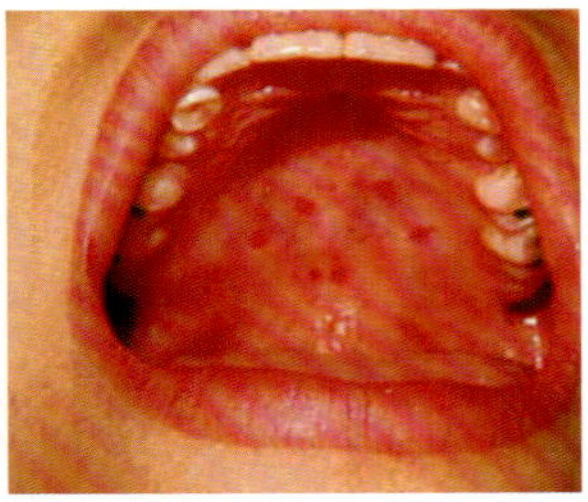

Coxsackie: Hand, foot, mouth disease

</td>
<td>

Hepatitis A (HAV)
Enterovirus
Acute viral hepatitis
Transmission: Fecal-oral
Asymptomatic, Self limiting in 6 weeks

Source: Shellfish, **oysters**, contaminated food, overcrowded conditions, **poor sanitation (travel).**

Higher risk: Prisons, anal sex, travel**.**

DX Marker: Anti-HAV IgM
Hepatocytes show ballooning and swelling (AKA: Councilman bodies). Councilman bodies = eosinophilic apoptotic hepatocytes.

Vaccination recommendations for HEP A: Travelers.
Vaccination recommendations for HEP B: Health care workers, diabetics/dialysis.
Vaccination recommendations for HEP A and B in adults: IV Drug users, close contacts of people with HEP A or B, homosexual men, chronic recipients of blood transfusions, liver disease, immunocompromised.

</td>
</tr>
<tr>
<td>

Asceptic (viral) Meningitis
MCC: Enteroviruses
MC meningitis in children (Asceptic Meningitis)
MC meningitis in adults (Herpes)

</td>
<td></td>
</tr>
</table>

Polio

Trendelenburg Gate: (aka: hip drop)

NOTE: The affected side is the side opposite of the lowered hip. When walking the body leans toward the affected side (EX: Compensation is by the upper body leaning to the left (in the case of right hip drop) in order to pull the right leg up and allow the foot to clear the ground. When standing, weakened abductor muscles allow the pelvis to tilt down on the opposite side. The pelvis sags on the opposite side of the lesioned superior gluteal nerve. (Example: If standing on the right leg, the left hip drops: meaning the contralateral side drops because the ipsilateral hip abductors do not stabilize the pelvis to prevent the hip dropping).

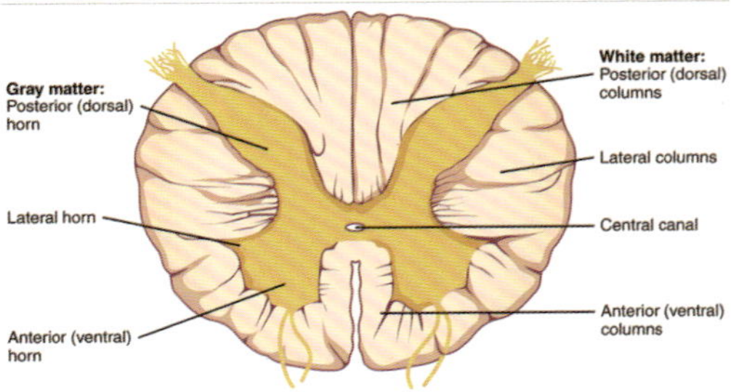

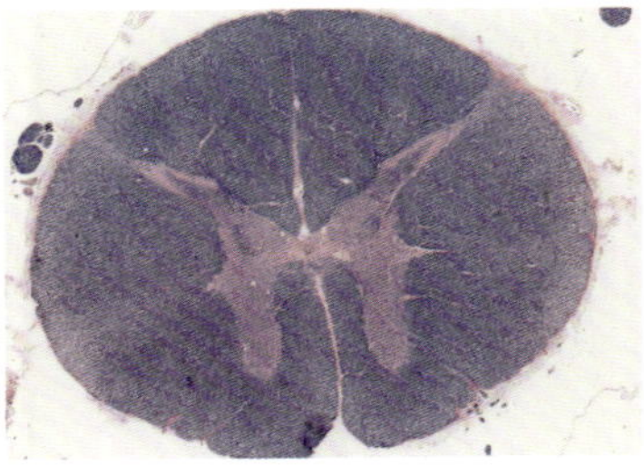

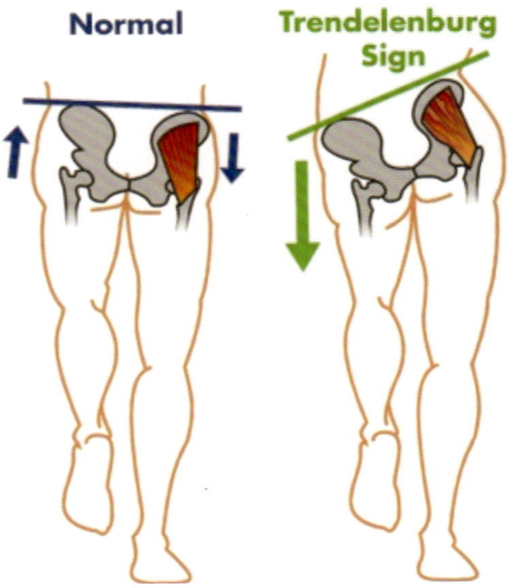

Reovirus

No Envelope **Only DOUBLE STRANDED RNA**, linear, Icosahedral **10 – 12 SEGMENTS** Wheel like shape 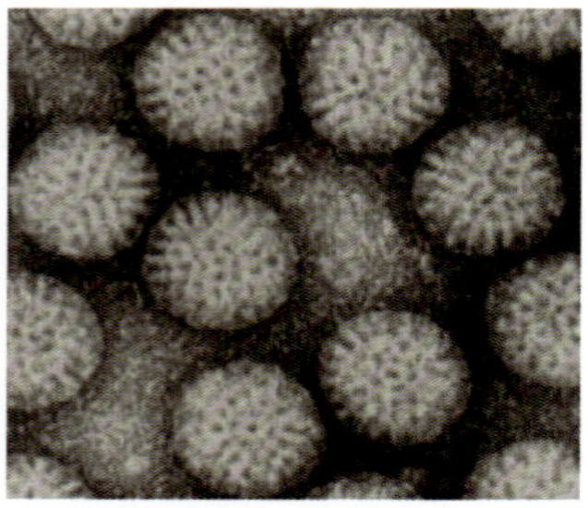 Reovirus (Wheel-like shape) **Coltivirus** (Colorado Tick Fever) Location: Rocky Mountain area. Transmission: Rocky Mountain Wood Tick SX: Headache, photophobia, myalgia, arthralgia, lethargy.	**Rotavirus** (**tip**: **ROTA** "**R**ight **O**ut **T**he **A**nus") **#1 MC fatal diarrhea in children** Transmission: **fecal/oral** Replicates in the gut and infects enterocytes of the villi (**villous destruction and atrophy**) of the small intestine causing decreased absorption of Na and loss of K. SX: Nausea, vomiting, watery diarrhea, low fever. Caution: **dehydration** is cause of death. TX: Supportive and insure of hydration

RNA ENVELOPED VIRUSES– ALL POSITIVE SENSE

Coronavirus

Enveloped Single stranded Helical Positive sense	**Common Cold** **SARS (Severe Acute Respiratory Syndrome)** Transmission: zoonotic SX: Flu-like, myalgia, sore throat, lethargy

Flavivirus

Enveloped Single stranded Icosahedral Positive sense	**Hepatitis C (HCV)** ↑varieties of HCV, so causes lower immunities due to antigenic structure. HCV is unstable, lacks 3' to 5' exonuclease proofreading. Transmission: **Blood** to blood in IV drug use, transfusions, poorly sterilized surgical instruments, tattooing. DX: ELISA, Confirmatory test: HCV RNA DX Cleared infection: Anti-HCV antibodies DX: Chronic HEP C: Fibrosis Labs: HEP C is ↓ C4 (**tip:** HEP C is 4 letters = C4) No vaccine and no prophylaxis available. SX: Jaundice, fatigue, loss appetite, joint pain. Can lead to cirrhosis and hepatocellular carcinoma. Associated with: **Cryoglobulinemia, Membranous glomerulonephritis,** Sjögren's, Porphyria Cutaneous Tarda, HIV TX: **Ribavarin, INFα, Sofosbuvir** (nucleotide analog) **Hepatitis C is the only treatable hepatitis.** **Liver transplant.**

Flavivirus cont'd

Yellow Fever Vector: Aedes mosquito. South America, Africa SX: Fever, liver damage, bleeding, black vomit **Dengue Fever** Vector: mosquito. Tropical. SX: Fever, dehydration, rash **Chikungunya Fever** (by the Chikungunya Virus) Vector: mosquito. Fever 2 – 7 days, joint pains lasting weeks to months. **Powassan Virus** SX: Flu-like symptoms. Affects the brain, causing infection and inflammation, neurological problems. (Viral encephalitis). Ticks: Ixodes, Dermacentor North America Flavivirus	**St Louis Encephalitis** Vector: mosquito. SX: Fever, headache, convulsions, paralysis **West Nile Virus** Vector: mosquito. SX: Headache, meningitis, encephalitis **Zika Virus** Vector: Aedes mosquito SX: Fever, dehydration, rash. Transmission: mosquito bite, human-to-human sexual contact, crosses the placenta. **Complications:** Microcephaly in newborns (mother to child transmission). Risk areas: Latin America, Caribbean, Africa, South America, Mexico, India, Eastern Pacific, extreme southern US.

Retrovirus (HIV-AIDS)

Enveloped Single stranded Icosahedral Positive sense Has reverse transcriptase (enzyme used to make complementary DNA (cDNA = double stranded DNA) from an mRNA template (reverse transcription)	**HIV-AIDS** **(See HIV chapter for all HIV details)** T cell leukemia

Togavirus

Enveloped Icosahedral, linear Single stranded Causes: Rubella, Eastern Equine Encephalitis, Western Equine Encephalitis	**Rubella (German Measles, 3 Day Measles)** SX: **Lymphadenopathy**, rash starting on head and moves to trunk, **arthritis (joint pain), thrombocytopenia** **Danger of congenital birth defects (See congenital birth defects chapter)**

RNA ENVELOPED VIRUSES – ALL NEGATIVE SENSE

Arenavirus

Enveloped **2 SEGMENTS** Helical, circular Single stranded	**Lassa Fever Encephalitis** Vector: mice Lymphocytic choriomeningitis (LCMV)

Bunyaviridae Virus

Enveloped **3 SEGMENTS** Helical, circular Single stranded **Hantavirus** SX: hemorrhagic fever, pneumonia Crimean-Congo hemorrhagic fever	California encephalitis Sandfly/Rift Valley fever **Heartland Virus** SX: High fever, fatigue, joint pain, maculopapular rash, SOB, joint pain, muscle aches, nausea, vomiting, diarrhea, low WBC and low platelets, loss of appetite. Ticks: Lone Star Tick Midwest USA: MO

Delta Virus (HEP D Virus)

Enveloped Circular Single stranded	Requires Hepatitis B (HBV) to co-infect. HBV must coat HDV with viral particles before it can infect. Causes a super infection.

Filovirus

Enveloped Helical, linear Single stranded	**Ebola Fever** Transmission: Direct contact with body fluids (blood) SX: Fever, sore throat, myalgia, headaches, vomiting, diarrhea, rash. Internal bleeding, liver and kidney failure. High death rate.

Orthomyxovirus

Enveloped **8 SEGMENTS** Helical, linear Single stranded **Bourbon Virus** SX: High fever, fatigue, joint pain, maculopapular rash, SOB, joint pain, muscle aches, nausea, vomiting, diarrhea, low WBC and low platelets, loss of appetite. Ticks Midwest USA: MO, KS, TN	**Influenza (Flu)** Highly variable due to **antigenic variation/antigenic shift.** Hemagglutinin (viral entry) Neuramidase (viral exit) (**tip**: **N**ever let a virus go) Resistance to flu is due to antibodies against hemagglutinin. SX: fever, **myalgia/arthralgias (aching muscles)**, headache, cough, sore throat, nausea, vomiting, diarrhea. Vaccines: Recommended annually TX: Self-limiting. Symptom relief: **Oseltamivir** (*Tamiflu*), **Zanamivir** a neuramidase inhibitor (flu) can be prescribed as long as patient has had flu symptoms **LESS THAN** 48 hours. If > 48 hrs: Symptomatic TX only: Hydration, antipyretics, analgesics.

Paramyxovirus

Enveloped Helical, linear Single stranded Causes: Parainfluenza, Measles, Mumps, RSV	**Parainfluenza (Croup, Laryngotracheobronchitis)** Viral infection of upper airway causing swelling of the throat. SX: **"Barking" cough**, stridor, rough voice, hoarseness, drooling, difficulty breathing (worse at night) DX: X Ray shows **"steeple sign"** TX: Oral steroids, inhaled/nebulized **(racemic) epinephrine and corticosteroids,** humidified oxygen. Do not use antibiotics, decongestants or antitussives. Self limited (1 weeks). 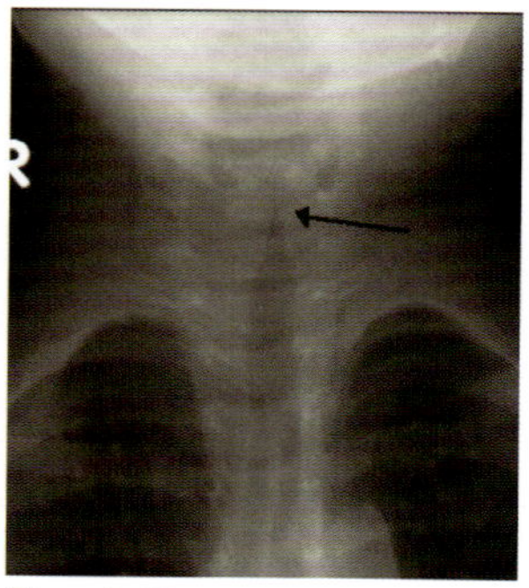 Steeple Sign

Measles (Rubeola Measles)
SX: **Koplik spots** (grey/white macules on buccal surface inside the mouth), maculopapular rash starting on head and moves down, "the 3 "C's": cough, coryza (inflammation of mucous membrane of the nasal cavities causing nasal congestion, loss of smell), conjunctivitis.
NO lymphadenopathy, NO arthritis (joint pain).

DX: Clinical. MAT: Measles IgM antibodies.

TX: Vitamin A, supportive.

RISK: Subacute Sclerosing Panencephalitis (SSPE)
Children that had the measles under 2 years old risk SSPE. Within 6 years the child begins **regressing in his/her milestones**. Ataxia, myoclonus, vision problems, IgG in CSF, behavior issues
(**NOTE:** remember that Rett's syndrome and Tay Sachs can also cause regression of milestones).

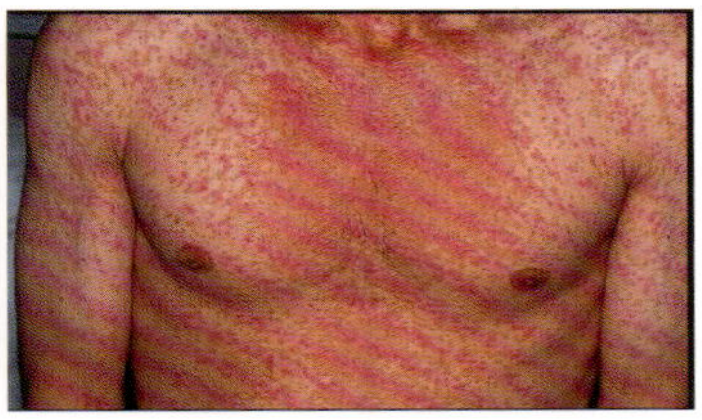

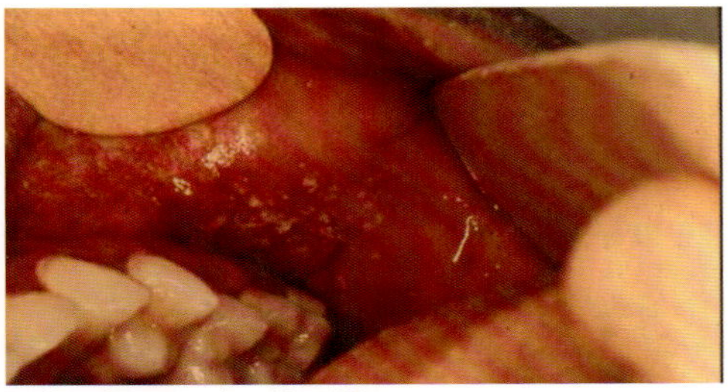

Rubeola measles Koplik spots

Mumps
SX: **Parotitis** (swollen parotid glands) preceded by fever, **orchitis** (inflammation of testes), aseptic meningitis.
DX: Clinical.
TX: Supportive.

Risk: **Orchitis can cause sterility** after puberty

Vaccine: MMR (live vaccine). Stimulates strong cell mediated immunity

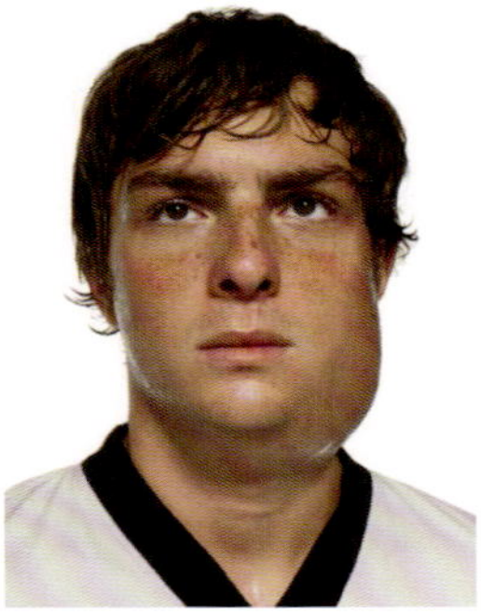

Parotitis

RSV
MC cause of bronchiolitis (inflammation of the small airways in the lungs) and pneumonia in children younger than 2 years old.

Contain **Surface F (fusion) protein** causing respiratory epithelial cells to bind and form multinucleated cells.
(**tip**: kids that get RSV are "F"abulous),

Transmission: respiratory secretions (mucus membranes) through close contacts or with contaminated objects or surfaces.

SX: Bad cold symptoms: Cough, runny nose, sore throat, earache, fever, lethargic, decreased appetite, wheezing, difficulty in breathing. Very contagious.

TX: Prevention of pneumonia: **Palivizumab** (monoclonal antibody). MOA: **Against F protein**.

Rhabdovirus

Enveloped Helical, linear Single stranded	**Rabies** Glycoprotein spikes. **Bind nicotinic ACh receptors in CNS** Transmission: bats, raccoons, skunks, dog bites. Once symptoms appear in CNS, without treatment, death is within 2 weeks SX: fever, agitation, photophobia, hydrophobia/hyper-salivation ("foaming at the mouth"), pharyngospasm, disorientation, paralysis, coma, death. DX: **Negri bodies (bullet shaped) cytoplasmic inclusion bodies** found in the brain. Migrate to the CNS in a retrograde direction up nerve axons. (**tip**: you always shoot a rabid animal with a bullet) Rabies vaccine: Killed vaccine of Rhabdovirus strains
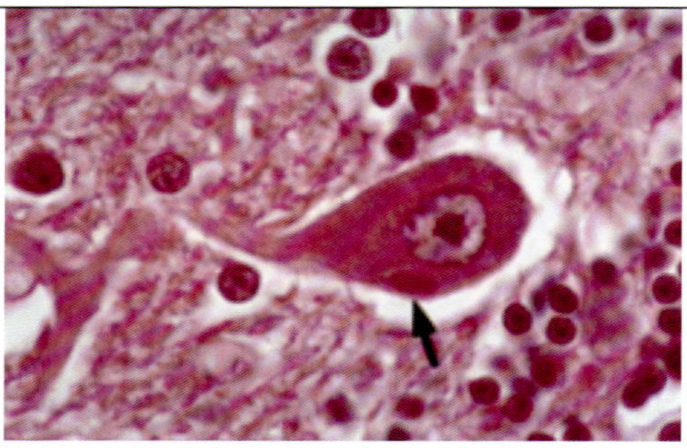 Rabies: Cytoplasmic inclusion bodies in neurons	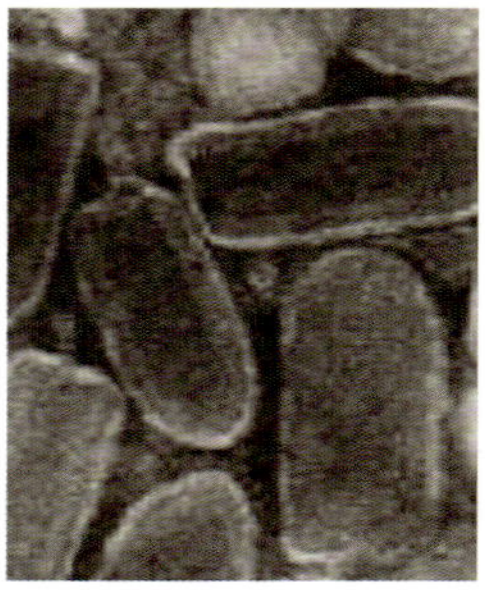 Rabies: Glycoprotein spikes
Rabies Prophylaxis (both active and passive immunity) 1) **Pre Prophylaxis: Rabies vaccine on days 0, 7, 21** 2) **Post exposure without previous vaccination: Rabies vaccine on 0, 3, 7, 14, Rabies Ig on Day 0** 3) **Post exposure with previous vaccination: Rabies vaccine on days 0, 3.**	**Rabies Propylaxis Determinants** 1) Any bite, capture animal if possible and obsverve for 10 days. If animal shows NO signs or symptoms, NO prophylaxis is needed. If animal shows signs, symptoms or dies the brain must be sent for evaluation (Florescent antibodies in the brain) show bullet shaped negri bodies. Must give post prophylaxis. 2) If the animal is not captured, you MUST assume rabies. Do Post Prophylaxis (Rabies + Ig) 3) Immediate prophylaxis for ANY bite to the head or neck 4) For bats: if a bat is found to be in a room/tent where someone has been sleeping, it MUST be assumed they have been bitten and prophylaxis must be given

HIV - AIDS
(AKA: Acute Retroviral Syndrome)

HIV
- Retrovirus
- Enveloped, single stranded, positive sense, linear, Icosahedral
- **Has reverse transcriptase**

HIV Diagnosis
- Normal CD4 count: 500 – 1500 cells/mm
- Immunocompromised ≤ 400
- **AIDS defining diagnosis ≤ 200 CD4 cells/mm**
- **BIT: ELISA** (antibodies to HIV protein)
- **Confirmatory test: Western Blot**

HIV Prognosis
- HIV PCR viral load (amount of viral RNA is in the plasma)
- High viral load: poor prognosis
- **CD4** is an indicator of **current immune status** (this damage has already occurred)
- **Viral load** is a marker of **disease activity** (this is damage about to occur).
  Goal: keep viral load < 50/μl.
  Patients that keep their viral load undetectable by PCR-RNA have the same life expectancy as a normal person.
  Viral load test are used to measure:
  - Measure response to therapy (↓ viral load is positive)
    Measure worsening or failure of treatment (↑ viral load is negative).
    Treatment failure = ↑ PCR-RNA viral load.
    Diagnose HIV in babies.
- **P24 and P41** are serological markers to diagnose HIV (HIV RNA)
- As CD4 counts decline, opportunistic infections increase.
  The goal of HAART therapy is to ↓ viral load which will then ↑ CD4.

HIV Presentation
Initial
- Presents like mono and the flu
- Night sweats, lymphadenopathy, diarrhea, abdominal cramps

Late
- Weight loss, fatigue, impaired memory, cortical and subcortical atrophy, **enlarged ventricles**

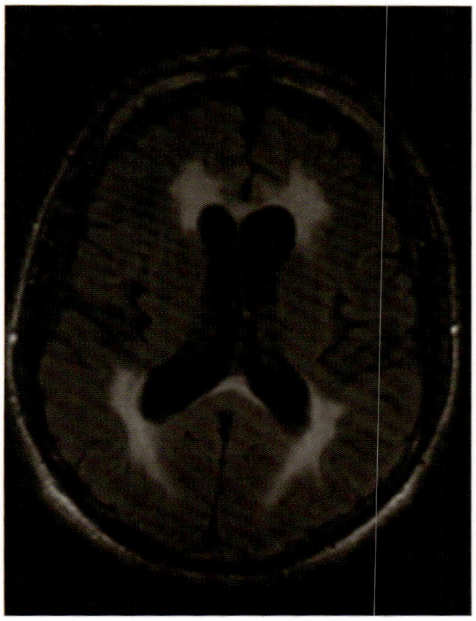

HIV Genes

- **Env gene**: gp160 is cleaved to form enveloped glycoproteins: gp120 and pg41. Envelopes come from the host cell plasma membrane.
  gp41 (transmembrane glycoprotein): **fusion** (entry into the cell)
  gp120 (glycoprotein): attaches (docking protein) to host CD4 and T cell so that virus can be **absorbed** by target cells.
- **gag gene: p24 and P17, capsid proteins and matrix proteins**
- **pol gene**: **reverse transcriptase, transcription, translation**
  pol gene provides **resistance** to anti-viral drugs (Reverse transcriptase inhibitors and protease inhibitors)
- Virus binds **CCR5** on the macrophages or binds the CXCR4 on T cells.
- CCR5 allows the HIV virus to enter cells
  Resistance (immunity) to HIV occurs when there is a mutation of CCR5 (homozygous)
- Reverse transcriptase: enzymes make dsDNA from RNA, then the dsDNA enters the host cell
- Retrovirus (HIV) envelope is acquired from **host cell plasma membrane**

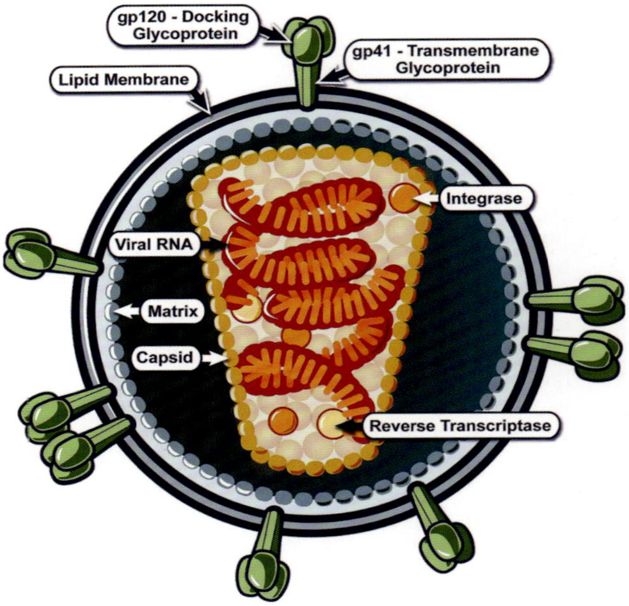

HIV in Pregnancy and Babies

- Pregnancy: If mother is already on HAART meds, she must continue throughout pregnancy.
  If mother contracts HIV during pregnancy, she must start on HAART meds.
  At birth, mother receives **AZT** during labor.
  At birth, infant receives oral **AZT** and continues on **AZT for 6 weeks**.
- Keeping viral loads undetectable (controlled) during pregnancy gives a < 1% transmission risk.
- Cesarean delivery for HIV-positive mothers when CD4 < 350 or if the viral load is high (above 1000/µl).
- HIV does not show up in babies until **after 1 month** old because anti-gp120 from the HIV mother crosses the placenta (↑ false negative results)
- SX of HIV in infants: **oral thrush**, pneumonia, lymphopenia
- **NO breastfeeding with aids**

HIV CD4 Counts and Diseases (See specific disease details under appropriate disease chapter)

- \> 200 Community acquired pneumonia: Strep pneumo
  < 200 Pneumocystis jiroveci (PCP)
  JC Virus
  PML (Progressive Multifocal Leukoencephalopathy)
  Cryptosporidium (Severe watery diarrhea)
- < 100 Histoplasmosis
  Candida esophagitis
  Toxoplasmosis
  CNS Lymphoma
- < 50 Mycobacterium avium
  CMV: Meningitis, Retinitis, pneumonia
  Aspergillus
  Cryptococcus meningitis
  TB
  Kaposi sarcoma

HIV Prophylaxis

- Pneumocystis Jiroveci Pneumonia (PCP): TMP/SMX. (If allergies to TMP/SMX: use Dapsone or Atovaquone)
- Mycobacterium Avium: Oral Azithromycin (1 per week).

HIV Diseases

Pneumocystis jiroveci Pneumonia (PCP)
Yeast
"Sporozoites" = Dark oval bodies
Stain: Methenamine **silver staining**

Highest Risk:
#1 AIDS defining disease. **CD4 <200**

BEWARE: if given ANY HIV patient with a CD4 count of **ANYTHING** over 200, the pneumonia is due to **Strep pneumonia**.
↑ pneumonia in premature infants
Immunocompromised
DX: Lung biopsy

SX: CXR shows: **Diffuse bilateral infiltrates** (interstitial pneumonia, "ground glass" appearance). Dry, **non-productive** cough.

Prophylaxis of Azithromycin for Mycobacterium avium should be started at this time.

TX: **TXP-SMX and add steroids** to aid in breathing
Prophylaxis for PCP can begin at CD4 of 200 with **Atovaquone or Dapsone**.

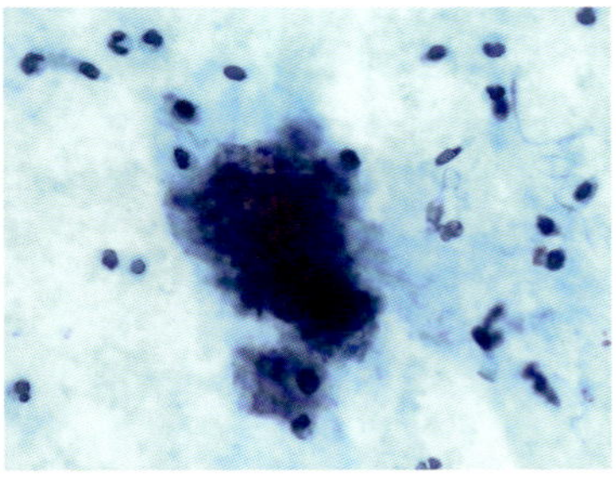

Pneumocystis jiroveci Pneumonia (PCP)
"Sporozoites"

Mycobacterium Avium
Pneumonia in HIV when the CD4 count reaches **<100**.

SX: Persistent cough, fever, night sweats, weight loss, diarrhea, malabsorption, anorexia, lymph node inflammation. It is common to find bronchiectasis involved. Can disseminate to the bone marrow.

Prophylaxis of Azithromycin **should be started when CD4 counts are at 200.**

Cryptococcus neoformans
Encapsulated yeast
Capsule **"halos" around budding yeast**
Budding yeast
ONLY fungus with a polysaccharide capsule

Cryptococcus meningitis
Spread: **hematogenous** dissemination to meninges.
Risk: HIV

Source: soil, pigeon droppings

DX:
Culture: Sabouraud agar
Stains: India Ink, stains red with mucicarmine
Capsule: Latex agglutination test against polysaccharide capsule

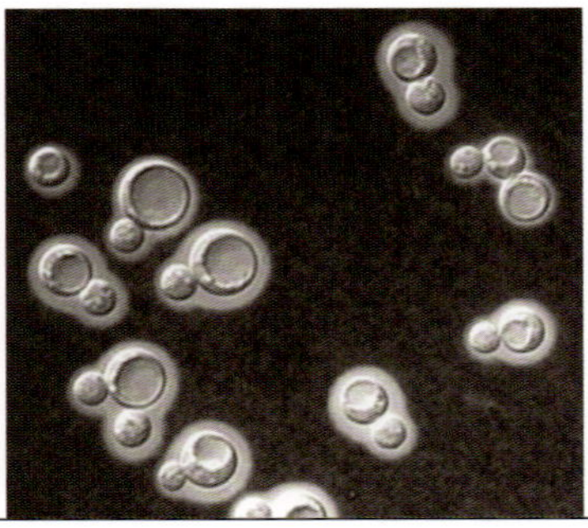

Toxoplasmosis gondii
Intracellular, parasitic protozoan
Source: Ingestion of oocysts (sporozoites). **Cat feces, deli meats,** skins of raw vegetables (peel vegetables).
Pregnant women must avoid these things – oocysts cross the placenta and infect the fetus.
Highest risk: HIV

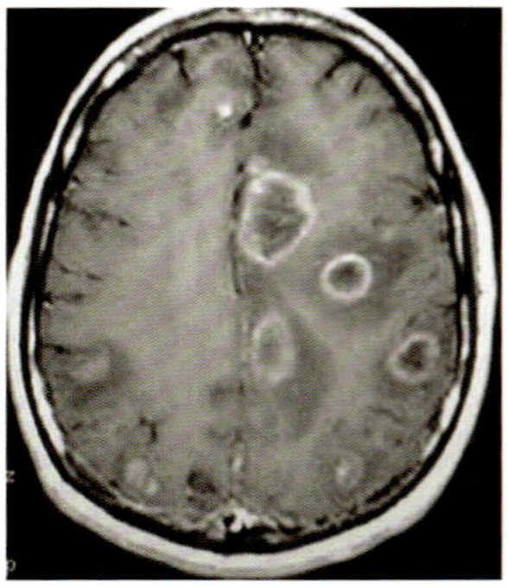

SX: Brain CT shows **Ring Enhancing Lesions (brain abscesses).**
Triad of: Chorioretinitis (cotton like- white/yellow lesions in the eyes), hydrocephalus, **intracranial calcifications**.
(**Tip**: tOxOplasmosis: the "O"s make a RING)

DX: Blood sample showing tachyzoites
TX: **Sulfadiazine (TMP) and pyrimethamine**
(If the TX of Sulfadiazine (TMP) and pyrimethamine does not work then the differential DX is Primary CNS Lymphoma

Cryptosporidium
Severe watery diarrhea in AIDS
Mild watery diarrhea in immuno**COMPETENT**
High risk of Sclerosing Cholangitis

Source: Oocysts (AKA: Red oocyst) in poor water supplies. Prevention: **Filtering water**

SX: Watery diarrhea (no blood), flatulence, bloating, increased Alk Phos

DX: Acid fast stain shows **Oocysts**

TX: **Nitazoxanide** in ImmunoCOMPETENT

Cytomegalovirus (CMV) – Herpes virus

Various forms of CMV infections can occur in HIV. Infections occur when CD4 counts <50 - 100.

MC form of infection is CMV retinitis – leads to blindness. (Patients will see "floaters" in their eyes and blurred vision).
Also causes CMV: pneumonia, meningitis, colitis, and esophagitis.

CMV retinitis: shows "Cotton wool spots" on fundoscopy.
CMV esophagitis shows **linear ulcers** on endoscopy.

TX: **Ganciclovir**

Progressive Multifocal Leukoencephalopathy (PML)
(AKA: JC Virus – Polyomavirus))

Inflammation of the white matter of the brain.
Caused by the JC virus.
Mortality rate of 30 – 50% in the first few months without treatment.
Other dz with a risk of PML: Hodgkin's lymphoma, multiple sclerosis, autoimmune dz, and psoriasis.

SX: Progressive weakness, clumsiness, difficulty in speech and vision, personality changes.

MRI shows nonenhancing areas of demyelination.

DX: JC virus in the CSF. CT shows white matter lesions.

Hairy Leukoplakia (EBV)
SX: White patches on lateral side of tongue.
Caused by EBV.
High risk in HIV.

Benign, white lesion cannot be scraped off, lytic lesions in the oropharynx.
White appearance is due to hyperkeratosis (overproduction of keratin) and epithelial hyperplasia.

TX: Self-limiting

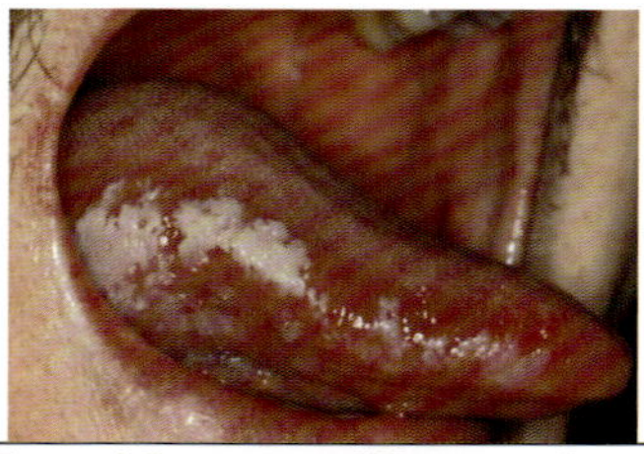

CMV Colitis (CMV)
Bloody diarrhea, abdominal pain, multiple mucosal eroding ulcers.
Microscopic findings: Large cells with eosinophilic and basophilic inclusions (Owl's eye)

TX: **Ganciclovir, Foscarnet**

Kaposi Sarcoma (Herpes virus, HHV-8)
Neoplasm of **endothelial** cells. (Vascular).
Biopsy: Spindle cells. Dark/purple flat/nodular skin lesions

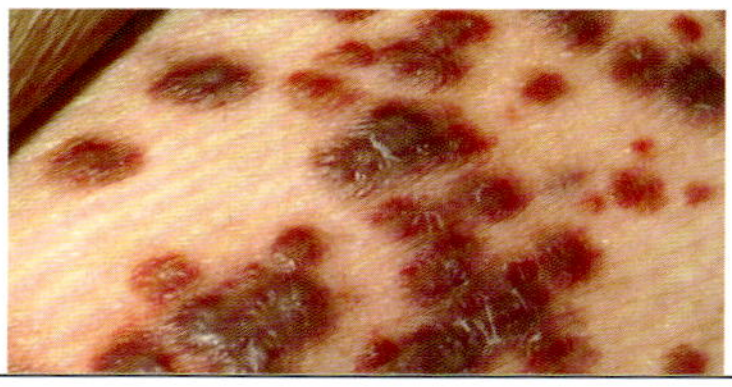

HIV Cryptococcosis Cutaneous
Multiple face and trunk reddish/purple papules with central umbilication (similar to molluscum contagiosum). Granuloma infection.
DX: cryptococcal antigens in serum or CSF. DX: Biopsy of lesions.

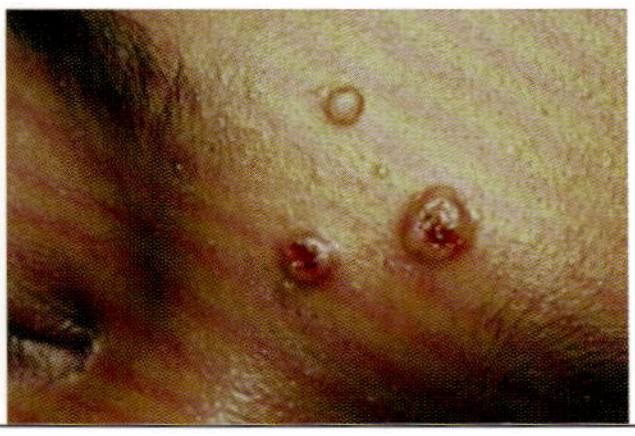

Squamous cell carcinoma from HPV
Women: cervix Men: anus

MC neurological complication of HIV:
Encephalopathy (progressive cognitive dysfunction with motor and behavioral changes).

Aspergillus fumigatus
45 ° branching, hyphae with septae
Spores (Conidiophore) with **"Chains" of spores**

"Fiber balls in lungs" or "**Colonizing** in lungs" (because it takes over old cavities, esp. after TB infection)
Mobile (moving ball)
Can show a **crescent** shape (moon) in the ball or "halo sign"

↑ Eosinophil's,
IgE response

SX: Hemoptysis, pleuritis pain.

CXR: infiltrates or cavitation.

EBV: B-Cell Lymphoma
Non-Hodgkin Lymphoma, CNS Lymphoma

If treatment for Toxoplasmosis **Sulfadiazine (TMP) and pyrimethamine** do not work, the pathology is most likely CNS Lymphoma. (Also with weak ring enhancing lesions).

Histoplasma capsulatum

Macrophage filled with Histoplasma
Spores with budding yeast
(**tip: "Histo hide**'s in macrophages)
AKA: Intracellular **macroconidia** with spikes.
AKA: **Ovoid cells** in macrophages
AKA: Yeast cells with thin walls
AKA: Huge hepatocytes
Found: **Ohio River valley, MS, MO.**

Infection Source: Wet/damp areas: Cave explorers due to contact with infected bat guano (AKA: spelunking), chicken farming, raccoons.
No person to person transmission

Acute Pneumonia
CXR: lungs show **reticulonodular** (**nodules**) pattern with hilar lymphadenopathy

SX: Fever, weight loss, **mouth ulcers**, **palate ulcers**, hepatosplenomegaly, night sweats.
Most common with HIV patients

DX:
BIT: **antigen in urine or sputum**
MAT: Biopsy with culture.

TX:
Local infections: **Fluconazole or Itraconazole**
Systemic infections: **IV Amphotericin B**

Candida albicans
Dimorphic yeast.
Pseudohyphae and budding yeast at 20° C
Germ tubes at 37°C
NO β 1-3 Glucan in the walls
↓ Glucan = osmotic instability

Candida Esophagitis: Oral and esophageal thrush in immunocompromised (esp. HIV with <50 cd4 counts and neutropenic patients).

SX: Difficulty and pain with swallowing, white coating will scrape off.

DX: White plaques in the mouth (can scrap off) and on endoscopy. Pseudohyphae and yeast on biopsy.

TX: Oral **Flucytosine** is BOTH diagnostic and therapeutic in Candida

HPV Squamous cell carcinoma. **Anal cancer in males** due to anal intercourse. SX: pain and pressure in the area of the anus, a lump or mass near the anus, change in bowel habits and anal discharge.	**Herpes Esophagitis** Similar to CMV esophagitis except the ulcers in the mouth are **"punched out".** (Remember CMV esophagitis has "linear" lesions).

HIV CNS Differentials

	Toxoplasmosis	CNS Lymphoma	PML/JC Virus	Herpes Encephalitis
Lesions	**MULTIPLE ring** enhancing lesions in basil ganglia (spherical shaped)	Weak **SOLITARY ring** enhancing	Multiple **NON-RING** enhancing lesions	
Location	Both cerebral hemisphere	Periventricular mass	Parietal/Occipital lobe	**Temporal lobe**
Effect	Mass effect	Mass effect	Focal lesions	
Fever			No fever	Acute onset
CSF Findings		**EBV DNA**		**RBC w/viral profile**
Misc Findings		(If TX for Toxo does not work then disease is CNS Lymphoma)	Vision, gate, speech affected. Hemiparesis	Acute onset: 2-3 days
Treatment	TMP/Pyrimethamine			IV Acyclovir

HIV Esophagitis Differentials

	Candida	CMV	Herpes (HSV)
CD4 Count	**CD < 100**	**CD < 50**	
Presentation	**Oral: White/Grey, pseudomembrane. Can scrape off.**	**LINEAR ULCERATION**, large, shallow ulcers, no thrush	Vesicles**, punched out** lesions. Multiple ulcers
Microscopic Findings	**Pseudohyphae, yeast**	**Intranuclear cytoplasmic** inclusion bodies (Owl's eye)	**Eosinophilic, intranuclear** inclusions. Cowdry Type A. Multi-nuclear squamous cells. Ballooning and degenerating cells.
Treatment	Fluconazole (Diagnostic and therapeutic)	Ganciclovir	Acyclovir

HIV Transmission

- **Transmitted by:**
  Bites from HIV positive persons, blood, semen, vaginal fluids, CSF, synovial, pleural, peritoneal, pericardial, and ANY other fluid with **VISIBLE blood.**
- Transfusion, perinatal (mom to child), vaginal transmission, needle stick, contaminated needles (IV drug use), sex (↑ with homosexual men), oral sex, anal sex.
- NO transmission danger as long as there is **NO VISIBLE BLOOD**.
  This is for: Urine, sweat, tears, sputum, vomit, nasal, and feces.
- NO transmission through kissing.
- Depletion of CD4 count takes from 5 – 10 years.

HIV Transmission Risk Without Prophylactic Treatment

- **#1: Mother to child: 25 – 30%**
- **#2: Anal sex: 1:100**
- Needle stick: 1:300
- Oral sex: 1:1000
- Vaginal transmission: 1:3000

HIV Post-Exposure Prophylaxis

- HAART therapy should begin within one hour of high risk exposure (unprotected anal or vaginal sex, needle stick injuries, sharing needles). After 72 hours the treatment may not be affective. The CDC recommends prophylaxis be given to any HIV negative person who was exposed to HIV for any reason.
- **Treatment last 4 weeks (28 days).**
- Side effects of HAART therapy: malaise, fatigue, diarrhea, headache, nausea, vomiting.
- Needle sticks: If the HIV status is unknown of the needle, post-exposure prophylaxis **is not indicated**. If the patient the needle stick occurs with is known to have HIV, prophylaxis is required.

HIV HAART Therapy (Highly active antiretroviral therapy)

- Initiated when:
  patient presents with aids defining illness, < 500 CD4 count, or high viral load > 100,000/μ., or opportunistic infection occurs.
- HAART Therapy = 3 drugs
  2 NRTI's (nucleoside reverse transcriptase inhibitors)
  1 NNRTI (non-nucleotide reverse transcriptase inhibitor) OR
  1 Protease inhibitor OR
  1 Integrase inhibitor
- MC drug used: ***Atripla*** (1 pill contains: **Emtricitabine, Tenofovir, Efavirenz**)

HIV Vaccine Recommendations (Same recommendations for ALL immunocompromised patients)

- **HEP B, 3 doses at 0, 1 and 6 months**
- **HEP A, 2 doses 6 months apart**
- **Annual influenza vaccine**
- **Pneumococcal with 1 booster shot at 5 years** (**Pneumovax**)
- **Tetanus every 10 years**
- **Meningococcal**
- **HPV**

ANTIVIRAL PHARMACOLOGY

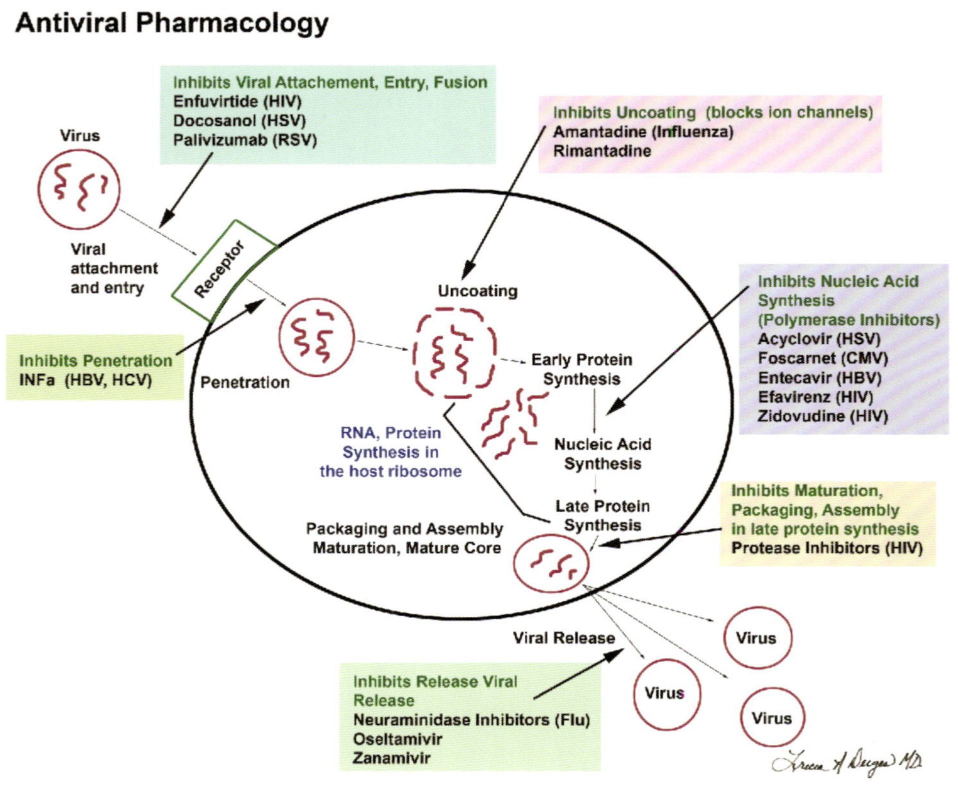

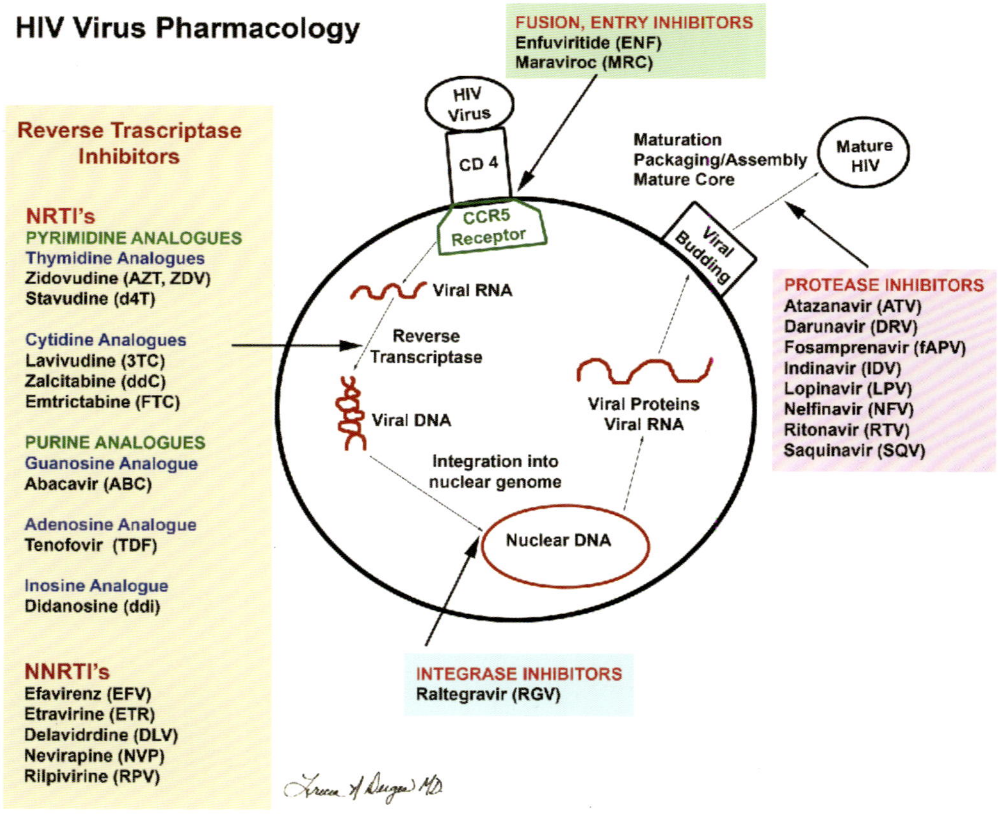

DRUG GENERIC name Trade name	Clinical Use	Mechanism of Action and Resistance	Toxicity and Notes
Amantadine	Parkinson's, No longer used to treat Influenza A due to a mutated M2 protein that allowed influenza's to become resistant. Fatigue in multiple sclerosis.	**Inhibits viral penetration and prevents uncoating of the M2 protein.** Releases dopamine from the nerve terminals.	Ataxia, dizziness, slurred speech. (**tip**: Aman "TO DINE". If you are going "to dine" you will need to take off your coat (uncoat).
Ribavirin	**RSV**, Chronic **Hepatitis C** (Use with **INFα** for HEP C)	Inhibits **duplication** of viral genetic material by **inhibiting** synthesis of **guanine** nucleotides by inhibiting **inosine** monophosphate dehydrogenase **(IMP)**	Teratogen. Hemolytic anemia.
Simeprevir Boceprevir Ledipasvir Telaprevir Sofosbuvir	Chronic Hepatitis C	Sofosburvir: RNA polymerase inhibitor. Simeprevir, Boceprevir, Ledipasvir, Telaprevir: **Protease inhibitors** (See all MOA's of protease inhibitors below under HIV meds).	None are used as a single agent.
Zanamivir **Oseltamivir** *Tamiflu*	**Influenza A and B**	**Inhibits neuraminidase** (Inhibits the release of the virus) (**tip**: MIVIR let a virus go)	Reduces the severity of the flu symptoms and **can only be given as long as the flu symptoms are less than 48 hours from onset**. The drug is not beneficial after 48 hours.
Interferons **IFN-α** **IFN-β** **IFN-Y**	Fight infections. **IFN-α: Chronic Hepatitis C and B** **(tip:** α, B, C) **IFN-β: Multiple sclerosis** (**tip**: β for Brain) IFM-Y: CGD (Chronic granulomatous dz)	Signaling cytokines (proteins) made by host cells to eradicate pathogens. **They "interfere" with viral replication.**	Neutropenia, myopathies, arthralgia, myalgia, leukopenia, thrombocytopenia, depression, flu-like symptoms. **Chronic Hepatitis:** Persistence of surface antigen for more than 6 months. Goal of chronic hepatitis therapy: Convert e-antigen to e-antibody. Reduce DNA polymerase to undetectable levels. TX for acute hepatitis C (with positive e antigen): treat with only one: Tenofovir, INFα, Adefovir, Lamivudine, Telbivudine, Entecavir.
Lamivudine INF-α Adefovir Tenofovir Entecavir Telbivudine	Chronic Hepatitis B		
Vitamin A	**Measles**		

The "Clovir's"			
Acyclovir **Famciclovir** **Valacyclovir**	**Acyclovir:** **Herpes (HSV),** **Herpes encephalitis** **Famciclovir:** Shingles (VZV) (**tip**: **FAM**ous for shingles)	**Terminates DNA chain by inhibiting DNA polymerase.** **Guanosine analog.** AKA: Incorporates into newly replicated viral DNA and **stops viral DNA chain synthesis.** **Requires thymidine kinase (enzyme) to phosphorylate drug.** Thymidine kinases/kinases cause differences in phosphorylation rates. Resistance: Mutated viral thymidine kinase.	Nephropathy due to **crystal deposits** leading to acute renal failure. TX: **Must stay hydrated**. Neurotoxic, phlebitis, confusion, nausea. Acyclovir is **SAFE in pregnancy**. Use if there are active lesions at 36 weeks. **Note:** the "clovir's" require viral **thymidine kinase** to be converted to acyclovir monophosphate. Host cell kinases then covert aciclovir monophosphate to aciclovir to triphosphate (ACV-TP). ACV-TP then inhibits and inactivates HSV DNA polymerases. This prevents any more viral DNA synthesis without affecting any of the other cell processes.
Ganciclovir, Valganciclovir	**CMV,** **CMV retinopathy in HIV.** **Hemorrhagic colitis in HIV.** Valganciclovir: product of ganciclovir and has better oral bioavailability.	**Inhibits DNA polymerase and terminates DNA chain.** CMV viral kinase forms 5" monophosphate. Resistance: Mutated CMV DNA polymerase or lack of viral kinase. **Requires kinase** (enzymes) to activate/phosphorylate.	Neutropenia (↑↑ PMN's if used with AZT), leukopenia, **agranulocytosis**.
Cidofovir	Alternative to Ganciclovir and Acyclovir	Inhibits DNA polymerase to terminate DNA chain. **DOES NOT require thymidine kinase/viral kinase phosphorylation.**	Nephrotoxicity (Administer with Probenecid and NaCl saline to decrease toxicity).
Foscarnet	Alternative to Ganciclovir and Acyclovir	Inhibits DNA polymerase in herpes and inhibits reverse transcriptase in HIV. **DOES NOT require thymidine kinase/viral kinase phosphorylation.** Resistance: Mutated DNA polymerase.	**↓ Mg, ↓ K (Hypomagnesia), (hypokalemia).** Chelates Ca so waste Mg. Seizures, arrhythmias.

HIV Therapy

- HAART Therapy (Highly Active Antiretroviral Therapy)
- 2 NRTI's (Nucleoside Reverse Transcriptase Inhibitors)
  - Plus 1 NNRTI (non-nucleoside Reverse Transcriptase Inhibitor), OR
  - 1 Protease Inhibitor OR
  - 1 Integrase Inhibitor
- HAART therapy is started once an HIV patients CD4 counts is < 500 cells/mm3 or has a high viral load.
- HAART therapy is used during pregnancy. If a woman already has HIV and is on HAART therapy she will continue it throughout the pregnancy. If a woman contracts HIV during pregnancy, she must start HAART therapy.
- HIV, Pregnancy, Fetus: AZT is given at **28 weeks** for prophylaxis and is given to the **newborn from birth until 6 weeks old**. (watch for a newborn that develops "thrush" (white coating) in their mouth a few weeks after birth).

DRUG GENERIC name Trade name	Clinical Use	Mechanism of Action and Resistance	Toxicity and Notes
NRTI's **Abacavir (ABC)** **Didanosine (ddi)** **Emtricitabine (FTC)** **Lamivudine (3TC)** **Stavudine (d4T)** **Tenofovir (TDF)** Zidovudine (AZT, ZDV)	HAART Therapy: HIV **AZT** is used at **28 weeks for prophylaxis** with HIV during pregnancy and is given to **the newborn at birth and continued for 6 weeks.** AZT: Treats HIV thrombocytopenia AZT: ↓ Kaposi symptoms, ↑ platelet production, ↓ opportunistic infections.	**Terminates DNA chain** by inhibiting nucleotide binding to reverse transcriptase (RT). DNA chain **lacks a 3' OH group.** **AKA: No 3' to 5' phosphorylation bond formation.** (RT: reverses normal 5' to 3' direction) **T**enofovir is a nucleo**T**ide, all other NRTI's are nucleosides and must be phosphorylated to be active.	**Lactic acidosis (nucleosides),** bone marrow suppression. **Didanosine, Stavudine: Acute pancreatitis and neuropathies.** (tip: it **DID** in your pancreas) **AZT: anemia** **Abacavir: Hypersensitivities**
NNRTI's Delavirdine (DLV) Efavirenz (EFV) Nevirapine (NVP) Etravirine (ETR) Rilpivirine (RPV)	HAART Therapy: HIV	**Inhibits replication of the HIV genome in host cells.** (Binds to reverse transcriptase at a different site than NRTI's)	Stevens Johnson, hepatotoxicity. Efavirenz: vivid dreams, CNS symptoms, drowsiness. **Delavirdine and Efavirenz: Do not use in pregnancy.** (**tip**: **NN**rti = **N**O **N**O in pregnancy)
Protease Inhibitors "the Navir's" **Atazanavir (ATV)** **Darunavir (DRV)** **Fosamprenavir (fAPV)** **Indinavir (IDV)** **Loprinavir (LPV)** **Nelfinavir (NFV)** Ritonavir (RTV) **Saquinavir (SQV)**	HAART Therapy: HIV (**tip**: NAVIR let a protease grow up)	Prevents **packaging, assembly and maturation** of new viruses. AKA: Lacks a **mature core**. AKA: Stops post translational processing of the polyprotein into a **core** protein. AKA: Stops proteins = **stops growth**. AKA: Inhibit viral **maturation** by **stopping protein synthesis.**	**Ritonavir: P-450 Inhibitor.** **Lipodystrophy (AKA: Hyperlipidemia = redistributes fat), Hyperglycemia. (Extra padding).** Hyperglycemia, GI, nephropathy, Diabetes mellitus II. Indinavir: **kidney stones**, hematuria
Integrase Inhibitor **Raltegravir (RGV)**	HAART Therapy: HIV	Inhibits HIV genome from integration into host cell by inhibiting HIV integrase. Host cells can't be used to process mRNA.	Hypercholesterolemia
Fusion Inhibitors **Enfuvirtide (ENF)** **Maraviroc (MRC)**	HIV Therapy	Enfuvirtide: Binds gp41 to inhibit HIV (virus) entry into the cell. Maraviroc: Binds CCR-5 on T cells (monocytes) inhibiting gp120.	Skin reactions at injection sites.

GENERAL PATHOLOGY CONCEPTS

Inflammation

- Characteristics: Redness (rubor), pain (dolor), heat (calor), swelling (tumor), loss of function (function laesa)
- Leukocyte extravasation
- Macrophages release IL-1, IL-6, TNFα, liver releases acute phase reactants
- Increased vascular permeability (allows more leukocytes to get through vessel walls)
- Increased vasodilation (allows more room in the vessel to get more leukocytes and other acute phase reactants to the damaged tissue for repair
- **Acute inflammation**: **Neutrophil,** eosinophil and antibody mediated. Rapid onset. Will result in either: complete resolution, abscess formation or progression to chronic inflammation (See infection time line below)
- **Chronic inflammation**: **Fibroblast** and mononuclear cell mediated. Granulomas. May result in scarring and amyloidosis

Margination (Leukocyte extravasation: Leukocytes exit blood vessels at sites of tissue injury)

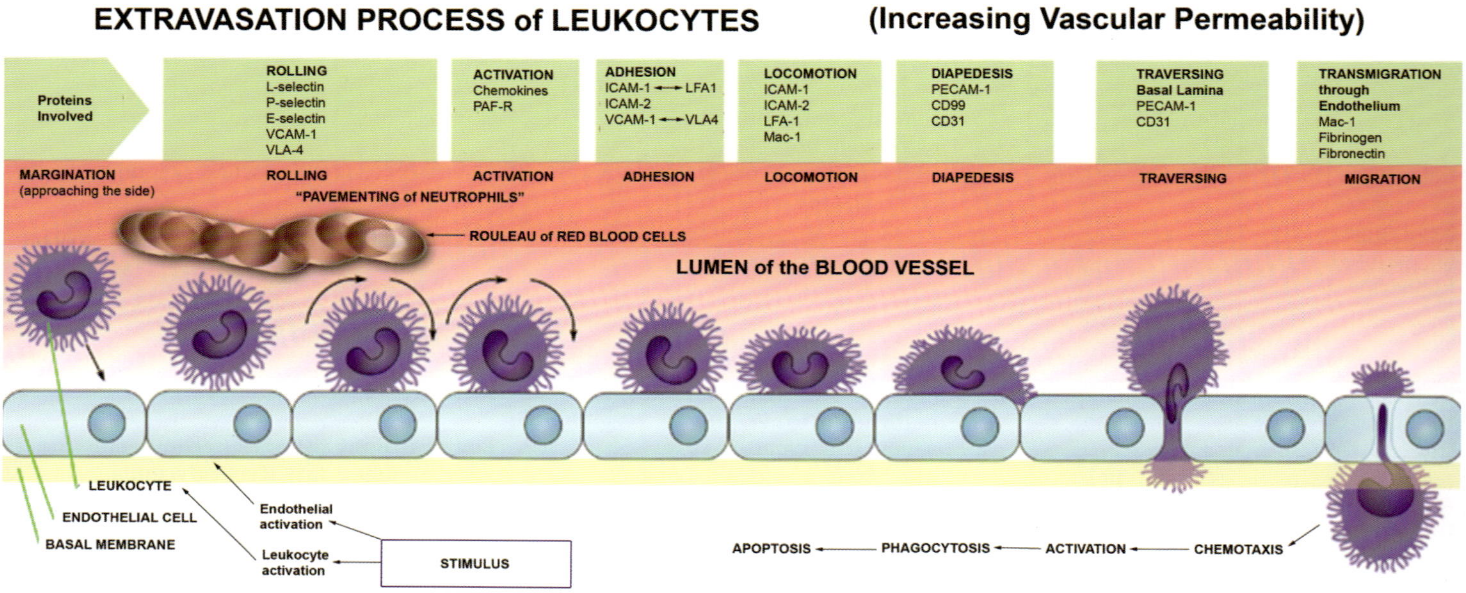

Margination/Leukocyte Extravasation Steps

STEP of Leukocyte extravasation	Process	Additional Molecules Involved
1) **Margination**	PMN's marginate to the sides of the blood vessel	Rouleau of RBC to the center of the vessel
2) **Rolling**	PMN's roll along vessel walls "**SELECTIN**" a spot to stop. **(E-selectin, P-selectin**)	GlyCAM-1 Sialyl-Lewis (AKA: Weibel Palade bodies/VWF), L-selectin (Sialyl-Lewis bodies are like the "glue factory" and VWF is the "glue" for adhesion.
3) **Adhesion (binding)**	PMN's adhere to the side of the blood vessel, ready to "INTO" (**INTEGRINS**) the tissues.	**ICAM-1 (CD54)** VCAM-1 CD11-18 INTEGRINS VLA-4 INTEGRIN
4) **Diapedesis** (AKA: extravasation, transmigration)	**PMN's exit** (squeeze through) the blood vessel endothelia cells.	**PECAM-1** (CD31)
5) **Chemotaxis**	**Chemotactic signals** guide leukocytes (by "TAXI") to the site of injury/infection	Signals sent to **liver** to release **Acute Phase Reactants**: C5a (PMN's), IL8 (PMN's), LTB4 (PMN's), **Kallikrein (Bradykinin).** Vasodilation occurs to increase vascular permeability.

WOUND REPAIR TIME LINE

Timeline	Reaction	Peaks
Immediate	Swelling due to vasodilation, clot formation (AKA: ↑ vessel permeability)	
24 hours	Neutrophils (PMS's), platelets	3 days
3rd day - Proliferative	T Cells & Macrophages (clear tissue)	7 days
7th day - Remodeling	Fibroblast (scarring) to ↑ tensile strength. Type III collagen replace by Type I	1 Month, finishes 3 – 6 months. **Note:** As wound healing continues into the weeks following the injury, there is ↑ in fibroblast migration and proliferation, ↑ synthesis in fibronectin (glycoprotein that binds extracellular matrix components) and collagen, there is ↓ degradation of extracellular matrix by metalloproteinases by Transforming Growth Factor – β. (TGF-β).

MACROPHAGES

- Antigen-presenting cells
- **Class II MHC** (major histocompatibility complex), **CD4, Helper T cells** and TcR (T cell receptor)
- Activated by interferon-y (gamma) and LPS (lipopolysaccharides from gram negative bacteria
- **Secrete: IL-1 (fever and mitosis of T lymphocytes); IL-6 (stimulates B lymphocytes into plasma cells, pyrogens (fever), TNFα (tumor necrosis factor – a (alpha); granulocyte=macrophage colony stimulating factor**

MACROPHAGE	ORGAN
Monocytes	Blood and Bone Marrow
Kupffer	Liver
Dust Cells/Alveolar Macrophage	Lungs
Microglia	Brain (CNS)
Hofbauer	Placenta
Sinusoidal or RES (reticuloendothelial system)	Spleen
Sinus Histocytes	Lymph Nodes
Giant Cell, Histocyte	Connective Tissues
Langerhans	Skin and Mucosa
Osteoclast	Bone
Granulomas	Epithelioid
Mesangial	Kidneys

Wound Healing Pathologies

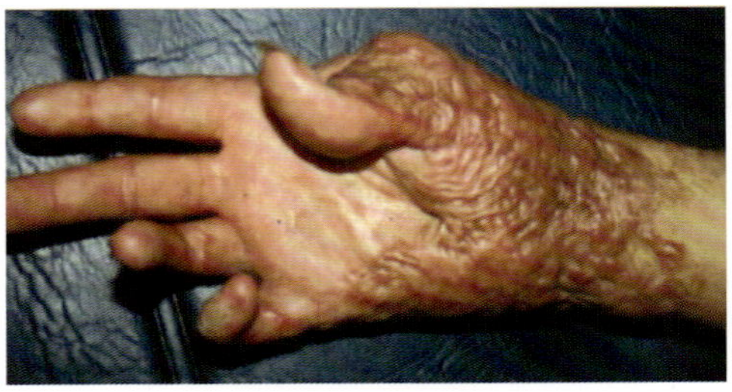

Contractures (AKA: Hypertrophic scars)

- Too much wound healing
- Too many metalloproteinase = deformity in wound healing
- Parallel collagen formation
- Confined to boarders of original wound
- MC seen on: **burn sites**, palms, soles

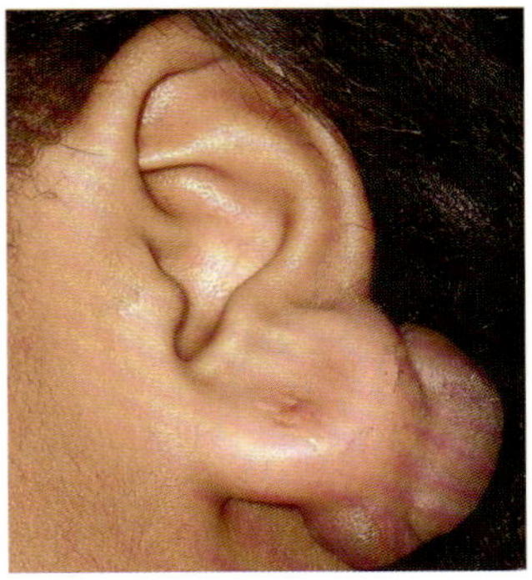

Keloids

- Excessive **collagen** formation
- Disorganized collagen formation
- Extends past the boarders of original wound
- Higher risk in African Americans
- MC location: ears due to ear piercing
- Can be removed but will grow back in most cases

Metalloproteinase

- Degrades collagen and proteins (AKA: tissue remodeling)
- Encourages wound healing
- Stimulates fibroblast and scar tissue
- Requires zinc (**tip**: to invade (dig) you need a metal shovel made of zinc)
- Too much metalloproteinase causes
    - a) causes contractures
    - b) causes **invasion leading to metastasis in cancers**

Growth Factors in Wound Healing

Growth factors: Receptor tyrosine kinase; Ras/Map kinase pathway. (Same as insulin)

Growth Factor	Action
VEG-F FGF	Angiogenesis
PDGF	Stimulates fibroblast for collagen synthesis. Secreted by platelets and macrophages.
TGF-β	Fibrosis, angiogenesis, cell cycle arrest.
EGF	Stimulates cell growth via tyrosine kinase.
Metalloproteinases	Tissue remodeling (Note: over activity is what allows a cancer to invade and metastasize. Requires zinc)

Granulomas

- **Granulomas, think macrophages (histocytes, epithelioid).** Macrophages make granulomas. Granulomas are on organized "collection" of macrophages. **(Think macrophages, think T cells, CD4, TH1, INFγ, IL-1, IL-6)**
- Immune system forms granulomas to "wall off" substances that it sees as foreign and are not able to eliminate.
- Granulomatous = "characterized by granulomas"
- **Granulomas secrete Vitamin D. Vitamin D ↑ absorption of Calcium and phosphorus in the gut**. So any pathologic process that involves granulomas can show an increased calcium level **(hypercalcemia).**
- **Anti**-TNFα drugs can cause granulomas to break down, releasing the disease they are holding. It is critical to do a PPD (latent TB) test before starting patients on any Anti-TNFα disease.

Granulomatous diseases

- Aspiration pneumonia: Granulomas form around food particles
- Blastomycosis
- Cat scratch disease (Bartonella): Granulomas in lymph nodes draining at site of scratch. Pus forming, ↑ PMN's
- Churg-Strauss syndrome
- Crohn's disease: Granulomas within the gut wall
- Cryptococcosis: Necrotizing or non-necrotizing granulomas
- Foreign-body granuloma: Splinters, glass, metal, etc, that penetrate the skin in which granulomas form around
- Francisella tularensis
- Histoplasmosis: Granulomas in biopsy
- Leprosy (Hansen's): Granulomas involve the nerves
- Listeria: Infections in infants can cause fatal disseminated granulomas (granulomatosis infantiseptica)
- Pneumocystis pneumonia: Occasionally seen in PCP (rare), seen in biopsy of lungs
- Rheumatic Fever: Granulomas caused by antibody cross-reaction
- Rheumatoid arthritis: "Rheumatoid nodules" (bumps) in the soft tissues around the joints or lungs
- Sarcoidosis: non-necrotizing (non-caseating) granulomas in lungs, lymph nodes and other organs
- Schistosomiasis: Granuloma formation in the liver
- Syphilis (tertiary): Treponema pallidum
- Tuberculosis: Granulomas show necrosis ("caseating tubercles") and also non-necrotizing
- Wegner's (c-ANCA), polyangiitis

Calcification

Dystrophic calcification

- Result of tissue damage (**tip**: " **D**"ystrophic = "**D**"amage)
- Precedes cell injury and cell necrosis
- MC location: stenosis of heart valves
- Labs: NORMAL calcium levels (normocalcemia)

Metastatic calcification

- Deposits of calcium in otherwise normal tissue
- Increased absorption or decreased excretion of calcium due to diseases (ie: hyperparathyroidism)
- Labs: Increased calcium levels (hypercalcemia)
  Normal calcium labs: 8.5 – 10.2 mg/dL
  High calcium: > 10.2 indicates a disease process
  Very high calcium: > 13 indicates cancer (mc: PTHrP from Squamous Cell lung cancer)
- (**tip**: "M"etastatic = "M" etastasis)

Amyloidosis

Deposition and accumulation of **misfolded** β-pleated proteins causing pathologies due to cell damage and apoptosis.

Amyloid Protein	Characteristics/Pathology
AL (Primary amyloidosis)	Deposits of **light chain** proteins from plasma cells in the kidneys. **Bence Jones proteins (shows M spike** on electrophoresis). Can also affect: heart (**restrictive cardiomyopathy**), liver (clotting cascade disruption = easy bleeding/bruising), GI (hepatomegaly), neurologic (neuropathies)
AA (Secondary amyloidosis)	Composed of Amyloid A. Accumulation of S amyloid A protein (SAA) in chronic infections: TB, **Rheumatoid arthritis**
Aβ amyloidosis	Deposition of amyloid β pleated sheet proteins from amyloid precursor protein APP. Aβ proteins can also cause **tau proteins** to be misfolded that form **neurofibrillary tangles. Alzheimer's**
Amylin	Deposits in the **pancreatic islet cells**

Lipofuscin

- **Normal aging**
- Accumulation of "**Wear and Tear**" **yellow-brown pigmented granules**
- Lipid residues of lysosomal digestion. Oxidation of unsaturated fatty acids.
- Found in: heart, kidney, liver, retina, nerve, ganglion cells

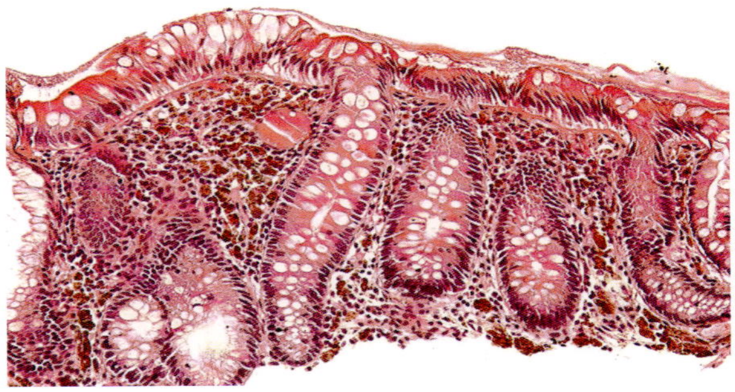

Cellular Changes

Cell Change	Description	Example
Hypertrophy	Increase in the SIZE of the cell. The cell does not increase its production of anything, it just becomes bigger.	Uncontrolled hypertension will cause left ventricular Hypertrophy. The size of the left ventricle increases: Displacing the apex of the heart to the left and causing high "R" waves on an EKG.
Hyperplasia	Increase in the NUMBER of cells. Because there are more cells there can an increase in production hormones in the glands or There can be an increased risk of cancer (ie: endometrial hyperplasia).	If the parathyroid gland enlarges (hyperplasia) the production of PTH increases which can lead to increased bone resorption.
Atrophy	Decrease in the size and/or number of cells which causes a decrease in tissue/muscle mass.	When a cast is removed after non-use of a limb, the muscles in that limb will be atrophied.
Metaplasia	Replacement of one cell type with another. MCC is due to an irritant. If the irritant is stopped the cell change is reversible. If the irritant is continued there is a risk of cancer. This is non-cancerous.	Barrett's Esophagus. Because of the acid that is refluxed into the esophagus from the stomach, the squamous cells will change into columnar with goblet cells to protect itself. If the reflex is not stopped, the metaplasia will become permanent leading to esophageal adenocarcinoma.
Dysplasia	Increased growth of immature cells with simultaneous reduction in growth of mature cells. This is considered cancerous.	Cervical Dysplasia. Result of cervical infection caused by the human papillomavirus (HPV).

Cell Injury

Reversible: ANY use of ANY of these words means the cell can still be revered/saved: Swelling, clumping, blebbing, fatty change, ATP depletion

Irreversible: ANY USE of ANY of these words or damage to ANY of these cellular organelles means the cell is dying of **necrosis or apoptosis** and can't be reversed/saved.

- **Nucleus**: pyknosis (condensation of chromatin – followed by karyorrhexis), karyorrhexis (fragmentation of nucleus), karyolysis (dissolution of chromatin due to enzymatic degradation by endonucleases)
- **Lysosome** damage
- **Mitochondrial** damage
- **Cell membrane (plasma)** damage (AKA: damage to phospholipids)

APOPTOSIS PATHWAYS: PROGRAMED CELL DEATH (natural) or NECROSIS (injury)

INTRINSIC APOPTOSIS PATHWAY (AKA: Mitochondrial Pathway)

- **BcL2 is anti-apoptotic** and prevents release of cytochrome by **binding Apaf-1**
- Apaf-1, if free, will **activate caspase 9**
- **CASPASES induce apoptosis**
- If **Cytochrome C** is released it allows **pro-apoptotic BAX, BAK and BIM out = apoptosis**
- If BcL2 (anti-apoptotic) is overexpressed or if Apaf-1 is overly inhibited, a cell can't be destroyed which will allow tumors/cancers to live (↓activity of caspases).

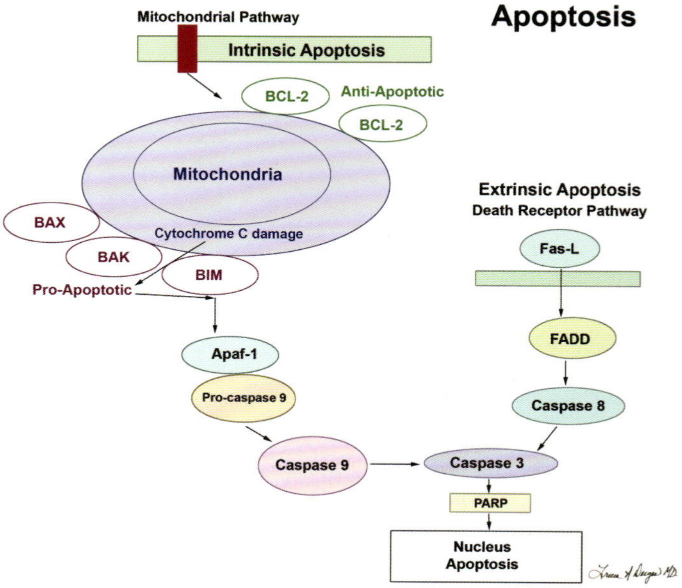

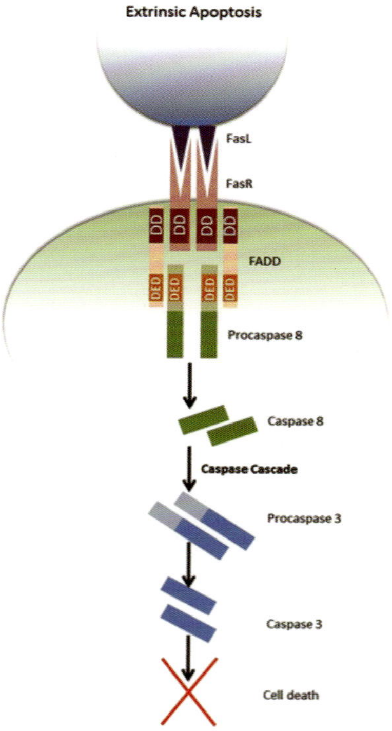

EXTRINSIC APOPTOSIS PATHWAY (2 paths) (AKA: Death Receptor Pathway)

- **Path 1: Fas Ligand binds with CD95** (Fas receptor) and activates caspases = apoptosis
- **Path 2:** Occurs in **negative selection in the thymus**. Negative selection requires Fas-FasL interaction. **Fas protects.** If Fas and FasL interact to form a complex they bind with FADD. **FADD binds inactive caspase 8 and activates them**, thereby allowing the apoptosis of lymphocytes that recognize "self" too much. If Fas is mutated, the Fas-FasL complex will not form, FADD is not able to bind caspases, so negative selection does not occur allowing lymphocytes out that recognize "self" too much to be released, which **causes autoimmune disorders**.

(**tip**: **E**xtrinsic = caspase **E**ight)

- **NECROSIS IS NOT programed cell death.** It is traumatic cell death that results from acute cell injury, disease or infection.

TIP: Apoptosis is heavily tested on the exams, be sure to recognize examples of apoptosis!

- Menstruation: Sloughing off of endometrial cells
- Embryo processes: spaces between digits
- Elimination of T cells that might cause an autoimmune attack
- Formation of proper synapses between neurons in the brain (requires surplus cells to be eliminated.

Pro and Anti-Apoptosis

Anti-Apoptosis	Pro-Apoptosis
Bcl-2	BAX
Bcl-LX	BAD
BCL-W	BID
Mcl-1	BOK
A1	BLK
	BAK

Necrosis

Enzymatic degradation and protein denaturation (proteins lose their structure and cease to function) = apoptosis of cells **due to injury**.

- Caseous necrosis: Lungs (TB, Nocardia, systemic fungi). This is **NOT the case** for abscesses caused by Klebsiella; this type of necrosis is considered liquefactive necrosis.
- Coagulative necrosis: Ischemia, infarctions: Heart, kidney, liver. Will usually cause a "wedge shape" infarct.
- Fatty Necrosis: Enzymatic (AKA: saponification): pancreas. Non-enzymatic: breast due to trauma
- Fibrinoid necrosis: Immune reaction in blood vessels (Temporal arteritis)
- Gangrenous necrosis: Dry (ischemic) and Wet (infection): diabetics, wounds
- Liquefactive necrosis: Brain, abscesses. **NOTE:** Abscesses can be anywhere. Necrosis by any abscess is considered liquefactive necrosis. Example: Klebsiella Pneumonia causes abscess in the lungs. So **BEWARE**: Abscesses caused by **Klebsiella** in the lungs in NOT caseous necrosis).

Necrosis verses Apoptosis

Feature	Necrosis	Apoptosis
Cell size	Enlarged (swelling)	Reduced (shrinkage)
Nucleus	**Pyknosis – karyorrhexis – karyolysis**	Fragmentation (round nucleosome)
Plasma membrane	Disrupted	Intact
Cellular contents	Enzymatic digestion – may leak out of cell	Intact – may be released in apoptotic bodies
Adjacent inflammation	Yes	None
Physiologic or pathologic	Pathologic	Physiologic and pathologic

Ischemia and Watershed areas

- Restriction of blood supply to the tissues. This causes a shortage of oxygen and nutrients needed to keep cells alive
- MC blockage of blood vessels or decreased supply by blood vessels to watershed areas (areas of the body that receive 2 blood supplies). These areas are the **most susceptible to ischemic damage** and are the **first areas to show damage.**

ORGAN	WATERSHED LOCATION and 1st Area to Show Damage
Brain	**Cortical area of ACA, MCA and PCA.** The first area of the brain to show ischemic damage: **Hippocampus** and Purkinje cells of the cerebellum.
GI	**Splenic flexure** of colon boarder at **SMA and IMA.** Distal sigmoid colon of IMA and hypogastric arteries, rectum.
Rectum	**IMA and the Internal iliac artery**
Heart	Left ventricle subendocardium. **Coronary Steal Syndrome** (AKA: Cardiac Steal Syndrome) = caused by narrowing of the coronary arteries and a coronary vasodilator is used which "steals" blood away from the ischemic parts of the heart, causing more ischemia. (Principal used in chemical stress testing to identify ischemic/decreased perfusion areas of the heart)
Kidney	**PCT** (Proximal tubule) in straight segment of the medulla). Thick ascending limb in the medulla.
Liver	**Zone III** of the central vein
Spinal cord	Anterior spinal artery (between T7 and T9). Upper thoracic (T1 – T4), first lumbar (L1)

Brain Inflammation

Chromatolysis (neurons)
Dissolution of the **Nissl bodies (AKA: Nissl substance)** in a neuron due to injury.
Nissl body/substance: large granular body in the neuron made of rough endoplasmic reticulum (RER) and free ribosomes for protein synthesis.

- Nucleus migrates to the periphery of the cell
- Increase in size of the nucleus, nucleolus causing swelling of the cell
- Nissl substance is throughout the cytoplasm

Red Neuron/Nuclei (12 – 24 hours)
Irreversible ischemic damage = cell death. Release of lysosomal enzymes/lysosomal digestion.

- Pyknotic nucleus (shrunken nucleus)
- High eosinophils in cytoplasm
- No Nissl bodies

Brain Repair Time Line

Timeline	Cell Reaction	Description
12 – 48 hours	**Red Nuclei (red neuron)**	Eosinophilic cytoplasm, pyknotic nuclei, **loss Nissl substance**
24 – 72 hours	Neutrophil infiltration	Necrosis
3 – 5 days	Macrophage **(Microglia)** infiltration	Phagocytosis by microglia
1 – 2 weeks	**Astrocytes "Reactive gliosis"**	Vascular proliferation, **liquefactive necrosis**
> 2 weeks	**Astrocytes "Glial Scar"**	Cystic area surrounded by **gliosis, astrocytes proliferate forming Glial scar**

Heart Injury Time Line

Timeline	Heart Description	Cellular	Complications
0 -4 hours	No change in heart tissue	**No change**	
4 – 12 hours	Dark mottling	**Wavy** fibers, **coagulative necrosis**, edema, eosinophils, hemorrhage	
1 – 3 days	Dark mottling	**Neutrophil** migration, coagulation necrosis	
1 – 3 days	Hyperemia	3 days: **T cells and Macrophages**	**Fibrinous pericarditis. EKG shows diffuse ST elevations. Friction rub on auscultation.** **TX: NSAIDS**
5 – 7 days	Yellow/brown	7 days: **Fibroblast.** **Granulation formation.** **(Scar)**	**Papillary muscle rupture (Chordae Tendineae): Acute flash edema.** **Free Wall Rupture: Tamponade** **Ventricular aneurysm** **Interventricular septal rupture: Hear a new murmur: VSD**
10 days	Yellow/brown	Fibroblast collagen: **Granulation tissue**	
2 weeks to months	Grey-white	**Scar formation (type 1 collagen)**	**Dressler's syndrome**: autoimmune inflammatory reaction to myocardial neo-antigens as a result of the MI. TX: **Colchicine**

Infarctions and Reperfusion Infarctions (free radical damage)
Red infarctions (wedge shape infarct)

- Hemorrhagic infarcts (coagulative necrosis)
- Lungs, liver, intestine (soft tissues with multiple blood supplies)

Pale infarctions

- Kidney, heart, spleen (solid tissues with single blood supplies)

Free Radicals

- Molecules with unpaired electrons. In searching to find another electron they "steal" electrons from nearest stable molecule. The molecule that lost the electron now looks for another one causing a chain reaction and damage to cells.
- Free radicals formed by: drugs, nitric oxide, leukocyte oxidative burst, radiation
- Free radical damage by: lipid peroxidation, DNA breaks and protein modification
- Antioxidants in the body protect against this damage unless there is an excess of free radicals or no antioxidants are available.
- Free radicals accumulate with age.
- **Vitamin E**: Antioxidant to defend against LDL oxidation and plaque in the **arteries**
- **Vitamin C:** Antioxidant to defend in the **GI system** (mouth, larynx, esophagus), pollution, cigarette smoke
- Best antioxidant source: 5 – 8 servings of fruits and vegetables per day
- **Free radicals also eliminated by enzymes: Superoxide dismutase, glutathione peroxidase, catalase**

Inhalation injury

MC: Exposure to fire (fire victims or fire fighters)
Primary concern: Swelling of throat due to inflammation, must be prepared to intubate.
Beware: If patient seems ok but shows **ANY sign of soot** around the mouth, red throat, etc, the patient **must be admitted** and monitored for **possible intubation**.

Lung Inflammation (Lobar Pneumonia)

Stage Timeline	Reaction	Description
Stage 1: 1st 24 hours	Congestion	Red and heavy. High in bacteria
2nd Stage	Red Hepatization	High in neutrophils and fibrin. High red exudate
3rd Stage	Grey Hepatization	Fibrin, neutrophils, dry, grey color, decrease in RBC's
Stage 4: Resolution	Macrophages and cough clear infection	Enzymatic digestion and exudate

Effusions
Exudate vs Transudate

(**tip**: "Trans" is transparent= **T**hin, like water)

Exudate vs Transudate Test in Thoracic Effusion Thoracentesis

Characteristic	**EXUDATE**	**TRANSUDATE (transparent, thin)**
Color	Cloudy	Clear
Protein content	↑↑ Protein content > 2.9 g/dL	↓ Protein content < 2.5 g/dL
Fluid sample protein/serum protein	> 0.5	< 0.5
Difference in fluid sample albumin/serum albumin	> 1.2 g/dL	< 1.2 g/dL
Specific gravity	> 1.02	< 1.02
LDH	> 0.6	< 0.6
pH	< 7.2	> 7.2
Cholesterol content	> 45 mg/dL	< 45 mg/dL
Glucose	< 60	> 60
Causes	Inflammation (increased vascular permeability), lymphatic obstruction, malignancy, pneumonia, PE, Rheumatoid arthritis, TB, Sarcoidosis, lymphoma, connective tissue dz	CHF, cirrhosis (ascites), Na retention CHF is due to ↑ hydrostatic pressure in pulmonary vessels Cirrhosis (ascites) is due to ↓ oncotic pressure

Exudate vs Transudate Test in Abdominal Paracentesis

- Albumin level in the serum minus the albumin level in the fluid sample.
  < 1.2 = exudate, > 1.2 = transudate.

  (NOTE: the exudate and transudate levels have OPPOSITE meanings in the abdominal vs thoracic test. Exudate is <1.2 in the abdominal labs and the exudate >1.2 in the thoracic labs).
  (**tip**: thoracic exudate is "above the belt" >1.2 and abdominal exudate is "below the belt" <1.2)

Edema

- **Oncotic pressure** (AKA: Colloid osmotic pressure) pressure exerted by proteins (albumin) in the plasma that pulls water into the capillaries. If there are less proteins in the plasma (in conditions such as proteins lost in the urine (proteinuria), malnutrition) then there is a ↓ in oncotic pressure and an ↑ in filtration across the capillaries into the surrounding tissue = edema (build up of excess fluid).
  Oncotic pressure is represented by the Π symbol in the Starling equation.
  MCC: nephrotic syndrome, liver failure.
- **Hydrostatic pressure:** The pressure that drives fluid out of the capillary (filtration). It is highest at the arteriolar end of the capillary and lowest at the venular end. It is determined by the interstitial fluid volume and the compliance of the tissue interstitium. The more fluid = ↑ hydrostatic pressure.
  MCC: cardiac failure
- **Starling Equation: (Pc – Pi) – (Πc – Πi)**
  Pc is the capillary hydrostatic pressure
  Pi is the interstitial hydrostatic pressure
  Πc is the capillary oncotic pressure
  Πi is the interstitial oncotic pressure

Edema Cause	Pathology
↑ Hydrostatic Pressure	Heart Failure (Left Ventricle or Cor Pulmonale), Primary renal sodium retention, ↓ GFR, venous obstruction, venous insufficiency
↓ Oncotic pressure (Hypo albumin)	Protein loss, nephrotic syndrome, ↓ albumin synthesis, cirrhosis, malnutrition
↑ Capillary permeability	Burns, trauma, sepsis, allergic reactions, ARDS, malignant ascites
↑ Interstitial oncotic pressure (Lymph obstruction)	Malignant ascites, hypothyroid, lymph node dissection

CSF Findings in Diseases (Lumbar punctures)

Disease	PMN's	Glucose	Lymphocytes	Protein	Pressure	RBC	Other
NORMAL	0 – 5	45 – 80		18 – 58		0	
Bacterial Meningitis	**↑↑ >1000**	**↓ <40**		> 400	↑		
Fungal Meningitis		**↓**	**↑↑**	↑	↑		
Viral Meningitis (AKA: Aseptic Meningitis)		**NORMAL**	**↑↑ > 90%**	Normal	↑		Note: there is a ↑ in WBC over the normal ratio of WBC and RBC in meningitis. In a subarachnoid hemorrhage the WBC is ↑ but the ratio is normal. **Normal ratio:** 1 WBC to every 500-1000 RBC
TB Meningitis	5 – 1000	**↓↓ <10**		↑↑ >400			
Lyme, Cryptococcus, Rickettsia		↓	↑↑	↑			
Guillain Barre	Normal	Normal		**↑↑ 45 - 1000**			
Tertiary Syphilis							**Positive VDRL**
Pseudo Tumor Cerebri					**↑↑**		
Multiple Sclerosis				**↑↑**			
Subarachnoid Hemorrhage (SAH)						**↑**	**Xanthochromia** Note: there is an ↑ in WBC but the WBC and RBC ratio is **normal**. In meningitis the WBC is ↑ than the normal ratio. **Normal ratio:** 1 WBC to every 500-1000 RBC.
Injury/improper stick technique						↑↑	
Herpes			**↑↑ > 90%**	↑	↑	**↑↑**	**(RBC with viral profile)**
HIV Toxoplasmosis							**EBV DNA**
Creutzfeldt-Jakob Disease				14-3-3 Protein			
Normal Pressure Hydrocephalus				Normal			
Subacute Sclerosing Panencephalitis							Antibodies to the measles virus

Enzymes with Numbers

(Enzymes named with numbers or letters are always a helpful tip)

Enzyme #/name	Association
5 (5α Reductase)	Converts testosterone to DHT
5 (5' Deiodinase)	Converts T4 to T3 in the periphery.
1 (1α Hydroxylase)	Converts 1,25 hydroxycholecalciferol into 1,25 dihydroxycholecalciferol
7 (7α Hydroxylase)	Converts cholesterol into bile acid. CYP**7**A1 gene. (Fibrates inhibit this enzyme to inhibit bile acid synthesis).
11 (11 beta-Hydroxylase).	Synthesis of glucocorticoids (cortisol) and mineralocorticoids (aldosterone). Deficiency: Congenital adrenal hyperplasia: loss of function mutation of the CYP**11**B1 gene)
14 (14α Demethylase)	Synthesis of lanosterol to ergosterol.
17 (17 Hydroxylase. 17-OH)	Synthesis of sex steroids and glucocorticoids (cortisol) and an increase in mineralocorticoids (aldosterone). Deficiency: Congenital adrenal hyperplasia: loss of function mutation of the CYP**17**A1 gene)
21 (21 Hydroxylase)	Synthesis of steroid hormones (steroids), glucocorticoids (cortisol) and mineralocorticoids (aldosterone). Deficiency: Congenital adrenal hyperplasia: loss of function mutation of the CYP**21**A2 gene)

MARKERS: CELL, TUMOR, CYTOKINES

CELL SURFACE MARKERS (Proteins)

CELL	MARKERS
Macrophages	CD14, **CD40** **MHC II, B7** (binds with CD28) APC (Antigen Presenting Cell)
B Cells	**CD19, CD20, CD21** (EBV), CD40 **MHC II, B7** (Binds with CD28), APC (Antigen Presenting Cell), Kills bacteria
T Cells	**TCR** (binds with MHC-antigen complex) **CD3** (Signals with TCR), **CD28** (Binds B7) APC (Antigen Presenting Cell) **Kills viruses, parasites, fungus, tumors, atypical bacteria**
Helper T Cells	**CD4**, CD40
Cytotoxic T Cells	**CD8** **MHC I**
NK (Natural Killer) Cells	**CD16, CD56**

CYTOKINES

CYTOKINE	RESPONSIBILITY
IL-1	FEVER, secreted by Macrophages, acute inflammation, secretions to recruit leukocytes
IL-2	Secreted by T cells. Stimulates: Helper T cells, Cytotoxic T Cells, regulatory T cells
IL-4	Differentiation into TH2 cells. Stimulates B cells, Class switches to IgG and IgE (tip: GE makes light bulbs 4 you)
IL-5	Class switch to IgA and eosinophils
IL-6	Stimulates Acute Phase reactants (C-Reactive protein, complement, fibrinogen, prothrombin, factor VIII, VWF, plasminogen, ferritin, hepcidin, haptoglobin, alpha 1-antitrypsin, serum amyloid A, ceruloplasmin)
IL-8	Chemotaxis for neutrophils (PMN)
IL-10	Inhibits TH1 and T cells
IL-12	Differentiates T cells into TH1, activates NK cells
TNF-α	Septic shock, increases vascular permeability
INF-γ	Activates NK cells (kills viruses, parasites, fungus, tumors, atypical bacteria)
Septic Shock	IL-1, IL-6, TNFα (septic shock: **must have the triad**: fever, low BP, tachycardia)

HLA ASSOCIATIONS WITH DISEASES

HLA	Disease Associations
HLA-A3	**Hemochromatosis**
HLA-B27	Most arthritis: Reactive arthritis (AKA: Reiter Syndrome), Psoriatic arthritis, **Ankylosing Spondylitis**
HLA-DQ2, DQ8	Celiac Disease
HLA-DR2	Goodpasture Syndrome, SLE, Multiple Sclerosis
HLA-DR3	**Graves** Disease, Diabetes Type I, SLE
HLA-DR4	**Rheumatoid Arthritis**, Diabetes Type I
HLA-DR5	**Hashimoto** Thyroiditis, Pernicious Anemia (B-12/Intrinsic Factor)

AUTOANTIBODIES

Pathology	Autoantibody
Graves Disease	Anti-TSH receptor
Hashimoto Thyroiditis	Antimicrosomal Antithyroglobulin
Myasthenia Gravis	Anti-Ach receptor
Lambert Eaton Syndrome	Antibodies against voltage-gated calcium channels
Polymyositis Dermatomyositis	Anti-Jo-1 Anti-SRP Anti-Mi-2
Mixed Connective Tissue Dz	Anti-U1 RNP (ribonucleoprotein)
Scleroderma, Limited (CREST)	Anticentromere
Scleroderma, Diffuse	Anti-Scl-70 Anti-DNA Topoisomerase I
SLE (Lupus) Antiphospholipid	Anti-cardiolipin Lupus anticoagulant
SLE (Lupus)	**Anti-dsDNA (specific)** Anti-Smith Antinuclear antibodies
Drug Induced Lupus	Antihistone
Rheumatoid Arthritis	**Anti citrullinated Protein Antibodies (anti-CCP) (specific)** IgM antibody against the IgG Fc region. Rheumatoid Factor (RF) (RF is NOT specific for Rheumatoid Arthritis. Several diseases are associated with RF).
Pemphigus Vulgaris	Anti-desmoglein
Bullous Pemphigoid	Anti-hemidesmosome
Sjogren Syndrome	Anti-SSA Anti-SSB anti-Ro, anti-La
Autoimmune Hepatitis	Anti-smooth muscle Antinuclear antibodies
Primary Biliary Cirrhosis	Antimitochondrial antibodies
Celiac Disease	Anti-gliadin IgA anti-tissue transglutaminase IgA antiendomysial Anti-reticulin
Wegner's Granulomatosis with polyangiitis	c-ANCA PR3-ANCA
Churg-Strauss Syndrome Microscopic Polyangiitis	p-ANCA MPO-ANCA
Goodpasture Syndrome	Anti-basement membrane
Type 1 Diabetes	Anti-glutamate decarboxylase
Primary Sclerosis Cholangitis	Anti-smooth muscle antibody
Dermatomyositis	Anti-Mi2 antibody
Primary Membranous Nephropathy	Anti phospholipase A_2 receptor

TUMOR SUPPRESSOR GENES: "Anti-oncogenes" **"LOSS of FUNCTION"** (Stops cell proliferation). Inactivation causes tumor development. Both alleles must be damaged/lost in order for development of disease.

GENE	TUMOR	GENE PRODUCT
BRCA1	Breast cancer Ovarian cancer	DNA repair protein
BRCA2	Breast cancer Ovarian cancer	DNA repair protein
PTEN	Breast cancer Prostate cancer Endometrial cancer	
CPD4 SMAD4	Pancreatic cancer	DPC – deleted in pancreatic cancer
DCC	Colon cancer	DCC – deleted in colon cancer
APC	Colorectal cancer	
Menin MEN1	MEN 1	
P53	Li-Fraumeni Syndrome	Transcription factor
P16	Melanoma	Cyclin dependent kinase
NF1	Neurofibromatosis 1	RAS GTPase protein
NF2	Neurofibromatosis 2	Schwannomin protein (Merlin)
TSC1	Tuberous Sclerosis	Hamartin protein
TSC2	Tuberous Sclerosis	Tuberin protein
Rb	Retinoblastoma Osteosarcoma	Inhibits E2F
VHL	Von Hippel-Lindau Dz	Inhibits factor 1a
WT1	Wilms Tumor (nephroblastoma)	
WT2	Wilms Tumor (nephroblastoma)	

ONCOGENES

"Proto-oncogenes" Pro Tumor/stimulates cell proliferation. Over **expression (amplification)** = ↑↑ growth.
"GAIN of FUNCTION" (Turns on tumor development)
One allele is already lost so there only needs to be damage/loss to the last remaining allele to develop the disease.
(**tip**: the on**GO**gene: **GO**es and turns on)

GENE	TUMOR	GENE PRODUCT
HER2/neu **c-erbB2**	Breast Ovarian	Tyrosine kinase
L-myc	Lung	Transcription factor
N-myc	Neuroblastoma	Transcription factor
c-myc	Burkett lymphoma	Transcription factor
BCR-ABL	CML AML	Tyrosine kinase
bcl-2	Follicular lymphoma	Anti-apoptotic
ras	Colon cancer Pancreatic cancer lung cancer	GTPase
c-kit	GIST tumor (Gastrointestinal stromal tumor)	Cytokine receptor
ret	MEN 2A, MEN 2B	Tyrosine kinase
BRAF	Melanoma	Serine-threonine kinase

TUMOR MARKERS

MARKER	TUMOR
α-fetoprotein	Yolk Sac tumor Testicular cancer Hepatocellular carcinoma Hepatoblastoma Mixed Germ Cell (secreted with β-hCG)
Alkaline phosphatase (ALP)	Paget's DZ Bone metastases Seminoma
β-hCG	Hydatidiform moles Choriocarcinomas (Gestational trophoblastic dz) Testicular cancer
CA-15-3 CA-27-29	Breast cancer
CA-19-9	Pancreatic cancer
CA-125	Ovarian cancer **NOTE:** CA-125 can be also be elevated with pancreatitis, cirrhosis, Endometriosis, peritonitis. (**tip**: women have 125 eggs)
Calcitonin	Medullary thyroid carcinoma (MEN)
CEA (Carcinoembryonic Antigen)	Colorectal cancer
PSA (Prostate Specific Antigen)	Prostate cancer (Can be elevated in BPH, prostatitis and after massaging the prostate in a prostate exam)
S-100	Melanomas (Neural Crest origin) Schwannomas Langerhans cells
TRAP (Tartrate Resistant Acid Phosphatase)	Hairy cell leukemia

CARDIOLOGY

Basic Concepts, Rules, Terminology

Myocardial Energy Sources

- Glycolysis
- Glucose Oxidation (Heart prefers Glucose Oxidation over Fatty Acid Oxidation because it uses less oxygen, therefor leaving more oxygen for the heart).
- Fatty Acid Oxidation (high oxygen requirement).

Cardiac Valves

- Atrioventricular (AV) Valves: Mitral Valve (Bicuspid Valve) and Tricuspid Valve
- Semilunar (SL) Valves: Aortic and Pulmonary Valves

Cardiac Muscle (Cardiac Myocytes)

- Cardiomyocytes (cardiac muscle cells)
- **Intercalated discs** connect individual cardiomyocytes, located in the Z line of the sarcomere.
- Normal cardiac striated muscle
- Cell junctions of intercalated disc: Fascia adherens, desmosomes, gap junctions.
  Fascia adherens: anchors actin.
  Desmosomes (AKA: Macula adherens) stop separation during contraction by binding intermediate filaments.
- **Gap junctions**: Allow action potentials to spread by allowing ions to pass between cells to depolarize.

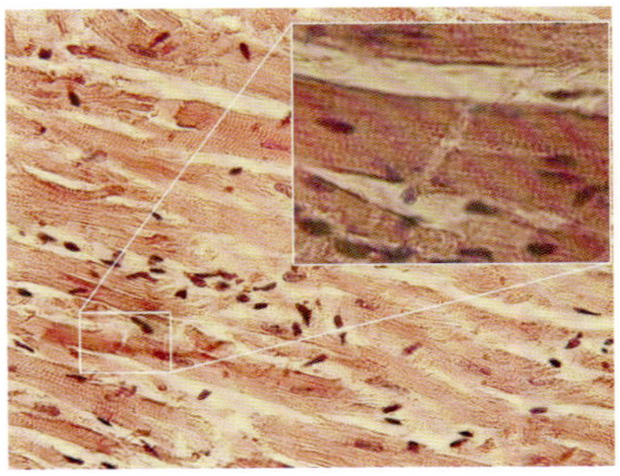

Normal cardiac striated muscle

Blood Volumes

- Males: 5 to 6 liters and Females: 4 to 5 liters

Systemic Circulation

- The part of blood circulation which carries oxygenated blood away from the heart, to the body, and returns deoxygenated blood back to the right side of the heart to be sent to the lungs via the Pulmonary Artery
- The atrium contributes 10% to 15% to cardiac output.
  Heart disease requires the atrial contribution to ↑ to 30% to 50%.

Pulmonary Circulation

- The part of the blood circulation which carries oxygen depleted blood away from the heart, to the lungs, and returns oxygenated blood back to the heart.

Normal Physiology of a Heart Beat

- Inspiration occurs
- ↓ in intrathoracic pressure (becomes more negative)
- ↑ of venous return to the RV
- ↑ RV stroke volume
- ↑ RV ejection time
- Delayed closure of pulmonic valve
- ↑ capacity of pulmonary circulation

Blood Supply to Organs

- Heart: **Has the greatest arteriovenous oxygen difference**. Oxygen extraction of the heart is 80%. Oxygen demand of the heart is **determined by coronary blood flow during early diastole** (not by oxygen extraction)
- Kidney: Has the highest blood flow. It filters approximately 160 liters per day
- Liver: Has the largest amount of the systemic cardiac output
- Lung: Has the largest blood flow: 100% of cardiac output
- Systemic blood flow is greater than the pulmonary blood flow. The largest amount of CO is due to systemic blood flow, not pulmonary blood flow

Autoregulation of Blood Flow to Organs

Brain: CO_2 regulates.
↑ CO_2 (hypoventilation) causes **vasodilation** in brain = ↑ **ICP.**
↓ CO_2 (hyperventilation) causes vasoconstriction
Heart: CO_2, adenosine, NO vasodilate
Kidneys: Tubuloglomerular and myogenic feedback and **peritubular cortical cells (erythropoietin)**
Lungs: Vasoconstrict when there is a hypoxia, diffusion or perfusion problem.
Lungs are unique from the rest of the body. When hypoxia is present the rest of the body will vasodilate, but the **lungs will vasoconstrict to shunt blood away from damaged areas** to areas that are able to do gas exchange.

Skeletal Muscle: Lactate, adenosine, K, H, CO2
Skin: Temperature control by sympathetic stimulation

Recoil
The ability of a hollow organ to distend with pressure and its ability to **recoil (elastance)** to its original shape after the pressure is removed.

- ↓ Compliance = ↑ systolic and ↓ diastolic
- LVH (Left ventricular hypertrophy, stiff) has LOW compliance, therefore will always have ↑ EDP with any EDV
- If ventricular relaxation is impaired (LVH) = ↓ function, ↓ compliance and ↓ ventricular filling
- Dilated hearts have high compliance, therefore will always have ↑ EDV and ↓ EF
- Compliance: C = Δ Volume/ Δ Pressure

Cardiac Rules

- **Systolic = pressure (S4)**
- **Diastolic = fluid (S3)**

Cardiac Output

- CO = SV
- ↑ HR = ↑ CO
- ↓HR = ↓ CO

Blood Volume, Blood Flow

- Blood volume: composed of RBC and blood plasma. RBC transport oxygen, plasma carries the RBC's. Plasma is composed of mostly water, proteins, hormones and minerals.
- Blood volume = blood pressure
- ↑ Volume = ↑ venous return to the heart
- Volume (diastolic) = ↓ TPR = ↑ venous return = ↑ flow
- Blood flow = Pressure
- ↑ Fluid = ↑ BP (why BP is checked closely during pregnancy)
- Resistance = Pressure
- If you ↑ diastole you ↑ filling time (ie: MOA Beta Blockers)

Venous Return

- ↑ Venous return = ↑ HR = ↑ stroke volume = ↑ cardiac output = ↑ blood pressure
- Venous return = CO and Mean systemic pressure.
  ↑ Venous return = ↑ fluid (Fluid infusion, sympathetic activity)
  ↓ Venous return = hemorrhage, spinal anesthesia

TPR, Pressure (AKA: Mean Arterial Pressure: MAP)

- Pressure (systolic) = pressure in the arteries (dilation = ↓ pressure and ↓ resistance); vasoconstriction = ↑ pressure and ↑ resistance)
- ↑ TPR = ↑ MAP = Afterload (AKA: blood pressure, mean arterial pressure)
- TPR is affected by viscosity (thickness) of the blood (ie: HCT)
  Thicker blood = slower
  Thicker blood (ie: polycythemia) has higher RBC
- If you ↑ diastole you ↑ filling time (ie: MOA Beta Blockers)
- ↓ TPR = ↑ blood flow to tissues and ↑ venous return to the heart
- ↑ TPR = ↓ blood flow to tissues and ↓ venous return to the heart
- TPR (↑ with vasopressors: Epi, N. Epi, Desmopressin)
  TPR (↓ with exercise or AV shunt (fistula)

Preload

- Preload is the amount of blood entering the heart (BOTH sides: left and right). ANYTHING that increases volume or venous return will increase preload
- Preload is estimated by EDV and by CVP (Central venous pressure)
- ↑Preload = ↑ volume (fluid)
- Vasodilators = ↓ Preload therefore ↓ fluid
- ↑ Preload = ↑ contractility = ↑ SV = ↑ CO
  Preload is decreased by **VENOdilators (dilates VEINS)** **(nitroglycerin) and ACE inhibitors, ARB's**
- ↓ Preload = ↓ contractility = ↓ SV = ↓ CO

Compliance: ↑ = Stretches easily. ↓ Difficult to stretch.

Afterload

- Afterload = MAP
- ↑Afterload = ↑ pressure = LVH
- Afterload is the pressure that is outside the heart that the valves must overcome in order to open and eject blood. If the pressure is high (high blood pressure) then it forces the heart to work harder, build its muscles (LVH) in order to force the valves open.
  Chronic hypertension = ↑ MAP = LVH
- Afterload is decreased by vasodilators (artery). **(Hydralazine) and by ACE inhibitors and ARB's.**
- **ACE inhibitors and ARB's** decrease BOTH preload and afterload

Contractility

- **Contractility goes hand in hand with stroke volume**
- ↑ Contractility = ↑ cardiac output = ↑ stroke volume = ↑ ejection fraction = ↑ blood pressure
- Contractility is increased with:
  Digitalis (blocks Na/K pump so ↑ intracellular Na and ↑ intracellular Ca by stopping Na/Ca exchange).
  Increase intracellular Ca.
  Decrease extracellular Na.
  Sympathetics/catecholamines (Increases Ca in sarcoplasmic reticulum)
  Anxiety
  Exercise
  Pregnancy
  ↑ Preload
  ↓ Afterload
- Contractility is decreased with:
  Beta Blockers (↓ cAMP)
  Systolic heart failure (dilated cardiomyopathy)
  Non-dihydropyridine Ca channel blockers (**Verapamil, Diltiazem**)
  Acidosis (pH < 7.4)
  Hypoxia (↓ PO2)
  Hypercapnia (↑ PCO2)
  ↓ HR, ↓ BP, ↓ contractility, ↑ TPR

Ejection Fraction

- Ejection fraction is the amount of blood that is ejected from the heart.
  Normal EF is ≥ 55%
  EF is ↓ in systolic heart failure (dilated heart)
  EF is normal in diastolic heart failure (stiff heart)

Inotropy

- ↓ Inotropy (heart failure) = ↓ SV = ↑ ESV
- ↑ Inotropy (contraction/sympathetic action) = ↑ SV = ↓ ESV

Cardiac Equations

- **CO = SV x HR**
- Fick's principle: CO = rate of O2 consumption / arterial O2 – venous O2
- MAP = CO x TPR
- MAP = 2/3 diastolic pressure + 1/3 systolic pressure
- **SV = EDV – ESV**
- **Pulse pressure = systolic pressure – diastolic pressure**
- **Blood flow: Q (flow) = Δ Pressure / Δ Resistance**
- Pressure = Q (flow) / Δ Resistance
- Resistance = Q (flow) / Δ Pressure
- Ejection Fraction: EF = SV / EDV
- **Net filtration: (Pc – Pi) – (πc – πi)**

Sympathetics verses Parasympathetic

Sympathetics

- β 1 Adrenergic receptors and increase sympathetic activity.
  Sympathetic activity can NEVER decrease. There must be an increase in parasympathetic stimulation (ie: CN X/Vegas)
- ↓ TPR = ↑ CO = ↑ contractility = ↑ HR = ↑ BP = ↑ venous return = ↑ afterload
  (arteries: vasoconstrict) (veins: vasodilate ie: nitric oxide (meds: nitrates - venodilate)

Parasympathetic

- CN X (Vegas nerve)
- ↓ CO = ↓ HR = ↓ BP = ↓ contraction
- To decrease sympathetic effects of the heart, parasympathetic effects must increase

Inotropy and Chronotropy

- Inotropy: Contractility of the heart (how hard is it beating)
  ↑ with sympathetics, catecholamines, digoxin
  ↓ with heart failure, narcotic overdoses
- Chronotropy: Heart rate (how fast is it beating)

Resistance

- **↑ Resistance is directly proportional to: longer vessels, higher viscosity (thickness), smaller radius, and higher pressure.**
  Viscosity (↑ RBC's) is related to HCT. ↑ in polycythemia, hyperprotein states (Multiple myeloma), Hereditary spherocytosis.
  Viscosity is ↓ in anemia (less RBC's)
- **Resistance is inversely proportional to the radius of the vessel to the 4th power**
  (↓radius = ↑ resistance)
  R4 = blood flow.
  EXAMPLE:
  If radius doubles (r2) then flow is ↑ 16 fold. (r = 4 x 4)
  If radius is reduced in ½ then flow is ↓ by 16 fold
- **Resistance in SERIES** (**tip**: **S**eries = **S**UM) is the SUM of the resistance in individual organs
  Organ R1 + Organ R2 + Organ R3 + Organ R4 = total resistance in series
- **Resistance in PARALLEL** is the total of all the systemic circulation
  1/R1 + 1/R2 + 1/R3 + 1/R4 = resistance in parallel

Cardiac Oxygen Requirements

- **Duration of DIASTOLE determines the coronary blood flow (oxygen delivery)**
- Things that ↑ the oxygen requirement for the heart
  (AKA: **INCREASED WORK LOAD ON THE HEART**)
  ↑ Afterload
  ↑ Contractility
  ↑ HR
  ↑ Heart size
  ↑ Wall tension
  ↑ Exercise

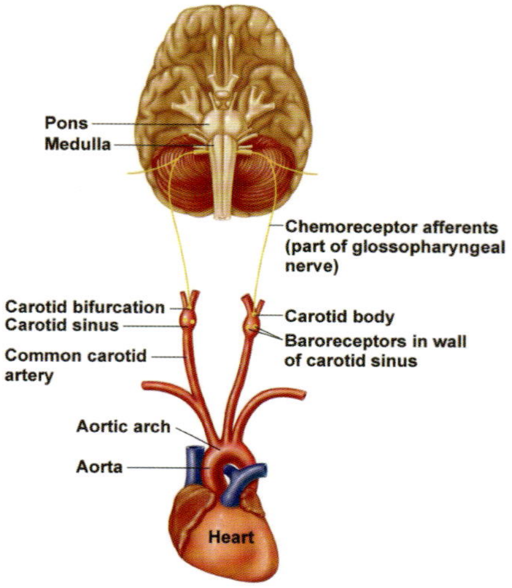

Receptors: Baroreceptors and Chemoreceptors

Receptor	Nerve Transmission	Nucleus	Function
Aortic arch	Vagus (CN X)	Solitary in medulla	↑ Blood pressure only
Carotid sinus	Glossopharyngeal (CN IX)	Solitary in medulla	↓ and ↑ Blood pressure

Baroreceptors

(AKA: Stretch receptors, sense a change in blood pressure)

- **↑ BP = ↑ baroreceptor firing frequency. If ↑ in firing = causes ↑ in parasympathetic activity**
- **↓ BP = ↓ baroreceptor firing frequency. If ↓ in firing = causes ↑ in sympathetic activity**
- **Hypotension (hemorrhage)/shock** = decreases BP = decreases the stretch in the vessel alerting the baroreceptor = decrease in afferent baroreceptor firing = sends message afferently on CN IX to solitary nucleus in medulla = ↓ efferent parasympathetic effects and ↑ in efferent sympathetic firing (β1 adrenergic) for sympathetic effects = vasoconstriction = ↑ HR = ↑ contractility = ↑ blood pressure.
- Tachycardia/palpitations: Perform **carotid massage**. Carotid massage = ↑ pressure on carotid sinus = ↑ stretch = increase in afferent firing so message sent via CN IX to solitary nucleus = ↑ CN X parasympathetic effects on the heart = ↑ AV node refractory period = ↓ HR
- Increase in parasympathetic activity = ↓ HR, SV, CO, BP (MAP)
- Decrease in sympathetic activity = Vasodilation = ↓ TPR, BP

Chemoreceptors

Receptor	Location	Function	Notes
Peripheral	Carotid and Aortic bodies	**↓ pH, ↓ PO2, ↑** PCO2	
Central (**tip**: **C**entral = **C**O2)	CNS	Changes in pH, **PCO2**	PCO2 determines blood flow in the brain. ↑ CO2 (hypoventilation) causes vasodilation in brain = ↑ ICP. ↓ CO2 (hyperventilation) causes vasoconstriction

Autoregulation of Blood Flow From Sitting to Standing

- Upon standing from a sitting position: gravity causes venous pooling in the lower extremities which ↓ preload and ↓ stroke volume.
- This decrease causes ↓ stretch (↓ firing) in the peripheral baroreceptor causing CN IX to send a message to the brain to stimulate the sympathetic system to cause a compensatory response (reflex).
- β-1 receptors are stimulated on the heart causing tachycardia and α-1 receptors are stimulated causing vasoconstriction.
- This reflex causes ↑ venous return and ↑ preload to the heart leading to ↑ cardiac output.
- **NOTE:** In normal aging, baroreceptors can slow down, decreasing the speed of the reflex response which can lead to orthostatic syncope. It is important for the elderly to sit up for a few minutes (after lying down) before standing or if sitting to stand slowing so that the baroreceptors are able to respond.

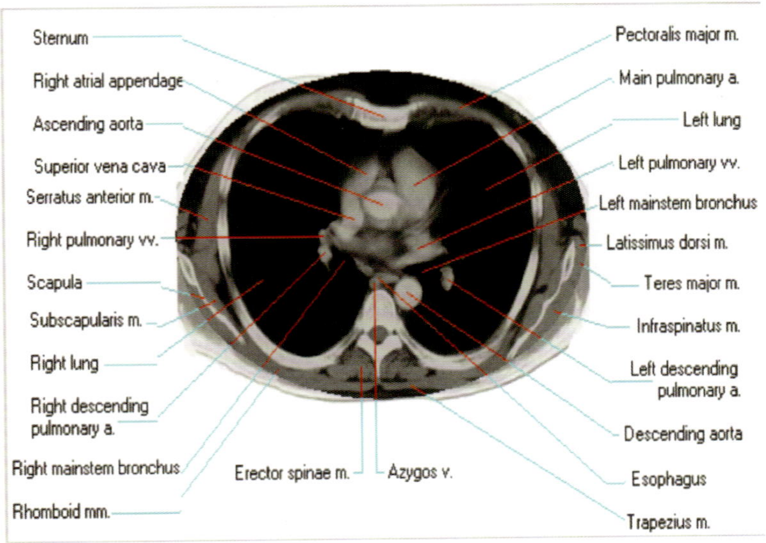

Normal Chest X-ray

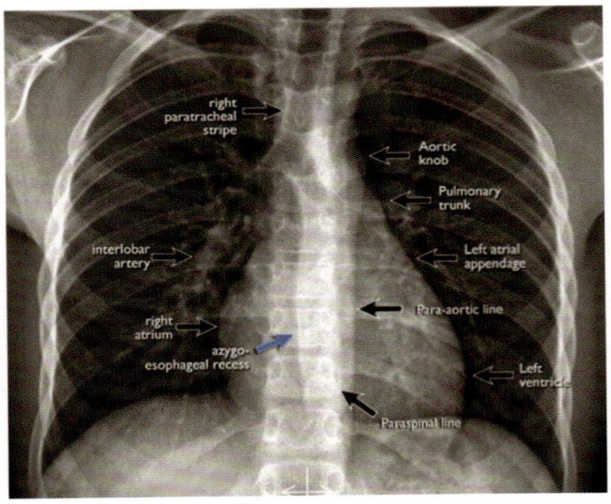

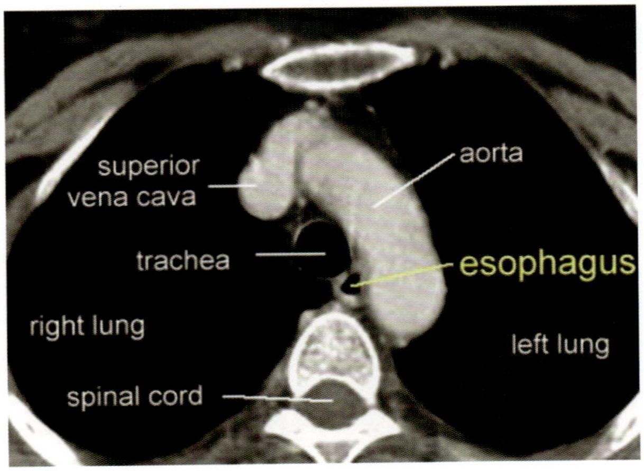

Normal Chest CT's

Aortic Arch and Tributaries

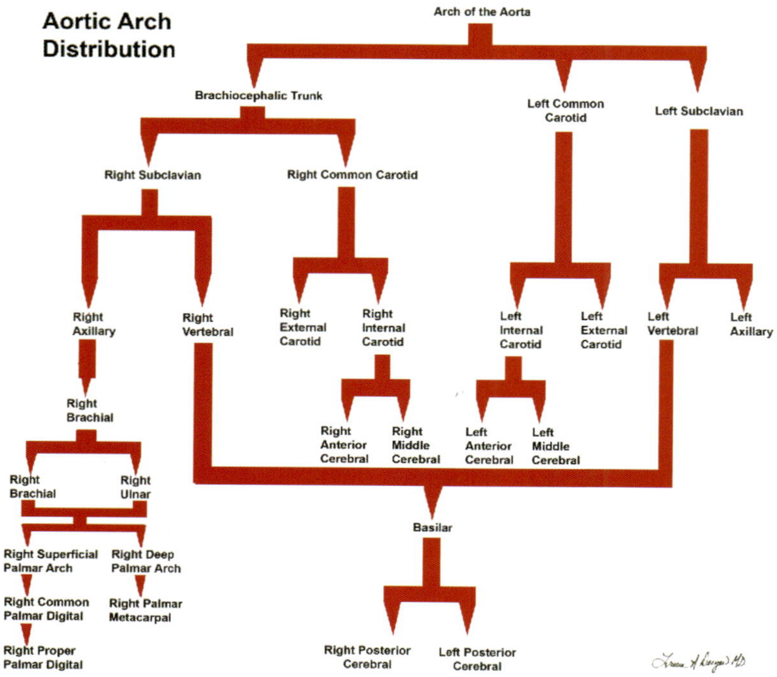

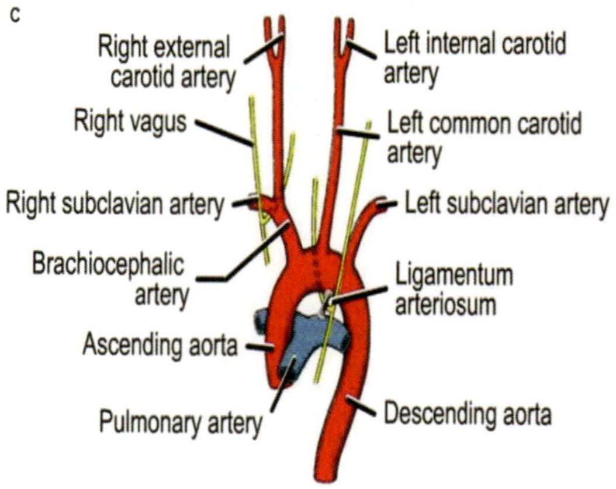

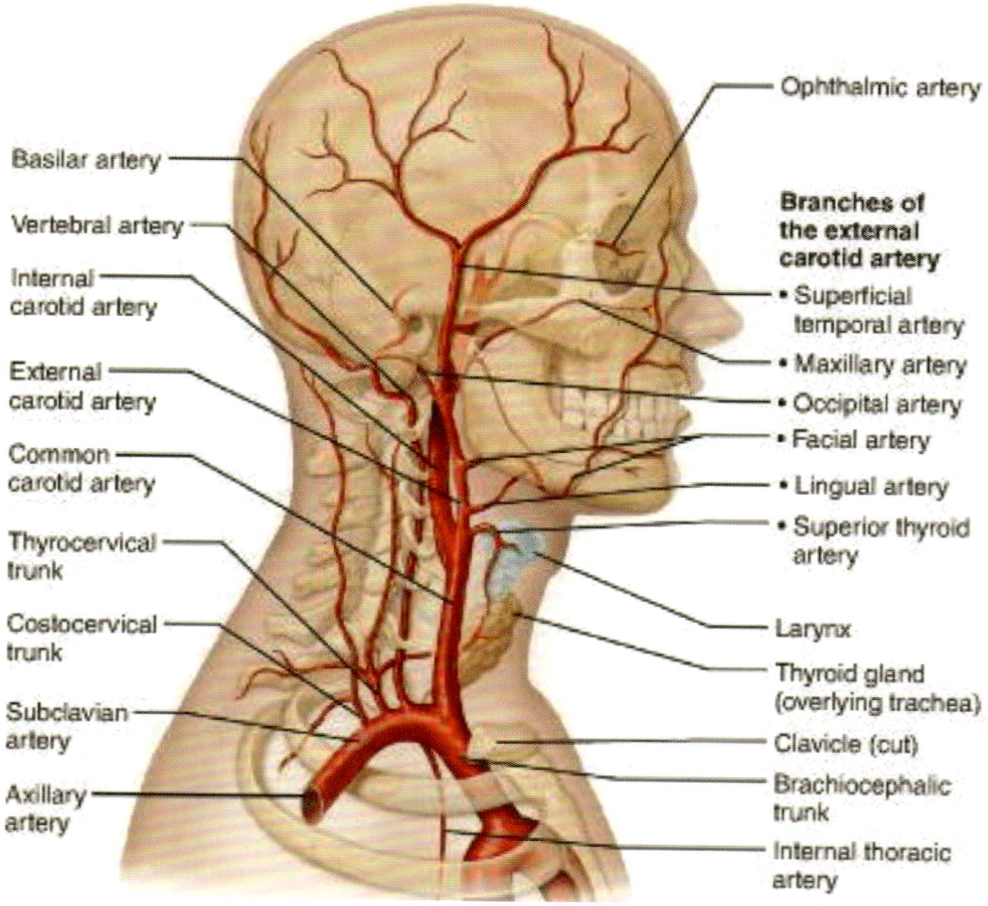

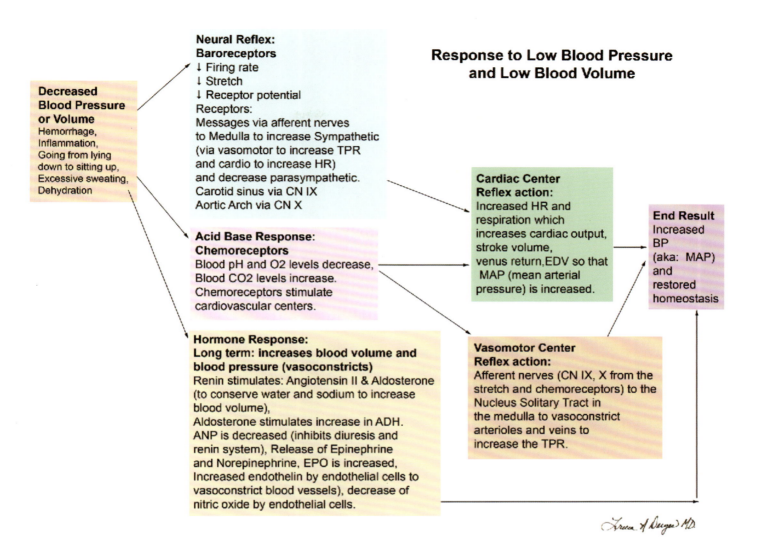

Response to Low Blood Pressure and Low Blood Volume

Decreased Blood Pressure or Volume
Hemorrhage,
Inflammation,
Going from lying down to sitting up,
Excessive sweating,
Dehydration

Neural Reflex:
Baroreceptors
↓ Firing rate
↓ Stretch
↓ Receptor potential
Receptors:
Messages via afferent nerves to Medulla to increase Sympathetic (via vasomotor to increase TPR and cardio to increase HR) and decrease parasympathetic.
Carotid sinus via CN IX
Aortic Arch via CN X

Acid Base Response:
Chemoreceptors
Blood pH and O2 levels decrease,
Blood CO2 levels increase.
Chemoreceptors stimulate cardiovascular centers.

Hormone Response:
Long term: increases blood volume and blood pressure (vasoconstricts)
Renin stimulates: Angiotensin II & Aldosterone (to conserve water and sodium to increase blood volume),
Aldosterone stimulates increase in ADH.
ANP is decreased (inhibits diuresis and renin system), Release of Epinephrine and Norepinephrine, EPO is increased,
Increased endothelin by endothelial cells to vasoconstrict blood vessels), decrease of nitric oxide by endothelial cells.

Cardiac Center
Reflex action:
Increased HR and respiration which increases cardiac output, stroke volume, venus return,EDV so that MAP (mean arterial pressure) is increased.

Vasomotor Center
Reflex action:
Afferent nerves (CN IX, X from the stretch and chemoreceptors) to the Nucleus Solitary Tract in the medulla to vasoconstrict arterioles and veins to increase the TPR.

End Result
Increased BP (aka: MAP) and restored homeostasis

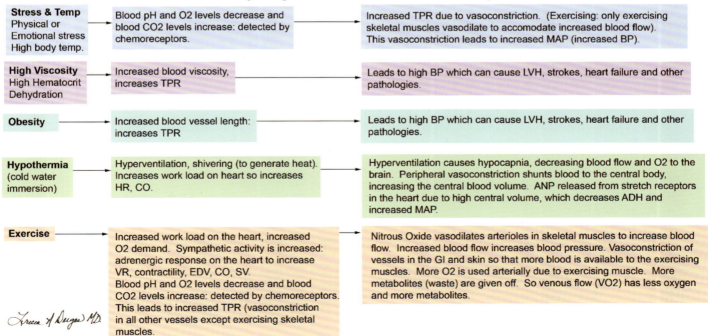

Additional Physiological Affects on the Cardiovascular System

Stress & Temp Physical or Emotional stress High body temp.	Blood pH and O2 levels decrease and blood CO2 levels increase: detected by chemoreceptors.	Increased TPR due to vasoconstriction. (Exercising: only exercising skeletal muscles vasodilate to accomodate increased blood flow). This vasoconstriction leads to increased MAP (increased BP).
High Viscosity High Hematocrit Dehydration	Increased blood viscosity, increases TPR	Leads to high BP which can cause LVH, strokes, heart failure and other pathologies.
Obesity	Increased blood vessel length: increases TPR	Leads to high BP which can cause LVH, strokes, heart failure and other pathologies.
Hypothermia (cold water immersion)	Hyperventilation, shivering (to generate heat). Increases work load on heart so increases HR, CO.	Hyperventilation causes hypocapnia, decreasing blood flow and O2 to the brain. Peripheral vasoconstriction shunts blood to the central body, increasing the central blood volume. ANP released from stretch receptors in the heart due to high central volume, which decreases ADH and increased MAP.
Exercise	Increased work load on the heart, increased O2 demand. Sympathetic activity is increased: adrenergic response on the heart to increase VR, contractility, EDV, CO, SV. Blood pH and O2 levels decrease and blood CO2 levels increase: detected by chemoreceptors. This leads to increased TPR (vasoconstriction in all other vessels except exercising skeletal muscles.	Nitrous Oxide vasodilates arterioles in skeletal muscles to increase blood flow. Increased blood flow increases blood pressure. Vasoconstriction of vessels in the GI and skin so that more blood is available to the exercising muscles. More O2 is used arterially due to exercising muscle. More metabolites (waste) are given off. So venous flow (VO2) has less oxygen and more metabolites.

Response to High Blood Pressure

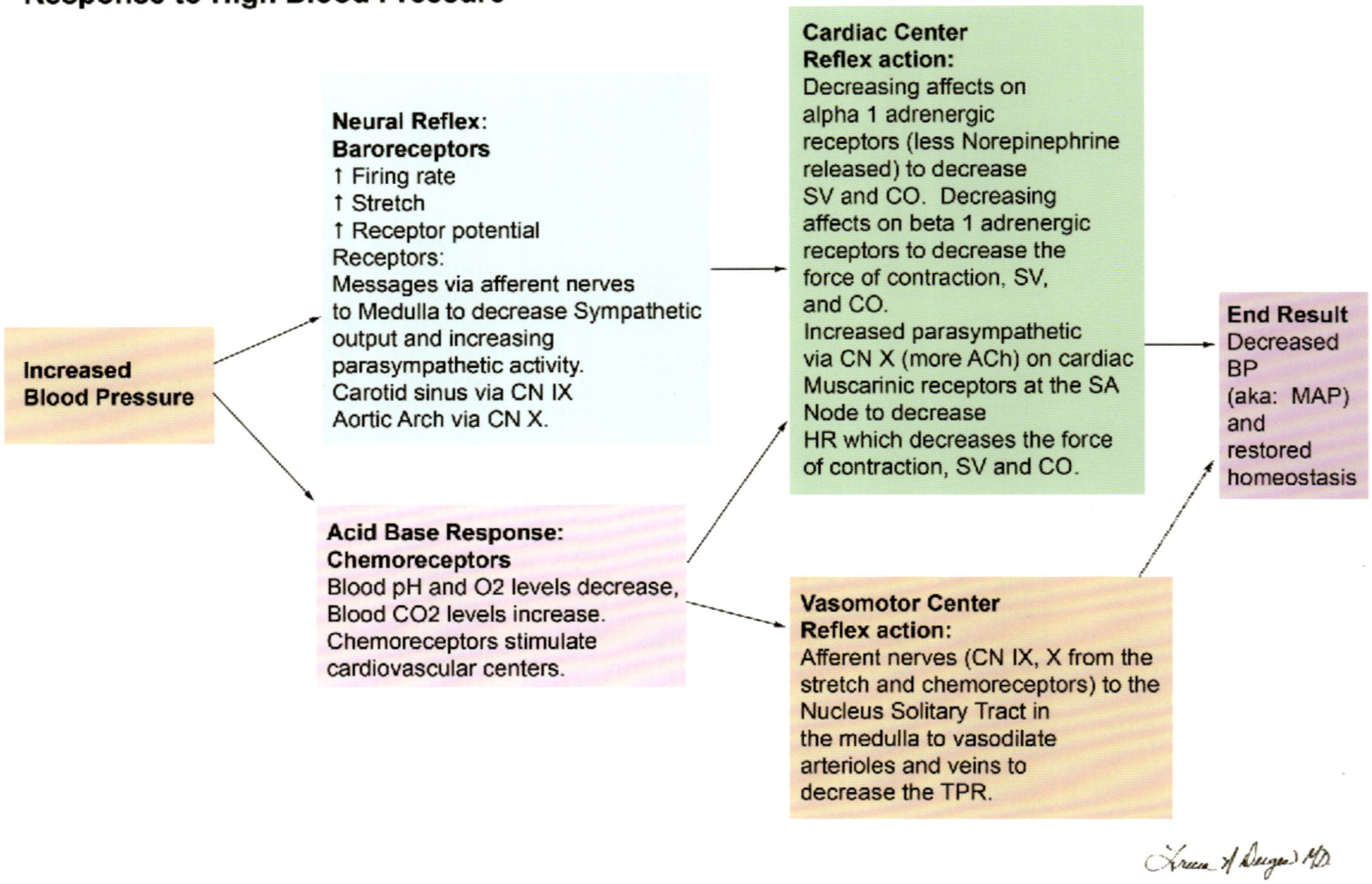

Physiologic and Pathologic effects on the heart

Exercise

- Thought of beginning the exercise automatically increases the HR, acting on β1 adrenergic receptors
- Exercise begins causing INCREASE WORK LOAD ON THE HEART (AKA: increased oxygen demand)
- This increases sympathetic activity:
  1) ↑ Venous return = ↑ EDV, ↑ CO, ↑ SV
  2) Vasodilation in skeletal muscles (so vessels are able to bring more oxygen to the exercising muscles) AND to increase the flow to be able to remove more metabolites (CO2, K, and H) from the cells.
  3) Vasoconstriction of viscera in GI and skin (this allows more blood to be sent to the muscles and increases the blood flow to the heart.
- Increases the activity of the cells therefore creates more metabolites (waste: CO2, K and H) – so vasodilation allows for this increase of metabolites to be taken away
- More metabolites in venous flow (↓ V O2) because more are made during exercise
- As body temperature increases with exercise, cutaneous arterioles dilate to radiate heat and ↓ body temp
- Aerobics dilates = ↓ TPR
- Isometric (weight lifting) = ↑ TPR, making heart muscles work harder = ↑ BP and ↑ risk of MI
- NO change in arterial content, ONLY venous. Venous content will show ↑ in metabolites (↑ CO2)
- Exercise = ↑ CO = ↓ TPR
- Cardio exercise also increases blood volume because it stimulates the release of ADH and aldosterone (both cause the kidney to retain water), therefore increasing blood plasma levels
- Exercise also increases the amount of proteins in blood plasma, therefore causing water retention and increased volume

Hemorrhage (Decreases blood volume)

- Baroreceptors sense change in ↓ BP due to ↓ blood volume, so there is ↓ venous return → ↓ cardiac output → so vessels vasoconstrict to ↑ TPR (Systemic Vascular Resistance) and ↑ pulmonary vascular resistance so that there is a ↑ venous return (preload) to ↑ SV and ↑ CO. When cardiac output is ↓ there is also a ↓ in hydrostatic pressure, which means less fluid leaves the capillaries, which causes the systemic capillary fluid to be reabsorb fluid from the tissue interstitium to ↑ the capillary plasma. In addition, because the baroreceptor firing rate is ↓ due to the decrease in BP → CN IX sends message to the brain to ↑ sympathetic effects (via adrenergic stimulation of B1 receptors on the heart) and to ↓ parasympathetic effect (CN X) → ↑ heart rate so that → ↑ CO.

Increasing Blood Volume

- Anything that increases blood volume (IV infusions, pregnancy, exercise, sympathetic activity, RAAS (renin-angiotensin-aldosterone, fluid intake, etc.), increases venous return. = ↑ CO = ↓ TPR

TPR (aka: Mean Arterial Pressure, MAP)

- Inversely related to CO.
  ↓ CO = ↑ TPR Anything that decreases CO: heart failure
  ↑ CO = ↓ TPR Anything that increases CO

Cold Water (immersion)/ Hypothermia

- **Shivering** (bodies way to produce heat), hyperventilation
- **↑ Metabolism (Venous O2), ↑ ventilation (hyperventilation), ↑ HR, ↑ CO, ↑ central blood volume, ↑ ANP (due to increase in central blood volume triggering the stretch receptors in the heart), ↑ MAP and ↓ ADH (due to increased volume).**
- Hyperventilation causes **hypocapnia** which causes decreased blood flow and oxygen to the brain
- Decrease in tissue metabolism
- **Peripheral vasoconstriction** of arterioles leading to increased central blood volume which causes the heart to work harder to pump the same amount of blood through the body
- Blood flow is directed away from non-essential muscles (extremities)
- ADH will decrease because of increased volume

Hypothermia: Cold Weather Exposure

- MC seen in alcoholics that fall asleep outside in the cold
- Can cause fatal arrhythmias.
- EKG shows J-Waves of Osborn (look like ST elevations)

Drinking Cold Water or Splashing Cold Water on the Face

(used to slow down heart rates in SVT)

- Drinking cold water constricts the vessels around the stomach which **activates the Vegas nerve**, which is in control of the parasympathetic system (runs by the heart, down the thorax and by the stomach)
- ↑ parasympathetic activity = ↓ decreased heart rate and ↓ CO
- Splashing cold water on the face also causes constriction of superficial vessels and activation of the Vegas nerve causing the same ↑ parasympathetic activity = ↓ heart rate and ↓ COV

Reactive Hyperaemia

- **When blood flow to a tissue is blocked for a period and then unblocked, blood flow through the tissue increases immediately 4 – 7 times normal**. This means that when the blood flow is allowed to be restored to an area that has been occluded of its blood supply, there is a sudden increase of blood flow. If the muscle in this occluded area has been exercising, the rate of blood flow once it is restored will be even greater. After this ischemia there will be a shortage of oxygen and a build up of metabolic waste.
  Vasocclusion → Decreased Oxygen → Vasodilation

Active Hyperaemia (aka: functional hyperaemia, metabolic hyperaemia)

- When any tissue becomes highly active (exercise, mental activity), blood flow is increased. Active cells use more oxygen and fuel (glucose or fatty acids) and they produce more metabolic waste (CO2, Hydrogen/protons, K, lactate, adenosine). When cells are active, local arterioles vasodilate so that more blood is able to reach the tissues.
  Increased local metabolism → accumulation of vasodilator metabolites → vasodilation

Cardiac Output – Pressure - Volume

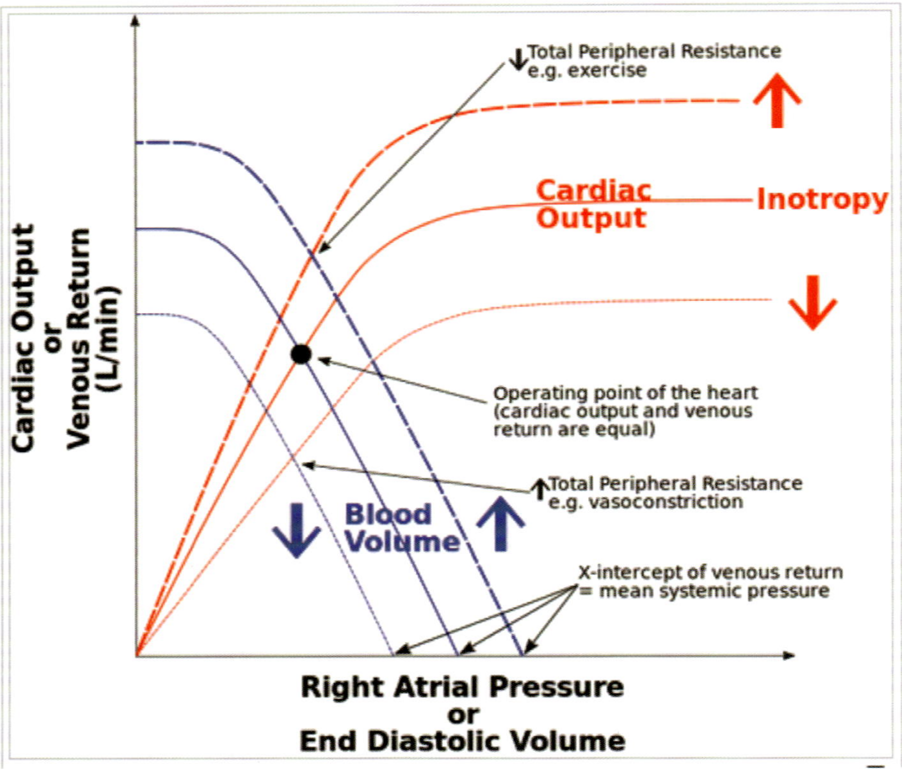

Cardiac Function Curve
(Frank-Starling law)

Y-axis = CO, SV
X-axis = EDV, PCWP, right atrial pressure.

Shifts along the same line indicate a change in preload. Shifts from one line to another indicate a change in afterload or contractility.

Maneuvers to increase or decrease blood flow to the heart will increase the volume of the murmur.

General rule for murmurs:
More blood = more murmur heard in MS, MR, AS, AR and less murmur in MVP and HCM.
Less blood = less murmur heard in MS, MR, AS, AR and more murmur in MVP and HCM.

Breathing Effect on Heart Sounds

- **Inhalation** (blood flows from the SVC and IVC into the right atrium) so all heart sounds (murmurs) are LOUDER on inhalation on the **RIGHT SIDE** of the heart
- **Exhalation** (blood is ejected from the heart) so all heart sounds (murmurs) are LOUDER on exhalation on the **LEFT SIDE** of the heart. Remember**: HCM and MVP do NOT increase during exhalation.**

Maneuvers to DECREASE fluid in the heart = **↓ venous return (flow) = ↓ preload = ↓ CO = ↓ EDV = ↑ TPR**

Valsalva maneuver and standing up

- **Increases intensity of HCM and MVP** (these murmurs get louder with less fluid in the heart, which is why the treatment for these conditions involves keeping more fluid in the heart. ie: **Beta blocker)**
- Decreases intensity of all other murmurs (AS, AR, MS, MR)
- **Use of diuretics is equivalent to the Valsalva or Standing up** = ↓ fluid, ↓ preload, ↓ venous return to heart, ↓ volume.

Maneuvers to INCREASE fluid to the heart = ↑ Venus return (flow) = ↑ preload = ↑ CO = ↑ EDV = ↓ TPR

Squatting or leg raise

- Increases the intensity of all other murmurs (AS, AR, MS, MR)
- Decreases the intensity of HCM and MVP because ↑ flow to the heart = ↑ fluid
- Squatting is the mechanism in Tetralogy of Fallot that increases venous return (decreasing TPR) and increases preload to the heart, which allows more blood to go into the heart and then sends more blood into the pulmonary (lungs) which provides for more oxygen delivery. Otherwise, with normal venous return, most blood is sent through the VSD (right to left shunt) sending deoxygenated blood to the left ventricle (by passing the lungs), which sends deoxygenated blood out into the body.

Maneuvers to INCREASE afterload

Handgrip or blood pressure cuff.

- **↑ afterload which causes ↑ blood to stay inside the left ventricle**
- ↑ blood = ↑ volume = ↑ pressure
- Has no affect on mitral stenosis

Amyl Nitrate (venodilator) DECREASES afterload

- **Same affect as ACE inhibitors/ARB's, Nifedipine**
- **↓ preload = ↓ afterload ↓ amount of blood inside of left ventricle = ↓ pressure**
- Amyl Nitrate, ACE Inhibitors/ARB's, Nifedipine have no affect on mitral stenosis

Cardiac Pacemakers – Electrical Conduction

- The heart can contract **without any innervation**
- **Gap junctions** (composed of two **conne**xins, (**tip**: gap junctions are "**connec**ted") conducts electrical signals so that heart muscle cells contract in unison
- Gap junctions connect each cardiac myocyte

SA Node (Sinoatrial node)

- Pacemaker of the heart and responsible for initiation of the heart beat
- Located on the wall in the right atrium at **the junction of where the SVC** enters. (**tip**: "S"A node = "S"VC)
- Innervated by the parasympathetic nervous system, CN X (Vegas nerve) and by the sympathetic nervous system, Spinal nerves T1 – T4)
- Stimulation of the Vegas nerve decreases the SA node rate causing a negative inotropic effect
- **Blood supply is MC right coronary artery** (60 – 70%: right side dominant) or a branch (Left circumflex) off the Left coronary artery (left side dominant)
- **Sick sinus syndrome**: occlusion of the arterial blood supply to the SA node so that the electrical pacemaker of the SA node is disrupted

AV Node (Atrioventricular node)

- Electrically connects the atrial and ventricle chambers to conduct the electrical impulses from the atria to the ventricles
- Located between the atria and ventricles near the opening of the coronary sinus: specifically: subendocardium of the interarterial septum
- Blood supply is MC right coronary artery (90%)
- **Slowest conduction**

Bundle of His

- Heart muscle cells that transmits electrical impulses from the AV node to the apex of the heart via bundle branches
- **Bundle branches** are off shoots that transmit action potentials from the Bundle of His to Purkinje fibres and are located in the interventricular septum. (Left and Right Bundle branches)
- Bundle branch blocks occur when a bundle branch becomes injured (heart disease, MI, cardiac surgery) and it stops conducting impulses appropriately
- **Right Bundle Branch Block (RBBB): impulses not being transmitted properly in the right ventricle. (Causes: Pulmonary embolism, RVH, rheumatic heart disease, myocarditis, cardiomyopathy, and ischaemic heart disease).**
- **Left Bundle Branch Block (LBBB): conduction of the left ventricle is delayed causing the left ventricle to contract after the right ventricle. (Causes: Aortic stenosis, dilated cardiomyopathy, Acute MI, Lyme disease)**
- **(tip: to distinguish between ECG patterns of a LBBB and a RBBB, is WiLLiaM MaRRoW. With a LBBB, there is a W in lead V1 and an M in lead V6, whereas, with RBBB, there is an M in V1 and a W in V6)**

Purkinje Fibers

- Located in the inner ventricular walls of the heart
- Creates synchronized contractions of the ventricles to maintain a consistent heart rhythm
- Carry the impulses from the Bundle of His to the myocardium of the ventricles which causes the ventricles to contract and eject blood from the heart
- **Fastest conduction**

Electrical Conduction Speed

- **Fastest to slowest:** Purkinje > atria > ventricles > AV node
  (**tip**: Park AT VENTura Avenue)

Conducting System of the Heart

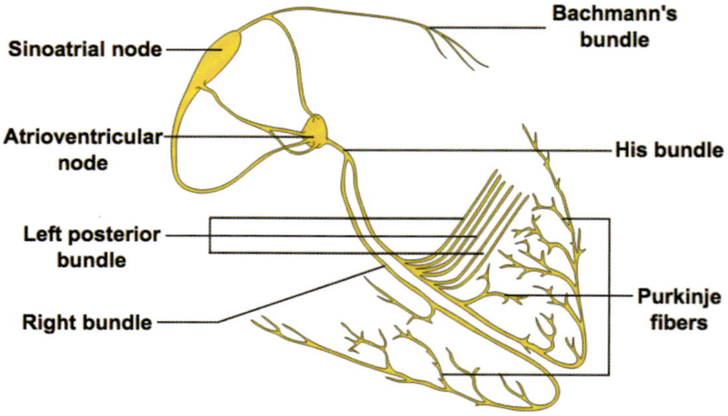

Pacemaker Cardiac Action Potential

Occurs in the SA and AV nodes

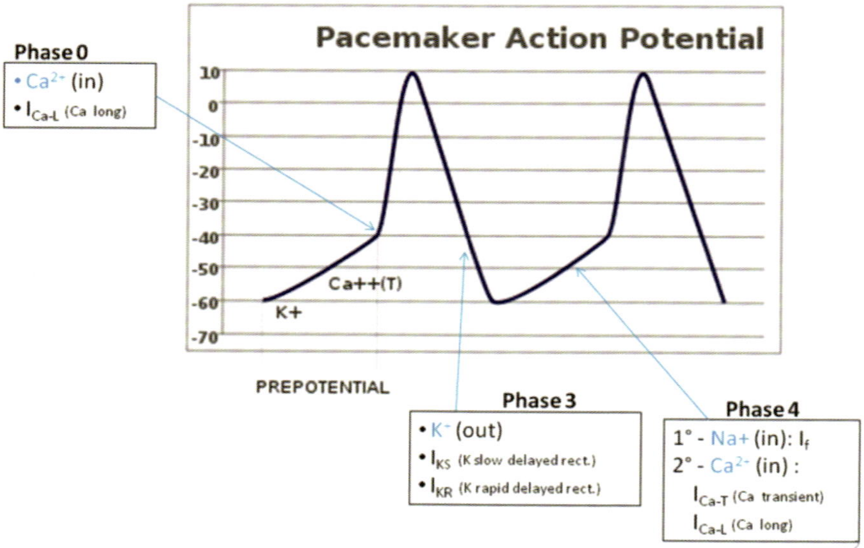

SA Atrial Action Potential	Ions	Action
Phase 0	Open **L-type voltage gate Ca channels**, Ca **influx**	Upstroke. Occurs in diastole and slows diastolic depolarization. **Stopping L-type calcium channels prolongs the time to reach threshold.**
Phase 3	Activation of K channels **= K efflux**, Inactivation of Ca channels	K leaves the cell
Phase 4	**Influx of Na**	Depolarization. Slope of Phase 4 = HR ACh and adenosine ↓ **depolarization and HR. This prolongs K flow so cell stays negative longer.** Catecholamines ↑ depolarization and HR

L-type Calcium Channel

- Voltage-dependent calcium channel
- "L" = Long length of activation
- Excitation (contraction) of cardiac, skeletal, smooth muscles and aldosterone secretion in adrenal cortex

Ventricular Cardiac Action Potential

Occurs in Bundle of His and Purkinje fibers

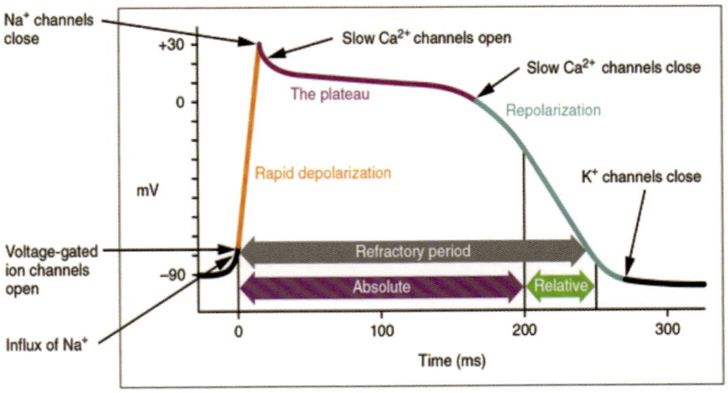

(a)

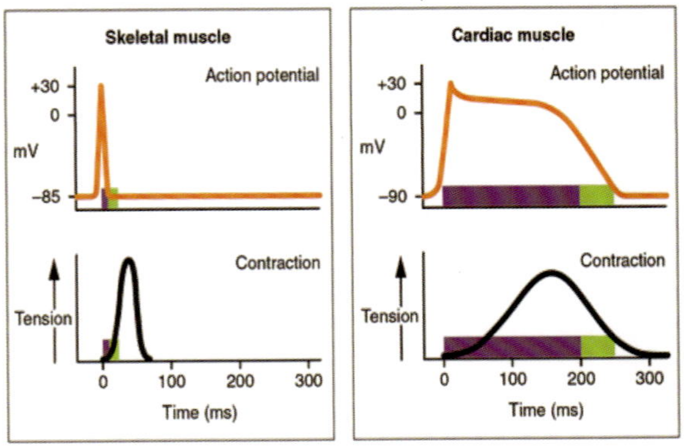

(b)

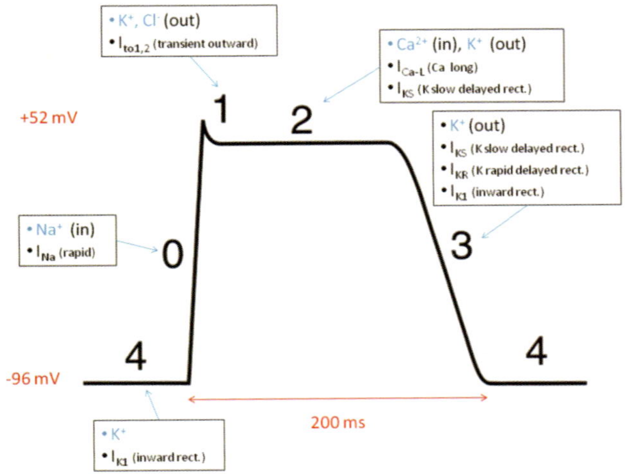

Ventricular Action Potential	Ions	Action
Phase o	Voltage gated **Na channels** open	Upstroke and depolarization
Phase 1	Inactivation of Na voltage channels	Initial ventricular repolarization
Phase 2	Plateau, **Ca influx** in voltage gated	Ca release from sarcoplasmic reticulum, myocyte contraction
Phase 3	**K efflux** in voltage gated channels, voltage gated Ca close	**Ventricular Repolarization, QT**
Phase 4	**K permeability** through **leaking** K channels	**Maintains resting potential of cell. K controls phase 4**

Parasympathetic and Sympathetic Effects on the Heart

- Sympathetic: Norepinephrine (AKA: noradrenaline) is released by sympathetic nerves and binds to the β1 receptors which couple with the Gs protein which stimulates the enzyme adenylate cyclase to increase the 2nd messenger cAMP (cyclic AMP). Adrenaline that is circulating in the blood also binds the β1 receptors. HCN channels (nonselective ligand-gated ion channels that open with increased levels of cAMP) open and the SA node action potential increases.
- Parasympathetic: Acetylcholine released by the Vegas Nerve (CN X) binds at the M2 muscarinic receptors which couple with Gi proteins which inhibit adenylate cyclase and decrease the cAMP levels, which close the HCN channels, decreasing the SA node action potentials.

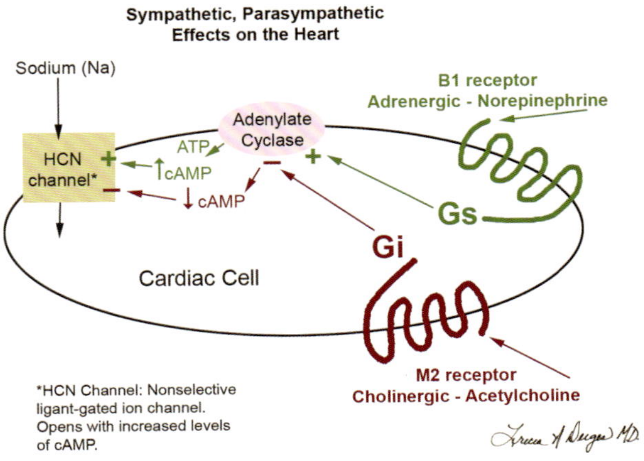

Cardiac Pressures

Left Atrial Pressure Determination

PCWP (Pulmonary capillary wedge pressure) = approximation of left atrial pressure. Measured with a Swan-Ganz catheter.
If there is an **increased PCWP** the problem is coming from the **left side of the heart** (not lungs, nor right side)

Right Atrial Pressure Determination

CVP (Central venous pressure) = approximation of the right atrial pressure. Is the pressure in the thoracic cava (at the right atrium). **Represents preload**.

Average, Normal Intracardiac and Vascular Pressures (mmHg)

Right Atrium	0 – 4 (varies with respiration)
Right Ventricle	25 sys/4 dias
Pulmonary Artery	25 sys/10 dias
Left Atrium	8 – 10
Left Ventricle	120 sys/10 dias
Aorta	120 sys/80 dias

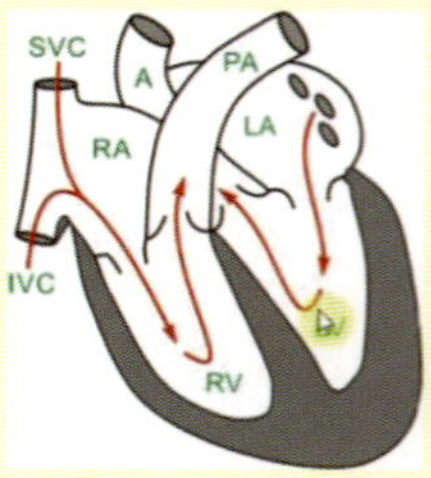

dys = systolic; dias = diastolic

Pressure-Volume Loop

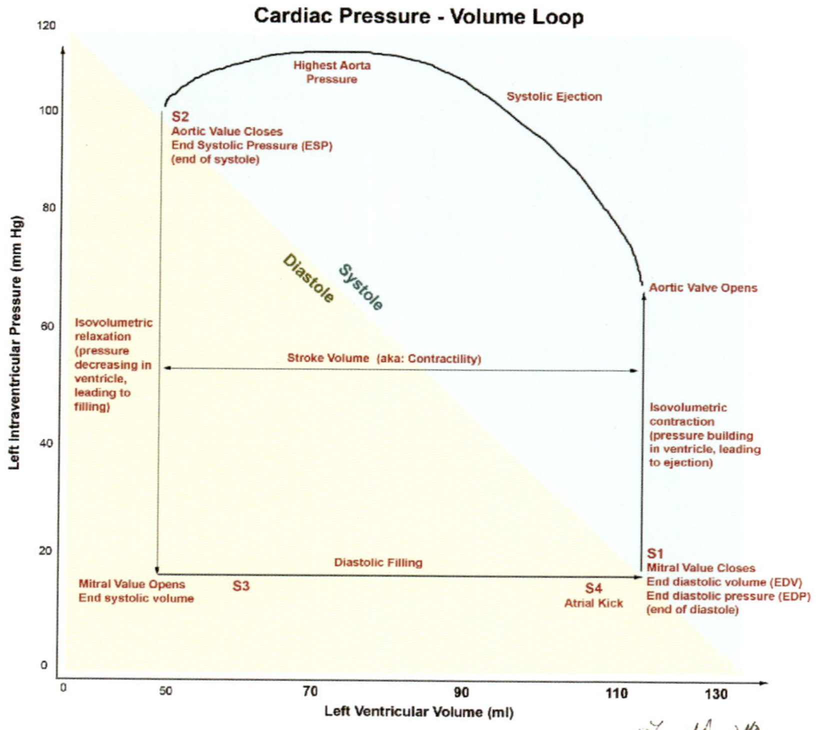

Note:
AV Valves: AKA: Mitral and Tricuspid Valves

Semilunar Valves AKA: Aortic and Pulmonic Valves

Heart Cycle

- **S1** = Mitral and tricuspid valves close (Point B). Ventricles have filled.
- **Isovolumetric contraction**: pressure is building.
- Aortic and pulmonary valves opens to allow ejection of blood.
- **Ejection**.
- **S2** = Aortic and pulmonary valves close (Point D).
- **Isovolumetric relaxation**: (between points D and A) Blood is filling the atria.
- Mitral and tricuspid valves open (Point A). Blood fills ventricles. This is also where **S3 occurs**.
- Rapid filling: (between points A and B), atrial kick.
- **S4** occurs **just before** S1 during atrial kick.
- Atrial kick: contraction of the atrium immediately before ventricular systole. It accounts for 5-30% of cardiac output. It is accentuated in cases of hypertrophic cardiomyopathy.

S3 Heart Sound

- During rapid filing phase (Point A)
- Associated with high fluid/volume
- Pathologic with CHF, dilated ventricles, mitral regurgitation
- Normal in children, young women in menses, pregnancy

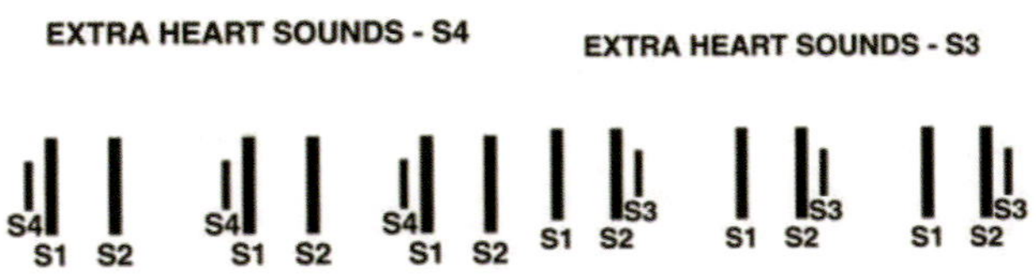

S4 Heart Sound

- During late diastole during atrial kick (just before Point B)
- Pathologic: Associated with high pressure and LVH

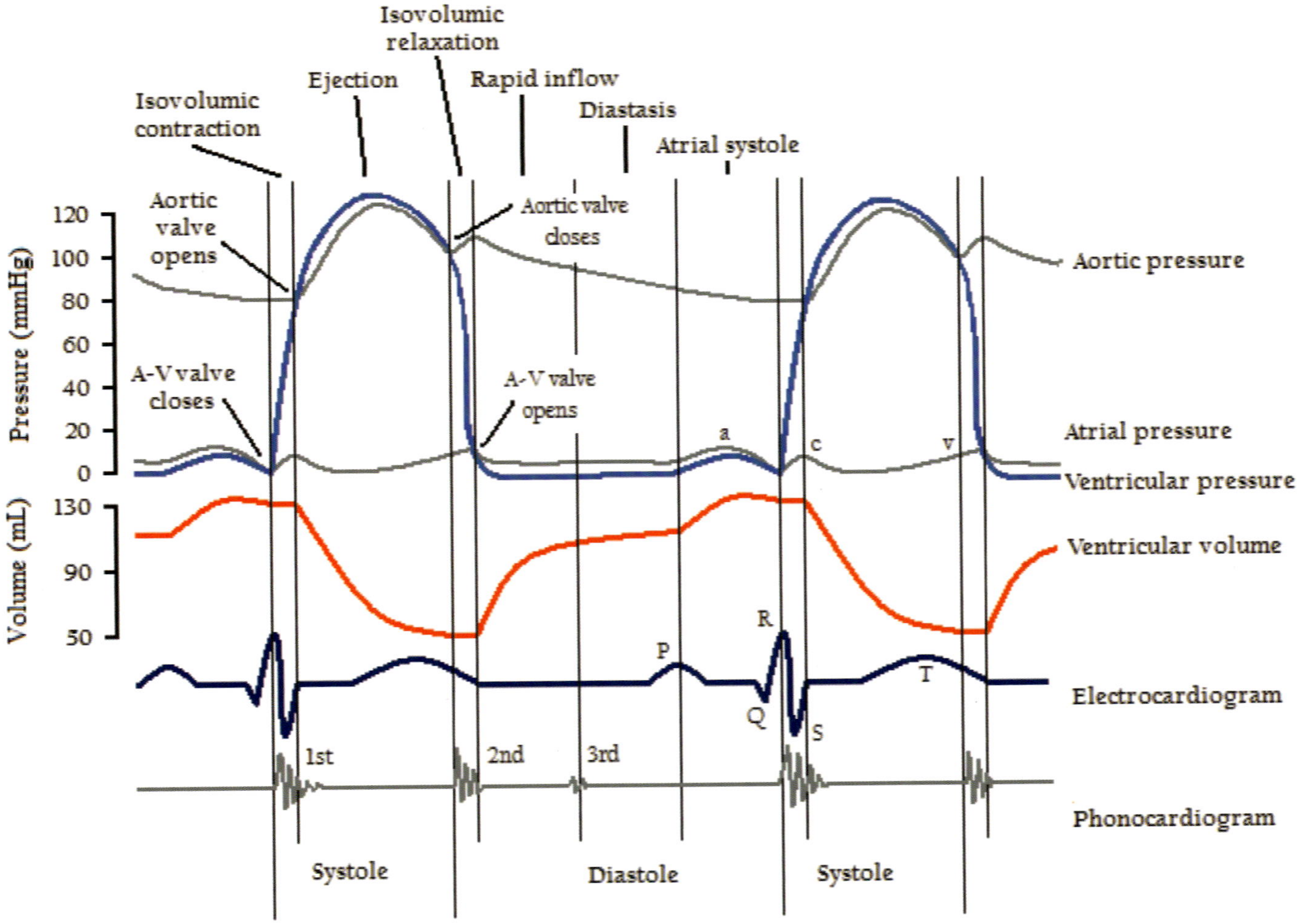

Changes in the Cardiac - Pressure Volume Curve

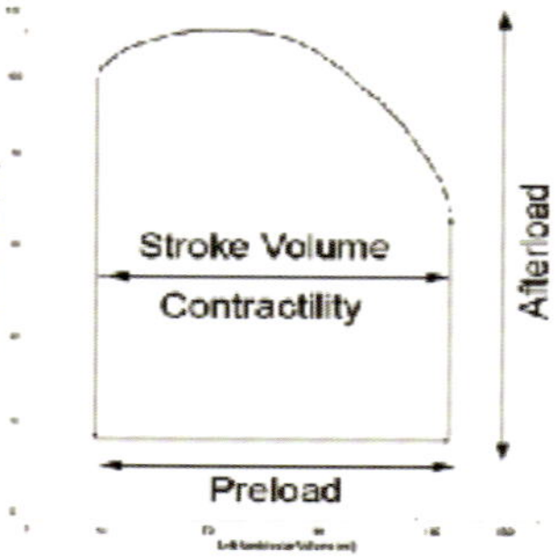

NORMAL

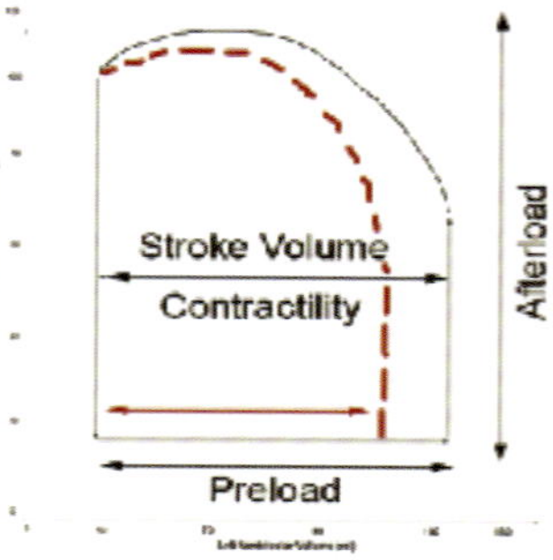

↓ Preload
Ex: Hemorrhage

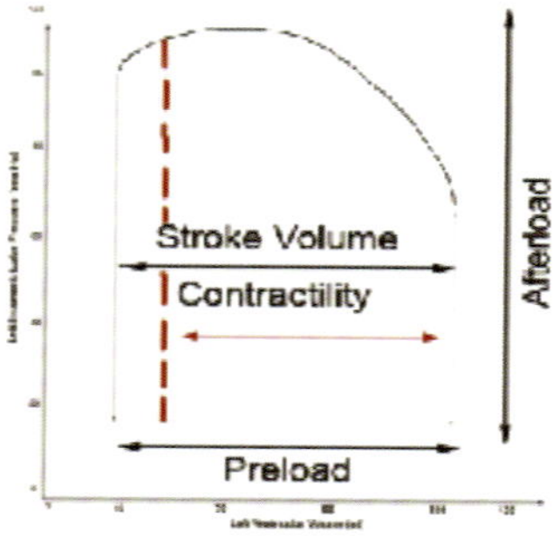

↓ Stroke Volume
Ex: Systolic Dysfunction, failing pump

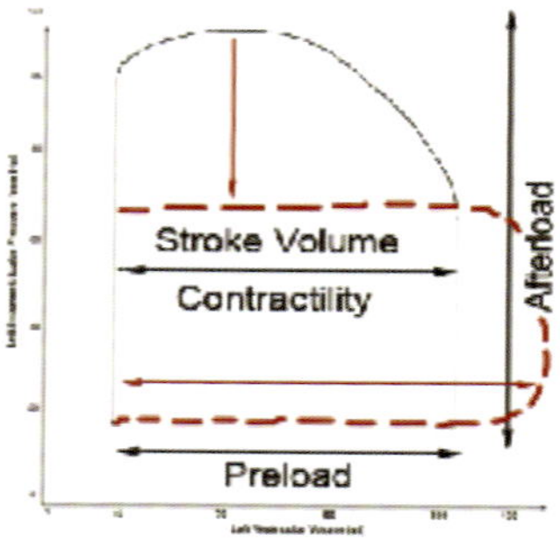

↑ Preload, Volume
↓ Afterload
Ex: AV Fistula

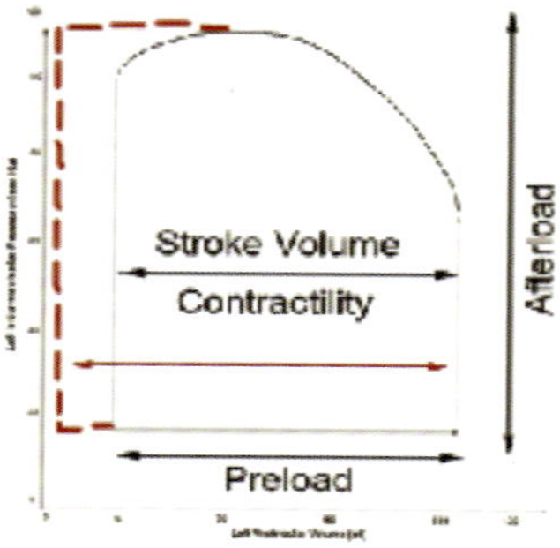

↑ Contraction, SV, EF
↓ ESV

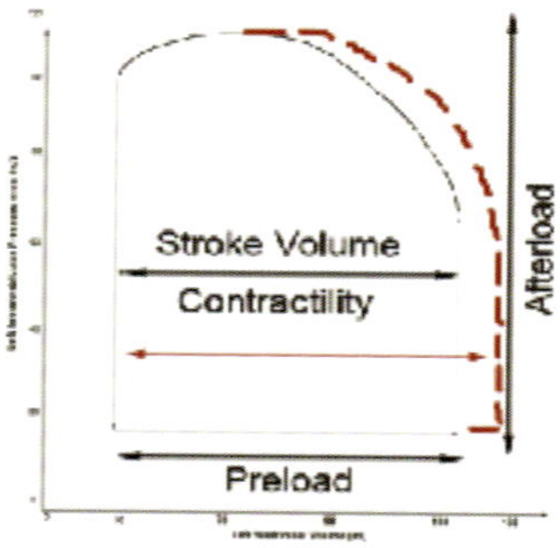

↑ Preload, Volume, EDV
Ex: IV Fluids, CHF, Renal Failure

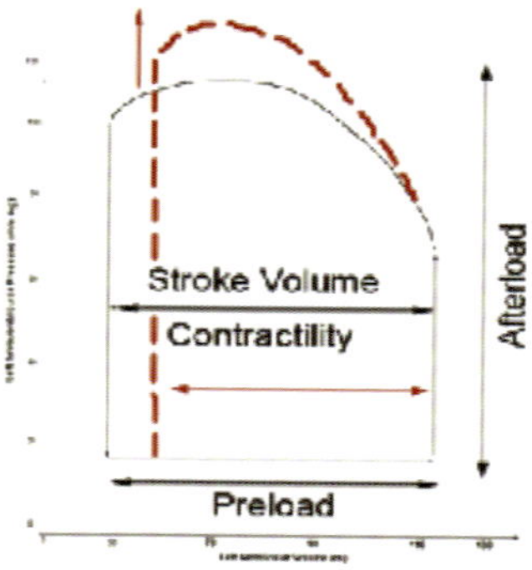

↑ Afterload, ESV, Pressure
↓ SV

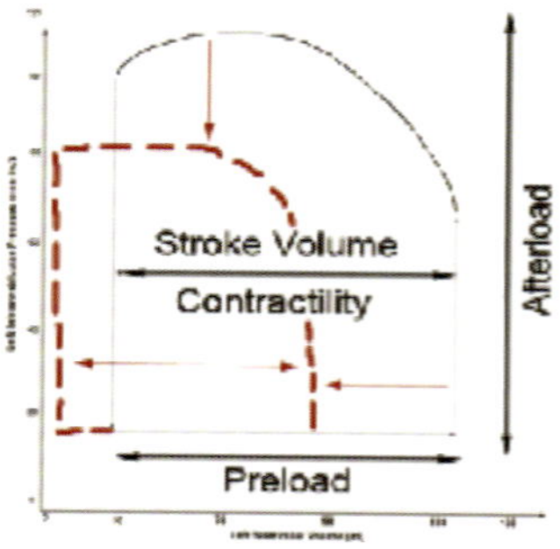

↓ Preload, Afterload
No Change: Contractility
Ex: Nitrous

Lorena A Dugan MD

Jugular Venous Pulse/Pressure (JVP or JVD)

- In normal inspiration blood fills (falls) into the right atrium. If there are no pathologies the blood falls in the atrium without meeting any additional pressure so the jugular vein stays under 3 cm. However, if there is a pathology that **inhibits or slows down the blood** that is supposed to fall into the atrium during normal inspiration, the blood **can't go forward so will back up into the jugular vein** causing it to enlarge causing JVD (or increased JVP)
- JVP/JVD is highest during right ventricular ejection (x wave)
- Pressure of the venous system visualized at the internal jugular vein
- **Normal CVP pressure assessment**: Patient positioned at 30° the observed height of the jugular vein should be **< 3 cm** above sternal angle

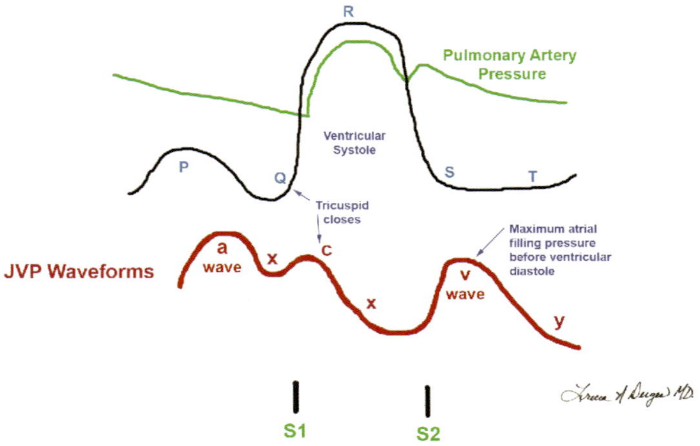

JVP Waveforms

- **a wave (upward) = atrial contraction.** It ends synchronously with the carotid artery pulse. The peak of a wave marks the end of atrial systole. This is absent in A-fib because there are no P waves in A-Fib
- **c wave (upward) = Right ventricle Contraction**. Pressure from RV contraction causes tricuspid to bulge into atrium
- **x** wave (downward) = Atrial rela**X**ation. Downward displacement of tricuspid value during RV contraction/systole. The x wave can be used as a measure of right ventricle contractility. JVD is highest during ejection of right ventricle. Absent in tricuspid regurgitation
- **v** wave (upward) = Increased pressure in right atrium due to **V**enous filling. This occurs during and following the carotid pulse.
- **y** wave (downward) = Rapid empt**Y**ing of blood from right atrium to right ventricle

Pathologies of JVD/JVP

Jugular Venous Distention (JVD)

- Bradycardia, fluid overload, right heart failure, pulmonary hypertension, tricuspid stenosis, heart failure.

Paradoxical JVP/JVD (AKA: **Kussmaul's sign: JVP rises with inspiration and drops with expiration**).

- Tamponade, constrictive pericarditis, pericardial effusion.

Absent a wave

- Atrial fibrillation (A-Fib: "Irregularly irregular heartbeat"). No P wave present.

Absent p wave

- Atrial fibrillation (no P wave present), A Flutter.

Cannon a waves (atria contracting against a closed tricuspid valve)

- Atrial flutter, 3rd degree heart block, tachycardia

Hepatojugular Reflex

- When pressure is applied to the abdomen and it causes a rise in JVD due to backed up fluid.

Pulse and BP Differentials

Pulse	Description/Notes
Pulsus paradoxus	Associated with cardiac tamponade and tension pneumothorax
Pulsus alternans	Associated with cardiac tamponade and indicates left ventricular systolic dysfunction. Alternating heights of the R peak on an EKG, indicating alternating strengths of a beat.
Pulsus tardus	Associated with aortic stenosis.
Pulsus bisferiens	Associated with aortic regurgitation.
Pulsus bigeminus	Associated with hypertrophic obstructive cardiomyopathy (HOCM)
Irregularly irregular	Associated with A-Fib
Different BP from one side to the other	Takayasu arteritis, tamponade, tension pneumothorax, vascular DZ
Different BP from upper body to lower	Coarctation of the aorta, PDA, vascular DZ

Heart Murmurs

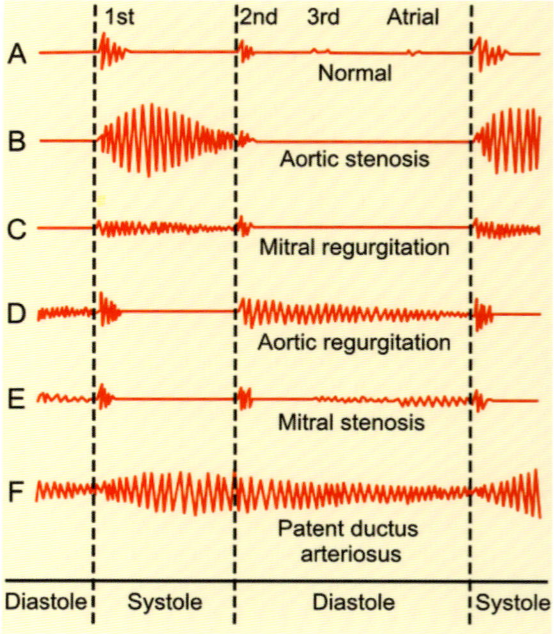

(**tip**: to easily remember what the opposing value is doing at the same time – think of the 4 main "big" heart murmurs (AS, AR, MS, MR) as 4 players that are going to divide into 2 teams (Systolic and Diastolic). The captains of the 2 teams are the "big" valves (the AORTICS) and each of these captains (AS and AR) . AS is the captain of the Systolic team and AR is the captain of the Diastolic team). Each captain can only pick one player for their team from the two remaining players (MS and MR) and that player **cannot** be the same murmur as they are (ie: can't put two stenosis or two regurg together). So that forces the team captain AS to have to pick MR for his team, leaving the other team captain (AR) left with the team member of MS. So if AS is happening, MR is its counterpart and if MR is happening its counterpart is AS and they are both on the systolic team. If AR is happening its counterpart is MS and if MS is happening AR is its counterpart and they are on the diastolic team).

Murmur's Not Considered Pathological

- When the murmur is only systolic. A diastolic murmur is pathologic.
- When it is < 2/6 grade.
- When there is infection, anxiety or fever involved.

MURMURS

Murmur	Systolic Diastolic	Character and EKG findings	Location best heard	Radiation and SX	Maneuvers to Exaggerate	Notes
Aortic Stenosis	Systolic Mid to late	**Crescendo-decrescendo** **EKG: LVH, S wave in V1, R**	**Right** 2nd ICS	**Radiates to: Carotids** SX: Chest pain, **syncope**, CHF and a HX of HTN. If AS presents as CHF, prognosis is 2 years.	Lean forward, louder on **exhalation**, ↑ intensity on squatting (anything adding more fluid), "Pulsus parvus et tardus" = weak pulses with delayed peak.	**Syncope**, MCC **calcified aortic valve** or bicuspid aortic valve. Do not use nitrates. **DX:** **BID: TTE (Transthoracic Echo).** **TEE (Transesophageal Echo) is more accurate than TTE.** **MAT: Left heart catheterization.** CXR: Left Ventricular Hypertrophy (LVH) TX: **Valve replacement.**

Murmur	Systolic Diastolic	Character and EKG findings	Location best heard	Radiation and SX	Maneuvers to Exaggerate	Notes
Mitral Regurgitation **Mitral Regurg cont'd**	**Holosystolic AKA: Pansystolic**	**High pitched, Blowing** murmur	Heard best at **apex.** Left 5th ICS, mid-clavicular line	**Radiates to: Axilla.** **SX: Dyspnea on exertion, S3**	Murmur worsens with hand grip (↑ TPR, ↑ afterload = pushes blood backward through valve). Squatting and leg raising will worsen murmur by ↑ venous return (↑ preload = ↑ more blood volume). Murmur becomes louder during **exhalation** Heard better by lying in **left lateral decubitus position.**	MCC: MVP, LV dilation, HTN, ischemic heart disease, papillary muscle rupture as post MI complication. TX: **ACE inhibitor/ARB's, Nifedipine.** **Surgery repair: Valve replacement when dilation of heart begins to occur. Once left ventricular ESV > 40 mm, damage irreversible or if EF < 60%.** **DX: ECHO** **BID: TTE (TEE is more accurate).**
Tricuspid Regurgitation (Insufficiency)	**Holosystolic AKA: Pansystolic**		Left lower sternal boarder	Radiates to: Right sternal boarder	**Inspiration** (↑ RA return)	MCC: RV dilation
Aortic Regurgitation (Insufficiency)	Diastolic	**Early diastolic, blowing, decrescendo** murmur, following S2	**Left 2nd** ICS, Left sternal boarder.	**Radiates to: Apex** SX: **Head bobbing** (Musset's sign, **Wide pulse pressure**, **bounding pulses** causes an ↑ upstroke to the carotid pulse (Hyperkinetic pulse: AKA: Water-hammer pulse: AKA Corrigan's Pulse), **Orthopnea**, **Paroxysmal nocturnal dyspnea**, **angina pectoris**, Murmur heard over femoral artery (Duroziez's sign), BP gradient higher in lower extremities (Hill sign), pulsations in the fingernails (Quincke Pulse sign), LVH, dilated aorta. ↑ carotid pulse and ↓ in carotid pulse downstroke, S3 hearts sound.	Murmur can be heard better by leaning forward. Become worse with handgrip (↑ afterload). Murmur becomes better (decreases in intensity) with Valsalva or standing (↓ fluid in the heart).	MCC: **bicuspid aortic valve,** aortic root dilation (dilated aorta), early rheumatic heart dz, HTN, endocarditis, cystic medial necrosis, **Syphilis (AKA: vaso-vasorum),** Ankylosing spondylitis, Reiter's syndrome. TX: Surgery repair if **EF is < 55%,** if Left Ventricular ESV is > 55mm, or acute valve rupture post MI. TX: **ACE inhibitors, ARB's, Nifedipine. Furosemide** if needed. **DX:** **BID: TTE (TEE is more accurate).** **MA: Left heart catheterization.** CXR: Left Ventricular Hypertrophy (LVH)

Murmur	Systolic Diastolic	Character and EKG findings	Location best heard	Radiation and SX	Maneuvers to Exaggerate	Notes
Mitral Stenosis	Diastolic	**Opening snap**, mid **Diastolic rumble** EKG: Biphasic P wave in leads V1 and V2. (P wave = atrial contraction)		SX: **Hemoptysis** (spitting up blood) – the **ONLY murmur that presents with hemoptysis**), **enlarged left atrium** causes: **Dysphagia** (pressing on the esophagus), **Hoarseness** (pressing on the left recurrent laryngeal nerve), **elevated left mainstem bronchus** and **straightening of left heart boarder** on CXR (due to left atrium pushing up on bronchus), **A-Fib** (potential of clots → stroke or arterial clots)	Squatting, leg raise, lying down ↑ venous return to heart = ↑ preload = volume = ↑ intensity of murmur.	MC: **Rheumatic fever** (patient will usually be an **immigrant**), Pregnant women (due to ↑ plasma volume). **DX:** **BID: TTE (TEE is more accurate).** **MAT: Left heart catheterization.** TX: **Diuretics.** **Rate Control: β-Blockers (Metoprolol), Calcium Channel Blockers (Diltiazem, Verapamil), Digoxin, Amiodarone.** **In pregnancy: Balloon Valvuloplasty.**
ASD	Systolic	**Fixed S2 splitting**	Left 2nd ICS	Radiates to: Back, neck, Shoulder. SX: Small ASD: asymptomatic. Larger Defects: Parasternal heave, shortness of breath.	No resolution of S2 with exhalation	MC: Downs Syndrome. DX: ECHO TX: Repair. MCC: Failure of fusion of the septum primum and secundum. Caused by different pressures on the two sides of the heart.
VSD	**Holosystolic**	Harsh sound	Tricuspid area, left lower sternal boarder	SX: Shortness of breath.	Hand grip; (↑ afterload). Worsens (becomes louder) with squatting, leg raise, exhalation.	Seen in **Tetralogy of Fallot or after septal rupture post MI.** DX: ECHO. Catheterization determines degree of shunt.
PDA	Continuos through systole And diastole	**Continuous, machine like murmur**	Left infraclavicular area (**just below the clavicle**)			MCC: **Congenital rubella**, prematurity

Murmur	Systolic Diastolic	Character and EKG findings	Location best heard	Radiation and SX	Maneuvers to Exaggerate	Notes
MVP	Systolic, Late systolic	**Mid-systolic click, crescendo**	Left 5th ICS, midclavicular line over apex	Radiates to: Axilla. SX: MC: asymptomatic. If symptoms: Palpitations, panic attack, atypical chest pain, no CHF symptoms. **NOTE: MVP and HCM do NOT increase with expiration.**	**Valsalva maneuver**, standing to decrease fluid (↓ preload, ↓ venous return to heart) will worsen murmur. Murmur improves (↓ in intensity) with more fluid (↑ preload): squatting, handgrip, lying down.	MC in **Marfan's, Ehlers-Danlos**, more common in women, rupture of **chordae tendineae.** DX: ECHO. TX: **B-Blocker: Propanolol.**
HCM AKA: HOCM Hypertrophic Obstructive Cardiomyopathy	Systolic	**Crescendo-decrescendo** **(Caution: do not get this confused with aortic stenosis – you must see where the murmur is heard. HCM is on the LEFT side, AS is on the RIGHT side)**	**Left** 5th ICS, Left lower sternal boarder	**Radiates to: Apex.** **NOTE: HCM and MVP do NOT increase with expiration.**	**Anything that ↓ fluid (↓ preload)** in the heart (Valsalva maneuver, standing, Ace Inhibitors, ARB's, Hydralazine, Digoxin) **or by anything that ↑ heart rate** (dehydration, exercise, diuretics) **or by anything that ↓ left ventricle chamber size** will make the murmur worse. Murmur improves with more fluid in heart (↑ preload), which is why **patient must be treated with β-blockers.**	Young athletes that drop dead on the field. AD, family history. DX: ECHO TX: **β-blockers. Allows heart to slow down to increase filling so that more fluid is maintained in the heart. Do NOT use** Ace Inhibitors/ARBs or diuretics in HCM because it will ↓ preload. **Ablation of the septum, Implantable defibrillator if patient experiences syncope.**
Pulmonic Murmurs			**Left 2nd** ICS			
S3 Gallop (FLUID)						Fluid overload. MC seen in CHF or Mitral Regurgitation. It is considered normal in young patients, athletes, young females starting menses, pregnancy.
S4 (Pressure)						Pressure. Left ventricular hypertrophy, ↓ compliance (ventricle will not stretch).

Murmur Volumes and Maneuvers

Murmur "team" tip: Murmur sounds (louder or softer) make up 2 teams. These 2 teams **always stay together** on sounds.

- Team 1: **HCM and MVP**. Get louder with ↓ fluid in the heart and softer with more fluid in the heart.
  These murmurs must be treated with **β-blockers** so that it **allows more time for the heart to fill with more blood.**
- Team 2: **Mitral and Aortic Stenosis, Mitral and Aortic Regurgitation.** Get softer with less fluid in the heart and louder with ↑ fluid in the heart (more fluid = more murmur).

Murmurs and Inspiration and Expiration

- Inspiration: Murmurs on the right side of the heart (Tricuspid, Pulmonic) ↑ in intensity
- Expiration: Murmurs on the left side of the heart (Mitral, Aortic) ↑ in intensity

- **Maneuvers that ↑ afterload (causes murmur to become louder)**
  Increases the sound of: VSD, Aortic Regurgitation, Mitral Regurgitation
  - **Handgrip** (Worsens all regurg (MR, AR) murmurs because it pushes blood back into the heart. It softens Aortic Stenosis because the arterial pressure is increased so that it makes it difficult for the aortic valve to open for blood to leave = no murmur sound). It worsens a VSD because it forces more blood from the left ventricle back to the right ventricle.
  - Blood pressure cuff
- **Drug that ↓ afterload**
  - **Amyl Nitrate** (Vasodilator. Decreases pressure in the aorta = ↓ afterload)
  - **ACE or ARB's** (vasodilators)

- **Maneuvers that ↓ preload (reduces blood volume inside the heart)**
  Increases the sound of HCM and MVP
  - Valsalva Maneuver
  - Standing up

- **Maneuvers that ↑ preload (increases blood volume inside the heart)**
  Increases the sound of Mitral and Aortic Stenosis, Mitral and Aortic Regurgitation (Insufficiency)
  (**tip**: MORE volume = MORE murmur sound)
  - Lying down
  - Leg raise
  - Squatting (increases venous return to the heart)

Murmur	↑ Afterload	↓ Afterload	↑ preload – more fluid	↓ preload – less fluid	Treatment
HCM	↓ intensity	↑ intensity	↓ intensity	↑ intensity	β -Blocker
MVP	↓ intensity	↑ intensity	↓ intensity	↑ intensity	β -Blocker
VSD	↑ intensity	↓ intensity	↑ intensity	↓ intensity	
Aortic Stenosis	↓ intensity	↑ intensity	↑ intensity	↓ intensity	Ace, ARB, Amyl Nitrate
Mitral Stenosis	----	----	↑ intensity	↓ intensity	
Aortic Regurg	↑ intensity	↓ intensity	↑ intensity	↓ intensity	Ace, ARB, Amyl Nitrate
Mitral Regurg	↑ intensity	↓ intensity	↑ intensity	↓ intensity	Ace, ARB, Amyl Nitrate

S2 Splitting Murmur Pathologies

Fixed Split	Wide Split with P2 Delay	Paradoxical A2 Delay
ASD	RBBB, Pulmonary HTN, RVH, Pulmonic Stenosis	LBBB, HTN, LVH, Aortic Stenosis

Grading of Intensity of Murmur

Grade	Murmur Description
Grade 1	Just audible with a good stethoscope in a quiet room
Grade 2	Quiet, but readily audible with a stethoscope
Grade 3	Easily heard with a stethoscope
Grade 4	Loud, obvious murmur with a palpable thrill
Grade 5	Very loud, heard over the pericardium and elsewhere in the body
Grade 6	Head with stethoscope off chest

Heart Injury Time Line

Timeline	Heart Description	Cellular	Complications
0 -4 hours	No change in heart tissue	**No change**	
4 – 12 hours	Dark mottling	**Wavy** fibers, **coagulative necrosis**, edema, eosinophils, hemorrhage	
1 – 3 days	Dark mottling	**Neutrophil** migration, coagulation necrosis	
1 – 3 days	Hyperemia	3 days: **T cells and Macrophages**	**Fibrinous pericarditis. EKG shows diffuse ST elevations. Frictions rub on auscultation.** **TX: NSAIDS**
5 – 7 days	Yellow/brown	7 days: **Fibroblast.** **Granulation formation**	**Papillary muscle rupture (Chordae Tendineae): :** **Acute flash edema.** **Free Wall Rupture: Tamponade** **Ventricular aneurysm** **Interventricular septal rupture: Hear a new murmur: VSD**
10 days	Yellow/brown	Fibroblast collagen: **Granulation tissue**	
2 weeks to months	Grey-white	**Scar formation**	**Dressler's syndrome**: autoimmune inflammatory reaction to myocardial neo-antigens as a result of the MI. TX: **Colchicine**

Lines of Zahn

Thrombi formed in the heart or aorta that have alternating lighter layers with fibrin and platelets with darker layers of RBC's. These indicate that the damage occurred before death. If the thrombi are a gel like consistency, the clot formed after death.

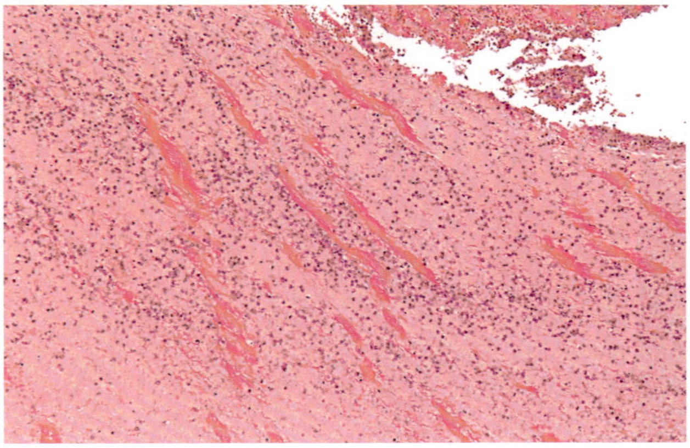

Shock

- Occurs anytime the bodies cells do not receive the oxygen and nutrients needed to function.
- SX: Triad: Severe hypotension, tachycardia, fever, altered mental status/confusion, ↑ LFT (ALT and AST), SOB, ↑ BUN/creatinine ratio, increased lactic acid, chest pain

SIRS Criteria (Systemic Inflammatory Response Syndrome): As of February 2016, SIRS criteria are no longer recommended for the diagnosis of sepsis.

***VO2:** Venous O2 drops because much of the oxygen has been downloaded and there is an increase in metabolites (waste) products.

Type of Shock	HR	CO	VO2	TPR SVR (Afterload)	EDV/P	PWCP LVEDP	Right Preload (CVP)	Cardiac Index =pump function	TX
Hypovolemic Shock Circulation is working but ↓ volume (hemorrhage). SX: Flat neck veins, **cool extremities**, **cold, clammy skin.** oliguria. Body releasing CATS, ATII, ADH to get fluid up. MCC: Massive hemorrhage, burns, dehydration.	↑ Tachy Is first visible sign of low BP	↓	↓	↑	↓	↓	↓↓	↓	Fluids and Pressors
Cardiogenic Shock Always has ↑ PWCP b/c ↑ left atrial pressure. SX: JVD, Pulmonary edema, pale, cold clammy skin. MCC: Myocardial infarction, valve dysfunction, arrhythmia, heart failure.	↑	↓	↓↓	↑	↑	↑	↑	↓↓	Treat heart problem with inotropes and diuresis.
Septic Shock (aka: Distributive shock) ↓ PWCP b/c no adequate filling of ventricles so ↓ EDV. **Warm and dry extremities**, faint pulses due to massive vasodilation. Gm negatives release **nitric oxide** and activate compliment. MCC: E. coli, S. aureus	↑	↑	NL, No use of O2	↓↓ **Vaso-dilation**, Pooling of blood, Hyper-dynamic flow so not enough time to extract O2	↓ No adequate filling of ventricles .	No change	↓	NL to slightly low. Heart pump is ok.	Fluids, Pressors, Anti-biotics ↑ **Body Temp.**

Type of Shock	HR	CO	VO2	TPR SVR (Afterload)	EDV/P	PWCP LVEDP	Right Preload (CVP)	Cardiac Index (pump function)	TX
EARLY Septic Shock	↑	↑		↓		↓			Hypo-tension, **↓ Body Temp.**
Neurogenic Shock Heart slows from unopposed vagal tone, loss of sympathetics and loss of ANS , causing vasodilation and ↓↓ blood pressure. (Brain or spinal injury). SX: Hyperreflexia, upgoing toes, warm skin. MCC: **CNS/Spinal cord** injury: cervical or thoracic.	↑	↓		↓↓		↓	↓	↓	Fluids and Pressors
Anaphylactic Shock. ↑ parasympathetic & ↓ sympathetic working In heart		↑	↓	↓		↓			
Pulmonary Embolism Have ↑ Right atrial & pulmonary pressure b/c ↑ preload.		↓		↑		NL			
Obstructive – Tamponade. All pressures are up. Aortic dissection, Tamponade. Skin is cold and clammy. Tamponade: Right ventricle collapse and impaired filling (↓ preload to left ventricle).		↓	↓↓	↑	↑	↑	↑	↓↓	Treat under-lying condition

Syncopes

Syncope (Fainting, passing out, swooning)	Description	Diagnosis/TX
Vasovagal	Fainting **proceeded** by dizziness, nausea. Caused by an identifying trigger: **emotional reaction**, uncomfortable situations, high stress or **prolonged standing**	Tilt table test
Orthostatic Syncope (AKA: Postural hypotension)	Due to a **change in body position**. BP **↓** and **↓** HR when standing up. Standing up, elderly urinating due to slow response of baroreceptors due to aging.	Can also be caused by diuretics, nitrates, alpha-blockers. "First dose hypotension"
Cardiac: Arrhythmias	Sudden, without warning. Due to structural or obstructive heart issues, MR, AV blocks, Thiazine (due to electrolyte disturbance), pulmonary embolisms. **Most common: Aortic Stenosis (elderly = calcified valve).**	**Implantable defibrillator**
Breath holding spells	Kids 6 – 18 months.	**Normal.** **No treatment – reassure**
Multi focal atrial tachycardia (MAT)	COPD	Do not give Beta Blockers, Give Calcium Channel Blockers
Deglutition (swallowing) syncope	Loss of consciousness on swallowing. Associated with ingestion of solid food, carbonated and ice-cold beverages, belching	
Sick sinus syndrome	Sinus node dysfunction. Alternating of brachycardia and tachycardia.	
Neurologic syncope	Caused by seizures, strokes, TIA's, migraines, normal pressure hydrocephalus	
Brainstem Stroke syncope	Caused by stoke of the brainstem circulation: vertebral or basilar.	

Syncope Criteria

- Most critical step: rule out cardiac causes.
- Sudden loss of consciousness
    - Neurologic: seizures
    - Cardiac origin
- Gradual loss of consciousness
    - Hypoxia
    - Hypoglycemia
    - Drug toxicity
    - Anemia
    - Toxic-metabolic problems
- Sudden regaining of consciousness
    - Cardiac origin
- Gradual regaining consciousness
    - Neurologic: seizures

Hypertension

- Defined as > 140 mmHg systolic pressure and > 90 mm Hg diastolic pressure. 140/90 mmHg.
  140/90 mmHg is the goal for diabetics.
  150/90 mmHg is the goal for patients > 60 years old.
- 90% causes of HTN are **"essential"** (no clear etiology).

- **2nd MCC of HTN** is **renal artery stenosis**
  DX: caused by **Fibromuscular dysplasia** (will usually be in young patients).
  SX: **Abdominal "bruit"**. Is heard throughout systole and diastole at the costovertebral angle.
  DX: Renal artery angiography shows **"string of pearls"** appearance, which is due to the alternating stenosis and arterial dilation.

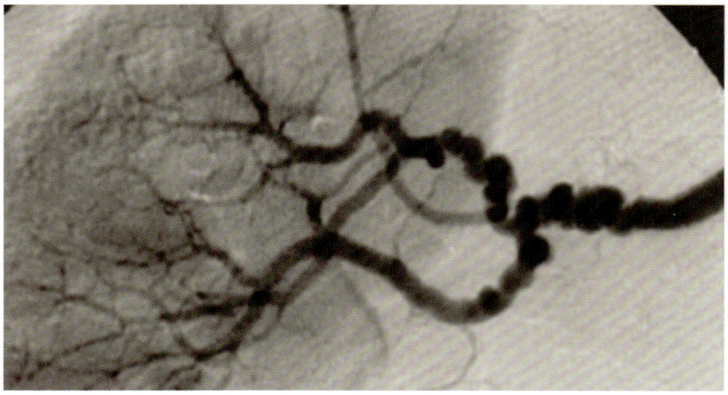

Fibromuscular dysplasia

- **Other causes of HTN**
  Nephritic DZ
  Stenosed renal artery (On just one side or both. So if one kidney is removed and the other kidney has a stenosed renal artery, the patient will still have HTN). **NOTE:** Don't forget, **anything** that causes the blood flow to the kidney to be reduced (whether due to a stenosed renal artery, dehydration, low blood pressure, decreased cardiac output (aka: low blood pressure), diuretics (hypovolemic), hemorrhage (hypovolemic) will cause the renin system to be activated.
  Pheochromocytoma: **Episodic** (AKA: Comes and goes, has been in the ED "before", wax and wane)
  Hyperaldosteronism: ↓ K (hypokalemia)= weakness
  Cushing's
  Coarctation of the aorta: Upper extremity pressure > lower extremity blood pressure
  Acromegaly
  Obstructive sleep apnea
  Acromegaly
  OCP's (can increase BP but **do not cause weight gain)**
  1° Hyperthyroidism
  Congenital adrenal hyperplasia
- Normal aging due to hardened, **non-compliant vessels.**
  Isolated HTN: MCC: Aortic stenosis and ↓ elasticity of arterial walls (wide pulse pressure) in the elderly
- Poorly controlled HTN can lead to an MI, stroke, aortic dissection, CHF, LVH, renal failure, retinopathy
- All cases of HTN must be repeated on 2 separate occasions, 1 week apart

Hypertension Treatment Protocol

- **Lifestyle changes for 3 to 6 months before initiating medications (unless BP is really high> 160/100)**
- **#1 most effective**: **Weight loss (↓ Calories)**
  For every Kg (2.5 lbs) lost = 1 mm Hg reduced
- Exercise (Improves HDL). Do aerobic physical activity three or four 40-minute sessions of moderate to vigorous activity per week. Caution: The most effective way to decrease HTN is to lose weight. If the vignette gives you both answers: weight loss and exercise in the answer choices, you must choose weight loss. Just because you exercise does not mean you lose weight. If exercise is in the answer choice and not weight loss, then choose exercise.
- Dietary modifications: DASH diet (Dietary Approaches to Stop Hypertension) (more fish, chicken, vegetables, fruits, whole grains, low-fat dairy, legumes, nontropical vegetable oils and nuts) (limit fat, red meat, sweets, sugar sweetened beverages)
- Sodium restriction to no more than 2400 mg of sodium per day. < 1500 mg per day = greater reduction in BP.
- Reduce alcohol intake
- Stop smoking helps reduce cardiovascular disease and cancer, but little effect on lowering HTN
- **Pharmacology therapy if lifestyle changes do not succeed.**
  - **If patient is over 60 years old and > 150/90 BP. (Goal is 150/90)**
  - **If patient is a diabetic or has Chronic Kidney Dz (CKD) and > 140/90 BP. (Goal is 140/90)**
- **Pharmacology therapy**
  - **Initial laboratory evaluation of HTN prior to medications: 12 lead EKG, Blood glucose level, Fasting cholesterol panel, Glomerular filtration rate, Hct level, Serum calcium level, Serum potassium level, urinalysis.**
  - **General non-African American population with/without diabetes: Initial treatment would be with one drug: Hydrochlorothiazide diuretic (HCTZ), ACE inhibitor, ARB or Calcium Channel Blocker (CCB)**
  - **General African Americans with/without diabetes: Initial treatment would be with one drug: Calcium Channel Blocker or Hydrochlorothiazide diuretic (HCTZ).**
  - **For pregnant patients: safe HTN medications: β Blockers (first line), Hydralazine, Calcium Channel Blocker, Methyldopa.**
  - **For patients with CKD initial treatment should be with an ACE Inhibitor or ARB to improve kidney outcomes.**
  - **If BP goal is not reached within one month of initiating treatment either increase the dose of the initial drug or add a second drug from the initial group of drug choices.**
  - **If BP can't be reached with two drugs, add and titrate a third drug from the initial group of drug choices.**
  - **Regularly monitor BP to evaluate needed changes in therapy.**
  - **If the patient has comorbidities, pharmacology treatment must take this into account and treat with the most appropriate drug.**

Pharmacology for HTN and HTN with Comorbidities

Comorbidity or Caution	HTN Pharmacology
Pregnancy	β Blockers (1st line), Hydralazine, CCB, Methyldopa
Black patients	CCB (Amlodipine), Thiazide diuretic (HCTZ)
Patients with CKD	ACE Inhibitor or ARB
Nonblack patients > 60 years old	ACE Inhibitor, ARB, Thiazide diuretic (HCTZ), CCB
Nonblack patients < 60 years old	ACE Inhibitor, ARB, do not give β Blockers
Nonblack patiens >75 years old with impaired kidney function	Thiazide diuretics (HCTZ), CCB
Depression	Do not give β Blockers
BPH	Alpha blockers
Nonblack Diabetics	ACE inhibitor or ARB (with good renal function)
Black Diabetics	Thiazide diuretic (HCTZ), CCB
Coronary artery disease	β Blockers, ACE inhibitor, ARB
Asthma, COPD or other respiratory problems	Do not give β Blockers
Hyperthyroidism	β Blockers
Osteoporosis	Thiazide diuretic (HCTZ)
Chronic Kidney Dz (CKD)	ACE Inhibitors, ARB
Post MI	β Blockers, ACE Inhibitor
Angina	β Blockers
Cerebrovascular disease	Thiazide diuretic (HCTZ), β Blockers, CCB
Atherosclerosis	ACE Inhibitor
Heart Failure	Thiazide diuretic (HCTZ), ACE Inhibitor, ARB, Spironolactone
CHF	ACE Inhibitor
HTN resistant to other medications	Alpha agonist (Clonidine)
History of Stroke	ACE Inhibitor, ARB
Migraine	β Blockers, CCB

Contradictions with HTN Pharmacology

HTN Medication	Contradictions
Thiazide diuretic (HCTZ)	Gout, hypokalemia, hypercalcemia
ACE Inhibitors, ARB's	Pregnancy, bilateral renal artery stenosis, hypovolemia, older patients, patients with impaired kidney function (increased risk of hyperkalemia, increased creatinine).
Hydralazine	Coronary artery disease
ACE Inhibitors and ARB's	Do not use these two medications simultaneously

Hypertension	Systolic Pressure (mm Hg)	Diastolic Pressure (mm Hg)
Normal	< 120	< 80
Pre-hypertension	120 – 139	80 – 89
Hypertension, Stage 1	140 – 159	90 – 99
Hypertension, Stage 2	≥ 160	≥ 100
Hypertensive Urgency	≥180	≥ 110
Hypertensive Emergency	≥ 200	≥ 120

Malignant Hypertension (AKA: Hypertensive emergency)

- Extremely high BP (>200/120)
- **Papilledema in the eyes must be present before considered malignant (end organ damage)**
- Mental status changes (end organ damage)
- Patient usually present to the ED
- **Vessels show "onion skinning"**
- TX: #1 = IV Labetalol, #2 = IV Nitroprusside
  Must **SLOWLY** reduce blood pressure over 24 – 48 hrs in HTN emergency.

  Nitroprusside side effect: Toxic = Cyanide poisoning.
    - **TX for cyanide poisoning**:
      Cyanide poisoning is a side effect of nitroprusside and nitric oxide.
    - **Hydroxocobalamin** combines with cyanide to form cyanocobalamin (Vitamin B-12), which is excreted.
    - **Sodium nitrate** induces methemoglobin in RBC's, which combines with the cyanide. Methemoglobinemia is then treated with Methylene Blue.
      Methylene blue inhibits Monoamine Oxidase. This changes the iron form Ferric (F^3 iron form) to Ferrous (F^4 iron form). Vitamin C can also assist in treating methemoglobinemia.
    - **Sodium thiosulfate** transforms cyanide (donates a sulfur atom) to thiocyanate by rhodanese, which is then excreted.

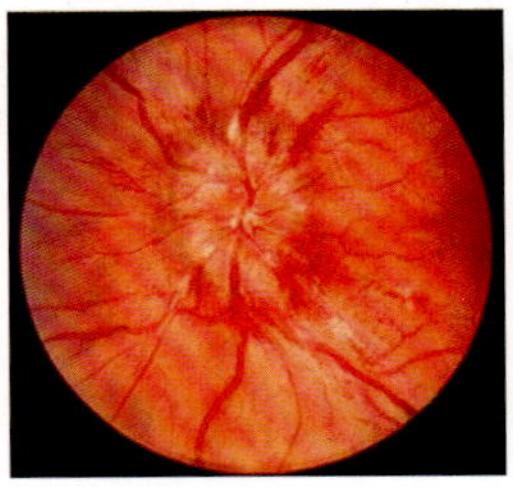

Papilledema

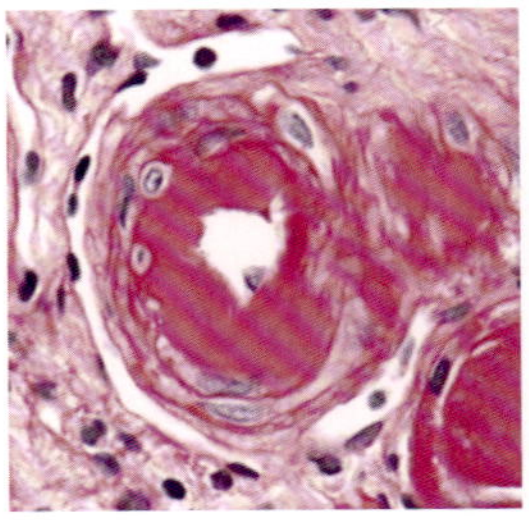

Onion skinning

Hypertensive Urgency (tip: It is **urgent** that you start getting the HTN under control)

- High BP (≥ 180 /110)
- Patient usually presents to your office. Patient not usually concerned or possibly even aware

Atherosclerosis (AKA: Arteriosclerotic vascular disease)

- **Initial cause: damage to the endothelial wall which exposes collagen (intimal layer)**
- Disease in which an artery wall thickens as a result of accumulation of WBC's (AKA: Fatty Streaks)
- **Fatty streaks**: Contains: Living WBC's, dead cells, cholesterol, triglycerides, and calcium.
  Fatty streaks are the beginning of the build up and are **normally found in children**.
- Fatty streaks reduce elasticity of artery walls (**takes years of build up** before affects blood flow)
- As atherosclerosis grows it forces the vessel to thicken and enlarge
- Rupture of **fibrous cap** of this fatty streak causes a thrombus which decrease or stop blood flow
- **If the Coronary arteries are affected = myocardial infarction**
- **If the arteries in the brain are affected = stroke**
- **If the arteries in the legs are affected = claudication**
- **THESE DZ are AKA's: DM (Diabetes) = CAD (Coronary Artery DZ) = PAD (Peripheral Artery DZ)**

Risk Factors: Modifiable

- Diabetes
- Smoking
- HTN
- Hyperlipidemia
- Hypothyroidism
- Dyslipoproteinemia (cholesterol, LDL)
- B6 deficiency

Risk Factors: Non-modifiable

- Advanced age
- Sex
  MI's are higher in men. Women become the same risk as men for MI's post menopausal (estrogen is heart protective)
- Genetics (family history)

Pathology of Atherosclerosis

- **Initial Cause: Endothelial cell/wall damage which exposes collagen = platelet aggregation = LDL = macrophages = fatty streak = fibrous cap**
- **Intimal Plaques/streaks**
- **Endothelial cells release PDGF = intimal hyperplasia and fibrosis by smooth muscle cells that migrate from media to intima.**
- Macrophages and LDL accumulate at the site of damage to for a foam cell
- Foam cells becomes a fatty streak
- Fibrous plaque and fibrous cap

MC Vessel Locations for Atherosclerosis Build Up

- Abdominal aorta > coronary artery > popliteal artery > carotid artery

Signs and Symptoms

Angina = Stable or Unstable

- **Cardiac: Stable angina:**
  When your heart **increases its work load** (ie: exercise) it demands more oxygen. When you increase work load on the heart the heart pumps faster and harder in order to bring in the additional oxygen requirement. If a plaque is located in the coronaries it will partially block the path of the blood delivering the oxygen to the heart. So your heart will "cry" (hurt) to tell you that it is not getting enough oxygen. Once you stop the added workload on the heart and resume a slower pace/rest, the pain goes away because the heart is now getting enough oxygen so has quit "crying".
  This is shown as **ST DEPRESSION on EKG. Meaning ≥ 70% blockage**. **Indicates ischemia = stress test.**
- **Cardiac Unstable angina:**
  When the fibrous cap of an atherosclerotic plaque ruptures the plaque moves, blocking the coronary artery. In this case oxygen delivery is compromised, causing pain at rest. This is unstable angina.
  This is shown as **ST ELEVATION on EKG: Meaning ≥ 90% blockage = MI**
- **Xanthomas:** Sign of hyperlipidemia. **Lipids (cholesterol**) accumulate in **foam cells creating nodules on tendons Tendinous xanthoma)**, Achilles tendon and dorsum of the hands.
- **Xanthelasma:** Sign of hyperlipidemia. Collection of cholesterol on or around the eyelids.
- **Corneal arcus:** Lipid deposits in cornea.

Lipid Levels and Goals

REMEMBER these are EQUIVALENTS: CAD = DM = PAD = Carotid Disease = Aortic Disease

ie: If you have Diabetes, you are automatically considered to have Coronary Artery Disease

Patient	Cholesterol	LDL (Low density)	Triglycerides	HDL (High density)
Normal	< 200	< 100	< 150	40 - 60
Borderline	200 - 239	130 - 159	159 - 199	Low < 40
High	≥ 240	> 160	> 200 (Very high > 500)	High ≥ 60
Diabetic GOAL		**< 70**		
CAD GOAL		**< 100**		

Risk Factors for ↑ Lipids

- Age: Males ≥ 45, Females ≥ 55
- Low HDL < 40
- Smoking
- High blood pressure ≥ 140/90
- Family history of Coronary Heart Disease (female relatives < 65, male relatives < 55)

Therapy Assessment

- **LDL Risk Factors and equivalents to Coronary Heart Disease.**
- **CHD (Coronary Heart DZ), Symptomatic CAD, Peripheral Artery DZ (PAD), Abdominal Aortic Aneurysm, Diabetes.**
- **Risk Factors other than LDL: Smoking, HTN, Low HDL, Family Hx of Heart DZ, Heart DZ in men < 45 and in women < 55.**
- **If 2+ risk factors (other than LDL) without CHD or CHD risk equivalents, this shows your 10-year CHD risk.**

Risk Category	LDL GOAL	LDL Level at Which to Initiate Therapeutic Lifestyle Changes (TLC)	LDL Level at Which to Consider Lipid lowering Drug Therapy
CHD or CHD Risk equivalents (10 year risk > 20%)	< 100 mg/dL	≥ 100 mg/dL	≥ 130 mg/dL
2+ Risk Factors (10 year risk > 20%)	< 130 mg/dL	≥ 130 mg/dL	≥ 130 mg/dL if 10 year risk is 10 – 20% ≥ 160 mg/dL if 10 year risk is < 10%
0 – 1 Risk Factor Anyone with a 0 – 1 risk factor have a 10 year risk of < 10% so a 10 year risk assessment in people with a 0 – 1 risk factor is not necessary)	< 160 mg/dL	≥ 160 mg/dL	≥ 190 mg/dL (160 – 189 mg/dL, LDL lowering drug optional)

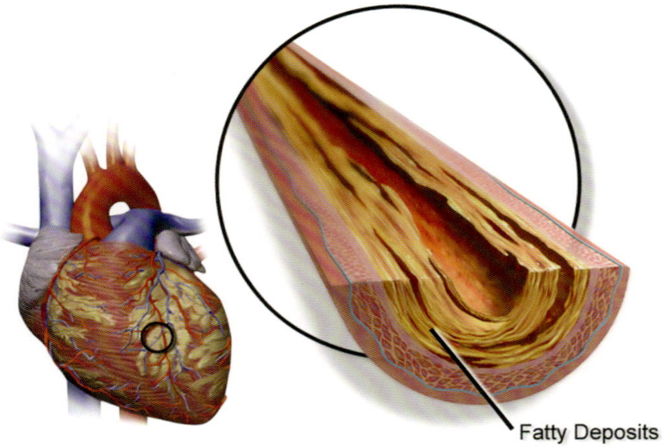

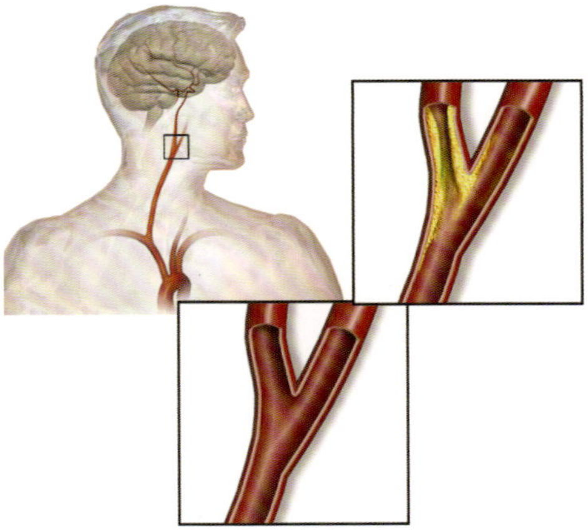

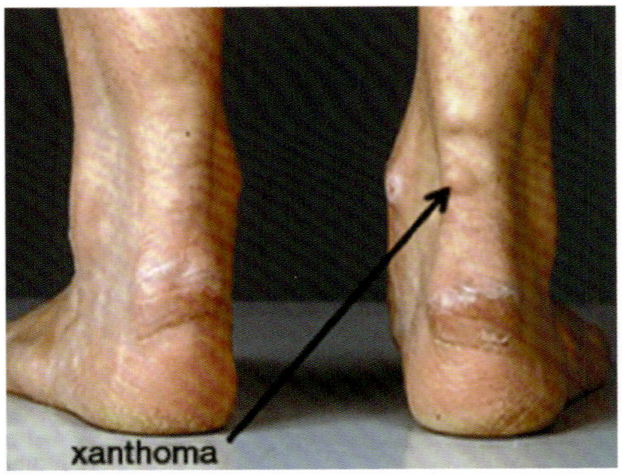

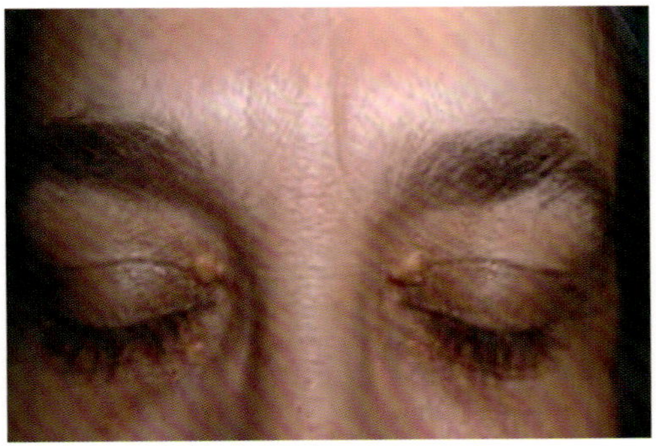

Xanthelasma

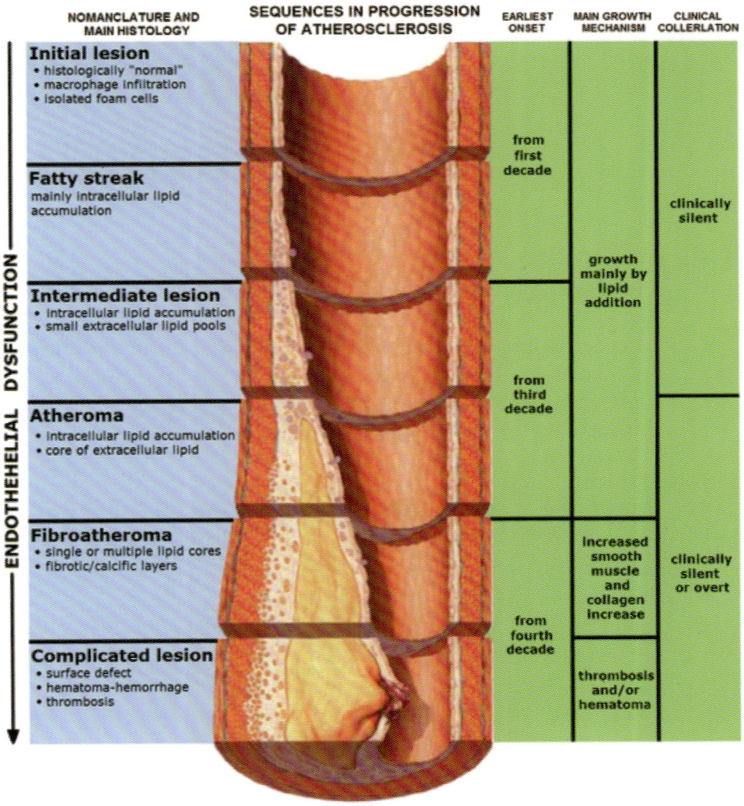

Aortic Aneurysms: Abdominal and Thoracic

- Dilation of the aorta

Complications (becomes painful in these situations)

- Leaking (could hear an abdominal bruit)
- Dissection
- Rupture (sudden hypotension)

Abdominal Aortic Aneurysm (AAA)

- **Associated with atherosclerosis**
- MC in hypertensive, male smokers > 50
- **Screening:** 1 ultrasound for any male > 60 if they have **EVER** smoked, even if they used to smoke but quit. Smoking degrades connective tissue in the walls of the artery
- TX: <5 cm in size: follow closely with yearly ultrasounds
  > 5 mm = surgical repair (stent)
  If it grows: > .5 cm in 6 months or > 1 cm in 1 year = surgical repair (stent)
- (**tip**: AAA = **A**therosclerosis. All A's)

Thoracic Aortic Aneurysm

- **Associated with HTN** which causes medial degeneration in older people
- Associated with Marfan's
- Associated with 3° Syphilis (AKA: obliterative endarteritis of the **vasa vasorum**)

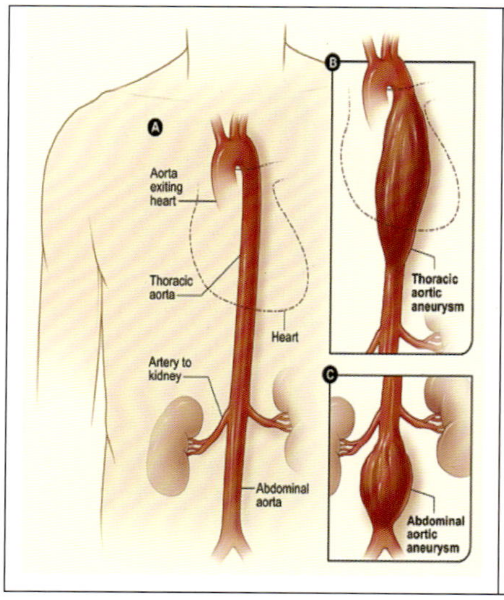

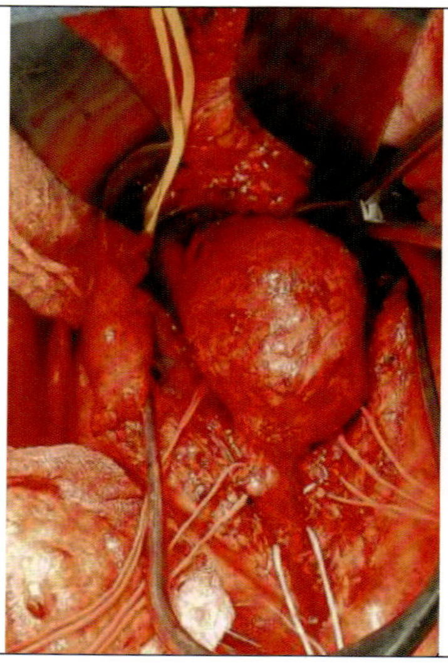

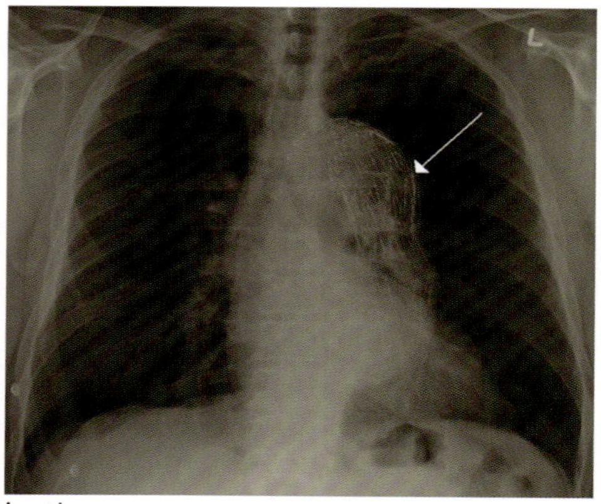

Aortic aneurysm

Aortic Dissection

- A **tear in the intimal layer** of the aorta (inner most layer) allows blood to flow between the layers of the aorta forcing the layers apart
- **3 Layers of aorta: outermost: adventitia, middle: media, innermost: intima**
- **Initial cause: "Intimal tear"**
  (Don't mix this up with initial cause of atherosclerosis. The **"initial cause" of atherosclerosis is endothelial damage, exposing collagen**, which leads to fatty streak, etc.).

Associated With

- **MCC: Blunt chest trauma in rapid deceleration (chest hits steering wheel) injuries and falls > 10 ft**
- **Chronic Hypertension**
- Thoracic aortic aneurysm
- Smoking
- Untreated tertiary syphilis
- Marfan's
- Ehlers-Danlos Syndrome
- Bicuspid aortic valve (congenital heart disease)
- Turners syndrome

Classifications

- Type A: Originates in the ascending aorta and extends to the aortic arch and on into the descending aorta (most dangerous). MC in younger patients
  TX: Emergency Surgery and medications
- Type B: Originates in the descending aorta. MC in elderly due to HTN and atherosclerosis
  TX: Medication (tip: Type B = Beta blockers)
- Meds for aortic dissection focus on decreasing blood pressure. DOC: Rapid acting beta-blockers: Propranolol, Labetalol, and Esmolol. Calcium channel blockers if Beta Blockers are contraindicated.

Complication

- Rupture

Diagnosis

- DX: TEE (trans-esophageal echocardiogram)
- BIT: CXR shows widened mediastinum
- MAT: CT Angiography

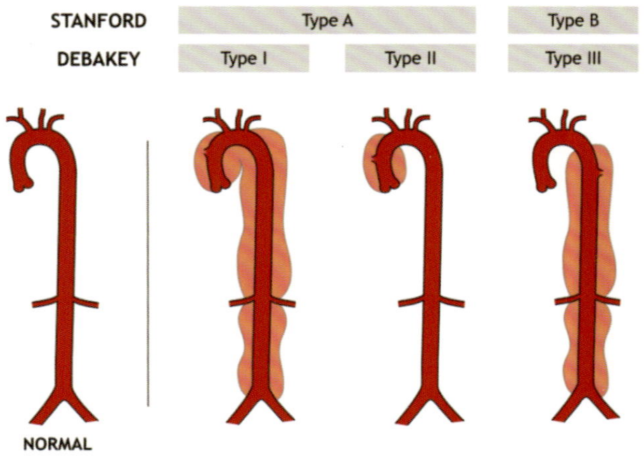

Symptoms

- Sudden onset of **severe, ripping pain to the back between the shoulder blades/scapula**
- Widening of the mediastinum or aortic arch on CXR
- Blood pressure is different between left and right arms
- Neck pain, intrascapular pain
- Decreased pulse in the upper extremities
- Shortness of breath

Treatment

- β-Blockers
- Nitroprusside (for HTN)
- Surgery
- Place in ICU

Complications

- Tamponade, aortic rupture, death

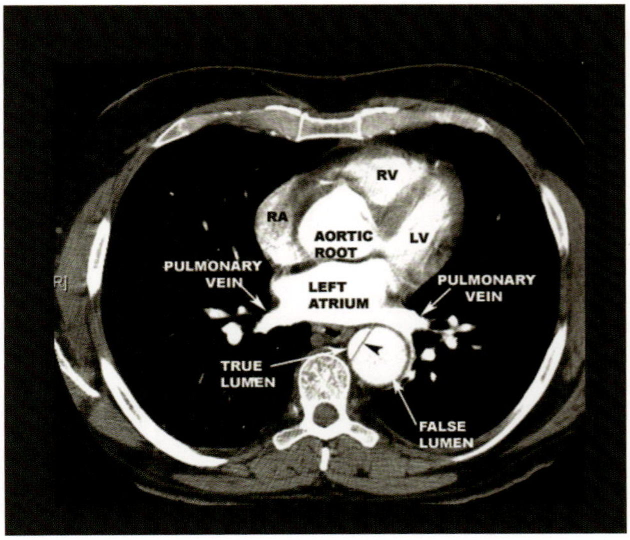

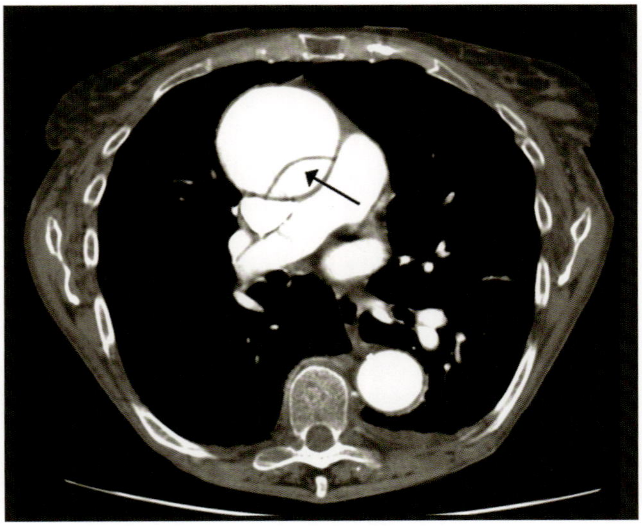

Coronary Artery Disease (CAD)

Coronary Artery Disease Risk Factors

- Hyperlipidemia (worst factor: high LDL. LDL is the most dangerous lipid)
- Diabetes (worst risk factor)
- Hypertension (most common risk factor)
- Smoking
- Family history of premature CAD (First degree: parents, siblings)
  Premature CAD: If first degree relative was male < 55, Female < 65
- Mens aged > 45 and Women aged > 55

Coronary Artery Disease Equivalents

- Diabetes
- Peripheral Artery Disease (PAD)
- Carotid Disease
- Aortic Disease
- Hypertension: Most common risk for CAD

Myocardial Infarctions (MI)

- "Heart attack", when blood flow stops to part of the heart causing damage to the heart muscle
- MI's = S4
- **1st Step: EKG**
- **Most common findings in a physical exam on an MI is a NORMAL PHYSICAL**
- ST Elevation MI (STIMI) or Non-ST Elevation (NSTEMI)
- **MI = Hypotension**

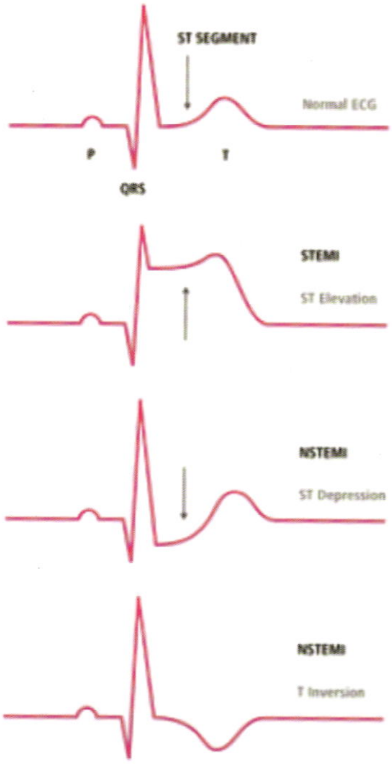

STEMI verses NSTEMI

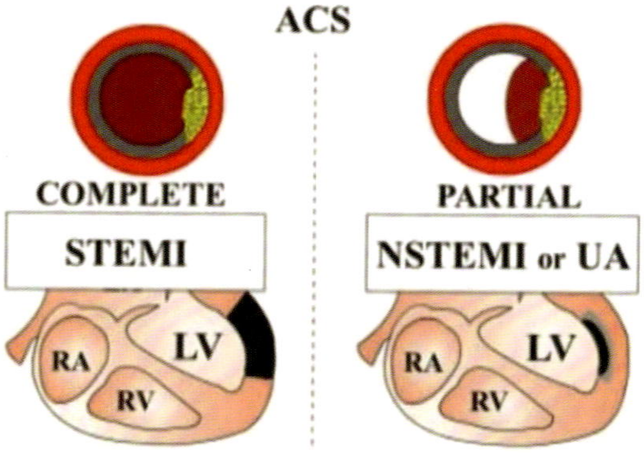

ST Elevation (STEMI)

- MI 90% blockage
- **Transmural = necrosis of entire thickness of myocardium**
- **BEST PROGNOSIS FOR ST ELEVATION: Amount of time that elapses until coronary blood flow is restored**
- **Unstable Angina** (Chest pain that does not improve with rest or new pain).
- **Cardiac enzymes are positive**
  Troponin (BEST marker) takes **4 -6 hours (peak: 12 hours)** to rise and the levels will remain high for up to **2 weeks**.
  CKMB levels rise can be detected between 3 – 6 hours (peak: 10 – 24 hours) and **return to normal in 48 – 72 hours, which** is why **this marker is used to detect a re-infarction.**
  LDH (Lactate Dehydrogenase) levels rise at 1 day and are gone in 3 days
  H-FABP (Heart-type fatty acid binding protein) cytoplasmic protein released from cardiac myocytes following an ischemic episode. Levels can be detected within 1 – 3 hours.
  GP-BB (Glycogen Phosphorylase Isoenzyme BB): levels rise between 1 -3 hrs.
  Myoglobin levels rise within 2 hours. (low specificity for MI, but is more rapid than troponin or CK-MB)
- **CKMB test are used to diagnosis a re-infarction**
- TPA's (AKA: Fibrinolysis, thrombolytics) must be given **within 30 minutes** upon presentation to the ED if PCI cannot be performed within 90 minutes.
- Cardiac Catheterization ("Cath Lab") shows which vessels are blocked **(AKA: Coronary Angiography).**
  Cardiac Catheterization is done through the femoral vein. (new routes, including the wrist, are now being used)

RESULTS and TREATMENTS of Cardiac Catheterization

- **#1 greatest efficacy in lowering mortality in a STEMI = Angioplasty (AKA: PCI)**
- **PCI must be done within 90 minutes of patient's arrival at the hospital**
- ≤ 2 vessels blocked = PCI **(Percutaneous Coronary Intervention)** AKA: **Coronary Angioplasty**, Balloon, Stent)
- 2 vessels blocked and patient is diabetic = CABG (Coronary Artery Bypass Graft) Diabetes = CAD.
- ≥ 3 vessels blocked = CABG
- Left (Main) Coronary Artery blocked (AKA: "widow maker") = CABG

MI Treatment (Acute Coronary Syndrome)

- **Best initial therapy: Aspirin to inhibit platelets**
- **Morphine**
- **Nitrates**
- **Oxygen**
- **Beta Blocker** (Metoprolol or Atenolol)*
  If the MI is due to COCAINE, do NOT use Beta Blockers, you MUST use Calcium Channel Blockers: Verapamil, Diltiazem
- **Clopidogrel or Ticagrelor** (anti-platelet) – ALWAYS added if a patient receives a stent and/or if patient is allergic to aspirin. **Prasugrel** can also be used and added to aspirin. Prasugrel has greater efficacy than Clopidogrel but can cause more bleeding in the elderly and those under 125 lbs. (**DO NOT** use Ticlopidine: associated with neutropenia)
- **Ace Inhibitor** (Helps prevent heart remodeling. Only lowers mortality in cases of left ventricular dysfunction or systolic dysfunction). Best when ejection fraction is < 40%.
- **Statin (Atorvastatin)** Use if the LDL of the patient is > 100, regardless of what an EKG or cardiac enzyme levels show. **LDL goal is < 100 and a goal of < 70 if the patient is a diabetic.**
  Additional risk factors for ↑LDL: Smoking, low HDL < 40, family history (if father was < 45 or mother < 55 when heart problems began), high blood pressure.
- **Spironolactone** (Aldosterone antagonist)
- **Glycoprotein IIb/IIIa Inhibitors (Abciximab, Eptifibatide, TIrofiban)**. Decrease risk of blood clot formation and are used when patient will be undergoing **PCI (stenting).** They decrease mortality in ST depression. **Used for Non-ST elevations**.
- **Thrombolytic Indications for Thrombolytics**: **Only used in ST elevation MI** ≥ 2 leads and chest pain or new Left Bundle Branch Block (LBBB)
- **Low Molecular Weight Heparin** Give after PCI and thrombolytics to prevent restenosis. Use in initial treatment with **ST depression (non-ST elevations)** and other **non-ST elevations** (ie: unstable angina). Heparin will prevent a clot from forming in the coronary arteries. LMWH is superior to unfractionated heparin.
- **Calcium Channel Blockers (Verapamil, Diltiazem) Used** when patient is unable to use a β-Blocker (ie: breathing issues: asthma, COPD), **COCAINE MI** (coronary vasospasms), Prinzmetal's angina, esophageal spasms, Raynaud's.
- **Amiodarone, Lidocaine** (**ONLY** used with there is V-Tach or V-Fib)
- **Pacemaker can be used as a treatment with an MI when there are: Heart Blocks, new Left Bundle Branch Blocks, and Symptomatic bradycardia.**
- **Lidocaine, Amiodarone (Cardio conversion): used for ventricular arrhythmias: ventricular tachycardia, ventricular fibrillation.**
- **Pacemaker:** Used in 2nd Degree Mobitz II Heart Block, 3rd Degree Heart Block, New left bundle branch block, Bifascicular block, symptomatic bradycardia.
- **CHF/Pulmonary edema/MI are always admitted to the ICU.**

Post MI Discharge Instructions

- **Drugs: Aspirin, ACE Inhibitor, β – Blockers, Clopidogrel (or Prasugrel), Statin**
  (Don't forget that ACE and ARB's keep Potassium = hyperkalemia)
- **May resume sexual relations in 2 - 6 weeks.** MCC erectile dysfunction is **anxiety** after an MI. Resuming sex after an MI is a common psychological concern due to the fact that patients are afraid it will cause another MI. Sex presents a very low risk of a recurrent MI. TX: **Sildenafil.**
  CAUTION: The patient will be on nitrates due to the MI. They must stop the nitrates (be at least 4 hours) prior to using the Sildenafil to avoid potentially fatal hypotension.

Treatments that **LOWER MORTALITY** in Acute Coronary Syndrome

- **Aspirin**
- **Thrombolytics** (if PCI can't be performed within 90 minutes). Thrombolytics must be given in within a few hours of onset of chest pain. **MOA: Thrombolytics** (tPA: Tissue plasminogen activator) activate plasminogen into plasmin. Plasmin breaks up the fibrin and platelet "mesh" into D-dimers. Within a few hours, Factor XIII stabilizes the fibrin/platelet mesh and plasmin can no longer break it down.
  - **Thrombolytics: Indications for Thrombolytics**: Only used in ST elevation ≥ 2 leads and chest pain or new Left Bundle Branch Block (LBBB)
  - **Thrombolytics** can only be used as long as there are **no contraindications**: past hemorrhagic stroke, non-hemorrhagic stroke < 6 months, brain bleeds, HTN > 180/110, recent surgery < 2 wks, bleeding ulcer, bleeding in the bowel, blood thinners, head trauma: anything that could increase the risk of bleeding.
  - **Thrombolytics must be given within 30 minutes of arrival in the ER.**

- **Angioplasty** (AKA: Percutaneous Coronary Intervention (PCI), Stent). MUST BE PERFORMED **WITHIN 90 MINUTES** of ARRIVAL AT THE ED.
  If PCI can NOT be performed within 90 minutes of arrival, thrombolytics must be given. This is common if the patient is in a small hospital not equipped with the ability for PCI.
- **Beta Blockers**: Are anti-arrhythmic and anti-ischemic. They slow the heart rate allowing for more time for **the coronary arteries to fill in diastole and more time for the left ventricle to fill, providing for more perfusion and increased cardiac output and stroke volume.**
- **Ace/ARB's Inhibitor:** Helps prevent heart remodeling. Only lowers mortality in cases of left ventricular dysfunction or systolic dysfunction). **Decreases afterload**.
- **Statin's (Atorvastatin)** (Used if patient is not within the appropriate LDL goal and used in ALL patients with ACS, regardless of what EKG or cardiac enzyme levels show).
- **Clopidogrel, Ticagrelor, Prasugrel:** Inhibits platelet aggregation.

DRUGS and TREAMENTS that DO NOT Decrease Mortality in STEMI's

- Nitrates
- Morphine
- Oxygen
- Lidocaine
- Calcium Channel Blockers
- Amiodarone

Non-ST Elevation (NSTEMI)

- **Stable angina**
- **ST depression**
- **Ischemia 70% blockage**
- **Ischemia is reversible, Infarction is irreversible**
- **Cardiac Enzymes are negative**
- **NO Thrombolytics** (AKA: TPA's) are given. TPA's are only for STEMI or new left bundle branch blocks within 12 hours of onset of chest pain/pressure.
- **Low molecular weight Heparin (LMWH)**
- **Glycoprotein IIb/IIIa Inhibitors (Abciximab, Eptifibatide, TIrofiban)**. Decrease risk of blood clot formation.
- **Stress test (Heart rate must reach 85% of maximum. Maximum HR = 220 minus the age of the patient)**
  - **Physical stress test**: Treadmill. Target heart rate is 85% of maximum heart rate so **you must be alert as to whether or not patient is able to run on a treadmill. Watch for older patients, patients with foot sores/ulcers/amputations, respiratory issues (COPD, asthma), patients with knee problems, obese patients (BMI > 30), out of shape, dementia – they will need a chemical stress test**
  - **Chemical stress test:** (**Dobutamine, Dipyridamole, Adenosine Thallium**)
    MOA: Thallium (nuclear isotope) looks like potassium to the heart. So healthy heart tissue will use (uptake) the thallium. So if there is a decrease in uptake it means that particular area of the heart is an unhealthy/damaged/under perfused area. Dobutamine, Dipyridamole (do not use in asthmatics, can cause bronchospasms): causes an ionotropic effect on the heart causing it to work harder, increasing oxygen demand. Echocardiogram will show areas of ischemia (damage or low blood flow).
  - **Echocardiography test:** Used with there is difficulty reading the EKG or other heart issues: Pacemaker, Left Bundle Branch Block, Left ventricular hypertrophy.

- **Based on the results of the stress test it may require coronary angiography to evaluate extent of blockage and number of vessels involved.**
- **Non-ST Elevations that still have symptoms and do not better after treatments must undergo angiography and possible PCI. Symptoms: Increasing cardiac enzyme levels (Troponin), continued angina, develop S3 gallop, develop CHF, EKG changes or sustained ventricular tachycardia. (If there is a sustained ventricular tachycardia it means that there is decreased oxygen being supplies so stenting is critical).**

Discharge Treatment for Stable Angina

- Aspirin (lowers mortality)
- β-Blocker (Metoprolol) (lowers mortality)
- Nitrates (pain)
- ACE or ARB to ↓ preload (vasodilate and ↓ afterload) in cases with ↓ ejection fraction

MI and EKG Readings – ST Elevations will be in specific leads, not diffuse

Area of Infarct	Coronary Artery	Leads – ST Elevations
Inferior wall (AKA: **Diaphragmatic surface, Inferior lateral)**	RCA (80%), LCX (20%)	II, III, aVF
Lateral wall	LCX	I, aVL, V5, V6
Anterior wall	LAD	V1 – V6
Anteroseptal wall	LAD	V1 – V4
Anterolateral	LAD or LCX	V4 – V6
Right Ventricle	RCA	V1 – V4
Atrial	RCA	I, V5, V6
Posterior	RCA or LCX	V7 – V9

Leads

Limb Leads		Precordial Leads	
I Lateral Left Ventricle	aVR	V1 Septal	V4 Anterior
II Inferior portion of Left Ventricle	aVL Lateral Left Ventricle	V2 Arterio-Septal	V5 Lateral Left Ventricle
III Inferior portion of Left Ventricle	aVF Inferior portion of Left Ventricle	V3 Arterio-Septal	V6 Lateral Left Ventricle

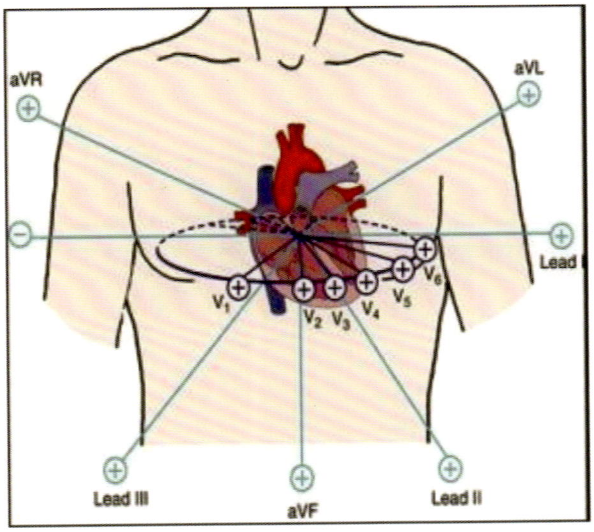

Pathologies Presenting With Diffuse ST Elevations (ST elevations in all leads)

Pericarditis
Prinzmetals Angina
Cocaine MI

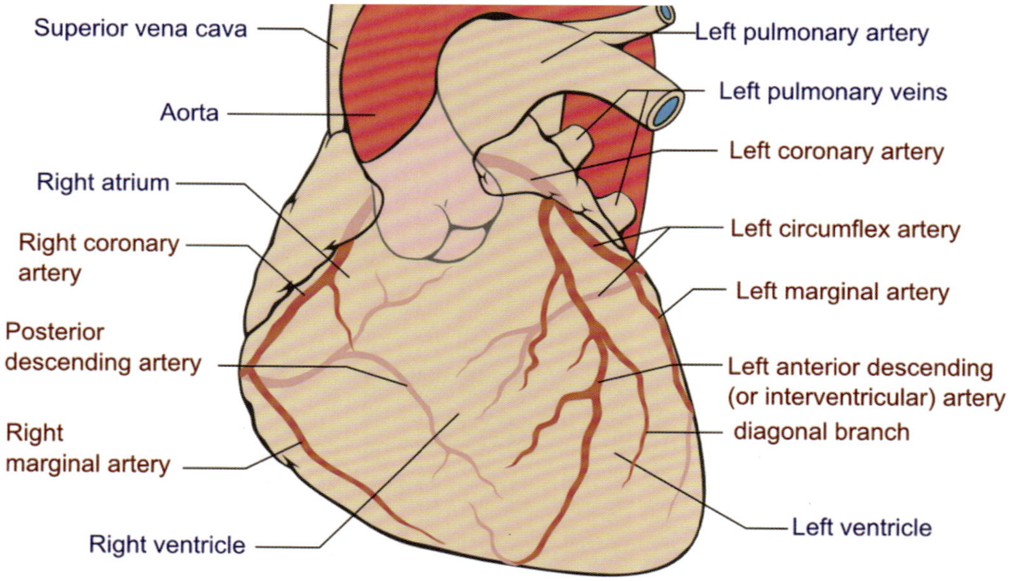

Superior vena cava
Aorta
Right atrium
Right coronary artery
Posterior descending artery
Right marginal artery
Right ventricle
Left pulmonary artery
Left pulmonary veins
Left coronary artery
Left circumflex artery
Left marginal artery
Left anterior descending (or interventricular) artery
diagonal branch
Left ventricle

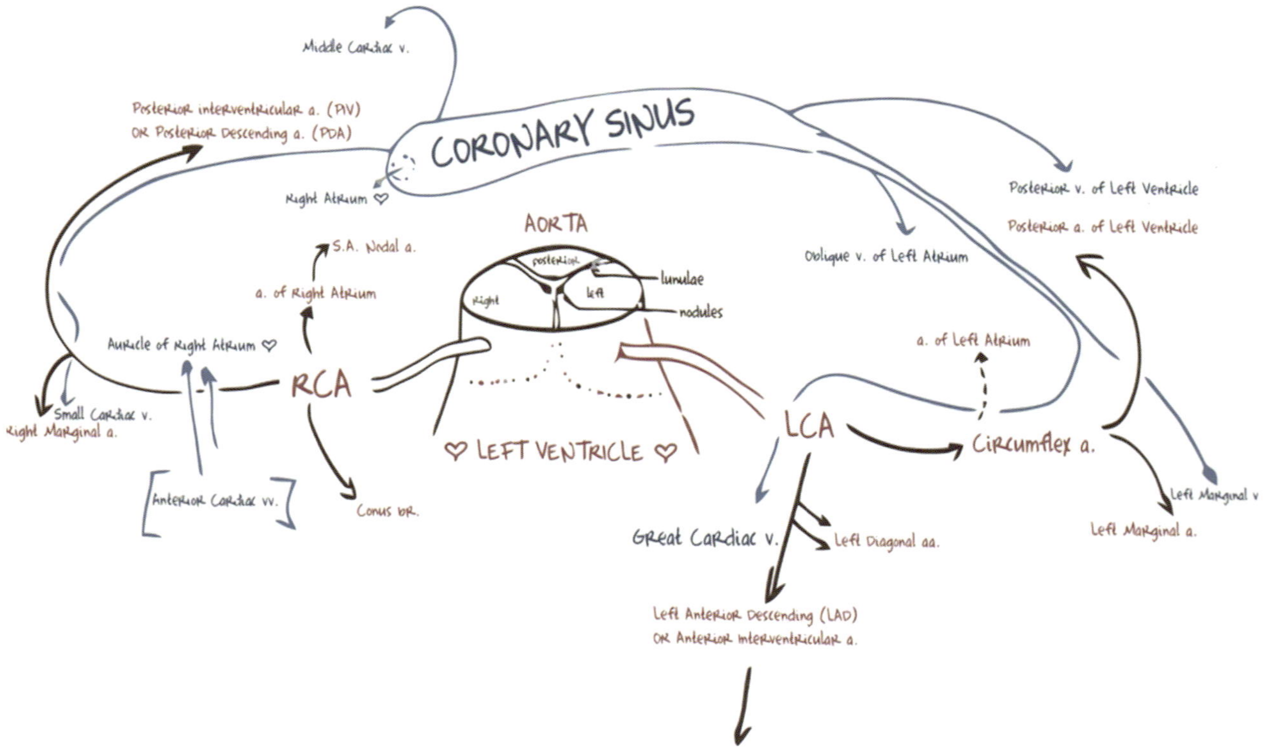

Middle Cardiac v.
Posterior interventricular a. (PIV)
OR Posterior Descending a. (PDA)
CORONARY SINUS
Right Atrium ♡
AORTA
posterior
right
left
lunulae
nodules
S.A. Nodal a.
a. of Right Atrium
Auricle of Right Atrium ♡
RCA
Small Cardiac v.
Right Marginal a.
Anterior Cardiac vv.
Conus br.
♡ LEFT VENTRICLE ♡
Posterior v. of Left Ventricle
Posterior a. of Left Ventricle
Oblique v. of Left Atrium
a. of Left Atrium
LCA
Circumflex a.
Left Marginal v
Left Marginal a.
Great Cardiac v.
Left Diagonal aa.
Left Anterior Descending (LAD)
OR Anterior Interventricular a.

Blood Supply of the Heart

Vessel	Heart Anatomy Supplied
Right Coronary Artery	Supplies: SA and AV nodes, Right atrium, Right Ventricle, Diaphragmatic surface (inferior) of the left ventricle and posterior surface of the interventricular septum. Supplies 15% of the blood to the myocardium.
Right Coronary Marginal	Supplies the right lateral wall of the left atrium and ventricle, Diaphragmatic surface (inferior).
Posterior Descending Artery (PAD)	Determines if the heart is right or left dominant, dependent upon which coronary supplies it (Left or Right Coronary). It is a branch most common off of the RCA (70% right dominant). If it is a branch off of the Circumflex Coronary Artery (CXA) it will be off of the LCA and be left dominant. **Note:** Meets the anterior interventricular artery (LAD) in the posterior interventricular sulcus. It supplies the posterior 1/3 of the **interventricular septum**. The remaining 2/3 of the interventricular septum is supplies by the anterior interventricular artery (branch of the LAD which is a branch of the Left Coronary artery).
Left Coronary Artery (AKA: Left Main, Widow Maker)	Branches into the Circumflex artery (LCX) and the Left anterior descending artery (LAD). Supplies left atrium posterior and anterior wall. Supplies 85% of the blood to the myocardium.
Left Circumflex Artery (LCX)	Comes off the Left Coronary Artery and supplies the left atrium, lateral and posterior wall of the left ventricle.
Left Anterior Descending (LAD)	Supplies the anterior and inferior wall of the left ventricle, the anterior surface of the interventricular septum, and the distal 1/3 of the posterior wall. LAD continues down to and around the apex and to the posterior side and anastomoses with the right coronary (Right Coronary Marginals) in the lower 1/3 posterior wall. **Artery travels in the Anterior Interventricular Sulcus.**

Right and Left Dominance of the Heart

- **The PDA (Posterior Descending Artery) determines the coronary dominance. Normally the PDA is a branch off of the Right Coronary Artery.**
- If the PDA is supplied by the RCA = Right-dominant (70%)
- **If the PDA is supplies by the LXA (Left Circumflex) = Left-dominant** (10%)
- If the PDA is supplied by both LXA and RCA = Co-dominant (20%)

Anastomoses of the Heart

- Branches of the LAD join the posterior interventricular branches of the RCA in the interventricular grove
- LXA (Left Circumflex) joins the RCA in the atrioventricular groove
- Between the septal braches of the RCA and LCA in the interventricular septum

Left Heart Failure vs Right Heart Failure

Left Heart Failure	Right Heart Failure
↑ Fluid (due to **hydrostatic pressure**) in the lungs (due to back up from failure of left side of heart). Bilateral crackles upon auscultation. ↑ **PWCP** due to backed up pressure. TX: Fluids, Na restriction (↓ BP), **Furosemide**	**No fluid in the lungs (no crackles).** ↓ **PWCP** (this has no affect on the left side of the heart/no backup from the left side of the heart). ↑ JVD, ↑ CVP (right atrial pressure due to back up) TX: Heavy fluids to maintain preload.

EKG and Myocardial Infarction Locations

MI	ST Elevation	Reciprocal ST Depression	Coronary Artery	Notes
Anterior MI	V2 – V4	None	LAD	Poor R wave progression. ST segment elevation. T wave inversion.
Septal MI	V1-V2	None	LAD	R wave disappears. ST segment elevation. T wave inversion.
Lateral Wall MI	**I, aVL, V5 – V6**	II, III, aVF (Inferior leads)	LCX	ST segment elevation.
Inferior MI	**II, III, aVF**	I, aVL (Lateral leads)	RCA (right side dominant 80%). LCX (left side dominant 20%)	Watch for bradycardia and heart blocks. T wave inversion. ST segment elevation.
Posterior MI	V1 – V4	Right R in V1 – V3 with ST depression in 1 – V3 > 2mm	RCA or LCX	Tall R and T waves in V1 – V2. ST depression in V1 – V3.
Right Ventricle MI	V1 – V4	I, aVL	RCA	**In right side MI's it is critical to give ↑↑ fluids to keep preload.**
Atrial MI	PTa in I, V5, V6	PTa in I, II or III	RCA	
Anterolateral	I, aVL, V2– V6		LCX, LAD	
Anteroseptal	I, aVL, V1 – V2		LAD	

Cocaine MI

- Vasospasms (Similar to Prinzmetals and Reynaud's)
- **Diffuse ST Elevations**
- SX: Dilated pupils, chest pain, ↑ coronary vasoconstriction, agitation, seizures, tachycardia, HTN
- Increased oxygen demand on the heart
- Pro-thrombotic state
- **DO NOT give Beta Blockers, MUST give Calcium Channel Blockers**
- TX: **Calcium Channel Blockers: Diazepam, Verapamil**
- For anxiety: **Lorazepam**

Post MI Cardiac Complications

- **Remember: the best prognosis for an MI is "Time blood flow is restored to the coronaries".**

Complication	Timeline	Signs	Artery	Notes
Right Ventricular MI (AKA: Acute Right Ventricle failure)		Hypokinetic right ventricle, Hypotension		DX: ECHO, Swan-Ganz. **TX: Must keep ↑ ↑ fluids (↑ Preload)**
V – Fib				**Most common cause of death BEFORE arrival at ED. Prognosis: TIME to DEFIBRILATION**
Fibrous Pericarditis	1 – 3 days post MI	**Friction Rub, Diffuse ST Elevations**, Relief if sitting forward.		TX: **NSAIDS**
Papillary Rupture (Chordae Tendineae) (Valve Rupture)	1 – 3 days post MI	**Flash pulmonary edema**, New murmur: MR due to "flail leaflet". Bi-basilar crackles		DX: ECHO (↑ in Oxygen saturation in right atrium as compared to right ventricle). TX: ACE Inhibitor, Nitroprusside, Balloon pump until surgery.
Ventricular aneurysm	1 week	Embolus from mural thrombus		
Free Wall Rupture	3 – 5 days	JVD, Chest pain, **tamponade,** shock, emboli, pericardial effusion		DX: ECHO. TX: Pericardiocentesis, surgery,
Interseptum Rupture	3 – 5 days	Left to right shunt, **new murmur VSD.** Higher pressure in the left ventricle causes a left to right shunt, so the oxygen saturation will be higher in the right ventricle than in the right atrium.	LAD/RCA	DX: ECHO. TX: ACE Inhibitor, Nitroprusside, surgery
Dressler syndrome	2 – 6 weeks	**Autoimmune reaction against antigens from MI**		TX: Colchicine
Complete Heart Block (3rd Degree)				DX: EKG shows Canon "a" Waves. TX: Atropine, Pacemaker
Sinus Bradycardia				DX: EKG. TX: Atropine, Pacemaker if symptomatic

Congenital Heart Pathologies (see congenital chapter for details)

Downs Syndrome: ASD, Endocardial Cushion, Intra Atrial Septum
Kartagener's: Situs Inversus
Tuberous Sclerosis: Cardiac rhabdomyoma
DiGeorge: Tetralogy of Fallot, Truncus Arteriosis
Marfan's: Necrosis of Aorta, MVP, Thoracic Aortic Aneurysm, Aortic Dissection
Fredericks Ataxia: HCM
Neonatal Lupus: Heart Block
Williams: Aortic Stenosis
Lang Neilson: Long QT Syndrome
Edwards: VSD
Congenital Rubella: PDA
Kawasaki: Coronary Artery Aneurysm
Turners: Coarctation of the Aorta, Bicuspid Aortic Valve
Infant of Diabetic Mother: Transposition of Great Arteries

Cardiac Pathologies

Left Heart Failure

- Due to any issues involving the left side of the heart or the heart pump as a whole: Aortic stenosis, Mitral stenosis (Rheumatic Fever – see hemoptysis), HTN, etc.
- Left heart issues cause the blood to back up (creating ↑ pressure at each step).
- **SX: Left Ventricular Hypertrophy (LVH).**
  Signs of LVH: Cardiac enlargement (heart that is > 50% of total transthoracic diameter), EKG show: high voltage R spike > 35mm in V5, S wave in V1, LBBB, left displacement of apex of heart, left axis deviation.

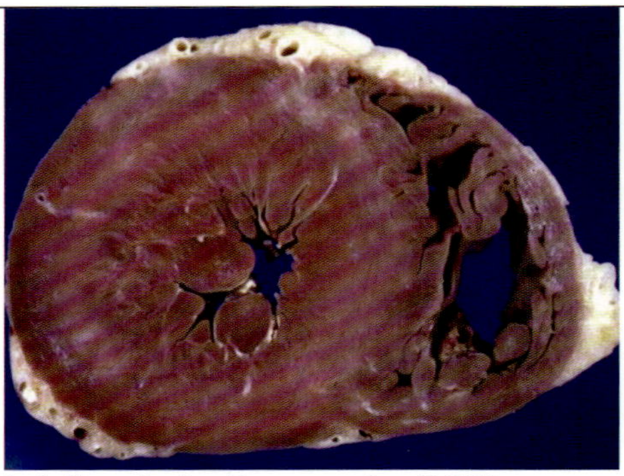
Left Ventricular Hypertrophy (LVH)

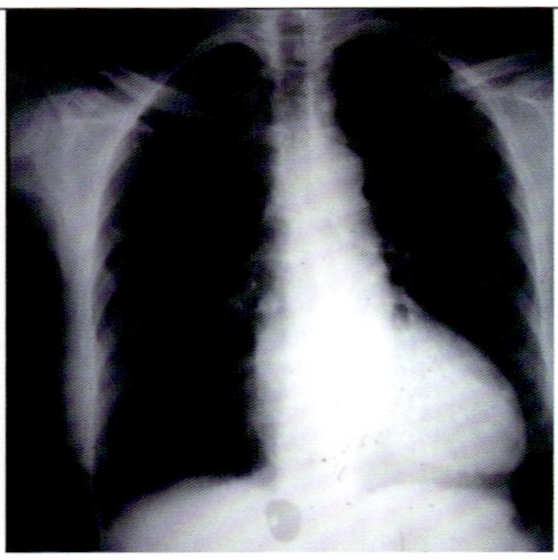

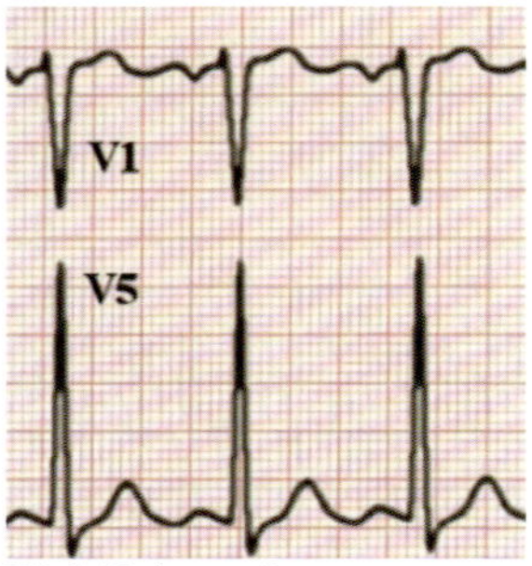

High Voltage R
"S" Wave

Pressure from the left ventricle (left ventricular hypertrophy (LVH) due to HTN or aortic stenosis) will back up increasing the pressure inside the **left atrium, enlarging it.**
Left atrium enlargement can present as: dysphagia (pressing on the esophagus), hoarseness (pressing on the left recurrent laryngeal nerve) or on CXR showing displacement (elevated) left main stem bronchi (due to heart pushing up on the bronchi), second bubble behind the heart.

Pulmonary edema: hydrostatic pressure from ↑ venous pulmonary pressure. Pulmonary edema comes from backup from the LEFT side of the heart so it will also show an increased PWCP. Indicated by presence of "**Heart Failure Cells**".

"Heart Failure Cells" in the alveoli. (Siderophages). (AKA: Alveolar macrophages, Dust cells). Hemosiderin-laden macrophages. Seen in patiens with left heart failure or chronic pulmonary edema. The left ventricle can't keep up with the pace of the incoming blood from the pulmonary veins causing a backup, which causes pressure on the alveolar capillaries causing RBC's to leak out. **Alveolar macrophages (dust cells) phagocytize the RBC's and become filled with hemosiderin.**

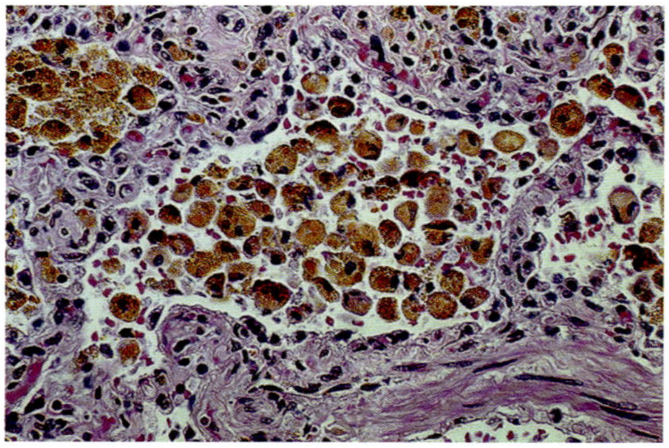

Orthopnea (need ↑ pillows at night or sleeps in a recliner to keep head level up above heart because there is so much fluid due to ↑ venous return that it makes it difficult to breath).

Paroxysmal nocturnal dyspnea (waking up out of a sleep short of breath due to increased fluid because of ↑ venous return).

Pulmonary Wedge Capillary Pressure (PWCP) (estimates pressure of left atrium).

- **PWCP is always HIGH when there are left sided heart problems because of back up which causes high pressure in the left atrium.** This back up will continue on into the lungs ➔ pulmonary edema (this is caused because of LEFT heart issues), so in pulmonary edema PWCP will also be increased because of the left heart involvement. If the problem/pressure is not corrected this backup will progress from the lungs into the right side of the heart and then into the systemic and portal systems (just as what would be seen in right heart failure).
- **PWCP is always NORMAL with any issues BEFORE the left atrium** (such as pulmonary HTN, pulmonary embolism, right sided heart problems). If the issue has never left the lungs and involved ANY part of the left heart, the PWCP is always normal because nothing has affected the left heart.
- **PWCP is LOW when there is hypovolemia**. If there is not enough fluid in the heart, then everything will be low.

Left sided heart failure "circle"

HTN = LVH = ↓ LV diastolic function (rigid walls on filling) = ↑ LV filling pressures so ↑ EDV and EDP to maintain CO and SV = Left atrial pressure rises which can enlarge the left atrium = ↑ PWCP = pulmonary venous congestion = ↑ hydrostatic pressure in lungs causing capillary leaks = ↓ pulmonary vascular compliance = pulmonary edema (bilateral bibasilar crackles) = alveolar collapse = ↓ ventilation = hypoxemia = vasoconstriction in lungs to shunt blood to areas to ↑ ventilation and ↓ venous congestion = pulmonary arterial HTN = ↑ afterload = ↑ Right ventricular dilation (right sided heart failure (Cor Pulmonale) = tricuspid regurgitation = ↑ JVD = peripheral edema (pitting) = hepatic congestion (portal congestion) = hemorrhoids.

Enlarged Left Atrium

An enlarged left atrium can result from left sided heart failure, mitral valve pathologies, myxoma, A-fib and anything that increases the pressure inside the left atrium (as indicated by an ↑ in PWCP).
Signs of an enlarged left atrium:

- Dysphagia due to compression or posterior displacement of the esophagus by the left atrium.
- Hoarseness due to compression of the left recurrent laryngeal nerve by the left atrium.
- Elevation or posterior displacement of the left main bronchus

CHF (Congestive Heart Failure)

AKA: Heart Failure Cardiac pump dysfunction – heart is unable to pump sufficiently to maintain blood flow. Is not able to push out the blood. CHF can be caused by systolic or diastolic pathologies and can only be distinguished with an ECHO. **Systolic dysfunction:** (dilated heart) = **low EF**, poor contractility, ↑ compliance. OR **Diastolic dysfunction:** (restricted heart, impaired relaxation, **normal EF** and contractility, ↓ compliance. Right heart failure = cor pulmonale. ↑ Compliance (stretches easily)	SX: **S3 gallop**, **progressive** shortness of breath (worse with exercise b/c ↓ oxygen delivery), **pitting edema in lower extremities**, excessive fatigue), cardiomegaly, **orthopnea** (dyspnea when lying flat, must be propped up to sleep: ie: # of pillows used), **JVD** (↑ JVD on inhalation **"Kussmaul sign" = respiratory alkalosis**), Cheyne stokes breathing (cyclic breaths), paroxysmal nocturnal dyspnea, ascites, **pulmonary edema** (rales/bilateral crackles upon auscultation due to hydrostatic pressure forcing fluid out of the capillaries into the alveoli). Chronic volume overload. **Pitting edema**: Is present **all the time in CHF.** If edema is due to **venous stasis** the swelling will be gone in the mornings b/c feet were raised all night, decreasing the effect of gravity.	Labs/Test **Labs: ↑BNP, Respiratory alkalosis.** **BNP: Natriuretic peptide that is released from the ventricles (ANP from Atria) when increased stretch due to ↑ fluid volume. BNP stops the Renin-Aldo system and causes diuresis.** **A normal BNP excludes CHF.** (Note: both BNP and ANP causes a ↓ systemic vascular resistance, ↓ central venous pressure, ↓ preload because of the ↓ in blood volume from the natriuresis and diuresis). **Respiratory alkalosis: Due to increased fluid in the lung, diffusion is ↓ causing hypoxia. The body compensates by hyperventilation leading to respiratory alkalosis.** ECHO: Dilated ventricle with **hypokinesia,** valve regurgitation, dilated (balloon shaped) heart. CXR: **Kerley B lines** Chest auscultation: **Pulmonary edema = bilateral bibasilar crackles. (Edema due to hydrostatic pressure)** ↑ Preload and afterload

Systolic TX:
Ace Inhibitors = ↓ Afterload.
β- Blockers (Metoprolol or Carvedilol) = ↑filling time in diastole = ↑ blood supply ↓ oxygen demand.
Spironolactone = stops Aldosterone = ↓ fluid.
Diuretics and Digoxin
(Calcium channel blockers are not beneficial in systolic dysfunction)

Diastolic TX:
β- Blockers (Metoprolol or Carvedilol) = ↑filling time in diastole = ↑ blood supply ↓ oxygen demand.
Diuretics. (Spironolactone and Digoxin do not help in diastolic dysfunction).

CHF exacerbation: **IV Furosemide**

DO NOT give fluids in CHF = will worsen

Drugs that ↓ mortality in CHF:
β- Blockers, ACE inhibitors or ARB's, Spironolactone.

CHF/Pulmonary edema/MI are always admitted to the ICU.
TX for CHF if there is a wide QRS (> 120 msec) on EKG (meaning ventricles are not beating together) and an ejection fraction < 35%: Biventricular Pacemaker. Will cause both ventricles to synchronize.

Must evaluate ejection fraction in CHF with ECHO. It is the only way to distinguish between systolic and diastolic dysfunction.

Drugs and treatments that ↓ mortality in CHF systolic dysfunction
ACE inhibitors/ARB's
Beta Blockers
Hydralazine/Nitrates
Implantable Defibrillator
Spironolactone or Eplerenone

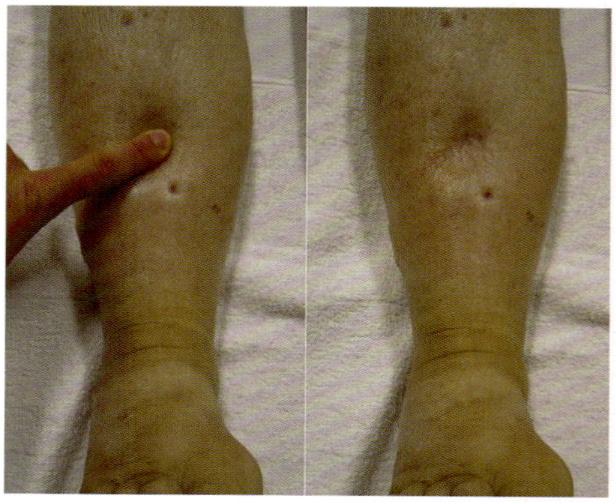

Pitting edema

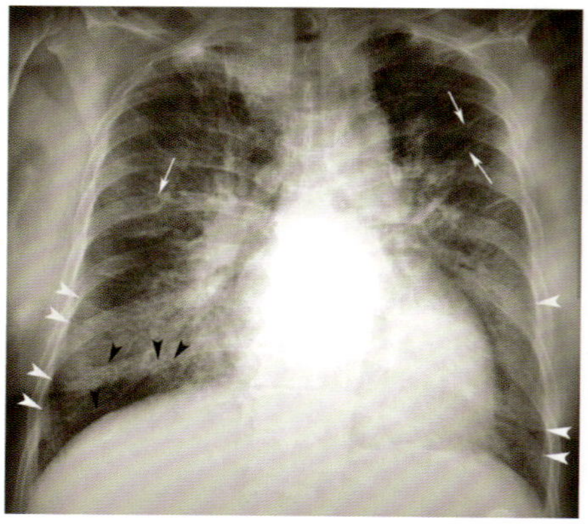

Kerley B lines

Cardiomyopathy

- Abnormal function of the heart muscle (contraction or relaxation)
- Forms of cardiomyopathy:
  - **Diastolic dysfunction** (concentric)
    Diastolic dysfunction is a **filling problem**. The ventricle is unable to be filled normally. **Normal EDV and EF, ↑ EDP (pressure). ↓ compliance.**
    Forms: **Hypertrophy (HCM or LVH).**
  - **Systolic** Dysfunction (eccentric)
    Systolic dysfunction is a **contraction/ejection/pumping problem**. The ventricle is unable to pump out blood, EF is low. **↑EDV, ↑ ESV, ↑ EDP, ↓ EF (< 50%), ↓ SV, ↓ CO, ↓ Contractility, ↑ Compliance.**
    Forms: Dilated.
- Symptoms
  - Shortness of breath, worsened by exertion, JVD, edema, rales.
- DX
  - ECHO

Concentric vs Eccentric Hypertrophy

- **Concentric Hypertrophy (AKA: Ventricular Hypertrophy – Diastolic dysfunction):** Hypertropic growth without overall enlargement of the heart. The walls of the heart (left or right ventricle) are thickened due to increased pressure overload of the heart. MC due to hypertension (systemic HTN for left ventricular hypertrophy and pulmonary hypertension for right ventricular hypertrophy). The result is diastolic dysfunction because there is little room left in the ventricle for the filling of blood. This ultimately causes ventricular failure, which then leads to systolic dysfunction.
  Histology: Enlarged myocardial cells with large nuclei.
- **Eccentric Hypertrophy (AKA: Dilated Hypertrophy – Systolic dysfunction)**: Due to volume overload causing Cardiomyocyte elongation (aka: wall thinning, dilated ventricles). This causes a systolic dysfunction because it is difficult to eject the blood from the heart.
  Histology: Addition of sarcomeres in series.

Dilated Cardiomyopathy
AKA: Eccentric Hypertrophy

Systolic Dysfunction (Dilated heart) **Eccentric** Impaired contraction **S3 beat** (↑ fluid)	**↑ EDV, ↑ ESV, ↑ EDP, ↓ EF (< 50%), ↓ SV, ↓ CO, ↓ Contractility.** Progressively **declining EF**. **Both EDV and EDP must stay up in order to maintain CO**	**Causes: Alcohol** abuse, Beriberi, Cocaine, **Chagas Dz, Coxsackie B, Doxorubicin, Adriamycin**, radiation, Amphetamines, Pregnancy, Thyroid Dz **Prevent cardiomyopathy** from Doxorubicin (Adriamycin) with **Dexrazoxane** (iron chelating agent)
TX: **Ace Inhibitors, ARB's** = ↓ Afterload. **Beta Blockers** = ↑filling time in diastole = ↑ blood supply ↓ oxygen demand. **Digoxin,** ICD (**implantable defibrillator for patients with an EF < 35%)**, heart transplant. BIT: ECHO (determines EF and wall motion)	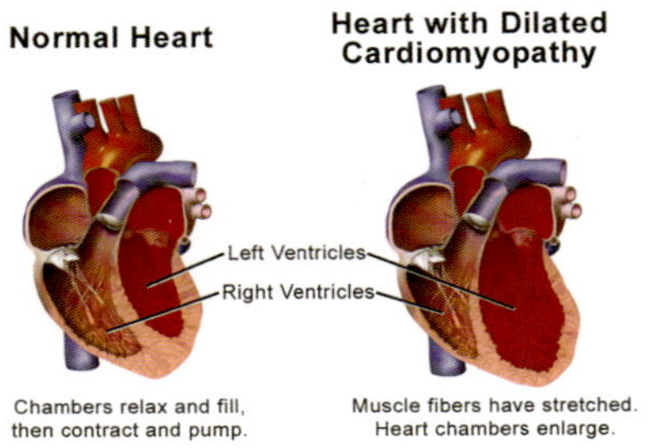 **Eccentric Hyper-trophy**: Due to volume overload causing Cardiomyocyte elongation (aka: wall thinning, dilated ventricles). This causes a systolic dysfunction because it is difficult to eject the blood from the heart. It is due to the addition of sarcomeres in series.	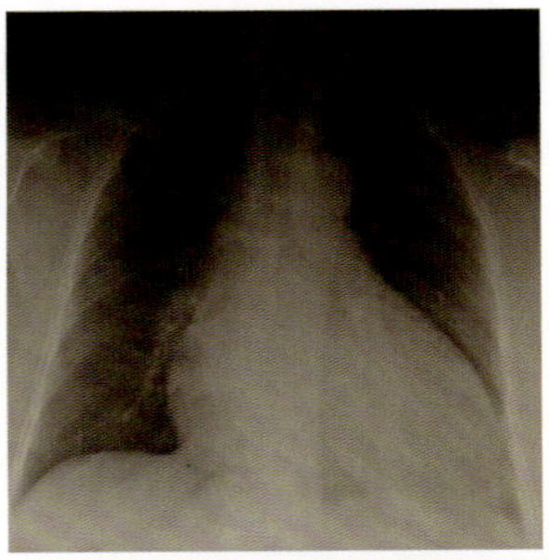 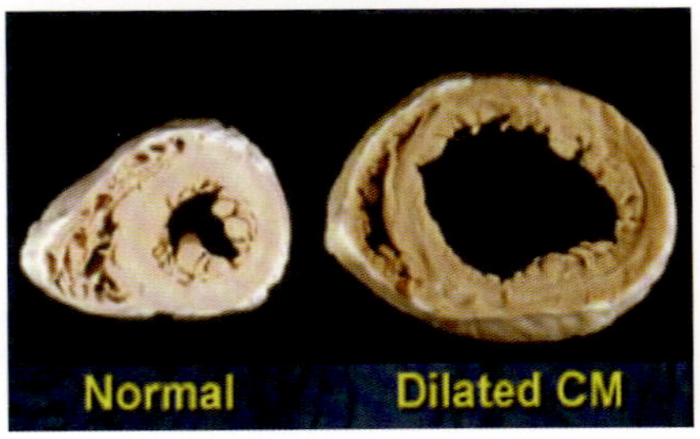

Hypertrophic Cardiomyopathies (HCM and HOCM)
Left Ventricular Hypertrophy (AKA: Concentric Hypertrophy)

Hypertrophic Cardiomyopathy (HCM) **Diastolic Dysfunction HCM (Stiff ventricle)** **Concentric (thickening of the ventricle walls, not the overall heart).** **LVH** Stiff ventricle – can't fill S4 (↑ Pressure) Pressure overload. ECHO: shows normal EF. **LVH can show on** EKG's as high R waves or inverted T waves, be **described as** "displaced apex", a LBBB, or left axis deviation. Right heart symptoms (JVD, ascites, hepatosplenomegaly, lower edema) are milder. **Note:** systemic HTN ↑ work on the heart causing myocyte growth due to expansion of the sarcomeres in order to ↑ contractility. ↓ Compliance (difficult to stretch)	**↑ EDP – ALL ELSE is normal, ↓ compliance.** **Mechanisms causing the hypertrophy** (cardiac remodeling): **Insulin-like growth factors, ↑ c-jun** is required for hypertrophy (promotes expression of the sarcomere proteins), **↑ β-Myosin Heavy Chain (MHC), ↑ Endothelin-1** (potent vasoconstrictor) activates hypertrophy due to ↑ HTN (systemic or pulmonary). NOTE: For right ventricular hypertrophy due to pulmonary HTN, ↑ pulmonary expression of Endothelin-1 (vasoconstriction). Causes: Chronic HTN, Aortic Stenosis DX: ECHO shows **LVH** SX: ↓ Exercise tolerance (↓ volume = ↓ Oxygen), Pulmonary edema (**hydrostatic pressure** from back up), Shortness of breath.	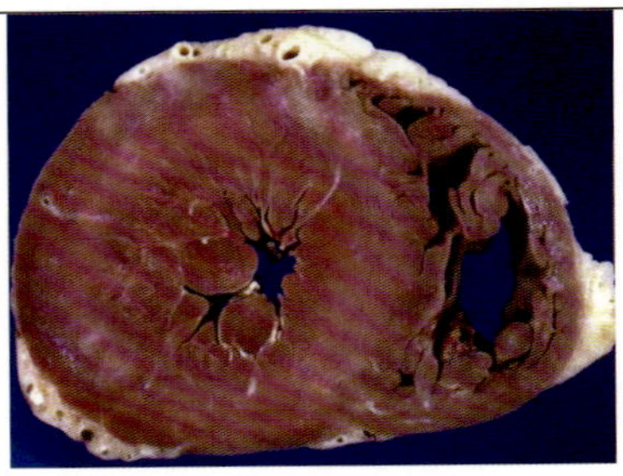 Left Ventricular Hypertrophy **Concentric Hypertrophy:** Hypertropic growth without overall enlargement of the heart. The walls of the heart (left or right ventricle) are thickened due to increased pressure overload of the heart. MC due to hypertension (systemic HTN for left ventricular hypertrophy and pulmonary hypertension for right ventricular hypertrophy). The result is diastolic dysfunction because there is little room left in the ventricle for the filling of blood. This ultimately causes ventricular failure, which then leads to systolic dysfunction. TX: **β-Blockers** (slows heart to allow it to **fill more.** More fluid in HCM decreases murmur. **Diuretics.** **DO NOT USE: Digoxin or Spironolactone.**

Hypertrophic Obstructive Cardiomyopathy (HOCM) Genetic: **Autosominal Dominant** Mitral valve **OBSTRUCTS outflow (AKA: Systolic anterior motion (SAM) of the mitral valve)** or hypertrophied septum **OBSTRUCTS outflow.** Hypertrophied intraventricular septum blocks the mitral valve leaf causing **obstruction** in ejection of blood. **Family History (AD)** Fredericks Ataxia Noonan's syndrome ("Turner-like" syndrome in the male) Anderson-Fabry Dz TX: **β-Blockers** (slows heart to allow it to **fill more.** More fluid in HCM decreases murmur. Ablation of septum. **Implantable defibrillator** if symptoms of syncope are present. If all TX fail = surgical myomectomy. **DO NOT USE: Ace Inhibitors and Diuretics**: this ↓ serum amount ↓ preload and fluid in heart = worsens murmur.	SX: Dyspnea, syncope, palpitations, dizziness, fainting, **sudden death in athletes.** **Murmur does not increase with expiration.** Symptoms **worsen with anything** that ↑ heart rate (heart must keep ↑ fluid inside the heart): exercise (sports), diuretics, and dehydration. (Remember diuretics, dehydration ↓ fluid = ↓ BP = reflex tachycardia). Symptoms **worsen with anything** that ↓ left ventricle size: Valsalva, standing suddenly, ACE inhibitor, ARB's, Hydralazine, Digoxin. Auscultation: **Crescendo – Decrescendo** systolic ejection murmur on **LEFT LOWER sternal boarder**. (don't mix up with aortic stenosis – upper RIGHT sternal boarder). Hear murmur better when **less fluid in heart = Valsalva maneuver.** **DX: BIT: ECHO (shows septum is 1.5 times thicker than the posterior wall). EKG shows: Septal Q waves. MAT: Catheterization.**	Biopsy: **Myofibrillar disarray (unorganized muscle fibers) and fibrosis** 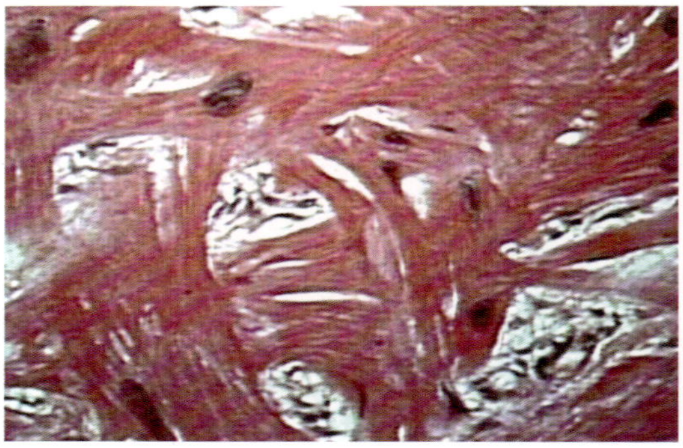 Disorganized cardiac muscle (HCM) 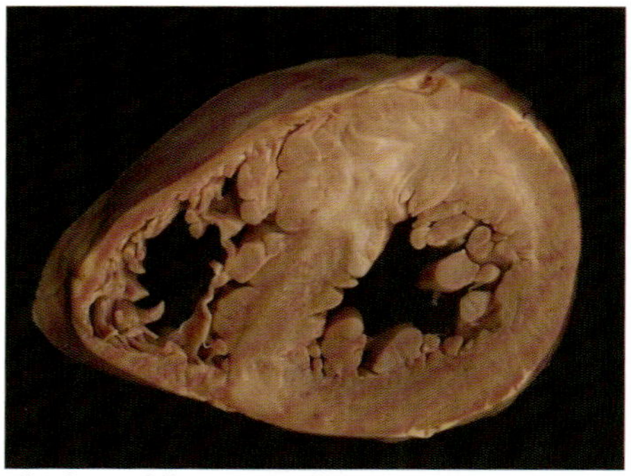 Thickened/hypertrophic septum.

Right Heart Failure

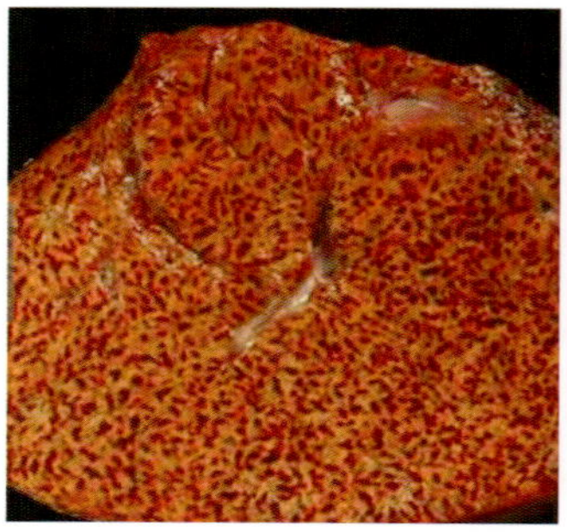

Nutmeg liver

- **Most common cause of right heart failure is left heart failure**
- **Death from right heart failure: cor pulmonale**
  SX:
  JVD (Jugular venous distention): Distended neck veins.
  Nutmeg liver (hepatomegaly) ↑ Central venous pressure = ↑ portal pressure.
  Peripheral edema (pitting edema of the lower legs) due to **oncotic pressure.**
- **Right ventricular hypertrophy (RVH): AKA: Concentric:** Due to pulmonary HTN. (AKA: Right axis deviation, RBBB)

Cor Pulmonale

(Death due to right sided heart failure, which includes anything, except pulmonary EDEMA, in the lungs. Because pulmonary edema is caused due to back up from the LEFT side of the heart)

- Common in: Women 20 – 40 years old due to **pulmonary HTN, obstructive sleep apnea, COPD**, pulmonary embolism
- Wide S2
- Chronic hypoxia = constricts pulmonary arteries = pulmonary HTN = right ventricular hypertrophy = right ventricular failure = **↑ JVD = hepatojugular reflux (↑ in JVD when pressure is applied over the abdomen is indicative of right heart failure)** = hepatosplenomegaly = ascites = lower pitting edema = ↑ lymph drainage.
- Everything backs up and increases pressure: ↑ IVC, ↑ hepatic vein, ↑ Central vein, ↑ sinusoidal, ↑ portal system.

Restrictive Cardiomyopathy

Combination of diastolic and systolic dysfunction: immobility due to no contraction and no relaxation due to deposition/infiltration of substances.

Symmetrical thickening of ventricular walls. NO THICK WALLS as seen in HCM. Preserved ventricular dimensions. Thick interventricular septum. **↓ Systolic dysfunction and ↓ Diastolic** (heart is stiff/restrictive = can't relax to fill and can't contract t eject. SX: Shortness of breath, **Kussmaul's sign** (↑ JVD upon inspiration), pulmonary hypertension (due to an ↑ in PWCP). **DX: BIT: ECHO.** **Cardiac Catheterization: Shows rapid x and y decent.** **MAT: Endomyocardial biopsy.** EKG: show low voltage. MAD: Endomyocardial biopsy.	Causes: **Sarcoidosis, amyloidosis** (excess protein deposits), Löffler syndrome (fibrosis with eosinophilic infiltrate), **hemochromatosis** (excess iron deposits), endocardial fibroelastosis (thick, elastic tissue in hearts of children), cancer, myocardial fibrosis, **glycogen storage diseases.** Hemochromatosis is the **ONLY** cause that is **reversible**: phlebotomy. TX: Correct underlying cause. **Diuretics.**	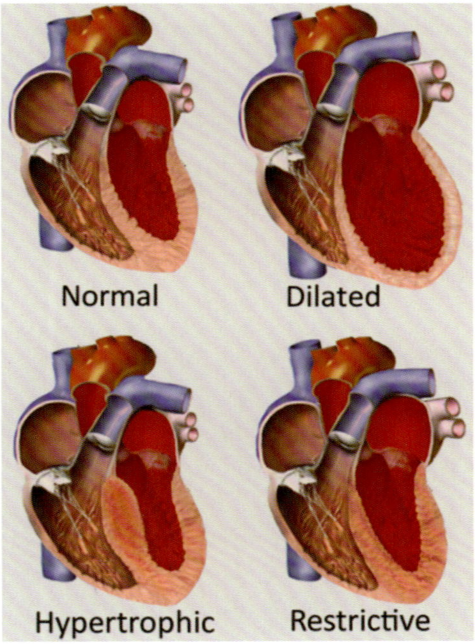

Pericarditis (Acute)

Inflammation of the pericardium **Acute Pericarditis** < 6 wks Acute Pericarditis Causes: **Viruses (MC: Coxsackie virus)** Fungal Bacteria (M. tuberculosis) Chagas Uremic pericarditis (Uremic TX: requires dialysis) Post infarct pericarditis **Dressler's syndrome (Fibrinous)** Drug Cause: **Doxorubicin**	SX: **Sharp, pleuritic pain**, pain can last for hours to days. Feels better when leaning forward. **Diffuse ST elevations** and/or PR depression in lead II. **Friction rub** on auscultation. Complications: pericardial effusion and cardiac tamponade. TX: **NSAIDS (Indomethacin, Ibuprofen, Naproxen)** **Colchicine ↓ reoccurrence.** (TX: Dressler's Syndrome with **Colchicine**)	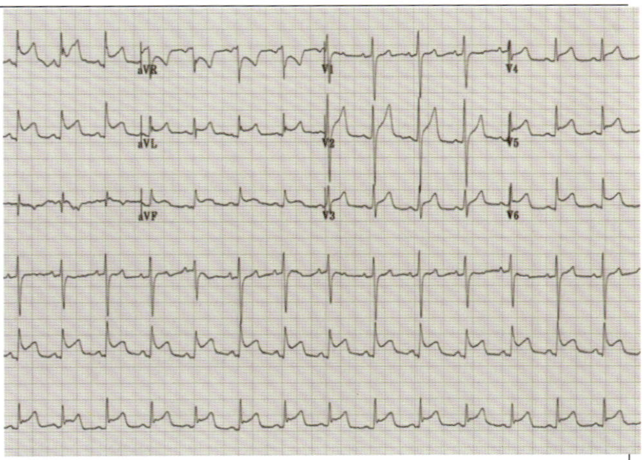 Diffuse ST elevations

Constructive Pericarditis (Chronic)

Chronic Pericarditis > 6 months. Thickened, fibrotic pericardium. Thick walls, ↓ CO, ↓ Filling. SX: **Pericardial knock (due to dystrophic calcification of pericardium),** Shortness of breath and **signs of right heart failure**: Kussmaul's sign (JVD upon inhalation), ascites, hepatosplenomegaly, lower pitting edema. DX: BIT: CXR shows calcification and fibrosis, pleural effusions. ECHO shows changes in cardiac chamber volume. EKG: show low voltage. MRI/CT: shows thickening of pericardium	Causes: MC Cause: **damage to myocardium** due to heart surgery or radiation treatment to the chest, TB, fungal or parasitic infections, pulmonary asbestos. (**tip**: Dystrophic calcification = "D" for due to "D"amage) TX: **Diuretics.** Surgical removal of pericardium (AKA: Pericardial stripping)	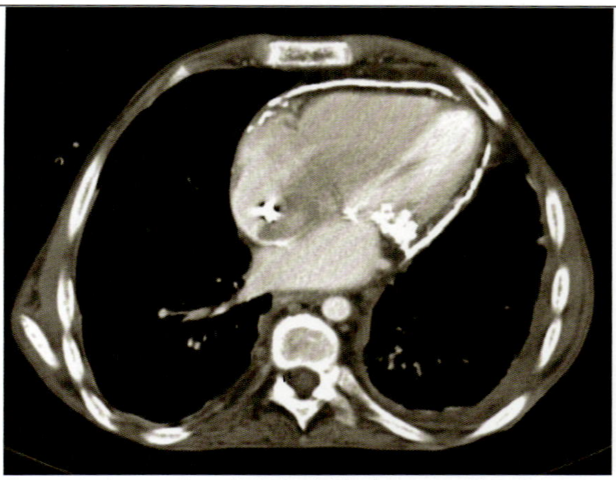 Constrictive pericarditis (calcified pericardium)

Takotsubo Cardiomyopathy

AKA: Stress induced cardiomyopathy
AKA: Broken heart syndrome
AKA: Apical ballooning cardiomyopathy

- Sudden, temporary weakening of the muscles of the heart triggered by major emotional stress (ie: death of a loved one, break up/divorce, financial problems, natural disaster, etc).
- SX: Heart pain, shortness of breath, ST segment elevation, and cardiac enzymes may/may not be increased.
- Causes: Sudden death, fatal ventricular arrhythmias, ventricular rupture, acute heart failure.
- MC found in post-menopausal women
- DX: Left ventricular ballooning. Part of the left ventricle contracts normally and the other part is dyskinetic (motion abnormalities).
- TX: Ace Inhibitors, Beta Blockers or Calcium Channel Blockers

Lyme Cardiomyopathy (aka: Lyme Carditis)

- Caused by infection with Borrelia burgdorferi (bite by the Ixodes dammini tick)
- MC SX: AV Conduction heart block
- Cardiac involvement occurs during the early disseminated phase of the disease (within weeks to a few months after the onset of Lyme disease
- Other cardiac complications: dilated cardiomyopathy
- Carditis is preventable: 10 – 21 days of oral doxycycline given during the early stages of Lyme disease. (Amoxicillin if the patient is <8 years old or is pregnant)

Eccentric Hypertrophy: Non-pathologic

- MC found in athletes
- Due to the exercising skeletal muscles increasing venous return to the heart, which causes a volume overload in the heart leading to eccentric hypertrophy. The hypertrophy causes an ↑ in ejection fraction

Pharmacology in Systolic and Diastolic Dysfunction

Pharmacology	Systolic Dysfunction (Dilated)	Diastolic Dysfunction HCM	Diastolic Dysfunction HCOM
ACE Inhibitors/ARB's	Yes	Unconfirmed benefit	No
β-Blockers	Yes	Yes	Yes
Digoxin	Yes	No	No
Diuretics	Yes	Yes	No
Spironolactone	Yes	No	No

Endocarditis

- **AKA: Deposit/aggregate of fibrin and platelets**
- Due to the infection or damage of the **endocardium** (**inner lining of the heart muscle** that also covers the heart valves)
- **Endocarditis can involve the heart muscles, heart valves or the lining of the heart (not just the valves)**
- **Complications:** Blood clots and emboli, brain abscess, CHF, glomerulonephritis, neurological problems, arrhythmias, stroke, severe valve damage.
- **Fever and new murmur**
- **Splinter hemorrhages**
- Flat, painless lesions (Janeway lesions)
- Raised, painful lesions (**O**sler nodes) (**tip**: **O** for **O**uch)
- Microemboli to brain, lungs, arterial vessels, eyes, kidneys
- **Roth spots in the eyes**
- If TIA's occur, check ECHO to see if an endocarditis is the source of the micro emboli
- Always get cultures **FIRST** before treatment. After culture, IMMEDIATELY start empiric treatment, **DO NOT WAIT** until result of culture come back. Once the culture results are back the treatment can be switched to the best-recommended treatment for that organism.
  Best empiric treatment: **IV Vancomycin and Gentamicin**
- Subacute Endocarditis: occurs on pre-existing damaged valve
- Acute Endocarditis: occurs on healthy valve

Endocarditis Diagnosis

Diagnosed by Duke's Criteria (must involve 2 major symptoms, or 1 major and 3 minor symptoms or 5 minor symptoms)
Diagnostic Test: Best Initial Test: TTE (Transthoracic Echocardiogram), If TEE is negative: perform TEE (Transesophageal Echocardiogram)
TX: Empiric TX: **Vancomycin and Gentamicin** combined.

Duke's Criteria

Major Symptoms	Minor Symptoms
• 2 positive blood cultures with: S. aureus, S. bovis, S. epidermis, Candida, Viridans, Streptococci, Enterococci, gram-negative rods. • Abnormal echocardiogram showing: Valvular vegetation, abscess, dehiscence of prosthetic valve, mass	• Fever • IV drug use • Prosthetic heart valve • Hx of endocarditis • Dental procedure with bleeding • Structural heart DZ • Janeway lesions (flat, painless) • Splinter hemorrhages • Osler's nodes (raised, painful) (tip: O = Ouch) • Roth Spots on retina • Arterial emboli • Mycotic aneurysm • Pulmonary infarcts (septic) • Conjunctival hemorrhage • Glomerulonephritis • Positive blood cultures (not falling under major SX)

Endocarditis Prophylaxis

The ONLY time that prophylaxis is given for endocarditis is:

(Prophylaxis: **Amoxicillin for oral/dental procedures**. **Cephalexin** *(Keflex)* if skin procedures. If patient is allergic to penicillin: Azithromycin, Clindamycin, Clarithromycin, Vancomycin)

- Prosthetic valve
- Unrepaired cyanotic heart disease
- Previous endocarditis
- Dental work involving blood
- Cardiac transplant with valvulopathy
- Respiratory tract surgery
- Transplant patients (recipients)
- Surgery of infected skin

Otherwise: NO prophylaxis is needed for: endoscopes, OB Gyn procedures, urology, all murmurs, MVP, valve heart disease, atrial or ventricular septal defects, pacemakers, implantable defibrillators, septal defects, dental fillings, flexible scopes, cystoscopy, urinary procedures.

Endocarditis Organisms – Characteristics - Treatments

Organism	Characteristics	Treatment
Staph aureus	IV Drug use, indwelling catheter (NOT central lines) Goes to healthy valves (MC: tricuspid valve) **CAUTION**: if murmur gets louder inhalation it is tricuspid if it gets louder on expiration it is the mitral.	**Nafcillin, Oxacillin, Cefazolin** **If prosthetic valve, add Rifampin**
Strep viridans (Mutans, other mouth organisms: ie: Eikenella, Kingella, Peptostreptococcus, Fusobacterium, Bacteroides, Actinomyces, H. aphrophilus, H. parainfluenzae, Actinobacillus, Cardiobacterium)	From poor dental hygiene. Normally goes to pre-damaged valves. MC: Mitral valve.	**Ceftriaxone (4 wks)**
Staph epidermidis	From prosthetic devices (valves, joints) and from central lines	**Vancomycin**
Enterococci (Group D) E. faecalis, E. faecium	Follows GI/GU manipulation procedures (AKA: **cystoscopy**) from contaminated instruments. **MC: Elderly men**	**Ampicillin and gentamicin**
Strep bovis (Group D) Clostridium septicum	Colonizes the gut. Indicates possible **colon cancer** or GI tuberculosis. **Next Step: Colonoscopy**	**Ampicillin and gentamicin**
Fungus		**Amphotericin** **Surgery: Valve replacement**
Culture Negative Endocarditis	MC: Coxiella, Bartonella Other culture negative: **HACEK:** H. aphrophilus, H. parainfluenzae, Actinobacillus, Cardiobacterium, Eikenella, Kingella.	**Ceftriaxone**
Non-bacterial Endocarditis (AKA: Marantic endocarditis)	Associated with terminal illness :(cancer or sepsis), SLE (Libman-Sacks), hypercoagulability, trauma. Sterile fibrin deposits. **NO bacteria**	
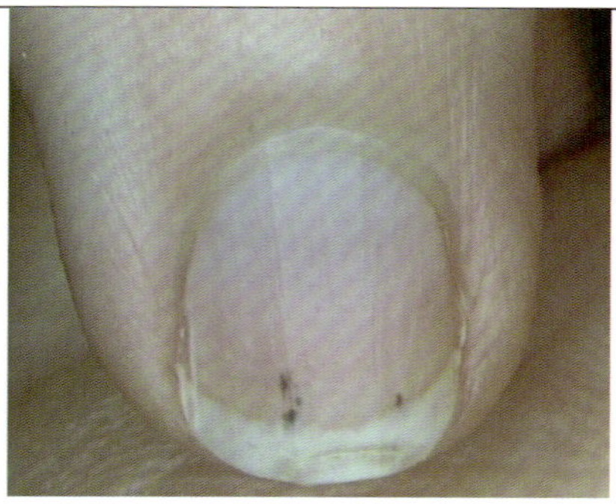 Splinter hemorrhages	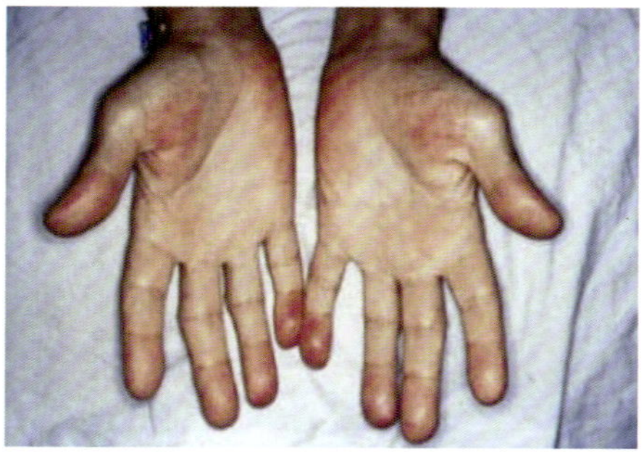 Osler's Nodes	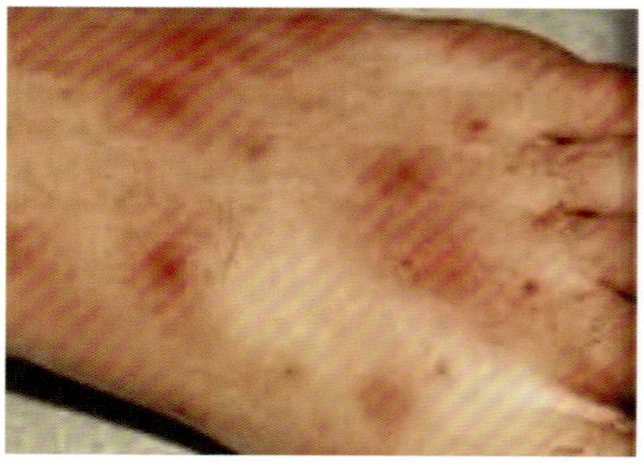 Janeway lesions

Rheumatic Fever

Rheumatic Fever **Group A Strep (Strep pyogenes)** MC: **Immigrants**, developing countries MCC: **Untreated strep throat** (AKA: Pharyngitis) Type II hypersensitivity **Antibodies against M protein**	SX: **Rash** (erythema marginatum), **chorea** (involuntary movements), **arthritis** (joint pain), cardiac. Labs: ↑ ESR, ↑ ASO titers DX: Aschoff bodies (granulomas with giant cells. Anitschkow cells (enlarged macrophages with ovoid, rod-like nucleus.	**Heart:** Most common valve affected: mitral. Young patients: Mitral regurg Older patients: **Mitral stenosis**. **Mitral stenosis causes hemoptysis** (due to backed up pressure in the lungs). **Note:** Mitral stenosis will also cause the **left atrium to enlarge**. Signs to indicate an enlarged atrium are: hoarseness (due to compression of left recurrent laryngeal nerve), elevation of the left main bronchus, dysphasia (compression of the esophagus). TX: Lifelong treatment of **penicillin** for prophylaxis so no reoccurrence.

Syphilis Heart Disease

- Tertiary Syphilis (3°)
- Disruption of the **vasa vasorum of the aorta causing Aortic Regurgitation (Insufficiency)**
  Vaso vasorum: network of small blood vessels that supply the walls of the large blood vessels (elastic arteries: aorta) and large veins (vena cava)

Cardiac Tamponade

Compression of the heart by a pericardial effusion (blood, fluid, pus, clots, gas) ↓↓ CO, **Equilibrium of diastolic** pressure in **all 4 chambers** (compression of the chambers begins on the right side: walls are thinner). ↓Filling (preload), shifting of the right ventricular septum into the left ventricle which ↓↓ filling = ↓ CO and ↓ SV, restricts venous return and ↓↓ blood pressure. **Diastolic collapse** of right atrium and ventricle. **CAUSE of DEATH: Lack of preload into the left ventricle.** TX: Emergency pericardiocentesis. Long Term TX: Pericardial window **DO NOT TREAT WITH DIURETICS.**	SX: **Beck triad (severe hypotension, distended neck veins, muffled, distant heart sounds),** ↑ HR, **pulsus paradoxus (↓ of BP > 10 mmHg on inhalation)**, Kussmaul sign, **tachycardia, JVD,** **Lungs are CLEAR** **Pulsus paradoxus** = ↓ in systolic blood pressure by ≥ 10 mmHg during inspiration. MOA: This because venous return is increased via inspiration so that the right ventricle expands. When it expands compressing the left ventricle causing a ↓ in blood pressure (≥ 10 mmHg). MAD: ECHO shows diastolic collapse of right atrium and right ventricle.	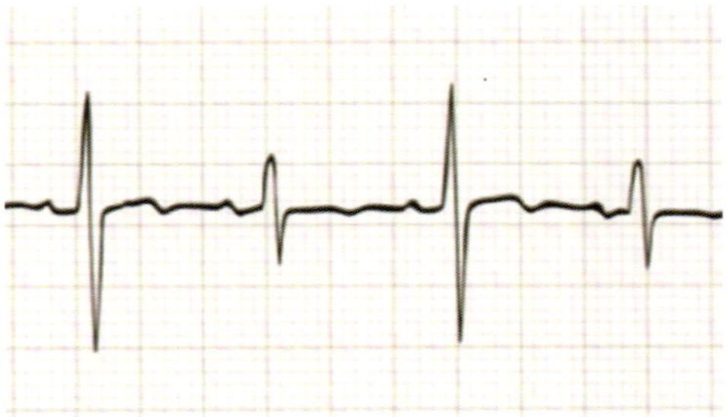 Electrical alternans EKG shows: **electrical alternans** (swinging of the heart in the pericardial sac) and low voltage. (**Variations of height of the QRS**). CXR: shows globular heart. Catheterization shows equal pressures in all chambers of the heart during diastole.
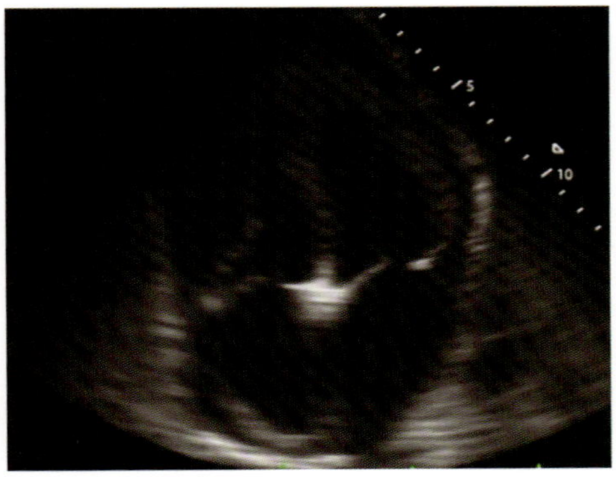	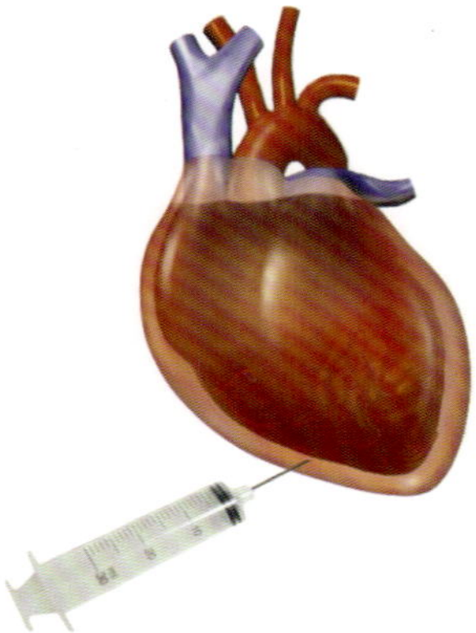	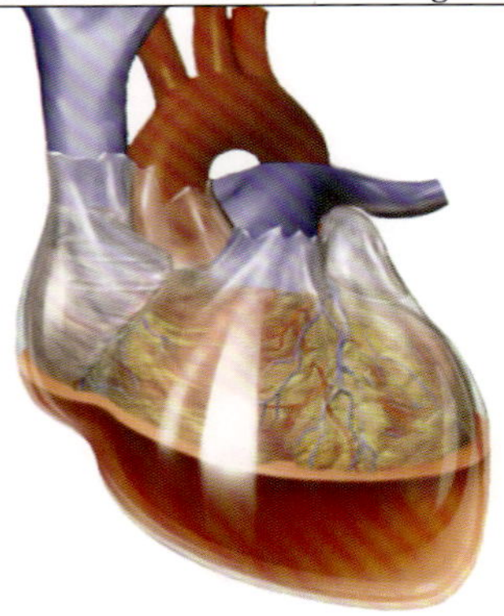

High Output Heart Failure (AV Fistulas)

Fistulas join arteries to veins bypassing capillaries so blood flow is increased dramatically. Heart can't meet the oxygen demand of the peripheral tissues because they are bypassed. So ↓ systemic TPR = ↑ blood flow to the heart. The ↑ blood flow = ↑ preload = ↑ CO = LVH = ↑ Mitral regurgitation.	SX: Wide pulse pressure, strong peripheral pulses (carotid upstroke), the area of the fistula is flushed and warm.

Prinzmetals Angina

Coronary Vasospasms (transient) **Diffuse ST elevations** on EKG in V4 - V6 MC: Young females High risk: **Smoking** Occurs between midnight and 8 am. Similar to Reynaud's	Treatment Stop smoking **TX: Calcium channel blockers** **Diltiazem** Do NOT give aspirin or will increase vasospasms **To invoke a vasospasm: Ergonovine** (constricts smooth muscle and stimulates α adrenergic and serotonin receptors

Cardiac Tumors

Most common heart tumor is metastasis (melanoma, lymphoma) **Myxoma** #1 MC cardiac tumor in **adults** MC: **Left atrium** SX: ↑ syncopal episodes, odd, beat on auscultation. Complication: emboli DX: **Scattered cells in a mucopolysaccharide stroma** Produce IL-6 Auscultation: Additional, odd sound **Rhabdomyoma** #1 MC cardiac tumor in **children** Associated with **Tuberous sclerosis**	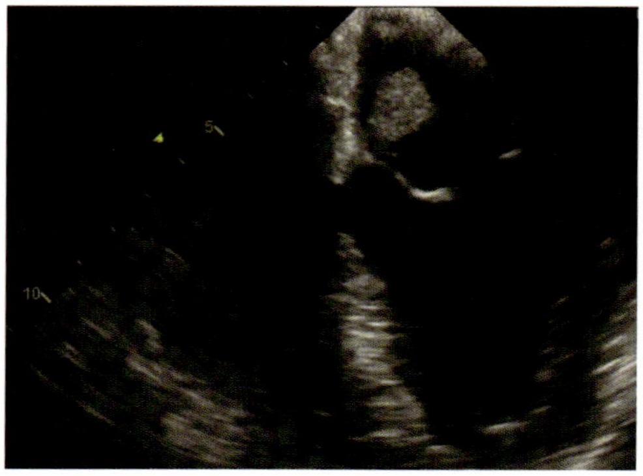 Myxoma

Heart Pathologies in Pregnancy

- Pregnancy ↑ plasma volume by 50%
- S3 heart sound: normal
- Mitral stenosis worsens in pregnancy
- Peripartum Cardiomyopathy and Eisenmenger Syndrome are dangerous cardiac pathologies in pregnancy

Peripartum Cardiomyopathy (PPCM) **Antibodies against the myocardium in pregnant women.** **Form of dilated cardiomyopathy.** **Systolic dysfunction and decrease of EF.** **Associated with CHF, arrhythmias, thromboembolism, and sudden cardiac death.** **Presents in last month of pregnancy or after delivery as a deterioration in cardiac function.** **SX: Orthopnea, dypsnea, pitting edema, nocturia, palpitations, chest pain.** **TX: same TX as for CHF (ACE inhibitors/ARB's, Diuretics, Digoxin, Spironolactone, β-blockers).** **If LV function does not improve: heart transplant is required.** **Subsequent pregnancies may worsen cardiac function.**	**Eisenmenger Syndrome** A left-to-right shunt switches to a **right-to-left shunt** due to pulmonary HTN in a person with a congenital VSD, ASD or patent ductus arteriosus (PDA). Can be present in infants and in pregnant women. Maternal mortality: 30% - 60% due to: syncope (fainting), thromboembolism, preeclampsia, hemoptysis, hypovolemia. SX: Cyanosis, high RBC (↑ HCT), syncope, arrhythmias, hemoptysis, heart failure, stroke. DX: ECHO TX: Hospitalization after 20th week (or earlier if condition worsens), surgical repair if caught before pulmonary HTN, transplantation

Cardiac, Chest Pain Differentials, Breath Sound Differentials

Cardiac Pathology	Description	Notes
Myocardial Infarction (MI) (AKA: Ischemic pain)	**Substernal Pain: Pressure,** squeezing, tightness, burning, aching, heaviness. **It can radiate** to neck, jaw, back, teeth, jaw, arm, or shoulders. Unstable angina (pain is not relieved with rest), shortness of breath, sweating (**diaphoresis**)	In elderly: Can present as abdominal pain. **ST elevations** in specific leads. Pain can be brought on by exercise, cold, stress. NOTE: This pain is NOT sharp, knifelike, stabbing,
Stable Angina	Pain caused by increase of oxygen demand on the heart (ie: exercising). Once patient rest, pain resides. Indicates ischemia. Pain last >2 minutes and < 10 minutes.	
Unstable Angina	Pain occurs at rest. Pain is not relieved by rest. New pain. Pain last > 10 min to 30 min.	
Pericarditis	**Sharp, positional** (pain changes with position change), pain better when leaning forward and worse when lying down.	**Diffuse ST elevations,** PR depression. Friction rub on auscultation. TX: **NSAIDS**
Costochondritis (AKA: musculoskeletal)	Pain upon inspiration, pain can be **reproduced upon palpation**, no radiation, chest wall tenderness, Last for hours	
Prinzmetals Angina	Palpitations Young women. Present in middle of night	Due to **vasospasms** of coronary arteries. Diffuse ST elevations TX: **Calcium channel blockers**
Cocaine MI	Same as an MI, but this is due to vasospasms	Diffuse ST elevations TX: **Calcium channel blockers. DO NOT use Beta Blockers**
Aortic Dissection	Tearing (ripping) **pain to the back** between shoulder blades	Unequal blood pressure in the arms. DX: Widened mediastinum.
Pulmonary Embolism	**Acute** shortness of breath, hypoxia (watch Oxygen Saturation, it will be in the low 90's), **clear chest x-ray**.	DX: Spiral CT, V/Q scan
Pneumothorax	Sudden shortness of breath, **decreased or no breath sounds unilaterally**, **hyperresonance**, possible tracheal deviation, sharp, pleuritic pain.	DX: Chest X-Ray
Asthma	Wheezing. Prolonged expiration.	
Pneumonia	Rales, rhonchi. Sputum, fever.	
Esophageal Spasms	Uncoordinated **spasms** in the esophagus. (AKA: Nutcracker esophagus)	TX: **Calcium channel blockers**
Intercostal Neuralgia	Spasmodic pain around the ribs. Pain caused by breathing, laughing, sneezing. Left sided pain in the back and left side of ribs, tingling, numbness, loss of appetite, atrophy of the muscles.	Nerve compression in the area of the ribcage. (Innervation of the muscles of the rib cage, skin and chest cavity). Nerves run under the rib with the vein and artery. **Nerve pain = burning**
Gallbladder	Pain radiates to the **right shoulder** (due to **phrenic** nerve)	
GERD	Epigastric pain Beware: heart attacks can present as GERD pain. Always check an EKG	Acid reflux, pain relief with antacids. **No sweating or shortness of breath.** **SX: Hoarseness, bad taste in mouth, cough (esp. night time cough).**
Diaphragm rupture	Abdominal pain referred to shoulder	CXR shows abdominal viscera above the diaphragm and loss of diaphragm contour
Peptic Ulcer	Epigastric pain. Pain worse with eating (patient will lose weight)	Epigastric pain in elderly must be evaluated for heart attack
Duodenal Ulcer	Epigastric pain. Pain less when food is kept on stomach (patient will usually gain weight).	DX: Endoscopy

MCC chest pain that is not due to ischemia is due to GI problems.		
Pleurisy	Inflammation of the pleura (membranes of the pleural cavity surrounding the lungs). Sharp, sudden (stabbing, burning, constant dull) pain on breathing (exhalation or inhalation). Pain can radiate to shoulder or back. Auscultation can also reveal a pleural friction rub (squeaking, grating sounds of the pleural linings rubbing together).	MCC: Viral infections (Coxsackie virus, RSV, CMV, Adenovirus, EBV, parainfluenza, influenza). Other causes: bacterial or fungal infections, effusions, cancers, pulmonary embolisms, chest injuries, autoimmune disorders, aortic dissection, heart surgery. TX: Underlying cause. Removal of air/blood/fluid from pleural space. Anti-inflammatories.

Reasons for Heart Surgery

- CABG (Coronary Artery Bypass Graft
- PACAB/Port CAB and MIDCAB (minimally Invasive Coronary Artery Bypass)
- Heart transplant
- Ablation for Wolf Parkinson-White, SVT's, tachyarrhythmias
- Atherectomy
- Percutaneous Coronary Intervention/Angioplasty, Stent
- Fungal endocarditis
- AV Block
- Ruptured valve/chordae tendineae
- Prosthetic valve replacement
- Abscess
- Myxoma

EKG's

EKG Heart rate Calculation

- Take a 6 second strip (Each large square is one second). Count the # R's in that 6 seconds. Multiply # of R's by 10 = HR
- Example below: (There are 8 R's in this 6 second strip. 8 x 10 = 80 BPM is the HR

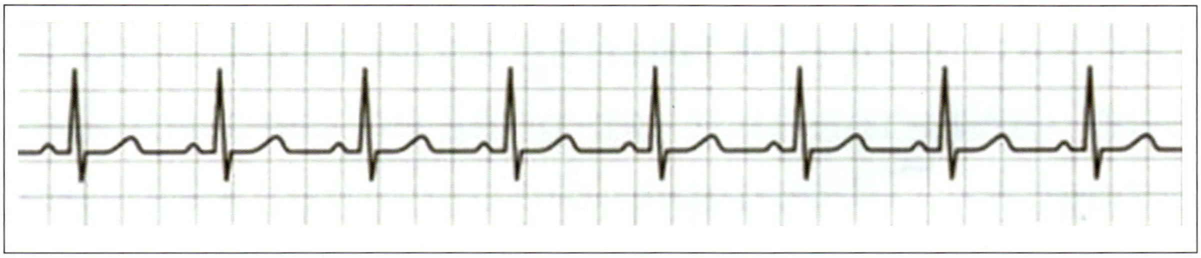

Normal Heart Rate: >60 to 100
Bradycardia: < 60
Tachycardia: > 100
EKG time key: 1 large block has 20 small squares (.20 seconds). Each small square is = .04 seconds.

EKG Leads

LIMB LEADS		PRECORDIAL LEADS	
Lead I Lateral left ventricle	Lead aVR	Lead V1 Septal	Lead V4 Anterior
Lead II Inferior portion of the left ventricle	Lead aVL Lateral left ventricle	Lead V2 Arterio-Septal	Lead V5 Lateral left ventricle
Lead III Inferior portion of the left ventricle	Lead aVF Inferior portion of the left ventricle	Lead V3 Arterio-Septal	Lead V6 Lateral left ventricle

Location in Heart	EKG Leads
Right Atrium	Lead II, AVR, V1
Right Ventricle	Lead II, AVF, V4
Left Atrium	Lead I, AVL, V2
Left Ventricle	Lead III, AVF, V4, V5, V6
Right Wall	Leads V1, V2
Anterior Wall	Leads V2, V3, V4, V5
Lateral Wall	Leads V5, V6

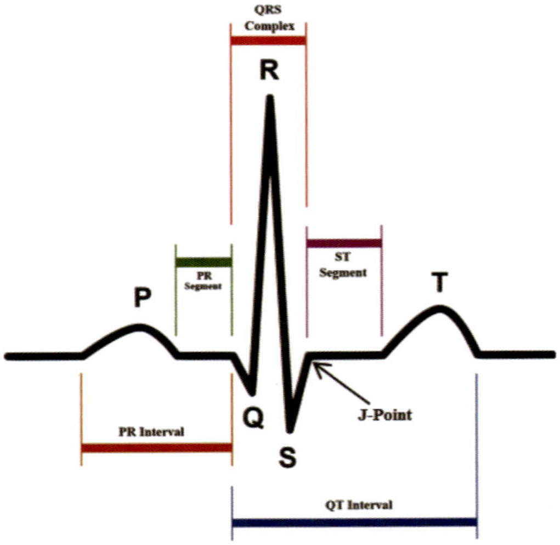

EKG Complex

EKG Structure	Key Ion starting action potential	Phase	Complex	Notes
P wave	Ca	Phase 0	Atrial Depolarization	Tall P wave = atrial hypertrophy. Absent in A-Fib, A Flutter Arrhythmias.
PR Interval	Ca	Phase 2	Atrial Contraction	Delay in the AV Node. See Cardiac Blocks for specific EKG signs and block treatments.
QRS Complex	Na	Phase 0	Ventricular Depolarization	Tall complex = LVH (left ventricular hypertrophy) = ↑ voltage. ↑ Width = ↑ duration
Q wave	Na	Phase 0	Ventricular Depolarization	Current in the septum
R wave	Na	Phase 0	Ventricular Depolarization	Current in the anterior wall
S wave	Na	Phase 0	Ventricular Depolarization	Current in the posterior wall
ST Segment	Ca	Phase 2	Ventricular Contraction	Hyperacute/ST elevation = MI > 90% occluded. Inverted/ST depression = Ischemia > 70%.
QT Interval	Ca	Phase 2	Ventricular Contraction	If prolonged can lead to torsades.
T wave	K efflux	Phase 3	Ventricular Repolarization	Peaked T wave: Hyperkalemia. (TX: **Calcium Gluconate**) Inverted or Flat T waves: Hypokalemia.
U wave	Na	Phase 4		Inverted U waves: CAD, HTN, Valvular heart dz, congenital heart dz, cardiomyopathy, hyperthyroidism. Prominent U waves: Brachycardia, severe hypokalemia, hypomagnesia, hypothermia, Digoxin, Class Ia, III antiarrhythmics.
Q wave				Old infarct. Patient has had a previous MI.

Ion Affects

Ion	Affect
↓Ca ↑ K	Short QT
↓ Ca	Long QT, Torsades
↓ Ca	Muscle cramps, tetany (**Chvostek's sign**: tapping side of face = twitch), perioral numbness, irritability, parathesis, depression, seizures, anxiety, fatigue
↑ Ca	Short QT, polyuria, nausea, **constipation**, dehydration, weakness, bone pain, confusion, stupor, coma
↓ K	Symptoms: Muscle weakness, respiratory failure, arrhythmias, tremor, muscle cramps, rhabdomyolysis, constipation, vomiting, diarrhea, hyporeflexia, flaccid paralysis. Causes: Inadequate potassium intake, Loop diuretics (Furosemide, Thiazides), Amp B, Cisplatin, DKA, Low Mg levels (Mg required for the processing of potassium), Increase of pH of the blood, high aldosterone levels, excess cola intake, TX: Replace the potassium, potassium-sparing diuretics, Saline with KCL, increase food high in potassium: leafy green vegetables, avocados, tomatoes, bananas, oranges, citrus fruits.
↓ K	EKG: Inverted T waves: AKA: flattened T wave, prominent U wave, ST depression, wide PR interval
↑ K	EKG shows: Peaked T wave. Wide QRS, Long PR, Short QT. Causes: ↑ with renal failure, low insulin, ACE inhibitors/ARB's, K Sparing drugs, some of the transplant rejection drugs. TX: **Calcium gluconate, glucose, insulin, dialysis, Kayexalate**

Arrhythmia's

Atrial Arrhythmias

- Atrial fibrillation
- Atrial Flutter
- Supraventricular Tachycardia (SVT)
- Multifocal Atrial Contraction (MAC)
- Premature Atrial Contraction (PAC)
- Synchronized shock for all Atrial arrhythmias – used when patient is unstable

Ventricular Arrhythmias

- Premature Ventricular Complex (PVC)
- Ventricular Tachycardia
- Ventricular Fibrillation

Prolonged QT Syndrome

- Caused by a delay in the outward flow of potassium (efflux) causing a delayed repolarization.
- Complications: Syncope, seizures, torsades de pointes or sudden death (irregular heartbeat that originates from the ventricles).
- Causes: Potassium and other imbalances, low serum magnesium, medications, bradycardia, family history (congenital long QT syndrome), liver disease, renal disease.
- Medicine causes: Class III anti-arrhythmics: Most likely: Sotalol, Ibutilide, less likely: Amiodarone. Class 1a anti-arrhythmics: Quinidine. Macrolides: Erythromycin. Antipsychotics: Haloperidol, Ziprasidone. Ondansetron, TCA's, SSRI's.

Hemodynamically Unstable Arrhythmias

Unstable patient: Synchronized cardioversion in acute atrial arrhythmias (A-Fib, A Flutter) to keep them from progressing to V-tach or V-fib. No anticoagulation is needed for acute A-Fib (< 2 days).
Chronic A-Fib (is an A-Fib lasting > 2 days). It takes several days for blood clots to begin forming so if cardio conversion becomes necessary because the arrhythmia did not return to a normal sinus rhythm on its own, anticoagulation must be done first. Initial Heparin therapy is NOT needed to start warfarin for A-Fib.
Unstable patient: Synchronized cardioversion in SVT and V-Tach. Must synchronize shock to keep the arrhythmia becoming V-fib or asystole.
All V-Fib: Unsynchronized cardioversion.

- **Chest pain (angina)**
- **Hypotension**
- **Confusion**
- **Dyspnea**
- **CHF**

Holter Monitoring

- **Helps to identify underlying rhythm abnormalities in a patient with frequent symptoms. Patient usually wears the monitor for 24 – 48 hours.**

Atrial fibrillation

- **"Irregularly irregular", variable R to R, palpitations.**
- **NO P waves**
- Rate must be controlled: 1) Beta Blockers, 2) Calcium Channel Blockers, 3) Digoxin, 4) Amiodarone

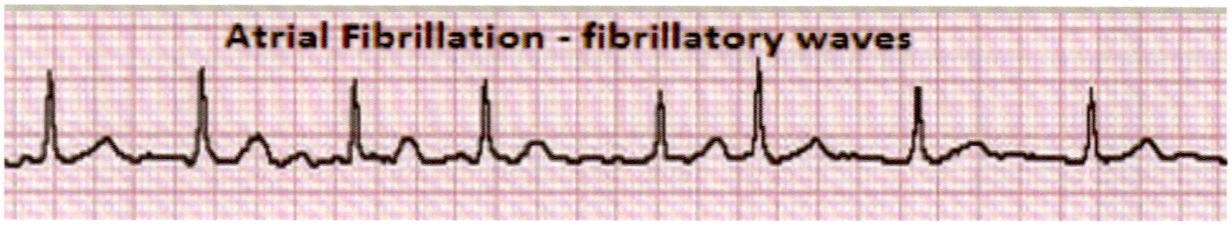

- **Must be on Warfarin therapy: Therapeutic PT/INR is 2 -3 (ideal 2.5) or high risk of throwing an emboli causing a stroke or acute arterial embolus. (Arterial embolus: sudden onset, extreme pain, loss of pulse, cold and discoloration of extremity).**
  (ONLY time PT/INR is 3.5 is if there is a prosthetic valve)
- **Originates in ectopic site: MC location: Pulmonary veins**
- **Anticoagulation determination: CHAD score (stroke risk)**
  Low: no anti-coagulation, use aspirin
  Intermediate: Anti-coagulate or aspirin
  High: Anticoagulate with Warfarin
- **Diagnosis: EKG.**
  If EKG does not show A-Fib: use telemetry monitoring for inpatients and use Holter monitoring for outpatients.
- **Additional test to order once A-Fib is diagnosed:**
  ECHO: check left atrium size, valve function, clots
  Electrolyte levels, TSH, Cardiac enzymes. (TSH: Hyperthyroidism is a common cause of A-Fib)
- **TX: Unstable patients: Synchronized cardioversion**
  Stable patients: Slow ventricular rate if > 100 - 110 bpm
  Rate Control: β-Blockers (Metoprolol, Esmolol), Calcium channel blockers (Diltiazem), Digoxin, Amiodarone.
  Anticoagulation: **Warfarin (INR/PT 2 – 3)**

CHADS2 - VASc Score

	CHAD	SCORE	Stroke Risk	THERAPY
C	Congestive Heart Failure	1	HIGH RISK 2 - 6	Warfarin (INR 2 - 3)
H	Hypertension > 140/90	1		
A	Age > 75	2		
D	Diabetes Mellitus	1	MOD RISK 1	Warfarin or Aspirin
S2	Prior TIA or stroke	2		
V	Vascular Disease	1		
A	Age 65 - 74	1	LOW RISK 0	Aspirin 100 - 300 mg daily
Sc	Sex category (female = 1)	1		

Atrial Flutter

150 bpm
Multiple P waves before QRS
3:1 conduction
"Sawtooth pattern", flutter waves.
Ectopic site: Re-entry circuit by Tricuspid

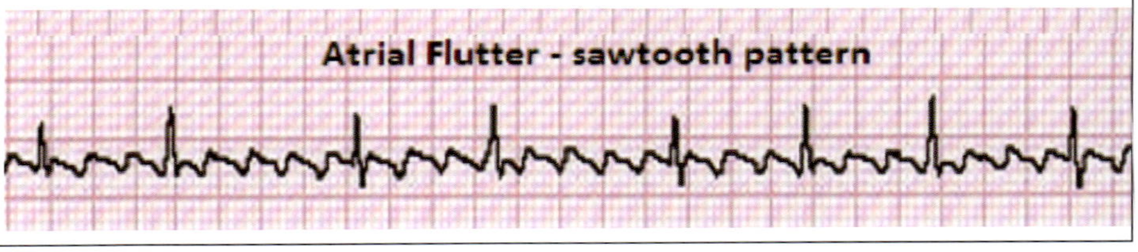

Rate Control drugs for A-Fib and A-Flutter

- Rate Control: **β-Blockers (Metoprolol, Esmolol), Calcium Channel Blockers (Diltiazem), Digoxin, Amiodarone.**

B-Blockers Metoprolol, Esmolol	**Calcium Channel Blockers Diltiazem**	**Digoxin**	**Amiodarone**
Use when patient has: Graves Dz Pheochromocytoma Migraines Ischemic Heart Dz	Use when the patient has/is: Migraine Asthma African American male	Use when the patient has: Hypotension	Use when all other rate control drugs do not work.

Multifocal Atrial Tachycardia (MAT)

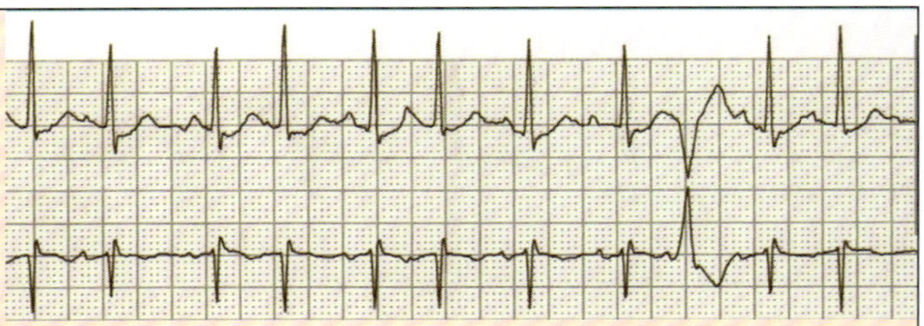

Polymorphic P Waves. Shows various atrial patterns before QRS complexes.
Tachycardia > 100 bpm.
Irregular chaotic rhythm that presents as an atrial arrhythmia.
Associated with COPD and emphysema, chronic lung diseases.
DX: TTE
TX: Treat the same as for A-Fib.
Give oxygen. DO NOT use β-Blockers.

SVT (Supra-ventricular Tachycardia)

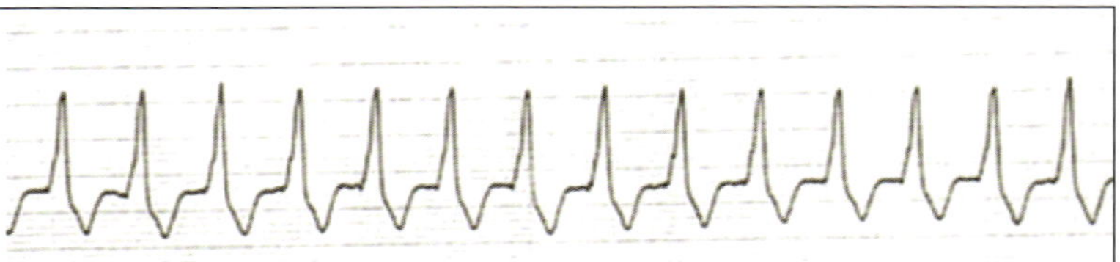

Narrow, Regular QRS
No P waves
Regular rhythm and ventricular rate of 160 – 180 bpm.
Ectopic site: re-entry via tricuspid
DX: Telemetry or Holter monitor if EDG does not show SVT.
TTE.
TX: Stable patient: Vagal maneuvers: **Carotid massage**, ice water face immersion, Valsalva.
Unstable patient: Synchronized cardioversion.

Adenosine: Produced endogenously by the body and is also a medication used in treating heart blocks.

IV Adenosine if vagal maneuvers do not work. It treats SVT's by working at the AV node to cause a transient heart block by inhibiting adenylyl cyclase, ↓ cAMP, ↑ potassium (K) influx causing hyperpolarization, which in turn inhibits Calcium. It is naturally released by the heart to vasodilates the smooth muscle of the arteries to ↑ **coronary blood flow**.
Side effects of Adenosine: Flushing, rash, diaphoresis, nausea, metallic taste, dizziness.

Long term TX of SVT's: Radiofrequency catheter ablation

Ventricular Tachycardia (VT)

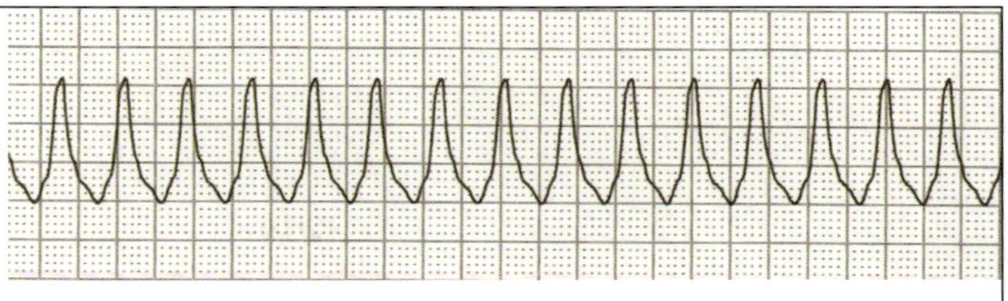

Monomorphic ventricular tachycardia. (All beats match).
Improper electrical activity originating in the ventricles.
HR of ≥ 150 bpm and ≥ 3 consecutive PVC's.
Can lead to: V-Fib, asystole, syncope, and sudden death.
Hemodynamically Stable: Conversion drugs: Lidocaine, Amiodarone, Procainamide, and Magnesium.
Hemodynamically Unstable: Synchronized cardioversion.
DO NOT use any anti-arrhythmic medications to prevent V-tach or V-Fib, makes it worse.

Ventricular Fibrillation (V-Fib)

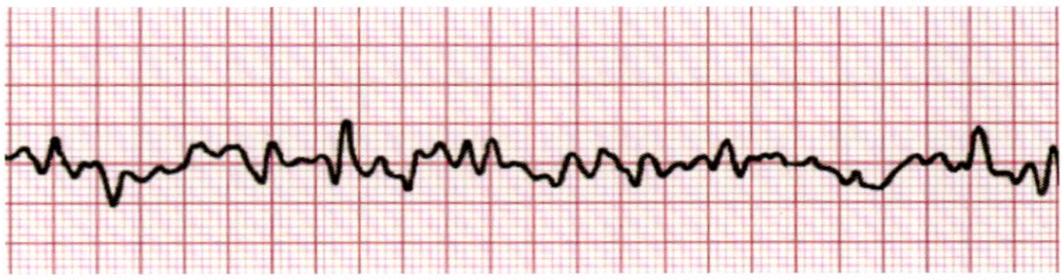

No identifiable pattern
Presents: **Sudden Death. MC reason that someone dies before arriving at hospital or shortly after arrival.**
No recognizable QRS complexes
#1 reason patients die before reaching the hospital or very shortly upon arriving at hospital
Prognosis: **Time to defibrillation.**
1st: Unsynchronized cardioversion. Do **NOT** intubate first – they are NOT breathing because they are dead.
Order of Treatment: CPR➔ unsynchronized cardioversion (defibrillate) ➔ IV epinephrine or vasopressin➔ Defibrillate ➔IV Amiodarone or Lidocaine ➔Defibrillate. (Perform CPR between each shock).
TX: **Implantable defibrillator (Best thing to ↓ deaths from V-Fib is to install defibrillators everywhere).**

Synchronized and Unsynchronized Cardioversion

Synchronized	Unsynchronized
Low energy shock that is synchronized with the peak of the QRS complex. Shock is delivered with or just after peak of the R wave. It does NOT deliver the shock during cardiac repolarization (T-Wave) otherwise the arrhythmia can precipitate V-Fib.	High-energy shock delivered as soon as the shock button is pushed on defibrillator. The shock falls randomly within the QRX complex. Used with there is no coordinated intrinsic electrical activity in the heart (pulseless V-Tach or V-Fib) or when the defibrillator fails to synchronize in an unstable patient. **Defibrillation Administration:** CPR (repeat CPR between each defibrillation) ➔ Defibrillate ➔ IV Epinephrine or Vasopressin ➔ Defibrillate ➔ IV Amiodarone or Lidocaine ➔ Defibrillate (repeat CPR between shocks)

PVC's (Pre-ventricular contractions)

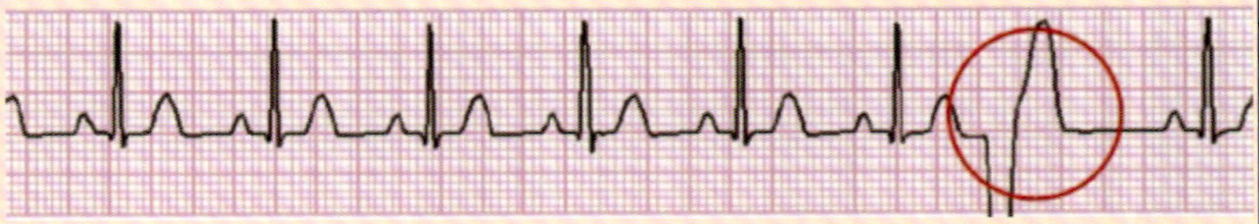

Wide QRS > 120 with bizarre morphology
Causes: Alcohol, smoking, caffeine, stress
Atrial PVC's are benign
EKG shows compulsory pause
No P wave, Widened QRS
Bigeminy: PVC after every other beat
Trigeminy: PVC every 3rd beat
Common post infarct
TX: Symptomatic: **Beta Blockers**
Asymptomatic: Observe

Torsades de pointes

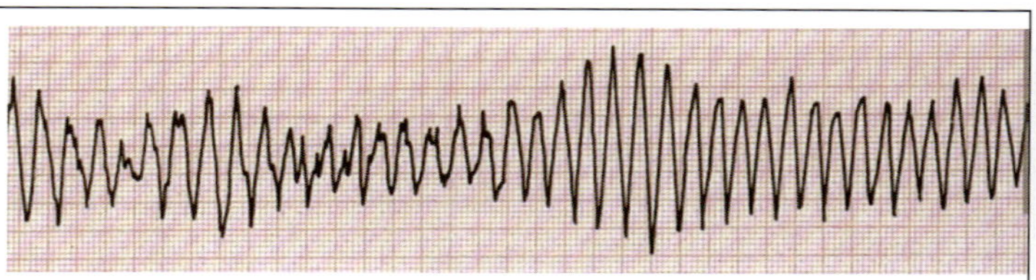

Polymorphic ventricular tachycardia, "winding" pattern
Can progress to ventricular fibrillation (V-fib)
Causes: Class Ia and III Anti-arrhythmics (**Sotalol, Ibutilide**, Dofetilide, Amiodarone), Erythromycin (Macrolides), Thiazides, Risperidone, Long QT Syndromes.
(**Note**: Amiodarone is the **least likely** of the Class III Anti-arrhythmic drugs to cause torsades).
Anytime ↓ in MG and/K there is an increased risk of ventricular arrhythmias and an increased risk of torsades.
Long QT can lead to Torsades
TX: **Magnesium sulfate**
Overdose of Magnesium: check for **decreased deep tendon reflexes.**
Magnesium sulfate also treats for pre-eclampsia and eclampsia.

Pulseless Electrical Activity (PEA)

- Cardiac arrest when a heart rhythm is seen on an EKG but is not producing a pulse (heart is not contracting or there are other reasons that cardiac output is insufficient enough to generate a pulse to supply blood to the body).
  AKA: Heart electrical activity is normal but there is no contraction.
- First line TX: CPR. (Do NOT shock, give CPR).
- Presents: Loss of consciousness, stops breathing spontaneously.
- EKG will show a normal EKG but there will be no pulse.
- **Causes: "6 H's and 6 T's"**
  Must treat the underlying cause.
- 6 H's: Hypovolemia, Hypoxia, Hydrogen ions (Acidosis), Hyper/Hypokalemia, Hypoglycemia, Hypothermia.
- 6 T's: Toxins (drug OD), Tamponade, Tension Pneumothorax, Tachycardia, Thrombosis, Trauma (Hypovolemia: blood loss).
- TX: CPR, IV Epinephrine (1 mg every 3 – 5 minutes)
- **Defibrillators can NOT be used. DO NOT SHOCK.**

Asystole

- **Flatline**. No cardiac electrical activity.
- No contraction = no CO and no blood flow.
- Check for underlying causes: **"6 H's and 6 T's"** (see conditions under PEA)
- TX: CPR or internal cardia massage, IV Epinephrine (AKA: Adrenaline) 1 mg every 3 – 5 minutes or IV Vasopressin 40 units every 3 – 5 minutes.
  Do NOT shock, give CPR alternating with administering vasopressors.
- **Defibrillators cannot be used.**
- **Asystole lasting ≥ 15 minutes, brain will have been deprived of oxygen long enough to cause brain death.**

Noise/Interference on EKG

Non-pathological waves on EKG.

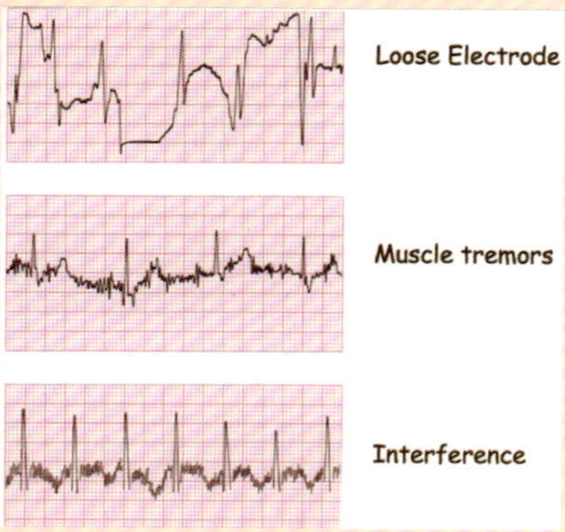

Wolff-Parkinson-White

AKA: Pre-excitation syndrome
Abnormal accessory electrical conduction pathway (AKA: aberrant electrical connection) through Bundle of Kent between the atria and ventricles. Ventricles contract prematurely because the electrical circuit bypasses the AV node. (The AV node is the "gatekeeper" that regulates the electrical activity going to the ventricles).
Reentry circuit.
Presents: SVT that alternates with V-tach. SVT worsens if use of Digoxin or Calcium Channel Blockers.
EKG shows **"Delta Wave"** with shortened PR interval.
SX: Palpitations, shortness of breath, syncope, SVT, dizziness.
DX: Cardiac electrophysiology (EP).
Do NOT use these meds, worsens the condition: Digoxin, Beta Blockers, CCB, Adenosine
Conversion: If unstable: Synchronised shock. If stable: Conversion drugs: Lidocaine, Amiodarone, Procainamide
TX: **Procainamide**, Radiofrequency catheter **Ablation**

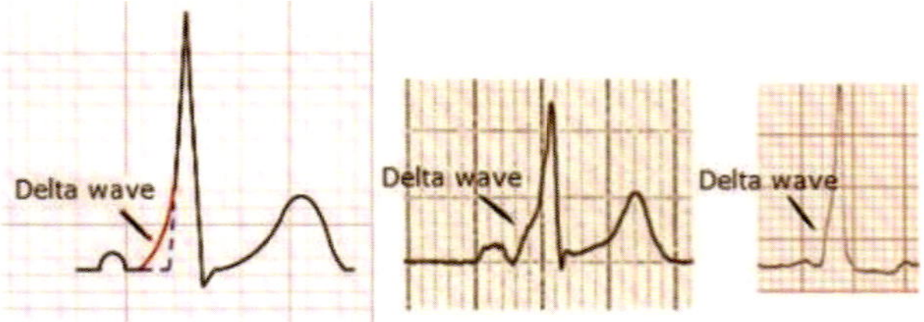

Long QT Syndrome (Congenital)

- Genetic: Inherited disorder of myocardial repolarization
- Mutation of K channels
  Cardiac myocyte action potential duration is determined by K channel proteins
- ↑ risk of sudden death due to torsades
- **Lange-Nielsen Syndrome**/Jervell Syndrome: **AR** Autosomal Recessive. **Deafness**, syncope, QT elongation, torsades. Family history of sudden cardiac death.
  TX: **Propanolol**
- Romano-Ward Syndrome: **AD** Autosomal Dominant. **NO deafness**.

Hypothermia Arrhythmia

- Hypothermia can cause fatal arrhythmias.
- EKG shows J-waves of Osborn. These are patterns that look like ST elevations
- **MC seen in alcoholics that fall asleep outside in the cold**

Heart Blocks

- **Causes: Bradycardia**, Salmonella, Lyme DZ, ANYTHING that slows down the heart (Beta blocker, CCB), Chagas, SA and AV nodal diseases, Digoxin.
  NOTE: Bradycardia (HR <60) can be a normal heart rate for some people. EKG will determine if the bradycardia is normal or pathologic.
- **β- Blockers are absolutely contraindicated in symptomatic heart block.**
  Do not use epinephrine: it may worsen conditions with ischemia (ischemia can cause bradycardia).

1st Degree Heart Block
PR interval is prolonged (> .20 sec)
Benign, No treatment

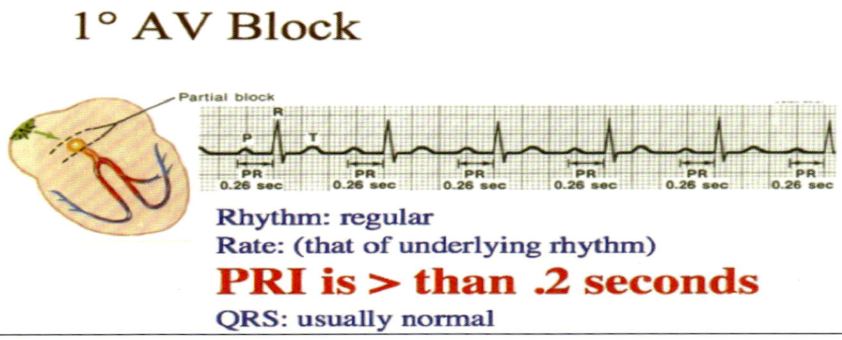

2nd Degree Heart Block
Mobitz Type I (AKA: Wenckebach)
Progressive lengthening of the PR interval until a beat is dropped (a P wave will not be followed by a QRS on the dropped beat)

TX: **Atropine**
If Symptomatic: Pacemaker

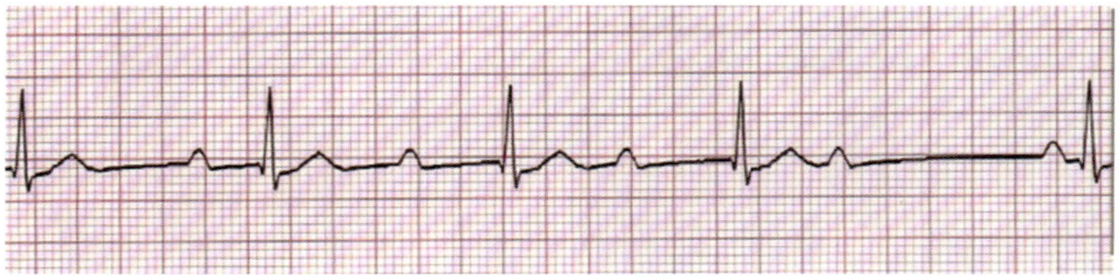

2nd Degree Heart Block
Mobitz Type II
Randomly dropped QRS.
No QRS following a P wave, normal PR intervals
Can progress to Type III
TX: Pacemaker

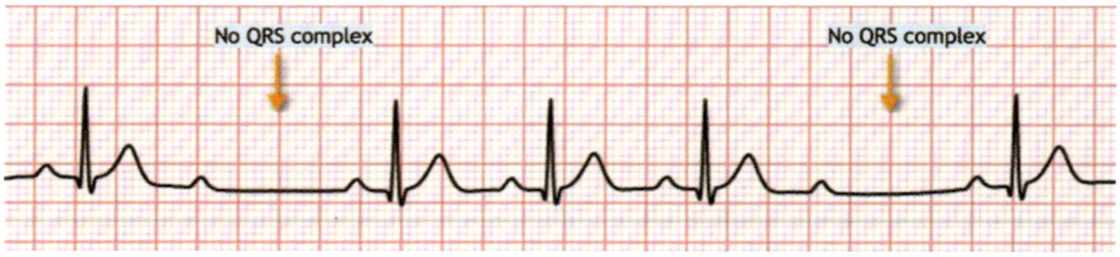

3rd Degree Heart Block
AKA: Complete
The **atria and ventricles beat independently of each other**

Canon A waves, bradycardia, P Waves and QRS are both present, but aren't related
TX: **Transvenous Pacemaker**

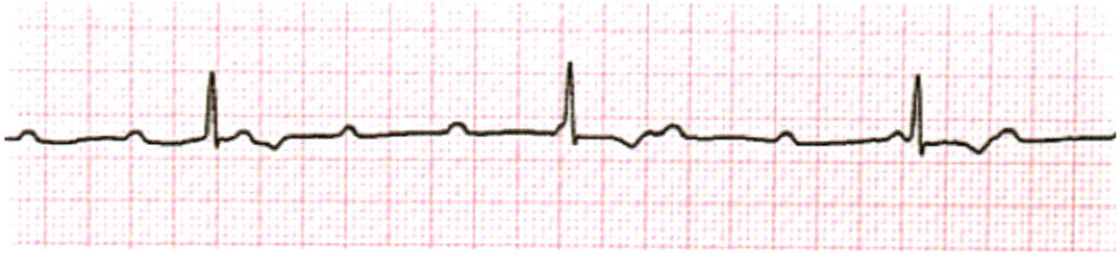

Sick Sinus Syndrome

- Heart switches back and forth from bradycardia to tachycardia
- MC in elderly
- SX: Syncope, dypsnea on exertion, angina
- TX: Pacemaker

Bundle Branch Blocks

Tip to identify EKG patterns of LBBB and RBBB:

LBBB: WiLLiaM MaRRoW (W in lead V1 and an M in V6)

RBBB: WiLLiaM MaRRoW (M in V1 and W in V6

LBBB
QRS > 120
T wave is opposite the QRS wave in V1
V6 (RsR) has "rabbit ears"
Left axis shift/deviation
Originates in the supra ventricle
Causes: Aortic stenosis, MI, CAD, AR, Dilated Cardiomyopathy, Lyme Dz, aortic root dilation

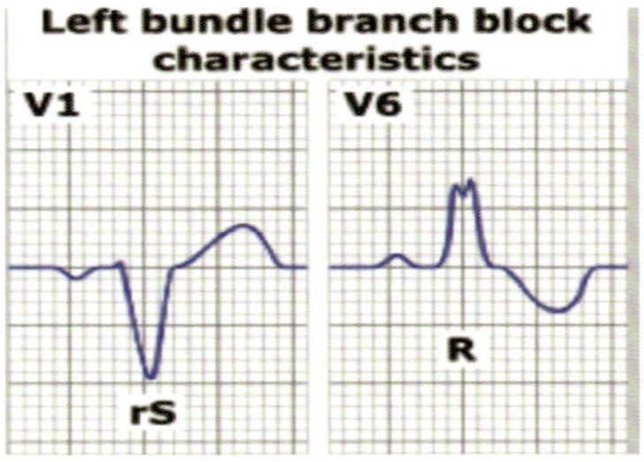

RBBB
Right axis deviation
V1 terminal R wave
V6 rabbit ears
Causes: PE, RVH, Rheumatic heart DZ, Myocarditis, Cardiomyopathy, HTN

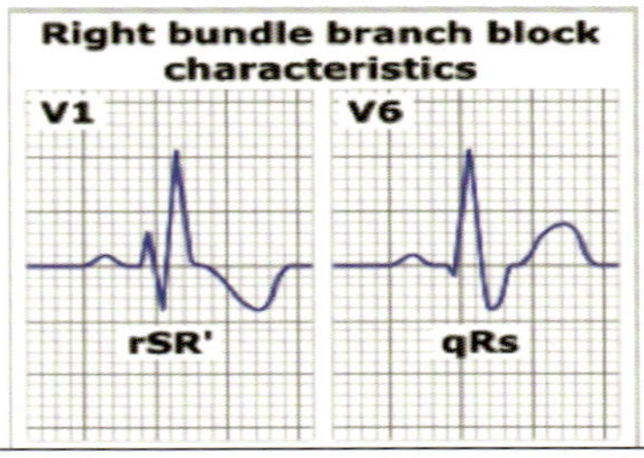

Vascular Pathologies

- All vasculitis present with: Arthralgia (joint pain), rash (skin lesions), fever, neuropathy, weight loss, fatigue.
- All vasculitis labs show: Thrombocytosis, ↑ ESR, normocytic anemia.
- MAT: Biopsy (except for Takayasu Arteritis)
- TX: Prednisone and glucocorticoids. Alternative medicines: Cyclophosphamide, Methotrexate, Azathioprine, 5-MP

Vasculitis

Vasculitis	Description	Symptoms/Diagnosis/Treatment
Large vessel Diseases		
Takayasu Arteritis (AKA: Aortic arch syndrome)	**Asian females** < 40 **Granulomatous** thickening of **Aortic arch**, intimal fibrosis, Vascular narrowing. Presents: Asian female with diminished pulses.	SX: **Weak upper extremity pulses**, night sweats, arthritis, fainting, weight loss, fatigue, anemia. Complications: TIA and stroke due to vascular occlusion. Labs: **↑ESR** HLA-B52 DX: Aortic arteriography or Magnetic Resonance Angiography (MRA) TX: **Steroids (Prednisone)** 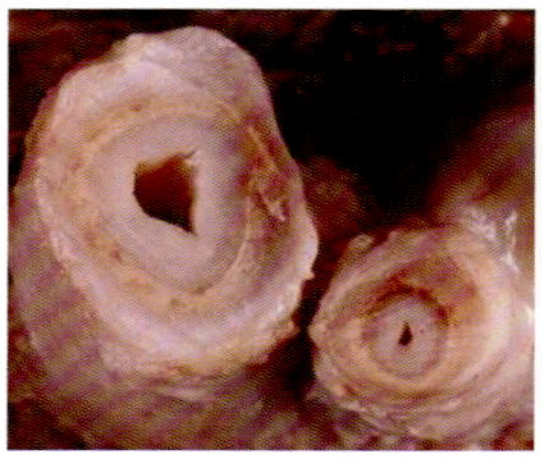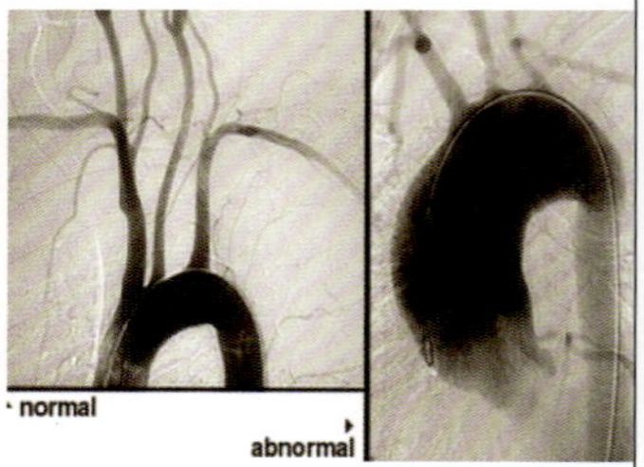
Temporal Arteritis (AKA: Giant Cell Arteritis)	MC: Elderly females MC: **Temporal artery, branch of the External Carotid.** Granulomatous inflammation	SX: Unilateral headache, scalp pain (hurts to brush hair), **jaw claudication** (pain in jaw when chewing), visual changes, symptoms in other arteries: bruits near the clavicle, aortic regurgitation, ↓ arm pulses, fever, weight loss, fatigue. Labs: **↑ ESR, ↑ CRP** **Note:** If the first ESR comes back elevated**, it is best to do a second test** to verify that it is positive for a high ESR before starting steroids, due to the serious side effects of steroids. **Associated with Polymyalgia rheumatic**. DX: **Biopsy of the temporal artery** TX: This is an **emergency. Immediate high dose corticosteroids** to prevent blindness (irreversible) – **do not wait for biopsy results.**
Medium Vessel Diseases		
Buerger Disease (AKA: Thromboangiitis obliterans)	**Heavy smokers**, men <40 **Intermittent (recurring) claudication, inflammation and thrombosis. Leads to gangrene and amputations.**	SX: Chronic inflammation and thrombosis of arteries and veins. Weak or absent peripheral pulses. Skin thin and shiny, reduced hair, skin color changes. Ulcerations gangrene. DX: **Cigar skin sensitivity test** TX: Smoking cessation slows progression. 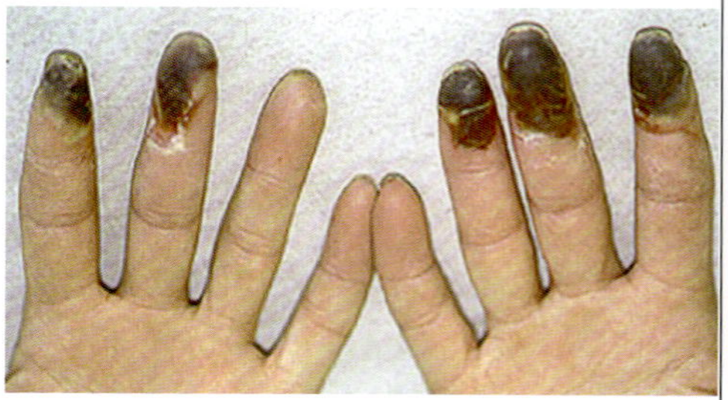 Don't confuse this with Berger's (kidney DZ). (**tip**: b**U**erger for **U**gly (gangrene)

Medium Vessel Diseases cont'd

Kawasaki Disease	MC: **Asian children < 4** **Autoimmune** disease which medium size vessels become inflamed. Risk: **Coronary artery aneurysms** without treatment. Myocarditis, Pericarditis. 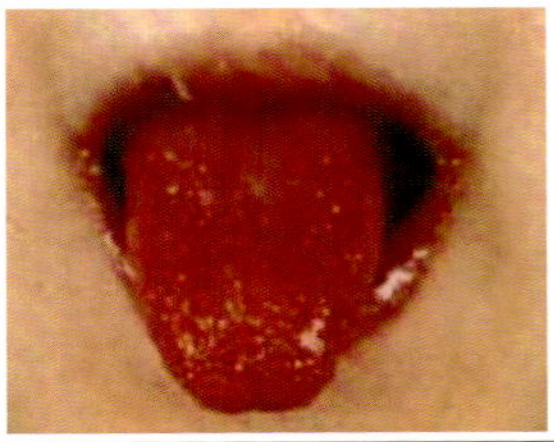	SX: **Must have a high fever (>104° for 4/5 days)**, conjunctivitis of the **eyes (red)**, swelling of hands and feet, **desquamating rash: peeling of the hands and toes**, swollen/painful lymph nodes in neck (cervical), **erythema of mucosal surfaces** in the mouth or lips ("Strawberry tongue") Labs: ↑ ESR, ↑ CRP (C-reactive protein), ↑ Platelets TX: High dose **Aspirin and IVIG.** No steroids. 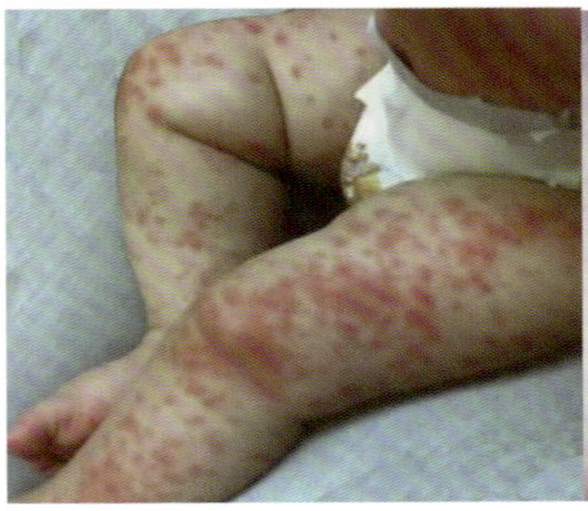 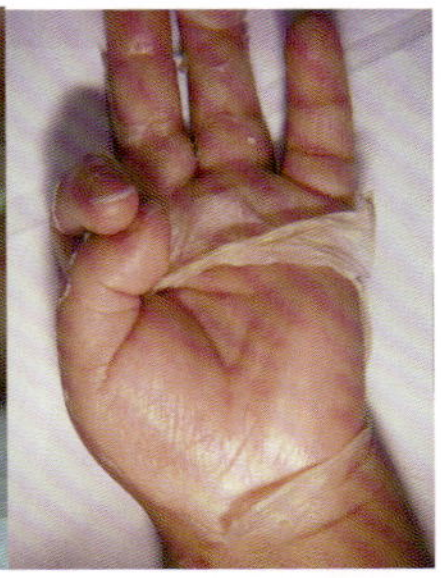
Polyarteritis Nodosa (PAN) (AKA: Kussmaul disease)	Inflammation of renal and visceral vessels. MC in lower extremities. **SPARES the lungs.** **Transmural inflammation** of the artery wall with **fibrinoid necrosis.** Arteriogram shows: microaneurysms and spasms. (Necrosis occurs at the branch points of the arteries). MC: occurs in the renal arteries. 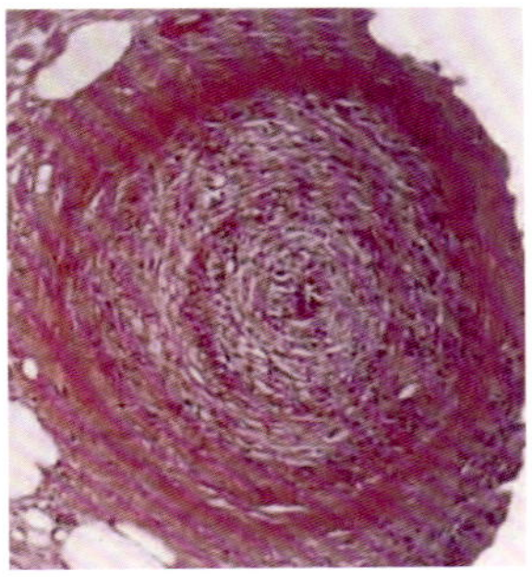 Fibroid necrosis of the vessel wall.	SX: Abdominal pain, HTN, melena, renal damage, fever, headache, weight loss. Skin shows rashes, ulcers and lumps: **Livedo reticularis** (skin with a mottled vascular pattern that appears like a net-like purplish discoloration and is aggravated by cold). GI: **abdominal pain** that is worsened by eating. (Vasculitis of the mesenteric vessels). Neurological: peroneal neuropathy that can lead to foot drop. Strokes, Cardio: Pericarditis. Testicular involvement. Renal involvement. HTN. Labs: Anemia, leukocytosis (↑ WBC). DX: MAT: Biopsy of symptomatic site. Angiography of the kidney shows "**Rosary sign**" (**small aneurysms like a string of beads**) Labs: **↑ ESR, ↑ CRP, P-ANCA.** Immune complexes. **TX: Prednisolone with cyclophosphamide or azathioprine** 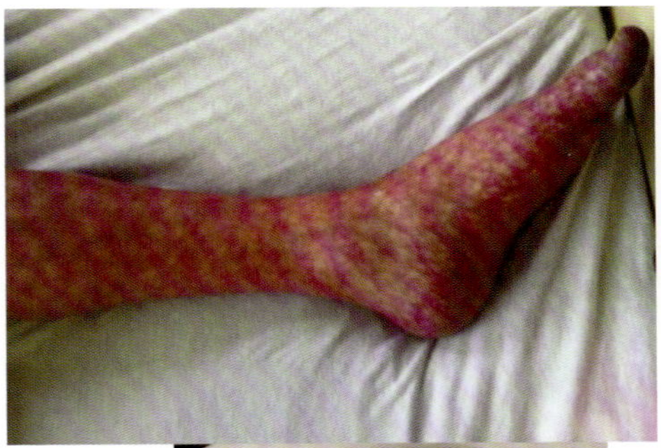 Livedo reticularis **Associated with: Chronic Hepatitis B.** NOTE: Must test all PAN patients for HEP B. (**tip**: "Poly" want a "B" cracker) 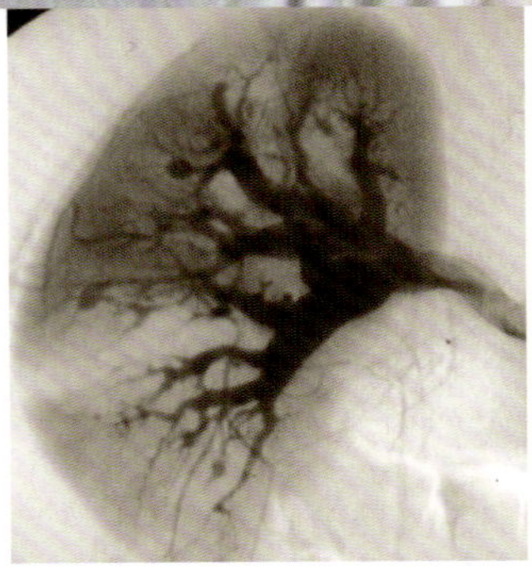 "Rosary Sign"

Small Vessel Diseases		
Churg-Strauss (AKA: Eosinophilic granulomatosis)	Autoimmune disease of medium vessels of patient with a history of allergic airway hypersensitivity. Triad of: Vasculitis, eosinophilia, asthma. **Granulomatous, necrotizing vasculitis with eosinophilia.**	SX: **Asthma or allergic rhinitis** (rhinorrhea and nasal obstruction, sinusitis), **Atopic Dermatitis (eczema like rash)**, **eosinophils, vasculitis** (inflammation of blood vessels), fever, weight loss, joint pain, rashes. **p-ANCA** (perinuclear anti-neutrophil cytoplasmic antibodies with a perinuclear staining and myeloperoxidase. (AKA: MPO-ANCA). **↑ IgE levels** **DX: MAT: Biopsy of lungs.** **TX: Prednisolone with cyclophosphamide or azathioprine**
Henoch-Schönlein Purpura	**Follows URI, usually in one week** 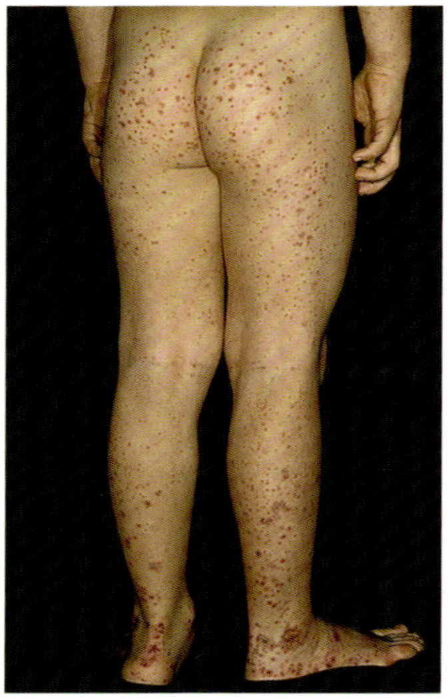 **(BEWARE:** The exam can make Post Strep Glomerulonephritis sound just like Henoch-Schönlein: LOOK at the time from the URI. If it has been **< 1 week it is Henoch**. If it is **> 1 week it is Post Strep** Glomerulonephritis.	SX: Triad of: Palpable **purpura on buttocks and legs (leukocytoclastic vasculitis), arthralgias** (joint pain) and **abdominal pain**, GI tract can present with pain and bleeding, **hematuria**. DX: MAT: **Biopsy** shows **leukocytoclastic vasculitis** (painless, palpable purpura on the buttocks and legs. Associated with **IgA nephropathy**. (**tip**: if you to buy a hen, it should be grade A) TX: Resolves spontaneously in most cases. **Steroids** (used for abdominal pain and/or renal insufficiency).
Microscopic Polyangiitis	**Necrotizing** vasculitis affects small vessels but has **NO granulomas**. Involves multiple organs. **Rapidly progressing glomerulonephritis – Crescents.** 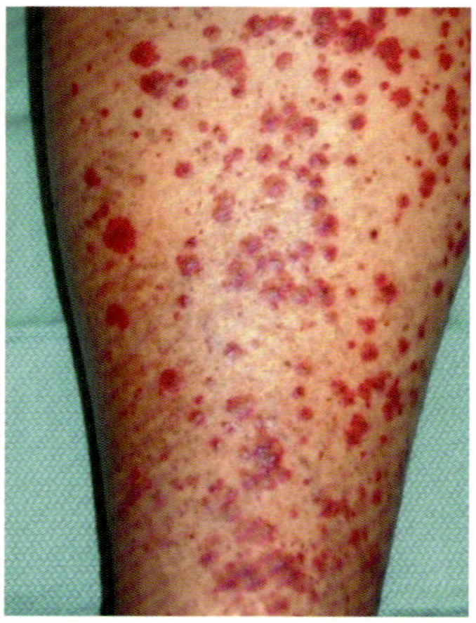	SX: Vasculitis can involve the **lungs and kidneys** (kidney failure). Presents like Wegner's but does **NOT** have any **nasopharyngeal (sinusitis or oral ulcers) involvement or granulomas.** **p-ANCA** (perinuclear anti-neutrophil cytoplasmic antibodies with a perinuclear staining and myeloperoxidase (PMN granule protein) specificity). Antimyeloperoxidase ↑ESR, ↑CRP **TX: Prednisolone with cyclophosphamide or azathioprine**

Wegener's (AKA: Granulomatosis with polyangiitis)	**Necrotizing vasculitis.** Involves lungs, kidneys and **WITH** nasopharyngeal problems (upper and lower respiratory problems), and **granulomas**. Can present as a pneumonia that does **not get better with antibiotics.** **Rapidly progressing glomerulonephritis – Crescents.**	Upper respiratory tract problems: **chronic sinusitis**, nasal septum perforation, **oral ulcers**, **otitis media**, mastoiditis, **necrotizing granulomas** in the lungs and upper airways and **tracheal stenosis**. 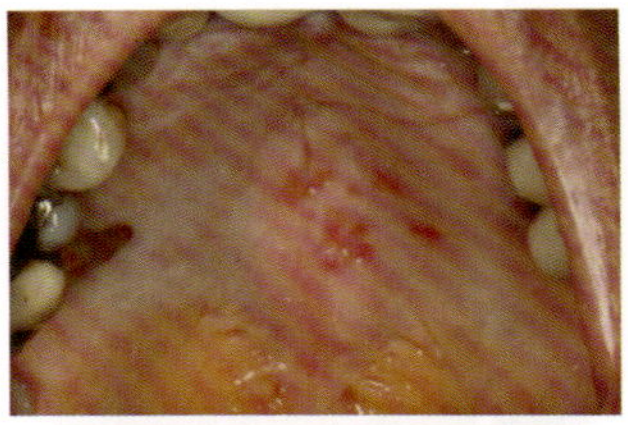 Lower respiratory tract problems: **hemoptysis**. Renal: Red cell cast, hematuria, **necrotizing glomerulonephritis** **(Must involve 3 areas: kidneys, lungs, and pharyngeal area).** (**tip**: The "W" has 3 points = involves 3 areas). 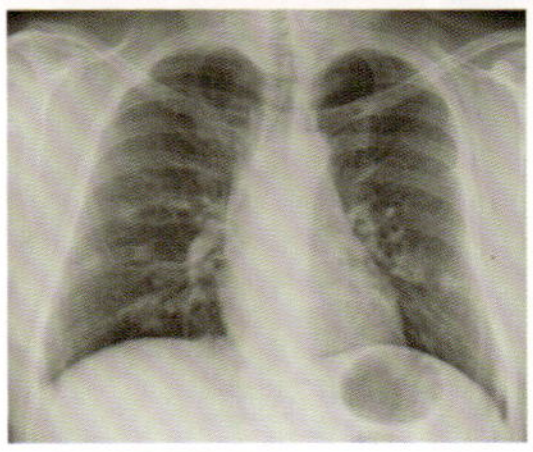 **DX: C-ANCA** (cytoplasmic antineutrophil cytoplasmic antibodies). (AKA: PR3-ANCA) MAT: Lung biopsy. **CXR: nodular densities** **TX: Prednisolone with cyclophosphamide or azathioprine** 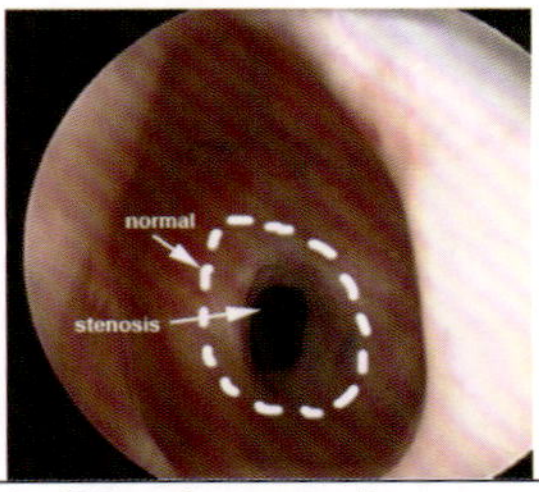
Cryoglobulinemia	Blood contains ↑ **cryoglobulins** (immunoglobulins) that become **insoluble at cold temperatures.** Associated with **HEP C, Sjogren** Syndrome and Multiple Myeloma, Waldenstrom macroglobulinemia, SLE, Rheumatoid arthritis. Labs: **IgM Antibodies against the Fc region of IgG, RF**, cold precipitable immune complexes.	SX: Joint pain, Neuropathy, **Glomerulonephritis (Membranous),** Purpuric skin lesions. Precipitated clumps can block blood vessels and cause toes and fingers to become gangrenous. (**tip**: Member of the "C" club: C = cancer, C = Cryoglobulinemia: C = HEP C) TX: Warm body/blood. Treat underlying causes: HEP C with **Interferon, Ribavirin.** **Caution:** Do not confuse this with cold agglutinins: this causes agglutination of RBC's. (EBV, Mycoplasma, Lymphoma, see hemolysis)
Behçet's Disease	Small vessel systemic vasculitis. MC seen in Asian or Middle Eastern persons.	SX: **Oral and genital ulcers**, **ocular** problems (optic neuritis, uveitis leading to blindness), skin involvement (**Pathergy**: hyperreactivity to needle sticks that result in sterile skin abscesses), lung involvement (hemoptysis, pleuritis), CNS involvement (mimics multiple sclerosis, meningoencephalitis), Cardiac involvement (pericarditis), GI involvement (abdominal pain, nausea, diarrhea, bloating). (**tip**: Behçet's is similar to a bidet toilet. The main feature of this dz. is genital ulcers and it is your genitals that are sitting on a bidet) TX: **Prednisone, Colchicine, Cyclophosphamide, Azathioprine**

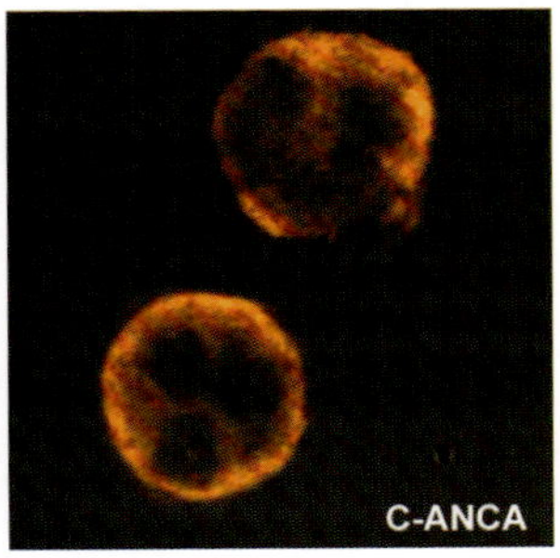

c-ANCA. Cytoplasmic staining of granulocytes

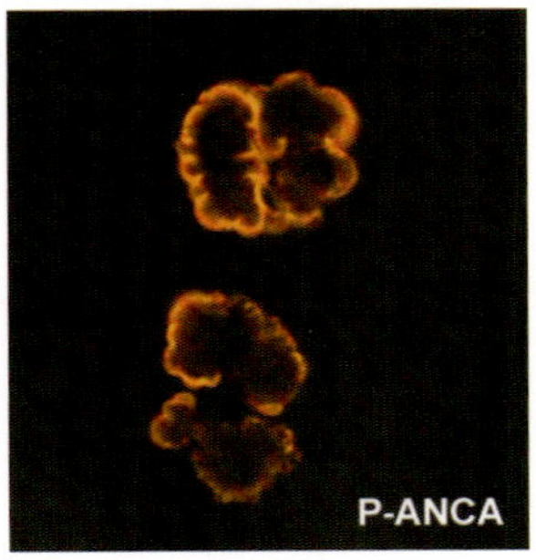

p-ANCA. Perinuclear staining of granulocytes

(**tip**: **c**-ANCA looks like **C**hocolate **C**hip **C**ookies and **p**-ANCA looks like **P**opcorn)

Misc. Vascular Pathologies
Venous Insufficiency (aka: Venous stasis, Stasis dermatitis)

Chronic disease in which the veins in the legs have difficulty returning blood back to the heart due to **incompetent valves and venous hypertension.**

SX: **varicose veins**, heavy pitting edema, swelling, erythema, high risk for cellulitis and cellulitis ulcers, hyperpigmentation, pruritis.

Causes: DVT's, phlebitis (inflammation of a vein), obesity, thrombophilia, arteriovenous fistula.

TX: **Compression stockings and elevation** of legs, lymphatic massage therapy, endovenous laser ablation, vein stripping.

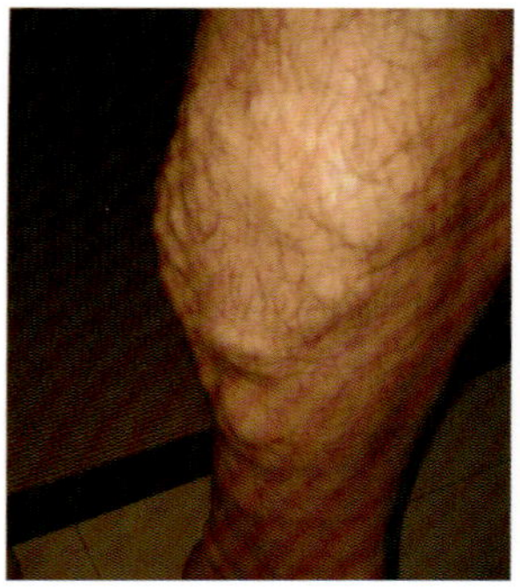

Varicose veins

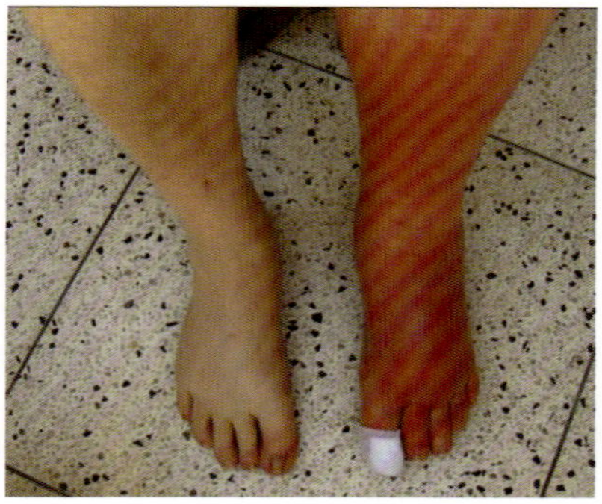

Hyperpigmentation and cellulitis due to venous insufficiency.

Note: The heavy pitting edema looks just like the heavy pitting edema seen with Congestive Heart Failure. A key differential is that the edema due to venous insufficiency will be significantly reduced upon awakening in the morning. Edema from CHF will still be present and **BNP labs will be elevated**. So if a patient states that their edema is decreased in the mornings, their edema is most likely due to venous insufficiency.

Post-thrombotic Syndrome

Complications in the legs due to damage and inflammation of deep vein thrombosis (DVT).
MC in lower extremities.

Cause: Venous valves are damaged b the DVT (thrombus) causing valve incompetence. Because of the continued obstruction from the thrombus the pressure in the veins are increased (venous hypertension).

SX: Similar to venous insufficiency but is due to damage from DVT's.
Pain, aching, cramping, swelling (edema), varicose veins, ulcers.

Risk increase if there is a history of DVT's (more than one in the same leg), obesity, poor anticoagulation therapy, a DVT that last more than one month, patient > 65.

TX: Compression stockings and elevation of legs.

Carotid Artery Stenosis

Narrowing (stenosis) of the carotid artery MCC: **Atherosclerosis** Internal carotid artery supplies the brain. (On the left, the Carotid artery arises from the arch of the aorta and on the right the Carotid artery arises from the brachiocephalic trunk (branch of the aorta. It then divides into the internal and external carotid) Plaque builds up at this division causing stenosis. **If pieces of this plaque break off (emboli) it can cause strokes or TIA's** (transient ischemic attack)	Risk: hyperlipidemia, HTN, smoking DX: Duplex ultrasound, Angiography TX: **If blockage is > 70%** or if patient **is symptomatic** (stroke/TIA) then **carotid endarterectomy** is performed. (surgical correction of the narrowing). This is superior to angioplasty. If blockage is < 70% angioplasty/stenting	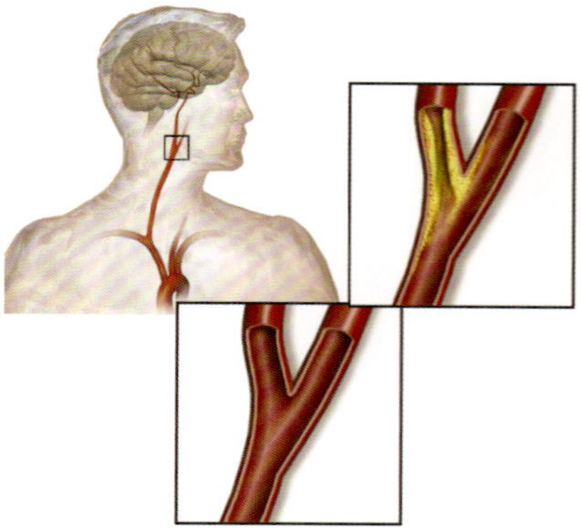

Peripheral Artery Disease (PAD)

(AKA: Peripheral vascular disease, peripheral artery occlusive disease)

Narrowing of arteries other than the heart or brain, most common are the **legs.** MC cause: atherosclerosis. **PAD = CAD = DM** (Narrowing of heart arteries = coronary artery disease, narrowing of the brain arteries = cerebrovascular disease) Main risk factor: **Smoking.** Other risk factors: Diabetes, HTN, and high cholesterol. Don't confuse this with **Spinal stenosis**. Spinal stenosis is worse walking downhill and is less when walking uphill or cycling. Pulses and skin will be normal. SX: **Leg pain when walking which resolves with rest.** (Same as stable angina in the heart), **bluish skin** (poor circulation), skin ulcers, little hair on skin.	DX: BIT: **Ankle-brachial index (ABI) of < 0.90** (normal ABI: ≥ 0.9) Greater than a 10% difference = obstruction. ABI = systolic blood pressure at the ankle divided by systolic blood pressure of the arm. MAT: Angiography. TX: Cilostazol (inhibits phosphodiesterase 3 (PDE3) stops platelet aggregation and vasodilates, **Aspirin, ACE inhibitors** (controls HTN), **Statins,** Target LDL goal < 100, **Stop Smoking**, exercise. **(Don't forget: Cilostazol is BOTH a vasodilator and a platelet aggregation inhibitor).** Calcium channel blockers do not work. They only expand the outside of the vessel, not the inside where the atherosclerosis is located.	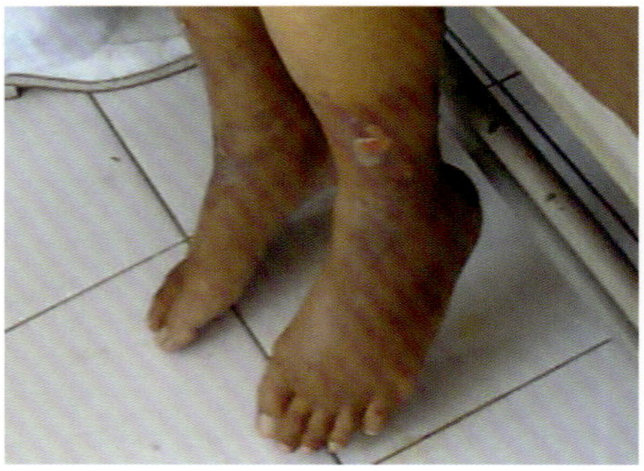

Raynaud's Phenomenon

Vasospasms that ↓↓ Blood flow in response to **cold or emotional** stress causing discoloration of fingers and toes. SX: Extreme pale discoloration of fingers or toes, numbness. MC: women Causes: Raynaud's Disease = idiopathic Raynaud's Syndrome = when **associated** with another disease process: **SLE or CREST** (limited Scleroderma) TX: **Calcium channel blockers** (Same treatment as for other vasospasm disorders: Prinzmetal angina, cocaine MI's)	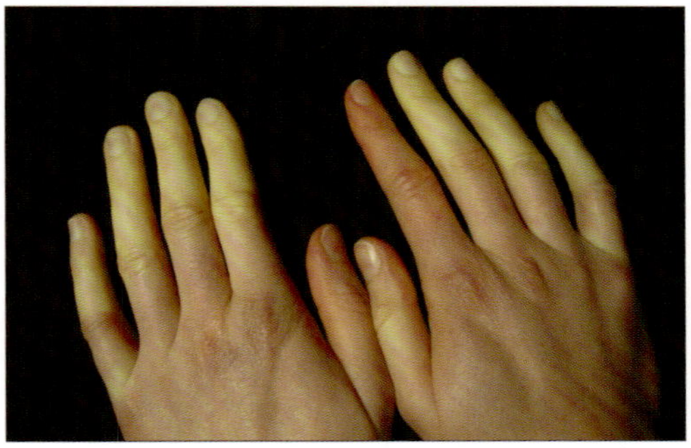

Leriche Syndrome (AKA: Aortoiliac occlusive disease)

Peripheral artery disease associated with the bifurcation of the **abdominal aorta at the bifurcation of the common iliac arteries**. AKA: Claudication at the femoral and common iliacs affecting the low back, hip, butt, thigh. MC: Smokers and with atherosclerosis SX: Claudication of the buttocks and thighs, erectile dysfunction, absent or decreased femoral pulse. Bruit in the iliac and femoral arteries. Atrophy of the lower extremities. (Triad of symptoms: claudication plus impotence and atrophy of lower extremities). TX: angioplasty or vascular bypass	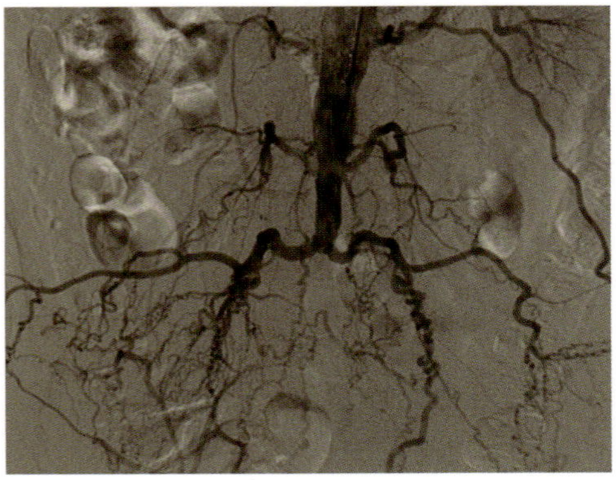

Osler-Weber-Rendu Disease
AKA: Hereditary Hemorrhagic Telangiectasia

Autosomal dominant **AVM Disease** (Arteriovenous malformation). Widespread AVM's (abnormal blood vessel formation) in GI, mucous membranes, skin, liver, brain, lung. Pulmonary AVM's can cause fatal hemorrhages. SX: **Telangiectasis** on the body (MC: lips), recurrent nosebleeds, clubbing, hematuria. Polycythemia (due to right to left shunting causing hypoxia).	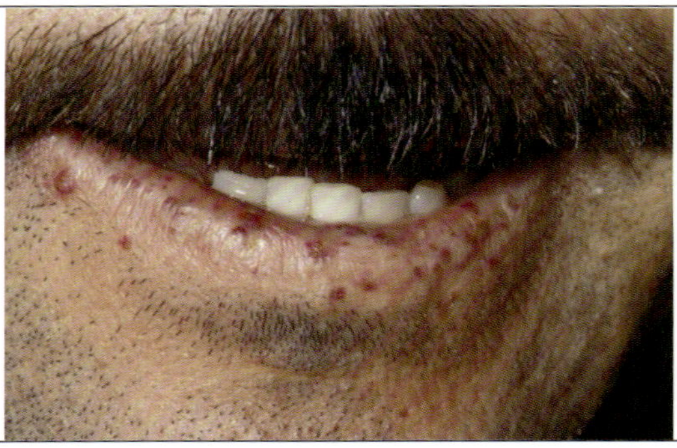

Vascular Tumors

Tumor	Description	Picture
Angiosarcoma	Vessel cancer – aggressive, poor prognosis MC: elderly and sun exposed areas, radiation, and arsenic.	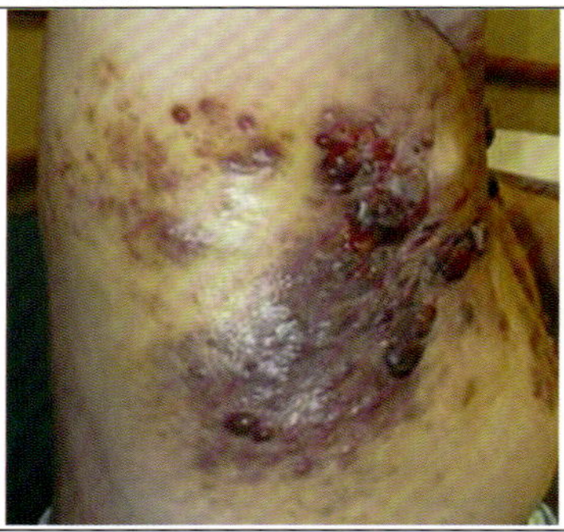
Bacillary Angiomatosis	Benign proliferation of **blood vessels forming tumor-like** masses on the skin and organs. (Can be mistaken for Kaposi sarcoma, biopsy to verify) Cause: Bartonella henselae (cat scratch/bite or ticks and fleas. Bartonella quintana is transmitted by lice. MC: assocated with HIV	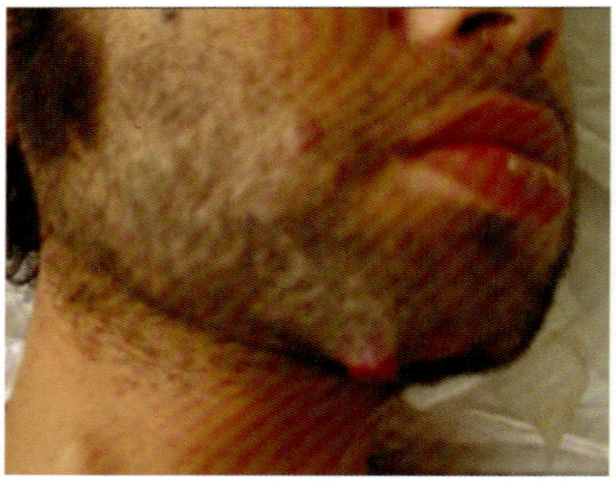
Cystic hygroma (AKA: lymphatic malformation)	Cavernous **lymphangioma on the neck**. Congenital lymphatic lesion. Contains large cyst-like cavities containing lymph Highly associated with **Turners syndrome** DX: prenatal ultrasound	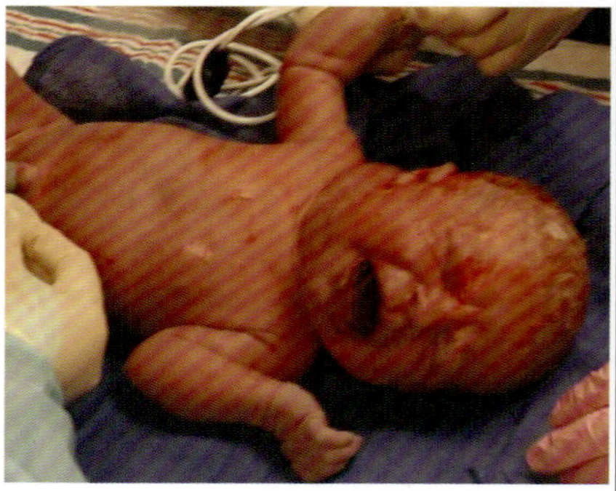

Glomus tumor	Benign tumor arising from the glomus body under the fingernail. Can also be found in the hand, foot, middle ear and wrist. SX: Painful, pain is reproduced in cold water. Glomus body = component of the dermis layer of the skin and is involved in temperature regulation. TX: Surgical extraction	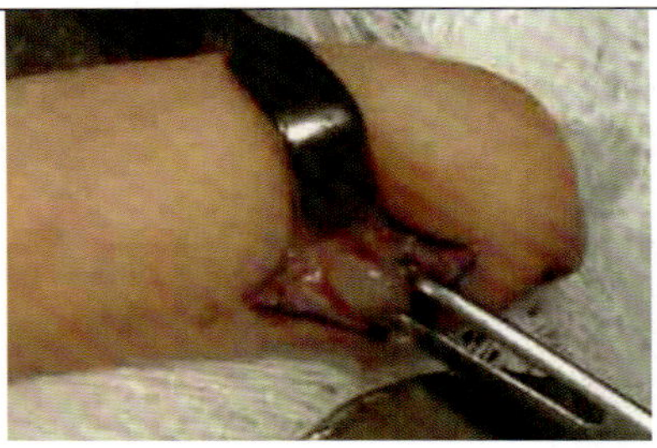
Kaposi sarcoma (HSV 8)	Tumor caused by infection with **herpesvirus 8.** **AIDS defining illness,** transmitted through **saliva**, (associated with deep kissing), organ transplants and blood transfusions **DX: skin biopsy** SX: **Nodules or blotch lesions** that are purple, red, brown or black in color. Can be on the skin, genitalia, mouth, GI or respiratory tract **Endothelial origin. (NOT epithelial)**	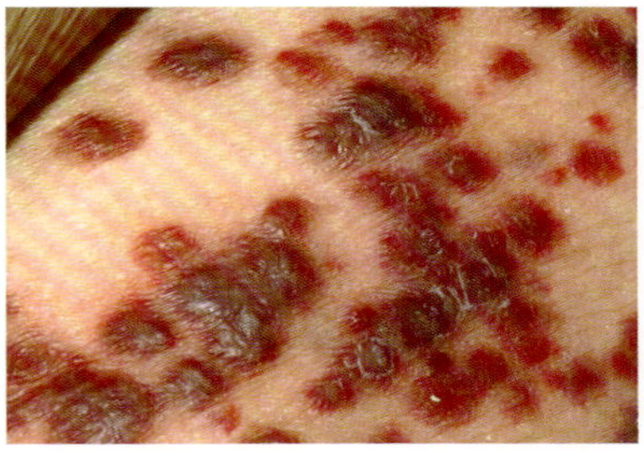
Lymphangiosarcoma	Malignant tumor associated with the **lymphatics**. **MC: post-radical mastectomy** SX: Massive lymphedema of the arm (following removal of the axillary lymph nodes), bruise mark on the skin that progresses to an ulcer and necrosis **TX: Compression sleeves**	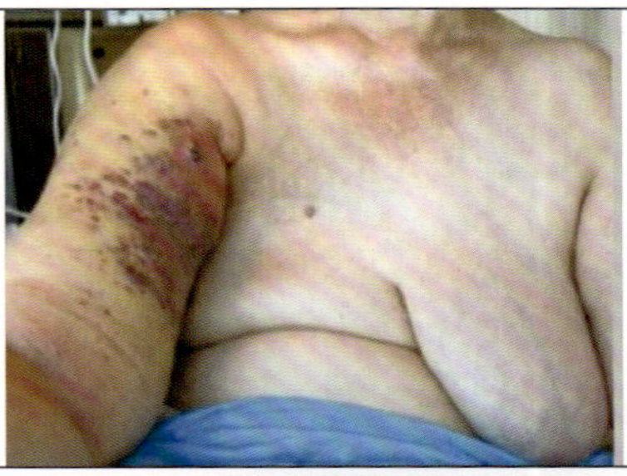
Pyogenic granuloma AKA: Granuloma gravidarum, Tumor of Pregnancy)	Vascular lesion that is due to an **overgrowth of a tissue** due to an irritation, physical trauma or hormones. MC in gums, skin and nasal septum. Look similar to a hemangioma but they appear after birth. SX: red/pink, purple granuloma, smooth or lobulated.	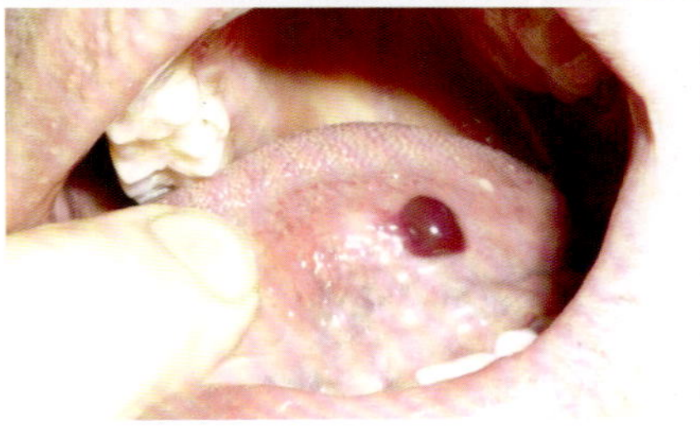
Cherry hemangioma	Benign capillary hemangioma of abnormal proliferation of blood vessels that increases with age (**elderly**) and does not regress. SX: Red or purple round dome on top of the skin. Can bleed profusely if injured. **Note:** the origin of hemangiomas are endothelial. This is not a skin problem, it is vascular. So do not choose epithelial or ectoderm origin.	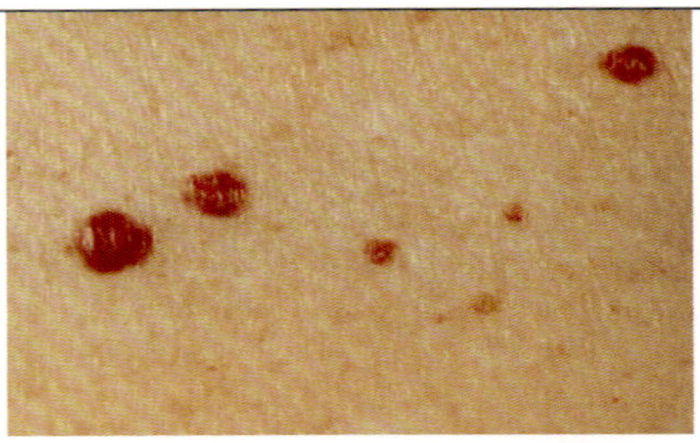
Strawberry hemangioma	Benign capillary hemangioma of endothelial cells of blood vessels in **infants/children**. Appears after birth, grows rapidly for first 6 months, and usually regresses between 5 and 12 years of age. (**tip**: children play with **S**trawberry shortcake). **Note:** the origin of hemangiomas are endothelial. This is not a skin problem, it is vascular. So do not choose epithelial or ectoderm origin.	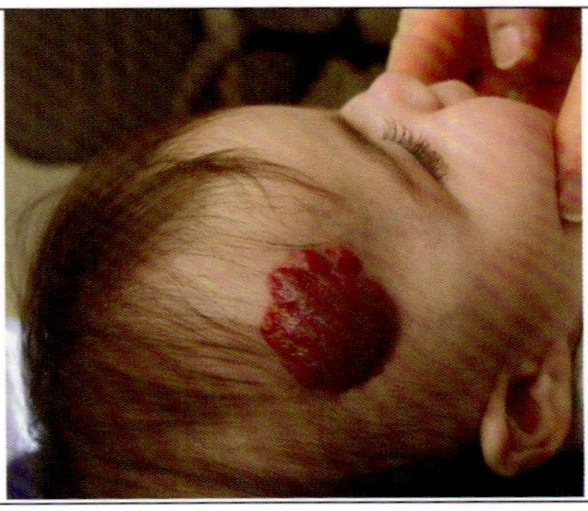

CARDIOVASCUAR PHARMACOLOGY

Antiarrhythmic Pharmacology

Class 1: Na Channel Blockers

- ↓ conduction of Na in depolarized cells
- ↓ slope of 0 Phase (AKA: Depolarization)
- ↑ threshold for firing
- ↓ SA node rate
- 1C > 1A > 1B (1B dissociates fast)
- Term: **ERP** (Effective Refractory Period): (AKA: Absolute refractory). Period of time that a new action potential can't be initiated. (**tip**: absolutely NO)
- Term: **Torsades de pointes** ("twisting of points"): Polymorphic QRS. Varied amplitude and cycle length. Irregular rhythm originating in the ventricles. Long QT.

Drugs Affecting the Cardiac Action Potential

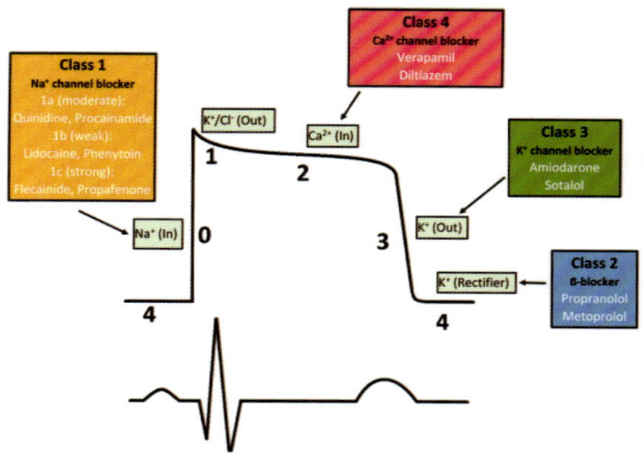

Torsade de Pointes

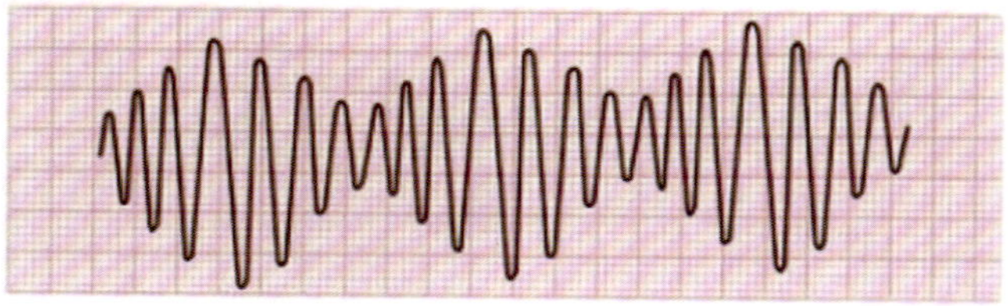

Class I Antiarrhythmic Drug Effects

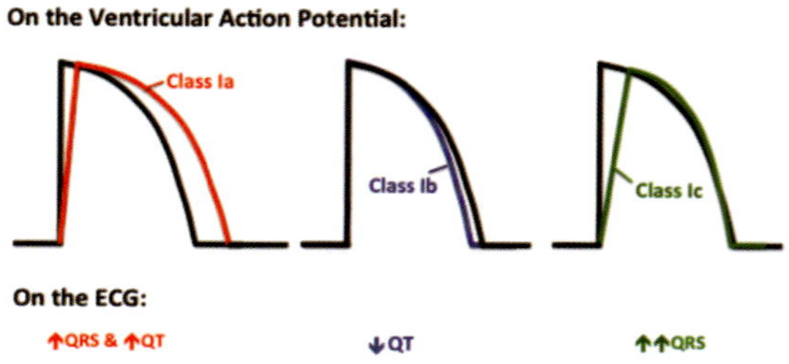

DRUG GENERIC name Trade name	Clinical Use	Mechanism of Action	Toxicity
Class 1A – Sodium (Na) Channel Blockers			
Disopyramide Quinidine **Procainamide** (**tip**: **D**ouble **Q**uarter **P**ounder)	Ventricular arrhythmias, recurrent A-fib, SVT. **Procainamide:** Wolff-Parkinson-White, Depressant action on SA and AV nodes. Cardio conversion.	**Blocks Na channels** in depolarized cells. (↓ Conduction velocity of depolarized cells) ↑ **AP duration** (lengthens the action potential). (AKA: Slows the upstroke of the AP). ↓ Conduction velocity. ↑ **QT Interval.** ↑ **Effective Refractory Period** (ERP) (prolongs ERP). Prolongs QRS. ↓ **Phase 0** depolarization Prolongs Phase 3.	All: ↑ **QT = torsades** (TX: **Magnesium sulfate**). Thrombocytopenia, ↑ K (hyperkalemia) Quinidine: Cinchonism (headache, tinnitus, vertigo) **Procainamide:** **Reversible SLE**-like syndrome (anti-histone antibody, antinuclear antibody)
Class 1B – Na Channel Blockers			
Lidocaine Tocainide Mexiletine Phenytoin (**tip**: **L**ettuce, **T**omato and **M**ayo **P**lease) Or: **P**eople **L**ove **M**exican **T**acos)	**Best for Ventricular arrhythmias.** **V-Tach.** (V-tach: arrhythmias that originate within the ventricular tissue). **Lidocaine:** **Best Post-MI drug**. and ventricular arrhythmias. Cardio conversion. Local anesthetic	**Blocks Na channels** in depolarized cells. (↓ Conduction velocity of depolarized cells) ↓**Phase 3 repolarization** ↓ **AP duration** Fast dissociation from Na Channels.	Lidocaine: CNS stimulation/depressant.

Class 1C – Na Channel Blockers			
Flecainide Encainide Propafenone (**tip**: **F**ries for **E**veryone **P**lease OR: **F**leas **E**at **P**eople)	SVT, A-fib	**Blocks Na channels** in depolarized cells. (↓ Conduction velocity of depolarized cells) No affect on AP. **Prolongs refractory period** in AV node. Prevents paroxysmal A-fib. Acts on His-Purkinje system.	Contraindicated with structural abnormalities: Post MI, ischemic heart dz. Proarrhythmic.

Class 2: β-Blockers*

- ↓ **HR and contractility** = ↓ **Oxygen demand** of the heart
- ↑ **Filling time in diastole (remember: diastole filling controls the coronary artery blood flow to the heart)**
- **Key: In Pheochromocytoma surgery you MUST give an α-1 blocker BEFORE a β-Blocker, otherwise you leave unopposed α-1 receptors = HTN emergency! In a Cocaine MI treatment (vasospasms/diffuse ST elevations)**
- **you must NOT use a β-Blocker because it leaves the α-1 receptor unopposed = HTN emergency. You must ONLY use a Calcium Channel Blocker.**
- ↓ **MI mortality**
  ***Drugs that ↓ mortality: β-Blockers, Ace Inhibitors, Aspirin, Spironolactone**
  Procedures that ↓ mortality: Implantable fibrillator, Angioplasty (balloon, PCI: Percutaneous Coronary Intervention)

DRUG **GENERIC name** **Trade name**	**Clinical Use**	**Mechanism of Action**	**Toxicity**
The "lol's" **Acebutolol** **Atenolol** **Betaxolol** **Bisoprolol** **Carvedilol** **Esmolol (short acting)** **Labetalol** **Metoprolol** **Nadolol** **Nebivolol** **Pindolol** **Propranolol** **Timolol** (**Tip**: **Selective: A – M.** **Non-Selective: N – Z** Exception: C and L Carvedilol Labetalol: These **both** selective **and** non-selective **and** work on α and β	SVT (↓ AV conduction velocity), V-Tach, Rate control (A-fib, atrial flutter), CHF (↓ progression of chronic heart failure), ↓ HTN (↓ CO = ↓ Renin (β-1 Receptor blockade on JG cells), MI (↓ mortality), angina pectoris (↓ HR and contractility = ↓ O2 consumption) **Timolol:** Glaucoma (↓ aqueous humor) **Propanolol:** Thyrotoxicosis, Essential tremors, migraines, portal HTN, Performance anxiety Nebivolol: combines β-1 and β-2 activate nitric oxide. Used to treat HCM because it allows the heart to slow so there is more time to fill. More blood in the heart is important for HCM.	↓ cAMP and ↓ Ca currents = ↓ SA and AV nodes activity. **↓ Afterload, ↑ EDV, ↓ BP, ↓ Contractility, ↓ HR.** Negative chronotropic effect. Negative inotropic effect. **↓ Phase 4 and ↓ conduction through AV node.** ↓ Conduction of AV node = ↑ **PR interval**. (**prolongs**) ↓ Ventricular rate and peripheral resistance (AKA: **Afterload**). **Inhibits release of renin** = ↓ vasoconstriction = ↓ Na and H_2O retention. Give with Nitrates to ↓ affects of reflex tachycardia.	All: **Bradycardia, AV block**, CHF, sedation, depression, **impotence**, **mask the signs of hypoglycemia**, weight gain. ↑ risk impotence in African American males. **Use CCB instead: Amlodipine.** **Do not use non-selective with ANY breathing problems** (asthma, COPD, etc)- must use only selective. Causes exacerbation. Metoprolol = dyslipidemia (↑ Cholesterol). **DO NOT GIVE in Cocaine MI's** (users) due to unopposed α-adrenergic activity and ↑↑↑ HTN. **Give ONLY CCB.** Prior to surgery for pheochromocytoma: must **give α-Blockers before β-Blockers** or will cause unopposed α-adrenergic activity. Propanolol: exacerbate vasospasms: Do not use in: Prinzmetal angina, Raynaud's. Pindolol, Acebutolol: Contraindicated in angina because they are partial beta agonist. **TX for OD: Glucagon** (↑ cAMP)

Class 3: Potassium (K) Channel Blockers

DRUG GENERIC name Trade name	Clinical Use	Mechanism of Action	Toxicity
Amiodarone Bretylium Dofetilide Ibutilide Sotalol	Atrial and ventricular arrhythmias. Are used as last resort. Amiodarone, Sotalol: Cardio conversion. **Ventricular fibrillation** (V-Fib): Treatment of choice: Defibrillation **before** conversion. **(Best prognosis for V-Fib is time to defibrillation)**	↑ **Phase 3** due to ↓ K current which causes: **↑ AP, ↑ ERP, ↑ QT**	ALL: **Torsades de pointes** due to ↑QT and bradycardia. (MCC: **Sotalol, Ibutilide**. All K channel blockers can lead to torsades de pointes). Least likely to proceed to torsades: Amiodarone. **Sotalol: Torsades de pointes**, excessive β blockade. Bretylium: New arrhythmias and ↓ blood pressure. **Amiodarone**: **Pulmonary fibrosis, hepatotoxic, hypo/hyperthyroidism** (**Amiodarone is 40% iodine**), photosensitivity, bradycardia, heart block, CHF, neurological effects, skin color changes, corneal deposits, constipation, gynecomastia. **MUST FOLLOW: LFT's, TSH, and PFT's. Do not use in patients with lung disease (Asthma, COPD, obstructive/restrictive pathologies).**

Class 4: Calcium (Ca) Channel Blockers (CCB)

- Block Calcium Channels (CCB)
- **Cardiac** Ca Channel Blockers: **Non-dihydropyridine** Calcium Channel Blockers: **Verapamil, Diltiazem** (**tip**: **Non**-di**HYDRO**pyridine = **Not hydro**, so **not for fluid** (blood)
- Cardiac and smooth muscle depend upon **extracellular Ca to L-Type Calcium channels**
- CCB do not affect skeletal muscles, they do not require the influx of Calcium for excitement
- **Slows conduction in the AV nodes to ↓ heart rate** (**Negative inotropic**)
- **Shortens Phase 2**
- ↓ contractility of the heart so do not use in heart failure

DRUG GENERIC name Trade name	Clinical Use	Mechanism of Action	Toxicity
Non-dihydropyridine Calcium Channel Blockers: For Cardiac.			
Verapamil Diltiazem Cardizem	Nodal arrhythmias, AV Nodal reentry, SVT, **Cocaine use/MI.** **Use with any vasospasm pathology: Cocaine MI, Prinzmetals angina, esophageal spasms, Raynaud's.** **Diltiazem:** (vasospasms): **Prinzmetal's Angina, Reynaud's** **Verapamil is best for the ventricles.** (**tip** = V = Ventricles)	↓ L-type voltage dependent Calcium channels in the AV nodal cells (cardiac) to ↓ contractility. (AKA: Stops voltage channels to the AV node → prolongs PR interval → slows heart rate). Calcium channel blockers **decrease intracellular calcium** = ↓ contractility. L-type Calcium channels are responsible for the plateau phase. **↓ Conduction velocity, ↑ ERP, ↑ PR Interval** **Note**: Cardiac glycosides (inotropes) ↑ contractility by ↑ intracellular calcium levels.	Antimuscarinic effects: Constipation, dizziness, flushing. Edema, negative inotropy, AV block, sinus node (SA node) depression. Verapamil: Gingival hyperplasia and causes ↑ prolactin levels. **DO NOT COMBINE CCB and β-Blockers = negative chronotropic effect, severe bradycardia and hypotension.**

Dihydropyridine Calcium Channel Blockers: (tip: diHYDROpyridine = hydro is fluid (blood). NOT FOR CARDIAC - DO NOT HAVE ANY EFFECT ON THE HEART			
Amlodipine **Nimodipine** **Nifedipine** Fenoldopam Clevidipine	**HTN Control** (vasodilates arteries) **Amlodipine**: Use for **HTN in African American males** instead of β-Blockers (↑ risk of impotence) **Nimodipine**: use for vasospasms in **Subarachnoid hemorrhage**. (**tip**: **NEMO** swims (in blood) **Nifedipine**: Best used with bradycardia because it causes reflex tachycardia (so gets HR up). **Fenoldopam**: Use in HTN emergencies. Artery dilation ➔ ↓ TPR ➔ ↑ Renal perfusion ➔ ↑ natriuresis. **Clevidipine:** Use with hypertensive urgency or emergency.	↓ L-type voltage dependent Calcium channels in the smooth muscle cells to ↓ contractility. **Act on vascular smooth muscle (arterials) ➔ vasodilation ➔ ↓ HTN.** (CCB do not work on venous smooth muscle)	Lower leg/ankle **edema**. Gingival hyperplasia. Dizziness, headache, red face (flushing).

Drugs Causing Prolonged QT (↑ risk of torsades)

- Amiodarone
- Methadone
- Procainamide
- Lithium
- Erythromycin
- Chloroquine
- Sotalol
- Quinidine
- Haloperidol
- Clarithromycin
- Cisapride
- SSRI

PR Interval Changes

- PR: Beginning of P wave to start QRS complex
- ↑ PR: 1st degree heart block, hypokalemia, acute rheumatic fever, lyme dz
- ↓ PR: **Wolfe-Parkinson White** (AKA: Pre-excitation syndrome)
  Wolfe-Parkinson White: Abnormal conduction b/t atria and ventricles = SVT, palpitations, dizziness, SOB, syncope, **delta wave** (slope in the rise of the QRS). TX: Obliteration.

Misc. Antiarrhythmics

DRUG GENERIC name Trade name	Clinical Use	Mechanism of Action	Toxicity
Adenosine	**Supraventricular Tachycardia (SVT)** when vagal maneuvers do not work, palpitations. SVT: arrhythmia originating at or above the atrioventricular node (AV node). **Vagal Maneuvers**: Carotid massage, Valsalva maneuver, submersing head in cold water. (**tip**: **ADD**enosine = **ADDs** to the **top of the ventricles**: SVT)	Hyperpolarizes cells and ↓ intracellular Calcium and ↑ K out of the cell.	Flushing, burning (pain) in the chest, hypotension. Effects are blocked by theophylline and caffeine.
IV Magnesium Sulfate **(AKA: Epsom salt)**	**Eclampsia, Torsades de pointes, Digoxin toxicity.** Replacement therapy for hypomagnesaemia,		Monitor for **overdose** (hypermagnesaemia): Shown by ↓ in deep tendon reflexes. TX: Stop medication.

Cardiac Glycosides

DRUG GENERIC name Trade name	Clinical Use	Mechanism of Action	Toxicity
Digoxin	**Rate control**: A-fib (↓ conduction at **AV node**), CHF (↑ contractility) **Caution**: Narrow therapeutic window. Must use cautiously in elderly, easy to OD. **Must ↓ dose in Digoxin in elderly**. (↓ clearance in the kidney's) and **slow acetylation.** Caution: Must ↓ warfarin dose if on digoxin	**Direct inhibition of Na/K ATPase pump. This indirectly inhibits Na/Ca exchanger (antiport) causing Ca to become trapped inside the cell and decreasing the influx of Na into the cell = ↑ contractility (positive inotropy), ↑ ejection fraction. It increases the intracellular calcium levels.** ↑ Parasympathetic activity of the heart by acting on the Vegas Nerve (CN X) = ↓ HR. ↑ Diastolic filing time. ↑ Contraction by ↑ intracellular Ca. ↓ ESV, ↑ EF Positive inotropic effect. Negative chronotropic effect. Cleared by **kidneys**. **Note**: Calcium channel blockers ↓ intracellular calcium levels which then ↓ contractility.	**GI symptoms**: anorexia, nausea, vomiting, diarrhea, abdominal pain, causes **vision problems (yellow-green halos, blurry vision**, problems with color perception), drowsiness, insomnia, agitation, depression, delirium. EKG changes: **T-wave inversion** (↓ K), ST depression, ↑ PR, ↓ QT. Overdose MOA: Digoxin "looks" like potassium (K) to the receptors. When hypokalemia occurs, digoxin binds the K (on the Na/K ATPase pump) = digoxin toxicity. **OD TX:** Anti-digoxin Fab fragments, Magnesium Sulfate, Atropine, activated charcoal in attempted suicides.

MISC Cardiac Pharmacology

DRUG GENERIC name Trade name	Clinical Use	Mechanism of Action	Toxicity
Nitrates Nitroglycerin **AKA: EDRF: Endothelium derived relaxing factor. (mimics nitric oxide)** **Isosorbide dinitrate (sublingual)**	Angina, Acute coronary syndrome, pulmonary edema **Isosorbide mononitrate is 100% bioavailable by mouth. (sublingual)**	Venodilation and arterial vasodilation. **Predominantly a venodilator.** **↓ Preload = ↓ EDV, ↓ BP, (reflex) ↑ Contractility, ↑ HR.** **↑ NO (nitric oxide) in vascular smooth muscle → ↑ cGMP smooth muscle relaxation. (NO is located in the meninges and skin)** EDRF: produced and released by the endothelium to promote smooth muscle relaxation. **↑cGMP** = ↓ Calcium → Myosin Dephosphorylase. ↓ ventricular stress = ↓ angina and ↓ blood pressure. ↓ Preload (decreased volume), ↓ Stretch of cardiac wall, ↓ heart size, ↓ Oxygen requirement, ↓ work load on the heart.	Hypotension, flushing, headache, reflex tachycardia. (TX: reflex tachycardia with β-Blockers) **DO NOT take with phosphodiesterase Inhibitors** (Sidena**fil**, (Viagra), Tadala**fil** (Cialis), Vardena**fil** (Levitra). This can lead to a fatally low blood pressure due to ↑↑ vasodilation. (**tip**: the "**fil**'s" **fill** the penis) **"Monday Disease" (Monday morning headache)** Severe headaches due to tolerance/dependence on nitroglycerin. Patient uses nitroglycerin during the week, and becomes dependent on it. He goes off of the nitroglycerin over the weekend (loss of tolerance). He starts back on the medication on Monday morning, which results in headache, dizziness, and tachycardia.
Clevidipine	Dihydropyridine calcium channel blocker. Use with hypertensive urgency or emergency.	↓ L-type voltage dependent Calcium channels in the smooth muscle cells to ↓ contractility. **Act on vascular smooth muscle (arterials) → vasodilation → ↓ HTN.** (CCB do not work on venous smooth muscle)	Lower leg/ankle **edema**. Gingival hyperplasia. Dizziness, headache, red face (flushing).
Hydralazine	**Methyldopa and Hydralazine: 1st line HTN in pregnancy.** HTN	Vasodilates arterioles and veins. Predominantly an **arterioles and arteries as a vasodilator by ↑ cGMP** = smooth muscle dilation. ↓ Afterload. Administer a β-Blocker in conjunction with Hydralazine to prevent reflex tachycardia.	**SLE-Like Syndrome**, headache, nausea
Abciximab TIrofiban Eptifibatide	Angioplasty (stents/balloon/PCI), Unstable angina. ↓ mortality with ST Depression.	**GPIIb/IIIa inhibitors.** Anti-platelet drugs. **Inhibit platelet aggregation.**	Bleeding, thrombocytopenia
Aspirin **(AKA: acetylsalicylic acid, ASA)**	Antiplatelet = ↓ platelet aggregation. **↓ Mortality in MI by 50%**	**Irreversibly inhibits cyclooxygenase (COX-1 and COX-2).** **↓ TXA_2**	↑ Bleeding time.

Clopidogrel	Antiplatelet = ↓ platelet aggregation. **Better drug than aspirin with stents. Aspirin allergies.**	**Inhibits the ADP receptor on platelet cell membranes.**	↑ Bleeding time. TTP
Atropine	Heart **Blocks** (2nd Degree Block: AKA: Mobitz Type 1, AKA: Wenckebach. Also for 3rd Degree heart block), Bradycardia (**tip**: meet me **AT** the **BLOCK**)	Blocks the Vagus Nerve (CN X). Muscarinic antagonist. (Vagus is parasympathetic, heart block is too parasympathetic)	Do not use in closed angle glaucoma.
IV Furosemide *Lasix*	**Diuresis in CHF, Acute pulmonary edema to ↓ Preload.**	Loop Diuretic. Inhibits cotransport of Na/K/2Cl of thick ascending limb of loop of Henle.	↓ K, ↓ Ca, ototoxic, sulfa allergy, gout (hyperuricemia), interstitial nephritis, acute pancreatitis
Ace Inhibitor	HTN, ↓ remodeling of heart after MI.	Vasodilates arteriole/arteries and venodilates: works on both sides of the heart. ↓ Peripheral vascular resistance. ↓ venous return. **↓ Preload and ↓ Afterload.** **Preserves K.**	Cough, angioedema
Dobutamine	Stress Test (Ischemia). Heart failure, cardiogenic shock	Inotropic = ↑ contractility. Sympathomimetic. $B_1 > B_2$ effects	
Dipyridamole	Stress Test (Ischemia)	Phosphodiesterase III inhibitor. ↑ cAMP in platelets = inhibits platelet aggregation, vasodilates, and causes **Coronary Steal Syndrome,** used to test for ischemia	
Dopamine **Nor-epinephrine** **("pressor 's")**	Hypotension		
Ranolazine	Angina when first line therapies are not effective.	Inhibits the late inward sodium current in cardiac muscle to ↓ intracellular calcium levels. This ↓ the tension on the heart wall to reduce the workload on the heart, thus decreasing the demand for oxygen.	Dizziness, constipation, headache, nausea, prolonged QT.

Hypertensive Emergencies (AKA: Malignant Hypertension)

- Hypertensive Emergencies: Blood pressure > 180/110.
  Patient presents to the ED.
  Must have end organ damage: **Papilledema MUST be present before diagnosis of malignant HTN can be made**.
  TX: Hypertensive emergency drugs (below)
  Blood pressure must be **lowered slowly**: Reduce no more than 25% within minutes to 1 - 2 hours. Then achieve a level of 160/100 mm Hg within 2 to 6 hours. Too rapid of reduction in blood pressure can cause ischemia or infarction to: coronaries, cerebrum, and kidneys.
- **Hypertensive Urgency** (Clinical situation – less urgent, not an emergency)
  Patient present to your office. May not even be aware of the ↑↑ HTN.
  TX: HTN control: meds, lifestyle changes, etc.

DRUG **GENERIC name** **Trade name**	**Clinical Use**	**Mechanism of Action**	**Toxicity**
Nitroprusside Fenoldopam Nicardipine Clevidipine Labetalol	HTN Emergency Causes of HTN Emergencies: Cocaine, amphetamines, preeclampsia, eclampsia, pheochromocytoma, Glomerulonephritis	**Nitroprusside: ↑ NO release increases cGMP.** **Fenoldopam (CCB):** Dopamine (D1) receptor agonist. Artery dilation → ↓ TPR → ↑ Renal perfusion → ↑ natriuresis.	Cyanide toxicity is a side effect of nitroprusside and nitric oxide. **Treatment Options:** Thiosulfate, Met Blue, Hydroxocobalamin. Hydroxocobalamin combines with cyanide to form cyanocobalamin (Vitamin B-12), which is excreted. Sodium nitrate induces methemoglobin in RBC's, which combines with the cyanide. Methemoglobinemia is then treated with Methylene Blue. Methylene blue inhibits Monoamine Oxidase. This changes the iron form Ferric (F^3 iron form) to Ferrous (F^4 iron form). Vitamin C can also assist in treating methemoglobinemia. Sodium thiosulfate transforms cyanide (donates a sulfur atom) to thiocyanate by rhodanese, which is then excreted.

Preload – Afterload Results

Drug	**Preload Results**	**Afterload Results**
Diuretics	↓ = ↓ volume = ↓ cardiac work	
Ace Inhibitor	↓ Preload Vasodilate: ↓ peripheral vascular resistance, ↓ venous return Preserves K	↓ Afterload Vasodilate: ↓ peripheral vascular resistance, ↓ venous return Preserves K
Phosphodiesterase Inhibitor	↓ Preload Vasodilates	↓ Afterload Vasodilates
Positive Inotropes		↓ Afterload = ↑ Contraction = ↓ Peripheral Vascular Resistance
Sympathometics		↓ Afterload = ↑ Contraction = ↓ Peripheral Vascular Resistance
Vasodilators	ACE Inhibitor/ARB, Hydralazine, Adenosine: ↓ BP, ↓ TPR, ↑ CO (when ↓ BP, heart ↑ CO to compensate	

CHOLESTEROL/LIPID PHARMACOLOGY

DRUG GENERIC name Trade name	Clinical Use	Mechanism of Action and Resistance	Toxicity and Notes
HMG-CoA reductase Inhibitors **The "statins"** **Atorvastatin** **Lovastatin** **Pravastatin** **Rosuvastatin** **Simvastatin**	**1st Line DOC to lower cholesterol.** ↓↓ cholesterol and ↓ triglycerides and ↑ HDL. ↓ mortality in coronary artery disease and post-MI.	↑ **(up regulates) LDL Receptors** (so they are out looking for more cholesterol to bring in). This ↑ in LDL receptors is the RESULT of the statins that causes the decrease in cholesterol (not the primary action of statins) Inhibits HMG-CoA reductase which ↓ liver cholesterol: Stops conversion of HMG-CoA to mevalonate so mevalonate can't convert into cholesterol, which ultimately increases transcription of HMG-CoA reductase. (**Cellular MOA:** Statins inhibit HMG CoA reductase leading to a decrease in cholesterol. The cell senses this decrease which causes cell signaling to increase the transcription and formation of HMG CoA reductase to try and meet cholesterol requirements)	**Hepatoxicity** **Rhabdomyolysis: Do NOT use fibrates (P-450 inhibitor)** or **niacin with Statin's**, they will ↑ muscle damage. (See myoglobin in the urine), Monitor CK. Note: Statins reduce hepatic cholesterol synthesis, lowering intracellular cholesterol, which stimulates upregulation of LDL receptors and increases the uptake of non-HDL particles from the systemic circulation.
Fibrates **Fenofibrate** **Gemfibrozil** **Bezafibrate** **Clofibrate**	↓ **Triglycerides**	**Inhibits 7 α-hydroxylase** (rate limiting enzyme to make bile acid from cholesterol) so cholesterol is unable to convert to bile. ↑ LPL to ↑ triglyceride clearance. Activates **PPAR-α** to ↑ HDL synthesis. (**tip**: Triglycerides are also called TAGS, so think of clothing (clothing is made of fiber), so all clothing has a price TAG on it, and the price on the tag is $7)	**P-450 Inhibitor.** **Do not use with Statins = ↑ muscle damage (rhabdomyolysis).** **Gallstones. Do not use with Bile Acid Resins = ↑ gallstones.** Hepatotoxicity, myopathy, gallstones. **(High triglycerides can lead to acute pancreatitis)**
Bile Acid Resins **Cholestyramine** **Colestipol** **Colesevelam**	↓ **Cholesterol**	**Inhibits absorption of bile acids in the intestine. By inhibiting the absorption of bile acids, the liver is forced to pull/use more cholesterol up in order to make more.** **Can be used synergistically with Statins.**	**Gallstones.** Bad taste. ↑ Triglycerides. ↓ absorption of fat-soluble vitamins.
Cholesterol Absorption Blockers. **Ezetimibe**	↓ **Cholesterol** Can also be used to Decrease pruritis in patients with partial biliary obstruction and in bile acid diarrhea.	**Inhibits cholesterol absorption at the brush border in the small intestine.** Specifically inhibits the transport Protein NPC1L1.	Diarrhea, abdominal pain, headache, Rash, angioedema. Note: Use when statins are contraindicated or inadequate.
PCSK9 Inhibitors Alirocumab Evolocumab	↓ **LDL** ↓ **Triglycerides** ↑ **HDL**	**Inactivates LDL receptor degradation** which increases the amount of LDL removed from the bloodstream.	Delirium, myalgia, demential

Niacin (Vitamin B3)	Hyperlipidemia ↑ **HDL** ↓ **VLDL** Also decreases LDL and triglycerides. Promotes weight loss. (**tip**: HDL is the “good” cholesterol. So it is NICE (Niacin) to be good)	**Inhibits lipolysis in adipose tissue. Inhibits triglyceride synthesis in the liver** which decreases production of VLDL and LDL. Niacin increases HDL.	Flushing (mediated by prostaglandins). Can TX cutaneous side effects (ie: flushing) by taking 325 mg aspirin 30 – 60 minutes prior to taking Niacin. **Do NOT use with statins** = ↑ muscle damage. Niacin causes insulin resistance (hyperglycemia) = **MUST ↑ diabetic medicines.** Niacin stimulates vasodilation = **MUST ↓ HTN medicines.** **Hyperuricemia = gout**
Orlistat	↓ Absorption of triglycerides	**Inhibits pancreatic lipase**	GI side effects. Steatorrhea (oily, loose stools), fecal incontinence, excessive flatulence. ↓ absorption of Vitamin A.

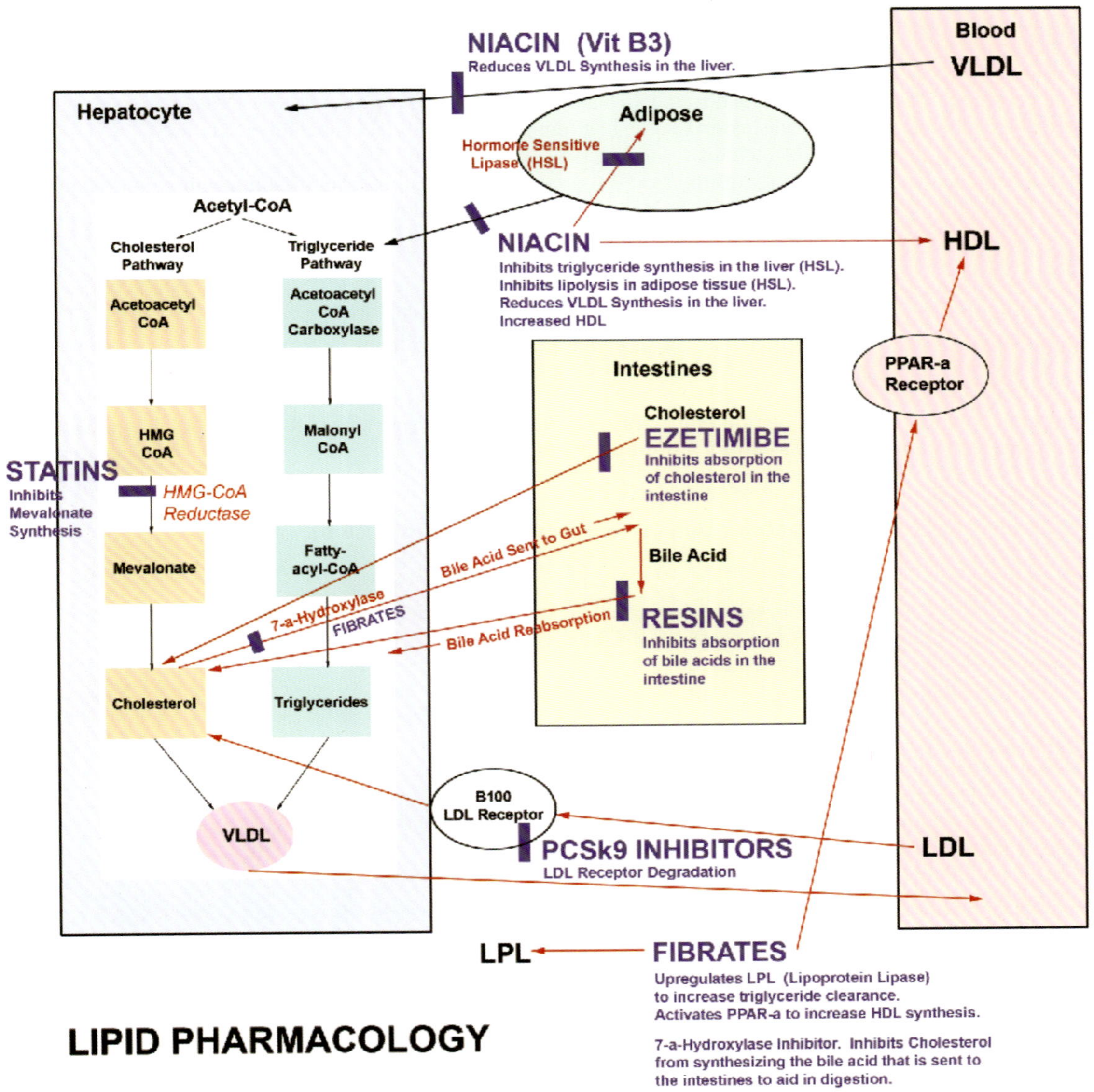

RESPIRATORY - PULMONARY

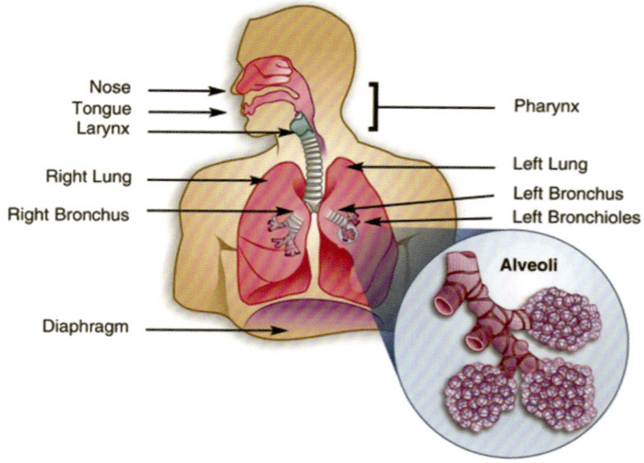

Muscles of breathing
Any use of accessory muscles means difficulty breathing

Inspiration
- Normal quiet inspiration: Diaphragm
- **Accessory** inspiration muscles: External intercostals, scalene muscles, sternomastoids

Expiration
- Normal quiet expiration: No muscles needed. It is passive.
- **Accessory** expiration muscles: Rectus abdominus, internal/extremal obliques, transverse abdominus, internal intercostals

Conducting Zone
- Large airway: nose, pharynx, larynx, trachea, bronchi
- Small airways: bronchioles, terminal bronchioles.
- **Medium bronchioles = highest resistance** (**tip**: **M**edium for **M**ost resistance)
- Dead space: where there is no gas exchange. (Pulmonary embolisms cause the lungs to vasoconstrict to shunt blood away to other working parts of the lung for gas exchange, so this area is now dead space)
- Cells
  Goblet cells extend to the beginning of the terminal bronchioles.
  Pseudostratified ciliated columnar cells extend to the beginning of the terminal bronchioles.
  Cuboidal cells start at the terminal bronchioles.
- Bronchioles: smallest airway (≤ 1 mm), terminate at the alveoli. Ciliated cuboidal epithelium over smooth muscle. The smooth muscle allows them to change in diameter so can increase or decrease airflow.

Respiratory Zone
- Respiratory bronchioles, alveolar ducts, alveoli.
- Cuboidal cells in respiratory bronchioles.
- Alveolar macrophages (AKA: Dust cell) (clear debris and are involved with immune response)

Dead space
- This is any area in which the alveoli (ventilation, diffusion) and capillaries (perfusion, flow) do not line up. There is **ventilation but there is no perfusion (flow). Example: Pulmonary Embolism.**

Shunt (aka: Physiologic shunt)
- Is the space where there is **perfusion (flow) but there is no ventilation (diffusion).**

Physiologic dead space
- The structures of the airway or blood vessels are normal, but there are other reasons why the alveoli and capillaries don't match up. Example: shunting of blood away from one area of the lungs (physicological obstruction).
  The total sum of the alveolar dead space and the anatomic dead space.

Alveolar dead space
- The difference between the anatomical dead space and the physiologic dead space. Represents the space in the alveoli occupied by air that does not participate in gas exchange (aka: alveolar ventilation). This can vary in different parts of the lungs and under different conditions.

Anatomical dead space
- The airways of the mouth, nose, pharynx, larynx, trachea, bronchi and bronchioles.
  An obstruction of either the airways or blood supply (ie: PE) or a foreign body inhaled.

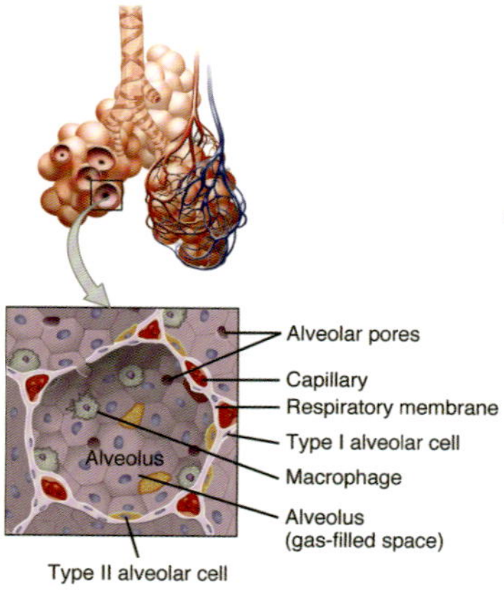

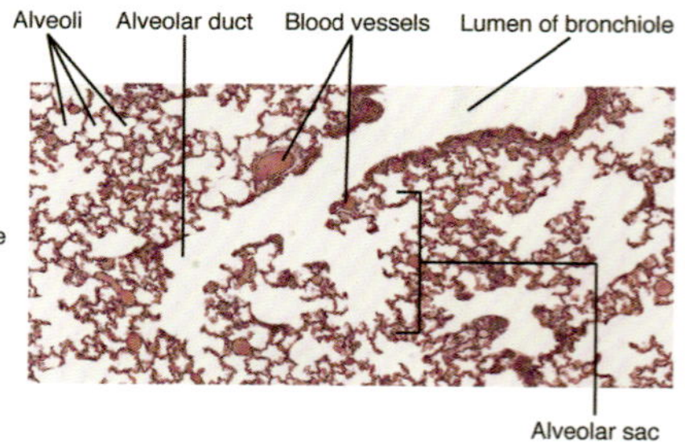

RESPIRATORY HISTOLOGY

- Nasopharynx: Respiratory epithelium
- Oropharynx: Striated squamous non-keratinized
- **Alveolar sac: Simple squamous**
- **Type I Pneumocytes: Simple squamous (thin). 97% of alveolar surface). Gas exchange. (AKA: the simple squamous epithelial cells of the alveolar walls). They are very thin to facilitate gas exchange.**
  Type I pneumocytes are unable to replicate and are affected by toxic substances. If there is lung damage, type II pneumocytes are able to proliferate and differentiate into type I pneumocytes.
- **Type II pneumocytes (AKA: the greater alveolar cells) large cuboidal type cells: Secrete surfactant (dipalmitoyl phosphatidylcholine) starting about the 24th week of gestation to decrease surface tension of the alveoli. It is not until 34 weeks that there is adequate enough surfactant to prevent RDS (respiratory distress syndrome, aka: hyaline membrane disease).**
  Type II pneumocytes can change into Type I pneumocytes to repair the lung.
  Type II pneumocytes are located at the blood-air barrier.
- **(tip: Type I Pneumocytes are thin and long – just like the number 1 and**
  Type II Pneumocytes are II (2) times the size of type I (cubed)

- Lobes of the lung: Right: Superior, Middle, Inferior. Left: Superior/upper **with lingula**, inferior.
- Pulmonary artery locations in respect to the bronchus: Right side: anterior. Left side: Superior (RALS)
- Gas exchange barrier/junction: Type 1 epithelial cells, tight junctions
- Trachea: (trunk of the branching tree): ciliated, pseudostratified columnar epithelium
- Bronchi (the 2 divisions of the trachea that go into each lung): ciliated, pseudostratified columnar epithelium
- Larger bronchioles: Divisions of the bronchi: ciliated, pseudostratified columnar epithelium.
  Smaller bronchioles leading to the alveoli: cuboidal epithelium.
- NOTE: Recurrent lung infections in Kartagener's is due to the dysfunction of the ciliated columnar epithelia cells.
- Alveoli (singular: alveolus): Bronchioles branch into the alveoli. Alveoli: simple squamous epithelium
- Intra-alveolar septum: simple squamous epithelium with capillaries in between. Each alveolus shares its wall with adjacent alveoli. Alveoli do not collapse individually, only as a group.
- **Clara Cells** (AKA: Club cells) dome shaped cells with microvilli of the bronchioles: ciliated simple epithelium. Protects bronchiolar epithelium by secreting the protein uteroglobin. They also detoxify the lungs by using P-450 enzymes and act as stem cells to regenerate bronchiolar epithelium.
- **Goblet Cells**: (goblet cup shape) Glandular simple columnar epithelial cells that gel-forming mucin, main component of mucus to protect mucus membranes. (Found in the respiratory, GI tract and conjunctiva in the upper eyelid). Goblet cells stop at the bronchi.
- **Alveolar macrophages (AKA: Dust cells)**
  Dust cells (AKA: Alveolar macrophages, AKA: Monocytes): located near the pneumocytes in the alveoli (clear debris and destroy foreign material).
- **Kerley B Lines**: Commonly seen on X-Ray in pulmonary edema, lymphomas, pneumonias, pulmonary fibrosis, sarcoidosis.
- Lung products that cause bronchoconstriction: Histamine, Bradykinin, ACE inhibitors.
- Lung products that cause bronchodilation: Prostaglandins, ACE (inactivates bradykinin)

Diaphragm

- Innervated by C3, C4, C5 (phrenic nerve). Which is what can refer pain from the abdomen to the shoulder)
  (**tip**: C3, 4, 5 keeps the diaphragm alive)
- **IVC enters the diaphragm at T8, esophagus at T10 and aorta at T12 (tip: I Ate 10 Eggs AT 12. This is for:** I (I for IVC) ate (8 – for level T8) 10 Eggs (Esophagus enters at level T10) AT twelve ("A" for Aorta enters at level T12).
- Is the main muscle used in **inspiration.** The diaphragm is pulled down to expand the size of the chest space, lowering the pressure inside the lungs and drawing air in from the environment.
- Caution must be used with any disorder that involves paralysis or weakening of the diaphragm. (**Myasthenia Gravis, Guillain Barre, asthma attack**). **If the diaphragm is impaired, breathing stops.** Must be prepared to intubate

Dust particle removal

- 10 – 15 microns = trapped and cleared from the upper respiratory tract (coughing, sneezing)
- 2.5 – 10 microns (inhaled particles) cleared by ciliate cells via mucous transport down to the beginning of the terminal bronchioles
- <2 microns = macrophages (dust cells) in the terminal bronchioles phagocytize particles

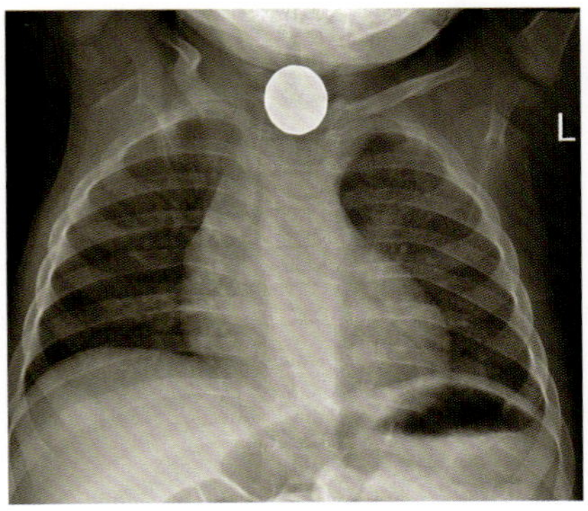

Aspiration of Foreign Object

- Will go down the right main bronchus because it is a shorter and straighter path
- If inhaled while upright, object will be in any section of the **right lower lobe.**
- If inhaled while lying down (recumbent), object will be in the **posterior segment of the upper (superior)** right lobe
- Removed by a **rigid** bronchoscopy
- ↓ V/Q ratio

Thoracentesis

- **Enter above the ribs (below the rib runs the Vein, Artery, Nerve (VAN)**
- **Can enter at:**
  7th rib mid clavicular
  9th rib midscapular
  11th rib post scapular

Order of layers for Thoracentesis and Pericardiocentesis:

- Chest Wall: Skin ➔ fatty tissue ➔ Intercostal muscle ➔ external intercostal muscle ➔ Innermost intercostal muscle ➔Parietal pleura ➔ Interpleural space ➔ Visceral pleura ➔ lung or pericardial sac

Lung Products

- **Surfactant = Type II pneumocytes (↓ alveolar surface tension = ↑ compliance = ↓ work of inspiration)**
- Prostaglandins
- Histamine = ↑ bronchoconstriction's
- ACE = changes ATI to ATII = inactivates bradykinin (Ace inhibitors ↑ bradykinin = cough, angioedema)
- Kallikrein: blood protein that participates in blood pressure control, coagulation, and pain
- Kallikrein and bradykinin are vasodilators
- Prekallikrein is the precursor of kallikrein. It is activated by **Factor XIIa** (intrinsic clotting factor)
- Kallikrein activates bradykinin
- Ace inhibitors ↑ bradykinin = dilates vessels = ↓ blood pressure
- Side affects of ↑ bradykinin from Ace inhibitors = angioedema and cough. Switch patient to ARB (Angiotensin II receptor blockers)

Lung Volumes

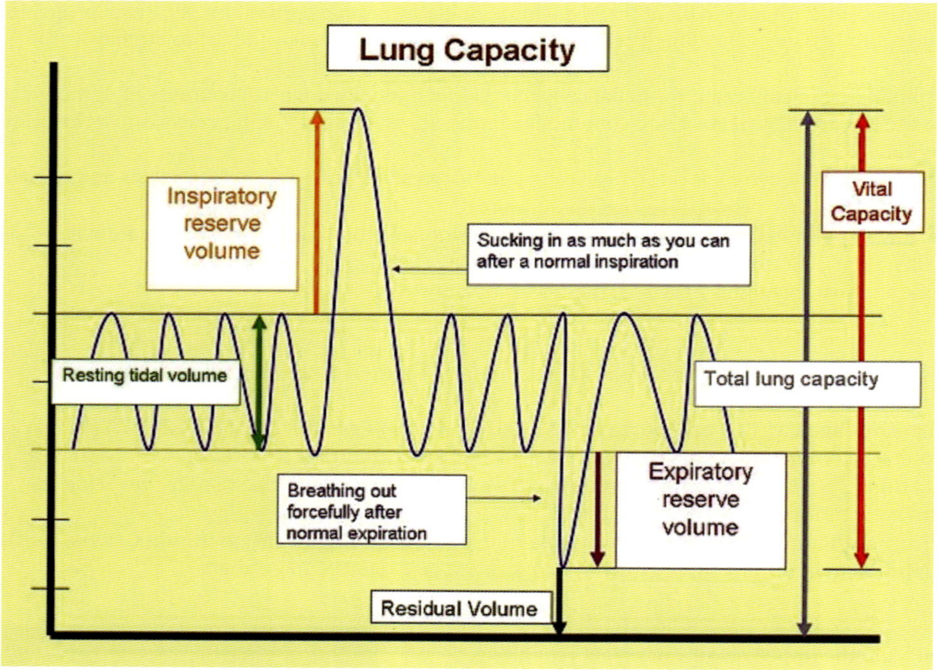

FRC

FRC: Point where the inward pull and outward pull of the lung is balanced.
FRC: Airway and alveolar pressure = 0 and Intra pleural pressure **= -5 (negative 5)** (Equal pressure at FRC)
Negative pressure = allows lung to expand

Oxygen and Oxygen Rules

- 1 Hb can bind 1.34 mL oxygen. (Normal Hb = 15 g/dL Cyanosis = deoxygenated Hb > 5 g/dL
- **PaO2 = Arterial oxygen PAO2 = Alveolar oxygen**
- Partial Pressure of oxygen (PO2) = part of the total gas volume/mixture that oxygen takes up/occupies. (Total pressure is the total of all gases that make up the mixture)
- PO2 Saturation (O2 Sat) = the amount of dissolved oxygen in the blood. (Hb has 4 "arms" to hold 4 oxygen molecules. If all 4 arms are filled with Oxygen molecules = 100% O2 saturation. The Hb is fully saturated (full). If anything else takes 1 or more of those "seats" (such as CO) then the O2 saturation ↓.
  O2 saturation ≤ 88% for COPD patients is when home oxygen is prescribed.
  O2 saturation much lower than 85% = intubation
- O2 Content = Total of all oxygen (the oxygen bound to Hb plus the oxygen dissolved in plasma)
- Oxygenation = when oxygen enters the tissue. Measure of % of Hb binding sites in the blood occupied by oxygen
- Exercise ↓ venous O2
- O2 Content ↓ when Hb ↓ = anemia
- Arterial O2 ↓ with chronic lung disease b/c of the physiologic shunt = ↓ O2 extraction rate
- ↓ O2 to tissues = reflex polycythemia (EPO) **ANYTHING** that ↓ O2 (hypoxia) = ↑ EPO
- Hypoxemia = ↓ PaO2 (Normal and increased A-a gradient
- Hypoxia = ↓ O2 to tissues (↓ CO, hypoxemia, anemia, CO poisoning)
- Ischemia = loss of blood flow (Impeded arterial flow, ↓ venous drainage)

Hypoxia Causes

- Alveolar hypoventilation (normal A-a gradient)
  High altitude, sedative, overdose, sleep apnea, obesity, Myasthenia Gravis
- Gas Diffusion (↑ A-a gradient)
  Thickening of capillary membranes, hyaline membrane disease
- V/Q Mismatch (↑ A-a gradient)
  Pneumonia, pulmonary embolism
- Right to left shunt (↑ A-a gradient)
  Congenital cyanotic heart diseases

Ventilation/Perfusion (V/Q)

Is the ratio between the amount of air getting to the alveoli (ventilation, diffusion) and the amount of blood that is reaching the alveoli (perfusion, flow).

There **must be a ventilation and perfusion match for gas exchange to occur** in the capillaries. If there is damage to the lungs that will not allow gas exchange (ie: PE), the lungs will vasoconstrict to send blood (AKA: perfusion) to another area of the lungs that are able to gas exchange). (This is opposite physio from the rest of the body, when there is damage the body vasodilates in order to send more blood to the damaged area).

V/Q mismatch is the most common cause of hypoxia.

- **PO2 in the lung is determined by the ratio of ventilation to blood flow (perfusion).**
- **Normal V/Q ratio = 0.8**
  Normal ventilation (V) is 4 L of air per minute.
  Normal perfusion (Q) is 5 L of blood per minute.
  So normal V/Q ratio is 4/5 = 0.8
  When V/Q is higher than 0.8 it means that the mismatch is poor perfusion. (Ventilation exceeds perfusion).
  (Example: PE is due to decrease in perfusion so the V/Q would be ↑ (> .8).
  When V/Q is less than 0.8 it means the cause of the mismatch is poor ventilation.
- **Ventilation (AKA: Diffusion, oxygen in) = gas (oxygen) = depends upon breathing**
- **Perfusion = blood flow = depends upon blood flow**
- **Parts of the lungs are higher than the heart and part of the lungs are lower than the heart. Therefore apex (top) of the lungs has a higher V/Q ratio and the base (lower) part of the lungs has a lower V/Q ration.**
- If there is a low PO2, to determine if the problem is with ventilation (diffusion) or perfusion (blood flow), if oxygen is administered and the PO2 improves, the problem was ventilation (diffusion). There was ↓ oxygen being breathed in which caused the V/Q mismatch, but once oxygen was given, the PO2 corrected itself.
  But if oxygen is given and the V/Q mismatch does not correct itself and the PO2 did not change, then the problem is not with lack of oxygen (because oxygen is being administered) the problem is with the blood flow. There is no flow, so no gas exchange is occurring. No matter how much oxygen is administered the can never be any gas exchange until the flow is restored.
- Greatest ventilation is in the apex of the lung (wasted). V/Q is highest at 3.0 = wasted ventilation. PaO2 is the highest and PaCO2 is the lowest. Organisms that thrive on oxygen live at the top of the lungs: ie: TB.
- Greatest perfusion is at the base of the lung (where gas exchange occurs). V/Q is the lowest at 0.6. Wasted perfusion. PaO2 is the lowest and PaCO2 is the highest.

V/Q Mismatch Pathologies

- **Low V/Q mismatch (< .8) = problem with ventilation (diffusion)**
  - Obstructive lung diseases (🡅 Aa, 🡅 Co2 and corrects with oxygen)
  - Asthma
  - Chronic bronchitis
  - Acute pulmonary edema
  - Foreign body aspiration
- **High V/Q mismatch (> .8) = problem with perfusion (flow)**
  - Pulmonary embolism
  - Emphysema

A-a gradient = A – a = A-a gradient (Normal = < 15)
(A = Alveoli O2 a = arterial O2)

Normal A-a Gradient

- COPD, Obesity, sleep apnea, scoliosis, drugs (narcotics, sedatives), anesthesia, CNS lesion (stroke), **hypoventilation,**
  high altitude, Myasthenia Gravis

🡅 A-a gradient

- Pulmonary embolism, atelectasis, restrictive lung dz (fibrosis), pleural effusion, Right to left shunt, diffusion limited, hypoxemia, RDS, pneumonia, congenital cyanotic heart diseases.

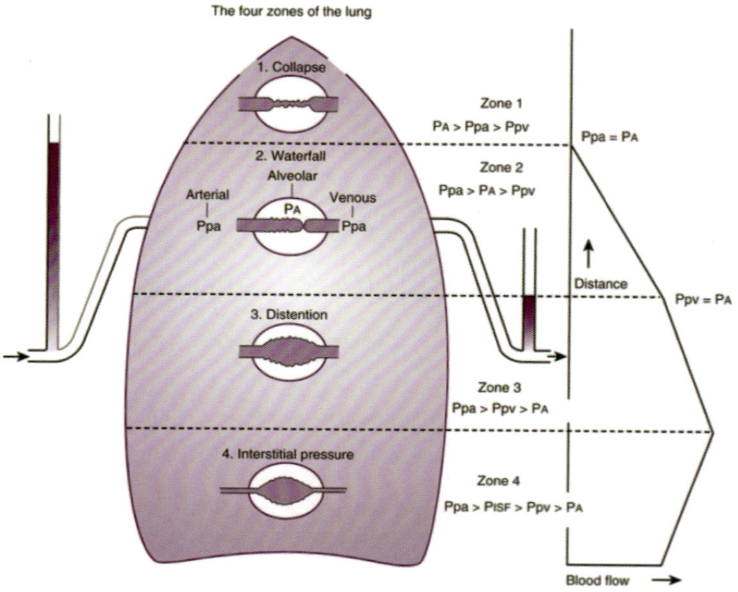

Zone Order:
(**tip**:

A > a > v
a > **A** > v
a > v > **A**

(**tip**: watch the big "A" and think **tic-tac-toe**. Once it moves, the others
drop will drop into the empty space)

A-a Gradient Differentials

Pulmonary Situation	A-a Gradient	CO2	Notes
Shunts	🡅 A-a	Normal CO2	Does not correct with oxygen. ARDS, cardiac shunt
V/Q Mismatch	🡅 A-a	🡅 CO2	Corrects with oxygen. Obstructive lung DZ, atelectasis, pulmonary edema, pneumonia, PE, pleural effusion.
Diffusion Limited	🡅 A-a	Normal CO2	Corrects with oxygen. Restrictive dz. Interstitial lung dz.
Hypoventilation	Normal A-a	🡅 CO2	Does not correct with oxygen. CNS depression.
Reduced inspired oxygen	Normal A-a	Normal CO2	Corrects with oxygen. High Altitude.

Resistance

- ↓ Lung volume = ↑ resistance = ↓ Compliance.
- Deflated lungs = ↓ radial traction on airways (AKA: Recoil)

Compliance

- How well a hollow organ is able to stretch
- High compliance (the organ is able to easily stretch) = Obstructive Disease: COPD, emphysema, asthma, CF, normal aging
- Low compliance (it is difficult for the organ to stretch) = Restrictive Disease: Pulmonary fibrosis, hemochromatosis, amyloidosis, pneumonia, pulmonary edema

Recoil

- The ability for the organ to return to its normal shape after being stretched.
- AKA: Elasticity, **Radial elasticity**
- Decreased recoil in α-1 Antitrypsin deficiency because elastase is not inhibited = elastin is destroyed
- ↓ in obstructive lung DZ

Radial Traction (aka: outward pulling)

- The connective tissue that surrounds the airways of the lungs = parenchyma. This forms a scaffold around the airways keeping them open with a force (radial traction). When inspiration occurs = traction ↑ as the fibers of the parenchyma stretch (AKA: elastic springs that anchor the airway lumen to the parenchyma (lung interstitium) = keeps airways open)
- **↑ in restrictive lung disease.**
  Restrictive lung DZ = interstitial fibrosis = ↑ radial tension (adds more elastic springs) between the airway and the parenchyma) = ↑ elastic recoil = ↑ expiratory flow rate.
- **↓ in obstructive lung disease.**
  Obstructive lung DZ = ↑ elastase activity = interstitium is broken down = ↓ elastic springs = ↓ recoil.
- Airways can collapse during exhalation b/c the ↓ radical tension to withstand the ↑ collapsing pressures = expiratory obstruction
- Radial traction = outward pull

Breathing Patterns

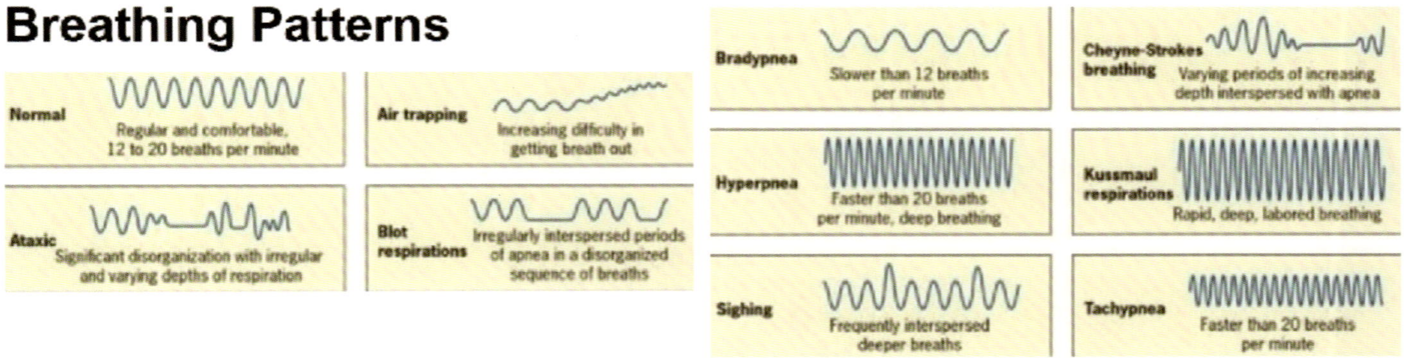

Lung Sounds (key words)

- Fremitus: Increased over areas of consolidation (sound waves transmit better in a solid/fluid medium) and decreased/absent over areas of pleural effusion or pneumothorax (sound waves decrease transmission through gas)
  - Tactile Fremitus: vibration felt on the chest wall
  - Vocal Fremitus: vibration heard on the chest wall from certain spoken words
- Percussion: Performed with middle finger striking the middle phalanges of the other middle finger on the other hand.
  The sound is "tympanic" if there is a pneumothorax (air stretches the pleural membranes).
  The sound is dampened/muffled if there is fluid between pleural membranes.
  - **"Hyper-resonant" (tympanic), ↓ breath sounds or no breath sounds = pneumothorax**
  - **"Dull to percussion": Pleural effusion**, atelectasis, **consolidation** (lobar pneumonia or pulmonary edema)
- Wheezing: Narrowed airways causing a continuous "musical" sound on inspiration and expiration = Asthma.
- Stridor: High pitched "musical" sound due to turbulent flow caused by epiglottitis, anaphylaxis, croup.
- Crackles (AKA: Rails): Can be soft (high pitched) or coarse (low pitched, rough) sounds during inspiration.
- Rhonchi: "bubbly" sound on inspiration or expiration

Normal Aging and Breathing Patterns

- ↑ Residual volume
- ↑ A-a PO2 difference
- ↓ Arterial PO2

Additional definitions

- Atelectasis: Collapse/closure of the lung = reduced or no gas exchange. (All or part of a lung)

Equations

Minute Volume = TV x RR (total volume x respiratory rate)
Alveolar Ventilation = (TV – 150 dead space) x RR
PVR = Pulmonary Artery Pressure – Pulmonary Wedge Pressure/CO (Pulmonary Vascular Resistance) (Pulmonary Wedge Pressure (PWCP) = Left Atrium Pressure)
Resistance in Series= R1 + R2 + R3
Resistance in Parallel = 1/R1 + 1/R2 + 1/R3
Total Lung Cap = IRV + TV + ERV + RV
Vital Cap = IRV + RV + ERV
FRC = ERV + RV
IC = TV + IRV

Obstructive DZ (COPD) always have high RV and TLC, low FEV1, and <80 FEV1/FVC, ↓ Radial traction, and ↓ Recoil.

Restrictive DZ (all others) have low RV and TLC, Normal to High FEV1/FVC ratio, ↑ Radial traction.

Oxygen Exchange

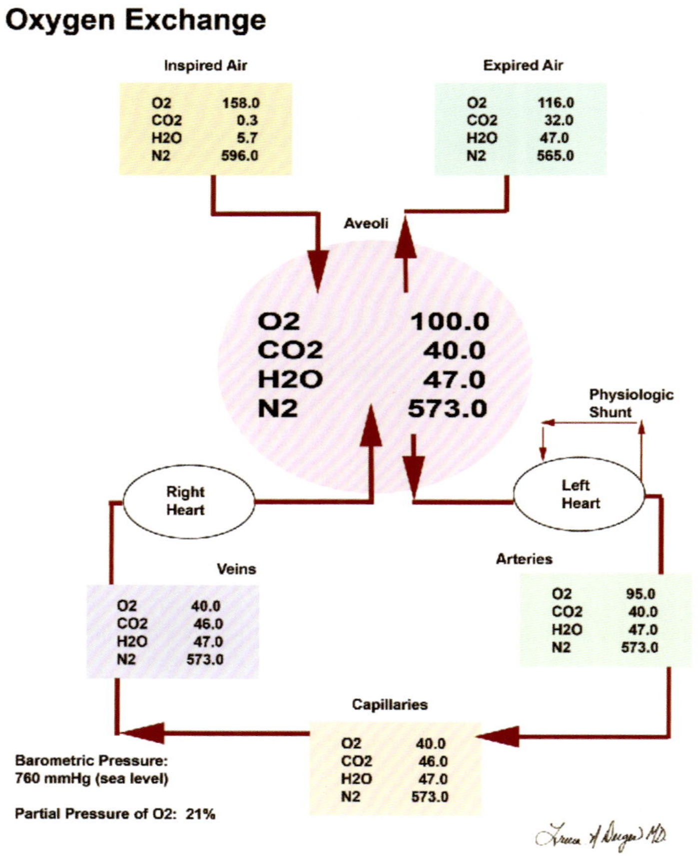

Oxyhemoglobin Dissociation Curve

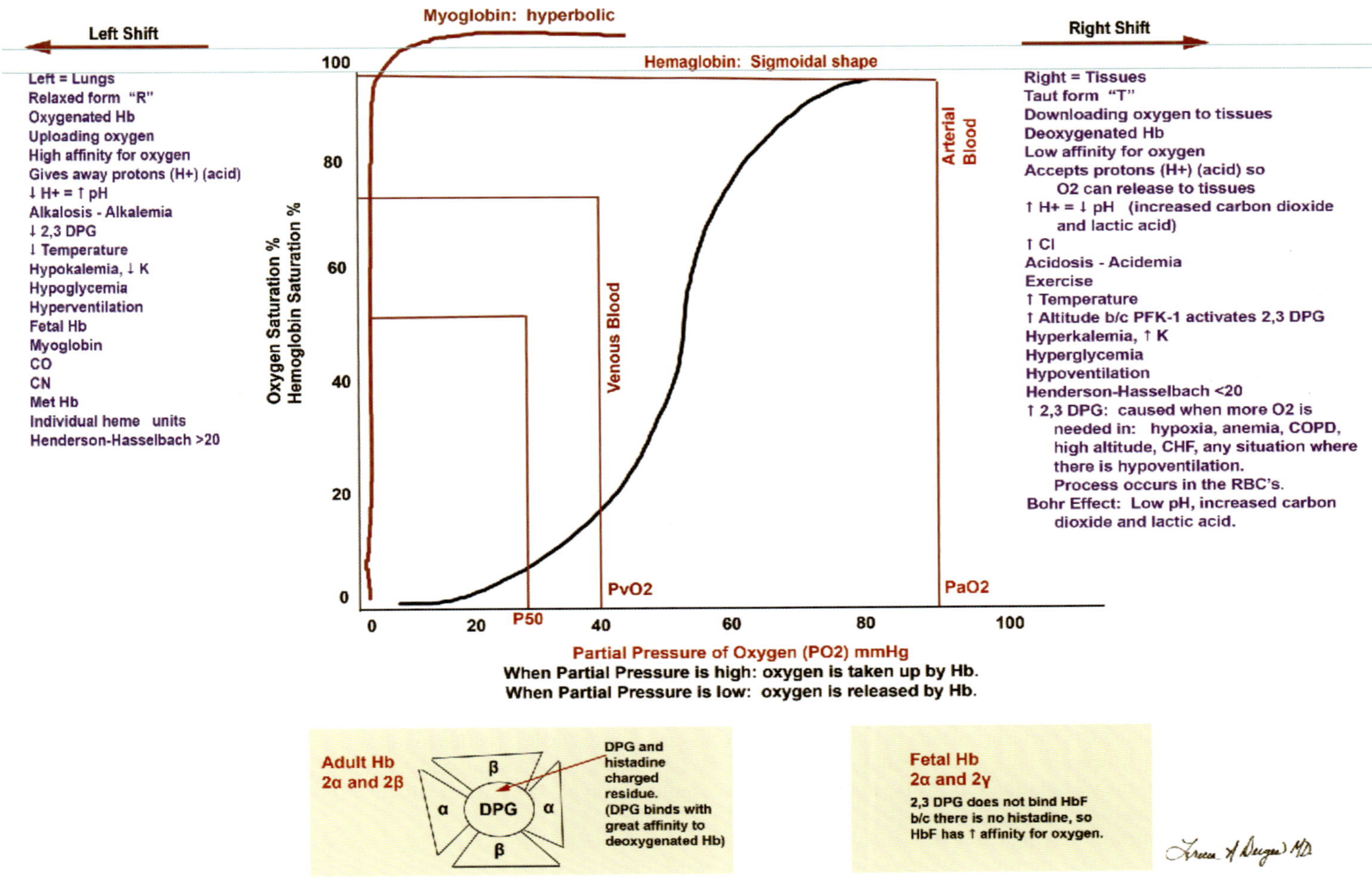

Hemoglobin

Fetal Hb

- 2α, 2γ
- Fetal Hb has a lower affinity for 2,3 BPG that adult Hb, therefore has a higher affinity for oxygen
  This is why Hydroxyurea is given to Sickle Cell. It ↑ the HbF in the patient = ↑ O2

Adult Hb

- 2α, 2β

Oxygen-Hemoglobin Curve

- P50 = Pressure of oxygen when 50% of the Hb is saturated. Normal 26.
- If there is a ↓ in P50 = Hb holds on to oxygen (left shift) so less oxygen is given off to tissues so there is a ↑ affinity for oxygen by Hb. If less oxygen is given off to tissues = hypoxia which causes a reflex polycythemia.

Hb affinity for oxygen

- Low affinity for O2 (wants to give it away to **T**issues) = **Taut (T) form** = **right** shift Oxy/Hb curve (AKA: Deoxyhemoglobin) (**tip**: **T** for **T**issues).
- High affinity for O2 (wants to hold on the O2, in the lungs) = **Relaxed (R) form** = **left** shift Oxy/Hb curve (AKA: Oxyhemoglobin, SO2, O2 Saturation) (**tip**: **L** for **L**oves oxygen, **L**ungs don't want to let it go)

2, 3 DPG

- 2, 3 BPG is a histadine charged residue – in the center of Hb. **It increases when there is an increased need for oxygen**. (Such as in: COPD, hypoxia, anemia, high altitude, CHF, hypoventilation) This occurs in the RBC's. Causes a right shift.
- HbF (Fetal Hb) has a high affinity for oxygen so it can't bind with 2, 3 BPG because HbF has no histadine.

Responses to ↓ Oxygen

High Altitude **Initial problem that starts this entire process: Hypoxia.**	**Exercise**	**CO2** **(AKA: hypercapnia)**
↓ atmosphere oxygen = ↓ PaO2 = Hypoxia = hyperventilation (respiratory alkalosis) = ↓ CO2 = ↑ erythropoietin (polycythemia if chronic) = ↑ Hct and Hb (if chronic) = ↑ 2,3,3-BPG (Binds Hb to release more oxygen = right shift to O/Hb curve) = ↑ mitochondria = ↑ renal excretion of HCO3 (metabolic acidosis). Chronic hypoxia leads to RVH and pulmonary vasoconstriction. TX: **Acetazolamide to** avoid altitude sickness	↑ HR (beta -1 sympathetic stimulation) = ↑ HR = ↑ CO = ↑ work load on heart = ↑ pulmonary blood flow = ↑ O2 consumption = vasodilation to send more O2 to exercising muscles = ↑ metabolite and CO2 production from muscles = **↓ venous O2 content and ↑ venous CO2 content and ↓ pH, but NO CHANGE in arterial readings** (same PaO2 and CO2)	Anything that ↓ breathing: COPD, hypoventilation, drug OD will cause ↑ CO2 and ↓ blood pH. CO2 is picked up by central chemo receptors so causes vasodilation of the vessels in the brain = ↑ ICP

COPD and CO2

CO2 (hypercapnia) is chronic in COPD.
Normal breaths are controlled by peripheral baroreceptors (Carotid bodies and Aortic Bodies) that monitor changes in pH and oxygen. PaCO2 is the main stimulator of the respiratory drive in healthy people. If there is any increase in PaCO2 (which causes decreased PaO2 = hypoxia = decreased pH) then a message is carried from the baroreceptor by cranial nerve IX to the solitary nucleus in the medulla to stimulate the need for respiration.
COPD: Patients with COPD are chronically hypoxic because of the retention of CO2. It is this hypoxia (reduced PaO2 and decreased pH) that stimulates the peripheral chemoreceptors (Carotid and Aortic bodies) that cause the stimulation (via CN IX) for respiration. Without this hypoxia a patient with COPD will lose the stimulation to breath.
It is critically important that high flow oxygen is never administered to a patient with COPD. This oxygen replaces the retained CO2, therefore taking away their hypoxia which then takes away their respiratory drive to breath. They will quit breathing.
Note: PaCO2 is the major stimulator of the central chemoreceptors in the medulla. These receptors are stimulated by the decrease in the pH of the CSF due to the diffusion of CO2 (H+) into the CSF. They are not stimulated by a decrease in pH in the blood because the blood brain barrier is impermeable to H+.
Therefore, the central chemoreceptors are the primary source for increased respiration due to Hypercapnia. Whereas the peripheral chemoreceptors are the primary source for increased respiration due to hypoxemia.

Methemoglobinemia

High levels of **ferric (Fe3) verses ferrous (Fe2)** form of hemoglobin in the blood. Ferric (Fe3) = ↓ ability to bind oxygen (impaired affinity for oxygen) = ↓ ability of the RBC to release oxygen to tissues = hypoxia. Ferrous (Fe2) has ↑ ability (affinity) to bind oxygen.
(**tip**: ferro"**US**" is the form that is good, it is in "US") (**tip**: the "2" of "us" and 3 is a crowd)

Methemoglobin binds cyanide so is used to treat cyanide poisoning caused by nitroprusside which is used in the TX of hypertensive emergencies.

Causes a Left shift in Oxy/Hb curve.
Labs: **Normal O2 Sat. ↓ affinity for O2, ↑ affinity for cyanide (CN)**

SX: **Chocolate colored blood** (oxidized Hb is **brown** and does not carry oxygen), cyanosis (AKA: dusky skin color), mental status changes, dizziness, exercise intolerance, fatigue, loss of consciousness.
Causes: Drugs, nitrates, nitroglycerin, chloroquine, primaquine, dapsone, sulfonamides, lidocaine, metoclopramide.
DX: Co=oximetry test
TX: **Methylene blue** (decreases the half life of methemoglobin) and **Vitamin C.**

Carbon Monoxide (CO)
MCC of death in house fires.

CO has a 200x greater affinity for hemoglobin than O2.
CO competes with oxygen for binding on Hb so ↓ oxygen available to tissues = hypoxia.
CO binds with Hb to form carboxyhemoglobin (HbCO).
No oxygen is released to the tissues.

No cytochrome oxidase: CO has ↓ affinity for cytochrome oxidase. ↓ aerobic metabolism and causes cells to switch to anaerobic metabolism = lactic acidosis and cell death.
No myoglobin: CO has ↑ affinity for myoglobin = ↓ cardiac output and hypotension = brain ischemia.

Labs: **Normal O2 Sat** (because some/all of the 4 arms of Hb is now filled with CO instead of O2), **↓ HCO3 and ↓ pH.** ↓ Total O2 content. **Normal PO2**. (Partial pressure)
Metabolic acidosis.

Left shift in Oxy/Hb curve.
Stops Complex IV of ETC.

SX: **First sign: Headache**, **cherry red** color to the blood, dyspnea, confusion, cardiac problems, seizures, and death due to MI.
(Always check to see if there are others in the household that are experiencing headaches).
DX: **Carboxyhemoglobin test**
Causes: automobile exhaust (garage in suicide attempts, underground parking attendant), house fires, wood-burning stoves, cigarette smoke (inside smokers), propane stoves, electrical generators, idling automobiles with exhaust pipe blocked by snow.

TX: BIT: **100% oxygen.**
Severe poisoning: hyperbaric oxygen. Hyperbaric oxygen better than 100% O2

Cyanide Poisoning

Cyanide stops cytochrome oxidase, stops Complex IV of the ETC = no ATP.
SX: Bitter **almond smell**

Causes: House fires, plastic, upholstery
Cyanide poisoning is also a side effect of nitroprusside and nitric oxide. **Nitrites (nitroprusside for HTN emergencies) can cause cyanide poisoning by oxidizing Fe2 (ferrous) to Fe3 (ferric)**

Cyanide TX options:
Thiosulfate, Met Blue, Hydroxocobalamin.
Hydroxocobalamin combines with cyanide to form cyanocobalamin (Vitamin B-12), which is excreted.

Sodium nitrate induces methemoglobin in RBC's, which combines with the cyanide. Methemoglobinemia is then treated with Methylene Blue. Methylene blue inhibits Monoamine Oxidase. This changes the iron form Ferric (F^3 iron form) to Ferrous (F^4 iron form). Vitamin C can also assist in treating methemoglobinemia.

Sodium thiosulfate transforms cyanide (donates a sulfur atom) to thiocyanate by rhodanese, which is then excreted.

TX: Nitrites.
Nitrites oxidize Hb to methemoglobin. Methemoglobin binds cyanide. Thiosulfate (sulfur) binds cyanide to form thiocyanate, which is then excreted.

CO2 Release from the RBC in the lungs

In the lungs:
Increase in oxygenation of Hb causes dissociation of H+ (protons), which shifts the bicarb to CO2 production and release.

In the tissues:
H+ (protons) shift the curve in the other direction, which causes the unloading of oxygen.

Aspirated Object

SX: **Sudden onset,** stridor, wheeze, cough dyspnea

TX: If inhaled: Rigid Endoscopy
(if ingested: Flexible endoscopy)

Location of inhalation
Sitting up: Lower right portion of the right inferior lobe
Laying down (supine): Superior portion of the right inferior lobe

Oxygen Saturation (94% - 99% normal)

- Hb binds 4 oxygen molecules.
- 1 g of Hb can bind 1.34 mL of oxygen
- ↓ Hb = ↓ Oxygen content of arterial blood but the oxygen saturation and PaO2 are normal

	PaO2 Dissolved Oxygen: (1.5% of O2 is dissolved in plasma; the rest is bound to Hb).	**O2 sat. Oxygen Saturation: (O2 bound to Hb)**	Total Oxygen Content: (Dissolved oxygen with Hb)	Hb Concentration
CO Carbon Monoxide	Normal	Normal	↓	Normal
Anemia (Low Hb)	Normal	Normal	↓	↓
Polycythemia (↑ Hb)	Normal	Normal	↑	↑

Restrictive verses Obstructive

RESTRICTIVE	OBSTRUCTIVE
↓ FVC, ↓ TLC, ↓ RV, ≥ 80% FEV1/FVC ratio ↓ Compliance **Rapid breathing** **↓ Tidal volume** **↓ Lung volume** ↓ Diffusing capacity ↑ Expiratory flow b/c ↓ compliance and ↑ elastic recoil **↑ Radial traction b/c fibrotic lung (Radial traction = outward pull)** ↑ Elastic resistance (they breath faster and more shallow to make breathing easier)	**↑ RV, ↑ TLC, ≤ 80% FEV1/FVC ratio** ↑ Compliance **Slow breathing** **↑ Tidal volume (to minimize the work of breathing)** **↑ Total lung volume** **↑ Residual volume** ↑ Airflow resistance (they breath slower and deeper to make breathing easier) ↑ CO2 = acidic (crosses BBB) ↑ Erythropoietin **↓ Radial traction** **↓ Recoil** ↓ Diffusing capacity ↓ PaO2 ↓ V/Q (COPD). (Note: Emphysema is ↑ V/Q) MCC Death: Bronchiectasis (↑ Reid index = Mucus) (Reid Index = Gland/Wall)
Causes Pulmonary fibrosis, CHF, ↓ Surfactant, pneumonias, Pulmonary edema (↑ hydrostatic pressure in pulmonary system = transudate = ↓ lung compliance = dyspnea (b/c no enough negative pressure to expand lungs), ARDS (AKA: hyaline membrane disease), Pneumoconioses, Drug toxicity (Bleomycin, Amiodarone, Methotrexate, Busulfan), Goodpasture's, Wegner's, Scoliosis, polio, morbid obesity, myasthenia gravis	**Causes** COPD, Emphysema, asthma, α-1 antitrypsin deficiency, Cystic Fibrosis, bronchiectasis, chronic bronchitis, obstructive sleep apnea

Restrictive verses Obstructive Breathing Patterns

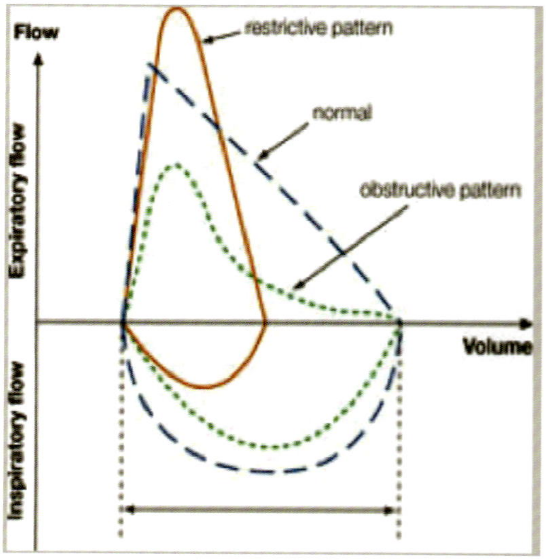

Flow-Volume Loop

Reid Index

- Mucus gland enlargement = ↑ wall thickness in chronic bronchitis (> 40% Reid Index)
  Ratio between the thickness the mucus/ mucus secreting glands and the thickness of the epithelium that covers the bronchi.
- Reid index: (B to C) / (A to D)

Restrictive Lung Diseases

- **Restrictive pattern: ↓ FEV1, ↓ FVC and a normal to increased FEV1/FEV ratio, ↓ TLC, ↓ RV, ↓ DLCO, ↑ Radial traction.**
- In interstitial lung diseases (alveolar wall injury) causes interstitial edema and accumulation of inflammatory cells. This causes an **↑ in type II pneumocytes, in type I pneumocytes and an ↑ in fibroblasts**. The proliferation in fibroblast results in fibrosis, destroying the normal lung architecture.

Pulmonary Fibrosis

Scar formation (excess fibrous connective tissue = fibrosis) in the lungs causing serious breathing problems. Gradual exchange of normal lung parenchyma with fibrotic tissue.
Non-compliant lung.

Causes: Autoimmune disorders, radiation therapy, connective tissue dz (scleroderma, SLE, RA, sarcoidosis, Wegner's, pneumoconiosis (occupational pollutants), interstitial pneumonia, and **medicines.**
Meds causing pulmonary fibrosis: Bleomycin, amiodarone, busulfan, methotrexate, hydroxyurea, nitrofurantoin

Spirometry shows: **Restrictive Patten**: **Normal FEV1/FVC is normal to high, ↓ RV, ↓ Total lung capacity, ↓ DLCO, ↓ compliance.**
↑ radial traction on the airways causes expiratory flow rate.

Difficult for the patient to breath air in, lungs can't expand due to decreased compliance → hypoxia → pulmonary HTN → right heart failure.

Restrictive Lung Diseases

(Please see appropriate chapters)
CHF, ↓ Surfactant, Amyloidosis, Sarcoidosis, Hemochromatosis, Tuberculosis

RDS, ARDS (AKA: hyaline membrane disease), Goodpasture's, Wegner's, Scoliosis, Polio, morbid obesity, Sarcoidosis, Myasthenia Gravis, Pneumoconioses, Pneumonias (see below).

SX: Pulmonary edema (↑ hydrostatic pressure in pulmonary system = transudate = ↓ lung compliance = dyspnea (b/c not enough negative pressure to expand lungs),

Idiopathic Pulmonary Fibrosis

Fibrosis of the lung (scarring), which causes a chronic, progressive decline in lung function.
Cause: Unknown. MC in patients who have smoked, MC > 50 years old.

SX: Restricted pattern on pulmonary function test, clubbing of the finger or toenails, progressive exertional dyspnea, dry non-productive cough on exertion.

Spirometry shows: **Restrictive Patten**: **Normal FEV1/FVC is normal to high, ↓ RV, ↓ Total lung capacity, ↓ DLCO, ↓ compliance.**
↑ radial traction on the airways causes expiratory flow rate.
CXR shows: Decreased lung volumes, Diffuse reticular opacities (ground glass appearance), "honeycombing" (clusters of cystic airspace).
Biopsy shows: Interstitial fibrosis
TX: no treatment.

Flow Volume Loop for Restrictive Lung Disease

Flow as compared to normal:

- Breaths are shorter and faster.
- It is difficult for restrictive lung dz to breath in: Inhalation loop will be smaller than the normal inhalation loop.
- Breathing out is not a problem so the exhalation loop will be the same as, or higher than the normal exhalation loop.

(See flow patterns in illustration above)

Pneumoconioses (Occupational lung pathologies)

Restrictive Lung Disease – Interstitial Lung Disease

- **PFT shows restrictive pattern: ↓ FEV1, ↓ FEV and a normal to increased FEV1/FEV ratio, ↓ TLC, ↓ RV, ↓ DLCO.**
- **Pulmonary HTN (loud P2 hear sound)**
- **Clubbing of finger**
- **Shortness of Breath**
- **Nonproductive cough**
- **Chronic hypoxia**
- **Hypertrophied right atrium and right ventricle**
- **No fever, no myalgia, no response to steroid treatment (except for Berylliosis)**
- **Presentation: Months to years**

Asbestosis
(AKA: Mesothelioma or Bronchogenic carcinoma)

Occupations: shipbuilding, plumbing, insulation, working with PVC, roofing

CXR: **Calcified pleural plaques** (Pleura) The pleura of the lungs is on the **periphery (lateral) – NOT centrally**.
It also shows **reticulonodular pulmonary infiltrates** (interstitial **fibrosis**), which are initiated by **alveolar macrophages**.

Histology: Psammoma bodies (AKA: pleural thickening with calcification).

PFT shows a restrictive breathing pattern.

MCC: **Bronchogenic carcinoma** – not mesothelioma.
(If the CXR shows a "mass", or a "central mass" it is Bronchogenic carcinoma. Mesothelioma is not a mass).

TX: Supportive

For it to be mesothelioma: YOU MUST SEE one or more of these: the word Pleural/pleura, periphery (lateral), MUST be at least 20 years from the time they worked in that job, or Ferruginous bodies (asbestos). IF THEY DO NOT USE THESE WORDS IT IS BROCHOGENIC CARNCINOMA!!

Ferruginous bodies: golden-brown rods (dumbbells)

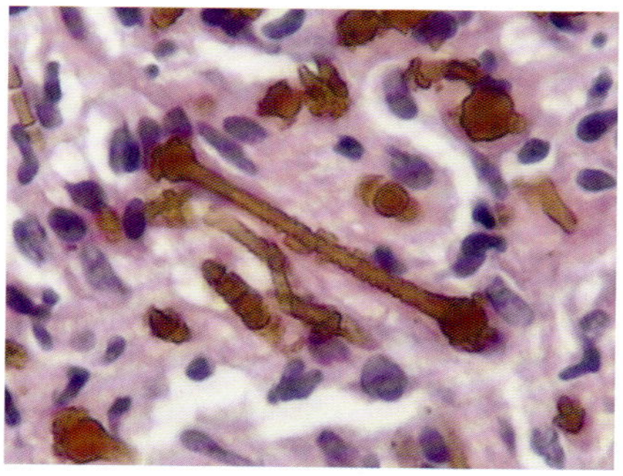

Ferruginous Bodies

Silicosis

Occupations: Glass blowers, sand blasters, mines, brickyards.

CXR: **"eggshell" calcification of hilar lymph nodes**

Cause: Inhalation of crystalline **silica dust**. Inflammation and scarring nodular lesions. (MOA: **Microphages** ingest silica and release **TNF, IL-1** stimulating **fibroblast** → collagen → fibrosis).

SX: Shortness of breath, cyanosis, cough, fever

TX: Supportive

Beryllliosis Exposure to beryllium (chemical element) Occupations: battery plant worker, aerospace manufacturing, beryllium mining, manufacturing of fluorescent light bulbs, electronic manufacturing CXR: **Non- caseating granulomas (inflammatory nodules)** SX: Shortness of breath, cough, chest pain, joint aches, weight loss, fever (SX are identical to sarcoidosis) TX: Steroids. **ONLY** pneumoconiosis that responds to steroids.	**Coal Workers Pneumoconiosis** (AKA: Black Lung disease) The lungs become black because the **macrophages** have phagocytized the coal dust with carbon causing the black color, inflammation, and fibrosis. This does NOT cause lung cancer. CXR: Nodules in the upper lobes
Byssinosis AKA: Brown Lung DZ, Monday Fever. Exposure to **cotton dust** in inadequately ventilated areas believed to be from endotoxins from gram-negative bacteria that grow on the cotton. Narrows the airways causes lung scarring and death from respiratory failure. SX: Wheezing, coughing, dyspnea, chest tightness. TX: Supportive	**Mercury** Mercury can poison from various sources: Indoor and outdoor released as a vapor, water, food. **Respiratory** exposure to vapor: dry cough, dyspnea, chest pain, pulmonary edema, **pulmonary fibrosis**, **pulmonary HTN (Loud P2 heart sound)**, respiratory failure, death. **GI:** metallic taste, nausea, emesis (vomiting), diarrhea, abdominal pain, dysphagia, and enteritis. **Renal:** Kidney failure. **Cardiovascular:** Tachycardia, HTN. **CNS:** headache, weakness, and vision changes. **Skin:** rash. TX: Respiratory and Cardiovascular: Supportive
Bagassosis Hypersensitivity pneumonitis due to exposure to **molasses or moldy cane sugar** due to Actinobacteria (MC: Streptomyces) (**tip**: think of a "BAG" of sugar). SX: Shortness of breath, cough, haemoptysis, low-grade fever, acute diffuse bronchiolitis.	

Pneumonia

Pneumonias: V/Q mismatch, ↑ A-a gradient

MC Community Acquired Pneumonias

Pneumonia	Treatment
Strep Pneumonia,	Ceftriaxone
	Azithromycin/Doxycycline MC used. (Macrolides)
	Fluoroquinolones (Levofloxacin, Moxifloxacin) Used if comorbidities or antibiotics used w/in past 3 months.
	Ampicillin/Sulbactrum

MC Nosocomial Pneumonias

Is NOT considered nosocomial unless patient has been an inpatient for ≥ 48 hours.

Pneumonia	Treatment
Klebsiella	Vancomycin
	Fluoroquinolones (Ciprofloxin, Levofloxacin, Moxifloxacin)
	Cefepime
	Ceftriaxone and Azithromycin
	NOTE: the use of PPI's ↑ risk of nosocomial pneumonias
Ventilator Pneumonia (Pseudomonas)	Piperacillin-Tazobactam, Cefepime, Imipenem, Meropenem, Gentamicin and Vancomycin, Gentamicin and Linezolid

Recurrent Pneumonias Occurring in the Same Location

- Anytime there is a recurring pneumonia at the same location there are two concerns that should be considered
  - Obstruction of some type: cancer/mass
  - Aspiration/swallowing problem
    (Zenker's diverticulum, post-stroke, altered mental status, seizures, etc.)

Recovery Prognosis of Pneumonia

- Depends upon the **integrity of the basement membrane**. If the basement membrane maintains its integrity it means there was no scaring and no edema.
- Stopping smoking
- Pneumococcal pneumonia vaccination
- Spirometry

Bacterial Pneumonia Presentation

- Acute onset, high fever, chills, cough, decreased breath sounds, pleuritic chest pain

Viral Pneumonia Presentation

- MCC: RSV
- Low-grade fever, tachypnea (fast breathing), URI symptoms (sore throat, headache, runny nose, cough, malaise, loss of appetite), can be wheezing

Pneumonias and their MC Causes

Pathogen	Description of Pneumonia
Chlamydia psittaci (Atypical pneumonia – not visible on gram stain)	Dry, non-productive cough. Associated with birds
Chlamydia trachomatis Seen in **infants** 1 – 3 months old.	Gradual onset. Staccato cough, peripheral eosinophilia, no fever or wheezing (differentiates from RSV), can also have chlamydia conjunctivitis shortly after birth.
Coccidioidomycosis	People that work or have been outside in the SW US.
Coxiella burnetii (Atypical pneumonia – not visible on gram stain)	Contact with placental fluids. Associated with farmers, veterinarians. Dry- nonproductive cough.
Haemophilus influenza	COPD
Klebsiella pneumonia	Aspiration: alcoholics, post-surgery, seizures, Zenker's, dysphagia, Diabetics, altered mental status, endotracheal intubation. Associated with inhalation of bacteria from mouth. Associated with anaerobes and hemoptysis ("currant jelly" sputum), and foul smelling sputum. **NOTE: The abscesses from Klebsiella cause liquefactive necrosis in the lungs – NOT caseous necrosis.** **MC nosocomial acquired pneumonia.**
Legionella (Atypical pneumonia – not visible on gram stain)	Associated with contaminated water sources (Air conditioning, water mist, ice machines, ventilation systems). Only pneumonia with GI symptoms (diarrhea, abdominal pain) and/or CNS symptoms (headache, confusion)
Mycoplasma pneumonia (Atypical pneumonia – not visible on gram stain)	Young, healthy patient. CXR looks worse than patient presents. Dry- nonproductive cough.
Pneumocystis (PCP)	HIV with CD4 counts < 200. Dry, nonproductive cough and diffuse bilateral infiltrates on CXR.
Pseudomonas	Associated with: **Diabetes, CF, ventilator patients, burn patients**. Must use pseudomonas drugs: **Piperacillin w/ Tazobactam or Cefepime; Imipenem or Meropenem.**
Staph aureus	Follows recent viral infection (influenza)
Strep pneumonia	**MC Community acquired pneumonia.** Consolidated lobular with ↑ fremitus.

Pneumonia hospitalization Indications (≥ than 2 symptoms = hospitalization)

- **Key requirements for hospitalization: Hypoxia and hypotension (systolic < 90 mm Hg)**
- **Confusion**
- **Uremia (↑ BUN)**
- **Respiratory distress (RR > 30/minute, pulse > 125/min) (AKA: Hypoxic)**
- **Low BP (systolic < 90 mm Hg)**
- **Temperature > 104°**
- **Age > 65 (Increased risk for pneumonia in elderly with lung diseases (causing hypoxia)**
- **Comorbidities: COPD, CHF, renal failure, liver DZ**
- **(TIP: CURB65)**
- **Any elderly patient that is hypoxic (with/without fever) should be admitted.**

Pneumonia Diagnosis

- **BIT: CXR**
- **MAT: Sputum gram stain and culture**

Effusions

Effusion is the escape of a fluid into a body part/cavity. The effusion is either an exudate or a transudate.
Albumin levels and ratios determine differentials between exudate and transudate.
Effusions can be either pleural or abdominal

- **Pleural Effusions** are effusions in the chest
  Excess fluid between the two pleural layers which causes ↓ in lung expansion and pain during inspiration
- **Abdominal Effusion** are effusions in the abdomen

Effusions can either be transudate or exudates

- **Transudate**
  Is due to ↓ oncotic pressure = liver failure or ↑ hydrostatic pressure = CHF.
  Transudate = "translucent" = ↓ protein content: CHF, ascites (cirrhosis), SBP (Spontaneous Bacterial peritonitis)
- **Exudate**
  Is due to ↑ capillary permeability that allows leakage of proteins.
  Exudate = Cloudy, ↑ protein content: Pneumonia, malignancies, collagen vascular disease, RA, Pulmonary embolism, TB, Sarcoidosis, connective tissue dz, infection, lymphoma (Must drain due to ↑ risk of infection), nephrotic diseases, infections (not SBP: Spontaneous Bacterial Peritonitis)

Chylothorax

- **Lymph** formed in the digestive system (AKA: chyle) that has accumulated in the pleural cavity (effusion) due to disruption or obstruction of the thoracic duct. Appearance: turbid, milky white due to **chylomicrons** and **high triglycerides**. (Associated with **Apo-E and B-48**)

Effusion Calculations

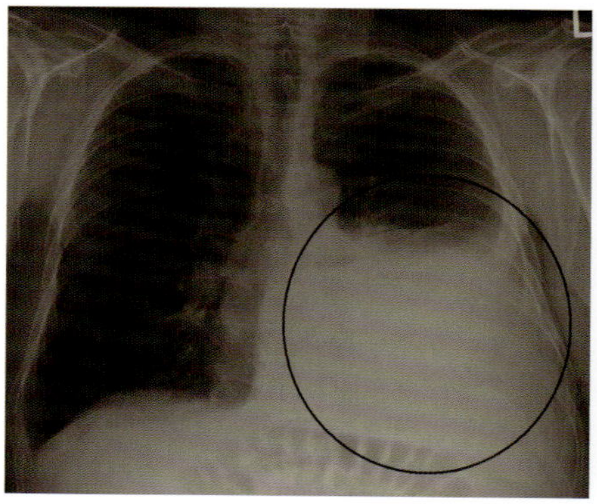

Pleural Effusion

NOTE: beware: The protein reading results in the thorax and the abdomen **is reversed**.
(**tip**: **B**elow the belt = a protein **B**elow 1 is **B**ad. Above the belt, the bad protein is high > 1)

Pleural Effusion Diagnosis	Ascites Sample Diagnosis
Effusion Sample Labs (done by thoracentesis) • Exudate: If ANY of these are present, it is an exudate: Glucose < 60 (glucose is being eaten for energy), pH < 7.2 (acidic), **LDH > .6**, Protein > .5 • If protein > 1 = exudate If protein < 1 = transudate	**Effusion Sample Labs (done by paracentesis)** SAAG (Serum ascites albumin gradient): Protein Analysis between serum protein and effusion proteins in ascites • Subtract the protein reading from the effusion sample from the serum protein content: • If the total is <1.2 = Effusion (cancer, nephrotic syndrome or infection: except for SBP (Spontaneous Bacterial Peritonitis) • If the total is > 1.2 = Transudate (CHF, Portal hypertension, hepatic vein thrombosis, constrictive pericarditis)

Pneumonia

Lobar Pneumonia	Mycoplasma	Bronchopneumonia
MCC: Strep pneumonia Legionella (Must include GI symptoms) Klebsiella SX: **Consolidation, ↑ fremitus,** dullness on resonance. (One localized spot in a lung lobe) **Watch for these S. pneumonia cases**: -**Elderly person** gets the flu and one week later begins to cough and run a fever = S. pneumo - HIV patient has a CD count of 275, it is NOT PCP. (**ANYTHING** above CD200 is S. pneumonia) 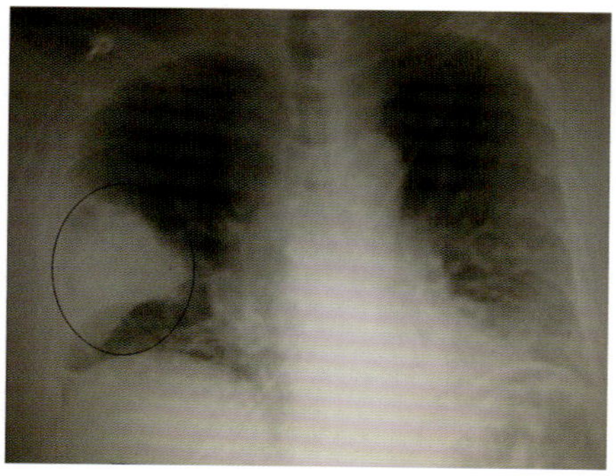	(AKA: Walking pneumonia) **Atypical Pneumonia** MC: young, healthy adult. SX: **Patchy**, diffuse inflammation. Slow to develop, short of breath, non-productive cough. CXR: **Ground glass** CXR in Mycoplasma will look much worse than the patient actually is. 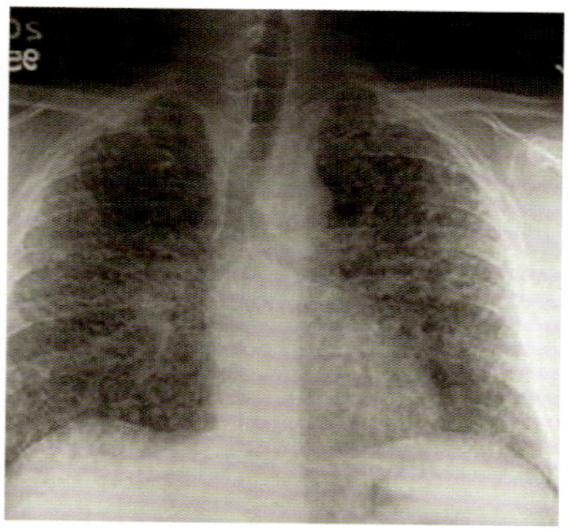	A. aureus Klebsiella Pseudomonas Associated with hospital-acquired pneumonia SX: Acute inflammation of walls of the bronchioles. Affects more than one lobe (unlike lobar, affecting only one lobe). Alveolar sacs are filled with pus/exudate. DX: PMN's in alveolar spaces 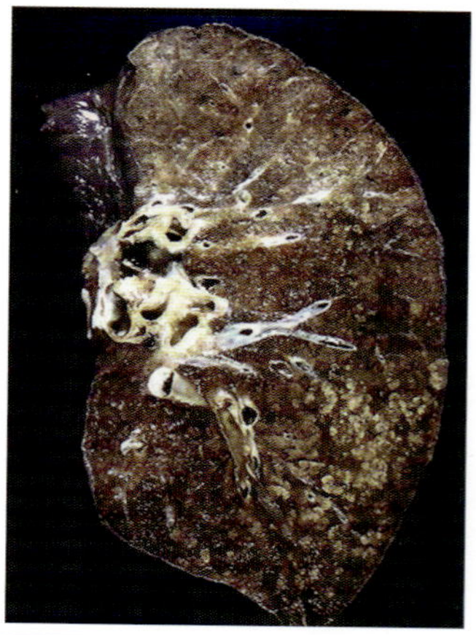

Strep Pneumonia

#1 MC Community acquired
(to be considered a nosocomial pneumonia, patient must have been in the hospital 48 hours)
Lobar pneumonia
Consolidated, only involves infiltrates in one lobe.
ENCAPSULATED

Vaccine:
Vaccine is against the **polysaccharide capsule**.
Vaccine: ⊘present to T cells, T cells independent and B cells respond.
Prophylaxis: Pneumococcal vaccine at age 65 or to all immunocompromised (HIV, chemo, asplenic, COPD). If given prior to age 65, must give booster at 5 yrs.

TX: Ceftriaxone (hotels, cruise ships, mist systems vegetables or outside theme parks whirlpools, fountains, ice machines, dental equipment)

Legionella Pneumonia
(AKA: Legionnaires disease)
Atypical Pneumonia

MC: in **older men that smoke and drink.**

Spread through **water systems**.

SX: **MUST have GI symptoms plus** pneumonia symptoms or **CNS symptoms (headache, confusion),** lobe **consolidation**, high fever.

DX: **Silver stain** or culture on **charcoal yeast with cysteine**.

Labs: **↑ PMN's in sputum**, hyponatremia

TX: **Fluoroquinolones, Azithromycin**

Pseudomonas Pneumonia

Nosocomial patients

Highest Risk Patients:
Cystic Fibrosis
Burn patients
Intubated ventilator patients
(NO flowers or plants allowed in intubated inpatient rooms!)
Diabetics
Immunocompromised
Neutropenic

Bronchiolitis (AKA: RSV)
Inflammation of the bronchioles (small airways that terminate at the alveoli).
MC in children < 2. Most severe in children < 2 months.

MCC: **RSV (Respiratory syncytial virus = Parainfluenza Virus: enveloped,, negative sense),** Adenovirus,

SX: Coughing, wheezing, shortness of breath, fever, tachypnea. Hyperinflation of the lung because air trapping due to the inflammation.

DX: BIT: CXR shows patchy atelectasis and hyperinflation.
MAT: ELISA (viral antigen testing) of nasopharyngeal secretions.

TX: Supportive unless fever, severe tachypnea (> 60/min) with use of accessory muscles in breathing.
β-agonist nebulizers.

Klebsiella Pneumonia

Klebsiella = in normal flora of mouth. Associated with **aspiration pneumonia** leading to abscesses in the upper lobe of the lungs.

Antigen: O antigen of LPS and K antigen w/polysaccharide capsule.
Encapsulated bacteria.

MC of hospital acquired pneumonia (AKA: nosocomial).
Due to aspiration of food particles, vomit (alcoholics, IV drug users, post surgical patients under anesthesia, stroke victims, **COPD**, renal failure, diabetics, malignancy, altered mental status, drug overdoses, esophageal fistulas in neonates, ANY weakened immune system, Zenker's diverticulum, etc.)

SX: Damages alveoli = bloody sputum (AKA: current jelly sputum), productive cough, fever, chills.

TX: **Ampicillin/sulbactam, piperacillin/tazobactam, cefepime, ceftazidime, 3rd Generation Cephalosporins**

Hypersensitivity Pneumonia
(AKA: Allergic alveolitis)

Inflammation of the alveoli caused by hypersensitivity to an inhaled antigen (dust) causing an immune response.

SX: 4 – 6 hours after exposure. Fever, cough, chills, rash, swelling headaches, chest tightness.

CXR: Interstitial **granulomas**, ground glass appearance.

Worsened by exercise.
Causes: **mold**, mist, compost, dust from seeds/beans, bird droppings, detergents

Allergic Bronchopulmonary Aspergillosis (ABPA)

Hypersensitivity response to **Aspergillus (A. fumigatus) spores**.

MC seen with **asthma or cystic fibrosis** patients.

SX: airway inflammation leading to bronchiectasis (abnormal dilation of airways), wheezing, shortness of breath, exercise intolerance, coughing.

DX: Sputum cultures for Aspergillus.

Type 1 (IgE) and Type III (IgG) hypersensitivity

Pneumocystis jiroveci (PCP, PJP) (AKA: Pneumocystis carinii)	**Coccidioidomycosis**	**Blastomycosis**
Yeast "Sporozoites" = Dark oval bodies Stain: Methenamine **silver staining** Highest Risk: **#1 AIDS defining disease. CD4 <200** (**tip:** if given ANY HIV patient with a CD4 count of **ANYTHING** over 200, the pneumonia is due to **Strep pneumonia**) ↑ pneumonia in premature infants Immunocompromised DX: BIT: **CXR shows diffuse bilateral infiltrates Interstitial pneumonia).** Labs: ABG showing ↑ A-a gradient., **↑ LDH levels** (if LDH levels are normal the DX is NOT Pneumocystis). **MAT: Bronchoalveolar lavage. Sputum stain: positive for pneumocystis. Lung biopsy** SX: Dry, **non-productive** cough, fever. **Prophylaxis of Azithromycin for Mycobacterium avium should be started at this time.** TX: **TXP-SMX. Add steroids** to aid in breathing if pO2 is < 70 or A-a gradient is > 35. **Caution: if patient has sulfa allergies to TMP/SMX or has G6PD you must use IV Pentamidine instead of TMP/SMX.** Prophylaxis for PCP can begin at CD4 of 200 with **Atovaquone or Dapsone**.	**Spherule filled with endospores** AKA: San Joaquin Valley Fever **Infection source**: Spores are in the dust and are breathed in most commonly after dust storms and earthquakes. Shows hyphae at 37° and single cells (**endospores** at 25°) Found: **Southwestern USA (CA, NM, AZ, UT)** No person to person transmission Pneumonia and meningitis Usually seen in **HIV only** CXR: lungs show **pulmonary infiltrate, hilar adenopathy**, pleural **effusions**. Can disseminate to skin and bones. SX: Night sweats, fever, cough, **granulomas**, pleuritic chest pain bone lesions, **maculopapular rash** (AKA: "desert bumps" = erythema nodosum), joint pain (AKA: "Desert Rheumatism" = arthralgia TX: Local infections: **Fluconazole or Itraconazole** Systemic infections: **Amphotericin B** Cells covered in budding **blastoconidia** Dimorphic fungus AKA: Budding yeast in a "Captains wheel" or wheel shape formation. **Paracoccidioidomycosis (AKA: Brazilian blastomycosis, South American blastomycosis)** Cells covered in budding **blastoconidia** Dimorphic fungus AKA: Budding yeast in a "Captains wheel" or wheel shape formation. Multiple buds differ from Coccidiomycosis Found: **Latin America** (South America, Brazil) Can affect immunocompetent host Begins as lobar pneumonia or pleurisy. SX: **Painful lesions on lips and on oral mucosa (cutaneous ulcers),** weight loss, fever, cough **TX:** **Sulfonamides, Itraconazole or Amphotericin B**	**Broad base budding** **Dimorphic fungi (cold = 20° is a mold) and (heat = 37° is a yeast in the body/tissues)** Found: **East of Mississippi river and Central America.** **Infection source**: soil, rotting wood. No person-to-person transmission. ↑ Pneumonia in **immuno COMPETENT (non-sick)** CXR: lungs show **dense consolidation and granulomatous nodules** that can disseminate to skin and bone. SX: Skin, bone lesions, fatigue, weight loss, **prostate** problems, joint/**bone** pain, **ulcers on skin** Heaped up lesions on skin with violet color with well-marked boarders. DX: check sputum with Potassium Hydroxide TX: Local infections: **Fluconazole or Itraconazole** Systemic infections: **Amphotericin B** **Mycobacteria avium** Pneumonia in HIV when the CD4 count reaches **<50**. Prophylaxis of **Azithromycin** should be started when CD4 counts are <200.

Chlamydia psittaci **Chlamydia atypical pneumonia** **AKA: Hypersensitivity pneumonia** Source: **birds, chickens, pigeons** High risk for: Veterinarians, pet shop workers, chicken farmers, farming molds. Transmission: aerosol SX: **dry cough, non-productive cough**, sore throat, fever, CXR shows **patchy** pneumonia If not treated, can become chronic leading to pulmonary fibrosis. TX: **Avoid the antigen (cause).** **Azithromycin IM or Doxycycline IM**	**Nocardia** Virulence factor: Cord factor Source: Soil SX: Pulmonary infections in immunocompromised Cutaneous infections after trauma in immunocompetent Risk of: Endocarditis, **slowly progressive pneumonia**, cough, dyspnea, fever, can spread to pleura of chest, subcutaneous abscesses. TX: **TMP/SMX (sulfonamides)**	**Histoplasmosis** **Macrophage filled with Histoplasma** **Spores with budding yeast** (**tip:** "Histo hide's in macrophages) AKA: Intracellular **macroconidia** with spikes. AKA: **Ovoid cells** in macrophages AKA: Yeast cells with thin walls AKA: Huge hepatocytes Found: **Ohio River valley, MS, MO.** **Infection Source**: Cave explorers (AKA: spelunking), chicken farming, raccoons. No person to person transmission **Acute** Pneumonia CXR: lungs show **reticulonodular** pattern with hilar lymphadenopathy, **calcified nodules.** SX: Fever, weight loss, **mouth ulcers**, **palate ulcers**, hepatosplenomegaly, night sweats. Most common with HIV patients DX: **antigen in urine or sputum** TX: Local infections: **Fluconazole or Itraconazole** Systemic infections: **Amphotericin B**

Bronchiolitis Obliterans Organizing Pneumonia (BOOP) AKA: Cryptogenic Organizing Pneumonia (COP) Non-infectious pneumonia. Is an inflammation of the bronchioles and surrounding lung tissues. MC: associated with rheumatoid arthritis or side effect of Amiodarone. SX: Cough, rales, fever, malaise, myalgia, and shortness of breath. Presents quickly: days to weeks. DX: CXR resembles pneumonia (patchy infiltrates) but there is no response to antibiotics and blood/sputum are negative for organisms. There will also be no exposure to occupational hazards. TX: Steroids.	**Ventilator-Associated Pneumonia (VAP)** MC cause: **Pseudomonas** infection. Patients are in ICU. SX: Typical SX of pneumonia may not present or be absent. Watch for fever, hypothermia, new purulent sputum, and hypoxemia. No plants/flowers allowed in with the patient. TX: **Pseudomonas: Piperacillin w/ Tazobactam or Cefepime; Imipenem or Meropenem.** **Gm positive/negatives:** **Vancomycin (Linezolid) and Ciprofloxacin or Gentamicin.**

Lung Inflammation - Stages (Lobar Pneumonia)

Stage Timeline	Reaction	Description
Stage 1: 1st 24 hours	Congestion	Red and heavy. High in bacteria
2nd Stage	Red Hepatization	High in neutrophils and fibrin. High red exudate
3rd Stage	Grey Hepatization	Fibrin, neutrophils, dry, grey color, decrease in RBC's
Stage 4: Resolution	Macrophages and cough clear infection	Enzymatic digestion and exudate

RDS (Respiratory Distress Syndrome) and ARDS (Acute Respiratory Distress Syndrome)

Respiratory Distress Syndrome
(AKA: RDS, Hyaline Membrane Disease).
Seen in neonates
Cause: Insufficient surfactant

- **Surfactant: Fetal Lung Maturation: L/S Ration 2:1**
- **Lecithin (AKA: Phosphatidylcholine) to Sphingomyelin**
- **Fetus lungs mature after 34 weeks**
- **Surfactant produced by Type II Pneumocytes in the lungs**
- **Surfactant decreases the surface tension of the lungs**
- **Hyaline membrane shows as pink on histology**
- Steroids given prior to **34 weeks** to mature lungs (causes stress = release surfactant)
  Betamethasone, Dexamethasone

Type II pneumocytes (AKA: the greater alveolar cells) large cuboidal type cells: Secrete **Surfactant = Type II pneumocytes (↓ alveolar surface tension = ↑ compliance = ↓ work of inspiration)**

Hypoinflated (underdeveloped lungs) can also be caused by oligohydramnios (amniotic fluid helps mature lungs) and by congenital diaphragmatic hernia (intestines crowding out the lung)

Acute Respiratory Distress Syndrome
Adult form of RDS, but his is not due to surfactant issues, it is due to atelectasis.
Can also be referred to as **hyaline membrane disease**.

Sudden respiratory failure due to diffuse lung injury secondary to other injuries:
Trauma (lung contusion), lung infection, sepsis, pneumonia, trauma, ↑ blood transfusions, aspiration, burns, pancreatitis, inhalation of chemicals/smoke/chlorine gas, near drowning, shock, systemic infection.

Disease of the alveoli causing ↓ gas exchange. The alveoli causing **atelectasis** (partial collapse of the lung) and hypoxemia leading to loss of surfactant = ↓ surface tension = ↑ fluid accumulation and ↑ fibrous tissue formation.

Complicated by infiltration of T lymphocytes and PMN's

SX: Within 72 hours of injury = shortness of breath, ↑ respiratory rate, ↓ O_2 Saturation.

DX:
CXR: infiltrates (opacities/fluid accumulation in lungs)
Histology: alveolar damage and **hyaline membrane** formation in alveolar walls.
Normal PWCP
Levels and severity:
PO2/FIO2 ratio < 300 = ARDS
PO2/FIO2 ratio < 200 = moderate
PO2/FIO2 ratio < 100 = severe

TX:
Positive end expiratory pressure (PEEP) to keep alveoli open, admit to ICU.
Mechanical ventilation with low tidal volume.
Prone positioning of body.
Dobutamine (positive inotrope), Diuretics.
Steroids are not effective.

Difference between ARDS and Pulmonary edema

- **Pulmonary edema** is due to a back up of pressure from the **left side of the heart**. High pressure on the left side of the hear means ↑ **PCWP** (high pressure in the left atrium)
- **ARDS** is a problem in the **lungs** (so the issue has not even reached the left side of the heart so no pressure has been built up in the left atrium) so **PCWP is NORMAL**

Obstructive Lung Diseases

COPD

(Chronic Obstructive Pulmonary Disease)
Lung destruction of alveoli that ↓ **elastic recoil** of the lungs. Chronically retain CO2.

MCC: **smoking.**
Other causes: air pollution exposure to chemicals and dust.

Best **prognosis factor is FEV1 percent.**
If it is ≤ 40% the prognosis is poor.

COPD is a combination of chronic bronchitis (long standing inflammation of large airways characterized by cough and sputum most days of 3 months of two successive years) and emphysema (loss of elastic recoil of lung, enlargement of the smallest airways (after the terminal bronchioles) and destruction of the alveoli walls).

↑ Compliancy of the lungs.
Radial traction and Recoil is **↓ in obstructive lung disease.**
Obstructive lung dz = ↑ elastase activity = interstitium is broken down = ↓ elastic springs = ↓ recoil.

Compensation:
COPD patients retain CO2 causing chronic respiratory acidosis with a compensatory metabolic alkalosis (increased PaCO2 and a decreased blood pH). Kidneys will compensate by ↑ HCO3 reabsorption (aka: decreasing renal HCO3 excretion) which will ↑ blood HCO3. It will also increase renal acid excretion in order to decrease the acidity in the blood by raising the blood pH). This will cause the urine to be come more acidic (decreasing the pH of the urine).

SX: Sputum production, shortness of breath (breath through **pursed lips** and worsened by exertion), ↑ deep cough, sputum, productive cough, muscle wasting, cachexia (loss of body mass that can't be reversed with nutrition), chronic cough, tripod positioning (arms resting on knees when leaning forward while sitting), use of accessory muscles in respiration, will have **polycythemia** (due to chronic hypoxia), **barrel chest** (due to air trapping), Pulmonary HTN (indicated with a loud S2), clubbing of fingers, respiratory acidosis with a metabolic compensation (↑serum bicarb).
Patient will also have emphysema.

COPD

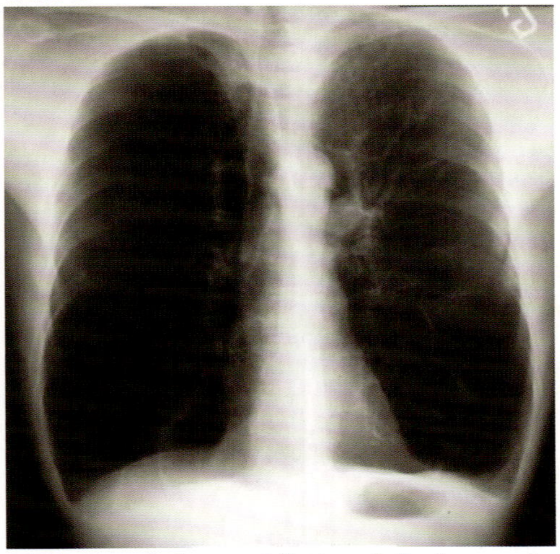

COPD: barrel chest and flattened diaphragm due to increased total lung capacity.

SX: If symptoms sound exactly like COPD but there is **NO smoking** involved, it is due to **Alpha-1 antitrypsin deficiency.**

Cor pulmonale: Pulmonary HTN (due to vasoconstriction in the lungs) causes strain on the right heart (RVH), which backs up = JVD, nutmeg liver, lower leg edema.

COPD patients depend upon **CO2** to stimulate their breathing response in the medulla via the **central chemical receptors**. High flow oxygen should **never** be administered to COPD patients or the oxygen will replace the CO2 and they will stop breathing. (AKA: it will remove the drive that allows them to breath).

DX:
BIT: **CXR: Barrel chest** (↑ Total lung volume, **↑ anterior-posterior diameter (AP)**, flattened diaphragm, bullae.

MAT: PFT (Pulmonary Function Test) shows **obstructive pattern:**
COPD Obstructive profile: ↓ FEV1/FVC ration (<80%), (FEV1 decreases more than FVC), ↓ FEV1, ↓ FVC, ↓ Radial Traction, ↓ Recoil.
↑ Reserve volume, ↑ Total lung volume.
↓ in DLCO (diffusion lung capacity for carbon monoxide). **↑ V/Q ratio, ↑ A-a ratio.**
Blood Gases:
Respiratory Acidosis (↓ pH, ↑ CO2, ↓ O2).

V/Q Mismatch: Inadequate ventilation due to damaged alveoli, but adequate perfusion.

COPD cont'd

Shows little improvement with Albuterol.
ECHO: Right atrial and ventricular hypertrophy and pulmonary HTN.
ABG: ↑ PCO2 and hypoxia. (ABG will indicate if patient is retaining CO2)
CBC: ↑ Hct (Polycythemia) and microcytic anemia. ↑ serum bicarb from compensation of respiratory acidosis.
EKG: Multifocal Atrial Tachycardia (MAT) or A-Fib, right axis deviation.

COPD Exacerbation: Severe shortness of breath, ↑ sputum production (green/yellow) and ↑ cough, ↑ HR and respiratory rate, blue tinge to the skin due to hypoxia, bilateral wheezing and crackles, use of expiratory muscles to prolong expiration.

TX: **Albuterol nebulizer, Ipratropium (most effective), corticosteroids (Beclomethasone, Hydrocortisone), systemic steroids (Methylprednisone).**
COPD not controlled with Albuterol should have Ipratropium or Tiotropium (inhaled anticholinergics are best), add inhaled steroids.
If not responding to treatment, use NIPPV (Non-invasive Positive Pressure Ventilation).

Best overall benefit to improve mortality in COPD patients:
#1 – stop smoking
#2 – home oxygen once O2 sat falls below 88% or pO2 ≤ 55.
#3 – Annual influenza and pneumococcal vaccinations
#4 – Albuterol, Ipratropium or Tiotropium inhaler.

Emphysema

Type of COPD
Difference between emphysema and COPD: Emphysema is just the loss of elastic recoil of lungs. COPD is loss of recoil coupled with airway inflammation.
(Air sacs are damaged)

Loss of elastic recoil of the lung and alveoli become damaged due to over inflammation and will burst. Ability to exchange gases is impaired or destroyed.

Patients can have emphysema without COPD but can't have COPD without having emphysema.

DX: Black carbon deposits, enlarged alveoli with thin septae.

MCC: Smoking

Emphysema is referred to as a **"pink puffer".**
Emphysema patients are able to get air and **do not retain CO2** (so the face is pink).
Due to enlargement of air spaces and a decrease in elastic recoil.
Causes:
Centroacinar = smoking.
Panacinar = α-1 AT deficiency (liver cirrhosis, PAS+, non-smokers)
Paraseptal: bullae/blebs that rupture causing pneumothorax.

A1AT is associated with **panacinar** emphysema and **no smoking.**
Smoking is associated with **centriacinar** emphysema and **smoking**. (**tip**: "S"entriacinar for "S"moking).

Chronic bronchitis is considered the **"blue bloater"** because of the constricted airways causing a **build up of CO2** leading to cyanosis (blue). Due to a hypertrophy of mucus-secreting glands in the bronchioles causing an ↑ **Reid index** > 50.
Chronic bronchitis must have a productive cough > 3 consecutive months for > 2 years. Small airways most affected.

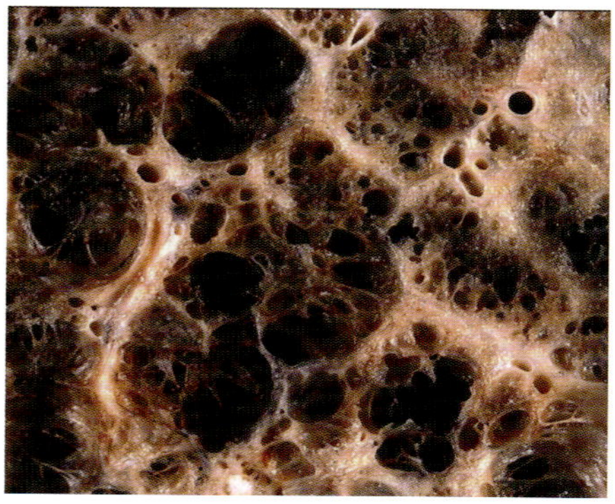

Emphysema

Alpha-1 Antitrypsin Deficiency

Genetic disorder.
Misfolded Protein.
Decreased A1AT in the blood and lungs.

Deficiency in the lungs is associated with **Panacinar emphysema or COPD, not associated with smoking**.
(Centriacinar emphysema)

A1AT protects the lungs against neutrophil elastase. Deficiency of this enzyme breaks down lung/connective tissue. It also deposits abnormal A1AT in the liver causing cirrhosis and liver failure.

DX:
CXR: Same as COPD: Barrel chest (↑ Total lung volume, **↑ anterior-posterior diameter (AP)**, flattened diaphragm, bullae.
Labs: ↓ albumin and ↑ PT due from cirrhosis of the liver (A1AT is made in the liver), **PAS +, ↓ A1AT.**

TX: infusion of A1AT

Bronchiectasis

Permanent enlargement/dilation of the large bronchi in the lung due to an anatomic defect. Chronic necrotizing inflammation of the lungs and inability to clear mucus.

SX: Reoccurring lung infections, chronic cough, fever, hemoptysis, **mucus production** (green/yellow), frequent lung infections (due to the mucus), **↑↑ volume of purulent sputum (> 100 mL/day)**, dysfunction of cilia, anemia of chronic DZ, weight loss, wheezing, clubbing, sinus congestion,

DX: BIT: CXR shows thickened, dilated bronchi that show "tram tracking" (parallel lines associated with dilated bronchi). Bronchi are larger than pulmonary artery branches.

MAT: CT scan.
Sputum culture: determines bacterial cause.

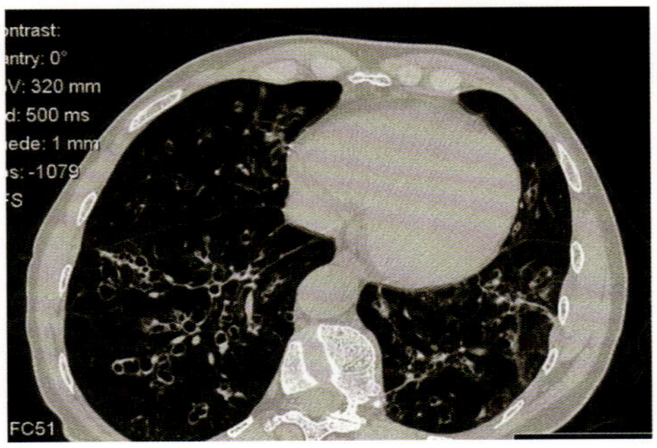

Causes: **MCC: Cystic Fibrosis**, pneumonia, TB, Kartagener, aspergillosis, foreign bodies, tumors, rheumatoid arthritis. Allergic bronchopulmonary aspergillosis (ABPA).

TX: Chest physiotherapy (cupping and clapping) to help dislodge mucus, controlling and treat infections with repeated courses of antibiotics (rotate antibiotics between infections to ↓ risk of resistance), vaccinations against pneumonia, influenza, pertussis, surgical resection if indicated.

Asthma

Reversible obstructive lung disease.
Chronic inflammation of the airways with recurring and variable symptoms.

SX: **Wheezing**, dyspnea, hypoxemia, mucus, cough, shortness of breath, chest tightness, nasal polyps,
sensitivity to aspirin, eczema/atopic dermatitis,
↑ length of expiratory phase (same profile as all obstructive diseases), will see use of accessory intercostal muscles.
Symptoms are worse at night.

Labs: CBC shows **eosinophil's**
↑ IgE levels.
(TX: **Omalizumab** = anti-IgE medication)
↑ IgE levels are associated with bronchopulmonary aspergillosis.

Triggers: exercise, cold air, aspirin, stress, viral URI's, environmental factors, emotional stress, NSAID's, histamine, β-Blockers, tobacco smoke, GERD, infection, pet dander, dust mites, pollen, cockroaches, nebulized medications, catamenial lung pathology (associated with endometriosis).

Eosinophils in the sputum show **Charcot-Leyden crystals.**
(Note: Eosinophil's kill parasites using **Major Basic Protein**).

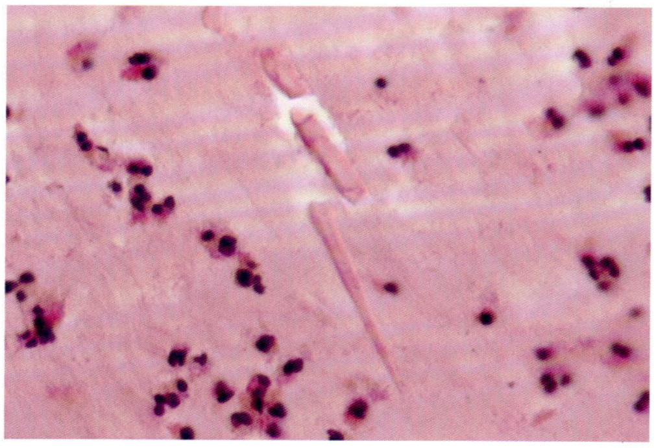

DX:
BIT: Peak expiratory flow (PEF) and/or Arterial Blood Gas (ABG). (NOTE: on ANY breathing problem, always order an ABG).
CXR: normal, hyperinflation.

MAT: Pulmonary Function Test (PFT).
Obstructive profile: ↓ FEV1/FVC ration (<80%), (FEV1 decreases more than FVC)
↑ Reserve volume, ↑ Total lung volume.
↑ FEV1 > 12% with use of Albuterol.
↓ FEV1 > 20% with use of Methacholine.
↑ in DLCO (diffusion lung capacity for carbon monoxide).
↓ V/Q Ratio

Asthma continued

Methacholine challenge test. (Induces an asthma attack in an asymptomatic patient). Test will show a decrease in FEV1.
Skin testing for allergens = ↑ broncho constriction.

TX:
Acute asthma: Inhaled short-acting β agonist (SABA):
Albuterol, Pirbuterol, Levalbuterol.
Long Term asthma: Low-dose inhaled corticosteroids (ICS) Beclomethasone, **Fluticasone, Triamcinolone**, Budesonide, Flunisolide, Mometasone.
Additional long term medications: Cromolyn, Nedocromil, **Montelukast, Zafirlukast, Zileuton**, Theophylline, **Omalizumab** (anti- IgE: stops degranulation of mast cells), Prednisone (oral).
Asthma not controlled with Albuterol should use inhales steroids.
Vaccinations recommended for asthma patients: Annual influenza, Pneumococcal.

TX: **Non-acute asthma**: 1) **Inhaled Albuterol, 2) Inhaled Methyl Prednisolone, 3) Salmeterol (long acting inhaled β-agonist).**

TX: **Exercised induced asthma: Use inhaled bronchodilator just prior to exercise.**

Aspirin-Induced Asthma
(AKA: Aspirin Sensitivity Syndrome)
Occurs 30 min. – 3 hours after taking aspirin.
Caused by increased production of leukotrienes in the arachidonic acid pathway.
SX: Persistent nasal block, episodes of periodic difficulty breathing.
TX: Desensitization to aspirin, surgery to remove nasal polyps.

Churg-Strauss: autoimmune disease with triad of eosinophil's, vasculitis, asthma. Associated with
P-ANCA.
AKA: **Atopic dermatitis**: eczema (itchy, inflammation of the skin) with asthma or allergies and eosinophils.

Allergic Bronchopulmonary Aspergillosis (ABPA) Hypersensitivity response of the immune system to Aspergillus spores (A. fumigatus) that colonizes the lungs.

To ↓ risk of complications during surgery and post-operative risk: Improve asthma control before surgery.

Asthma Exacerbation

SX: Hyperventilation (↑ RR), hypoxia, respiratory acidosis, ↓ PEF (Peek Expiratory Flow), there may or may not be wheezing present.

NOTE: **Asthma exacerbation: Indications that the patient may be about to quit breathing:** A high respiratory rate (normal RR is 10 – 16 bpm) AKA: shortness of breath, lack of wheezing, hypoxia (low O2 Sat on oximeter), decrease in peak flow, respiratory acidosis. Be prepared to intubate and admit to ICU.

Test for severity of an asthma exacerbation:
↓ Peek Expiratory Flow (PEF), Arterial Blood Gas (ABG) with an ↑ A-a gradient.

TX Asthma Exacerbation: **Oxygen, Inhaled Albuterol, Bolus of Methyl Prednisolone, Inhaled Ipratropium, Magnesium** (relieves bronchospasms).
↑ FEV1 > 12% with use of Albuterol.
↓ FEV1 > 20% with use of Methacholine.
↑ in DLCO (diffusion lung capacity for carbon monoxide).

Raise the head of the bed. (In ALL issues with breathing problems: ER, after surgery, etc., raising the head of the bed can ↑ oxygenation by as much as 50%. #1 best thing to ↑ oxygenation.
ALL patients presenting with shortness of breath must receive: Raise head of bed, oxygen, Chest X-ray, Arterial Blood Gas (ABG), continuous oximeter.

Medications **not effective** in acute asthma exacerbations: **Salmeterol, Omalizumab, Terbutaline, Theophylline, Cromolyn, Leukotriene drugs, Epinephrine, Inhaled corticosteroids.**

Chronic Bronchitis

Form of COPD
Long-standing inflammation of large airways characterized by cough and sputum most days of 3 months of two successive years. Inflammation causes narrowing of the air tubes affecting respiration.
(Air sacs are not damaged)

Referred to as the "blue bloaters" because it is difficult to get air in the constricted airways causing retention of CO2 leading to cyanosis.

Reid Index: > 40%

CYSTIC FIBROSIS, AR

Normal: CFTR protein secretes Cl in lumen and no Na absorption

Abnormal: CFTR protein does not secrete Cl and increased Na absorption

- Defect of **CFTR gene on chromosome 7**
- **Deletion of PHE at position 508 in CFTR protein**
- **Frameshift** mutation +/- base pair
- AKA: **Misfolded protein**
- AKA: Defect in cellular transport of Cl
- AKA: Decreased Cl secretion = increased intracellular Cl = increased Na reabsorption = increased H2O reabsorption = thick mucus excreted into lungs and GI
- AKA: Increased concentration of Cl ions in sweat
- AKA: Defective ion transport at epithelial surfaces
- AKA: No intracellular folding
- AKA: No glycosylation of protein
- AKA: CFTR encodes an ATP gated CL channel that secretes Cl in lungs and GI and reabsorbs Cl in sweat glands.
- **Number one cause of malabsorption in Caucasians**
- DX:
  MAT: **Sweat chloride test**: shows increased Cl in sweat. (Pilocarpine ↑ ACh which ↑ sweat. Chloride levels in sweat > 60 mEq/L = CF)
- CXR: Atelectasis, bronchiectasis, pneumothorax, hyperinflation.
- PFT: Show obstructive pattern.
- Pancreas: Beta islet cells function is not affected until patient is older.
- SX: recurrent pulmonary infections (esp. Pseudomonas), **infertility in males** (azoospermia due to **lack of vas deferens** = no sperm), infertility in females due to thickened mucus on cervix blocks sperm entry and chronic lung dz alters menstrual cycle), **malabsorption** = steatorrhea, malabsorption leads to deficiency of fat soluble vitamins D, E, A, K, **nasal polyps**, **meconium ileus** in newborns (abdominal distention), chronic bronchitis, bronchiectasis, **biliary cirrhosis,** recurrent **pancreatitis.**
- TX: **N-acetylcysteine**
  MOA: mucolytic – cleaves disulfide bonds, replace pancreatic enzymes, antibiotics to treat bacterial infections (rotate antibiotics to prevent resistance), all CF patients should get influenza and pneumococcal vaccinations. Lung transplant if no response to treatment.

NOTE: don't forget that Pseudomonas infections are the most common in CF patients.

Allergic Bronchopulmonary Aspergillosis (ABPA)

Hypersensitivity response of the immune system to **Aspergillus spores** (A. fumigatus) that colonizes the lungs. Causes **inflammation** of the airways, which can lead to bronchiectasis (permanent dilation of the bronchi).

MC in cystic fibrosis or asthma.

SX: Presentation: asthmatic patient with worsening asthma symptoms. Wheezing, hemoptysis, productive cough, fever, malaise. Airway inflammation leading to bronchiectasis (abnormal dilation of airways), shortness of breath, exercise intolerance.

DX:

Labs: ↑ IgE, **eosinophils**, A. fumigatus-specific antibodies.

CXR or CT: shows pulmonary infiltrates and central bronchiectasis.

Sputum: shows brownish (brown specs) in mucus.

Sputum cultures: Positive for Aspergillus.

Type 1 (IgE) and Type III (IgG) hypersensitivity.

TX: Oral **prednisone** (corticosteroids). (Inhaled steroids are not effective). Oral **Itraconazole** for recurrent ABPA.

Post Operative Atelectasis

Surgery can ↓ FRC by 30% and VC by 50%. Other factors that ↓ respiratory drive are postoperative pain (results in shallow breathing) and narcotics for the pain.

Fastest way to ↑ FRC from 20 – 34% and prevent atelectasis is to raise the head of the bed. This ↓ intra abdominal pressure on the diaphragm. (Note: for ANY breathing problem, raising the head of the bed is the fastest way to improve breathing).

Lobar segment collapse causing ↓ lung volume. Retained secretions ↓ lung compliance. Anatomy shifts toward atelectasis.

(**Note:** pneumonia has normal lung volume and there is no shifting of the anatomy).

↑ risk from post op day 2 – day 5. MC with abdominal or thoraco-abdominal surgery.

↑ risk with the elderly and smokers.

SX: Low oxygen saturation, pleural effusion (transudate), fast and shallow breathing, ↑ heart rate and temperature, poor cough (due to pain when coughing), hypoxia

Causes: Respiratory alkalosis: ↑ pH, ↓ CO2, ↓ O2, ↓ respiratory rate.

Prevention: Incentive spirometry, deep breath breathing exercises, pain control.

Obstructive Sleep Apnea

Central Sleep Apnea
(AKA: Cheyne-Stokes respiration)
Decreased respiratory drive from the CNS.
No effort made to breath.

Malfunction of neurological controls for breathing causing **failure of inhalation** causing the % of O2 to drop (hypoxaemia) and CO2 (hypercapnia) to increase.
After a long pause (**Cheyne-stokes**) breathing occurs in shallow to deeper cycles.

TX: CPAP (senses when you do not breath and breaths for you), **No use of alcohol and/or sedatives.**
Acetazolamide (Causes metabolic acidosis to help drive respiration. Bicarb is eliminated out of the body because there is no carbonic anhydrase to reabsorb it, making the body acidotic).

Obesity Hypoventilation Syndrome
BMI ≥ 30
Hypoventilation.
Unlike OSA, there is ↓ PaO2 and ↑ CO2 during the day

Obstructive Sleep Apnea (OSA)
Efforts are made to breath but because of collapse in the upper airways (**blockage/obstruction**), air can't get into the lungs so patient is unable to get the air they need to breath.

Causes: **Obesity**, thick necks, nasal deformation, large adenoids, allergies, large tonsils, sleeping in awkward positions, large uvula.

SX: **Snoring**, nocturnal hypoxia, ↑ night time awakenings, **daytime somnolence**, **headaches in the mornings** (due to ↑ CO2 at night), fatigue, sore throats (snoring), **orthopnea** (dyspnea when lying flat, must be propped up to sleep: ie: # of pillows used), systemic and pulmonary HTN, arrhythmias, polycythemia (due to hypoxia and ↑ EPO), right heart failure (Cor Pulmonale), fat neck, erectile dysfunction.
(Normal PaO2 during the day, ↓ PaO2 and ↑ CO2 during the night)

DX: **Polysomnography** (sleep study).
Mild apnea: 5 – 20 apneic episodes/hour.
Severe apnea: > 30 episodes/hour.

TX: **Weight loss**, CPAP or BiPAP (Continuous Positive Airway Pressure)

Differentials in Obstructive Lung Disease

Disease	**DLCO** (Diffusion capacity for carbon monoxide) Measures the partial pressure difference between inspired and expired carbon monoxide.	**Notes**
COPD/Emphysema	**↓ DLCO**	FEV1 in COPD and Emphysema does not improve after use of bronchodilator
Chronic Bronchitis	Normal DLCO	
Asthma	**↑ DLCO**	FEV1 in asthma improves after use of a bronchodilator. Reversible after bronchodilation.

Pulmonary Embolism

Pulmonary Embolism and DVT and Arterial Embolisms and Superficial Clots and other Emboli

Virchow's triad

- **Venous stasis** = **slow blood flow**. Causes: driving, flying, pregnancy, OCP's, hormone replacement therapy, bed rest/hospitalization, orthopedic cast, obesity, sitting in wheel chairs (**Caution**: Beware of the patient that is wheel chair bound and **be aware of the diver that is NOT ascending**. If the diver becomes acutely short of breath while swimming, it is **not** nitrous bubbles, it is a PE due to a DVT because the diver probably flew to the diving destination. If the diver **IS ascending** then the shortness of breath is due to nitrous bubbles.)
- Hypercoagulability = abnormal blood coagulation (Factor V Leiden, antithrombin deficiency, Protein C and S deficiency, polycythemia vera, nephrotic syndrome, cancers)
- Turbulence caused by endothelial blood vessel lining damage (surgeries, IV drugs)
- Considered: Dead space.

Pulmonary Embolism

Sudden/acute onset shortness of breath.
(Pulmonary edema with CHF is not acute, this take a couple of hours, PE shortness of breath is immediate), ↓ O2 sat (look for it in the low 90's), normal CXR. ABG shows ↑ A-a gradient. Pleural effusion can be an exudate and transudate. Can see hemoptysis.
No specific physical findings.

Shows a respiratory alkalosis due to hyperventilation (↑ pH, ↓ PaO2, ↓ PaCO2)

V/Q Mismatch. Good ventilation but poor perfusion (clot in pulmonary artery). ↑V/Q ratio.

↑ Risk: Fat embolus, Air (scuba), DVT (deep leg veins), bacterial endocarditis, amniotic fluid, tumors**., immobility**, surgery (higher risk in orthopedic/joint replacement or abdominal surgery), trauma, Factor V mutation, Protein C and S deficiency, malignancy, lupus anticoagulant.

Pathway of a PE: Thrombus ↑ pulmonary vascular resistance → ↑ Right ventricular pressure → hypokinesis and dilation of the right ventricle → ↓ preload (pushes septum into the left ventricle) → hypotension = ventricular dysfunction, ↑ BNP and troponin.

DX: BIT: Spiral CT (AKA: pulmonary angiography), V/Q scan. D-Dimer (sensitive but poor specificity). Negative D-Dimer test = PE is unlikely.
Chest X-Ray is normal, it may show atelectasis.
EKG: Sinus tachycardia, nonspecific ST-T wave changes, Right axis deviation, right bundle branch block.
MAT: Angiography (invasive test with a high risk of death).

TX: Start Heparin immediately, do not wait for result of the CT or V/Q scan. Oxygen, Heparin to bridge to Warfarin.
If patient is at **risk for bleeding: use IVC Filter**. (Bleeding ulcer, recent major surgery, previous hemorrhagic stroke).
Thrombolytics for patients that are hemodynamically unstable (AKA: hypotension).

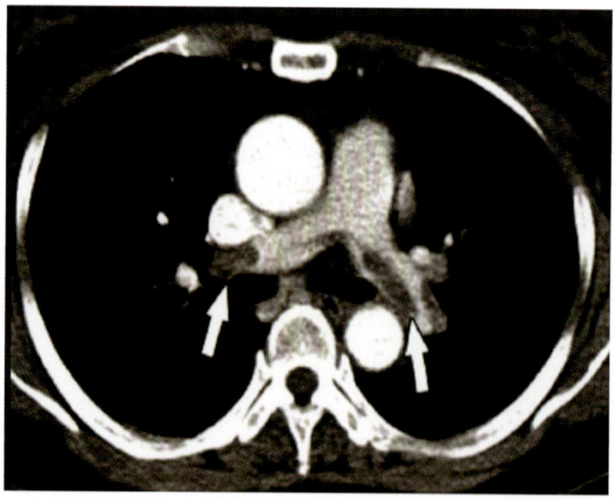

DVT (Deep vein thrombosis)

Formation of a blood clot in the deep veins.
Slow onset
Causes: See above

SX: Clot in the calf = **positive Homans sign (pain on dorsiflexion of leg), pain, swelling, redness (erythema).**

DVT's can anywhere in the deep veins.
The larger and closer to the heart, the more dangerous.
Most are in the calf (popliteal vein), clots in the femoral vein, iliofemoral vein or IVC are dangerous

DX: Doppler ultrasound to locate DVT in lower leg.
Labs: **D-Dimer (fibrin degradation product) and indicates clotting (PE, DVT).**
Wells Criteria (see below)

TX: Anticoagulation: **Heparin** (low molecular weight) followed by 6 months of **warfarin** for first clot.
> 1 clot history = lifetime warfarin therapy.
Warfarin: Must follow **PT/INR; keep between 2 – 3 (2.5 ideal).**
If patient has a prosthetic valve then PT/INR 3 – 4 (3.5 ideal).
(Warfarin toxicity: active bleeding requires **fresh frozen plasma**)

IVC Filters: (Inferior vena cava filter) used when the patient is not able to be anti-coagulated: Recent hemorrhagic stroke, bleeding ulcer, recent surgery, **anything** that would cause the patient to bleed more.

Arterial Embolism Comes from left side of heart and blocks blood flow to an organ or body part. (brain = stroke, heart = heart attack, kidneys, intestine (mesenteric ischemia), eyes) Causes: A-Fib, myxoma, patent foramen ovale, obesity, smoking, diabetes, sedentary lifestyle, HTN, stress, increased age, recent surgery SX: **Immediate onset**, severe pain, cyanosis of distal tissue from the clot, ↓ or no pulse, muscle spasms, numbness, paralysis, cold limb Emergency.	**Superficial Thrombophlebitis:** thrombus develops in a vein near surface of the skin, usually in the lower legs. SX: inflammation, redness, pain, **palpates a hard, tender "cord"** under the skin. Complication: can progress through perforating veins into the deep veins to become a DVT and PE **Trousseau's Syndrome**: Recurrent, migratory thrombophlebitis can indicate malignancy (Associated with: pancreatic, lung, gastric cancers) **Amniotic Fluid Emboli:** amniotic fluid or fetal cells enter mother's bloodstream leading to hypotension, cardiac failure and DIC. Emergency, high mortality rate. **Gas/Air Emboli:** Nitrogen gas bubbles that precipitate in the brain from a diver ascending to quickly. (**Caution**: beware of the diver that is NOT ascending, just swimming along and becomes short of breath, this is a PE from a DVT due to him flying to the dive spot) TX: Hyperbaric chamber **Fat Emboli:** Due to long bone fractures, trauma, liposuction, and burns. (MC: closed fractures of the pelvis). **Cholesterol Emboli:** Cholesterol emboli that are released from atherosclerotic plaque. These emboli can also be released after procedures, which clean out atherosclerotic plaques in the carotid artery or coronary arteries, angiography, vascular surgery, coronary catheterization and administration of anticoagulants.

Wells Criteria for DVT (probability of having a DVT)

Wells score or criteria: (possible score −2 to 9)

1. **Active cancer (treatment within last 6 months or palliative): +1 point**
2. **Calf swelling ≥ 3 cm compared to asymptomatic calf (measured 10 cm below tibial tuberosity): +1 point**
3. **Swollen unilateral superficial veins (non-varicose, in symptomatic leg): +1 point**
4. **Unilateral pitting edema (in symptomatic leg): +1 point**
5. **Previous documented DVT: +1 point**
6. **Swelling of entire leg: +1 point**
7. **Localized tenderness along the deep venous system: +1 point**
8. **Paralysis, paresis, or recent cast immobilization of lower extremities: +1 point**
9. **Recently bedridden ≥ 3 days, or major surgery requiring regional or general anesthetic in the past 12 weeks: +1 point**
10. **Alternative diagnosis at least as likely: −2 points**

Wells scores ≥ 2 have a 28% chance of having DVT, score < 2 chance is 6%.

Wells Criteria for Pulmonary Embolism (probability of having a PE)

- **Clinically suspected DVT = 3.0 points**
- **Alternative diagnosis is less likely than PE = 3.0 points**
- **Tachycardia (heart rate > 100) = 1.5 points**
- **Immobilization (≥ 3d)/surgery in previous four weeks = 1.5 points**
- **History of DVT or PE = 1.5 points**
- **Hemoptysis = 1.0 points**
- **Malignancy (with treatment within 6 months) or palliative = 1.0 points**
- **Score >6.0 = High probability of PE**
- **Score 2.0 to 6.0 = Moderate probability**
- **Score <2.0 = Low probability Score > 4 = PE likely do diagnostic imaging.**
- **Score ≤ 4 = PE unlikely. Check D-Dimer to rule out PE.**

Pneumothorax

Accumulation of air in the pleural space.

Causes: injury to chest wall, stab or bullet wounds, fractured rib (**Stab wounds:** Remember, the lungs extend above the clavicle. So beware of the stab wound that occurs above the clavicle – it hits the lungs)

SX: **Hyperresonance and diminished breath sounds** (on affected side), ↓ **fremitus**, unilateral chest pain, dyspnea. Trachea can deviate **toward the side of the insult (vacuum pulling the trachea in).**

TX: Small pneumothorax: self-resolving.
Larger pneumothorax: chest tube connected to a one-way valve system

NOTE: When you look at a CXR, the area with the pneumothorax will look very black (just air). Areas of lung tissue will always have small lines; they will not appear solid black. If you look closely, sometimes you can also see the outline of the collapsed lung.

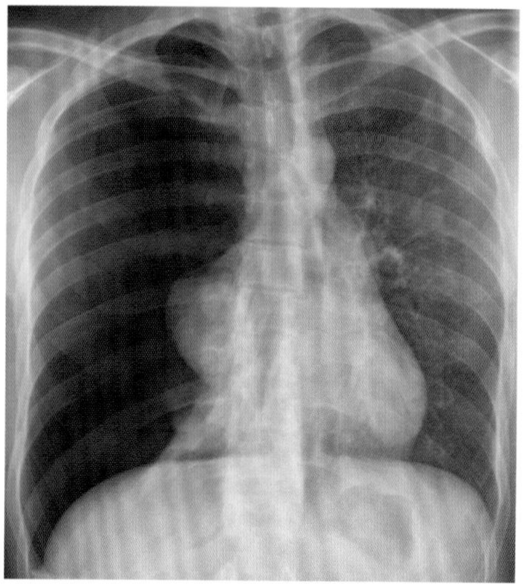

Spontaneous Pneumothorax

Accumulation of air in the pleural space due to rupture of apical **blebs.**

MC: COPD, **Marfan's,** smoking, family history
(watch for a tall, thin male that reports to the ER short of breath and chest pain).

Tension Pneumothorax

Air enters the chest but is unable to exit, therefore building up pressure, which can compress the lungs and heart (**tamponade**). Impairs respiration and/or blood circulation.

Emergency: **Immediate thoracentesis and chest tube placement.**

SX: shortness of breath, chest pain. **Hyperresonance** and decreased or **no breath sounds, tamponade**, JVD

MC: due to trauma to the chest, lung infection, mechanical ventilation.

Trachea can deviate away from the insult (due to the pressure pushing it away)

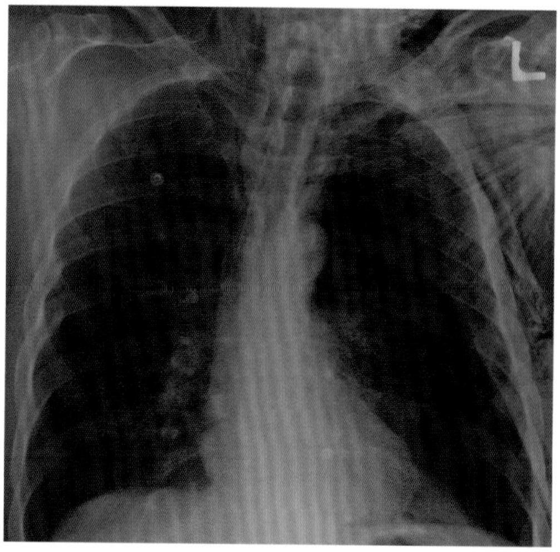

On chest x-rays for pneumothorax:
Watch for the really dark/black areas. Remember you should see "fuzzy – little tiny lines" areas – not black- on a chest x-ray. Lung tissue shows up. If it is dark/black, there is no lung there. You can also see a very faint line of the collapsed lung if you look close enough.

Hemothorax
Pleural effusion that contains blood.
MCC penetrating or blunt trauma to the chest. Other causes: surgery, spontaneous, aortic dissection, thoracic aortic aneurysms, endometriosis (endometrial tissue on the pleural surface that bleeds).
SX: Dyspnea, tachypnea, chest pain.
TX: Treat underlying cause of bleeding.

Hemopneumothorax
Combination of a hemothorax and a pneumothorax.
MCC: penetrating injury causing air and blood to enter the pleural space.
CXR shows air-fluid levels and collapse of the lung.
This can be under tension or not under tension. If the mediastinum is deviated away from the injury, it is under tension. If the mediastinum is midline, there is no tension.

Additional Lung Injuries and Diseases

Mycobacterium tuberculosis Gm +, Bacillus/rod Cell wall: contains **Mycolic Acid.** **Lowenstein-Jensen media** It will not gram stain because of mycolic acid, must use carbolfuchsin (aniline dye). **Sputum culture: Acid Fast Bacilli by Ziehl-Neelsen stain** MC: Immigrants or developing countries. Primary Infection: Mid to lower lung, **Ghon complex**. Secondary Infection*: **Upper** lobes of lung, fibrous cavity. **Caseating granulomas** (Central necrosis with multinucleated Langhans cells). Causes caseous necrosis in the lungs. Virulence: **Cord Factor**: grows in serpentine cords (**parallel**) with cord factor. **Inhibits macrophage maturation** stimulates release of TNFα Spreads: Respiratory droplets SX: Intermittent fevers, night sweats, weight loss, hemoptysis, chronic cough, weight loss. CXR shows **upper lobe lesions** surrounded by alveolar infiltration. DX: PPD test (Purified Protein Derivative), Test for latent TB: IGRA (Interferon Gamma Relase Assay: QuantiFERON) blood test. **PPD: Positive if:** **5mm** for immunocompromised (HIV, steroid, transplants) and those in close contact with person's with TB. **10mm** for health care workers, alcoholics, immigrants, homeless, and prisoners. **15mm** for the general public with no risk. (Once PPD is positive, PPD test should not be given again). If PPD is positive, CXR is done. If it is negative then patients takes INH and B6 for 9 months. *(Mycobacterium tuberculosis cont'd)* If PPD is positive and CXR is positive. Requires 4 drug treatment of: **TX: Isoniazid plus B6** (6 months), **Rifampin** (6 months), **Pyrazinamide** (2 months), **Ethambutol** (2 months). Isolation: **Negative pressure room** ***Infliximab**: (TX: Crohn's and Ulcerative Colitis). Can **reactive TB** so you must do a **PPD test** before starting this drug.	**Pulmonary Hypertension** MC: **young women**. **High blood pressure in the pulmonary artery, pulmonary vein and pulmonary capillaries** SX: (similar symptoms to CHF) shortness of breath, (AKA: orthopnea or paroxysmal **nocturnal dyspnea**: lying flat/sleeping), exertional breathlessness, dizziness, clubbing, fainting (↓ preload to the left atria/ventricle = ↓ CO = ↓ oxygen to the brain = fainting/syncope), JVD, nutmeg liver, portal HTN (hemorrhoids, esophageal varices, ascites), lower extremity edema, lungs are clear on auscultation, weakness, fatigue, hoarseness (due to compression of the left recurrent laryngeal nerve). Heart SX: **Loud P2 (P2 is louder than A2),** Tricuspid regurgitation, right ventricular hypertrophy and right atrial enlargement, right displacement of apex of heart, Raynaud's, right axis deviation, right heart failure, Cor Pulmonale. MOA: ↑ pulmonary vasculature which causes ↑ HTN in pulmonary vasculature which makes it difficult for the right ventricle to send blood into the lungs, causing the back up of blood from the right ventricle into the right atrium and then into the systemic system. Ultimately causes **right heart failure (Cor Pulmonale).** Causes: Mitral stenosis, COPD, Polycythemia vera, Restrictive/Interstitial lung disease. **DX: TTE (Transthoracic echo) shows right ventricular and atrial enlargement.** **EKG shows right axis deviation.** **CXR shows enlarged pulmonary arteries.** **MAT: Right heart catheterization (Swan-Ganz) with ↑ pulmonary artery pressure.** **TX: Polysomnography to rule out obstructive sleep apnea.** **Bosentan (prevents vasculature in the pulmonary system).** **Prostacyclin (Epoprostenol, Treprostinil) pulmonary vasodilators.** **Curative TX for pulmonary HTN: lung transplantation.**

Burn Victims – Inhalation Injury

Any burn victim that is brought into the ER, even if they look just fine and want to go home, **you must keep them** for observation 24 hrs. to insure swelling does not occur that blocks their airway. Patient will usually have **soot around their mouth or a red throat.**

Burn victims can have numerous **complications**:
Edema that blocks their airway, curling's ulcers, sepsis, atelectasis, pseudomonas lung infections, wound contractures.

Complications: **Pseudomonas** infection.

TX: Early intubation if needed. ↑↑ fluid replacement with 9% normal saline, ↑ flow oxygen.
Do not give steroids b/c it will make them immunocompromised and increase the risk of infection.

Pleurisy

Inflammation of the **pleura** (lining surrounding the lungs). Inflamed layers rub against each other.

Causes: viral/bacterial infections, SLE, RA, chest injuries, aortic dissections, cancers, PE, IBD, cardiac problems, parasite or fungal infections

SX: **Pain upon breathing** (due to chest expansion – if patient does not breath = ↓ or no pain), fever, chills, rapid, shallow breaths. Hurts worse with inhaling, sneezing, laughing, coughing

Pain: sharp, stabbing

Lung Contusion (bruise)

Cause: **chest trauma** (blunt force, penetrating, blast, rapid deceleration injury. MCC: motor vehicle accidents).
Leaking fluid from injury eventually leads to hypoxia and respiratory distress.
MC develops within the first 24 hours. It is not apparent immediately after trauma.

Complications: Pneumonia, ARDS

SX: Initial symptoms mild (takes several hours to a day or more for it to appear) then progressing to cyanosis, low oxygen saturation, dyspnea, rapid breathing and heart rate, hemoptysis, hypotension, chest pain, ↓ breath sounds on the affected side, chest all bruising, normal blood pressure. Worsens when IV fluids are given.

DX: CXR shows patchy-irregular alveolar infiltrates. AKA: homogenous opacification.

TX: Admit and monitor for 24 – 48 hrs. Resolves in 3 – 5 days.

Flail Chest

Segment of a rib breaks and becomes detached from the chest wall causing the chest wall to have **paradoxical breathing** (the area of the broken, detached rib moves inward while the rest of the chest if moving outward due to pressure changes).

SX: chest pain, chest bruising, peripheral cyanosis, dyspnea (shallow and rapid respiration), paradoxical breathing, pulmonary contusion, vitals are stable.

Causes: motor vehicle accidents, falling.

TX: **PAIN CONTROL** (in ALL rib injuries **pain control is critical**. Due to the pain the patient will not breath deep and can lead to atelectasis. Positive pressure ventilation, surgery if indicated.

Invasive Aspergillosis
Infection of the lung by Aspergillus.

↑ risk when patient has other underlying lung diseases: ie: Tuberculosis or COPD, ABPA (Allergic Bronchopulmonary Aspergillosis), stem cell transplants, leukemia, chemotherapy, immunocompromised, neutropenia.

MCC: Aspergillus fumigatus.

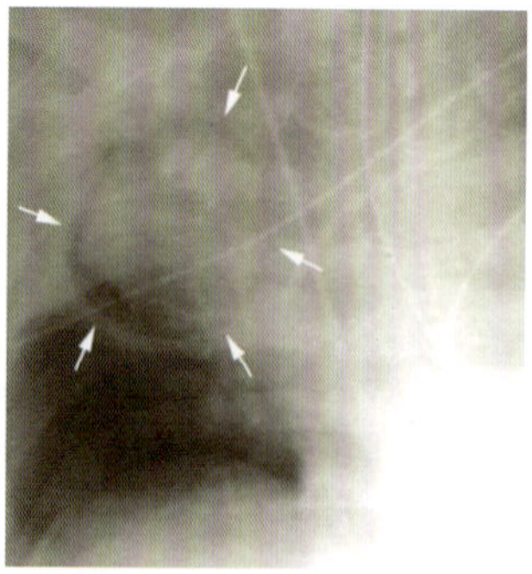

SX: Fever, cough hemoptysis, chest pain, difficulty breathing.
If not treated Aspergillosis can disseminate through the blood stream and cause widespread organ damage.

DX: CXR shows **fungus ball (cavity mass) that is mobile**.
Can show a **"halo sign"** and it later stages a **"crescent sign"**.
Silver stain shows Aspergillus.

TX: **Amp B**, with surgical debridement, **Voriconazole.**

Acute Pulmonary Edema
Fluid accumulation in the air spaces and parenchyma of the lungs causing impaired gas exchange and may lead to respiratory failure or cardiac arrest due to hypoxia.

Test: V/Q mismatch, ↑ A-a gradient, ↑ CO_2. If oxygen is given all readings are corrected.
↓ Compliance. ↓ Compliance = dyspnea.
↑ Hydrostatic pressure in pulmonary system. (Transudate)

Exacerbated by anything that retains sodium (ie: Aldosterone). This includes drugs that hold sodium (ie: Pioglitazone/PPAR receptor). Use drugs that inhibit Aldosterone (ie: **Spironolactone**).

Cardiogenic pulmonary edema: Due to the failure of the left ventricle of the heart. It is not able to take in blood from the pulmonary circulation (lungs).
MCC: Congestive heart failure. (Labs will show **↑ BNP** if it is due to CHF). Other cardiac causes: arrhythmias, fluid overload from kidney failure or IV therapy, HTN crisis due to ↑ in blood pressure.
PWCP > 18.

Non-cardiogenic pulmonary edema: Due to an injury of the lung parenchyma or vasculature of the lung. Other causes: neurogenic (seizures, electrocution), strangulation, head trauma, negative pressure in the chest (ruptures capillaries and floods the alveoli), multiple blood transfusions (fluid overload), ARDS.
PWCP < 18.

TX: **IV Furosemide, nitrates, oxygen, morphine initially**. After 30 minutes administer an ionotropic (**Dobutamine, Amiodarone or Milrinone**).

Massive Hemoptysis

- > 600 mL loss over 24 hours or > 100 mL/hour
- ↑ danger of asphyxiation b/c airway filled with blood
- Rule out GI bleed
- TX: Intubate/establish airway
  Place patient so that bleeding lung is in dependent (lateral) position to stop collection of blood in opposite lung.
  Bronchoscopy to find source of bleeding, suction, treat

Incorrect Endotracheal Placement

- ETT (Endotracheal tube) should be 2 – 6 cm above carina
- If the ETT goes to far it will do into the right lung and over inflate and under ventilate the left lung causing an asymmetrical chest
- After intubation listen to left lung sounds. If left lung sounds are ↓↓ then reposition tube

Diaphragmatic Hernia
MC on the left side.
MCC: Blunt trauma to the abdomen.

SX: Mild respiratory distress, elevated hemi-diaphragm, hypotension, tachycardia, JVD, tamponade

DX: CXR is abnormal. Heart shows as a global silhouette.

Lung Sounds

Pathology	Fremitus	Resonance	Breath Sounds	Note
Tension Pneumothorax	Absent	Hyperresonance	↓	Tracheal deviation away from lesion
Pneumothorax	Absent	Hyperresonance	↓	Tracheal deviation towards lesion
Pleural Effusion	↓	Dullness to percussion	↓	
Atelectasis	↓	↓	Absent	Tracheal deviation towards lesion
Lobar Pneumonia	↑	Dullness to percussion	Bronchial	

Mediastinum Location for Differential Lung Pathologies

Posterior Mediastinum	Mid Mediastinum	Anterior Mediastinum
All neurogenic tumors	Aortic arch aneurysm	Thymoma (Myasthenia Gravis)
Meningocele	Bronchogenic cyst	Retro-sternal thyroid
Diaphragmatic hernia	Tracheal tumors	Teratoma
Aortic aneurysm	Pericardial cyst	Lymphoma
Lymphoma	Lymphoma	
Enteric cyst	Lymph node enlargement	

Swan-Ganz Catheterization (Pulmonary artery catheter)

Catheter inserted into the pulmonary artery that measures pressures in the right atrium, right ventricle, pulmonary artery and the PCWP of the left atrium. It detects heart failure, monitors therapy, evaluates the effects of drugs and sepsis.
Ie: Differentiates between types of shock, cardiogenic verses non-cariogenic pulmonary edema, 1° and 2 pulmonary edema, fluid requirements, types of shock, management of myocardial infarctions.

Shock

Type of Shock	HR	CO	VO2	TPR	EDV/P	PWCP	Right Preload (CWP)	Cardiac Index (pump function)
Hypovolemic. Circulation is working but ↓ volume (hemorrhage). SX: Flat neck veins, **cool extremities**, **cold, clammy skin.** oliguria. Body releasing CATS, ATII, ADH to get fluid Up.	↑ Tachy Is first visible sign of low BP	↓	↓	↑	↓	↓	↓	↓
Cardiogenic. Always has ↑ PWCP b/c ↑ left atrial pressure. SX: JVD, Pulmonary edema	↓	↓	↓	↑	↑	↑	↑	↓↓
Septic Shock. ↓ PWCP b/c no adequate filling of ventricles so ↓ EDV. **Warm extremities**. Gm negatives release **nitric oxide** and activate compliment		↑	NL, No use of O2	↓ **Vasodilation**, Pooling of blood, Hyperdynamic flow so not enough time to extract O2	↓ No adequate filling of ventricles.	NL to ↓ No pressure produced b/c infection, even when ↑ preload, So causes end organ damage. No adequate filling of ventricles.	NL to ↓	NL to slightly low. Heart pump is ok.
Neurogenic Heart slows from unopposed vagal tone, loss of sympathetics and loss of ANS , causing vasodilation and ↓↓ blood pressure. (Brain or spinal injury)	↓	↓		↓				↓
Pulmonary Embolism Have ↑ Right atrial & pulmonary pressure b/c ↑ preload		↓		↑		**NL**		
Tamponade, **Aortic dissection** All pressures are up because tamponade constricts		↓		↑	↑	↑	↑	↓↓
Anaphylactic Shock. ↑ parasympathetic & ↓ sympathetic working In heart		↑	↓	↓		↓		

Anatomical Locations for Penetrating Injuries to the Chest

- **Above clavicle**: apex of lungs and subclavian artery
- 2nd intercostal space
  L – Aortic arch
  R – Right lung
- 3rd intercostal space
  L – Pulmonary trunk, ascending aorta, SVC
  R – Right lung
- **4th and 5th and 6th intercostal space**
  L – Left sternal boarder: Right Ventricle
  L – 4th intercostal midclavicular – Left lung
  L – 5th medial to left mid-clavicular – Left Ventricle
  R- Right atrium
- 4th and 5th midaxillary line
  liver
- 9th intercostal space
  L – Spleen

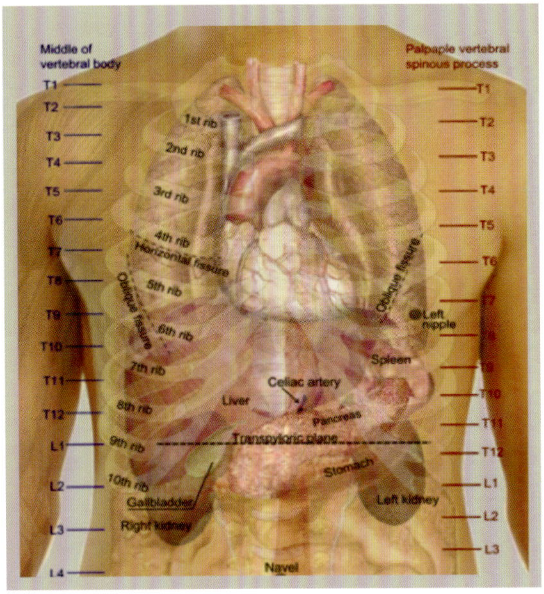

When To Intubate and Send to ICU

Situation	Notes
Asthma patient with ↑ CO2	Respiratory alkalosis with ↓ CO2 is normal in an asthma exacerbation. If CO2 is rising, the patient is tiring and may stop breathing. CO2 retention causes muscle fatigue.
Persistent hypoxemia	
Increasing oxygen demands	
Upper airway injury.	Burns within 24 hours (beware of soot around the mouth or a red throat) this indicates inflammation and swelling/edema so the patient must be monitored for 24 hours. Laryngeal edema causing inspiratory stridor.
Altered Mental Status	Drug OD, end stage renal DZ, seizures → due to aspiration risk
Neurologic depression	Neuromuscular weakness develops causing ↑ retention of CO2 (hypercapnia) in Myasthenia Gravis, Guillain Barre.

Mechanical Ventilation

Indications: Compromised airway, hypoxia (PaO2 < 50%), ↑↑ CO2 (PaCO2 > 50%), airway obstruction, respiratory distress (RR > 30 and use of accessory muscles), atelectasis, post operative pain, surgery (surgery can ↓ FRC by 30% and VC by 50%), narcotics post surgery (↓ respiratory drive).

To decrease/prevent atelectasis and ↑ FRC 25 – 30% = RAISE HEAD OF BED. This ↓ intra abdominal pressure on the diaphragm. This is for post surgical or ANY breathing difficulties (esp. in the ED for breathing exacerbations or other conditions that the patient has ↓ respirations)

Cricothyrotomy (Surgical opening in the cricothyroid membrane directly into the trachea). Emergency airway access when intubation is not successful or not available.

Tracheostomy (surgical passage into the trachea). Patients requiring prolonged ventilation.

Pseudomonas is the MC infection (pneumonia) on patients on ventilation. Patients on ventilation should not have flowers, plants, etc. in the room.

Positive Pressure Ventilation (AKA: PEEP) (gas is pushed into the trachea)

- Airway pressure = pulmonary compliance
- PEEP improves oxygenation by not collapsing alveoli at the end of respiration (keeps them open so more surface area for gas exchange) = ↑ functional residual capacity and ↓ work of breathing.
- ↑ PEEP = ↑ oxygenation
- Goal is to keep FiO2 < 40%
- If FiO2 (inspired oxygen) drops < 90% → ↑ PEEP setting
- If FiO2 (oxygen) is too high → ↓ PEEP (Keep FiO2 low to avoid Oxygen toxicity)
  Oxygen toxicity occurs if patient gets to much oxygen.
- If ↓ ↓ oxygen → ↑ FiO2 and/or add PEEP
- Oxygen = FiO2
- Lower PEEP = Higher FiO2
- Higher PEEP = Lower FiO2
- Hyperventilating patients (respiratory alkalosis) → ↓ respiratory rate on the ventilator
- Tidal Volume

Negative Pressure Ventilation (air is sucked into the lungs) (AKA: iron lung)

Respiratory Quotient (RQ)

- RQ Ratio = CO2 eliminated/O2 consumed. Normal = 1.05
- Amount of CO2 produced to the amount of oxygen consumed. (Shows major fuel being used for ATP production)
- RQ value corresponds to a caloric value for each liter of CO2 produced
- The higher the ratio of CO2 produced to the oxygen uptake is due to excess carbs in the diet
- RQ Values:
  Carbs = 1.0
  Proteins = .8
  Fatty Acids = .7

Lung Cancers and Tumors

- Lung cancer is MCC of cancer deaths
- Single nodule: primary cancer
- Multiple lesions: metastasis
- Presents with: Coin lesions, noncalcified nodule, cough hemoptysis, wheezing
- MC metastasis to lung from: breast, colon, prostate, bladder
- MC lung metastasis to: adrenal glands, brain, bone, liver
- **Procedure when a nodule is found in the lung**
  - **BIT: Refer (find) a previous CXR to compare**
  - If nodule was on previous CXR and there has been no change, follow up every 6 months
  - Biopsy all enlarging lung lesions, lesions that were not on the previous CXR or if a previous CXR can't be located
  - **NOTE: MC adverse effect of a lung biopsy is a pneumothorax**
- Squamous and Small cell cancers = **centrally located**, due to smoking.
  Squamous can release PTHrp and Small Cell can release PTHrp or ACTHrp.

  (**tip**: think all "S" sounds: **S**quamous, **S**mall, "**S**"entral (central), **S**moking)
  Adenocarcinoma and Large cell cancers = **peripheral**

- Test for Malignancy
  - PET Scan (Positron Emission Tomography): Malignant lesions have an ↑ uptake of tagged glucose so a positive PET scan = ↑ risk of malignancy. Test for malignancy without a biopsy.
  - Sputum Cytology: Positive test = ↑ risk of malignancy. Next step: resect the lesion. A negative test does not exclude malignancy.
  - Transthoracic Needle Biopsy used for peripheral lesions
  - Bronchoscopy used for central lesions
- TX: Surgical resection if the nodule is localized without any contradictions.
  Contradictions: Metastases, Involves the vessels: IVC, SVC or aorta, malignant pleural effusion, nodule located within 1 cm of the carina (bifurcation of the two primary bronchi) or is bilateral.

Characteristics of Benign and Malignant Lung Nodules

Benign	Malignant
• No change in size of lesion • Nonsmoker • Small, **smooth** < 1 cm lesion • No adenopathy • < 30 years old • **Central, dense calcification. Popcorn lesions.** • Normal PET scan • Normal lung	• Enlarging lesion • Smoker • Large, speculated (irregular/spikes) > 2 cm, poorly defined and **irregular boarders** • Adenopathy • > 50 years old • Eccentric, sparse calcification. **Microcalcification.** • Abnormal PET scan • Abnormal PET scan • No calcification • Unintentional weight loss • Low density • Previous cancer

Small Cell Carcinoma

(AKA: Oat Cell Carcinoma)
Paraneoplastic syndrome (Neuroendocrine)

Centrally located (hilar mass), narrows bronchial airways.
Neuroendocrine: + for **chromogranin, synaptophysin (specific to neurons).**
Amplification of L-myc oncogene.
Associated with smoking.
Very aggressive.

Histology: **Aggressive**: ↑ mitotic rate, **necrosis**, sheets of **undifferentiated**, primitive, **small blue tumor cells** with nuclear molding.
(AKA: **Kulchitsky cells**) and "salt and pepper" chromatin.

Associated with **Lambert Eaton** (autoimmune reaction: antibodies against presynaptic voltage-gated **calcium channels** in the neuromuscular junction).

Can produce: ACTH rP, ADH rP
(**caution:** beware on the exam if the answer leads to a lung cancer producing either ACTH or ADH and you note in the answer both choices: ACTH or ACTH rP. You MUST chose ACTH rP. ACTH is not from the lung cancer, ACTH rP is. But if they only give you one choice ACTH: then it is ok to choose it.

TX: Small Cell has good response to radiation therapy

Squamous Cell Carcinoma

Centrally located (AKA: hilar mass)
Associated with smoking

Histology: Large sheets of squamous cells (AKA: keratin pearls). (Squamous = keratin).
Keratin pearls stain dark pink.

Can produce: PTHrP

(**tip:** to remember which related hormone is produced from Small Cell or Squamous: Remember:
"P" is next to "Q" in the alphabet. PTH = squamous)

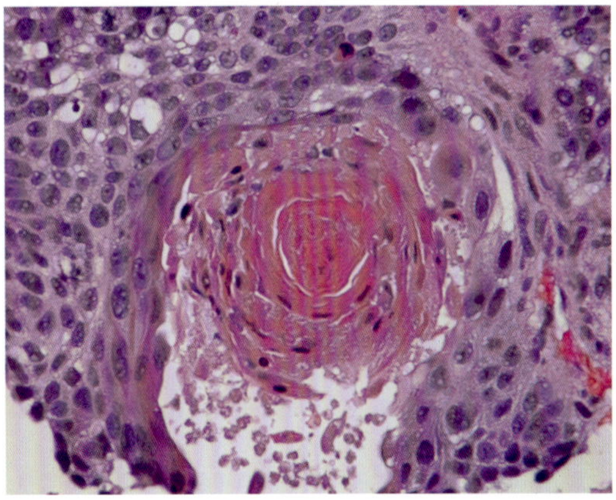

Keratin Pearls

Adenocarcinoma

Peripheral location
MC in non-smokers
Neoplasia of epithelia tissues with a glandular origin producing mucus. Presents like pneumonia and develops at a site of prior injury or inflammation.
Stains + for mucin and TTF-1 (cell marker)
Gene mutations: k-ras, HER2, BRAF, EGFR, ALK
CXR: multiple densities

TX: Surgery

Large (Giant) Cell Carcinoma

Peripheral location. Worst prognosis.

Histology: Transformed pleomorphic giant epithelial cells

Poor prognosis

Pulmonary Carcinoid Tumor Neuroendocrine tumor 2 Types: Typical and Atypical (both low grade) MC tumor of the appendix. Typical Histology: Stippled chromatin with increased amounts of cytoplasm. Primary tumor begins in the GI tract (referred to as the "appendix tumor"). Symptoms do not appear until after metastases. Secretes Serotonin and kallikrein. Can cause pulmonary stenosis and right heart failure. SX: Flushing, diarrhea. DX: **5-HIAA** (5-hydroxyindoleacetic acid) in the urine. TX: Surgery	**Mesothelioma** **Asbestosis (Exposure to asbestos)** **(Caution: do not confuse this with Bronchogenic carcinoma, the most common cause of asbestosis)** Occupations: shipbuilding, plumbing, insulation, working with PVC, roofing CXR: **Calcified pleural plaques** (Pleura) The pleura of the lungs is on the **periphery (lateral)** – NOT centrally. Hemorrhagic pleural effusions. Histology: Psammoma bodies (AKA: pleural thickening with calcification) MCC: **Bronchogenic carcinoma** – not mesothelioma. (If the CXR shows a "mass", or a "central mass" it is Bronchogenic carcinoma. Mesothelioma is not a mass) **For it to be mesothelioma: YOU MUST SEE one or more of these: the word Pleural/pleura, periphery (lateral), MUST be at least 20 years from the time they worked in that job, or Ferruginous bodies (asbestos). IF THEY DO NOT USE THESE WORDS IT IS BROCHOGENIC CARNCINOMA!!** 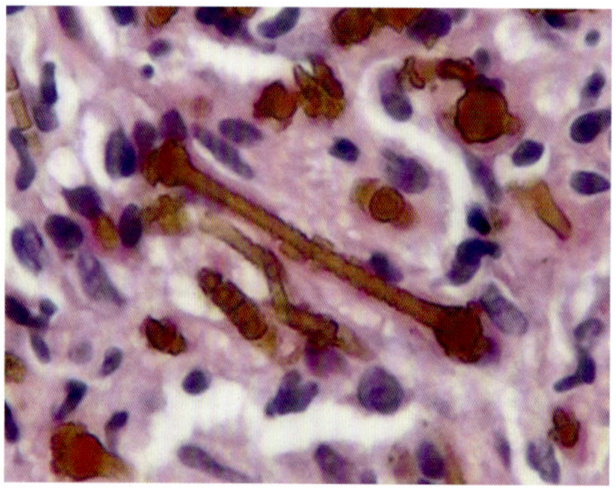 Ferruginous bodies: golden-brown rods (dumbbells)
Superior Vena Cava Syndrome Obstruction of the SVC (usually a tumor compress the SVC) = ↓ blood flow from the head (backing up blood), neck and arms causing a back up of blood = swelling, erythema and edema SX: Face swelling and erythema (facial plethora), JVD, and edema (face, arms, neck), ↑ ICP, dizziness, headaches Complications: rupture or aneurysm of intracranial arteries	**Pancoast Tumor** Tumor of the pulmonary apex. Mass/tumor compressing the cervical sympathetic ganglion causing **Horner syndrome** (Miosis, anhidrosis (no sweating) and ptosis). **Compression** by mass can also occur and cause: SVC syndrome, hoarseness (due to compression on the left recurrent laryngeal nerve), damage to the brachial plexus, Vagus nerve, phrenic nerve, brachiocephalic vein.

Pulmonary Hamartoma
MC benign lung tumor.
Usually are incidental findings on CXR.

CXR: Round or coin lesion with "popcorn calcification" containing hyaline cartilage, fibrous and adipose tissues.
Complications: obstruction if occur near an airway → pneumonia or bronchiectasis

RESPIRATORY – PULMONARY PHARMACOLOGY

Asthma, COPD Pharmacology

- Bronchoconstriction exacerbates asthma (and all other breathing disorders).
- Bronchoconstriction mediated by:
  Parasympathetic and inflammatory processes

DRUG GENERIC name Trade name	Clinical Use	Mechanism of Action and Resistance	Toxicity and Notes
Albuterol	Rescue inhaler (emergency) for **acute/short term asthma and COPD attacks.**	**β-2 agonist.** Relief of bronchospasm. Relaxes bronchial smooth muscle. Vasodilates.	Anxiety, headache, dry mouth, palpitation.
Salmeterol **Formoterol**	Long term/acting asthma and COPD treatment	**β-2 adrenergic agonist.** Relieve of bronchospasm. Relaxes bronchial smooth muscle. Vasodilates.	Dizziness, migraine headaches, sinus infection.
Fluticasone **Beclomethasone**	Prophylaxis of asthma, chronic asthma. Nasal spray for allergic rhinitis. TX of nasal polyps.	Glucocorticoids. Agonist at the glucocorticoid receptor. Inhibit cytokines. Reduces inflammation in the airways (and skin).	Nasal spray: headache, GI symptoms, nosebleed and cough. **NOTE: Must rinse mouth with Nystatin after using the inhaler to prevent candidiasis (white coating) on the tongue and throat.**
Mometasone *Nasonex*	Allergic rhinitis (hayfever, seasonal allergies), asthma, nasal polyps.	Corticosteroid. Reduce allergic reactions in mastocytes and eosinophil's (cells responsible for allergic reactions)	Headaches, sore throat, nosebleeds, coughing, throat dryness, mucus/phlegm may contain small amounts of blood.
Cromolyn Nedocromil	Prophylaxis against asthma, Rhinitis.	Inhibits release of histamine (by inhibiting tryptase to stop degranulation) of mast cells.	Does not treat an asthma attack – only for prophylaxis.
Ipratropium *Atrovent*	COPD	Muscarinic antagonist. Inhibits ACh so that it inhibits bronchoconstriction.	Minimal anticholinergic affects. Dry mouth, sedation. (**tip**: with COPD, I "PRAY" I can breath)
Theophylline	COPD, Asthma	Methylxanthine is a drug that bronchodilates. Inhibits phosphodiesterase → ↑ cAMP.	**Narrow therapeutic window.** Caution when used with P-450 inhibitors = ↑ toxicity.' CNS symptoms, GI symptoms, seizures, cardiac issues, headaches. Member of the Xanthine family: similar to caffeine.
Omalizumab	Allergies, asthma that does not respond to corticosteroids or β-2 agonist.	Humanized monoclonal IgE antibody. Blocks binding to FcεRI receptor on mast cells, basophils and dendritic cells. **Anti-IgE.**	**Anaphylaxis.** Slight ↑ risk of strokes and heart disease.
Montelukast *Singulair* **Zafirlukast** *Accolate*	Aspirin induced asthma. Asthma, Seasonal allergies.	**Leukotriene D4 receptor antagonist.** Reduces bronchoconstriction, ↓ inflammation.	Best for long term TX of atopic asthma. GI symptoms, headaches, hypersensitivity, sleep disturbances, ↑ bleeding tendency. ↑ incidence of Churg-Strauss
Zileuton	Maintenance treatment of asthma.	**Inhibitor of 5-lipooxgenase,** inhibiting leukotriene formation.	Best for long term TX of atopic asthma. Sinusitis, nausea. Can ↑ concentrations of warfarin, propranolol, theophylline.
Methacholine	Asthma challenge test to DX asthma	**Muscarinic agonist.**	

H1 Blockers (Antihistamine)

DRUG GENERIC name Trade name	Clinical Use	Mechanism of Action and Resistance	Toxicity and Notes
1st Generation			
Diphenhydramine *Benadryl* **Chlorpheniramine** **Diphenhydramine** **Meclizine** **Pheniramine** **Promethazine** *Phenergan*	Allergies, sleeping aid, motion sickness Meclizine treats Ménères disease by ↓ endolymph. ↓ vertigo. ↓ motion sickness.	Reversible inhibitor of H1 histamine receptors. H1 antagonist.	Sedation, antiserotonergic, anti-muscarinic, anti-α- adrenergic, bradycardia. CNS depressant.
2nd Generation			
Loratadine *Claritin* **Fexofenadine** *Allegra* **Desloratadine** *Clarinex* **Cetirizine** *Zyrtec*	Allergy	Reversible inhibitor of H1 histamine receptors.	**Much less sedating** that 1st generation H1 Blockers because of ↓ entry into the CNS. Better to use for those that operate machinery, drive distances, etc.

Mucolytics, Expectorants, Antitussive (cough), Decongestants

DRUG GENERIC name Trade name	Clinical Use	Mechanism of Action and Resistance	Toxicity and Notes
Mucolytic			
N-acetylcysteine	**Mucus breakdown** in Cystic Fibrosis, COPD, bronchitis, bronchiectasis, amyloidosis. Antidote for acetaminophen overdose.	**Increases glutathione levels** and binds with the toxic break down products of acetaminophen.	GI symptoms, skin allergy, non-immune anaphylaxis.
Expectorants			
Guaifenesin *Robitussin* *DayQuil* *Mucinex*	**Expectorant**	Thins respiratory secretions so that phlegm can be bought up.	Not a cough suppressant.
Antitussive			
Dextro-methorphan *NyQuil, Dimetapp, Vicks, TheraFlu* *Robitussin*	Antitussive. Cough suppressant.	NMDA receptor antagonist. Synthetic codeine analog.	High doses are used for recreational effects (hallucinogenic states similar to PCP or ketamine). GI symptoms, drowsiness, dizziness, constipation, sedation, confusion, nervousness, closed eye hallucinations. High dose side effects: Dilated pupils, sweating, hallucinations, euphoria, muscle spasms, tachycardia, HTN Overdose: Naloxone

Decongestants			
Pseudoephedrine **Phenylephrine** *Allegra D, Claritin D, Mucinex D, Sudafed, Zyrtec D, Benadryl Plus, Actifed, Aleve D*	Nasal congestion, open Eustachian tubes. Promotes wakefulness. First line prophylactic for recurrent priapism.	Sympathomimetic drug (adrenergic) of the Phenethylamine and amphetamine class. Acts on α and β-2 adrenergic receptors to vasoconstrict and relax smooth muscle in the bronchi. Shrinks swollen nasal mucous membranes.	HTN, CNS stimulation, insomnia, nervousness, dizziness, anxiety, tachycardia, palpitations, mydriasis. **Rebound nasal congestion.** Also used in the illicit manufacture of methamphetamine and methcathinone.

Angioedema Pharmacology

DRUG GENERIC name Trade name	Clinical Use	Mechanism of Action and Resistance	Toxicity and Notes
Ecallantide	Acute angioedema, Hereditary angioedema	Inhibits kallikrein (protease), which then inhibits bradykinin from being released from its precursor kininogen. If it can't be released = no vasodilation.	Nausea, headache, fatigue, diarrhea.

Pulmonary Hypertension Pharmacology

DRUG GENERIC name Trade name	Clinical Use	Mechanism of Action and Resistance	Toxicity and Notes
Bosentan Ambrisentan Darusentan Sitaxsentan	Pulmonary Hypertension	Endothelin-1 receptor antagonist at the endothelin-A and endothelin-B receptors. Inhibits the constriction of the pulmonary blood vessels.	Teratogenic. Anemia: must monitor Hct. Hepatotoxicity: must monitor LFT's.
Sildenafil Tadalafil	Pulmonary Hypertension, Erectile dysfunction.	Phosphodiesterase-5 inhibitor. Inhibits the degradation of cGMP.	Headaches, flushing, nasal congestion, photophobia. Caution: do not use with nitrates or alpha blockers. Must also be cautious when using with P-450 inhibitors. **Note**: Must wait a minimum of 4 hours between use of nitrates and the phosphodiesterase-5 inhibitor due to the possibility of a severe drop in blood pressure that could result in death.

GASTROINTESTINAL

GI Development

Area of Development	Organs Included	Blood Supply
Foregut	Pharynx to duodenum	Celiac artery **(Celiac also supplies spleen, spleen is in the midgut)**
Midgut	Duodenum to transverse colon	Superior Mesenteric Artery (SMA)
Hindgut	Distal transverse colon to rectum	Inferior Mesenteric Artery (IMA)

Retroperitoneal Organs (SAD PUCKER)

- Suprarenal (adrenal) gland
- Aorta and IVC
- Duodenum (2nd, 3rd parts)
- Pancreas (head), NOT tail
- Ureters
- Colon (ascending and descending)
- Kidneys
- Esophagus, lower 2/3
- Rectum

GI Ligaments

GI Ligament	Connects	Structures Contained	Additional Anatomy
Falciform	**Liver to anterior abdominal wall**	**Ligamentum teres (derivative of fetal umbilical vein)**	
Gastrocolic	Greater curvature of stomach and transverse colon	Gastroepiploic arteries	Part of greater omentum
Gastrohepatic	Lesser curvature of stomach to liver	Gastric arteries	**Left gastric involved in esophageal varices** **(left gastric is off the Azygos)**
Gastrosplenic	Greater curvature of stomach and spleen	Short gastrics, left gastroepiploic vessels	
Hepatoduodenal	Duodenum to liver	Portal triad: Proper Hepatic Artery, Portal Vein, Common Bile Duct	
Splenorenal	Spleen to abdominal wall	Splenic artery and vein, tail of pancreas. Splenic artery runs beneath the stomach.	Concerns of **stomach ulcers eroding into the splenic artery**

GI Organs: Histology: Absorption

Organ	Histology	Function	Notes
Oral Cavity	Squamous Cell	1st step of digestion with amylase	
Tongue	Stratified squamous epithelium. **Taste buds**: Columnar epithelial sensory cells on the **fungiform and circumvallate papillae**.		Sensory cells replaced every 10-14 days by differentiation of stem cells.
Pharynx	Squamous Cell		
Larynx	Squamous Cell		

Organ	Histology	Function	Notes
Esophagus	Upper 2/3: Nonkeratinized **Stratified, striated squamous** epithelium. Muscle: Majority is smooth muscle innervated by sympathetic nerves **(involuntary)** via sympathetic trunk. **Striated muscle** is innervated by Vegas nerve carried by LMN	Passes food via peristaltic contractions from the pharynx to stomach. Epiglottis prevents food from going down the larynx during swallowing. Lower 2/3 = retroperitoneal.	Three esophageal sphincters: 1) Upper Esophageal Sphincter (UES) is triggered by swallow reflex. Skeletal muscle that is motor control = cricopharyngeal. 2) Inferior pharyngeal constrictor 3) Lower Esophageal Sphincter (LES) is between stomach and esophagus. **Barrett's Esophagus**: when metaplasia occurs and squamous cells transition into columnar cells in lower 1/3 of the esophagus.
Stomach	Columnar cells	**Parietal Cells** (AKA: oxyntic cells) in fundus/body, acidophilic, secrete HCL (H+ ions), Intrinsic factor. **Chief Cells** (pepsinogen), basophilic. R-Protein binds Vitamin B12 to escort to the ileum where it frees B12 in order for it to bind to Intrinsic Factor to be absorbed.	Peristalsis: 3 waves/min. pH 2.0
Duodenum	Villi, Microvilli ↑ absorption area	Absorbs: **iron (Fe2) and Vit C** helps improve iron absorption. Absorption carbs, lipids, AA **Brunner Glands** (submucosa) secrete alkaline mucus. Crypts of Lieberkuhn.	Peristalsis: 12 waves/min.
Jejunum	Crypts of Lieberkuhn. Plicae circulares (valvular flaps projecting into lumen)	Absorbs Folate	(**tip**: "Foals" are born in "June")
Ileum	Peyer Patches (lamina propria, submucosa) contain M cells = present antigens. Crypts of Lieberkuhn. Goblet cells.	**Absorbs B12 and Intrinsic Factor, bile salts,** Folate.	Peristalsis: 9 waves/min. Separated from the cecum by the ileocecal valve.
Cecum		Intraperitoneal. Separates the ileum to the ascending colon via ileocecal valve.	Appendix is connected to cecum
Ascending colon	Crypts of Lieberkuhn. Goblet cells. No villi.	Retroperitoneal	Parasympathetic innervation: Vegas. Sympathetic: thoracic splanchnic nerves.
Transverse colon	Crypts of Lieberkuhn. Goblet cells. No villi.	Peristalsis of food. Intraperitoneal.	
Descending colon	Crypts of Lieberkuhn. Goblet cells. No villi.	Junction of transverse and sigmoid = **splenic flexure** (watershed). Retroperitoneal Stores remains of digested food to be emptied into rectum.	
Sigmoid colon (S shape)		Expel solid and gaseous waste from GI tract. Intraperitoneal. "S" curve allows gas to be trapped and expelled without expelling feces.	Connects descending colon to rectum. High risk area: Diverticulosis, Volvulus (twisting bowel)
Rectum		Temporary storage site for feces. Once full increase in intrarectal pressure causes defecation. Controlled by internal and external sphincter. Intraperitoneal.	Terminates at dentate line (puborectalis sling). Followed by anal canal. Internal hemorrhoids: above dentate (pectinate) level, external hemorrhoids below dentate level.

GI Tract Anatomy

- Mucosa (nearest the lumen of the gut)
  Epithelium = absorption, lamina propria, muscularis mucosa
- Submucosa: Meissner's plexus, parasympathetic fibers (CN IX/Vegas) innervate the mucosa
- Muscularis externa: Auerbach (Myenteric nerve plexus), circular muscle layer. Parasympathetic and sympathetic input to both layers of the muscular layer, peristalsis
- Serosa if located intraperitoneal: Adventitia if located retroperitoneal.
- Crypts of Lieberkuhn (gland) in epithelial lining of the small and large intestine. Contain: enterocytes, goblet cells, enteroendocrine cells, stem cells, Paneth cells (found: in small intestine but not in the colon).
- Peritoneum: Parietal: lining of the internal surface of the abdominopelvic wall.
  Visceral peritoneum: lining the viscera (organs).
- Peritoneum cavity: Greater and Lesser sac (AKA: Omental bursa).
- Omentum: fold of peritoneum that connects the stomach with other abdominal organs.
- **Lesser omental bursa** (lesser sac): smaller portion of the peritoneal cavity. This is the area that will collect fluid in the abdomen (**ascites**).
- **Villi:** Located in the small intestines. They increase the **surface area to allow for increased absorption.**

Layers of the abdomen that a scalpel must cut through during surgery

- Skin ➔Superficial fascia (fatty layer, AKA: Camper's fascia) ➔ Superficial Fascia membranous layer (Scarpa's fascia) ➔External oblique muscle ➔ Internal oblique muscle ➔ Transversus abdominis muscle ➔ Transversalis fascia ➔ Extraperitoneal fat ➔ Parietal peritoneum

Boundaries of the Omental Foramen

- Anterior: Hepatoduodenal ligament, Posterior: IVC, Superior: Caudate lobe of the liver and Inferior: 1st part of the duodenum.

Cells types of the GI

Stem cells are located in the crypts of the small intestine. They are responsible for repair and are the location of the most active cell division.

Stem cells in the crypts differentiate into these cell types:

- Enterocytes: simple columnar, **microvilli**. They increase surface area for absorption of vitamins, lipids, amino acids, peptides, water, electrolytes and simple sugars. The apical surface is the glycocalyx (oligosaccharides), which aid in the digestion of carbohydrates (monosaccharides) and proteins (amino acids).
- Enteroendocrine cells (enterochromaffin-like cells): secretes hormone serotonin, CCK, histamine, secretin, enteroglucagon (decreases motility so that there is sufficient time for nutrients to be absorbed).
- Goblet cells: glandular simple columnar epithelial cell, secrete mucus (composed of mucins) for protection.
- M Cells (Microfold cells) send samples of foreign antigens to lymphoid tissue in the mucosa (MALT). Associated with Peyer's patches (lymphoid nodules) in the ileum.
- Paneth cells: located in Crypts of Lieberkuhn (intestinal glands), contain eosinophilic granules (anti-microbial) for host-defense and immunity.
- Cup cells and Tuft cells (associated with immunity)

Other Cells Types of the GI

- Parietal cells: secretes HCL (H+/protons), intrinsic factor
- Chief cells: secretes pepsinogen
- Brunner Glands: Located in the duodenum: secretes an alkaline, bicarb mucus
- D Cells: Somatostatin
- G Cells: Gastrin (antrum of stomach)
- I Cells: CCK (Duodenum, jejunum)
- **Duodenum has Brunner's glands. The jejunum does NOT have any Brunner's glands or Peyer's patches. The ileum has Peyer's patches.**
- **Duodenum absorbs iron. The jejunum absorbs folate. The ileum absorbs B-12.**

Enteric Nervous System

- Governs function of GI system
- Neural crest cells
- ACh, dopamine (contains 50% of dopamine of body), serotonin (contains 90% of serotonin of the body)
- Two types of ganglia: Myenteric (Auerbach's) in muscularis externa and submucosal (Meissner's plexus) in submucosa
- Communicates with CNS via: parasympathetic (vagus nerve) and sympathetic (prevertebral ganglia)

Ion Transport

- H+ (proton) is converted to CO2 in the blood ➔ CO2 diffused into parietal cell ➔ CO2 converted back to H+ ➔ H+ is transported into GI lumen by H+K+ATPase pump
- CL – is transported into parietal cells by CL-/HCO3 transporter ➔ CL diffused into GI lumen via CL- channel

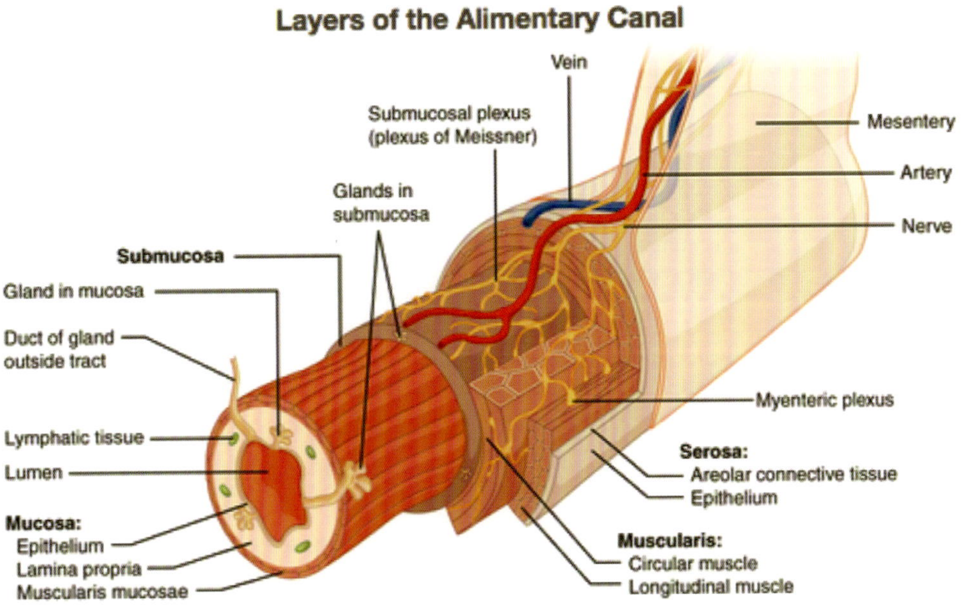

GI Enzymes, Hormones

Substance	Location	Function	Regulated By	Notes
Amylase	Begin in mouth	Starch digestion		Esophageal ruptures will result in amylase detected in effusions
Bicarb (HCO3)	Mucosal cells throughout upper GI, salivary glands, pancreas, **Brunner's glands (duodenum)**	Neutralizes HCL	Stimulated by ingestion of food which stimulates **secretin** in the S Cells of duodenum	Brunner's glands in duodenal secrete alkaline mucus. Brunner's glands hypertrophy when ulcers are present trying to provide protection.
Bile	Produced in the liver and stored in the gallbladder. **Note**: Bile salts are made from cholesterol via **7α-hydroxylase**. Bile sales form **micelles** that emulsify fats so they can be digested and absorbed.	Emulsifies lipids (acts as a surfactant). Helps absorb lipids and fat-soluble vitamins. Excretion of cholesterol.		Composed of: Water, **bile salts**, bilirubin, cholesterol, fatty acids, lecithin. Note: without bile, fats can't be digested and are excreted in the stool (aka: steatorrhea: white/gray/greasy stools).
Cholecystokinin (CCK)	Produced by the **enteroendocrine cells (I Cells) in duodenum**, Jejunum. Composed of amino acids in post-translational modification of preprocholecystokinin.	Stimulates digestion of proteins and fats**.** **Increases** pancreatic secretions, stimulates **gallbladder contraction** and causes relaxation of Sphincter Of Oddi so that bile can enter the duodenum. Suppresses hunger. ↓ gastric acid, inhibits gastric emptying and stimulates the acinar cells (pancreas). It also stimulates production of hepatic bile. **Decrease**: gastric Emptying.	Stimulated by Ingestion of food	Acts on muscarinic M3 receptors = Increase pancreatic secretions (**tip**: KIS your duodenum = K, I and S cells) CCK is inhibited by somatostatin and pancreatic peptide.

Substance	Location	Function	Regulated By	Notes
Chymotrypsin	Pancreas	Breakdown of proteins and polypeptides		Precursor: chymotrypsinogen cleaved by trypsin, connected by disulfide bonds.
Colipase	Pancreas	Activates pancreatic **lipase** which ↓ the **hydrolysis of triglycerides.**		
Endocannabinoid (Endocannabinoid system: ECS)	Brain, CNS and PNS.	Endogenous cannabinoid receptors in the brain (hypothalamus, nucleus accumbens). Stimulates food-seeking behavior. ↑ appetite.		Note: Increases signaling for sweet taste. The ECS also is involved with pain-sensation, memory, mood and the psychoactive effects of cannabis.
Elastase		Breakdowns proteins and elastin		
Enterochromaffin cells (AKA: Kulchitsky cells)	Neuroendocrine cells in the epithelial lining of lumen of GI tract	Secretes 90% of the body's supply serotonin		**Neuroendocrine** progenitors to enterochromaffin cells in the bronchial epithelium associated with **small cell lung cancer.**
Enterochromaffin-like cells	**Neuroendocrine** cells in the gastric glands of fundus	Assist in production of gastric acid via release of histamine.		
Gastric Inhibitory Polypeptide (GIP)	Mucosa of the duodenum and jejunum	↑ insulin release and ↓ H+ secretion	Stimulated by ingestion of food	
Gastrin	**G Cells in pyloric antrum** of stomach, duodenum and pancreas	Increase: H+ (gastric acid), gastric motility	Stimulated by Stomach distention, Vagal stimulation, Amino acids, proteins, hypercalcemia, alkalinization. Inhibited by: stomach pH < 1.5, secretin, VIP, glucagon, GIP, calcitonin, Somatostatin.	**Stimulates chief cells to secrete pepsinogen.** High association with **Zollinger Ellison and MEN syndrome.** (many ulcers in stomach and/or duodenum)
Gastric Acid	**Parietal Cells** in body of stomach	↓ pH in stomach	**Stimulated by ACh, gastrin, histamine via the Vegas Nerve.** (**NOTE**: This is why PPI's are more effective than H2 Blockers in GERD. H2 blockers only block 2/3 of the acid production). Inhibited by Somatostatin, GIP, secretin, prostaglandins.	**Gastrinoma**: gastrin secreting tumor in the pancreas causing ulcers. High association with Zollinger Ellison and MEN syndromes.
Ghrelin	Stomach	Appetite regulation: Stimulates hunger and GH release. Hunger hormone that opposes leptin.		↑ ghrelin production in Prater-Willi and sleep deprivation.
Intrinsic Factor	**Parietal cells** in fundus/body	Required to bind with **Vitamin B12** in terminal ileum. B12 must bind to **R-Protein** to be transported to the ileum to then be released to bind with Intrinsic factor.		**Pernicious anemia:** caused by auto-antibodies against parietal cells (anti-parietal cells antibodies), deficiency of B12, Diphyllobothrium latum parasite, ANY malabsorption pathology. **Highly associated with Hashimoto's** hypothyroidism.

Substance	Location	Function	Regulated By	Notes
Leptin	Appetite regulation. Produced in adipose tissue. **Note:** Remember that when calorie intake is decreased, β oxidation (hepatic lipid oxidation is ↑)	Acts on arcuate nucleus in hypothalamus to indicate we are full = stops hunger. Suppresses appetite.	Satiety hormone. Tells us we are full. **↑ Leptin = no hunger = weight loss.** **↓ Leptin = hunger = weight gain.** (**tip**: "Leps" me loose weight)	Ghrelin (hunger hormone that **opposes leptin**). Secreted when the stomach is empty and inhibited when the stomach is stretched. Leptin decreases the signaling for sweet taste.
Lipase	Pancreas	Breaks down and transports dietary lipids (fats)		**Specific to pancreas** (can determine the location of abdominal injury (seat belt) between spleen and pancreas. Spleen will show amylase.
Motilin	Small intestine	Produces **migrating motor complexes (MMC)**	Increased in fasting state	Motilin receptor agonists stimulate intestinal peristalsis (ex: **erythromycin**)
Nitric Oxide	Endothelial cells of smooth muscle	Relaxes smooth muscle: vessels and lower esophageal sphincter	**cGMP**	
Pepsin	Chief cells in the body of the stomach	Digestion of **proteins**	**Gastrin and Vagus nerve trigger release of HCL and pepsinogen.** (Pepsinogen activates pepsin)	Pepsinogen is the zymogen (precursor) of pepsin. Stimulated by HCL. (**Gastrin and Vagus nerve trigger release of HCL and pepsinogen at M3 receptors**). Pepsin cleaves the N-terminal of phenylalanine, tryptophan and tyrosine.
Phospholipase A		Digestion of fats		
R-Protein (AKA: Haptocorrin, Transcobalamin I, TCN1)	Stomach	Glycoprotein produced by the salivary glands. Binds Vitamin B12 in the stomach and escorts it to the ileum where pancreatic enzymes frees the B12 so that it can bind to intrinsic factor and be absorbed.		Dysfunction leads to pernicious anemia.
Secretin	S Cells in the duodenum	↑ Pancreatic **HCO3 and bile** secretion, ↓ gastric acid secretion	Stimulated by ingestion of food	(**tip**: KIS your duodenum = K, I and S cells)
Somatostatin	**Delta of the pancreatic islets of Langerhans**, GI mucosa and **D cells** in the pyloric antrum	Decreases: gastric acid, pancreatic secretions, insulin, glucagon, gallbladder contraction (CCK)	Stimulated by gastric acid. Inhibited by vagal innervation	Octreotide (Somatostatin analog): inhibits secretion and absorption of pancreatic and digestive enzymes and inhibits growth
Substance P	Pain (Nociception)	**Processes pain and harmful stimuli for the CNS.** Located in: skin, somatic (joints and bones) and visceral (body organs). **Fast pain (sharp pain)** and **cold** = travels on **A Delta (δ) fibers.** **Slow/dull (aching) pain** and **warmth** travels on **C fibers.**		Neuropeptide, receptor is neurokinin 1 (nociceptor) Coexist with glutamate. Nociceptors are free nerve endings with cell bodies in the dorsal root ganglia (outside spinal cord)

Substance	Location	Function	Regulated By	Notes
Trypsin	Pancreas	Enzyme that aids protein digestion. Trypsinogen via enteropeptidase (AKA: enterokinase) is cleaved into trypsin which then stimulates: Chymotrypsin, Carboxypeptidase, and Elastase.		Trypsin: CCK stimulates trypsinogen, which activates **enterokinase** (AKA: **enteropeptidase)**, which cleaves trypsinogen into trypsin. (**Tip**: to go on a Trip, rent a car from Enterprise). Trypsin cleaves the amino acids: arginine and lysine on the carboxyl side.
Trypsinogen	Pancreas	Stimulated by CCK to form trypsin by activating **enteropeptidase (enterokinase)** to cleave trypsinogen to trypsin. (**Tip**: to go on a Trip, rent a car from Enterprise)		Precursor (zymogen) of trypsin. One of the pancreatic juices: amylase, lipase, chymotrypsinogen.
Vasoactive Intestinal Polypeptide (VIP)	Parasympathetic ganglia in small intestine, gallbladder and sphincters	Increases water and electrolyte secretion and relaxation of GI smooth muscle	Stimulated by vagal innervation. Decreased by sympathetic stimulation	**VIPomas:** non-islet cell pancreatic tumor that secretes VIP (>3L/day copious watery diarrhea) **High association with MEN.** TX: Octreotide

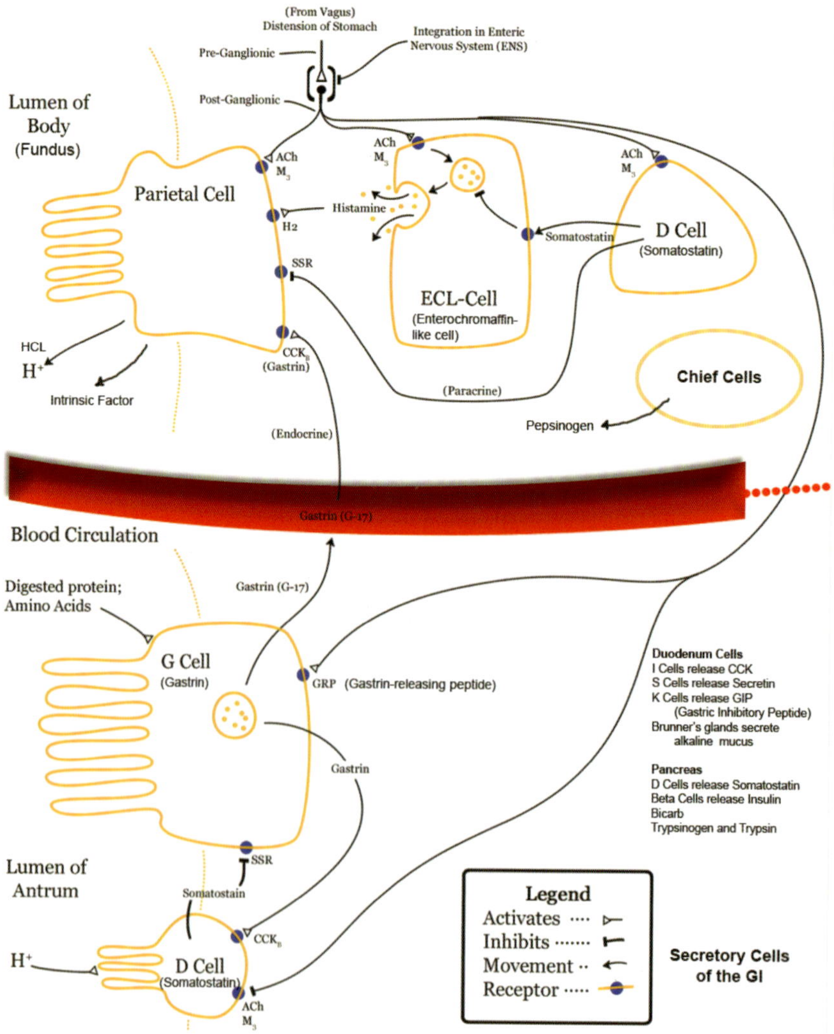

GI Blood Supply

GI Blood Supply and Innervation

Artery	Innervation	Organs Supplied	Embryonic GI Region	Notes
Celiac	Vegas CNX	**Spleen** (mesoderm), liver, **pancreas**, Proximal duodenum, gallbladder	Foregut	Celiac Trunk branches: Splenic artery, Common Hepatic, Left Gastric
Superior Mesenteric Artery (SMA)	Vegas CNX	Distal duodenum, 2/3 transverse colon. (Small bowel). Arises from the aorta directly posterior to the neck of the pancreas.	Midgut	The SMA is the artery that wraps around the ileum due to malrotation during embryonic development = "**Apple Peel Atresia**" Splenic flexure = watershed area (where the IMA and SMA meet
Inferior Mesenteric Artery (IMA)	Pelvic	Distal 1/3 transverse colon to upper rectum (Splenic Flexure). Arises from the abdominal aorta directly posterior to the 3rd part of the duodenum.	Hindgut	Splenic flexure = watershed area (where the IMA and SMA meet) IMA can inhibit the ascension of the kidney in an embryo (Horseshoe Kidney/Turners)
Right gastrics		Distal lesser curvature of the stomach		
Left gastrics				Backup into the left gastrics cause esophageal varices. The left gastric branches from the azygos.
Cystic Artery				Branch of the right Hepatic Artery
Azygos venous system		Connects the superior vena cava system with the inferior vena cava system. Serves as **anastomoses** for blood to the **right atrium** if either of the SVC or IVC are blocked. Serves as part of the esophageal anastomoses. **Left gastric vein (arising from the portal vein in the portal system) goes to the esophagus and enters into the systemic circulation at the azygos vein, which dumps into the superior vena cava.** Two parts of the system: Right side: Azygos vein. Left side: Hemiazygos vein.	Runs up the side of the thoracic vertebral column and drains into the SVC.	Azygos if formed at the 12th thoracic vertebra where the lumbar veins and subcostal veins join (AKA: "Arch of the azygos vein"). It sends deoxygenated blood from the posterior walls of the thorax and abdomen into the SVC.

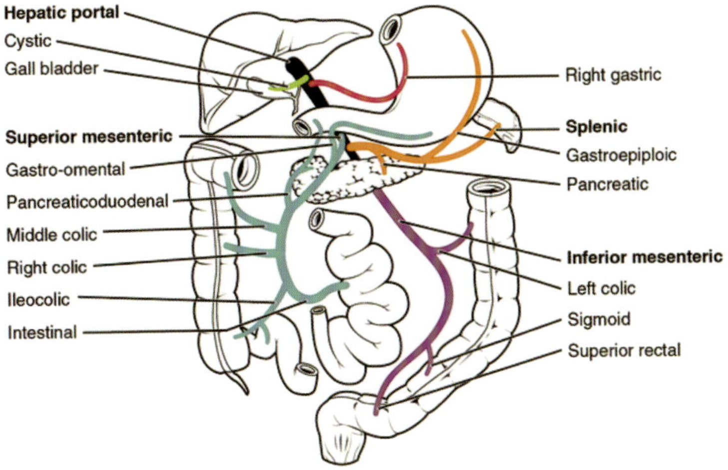

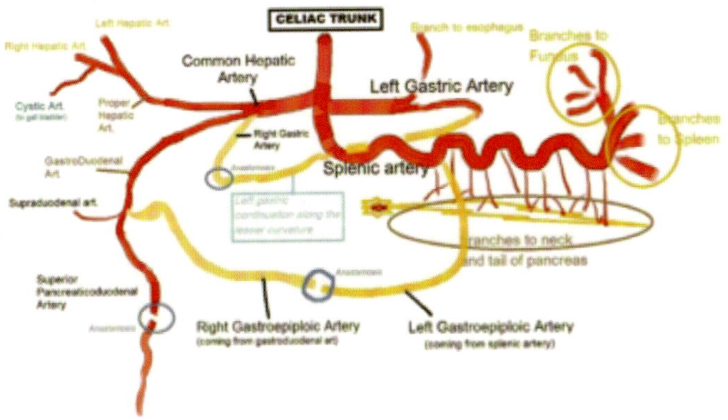

IVC and Portal Systems

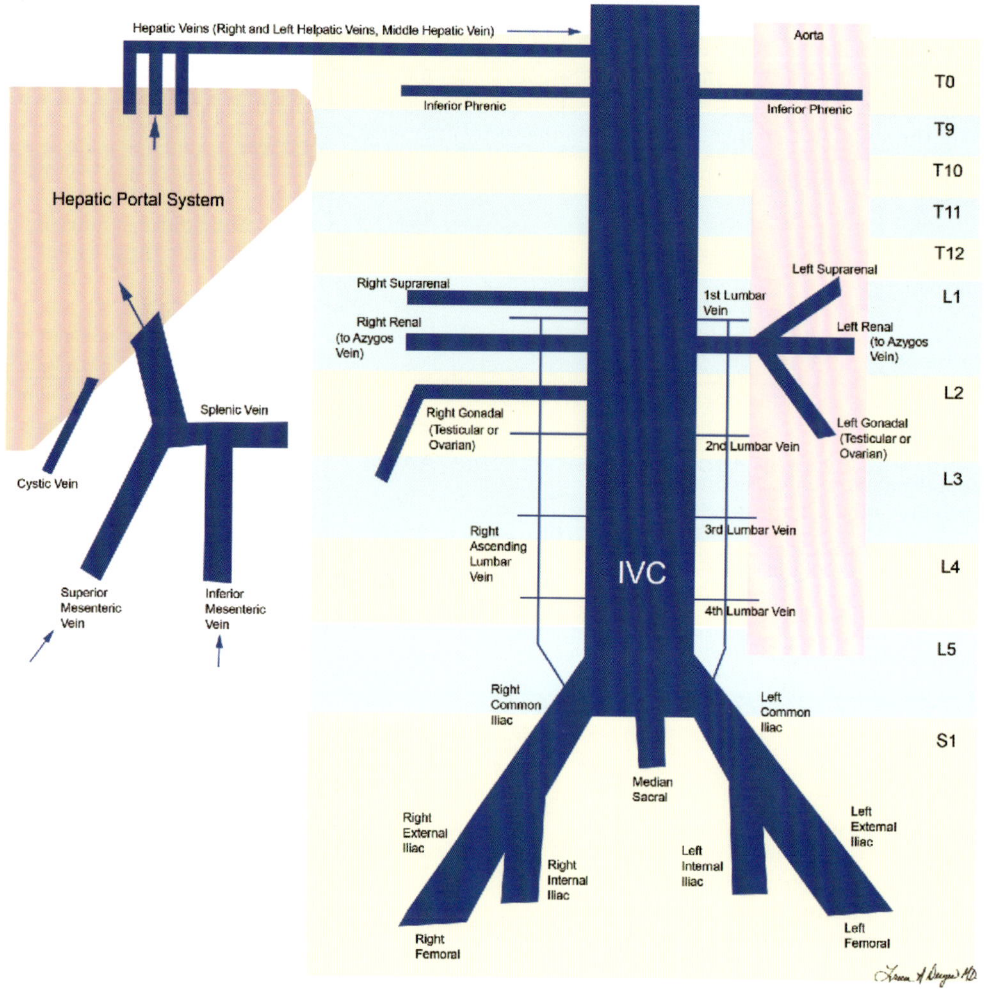

Anal Canal: Blood Supply and Lymphatics

Upper ½ of the Anal Canal	Lower ½ of the Anal Canal
Artery: Superior rectal artery which is a branch of the IMA	Artery: Inferior rectal artery which is a branch of the Internal pudendal artery
Veins: Superior rectal vein into the inferior mesenteric vein	Veins: Inferior rectal vein into the internal pudendal vein. **(The Inferior rectal vein is involved with hemorrhoids)**
Lymph: Pararectal nodes then into the Inferior mesenteric nodes	**Lymph**: Superficial inguinal nodes

Portal Venous System Anastomoses

(AKA: Portocaval anastomosis: connections between the portal circulation and the systemic circulation)
Any blockage of the liver (ie: cirrhosis) will decrease the ability of blood to flow through the portal system (liver) causing back up and increased pressure (ie: portal hypertension). This high pressure will force the blood to find other routes (anastomoses) back to the systemic circulation. If this pressure becomes too great the vessels will enlarge and potentially rupture (bleeding and varices).

Site of Anastomosis	Clinical Sign	Portal Vessel to Systemic Vessel
Esophagus	Esophageal varices	**Left gastric vein (arising from the portal vein in the portal system) goes to the esophagus and enters into the systemic circulation at the azygos vein, which dumps into the superior vena cava.** TX: If banding esophageal varices is unsuccessful then **TIPS** (intrahepatic portosystemic shunt) is used. Decreases portal HTN by shunting portal blood to systemic circulation.
Umbilicus	Caput medusa	**Paraumbilical veins (arise from the left branch of the portal vein) in the portal circulation meet the superficial epigastric** vessels of the systemic circulation (off the great saphenous vein) and then drains into the femoral vein.
Rectum	Anorectal varies (Hemorrhoids)	Superior rectal (off of the inferior mesenteric) of the portal circulation goes to the middle and inferior rectal veins (off of the internal iliac vein).
Retroperitoneal		Portal system: Inferior mesenteric gives way to the superior mesenteric and left colic veins which give way to the right and middle colic veins then meet the systemic system at the gonadal veins (ovarian or testicular) which arise from the IVC on the right and the renal vein on the left and then also meet with the lumbar veins (aka: azygos vein).

Collateral Arterial Circulation Compensation for Blockage of Abdominal Aorta

- Superior epigastric (off internal thoracic) communicates with Inferior epigastric (off external iliac)
- Superior Pancreaticoduodenal (off celiac trunk) with
  Inferior pancreaticoduodenal (off SMA)
- Middle colic (off SMA) with Left Colic (off IMA)
- Superior rectal (off IMA) with Middle and inferior rectal (off internal iliac)

Innervation of GI

- Splanchnic Nerves: Innervates the visceral structures of the abdomen and pelvis.
- Splanchnic nerves made up of: sympathetic and parasympathetic preganglionic fibers. From T5 – T12.
- Sympathetic preganglionic fibers: Thoracic, lumbar and sacral.
- Parasympathetic preganglionic fibers: Pelvic splanchnic nerves.
- Thoracic splanchnic nerves (lie medial to the sympathetic trunks)
  Greater: T5 – T9 (foregut and midgut); lesser: T10 – T11 (foregut and midgut); and least splanchnic nerves: T12 (kidneys and gonads).
- Lumbar splanchnic nerves: composed of upper and lower.
  Upper: L1 – L2 (hindgut)
  Lower: L1 – L2 (rectum, bladder, male genital tract).
  Actions: Inhibits peristalsis, vasoconstriction, release of glucose, adrenalin secretion, ↑ sphincter tone, ejaculation (pudendal nerve also innervates this).
- Sympathetic postganglionic of thoracic nerves: Celiac, superior mesenteric, aorticorenal.
- Sympathetic postganglionic of the lumbar nerves: Inferior mesenteric, inferior hypogastric.
- Parasympathetic splanchnic nerves: Pelvic splanchnic nerves.
- Parasympathetic preganglionic nerves: S2 – S4 (hindgut, pelvis, perineum). Innervate: rectum, bladder, erectile tissues (penis, clitoris). Actions: Decrease tone of sphincters (micturition), erection, increase peristalsis (digestion).

	Presynaptic Sympathetic (Sensory innervation)	Presynaptic Sympathetic Ganglion (pre-ganglionic)	Postsynaptic Sympathetics (post-ganglionic)	Preganglionic Para-sympathetic	Postganglionic Parasympathetic	Artery	Referred Pain
Foregut	T5 – T9	T5 – T9 Greater Splanchnics	Celiac ganglion	Vagus (CN X)	Vagus (CN X) Terminal ganglion	Celiac	Epigastrium
Midgut	T10 – T12	T10 – T11 Lesser splanchnics	Superior mesenteric ganglion	Vagus (CNX)	Vagus (CN X) Terminal ganglion	SMA	Umbilical
Hindgut	L1 – L2	L1 – L2 Lumbar splanchnics	Inferior mesenteric ganglion	S2 – S4 Pelvic splanchnics	Terminal Ganglion	IMA	Hypogastrium
Pelvic Viscera	L1 – L2	L1 – L2 Lumbar splanchnics	Superior hypogastric plexus	S2 - S4 Pelvic splanchnics			

Pancreas

- Performs both endocrine (acinar and duct cells) and exocrine rolls
- Produces: Insulin, glucagon, somatostatin, pancreatic polypeptides
- Secretes digestive enzymes to help digest and absorb nutrients in the small intestine and to release B12 from R-Protein:
  Bicarb from centroacinar cells stimulated by secretin
  Digestive enzymes from basophilic cells stimulated by CCK
- Digestive enzymes:
  Trypsinogen and Chymotrypsinogen (**Enteropeptidase (enterokinase) cleaves trypsinogen to form trypsin**)
  Pancreatic Lipase
  Pancreatic Amylase
  Phospholipase A2, lysophospholipase
  Cholesterol esterase

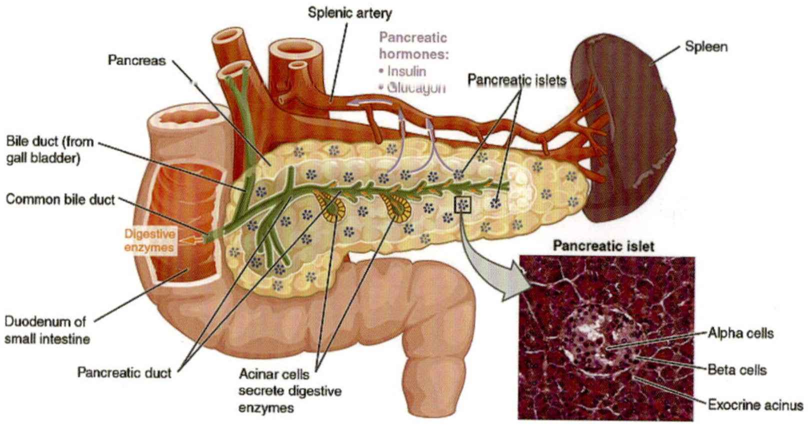

- Blood supply:
  Splenic artery supplies the neck, body and tail.
  Superior and inferior pancreaticoduodenal artery supply the anterior and posterior surfaces and head
  Drainage of the body and neck into the splenic vein
  Drainage of the head into the superior mesenteric and portal veins
- Make up:
  Islets of Langerhans composed of:
  α (alpha) cells on periphery secrete glucagon
  β (Beta) cells in the central secrete insulin
- (**tip**: INsulin is on the INside)
  δ (Delta) cells interspersed secrete somatostatin
  F cell secrete pancreatic polypeptide (Amylin)

Pancreatic Cell

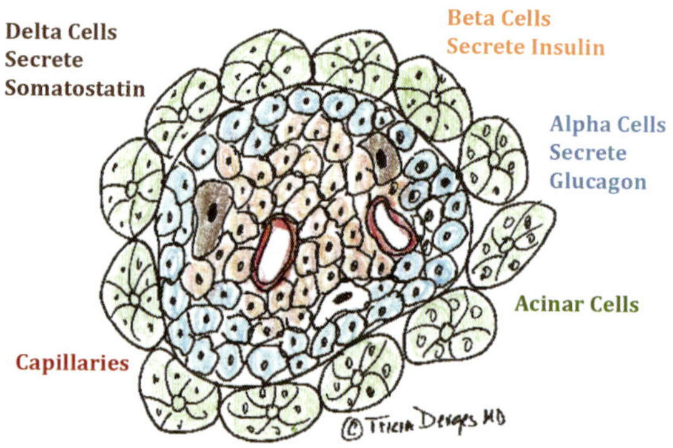

- Structure
  Head
  Body
  Tail
  Ampulla of Vater (aka: hepatopancreatic duct): formed by the union of the pancreatic duct and common bile duct, it is located at the duodenal major papilla. It marks the transition from the foregut to the midgut (at the SMA).
  Pancreatic duct (aka: duct of Wirsung) joins the pancreas to the ampulla of Vater to supply pancreatic enzymes that help in digestion.
  Accessory pancreatic duct (aka: Duct of Santorini): an additional pancreatic duct found in some people.
  Sphincter of Oddi (aka: hepatopancreatic sphincter): muscular valve that controls the flow of bile and pancreatic enzymes (juices) through the ampulla of Vater into the 2nd part of the duodenum. (Note: CCK relaxes the sphincter of Oddi by vasoactive intestinal peptide).

Liver

- Kupffer cells = macrophages in the liver
- Development: 3rd to 8th week of embryogenesis
- Foregut development
- Umbilical vein supplies nutrients in fetus
- Ductus venosus carries blood from left portal vein to left hepatic vein and IVC (allows placental blood to bypass the liver
- Falciform ligament (attaches liver to anterior abdomen) is remnant of umbilical vein
- Umbilical vein becomes the ligamentum teres (AKA: round ligament of the liver) after birth. The remaining small paraumbilical veins (in the ligament) act as one of the portal anastomosis sites in severe portal HTN causing caput medusae
- Ductus venosus becomes the ligamentum venosum after birth. Can be continuous with round ligament of the liver and is surrounded by the lesser omentum
- Adult blood supply: hepatic portal vein and hepatic arteries. Blood flows through liver sinusoids and empties into the central veins ➔ hepatic veins ➔IVC
- Tends to experience "graft vs host" rejection in transplants (as does bone marrow transplants)

Liver Functions

- Conjugates bilirubin (breakdown of bilirubin via glucuronidation)
- Gamma carboxylation of clotting factors of 2, 7, 9, 10, proteins C, S
- Urea Cycle (breaks down ammonia into urea)
- Stores glycogen, 1 – 2 yrs supply of **Vit A** in hepatic **Stellate cells**, 1 – 4 months supply of Vit D, 3 - 5 yrs supply Vit B12, Vitamin K, Iron, Copper. (B12 is found in all animal foods, except honey)
- Glycogenesis
- Gluconeogenesis
- Glycogenolysis
- P-450, Detoxification (Smooth Endoplasmic Reticulum)
- First pass metabolism
- Produces: Thyroid Binding Globulin,
- Produces: Albumin (most abundant protein in the blood). Albumin maintains oncotic pressure (pressure exerted by proteins in vessels plasma that pulls water into the circulatory system). It is an opposing force to capillary filtration pressure and interstitial colloidal osmotic pressure). GFR is tremendously affected by osmotic pressure.
  (Rough Endoplasmic Reticulum = ribosomes)
- A1 antitrypsin production
- Produces bile
- Cholesterol and triglyceride synthesis (VLDL, LDL)
- Synthesizes angiotensinogen (which is activated by renin from the kidneys).
  ATI is sent to the lungs where ACE converts ATI to ATII
- IGF-1 Insulin-like Growth Factor (growth hormone)
- Releases acute phase reactants

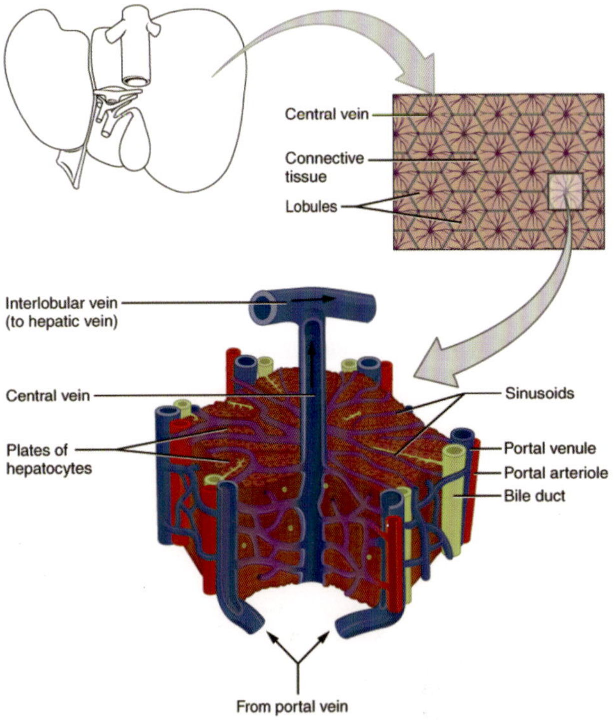

Hepatic Zones

Zone	Notes
Zone 1 (periportal)	Affected most by **toxins/drugs** (cocaine) and **hepatitis**
Zone 2 (intermediate zone)	
Zone 3 (pericentral vein – centrilobular)	First zone affected by **ischemia.** (Centrilobular necrosis). **Contains cytochrome P-450 system**. Affected most by **alcoholic hepatitis** and metabolic toxins.

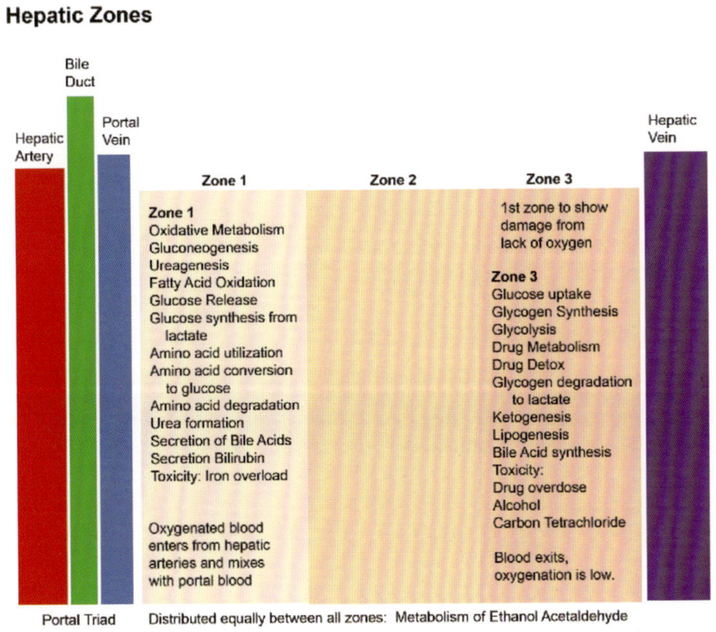

Gallbladder (AKA: cholecyst)

- Foregut development
- Storage and concentration site for bile (made in the liver)
- Part of the biliary system
- Released into the small intestine
- Hartmann's pouch (out-pouching of gallbladder) where gallstones tend to get stuck
- Cells: Innermost surface: columnar cells with brush boarder of microvilli
- No muscularis mucosae layer
- Bile is sent to gallbladder from liver. Once in gallbladder it is concentrated by removing water and electrolytes via active transport creating osmotic pressure that causes water and electrolytes (chloride) to be reabsorbed
- Cholecystokinin (CCK) stimulates the gallbladder to contract to drain bile into common bile duct and then into the duodenum.
- Bile = bile salts and water
- Bile = emulsifies fats to aid in absorption
- Bile aids in eliminating bilirubin (product of hemoglobin metabolism)

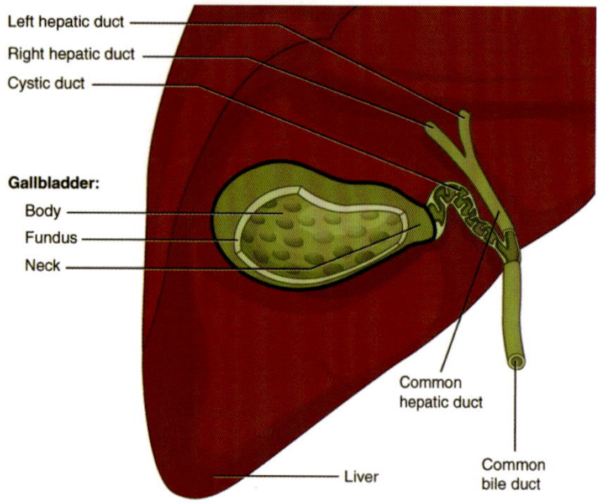

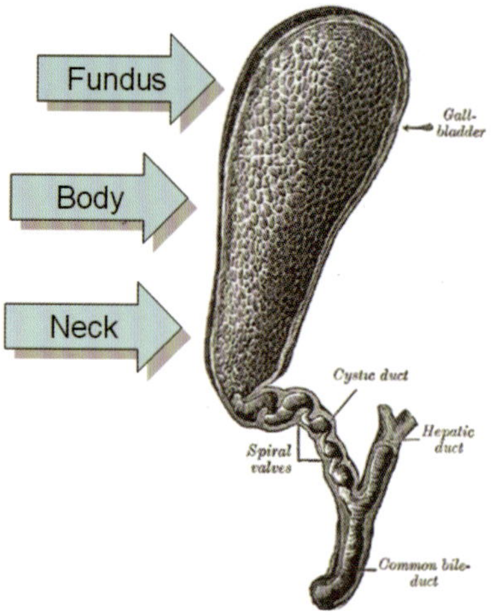

Stomach

- Secretes proteases (protein-digesting enzymes) and gastric acid to aid in food digestion
- Lower esophageal sphincter (LES) in the cardiac region of stomach, keeps HCL from regurgitating back up the esophagus (Relaxation of LES = GERD)
- At cardiac region: cells change from stratified squamous (esophagus) into column
- **Blood supply:**
  Lesser curvature: right gastric artery (inferiorly), left gastric artery (superiorly)
  Greater curvature: right gastro-omental artery (inferiorly), left gastro-omental artery (superiorly)
  Fundus and upper portion of greater curvature = **short gastric arteries** via the splenic artery
- **Innervation:**
  Pain sensation from the stomach is via the sympathetic plexus in the celiac plexus.
  Parasympathetic innervation: CN X
- **Flow of food**: Mouth (**amylase begins breakdown of starch**) ➔ bolus of food is swallowed through UES ➔ descends down esophagus via peristaltic movements ➔ LES into stomach ➔stomach digest food into chyme (takes from 40 minutes to a few hours. Average person holds 1 liter of food) ➔ 1st part of duodenum to be absorbed (some absorption is done in the stomach if they are small molecules: water, aspirin, amino acids, ethanol, caffeine)

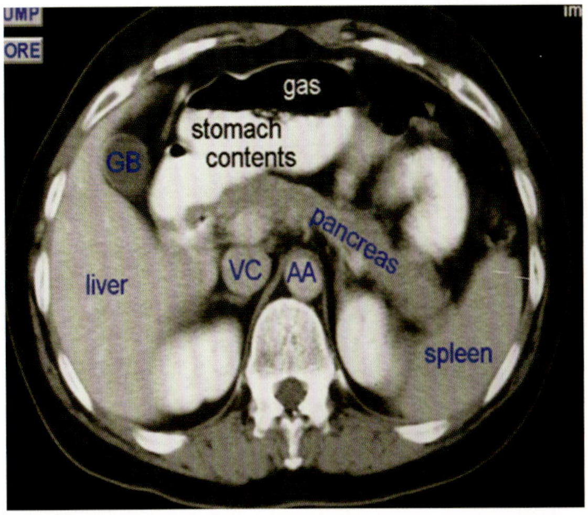

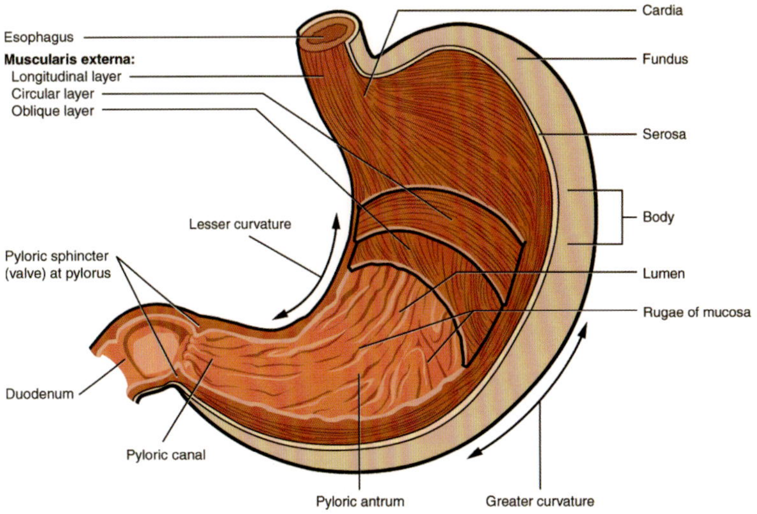

GI Pathologies: GI Pain Location Differentials

Pain Location	Most Probably Pathology	Notes	Differentials
LLQ	Diverticulitis	Due to history of pressure, can present with bleeding	Ovarian torsion, ectopic pregnancy, Sigmoid volvulus
RLQ	Appendicitis	+ McBurney's Sign (**tip**: mc "B"urney's is the sign that is "B"elow the McMurphys)	Ovarian torsion, ectopic pregnancy, Cecal diverticulitis
URQ	Gall Bladder (Cholecystitis, Cholelithiasis)	+ Murphy's Sign: Pain can radiate to upper right shoulder	Liver pathologies, Subphrenic abscess, Biliary colic, Cholangitis, Perforated duodenal ulcer
ULQ	Stomach Ulcer, Spleen		Spleen rupture, Splenic flexure syndrome
Mid-Epigastric Pain	Pancreatitis	Lipase: specific to pancreas	Peptic ulcer, Aortic dissection, Pancreatic cancer
Severe pain radiating to the back	Acute pancreatitis	MCC: Alcohol, Stones	
Diffuse abdominal pain with distension	Ruptured organ (MC: Stomach)	See air under the diaphragm on an upright abdomen/chest X-ray	Obstruction (will see air/fluid levels in the bowel on X-ray)
Suprapubic Pain	UTI		
Pain radiating to the groin	Kidney Stone		
Colicky Pain	Intussusception		Gastroenteritis
Costovertebral pain, flank pain	Pyelonephritis	White cast in the urine	Any pain in this area indicates a kidney pathology
Crampy abdominal pain	Ischemic colitis	Watershed area, can have blood in the stool	

GI Pathologies and Pain Differentials

GI Pathology	Symptoms and Description
Pancreatitis:	Constant pain, gradual in onset, severe pain radiating to the back, ↑ drinking
Gastroenteritis (Food Poisoning)	Vomiting, diarrhea, colicky pain (comes and goes)
Cholangitis (Common Bile Duct)	Charcot Triad Symptoms: Fever, Chills, Jaundice, RUQ pain
Choledocholithiasis (Common Bile Duct)	Jaundice, pale stools, dark urine
Duodenal Ulcer	Sudden severe burning pain, relieved with food
Alcoholic Gastritis	Pain relieved by vomiting, bleeding
Perforation of lower esophagus	Vomiting precedes pain
Pancreatic Cancer	Constant, gnawing epigastric pain

Epigastric Pain Differentials

Pathology	Symptoms
Non-ulcer dyspepsia (functional indigestion)	Symptoms without any pathology
GERD (Gastroesophageal reflux)	Nocturnal cough, wakening with acid/bitter taste and hoarseness
Gastric Ulcer	Pain worsens with food, weight loss
Duodenal Ulcer	Pain is better with food, weight gain
Gastroparesis	Neuropathy and bloating: MC in diabetics
Gastric Cancer	Weight loss
Pancreatitis	Tender to palpation in midepigastric area, pain radiates to the back

Referred Pain Differentials

Pathology/Cause	Site of Referred Pain
Gallbladder	Right shoulder/scapula
Pancreas	Back
Appendix	RLQ
Pyelonephritis, hydronephritis	Costovertebral angle/Flank
Nephrolithiasis	Groin
Prostate	Perineum, glans penis
Gastric perforation	Epigastric pain to right shoulder
Esophagus	Substernal chest pain
Esophageal rupture	Left shoulder
Pharynx	Ears
Cold foods/drinks (AKA: brain freeze)	Due to rapid temperature changes in the sinuses
Myocardial infarction	Left jaw, arm chest

GI Blood Loss Source

- Blood loss of > 30% can present with a systolic blood pressure < 100 or heart rate > 100
- Most critical step in severe GI bleed is fluid resuscitation (bolus of 9% normal saline, AKA: Lactate ringers)
- Stool color indicates location of bleed
  Heme positive stool can occur from as little as 5 – 10 mL of blood loss.
  - Red, bright red: From the left side (descending colon, sigmoid, rectum), lower GI bleeds.
  - Maroon, burgundy: From the right side (ascending colon), lower GI bleeds.
    Lower GI bleeds due to: Cancer, Ischemic colitis, polyps, inflammatory bowel disease, Angiodysplasia, Diverticular disease.
  - Black, tarry: **Upper GI bleeds**
    Upper GI considered proximal to the **ligament of Treitz** (where the duodenum and jejunum meet).
    Coffee ground emesis (vomited blood: Bleeding from the duodenum, stomach or esophagus. This can occur with as little as 5 – 10 mL of blood loss.
    Upper GI bleeds: due to: Ulcer disease, cancer, varices, esophagitis, gastritis, duodenitis
- Test: Stood Guaiac Card (AKA: Hemoccult, Occult)
  - Only the iron in Hb or myoglobin will make the Guaiac card positive.

Vomiting

Occurs due to the stimulation of either the vomiting center in the medulla (near the respiratory center) or the chemoreceptor trigger zone in the area postrema on the floor of the fourth ventricle.

Paths:

- Vomiting due to psychological stress occurs via the cerebral cortex and limbic system to the vomiting center.
- Anticipatory vomiting occurs via the cerebral cortex and limbic system to the vomiting center.
- Vomiting due to motion sickness occurs via the vestibular/vestibulocerebellar system from the labyrinth of the inner ear to the vomiting center.
- Vomiting due to chemical (drugs, chemotherapy drugs, toxins) occurs via the chemoreceptor trigger zone in the area postrema when chemical signals are detected in the bloodstream and cerebrospinal fluid.
- Gastrointestinal distention, irritation and delayed gastric emptying stimulate the vagal and visceral nerves.

Causes of vomiting

Due to anything that can obstruct the GI tract or any of its tributary's.

- Hirschsprung's' disease
- Small bowel atresia (aka: duodenal atresia). MC: Down's Syndrome (aka: double bubble sign)
- Biliary atresia
- Intestinal malrotation
- Volvulus
- Meconium ileus
- Meconium plug
- Colonic atresia
- Intussusception
- Appendicitis
- Hepatitis
- Gall bladder disease
- Pancreatitis or pancreatic cancer of the head of the pancreas
- Indirect hernia
- Lactobezoar (aka: Inspissated Milk Syndrome): Obstruction of the small bowel by milk curds.
- Foreign bodies
- Pyloric stenosis (hypertrophy of the muscle surrounding the opening of the pylorus: pyloric sphincter).
- Foreign bodies: MCC: swallowed coins. MC places of obstruction: cricopharyngeus and the lower esophageal sphincter.
- Gastroesophageal reflux (aka: GERD: poorly coordinated swallowing and delayed gastric emptying), Peptic ulcer disease
- Esophagitis
- Acute gastroenteritis (MCC: Rotavirus)
- Concussion/head trauma
- Migraine headaches
- Viral meningitis
- Increased intracranial pressure
- DKA
- Strep throat (Streptococcal pharyngitis)
- Asthma
- Anorexia nervosa and bulimia
- Pregnancy
- Stress

Salivary Gland Pathologies

- **Chorda tympani controls salivation from the sublingual and submandibular glands**
- **Parotid gland is innervated by the glossopharyngeal nerve (CN IX)**

<table>
<tr>
<td>Mucoepidermoid Carcinoma
Malignant
MC: Salivary gland malignancy in adults
Painless, firm/hard, slow growing.
Squamous, mucus secreting cells.

Peak: 20 – 40 yrs

Associated with CMV</td>
<td>Warthin Tumor
(AKA: Papillary Cystadenoma)
MC: Parotid gland.
Peak: 60 – 70 years.
Benign cystic tumor of salivary glands.

Histology: Abundant lymphocytes and germinal centers.

Associated with smoking.</td>
<td>Pleomorphic Adenoma
Potential to be malignant.
Mixed tumor of salivary gland.
Slow growing, painless.
Firm single nodular mass.
Mixture of polygonal epithelial and spindle shaped myoepithelial elements in a variable stroma: can be mucoid, cartilaginous, hyaline or myxoid.
TX: Surgery (can reoccur if incorrectly excised)</td>
</tr>
<tr>
<td>Sjögren Syndrome

Associated with Rheumatoid arthritis and SLE.

Autoimmune: WBC destroy exocrine glands (salivary and lacrimal).

Labs: Anti-Ro, Anti-La, Anti-SSA, and Anti-SSB. Autoantibodies to snRNP's (AKA: Ribonucleoprotein antigens, spliceosome, introns and exons).
↑ CSF levels of IL-1.
Associated with other autoimmunize disorders: SLE, RA.</td>
<td colspan="2">Sjögren SX: Xerostomia (dry mouth), dry eyes (Xerophthalmia. Feels like grains of sand in the eye), Dental cavities/caries (no saliva so can't help clean the teeth), vaginal dryness, dry skin, fatigue, bilateral parotid enlargement, dysphagia (no saliva to help swallow).

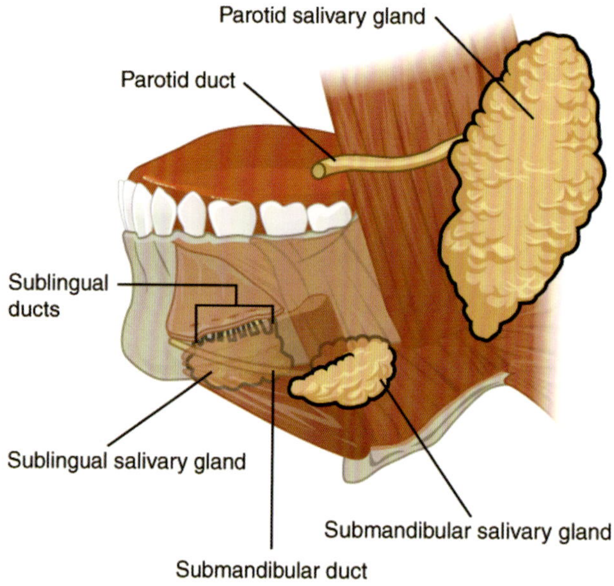

TX: Keep eyes and mouth moist.</td>
</tr>
</table>

Muscles of Mastication

Muscle of Mastication	Origin	Insertion	Action
Masseter	Zygomatic arch	Mandible	Closes jaw
Temporalis	Temporal bone	Coronoid process	Closes jaw
Medial Pterygoid	Sphenoid, Palatine, Maxillary bones	Medical ramus	Closes jaw
Lateral Pterygoid	Sphenoid bone	Anterior mandibular condyle	**Opens jaw**, allows grinding side to side, protrudes mandible. (**tip**: "L"ateral or "L"oser: if you say the wrong things when you open your mouth"

Sinuses

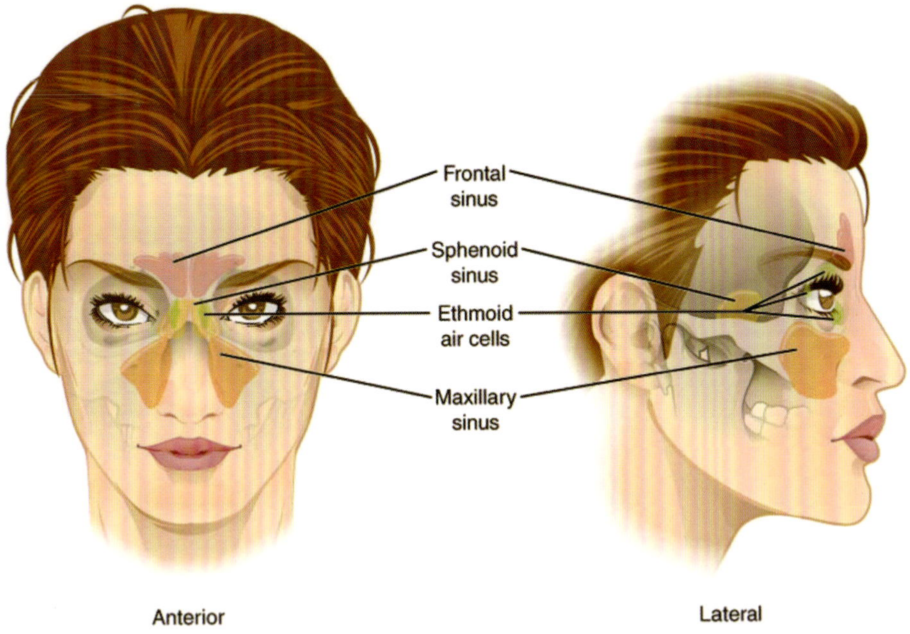

Transsphenoidal Tumor Resection

- Removal of a pituitary tumor is done through the sphenoid sinus: **Transsphenoidal surgery.**

Sinusitis (AKA: Rhinosinusitis)

- Inflammation of the sinuses. MC due to bacterial infection, allergies, viral infection, infection, air pollution.
- Higher risk with asthma, cystic fibrosis, immunocompromised.
- Acute sinusitis: last < 4 weeks.
  Chronic sinusitis: last > 12 weeks.
- SX: headaches, sore throat, cough, decreased smell, plugged nose, thick nasal mucus, fever, pain/pressure over the sinuses. Cough is worse at night.
- Pain/pressure over the sinuses.
- MC: Viral causes. Consider bacterial infection is: Symptoms last more than 10 days, pain develops over the sinus, blowing up dark green mucus.

Sinus	**Location/Description of Pain/Pressure**
Maxillary	Cheek area
Frontal	Above the eyes, headache in the forehead
Ethmoidal	Between/behind the eyes, upper part of the nose, headaches
Sphenoidal	Behind the eyes, radiates to the top of the head, over the mastoid process, back of the head.

Esophagus and Pharyngeal Pathologies

- Most present with dysphagia and weight loss.
  Dysphagia: difficulty swallowing.
- Progressive dysphagia: solids first then liquids. (MCC: cancer)
- Dysphagia with weight loss is generally an esophagus problem.
  Dysphagia with weight loss, blood in the stool and anemia is generally due to cancer.
- DX: BIT: Barium studies first (Cause of dysphagia must be determined first before an endoscopy is done due to the risk of esophageal rupture)
- Endoscopy used to diagnose Barrett's esophagus and esophageal adenocarcinoma
- Only esophageal cancer and Barrett's esophagus is diagnosed by biopsy
- MAT: Esophageal manometer
- Odynophagia: painful swallowing. MCC: Due to infection process (HIV, CMV, HSV, Candida)
- Esophagus disorders can mimic Prinzmetal's angina.
  Prinzmetal's angina presents with diffuse ST elevations and coronary vasospasms. Esophageal disorders (in particularly esophageal spasms) do not present with any EKG abnormalities nor coronary spasms.
  However, treatment is the same for both: Calcium channel blockers and nitrates.
- Frontal sinuses do not open until 7 years old.

Eosinophilic Esophagitis
Food allergies.

SX: Heartburn, dysphagia.

DX: Endoscopy and biopsy shows Eosinophil's

TX: PPI's and Budesonide steroids *(Pulmicort)*

Esophagitis
Immunocompromised.
↑ CMV (**linear ulcers**)
↑ HSV (**punched out** ulcers)

SX: Candida: white pseudomembrane, Odynophagia (especially if CD4 count is < 100), dysphagia.

TX: **Fluconazole** (Diagnostic and therapeutic)

Achalasia
Loss of **myenteric (Auerbach)** plexus.
Causes: ↑ amplitude/tone/pressure at the LES (LES can't relax) with **absent** peristoltic waves.
AKA: Hypertrophy of circular muscles with absence or degeneration of ganglia in Auerbach plexus.

SX: progressive **dysphagia** from solids to liquids, regurgitation of food.

Cause: Loss of Auerbach plexus, Chagas disease (Trypanosoma cruzi)

DX: BIT: Barium swallow shows "Birds Beak" appearance.
MAT: Esophageal manometer shows absence of normal peristalsis and low tone (unable to relax) LES.
Normal mucosa.

TX: Balloon dilation/pneumatic dilation of LES or myotomy surgery.
Botulinum toxin injection if surgery or dilation is not possible.

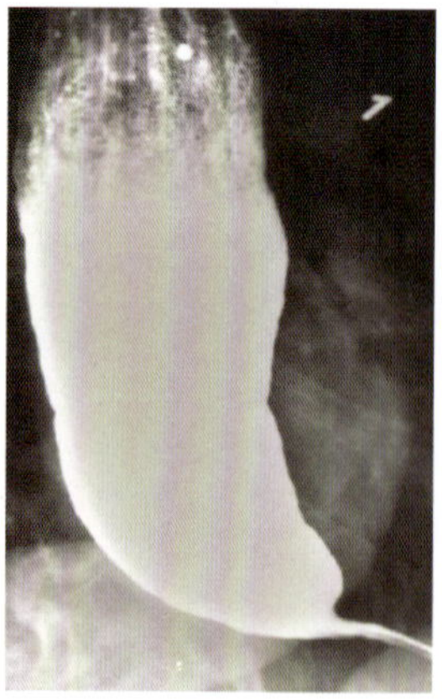

Esophageal Strictures
(AKA: Schatzki's Rings)
Distal strictures.

Causes: Acid reflux or lye ingestion. (Injury), can also due **to high acid reflux** during pregnancy or continual acid damaging the esophagus.

SX: Intermittent dysphagia.

Heals and leaves **strictures** (scarring that makes circular bands narrowing the esophagus = stops food = pain.

DX: Barium study.
TX: Pneumatic dilation and/or surgery.

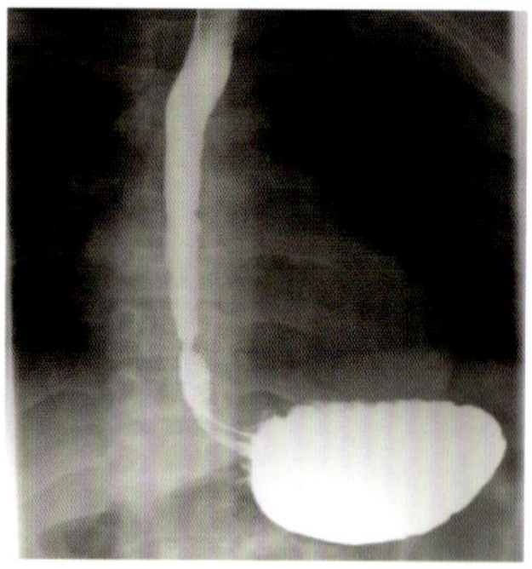

Esophageal Varices Painless bleeding in lower 1/3 of esophagus from **left gastrics** due to **portal HTN.** Path: **Left gastric vein (arising from the portal vein in the portal system) goes to esophagus into the systemic circulation at the azygos vein which dumps into the superior vena cava.** **TX: If banding esophageal varices is unsuccessful then TIPS (intrahepatic portosystemic shunt) is used. Decreases portal HTN by shunting portal blood to systemic circulation.** **TX: Banding** **If banding does not work: TIPS** **Propanolol for ↓ portal HTN**	**Mallory-Weiss Syndrome** Mucosal/submucosal lacerations at the gastroesophageal junction in the proximal stomach. It does **not** penetrate the esophagus, only the mucosa. MCC: Vomiting/retching (alcoholics). SX: Hematemesis, painful swallowing (odynophagia). DX: Esophagogram shows no leakage. TX: Supportive.	**Boerhaave Syndrome** **Emergency** Distal **esophageal rupture**. MCC: Iatrogenic (due to endoscopy), **violent** vomiting. Amylase seen in chest effusions. SX: Severe, acute onset, radiates to left shoulder, gas/air under the skin (subcutaneous emphysema). DX: CXR shows mediastinal widening. Esophagogram shows leakage. TX: Emergency surgery: high mortality.
GERD (AKA: Gastroesophageal Reflux Disease) SX: Heartburn, regurgitation, bitter taste in the morning at back of mouth (bitter taste receptors are in the back of the mouth: CN Ix, X), dysphagia which can lead to: hoarseness in the morning, nocturnal **cough**. (**MCC of nocturnal cough**: #1: post nasal drip and #2: GERD). Cause: lower tone in the LES (lower esophageal sphincter) TX: **PPI** (Proton pump inhibitors) **H2 Blockers** (Not as effective as PPI's because they only stop 2/3 of gastric acid production, where as PPI's stop all production).	**Sclerodermal Esophageal Dysmotility (AKA: CREST syndrome)** E = Esophagus Esophageal smooth muscle atrophy = **↓ LES tone** and dysmotility (peristalsis) = dysphagia due to acid reflux. **No peristalsis in distal esophagus** (AKA: **Fibrosis and atrophy** of esophageal smooth muscle, **LES is incompetent** = it is loose and decreased tone) High risk: Barrett's Esophagus and aspiration (due to dysphagia). SX: Presents with ↑ reflux. TX: **PPI's**	**Esophageal Spasms** (AKA: Corkscrew esophagus or Nutcracker esophagus) **Vasospasms** of esophagus. SX: Sudden, **episodic retrosternal severe chest pain** that radiates to **interscapular** (easily mistaken for MI), dypsnea, dysphagia. (There is always pain present but dysphasia may or may not be present). Last approximately 15 min. Patient feels like they are having a heart attack, presents like Prinzmetal's angina. Cause: ↑ with emotional stress, hot or cold foods or drinks. DX: MAT: Manometry with **Ergonovine** Shows abnormal patterns. Barium study is done while a spasm is occurring: corkscrew pattern. Endoscopy and esophagram are normal. TX: **Nitro tablets for pain and CCB**
Oropharyngeal Dysphagia Upper esophagus does not initiate swallowing. Occurs above the UES. SX: cough, drool, aspiration. Patient can cough up undigested food. DX: Nasopharyngeal laryngoscopy	**Plummer-Vinson Syndrome** Proximal strictures. Triad of symptoms: **Dysphagia** (due to esophageal webs)**, iron deficiency anemia and glossitis (shinny, smooth tongue).** MC: in women. TX: Iron replacement	**Esophageal Dysphasia** SX: Sensation that food is sticking in the upper or lower chest DX: Esophagogastroduodenoscopy

Drug Induced Esophagitis (AKA: Pill induced esophagitis) **MC: Bisphosphonates, Potassium Chloride, Quinidine, Iron, Aspirin, NSAIDS, Tetracycline, Doxycycline** **Complications: Esophageal burns, retrosternal pain.** SX: Epigastric pain, retrosternal pain, food and beverages make it worse. **To ↓ risk of complications:** Drink full glass of water when taking the medications, sit or stand upright for at least 30 minutes after taking the pill. TX: Stop drug until esophagus heals. Then restart drug, take with full glass of water and sit upright when taking.	**Zenker Diverticulum** **Motor dysfunction of cricopharyngeal. Causes a dilation/pouching of the posterior pharyngeal constrictor muscles.** **False diverticulum**. **Crycopharyngeal** sphincter dysfunction Occurs above the **upper esophageal sphincter**) does **not relax** when swallowing = dysphasia. Cryopharyngeal muscle function is to start peristalic waves to push food bolus down to the stomach. High risk: elderly males > 50 SX: Dysphagia, **foul breath** (halitosis) food is trapped in the diverticulum). Choking on food causing pain. ↑ risk of aspiration pneumonia. (Food will be undigested food) Complications: **Pulmonary aspiration** Zenker's DX: Esophagram (AKA: Z-gram), Barium study, surgical resection. DO NOT do an endoscopy due to risk of rupture. TX: Excision: Cricopharyngeal myotomy	**Peritonsillar Abscess** Collection of pus around the tonsils. Usually a complication of tonsillitis. Occurs in children and adults. SX: **Muffled voice** ("hot potato" voice), **deviated uvula**, pain in the tonsillar area, headache, fever, swollen lymph nodes, halitosis, salivation, ipsilateral earache trismus (can't open mouth completely), **odynophagia** (pain on swallowing) TX: Incision and drainage (needle aspiration), IV antibiotics: **Clindamycin or Metronidazole combined with Benzylpenicillin (Penn G)** **Tonsillitis**: Does **NOT** have a deviate uvula and no muffled voice. MC: in children, group A Strep.
Esophageal Rupture Common complication with Boerhaave's (forceful or recurrent vomiting. Can be due to alcohol, flu, and morning sickness during pregnancy, etc.). SX: Effusion shows ↑↑ **amylase** (>2500) in unilateral pleural effusion, vomiting, dyspnea, cyanosis, tachypnea, shock, pain radiating to left shoulder. DX: CT or esophagraphy/esophagram (with water contrast). CXR: **Mediastinal widening (mediastinitis)** , crepitus (subcutaneous emphysema), pleural effusion, pneumomediastinum	**Botulism Toxin** Can be pathologic or theraputic. MOA: Botulism inhibits the release of acetylcholine at the neuromuscular junction inhibiting the nicotinic receptors and ↓ action potential to relax the skeletal muscles. Pathologic: Clostridium botulinum (spore) Descending paralysis. Loss of gag reflex (CN IX). Ingestion or Inhalation of the spore. Theraputic: Botulism toxin is given to relax the gastroesophageal sphincter.	**Esophageal Adenocarcinoma (lower 1/3 esophagus), MCC: Barrett's Esophagus** **or** **Squamous Cell Carcinoma (upper 2/3 esophagus), MCC smoking.** **This ALSO includes squamous cell carcinoma in the mouth/lips due to smoking and/or chewing tobacco.** SX: **Progressive dysphagia**: First difficulty with solid foods, progressing to liquids. Anemia, heme-positive stool. Risk: Alcohol, achalasia, Barrett's Esophagus, smoking, Zenkers, obesity, GERD, hot liquids. TX: 5-fluorouracil after surgical resection.

Retropharyngeal Abscess (RPA)

Abscess behind the posterior pharyngeal wall (retropharyngeal space).
Common in infants and children.

SX: Stiff neck (AKA: torticollis), dysphagia, stridor, drooling, enlarged cervical lymph nodes

DX: X ray of neck shows swelling of retropharyngeal space.
CT definitive.

Complications: Airway obstruction and/or both.

TX: Surgery

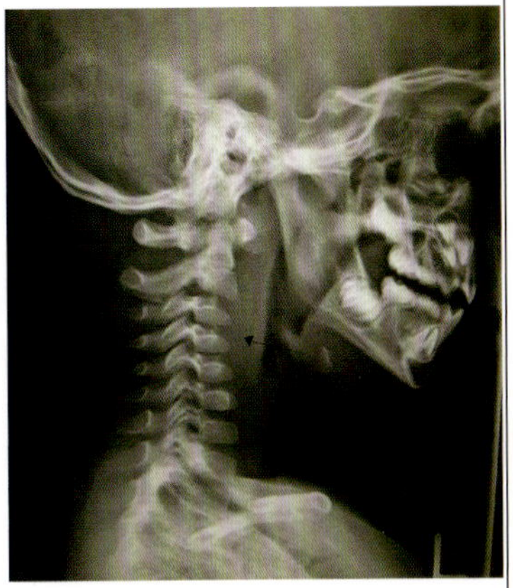

Barrett's Esophagus

Metaplasia of stratified **squamous** epithelium with nonciliated **columnar** cells and **goblet** cells.
Esophagus has peptic **strictures due to:** GERD, scleroderma or radiation causing caustic ingestion

AKA: Symmetric circumferential ring at LES.
SX: Esophageal dysphasia: sensation food is stuck in the chest.
Dysphagia for solids (fluids are ok).
No weight loss.

DX: Endoscopy with biopsy.

TX: **PPI's.**

- **Biopsy shows metaplasia: PPI's and follow with endoscopy every 2 years.**
- **Biopsy shows low-grade dysplasia: PPI's and follow with endoscopy every year.**

Biopsy shows high-grade dysplasia: Ablation, mucosal resection.

Swallowing Foreign Body

Coin or object Ingestion:
Initical TX: X-ray.
If asymptomatic: watch inpatient for 24 hours and re x-ray.
If symptomatic (difficulty swallowing, vomiting, refusing to eat) or has not passed the coin in 24 hours, must remove object by endoscopy.

Battery Ingestion:
Tx is based on location.
DX: X-ray

If battery is still in the esophagus it must be immeidately removed by flexible endoscopy so that there is no mucosal damage.
If the battery is past the esophagus, allow it to pass naturally.

Immature Esophagus
Gastoresophageal reflux (GER) in babies < 3 months.
AKA: Spitting up.

Causes: Immature esophageal sphincter.

TX: Keep baby sitting up for 30 minutes after feedings.

Glossitis

Condition seen in iron deficiency, zinc deficiency, B1, B2, B3 deficiency, infections

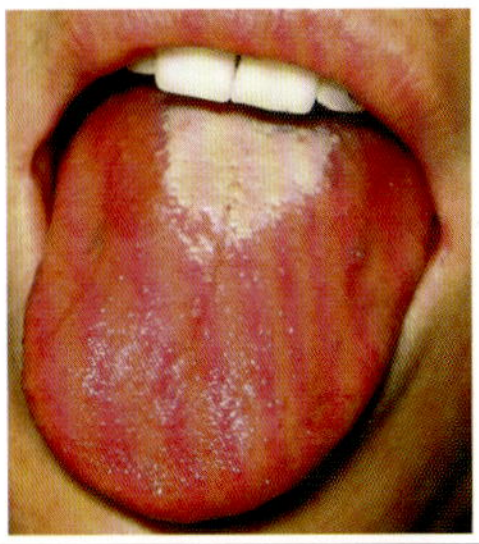

Esophageal manometry

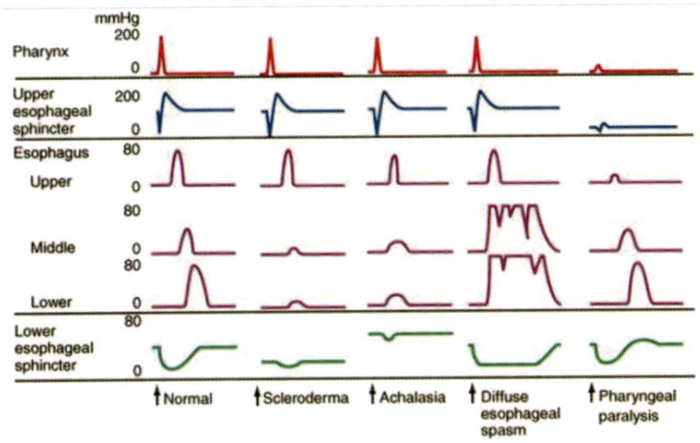

Stomach Pathologies

"Alarm Symptoms" = Unintentional weight loss, dysphagia, anemia. For all patients that present with "alarm symptoms", endoscopy and biopsy are required to evaluation for cancer.

Gastritis - Chronic Gastritis **Inflammation** of the lining of the stomach. SX: Abdominal pain, heart burn, nausea, vomiting Complications: ulcers, bleeding, pernicious anemia (if due to an autoimmune disease against parietal cells) **Histology of antrum and fundus:** Hyperplasia of the enterochromaffin-like cells, mucosal atrophy, epithelial metaplasia (metaplastic goblet cells), usually no erosions. Causes: **Helicobacter pylori**, NSAIDS, alcohol, trauma, sepsis, cocaine, smoking, radiation, uremia (from multiple organ failures), Crohn's, autoimmune disorders, **burns (Curling Ulcers)** TX: **PPI: Omeprazole, H2 Blockers: Ranitidine** If due to H. pylori **(triple therapy): Requires a PPI and 2 antibiotics: Amoxicillin and Clarithromycin**. If due to pernicious anemia: supplement with B-12	**GERD (Gastroesophageal Reflux Disease)** Cause: **↓ in lower esophageal sphincter tone** (relaxation) allowing stomach acid to reflux into the esophagus or can be caused by a hiatal hernia (herniation of stomach into the esophagus) SX: Heartburn, **nocturnal cough, hoarse voice** in the mornings (from acid), dyspnea, reflux. Complications: Esophageal strictures, **Barrett's esophagus** (metaplasia: squamous epithelial cells changing to intestinal columnar epithelium), reflux esophagitis (necrosis of esophagus), esophageal adenocarcinoma. Note: Lifestyle changes; Lose weight and ↓ of foods: coffee, chocolate, fatty, acidic, spicy foods help symptoms. Stopping smoking **DOES NOT** make a significant difference. TX: **Omeprazole (PPI), H2 Receptor Blockers** Severe Cases/Surgery: Nissen fundoplication. (**Beware:** watch for the "casual" case history of someone with heartburn listed among other misc. issues. You must assume they are being treated for GERD, so watch for a **P-450 inhibition** regarding **Cimetidine**).
Autoimmune Atropic Gastritis **Autoimmune: Antiparietal Cell Antibodies (AKA: Oxyntic cells) and/or** **Autoimmune: Autobodies against Intrinsic Factors** Antibodies against **parietal cells** or **intrinsic factor** of the stomach (fundus/body) cause inability of parietal cells to produce intrinsic factor. **Intrinsic factor is required for Vitamin B-12** to be absorbed in the ilium. SX: Gland **atrophy** (not working), intestinal metaplasia, inflammation, absent rugae in fundus. Mucosa can become "**villiform**" (AKA: Looks like the small intestine) Autoimmune Atrophic Gastritis are at a higher risk of developing **Hashimoto's thyroiditis**, gastric carcinoma and **achlorhydria** (low production of HCL leading to a higher pH in the stomach which can cause: bacterial overgrowth, increase risk of infections from Vibrio vulnificus in seafood, decreased absorption of iron (leading to **iron deficiency anemia**/microcytic anemia), decreased absorption of electrolytes and vitamins: including B-12 which then leads to ataxia, paresthesias, mood and personality changes, memory problems and **pernicious anemia**).	**Ménétrier Disease** (AKA: Hypoproteinemic hypertrophic gastropathy) Premalignant disease of the stomach. Can lead to gastric adenocarcinoma. Cause: Excessive secretion of protein **TGF-α** (Transforming growth factor alpha = tyrosine kinase activity) SX: TGF-α inhibits gastric acid secretion = parietal cell atrophy, ↑ mucus cells, protein loss, hypertrophy of the rugae of the stomach causing huge gastric folds with antrum normally spared.

Non-Ulcer Dyspepsia	Atrophic Gastritis
(AKA: Functional indigestion) • MCC of epigastric pain in patients < 50 years old. • Indigestion for > 6 months **without evidence of a disease to explain the symptoms** of heartburn, belching, epigastric pain, early satiety. • Patients > 55 presenting with dyspepsia must be evaluated by endoscopy and biopsy to rule out ulcers or malignancies. • Any patient presenting with "alarm symptoms" weight loss, dysphagia, anemia must be evaluated by endoscopy and biopsy to rule out ulcers or malignancies. • Dyspepsia will have a **normal** endoscopy. • TX: **PPI's, H2 receptor antagonist**, lifestyle modification.	Inflammation of the stomach mucosa causing loss of gastric glandular cells so that they are replaced by fibrous tissue. So secretions from glands (HCL, intrinsic factor, pepsin) is impaired leading to digestive problems (malabsorption). Without intrinsic factor, B-12 can't be absorbed in the ileum, leading to pernicious anemia. Iron is unable to be absorbed leading to iron deficiency anemia.

Peptic Ulcer Disease (PUD): Gastric Ulcer and Duodenal Ulcer
(AKA: Dyspepsia)

SX: **Epigastric pain**, fullness, early satiety, abdominal burning, nausea
DX: Endoscopy, Barium studies.

TX Rules: < 55 and NO alarm symptoms= treat with medications, <55 with alarm symptoms = endoscopy, >55 = Endoscopy
"Alarm Symptoms": Weight loss, early satiety, vomiting, hematemesis, abdominal mass, anemia, lymphadenopathy, family history of gastric cancer, odynophagia with heartburn (GERD)

Gastric Ulcer	Duodenal Ulcer
(AKA: Acute erosive gastritis) SX: **Weight loss = Painful to eat** MC Cause: Decrease in mucosal protection, H. pylori, **NSAIDS** (cause pain not necessarily bleeding) (**Caution**: ALWAYS be careful when ANY question mentions patient has "chronic pain" = this means they are **taking painkillers (NSAIDS) chronically)** **Note:** In patients >55 or in cases that there is no response to medications, endoscopy is required to rule out cancer by biopsy.	SX: **Weight gain = ↓ pain with food on stomach** Pain worsens at night (no food on stomach), hypertrophy of Brunner's Glands MC: **H. pylori,** Zollinger-Ellison DX Test for H. pylori: H. pylori **stool antigen** (positive in active infection). **Urea breath test** (positive in active infection. H. pylori is urease positive). **Endoscopic biopsy** (most accurate). Note: Capsule endoscopy can't detect H. pylori. TX: See below.

Ulcer Complications (Gastric or Duodenal)

Perforation: Can perforate the posterior of the stomach into the **splenic artery.**

Stomach perforation:
DX: **Upright abdominal-chest X-ray**: will show **air under the diaphragm**.
SX: DIFFUSE abdominal pain.
TX: Emergency surgery

Hemorrhage (GI Bleeds):
SX: **Hematemesis of 5 – 10 mL of bleeding ("coffee grounds"), melena of 50 – 100 mL of bleeding (dark/black/tarry stools) =** (sign of an **upper GI bleed**, the blood has oxidized as it goes through the GI system.
Guaiac/Occult (heme) positive stool = > 5 mL of bleeding (sign of a **lower GI bleed**).
Bright red stool = left colon bleed; burgundy/maroon stool = right colon bleed.
Bleeding from the lesser curvature = left gastric artery.
Bleeding from the posterior wall of duodenum = gastroduodenal artery.

Ulcer Complications cont'd

(**Remember**: any chronic bleeding = anemia (RBC breakdown) ➔ ↑ urea ➔ ↑BUN/Creatinine ratio)
MCC: Upper GI Bleed: Ulcers. Other causes: Esophageal varices, cancer, esophagitis, gastritis, duodenitis.
MCC: Lower GI Bleed: Diverticulosis. Other causes: Hemorrhoids, angiodysplasia (AVM), upper GI bleed, Ulcerative colitis, Crohn's, Polyps, colon cancer.

Complications in GI bleeds:

- **Iron deficiency anemia (Microcytic anemia). Labs: ↓ serum iron, ↓ TIBC, ↓ Ferritin**
- **↓↓ in blood pressure. TX: Normal saline (9% NaCL) or Ringer lactate.**
- **Blood loss of 15% - 20% causes orthostasis (↓ > 20 pts in Systolic pressure when sitting up or > 10 pts ↑ in pulse when sitting or standing from lying down.**
- **Blood loss of 30% causes tachycardia (> 100 bpm) and ↓ in systolic pressure to < 100 mm Hg.**

Treatment for GI bleeds:

- **Normal saline (9% NaCl) or Ringer lactate**
- **For active variceal bleeding: Somatostatin analog: Octreotide (↓ portal pressure), banding by endoscope, and TIPS (Transjugular intrahepatic portosystemic shunting) if banding and Octreotide do not work.**
- **Prevention of bleeds: Propanolol (decreases portal pressure)**
- **Transfusion of packed red blood cells if Hct is < 30 in elderly and CAD patients or if Hct is <20 in young patients.**
- **If platelet count < 50,000 and there is active bleeding: Platelet transfusion. (Platelet transfusion for spontaneous bleeding when platelet count < 10,000)**
- **If ↑ PT/INR: Fresh frozen plasma**

Use of NG Tube (Nasogastric tube) in Bleeding

- **Assist to determine if there is an upper or lower GI bleed.**
- **If the pyloric sphincter is open, the duodenum can be visualized for blood (there will also be bile present if the sphincter is open).**
- **If the pyloric sphincter is closed, the duodenum cannot be visualized so duodenal bleeding cannot be ruled out.**

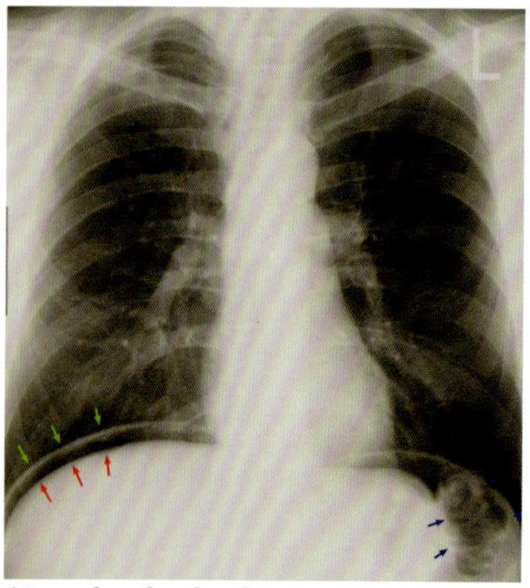

Air under the diaphragm
(indicates a perforation: stomach ulcer, bowels)

Ulcer Treatments if due to H. pylori

DX: **Urea breath test (H. pylori is urease + and loves alkaline environments), H+ breath test, or check H. pylori fecal antigens. Use the same test to check for eradication of H. pylori after treatment.**
TX: **2 antibiotics and 1 PPI.** **Omeprazole, Clarithromycin and Amoxicillin.**
If allergic to Penicillin: Omeprazole, Clarithromycin and Metronidazole.
MCC of failure of treatment for H. pylori: Alcohol, tobacco, NSAID's, non-compliance to the medications.

Gastroparesis
(AKA: Delayed gastric emptying)

Paresis (partial) of the stomach.

SX: ↓ contractions causes food to remain in the stomach for a long time, vomiting, abdominal pain, nausea, **early satiety** (feeling full after just a small amount of food), bloating, anorexia (lack of appetite), **succussion splash** (sloshing sound in stomach heard on auscultation due to retained gastric contents due to paresis or gastric outlet obstruction)

MCC: Damage to the vagus nerve, neuropathy **due to diabetes**

TX: Metoclopramide, Erythromycin

Gastric Outlet Obstruction (GOO)

Obstruction at level of pylorus.

SX: recurrent vomiting of accumulated food in the stomach, early satiety, succession splash (sloshing sound in stomach heard on auscultation due to retained gastric contents due to paresis or gastric outlet obstruction), postprandial pain, weight loss, postprandial pain, weight loss.

Causes: MCC: PUD, tumor/malignancy, Crohn's, Pyloric stenosis, strictures due to caustic chemical damage (MC due to caustic damage from ↑ aspirin ingestion due to suicide attempt).

DX: Upper endoscopy. If this test is negative, perform a scintigraph to check for gastroparesis (↓ nerve innovation (neuropathy). MC: due to diabetes.

Gastric Dumping Syndrome

Ingested foods rapidly bypass the stomach and enter the small intestine not fully digested.

SX: Nausea vomiting, bloating, cramping, diarrhea, fatigue, weakness, dizziness, abdominal pain, dypsnea, sweating.

MCC: gastric bypass

TX: ↓ speed of food passage. Eating more often with smaller meals low in carbs and higher in proteins, ↓ simple sugars and drink liquids between meals (not with them), ↑ fiber to delay emptying and ↓ insulin peaks.

After gastric bypass: you must supplement: Iron (Ferrous sulfate), folate, B-12, Intrinsic Factor and fat soluble vitamins D, E, A, K due to malabsorption problems.

Surreptitious Vomiting (Chronic vomiting)
Causes: ↑ vomiting in pregnancy (Hyperemesis Gravidarum), bulimia, any condition with ↑↑ vomiting.

Vomiting (vomiting out HCL) = loss of H+ (↓ Protons, K (Potassium) and Chloride (hypochloremia).
Due to hypochloremia, kidneys will be reabsorbing Chloride from the urine. (Bicarb HCO3) is also being reabsorbed with Chloride = metabolic alkalosis.

Labs: Normal BP with ↓ **urine Chloride** (Normal chloride: 20 – 250 mEq/L)

Note: Patients with vomiting (gastric loss) must reabsorb chloride from urine (hypochloremia = volume depletion).
Metabolic acidosis (↓ K, hypokalemia) can be caused by abnormal Na handling (ie: Bartter or Gitelman, diuretic use). Will see ↑ K in the urine. Bartter or Gitelman or diuretic use: unable to reabsorb Cl because it is lost in the urine, therefore will see ↑ Cl in the urine.

Gastrostomy Tube Feeding.
Enteral feeding delivers nutrition through a catheter inserted directly into the GI tract.
Has fewer side effects and is preferred over parenteral feeing.
Enteral Feeding:
30 Kcal/Kg/Day with 1 gm/Kg protein.

Parenteral Feeding.
Provides nutrition intravenously which goes directly into the bloodstream.

Note: Parenteral feeding runs a risk of gallstones due to the inactivity/stasis of the gallbladder because of no stimulation from CCK.

Subphrenic Abscess

Occurs after 1 week after abdominal surgery that is done close to the diaphragm.

SX: Fever and pain radiating to the shoulder.

Delayed Gastric Emptying

MCC: Neuropathy (diabetes)

SX: Early satiety, feeling of fullness, succession splash, nausea, bloating,
↓ appetite

DX: Upper endoscopy to rule out obstruction. If test is negative perform a scintigraph to check for gastroparesis (shows ↓ nerve innovation. This is ↑ in diabetes).

TX: Smaller, more frequent meals, ↓ fiber and fat intake.
Metoclopramide, Erythromycin, Cisapride

Gastrinoma
(AKA: Zollinger-Ellison Syndrome)
Distal, multiple duodenum ulcers caused by a tumor in the pancreas or duodenum that secretes ↑↑ gastrin.

SX: ↑ gastrin → ↑ gastric acid → parietal cell proliferation.
Severe diarrhea occurs because pancreatic enzymes are inactivated by gastric acid.

Highly associated with MEN syndrome. If associated with men, labs may show ↑ calcium due to hyperparathyroidism.

DX: High gastrin levels even after administration of secretin or secretion of high gastric acid.
Somatostatin Scintigraphy shows a significant increase in the number of somatostatin receptors.

TX: Lifelong **PPI's**

Stress Ulcers
Ulcers, mc found in the fundus of the stomach, due to the physiologic stress of a serious illness or trauma.

Cushing Ulcer: Gastric ulcer due to **↑ intracranial pressure.** High ICP stimulates the vagus nerve to release acetylcholine → stimulates M3 receptors on the stomach → parietal cells → IP3/Ca → H/K ATPase pump → increasing gastric acid production.

Curling Ulcer: Gastric ulcer due to complications from **severe burns**. Decreased plasma volume causes ischemia and necrosis of the gastric mucosa. They can also lead to perforation and hemorrhage causing death. (**tip**: "Curl"ing iron burns)

SX: Bleeding, hemodynamic instability, ↓ Hb (requiring transfusion).

Risk factors: Critically ill patients on mechanical ventilation > 48 hrs, or patients with >2 of: sepsis, heart or renal failure, stroke, hepatic encephalopathy, HTN, blood thinners.

Prophylaxis: In cases of burns, head trauma, intubation and mechanical ventilation and combination use of blood thinners (heparin and warfarin): **PPI or H2 Blocker**

Stomach Cancers

Stomach Cancer (AKA: Gastric Cancer)
MC: Adenocarcinoma

Associated with: **Acanthosis nigricans**
Metastasis to: liver, lymph nodes, lungs, bones

DX: Endoscopy

SX: indigestion, heartburn, weight loss, anorexia (loss of appetite, abdominal pain, fatigue, bloating, vomiting blood, blood in stool, anemia.

Histology: **Signet Ring Cells (Clear cell filled with mucus with nucleus pushed to the side)**

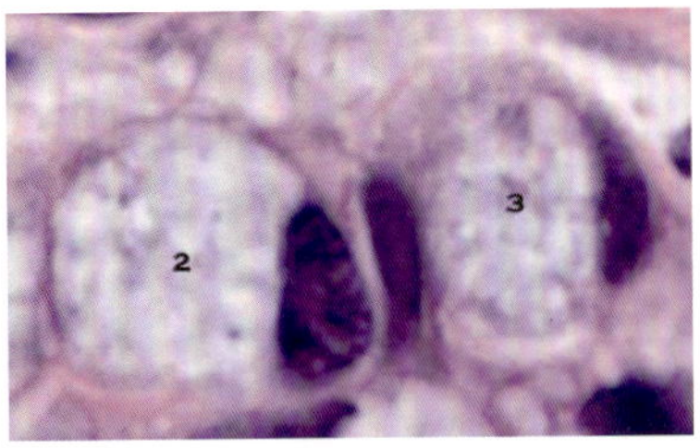

MCC: Multifactorial
H. pylori, smoking, dietary foods (smoked foods/nitrosamines), salt rich foods, red meat, pickled vegetables, nitrates, nitrites.

Lower risk: fresh fruit and vegetables, citrus, antioxidants, Mediterranean diet, garlic, mushrooms.

Prognosis:
Best: if contained within the mucosa and submucosa.
Worst: If extends into the muscularis layer

Stomach Cancers and Metastasis

Diffuse Gastric Cancer
MC: glandular cells lining the stomach
Histology: Signet Ring Cells. Thick, leathery stomach wall (AKA: **Linitis plastica**).
Is **NOT** associated with H. pylori.

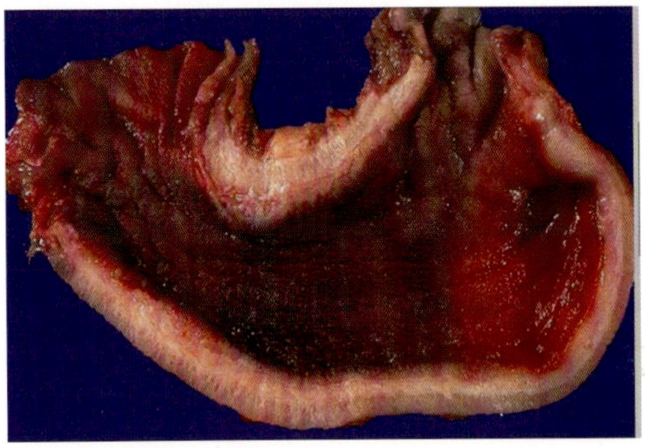

Intestinal Gastric Cancer
MC: **H. pylori, nitrosamines (smoked foods), smoking**, chronic gastritis, achlorhydria (no HCL production)

Krukenberg Tumor Metastasis
Metastasis to the ovaries.
SX: Bilateral, signet ring cells, ↑ mucus

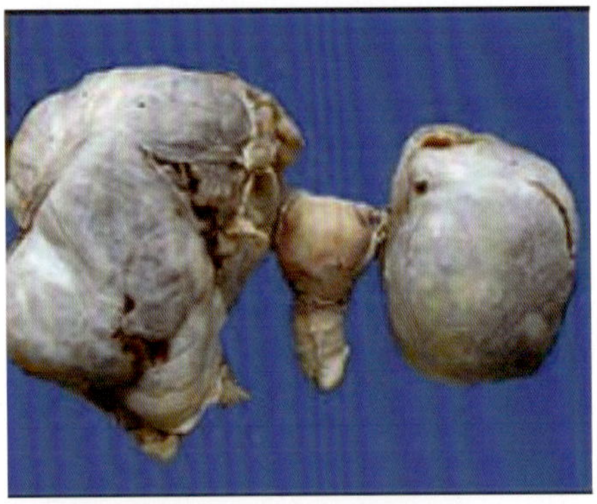

Sister Mary Joseph Nodule
Metastasis to umbilical area. Nodule bulging into the umbilicus.

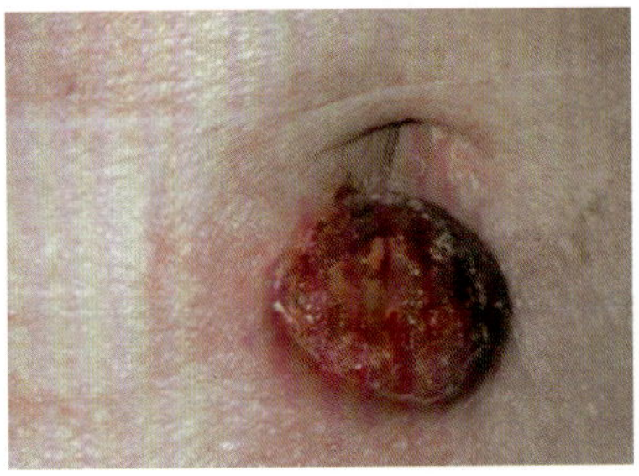

Virchow Node
Metastasis to **left** supraclavicular lymph node

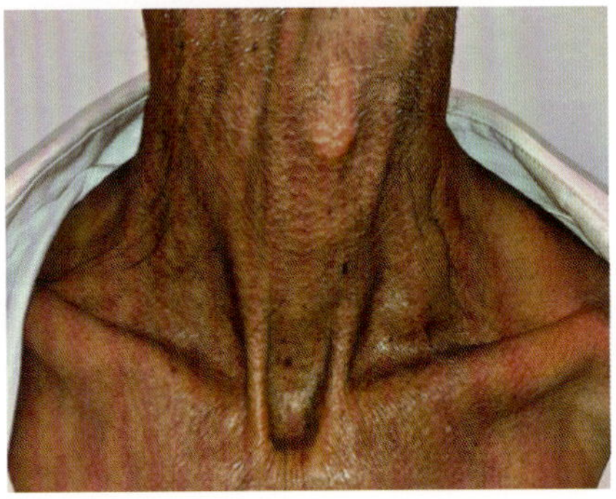

MALT lymphoma (Mucosa Associated Lymphoid Tissue)
MCC: H. pylori

Initial TX: 2 antibiotics (**Clarithromycin, Amoxicillin**) and a PPI (**Omeprazole**)
If initial TX fails: CHOP or CHOP plus Bleomycin.
(CHOP: Cyclophosphamide, Vincristine, Adriamycin, Prednisone)

Pancreas Pathologies
(Diabetes Mellitus: See Insulin under the Endocrine Chapter)

Acute Pancreatitis

MCC: Alcohol and obstruction by gallstones
Other causes: **Hypertriglyceridemia** (> 1000 mg/dL), abdominal trauma, carcinoma of the head of the pancreas, scorpion venom, fat necrosis, Cystic Fibrosis,
eating disorders (anorexia, bulimia), Chinese liver fluke, post ERCP, hyperparathyroidism (↑ calcium), mumps, varicella zoster.
Drugs: Valproic acid, Didanosine, Corticosteroids, Azathioprine, Sulfa drugs, Diuretics (Thiazides, Furosemide), Tetracycline, Metronidazole, OCP's.

Cause: Activation of pancreatic enzymes that cause necrosis and apoptosis (caspases):
Path: **Trypsinogen is converted to trypsin** by **enterokinase**, which then stimulates proteolytic enzymes (amylase and lipase).
Lipase is specific to pancreas.
(**tip**: if you are going on a "TRIP"sinogen or a "TRIP"sin, then you need to rent a car from "ENTER"prise).

SX: **Severe epigastric pain radiating straight to the back** (Cholecystitis pain radiates to the side and then to the back), nausea, chills, anorexia, vomiting, hiccups, tachycardia, fever.

DX:
BIT: ↑ **serum amylase and lipase (**amylase is sensitive, **lipase is specific to the pancreas).**
MAT: Abdominal CT
ERCP (Endoscopic Retrograde Cholangiopancreatography): Used to evaluate for detects stones in the common bile duct, scars (strictures) or leaks in the pancreatic duct, Sphincter of Oddi dysfunction, cancer.
ERCP is also therapeutic: it can remove stones, place stents in the bile duct, dilate strictures.

Detection of trypsinogen in the urine (AKA: Trypsinogen Activation Peptide test).

Acute Pancreatitis cont'd

APACHE II score used to give prognosis.

TX: Pain = **Meperidine or Fentanyl**. No morphine due to ↑ pain by aggravation of sphincter of Oddi.
NPO (bowel rest), aggressive hydration (9% NS or lactated Ringer's), TPN (total parenteral nutrition) until symptoms resolve. ERCP.
Antibiotics if ↑ WBC: Imipenem, Meropenem
If due to gallstones: Cholecystectomy.

If CT shows > 30% necrosis, must administer antibiotics. If necrotic, requires surgical debridement to prevent ARDS and death.

Pancreatic Pseudocyst

Complication of acute pancreatitis. Collection of pancreatic enzymes, blood and necrotic tissue.

False cyst: there is **no epithelial lining**. Wall is fibrotic, lined by **granulation tissue** and encapsulated close to the pancreas.

Complication: hemorrhage, obstruction, rupture.

TX: Surgery.

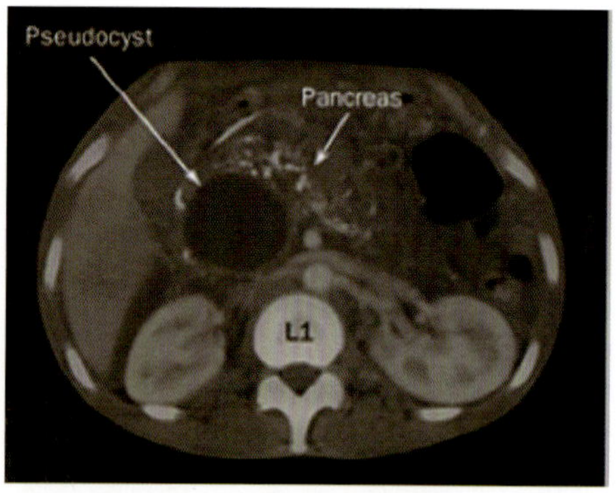

Chronic Pancreatitis

Chronic inflammation and calcification of the pancreas.
Histology: Calcifications, destruction of α and β pancreatic cells.

MC: Alcohol abuse.

Complications: **malabsorption** (no amylase or lipase is able to be released in the duodenum to breakdown fats and aid in digestion) so all signs and symptoms relating to malabsorption (steatorrhea) pathologies can apply. ↑ risk of **pancreatic cancer.**
If due to alcoholism: SX can also include mega-blastic anemia (↑ MCV, ↓ Hb) due to **folate deficiency**. (Folate deficiency causes a defect in DNA synthesis. There is no synthesis of purines or pyrimidines (↓ thymidine base synthesis).

Labs: Amylase and lipase are not usually elevated as seen in acute pancreatitis.

BIT: Abdominal x-ray shows calcifications.
MAT: Secretin stimulation test (normal test: response to injection of secretin is release of bicarb).

TX: Cessation of alcohol, ↓ fat in diet, eat smaller meals, replace pancreatic enzymes (oral amylase and lipase).

Pancreatic Adenocarcinoma

MCC: Smoking
Other causes: Chronic pancreatitis, diabetes, family history, ↑ age, ↑ men and African Americans, obesity.

SX: Constant, gnawing epigastric pain, abdominal pain radiating to the back, unintentional weight loss, feeling of fullness, obstructive jaundice, daytime fatigue, Trousseau syndrome (spontaneous blood clots and superficial thrombosis), malabsorption, pain interferes with sleep.

SX: If in the head of the pancreas = **painless**, jaundice, unintentional weight loss, malabsorption (steatorrhea)
SX: If in the body of the pancreas = **pain**, unintentional weight loss

Metastasis to: lymph nodes, liver, lungs

DX: CT, palpable, non-tender gallbladder

Tumor marker: **CA 19-9**

Labs: ↑↑ ALP, ↑ Conjugated bilirubin (due to obstruction of the biliary duct system by the head of the pancreas)

Necrotic Pancreatitis

DX:
If CT shows > 30% necrosis of the pancreas then biopsy of pancreas and TX with Imipenem.
If biopsy shows necrosis: TX: surgical debridement.

Pancreatic Laceration
MC: Blunt abdominal trauma. Patient can present without any SX and then return a week later with problems.

SX: Fever, chills, deep abdominal epigastric pain.
NOTE: The spleen and pancreas can present similarly and an automobile accident can cause damage to either. The spleen will present with LUQ pain and show Amylase. Beware, because the spleen is the MC organ damaged in an automobile accident due to the seat belt, watch the Lipase and pain presentation, they may be describing a pancreas injury.

Complications: Retro peritoneal abscess that leads to pseudocyst.
DX: Abdominal CT
Labs: Lipase is specific to the pancreas. Amylase is NOT specific to the pancreas.
TX: Drain and surgical debridement

Insulinoma AKA: Islet cell adenoma. Pancreatic PanNET tumor (pancreatic neuroendocrine tumor) derived from the beta cells (islets of Langerhans cells) that continue to secrete insulin despite normal blood glucose levels causing hypoglycemia. High risk associated with MEN syndrome. DX: Hypoglycemia can be caused by several things: Insulinoma, injection of insulin or excessive intake of **sulfonylurea drugs**. Blood test will show: ↓ blood glucose (< 45 mg/dL), ↑ **insulin, proinsulin, C-peptide** with both an insulinoma and abuse of a sulfonylurea drug because the body is making it. Injection of insulin will not show proinsulin or C-peptide because the body did not make it. Sulfonylurea drugs as the cause can quickly be ruled out by checking a UA. The drug will show up in the urine. MRI will show a tumor if it is due to an insulinoma. SX: Symptomatic fasting hypoglycemia: headaches, lethargy, diplopia, tachycardia, palpitations, anxiety, seizures, and coma. TX: Surgical removal	**Glucagonoma** Pancreatic neuroendocrine tumor. Presents with diabetes. SX: Triad: Red plaques/rash with central clearing and eroded boarders: boards have blistering crusting and scaling. (MC: perioral, perineum, extremities, face), diabetes and anemia. Can also see diarrhea, weight loss, DVT, ulcers in the GI tract, hyperglycemia. DX: Glucagon level > 500 confirms. (<500 indicate other diseases). CT/MRI TX: **Octreotide** **VIPomas** Non-β cell pancreatic tumor producing Vasoactive Intestinal Peptide. Endocrine tumor. Associated with **MEN type I.** SX: **Excessive watery diarrhea** (> 750-1000 mL/day). **Dehydration**, lethargy, muscle cramps (due to ↓ K), nausea, vomiting, colicky abdominal pain. Labs: ↓ K (**hypokalemia**), achlorhydria, vasodilation (which causes flushing and hypotension), hypercalcemia, hyperglycemia, ↑ VIP level in the serum. TX: **Octreotide.**
Hemorrhagic Pancreatitis SX: Retroperitoneal hemorrhage and pancreatic necrosis. Bluish discoloration on the flanks or peri-umbilical region.	**Gastrinoma** **(AKA: Zollinger-Ellison Syndrome)** Distal, multiple duodenum ulcers caused by a tumor in the pancreas or duodenum that secretes ↑↑ gastrin. SX: ↑ gastrin → ↑ gastric acid → parietal cell proliferation. Severe diarrhea occurs because pancreatic enzymes are inactivated by gastric acid. Highly associated with **MEN syndrome**. If associated with men, labs may show ↑ calcium due to hyperparathyroidism. DX: High gastrin levels even after administration of secretin or secretion of high gastric acid. Somatostatin Scintigraphy shows a significant increase in the number of somatostatin receptors. TX: Lifelong **PPI's, Octreotide**

Small Intestine and Colon Pathologies

Malabsorption

- **Any pathology** that affects the intestines can cause malabsorption: MCC: Cystic fibrosis. Other causes: Celiac DZ, Ulcerative colitis, Crohn's, Whipple DZ, Tropical sprue, chronic giardia, IgA deficiency, any type of mucosal damage (enteropathy), defects of ion transport, pancreatic insufficiency, impaired enterohepatic circulation, bariatric surgery, dairy intolerance, parasites (Giardia, roundworm, hookworm), Carcinoid, hypo/hyperthyroidism, malnutrition, etc.
- Malabsorption affects the absorption of: Iron, folate, fat-soluble vitamins (DEAK), Vitamin B12.
- Malabsorption signs present with: **steatorrhea** (greasy, floating, foul smelling stool), weight loss, flatulence, abdominal discomfort and any specific symptom due to what is not being absorbed (below):
- Signs and symptoms will be associated with what is not being absorbed:
  Vitamin B12: Neuropathy, macrocytic anemia (will show hypersegmented neutrophils), pernicious anemia.
  Vitamin D: Osteoporosis, hypocalcemia.
  Vitamin E: Neuromuscular (myopathies) and neurological problems (dysarthria, absence of deep tendon reflexes, loss of proprioception, vibratory sensation, positive Babinski sign, retinopathy, anemia (oxidative damage to RBC)
  Vitamin A: Vision problems (night blindness).
  Vitamin K: Easy bruising and bleeding (Vitamin K is not able to gamma carboxylate the clotting factors).
  Folate: Depression, anemia (macrocytic/megaloblastic), behavior disorders, palpitations, weakness (↓ production of DNA), neural tube defects.
  Iron: Iron deficiency anemia (Microcytic), Restless leg syndrome, irritability, hair loss, brittle/spoon nails, PICA.

Pancreatic Insufficiency

Causes: MCC: Cystic Fibrosis, chronic pancreatitis, cancer

DX: D-xylose Absorption Test.
Normal test = ↑ D-xylose in urine and ↓ in stool (it is absorbed in the veins and excreted in the urine).
Abnormal test = ↑ D-xylose in stool and ↓ in urine (meaning the intestines were not able to absorb it like they should have = malabsorption/problems with the mucosa wall.)

Lactase Deficiency
(AKA: Lactose Intolerance)

Inability to digest lactose (disaccharide of **galactose and glucose**, found in milk and dairy products) due to lactase deficiency in the lining of the duodenum.

SX: Osmotic diarrhea, bloating, cramps, flatulence, borborygmi (rumbling stomach), vomiting.

Histology: **Normal villi**

DX: **Hydrogen breath test**, **Stool acidity test** (if patient is lactose intolerant, lactose will not be absorbed, mix with the bacteria in the colon causing acid stools)

TX: Ingesting live yogurt cultures of lactobacilli or stop intake of lactose containing foods.

Whipple Disease

Infection with **Tropheryma whipplei**. Combination of malabsorption and pathologies in other parts of the body (brain, eye, heart, lungs, skin)

SX: Weight loss, joint pain, arthritis, steatorrhea, flatulence, abdominal distention, uveitis, endocarditis, confusion, headaches, seizures.

DX: Biopsy of intestine, PCR. **PAS + (Periodic Acid-Schiff stain,** detects polysaccharides (glycogen) and mucosubstance (glycoproteins and glycolipids, mucins) in tissues)

(**tip**: Mr. Whipple says "PASs the Charmin")

TX: **Penicillin, Ampicillin, Tetracycline.**

Abetalipoproteinemia

Mutation in **MTTP gene** (microsomal triglyceride transfer protein) that causes deficiencies of apolipoproteins **B48 and B-100.** B-48 and B-100 are needed for synthesis and export or **chylomicrons, VLDL** and cholesterol.

SX: Usually appears in the first few months of life as failure to thrive. Other symptoms of babies and all other ages: steatorrhea, difficulty in coordination and balance, progressive decreased vision.

SX: **Acanthocytes** (AKA: RBC with spiny or thorny projections), hypocholesterolemia, Retinitis pigmentosa (rod degeneration)

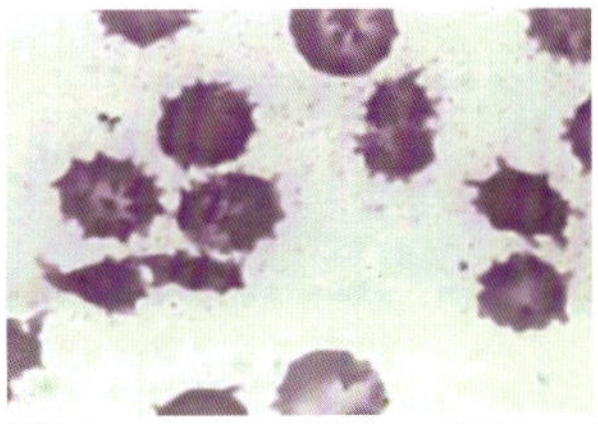

TX: Large quantities of Vitamin E, dietary restriction of triglycerides.

Celiac Sprue Autoimmune **Autoantibodies (Anti-gliadin, IgA anti-endomysial, IgA anti-tissue transglutaminase, Anti-IgA, IgG antibodies against gluten, Anti-Reticulin)** **Gluten: Wheat, rye, barley, oats** Associated with HLA-DQ2, HLA-DQ8 Histology: **Blunting/flattening of the villi and crypt hyperplasia.** Inflammatory process mediated by **T cells.** ↓ surface area of absorption. SX: Chronic, non-bloody diarrhea, abdominal pain and cramping, mouth ulcers, **steatorrhoea** (foul and greasy stool), weight loss or failure to gain weight (children), pre-tibial edema, protruding belly Associated with **Dermatitis Herpetiformis**. Vesicular, erythematous, pruritic, linear rash, resembling herpes, on extensor surfaces: **elbows, knees**. (it will NOT be on the mouth or genitals). TX: **Gluten free diet**. (Change diet) Antibiotics **DO NOT** improve Celiac (as Tropical Sprue does) (Foods that are ok to eat: beans, rice, corn, potatoes) Treatment failure: If no improvement with gluten free diet, must consider T Cell intestinal lymphoma: abdominal pain, weight loss, anemia, diarrhea.	**Tropical Sprue** Similar symptoms to Celiac Sprue. Histology: Flattening and inflammation of the villi in the small intestine. MC: **Contracted in the tropics**. Prevention: bottled water for drinking, brushing teeth and washing food. Consuming only peeled fruits. TX: **Does respond** to: **Antibiotics: Tetracycline, TMP/SMX, supplement B_{12} and folic acid** 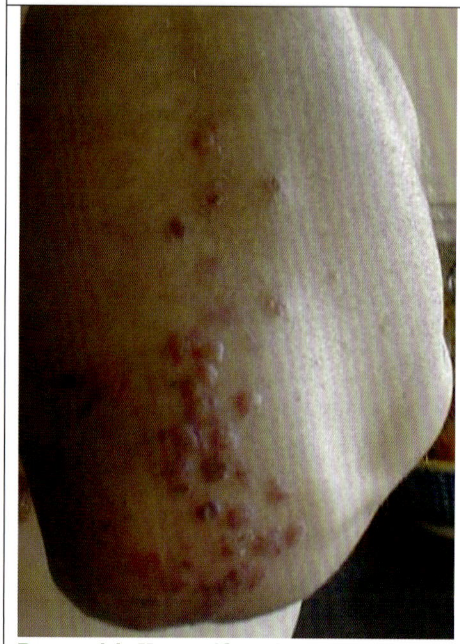 **Dermatitis Herpetiformis (Associated with Celiac Sprue)**
Chronic Giardiasis Protozoan Source: Cysts in water. **Mountain streams,** campers/hikers SX: **Foul-smelling stools**, fatty diarrhea, bloating, gut inflammation and **villous atrophy (no invasion), malabsorption** DX: Trophozoites or cyst in stool **Chronic Giardia: due to IgA DEFICIENCY**. Normal: IgA protects the gut wall and stops adhesion/attachment of Giardia. TX: **Metronidazole**	**Diphyllobothrium latum** Source: Ingestion of larvae from raw freshwater fish Pathology: **Pernicious anemia** due to Vitamin B12 deficiency. D. latum completes for the B12 so it is not available to bind with intrinsic factor in the ilium. TX: **Praziquantel**

Crohn's Disease	Ulcerative Colitis
MC: Terminal ilium and colon, **spares the rectum**. Can occur anywhere between the mouth and rectum. Defective NFKB cytokine, which allows the inflammation from the microbes to exist. Histology: Skip (**non-continuous**) lesions, "cobblestone mucosa", **transmural non-caseating granulomas (TH-1** and macrophage, T cell mediated). **ASCA positive** (anti Saccharomyces cerevesiae antibody), ANCA negative. SX: **Secretory** diarrhea (due to poor absorption and loss of inflamed mucosa and increased electrolyte content). Complications: **Transmural Fistulas** (connecting bowel with bladder), fistulas or abscesses around anus, anal fissures, perianal skin tags, malabsorption, Fibrotic Strictures (fistulas leave strands of connecting tissue allowing intestines to become entangled and strangulate/**obstruction** = "air – fluid levels on x-ray), colorectal carcinoma, risk for cholesterol gallstones (due to ↓ in bile acid resorption in the ileum so the bile is excreted in the stool causing an increase of cholesterol/bile ratio in the gallbladder leading to gallstones), hypocalcemia (due to malabsorption of Vit D = ↓ reabsorption of Ca and Phosphate), ↓ absorption of B12 leading to pernicious anemia. TX: Surgery will not cure, Crohn's recurs. **Infliximab*, Mesalamine, Methotrexate, Azathioprine** (**tip:** I am "fixin" my Crohn's and UC) ***Be sure to do a PPD test before starting Infliximab due to potential of reactivating TB.**	Autoimmune, ↑ family history MC: **Always rectal** involvement Histology: **Continuous** lesions, crypt abscesses, **TH-2** antibody mediated, loss of haustra ("lead pipe" appearance on x-ray), **pseudopolyps** (areas on the colon that look like "polyps" but are actually what is left of the mucosa that has not been ulcerated away, "**clumps** of mucosal surface"). **P-ANCA positive** (antineutrophil cytoplasmic antibody), ASCA negative. SX: **Bloody** diarrhea, abdominal pain. (**tip:** anytime the question mentions "rice" or "something/particles" seen in the diarrhea (bloody or watery) this is simply pieces of the epithelia colon surface) Complications: **Colorectal carcinoma, 1° sclerosing cholangitis**, megacolon, malabsorption. TX: Surgery is curative: resection of the large intestine (colectomy) **Infliximab*, Mesalamine, Sulfasalazine, 6-mercaptopurine** (**tip:** I am "fixin" my Crohn's and UC) ***Be sure to do a PPD test before starting Infliximab due to potential of reactivating TB.**
Ischemic Colitis (AKA: Mesenteric Ischemia) Injury of the colon due to ischemia. MC location: **Splenic Flexure "Watershed areas" (rectosigmoid junction)** due to decreased flow to the **SMA.** (rectum is rarely involved because of dual blood supply: IMA and internal iliac artery) Causes: **Anything that decreases the oxygen (blood supply) to the intestines:** Atherosclerosis of mesenteric arteries, low blood pressure, vasoconstricting drugs, thrombosis of the SMA = bowel infarction, emboli (after surgery, recent MI, A-Fib, abdominal malignancy, cardiac arrhythmia) Can progress from mild, non-occlusive to an occlusive emergency. SX: **Abdominal angina**: MC: elderly. **Severe postprandial pain about 1 hour after eating**, dyspepsia, weight loss (DX: by angiography or doppler). This is the same principal as stable angina in the heart. The intestines are asked to increase workload → ↑ the need for oxygen → pain. Once "work" is done, pain subsides. Note: Patient may have a history of TIA's or strokes (atherosclerosis will be in all vessels, not just heart). **Severe due to total ischemia:** SX: abdominal pain, **bloody diarrhea**/rectal bleeding within 24 hours. High risk: Post operative due to clot	**Appendicitis** Acute inflammation of appendix due to **fecalith obstruction** (AKA: Obstruction of lumen by fecalith). **Labs:** Polymicrobial infection (MC: E. coli or B. fragilis). ↑ WBC with left shift. **Perforation** of appendix shows: ↑ WBC (> 18,000) Ultrasound shows: Thickening of appendix walls. SX: Fever, right lower quadrant pain (beginning initially in the umbilical region and migrating to the RLQ), anorexia, nausea, vomiting. DX signs: Positive **McBurney's Point** (rebound pain in RLQ), Positive **Rovsing's Sign** (palpation of the LLQ produces pain in the RLQ), Obturator Sign: pain with flexing or internal rotation of the right thigh. Positive **Psoas Sign:** pain with extension of the hip/thigh due to irritation of the **iliopsoas hip flexors** in the abdomen. The right iliopsoas lies under the appendix. MAT: CT Complications: Ruptured appendix → peritonitis (abscess formation, gangrenous perforation). TX: Appendectomy (Laparoscopic surgery)

Diverticulitis/Diverticulosis

False diverticulum (only involves mucosa and submucosa)
MC: Sigmoid
Commonly called: "Left sided appendicitis"

SX: MCC of Left lower quadrant pain, fever, **leukocytosis** (↑ WBC), can have non-inflammatory painless, rectal bleeding (hematochezia).

Cause: "pressure" or "high intraluminal pressure" inside the colon that causes "outpouching" of the colon wall and **impaction by fecalith. MCC: chronic constipation**. Other causes**: low fiber diets.**

Note: Diverticulitis can bleed (bright blood) due to diverticulum that has eroded into a vessel. Internal and external hemorrhoids and angiodysplasia can also bleed. Internal hemorrhoids and angiodysplasia are not painful. Angiodysplasia presents with a substantial amount of bleeding).

DX:
BIT: CT scan
Note: Do **NOT** do colonoscopy to dx diverticulitis due to potential of perforation.

TX; NPO and IV fluids for bowel rest, antibiotics, ↑ exercise and **fiber intake**. Bowel resection surgery in severe cases.
TX: Oral outpatient: **Ciprofloxacin and Metronidazole.**
Inpatient **IV: Ceftriaxone and Metronidazole**
Surgery required if: continued recurrences, no response to medicine, perforation.

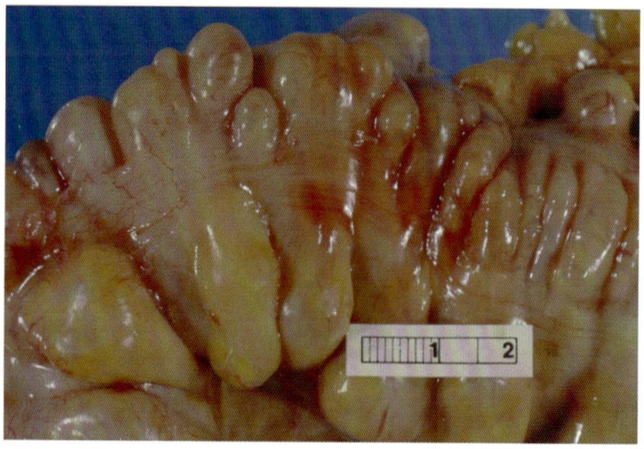

Small Bowel Obstruction

MCC: Adhesions from prior abdominal surgery
(**Beware:** watch for ANY mention of previous surgeries in the patients history when indicating abdominal pain or air/fluid levels on x-ray), Fitz Hugh Curtis Syndrome (PID), constipation, hernias, tumors.

SX: Abdominal distension, colicky abdominal pain, nausea, vomiting, **hyperactive bowel sounds** (high pitched bowel sounds, tinkling bowel sounds), tympany

SX if complete obstruction/strangulation: loss of blood supply to bowel, tachycardia, ↑ WBC, rigid abdomen, shock.

DX: **Air – fluid levels on x-ray.**
If there are no air/fluid levels after an area that show air – fluid levels = complete obstruction. AKA: Dilated loops of bowel.
Air – Fluid levels all the way through bowel = partial obstruction.

TX:
Partial obstruction = Bowel Rest (NPO, IV fluids), nasogastric tube.
Complete obstruction: Surgical emergency.

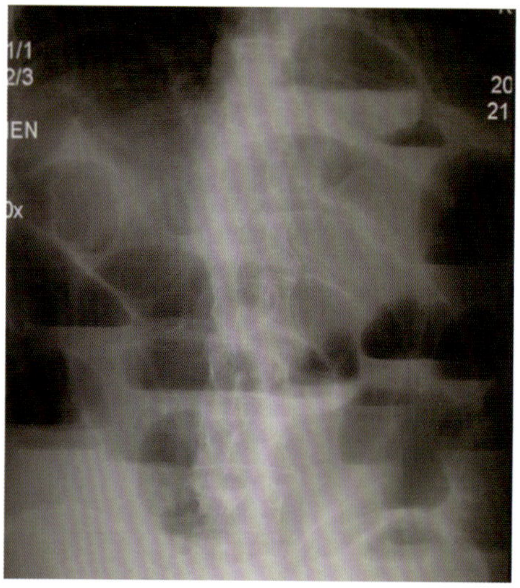

Small bowel obstruction

Gallstone Ileus

Small bowel obstruction due to gallstones blocking lumen of the small intestine via a **fistula**.

DX: Radiographic studies: Rigler's triad: pneumobilia (air in the biliary tree), gallstones, small bowel obstruction.

Anal Fistula

Originates in the anal glands (between internal and external anal sphincter) and drain into the anal canal.

Cause: Blockage of gland outlet causing formation of an abscess that exits to the outside skin in the vicinity of the anus through a **fistula** it forms.

SX: Pain, bloody or purulent discharge, pruritus, erythema, opening of a fistula on the skin.

Carcinoid Tumor **(**AKA: Appendix tumor) Originates in the small bowel Tumor of neuroendocrine cells. Secretion of **serotonin (5-HT) and kallikrein**. (note: kallikrein is facilitated by factor XII) Asymptomatic until metastasis outside the small bowel to the liver. SX: **Flushing** (due to **kallikreins** conversion to **bradykinin** ➔ powerful vasodilation), **wheezing** (asthma), **secretory diarrhea**, syncope, **right-sided endocardial thickening (heart failure),** fibrosis of tricuspid and pulmonary valve (stenosis). DX: **🡅 Urinary excretion of 5-HIAA** (5-hydroxyindoleacetic acid) a degradation produce of serotonin. TX: **Octreotide** (Somatostatin analog)	**Irritable Bowel Syndrome** Chronic diarrhea. **Alternating diarrhea and constipation**, no fever, no weight loss, abdominal pain relieved by a bowel movement and 🡇 pain at night, no blood in the stool. DX: All DX test will be **normal** (ie: O & P, Stool white cells, occult, abdominal CT, colonoscopy) TX: 🡅 Fiber, exercise. TX: if no relief from 🡅 fiber: **Dicyclomine, Hyoscyamine** (anticholinergic agents that relax the bowel). TX: if no relief from anticholinergic agents: **Amitriptyline**.
Fecal Incontinence Uncontrolled passage of fecal material. > 10 mL for > 1 month in patients > 3 years of age. DX: Clinical Hx. BIT: Flexible sigmoidoscopy. MAT: Anorectal manometry. TX: Medical TX: 🡅 fiber. Muscle strengthening exercises. Injections of Dextranomer/hyaluronic Acid (*Solesta*). If treatments fail: surgery.	**Spontaneous Bacterial Peritonitis (SBP)** Infection in the abdomen without a perforation of an organ. Paracentesis shows: **PMN's > 250 and ascites**. (Ascites albumin > 1.1 = transudate) Causes: Infection in the ascites fluid, colonic perforation, peptic ulcer perforation (Abdominal/chest x-ray shows air under the diaphragm). MCC: E. coli and Klebsiella SX: MC in patients with cirrhosis, ascites, low fever, abdominal discomfort, distension, flapping tremor, altered mental status. Abdominal X-ray shows: Layered waves TX: **Cefotaxime, Ceftriaxone** and lifelong prophylaxis against recurrence.
Diaphragmatic Hernia (not congenital) MCC: Blunt abdominal trauma, MC on left side. X-ray shows: **elevation hemi-diaphragm**, deviated mediastinum and global heart silhouette SX: Respirator distress, JVD, tachycardia, hypotension	**Angiodysplasia** MC: > 60 years Vascular malformations that dilate vessels in the gut. (AVM) MC cause is due to aging and strain on the gut. SX: **Painless 🡅🡅 hematochezia**. (Blood can present bright red (if from the rectal, sigmoid region) or maroon/burgundy if from the right sided colon or melena (black/tarry) if from the upper GI tract), **anemia**. **NO PAIN** as you would see in diverticulitis. FOBT is positive if current bleeds. MC: ascending colon or cecum. **Note:** Strain can be caused by increase in blood pressure due to emotional outburst (arguing, sudden rise in BP). Associated with aortic stenosis and end stage renal disease.

Internal Hemorrhoids	External Hemorrhoids
• **Above the pectinate line** • Occur when there is ↑ pressure on the veins in the lower rectum and anus. • Not painful, can bleed, itching • Covered by mucosa • Causes: straining when having a bowel movement, sitting for prolonged periods of time, pregnancy, aging, cirrhosis, chronic constipation or diarrhea, obesity, high fat/low fiber diet. • **Involves the inferior rectal veins** located in the hemorrhoidal plexus. **Involves the superficial inguinal nodes.**	• **Below the pectinate line** • Extremely painful, can bleed, itching • Covered by skin • Causes: straining when having a bowel movement, sitting for prolonged periods of time, pregnancy, aging, cirrhosis, chronic constipation or diarrhea, obesity, high fat/low fiber diet. • **Involves the inferior rectal veins** located in the hemorrhoidal plexus. **Involves the superficial inguinal nodes.**

Toxic Megacolon

Extreme expansion, dilation and distension of the colon.

SX: Dilated colon, abdominal distension (bloating), abdominal pain, fever, shock, bloody diarrhea, tachycardia, dehydration, painful bowel movements.

Complications: Perforation, sepsis, shock, coma, death.

Risk factors: Complication from Crohn's disease, Ulcerative colitis, Hirschsprung disease, Clostridium difficile infections (which lead to pseudomembranous colitis which progressed to toxic megacolon), Entamoeba histolytica, Shigella, Trypanosoma cruzi (Chagas disease), Campylobacter jejuni, colorectal cancer, Salmonella, Typhoid fever, Reiter's syndrome.

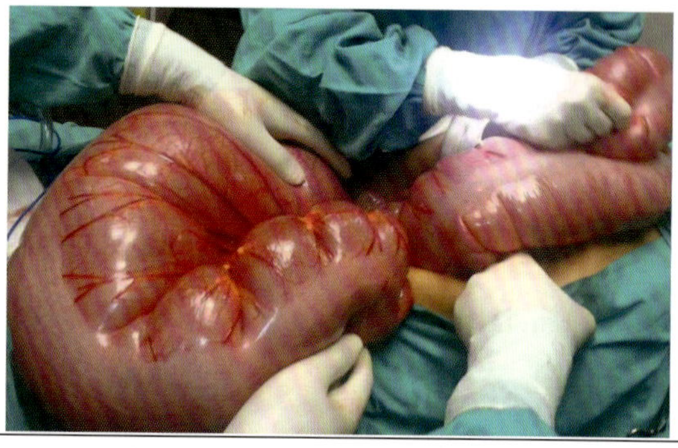

DX: X-ray shows dilated colon.

Labs: elevated WBC.

TX: Colectomy. IV antibiotics for infection and fluids for dehydration

Watershed Areas of the GI

- Splenic flexure: **Superior (SMA) and Inferior (IMA) mesenteric arteries.**
- Rectum: **Inferior (IMA) and the Internal Iliac artery**

Please see Congenital and Embryo Chapters for additional intestinal disorders:

Meconium Ileus (Cystic Fibrosis)
Necrotizing Enterocolitis
Hirschsprung Disease

Differentials between Ulcerative Colitis and Crohn's Disease

Crohn's	Ulcerative Colitis
Occurs in young and adults, male and female at any age. 10x higher if family Hx. Onset between 15 and 30 years old. Increased risk with smoking.	Occurs in young and adults, male and female at any age. 10x higher if family Hx. Peak incidence: between 15 – 30 years old. Not an increased risk for smokers.
Cause: multifactorial	Cause: multifactorial
Occurs anywhere between the mouth and anus. Can include mouth sores. MC in terminal ileum.	Limited to the colon and rectum (MC on the right)
Non-continuous lesions: AKA: "Skip" lesions AKA: Cobblestones	**Continuous** lesions **Note:** If the exam shows you a slide that looks like clumps sitting on the mucosa wall (similar to polyps) this is actually all that is left of the **mucosal wall**, the rest has been eroded away.
Affects **all the layers** of the bowel walls	Affects only the inner most lining of the colon
Transmural **noncaseating** granulomas	No granulomas
Forms **transmural fistulas** between the colon and other organs (bladder: anus, etc.). Causing a high risk of **adhesions, strictures and obstructions**	No fistulas
Bloody stools, weight loss (monitor for anemia)	Bloody stools, weight loss (monitor for anemia)
Can lead to colon cancer	Can lead to colon cancer
Seldom risk of 1° sclerosing cholangitis	Can lead to **1° sclerosing cholangitis**
DX: Colonoscopy	DX: Colonoscopy
Colon cancer screen: First colonoscopy after 8 – 10 years of first diagnosis and then every 1 – 2 years after this.	Colon cancer screen: First colonoscopy after 8 – 10 years of first diagnosis and then every 1 – 2 years after this.
ASCA positive (anti Saccharomyces cerevesiae antibody), ANCA negative	**p-ANCA positive** (antineutrophil cytoplasmic antibody), ASCA negative
No cure. No surgery, disease recurs.	Generally cured by surgery: removal of the large intestine (colectomy).
Tenesmus is uncommon	Tenesmus is common (feeling of incomplete defecation)
HLA-B27, arthritis, uveitis	HLA-B27, arthritis, uveitis
Associated with **TH1** (macrophage, T cell mediated)	Associated with **TH2** (antibody mediated)
TX: **Infliximab, Sulfasalazine, Mesalazine**	TX: **Infliximab, Sulfasalazine, Mesalazine**

Diarrhea

- Excessive loss of stool and fluids (> 3 times per day)
- **Normal anion gap acidosis**
- Can cause pre-renal azotemia
- Loses K

Acute

- Fecal/oral transmission
- Due to: bacteria toxins, viruses, protozoa
- Last a couple of days

Chronic

- MCC: Irritable bowel syndrome.
  SX: alternating between diarrhea and constipation, mucus in stool, no blood,
- ↑ diarrhea before and after breakfast
- Malabsorption
- Dz of the small bowel, colon
- Can last weeks

Watery Diarrheas

- Vibrio cholera: "Rice Water" diarrhea
- Listeria
- Giardia: from swimming/drinking fresh water
- Cryptosporidium: HIV with CD4 < 100.
  TX: **Nitazoxanide**.
- Viruses: Norovirus, Rotavirus
- Medications, laxatives, alcohol, antacids with Mg, NSAIDS, chemo drugs, HTN meds
- Staph aureus: presents with vomiting and diarrhea
- Bacillus cereus: Vomiting and diarrhea. Associated with refried/reheated Chinese rice or pasta
- Scombroid: Histamine fish poisoning. (Mahi-mahi, tuna, mackerel), presents with wheezing, flushing, vomiting, diarrhea. TX: **Diphenhydramine**

Bloody Diarrheas (AKA: Infectious diarrhea)

- E. coli: Abdominal pain, **NO fever**
- Campylobacter: **Fever**, NO abdominal pain. **Starts watery and turns bloody in 2 – 3 days.** Associated with Guillain-Barre and reactive arthritis.
- Shigella: **Fever**, NO abdominal pain. Associated with reactive arthritis.
  MCC: daycares
- Salmonella: **Fever**, NO abdominal pain. Associated with chicken and eggs.
- Entamoeba (parasite picked up during travel), causes liver abscesses
- Vibrio parahaemolyticus: Associated with seafood
- Vibrio vulnificus: Associated with shellfish (oysters, clams), presents with liver dz and skin lesions
- Yersinia: Food (vegetables, meat and milk products) that have been contaminated by infected urine or feces of rodents.

DX: BIT: Fecal leukocytes
MAT: **Stool culture** (O & P)

TX: Hydration for both mild and severe. Mild cases will self-resolve. Severe cases: **Ciprofloxacin**. (Severe: hypotension, tachycardia, abdominal pain, blood, fever).

Secretory

- ↑ secretion or no absorption. Secretes chloride and Na anions continuously even without food intake. ((**↑cAMP**)
- Persistent, odorless, tea-color
- Loss of H2O, Na, K
- No structural damage
- MC: **Vibrio cholera** (Cholera toxin)
- **Prevention: Improved sanitation**
- Other causes: **VIPomas** (associated with MEN)
- Isotonic to plasma
- **Diarrhea continues even with ↓ of food intake or change of diet**
- "Rice water stools" (parts of the gut endothelial lining)
- SX: Severe dehydration. Death is usually due to dehydration

TX: **Octreotide**

Osmotic

- ↑ water drawn into the bowels. Things that are in the bowel are pulling water into the bowel
- **Diarrhea stops when offending agent is stopped or diet is changed**

Causes: **lactose intolerance**, drinks ↑ sugar, ↑ salt, ↑ Mg, ↑ Vitamin C, laxatives, undigested lactose intolerance, fructose malabsorption, sorbitol (sugar-free foods), pancreatic DZ

Inflammatory • Ulcerative colitis, Crohn's DZ • Chronic diarrhea. • Due to damage to the mucosal lining on the brush boarder causes loss of protein rich fluids and ↓ ability to reabsorb • Causes: bacterial/viral/parasitic infections, autoimmune, IBD, TB, colon cancer, enteritis • SX: Blood, pus, weight loss, fever	**Exudative/Invasive** • **Blood and pus** • Causes: E. coli 0157:57, Ulcerative colitis, some food poisoning, IBD, Crohn's
Dysentery • Bloody, invasion of the bowel tract • Causes: Shigella, Salmonella, Entamoeba (protozoan) • MCC diarrhea in children < 5 (day care centers): Rotavirus	**Motility** • **Hypermobility**. Rapid movement of food through the intestines because there is not enough time for water and nutrients to be absorbed. • Causes: Vagotomy, Diabetic neuropathy, bowel resection, hyperthyroid
Rotavirus (Reo virus) • **MC fatal diarrhea in children** • Fecal/oral transmission • Toxic rotavirus protein NSP4 causes Calcium and Chloride secretion • DX: look for virus in the stool by enzyme immunoassay **WARNING**: Do NOT give children <2 years old **Loperamide** (can be fatal)	**Laxative Abuse** (AKA: Factitious diarrhea) • Frequent watery stools 10 – 20 times/day, nocturnal diarrhea • **Dark brown colon discolor** • Lymph follicles show through as pale patches (melanosis coli)
Post-cholecystectomy Diarrhea • Bile salt (bile acid) induced because of ↑ bile acids. • TX: **Cholestyramine** (bile salt binding agent)	**Carcinoid** • Chronic diarrhea • **Serotonin** secreting tumor due to excess excretion of serotonin = causes flushing and hypotension. • **DX: urinary 5-HIAA level** • TX: **Octreotide** (Somatostatin analog)
Antibiotic-Associated Diarrhea: Clostridium difficile (C. diff) • MCC: **Ampicillin, Clindamycin, Fluoroquinolones, Cephalosporins**, antibiotics, NSAIDS • PPI's increase the risk of C. diff in hospitalized patients DX: Stool toxin assay TX: Metronidazole. If Metronidazole fails use: oral vancomycin.	**Lactose intolerance** • Chronic diarrhea • MCC of chronic diarrhea and flatulence. Remove all milk and milk-related products from the diet • Yogurt may be used in the diet.

Fat Malabsorption Diarrhea	Irritable Bowel
• Chronic diarrhea • SX: Weight loss, steatorrhea (oily, greasy stools that float, foul smell) • Types: Celiac, Chronic pancreatitis, Tropical sprue, Whipple DZ • Complications: Vitamin B12 malabsorption, easy bruising (due to Vit K malabsorption), Hypocalcemia (Vit D malabsorption), oxalate over absorption leading to kidney stones. **DX:** Sudan black stain of the stool, 72 hour fecal fat • **Celiac:** blunted villi on small bowel biopsy, antibodies to wheat, rye, barley, oats (Antigliadin, antiendomysial, antitissue transglutaminase), **D-xylose is not absorbed because villous lining has been destroyed.** TX: Eliminate these grains from diet. Does not respond to antibiotics. • Tropical Sprue: Presents like Celiac DZ but history of patient visiting the tropics. Antibody test are negative. Small bowel biopsy shows microorganisms. Responds to antibodies: TX: **TMP/SMX or Tetracycline** for 3 – 6 months. • Whipple Dz: Joint pain, ocular issues, neurological findings. Small bowel biopsy PAS positive, PAS of stood is positive for T. whippelii. TX: **TMP/SMX or Tetracycline** for 12 months. • Chronic Pancreatitis: MC: alcoholics with multiple presentations of acute pancreatitis. Malabsorption does not begin until the pancreas enzymes are unavailable due to the fibrosis and calcification of the pancreas. DX: BIT: Abdominal X-ray shows calcifications in the pancreas. MAT: Secretin stimulation test. Labs: iron and folate normal b/c pancreatic enzymes are not needed for absorption and D-xylose test will be normal: it will be absorbed.	• Chronic diarrhea • **Alternating diarrhea and constipation**, abdominal pain relieved by a bowel movement and ↓ pain at night • DX: All DX test will be **normal** (ie: O & P, Stool white cells, occult, abdominal CT, colonoscopy) • TX: ↑ Fiber, exercise. • TX: if no relief from ↑ fiber: **Dicyclomine, Hyoscyamine** (anticholinergic agents that relax the bowel). • TX: if no relief from anticholinergic agents: **Amitriptyline**.

Diarrhea Differentials

Symptom	Cause	Notes
Blood, NO fever, abdominal pain	E. coli	
Blood, fever, NO abdominal pain	Campylobacter, Shigella, Salmonella	
HUS, TTP	E. coli	
Immunocompromised or travel	Protozoa, parasites, giardia, Cryptococcus, entamoeba	
Viral, Gastroenteritis		Vomiting

Constipation

Correct the underlying cause.

- **Opiates (narcotic) medications (common post-op)**
- Calcium channel blockers
- ↑ Calcium levels
- Dehydration (NOTE: be aware of urine output. Dehydration can lead to kidney failure, especially in the elderly. Monitor the BUN/Creatinine ratio: > 20:1)
- Ferrous sulfate
- Diabetes due to neuropathy: loss of sensation in the bowels = ↓ stretch sensation = ↓ GI motility
- Anticholinergic medications
- Tricyclic antidepressants
- **Dysfunction of the pelvic splanchnic nerves: MC due to diabetes**
- TX: ↑ Hydration, ↑ exercise (exercise moves the bowels), ↑ fiber

Chronic Constipation Treatments

Management: Evaluate 2° (ie: meds) causes of constipation and treat appropriately.
If no 2° causes found: ↑ dietary fiber to 20 – 35 mg/day. If increasing fiber does not work: start bulk forming laxative (ie: psyllium). If bulk forming laxative does not work: start osmotic or stimulate laxative. If osmotic or stimulate laxative does not work: colectomy/hemicolectomy.

Type of Laxatives	Laxatives	Method of Action
Bulk form laxatives	Psyllium, Methycellulose, Polycarbophil	MC used, safe and effective. ↑ bulk stool, softens stool, maintains stool water.
Osmotic Laxatives	Polyethylene glycol (used as prep for colonoscopy), lactulose (used in hepatic encephalopathy), sorbitol.	↑ intestine water secretion and stool volume. Long-term use may cause: electrolyte issues by ↓ potassium in kidney disease.
Saline Laxatives	Milk of Magnesia, Magnesium citrate.	↑ intestine water secretion causing ↑ Mg. Avoid in kidney damage.
Stimulant Laxatives	Dicacodyl Senna	↑ intestine peristalsis and H2O electrolyte secretion. Long-term use may cause electrolyte abnormalities: ↓ K.
Chloride Channel Activator	Lubiprostone	↑ Chloride rich intestinal fluid secretion. May cause severe constipation. Use only when no response to other treatments. Side effects unknown with long-term use.

Colorectal Cancer

Colon Cancer Risk

- Family history, genetics
- Intake of > 45 gms of alcohol per day (45 gms = 3 beers. A 12 oz beer = 13 gms)
- Cigarette smoking

Heterotopic Gastric (Fundic) Mucosa (HGM)

NOT TO BE CONFUSED WITH COLORECTAL CANCER

Gastric epithelium (mucosa) anywhere within the GI tract. It is mature gastric tissue located where it is normally not found. The polypoid (multiple polyps) mass usually consist of fundic mucosa with parietal and chief cells, lined by foveolar epithelium with a full mucosal thickness. These are not polyps associated with colorectal cancer. MC location: duodenum.
If it is congenital it is referred to as heteroplasia. If it is acquired it is referred to as **metaplasia**. It can be located in the colon, rectum, duodenum, esophagus or stomach. The polypoid mass usually consist of fundic mucosa with parietal and chief cells.
Complications: Obstruction, ulceration, diarrhea, perforation, pain, intussusception.
NOTE: Gastric metaplasia due to chronic inflammation is MC due to H. pylori. If due to H. pylori there will be no parietal cells. If due to peptic ulcer disease (PUD) there will be no goblet cells.

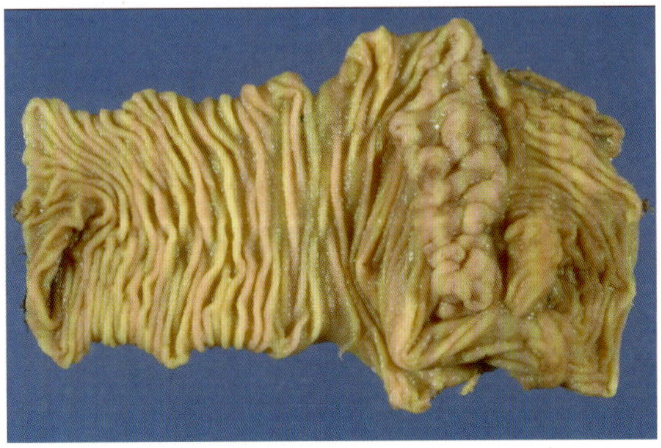

Heterotopic Gastric Mucosa in the gut

Colonic Polyps (abnormal growths from a mucus membrane)

Benign

- **Hyperplastic:** Benign (non-neoplastic). MC located in the rectosigmoid region. Well differentiated mucosal cells.
- **Tubular Adenoma** (AKA: **Hamartomas** = **non-neoplastic** polyp, asymptomatic. 90% of most polyps in the bowel. Uniform pattern, organized. Low risk of malignancy. Common with Peutz-Jeghers and juvenile polyposis).
- Submucosal polyps (lipoma, lymphoid aggregates)
- Inflammatory polyps (Ulcerative Colitis, Crohn's)
- Mucosal Polyps: Resemble polyps but are normal mucosa.

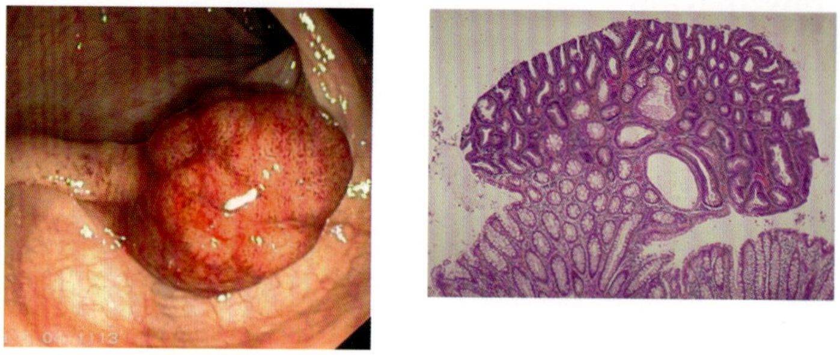

Tubular Adenoma (polyp)

Malignant: High Risk

- Tubulovillous Adenoma: Elongated crypts, few pits, projections.
- Have a **higher risk** of progressing to adenocarcinoma than tubular adenomas.
- **Villous Adenoma (AKA: Dysplastic polyps = malignant)** (**tip**: Villous = Villain = bad)
  AKA: **Adenomatous** (MC: precancerous) Precursor to Colorectal Cancer, high chance of developing into colorectal adenocarcinoma. Mutations in APC and KRAS. Multiple projections, haphazard and irregular pattern, lobules.
- Associated with lower GI bleeds.
- Serrated: Mutations in BRAF and hypermethylation of CpG

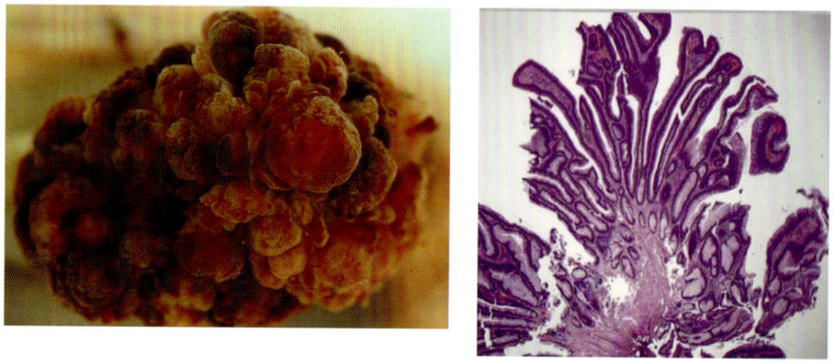

Villous Adenoma (Dysplastic polyp)

Colorectal or Anal Cancer Metastasis to the Liver (MC site of metastasis)

- Pathway from the cecum: Ileocolic vein → Superior Mesenteric vein → Portal vein →Hepatic vein
- Pathway from the ascending colon: Straight Veins → Right Colic vein → Superior Mesenteric vein → Portal vein →Hepatic vein
- Pathway from the transverse colon: Marginal Veins → Middle Colic vein → Superior Mesenteric vein → Portal vein →Hepatic vein
- Pathway from the rectum: Inferior/Middle rectal vein → Superior rectal vein → Inferior Mesenteric vein → Splenic vein → Portal vein → Hepatic vein
- Pathway from the Sigmoid colon: Sigmoid veins → Inferior Mesenteric vein → Splenic vein → Portal vein → Hepatic vein
- Pathway from the descending colon: Left Colic vein → Inferior Mesenteric vein → Splenic vein → Portal vein → Hepatic vein

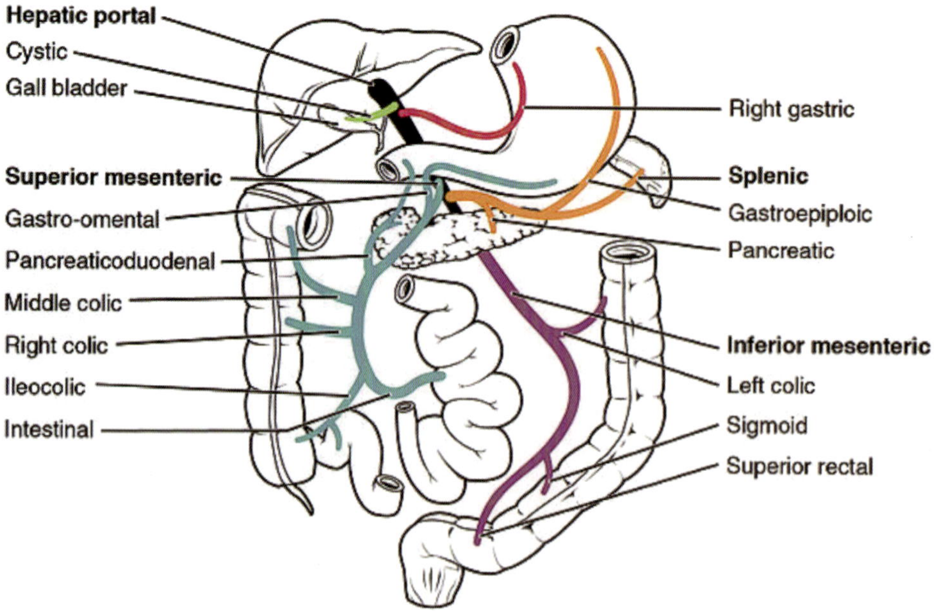

Colorectal Cancer and Benign Polyps

Hereditary Nonpolyposis Colorectal Cancer (HNPCC)
(AKA: **Lynch Syndrome**)

Autosomal Dominant
Cause: mutation of **DNA Mismatch Repair Tumor Marker: CEA** (used for monitoring recurrence not for screening)

Ascending colon right side:
SX: Burgundy/maroon stools (due to bleeding), iron deficiency anemia, weight loss.
Descending colon left side:
SX: Partial obstruction from mass (Barium studies show "**apple core lesion**"), hematochezia, colicky pain.

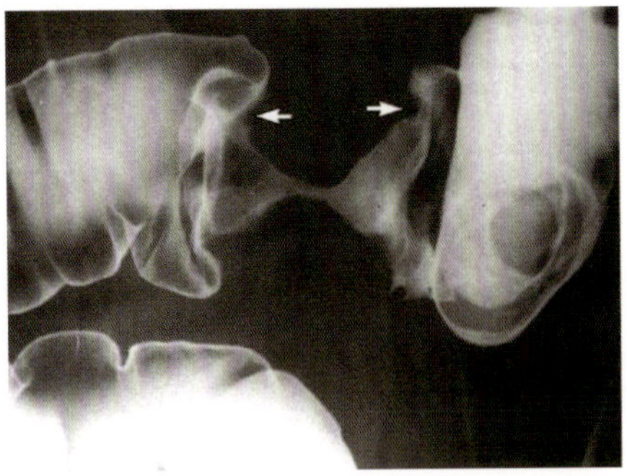

Metastasis to liver.
Metastasis via Inferior Mesenteric nodes.

S. bovis Endocarditis and Clostridium septicum is associated with colon cancer.
First step after S. bovis identification = **colonoscopy**.

Familial Adenomatous Polyposis (FAP)

Autosomal Dominant
Always involves the **rectum**
Cause: **Inactivation of tumor suppressor gene, mutation of APC gene on chromosome 5q.**

2 Hit Hypothesis

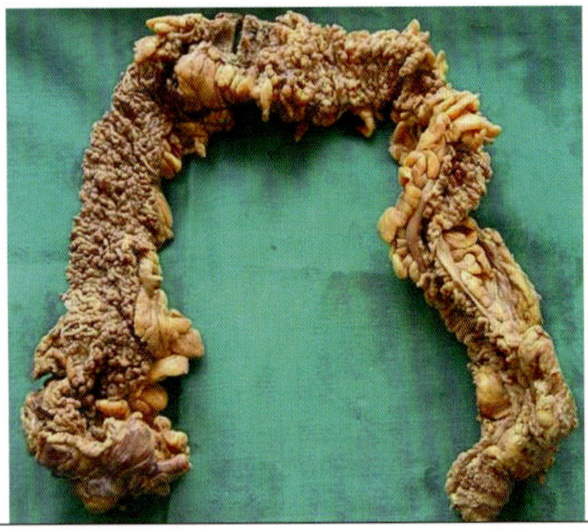

DX: Colonoscopy shows 1000's of polyps. Start colonoscopy screening at the age of 12.

TX: Colectomy once polyps are found

Gardner Syndrome
Colon cancer associated with benign bone tumors (osteomas), desmoid tumors or other benign soft tissue tumors.

Autosomal Dominant
Mutation in the **APC gene** on chromosome 5q
Multiple polyps inside the colon with tumors outside the colon (**extracolonic tumors**).
Extracolonic tumors: Fibromas, dermoid cyst, osteomas

DX: No special screening

Turcot Syndrome
Colon cancer associated with brain cancer.

Autosomal Dominant
DNA mismatch repair mutation.
Multiple polyps in the colon and increased risk of **brain cancer** (Glioblastoma or Medulloblastoma)

Peutz-Jeghers Syndrome
Hamartomatous polyps throughout the GI tract.
Autosomal Dominant.
10% increased risk of colon cancer.

Presents with hyperpigmented spots (melanotic spots) on the lips, mouth, hands, feet.

DX: No special screening

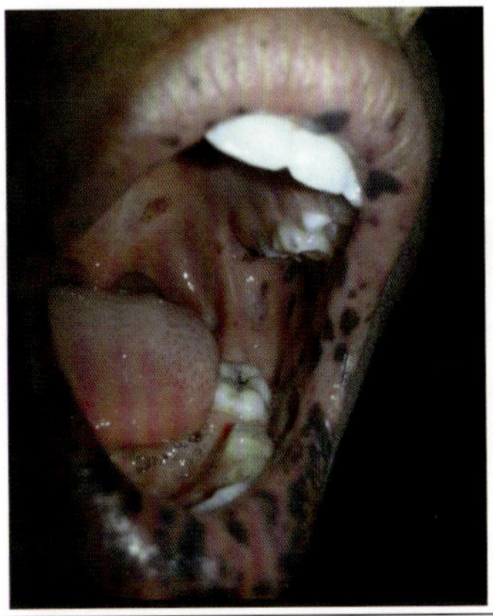

Juvenile Polyposis (Juvenile Polyps).
Colon cancer associated with hamartomatous polyps.

Multiple polyps (>5 polyps) in the colon or rectum of the GI tract, most are benign and self-limiting.
Can lead to increased risk of adenocarcinoma.

DX: No special screening

Inflammatory Polyp
Benign, painful.
Whitish in appearance (few spots or covering entire polyp) is pus (WBC fighting the inflammation)
Self-limiting

Screening for Colon Cancer

- Normal patient: Begins screening by **colonoscopy at age 50**. Normal test results: **repeat every 10 years**.
- Adenomatous polyps: Repeat colonoscopy every 3 to 5 years.
- **CEA** (Carcinoembryonic antigen) marker is used to monitor therapeutic response. It is not used for screening.

Sigmoidoscopy (similar to a colonoscopy): Exams only up to the sigmoid (most distal part of colon). Colonoscopy exams the entire large bowel. Positive test: If polyps or abnormal tissue is found the test will be followed up by a colonoscopy. Negative test (no cancer risk found): repeat sigmoidoscopy every five years.

Patient with family history of one member of the family:
Colonoscopy starting at age 40 or 10 years before the age of the family member that had cancer.
(which ever comes first)

Patient with family history of either 3 family members, 1 member with cancer < 50 or family history involving 2 generations:
(AKA: Lynch syndrome, Hereditary nonpolyposis colon cancer)
Colonoscopy every 1 – 2 years starting at the age of 25.

Patient with ulcerative colitis: start screening within 8 years of diagnosis of ulcerative colitis, then screen every 1 – 2 years later.

Patient with FAP (Familial Adenomatous Polyposis) Autosomal Dominant. Must start colonoscopies at 12 years old and then every 1 – 2 years.

If a dysplastic polyp is found:
Repeat colonoscopy 3 – 5 years after the polyp was found.

Progression to Colorectal Cancer

Pathways to Colorectal Carcinoma: DNA mismatch repair gene mutation

Steps from adenoma to carcinoma
APC (suppressor mutation of epithelial cells, inactivation)/early adenoma ➔ COX-2 (overexpression causes ↑ proliferation of the epithelium) ➔ K-RAS (proto-oncogene that ↑↑ cell proliferation) late adenoma. Mutation of KRAS proto-oncogene leads to ↑ growth proliferation and growth of tumors to an adenoma ➔ Loss of tumor suppressor P53 (final step: suppressor mutation) leads to carcinoma (aka: adenocarcinoma). NOTE: Tumor suppressors inhibits proliferation, mutation will lead to proliferation.

↓ activity of tumor suppressor (P53) leads to neoplasm ➔ DCC (Deleted colon cancer).

Treatment: Colectomy (surgical resection of the colon) and **F-fluorouracil** chemotherapy.
(**tip**: if you have colon cancer, you are F....d)

Adenoma to Carinoma in Colon Cancer

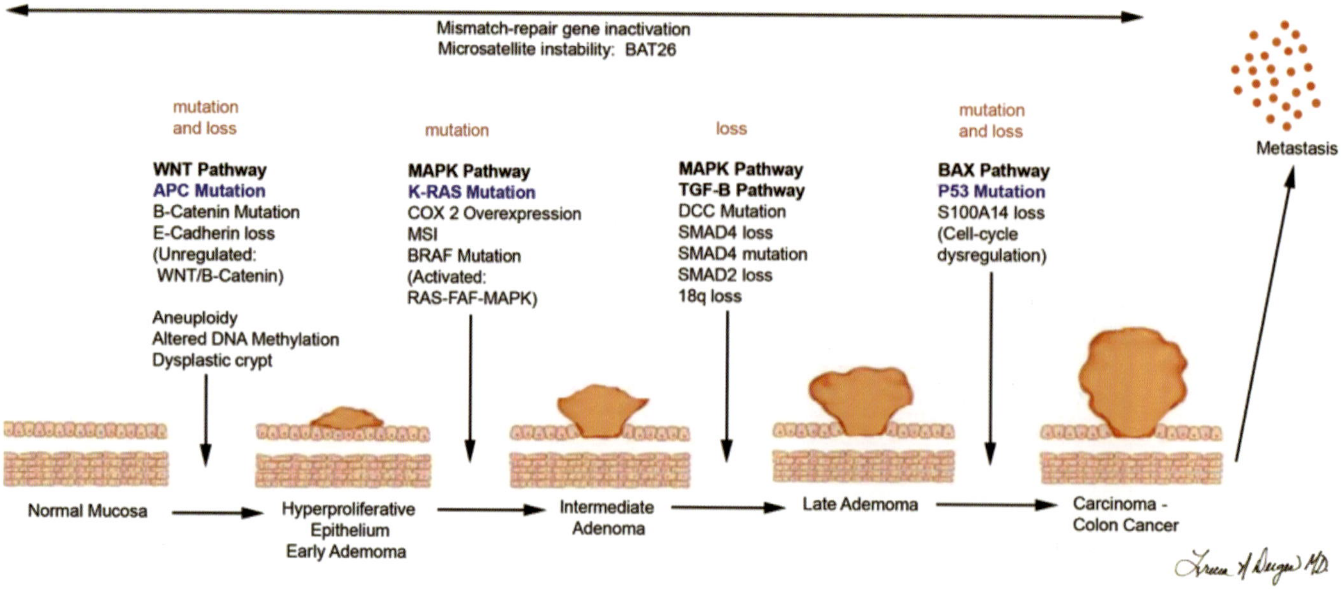

Liver Pathology

Liver Pathologies

- **Anything** that affects/damages the liver (hepatocytes) can affect any of the functions the liver is responsible for: clotting factors, estrogen, protein synthesis (albumin, thyroglobulin, A1AT, ceruloplasmin), bilirubin conjugation, bile synthesis, copper and iron mineral functions, cholesterol synthesis, urea cycle, glycogen synthesis and breakdown, gluconeogenesis, P-450 system, Vit D conversion, Storage of Vitamin A and Vitamin B-12, Acute Phase Reactants (to mount bodies defenses), first pass drug metabolism, etc. Any of these can lead to many different pathologies.
- Jaundice is an immediate indicator of liver dysfunction
- Hepatic encephalopathy is an indicator of liver failure. The urea cycle is not working so ammonia is allowed to build up in the brain (confusion, lethargy, coma, death). TX: **Lactulose**
- **Key factors to monitor in liver failure: Albumin and PT**
- **NOTE: Elevations of ALT, AST and GGT are indications of liver damage. Elevations of AST (2:1) indicate alcohol pathologies. Elevations of ALT indicated viral pathologies. Elevations of ALT and AST (into the 100's) indicate hepatitis. Extreme elevations of ALT and AST (into the 1000's) indicate drug toxicity.**
  Elevations of ALP and GGT indicate cholestatic disease.

Drugs Causing Liver and Gal Stone Pathologies

Pathology	Drugs
Fatty Liver	Valproic Acid, Tetracycline, Anti-virals
Fulminant Liver Dz (toxic)	Acetominophen, Aspirin, Carbon Tetrachloride
Hepatitis/Liver Failure	Halothane, INH, Phenytoin, Methyldopa, Metformin
Granulomas	Allopurinol, Phenylbutazone
Cholestasis	Chlorpromazine, Nitrofurantoin, Erythromycin, Steroids

Portal Anastomosis

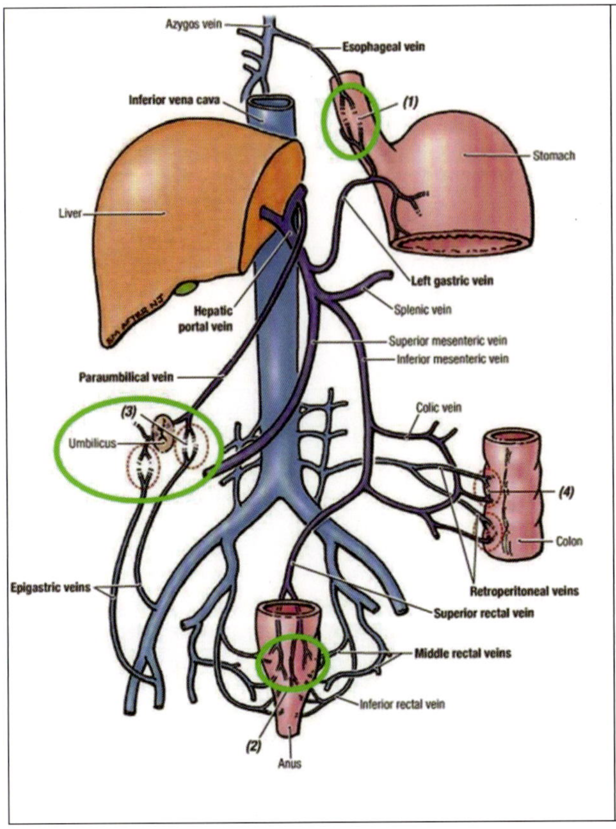

Portal Anastomosis

Esophageal Varices:
Left Gastric and Esophageal Veins
(branch of the **Azygos venous system**. The azygos vein transports Deoxygenated blood from the posterior walls of the thorax and abdomen into the **Superior Vena Cava vein**).

Hemorrhoids:
Superior rectal vein and Middle/Inferior Rectal Veins

Caput:
Paraumbilical and Superior and Inferior Epigastric Veins

Liver Serum Markers, Proteins, Hormones

Acute Phase Reactants (APR)	Proteins that respond to inflammation via stimulation by cytokines (IL1, IL6, IL8, TNFα) released by PMN's and macrophages. C-reactive protein, amyloids, compliment, fibrinogen (coagulation factors), plasminogen, ferritin, hepcidin, haptoglobin, ceruloplasmin, A1AT. APR correlate with ESR (erythrocyte sedimentation rate)
Albumin	Most common protein found in the body and main protein of human blood plasma (50%). Main function: regulate the colloidal osmotic pressure of the blood. Normal plasma level: 3.5 – 5 g/dL. (Under 3 yrs old 2.9 – 5.5 g/dL) Low albumin: Due to liver disease, nephrotic syndrome, burns, malabsorption, malnutrition, and malignancies. High albumin: Due to dehydration, retinol (Vitamin A) deficiency.
Alkaline phosphatase (ALP)	Enzyme responsible for removing phosphate groups. Normal level: 20 – 140 IU/L (levels higher in children and pregnant women). **High ALP can indicate**: **bile duct** obstruction, untreated Celiac DZ, **liver and bone** diseases/tumors, Sarcoidosis, hyperthyroidism, hyperparathyroidism, lymphoma, leukemia. Placental ALP is elevated in **seminomas**. **Elevations of ALP and GGT indicate cholestatic disease.** Differential between bone and liver disease is determined by heat stability ("bone burns, liver lasts").
AST (aspartate transaminase) ALT (alanine aminotransferase) (AKA: Liver Enzymes)	AST: found in liver, heart, skeletal muscle, kidneys, brain. ALT: plasma, mainly in liver AST and ALT normal levels: 8 – 20 U/L Alcoholic hepatitis: AST > ALT (**tip**: a**S**t, **S** = **S**cotch) Viral hepatitis: ALT > AST Liver damage due to drugs: ↑↑↑ ALT and AST (massive #'s cells being killed off)
Alpha 1-antitrypsin	Protease inhibitor. Inhibits neutrophil elastase from breaking down elastin
Angiotensinogen	Precursor for angiotensin
Betatropin	Stimulates the proliferation of insulin-secreting beta cells in the pancreas.
C-Reactive Protein	Activates compliment system and binds to phosphocholine on the surface of dead/dying cells. This allows for phagocytosis by macrophages.
Ceruloplasmin	Copper carrying protein along with transferrin in the blood. Low levels are seen with: Wilson's DZ, Menkes DZ, overdose of Vitamin C, copper deficiency, Aceruloplasminemia (brain pathologies). High levels are seen with: Pregnancy, OCP use, RA, Alzheimer's, schizophrenia.
Coagulation Factors	Factors: 2, 5, 7, 10, Protein C & S
Complement Factors	Allows for chemotaxis, opsonization and lysis of cells. It "complements" antibodies and macrophages in the clearing of pathogens. Part of the innate immune system.
Ferritin	Binds iron (puts in storage) to keep microbes from using the iron (they need iron)
Fibrinogen	Fibrinogen is converted to fibrin = forms clots
Gamma-glutamyl Transpeptidase (GGT)	Transfers glutathione to an amino acid to make glutamate. Located in cell membranes and transfers amino acids across the membrane and is involved in glutathione metabolism. Increased levels indicate: heavy alcohol use, biliary disease, (GGT is NOT increased in bone disease), certain drugs (NSAIDS, barbiturates, phenytoin, St. John's wort, Kava), liver diseases. **Elevations of ALP and GGT indicate cholestatic disease.**
Haptoglobin	Binds with hemoglobin after RBC breakdown and to keep microbes from using the iron
Hepcidin	Blocks release of iron from intracellular stores (ferritin) inside the intestinal enterocytes and macrophages so microbes can't use the iron
Insulin-like Growth Factor-1 (IGF-1)	Growth hormone released from anterior pituitary and binds to cell surface, **tyrosine kinase receptors** on the liver, which stimulates release of IGF-1. Binding of IGF-1 to cells with IGF receptors stimulates them to move from G_1 of the cell cycle to S phase and then into mitosis. Highest levels of IGF-1 found in puberty.
Plasminogen	Plasminogen is converted to plasmin = lyses fibrin and clots
Thyroid Binding Globulin (TBG)	Binds with thyroid hormones Thyroxine (T4) and Triiodothyronine (T3) in the bloodstream. Production levels can be modified by: estrogen, corticosteroids and liver failure. Estrogen (pregnancy) causes ↑ TBG = will bind more hormones (T3 and T4) = ↓ free T3 and T4 levels in the blood = **normal** stimulation of TSH = production of more T3 and T4. **TBG levels will always increase during pregnancy. It is the only situation where the T4 levels will be ↑ but will show a normal TSH.** Steroids causes ↓ TBG = ↓ bound and free T3 and T4 in the blood.
Thrombopoietin	Stimulates precursor cells in the bone marrow to differentiate into megakaryocytes, which generate platelets.

Effusions

Effusion is the escape of a fluid into a body part/cavity. The effusion is either an exudate or a transudate.
Albumin levels and ratios determine differentials between exudate and transudate.
Effusions can be either pleural or abdominal

- **Pleural Effusions** are effusions in the chest
  Excess fluid between the two pleural layers which causes ↓ in lung expansion and pain during inspiration
- **Abdominal Effusion** are effusions in the abdomen

Effusions can either be transudate or exudates

- **Transudate**
  Is due to ↓ oncotic pressure = liver failure or ↑ hydrostatic pressure = CHF.
  Transudate = "translucent" = ↓ protein content: CHF, ascites (cirrhosis), SBP (Spontaneous Bacterial peritonitis)
- **Exudate**
  Is due to ↑ capillary permeability that allows leakage of proteins.
  Exudate = Cloudy, ↑ protein content: Pneumonia, malignancies, collagen vascular disease, RA, Pulmonary embolism, TB, Sarcoidosis, connective tissue dz, infection, lymphoma (Must drain due to ↑ risk of infection), nephrotic diseases, infections (not SBP: Spontaneous Bacterial Peritonitis)

Effusion Calculations

Pleural Effusion Diagnosis	Ascites Sample Diagnosis
Effusion Sample Labs (done by thoracentesis) • Exudate: If ANY of these are present, it is an exudate: Glucose < 60 (glucose is being eaten for energy), pH < 7.2 (acidic), LDH > .6, Protein > .5	**Effusion Sample Labs (done by paracentesis)** SAAG (Serum ascites albumin gradient): Protein Analysis between serum protein and effusion proteins in ascites • Subtract the protein reading from the effusion sample from the serum protein content: • If the total is <1.2 = Effusion (cancer, nephrotic syndrome or infection: except for SBP (Spontaneous Bacterial Peritonitis) • If the total is > 1.2 = Transudate (CHF, Portal hypertension, hepatic vein thrombosis, constrictive pericarditis)

NOTE: beware: The protein reading results in the thorax and the abdomen **is reversed**.

Liver Protein and Mineral Pathologies

Alpha-1 Antitrypsin Deficiency	Hepatitis A (HAV)
Genetic disorder. Decreased A1AT in the blood and lungs. A1AT deficiency in the lungs is NOT associated with smoking and is considered **Panacinar emphysema**. (Centriacinar is associated with **COPD** and IS **associated with smoking**). A1AT protects the lungs against neutrophil **elastase**. Deficiency of this enzyme breaks down lung/connective tissue. It also deposits abnormal A1AT in the liver causing cirrhosis and liver failure. Patient may mention having had jaundice problems as a baby. DX: **PAS +**	Enterovirus, no envelope **Acute** viral hepatitis Transmission: Fecal-oral Asymptomatic, no treatment, self limiting in 6 weeks Source: Shellfish, **oysters**, overcrowded conditions, **poor sanitation (travel)** DX Marker: Anti-HAV IgM **Hepatocytes show ballooning and swelling (AKA: Councilman bodies). Councilman bodies = eosinophilic apoptotic hepatocytes.** Source: **Contaminated food, oysters** Higher Risk: Prisons, anal sex, travel

Hemochromatosis AD and AR
(AKA: Iron overload)
Genetic disorder: can be autosomal recessive or autosomal dominant.

Mutation of **HFE (C282Y) gene** on chromosome 6, which stops regulation.
Associated with **HLA-A3.**

Accumulation of iron in organs (liver, heart, endocrine organs, pituitary) throughout the body due to an **overload of iron** that leads to end organ damage. (Can set metal detectors off).
(Remember: Vitamin C helps to absorb iron in the intestine).

Hemochromatosis is the **ONLY** restrictive heart disease that is reversible by phlebotomy.

Labs: ↑ serum iron saturation, ↑ ferritin levels, ↓ TBIC, ↑ AFP, ↑ LFT's.

Caused: genetic or multiple **blood transfusions** (seen with **beta thalassemia major**, sickle cell, Diamond-Blackfan) and ↑↑ **absorption of iron in the intestine**.

SX: Cirrhosis of the liver, diabetes (AKA: "Bronze" diabetic) (look for **any NEW diagnosis of diabetes** in someone older – deposits of copper in the pancreas = ↓ function of pancreatic islet beta cells = diabetes), restrictive cardiomyopathy, arthritis (calcium pyrophosphate deposition in joints), impotence (erectile dysfunction, ↓ libido), infertility, Sick Sinus Syndrome (due to conduction defects), panhypopituitarism. skin darkening (deposits in the skin).

DX: MRI show iron deposition in the liver and genetic testing, liver biopsy.

NOTE: women are usually not affected until **after menopause**.
Monthly periods act as phlebotomy.
MCC death is due to cirrhosis.

Complications: Increased risk of hepatocellular carcinoma, ↑ risk of infections from Listeria, Vibrio, and Yersinia.

TX: weekly phlebotomy, ↓ intake of iron rich foods.
Note: if phlebotomy is started before the liver becomes cirrhosis, liver damage can be reversed.
Deferoxamine (if phlebotomy not possible)

Wilson's Disease AR
(AKA: hepatolenticular degeneration)

Accumulation of copper in organs throughout the body due to ↓ hepatic copper excretion (ceruloplasmin).
Copper is transported into the bile by **ATP7B gene** (hepatocyte copper transporter).
Cystic degeneration of the putamen.

Labs: ↑ **Free copper,** ↑ **urine copper,**
↓ **ceruloplasmin**
(note: Menkes, associated with collagen synthesis, has ↓ Free copper and ↓ urine copper)

Causes: damages/degeneration with free radicals, hepatocyte degeneration.
MC in young adults <30.

SX: Jaundice (yellow sclera), rigid muscles, flapping tremors (asterixis), hepatomegaly, ataxia, **Kayser-Fleischer rings** (corneal deposits), dementia, **choreiform movement** disorder, neuropsychiatric abnormalities: **psychosis and delusions**, **hemolysis.**
Can lead to hepatocellular carcinoma.

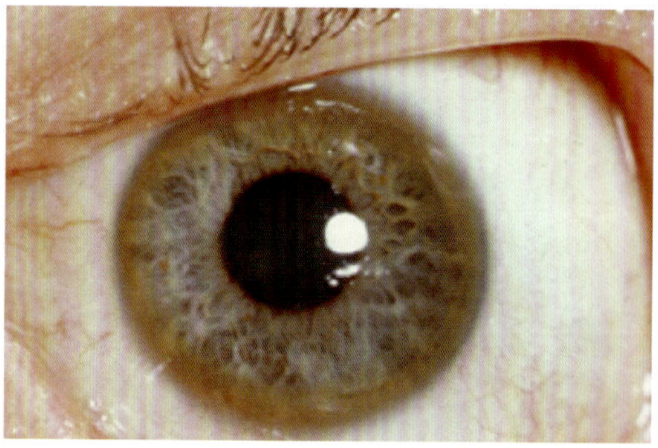

Kayser Fleischer Rings

DX: BIT: Slit lamp to confirm **Kayser Fleischer rings**.

MAT: ↑ copper urinary excretion after administration of penicillamine.

TX: **Penicillamine** (binds copper (chelation) to ↑ excretion of copper in the urine), **Trientine** or **zinc** (zinc ↓ absorption of copper in the intestine.
(**tip**: a "penny" is made out of copper)
↓ consumption of copper containing foods: nuts, chocolate, mushrooms, dried fruit, liver, and shellfish.

Hepatitis D
Delta Virus
Enveloped, Circular, Single stranded
Requires Hepatitis B (HBV) to co-infect.
HBV must coat HDV with viral particles before it can infect.
Causes a super infection.

Hepatitis E
No Envelope, Single stranded, linear, **Positive Sense**, Icosahedral
Associated with **pregnancy**
Causes death

(**tip**: **E** for **E**mbryo (pregnancy)

Hepatitis B	Hepatitis C (HCV)
Hepatitis B Hepadnavirus **Enveloped with Spheres and Tubes,** Double stranded, circular **Has: Reverse Transcriptase** **ONLY DNA Hepatitis** Replicates DS DNA ➔template ➔progeny DS DNA Viral hepatitis: 1st stage: Viral prodrome = fever, malaise, nausea, vomiting 2nd stage: ↑ ALT verses AST High risk for **hepatocellular carcinoma**. Show high LFT's: ↑ ALT and ↑AST. (Viral liver causes usually show a higher ALT while liver problems due to alcohol show a higher AST **(tip:** "S" = scotch) Acute hepatitis infections show ↑↑ ALT and ↑ AST with normal Alk Phos Associated with: **Polyarteritis Nodosa**, Membranous Glomerulonephritis TX: **INF- α**	**Hepatitis C (HCV)** Flavivirus **Enveloped,** Single stranded, Icosahedral, Positive sense ↑varieties of HCV, so causes lower immunities due to antigenic structure. HCV is unstable, lacks 3' to 5' exonuclease proofreading. Transmission: **Blood** to blood in IV drug use, transfusions, poorly sterilized surgical instruments, tattooing. DX: ELISA, Confirmatory test: HCV RNA DX Cleared infection: Anti-HCV antibodies DX: Chronic HEP C: Fibrosis Labs: HEP C is ↓ C4 (**tip:** HEP C is 4 letters = C4) No vaccine available. SX: Jaundice, fatigue, loss appetite, joint pain. Can lead to cirrhosis and hepatocellular carcinoma. Associated with: **Cryoglobulinemia, Membranous glomerulonephritis,** Sjögrens, Porphyria Cutaneous Tarda, HIV TX: **Ribavarin, INFα, Sofosbuvir** (nucleotide analog)
Autoimmune Hepatitis Chronic autoimmune disease of the liver. MC in young woman with other autimmune dz (MC: ITP, Thyroiditis, Hemolytic anemia). Antibodies: **Anti-smooth muscle antibodies**, positive ANA, liver-kidney microsomal antibodies, anti-liver/kidney microsomal antibodies. SX: acute liver inflammation, jaundice, right upper quadrant abdominal pain, fatigue, myalgias, arthralgias, thrombocytopenia. Labs: BIT: ANA autoantibodies, Anti-smooth muscle (SMA), ↑ IgG, elevated ALT, AST. MAT: Liver biopsy. TX: **Prednisone, Azathioprine**	

HEPATITIS

Virus	Classification	Transmission	Carcinoma Risk	Additional Facts
HEP A (HAV)	RNA - Picornavirus	Fecal-oral	No	Acute – self limiting Vaccine: 2 doses
HEP B (HBV)	DNA - Hepadnavirus	Sexual	Yes	Vaccine: 3 doses
HEP C (HCV)	RNA - Flavivirus	Blood	Yes	No vaccine
HEP D (HDV)	RNA – Delta Virus	Sexual, Parenteral	Yes	Must HEP B
HEP E (HEV)	RNA Hepeviridae Virus	Fecal-oral	No	↑ mortality in pregnant women

Additional Liver Pathologies

Hepatic Encephalopathy

Altered level of consciousness (confusion), which can lead to coma and then death.

MCC: Accumulation of **ammonia** in the bloodstream because normal routes of clearing the ammonia in the liver are failing. (Urea cycle in the liver)

Other causes: Excessive nitrogen load (↑ protein intake, GI bleeds (esophageal varices), renal failure (↓ excretion of urea), constipation, Hyponatremia, Hypokalemia (diuretic usage), dehydration, infections (UTI's, SBP), drugs (benzodiazepines, narcotics, antipsychotics, alcohol).

SX: Somnolence, ↓ level of consciousness, jaundice, + Babinski sign, seizures, cerebral edema, asterixis ("flapping tremor")

TX: **Lactulose** (Metabolized in the colon by bacterial flora which allows it to convert NH3 to a nonabsorbable NH4 and be excreted).
Spironolactone: ↓ ammonia forming organisms and ↑ clearance of protein in the gut.
↓ high protein foods

Nutmeg Liver

(AKA: Congestive Hepatopathy)

Venous backup into the liver from right-sided heart failure or Budd-Chiari syndrome.

Complications: Persistent congestion will cause fibrosis of the liver causing cardiac cirrhosis.

SX: Fullness in the RUQ, ascites, light/grey stools, hepatomegaly.

Pathway:
Right heart failure causes backup of blood (see JVD) into IVC → hepatic veins → liver → causing centrilobular necrosis.

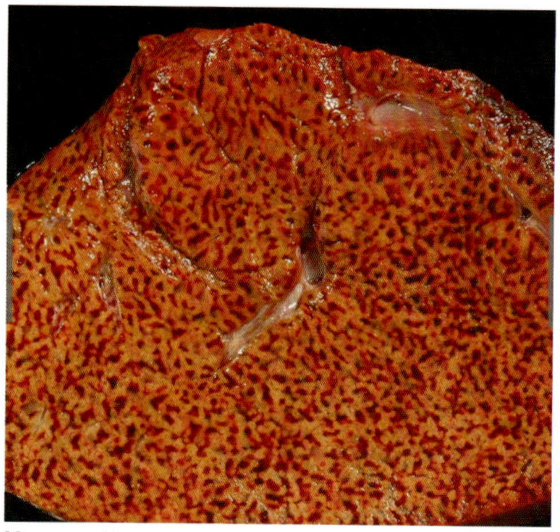

Nutmeg Liver

Budd-Chiari Syndrome

Occlusion of the hepatic veins.
MCC: blood clot.

SX: **No JVD** (this is occurring before the heart so no back up of blood above the heart, only backs up into the liver and portal system), abdominal pain, jaundice, hepatosplenomegaly, ascites, ↑ LFT's, hepatic encephalopathy.

Other causes:
Polycythemia vera, pregnancy, OCP's, hepatocellular carcinoma, hypercoagulable states.

TX: **Heparin, Warfarin, diuretics**, sodium restriction

Reye Syndrome

Rapid progressive encephalopathy after a viral illness (**influenza**) that has been treated with **aspirin.**

SX:
1: Rash on hands and feet, vomiting, lethargy, confusion, nightmares
2: Fatty liver, hyperactive reflexes, hyperventilation
3: ↑↑↑ ALT and AST
4: Coma, cerebral edema
5: Dilated pupils, liver dysfunction
6: Seizures, multiple organ failure, flaccidity, hepatic encephalopathy, death

MOA: Aspirin ↓ β-oxidation and damages cellular mitochondria = apoptosis.

(Only use for aspirin in children is to treat Kawasaki disease)

Acetaminophen Toxicity MCC acute hepatic failure and 2nd MCC liver failure requiring transplantation. SX: Initially: asymptomatic. End organ damage does not present until 24 – 48 hours. **Minimum toxic single doses:** **Adult: 7.5 – 10g or > 4 grams (4,000 mg) in one day.** **Children (healthy, 1 – 6 yrs) 150 mg/kg – 200 mg/kg.** **SX: Up to 24 hrs after ingestion: asymptomatic or could show nausea, vomiting, fatigue, sweating.** **24 – 72 hrs: RUQ pain, tachycardia, hypotension, oliguria, dark urine.** **72 – 96 hrs: Hepatic necrosis, jaundice, coagulopathy, hematuria, hypoglycemia, hepatic encephalopathy, renal failure, confusion, death.** **DX: Rumack-Matthew nomogram (interprets the acetaminophen plasma concentration as correlated with time since ingestion to determine whether treatment is necessary).** **Test given after 4 hours after ingestion.** **If acetaminophen levels have not reached toxic levels by 4 hours, the patient is discharged. No need of treatment. If the levels have reached toxic levels, OD treatment is administered.** **Ingestion of 8 – 10 g of Acetaminophen can be toxic. 15g can be fatal.** **If the OD occurred more than 24 hours ago = no TX.** **NOTE: If they have ingested a bottle: treat them.** TX: **N-Acetylcysteine**	**Halothane Hepatitis** Severe liver disease from the inhaled anesthetic, Halothane from the metabolism of halothane to trifluoroacetic acid via oxidative reaction in the liver causing lethal hepatotoxicity. MC in the 1950's, replacing ether and chloroform as surgical anesthetics, in the United States, now found mainly in developing countries. SX: Fever, anorexia, nausea, myalgia, arthralgia. Labs: ↑↑ ALT and AST. TX: Supportive **Note**: On the exam, watch for someone that has gone in for a very common general surgery (cholecystectomy) and a few days later presents with fever, nausea, myalgias and increased LFT's.

Liver Cyst

Entamoeba histolytica Anaerobic protozoan Source: Cyst in water SX: Dysenteric **Bloody diarrhea**, liver abscess (thick exudate). Ultrasound shows a hypoechoic lesion (dark area) in the liver. Weight loss, fatigue, abdominal pain, ameboma (amebic granuloma, lesions inside the bowel) DX: Needle aspiration shows brown fluid. Trophozoites with RBC's or Cysts with **4 nuclei** in the stool. Cyst shows a "Cartwheel" distribution in the nucleus. No microorganisms are seen. **DO NOT BIOPSY the LIVER or RUPTURE CYST** TX: **Metronidazole** in the liver **Nitroimidazole** in the intestine	**Echinococcus granulosus** (AKA: **Hydatid Cyst**) Source: Host: Sheep and dogs with sheep. Ingestion of eggs from dog feces (fecal/oral). SX: **Hydatid cyst in liver**, lung, kidneys and spleen with daughter cyst inside, granulosus TX: Surgery. **DO NOT BIOPSY or CUT OPEN THE CYST, ANTIGENS WILL BE RELEASED CAUSING ANAPHYLAXIS AND DEATH.** Ethanol must be injected into the cyst to kill it before it can be removed. TX: **Albendazole**

Malaria **(For all details: see parasites in the Microbiology section)** RBC lysis by parasites **Anopheles** mosquito SX: Fever, headache, anemia, splenomegaly DX: Blood smear shows trophozoites inside of RBC **Life cycles:** sporozoites (injected by saliva of mosquitoes into the host's blood and then invade the hepatocytes in the liver); Merozoites (infect the RBC's); Trophozoites (grow in the RBC's); Schizonts (divide in the RBC's); **Hypnozoites (stay latent in the liver for up to 30 years: P. vivax, P. ovale** For Chloroquine resistance, use: **Mefloquine, Atovaquone, Proguanil** Side effect of Mefloquine: psychedelic nightmares. **For P. vivax and P. ovale must add Primaquine to kill the hypnozoites in the liver.**	

Hepatocellular Carcinoma and Tumors

Hepatocellular Carcinoma (HCC)	**Hepatocellular Adenoma (AKA: Hepatic Adenoma)**
MC malignant liver cancer. Associate with: **HEP B and C**, Hemochromatosis, A1AT deficiency, Wilsons Disease, alcoholic cirrhosis, Aflatoxin (from aflatoxins: dust from peanuts/nuts), non-alcoholic fatty liver disease causes, alcoholism SX: jaundice, ascites, blood clotting abnormalities (easy bleeding/bruising), unintentional weight loss, URQ pain, nausea, lethargy Labs: ↑ **AFP,** ↑ DCP (Des-gamma carboxyprothrombin – protein induced by vitamin K absence) DCP = marker for HCC DX: CT shows: Single tumor = primary Multiple tumors = metastasis Prevention: **Vaccination against HEP B.** TX: Surgery resection, liver transplant, radiation	Benign liver tumor associated with **OCP's** (high estrogen). MC in young to middle age women 20 - 40. Can also be associated with glycogen storage diseases type 1 and anabolic steroid use. SX: RUQ or epigastric pain, can sometime palpate a mass in the right lobe, jaundice. Most are asymptomatic and are discovered incidentally on imaging. Can progress to hepatocellular carcinoma. Histology: Well-circumcised nodules with sheets of hepatocytes with vacuolated cytoplasm. Normal hepatic architecture is absent. Portal and bile ducts are absent. Enlarged hepatocytes with glycogen and lipid deposits. Reticulin staining shows well-circumscribed nodules consisting of sheets of clear cytoplasm. Labs: ↑ ALP, ↑ GGT DX: MRI. **No biopsy**: cyst can rupture and patient can hemorrhage inside the abdomen. TX: **Discontinue OCP's**. If adenoma does not disappear after discontinuation of OCP, cyst can be surgically removed

Cavernous Hemangioma	**Angiosarcoma**
Collection of dilated blood **vessel** malformations (hemangioma) that form a benign tumor that slowly leaks blood (hemorrhage) out around the smooth muscle. DX: **Do not biopsy**: risk of hemorrhage 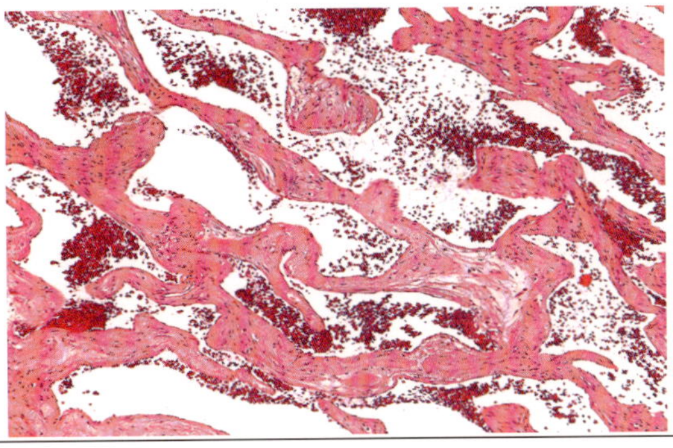	Malignant, fatal. Cancer of endothelial origin that lines vessel walls. Histology: Hemorrhage and necrosis. Increased nuclear to cytoplasm ratio. MCC: exposure to the gas **vinyl chloride**, which is used in producing **polyvinyl chloride (PVC – synthetic plastic, plastics)** plants. Also associate with exposure to **arsenic**-containing insecticides.

Alcohol and the Liver

- Liver metabolizes alcohol – the alcohol circulates in the bloodstream until metabolized (zero order)
- Alcohol is metabolized ½ oz per hour.
  Bottle of beer: 12 oz; ¼ glass wine: 6 oz; shot: 1 ¼ oz
- Pyruvate (from glycolysis) is unable to enter the TCA cycle or initiate gluconeogenesis (Oxaloacetate via Pyruvate carboxylase). It is shunted via **Pyruvate decarboxylase to Acetaldehyde and then to Ethanol via Alcohol dehydrogenase.** This creates and increased NADH: NAD ratio
- Pyruvate is unable to enter the TCA or initiate gluconeogenesis, **blood glucose levels cannot be maintained** causing hypoglycemia
- **↑ NADH/NAD ratio** is what leads to hepatic steatosis (AKA: Fatty liver dz)
- **Alcohol and stones are the #1 causes of acute pancreatitis**
- **Fomepizole** (antidote for methanol/ethylene glycol poisoning) inhibits Alcohol dehydrogenase
- **Disulfiram** inhibits Acetaldehyde dehydrogenase so allows Acetaldehyde to accumulate causing hangovers (Acetaldehyde dehydrogenase converts Acetaldehyde to Acetate.
  Antabuse Drugs cause a Disulfiram affect: **Metronidazole, Griseofulvin, Procarbazine, 1st generation Sulfonylureas (Chlorpropamide, Tolbutamide), Some Cephalosporins (Cefotetan, Cefoperazone, Cefamandole).**
  Cephalosporins: MOA: Methylthiotetrazole side chain blocks Aldehyde dehydrogenase and also block Vitamin K epoxide reductase causing hypoprothrombinemia (deficiency of prothrombin (Factor II) which ↑ risk of bleeding).

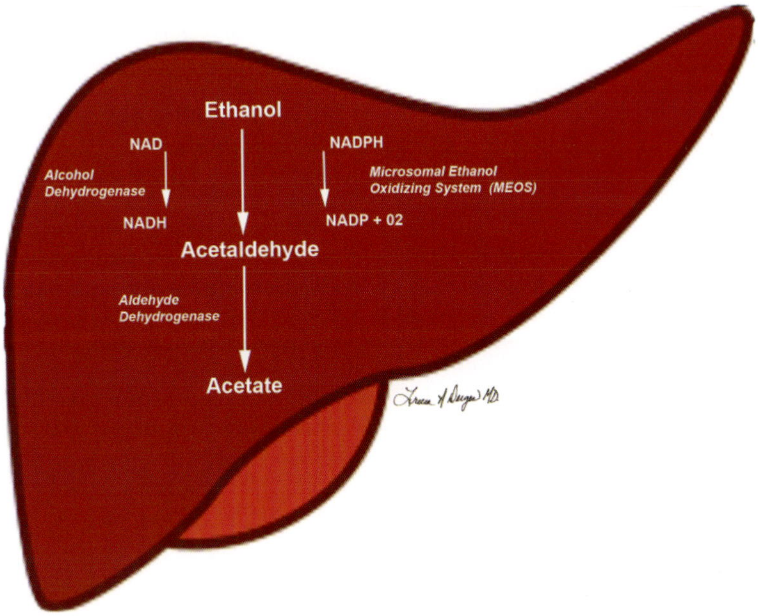

Alcoholic Liver Pathologies

All alcoholic steatosis, hepatitis and cirrhosis are reversible with ↓ or cessation of alcohol.

Alcohol and stones are the #1 causes of acute pancreatitis.

Hepatic Steatosis

(AKA: **Fatty Liver**, **Macrovesicula**r steatosis)
MCC: Excess alcohol intake (More than 2 drinks/day).

Large vacuoles of triglycerides (fat) accumulate in liver cells causing fatty liver.

Cause: **↑ NADH/NAD ratio**. (Alcohol causes ↑ NADH). NAD is required for the first complex in the ETC.

Alcohol intake → alcohol dehydrogenase → Acetaldehyde = NADH = ↑ NADH/NAD ratio.

Pathway: ↑ NADH = ↑ fatty acid synthesis → ↓ NAD → ↓ fatty acid oxidation (breakdown) → ↑ triglycerides = Fatty Liver

Histology: **Macrovesicular** fatty change. (Hepatocytes filled with fat giving a signet ring appearance). (**tip**: fat is big: macro)

Labs: AST > ALT

10% of patients will develop hepatocellular carcinoma.

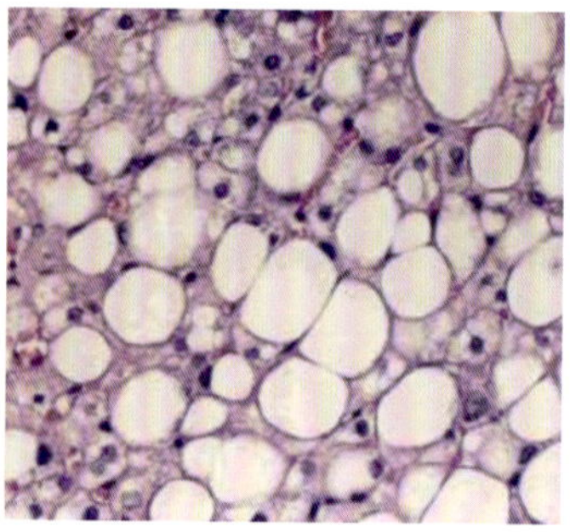

Non-alcoholic Fatty Liver Disease

AKA: Nonalcoholic Steatohepatitis (NASH)
MCC: Obesity
Other causes: Drugs: Amiodarone, methotrexate, expired tetracycline, HAART therapy, tamoxifen, mushroom poisoning, malnutrition, parenteral nutrition, gastric bypass, abetalipoproteinemia, glycogen storage diseases, fatty liver of pregnancy, metabolic syndrome.

Excess accumulation of fats in the liver (steatosis) due to other causes than alcohol.
(look for the same symptoms as in Hepatic steatosis but the patient does not drink)

Associated with Diabetes Type II (insulin resistance), metabolic syndrome (obesity), HTN.
(see other causes below).

SX: URQ pain/discomfort, mild jaundice, fatigue

Labs: Abnormal LFT's.

DX: Liver biopsy showing fatty infiltration.

TX: Diet, exercise, anti glycemic drugs, avoiding high-fructose corn syrup and trans-fats, gradual weight loss.

Other causes of non-alcoholic fatty liver: Metabolic (Abetalipoproteinemia, glycogen storage diseases, pregnancy, lipodystrophy); Nutrition (malnutrition, total parenteral nutrition, severe weight loss, gastric bypass); Drugs/toxins (Amiodarone, Methotrexate, Diltiazem, expired Tetracycline, HIV therapy, Glucocorticoids, Tamoxifen, mushroom poisoning); Inflammatory bowel disease, HIV, HEP C, A1AT deficiency, soft drinks high in fructose, genetics.

Alcoholic Hepatitis

Inflammation of the liver due to excess alcohol intake.

Associated with fatty liver and alcoholic liver disease.

Progressive: Fibrosis to cirrhosis.

SX: Jaundice, ascites, hepatic encephalopathy, hepatomegaly, fatigue.

Labs: AST > ALT (AST is usually 2 times higher than ALT), ↑ prothrombin time, can see ↑ bilirubin

Histology: **Ballooning** degeneration of hepatocytes (cells swelling with excess fat, water, protein) causing **necrosis**, PMN infiltration, and **Mallory Hyaline Bodies** (AKA: **pre-keratin** filaments accumulating in hepatocytes, (AKA: **eosinophilic inclusion bodies).**
Mallory bodies are intermediate cytokeratin filament proteins that are bound by other proteins (heat shock proteins) or are ubiquinated.

Mallory bodies are also seen in: Wilson's disease, hepatocellular carcinoma, morbid obesity, primary biliary cirrhosis and non-alcoholic cirrhosis.

Alcoholic Cirrhosis

Continual abuse of alcohol replaces healthy liver tissue with fibrosed scar tissue that destroys the liver: blocks flow of blood/nutrients, hormones and inhibits the filtering of drugs and toxins.
Blockage of blood flow causes ↑↑ portal HTN leaving to many pathologies (See complete list below)

Higher risk: HEP B and HEP C, alcohol, any of the non-alcoholic fatty liver diseases.
(2 – 3 drinks/day for several years ↑ risk)

SX: Pruritis, fatigue, lower leg edema, jaundice, portal HTN, esophageal varices, gastric varices (dilated stomach veins), telangiectasis (spider angioma), **ascites (due to low oncotic pressure)**, hepatic encephalopathy, splenomegaly, palmar erythema, thrombocytopenia (due to splenic sequestration).

Labs: Paracentesis of ascites fluid: SAAG (Serum-to-ascites albumin gradient. >1.1 is a transudate due to ascites (from portal HTN).

DX: Liver biopsy

Cirrhosis cont'd

Histology: **Micronodular** shrunken liver. (Hobnail and irregular appearance). Sclerosis around Central Vein in Zone III. (**tip**: with cirrhosis, your liver is tiny = micro).

TX: Not reversible, no cure. Alcohol abuse makes it difficult to be approved for transplant.

TX for Portal HTN: **Propanolol**
TX for ascites: **Spironolactone**
TX for **hepatic encephalopathy**: **Lactulose**
TX for ↓ work load on heart: **Nitrates**

Complication: Spontaneous Bacterial Peritonitis (SBP). SBP lab's will show cell count > 250 of neutrophils.

TX: **Cefotaxime**

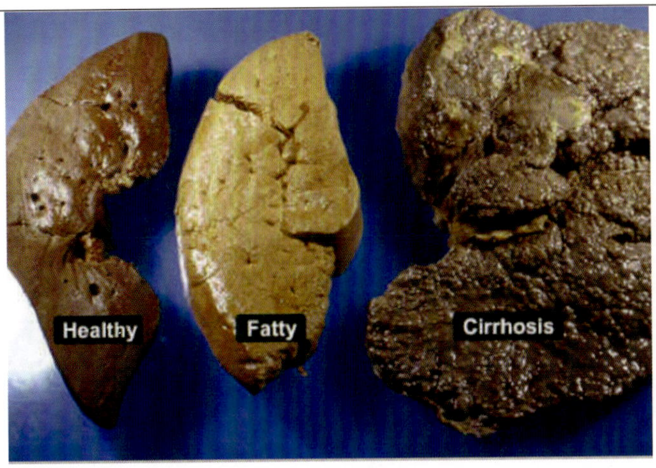

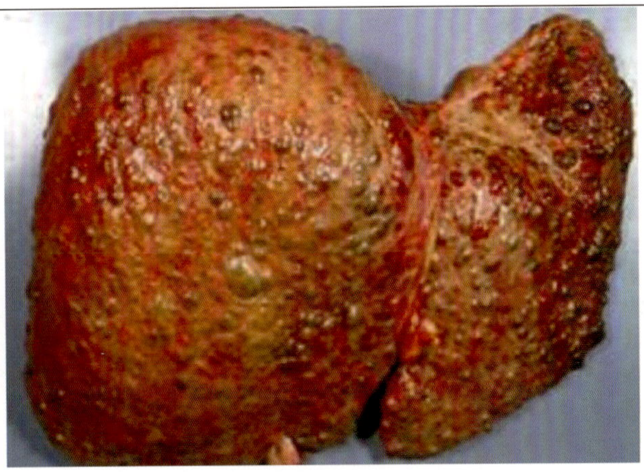

Cirrhosis of the liver

Additional affects of Cirrhosis and Portal HTN on the body:

- Esophageal varicies (left gastrics stemming from azygos)
- Caput medusae
- **Ascites**
  TX: Spironolactone
- Hemorrhoids
- Hepatic encephalopathy
- Jaundice
- Asterixis ("flapping" tremor of the hands)
- Bleeding due to ↓ in clotting factors and ↑ prothrombin time
- Lower leg edema
- ↓ body hair
- Palmar erythema
- Telangiectasis (AKA: spider amnioma, spider nevi)
- Fetor hepaticus (malodorous breath)
- Gynecomastia
  Due to the failure of liver to degrade estrogen
- Testicular atrophy, ↓ libido, impotence
- Sepsis (blood poisoning)
- Peptic ulcers
- Melena (due to peptic ulcer bleeds)
- Anemia
- Hypoglycemia

Alcoholics

- **Megaloblastic anemia with hypersegmented neutrophils.**
  This **differentiates between** deficiencies in Vitamin B-12 and Vitamin E as to the cause of dorsal column symptoms and differentiates whether it is deficiency in B-12 or Folate and drug/alcohols as being the cause of megaloblastic anemia. Only Vitamin B-12 and Folate show megablastic anemia and hypersegmented neutophils.
- Most common deficiency: **Vitamin B-1 (Thiamine).**
  Without Vitamin B-1, the Pyruvate dehydrogenase complex can't be formed so Pyruvate is not able to proceed into the TCA cycle or initiate gluconeogenesis. It is shunted via Pyruvate decarboxylase to Acetaldehyde.
- Alcoholics are also deficient on **folate.** Without folate there is ↓ purine and pyrimidine synthesis = ↓ Thymidine synthesis.
- Must supplement with **Vitamin B-1 and Folate** (AKA: "Banana Bag") before given before giving any carbohydrate containing fluids or food to stop complications (Wernicke's syndrome). **"Banana Bag":** IV fluids containing thiamine, folic acid, magnesium sulfate.
- Complications: Wernicke's and Korsakoff syndrome.

Wernicke's Encephalopathy
Deficiency in Vitamin B-1.
Wernicke's area; Posterior section of the Superior Temporal Lobe in the left cerebral hemisphere.

Ophthalmoplegia (nystagmus)
Dementia (altered mental state, confusion, decrease in awareness)
Ataxia (gate, balance disturbance)
Hypotension
Tachycardia
Hypothermia

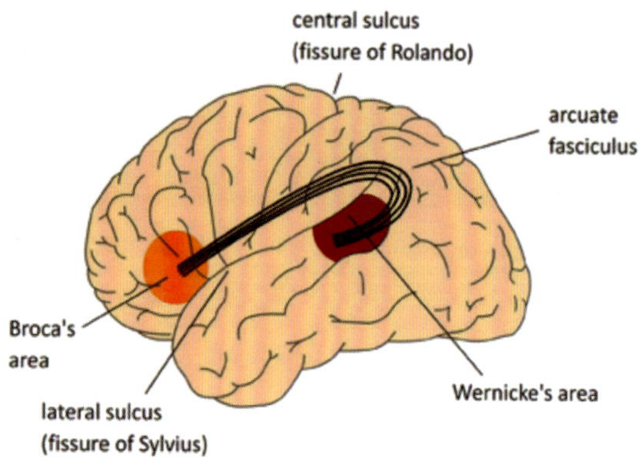

Korsakoff's Syndrome
Severe memory impairment.
Damages the **mammillary bodies.**

Anterograde amnesia (loss of ability for making new memories)
Retrograde amnesia (loss of previous memories)
Aphasia (speech)
Apraxia (motor disorder, can't perform task)
Agnosia (sensory disorder, can't recognize objects, persons, shapes, sounds, smells)
Deficit in executive functions

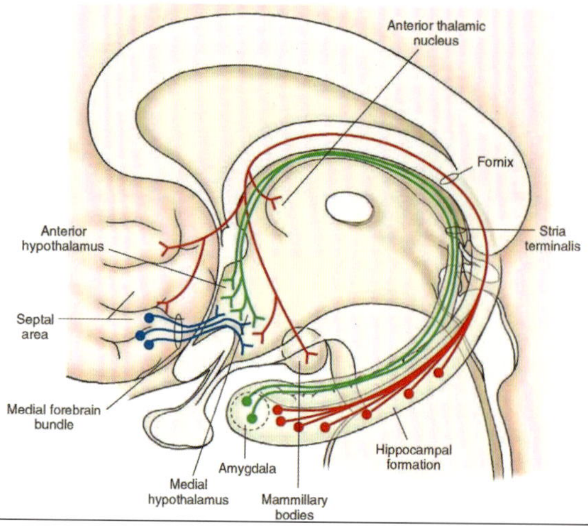

Alcoholism: Alcohol Dependence

- Alcohol **Dependence**: Individual feels that they need the drug in order to make it through the day. They develop physical and psychological dependence upon the alcohol.
- Alcohol **Abuse**: individual is so dependent upon the alcohol that it leads to harmful consequences. Relationships are impacted. Failure to fulfill obligations. Individual has strong cravings to use alcohol and may put themselves in dangerous situations, physical or illegal. If they discontinue the alcohol they will suffer withdrawal symptoms and potentially death.

Stages of Overcoming Substance Addiction

- **Pre-contemplation**: Individual does **not** recognize there is any problem.
- **Contemplation:** Individual now realizes there is a problem but has **no interest** in changing the behavior. (This usually occurs when a partner leaves.)
- **Preparation**: Individual now realizes they **need/want to change** their behavior. (this usually happens when someone is harmed: emotionally or physically).
- **Action:** Individual is actively taking steps to change their behavior.
- **Maintenance**: Individual is maintaining the change in behavior.
- **Relapse**: Individual stops maintaining behavior changes and returns to old behaviors.

Alcohol Withdrawl (AKA: DT's)

- Withdrawl begins between **6 and 24 hours** after the last drink.
  (**Beware** of the patient that has been admitted for routine work/surgery that becomes aggitated, aggressive or difficult.)
  SX: Insomnia, anxiety, diaphoresis, headaches, palpitations.
  TX: Thiamine, folate, glucose, **Diazepam, Lorazepam or Chlordiazepoxide**
  (**tip**: give "DIE"zepam to an alcoholic so they won't "DIE") or (**tip**: picture a mercedes "BENZ" with a bottle of alcohol in it).
- 12 – 24 Hours after last drink
  SX: Visual and tactile hallucinations (feeling or seeing bugs crawling on them).
- 48 Hours after last drink: Seizures
- 48 – 96 Hours after last drink
  SX: **Delirium tremens (rapid onset of confusion)**, Hallucinations continue, HTN, diaphoresis, disorientation, fever, seizures, shivering, agitation, death

Alcohol Management

Acute Outpatient Management

- Refrain from leaving until alcohol level returns to the legal limit
- Do not allow more intake of alcohol
- Do not allow the patient to drive or operate any machinery
- Sedate patient if they become agitated or aggressive (do not give Haldol: reduces seizure threshold).
- Consider admission into detox/inpatient

Acute Inpatient Management

- Be aware of withdrawal symptoms (begins between 6 and 24 hours after the last drink).
- Administer: IV or IM **Thiamine, magnesium, potassium, folate, B12** ("Banana Bag") to prevent Wernicke-Korsakoff.
- Administer **Chordiazepoxide or Diazepam** (Benzodiazepines).
  If patient has severe liver disease give short acting benzodiazepines**: Lorazepam or Oxazepam**.

Chronic Management

- Involve patient in a rehabilitation group (such as AA: Alcoholics Anonymous).
  NOTE: The most affective management of alcohol abuse and prevention of relapse is **Alcoholics Anonymous** (AA).
- Provide psychotherapy and medical therapy together.
  Note: Disulfiram (Antibuse) has poor compliance.

Biliary Tract

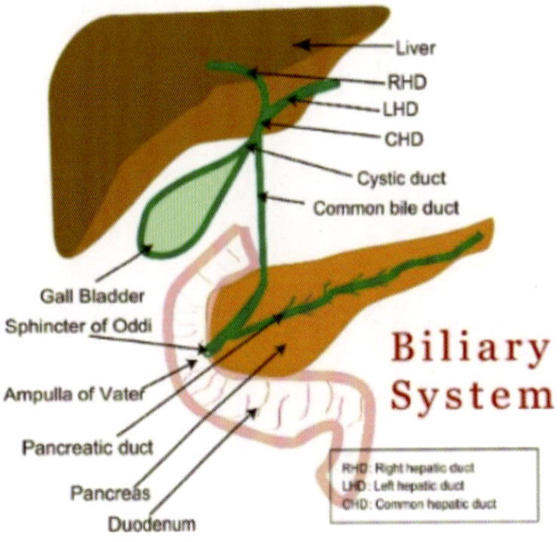

- Biliary tract = liver, gall bladder and bile ducts.
- Bile is synthesized in the liver.
- Bile is stored in the gall bladder until CCK stimulates gallbladder contraction releasing bile into the duodenum to aid in the digestion/absorption of lipids and fat-soluble substances (ie: fat soluble vitamins DEAK).
- Composition of bile in the gallbladder: Water, bile salts, conjugated bilirubin, electrolytes, fats (cholesterol, fatty acids, lecithin)
- Bile also aids in the excretion for bilirubin
- Without bile fats can't be digested and will be excreted in the feces (steatorrhea)
- Bile salts (AKA: bile acids) synthesis occurs in the liver via the cytochrome P450 oxidation of cholesterol via the enzyme 7 alpha-hydroxylase. Bile acids are conjugated with either glycine or taurine. Conjugated bile acids = bile salts. Synthesis of bile acids is a major function of cholesterol.
- Biliary obstruction: usually due to gallstones in the bile ducts. Bile ducts carry bile from the liver and gall bladder to the duodenum. Extra bile is stored in the gall bladder.
- Pathway of bile: Bile canaliculi (tube that collects bile secreted by hepatocytes) ➔ Canals of Hering (destroyed in biliary cirrhosis) ➔merge with other bile canaliculi to form the intrahepatic bile ductule ➔interlobular bile ducts ➔left and right hepatic ducts ➔ merge to form common hepatic duct ➔exits liver and joins cystic duct (from gall bladder) ➔ merge to form the common bile duct ➔ merges with pancreatic duct at Ampulla of Vater ➔ entering duodenum
- Common bile duct is part of the portal triad (hepatic artery, hepatic vein, common bile duct, lymphatic vessels, branch of vagus nerve) carried in the hepatoduodenal ligament
- Bile flows the opposite direction from blood
- Obstruction always shows light stools and dark urine and labs always show ↑ bilirubin, ↑ ALP, ↑ GGT

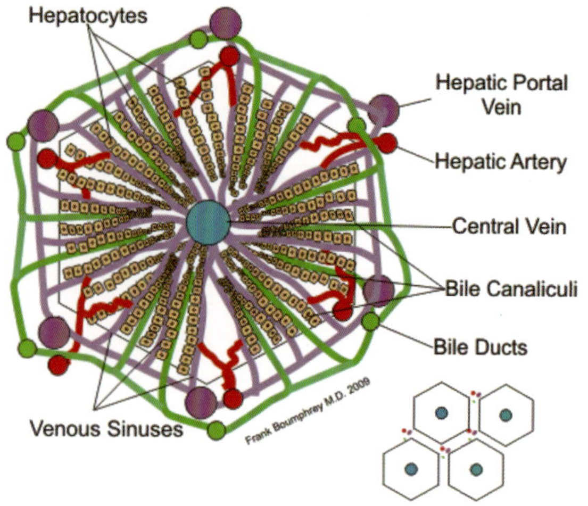

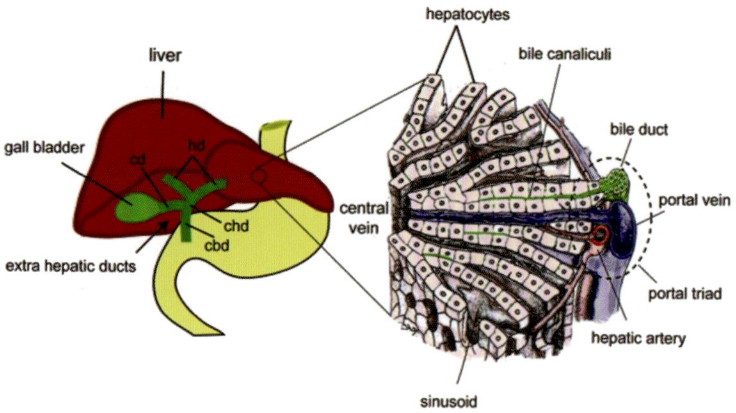

Biliary Tract Pathologies

Primary Sclerosing Cholangitis	Primary Biliary Cirrhosis	Secondary Biliary Cirrhosis
Fibrosis of the bile ducts inside and outside of the liver. (AKA: **intra and extra hepatic).** **Anti-smooth muscle antibody (ASMA)** Associated with **ulcerative colitis**. SX: **Severe pruritus**, fatigue, jaundice, episodic acute cholangitis (infection within bile ducts), malabsorption (steatorrhea), cirrhosis, portal HTN, hepatomegaly, hepatic encephalopathy. Labs: **P-ANCA**, ↑ IgM, ↑ ALP, ↑ Bilirubin DX: **ERCP** (endoscopic retrograde cholangiopancreatography) shows **"beading"** (alternating strictures and dilation) of the bile ducts inside and outside of liver. 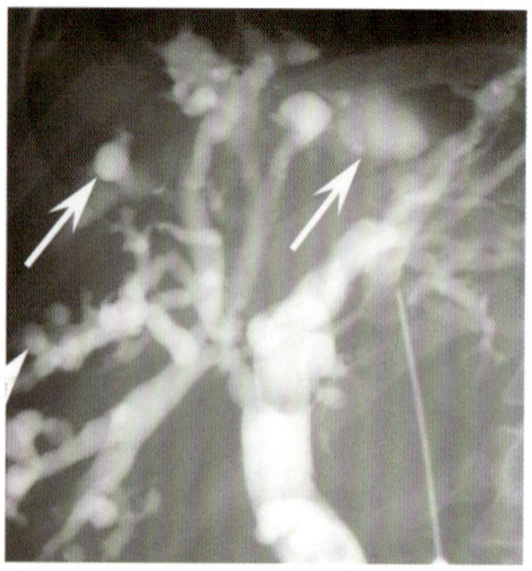 TX: Liver transplant Ursodeoxycholic acid can help improve LFT's and improve bile flow (bile salts) Note: ERCP test deal with the common bile duct and pancreas pathologies. HIDA test is assocated with the gal bladder (ejection fraction of the bile).	Autoimmune **Anti-mitochondrial** antibodies against the pyruvate dehydrogenase complex. MC: Middle-aged woman. Slow, progressive destruction of **intrahepatic bile ducts** (Canals of Hering) allowing bile and toxins to build up in the liver (cholestasis) causing **fibrosis and cirrhosis**. Histology: granulomas and lymphocyte infiltration SX: Pruritus, jaundice, cirrhosis, portal HTN, xanthoma (cholesterol deposits), hepatosplenomegaly, hepatic encephalopathy. Common with other autoimmune dz. Associated with RA and Sjögren's syndrome, CREST, Celiac dz Labs: ↑ LFT's, ↑GGT, ↑ALP, IgM BIT: ↑ ALP and normal bilirubin, ↑ IgM. MAT: **Anti-mitochondrial antibody** (AMA) TX: Liver transplant Ursodeoxycholic acid can help reduce the cholestasis and improve LFT's.	Bile ducts are unable to transport bile effectively due to a secondary **extrahepatic** cause that results in blockage, scarring or inflammation. Secondary causes: Congenital: biliary atresia, cystic fibrosis, gallstones, cancer of the pancreatic head. SX: Pruritus, jaundice, fatigue, xanthomas, dark urine, light stools, easy bruising, arthritis, fluid retention. Labs: ↑ cholesterol, ↑ conjugated bilirubin, ↑ ALP

Gallbladder Pathologies

Acute Cholecystitis	**Cholelithiasis: gallstones**	**Cholestasis**
Cholecystitis: Inflammation of the gallbladder (cystic duct inflammation/infection due to retention of bile in the gallbladder and 2° infection by bacteria: e. coli, Klebsiella, Enterobacter or Bacteroides) MCC: blockage of **cystic duct** by gallstones (cholelithiasis) SX: + Murphy sign, sudden RUQ pain, **fever, No jaundice**, radiation to the right shoulder, vomiting, anorexia, thick gallbladder wall. **Note**: Cholecystitis pain radiates to the side and then to the back, but pain from acute pancreatitis goes directly, straight to the back. Pain can also occur after eating. (stimulation of an inflamed gallbladder is painful). Labs: No ALP, ↑ WBC Chronic cholecystitis: Same SX plus: repeated gall bladder attacks, gallbladder with thick wall, shrunken and fibrosis. DX: Ultrasound or **HIDA** scan to check for stones/obstruction in **cystic duct**. HIDA scan: radioactive isotope injected. If the gallbladder is visualized within 1 hour = no disease. If gallbladder is **not visualized** within 4 hours due to accumulation of the isotope = cholecystitis or cystic duct obstruction. (**tip:** NOT visualized is NOT good) ERCP to check for stones/obstruction in the **common bile duct (pancreas)**	MCC: Cholecystitis due to blockage of the cystic duct causing **Acute Biliary Colic**: **Acute Biliary Colic** Type of pain from the gallbladder contracting against gallstones. SX: **No fever**, **No jaundice**, + Murphy's sign, RUQ pain, that can radiate to right shoulder, nausea, vomiting, anorexia, **Pain occurs after eating (esp. with spicy and greasy foods)** Pain resolves between meals. Labs: No increase in WBC High risk for developing gallstones: female, age, race, obesity, OCP's, prolonged fasting, rapid weight loss, total parenteral nutrition, cirrhosis, family history, pregnancy. DX: Ultrasound TX: Cholecystectomy (Gallbladder removal)	Bile is not able to flow from the liver to the duodenum (due to obstruction, gallstone, tumor, metabolic, genetic, medicine side effect) causing malabsorption. SX: Jaundice, dark urine, light stool, pruritis. (Obstruction always shows light stools and dark urine and labs always show ↑ bilirubin, ↑ ALP, ↑ GGT). Histology: **hepatocytes show brown/green plugs** because bile can't be excreted causing **bile lakes** leading to hepatic necrosis. Intrahepatic causes: Drugs (Erythromycin, OCP's, steroids, Cimetidine, Chlorpromazine, estrogen, gold salts, nitroglycerin), 1° Biliary Cirrhosis, Cholestasis of pregnancy, 1° Sclerosing Cholangitis, **parenteral nutrition** (IV feeding that bypasses eating and digestion: therefore the gallbladder is not stimulated by CCK, so it remains in stasis: which can lead to gallstones). Extrahepatic: 1° Sclerosing Cholangitis, Choledocholithiasis, biliary dilation, malignancy (pancreatic or gallbladder) Malabsorption: No emulsification = ↓ fat-soluble vitamins (DEAK) and no biliary dilation.

Ascending Cholangitis **Ascending infection of the bile duct from bacteria** at the junction of the duodenum. Bile duct is usually already obstructed with gallstones. Medical emergency. Labs: ↑ WBC, ↑ C-reactive protein, abnormal LFT's, ↑ bilirubin, ↑ ALP, ↑ GGT. Bacteria: MC: E. coli. Others: Klebsiella, Enterobacter. SX: **Charcot's triad: Pain, jaundice and fever. (Chills).** Abdominal pain, low blood pressure, confusion, rigors (uncontrolled shaking). Progression to **Reynold's Pentad**: Charcot's triad **plus** septic shock and mental confusion. Can lead to death. TX: ERCP to unblock the bile duct **Ampicillin and Gentamicin**	**Choledocholithiasis** Gallstone obstructing the common bile duct or gallstones in the gallbladder. SX: SX: Fever, pain, **jaundice**, anorexia, no inflammation, nausea, vomiting. Labs: ↑ ALP, ↑ direct bilirubin **Cholecystectomy** Surgical removal of gallbladder.	**Acute Acalculous Cholecystitis** Development of cholecystitis in a gallbladder without gallstones. Complication of various other medical or surgical conditions. MC occurs in critically ill patients. Cause: Ischemia or reperfusion injury to the gallbladder, bile stasis, opioids, ventilators, total parenteral nutrition, burns, severe trauma, HIV. DX: Ultrasound shows: distended, thickened gallbladder with or without pericholecystic fluid. Labs: ↑ WBC
Post Cholecystectomy Syndrome Abdominal symptoms after removal a cholecystectomy. SX: nausea, vomiting, gas, bloating, diarrhea, URQ pain. (Experiences same pain prior to the gallbladder surgery) Symptoms can be temporary to lifelong. Chronic diarrhea (bile acid diarrhea) that can be treated with: **Cholestyramine** (bile acid sequestrant) DX: Ultrasound shows: dilated common bile duct.	**Choledochal Cysts** (AKA: bile duct cyst) Congenital cystic dilation of the bile ducts. MC in first year of life. SX: Jaundice, intermittent abdominal pain, URQ mass. TX: Surgery	**Porcelain Gallbladder** **Dystrophic calcification** (calcium salt deposits) and inflammatory scarring of the gallbladder wall. MC: middle age, obese females Associated with gallbladder cancer. SX: Abdominal pain (AKA: Biliary colic) (esp. after meals), jaundice, vomiting. TX: Cholecystectomy 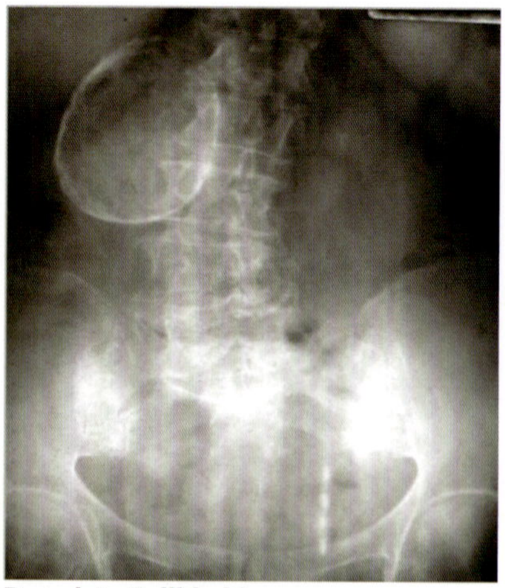 Porcelain Gallbladder

Emphysematous Cholecystitis	Vanishing Bile Duct Syndrome	Postoperative Cholestasis
(AKA: Clostridial Cholecystitis) Acute infection of the gallbladder by gas forming organisms (Clostridium, E. coli) Medical Emergency. CT shows air-fluid levels in gallbladder (AKA: Crepitus) High risk: Elderly males (esp. Diabetics), immunocompromised Complications: Compromise of cystic artery (obstruction or stenosis), gangrene perforation. TX: Cholecystectomy, fluids, parental antibiotics: **Ampicillin plus Sulbactam, Piperacillin plus Tazobactam, Clindamycin plus Metronidazole**	↓ quantity of bile ducts (Ductopenia) MCC: 1° Biliary sclerosis	Benign Transient jaundice after major prolonged abdominal or cardiovascular surgery that had a hypotensive episode with extensive blood loss and transfusions. It can also be due to extra hepatic biliary obstruction due to intra-abdominal complications or drugs given postoperatively. SX: Hypotension, jaundice in 2 – 3 days, no fever Labs: ↑↑ ALP, normal ALT/AST TX: Self-resolving.

Cholelithiasis (Gallstones)

- Calculus (stone) formed within the gallbladder as a congregation of bile components
- Stone can pass from the gallbladder and cause obstruction in the cystic duct, common bile duct, pancreatic duct, ampulla of Vater
- **CCK stimulates contraction of the gallbladder** (compressing against the stones causing pain. After digestion is complete, pain subsides)
- Gallstones obstructing bile ducts can lead to ascending cholangitis and/or pancreatitis (medical emergencies)
- Asymptomatic ("silent stones") require no treatment
- Symptomatic gallstones: RUQ pain that can radiate to the right shoulder or between shoulder blades, nausea, vomiting. Pain usually occurs after eating spicy/greasy foods or after drinks
- + Murphy's sign on physical exam
- **NOTE: Cholesterol synthesis (HMG CoA Reductase) is ↑** when there are cholesterol gal stones (stones are due to too much cholesterol).

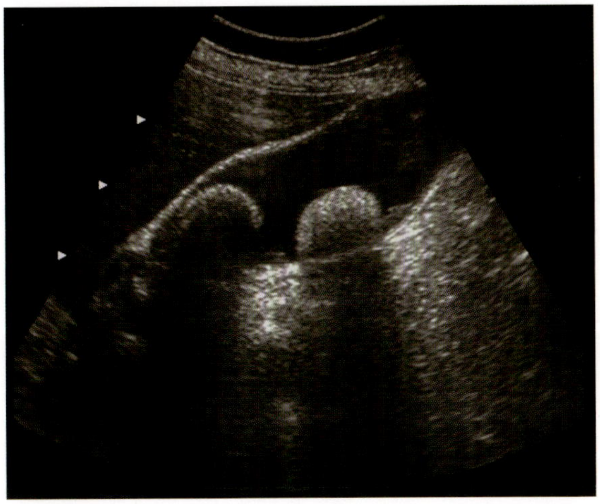

Cholesterol Gallstones
80% of stones in the Western world.
Radio**L**ucent
(tip: **L** = **L**ost)

Appearance: 2 – 3cm, Light yellow, dark green, brown, chalk white.

Composition of the stones: ↑ cholesterol, ↓ bile acid content and ↓ phosphatidylcholine.

Cholesterol Stones: ↑ Risk: Women, overweight, reproductive years, pregnancy, ↑ age, estrogen therapies (OCP or pregnancy), rapid weight loss, Crohn's, Cystic Fibrosis, **Bile Acid Resin Drugs (Cholestyramine, Colestipol, Colesevelam), Fibrate drugs (Clofibrate, Bezafibrate, Fenofibrate**), total parenteral nutrition (TPR).

Note: Anytime that cholesterol is not being used to synthesize other products (bile salts) it builds up ↑ the risk of gallstones.
Example: Fibrates: Fibrates inhibit the enzyme 7-α hydroxylase, which converts cholesterol into bile. If cholesterol is not allowed to be converted to bile it builds up = ↑ risk of gallstones.

↓ Risk: low carb diet, exercise, decaffeinated coffee

DX: Ultrasound

TX: Cholecystectomy
Ursodeoxycholic Acid for patients that are not good surgical candidates (elder, sick, pregnant)
Surgery can be performed during the 2nd trimester of pregnancy.

NOTE: HIDA scan (Hepatobiliary Iminodiacetic Acid) is the test that measures the ejection fraction of bile from the gallbladder. Usually required before insurance will approve gallbladder surgery. HIDA is used for gallstones in the gallbladder and the cystic duct.

NOTE: ERCP test looks for stones in the bile ducts or pancreatic duct. It is also used to view pancreas pathologies. (not used for stones in the gallbladder or cystic duct).

Pigment Gallstones

Black and Brown Pigment Stones

Black Stones: Radiopaque
Composed of: Bilirubin and calcium (calcium phosphate salts)

Brown (Mixed) Stones: Radiolucent
Composed of calcium carbonate, palmitate phosphate, bilirubin, bile pigments.

Causes: chronic hemolysis (sickle cell and hereditary spherocytosis), cirrhosis, biliary tract infections, (parasitic infections: MC: Asians)

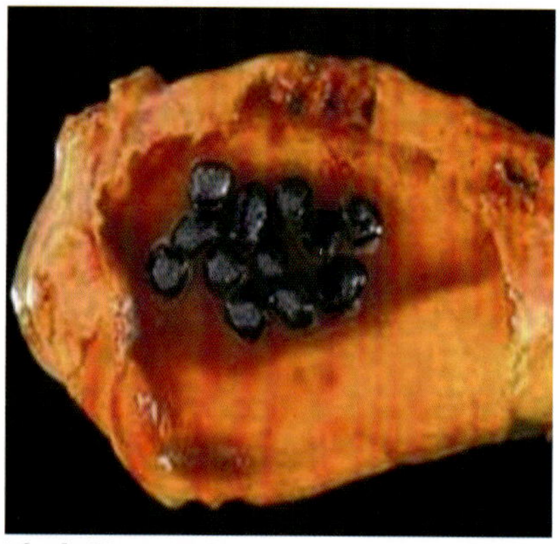

Black Pigment Stones

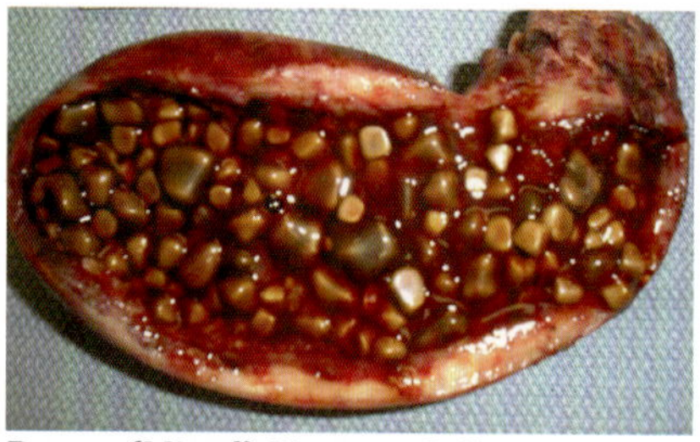

Brown (Mixed) Pigment Gallstones

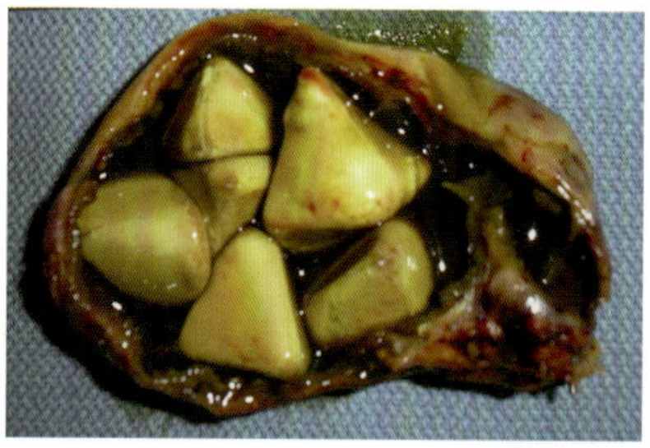

Cholesterol Gallstones

Choledocholithiasis

Stone obstructing the common bile duct.

SX: Fever, pain, jaundice, anorexia, no inflammation, nausea, vomiting.

Labs: ↑ ALP, ↑ direct bilirubin

Gallstone Ileus

Bowel obstruction due to a gallstone in the lumen most commonly at the ileocecal valve because of a fistula that formed between the gallbladder and small intestine.

Abdominal x-ray shows air in the gallbladder. (Air from the intestine coming through the fistula and into the gallbladder).

Gallbladder/Bile Differentials

Pathology	Differential	Notes
Bile Duct Pathology		
Primary Sclerosing Cholangitis	Extra and intrahepatic. Involves bile ducts between liver and intestine. Associated: Ulcerative colitis. p-ANCA. No antibodies.	
Primary Biliary Cirrhosis	Intrahepatic. Involves bile ducts in the liver and outside the liver (between liver and intestines) **Anti-mitochondrial antibodies**.	
Painful Gallbladder Pathology: ALL have URQ pain		
Acute Cholecystitis	Pain (acute biliary colic), fever and NO jaundice	Due to inflammation of the gallbladder.
Cholelithiasis (Gallstones)	Pain (acute biliary colic), NO fever and NO jaundice	Due to stones in the gallbladder or cystic duct.
Choledocholithiasis	Pain, jaundice and NO fever	
Ascending Cholangitis	Pain, Jaundice, Fever and Chills	Reynold's Pentad: when Cholangitis progresses: Hypotension, confusion.

Bilirubin

- Bilirubin is the breakdown product of heme (RBC that have died or been lysed).
- Bilirubin is from the normal clearance of old RBC's
- Hyperbilirubinemia is due to many factors: hemolysis, liver pathologies, drugs, hepatitis, chemotherapy, biliary obstruction
- Bilirubin is responsible for the yellow color in bruises, brown color in feces (converted to **stercobilin**) (**tip**: "S" = stool), yellow color of urine (converted to **urobilin**) (**tip**: "U" = urine) and yellow color in jaundice.
- Bilirubin is excreted in the bile and urine.
- Biliverdin (green bile pigment, a product of heme catabolism) is converted to bilirubin via biliverdin reductase.
- Unconjugated (AKA: Indirect) is fat soluble
- Conjugated (AKA: Direct) is water and goes into bile and excreted into the small intestine. Bile acid resorbed in the terminal ileum and bilirubin is not reabsorbed and goes into the colon. Bacteria in the colon metabolize it into urobilinogen, which is then oxidized into stercobilin (brown feces color) and excreted in the feces. Some of the urobilinogen is reabsorbed and processed by the kidneys (urobilinogen is oxidized into urobilin (yellow urine color) and excreted in the urine.
- Conjugation: Occurs in the liver. Unconjugated bilirubin is conjugated to glucuronic acid via glucuronyltransferase (UDP-glucuronosyltransferase, UGT).
- **Jaundice**: yellowish tinge of the skin and whites of the eyes (sclera) due to high bilirubin levels. Normal levels of bilirubin: < 1.0 mg/dL. Levels > 2 – 3 mg/dL result in jaundice. High bilirubin levels in babies may cause **kernicterus.**
  Caution: yellow skin can also be caused by **carotenemia** (excess intake of carrots) causing increased serum carotenoids and by certain medications: ie: **Rifampin.**

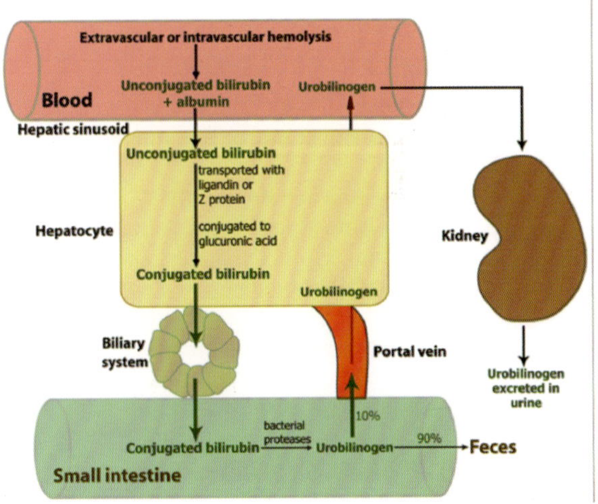

Bilirubin Lab Levels

Elevated serum bilirubin levels or elevated conjugated bilirubin in the urine indicates a pathological process.
Total bilirubin levels are the total of both conjugated (direct) and unconjugated (indirect) together
Indirect bilirubin levels are calculated from the Total Bilirubin minus the Direct Bilirubin
Urine test: Bilirubin is not normally found in the urine. Presence of bilirubin and urobilinogen can indicate an obstructive liver disease pathology. When there is liver disease, the urobilinogen cycle is inhibited which increases urobilinogen levels. (Urobilinogen gives urine its yellow color (**urobilin**).

Hyperbilirubinemia

Mild elevation of bilirubin: Gilbert's syndrome, Rotor syndrome, Hemolysis
Moderate elevation of bilirubin: Hepatitis, chemotherapy, some drugs (Sulfonamides, Antipsychotics)
High elevation of bilirubin: Crigler-Najjar syndrome, Dubin-Johnson syndrome, choledocholithiasis, bile duct obstruction (stones), cirrhosis, primary biliary cirrhosis, neonatal hyperbilirubinaemia (newborn liver is not processing the bilirubin)

Bilirubin Pathologies

UNCONJUGATED (INDIRECT) PATHOLOGIES (Fat Soluble)

Crigler-Najjar Syndrome, Type I, AR • Unconjugated • Bilirubin levels of >20 umol/l (very high levels of bilirubin) • **Absence of UDP glucuronosyltransferase. They are not able to conjugate.** • Extreme jaundice and high levels of serum bilirubin in first few days of life • **Kernicterus** • Treatment with phenobarbitol will not decrease levels of bilirubin • Death unless liver transplant	**Crigler-Najjar Syndrom, Type II, AR** • Unconjugated • **NO Kernicterus** • Bilirubin levels of <20 umol/l • Treatment with phenobarbitol WILL decrease levels of bilirubin
Gilbert's Syndrome • Unconjugated • **Reduced** activity of UDP glucuronosyltransferase. • Patient leads normal life, basically asymptomatic • Jaundice only occurs when patient is **stressed** (ex: exams, break up, etc.), exertion, fasting's or infections	**Unconjugated Bilirubin (Indirect) Complication and treatment** • **Kernicterus**: build up of unconjugated bilirubin into the brain = bilirubin encephalopathy. • Bilirubin is neurotoxic = severe brain damage or death • Labs: high levels of serum bilirubin • SX: lethargy (won't wake up to feed), decreased feeding, hypotonia, high pitched cry, spasmodic torticollis (AKA: cervical dystonia) are involuntary neck movements, opisthotonus (muscle spasms), vertical gaze palsy, fever, seizures • TX: **Exchange transfusion (AKA: Plasmapheresis)** (patients blood is removed and replaced)
Physiologic Jaundice • Unconjugated • **Appears after first day of life, during the first week** • Due to decreased activity of UDP-glucuronosyltransferase because the liver is **immature** and is not conjugating adequately and that Fetal Hb is being broken down and replace by adult Hb • Last about 2 weeks in term infants, and up to one month in premature and exclusively breastfed infants • Higher risk with premature babies • **Mildly** elevated **serum indirect bilirubin** • Higher risk with diabetic mothers, Asian and Native American infants • TX: **Phototherapy: converts unconjugated bilirubin to water-soluble form**	**Hemolytic Disease of the Newborn (ABO)** • Unconjugated • **AKA: Erythroblastosis fetalis (Parvo B19)** • **Maternal IgG antibodies** pass into the fetal circulation and cause hemolysis to the fetal RBC's Anti-A and anti-B antibodies are usually IgM and do not pass through the placenta • Can cause hydrops fetalis (heart failure) • **Can occur in a first born baby** (Unlike Rh Disease which first occurs in the 2nd baby) • More common in mother's with blood type O, very seldom to mother's with A or B • Jaundice develops in the first day of life • Fetal anemia TX: High bilirubin levels = exchange transfusion

Breast Milk Failure • Unconjugated due to a "biochemical" problem • Develops **after the first week (between 1 and 2 weeks)** • Due to interaction between hormone and enzymes in breast milk affecting conjugation • Stop breast feeding for a few days, use formula, then restart breastfeeding • Self Limiting	**Breast Feeding Failure** • Unconjugated due to a "mechanical" problem • Occurs **within the first week of life** (overlaps with physiologic jaundice) • Due to **inadequate breast milk volume or intake** = bowel movements to remove bilirubin from the body. • Failure to thrive • Work with mother on longer for more frequent feedings to stimulate adequate milk production. Can also supplement with formula. • (**tip**: "F"eeding goes "F"irst. Its in the first week whereas breast milk failure is after the first week).
Rh Disease (AKA: Rhesus, Rhesus Hemolytic Disease of the Newborn) • Unconjugated • **Mother is Rh negative, father is Rh positive and baby is Rh positive** • **Mother's antibodies (IgG) against Rhesus D antigen on babies RBC's** • In first birth mother is exposed to infants blood causing development of antibodies so that all **subsequent pregnancies are in danger** • Severe disease causes erythroblastosis fetalis (AKA: hemolytic disease of the newborn), hydrops fetalis or stillbirth • DX: **Indirect Coombs test for IgG in the mother** TX: Rhesus D negative mothers given an anti-RhD IgG immunoglobulin injection (AKA: **RhoGAM**) **at 28 weeks gestation** Non-sensitized mothers are given **RhoGAM** immediately (within 72 hrs) after birth	Other pathologies that cause unconjugated bilirubin: Spherocytosis, Arteriovenous malformations, G6PD deficiency, Pyruvate Kinase deficiency, Sickle Cell Disease, Alpha-Thalassemia, Polycythemia, Hypothyroidism, Sepsis, UTI

CONJUGATED (DIRECT) BILIRUBIN (Water soluble)

Biliary Atresia • Conjugated (water soluble) • Occurs about 2 weeks of age • **Light stools and dark urine** (sign of conjugated bilirubin) • **Extrahepatic**: bile duct is blocked or absent • **NO kernicterus** • Leads to Neonatal Cholestasis • **Negative coombs test**	**Dubin-Johnson*** • Conjugated • High bilirubin levels • Problem is with **excretion** of conjugated bilirubin • **Liver is black** • Deposits of **epinephrine metabolites in hepatic lysosomes** • Normal LFT's • **Increased urinary coproporphyrin**
Rotor Syndrome* • Conjugated • Mildly elevated bilirubin • Problem is with **storage** (milder form of Dubin-Johnson) • Jaundice triggered by: Stress, OCP's, Pregnancy • **Liver is NOT black** • Deposits of epinephrine metabolites in hepatic lysosomes • Normal LFT's • Increased urinary coproporphyrin	***Excretion of conjugated bilirubin**: **Active ATP transport**. If these channels are blocked the conjugated bilirubin can not go to the biliary system but will go into the plasma (water soluble) and will increase the urinary excretion of bilirubin (**UA = increased levels of coproporphyrin**). If the active ATP transport is not working, the bilirubin can still be excreted from the liver into the plasma by **passive organic ion diffusion.** UA = normal urinalysis should never show bilirubin. If bilirubin shows in urine, urine will be dark and the bilirubin will be conjugated (water soluble). Other pathologies of conjugated bilirubin: TORCH infections, HEP A and B, Alpha-1-antitrypsin deficiency, Cystic Fibrosis, TPN (total parenteral nutrition), Bile duct obstruction, Choledochal cyst

Hernias

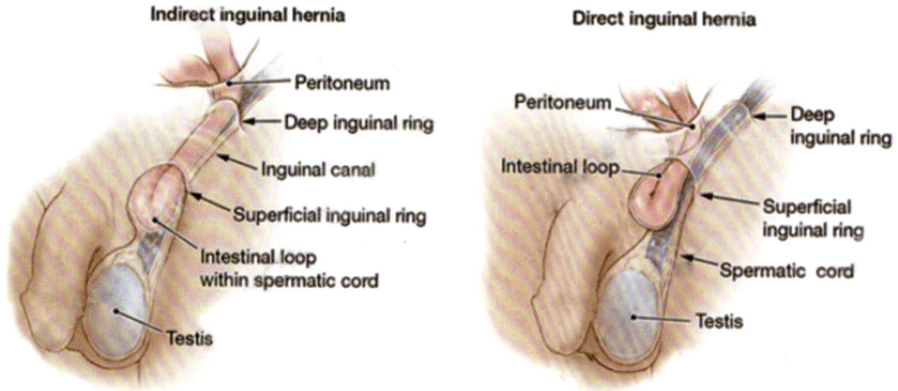

Direct Hernia	**Indirect Hernia**
• Loop of intestine protrudes through Hesselbach's triangle in the abdominal wall through the superficial inguinal ring • **Medial to inferior epigastric vessels** • MC in older men due to weakness in abdominal wall: breakdown of the **transversus abdominalis aponeurosis and transversalis fascia.** (**tip**: "M"en = "M"edial to the vessels) • MC acquired. **Hesselbach Triangle boarders:** **Medial boarder: Lateral margin of rectus sheath.** **Superolateral boarder: Inferior epigastric vessels.** **Inferior boarder: Inguinal ligament (AKA: Poupart's ligament**)	• Loop of intestine extends through the deep (internal) inguinal ring, the superficial (external) inguinal ring and into the scrotum. (same path as the decent of the testes) • **Lateral to the inferior epigastric vessels** • MC in infants and children due to failure of closure of process vaginalis (can cause hydrocele) • Infant ↑ risk due to a **patent processus vaginalis.** • MC congenital. (**tip**: Indirect ➔ lateral to vessels: you go **IN**to the **LAT**rine to pee) (**tip**: "L"ateral = "L"ittle kid) (**tip**: "IN"direct = "IN"fant)
Diaphragmatic Sliding Hiatal Hernia **Type 1** Stomach herniates upward through the gastroesophageal junction into the esophagus. MCC: obesity. Other causes: congenital, pregnancy, coughing, straining during bowel movements. SX: Heartburn, GERD, chest pain, pain with eating because food collecting in lower esophagus until it passes to stomach), heart palpitations (due to irritation of vagus nerve) DX: endoscopy, barium swallow TX: Weight loss, PPI or H2 blockers, raising head of bed, life style changes.	**Diaphragmatic Paraesophageal Hernia** **Type II** Weakness or tear in diaphragm that allows part of the stomach to protrude into the thorax. The gastroesophageal junction is normal. Complications: Stomach can become strangled and have its blood supply shut off. MCC: obesity. Other causes: congenital, pregnancy, coughing, straining during bowel movements. SX: Chest pain (can be confused with heart attack), GERD, heartburn TX: Surgery DX: Barium swallow

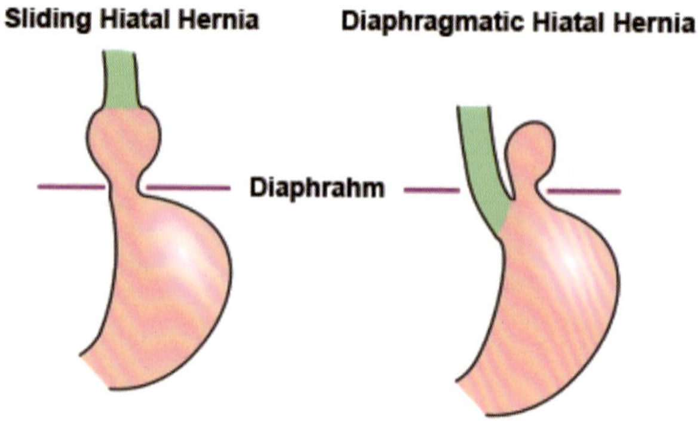

Femoral Hernia
Protrusion of bowel through a weakness in the abdominal wall through the femoral ring (just **below the inguinal ligament on the lateral aspect of the pubic tubercle)** and into the femoral canal.
MC: **older women** (can occur in males also).
(**tip**: "F"emale = "F"emoral)
Complication: strangulation of bowel.
TX: Surgery

Boarder of femoral triangle:
Anterior/Superior: cribriform fascia.
Posterior: adductor longus, pectineus, iliopsoas
Medial: medial boarder of adductor longus.
Lateral: medial boarder of Sartorius

Boarder of femoral canal (medial compartment of the femoral sheath. Allows expansion of the vein during exercise):
Anterior/Superior: Inguinal ligament
Posterior: Pectineal ligament
Medial: Lacunar ligament
Lateral: Femoral vein

Femoral sheath: formed by fascia's: transversalis and iliaca. Contains 3 compartments: Medial (Femoral canal), Middle (femoral vein), Lateral (femoral artery, femoral branch of genitofemoral nerve)

Femoral triangle (sheath) contains:
Femoral artery, femoral vein, lymphatic vessels (lymph node of Cloquet), femoral nerve
(**tip**: NAVeL) nerve, artery, vein, e=empty, lymph)

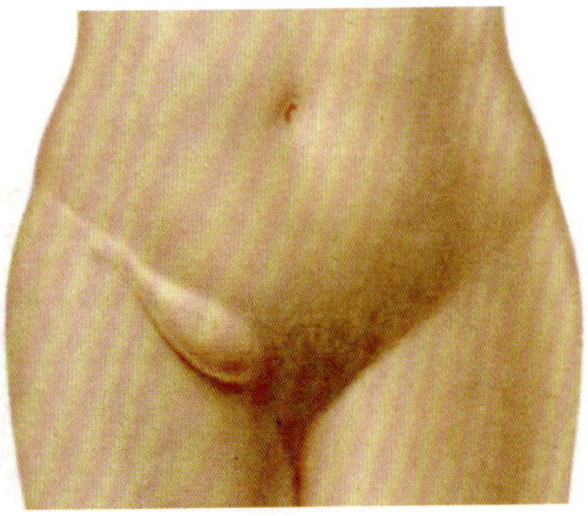

Umbilical Hernia
Protrusion of the bowel through the umbilicus (navel/belly button) due to congenital malformation of the navel or increased intra-abdominal pressure due to obesity, heavy lifting, multiple pregnancies, hx of coughing.

Complication: strangulation of bowel.
TX: Surgery
(Note: an umbilical hernia on a new born is associated with hypothyroidism/cretinism).

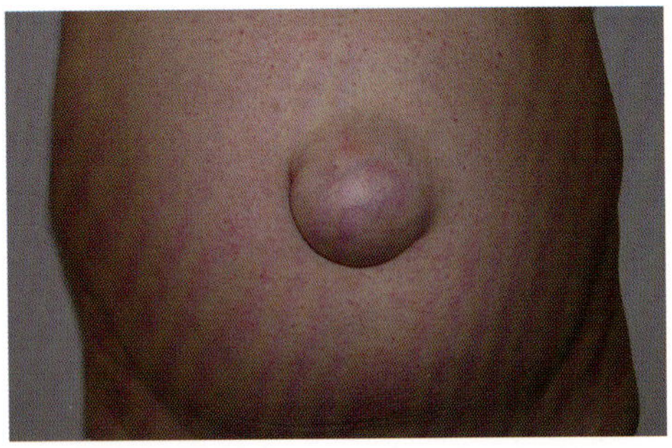

Incisional Hernia
Protrusion of bowel through the abdominal wall due to weakness in the fascia.

MCC: Previous surgical incisions. Can also be due to increased intra-abdominal pressure (chronic coughing, constipation, pregnancy, ascites, urinary obstruction), obesity.

TX: Surgery

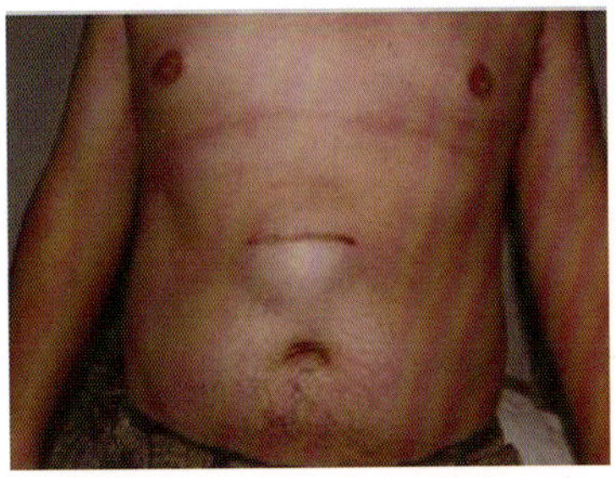

Hernia Surgery Layers

Skin ➔ Superficial fascia (contains 3 fascia: Camper's, Scarpa's) ➔ Camper fascia (adipose tissue) (tip: the camper is the fat guy**) ➔ Scarpa fascia** (fibrous tissue that helps form the fundiform ligament of the penis and contains 3 fascias: Colles: posterior perineum; Dartos: scrotum/labia majora; Deep superficial fascia: penis/clitoris) ➔ **External oblique** (inguinal ligament, superficial inguinal ring, external spermatic cord, anterior rectus sheath) ➔ **Internal Oblique** (cremasteric and muscle fascia, medial rectus sheath) ➔ **Transverse abdominis** (conjoining tendon, posterior rectus sheath) ➔ **Transversalis fascia** (deep inguinal ring, internal spermatic fascia, posterior rectus sheath, femoral sheath (femoral canal: femoral artery, vein) ➔ **Extraperitoneal layer** (testes) ➔ **Parietal Peritoneum**

GASTROINTESTINAL PHARMACOLOGY

DRUG GENERIC name Trade name	Clinical Use	Mechanism of Action and Resistance	Toxicity and Notes
PROTON PUMP INHIBITORS			
The "prazoles" **Omeprazole** *Prilosec* **Lansoprazole** **Esomeprazole** **Pantoprazole** **Dexlansoprazole**	Peptic ulcers, GERD, Zollinger-Ellison (Associated with MEN I), esophageal reflux IV Use: prevention of Cushing's Ulcers (↑ ICP) and Curling's Ulcers (burn victims)	**Irreversibly inhibit H/K ATPase pumps on the secretory surface of the parietal cells in the fundus/body of the stomach, so that HCL release is suppressed (aka: proton, H^+, acid).**	**Creates an ↑ pH/alkaline environment so will causes Vibrio cholera to worsen because Vibrio prefers an alkaline environment.** **Drugs that depend upon an acidic stomach environment (Ketoconazole, Itraconazole, Atazanavir) are poorly absorbed.** **Intestinal absorption of drugs that depend upon the acid nature of the stomach (aka: acid-labile) have increased absorption. (Erythromycin).** ↑ risk of C. difficile, ↓ serum Mg. NOTE: Anyone on a PPI or H2 blocker will have an increased gastrin level.
H2 BLOCKERS			
Cimetidine Ranitidine Famotidine Nizatidine (**tip**: tidine = It takes **2**, to **DINE**)	Peptic ulcers, esophageal reflux, gastritis. Proton Pump Inhibitors are DOC, more effective than H2 Blockers. IV Use: prevention of Cushings Ulcers (↑ ICP) and Curlings Ulcers (burn victims)	Reversibly bock histamine H2 receptors so ↓ H^+ secretion by parietal cells in the fundus/body of the stomach.	**Cimetidine: P-450 inhibitor.** Antiandrogenic effects: stops sex hormones, gynecomastia, ↓ libido, impotence, prolactin release. Cimetidine and Ranitidine ↓ renal excretion of creatinine. NOTE: Anyone on a PPI or H2 blocker will have an increased gastrin level.
H. pylori	**Triple Therapy** for H. pylori: **Omeprazole, Clarithromycin, Metronidazole**		

PROTECTION, DIARRHEA and LAXATIVES			
Bismuth Sucralfate *Pepto Bismol*	Diarrhea, healing of ulcers.	**Protects** ulcer epithelium. Adheres to ulcer to provide physical protection while pH is reestablished in the mucus by HCO_3 secretion.	**Black stools** **Reyes Syndrome** (Bismuth Sucralfate = salicylic acid= aspirin)
Antacids *Alka-Seltzer, Maalox, Milk of Magnesia, Pepto-Bismol, Rolaids, Tums, Mylanta, Gaviscon* *(Specific categories below)*	Neutralizes stomach acid, relieves heartburn	Alkaline ions neutralize gastric acid in the stomach.	**Hypokalemia.** Antacids containing calcium or aluminum = Constipation. Long-term use may cause kidney stones. Antacids with Mg = diarrhea. Antacids with aluminum = osteoporosis. Can affect efficacy of other drugs.

DRUG **GENERIC name** **Trade name**	**Clinical Use**	**Mechanism of Action and Resistance**	**Toxicity and Notes**
Calcium Carbonate *Maalox, Rolaids, Tums, Mylanta*	Gastric antacid. Treats diarrhea. Use with Irritable Bowel Syndrome, hyperphosphatemia in chronic renal failure.	Phosphate binder.	Hypercalcemia, rebound acid. Do not take with **tetracycline**. Can chelate and decrease efficacy of other drugs. Interactions with **Ciprofloxacin**.
Magnesium Hydroxide *Milk of Magnesia*	Treats constipation. TX for stress ulcers. Laxative. Antacid.		Osmotic diarrhea. Draws fluid from the body to put into the GI. Diarrhea also gets rid of potassium = hypokalemia (cardiac problems: arrhythmias/arrest). Hypotension, hyporeflexia. TX: Must take extra potassium to avoid muscle cramps.
Aluminum Hydroxide *Gaviscon*	Antacid relieves symptoms of ulcers, heartburn, and dyspepsia.		Constipation, Hypophosphatemia, seizures, osteodystrophy. Can be used with Magnesium Hydroxide as a laxative.
Diphenoxylate (opiate)	Anti-diarrheal by decreasing motility.	Agonist at Mu opioid receptors in the GI tract. Opens K channels, closes Ca channels. Low chance of addition.	Addiction, dependence, euphoria.
Loperamide (opioid) *Imodium*	Anti-diarrheal. Inflammatory bowel dz	Opioid-receptor agonist. Act on the Mu receptors in the myenteric plexus of the large intestine. Slows contraction/tone of the intestines so increases the time the waste stays in the intestine, allowing more water to be absorbed from the waste/fecal matter. Have little CNS effects.	Constipation, dry mouth, sleepiness, nausea, risk of megacolon, Stevens-Johnson syndrome. Do not use in cases of bloody diarrhea. **Do NOT use in children < 3 years old – can cause paralytic ileus leading to death.**
Misoprostol	Prevention of NSAID-induced peptic ulcers. **Keeps PDA's open.** ↑ **Contractions:** can **induce labor** or act as an **abortient** in an ectopic pregnancy.	PGE_1 analog (Prostaglandin). ↑ production of mucus and ↓ HCL production.	Diarrhea. **Do not use** in women that may be childbearing as Misoprostol is used as an **abortient.**
OSMOTIC LAXATIVES			
Magnesium Hydroxide Magnesium Citrate **Polyethylene Glycol** **Lactulose**	Chronic constipation. Polyethylene Glycol: Bowel prep for colonoscopy. **Lactulose**: Hepatic Encephalopathy	Draws water from the body to put into the bowel lumen to soften stools. **Lactulose:** traps ammonia in the colon by acidic metabolites of lactulose to ↓ hepatic encephalopathy. It binds ammonia (NH3) and converts it to NH4 (non-absorbable form) so that it can be excreted.	Diarrhea, dehydration. **People with bulimia commonly abuse osmotic laxatives.** Lactase deficiency cause osmotic diarrhea.

BOWEL DISEASE

Note: Natural or synthetic opioid agonists (drugs that work on the μ opioid receptor (MOR) are beneficial in the treatment and possibly prevention of intestinal inflammation. The activation of MOR suppresses lymphocyte and antibody production and decreases macrophage-mediated immunity. MOR deficiency can lead to intestinal inflammatory conditions. Tumor necrosis factor α (TNF- α) can affect the expression of MOR. MOR has anti-inflammatory properties.

DRUG GENERIC name Trade name	Clinical Use	Mechanism of Action and Resistance	Toxicity and Notes
Infliximab *Remicade*	**DOC: Ulcerative Colitis, Crohn's DZ, Rheumatoid Arthritis**, Ankylosing Spondylitis, Psoriasis	Monoclonal antibody against TNF-α **Note:** TNF-α is produced by macrophages and T lymphocytes and is proinflammatory. It induces PMN chemotaxis to sites of inflammation, activates coagulation and fibrinolysis and induces granuloma formation.	**MUST do PPD test. Drug may reactivate latent TB.**
Sulfasalazine	**Use if Infliximab does not work.** Ulcerative Colitis, Crohn's DZ, Rheumatoid arthritis.	Anti-inflammatory drug inside the intestines. Decreases eicosanoids (signaling molecules derived from Omega-3 or Omega-6) and inflammatory cytokines.	Sulfa toxicities, malaise, nausea, reversible oligospermia. Note: Sulfasalazine is a sulfa drug derived from Mesalazine.
Ciprofloxacin **AND** Metronidazole *Flagyl*	**Diverticulitis**	Ciprofloxacin: Inhibits DNA gyrase (topoisomerase II) Metronidazole: Free radicals damage DNA.	Cipro: Do not take with antacids. Tendon/cartilage ruptures, tendonitis. Teratogen. Metronidazole: Disulfiram-like reaction. Metallic taste.
Eluxadoline *Viberzi*	Irritable bowel syndrome (IBS)	μ opioid myenteric plexus receptor agonist that acts on the enteric nervous system.	Constipation

SOMATOSTATIN ANALOG

Octreotide	VIPomas Gastrinoma Carcinoid Syndrome Acromegaly, Acute variceal bleeds Insulinoma Secretory diarrhea	**Somatostatin analog**	Steatorrhea, nausea, cramps

ANTIEMETIC (Nausea)

Ondansetron	Stop nausea and vomiting in **chemotherapy,** post operative surgery and gastroenteritis. **Travelers diarrhea.**	**5-HT antagonist (Serotonin antagonist). ↓ Vagal stimulation.**	Constipation, headache, **Torsades de pointes**
Scopolamine	Antiemetic: Motion sickness	**Muscarinic antagonist (AKA: Anti-cholinergic)**	Dry mouth, tachycardia, pruritus, constipation, urinary retention, and drowsiness.
Diphenhydramine *Benadryl*	Antiemetic: motion sickness	Antihistamine, antimuscarinic.	Sedation

MOTILITY

DRUG GENERIC name Trade name	Clinical Use	Mechanism of Action and Resistance	Toxicity and Notes
Metoclopramide	Antiemetic. **Gastric motility** disorders. Promotes gastric emptying. Post-surgery gastroparesis. Pre-op to ↓ regurgitation.	**Dopamine antagonist in medulla oblongata.** **D_2 receptor antagonist. ↑ Motility, ↑ Lower esophageal tone, ↑ contractility.**	Parkinsonian effects. Fatigue, depression, restlessness, drowsiness. **Do NOT use in patients with small bowel obstruction.** **Do not use with Parkinson's Dz (D1-receptor blocker)**
Cisapride	Gastric motility/gastric emptying and increases LES tone.	Stimulates release of acetylcholine from the myenteric plexus.	Arrhythmias

WEIGHT LOSS

Orlistat *Xenical*	Obesity	**Inhibits gastric and pancreatic lipases.** (lipases breakdown triglycerides/fats). Triglycerides that are not broken down are excreted.	Explosive diarrhea, steatorrhea, flatus. (Reducing intake of fats can reduce this side effect). Reduces levels and absorption of amiodarone and cyclosporine.
Cisapride	Gastric motility/gastric emptying and increases LES tone.	Stimulates release of acetylcholine from the myenteric plexus.	Arrhythmias

GALLBLADDER

DRUG GENERIC name Trade name	Clinical Use	Mechanism of Action and Resistance	Toxicity and Notes
Ursodeoxycholic Acid	**Dissolve cholesterol gallstones** in patients that are not good surgical candidates. Prevents gallstones in patients who are losing weight quickly. Primary Biliary Cirrhosis. **Biliary stasis in pregnancy.**	Reduces cholesterol absorption. Improves bile flow (bile salts).	Constipation, dizziness, muscle/joint pain, diarrhea, vomiting, hair loss.

DRUG **GENERIC name** **Trade name**	**Clinical Use**	**Mechanism of Action and Resistance**	**Toxicity and Notes**
INF-α	**Hepatitis B and C (chronic)**	Anti-viral	Neutropenia, myopathy
Ribavirin	**Hepatitis C (chronic)**	Inhibits IMP (Inosine Monophosphate). Inhibits duplication of viral genetic material.	Hemolytic anemia. Teratogen
Simeprevir Telaprevir Boceprevir Sofosbuvir	Hepatitis C	Protease Inhibitor. Binds to the HCV nonstructural protein active site. Inhibits RNA polymerase that the HEP C virus uses to replicate its RNA.	Irritability, headache, fatigue, nausea, rash.
Disulfiram *Antabuse*	**Treatment of alcoholism**	Produces acute sensitivity to ethanol (alcohol). Inhibits Acetaldehyde dehydrogenase causing a hangover.	Headache, garlic taste, neurotoxicity, extrapyramidal effects. Disulfiram-like side effects are caused by certain drugs: Metronidazole, Griseofulvin, Procarbazine (chemo drug for Hodgkin's lymphoma and glioblastoma), 1st Generation Sulfonylureas: Tolbutamide, Chlorpropamide, Some Cephalosporins: Cefoperazone, Cefamandole and Cefotetan.
Spironolactone	**Ascites** **One of the 4 drugs that DECREASES MORTALITY**	Competitive aldosterone receptor antagonists in the cortical collecting tubule (distal nephron). (Potassium sparing diuretic)	**Electrolyte abnormalities (Hyperkalemia = arrhythmias), urinary frequency, ↓ libido (↓ testosterone and DHT), erectile dysfunction, GI symptoms, gynecomastia, anti-androgen effects.**
Penicillamine, Trientine	**Wilson's Disease** (copper accumulation)	Copper chelator. Binds to accumulated copper and eliminates it in the urine.	Nephropathy, hepatotoxicity, aplastic anemia, Membranous glomerulonephritis.

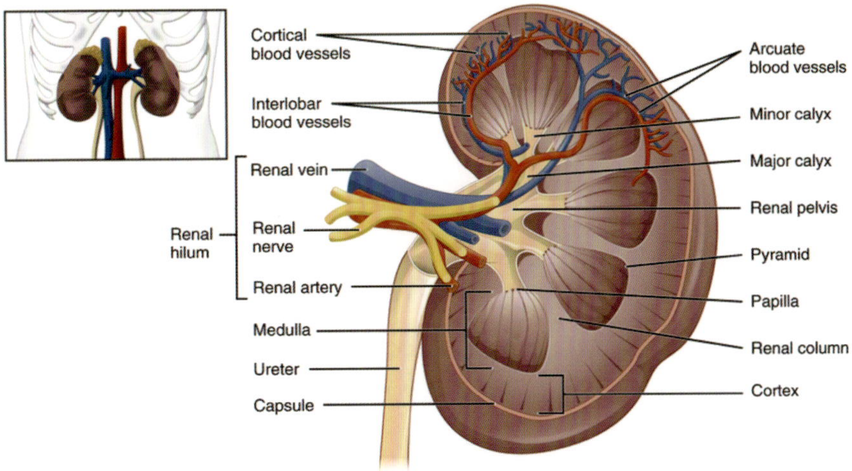
Cortical
blood vessels
Interlobar
blood vessels
Renal hilum
Renal vein
Renal
nerve
Renal artery
Medulla
Ureter
Capsule
Arcuate
blood vessels
Minor calyx
Major calyx
Renal pelvis
Pyramid
Papilla
Renal column
Cortex

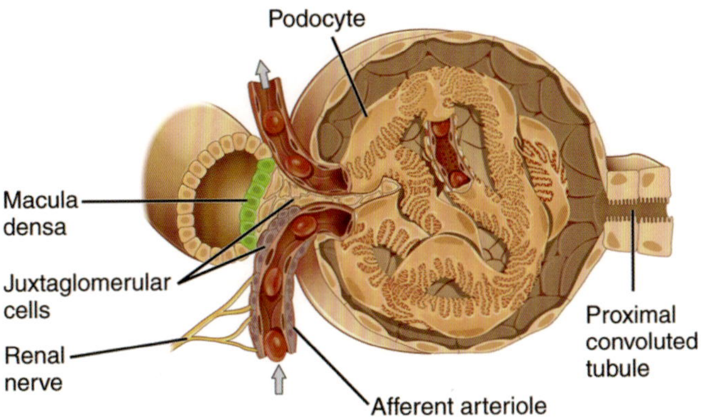
Podocyte
Macula
densa
Juxtaglomerular
cells
Renal
nerve
Afferent arteriole
Proximal
convoluted
tubule

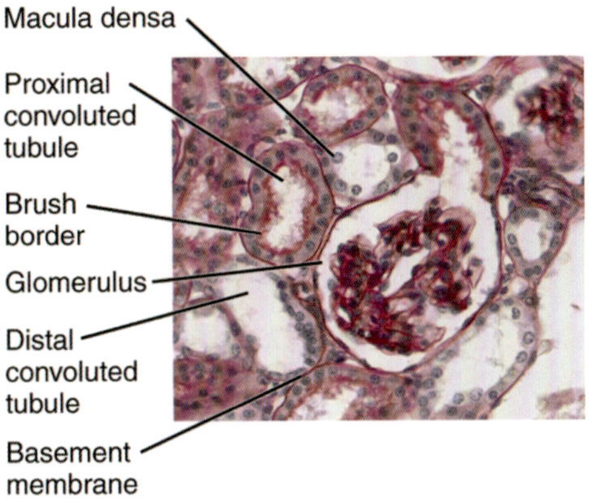
Macula densa
Proximal
convoluted
tubule
Brush
border
Glomerulus
Distal
convoluted
tubule
Basement
membrane

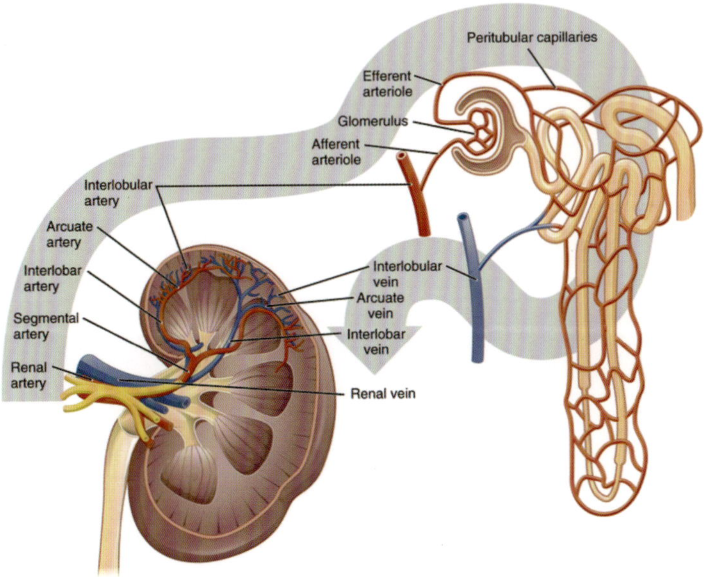
Peritubular capillaries
Efferent
arteriole
Glomerulus
Afferent
arteriole
Interlobular
artery
Arcuate
artery
Interlobar
artery
Segmental
artery
Renal
artery
Interlobular
vein
Arcuate
vein
Interlobar
vein
Renal vein

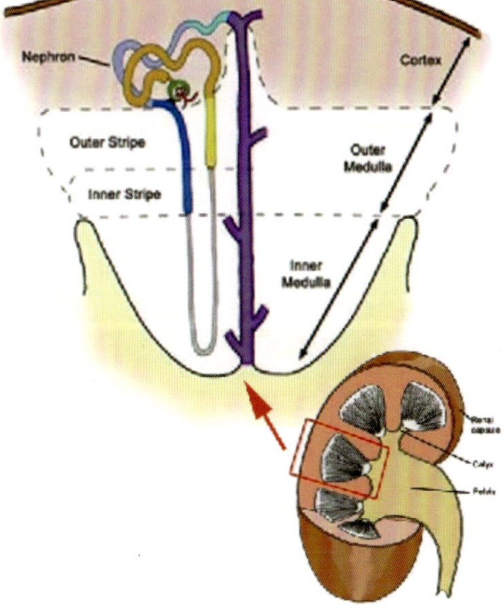
Nephron
Cortex
Outer Stripe
Outer
Medulla
Inner Stripe
Inner
Medulla

Renal Equations

Clearance = Urine Concentration/Plasma Concentration (What is clearing thru the tubes)
GFR = Inulin in urine x Volume (flow or rate)/Inulin in Plasma (GFR aka Inulin)
RBF = RPF/1 – Hct (RPF aka PAH) Must calculate PAH first
RPF = PAH
PAH = PAH in urine x Flow Rate/PAH in Plasma
Filtration Fraction = GFR/RPF aka (Inulin/PAH)
Starling (AKA: Net Filtration) = (Pc – Pi) – (^c - ^i)
c = capillary I = interstitial (Everything is MINUS)

GFR = inulin clearance, creatinine
Creatinine clearance and glomerular filtration rate (GFR) are inversely proportional to serum creatinine. GFR can be estimated from the measurement of serum creatinine*. (This is a good estimate as long as the GFR is not changing rapidly).

Blood Glucose Balance

The kidneys, in addition to the liver, help to **maintain blood glucose** levels in the starvation state. They release glucose through **gluconeogenesis**.

Fluid Distribution in the Body

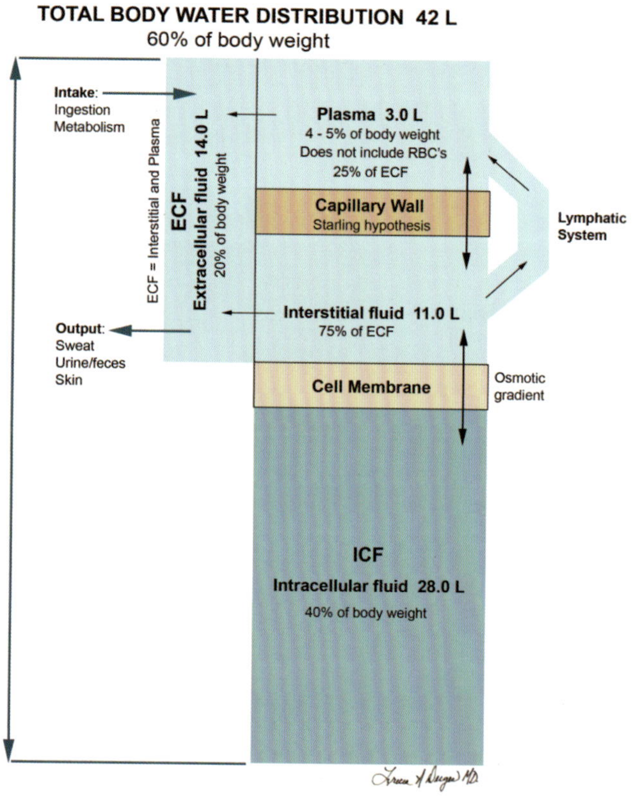

Osmolality

- Normal: 275 – 295 mOsmol/kg
- Water flows/follows where the most solute is (↑ OSM)
- Hypotonic: water leaves the ECF and comes into the cell so the cell swells. (More solute on the inside of the cell than in the ECF, so the water follows the ↑ solute/OSM).
- Hypertonic: water will leave the cell and enter the ECF so the cell shrinks. (More solute in the ECF than inside of the cell, so the water will follow the ↑ solute/OSM).

Osmolar Gap

Difference between measured serum osmolality and calculated serum osmolality.

- OSM Gap = (2 x Na) + glucose/18 + BUN/2.8 + Ethanol/3.7
- **Normal OSM gap = < 10 mOsm/Kg**
- Osmolar gap due to alcohols, sugars lipids, proteins.
  - Alcohols: Ethanol, methanol, ethylene glycol, acetone, isopropyl alcohol
  - Sugars: Mannitol, sorbitol
  - Lipids: Hypertriglyceridemia
  - Hypergammaglobulinemia (M. Waldenstrom)

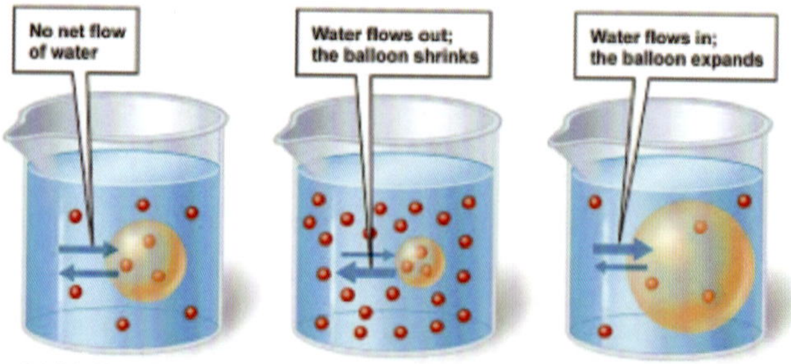

(a) A balloon in an isotonic solution (b) A balloon in a hypertonic solution (c) A balloon in a hypotonic solution

Transport

Type Transport	Gradient	Energy	Carrier	Saturation
Passive diffusion	Moves down gradient	No ATP needed	No carrier needed	Does not saturate
Facilitated diffusion (carrier mediated)	Moves down gradient	No ATP needed	Needs carrier protein	Can saturate
Active transport	Moves against gradient. (Concentration or electrical)	ATP needed. Requires ATPase pumps.	Needs carrier protein	Can saturate

OSM and Fluid Volume Shifts

OSM in steady state = ICF + ECF

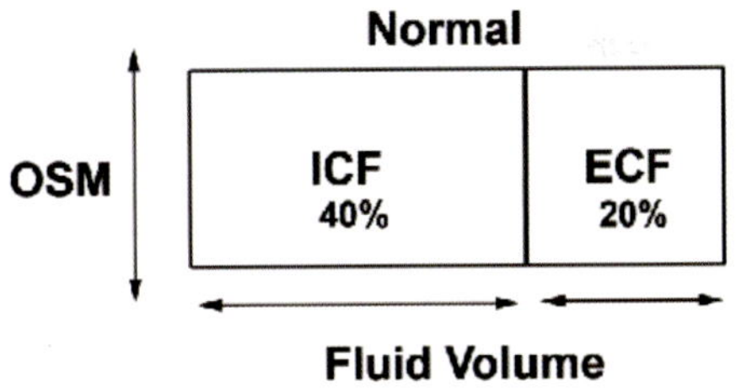

Shows the change in OSM and fluid volumes from the normal

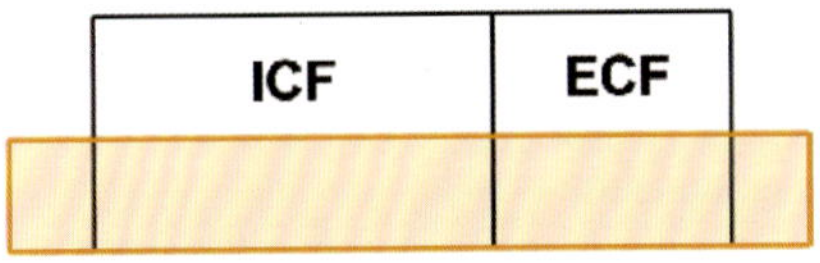

Note: OSM reduced and volume expanded in both compartments.

Causes: SIADH, Edema (right heart failure), Psychogenic polydipsia, cirrhosis, decreased OSM,nephrotic syndrome, high ingestion of hypotonic fluid (decreases OSM).

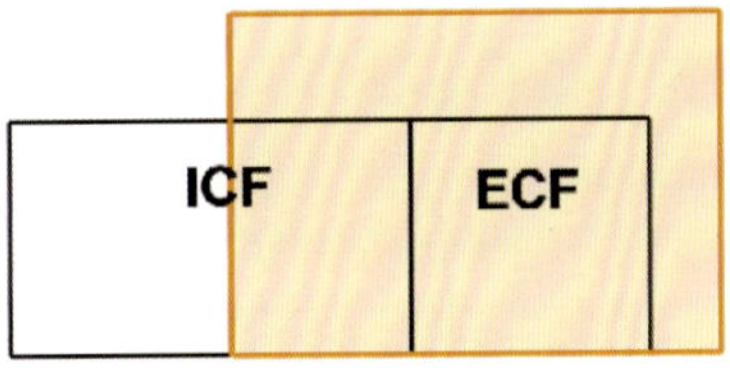

Note: OSM increased, fluid volume decreased in ICF and increased in the ECF. Fluid in ICF shifts to ECF because of increased OSM.

Causes: Hypertonic saline infusion, Hypertonic volume expansion, increased OSM, HCO3 (bicarbonate).

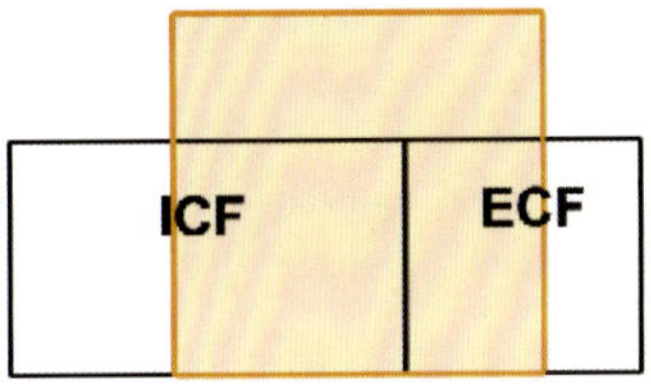

Note: OSM increased, fluid volume decreased in both ICF and ECF.

Causes: Dehydration, high sweating, Loss of water, Osmotic diuresis, Decrease of volume, Fever, High OSM, Hyperosmotic.

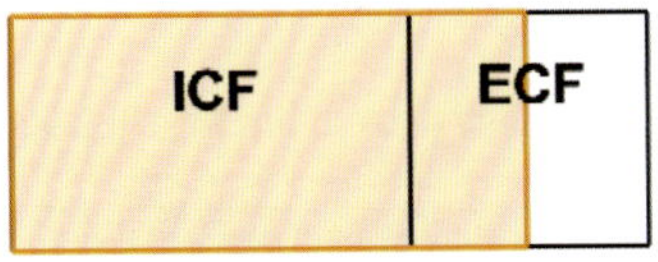

Note: OSM stayed the same, fluid volume in the ICF stayed the same and fluid volume in the ECF decreased.

Causes: Loss of isotonic fluid, Secretory diarrhea, Vomiting, Whole blood loss, Bleeding, GI Hemorrhage, Iso-osmotic volume contraction.

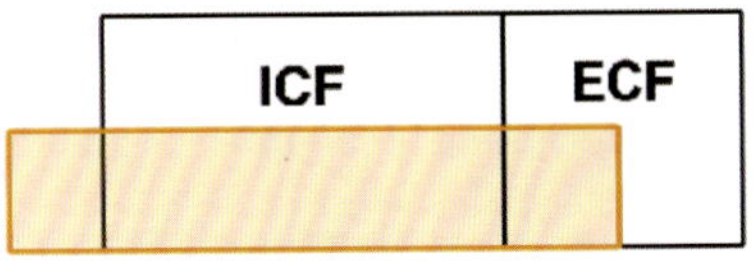

Note: OSM decreased, fluid volume increased in the ICF and decreased in the ECF.

Causes: Diuretics

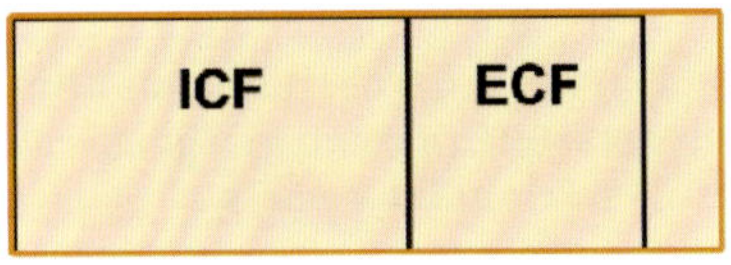

Note: OSM remains the same, fluid volume remains the same in the ICF and fluid volume increases in the ECF.

Causes: Excessive infusion of normal saline.

Affects on Diffusion

- Diffusion moves from areas of high concentration to low concentration in an effort to attain equilibrium.
- Rate of diffusion is directly proportional (positive correlation) to the concentration gradient (↑concentration difference = ↑ the rate of diffusion, temperature (↑ temperatures = ↑ rate of diffusion), pressure (↑ pressure = ↑ speed of diffusion), surface area (↑ Surface area = ↑ diffusion).
- When both areas are equal (zero gradient) = no net diffusion.
- Diffusion is inversely proportional (negative correlation) to membrane thickness (thicker membranes = slower diffusion), distance (short distances = ↑ diffusion. Long distances = ↓ diffusion), and molecular weight (heavier particles = ↓ diffusion), resistance (↑ resistance = ↓ diffusion).

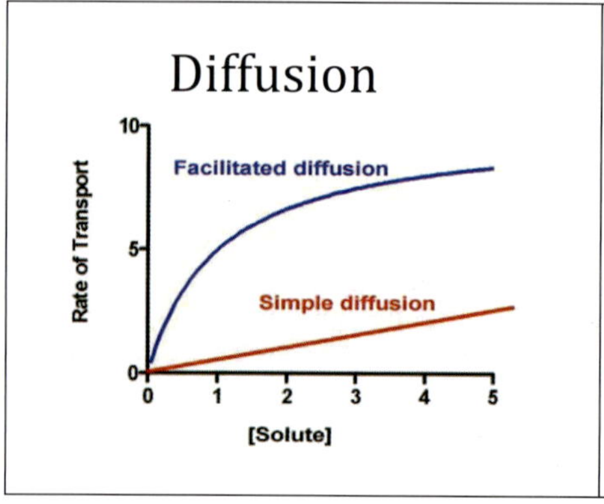

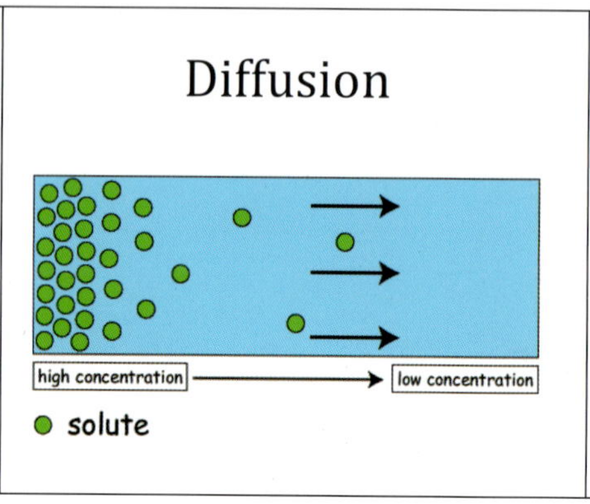

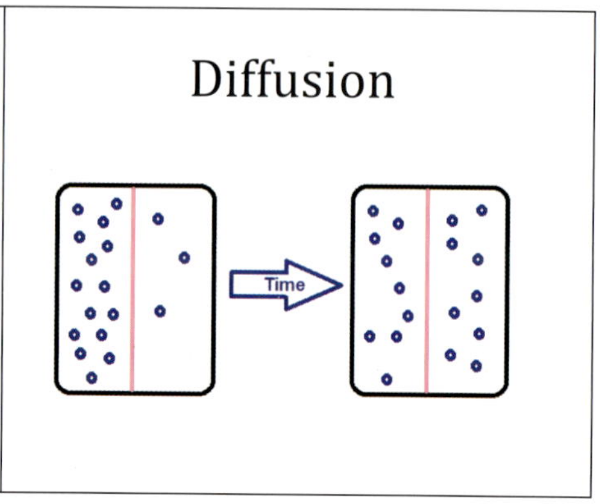

Renal Histology and Terminology

- Macrophages of the kidney = **mesangial cells**
  Mesangial cells are in the vascular pole of the glomerulus
- Renal Pelvis, ureters, bladder, urethra = transitional epithelium containing smooth muscle
- Composition of the kidney: specialized secretory cells and ducts made up of secretory epithelial cells
- Secretory cells of the kidney are the nephron. The nephron is the function unit of the kidney and is composed of **renal corpuscles, each having a renal tubule**
- **Renal corpuscles** secrete (produce) a filtrate of blood plasma that drains into its own renal tubule.
  Renal tubules modify this filtrate by reabsorbing everything that is not waste.
  Renal corpuscle have two poles: Vascular and Urinary
  Vascular pole: afferent and efferent arterioles, juxtaglomerular complex (JG cells. JG cells line the smooth muscle cells of the afferent arteriole) and are located between capillaries.
  Urinary pole: PCT (the outflow for the glomerular filtrate)
- **Renal tubules** consist of: convoluted tubules (PCT, DCT), loops of Henle (straight segments) and collecting ducts
- Kidney has an outer cortex and a deep medulla comprised of millions of individual nephrons
- **Cortex** consist of: convoluted tubules and renal corpuscles
- **Medulla** consist of loops of Henle and collecting ducts
- The kidney (cortex and medulla) drain into the pelvis (beginning of the ureter) which drains into the ureter
- Pelvis and ureter are **transitional epithelium**
- **Afferent arteriole** (incoming) = glomerular capillaries). Incoming blood into the glomerulus and they arise from interlobular arteries. (**Interlobular vessels** ascend from the arcuate vessels).
- **Efferent arteriole** (outgoing) = Blood leaving the glomerulus that enters the peritubular capillaries or vasa recta
- **Peritubular capillaries**: Enclose the PCT and DCT in the cortex and receive the water, ions, molecules that are pumped across the tubular epithelium. Their flow returns back to the interlobular veins.
- **Vasa recta**: Parallel grouping of vessels (arterial and venous) that carry blood in and out of the medulla. They return blood to the arcuate veins. (Arcuate vessels arch in the boundary between the cortex and medulla).
- **Interlobar vessels** (arteries and veins) are off of the renal artery and vein and ascend between lobes.
- **Juxtaglomerular apparatus**: Located at the vascular pole of each renal corpuscle. It consist of two structures (JG cells and the macula densa and lacis cells (extra-glomerular mesangial cells)
  - Juxtaglomerular cells (JG cells) in the wall of the **afferent arteriol (smooth muscle cells with secretory granules that secrets the hormone renin)**
  - **Macula densa**: Epithelial cells nuclei along the DCT tubule (adjacent to the afferent arteriole) located at the vascular pole of the corpuscle. It is a sensor for **sodium and chloride** concentration. The macula densa also contains Na-K-Cl symporter (aka: cotransporter). (See detailed explanation under the "thick ascending segment" of the Loop of Henle below).

- **Renal corpuscles** consist of:
  - Bowman's capsule/space is the outer, epithelial wall that encloses Bowman's space: **Simple squamous epithelium**. It is the outer "parietal" epithelium of the renal corpuscle.
  - **Bowman's space** (AKA: urinary space), lies within Bowman's capsule and surrounds the loops of the glomerulus. This space is where plasma filtrate collects as it leaves the capillaries through the filtration membrane
  - **Glomerulus** (comprises most of the corpuscle) is a small "knot" of capillaries suspended in Bowman's capsule comprised of:
    - Glomerular capillaries that have a **fenestrated (full of holes) endothelium**. Fenestrated capillaries are lined with capillary endothelial cells. Fenestrations are too small for blood cells to pass but plasma passes freely out of the holes and into the filtration membrane
    - **Podocytes** (AKA: Footed cells): epithelial cells covering the glomerular capillaries. They are the inner "visceral" epithelium located on the outside edge of the glomerular capillaries that support the filtration membrane. Each podocyte has a pedestal (foot) that sits on top of the filtration membrane that allows fluids to pass through filtration slits (gaps).
      Podocytes make up/synthesizes the glomerular basement membrane (GBM).
      GBM contains **heparin sulfate (a GAG: glycosaminoglycan)** that have negative charges. This negative charge keeps albumin from going into the urine.
      The loss of this negative charge is what causes protein loss (albumin) and for protein to be found in the urine = ↑ urine protein which leads to **↑ oncotic pressure (edema).**
      > 3.5 gms protein in urine in 24 hours: nephrotic
      < 3.5 gms protein in urine in 24 hours: nephritic

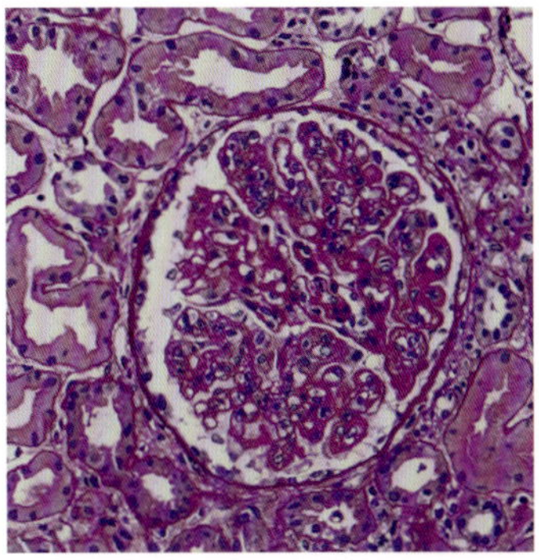

    - Filtration membrane: Outside the glomerular capillary endothelium between the podocytes and capillary endothelium. Composed of **END**othelial and podocyte (**EPI**thelial) basement membranes. It is where the endothelial basement membrane fuses with the podocytes.
      (**tip**: note the END and the EPI, these tie to the deposit pathologies in nephrotic vs nephritic dz).
      Filtration membrane holds back cells and plasma proteins while allowing water, small molecules and mineral ions to pass into Bowman's space and into the renal tubule.
      Filtration membranes can only be visualized using PAS or silver stain.
    - Mesangium: supporting tissue consisting of mesangial cells (macrophages) and matrix (connective tissue)
  - Beginning of the **proximal tubule** ("drain" carrying fluid away from Bowman's space). Proximal tube is **cuboidal epithelium**

- **Renal tubules** consist of:
  - **PCT: Proximal convoluted tubule** (Cortex) reabsorbs the majority of minerals/nutrients from the tubular fluid and brings them back into the blood via the peritubular capillaries. It is **isotonic.**
    Lined by: **Simple cuboidal epithelium**. Apical end of the PCT: **brush boarder of microvilli** that increases surface area for reabsorption. Contain ↑ **mitochondria** to provide energy to pump ions/molecules against their concentration gradient. ↑ mitochondria create an **acidophilic** environment.
    PCT reabsorbs bicarbonate. Damage to the PCT decreases ability to reabsorb bicarb so it is lost in the urine, which causes the urine pH to decrease (< 5.5).
  - **Loop of Henle** drops into the medulla to create a hypertonic environment in order to conserve water. This section is impermeable to water. This area is **Hypertonic.**
    Descending thick segment: **simple cuboidal epithelium** (AKA: pars recta)
    Descending thin segment: **simple squamous epithelium**
    Ascending thin segment: **simple squamous epithelium**
    Ascending thick segment: **simple cuboidal epithelium** (AKA: pars recta). The ascending thick segment contains the **NA-K-Cl symporter (aka: cotransporter) on the apical side.** (NOTE: Symporter moves solutes in the same direction). This transports sodium, potassium and chloride ions across the cell membrane. This is where loop diuretics work, inhibiting the reabsorption of sodium. By inhibiting sodium reabsorption the OSM is increased in the urine, causing diuresis and decreasing blood pressure. The thick ascending segment is impermeable to water.
  - **DCT: Distal convoluted tubule** returns back to vascular pole region (afferent arteriole and JG apparatus). Acts like the PCT by reabsorbing molecules out of the tubule and returning them back to the blood. through the peritubular capillaries. **Contains the macula densa** that is a sensor for **sodium and chloride** concentrations (**Na-Cl symporter, SLC12 cotransporter family**). DCT lined by **simple cuboidal epithelium** but **does NOT have a brush boarder** like the PCT. Distal tube acts under the influence of aldosterone in order to **generate new bicarbonate.**
    Sodium, chloride and Calcium are reabsorbed here (Na-Cl symporter, SLC12 cotransporter family). This is where thiazide diuretics work. They inhibit the Na-Cl symporter so that sodium and chloride is not reabsorbed, thereby increasing diuresis and decreasing blood pressure. Thiazides also increase the reabsorption of calcium at the DCT by increasing the action of the Na-Ca antiporter on the basolateral membrane (antiporter: moves solutes in the opposite directions). This causes more calcium to be reabsorbed and move into the interstitium, which then decreases intracellular calcium. When there is less calcium in the cell, it causes the reabsorption of more calcium from the lumen.

- **Collecting Duct** (tubule) returns back through the medulla to drain into the pelvis, which drains into the ureter, and collect the urine from the DCT. Lined by **simple cuboidal epithelium**. The duct is able to adjust the **permeability to water** (controlled by **ADH**). **High permeability** = water diffuses out into the medulla causing the urine in the duct to become **concentrated**. **Low permeability** = water is retained in the duct causing the urine to become **diluted** and is excreted from the body

- **Renal Tubule anatomy**
  - **Apical membrane** of the renal tubules and urinary collecting ducts **face the lumen** of the tubule, in contact with tubule fluid. Apical cells are connected to the lateral membranes by **E-cadherin** molecules.
  - **Basolateral membrane** is made up of basal and lateral membranes. Basal membranes connect epithelial cells to the basement membrane. Lateral membranes are on the lateral sides of the membrane where the cells connect to each other. These are located in the renal tubules and urinary collecting ducts and **face away from the lumen** of the tubule (face the plasma/blood/peritubular fluid, interstitium), they are connected to the extracellular matrix by **integrins**. The epithelial cells take up metabolic waste products for disposal into the lumen so that they can be transported out in the urine. They also allow the recycling of substrates (glucose) by pulling them from the lumen of the tubule and secreted back into interstitial fluids.

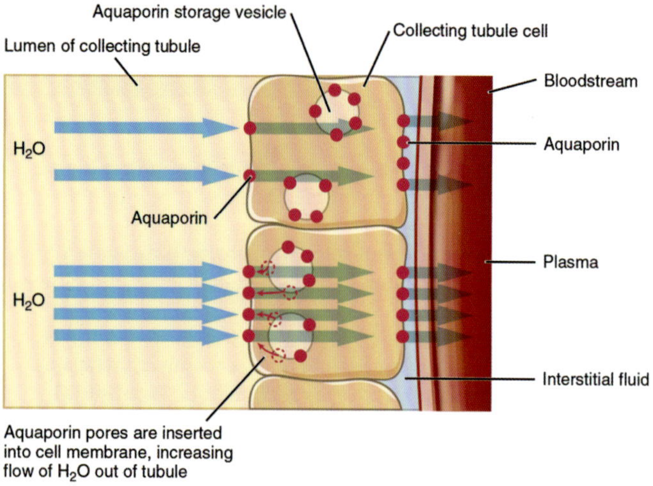

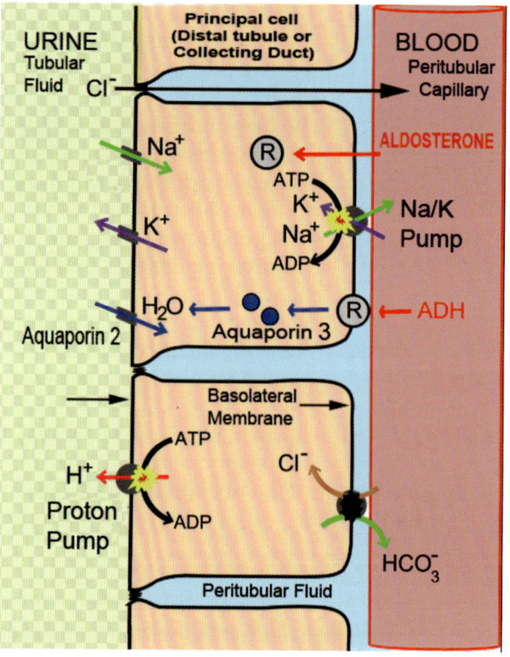

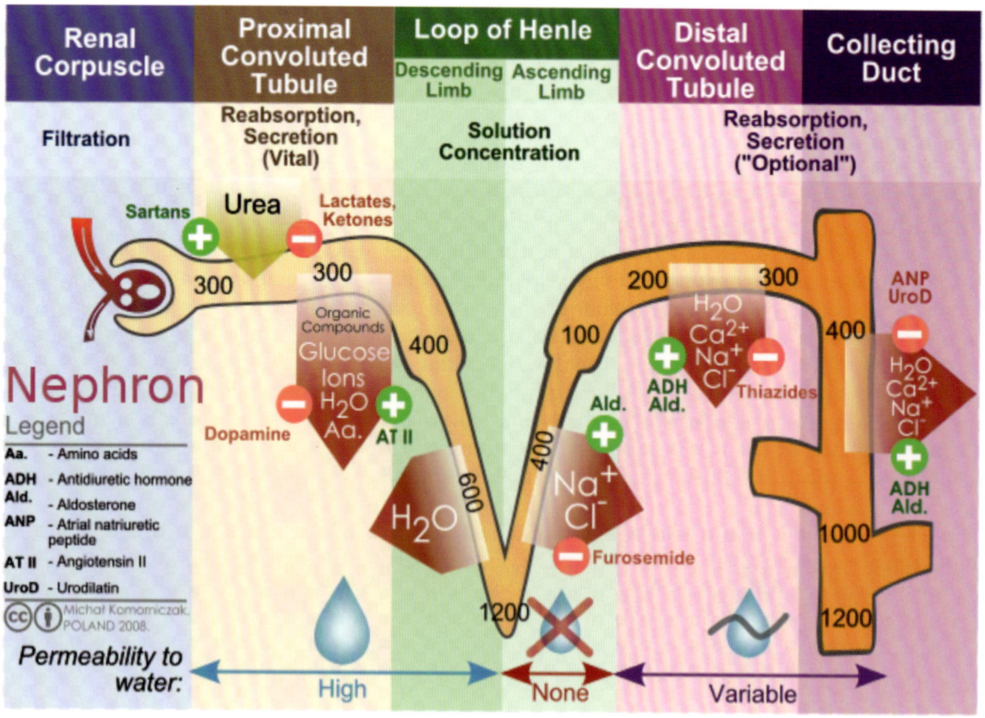

Specific Gravity: Evaluation of kidney function. Normal range: 1.000 to 1.030. It indicates if the kidney is able to concentrate urine. **Failure to concentrate urine is the first thing to disappear in renal failure**. This occurs before a change in Cr/BUN ratios. Urine is tested first thing in the morning because the urine should always concentrate overnight. If it concentrates, then kidney function is normal.

- **↑ Specific gravity > 1.023 = normal kidney function:** (hypersthenuria) = increased concentration of solutes in the urine. Causes: diarrhea, dehydration, emesis, UTI, renal artery stenosis, excessive sweating, SIADH, hepatorenal syndrome, hypovolemia
- **↓ Specific gravity < 1.01** (hypotonic urine = not concentrating urine = **renal failure**): (hyposthenuria) = decreased concentration of solutes in the urine. Causes: pyelonephritis, ATN (acute tubular necrosis) interstitial nephritis, psychogenic polydipsia (excessive fluid intake), renal failure

Filtration

- FF does not change if tube diameter is normal
- FF ↓ if tube diameter is dilated
- FF ↑ when dehydrated or a decreased flow (constricted efferent) is leaving thru the efferent arteriole
- FF = amount of fluid in Bowman's. ↑ Fluid = ↑ GFR, ↓ Fluid = ↓ GFR
- Low flow (↓ RPF) into kidneys (afferent arteriole) from ↓ BP, dehydration @ JG cells = renin system
- ATII constricts efferent arteriole = backup fluid into Bowman's = ↑ hydrostatic pressure in Bowman's = ↓ plasma flow through capillaries = ↑ FF
- **GFR = hydrostatic pressure (↑ GFR = ↑ hydrostatic pressure. ↓ GFR = ↓ hydrostatic pressure)**
- Only time GFR is ↑ is when efferent is constricted b/c of ↑ pressure forcing blood to stay in the glomerulus to be filtered
- ↓ GFR = ↓ glomerulus capillary pressure. If pressure ↓ = ↑ RPF (↓ resistance = better flow)
- ↑ GFR = ↑ urine output and can lead to dehydration and electrolyte depletion
- ↓ GFR = ↑ wastes reabsorbed and can lead to azotemia
- ↓ GFR and RBF (sympathetic nerves (Epinephrine and norepinephrine), Angiotensin II, Endothelin
- ↑ GFR and RBF (Prostaglandins, Nitric Oxide, Bradykinin, ANP
- Vasoconstriction: ↑ vascular resistance = ↓ RPF, ↓ GFR, ↓ Hydrostatic pressure
- Vasodilation: ↓ vascular resistance = ↑ RPF, ↑ GFR, ↑ Hydrostatic pressure
- If arterial pressure is ↑ = ↑ afferent resistance and ↓ efferent resistance
- ↑ flow (speed) into glomerulus = little time to filter = ↓ FF
- ↓ flow (speed) into glomerulus = more time to filter = ↑ FF

Constricting Afferent (lower amount of blood enters glomerulus) ↓ RPF, ↓ GFR, ⦸FF **NSAIDS constrict afferent (can lead to renal failure).**	**Constricting Efferent** (↓ blood flow leaving the kidneys forcing more blood to go through filtration in the glomerulus)" ↑ **Hydrostatic** pressure. If ↑↑ hydrostatic pressure occurs, can lead to hydronephrosis. ↓ RPF, ↑ GFR, ↑ FF **ATII constricts efferent.**	**Dilating Efferent** (decreases pressure in glomerulus) ↑ RPF, ↓ GFR, ↓ FF **Ace Inhibitors dilate efferent.**	**Dehydration, Renal Artery Stenosis, Endothelin-1, Adenosine, ADH.** (**decreased flow** in and out of glomerulus) ↓ RPF, ↓ GFR, ↑ FF
Dilating Afferent (allows more RBF) ↑RBF, ↑ GFR, ↓ FF **Prostaglandins,** Kinins, ANP, NO, CCB, Dopamine **dilate afferent.** Prostaglandins are blocked by **NSAIDS** = constrict afferent which can lead to renal failure in patients with poor renal function.	**ANP:** **Dilates afferent and constricts efferent:** ↑RBF, ↑ GFR, ↓ FF **↑ Plasma Proteins** RPF: no change, ↓ GFR, ↓ FF **↓ Plasma Proteins** RPF: no change, ↑ GFR, ↑ FF **Constriction of Ureter** RPF: no change, ↓ GFR, ↓ FF	**NEpi, Epi** (Catecholamines) (**α1 constricts afferent and efferent**) – Sympathetic. ↓↓ RPF, ↓ GFR, ↑ FF **Mannitol** ↑ RPF, maintains FF **Diuretics** (loops & thiazides) ↓ FF ↑ NcCl at Macula Densa ↑ RPF, ↓ GFR	**Sympathetic Actions: Constrict afferent.** **↓ RPF, ↓ GFR, ↑ FF** **↓ Hydrostatic pressure** **Sympathetic Actions:** ↓ Blood pressure Hemorrhage Emotion Pain Fear Adenosine

Hormone/Drugs Actions On the Kidney

Afferent Arterioles

- **ANP (BNP) responds to ↑ stretch in the atria due to increased stretch due to ↑ fluid = dilates afferent arteriole smooth muscle via cGMP to ↑ GFR to ↑ diuresis and inhibit renin/aldosterone system.**
  Provides: "Aldosterone Escape"
- **NSAIDS** constrict afferent arterioles

PCT

- PTH ↓ plasma Ca and ↑ plasma phosphate

Efferent

- Ace Inhibitors dilate efferent arterioles
- ATII constricts efferent arterioles

Collecting Tubules/Ducts

- Aldosterone ↑ Na reabsorption, ↑ K and H secretion (excretion).
  Activated due to ↓ blood volume/ BP.
  K is secreted by Principal Cells.
  H is secreted by Intercalated Cells.
  ADH (Vasopressin) binds principal cells = ↑ water channels and water reabsorption (aquaporin channels).
  Activated due to ↑ plasma OSM and ↓ blood volume/BP

Hormones of the Kidney

Erythropoietin (AKA: **Interstitial fibroblast of the kidney, Peritubular capillaries in the renal cortex**) **NOTE: Erythropoietin can also be produced in the liver.** Jak 2 Signaling. **Responds to hypoxia** to stimulate synthesis of Hb. (RDS in newborns, high altitude, COPD (chronic), ANY situation that has ↓ oxygen) Released by interstitial cells in the peritubular capillaries. Exogenous EPO: Athletes doping. Renal failure. **Polycythemia Absolute** = due to an EPO secreting tumor. EPO is continually secreted despite high Hb levels.	**Renin** **Secreted by JG cells** (juxtaglomerular apparatus, **smooth muscles cells on the afferent arterioles**) in **response to ↓ blood flow/BP, (dehydration, hemorrhage), ↓ CO to activate the renin-angiotensinogen-aldosterone system.** (**Remember**: if renin is elevated in the presence of high blood pressure = evaluate for a renin secreting tumor).	**1,25 Vitamin D** **25-OH Vitamin D from the liver (calcifediol /ergocalciferol) is transported to the kidney to be converted to the active form of Vitamin D (Calcitriol) via the enzyme 1α Hydroxylase (stimulated by PTH).** The active form of Vitamin D is then transported to the gut to reabsorb Calcium and Phosphate. To much Vitamin D = ↑ Calcium. To little Vitamin D = ↓ Calcium and Phosphate. Vitamin D is also secreted from granulomas = ↑ Calcium blood levels.	**Prostaglandins** **Vasodilate the afferent arterioles to ↑ RBF** **NSAIDS** block prostaglandins which causes constriction of the afferent arteriole and ↓ GFR. In patients with poor renal function, this can lead to renal failure.

Ions/Electrolytes in the Kidney

- Na, Cl, HCO3 move together
- K, H (protons/acid) move together (Caution: In vomiting, CL follows H (AKA: H, acid)
- **Na, Cl, HCO3 move opposite of K, H (If Na, Cl and HCO3 are reabsorbed (kept in the body, then K and H are excreted from the body**
- ↑ Cl causes: dehydration, ↑ salt, ↓ cortisol
- ↓ Cl causes: Cushing's, ↑ cortisol, SIADH, Metabolic alkalosis, ongoing vomiting

Abnormal Electrolyte Symptoms/Pathologies

- Low Ca = QT prolongation, tetany, seizures
  High Ca = Renal stones, bone pain, abdominal pain, constipation, anxiety, altered mental status
- Low Mg = Torsades de pointes, tetany, muscle cramps, depression, irritability of the CNS, epileptic fits. EKG shows: Tachycardia, prolonged QT
  High Mg = Bradycardia, heart block, cardiac arrest, hyporeflexia of deep tendons, loss of patellar reflex, hypotension, low heart rate, sleepiness, decreased respiration.
- Low Phosphate (PO4) = Osteomalacia, bone loss
  High Phosphate (PO4) = Renal stones, hypocalcemia
- Low K = EKG shows Flattened or inverted T waves and U, wide PR interval = arrhythmias.
- High K = EKG shows: Peaked T waves, loss of P wave, wide QRS = arrhythmias. Muscle weakness (excess K inhibits contraction leading to rhabdomyolysis, palpitations, fatigue.

HIGH POTASSIUM (Hyperkalemia) (Normal 3.5 – 5.0 mE/L)

- Severely high K (≥ 6.0 mE/L) **Must be brought DOWN immediately**, **EVEN before** administering fluids (NaCl) due to severe hypovolemia due to potential of cardiac arrhythmias or sudden cardiac death.
- **Causes**: Very common in tumor lysis syndrome (seen in cancer treatments due to high numbers of dying cells releasing potassium), metabolic acidosis (K shifts out of cells), Digoxin toxicity (Digoxin "looks" like K), Beta Blockers (decreases the activity of the Na/K ATPase pump so K is forced to stay outside of the cell), Addison's dz (no Aldosterone, so sodium is lost and K remains), prolonged immobility, Renal Tubular Acidosis (Type IV), renal failure (kidneys lose ability to excrete K), DKA (Insulin deficiency), seizures, crush injuries (destroys cells releasing K. AKA: rhabdomyolysis). Drug causes of 🡑 potassium: Diuretics (Potassium sparing: Spironolactone, Eplerenone, Amiloride, Triamterene), ACE inhibitors and ARBS (Angiotensin Receptor Blockers) (inhibit aldosterone).
- **EKG shows**= **Peaked T waves**, loss of P wave, wide QRS = arrhythmias.
- **Symptoms**: muscle weakness, palpitations, fatigue.

Treatments to reduce Potassium

#1 = **calcium gluconate** (does not have an effect on K levels, it reduces the excitability of cardiomyocytes so 🡓 risk of arrhythmias.
Other methods: **IV Insulin and glucose** to drive K into the cells, dialysis to filter K from the blood if kidney function impaired, water pills to remove K via urinary tract, **Kayexalate (AKA: polystyrene sulfonate**) helps excrete K in the feces – this is a slower method – **always** choose calcium gluconate over Kayexalate), **Bicarbonate** causes K to go into the cells (not normally used).
Non-emergency situations K can be lowered by altering diet to reduce potassium rick foods:
bananas, nuts and beans, milk, apricots, salmon.

Low Potassium (Hypokalemia)

- Low K (< 3.5 mE/L). K must be replaced to 🡓 potential of arrhythmias.
- **Causes:** Insufficient potassium intake, starvation (MC: anorexia nervosa and people on ketogenic diets), Conn's Syndrome (High aldosterone pathologies), vomiting (causes metabolic alkalosis due to loss of K), Renal Tube Acidosis of PCT and DCT, diarrhea, excessive perspiration, Bartter syndrome (kidneys can't reabsorb Na and Cl in the loop of Henle leading to loss of K), low levels of magnesium (Mg is required to process potassium), alkalosis (increased pH in the blood), Bartter's or Gitelman syndrome, renal artery stenosis.
  Drugs: **Diuretics (Loops or Thiazides), Amphotericin B, Cisplatin, Foscarnet.**
- **EKG shows:** Flattened or inverted T Waves and U waves, wide PR interval.
- **Symptoms: Arrhythmias, Muscle cramps** (🡓 function of skeletal muscle), fatigue, muscle weakness, constipation. (🡓 function of smooth muscle), hyporeflexia, respiratory depression (🡓 function of skeletal muscle).
- **TX:** Replace potassium

Magnesium

- Mg = cofactor for many reactions. Most important reactions involve ATP.
- Mg directly affects K, Na, Ca.
- Potassium efflux in inhibited by Mg. Without Mg, K excretion is increased in the kidney causing hypokalemia.
- Magnesium inhibits the release of calcium from the sarcoplasmic reticulum causing an increase of intracellular calcium ➔ release of PTH ➔ hypoparathyroidism and hypocalcemia.
- Magnesium is required for the Na/K ATPase pump in the skeletal muscles (myocytes) of the heart. If there is 🡓 Mg there will be an 🡑 in potassium loss ➔ intracellular increase of potassium ➔ tachycardia.
- Magnesium increases prostaglandins ➔ 🡓 thromboxane (inhibits platelets) causing microvascular leakage and vasospasms leading to convulsions = **pre-eclampsia**.
- Magnesium stimulates bronchodilation.

High Magnesium (Hypermagnesemia)

- High Mg levels in the blood (Normal: 1.5 – 2.0 mDq/L)
- Magnesium levels depend upon uptake of Mg in the intestine, excretion in the kidney, and storage in the bone.
- **Causes:** Renal insufficiency ↓ excretion of magnesium (is impaired once creatinine < 30 ml/min), DKA, lithium toxicity, hyperparathyroidism, hypothyroidism, adrenal insufficiency, excessive hemolysis.
- **Symptoms:** Bradycardia, heart block, cardiac arrest, hyporeflexia of deep tendons, loss of patellar reflex, hypotension, low heart rate, sleepiness, decreased respiration.
- **TX:** **IV calcium gluconate**, increase renal excretion by: **IV diuretics** (with normal renal function), dialysis (used when there is kidney failure).

Low Magnesium (Hypomagnesemia)

- Low Mg levels in the blood
- **Causes:** Inadequate intake of magnesium, malabsorption, alcoholism, chronic stress, chronic diarrhea, acute pancreatitis, Bartter's and Gitelman Syndromes, parathyroid surgery, pre-eclampsia (Magnesium increases prostaglandins → ↓ thromboxane causing microvascular leakage and vasospasms leading to convulsions = pre-eclampsia).
  Drugs: **diuretics (Loops and Thiazide), Omeprazole, Aminoglycosides, Amphotericin B, Foscarnet, Cisplatin, Adrenergic's, Digitalis.**
- **EKG shows:** Tachycardia, prolonged QT
- **Symptoms:** Torsades de pointes, tetany, muscle cramps, depression, irritability of the CNS, epileptic fits.
- **TX:** Replacement of magnesium.

Acid – Base

Buffers

- Extracellular Buffer: **Bicarbonate** (HCO_3). Bicarbonate combine with excess hydrogen ions (protons) to form carbonic acid.
- Intracellular Buffer: Proteins (such as hemoglobin, histadine), organic/inorganic phosphates, RBC's. **Hemoglobin** is the most important buffer in the RBC because it buffers the carbonic acid.
- Note: Bone is also a buffer for acid. Excess hydrogen ions are taken up the bone in exchange for Na and K and bone mineral resulting in the release of buffering compounds: $NaHCO_3$ and others.

Compensation Response

- Reduce the effects of a specific disorder on the pH. They do not restore pH back to a normal value.
- Correcting underlying causes is the only thing that can return pH back to a normal value.
- A respiratory problem can only be compensated with a metabolic (kidney) response. Slower: takes several days.
- A metabolic problem can only be compensated with a respiratory (alveolar ventilation) response. Immediate.
- The direction of a compensatory response is always the same as the initial change.

Acid – Base

ABG	pH	$PaCO_2$	HCO_3
Respiratory Acidosis	↓	↑	normal
Respiratory Alkalosis	↑	↓	normal
Metabolic Acidosis	↓	normal	↓
Metabolic Alkalosis	↑	normal	↑

- Normal pH = 7.35 – 7.45 (**average 7.4**)
  Normal PCO_2 = 36 – 44 (**average 40**). PCO_2 is regulated by respiration. Abnormalities that alter the PCO_2 are respiratory alkalosis (low PCO_2) and respiratory acidosis (high PCO_2).
  Normal HCO_3 = 22 – 26 (**average 24**) HCO_3 is regulated by the renal system. Abnormalities that alter the HCO_3 are metabolic alkalosis (high HCO_3) and metabolic acidosis (low HCO_3).
- **Metabolic Acidosis**: pH < 7.4, ↓ HCO_3, ↑ PCO_2 due to compensatory alveolar hyperventilation (respiratory response). The drop in arterial pH stimulates the peripheral and central chemoreceptors that control respiration causing an increase in ventilation.
  Due to loss of bicarbonate: diarrhea, Carbonic anhydrase inhibitors, Type 2 RTA in the PCT, pancreatic pathologies, administration of HCL or ammonium chloride, decrease in renal acid excretion in Type 1 RTA in the DCT, renal failure, hyperkalemia, recover from DKA, lactic acidosis, uremia, DKA, starvation, alcohol, intoxication from methanol, ethylene glycol, salicylates, INH.
- **Metabolic Alkalosis**: pH > 7.4, ↑ HCO_3, ↓PCO_2 due to a compensatory hypoventilation (↓ alveolar ventilation). Accompanied by hypochloremia and hypokalemia. The increase in arterial pH stimulates the peripheral and central chemoreceptors that control respiration causing a decrease in ventilation.
  Due to loss of hydrogen ions (AKA: protons, potassium, acid): vomiting, hypokalemia, dehydration (ANY volume depletion kicks in the renin system → aldosterone → retains Na and Cl and excretes K = metabolic alkalosis), nasogastric suction, chloride losing diarrhea, vomiting (loss of H/acid and volume depletion), villous adenoma, antacid therapy, renal loss due to loop or thiazide diuretics, excess mineralocorticoids, hypercalcemia, hydrogen movement into cells (hypokalemia), massive blood transfusion, antacids, administration of $NaHCO_3$, sweat loss in cystic fibrosis, gastric loss in achlorhydria, Bartter's syndrome, Gitelman 's syndrome, Conn's, Cushing's Syndrome.

- **Acute: Respiratory Acidosis** = abrupt failure of ventilation: Depression of CNS respiratory center by drugs, neuromuscular dz (ALS, Guillain-Barré, MG), airway obstruction.
- **Chronic: Respiratory Acidosis** = Secondary to a pathology: COPD (hypoventilation), V/Q mismatch, obesity (Pickwickian syndrome), decreased diaphragm dysfunction.
- **Acute Respiratory Acidosis**: pH < 7.4, ↑ pCO_2 increases carbonic acid in the plasma, which can't be buffered by HCO_3, so there is **no decrease** in HCO_3 levels.
- **Chronic Respiratory Acidosis**: pH < 7.4, ↑ pCO_2, ↑ HCO_3 (bicarb) due to compensation by Metabolic Alkalosis (kidney is excreting hydrogen ions and ammonium and the reabsorption of bicarbonate is increased to raise the serum HCO_3 levels. **Takes 3 – 5 days.**
- **Respiratory Alkalosis** (Hyperventilation = ↑ frequency in alveolar respiration and tidal volume which ↑ minute ventilation = hypocapnia = ↓ serum levels of potassium and phosphate): pH > 7.4, ↓ CO_2, ↓ HCO_3 (bicarb) due to compensation by the kidneys to ↓ **excretion of renal acid (hydrogen) and ammonium and ↑ excretion of HCO_3**. **This takes 2 – 3 days**.

Acid Base Table

Primary Disorder	Initial Chemical Change	Compensatory Response	Compensatory Mechanism
Metabolic Acidosis	↓ HCO_3	↓PCO_2	Hyperventilation
Metabolic Alkalosis	↑ HCO_3	↑PCO_2	Hypoventilation
Respiratory Acidosis	↑PCO_2	↑HCO_3	
Acute			Intracellular buffering (hemoglobin, intracellular proteins)
Chronic			Making new HCO_3 due to increased excretion of ammonium and hydrogen ions.
Respiratory Alkalosis	↓PCO_2	↓HCO_3	
Acute			Intracellular buffering
Chronic			Decreased reabsorption of HCO_3 and decreased excretion of ammonium and hydrogen ions.

Acid Base Calculation (naming)

- Look at pH
  Acidic (<7.4) or Alkalotic (>7.4) = give you the last "name"
  Now change the pH to an arrow ↑ or ↓. Acidic = ↓ Alkalotic = ↑
- Look at CO_2 (change the number to an arrow ↑ or ↓
- If arrows in the above 2 steps are going the SAME direction = metabolic
  If arrows in the above 2 steps are going the OPPOSITE direction = respiratory
  (**tip**: **R**espiratory = **R**everse)

- **Mixed Acid Base:**
  MCC: **Aspirin toxicity**. Other causes: Gram-negative sepsis, acute cardiopulmonary arrest, severe pulmonary edema.
  Both CO_2 and HCO_2 will be **very low at the same time** and **pH will be NORMAL**: Metabolic acidosis will present first and then a short time later
  (due to hyperventilation) respiratory alkalosis will present.
  - **Phases of salicylate (aspirin) toxicity**
  - Phase 1: hyperventilation causing respiratory alkalosis and compensatory alkaluria (Potassium and sodium bicarbonate are excreted in the urine). Phase last approximately 12 hours.
  - Phase 2: Paradoxic aciduria along with respiratory alkalosis once enough potassium has been lost. Phase last from 12 - 24 hours.
  - Phase 3: Metabolic acidosis along with hypokalemia and dehydration. Phase begins within 4 – 6 hours after ingestion for child and within 24 hours after ingestion for teen or adult.
  - Symptoms: Diaphoresis, tinnitus, nausea, vomiting: early signs.
    As it progresses: hyperventilation, vertigo, tachycardia, hyperactivity.
    When it becomes severe: agitation, hallucinations, convulsions, lethargy, hyperthermia, and delirium.

General Rules for Mixed Acid Base Disorder

- You do not see the compensatory response that would be expected.
- The compensatory response is extreme.
- The pH is normal but the HCO3 or PCO2 is abnormal.
- Normal compensatory responses should always be in the same direction as the initial abnormal change, mixed acid base occurs when the HCO3 and the PCO2 both are abnormal but are going in the opposite directions (one is high and the other low).

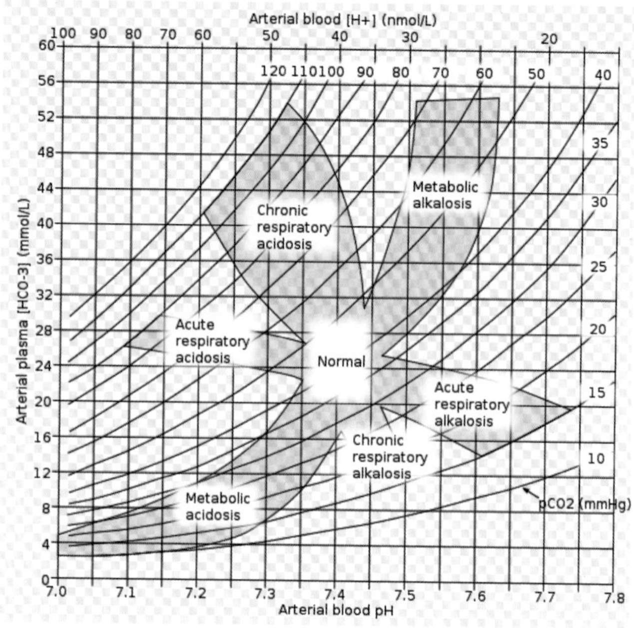

Anion Gap and Non-Anion Gap Metabolic Acidosis (pH < 7.4)

- **Formula: Na - (HCO3 + Cl)**
- If total is 6 – 12 mEq/L, it is a **normal anion gap acidosis** (non-anion gap)
  If total is > 12, it is an **anion gap acidosis**
- **Anion Gap Acidosis:**
  Anion gap is due to decreasing chloride levels.
  Causes: (MUDPILES): Methanol, Uremia, **DKA**, Propylene glycol, Iron tablet/INH, Lactate (**Lactic acidosis**), **Ethylene glycol** (oxalic acid), **Salicylates (aspirin** in the later states of OD)

- **Non-Anion Gap Acidosis** (AKA: hyperchloremic metabolic acidosis)
  Anion gap is normal because the chloride level rises.
  Causes: (HARD-ASS): Hyperalimentation (overdose of nutrients), Addison's Dz, **RTA (renal tube acidosis)**, **Diarrhea**, Acetazolamide, Spironolactone, Saline infusion.
  - **Most common cause of non-anion gap acidosis: RTA and diarrhea**. To differentiate between these two causes you must look at the Urine Anion Gap (UAG). **UAG = Na minus the Cl (Sodium minus the chloride).**

  - **Diarrhea as the cause: UAG will be a positive number.** (Kidneys are able to excrete acid into the urine so urine chloride ↑).
    Diarrhea loses bicarb and potassium causing low bicarb, hypokalemia. It causes an increase in chloride reabsorption leading to hyperchloremia. (Low bicarb and high chloride = normal anion gap).

  - **RTA as the cause: UAG will be a negative number.** (RTA is a defect in excreting acid into the urine so urine chloride ↓).

Anion Gap Metabolic Acidosis

Acidosis	Type of Acid - Mechanism	Cause	Diagnosis/Symptoms	Treatment/Notes
Methanol Alcohol (**tip**: "M" for "Mind" issues (eye/CNS)	Metabolized into formaldehyde and then to formic acid. **Formic acid** inhibits cytochrome c oxidase = hypoxia.	Ingestion, inhalation, absorption. Found: paints, solvent, antifreeze, explosives, gasoline,	CNS depression, headaches, nausea, headache, loss of vision.	**Fomepizole, Ethanol**. Dialysis if severe. Inhibits alcohol dehydrogenase.
Ethanol Alcohol	Metabolized into alcohol dehydrogenase by **acetaldehyde** and then into acetyl (in acetyl CoA) by acetaldehyde dehydrogenase. (Acetyl CoA final product of carbs and fat metabolism used to make ATP). **Acetaldehyde** is the toxic cause of the effects. Converts NAD to NADH.	Ingestion	CNS depressant, slowed cognition, impaired motor and sensory function, loss of consciousness, delirium tremors, death. Addiction. Binds NMDA (Glutamate) receptors and enhances GABA.	**Fomepizole, Ethanol**. Dialysis if severe. Inhibits alcohol dehydrogenase. **Note:** Used as an antidote to methanol and ethylene glycol overdose. It is an antitussive, used an as antibacterial in hand sanitizer gels (dentures proteins) **Note: Must give alcoholic B-1 replacement before giving any glucose.** "Banana Bag"
Ethylene Glycol	Metabolized into **glycolic acid and then to oxalic acid.** Oxalic acid binds with calcium to form **calcium oxalate crystals** that deposit into the kidneys, heart, brain, lungs.	Antifreeze ingestion	Nausea, vomiting, cardiovascular kidney failure, seizure, lack of coordination, headaches, confusion, encephalopathy, cerebral edema.	**Fomepizole, Ethanol**. Dialysis if severe. Inhibits alcohol dehydrogenase.
Lactic Acidosis	Build up of **lactate** (levels >5 mmol/L and serum pH < 7.35). ANY ↓ in perfusion in the kidneys results in anaerobic metabolism which causes a ↑ in glycolysis, which leads to excess of pyruvate, so is then converted to lactate and released into the bloodstream. This also causes a build up of hydrogen cations (because lactate was not able to produce the ATP for them to bind) so hydrogen cations build up causing acidosis.	Very ill people: Sepsis, excessive exercise, hypoperfusion, hypotension, ethanol toxicity, DKA, hemorrhage, hypoxia, genetic deficiencies, drugs: **Metformin, INH, NRTI's.**	Nausea, vomiting, high respiratory rate, muscle weakness. DX: Blood lactate levels.	Correct underlying condition.

Lack of Insulin	**Ketoacids.** Lack of insulin (glucose) ➔ ↑ glucagon ➔ gluconeogenesis, glycogenolysis, release lipolysis (releases free fatty acids via beta oxidation into ketone bodies: β-hydroxybutyrate, acetoacetate) ➔ acidic ketone bodies make the blood acidic.	**DKA (Diabetics),** starvation	**Kussmaul breathing** (hyperventilation = respiratory alkalosis), nausea, vomiting, **abdominal pain**, excessive thirst, dehydration (dry mouth, decreased skin turgor), **ketotic breath** (fruity breath), low blood pressure, tachycardia, cerebral edema, loss of pupillary light reflex, coma, death. Labs: ↓ Na, K, Cl, phosphate, Mg, Ca. **Glucose levels > 250** mg/dL, **ketones in the urine** (acetoacetate) and ketones in the blood (β-hydroxybutyrate).	Insulin, potassium replacement and normal saline (9% NaCl)
Salicylates	**Salicylic Acid** uncouples oxidative phosphorylation, leading to an increased ADP: ATP ratios. Causes a **mixed acid/base** with metabolic acidosis with compensatory respiratory alkalosis.	**Aspirin toxicity.** Ingestion of aspirin or aspirin containing products (including topicals such as Ben-Gay, oil of wintergreen or methyl salicylate).	Early stages: diaphoresis, nausea, vomiting, **tinnitus**. Progression: **hyperventilation (respiratory alkalosis)**, vertigo, hyperactivity, tachycardia. Severe: delirium, hallucination, agitation, convulsions, lethargy, hyperthermia.	Note: It is also ototoxic due to the inhibition of Prestin (motor protein of the hair cells in the cochlea).
Uremia (urea in the blood)	Urea is a component of urine composed of excess amino acids and protein metabolites. In a normally functioning kidney it is excreted out in the urine. But when the kidney is failing, it backs up into the blood stream.	**Kidney failure.**	CNS symptoms: fatigue, nausea, vomiting, confusion, seizures, encephalopathy, coma. DX: Elevated BUN, creatinine.	Dialysis to remove nitrogen waste

Physiologic Effects of Acidosis and Alkalosis on the Body

Effects of Acidosis	Effects of Alkalosis
CNS • Cerebral vasodilation = ↑ in cerebral blood flow and intracranial pressure • High PCO2 causes central depression	CNS • Cerebral vasoconstriction causes a decrease in cerebral blood flow which causes confusion, asterixis, seizures, loss of consciousness • Increase in neuromuscular excitability causing paraesthesias, numbness, carpopedal spasm
Respiratory • Kussmaul respirations (hyperventilation) • Initially (< 6 hours) causes the oxyhaemoglobin dissociation curve to shift right (taut form) • After 6 hours, there is a decrease in 2,3 DPG levels in RBC which causes the oxyhaemoglobin dissociation curve to shift back to the left (relaxed form)	Respiratory • Impaired unloading of oxygen which shifts the oxyhaemoglobin dissociation curve to the left (relax state) • Then there is an increase in 2.3 DPG in the RBC's which shifts the oxyhaemoglobin curve back to the right (taut state) • Central and peripheral chemoreceptors inhibit the respiratory drive

Physiologic Effects of Acidosis and Alkalosis on the Body cont'd

Acidosis	Alkalosis
Cardiovascular • At a pH < 7.2 there is a decrease in contractility • Sympathetic over activity: tachycardia, increased risk of arrhythmias, vasoconstriction • When severe acidosis, there is resistance to the effects of catecholamines • Venoconstriction of peripheral veins • Peripheral arteriolar vasodilation • Vasoconstriction of pulmonary arteries • Hyperkalemia, which affect the heart	Cardiovascular • Arrhythmias • Decrease in contractility
Misc Effects • Increase in bone resorption • Increase in extracellular phosphate concentration • Hyperkalemia because potassium is shifted out of cells	Misc Effects • Hypokalemia because the hydrogen ions shift into the cells

Alkalemia (pH > 7.4)
- Respiratory Alkalosis
  Hyperventilation, Hypoxemia, High Altitude, Tumor, Pulmonary embolism, Salicylates (aspirin in the early stages of OD), Anxiety/hysteria
- Metabolic Alkalosis (compensated with respiratory hypoventilation)
  Vomiting, Loop diuretics, Antacids, Hyperaldosteronism

Net Reabsorption (fluid pulled back in from tubules to bring back into body so it is not excreted)
- Filtered > excreted
- More reabsorbed so less excreted out
- ↑ reabsorbed: Glucose, Sodium Urea
- Amount of fluid entering glomerulus minus amount excreted = how much was reabsorbed

Net Secreted (Filtered) (fluid put out into tubules from body to be excreted)
- Excretion > filtered
- More is added into tubes after filtration
- ↑ secreted: PAH, creatinine)
- Amount of fluid excreted minus the fluid entering the glomerulus

Reabsorption

PCT
- Main location of reabsorption (Main points location for: Ca reabsorbed in DCT and Urea in collecting tubules)
  - Reabsorbs: glucose, amino acids, bicarb (HCO_3), phosphate, Chloride, Potassium, Sodium, Urea (majority of urea absorbed in the **collecting tubules**)
- **Isotonic**
- PTH inhibits Na/PO4 cotransport → excretion of PO4
- ATII activates Na/H exchange to ↑ Na, water and HCO3 reabsorption

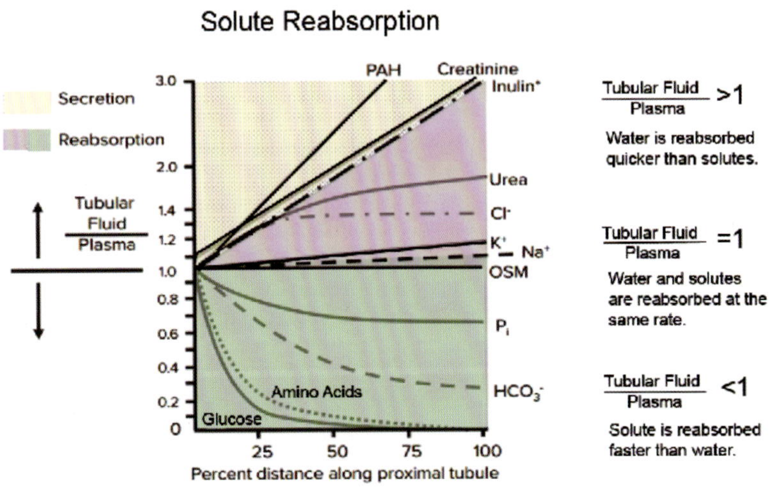

Thick ascending loop of Henle
- Reabsorbs Na, K, Cl
- Impermeable to water (water is not able to dilute down urine at this point)
- No presence of ADH
- **Hypertonic**

DCT

- Reabsorbs Na, CL
- PTH = absorption of Ca through Ca/Na exchange
- Generates bicarbonate (whish is then reabsorbed in the PCT)
- **Hypotonic**

Collecting tubule

- Reabsorbs Na
- Secretes K and H (regulated by Aldosterone)
- Aldosterone acts on luminal side (side next to tubule
- ADH acts on V2 receptors which then work with aquaporin H2O channels on luminal side
- Uric acid reabsorbed (**Main site**. Some reabsorbed in PCT)

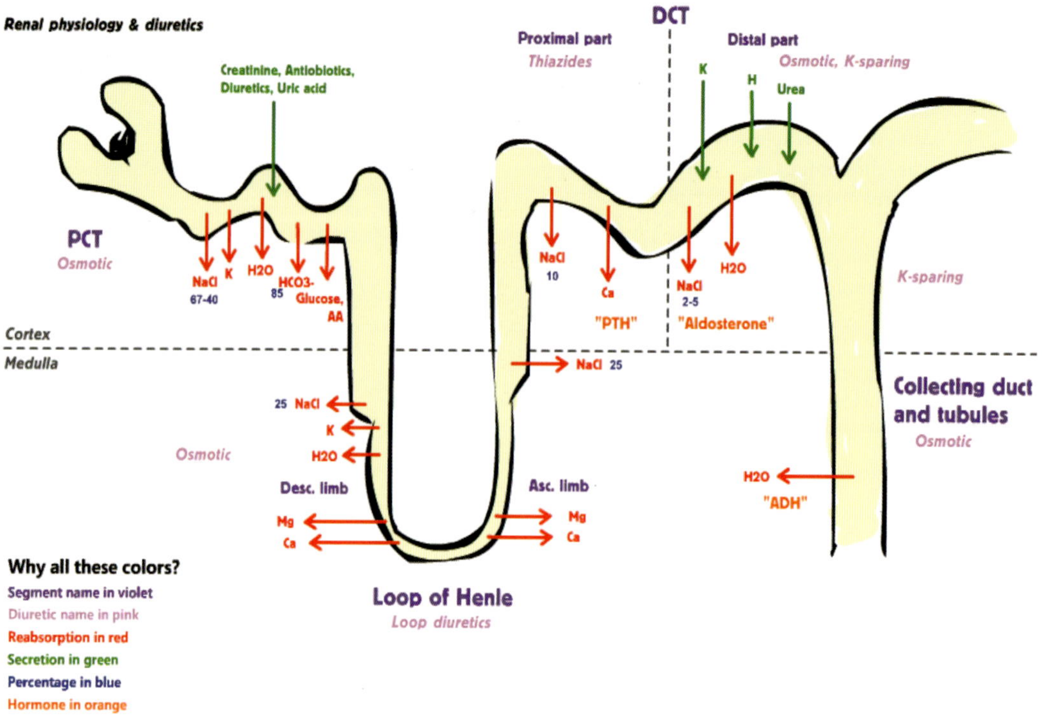

Clearance

Glucose Clearance and Reabsorption

- Glucose is 100% reabsorbed in the **PCT by Na/Glucose** cotransport as long as the glucose level is at normal plasma level
- Once plasma glucose is **200 mg/dL, glucose spills over** into the urine (glucosuria)
- All Na/Glucose transporters are totally saturated once plasma glucose reaches 375 mg/dL
- Glucosuria is an indication of diabetes mellitus
- Pregnancy = ↓ reabsorption amino acids (aminoaciduria) and ↓ reabsorption of glucose (glucosuria)

Renin-Angiotensin-Aldosterone System

- **JG cells (Juxtaglomerular apparatus)** of the afferent arteriole respond to hyperperfusion
  JG Cells **(AKA: modified smooth muscle of afferent arteriole)**
- **Macula densa** cells respond to ↓ Na
- β1 receptors respond to ↑ sympathetic tone
- AT II = most potent vasoconstrictor in the body.
  Method of Action:
  ↓ RPR (Renal Plasma Flow) (ie: Hypoperfusion/↓ BP due to CHF, hemorrhage, dehydration, renal artery stenosis, adrenal insufficiency) → ↓ GFR ↑ →JG cells sense decreased flow/pressure → If decrease is due to systemic reasons (not renal artery stenosis) then carotid arch and aortic arch receptors are activated → sympathetic response on β 1 receptors to release renin from granules in the JG cells into the blood → Renin acts as protease to convert angiotensinogen to angiotensin I in the liver → ATI goes to lungs to be converted to Angiotensin II by ACE (angiotensin converting enzyme) → **ATII stimulates several factors** (below) in order to ↑ volume and pressure.
  ATII stimulates receptors on vascular smooth muscle to vasoconstrict vessels. It constricts the efferent arteriole = ↑ FF when RPF is decreased in low volume states to preserve renal function (GFR).
  ATII stimulates release of aldosterone = ↑ Na absorption, ↑ K+ (Principal Cells) and H+) Intercalated Cells) secretion.
  ATII stimulates ADH to act on medullary collecting duct = ↑ water reabsorption (↑ water channels (aquaporin) in Principal Cells).
  ATII stimulates sympathetic nervous system = PCT reabsorption of Na, water, urea (BUN), uric acid, calcium. This causes creatinine to be secreted in the PCT (excreted) causing **> 20 BUN: Cr ratio**, ↑ urine OSM (>500) and fractional excretion of Na of < 1% (% of Na filtered by the kidney which is excreted in the urine).
  ATII Stimulates hypothalamus = to ↑ thirst.

Renin-angiotensin-aldosterone system

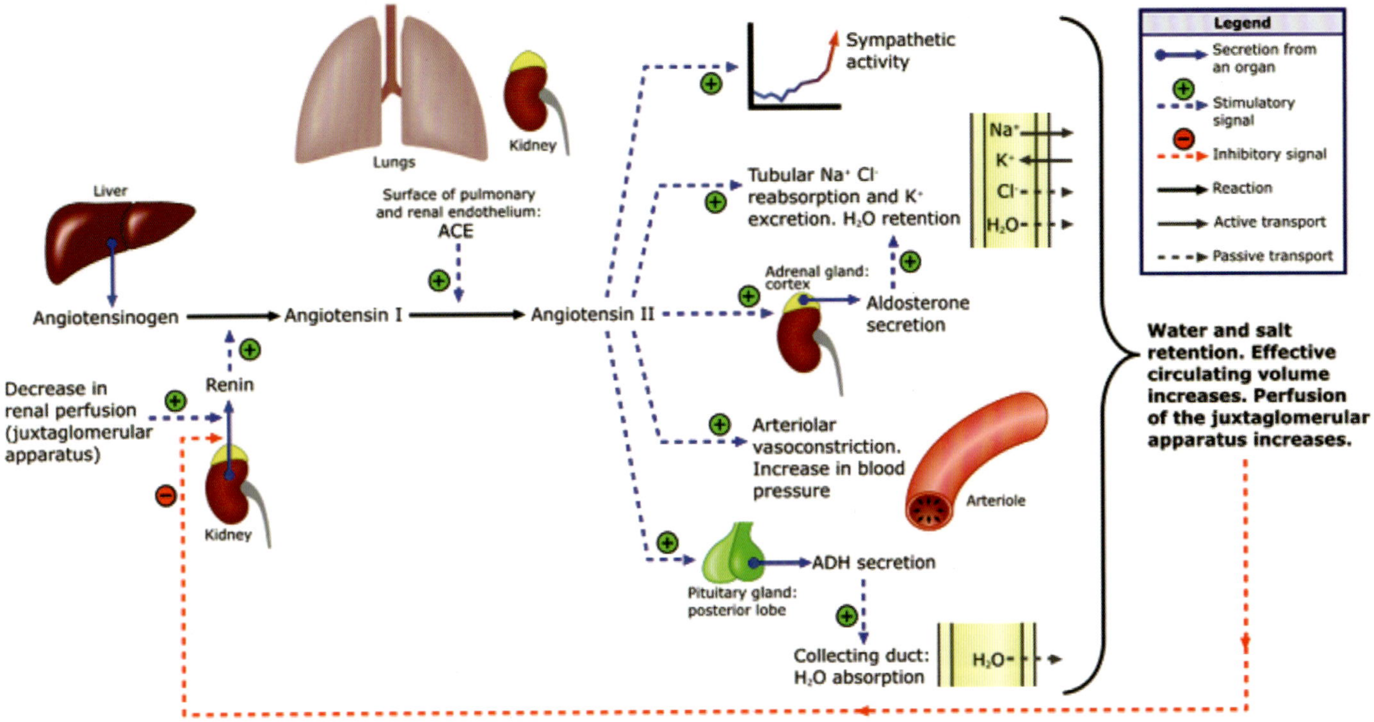

Angiotensinogen System Review:

- Angiotensinogen (α-2-globulin) produced and released into plasma from the liver. Levels are increased by estrogen, thyroid hormones, steroids and ATII levels. It is also a renin substrate.
- Renin is produced in the kidneys (juxtaglomerular cells/JG cells/smooth muscle cells on the afferent arteriole) in response to renal sympathetic activity due to: pre-renal delivery of ↓ blood flow/volume/pressure or ↓ delivery of Na and Cl to the macula densa.
- Angiotensin I formed by action on renin on angiotensinogen. It cleaves peptide bond between leucine and valine on angiotensinogen, which produced ATI.
- ATI is converted to ATII by ACE (angiotensin-converting enzyme) in the lungs by removing C-terminal residues on ATI. (ACE is found in the lung predominantly, but is also found in endothelial cells or the kidney epithelial cells).
- ATII is an endocrine (secretes hormones), paracrine (influences near-by cells), autocrine (same cell) and intracrine (intracellular) hormone.
- ATII is degraded by ATIII by angiotensinase in RBC's and vascular areas of tissues.
  ATII half-life is 30 seconds in circulation and 30 minutes in tissues.

Effect of ATII on the Kidneys:

- Renal artery, Afferent arterioles → vasoconstriction (Gq = ↑ PLC → IP3 → ↑ intracellular Ca)
- Efferent arterioles → vasoconstriction (Gq = ↑ PLC → IP3 → ↑ intracellular Ca)
- Mesangial cells: Contraction and ↓ filtration (Gq = ↑ PLC → IP3 → ↑ intracellular Ca)
- PCT: ↑ Na reabsorption. Starling forces in peritubular capillaries → ↑ reabsorption.
  Efferent, afferent arteriole contraction = ↓ hydrostatic pressure in peritubular capillaries
  efferent arteriole contraction = ↑ filtration fraction → ↑ colloid osmotic pressure in peritubular capillaries
- Tubuloglomerular feedback: ↑ afferent arteriole sensitivity from signals from macula densa
- Medullary blood flow is ↓

Creatinine

- **Normal renal function declines 1% for every year past the age of 40.**
- Creatinine measures overall kidney function
- It is a waste product in the blood that is produced after muscle activity and is normally removed by the kidneys, but when the kidney fails to function the creatinine level rises.
- Rising creatine levels indicate declining renal function
- Decrease of creatinine filtration causes higher amounts of creatinine in the blood

Chronic Renal Failure/End Stage Renal Disease

Patient has a BUN/Cr ratio of 10:1 > 3 months = kidney failure.

- Waxy Cast
- **↓ CA in serum, ↑ Phosphate in serum, ↑ PTH** (Without active Vitamin D, calcium can't be reabsorbed in the gut. **This is the cause of 2° Hyperparathyroidism.**
  TX: Replace Vitamin D and Calcium.
- Decreased or no production of EPO (Causes anemia. EPO must be exogenously administered)
- **↓ Calcitriol (active Vitamin D)** (Inability to covert vitamin D3 into its active form calcitriol (1,25)
- Anion gap metabolic acidosis (can't get rid os organic acids) = ↓ pH
- Muscle wasting due to acidosis which causes protein catabolism
- Bone loss due to bone bufering of acid (build up of H+ ions)
- **↓ pH, ↓ CO2, ↓ HCO3**
- **↓ EPO production**
- Hyperkalemia
- Hypocalcemia
- Pruritus (TX: Dialysis, UV light)
- Uremia (Leads to uremic pericarditis. Can only be treated by dialysis, not NSAIDS).
- Dyslipidemia (Lymphocytes help ↓ lipid accumulation, lymphocytes are unable to function in a uremic environment.
  TX: Dialysis)
- **A non-functioning kidney will show tubular atrophy**
- Infection (Neutrophils can't degranulate in a uremic environment so can't fight off infections)
- Water and sodium retention complicating HTN, CHF, pulmonary edema
- Growth retardation, developmental delays
- Hypertension
- Renal osteodystrophy. (Abnormal bone mineralization resulting from hyperparathyroidism, calcitriol deficiency, increased serum phosphate.
- Osteomalacia and Osteopenia can be caused by calcitriol deficiency
- Normocytic anemia
- Bleeding (Platelets can't degranulate in a uremic environment. TX: **DDAVP** ↑ platelet function).
- Hyperphosphatemia (Phosphate should be excreted in normally functioning kidneys, failing kidneys can't excrete it)
- Hypermagnesemia (Magnesium is unable to be excreted in failing kidneys. TX: Restrict foods/medicines containing Mg)
- ↑ Insulin levels (Insulin is normally excreted by normally functioning kidneys)
- Endocrine problems: ↓ testosterone in men = ↓ libido and erectile dysfunction.
  ↓ estrogen causes anovulation in women. (TX: Dialysis, hormone replacement: testosterone and estrogen)
- **2° hyperparathyroidism** due to ↑ PTH because of chronic hypocalcemia (which also continues to breakdown bone)

Urine Chloride Differentials

- Normal urine chloride labs: 20 – 250 mEq/L
- ↑ Chloride in urine = ↑ acid in the urine
- ↓ Chloride in the urine = ↓ acid in the urine

Pathology	Urine Chloride Levels	Notes
Surreptitious Vomiting (Chronic vomiting)	**Decreased ↓**	**Normal BP** Vomiting out HCL. So losing H+, Chloride, K. Kidneys will be reabsorbing Chloride (and HCO3) from the urine = Metabolic **alkalosis**
Hyperemesis Gravidarum (Severe vomiting in pregnancy)	**Decreased ↓**	**Normal BP** Vomiting out HCL. So losing H^+, Chloride, K (hypokalemia) Kidneys will be reabsorbing Chloride (and HCO3) from the urine = Metabolic **alkalosis**
Diuretic Use	**Increased** with + urine test for diuretics	Kidneys are not reabsorbing chloride = ↑ urine chloride
Bartter's Syndrome Defect in thick ascending limb of loop of Henle or DCT. Excessive urinary loss of Na, Cl, and K. Mutation of CLCNKB gene	**Increased**	Kidneys are not reabsorbing chloride = ↑ urine chloride. **Urine labs**: ↑ urine chloride, ↑ urine sodium, and ↑ urine potassium. **Plasma labs**: ↓ K (hypokalemia), ↑ plasma renin and ↑ aldosterone with normal BP, Metabolic alkalosis (Present same SX as people on loop diuretics)
Gitelman 's Syndrome Defect in Sodium-chloride symporter in the DCT. Mutation in NCCT gene.	**Increased**	Kidneys are not reabsorbing chloride = ↑ urine chloride. Urine labs: ↑ urine chloride, ↑ urine potassium, ↓ urine calcium, ↓ urine Mg, metabolic alkalosis. **Plasma Labs:** Hypochloremia, hypokalemia, hypercalcemia, hypermagnesemia (Presents with same SX as people on thiazide diuretics)

Chloride Shift

(AKA: Hamburger shift)

- **Exchange of bicarbonate (HCO_3) and chloride across the membrane of RBC's.**
- PATHWAY: CO2 in circulation enters RBC via passive diffusion. Carbonic anhydrase inside the RBC converts CO2 into carbonic acid (H_2CO_3). The carbonic acid then dissociates and forms bicarbonate and a hydrogen ion (H^+). This conversion decreases the CO2 inside the cell so more extracellular CO2 enters the cell. RBC's then exchange these bicarb ions for chloride ions with an anion exchanger. So bicarb is sent out of the cell and chloride is brought into the cell. Because there is more CO2 in the venous system verses the arterial system, more bicarb can be exchanged, so the blood chloride levels in the venous system are lower than that of the arterial system because more chloride ions are being brought inside the cells out of the blood system.

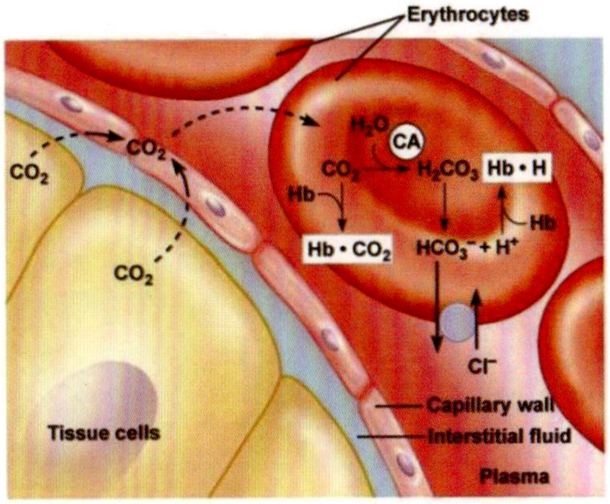

Chloride Shift (Hamburger Shift)

Micturition (voiding, urination)

- Storage phase (urine stored in bladder)
- Voiding phase (urine passes from bladder through urethra).
- **Low bladder volumes: ↓ afferent firing → tightening of the sphincter and urethra.**
- **High bladder volumes: ↑ afferent firing → conscious urinary urge → bladder contracts (detrusor) and sphincter and urethra relax → urination (micturition). Aided by the voluntary contraction of the abdominal muscles.**
- **Sympathetic effect: Internal urethral sphincter tense, detrusor relaxed**
- **Parasympathetic effect: (micturition) detrusor muscle contracts and internal urethral sphincter to relax.**
- Normal bladder holds 400 – 600 ml (14 oz – 20 oz)
- Normal residual volume (post-urination) is < 50 ml. >65 ml is considered urinary retention.

Renal Pathologies

Definitions in kidney disease

- Diffuse: means every glomerulus is affected
- Focal: means that not all glomeruli are involved
- "itis" If kidney pathology ends in "itis" is means immunologic pathology (ex: Diffuse glomerulonephritis, IgA glomerulonephritis). "Itis" are Type III hypersensitivity (Immune-complexes) (ie: Goodpasture's, Post Strep GM)
- If pathology is both diffuse and focal: it is Focal Segmental Glomerulus
- Proliferative: means "many". (ex: Diffuse proliferative means all the glomeruli have many nuclei
- Thick membranes: membranous glomerulonephritis
- Thick membranes and increased numbers of cells: means Membranoproliferative glomerulonephritis

Diagnostic test in kidney disease

- Immunofluorescent stain: (only shows 2 patterns) Linear and granular (AKA: bumpy, lumpy) which are immune complexes
- Electron Microscope (EM) is used for seeing podocytes

Urine Casts

Casts	Pathology
Fatty Casts (AKA: Oval Fat Bodies)	Nephrotic syndrome. ↑ **Cholesterol**. Maltese cross
Granular Casts (AKA: Muddy brown cast)	**Acute tubular necrosis (ATN)** Location: **PCT** Urine: see pieces of tubular epithelium. Causes: ↓ blood flow/BP, drugs After healing, tubes regenerate and show as **normal** tubules
Hyaline Casts	Kimmel-Wilson (Diabetics) Shows pink with stain. Can also be caused by dehydration: Tamm-Horsfall protein precipitates.
RBC Casts	**Glomerulonephritis**, malignant HTN Hematuria in urine but **no casts**: Bladder cancer, kidney stones
Waxy Casts	Renal Failure (advanced or chronic) BUN/creatine > 15
WBC Casts	**Pyelonephritis,** transplant rejection No casts: pyuria, cystitis

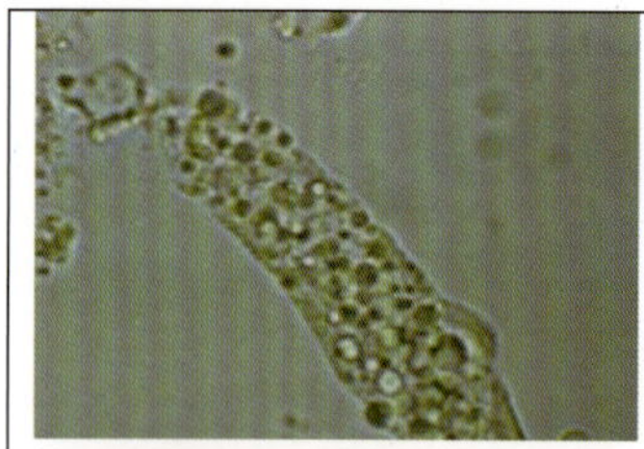
Fatty Casts

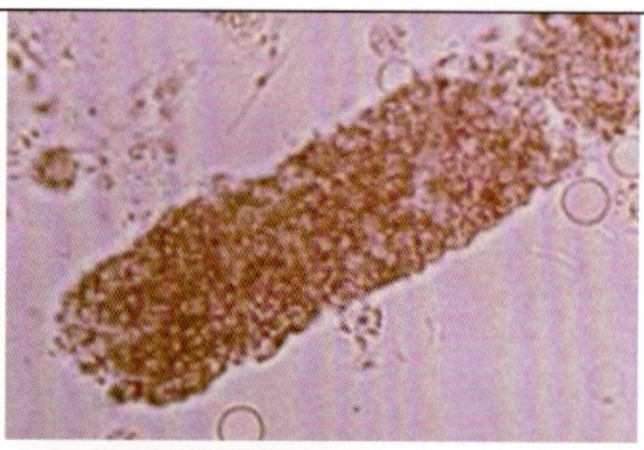
Granular Casts

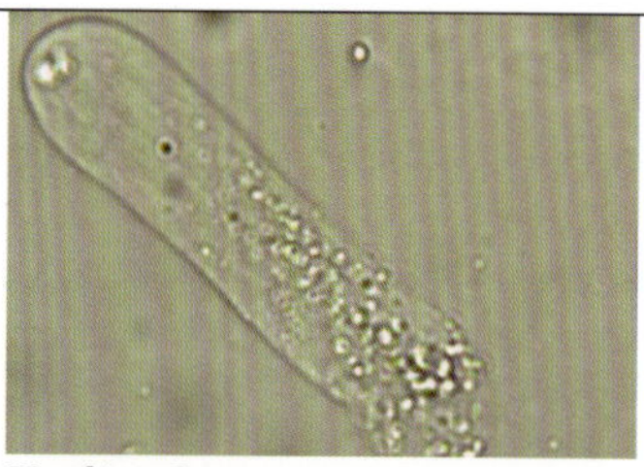
Hyaline Casts

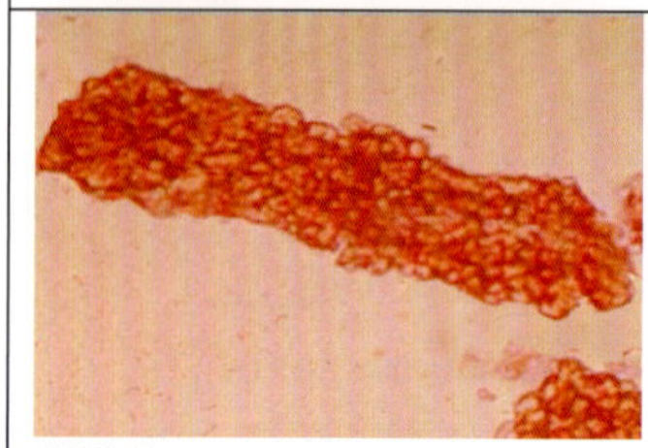
RBC Casts

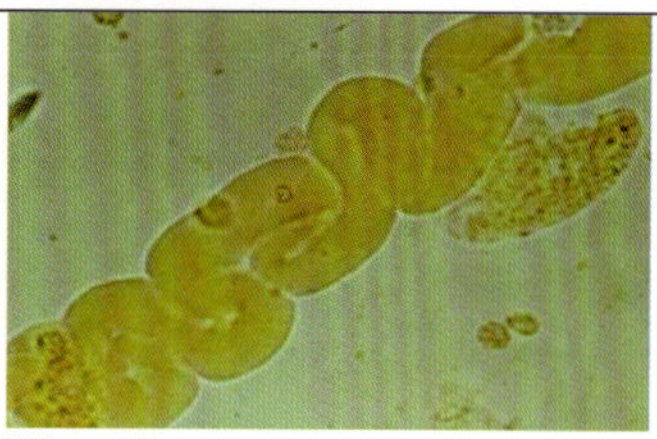
Waxy Casts

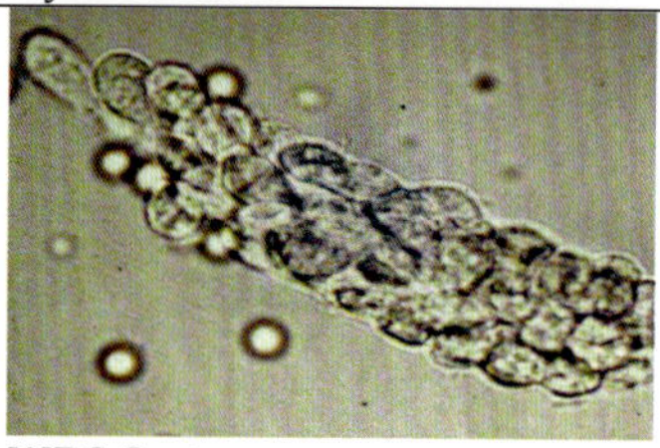
WBC Casts

Additional Test

- Proteinuria (BIT: Urinalysis. MAT: Protein: Creatinine ratio)
  - Normal protein in the urine: < 300 mg in 24 hours
  - Normal protein excretion: Tamm-Horsfall protein: most abundant, normal glycoprotein excreted in urine
  - Transient proteinuria: temporary, benign protein in the urine
    - **Causes**: Fever, exercise, cardiac failure, extreme cold, seizures, dehydration, stress
    - DX: UA shows mild proteinuria,
  - Orthostatic proteinuria: transient proteinuria due to being a person being on their feet for long periods: teachers, waiters, etc.
  - Bence-Jones proteins cannot be detected by urinalysis, immunoelectrophoresis is required
  - Activity and prolonged standing ↑ protein in the urine
  - DX: Biopsy to determine the cause
- Macroalbuminuria
  - Tiny proteins to small to be detected by urinalysis: Normal: 30 – 300 mg/24 hours
  - Macroalbuminuria is monitored to track the progression of diabetes, it indicates worsening renal function
  - Diabetics, with good renal function, should be put on ACE inhibitors or ARB's to slow the progression of diabetic nephropathy
- Hematuria
  - Normal urine has < 5 RBC per microscope field
  - Glomerulonephritis (dysmorphic RBC's)
  - Causes: kidney stones, bladder cancer or other renal cancers (painless hematuria), cystitis, pyelonephritis, trauma to the kidney, medicines (MC: Cyclophosphamide: hemorrhagic cystitis), bleeding disorders, IgA Nephropathy
  - False positives for hematuria can be caused by myoglobin or Hb
  - Cystoscopy used to DX hematuria if there is no history of infection or trauma or if a mass is present in the bladder. Beware if signs in the vignette point to **endocarditis** after a cystoscope due to unclean instruments
- White Blood Cells
  - Indicates presence of inflammation or infection
  - Can indicate acute interstitial nephritis or allergic interstitial nephritis. Eosinophils are always a good clue in any test that indicates the problem is due to an allergy or allergic reaction to a drug. Exception: NSAID's pathology does not show eosinophils
- Osmolality Rules
  - Osmolality = urine concentration.
    ↑ OSM = ↑ concentrated = urine Na > 20 and urine OSM < 300.
    ↓ OSM = dilute = urine Na
  - OSM Physio: When intravascular volume is down due to dehydration, hemorrhage, etc., ADH will be released (increase) so that the renal tubes will reabsorb more water (pulling it out of the urine) to bring back into the vasculature leaving the urine more concentrated.
    If a person has an overload of fluid, the body will diurese causing the kidneys to resorb (secrete) more water from the vasculature into the urine, which then causes the urine to become dilute.
  - Dehydration = will increase OSM (urine concentration). Dehydration will cause ADH to be released so that it tries to bring in and preserve what water it can in order to replenish the vasculature, leaving the urine concentrated.
    Dehydration is a prerenal cause, which can lead to ATN (acute tubular necrosis). In ATN (cell death), the cells are not able to absorb sodium or water (↑ OSM) so they are excreted in the urine.
  - Specific gravity is relative to urine osmolarity. High urine OSM = high specific gravity.

Renal Failure

Azotemia

Abnormally high levels of nitrogen containing compound urea in the blood due to insufficient filtering of blood in the kidneys, which can lead to uremia. (Urea is a component of urine composed of the end products of metabolism of the amino acids and proteins urea and creatinine. Uremia is the excess of these end products because they are not being filtered and excreted in the kidneys).

BUN/Cr Ratio: Normal: between 10:1 and 20:1
(example: BUN of 14 and a creatinine of 1.2 is a ratio of 12:1).
Both kidneys must be affected before the creatinine rises.

- BUN (Blood Urea Nitrogen) is the amount of nitrogen from the waste product urea that is in the blood. It indicates how well the kidneys are working. If the kidneys can't remove the urea from the blood, BUN levels will rise. Other factors can increase the BUN: heart failure, high protein diet, and dehydration. Other factors can decrease the BUN: liver disease and pregnancy.
- BUN: Blood Urea Nitrogen (normal: 7 to 20 mg/dL)
- Creatinine: end product of creatine metabolism (normal 0.5 – 1.2 mg/dL)
- Dehydration or ↓ CO: causes ratio to > 20:1
- Pregnancy, liver disease or diets low in protein can cause low BUN/Cr ratio
- The creatinine ratio can rise as a result of chemotherapy treatment due to tumor lysis syndrome. Tumor lysis syndrome can lead to hyperuricemia → gout. TX: **Allopurinol.**

Location	Description
Prerenal Azotemia	**ANYTHING that decreases perfusion entering the kidney** (AKA: BEFORE entering the kidney) that is not due to renal diseases/causes. **NOTE:** Anytime there is hypoperfusion to the kidney, the kidney will respond by trying to **conserve water**. If perfusion is not restored, then the result will be acute tubular necrosis (due to ischemia). **Indicates decrease in renal function.** Causes: **Hypoperfusion or dehydration, hypotension (↓ BP due to CHF, hemorrhage, dehydration, renal artery stenosis, adrenal insufficiency, sepsis, anaphylaxis), renal artery stenosis, diuretics, pancreatitis, low oncotic pressure (low albumin), burns. Anything that ↓** Cardiac Output will lead to prerenal azotemia → ↓ GFR due to ↓ renal blood flow (tamponade, constrictive pericarditis), NSAID's which constrict the afferent arteriole, cirrhosis (oncotic pressure). **BUN Increase Physiology:** BUN reabsorption is increased so BUN is elevated as compared to the creatinine. BUN is increased do to the effects of ADH on the collecting duct. Hypoperfusion/hypotension stimulate renin which stimulates aldosterone which stimulates ADH. **ADH acts on the distal tube and collecting ducts**. ADH also causes increased urea absorption at the urea transporter at the collecting ducts, which causes the increase in BUN. **BUN/Creatinine > 20, ↓ GFR, ↓ RPF** **Urine OSM >500**, Urine Na < 20, **Fractional excretion of Na <1%.** TX: Treat the underlying cause.

Intrinsic (Primary) renal azotemia, **Acute Tubular Necrosis.**

Due to issues that arise inside the kidney (parenchymal).
Causes: **Acute tubular necrosis**, ischemia, toxins (drugs: NSAID's, Cisplatin, Sulfa drugs, Cyclosporine, Amphotericin B, Aminoglycosides, Penicillin), renal failure, glomerulonephritis (Strep infection), crystal deposits, amyloid deposits (Bence-Jones), radiographic **contrast dyes, ethylene glycol** (causes build up of calcium oxalate in renal cortex).

Causes: ↓ GFR = ↓ filtration so that nothing is filtrated as it should be causing higher levels of urea in the blood and low levels of urea in the urine as compared to creatinine.
BUN/creatinine <15, Urine Na >40, Urine OSM < 350, Fractional excretion of Na >1%.
SX: Eosinophilia. Protein and blood in the urine = **brown/granular casts.**
NOTE: PCT will repair itself once the offending cause is stopped. If the vignette ask what will be seen on histology a couple of weeks after the ATN, it will be regenerating cells.

TX: Correct the underlying cause in ATN.
Dialysis is only used when there is: **Uremic Pericarditis**, Hyperkalemia, Encephalopathy, Metabolic Acidosis. (Do not do dialysis in the case of hypokalemia: treat with Vitamin D and calcium).

Contrast Dyes NOTE: Do NOT use contrast dyes in any patient with poor renal function. Contrast dyes are toxic to the kidney tubules. Contrast dyes cause the afferent arteriole to spasm, which leads to ATN causing the specific gravity to become high. Renal damage from contrast dyes rapid (< 24 hrs) verses other causes (medicines), which take several days. It is important to stop **Metformin** before undergoing any type of contrast dye testing. **Prior to undergoing testing with contrast dyes**, patient must **be well hydrated (saline hydration) to prevent renal toxicity.**

Rhabdomyolysis NOTE: Due to trauma/crush injuries, seizures, venomous bites, prolonged immobility. **Beware** of the vignettes that have a patient on a **Statin drug**. They will have "red" urine (myoglobin due to rhabdomyolysis) because of either excessive exercising/running or because a fibrate or niacin has been added to the statin.
In myoglobin no RBC are noted because this is **myoglobin. Myoglobin is very toxic to the kidneys and ↓ serum calcium levels. (Causes a left shift to the oxy-heme curve**).

Rhabdomyolysis and low serum calcium physiology:
In the normal contraction process of muscles, an action potential travels down the T tubules (transverse tubules). The depolarization activates L-type voltage dependent calcium channel (dihydropyridine receptors) in the terminal cisternae. Then intracellular ryanodine receptors then release the calcium from the sarcoplasmic reticulum where it then binds to the troponin C on the actin thin filaments of the myofibrils. Troponin causes an allosteric change in the tropomyosin so that the actin binding sites are exposed for the binding of the myosin heads. Myosin (thick filaments) along with ADP then binds with actin to form a cross bridge and then actin acts as a cofactor to myosin to releases the ADP. This causes a power stroke (shortening the I-band and sarcomere). Once the power stroke occurs, the ADP is released from the myosin head causing the power stroke to stay in place until ATP binds to the myosin so that the cross bridge with actin can be released. If there is no ATP, the myosin and actin are unable to break the cross bridge, resulting in a sustained power stroke (rigor mortis). Once the cross bridge is broken the muscle returns to its resting state and the calcium is pumped back out of the cytosol into storage in the terminal cisternae in the sarcoplasmic reticulum by sarco/endoplasmic calcium-ATPase pumps (SERCA) to begin the process all over again.
When muscle is damaged (due to any of the causes listed above) it damages the sarcolemma (cell membrane of a striated muscle fiber cell). It is the barrier (plasma membrane) between extracellular and intracellular compartments. In these plasma membranes are the sarco/endoplasmic calcium ATPase pumps (SERCA the T-tubules (transverse tubules) which connect to the terminal cisterna (stores for calcium) in the smooth endoplasmic reticulum (AKA: sarcoplasmic reticulum). If this membrane is damaged it allows the SERCA to pull calcium out of the serum, thereby causing a decrease of serum calcium when there is muscle damage.

Labs: Myoglobin (from rhabdomyolysis), ↑↑ CPK (Creatine Phosphokinase), **Hyperkalemia** (dying cells release K. K is located intracellularly), Hyperuricemia (nucleic acids are released when the cells die and are then metabolized to uric acid), ↑ phosphate (due to the damaged muscle), ↓ Ca (Ca binds to the damaged muscle. The Ca will release from the muscles once healed and return calcium levels back to normal). If hypocalcemia is severe it can causes a prolonged QT or seizures. Treat with Vitamin D and calcium. (do not do dialysis).

DX: BIT: Urinalysis: shows positive for blood but no RBC's on microscopic exam.
MAT: Urine myoglobin.

NOTE: Beware of ANY situation that has ↑ potassium levels = fatal arrhythmia's. You MUST monitor the EKG when potassium is abnormal (high or low). Do **NOT replace potassium in hyperkalemia**. There is already too much extracellularly and any additional potassium will potentially cause a fatal arrhythmia.

TX: Normal 9% NaCl fluid, bicarbonate (drives K back into the cells) or **Calcium Gluconate, Mannitol** (osmotic diuretic). Urine alkalinization.

Postrenal azotemia	Due to blockage of urine flow below the kidneys. Not due to renal disease. Causes: Blockage of ureters by kidney or bladder **Stones, BPH**, cancer, congenital anomalies, pregnancy, cervical cancer, neurogenic bladder, chemotherapy. SX: **Bilateral** or unilateral obstruction leading to hydronephrosis (DX: ultrasound), distended bladder and large volume of urine eliminated upon placement of a urinary catheter. Renal damage causes reduced absorption of BUN so BUN/Cr ratio is lowered. **BUN/creatinine >15**, Urine Na > 40, Urine OSM < 350. TX: Treat the underlying cause.

Tubular Pathologies

Acute Drug-Induced Interstitial Nephritis (AKA: Nephrotoxic ATN, Tubulointerstitial nephritis) Occurs in the PCT. Pyuria, **Eosinophils**, Azotemia (high blood level of urea/nitrogen) SX: Costovertebral pain, hematuria, **rash, fever**. Labs: Pus and PMN's in urine, ↑ BUN/Creatine Cause: Drugs (MC: Aminoglycosides, Gentamycin and IV Pyelograms) (**Diuretics, sulfonamides, penicillin derivatives, rifampin, NSAIDS**)	**Acute tubular necrosis** **MCC: not treating prerenal azotemia.** Normal anion gap metabolic acidosis ↓ HCO3, ↑ Cl, ↑ H Pre-renal (↓ CO = ↓ renal blood flow = oliguria. Granular (muddy brown) casts. AKA: **Coagulation necrosis**. MC location: **#1: PCT.** #2: Thick ascending limb (Na/K/2 Cl transport pumps) Stages: **1)** Initial injury to **PCT (Most common)** **2)** Maintenance phase: oliguria, edema, cast, metabolic acidosis, ↑ K, ↑ **BUN/Creatinine** 3) Recovery: Decrease in BUN/Creatinine, hypokalemia Causes: **Ischemia, ↓ renal blood flow**, sepsis, hemorrhage, CHF, **hypotension, shock**, drugs, radio contrast dyes, myoglobinuria, hemoglobinuria**.** **Radio contrast dye:** Do not use in patients with renal failure. Prior to use, all other patients must **hydrate** well.
Bartter Syndrome Inherited reabsorptive defect (Na/K/2Cl cotransporter) in the ascending loop of Henle. Labs: Normal sodium, hypokalemia, hypercalciuria, metabolic alkalosis	**Liddle Syndrome** Autosomal dominant ↑ Na reabsorption in DCT and collecting tubules. SX: HTN, hypokalemia, metabolic alkalosis, ↓ aldosterone TX: **Amiloride**
Gitelman Syndrome Inherited defect in reabsorption of NaCl in DCT. Similar to Bartter Syndrome: hypokalemia, metabolic alkalosis, **NO hypercalciuria**	**Fanconi Syndrome** PCT absorptive defect. (PCT tubular transport dysfunction) ↑ excretion of amino acids, HCO3, PO4 and glucose and HCO3 wasting. SX: PCT acidosis, hypophosphatemic rickets, hypokalemia, polyuria, polydipsia. Causes: Genetic and may occur along with Wilson's Dz, Galactosemia, glycogen storage dz, hereditary fructose intolerance. Acquired causes: **Taking outdated tetracycline**, chemotherapy drugs (Streptozocin, Ifosfamide), HIV drugs (Didanosine, Cidofovir). TX: replacement of substances lost in the urine (esp. bicarbonate)

Analgesic Nephropathy Free radical damage and ischemia leading to **renal papillary necrosis** and chronic interstitial nephritis. Acetaminophen: produces free radicals. **Aspirin blocks PGE2 (vasodilator) to ATII (vasoconstrictor is in charge of renal blood flow = ischemia).** Heavy/chronic long term use of **NSAIDS, acetaminophen**, phenytoin DX: Chronic necrosis of renal papilla, Sudden renal colic **Note:** Always watch the vignette that is experiencing some type of chronic pain. It will not mention that they are taking NSAIDS, but anytime someone is in pain – assume they are taking pain meds.	**Renal Papillary Necrosis** Sloughing off of renal papillae Benign. SX: Rapid onset (hours). Flank pain, hematuria and proteinuria. May also see necrotic debris in the urine (renal papillae). (Resembles pyelonephritis symptoms. Pyelonephritis will also have flank pain but takes several days to present and will have a positive urine culture. CT shows a swollen kidney and can be treated with antibiotics). Associated with DM, chronic pyelonephritis, **Sickle Cell** Anemia, heavy **NSAID** use especially when NSAID's are used with one of the other pathologies listed here. BIT: Urinalysis. Negative urine culture. MAT: CT scan shows loss of papillae. TX: No treatment. Benign.

Nephrosclerosis **Patient with chronic essential, uncontrolled HTN causes hyaline arteriolosclerosis.** **Physio:** Arteriolosclerosis (thickened arteries) causes ↓ blood flow to the kidneys → tubular atrophy → fibrosing off of glomeruli → renal failure. Histology: Kidney has a cobblestone appearance, petechial on the surface of the kidney (AKA: flea bitten kidney/ coagulation necrosis) → malignant HTN→ HTN emergency if BP is not lowered (must see papilledema). TX: **Nitroprusside**	

Renal Tubular Acidosis (RTA)
Metabolic acidosis with a **normal anion gap**.
MCC of non-anion gap acidosis: **RTA and diarrhea.**

Type I: Distal RTA
DCT is unable to excrete hydrogen ions and unable to make new bicarb which raises the pH of the urine (>5.5), causing **alkaline urine**. This increases the risk of **calcium oxalate kidney stones**.
Potassium is also lost in the urine = **hypokalemia.**
TX: IV Ammonium Chloride to replace the bicarb so that PCT will absorb it and correct the alkaline urine.

Type II: Proximal RTA
PCT is unable to reabsorb the bicarb made by the DCT. So bicarb is lost in the urine causing the urine pH to decrease (<5.5) and become **acidotic** (↓ risk of stones).
Potassium is also lost in the urine = **hypokalemia.**
Loss of bicarb in the urine causes low serum bicarb so calcium is pulled out of the bones leading to soft bones (osteomalacia).
TX: **Thiazide diuretics**. (Cause volume depletion, which increases bicarb reabsorption).

Type IV: Hypoaldosteronism, Hyporeninemia RTA
MC: Diabetics
Due to **decrease in aldosterone or stimulation of aldosterone**. Anytime there is a decrease in aldosterone there is loss of sodium and retention of potassium (AKA: hydrogen/protons), which causes **hyperkalemia**.
TX: **Fludrocortisone** (mineralocorticoid effect = increases aldosterone)

Nephritic vs Nephrotic

Nephritic	NephrOtic
• **Proteinuria < 3.5 g/day** (hypoalbuminemia) • Hematuria • **RBC casts** • **HTN** (due to salt retention) Azotemia (high urea due to poor filtration) Oliguria • Inflammation • Milder edema	• **Proteinuria > 3.5 g/day** (hyperalbuminemia) ↑ Permeability in vascular walls = ↑ loss of proteins = proteinuria. • **Hyperlipidemia** (↑ lipid panels, ↑ atherosclerosis, ↑ risk of CAD, DM) Due to ↑ **loss of albumin (due to loss of negative charge in the basement membrane/heparin sulfate),** the liver compensates by increasing production of proteins: lipoproteins = ↑ cholesterol, triglycerides, VLDL, LDL causing ↑ serum lipoproteins causing lipiduria. • **Fatty Cast** (Maltese cross) • Foamy urine (due to ↑ protein) • Edema due to ↓ oncotic pressure. ↓ volume (↓ renal perfusion) activates renin = sodium retention = worsens edema. • **Hypercoagulability (thromboembolism)** due to **loss of anti-thrombin III loss in the urine** • Loss of immunoglobulins (↑ risk of infections) (**tip**: think of the big O as big and FAT)

Nephritic Syndromes

Key points: Protein < 3.5 gm/day (still can cause edema), hypertension and RBC cast (blood in urine).

Acute Post Streptococcal Glomerulonephritis (APGN)

MC: children. **AGE determines prognosis**.

Occurs in the 3 - 6 weeks following a skin (impetigo) or 1 -2 weeks after a pharynx (strep throat) infection, or scarlet fever, due to Streptococcus.

Type III hypersensitivity (Immune complexes: Ag-Ab complexes)

SX: Brown or **cola colored urine** (due to **hematuria**), periorbital and peripheral **edema** (↑ hydrostatic pressure), **hypertension**, RBC cast, mild proteinuria.

DX: BIT: **ASO titers (anti-streptolysin O titre)**,
anti-DNase B titres, ↓ C3 Compliment levels
Deposits of IgM, IgG and C3 in glomerular basement membrane and mesangium.
MAT: Anti DNase Antigen

TX: Penicillin (Erythromycin in penicillin allergies). Supportive. Monitor electrolytes and fluids.

Immune complexes (antigen-antibody complexes formed during the Strep infection) become lodged in glomerular basement membrane below podocyte foot processes leaving a **lumpy bumpy appearance on light microscopy** and **subEPIthelial humps on electron microscopy.**

NOTE: Caution! The question can make Henoch Schonlein sound exactly like Post strep Glomerulonephritis. To decide which is the answer: **LOOK AT THE TIME SINCE the PREVIOUS INFECTION**. If it is only 1 week, it is Henoch Schonlein, if it is 10 days or more it is Post strep.

(**tip**: "S"kin = goes to a "S"ingle location = post strep Glomerulonephritis . "T"hroat goes to "T"wo locations = Post strep glomerulonephritis and rheumatic fever).

Alport Syndrome	Diffuse Proliferative Glomerulonephritis (DPGN)
Genetic disorder (MC: X link) Slow to renal failure: MC in males 15 – 20 years. SX: Glomerulonephritis, intermittent hematuria, end-stage kidney disease, **hearing loss**, eye problems (cataracts, collagen in the eye lens). Presents after a URI a young boy will have hematuria and **hearing** problems. Note: family history may show males with renal problems and hearing loss. Mutation in type **IV collagen** causes **splitting** of the glomerular **basement membrane**.	**(Lupus Glomerulonephritis – Type IV)** **Lupus Nephritis** MCC: **SLE** (MC of death in SLE) MAT: Biopsy. **"Wire looping" of capillaries** on light microscopy. **SubENDothelial IgG immune complexes, C3 deposition.** (**tip**: Lupus = LOOPing) (**tip**: we need to **END** lupus = sub**END**othelial) TX: **Cyclophosphamide, Mycophenolate**

Berger Disease
IgA Glomerulonephritis, IgA Nephropathy
(is a variant of Henoch Schonlein)
(it is an "itis" so it is an immune complex, type III HS)

(**tip**: If you eat a Berger, you want it to be grade A)

Occurs after a URI or acute gastroenteritis infection.
MC in 20 – 30 year old patients.
SX: hematuria, protein in urine, edema, hematuria, ↑ BP.

DX**: IgA and immune complex** deposits in mesangium.
NORMAL compliment levels.
MAT: Kidney biopsy.
TX: Control blood pressure.

(**Don't mix this up** with Buerger's DZ: Buerger's is a vascular DZ related to older men that smoke causing gangrene in their hands and feet due to clotting of the small /medium arteries)

Rapidly Progressive Glomerulonephritis Diseases
CRESCENTIC (Crescent)
(RPGN)
Crescent cells due to: **fibrin and plasma**.
Poor prognosis, rapid renal failure (days – weeks)
Goodpasture Syndrome
Wegner's Polyangiitis
Microscopic Polyangiitis

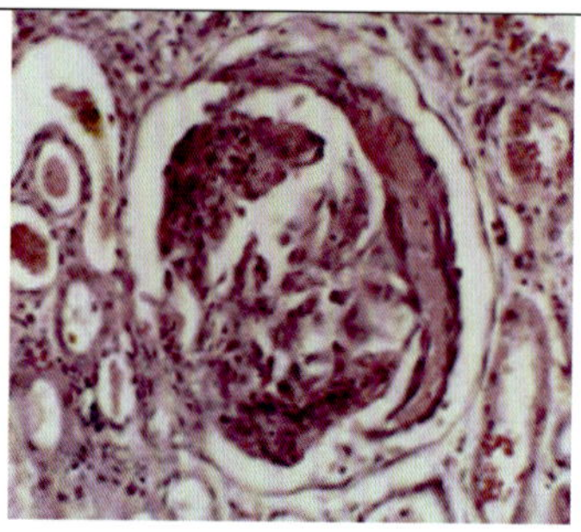

Crescent Cells in the Glomerulus
Composed of fibrin and plasma

Goodpasture Syndrome
Autoimmune (anti-glomerular basement antibody, anti-GMB)
Abnormal antibodies by the plasma cells against basement membrane **Type IV collagen** in the alveolar basement membrane of the **lungs** (hemoptysis) and **kidneys** (kidney failure/hematuria). There is NO upper respiratory involvement.

DX: **Linear deposits** of **IgG and C3** in basement membrane. (**tip**: "**G**"oodpastures – Ig"**G**")
(**tip**: the **pastures** out in the country are always lined with a long **LINEAR** fence)

TX: Plasmapheresis (antibodies are filtered out)

(**tip**: out in the country there are many **pastures** along the road and all of them are lined with **LINEAR** fences)

Wegener's Granulomatosis (WG)
Disease affecting multiple organs: **Vasculitis** affecting small/medium vessels, **kidney** with rapidly progressive glomerulonephritis, **lung** (pulmonary) nodules ("coin lesions") in the lungs and ulcerations throughout **oral** mucosa (**nasopharyngeal** problems).

SX: oral ulcers, hemoptysis, renal failure (crescent cells).
Nosebleeds, deformity of nose (saddle nose) due to perforated septum, loss of hearing, **stenosis of the trachea**, arthritis, **sinusitis**. Renal: Red cell cast, hematuria, **necrotizing glomerulonephritis.**

DX: **c-ANCA** (cytoplasmic anti-neutrophil cytoplasmic antibodies). (Cytoplasmic stain that reacts with proteinase 3 enzyme in PMN's)
CXR: nodular densities
TX: Prednisolone with cyclophosphamide or azathioprine

Microscopic Polyangiitis
(Vasculitis associated with ANCA)

Autoimmune DZ
Idiopathic, limited to the kidneys

Necrotizing vasculitis affects small vessels but has **NO granulomas**.
Lack of anti-glomerular basement membrane antibodies.
Involves multiple organs.
Rapidly progressing glomerulonephritis – Crescents.

SX: Vasculitis can involve the **lungs and kidneys** (kidney failure).
Presents like Wegner's but does **NOT** have any **nasopharyngeal (sinusitis or oral ulcers) involvement or granulomas.**

p-ANCA (perinuclear anti-neutrophil cytoplasmic antibodies with a perinuclear staining and myeloperoxidase (PMN granule protein) specificity).
Antimyeloperoxidase
↑ESR, ↑CRP

TX: Prednisolone with cyclophosphamide or azathioprine

Churg-Strauss
AKA: Eosinophillic granulomatosis
AKA: Atopic dermatitis
(Vasculitis associated with ANCA)

Autoimmune DZ of medium vessels.
Granulomatous, necrotizing vasculitis with eosinophilia.
Triad: Vasculitis of medium sized vessels in persons with airway allergic hypersensitivity, asthma or allergic rhinitis.
3 stages of development: 1) **Allergic** stage (asthma and/or allergic rhinitis), 2) **Eosinophilic** stage = high levels of eosinophils in blood/tissue causing damage to lungs and digestive tract, 3) Vasculitis stage: inflammation of blood vessels.

Must see the **triad** of: Allergies or asthma + eosinophils + Skin rash (eczema or **atopic dermatitis**).

DX: Eosinophils, p-ANCA
p-ANCA (perinuclear anti-neutrophil cytoplasmic antibodies with a perinuclear staining and myeloperoxidase (PMN granule protein) specificity)
↑ IgE levels

TX: Prednisolone with cyclophosphamide or azathioprine

Henoch-Schönlein Purpura

Vasculitis of small/medium vessels due to deposits of IgA and C3.
Follows URI or gastroenteritis within a week.
MCC: Campylobacter
MC in children < 8.

SX: Triad of: Palpable, raised, non-painful **purpura on buttocks and/or legs, arthralgias** (joint pain) and **abdominal pain**, fever.

Associated with **IgA nephropathy**.
IgA and C3 deposits in kidney, skin and GI tract.
Labs: Increased IgA and IgM, Anticardiolipin or Antiphospholipid antibodies, ↑ WBC and ESR.

(**BEWARE:** The exam can make Post Strep Glomerulonephritis sound just like Henoch-Schönlein: LOOK at the time from the URI. If it has been **< 1 week it is Henoch**. If it is **> 1 week it is Post Strep** Glomerulonephritis.

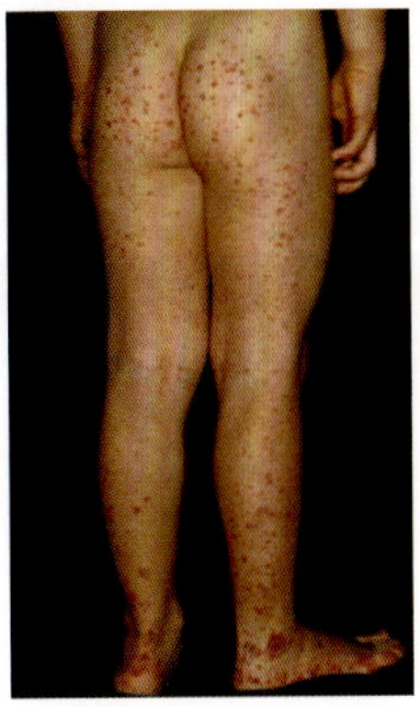

TX: **Corticosteroids.**
Self-limiting. Aspirin when Anticardiolipin or Antiphospholipid antibodies are present.

(**tip**: if you to buy a hen, it should be grade A)

Cryoglobulinemia

Blood contains large amounts of cryoglobulins (immunoglobulin proteins) that become insoluble at reduced temperatures.

Acute inflammation
Cold agglutinin (IgM) (IgM = Acute)
IgM directed against the Fc region of IgG
Non-bacterial infection

Associated with HEP C, multiple myeloma. (Look for someone with HEP C and kidney problems).

SX: RBC casts, palpable purpura, proteinuria, hematuria, ↓ compliment

Note: Associated with the "C" Club (**Membra**nous and **Membra**no Nephritis)
Tip: I am a "**Member**" of the "**C**" club: Most all of the pathologies that cause the Membranous and Membrano Nephritis Syndromes all begin with C:
Hep **C** (so include Hep B), **C**ryoglobulinemia, **C**ancer, **C**old agglutinations.

Subepithelial and Subendothelial Humps

	Subepithelial Humps	Subendothelial Humps
Nephritic Syndrome	Acute Post Streptococcal Glomerulonephritis	Diffuse Proliferative Glomerulonephritis. (Lupus). (**tip**: **END** Lupus)
Nephrotic Syndrome	Diffuse Membranous Nephropathy	Membrano Proliferative Glomerulonephritis

Nephrotic Syndromes

Key Points: Protein > 3.5 gm/day (edema), hypercoagulable (↑ risk of clots due to loss of **Antithrombin III**, Protein C, Protein S in the urine), ↑ lipids: cholesterol, triglycerides, LDL and low HDL (lipoprotein's are lost in the urine so VLDL and LDL are not able to be removed from the serum), fatty cast.
MAT: Renal biopsy.

Minimal Change Disease

(AKA: Lipoid nephrosis)
Idiopathic
(**tip**: minim"**O**" change = nephr**O**tic)

MCC of nephrotic syndrome in children ages 2 – 6

DX: **Effacement (thinning) of foot processes** seen on electron microscopy. Thinning allows loss of albumin **due to loss of negative charge** of the basement membrane.
(Heparin sulfate is found in the basement membrane).
Normal compliment, hypoalbuminemia, hyperlipidemia.

SX: **Foamy urine, puffy face** (edema)

Triggered by recent illness, infection, and vaccination.

Does **NOT** involve: Complexes, compliment, immunoglobulins, fatty cast, and secretions of T cells.

TX: **Steroids (Prednisone)**

Diabetic Glomerulonephropathy

Progressive disease.

Light microscopy show **thickening** of the glomerular basement membrane (diffuse scarring of the glomeruli), **eosinophilic nodular** glomerulosclerosis.

DX: **Hyaline arteriosclerosis** (thickening of the arterioles), fatty cast, **positive PAS stain**. (**Nonenzymatic glycosylation** of the GBM)
Nodules in the glomerulus (AKA: oval/ovoid hyaline mass)

Damage due to **nonenzymatic glycosylation** of **efferent** arterioles causing mesangial expansion leading to ↑ GFR.
Nodules (AKA: Kimmelstiel-Wilson nodules).

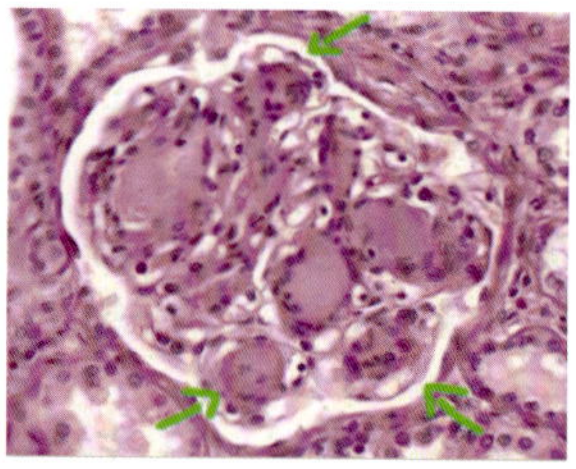

Track progression by monitoring microalbumin levels.

TX: **ACE Inhibitors (or ARB's)**. ACE is used to slow down (not stop) progression. It will **dilate the efferent arterioles so that GFR and FF is decreased** so there is not so much pressure pushing against the glomerulus to push proteins through the basement membrane and into the urine, destroying the glomerulus. **ALL diabetics MUST be put on an ACE Inhibitor (or Arb) to stop this progression unless they have renal problems.**

Diffuse Membranous Nephropathy

MCC nephrotic syndrome in adults.

Cause: **Immune complex** deposition.

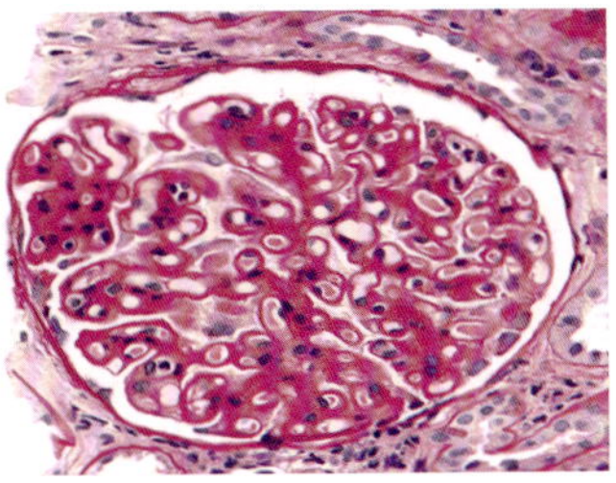

Electron microscope shows **"spike and dome"** appearance and and **subEPIthelial immune complex** deposits. Basement membrane is diffusely thickened.
NO compliment problems.

Silver stain of the glomerulus shows a **fatty cast (Maltese cross)**
Fatty cast = cholesterol

Associated with: HEP C, HEP B, Cancer
(**tip**: For BOTH of the Membranous Nephropathy's: think:
A **MEMBER** of the **C** club: HEP C, Cancer (then HEP C will trigger HEP B), Cryoglobulinemia, Cold Agglutins.

Membrano Proliferative Glomerulonephritis (MPGM)
(is an "itis" so is an immune complex: type III hypersensitivity)

Immunofluorescence shows "tram-track" glomerular basement membrane **"splitting"** and **subENDthelial immune complex** deposits.
↓ C3 Compliment

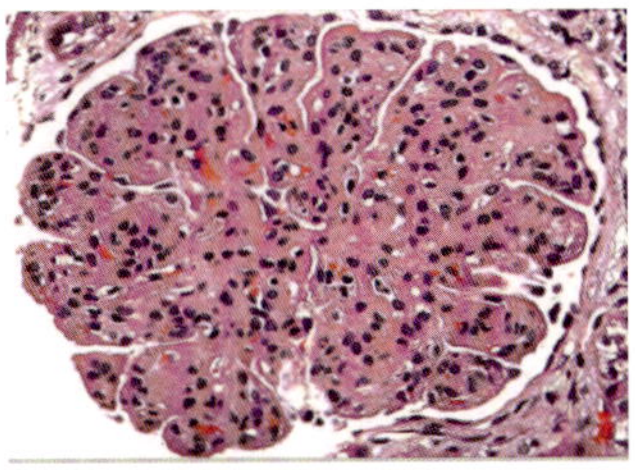

They are **"splitting"** because of **mesangial growth/proliferation**: remember: **mesangial cells are the macrophages of the kidney.** They job is to "eat". In this case they are "eating" way to much, are getting to fat, so they "Split" open. When they split open it looks like train tracks.

Associated with HEP C, HEP B and Cancer
(**tip**: For BOTH of the Membranous Nephropathy's: think:
A **MEMBER** of the **C** club: HEP C, Cancer (then HEP C will trigger HEP B), Cryoglobulinemia, Cold Agglutins.

Focal Segmental Glomerulosclerosis

MCC in African Americans and Hispanics

Light microscope shows: Segmental **fibrosis (sclerosis)** and hyalinosis of the glomerulus
(AKA: **Scarring** of the glomerulus)

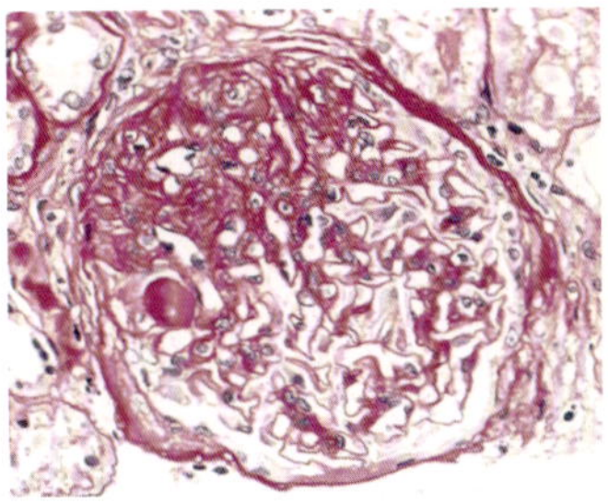

Electron microscope shows: effacement of foot processes

Associated with **HIV, heroin, IV drugs**, sickle cell

Amyloidosis
Deposition of amyloid proteins in the kidney due to other pathologies.

MC: **Multiple myeloma** (AL proteins: AKA: Bence Jones).
Others: Rheumatoid arthritis, TB.

DX: **Congo red stains** shows **apple-green birefringence** under polarized light
(**tip:** anytime you see "Congo red stain" always think proteins)

Renal Infections

Cystitis
Inflammation of bladder.
↑ PMN infiltrate into renal interstitium. Over 1000 colonies of PMN's.

SX: **Suprapubic pain**, urinary frequency and urgency, dysuria (painful urination).

MCC: e. coli due to virulence factor of fimbria (ascends the urinary tract by adhering to the mucosal wall)
Other causes:
S. saprophyticus: "honeymoon cystitis". Common in young girls (<8) and in sexually active adolescents.
N. gonorrhea or Chlamydia causes **urethritis** (STD) will show pyuria (pus) and negative urine culture (remember: Chlamydia is intracellular – can't be seen)

Labs: Positive leukocyte esterase (an enzyme released by WBC. So presence of this shows WBC=PMN's) (PMNs are most abundant type of WBC). **Positive for nitrates** (indicate presence of **gram-negative organisms (ie: e.coli).**
(**tip**: **N**egative bugs = **N**itrates)

TX: **TMP/SMX** (Bactrim)
Pregnancy: **Nitrofurantoin, Cephalexin, Amoxicillin** (**DO NOT use TMP/SMX during pregnancy**)

For UTI's in pregnancy. Antibiotics should be prescribed if any symptoms occur or an increase in WBC on routine labs during check ups. Do not wait to see if an infection develops. Treat now.
Chronic cystitis: antibiotics (TMP/SMX)

Pyelonephritis

Infection of the kidney cortex.
Cause**: Ascending infection due to an incompetent vesicouretal junction.** (Physio: the ureterovesical junction (ureter meets the bladder) is incompetent and allows the urine from the bladder infection (via: vesicouretal reflux) to be refluxed back into the ureters and back up into the kidney).

SX: Flank tenderness, costovertebral angle tenderness, nausea, vomiting, fever, dysuria, chills.

MCC: **Ascending UTI infection with e. coli** (due to untreated UTI).
Other causes: vesicoureteral reflux (abnormal backward movement of urine from the bladder into ureters or kidneys), hematogenous spread to kidneys.

Acute Pyelo Labs: **White blood cell casts** in urine. **Bacteria and pyuria** in urine, CT shows striated parenchymal enlargement due to **massive infiltrates of PMN's**.

Chronic Pyelo Labs:
Blunting of the calyces.
Cause: recurrent acute infections.

Histology: Scarring and blunting of calyx. Tubules can contain lymphocytic infiltrate, eosinophilic cast in the tubules resembling thyroid tissue (AKA: thyroidization of the kidney)
Over 10,000 colonies of PMN's.

Sodium Pathologies

Hypernatremia
MCC: Nephrogenic or Central Diabetes Insipidus.
Hypernatremia due to loss of water due to sweating, fever, diuretics, diarrhea, pneumonia, burns, **Diabetes Insipidus** (DI).

Symptoms: Polyuria and nocturia (similar presentation as Diabetes Mellitus), lethargy, confusion, seizures, brain damage.

TX: Treat specific cause and normalize sodium levels. Do **NOT** reduce sodium levels to rapidly or it will cause cerebral edema.
Nephrogenic Diabetes Insipidus
Inability to reabsorb water and concentrate urine at the collecting ducts due to insensitivity to ADH hormone released by the pituitary.
Causes: Chronic kidney dz, hypercalcemia, hypokalemia, drugs: **Lithium, Demeclocycline**.
Labs: ↓ Osm (dilute urine), high urine volume, ↑ ADH (build up because receptors are insensitive to it).
TX: Replace potassium and calcium. If due to lithium: stop drug.

Central Diabetes Insipidus
High water loss does to defective production in the hypothalamus or release of ADH (antidiuretic hormone) from the posterior pituitary.
Causes: tumors, strokes, trauma, infection, hypoxia).
Labs: ↑ Osm (concentrated urine), low urine volume, ↓ ADH (not being produced/released).
TX: Replace **ADH** (AKA: **Vasopressin, DDAVP**)

Water Deprivation Test
Water is withheld from patient to evaluate urine output and urine OSM.
DI = ↑ Volume of urine and ↓ urine OSM.

Desmopressin (ADH) Test (administration).
Determines the difference between Central, Nephrogenic and polygenic causes.
Central DI: shows an increase in OSM and ↓ in urine volume, and ↓ ADH. (Serum sodium ↑).

(**tip**: "**C**"entral shows a "**C**"hange in OSM)
Nephrogenic DI: Shows no change in either: urine or OSM, and ↑ ADH. (Serum sodium ↑).
Polygenic: Dilute urine and there will be no abnormalities in the serum sodium.

Hyponatremia
Hyponatremia can occur in 3 states: Hypervolemia, Hypovolemia and Euvolemia.
SX: CNS symptoms. Anorexia (loss of appetite), confusion, irritability, muscle weakness, cramps, headache, seizures, lethargy, coma.
Sodium must be corrected slowly.
Normal plasma Osm: 280 – 300 mmol per kg.

A **hypervolemic state** (high volume) because of ↑ ADH.
MCC: CHF, cirrhosis, nephrotic syndromes.
Physiology: ↓ intravascular volume causes the
pressure receptors in the atria and carotids to sense the ↓ in volume (↓ stretch) and stimulate ADH release so as to try and increase water reabsorption so the intravascular volume increases.
TX: Correcting the underlying conditon.

A **hypovolemic state** (low volume) is due to Addison's disease (loss of Aldosterone = ↓ Na) or ↑ or chronic free water intake.
Other causes are the same as which can cause hypernatremia (sweating, fever, diuretics, pneumonia, burns, vomiting, diarrhea).
Hypernatremia occurs if there is not water replacement.
TX: Normal isotonic saline solution.

A **euvolemic state** (normal volume) is due to psychogenic polydipsia, hyperglycemia, SIADH, hypothyroidism.

- **Psychogenic polydipsia** (AKA: Primary polydipsia): Excessive intake of free water. MCC: dry mouth.
  The kidneys are unable to handle the fluid overload.
  Serum sodium can become so diluted that seizures and cardiac arrest can occur. Weight gain is also seen.
  No sodium correction required. Whereas in
  Note: Often seen in bipolar disorders or schizophrenia because of the phenothiazine in their medications, which can cause a dry mouth.
  Labs: ↓ urine volume, dilute urine (50 – 100 mOsm/kg)
- **Hyperglycemia**
  High glucose causes an osmotic pull on fluid inside the cells. Water is pulled from the cells (water follows sodium, sugar and protein) into the higher Osm surroundings (high glucose), dropping the sodium levels.
  Labs: For every 100 mg/dL of glucose above normal there is a 1.6 mEq/L decrease in sodium levels.
  TX: Correct glucose levels.

- **SIADH** Normal control of ADH is lost and ADH hormone is secreted independently.
  Labs show normal BUN/Creatine, bicarb, ↓ serum uric acid, ↓ serum OSM (< 290 mOsm/kg), urine OSM (> 100 mOsm/kg) and urine sodium (> 20 mEq/L).
  TX:
  Mild (asymptomatic): Restricting fluids.
  Mod/Severe (seizures, altered mental status): 3% hypertonic saline, **ADH blockers (Conivaptan).**
  Demeclocycline if SIADH is due to Small Cell.
  Complications: **Central Pontine Myelinosis** may occur if sodium levels are corrected too quickly. Do not correct sodium > 8 – 10 mEqL in 24 hours or > 18 mEq/L in first 48 hours.
  SIADH: MCC: lung (**Small Cell Cancer produces ADH**).
  Other causes: brain pathologies.
  Drug induced SAIDH: ADH analogs (DDAVP, Oxytocin, Vasopressin), anticonvulsants, antiparkinson agents, antineoplastics, antipsychotics, hypoglycemic agents, analgesics (Fentanyl, Ibuprofen, Diclofenac, Trazodone), Cardiovascular agents, diuretics, INFα, Ecstasy (MDMA), Nicotine, Omeprazole, SSRI's, Cyclophosphamide, tricyclic antidepressants, sulfonylureas.

Hypothyroidism
Thyroid hormones are needed in order to excrete water.
↓ thyroid hormone = ↓ excretion

Correction of Sodium in Hyponatremia

- Normal serum sodium: 135 – 145 mEq/L.
- When sodium levels decrease water is able to enter the brain cells and cause swelling. This can occur at sodium levels of <115 mEq/L.
- Complications if sodium levels are corrected to quickly: **Central Pontine Myelinolysis**. Breakdown of the myelin sheaths on the CNS nerve cells in the pons in the brainstem. SX: quadriparesis, dysphagia, loss of consciousness, **"locked-in syndrome"** (cognitive function is intact but all muscles are paralyzed except for the blinking of the eye).

Severity of the Hyponatremia	Sodium Level	Symptoms	Treatment
Mild	> 125 - < 135 mEq/L	Asymptomatic	**Withhold fluids**
Moderate	>115 – 125 mEq/L	Confusion, short term memory loss	Normal saline fluid with loop diuretic
Severe	≤ 115 mEq/L	Seizures, Coma	Hypertonic saline, **Conivaptan** (V1A selective), **Lixivaptan**, **Tolvaptan** (V2 selective). **Correction Rate: Serum sodium must NOT raise more than 8 mmol/L over 24 hours. (0.33 mmol/L/hour).**

ADH Differentials

Syndrome	Plasma OSM	Urine OSM	Plasma ADH	Pathology	Association
SIADH	↓	↑↑	↑	ADH causes ↑↑ water to be reabsorbed in the kidneys leading to hyponatremia (hypo-osmolarity in the plasma and concentrated urine	Small Cell Lung Cancer ADH rP
Psychogenic Polydipsia	↑	Dilute ↓↓	↓	Extremely high water intake prevents the Kidneys from excreting free water which Causes a tremendously diluted urine (≤50 mOsm)	Psychiatric problems. MC: Schizophrenia
Central Diabetes Insipidus*	↑	↓	↓	↓ in secretion of ADH from the hypothalamus/posterior pituitary causing hyperosmolar plasma because of the wasting of free water.	Head trauma causing damage to the pituitary stalk.
Nephrogenic Diabetes Insipidus*	↑	↓	↑	Kidneys do not respond (aquaporin channels) to ADH, which results in wasting of free water and hyperosmolar plasma.	Lithium toxicity

Note: To determine whether the DI was caused by a central cause or a nephrogenic cause: Look at the results of the OSM from the Desmopressin test. If results show that the OSM changed after the test, then the cause of the DI is due to a central problem (Hypothalamus/pituitary). (**Tip**: "**C**"hanged = "**C**"entral).

Misc Renal Pathologies

Hydronephrosis	Medullary Sponge Kidney
↑ Hydrostatic pressure (GFR) in Bowman's capsule Dilation of the renal pelvis and calyces (cortex and medulla) due to build up of pressure (backup of urine). AKA: Compression atrophy. MCC: urinary obstruction due to: **Renal stones**, cancers, BPH, injury to ureter, vesicoureteral reflux, retroperitoneal fibrosis. Complications: atrophy of renal cortex and medulla	Dilated collecting ducts Causes: kidney stones, UTI's SX: Painless hematuria

Vesicoureteral Reflux (VCR)	Renal Artery Stenosis
MCC: urologic problem in kids. Abnormal backward movement of urine from the bladder into ureters or kidneys causing renal failure and renal scarring SX: Pyrexia (fever), dysuria, frequent urination, malodorous urine, GI symptoms. Can also present with abnormal genital. Cause: Anatomical causes: **Posterior urethral valves** (males), urethral stenosis Functional causes: Neurogenic bladder, bladder instability DX: Voiding cystourethrogram (VCUG) **Voiding cystourethrograms protocol** **Children 2 – 4** with 1st UTI: check renal ultrasound to check for **abnormal anatomy** that could lead to VCR. **Recurrent febrile UTI's**: perform a voiding cystourethrogram	**MCC: 2° HTN** SX: **Abdominal bruit** Cause: See in young adult patients due to **fibromuscular dysplasia** DX: Angiography of renal vessels
Hemolytic Uremic Syndrome (HUS) **Cause: E. coli O157:H7 (Verotoxin, AKA: Shiga-like toxin).** **Intravascular hemolysis.** **MC in children.** **MOA: Shiga-like toxin** causes endothelial cells to become thrombogenic (making clots) and inactivate the **metalloproteinase ADAMTS13** (the deficiency that causes TTP). Once ADAMTS13 inactivates multimer 's of VWF activate platelets causing microthrombi. The activated platelets clog the arterioles and capillaries of the body destroying RBC and creating schistocytes. The clogged vessels (micro vascularization) reduce blood flow to vital organs causing ischemia leading to DIC. (DIC in HUS does not consume coagulation factors, only consumes the platelets) so the fibrin degradation products (D-Dimers), fibrinogen and coagulation labs are normal. (**TTP is a close pathology** and MOA to HUS caused by deficiency in ADAMTS13. TTP causes more CNS problems and is more common in adults, HUS causes more renal problems and is more common in children). **SX:** Triad of: **Microangiopathic Hemolytic anemia** (destruction of RBC) = **schistocytes** **Thrombocytopenia** (low platelets) **Acute kidney failure** (uremia) **Labs:** Increased serum: ↑ LDH, ↑ indirect bilirubin, ↑ BUN/creatinine Urine Labs: Hb, hemosiderin, albumin, RBC and WBC casts TX: Plasmapheresis (plasma exchange) **DO NOT** transfuses platelets into TTP (or HUS) → worsens.	**Paroxysmal Nocturnal Hemoglobinuria (PNH)** • PNH: Stem cell defect. • Destruction of RBC by **over activation of complement**. • **DAF** (Decay-Accelerating Factor) protects RBC's, displays cell markers: **CD55 and CD59** • AKA: **GPI anchored** enzyme deficiency • Mutation in the **PIG A gene (leads to absence of GPI anchors on cell membrane)** • Without **GPI anchor** on membrane complement lyse the RBC's • MCC death: Thrombosis (MC site: Hepatic and Mesenteric Veins) • SX: red discoloration of the urine due to presence of Hemoglobin and hemosiderin from breakdown of RBC's, seen mostly in the morning from concentrating overnight. • Complications: Aplastic anemia, acute leukemia, myelodysplasia. • DX: Flow cytometry shows ↓ CD55/CD59. • Labs: hemolytic anemia, low Hb, increased LDH (Lactate dehydrogenase),↑bilirubin, ↓ haptoglobin, ↑ reticulocytes, pancytopenia, iron deficiency anemia. • TX: **Prednisone. Eculizumab** (inactivates C3). Folic acid replacement. **Transfusions if necessary.** **Cure: Allogenic bone marrow transplant.**

Fanconi Syndrome Disease of the PCT (proximal renal tubules). Glucose, bicarb, phosphate, uric acid and amino acids are secreted into the urine instead of being absorbed. Causes: Cystinosis (abnormal accumulation of cysteine), Wilson's DZ, galactosemia, hereditary fructose intolerance, glycogen storage diseases, expired tetracycline, lead poisoning, multiple myeloma, tyrosinemia, **outdated tetracycline**. SX: Polyuria, polydipsia, dehydration, acidosis, hypokalemia, hypophosphatemia/hyperphosphaturia, proteinuria, hyperchloremia. Complications: Rickets (children) and osteomalacia (adults). Phosphate is required for bone development in addition to vitamin D and calcium. TX: Replace the lost substances excreted in the urine and hydration.	**Fibromuscular Dysplasia** **2nd MCC of HTN** is **renal artery stenosis** DX: caused by **Fibromuscular dysplasia** (will usually be in young patients). SX: **Abdominal "bruit"**. Is heard throughout systole and diastole at the costovertebral angle. DX: Renal artery angiography shows **"string of pearls"** appearance, which is due to the alternating stenosis and arterial dilation. 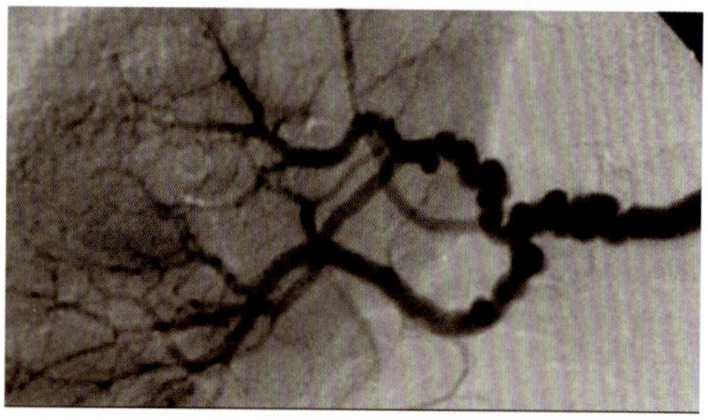
Cholesterol Embolism AKA: Atheroemboli AKA: Atheroembolic Renal Disease (AERD) **Cholesterol emboli** that are released from cholesterol plaques in the aorta or coronary arteries during catheter procedures and obstruct smaller blood vessels in the body. In the kidneys they can cause kidney damage. SX: **Livedo reticularis** on the skin (mottled reticulated vascular pattern that looks like a purplish lace pattern on the skin), gangrene, renal failure. Labs: ↑ **Eosinophils** in the urine, RBC cast can be seen occasionally, ↑ ESR, ↑ C-reactive protein, BUN/Creatinine ratio, ↓ compliment.	**Hepatorenal Syndrome** Individual with **cirrhosis** (portal HTN), fulminant liver failure, or alcoholic hepatitis that develops **kidney failure**. Failing liver function changes the blood supply circulation that supplies the kidney. SX: liver failure, kidney failure, abnormal circulation. Jaundice, altered mental status, ascites, oliguria and any other signs seen with portal HTN. Labs (same as in prerenal): BUN/Creatinine > 20, Fractionalized excretion of sodium <1%, low urine sodium < 15 mEq. TX: Liver transplant. **Octreotide, Midodrine** (alpha-agonist). While waiting on transplant other TX: TIPS (transjugular intrahepatic portosystemic shunt) to decrease blood pressure in the portal vein, hemodialysis (kidneys) and liver dialysis (liver)
Renal Osteodystrophy Bone mineralization deficiency due to electrolyte and endocrine dysfunctions because of chronic kidney dz. SX: bone pain, joint pain, bone fracture or deformation.	

Renal Cyst Pathologies

Polycystic Kidney Disease
(ADPKD)

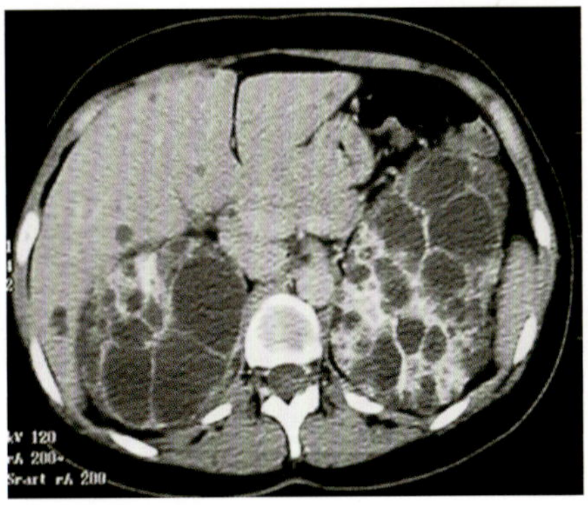

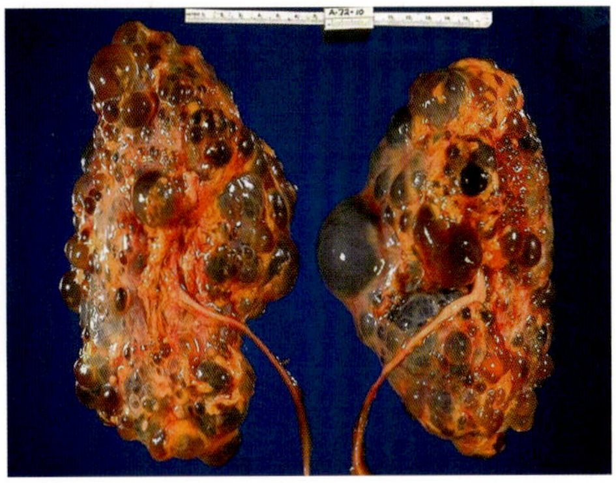

Autosomal Dominant mutation in PKD1 (chromosome 16) or PKD2 (chromosome 4)

Multiple Cysts develop and grow in the kidneys.

SX: hematuria, excessive urination, HTN, headaches, abdominal pain, **palpable abdominal masses**

MCC death: Chronic kidney DZ or HTN due to ↑ renin production.

Associated with: **SAH (berry aneurysms), mitral valve prolapse**, hepatic cysts (benign cyst)

Medullary Cystic Kidney Disease (MCKD)
(AKA: Medullary kidney disease)
Autosomal Dominant.

Tubulointerstitial sclerosis leading to end stage renal dz.
Small cyst in the center of the kidney causing **scars and fibrosis.**

MCKD causes kidneys to produce urine that is not concentrated (too watery, lacking the normal waste) and causing polyuria. When the kidneys make too much urine then sodium and other vital ions and chemicals are lost leading to kidney failure.

Renal Cancers and Tumors

Renal Cell Carcinoma (in an adult)
AKA: Renal Adenocarcinoma
(Wilm's tumor: in a child)

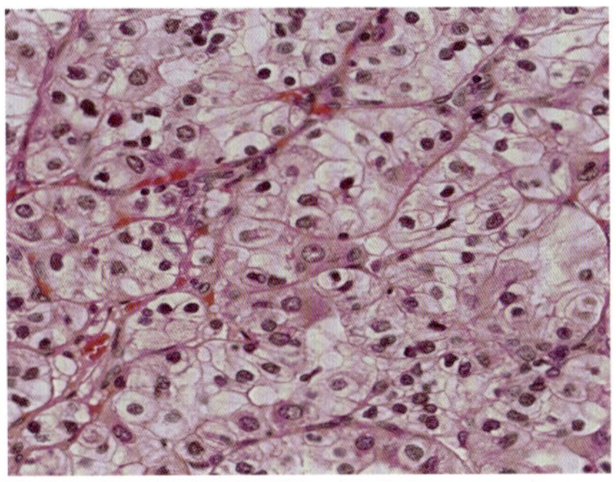

Clear cells of glycogen

Polygonal **clear cells filled with lipids and carbohydrates (aka: Glycogen)**.
Hypervascular mass.
Originates in the lining of the **PCT**.

Risk: **MCC: Smoking**, obesity

SX: Hematuria, **palpable mass**, flank pain, fever, weight loss, **secondary polycythemia**

Metastasizes to lung and bone (hematogenous spread via renal vein).
Produces ectopic hormones: EPO, PTH (leading to hypercalcemia).

Histology: **Cells are clear, full of glycogen**.

Associated with: Von Hippel-Lindau, paraneoplastic syndromes caused by hormones produced by the tumor (Paraneoplastic syndromes are cancers in the body that are not due to the local presence of cancer cells. It is mediated by hormones and cytokines. Ie: ADH, ACTH, PTH)

Staging:
Stage 1 = confined to **capsule**
Stage 2 = has **extended through the capsule** (Gerota's facia)
TX: if Stage 2 = radical nephrectomy

Bladder Cancer
Most common type: **Transitional cell carcinoma**.
Additional types of bladder cancer: Squamous Cell Carcinoma, Small-cell carcinoma, Sarcoma, Adenocarcinoma, Flat Carcinoma.

MC cancer of the urinary tract

Papillary growth lined by transitional cells. (AKA: **Papillary lesion**)

SX: **Painless hematuria**, no RBC casts

Causes of **transitional cell carcinoma**: **MCC: Smoking**, aniline dyes, **Cyclophosphamide**.
Causes of **squamous cell carcinoma** of the bladder: **schistosoma haematobium.**

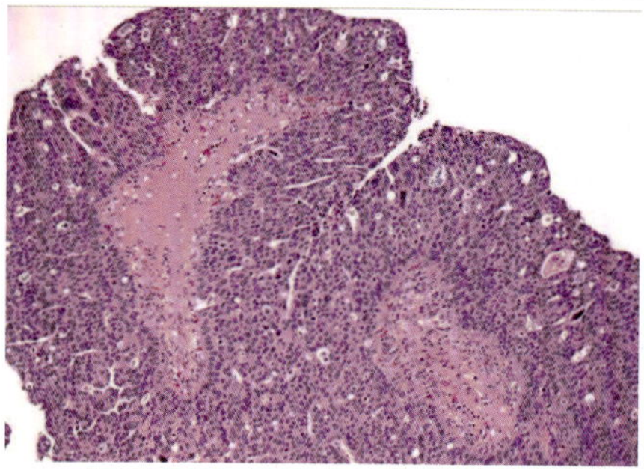

Transitional Cell (Bladder) Carcinoma

Note: Schistosomiasis (aka: snail fever) is caused by schistosoma haematobium. Schistosoma (helminth) is a parasite from infected **freshwater snails. MC in developing countries** (Africa, Asia, South America). Infection is by contact with contaminated water: children playing in the water, farmers, fishermen, anyone using unclean water.
SX: abdominal pain, bloody stool, blood in the urine, diarrhea.
Causes: **bladder cancer**, kidney failure, infertility, liver damage. It can cause delayed growth and learning disabilities in children.
DX: O & P will show parasite eggs in the **stool** or antibodies against the disease in the blood.
TX: **Praziquantel**.

(**Caution**: do not confuse S. haematobium with S. mansoni which is in the liver)
(**tip**; haemato**B**ium, **B** = **B**ladder or "Heme" for painless hematuria in bladder cancer)

Wilm's Tumor
(AKA: **Nephroblastoma**, Renal Adenocarcinoma in children)
MC renal neoplasm in children.
Primitive tumor.

MC: Children ages 2 – 4
SX: **Palpable flank mass**, hematuria, **aniridia (no iris)**, genitourinary malformations, mental retardation, hemihypertrophy of an extremity (one extremity is bigger than the other), HTN (because tumor is making renin), unilateral.

AKA: Immature epithelial cells
AKA: Ribbons of fibroblastic stroma cells

Can be unilateral or bilateral, does **NOT** cross the **midline** (they are in the kidneys which are on the sides and in the back)

(Caution: do not confuse this with neuroblastoma. Neuroblastoma normally presents in children **< 1 year old** and **CAN cross the midline).**

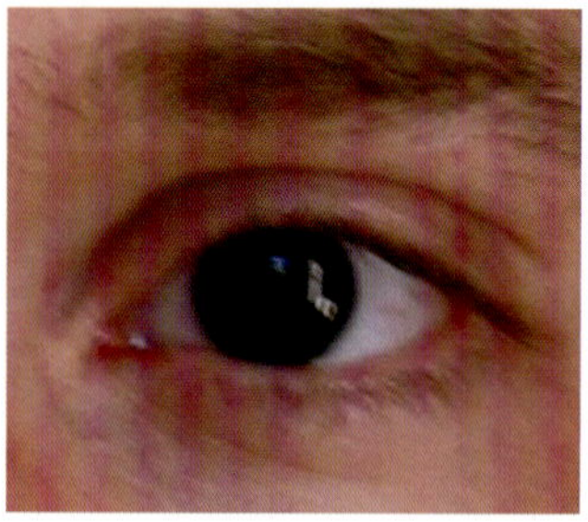

Aniridia (no iris)
Associated with Nephroblastoma

Neuroblastoma
MC Extracranial solid cancer in children.
Neuroendocrine tumor (neural crest/sympathetic nervous system). **pNTs** (neuroblastic tumor).
MC: Primary tumor in the adrenal glands (but also can appear in other nerve tissues in the neck, pelvis, abdomen, chest). Anywhere in the sympathetic nervous system chain from neck to pelvis.
Associated with: n-myc oncogene

SX: If in the abdomen: swollen abdomen, constipation.
In the chest: breathing difficulties.
In the bone marrow: anemia.
In the spinal cord: weakness, difficulty walking, crawling, and standing.
In the bone (legs/hips) pain and difficulty walking, standing.

Histology: Small, round blue cells, **Homer Write rosettes patterns (cells surrounding the neuropil** (unmyelinated axons, dendrites, glial cells).

DX: **↑ HVA and VMA in urine.**

(Caution: do not confuse this with nephroblastoma. Nephroblastoma normally presents in children **2 – 4 years old** and **does NOT cross the midline).**

Renal Oncocytoma MC: Benign but can become malignant Tumor in the kidney made of **oncocytes** (Oncocytes: epithelial cell containing an excessive amount of **mitochondria**) resulting in acidophilic granular cytoplasm) (Remember: Mitochondria create an acidophilic environment)	

Kidney Stones

- Obstruction can cause hydronephrosis or pyelonephritis
- Colicky, radiating pain to the groin
- Unilateral flank tenderness, hematuria
- Fat malabsorption increases risk for stones
- **Good Hydration is TX unless larger stone**
  Stone Treatment protocol:
  Stones < 5 mm (0.5 cm) (0.2 inches) = hydrate and pass
  Stones 6 – 9 mm (0.6 – 0.9 cm) = lithotripsy (extracorporeal shock wave). Can also give Nifedipine and Tamsulosin to try and pass.
  Stones > 9 mm (0.9 cm) (0.35 inches)= Removal/surgery: Ureteroscopy or nephrolithotomy
- Radiopaque (can see the stone)
  Radiolucent (can't see the stone: **tip:** radio**L**ucent = **L** = **L**ost)

Calcium Oxalate Stones

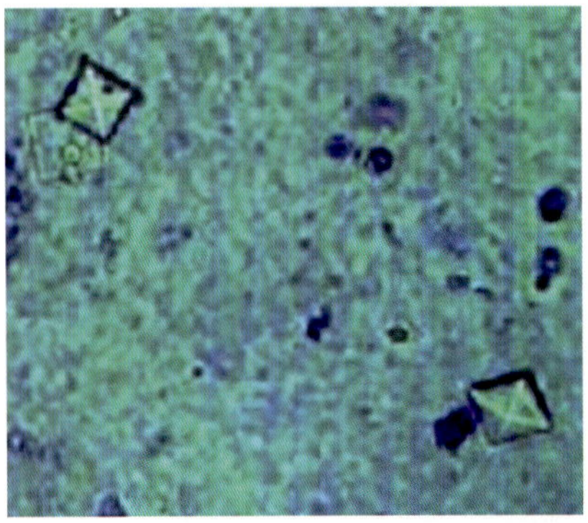

Occurs when urine is **acidic** (↓ pH)
MC: 80% of stones
Radiopaque
Stone color: dark brown/black
Stone shape: envelopes, dumbbell

Labs: **↑ Ca in urine, normal serum Ca**

Causes: **↑ oxalate**. High oxalate can be caused by IBD (Crohn's), bowel resections, bypass procedures, patients consuming foods high in oxalate (dark vegetables, vitamin C, chocolate, nuts, potato chips, French fries, beets), ethylene glycol (antifreeze consumption)

(MOA of oxalate: oxalate binds with calcium and forms small crystals and are excreted in the urine. If there is an excess of free oxalate (not bound to calcium) due to an excess of oxalate, it has no calcium to bind with. So it is absorbed alone and sent to the kidneys and builds up in the urine. The excess concentration of oxalate in the urine then causes oxalate stones)

TX: ↑ Hydration, ↑ **Citrate** intake (AKA: **potassium citrate**). AKA: **Celation** therapy. Citrate inhibits crystal formation/growth. **Thiazide diuretics** (It reabsorbs calcium from the urine in the DCT. The calcium that is pulled out is then able to bind with the free oxylate and decreases the risk of stones).

Calcium Phosphate Stones

Occurs when urine is **alkaline** (↑ pH)
<10% of stones

Radiopaque
Stone color: dirty white

Causes: hyperparathyroidism, renal tubular acidosis

Struvite Stones (AKA: Ammonium magnesium phosphate, Staghorn stones, Urease stones)	**Cysteine Stones**	**Uric Acid Stones**
Occurs when there are infections in the kidney by **urease +** organisms that hydrolyze urea to ammonia causing urine alkalization. Organisms like **alkaline urine (↑ pH)**. Urine smells like ammonia = caused by urease. Radiopaque Stone color: dirty white Stone shape: coffin lid Causes: Infection by urease + bacteria. MC: **Proteus mirabilis**, Proteus vulgaris, Morganella morganii, Klebsiella, Serratia, Enterobacter TX: Treat underlying infection and surgical removal 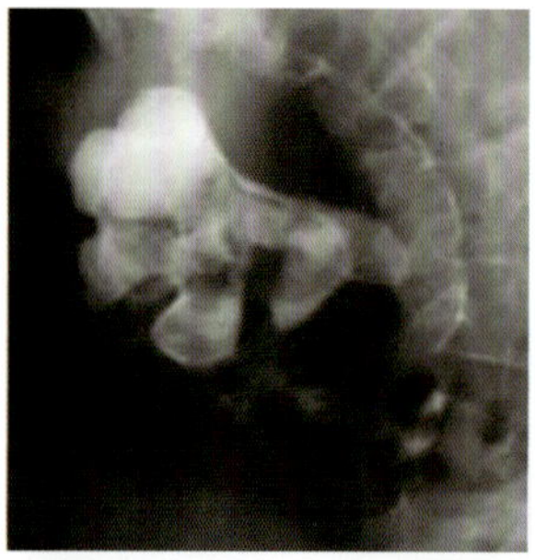 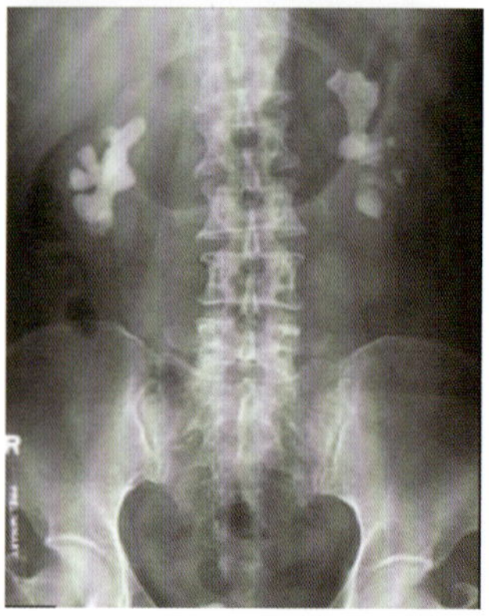	**Genetic** disorder. Amino acid **cysteine** leaks through the kidneys into the urine to form crystals. Acidic urine (↓ pH) Rare. Radiopaque Stone color: pink/yellow Stone shape: hexagonal 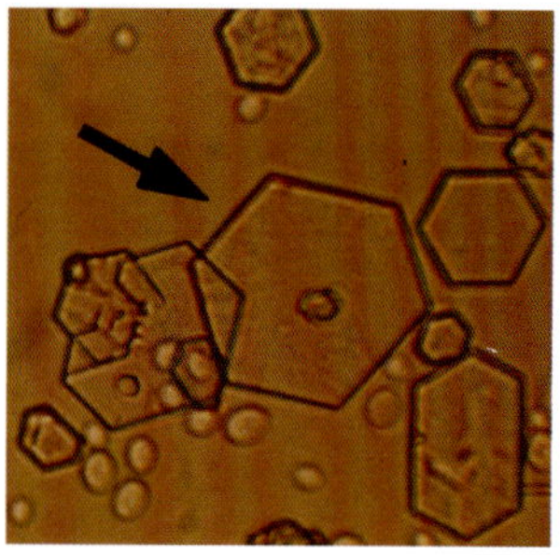 Causes: **Dysfunction of amino acid transport** of COLA (**cysteine**, ornithine, arginine, lysine). PCT can't absorb cysteine Patients with Fanconi syndrome, cystinuria, cystinosis are at risk. Labs: Aminoaciduria DX: Sodium cyanide/Nitroprusside test TX: **Alkalization of urine**, hydration	Occurs when urine is persistently acidic (↓ pH) ↑ acid = ↑ stones <5 % of stones **Radiolucent** **Can't be seen on x-ray.** (**tip**: radio**L**ucent – "**L**" for **L**ost) Stone color: yellow/reddish brown Stone shape: **Rhomboid**, diamond shape, rosettes Causes: Diets **high in protein**, esp: meats, fish, shellfish, obesity TX: **Potassium citrate or potassium bicarb**, **Allopurinol** will reduce urate formation. **Urine alkalization** 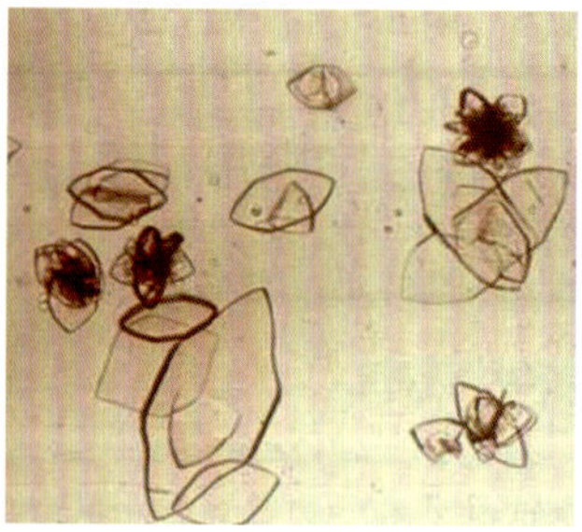

Incontinence

- **Detrusor muscle = main part of bladder.**
  Parasympathetic (allows urination).
  It stretches to accommodate urine and contracts to expel urine.
  ↑ detrusor activity means ↑ contractions = urgency (need to urinate often)
- **Sphincter**
  Sympathetic control (stops urination)
- If patient is dribbling (going to much) that is too much parasympathetic, so treat it with sympathetics to stop it
- If patient is not able to urinate (post surgery) that is too much sympathetic, so treat with parasympathetic 's
- The ureters come into the bladder at the **trigone** (triangular area in the detrusor)
- Normal post-void residual urine 20 – 25 mL. Abnormal > 50 ml
- Normal bladder capacity: 16 – 24 oz urine. 400 – 600 ml
- Urethra length (average): males 8 inches, females 1.5 inches
- S3 – S4 innervate the muscles of the perineum. This is the group of muscles that is weakened from multiple childbirths.

Overflow Incontinence

Involuntary release of urine from an overly full bladder, without the urge to urinate.
Small volume, continuous leakage causing **incomplete emptying of bladder because of ↓ detrusor contraction**.

Causes: outlet obstruction (BPH, prostate cancer, narrowing of urethra) a weak detrusor (underactive detrusor), or medication side effects (anticholinergic, antipsychotics, antidepressants).

SX: constant dribble, even after urinating.
DX: Check post-void residual volume.
Abnormal test if > 50 mL of residual urine.

Causes: Diabetic neuropathy

TX: **Bethanechol** activates muscarinic receptors stimulating contraction.
(Must rule out any urinary obstruction as the cause prior to using medication)

Stress Incontinence

↑ in abdominal pressure (laughing, coughing, sneezing) cause loss of urine due to **↓ strength of pelvic floor muscles**

Cause: **Dysfunction of urethral sphincter**

Risk: Multiple pregnancies

TX: **Kegel** exercises. If not successful urethropexy (bladder "sling", bladder neck suspension)

Urge Incontinence

Involuntary, no reason the patient suddenly feels the need to urinate.

Cause: Hyperactive detrusor muscle

TX: **Oxybutyn** (urinating too much (parasympathetic) so moves it into sympathetic so that it will stop)
Other agents: Solifenacin, Tolterodine.
Surgical tightening of the urethra.

Cystocele

When the bladder herniates into the vagina.

Risk: injury during childbirth, weak pelvic muscles, post-menopausal (estrogen helps keep the elastic tissues around the vagina strong, estrogen decreases after menopause)

SX: Discomfort and difficulty emptying bladder.

Grade 1: bladder droops a short distance into the vagina
Grade 2: Bladder falls enough to reach the opening of the vagina.
Grade 3: Gladder bulges out through the opening of the vagina

TX: Mild cystocele or poor surgical candidates: **Pessary** (a small device inserted into the vagina to hold the bladder in. It must be removed and cleaned regularly)
Severe cystocele: surgery

Neurogenic Bladder

Dysfunction of the bladder due to disease of the CNS or peripheral nerves involved in control of micturition (urination).
Patients are not able to pass urine without a catheter.

Causes: Spinal cord diseases (syringomyelia), spina bifida, neural tube defects, brain tumors, diseases of the brain, pregnancy, Diabetes, alcoholism, Vitamin B-12 deficiency.

SX: Bladder atony with urinary retention and overflow incontinence.
↑ post void volume (retention)

Post-operative Incontinence

Inability to urinate after surgical procedures.
Risk with urogenital surgeries.

TX: **Bethanechol**

RENAL PHARMACOLOGY

Diuretics

Electrolyte Changes

- **ALL diuretics can cause 1st dose hypotension**
- **NOTE: Remember the trade off: If H and K go out HCO3, Na, Cl stay in. If HCO3, Na, Cl stay in, then H and K go out.**
- **All diuretics lower ECF (extracellular fluid) volume by inhibiting tubular reabsorption of sodium, which causes its excretion.**
- Potassium (K) sparing aldosterone antagonist diuretics ➔ academia by retaining K^+ and H^+. By retaining K = buildup of K in the blood (hyperkalemia) ➔ cells then uptake K by exchanging it for an H (K/H exchanger), sending more H+ into the blood ➔ academia (🡻 pH).
- Loop and thiazide diuretics ➔ alkalemia (🡹 blood pH):
  If K is excreted, the cells send out the K in exchange for bring in an H causing less H (protons) in the blood = 🡹 blood pH.
  In diuresis = 🡻 volume = enacts the renin system = angiotensin II = Aldosterone = keeps Na, HCO3, Cl = 🡹 blood pH (alkalemia).
- Loop diuretics 🡻 Ca reabsorption so Ca levels rise in the urine and 🡻 in the serum = hypocalcemia.
- Thiazide diuretics 🡹 Ca reabsorption from the urine so Ca levels 🡻 in the urine and 🡹 in the serum.
- All diuretics (except Acetazolamide) 🡻 serum NaCl = hyponatremia
- All thiazide and loop diuretics lose serum Potassium = hypokalemia
- Acetazolamide ➔ acidemia (🡻 blood pH) due to 🡻 in HCO_3 reabsorption.

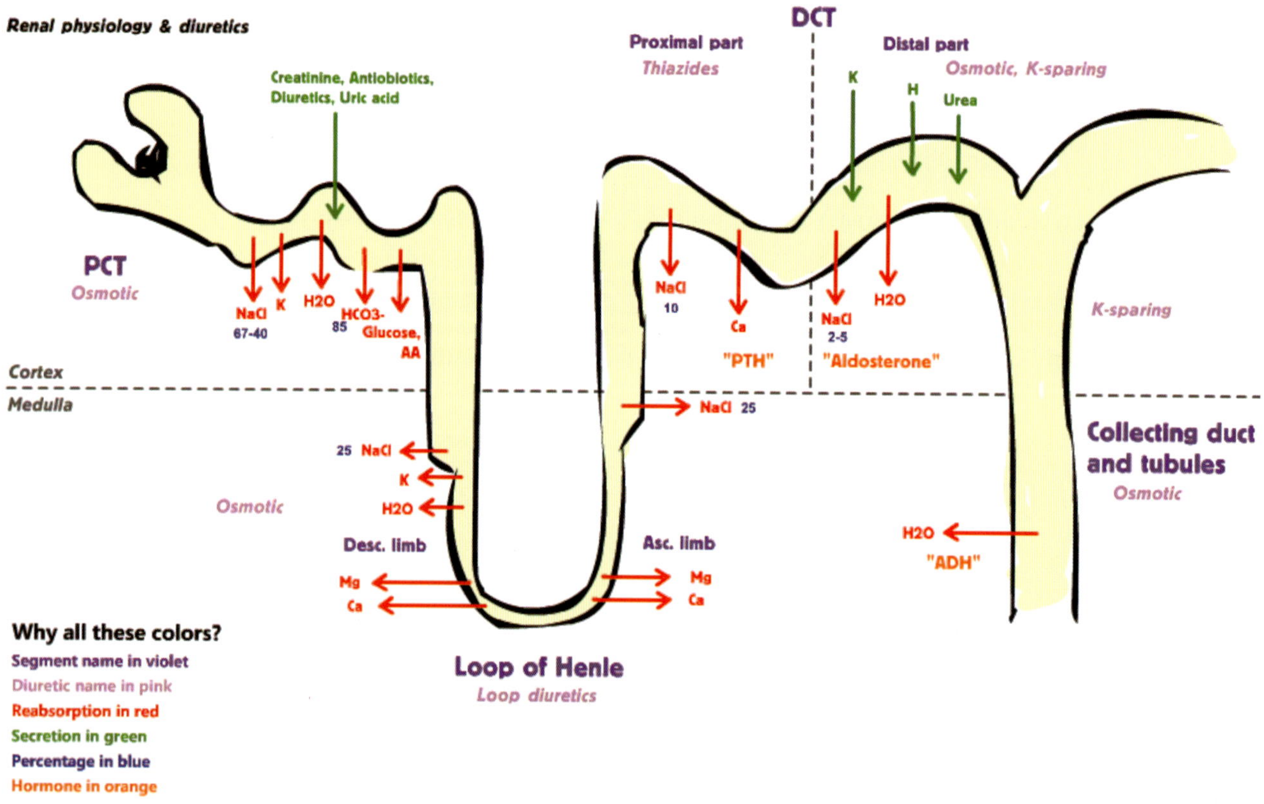

DRUG GENERIC name Trade name	Clinical Use	Mechanism of Action and Resistance	Toxicity and Notes
Acts on the PCT (Isotonic region)			
Acetazolamide	**Pseudotumor cerebri** (to ↓ ICP), **altitude sickness**, **glaucoma** (to ↓ eye pressure), alkalinize the urine.	Inhibits **Carbonic anhydrase**. Moves HCO_3 out of the body. **Decreases ICP:** Acts on the macula densa to vasoconstrict the afferent arteriole to ↓ CSF synthesis to ↓ ICP. CSF synthesis requires carbonic anhydrase and Vitamin A.	**Sulfa allergies**. Metabolic acidosis. Ammonia (NH_3) toxicity.
Mannitol	**Head trauma** (↓ ICP by getting rid of fluid), **drug overdose.**	Osmotic diuretic (↑ tubular OSM causing ↑ diuresis) which ↓ ICP and intraocular pressure.	Hypernatremia due to ↑↑ water loss. CHF because of volume expansion. Dehydration, pulmonary edema. Do not use in anuria (↓ urine output)
Acts on the Loop of Henle (Impermeable to water = hyperosmotic region)			
Furosemide	**CHF**, pulmonary edema, HTN, hypercalcemia, nephrotic syndromes, cirrhosis. **CHF Exacerbation or pulmonary edema**: must use **IV furosemide**.	Inhibits the cotransport of Na/K/2 Cl in the thick ascending limb preventing the concentration of urine. Stimulates PGE so that the afferent arteriole vasodilates. (allows larger entry of fluid so ↑ diuresis). Note: that PGE's are inhibits by NSAIDS.	**Loses Ca, K.** **Hypokalemia.** Hypocalcemia. Hyperuricemia (causes Gout), **Sulfa allergies** (it is a sulfonamide derivative), **Acute Tubular interstitial nephritis (ATN), ototoxic** (do not use with other drugs that ↑ ototoxicities: Aminoglycosides, aspirin, Cisplatin, some cephalosporin's), **acute pancreatitis.**
Bumetanide	Use with Furosemide to ↑ its efficacy.	Helps ↑ absorption.	
Ethacrynic Acid	**Same use as Furosemide but used in patients with sulfa allergies.**	Phenoxyacetic acid derivative. (Furosemide is a sulfonamide derivative).	**Same as furosemide.**
Acts on DCT (Hypertonic region)			
Hydro-chlorothiazide **(AKA: Thiazide,** HZT, HCT, HCTZ)	**HTN, CHF, Hypercalciuria, nephrogenic diabetes insipidus, osteoporosis (retains Ca), to ↓ renal stone formation by ↓ the excretion of calcium.**	Inhibits **NaCl reabsorption** in the DCT. Decreases dilution of urine (makes urine hypertonic) and **reabsorbs/retains Ca.**	**Sulfa allergies.** **Loses: Na, K, Cl = hyponatremia, hypokalemia.** **Retains: Ca.** **Causes: "GLUC"** **↑ Cholesterol, ↑ LDL (hyperlipidemia),** **↑ uric acid (hyperuricemia = gout),** **↑ Ca (hypercalcemia)**

Acts on the Cortical Collecting Tubule

Potassium Sparing Drugs (K sparing)

Spironolactone	**Hyperaldosteronism (Aldosterone secreting adrenal tumor), CHF, Potassium depletion, Ascites**	Competitive **aldosterone receptor antagonist.**	**NOTE: Spironolactone is one of the 4 drugs that ↓ morality rates! (Aspirin, β-Blocker, Ace Inhibitor, Spironolactone)** **Retains Potassium.** **Do not use in renal failure.** **Hyperkalemia = arrhythmias, Antiandrogen effects = gynecomastia** (↓ testosterone → ↓ DHT = ↓ **libido, erectile dysfunction)**
Eplerenone	Same as Spironolactone	Competitive **aldosterone receptor antagonist.**	Hyperkalemia = arrhythmias.
Triamterene	Same as Spironolactone	**Blocks Na channels** in collecting tubule	Hyperkalemia = arrhythmias.
Amiloride	Same as Spironolactone	**Blocks Na channels** in collecting tubule	Hyperkalemia = arrhythmias.

Ace Inhibitors

DRUG **GENERIC name** **Trade name**	**Clinical Use**	**Mechanism of Action and Resistance**	**Toxicity and Notes**
The "pril's" Enalapril Lisinopril Captopril Ramipril	**HTN, CHF, Diabetic nephropathy, post MI to prevent heart remodeling due to chronic HTN.** **Used with ALL patients with proteinuria.** **NOTE: Ace Inhibitors are one of the 4 drugs that ↓ morality rates! (Aspirin, β-Blocker, Ace Inhibitor, Spironolactone)**	Inhibits ACE in the lungs. Inhibiting ACE in the lungs prevents angiotensin II conversion from angiotensin I (from the liver). Acts on the efferent arterioles by inhibiting vasoconstriction (keeps the exit route open from the glomerulus = **↓ GFR (pressure).** ↓ GFR keeps proteins from causing damage as they are forced through the glomerular basement membrane (foot processes) and slows GMB thickening → so helps ↓ progression of diabetic nephropathy. (Monitored by microalbumin levels). By inhibiting ACE, bradykinin (product of Kallikrein via Clotting factor XII) is not able to be inactivated → vasodilation (responsible for causing the side effects of ACE inhibitors)	Dry, non-productive, hacky **cough, angioedema.** **Teratogen** (do NOT use in pregnancy) (**tip**: mom's do not shop in ACE hardware) **Retains K** (since ATII is not synthesized, aldosterone can't be activated = ↓ Na and ↑ K). = **Hyperkalemia.** With ↓ Na = ↓ volume = **hyponatremia and hypovolemia.** First dose hypotension. Do NOT use in renal failure, renal artery stenosis or **anyone that depends on ↑ GFR for renal function.** **Do not use in individuals with hereditary angioedema** (AKA: C1 esterase inhibitor deficiency = deficiency causes ↑ levels of bradykinin. By adding ACE inhibitors, the levels of bradykinin ↑↑ = angioedema).

Angiotensin II Receptor Blockers (ARBS)

DRUG GENERIC name Trade name	Clinical Use	Mechanism of Action and Resistance	Toxicity and Notes
The "sartan's" **Losartan** **Valsartan** Candesartan	Same as ACE inhibitors. Use in patients that develop **side effects from ACE inhibitors.** **HTN, CHF, Diabetic nephropathy, post MI to prevent heart remodeling due to chronic HTN.**	Selectively blocks binding of Angiotensin II to the angiotensin receptor so the same effects are achieved as with an ACE inhibitor except that bradykinin levels are not increased (**they stay normal**).	**Teratogen** (do NOT use in pregnancy), Weight gain. **Retains K** (since ATII is not synthesized, aldosterone can't be activated = ↓ Na and ↑ K). = **Hyperkalemia.** With ↓ Na = ↓ volume = **hyponatremia and hypovolemia.** First dose hypotension. Do NOT use in renal failure, renal artery stenosis or **anyone that depends on ↑ GFR for renal function.** **NOTE: Ace Inhibitors are one of the 4 drugs that ↓ morality rates! (Aspirin, β-Blocker, Ace Inhibitor, Spironolactone)**

Renin Inhibitor

DRUG GENERIC name Trade name	Clinical Use	Mechanism of Action and Resistance	Toxicity and Notes
Aliskiren	HTN	Inhibits renin by blocking conversion of angiotensinogen to angiotensin I.	Do NOT use with individuals on ACE inhibitors or ARBs. **Retains K** (since ATII is not synthesized, aldosterone can't be activated = ↓ Na and ↑ K). = **Hyperkalemia.** With ↓ Na = ↓ volume = **hyponatremia and hypovolemia.** First dose hypotension. Do NOT use in renal failure, renal artery stenosis or **anyone that depends on ↑ GFR for renal function.**

Urinary Incontinence

DRUG GENERIC name Trade name	Clinical Use	Mechanism of Action and Resistance	Toxicity and Notes
Bethanechol	**Bladder (urinary) retention,** postoperative ileus, neurogenic ileus.	Neurotransmitter binds directly to the muscarinic receptors. Direct agonist.	Activates bladder and bowels.
Oxybutynin Tolterodine Darifenacin Fesoterodine Solifenacin Trospium	↓ urinary (bladder) urgency. ↓ bladder spasms (detrusor muscle).	Anti-Muscarinic. Antispasmodic effect on smooth muscle. ↑ sympathetic affects	Do not use in: closed-angle glaucoma, GI obstruction, hiatal hernia, GERD, Myasthenia Gravis, Ulcerative colitis.

Misc Renal Drugs

DRUG **GENERIC name** **Trade name**	**Clinical Use**	**Mechanism of Action and Resistance**	**Toxicity and Notes**
Calcium Carbonate *Maalox, Rolaids, Tums, Mylanta*	**Hyperphosphatemia in chronic renal failure,** Gastric antacid treats diarrhea, IBS.	Phosphate binder.	Hypercalcemia, rebound acid. Do not take with **tetracycline**. Can chelate and decrease efficacy of other drugs. Interactions with **Ciprofloxacin**.
Erythropoietin	Anemia in chronic renal failure, chemotherapy induced anemia, IBD, Myelodysplasia (due to chemotherapy and radiation).	Binds to the erythropoietin receptor on the RBC progenitor and activates JAK2.	Myocardial infarction, DVT, recurrence of tumors, stroke.

REPRODUCTIVE

Embryo: see embryo chapter
Lymph drainage: see immunology chapter

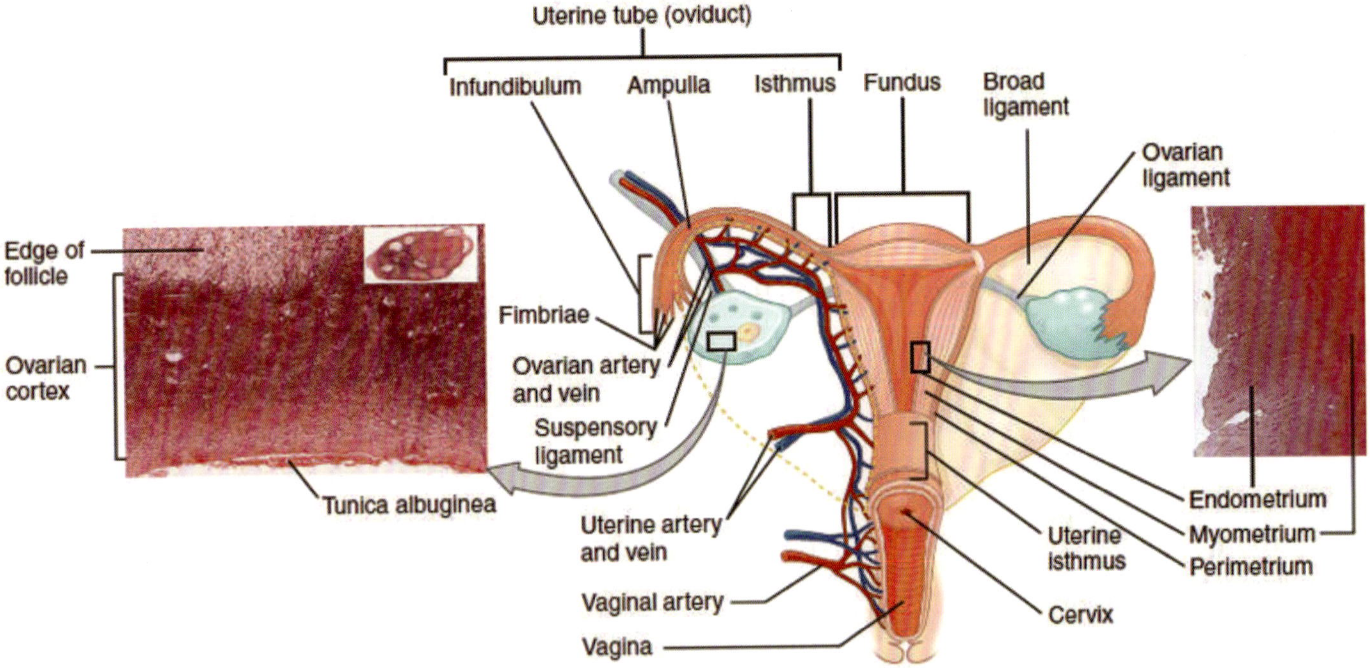

Female Histology

Structure	Histology
Oocytes	Yolk Sac
Ovary	Cuboidal
Fallopian tube (Oviduct)	Ciliated, Simple Columnar
Uterus	Simple Columnar w/glands
Transformation Zone	Squamocolumnar junction (Most common area for cervical cancer)
Endocervix	Simple Columnar
Ectocervix	Non-keratinized Stratified Squamous
Vagina	Non-keratinized Stratified Squamous

Female Anatomy: Ligaments, Vessels, Nerves, Lymph

Structure	Function	Make Up of Structure	Notes
Broad Ligament	Wide fold of peritoneum connecting uterus, fallopian tubes, ovaries to pelvic floor and lateral wall. Maintains the position of the uterus.	Contains: Ovaries, fallopian tubes, Round ligament, Ovarian ligament, Suspensory ligament	**3 Subdivisions:** Mesometrium: uterus. Mesosalpinx: fallopian tube. Mesovarium: ovaries.
Cardinal Ligament (AKA: transverse or Lateral cervical Ligament)	Connects cervix to lateral pelvic wall (located at base of broad ligament)	**Contains the uterine and vaginal arteries, veins and nerves.**	**Ureter (retroperitoneal) can be cut during ligation of uterine vessels during a hysterectomy.** (**tip**: the water flows under the bloody bridge)
Ovarian Ligament	Connects the ovaries to lateral wall of uterus	Composed of fibrous and muscular tissues.	Develops from the **gubernaculum**

Female Anatomy: Ligaments, Vessels, Nerves, Lymph

Structure	Function	Make Up of Structure	Notes
Round Ligament of the uterus	Connects uterine fundus to Labia majora.		Remnant of the **gubernaculum** (Attaches the gonad to the labioscrotal swellings in the embryo). Round ligament leaves pelvis thru deep inguinal ring and inguinal canal to the labia majora. Maintains the anteverted position of the uterus.
Suspensory Ligament of the ovaries (AKA: Infundibulopelvic Ligament)	Connects ovary to the lateral wall of the pelvis.	Contains **Ovarian vessels, nerves and lymph:** Ovarian artery, Ovarian vein, ovarian nerve plexus, Lymphatic vessels	Located over the iliac vessels. Suspensory ligament originates from the mesonephros from the mesoderm. Ovarian artery is off of the abdominal aorta. **Ureter (retroperitoneal)** can be cut during ligation of uterine vessels during a hysterectomy. (**tip:** the water (ureter) flows under the bloody bridge (ovarian vessels).
Uterosacral Ligament	Extends from the **cervix to the sacrum**. Provides support to the uterus.		
Vagina	Receives the penis during sexual intercourse. Canal for delivery of a newborn baby. Canal for menstrual fluid and tissue to leave the body.	Anterior to the vagina: bladder and urethra. Posterior to the vagina: Rectum and anus. Laterally: ureter and uterine artery.	**Blood supply**: Vaginal Artery, which travels with the uterine arteries/veins and nerves in the **Cardinal Ligament (aka: Lateral cervical ligament)**. The Vaginal and Uterine arteries branch off the Internal Iliac Artery (which is off of the Common Iliac artery which is off of the abdominal aorta). **Venous return**: vaginal venous plexus that drains into the uterine vein to the internal iliac vein. **Nerves**: ANS. Sensory from the deep pudendal nerve. Pain fibers from the sacral nerve roots. **Lymph:** Upper 1/3: External iliac, Middle 1/3: internal iliac, Lower /1/3: **Superficial inguinal.**
Cervix	Connect the vagina with the uterus, acting as a gate. Facilitates the passage of sperm into the uterine cavity (dilation of the external and internal os). Maintains sterility of the upper female reproductive tract.	2 regions: Ectocervix: portion of the cervix that projects into the vagina. Lined by stratified squamous non-keratinized epithelium. The opening is the external os. Endocervix (endocervical canal): proximal and inner part of the cervix. Lined by mucus-secreting simple columnar epithelium. The internal os is located where the uterine cavity begins.	Blood-Vein-Nerve supply: **Uterine artery** (which travels with the vaginal arteries/veins and nerves) in the **Cardinal Ligament** (AKA: Lateral cervical ligament). Venous drainage by the uterine veins. **Lymph:** by the iliac, sacral, aortic and inguinal lymph nodes.
Uterus	Secondary sex organ: mature during puberty under influence of hormones produced by the primary sex organs (ovaries). Maintenance and transportation of gametes. **Ureter (retroperitoneal)** can be cut during ligation of uterine vessels during a hysterectomy. (**tip:** the water (ureter) flows under the bloody bridge (ovarian vessels).	Anteverted: Rotated forward towards the anterior body. Anteflexed: Flexed towards the anterior body. Posterosuperior to the bladder. Anterior to the rectum. **3 Layers**: Peritoneum, myometrium (thick smooth muscle layer. These cells undergo hypertrophy and hyperplasia during pregnancy and childbirth), endometrium (inner mucous membrane lining the uterus composed of the stratum basalis and stratum functionalis)	**Blood-Vein-Nerve supply** travel through the **Cardinal ligament** (**aka: Lateral cervical ligament**) carries the Uterine and Vaginal arteries/veins and nerves. The arteries branch off of the internal iliac artery (which branches off of the Common Iliac artery which branches off of the AA). **Venous drainage** is via a plexus in the broad ligament that drains into the uterine veins. **Lymph**: Iliac, sacral, aortic and inguinal lymph nodes. **Nerves**: Sympathetic from the uterovaginal plexus (inferior hypogastric plexus). Parasympathetic fibers from the pelvic splanchnic nerves (S2-S4).

Female Anatomy: Ligaments, Vessels, Nerves, Lymph

Vulva (AKA: pudendum)	Sensory tissue during intercourse. Micturition: directs flow of urine. Helps protects the internal reproductive tract from infection.	Mons pubis: fat pad, anterior to the vulva, covered in pubic hair. Labia majora: Two hair bearing external folds, derived from the labioscrotal swellings. Labia minora: Two hairless folds, derived from the urethral folds. Fuse anterior to form prepuce (hood) of the clitoris and posterior to the vaginal opening. (Fourchette). Vestibule: External vaginal orifice/opening. **Bartholin's Glands** (AKA: vestibular nerves): Glands on each side of the vaginal opening. They secrete lubricating mucus during sexual arousal. Clitoris: Under the prepuce and derived from the genital tubercle. Formed of erectile corpora cavernosa tissue (analogous to the penis) which becomes engorged with blood during sexual stimulation.	**Blood supply**: Pudendal arteries. Venous drainage by the pudendal veins. **Lymph: Superficial inguinal lymph** nodes. **Nerves**: Anterior vulva: by the ilioinguinal nerve and the genitofemoral nerve. Posterior vulva by the pudendal nerve and the posterior cutaneous nerve of the thigh. Clitoris and vestibule nerves: parasympathetic innervation from the cavernous nerves from the uterovaginal plexus.
Ovaries	Primary sex organs. (female gonads). Produces oocytes for fertilization and produces the sex steroid hormones estrogen and progesterone in response to LH and FSH.	3 parts: Surface: Simple cuboidal epithelium (ie: germinal epithelium), Cortex: (connective tissue) containing primordial follicles which contain an oocyte, Medulla: Inner part contains neurovascular network.	**Blood supply**: Ovarian arteries arise from the abdominal aorta (just below the renal artery). Venous drainage by the ovarian veins. The left ovarian vein drains into the left renal vein and the right ovarian vein drains directly in to the Inferior vena cava. **Lymph: Para-aortic nodes**. **Nerves:** Runs through the suspensory ligament of the ovary and enters at the hilum. Sympathetic and parasympathetic nerve fibers are from the ovarian and uterine (pelvic) plexuses.
Fallopian Tubes (aka: Oviduct, Salpinges (Salpinx), Uterine Tubes)	Allows passage of the egg from the ovary to the uterus.	Segments: **Infundibulum** with fimbriae (near ovary), **Ampulla** (major portion of the lateral tube), **Isthmus** (narrow part that links the tube to the uterus), **Ostium** (thick point where the tube meets the peritoneal cavity, **uterotubal junction** (where the tube enters the uterine cavity).	**Cells:** Simple columnar epithelium. Ciliated cells are heaviest in the infundibulum and ampulla. Estrogen increases the production of cilia on these cells. **Peg Cells** produce tubular fluid which provide nutrients for the oocytes, zygotes and spermatozoa. Progesterone increases the number of Peg Cells and estrogen increases their secretory activity. The tube is made of layers of smooth muscle.

Rectouterine Pouch (AKA: Pouch of Douglas)

- Located between the uterus and rectum
- When female stands, fluid from the abdomen collects in the pouch
- Should drainage be necessary: access to the pouch is **obtained through the vagina**

Male Anatomy

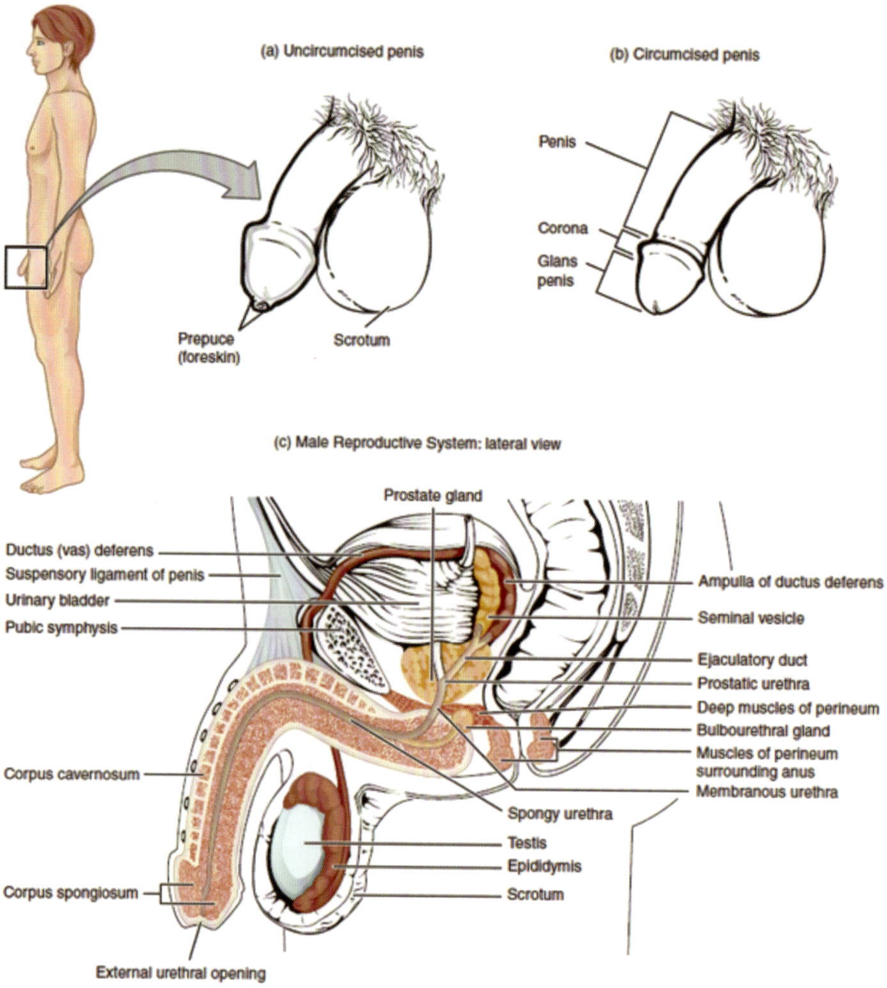

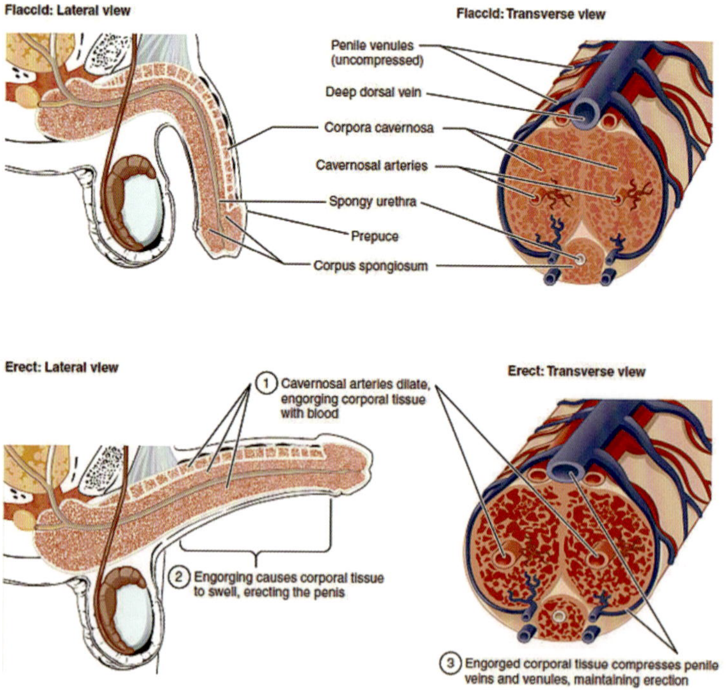

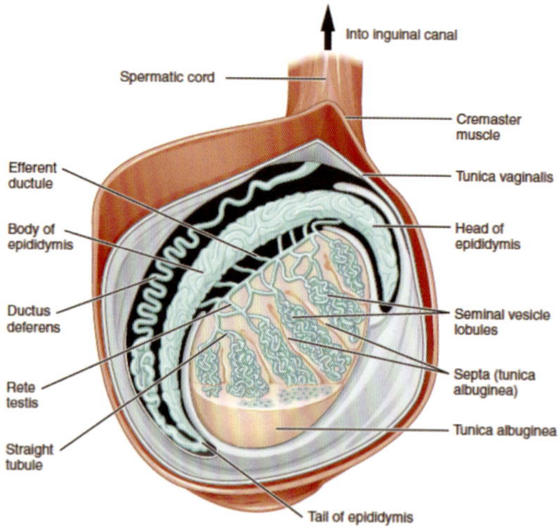

Testicle

Male Anatomy: Histology, Blood Supply, Innervation, Lymph

Structure	Histology, Anatomy, Blood Supply, Innervation
Penis	**Root of the penis supported by: suspensory ligament (connects to the pubic symphysis) and the fundiform ligament.** **Blood supply: Dorsal artery of the penis, Deep arteries of the penis, Bulbourethral artery: all 3 are branches of the internal pudendal artery off of the internal iliac artery.** **Venous drainage is by the deep dorsal vein of the penis and the superficial dorsal veins.** **Innervation: Supplied by S2 – S4 of the spinal cord and the spinal ganglia.** **Sensory and sympathetic innervation supplied by the dorsal nerve of the penis a branch of the pudendal nerve. Parasympathetic innervation is from the prostatic nerve plexus (this is responsible for the vascular changes which cause erection).** **Lymph drainage: Skin: Superficial Nodes. Glans Penis: Deep Inguinal Nodes.** **Body and Root drainage: Internal Iliac Nodes.**
Seminiferous Tubule	Seminiferous tubule is inside the testes and are the **site of meiosis for spermatozoa**. Spermatogenic cells lie between the Sertoli cells. These cells differentiate into sperm cells). Regulate spermatogenesis from germ cells.
Sertoli Cells	Columnar type cells that line the seminiferous tubule. Respond to FSH. Responsible for spermatogenesis, secreting **inhibin, Mullerian inhibitory factor, Androgen binding proteins.**
Spermatogenic Cells	Spermatogenic cells lie between the Sertoli cells. They differentiate into sperm cells
Epididymis	**Storage of sperm**. Outside is pseudostratified epithelium. Made up of: Main cells: columnar cells, Basal cells: pyramid shaped cells, Apical cells in the head region, Clear cells in the tail region. It is the tube that connects the testicle to the vas deferens. The head receives spermatozoa through efferent ducts of the testes. The tail absorbs fluid to concentrates the sperm. Epithelia cells contain sterocillia (cilia like/microvilli like).
Vas deferens (AKA: Ductus deferens)	Ducts that transport sperm **from the epididymis to the ejaculatory ducts**. Lined by stereocilia. These are the structures that are ligated during a vasectomy.
Leydig Cells	Produce testosterone. Respond to LH. Quiescent until puberty.
Corpus cavernosum	Two "Sponge like" areas of erectile tissues along the penis shaft. Contain most of the blood during an erection. (Homologous to the corpus cavernosum clitoridis in the female)
Corpus spongiosum	Erectile tissue that contains the urethra and forms the glans penis. (**tip**: you use a SPONGE to hold water (urine)
Penile Artery (AKA: Common penile artery)	Artery that supplies blood to the penis. Comprised of 3 arteries: Dorsal artery of the penis, cavernosal artery, bulbourethral artery. Damage to this artery may cause erectile dysfunction.
Dorsal artery of the penis	Artery that fills to cause an **erection**.
Dorsal veins of the penis	Engorgement of the filled dorsal artery compresses on the tissues (tunical albuginea) around the dorsal veins, compressing them so that blood can't flow out of the penis so that the erection is sustained until ejaculation.
Cavernosal artery	Small artery that runs through each of the corpus cavernosum and fills during an erection.
Bulbourethral artery	Artery that arises from the internal pudendal artery and flows down each side of the urethra in the corpus spongiosum
Bulbourethral gland (AKA: Cowper gland)	Two exocrine gland that secretes mucoproteins into ejaculate mixture and produces some of the PSA. Lubricates distal urethra. Lie posterior and lateral to the urethra at the base of the penis. (Homologous to the **Bartholin's glands** in the female)
Prostate Gland	Gland that surrounds the ejaculatory ducts and **secretes PSA and a white alkaline fluid into the ejaculate containing sperm and seminal vesicle fluid.** Alkaline fluid helps **neutralize the acidic environment of the vagina** to prolong the lifespan of the sperm. The urethra passes centrally through the prostate. This is subject to BPH, prostate cancer and prostatitis (inflammation of prostate gland). (Homologous to Skene's gland in the female)
Cremaster Muscle	Skeletal muscle that covers the testis and spermatic cord. Blood supply by the cremasteric artery. Innervated by the **genital branch of the genitofemoral nerve**. Function: Raise and lower the testes to regulate temperature to protect spermatozoa. Control can be involuntary (during sex, cold/warm temps, **"cremasteric reflex"** (stroking of the thigh raises the testicle) or voluntary (Kegel exercise) via the pubococcygeus muscle. **Loss of decrease of cremasteric reflex is an indication of a testicular torsion.**
Tunica vaginalis	Serious membrane covering of the testes and spermatic cord. Derived from the processus vaginalis (fetal development). This is an extension of the peritoneum.
Pampiniform (venous) plexus	Network of small veins in the spermatic cord. It drains the testis and helps in temperature control of the testes. (In females it drains the ovaries). Obstruction of these veins leads to a **varicocele.**
Spermatic Cord	Structure formed by the vas deferens. It extends from the deep inguinal ring down into each testicle. It is covered by a serious membrane (tunica vaginalis). It contains: Testicular artery, deferential artery, cremasteric artery, genital branch of the genitofemoral nerve, ilio-inguinal nerve, vas deferens, pampiniform plexus, lymphatic vessels, tunica vaginalis (remains of processus vaginalis). Injury to this structure can cause testicular torsion.

Inguinal Ring	Entrance to the inguinal canal. The spermatic cord passes through it in the male. (Round ligament of the uterus passes through it in the female). **Boundaries:** Superior and lateral: transversalis fascia; Inferior and medially by the inferior epigastric vessels.
Inguinal Canal	Passage in the abdominal wall in which the **ilioinguinal nerve, the spermatic cord (men) or round ligament of the uterus (woman) passes through. Site of indirect hernias.**

LYMPH DRAINAGE

Four main groups of lymph nodes

Sacral Nodes	Internal Iliac Nodes	External Iliac Nodes	Common Iliac Nodes
Lie in the hollow of the sacrum. Receive drainage from: pelvic, perineal and gluteal regions. Drain to the **internal iliac or common iliac nodes**.	Lie around the internal iliac artery. Receive drainage from the pelvic viscera, perineum and buttock. Drain to the **common iliac nodes.**	Lie around the external iliac artery. Receive drainage from the **superficial and deep inguinal nodes**, some of the pelvic viscera and abdominal wall below the umbilicus. Drain to the **common iliac** nodes.	Receive drainage from the **external and internal iliac nodes** and the **sacral nodes**. Drain to the lumbar nodes.

Lymph Node	Drainage
External Iliac Nodes Along the external iliac vessels and *drains into common iliac nodes.* *Receives drainage from the superficial and deep inguinal nodes.*	**Superior bladder**, upper 1/3 vagina**, anterior cervix** and lateral cervix (drains with uterine arteries and cardinal ligaments at base of broad ligament) legs, buttock, ductus deferens, superior uterus, and **ultimately drains into the Paraaortic/Aortic nodes.**
Internal Iliac Nodes Along the internal iliac vessels and *drains into the common iliac nodes.* *Receives drainage from the sacral nodes.*	**Prostate, base of the bladder,** middle 1/3 vagina, **lower uterus, posterior cervix,** lateral cervix (drains with uterine arteries), all pelvic structures, upper anal canal (above pectinate line), and **ultimately drains into the Paraaortic/Aortic nodes.**
External and Internal Iliac Nodes	Seminal vesicle, bladder, urethra, ureter, vagina
Deep Inguinal Lymph Nodes Between the leg and pelvis under cribriform fascia. Affected due to infections of STD's, leg and foot infections. *This drains into the external iliac nodes.*	**Penis,** scrotum, **vulva, clitoris,** perineum, gluteal region, lower abdominal wall, lower anal canal (below the pectinate line)
Superficial Inguinal Nodes Beneath inguinal ligament and **drain into the deep inguinal** lymph nodes. *This drains into the external iliac nodes.*	**Scrotum**, tunica vaginalis, **rectum**, **lower 1/3 vagina**, **vulva**, perineum, (below the hymen), lower anal canal (below the pectinate line).
Paraaortic (Lumbar)/Aortic Nodes *Receives drainage from the internal and external iliac nodes.*	Upper uterus, fallopian tubes, **ovaries, testes**, kidneys
Common Iliac Nodes *Receives drainage from the external and internal iliac nodes and the sacral nodes.*	
Lumbar Nodes (AKA: lateral aortic nodes) Between the diaphragm and pelvis along the IVC and aorta. *Common iliac drains into the Lumbar nodes and converge to become the* **THORACIC DUCT**	Intestinal trunk
Axillary Nodes Underarm to the collar bone	**Breast**, upper chest wall, upper limbs

(**tip:** You have a "**Para**" testes and ovaries, **S**crotum is **S**uperficial and the penis goes **Deep**)

Female Lymph Drainage

Uterus/Ovaries: Paraortic/Ext Iliac/Superficial
Vagina: upper: Ext Iliac lower: Common Iliac

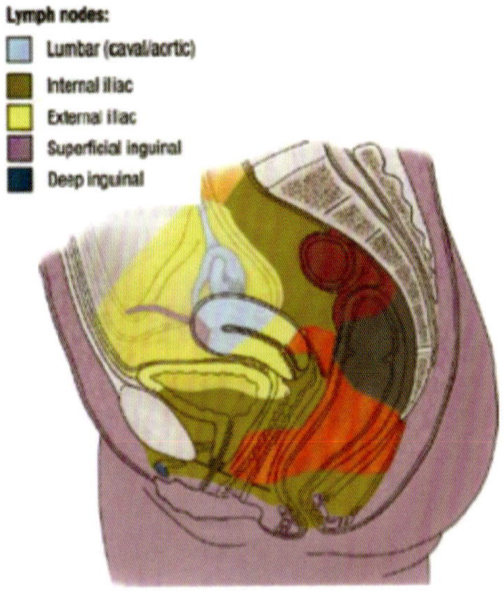

- Ovary and uterine tubes – to Lumbar lymph nodes
- Uterus:
  - lateral angle and teres ligament – Superficial inguinal lymph nodes
  - fundus and upper part of the body - Lumbar lymph nodes
  - lower part of the body - External iliac lymph nodes
  - cervix - External & Internal iliac
- Vagina:
  - Superior to hymen - to External & internal iliac
  - Inferior to hymen - to Superficial inguinal nodes
- All external genitalia (with exception - glans clitoris) - Superficial inguinal lymph nodes
- Glans clitoris – Deep inguinal

Male Lymph Drainage

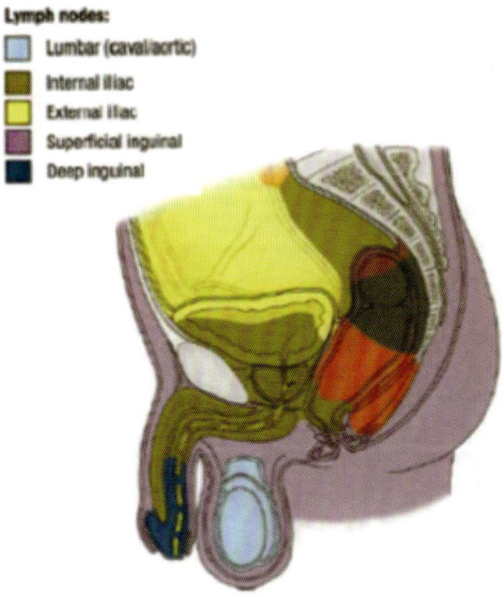

- Testis & epididymis – lumbar lymph nodes Para Aortic
- Scrotum – superficial inguinal nodes
- Penis:
  - skin - superficial inguinal nodes
  - glans – deep inguinal nodes
  - body and roots – internal iliac nodes
- Prostate gland & bladder - internal iliac nodes
- Anal canal:
  - above pectinate line - internal iliac
  - below pectinate line - superficial inguinal nodes

Tanner Scale (Stage) of Sexual Development

Tanner Stage	Description
Stage 1	Prepubertal (child – usually under 9 years old) Testicular volume < 1.5 ml, penis < 3cm No pubic hair Breast – no glandular tissue
Stage 2	Pubic hair appears: **light, fine, downy.** **Breast buds forms** (**Breast formation requires estrogen** = Hypo-pituitary axis is working and if the female starts menarche early, this is normal development) Testicular volume 1.6 – 6 ml
Stage 3 (growth spurt)	Pubic hair becomes **dark, curly and course.** Penis length increases. Breast enlarge and become more elevated, areola begins to widen. Testicular volume 6 – 12 ml This is the stage with ↑ growth. It is also not uncommon to have some mild scoliosis during this stage due to the fast growth.
Stage 4	Penis increases in width and scrotal skin darkens. Development of glans. Increased breast size and elevation. Areola and papilla (nipple) form a secondary mound. Testicular volume 12 - 20 ml Hair extends across pubis but spares medial thighs.
Stage 5	Adult. Areolae no longer raised, papilla project centrally, full breast. **Testicular volume > 20 ml** Hair extends to medial surface of thighs.

Female Physiology

Hormones

	Estrogen	Progesterone
Source	Ovary (17 β **estradiol**), placenta (**estriol**), Adipose tissue (**estrone** via aromatization)	**Corpus luteum**, placenta, adrenal cortex, testes
Function	Development and regulation of the female reproductive system and secondary sex characteristics. Stimulates endometrial proliferation. Development: breast, genitalia, fat distribution. Follicle growth. FSH stimulates the ovaries to produce estrogen by the granulosa cells (in the ovarian follicles) Breast tissue will not grow without estrogen (Tanner stage 2) **Production** Starts in the **Theca cells** in the ovary due to stimulation by **LH**. Estrogen is made when **Cholesterol is converted to Androstenedione via the enzyme Desmolase.** **Androstenedione crosses** into the **Granulosa cell** where **FSH stimulates** this to convert to **estrogen via the enzyme Aromatase**.	Progesterone = PRO pregnancy. Corpus luteum produces progesterone. **B HCG maintains corpus luteum** until placenta takes over. Maintains endometrium to support implantation. Prepares uterus for fertilized egg: Stimulates endometrial glandular secretions and **spiral, tortuous artery development**. ↓ myometrial excitability (inhibits contractions). Produces thick mucus over cervix to prevent entry by sperm. Inhibits LH and FSH Prevents endometrial hyperplasia. ↓ in progesterone after delivery disinhibits prolactin = lactation. If no implantation: ↓ progesterone = apoptosis of endometrial cells = menstruation.

Additional Hormones

Human Chorionic Gonadotropin (hCG)	**Human Placental Lactogen (HPL)**
Glycoprotein (oligosaccharides attached to polypeptides) that is 237 amino acids long. Composed of: α subunit (92 amino acids long) and shares the same α subunit as LH, FSH and TSH. β subunit (145 amino acids long), which is specific to the embryo (this is why the β hCG is used for pregnancy test). βHCG (Beta sub unit) secreted from **Syncytiotrophoblasts** (epithelial covering of the embryonic placental villi which goes into the wall of the uterus to establish circulation between the mother and the fetus). βHCG is detectible in blood in 1 week and **in urine at 2 weeks.** Maintains the corpus luteum (which secretes progesterone until the placenta takes over after the first trimester. βHCG doubles every day until 16 weeks in normal pregnancy then recedes. **Levels that remain high or increase could indicate a molar pregnancy, multiple gestations, choriocarcinoma.** **Note:** βHCG is also a **tumor marker**. It is secreted in some cancers: choriocarcinoma, seminomas, hydatidiform mole pregnancies, teratomas and germ cell tumors. When βHCG is combined with AFP (alpha-fetoprotein) it is a marker for germ cell tumors.	Polypeptide placental hormone secreted by the syncytiotrophoblast during pregnancy. It increases the metabolic state of the mother during pregnancy to meet the energy needs of the fetus

Desmolase (enzyme responsible for converting Cholesterol into Androstenediol) in the Theca cell. Stimulated by LH.

Aromatase (enzyme responsible for converting Androstenediol to Estrone) in the Granulosa cell. Stimulated by FSH.

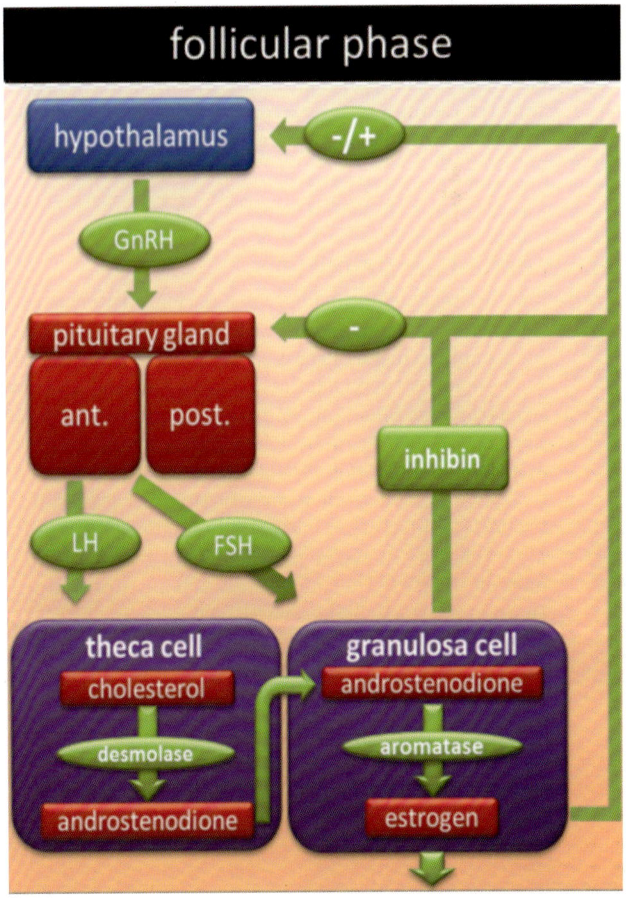

Menstrual Cycle

- Cycle: 28 days.
- **Follicular phase (AKA: Proliferative phase)** = Phase ends with ovulation. Last day 1 – 14 of the menstrual cycle.
  FSH secretion begins to rise at the end of the previous menstrual cycle and is the highest during the first week of the follicular phase. This rise starts the maturation of 5 – 7 ovarian follicles.
  FSH stimulates proliferation of the granulosa cells and LH receptors in the developing follicles.
- **FSH activates aromatase in the granulosa cells to secrete estrogen**. This increased level of estrogen stimulates GnRH which then increases production of LH.
- **LH stimulates the thecal cells to produce androgens** which cause proliferation, differentiation and secretion of the follicular thecal cells and increase LH receptors on the granulosa cells.
- Rising estrogen levels during the follicular phase stimulates the growth of the myometrium and endometrium of the uterus. It also stimulates progesterone receptors on endometrial cells so they are ready to respond to progesterone in the luteal phase.
- Rising estrogen just prior to the LH surge decrease the acidity of the vagina > 6.5 pH (creating a more hospitable environment for sperm) and causes the cervical mucus to become thin and clear (AKA: Ferning) all to allow for easier entry by the sperm.
- Estrogen levels are the highest just before the LH surge.

- **LH Surge = ovulation of the follicle.**
  Mid-cycle (14 days)
- At this stage the first meiotic division of the oocytes is complete.
- **Luteal phase (AKA: Secretory phase)** = follows LH surge. Days 15 – 28 of cycle.
  Mucus over cervix becomes heavy, thick, and acidic to prevent sperm entry.
- Luteal phase begins with formation of corpus luteum and ends with either pregnancy or menstruation.
- The **corpus luteum** is the remaining parts of the follicle, it **produces progesterone**.
- Progesterone prepares the endometrium for implantation of the blastocyst (cell mass that forms the embryo. The outer layer of cells of the blastocyst are the trophoblast cells. The trophoblast cells give rise to the placenta). It also raises the woman's basal body temperature.
- Progesterone from the corpus luteum suppresses production of FSH and LH. If FSH and LH continue to stay suppressed the corpus luteum will atrophy and die. If the corpus luteum dies, progesterone and oestrogen levels fall which stimulate FSH to begin readying follicles for the next cycle and triggers menstruation.
- If pregnancy occurs then the corpus luteum does not die. **β-hCG (from the syncytiotrophoblast: epithelial covering of the embryonic placental villi that invade the wall of the uterus to establish nutrient circulation between the embryo and other) then supports the corpus luteum** so that **progesterone is produced. The corpus luteum continues to produce progesterone for up to 12 weeks at which time the syncytiotrophoblast in the placenta are mature enough to take over the progesterone production, at which time the corpus luteum dies.**

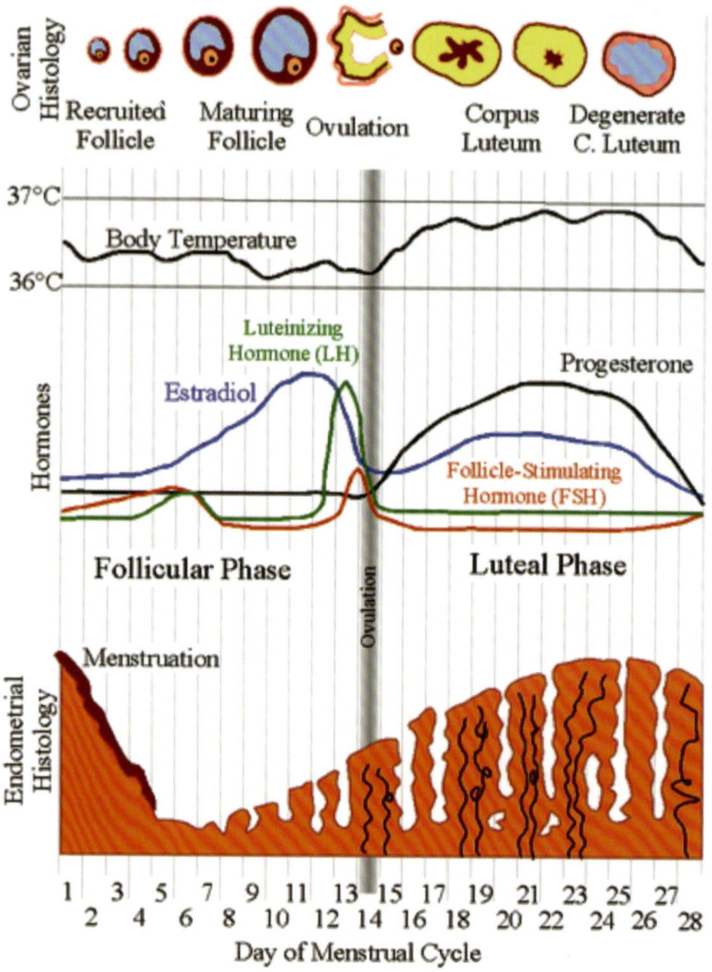

Menses Pathology Definitions

- Metrorrhagia: Spotting between periods (uterine bleeding at irregular intervals). Causes: Endometrial/cervical cancer (especially if postmenopausal), endometrial polyps, exogenous estrogen administration.
- Menometrorrhagia: Prolonged, excessive, irregular bleeding in regards to duration, amount of bleeding and time intervals. Causes: Exogenous estrogen administration, endometrial/cervical cancer, malignant tumors, endometrial polyps.
- Breakthrough bleeding: Mid-cycle bleeding. MCC: OCP users due to insufficient estrogens and excessively thick endometrium lining
- **Mittelschmerz**: Mid-cycle abdominal pain due to ovulation. Occurs 2 weeks after last period. Unilateral pain on the side of the ovary where ovulation occurred. No other issues of concern present. **Must rule out**: Appendicitis (if on right side) and ovarian torsion (Sudden onset lower abdominal pain that radiates to the back with nausea and vomiting.
- Menorrhagia: Heavy menstrual bleeding with/without clots (>80 mL blood loss or > 7 days of bleeding. High risk: iron deficiency anemia. Causes: Uterine fibroids, Dysfunctional uterine bleeding (DUB), IUD's, endometrial hyperplasia.
- Hypomenorrhea: Light menstrual flow, may just be spotting. Causes: OCP's (Oral Contraceptive Pills), Obstruction (hymen or cervical stenosis).
- Oligomenorrhea: Menstrual cycles lasting > 35 days. Causes: Pregnancy, anorexia, menopause, estrogen secreting tumor.
- Polymenorrhea: < 21 day cycle
- Menarche: Beginning of periods/ovulation
- Dyspareunia: painful intercourse
- Postcoital bleeding: Bleeding after intercourse. Causes: Cervical dysplasia, atrophic vaginitis, cervical cancer, cervical polyps, STD (Gonorrhea/Chlamydia/Trichomoniasis), Cervicitis/Vaginitis, vaginal yeast infection, uterine polys.

Ovulation	Pregnancy	B HCG	Lactation	Breast Milk
↑ Estrogen from ovaries = ↑ GnRH receptors on anterior pituitary = Estrogen surge **(LH surge)** = ovulation	MC Site fertilization: Ampulla within 1 day of ovulation. Implantation on wall of uterus = 6 days after fertilization. **MCC of amenorrhea.**	βHCG (Beta sub unit) secreted from **Syncytiotrophoblasts:** detectible in blood in 1 week and **in urine at 2 weeks.** βHCG doubles every day until 16 weeks in normal pregnancy, the recedes. **Levels that remain high or increase could indicate a molar pregnancy, multiple gestations, choriocarcinoma.** **Ectopic pregnancies have lower levels of β–hCG and levels do not double every 48 hours.** **B-hCG subunit Alpha is shared by LH, FSH, TSH.** **B HCG maintains corpus luteum till placenta can produce its own progesterone.** (**Tip**: Beta (β) is for Baby)	↓ Progesterone stimulates lactation. **Prolactin** (dopamine is inhibited) maintains lactation. **Oxytocin** (posterior pituitary) assist in milk let down. .	**IgA (requires "J" chain secretory piece on IgA).** **IgA and IgG = passive immunity. Baby is protected until 2 months old. (vaccinations start). Baby does not start making its own IgG till 6 months.** Colostrum: first milk produced after birth. Contains antibodies to protect the newborn and mild laxative to help baby pass meconium (first stool). ↓ infant infections and decreases risk of development of allergies, asthma, diabetes mellitus and obesity. Breast milk fed babies: must supplement: Vitamin D. Breast milk fed babies of vegan moms must supplement: Vit. B12, iron, zinc, calcium and omega-3-fatty acids. Goat's milk fed babies: must supplement folate. Breastfeeding ↓ risk of breast and ovarian cancer due to ↓ exposure to estrogen Vitamin D. Breast milk fed babies of vegan moms must supplement: Vit. B12, iron, zinc, calcium and omega-3-fatty acids. Breastfeeding ↓ risk of breast and ovarian cancer due to ↓ exposure to estrogen

Menopause	Premature Ovarian Failure (early menopause before age of 40)	Morning Sickness	Normal Changes in Pregnancy	↑ AFP
Average age = 51 ↓ Estrogen, ↑ LH, ↑↑ FSH ↓ Ovarian follicles DX: ↑↑ FSH is confirmatory for menopause. (Loss of negative feedback on FSH due to ↓ estrogen)	Not pathologic. SX: Same as menopause: Hot flashes, atrophy of vagina, osteoporosis, sleep difficulty, coronary artery disease (no longer estrogen protective)	Metabolic alkalosis. (Loss of H+ and K) ↑ pH, ↑ CO_2, ↑ HCO_3 **Hyperemesis Gravidarum** (4 – 10 weeks) **Severe vomiting** = wt loss, ketonuria	↓ BUN/creatinine due to ↑ renal flow. ↑ TBG (thyroid binding globulins) = ↑ T4, normal TSH. ↑ Fluid = S3 heart sound.	(Alpha Fetal Protein levels) **MCC: Incorrect dating error** Multiple gestations Abnormal "openings" of the fetus: Spina bifida Neural tube defects Gastroschisis Omphalocele Anencephaly

Oogenesis

- **Primary oocytes are arrested in Meiosis I in Prophase I until ovulation (menarche)**
- **Secondary oocytes: Meiosis II is arrested in metaphase II until fertilization**
- Meiosis = 1 haploid ovum: (1N, 1C) (**tip**: 1 happy (haploid) egg) (**tip**: when a sperm MET and egg)
- N = chromatids (individual pieces)
  C = # Chromosomes
  Polar Body: Haploid cells that are formed at the same time as an egg cell during oogenesis but does not have the ability to be fertilized. When they divide, they only get cytoplasm.

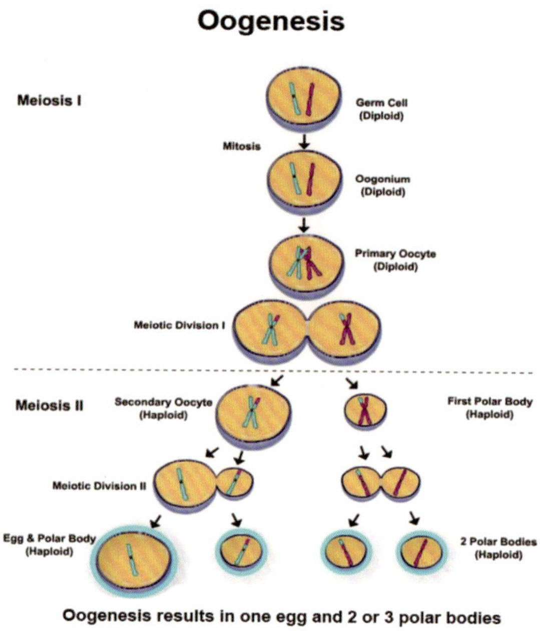

Spermatogenesis

- Begins at puberty = spermatogonia
- Occurs in seminiferous tubules producing spermatids that undergo spermiogenesis (gain of **acrosomal cap**) and form mature spermatozoon.
- End result: **Meiosis = 4 haploid spermatids (1N, 1C)**
  (**tip**: 4 happy sperm)
  N = chromatids (individual pieces)
  C = # Chromosomes
  (Cells always have pairs of chromosomes: each chromosome = 1N, so a complete set is 2N).
  (Diploids divide in half so each chromosome has its own cell with ½ of the pair so it can meet up with a mate and reproduce).

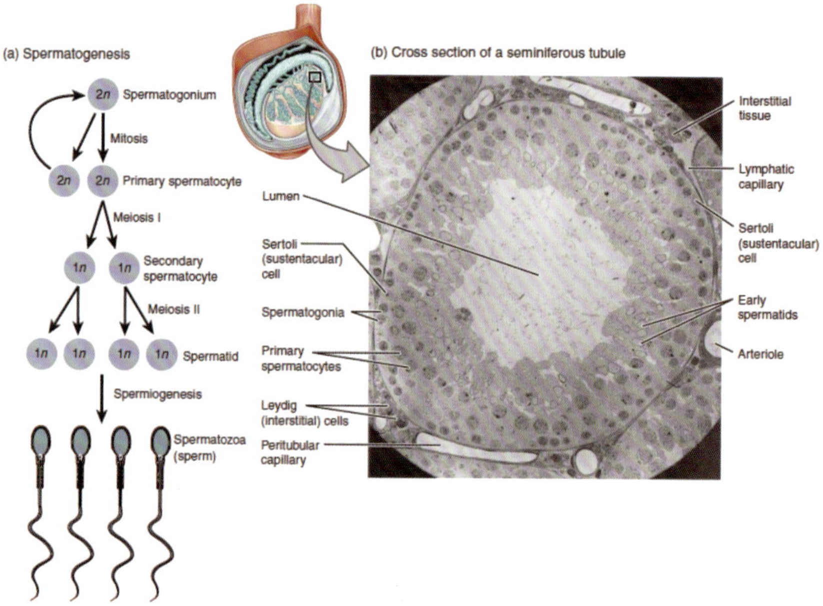

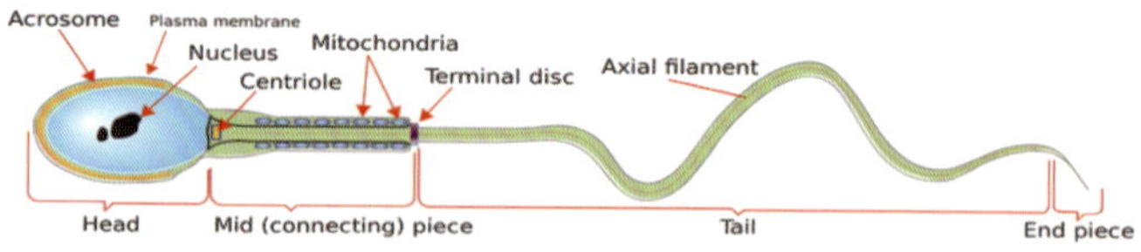

Sperm

- **Spermatogonium and primary spermatocyte = Diploid (2N, 2C)**
- **Secondary spermatocyte = Haploid (1N, 2C)**
- **Mature Spermatid = Haploid (1N, 1C)**
- (**tip**: mature sperm is a HAPpy sperm)
- **Zinc** is required
- **Fructose** (energy) is required

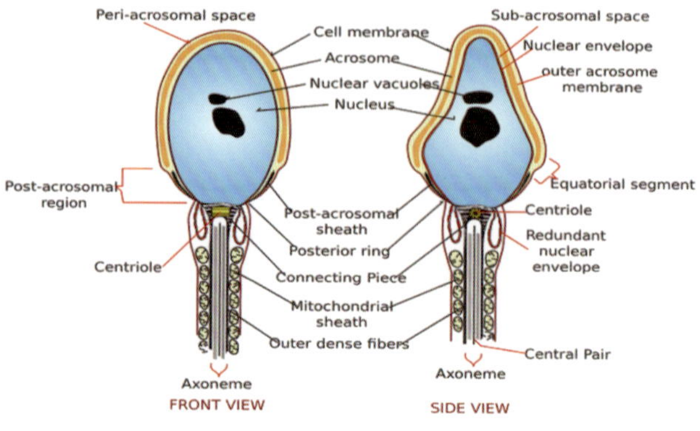

Androgens

- Testosterone, DHT (dihydrotestosterone, androstenedione
- Aromatase converts androgens to estrogen (in males: occurs in **testes and adipose**, in females: occurs in ovaries and adipose tissue)

Testosterone

- Responsible for **internal** male sex organs:
  Epididymis, vas deferens, seminal vesicles (**Not prostate**)
- Growth spurt: penis enlargement, seminal vesicles, sperm, muscles, deepening of voice, libido
- **Closes epiphyseal plate**. (Precocious puberty = short)

DHT

- Responsible for **external** male sex organs:
  Penis, scrotum, **prostate**
- Testosterone is converted to DHT via **5α-reductase** (**Finasteride** inhibits 5 α-reductase)
- Later in life contributes to: **balding, prostate growth (BPH)**,
  sebaceous gland

Male Feedback

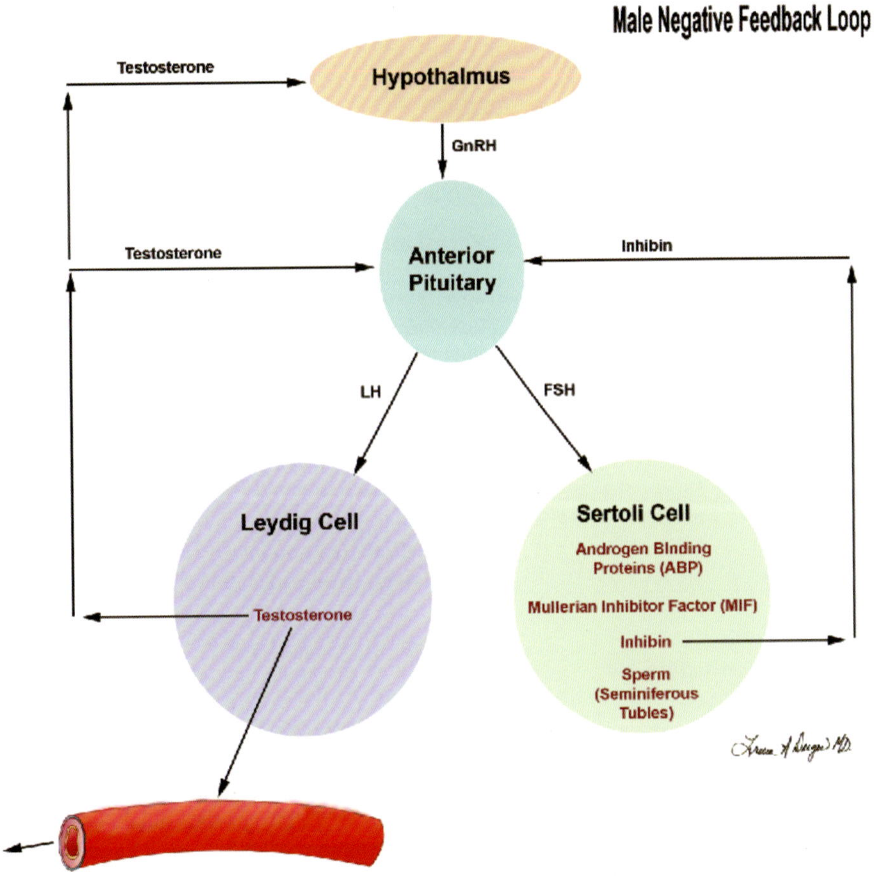

- LH ➔ Leydig cells ➔ Testosterone ➔ Blood vessels and feedback to pituitary and hypothalamus
  (**Tip**: **T**estosterone = **T**wo feedbacks)
- FSH ➔ Sertoli cells ➔ ABP (Androgen Binding Proteins), Inhibin, Mullerian Inhibitory Factor (MIF) ➔ Inhibin feedback to pituitary
  (**Tip**: **1**nhibin = **1** feedback)

Cell	Function	Notes
Leydig Cells (Endocrine cells)	**LH** stimulates to secrete **testosterone**	Contains **aromatase.** Testosterone unaffected by temperature
Sertoli Cells (non-germ cell)	**FSH** stimulates to secrete: **ABP** (Androgen Binding Proteins: maintains testosterone levels) **MIF** (Mullerian Inhibitory Factor: inhibits female organs **Inhibin:** Provides feedback to pituitary (FSH) **Tight Junctions** form blood-testis barrier. Sertoli cells line the seminiferous tubule. (Seminiferous tubule are inside the testes and are the site of meiosis for spermatozoa. Spermatogenic cells lie between the Sertoli cells. These cells differentiate into sperm cells). Regulate spermatogenesis. Convert testosterone and androstenedione to estrogen via aromatase.	**Sensitive to temperature.** **↑** temps = **↓** sperm production and inhibin
Spermatogonia (Germ cells)	Maintains **germ pool** of primary spermatocytes	Line seminiferous tubules

Sexual Response Cycles

Female	Male : Erection and Ejaculation
Excitement Phase: vaginal **lubrication**, uterus elevates, (foreplay = enhances this stage). **Plateau** Phase: expansion of inner vagina Orgasm: **Contraction** of uterus Resolution: Skin flushing, tachycardia by ANS	(**tip**: Point and Shoot. Point: parasympathetic and Shoot: sympathetic) **Parasympathetic (pelvic nerve) = Erection** **Nitric Oxide ➔ ↑ cGMP ➔** smooth muscle relaxation ➔ vasodilation of **dorsal artery** which then fills and dilates the **Cavernosal arteries** (in the Corpora cavernosa) in the penis. This engorges the **corpora cavernosa**, which compresses the tissue around the **veins (tunica albuginea)** of the penis causing them to constrict, preventing blood from leaving the veins which causes the penis to become rigid and maintains the erection. **Norepinephrine ➔ ↑** Ca ➔ smooth muscle contraction ➔ vasoconstriction. **Sympathetic (hypogastric nerve)** = Emission **Ejaculation (pudendal nerve)**

Erection

Arterial inflow without venous outflow = erection

Ejaculation pathway

Sperm flow from the lower epididymis (Storage department. Stores sperm 2 – 3 months) through the vas deferens via peristaltic actions. Sperm aren't able to swim yet because they haven't gone through the prostate. ➔ excretory duct of the seminal vesicle joins the vas deferens to form the ejaculatory ducts ➔ sending sperm through the prostate gland which adds a milky white alkaline fluid (helps neutralize the acidity of the vaginal tract to prolong the life of the sperm) to the sperm and fluid from the seminal vesicles to create semen ➔ urethra (corpus cavernosa) ➔ ejaculation.

Pathway of the sperm: Seminiferous tubules ➔ epididymis ➔ vas deferens ➔ ejaculatory duct ➔ urethra ➔ urethral meatus.

Pudendal nerve (sympathetic fibers)

- Sensory function: external genitalia (penis and clitoris), and skin around the perineum and anus of both males and females.
- Motor function: pelvic muscles, external urethral and anal sphincter.
- Pudendal block used to anesthetize the perineum during labor.
- Exits the pelvis through the lower greater sciatic foramen and reenters the pelvis through the lesser sciatic foramen.
- Innervated from S2, S3 and S4 in the sacral nerve roots. (**tip**: 2, 3, 4 keeps the penis off the floor)
- Gives rise to the inferior rectal nerve, perineal nerve and the dorsal nerve of the penis or clitoris.

Fertilization

- Sperm undergo **capacitation** in female reproductive tract. ↑ motility, **acrosome reaction** (acrosome = cap structure over head of sperm) allow for the sperm to break through the **zona pellucida,** surrounding the ovum (egg)
- Sperm binds to the corona radiate (layer of follicle cells attached to the oocyte, adjacent to the zona pellucida – the outer protective layer of the ovum)
- Sperm reach the zona pellucida (matrix of glycoproteins) and bind with a ZP# glycoprotein in the zona pellucida, triggering the acrosome to burst releasing enzymes that aid the sperm penetrate
- Once past the zona pellucida a cortical reaction occurs. Granules inside the secondary oocyte fuse with the plasma membrane so that enzymes can be expelled by exocytosis to the zona pellucida to prevent entry by other sperm. Prevents fertilization by more than one sperm.
- Once the sperm enters the cytoplasm of the oocyte, the oocyte undergoes its **second meiotic division**

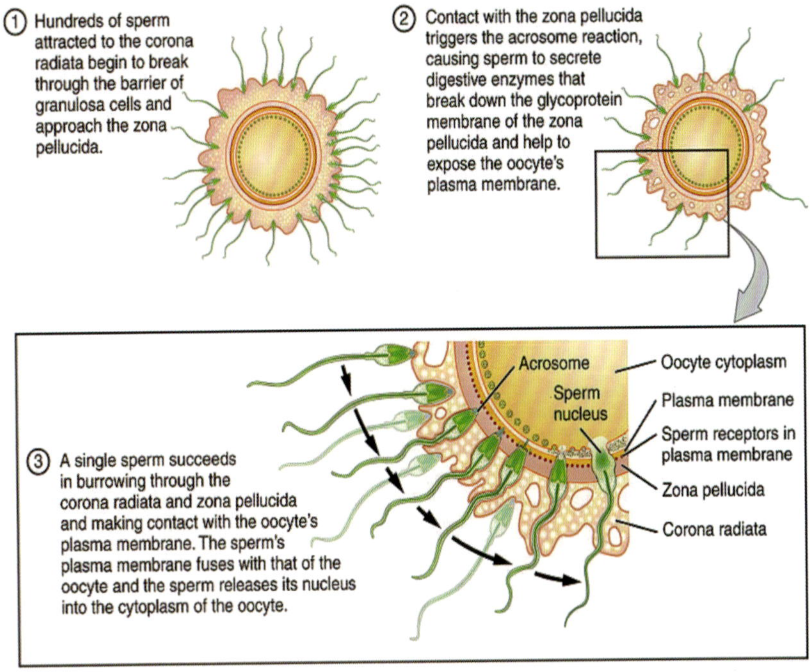

Reproductive Pathology
Sex Chromosome Disorders

Turner Syndrome (45XO) Monosomy

- 45XO/46XX due to mosaicism
- **SHOX gene**
- Nondisjunction in **paternal** meiosis I
- No Barr body
- Decreased estrogen = **increased LH and FSH**
- SX: **Absent ovaries (AKA: streak ovaries)** (no menses because no estrogen, but they can still carry a fetus with in-vitro), **coarctation** of the aorta (different BP in upper body verses lower body), notched ribs, cystic **hygroma** (posterior neck swelling and extra skin at birth), **dactylitis** (swelling of hands and feet due to lymphedema due to dysgenesis of lymphatic network), low hairline, short 4th metacarpal, **horseshoe kidney (due to inferior mesenteric artery)**, nail dysplasia, discolored spots on skin (nevi), web neck, wide chest (AKA: shield chest), bicuspid valve, arched palate
- Note: **There is a small percent of Turners that do have ovaries**, therefore they will have normal cycles and are able to get pregnant. So if your vignette describes a girl who has the other signs of Turner's but has periods or was **able to get preg**nant, it still is Turners.

Klinefelter's Syndrome (47 XXY, or XXY)

- Inactivated Barr body (X chromosome)
- Dysgenesis of seminiferous tubules (no sperm) = **decreased inhibin = increased FSH**
- Dysfunction of Leydig cells = decreased testosterone = **increased LH = increased estrogen**
- SX: **Infertility**, testicular atrophy, long extremities, **gynecomastia,** decreased libido, impotence
- Labs: **↑ FSH, ↑** LH
- Histology: Shows many Leydig cells, few Sertoli cells and **absent germ cells.**
- XXY males can also have health problems that typically affect females: breast cancer, osteoporosis and autoimmune disorders.
- Due to a **nondisjunction during paternal or maternal meiosis I.** (Nondisjunction: when homologous chromosomes (X and Y or two X chromosomes) fail to separate).
- Error in chromosome **segregation in anaphase** during the **primary spermatocyte** stage of spermatogenesis.

True hermaphroditism (46XX/46XY, 47XXY, 46XX/47XXY) • Individual born with both testicular and ovarian tissue • Ambiguous external genitalia depending upon amount of testosterone produced between 8 and 16 weeks of gestation	Female Pseudohermaphrodite (XX) • Ovaries present, external genitalia virilized • Due to excessive exposure to androgens during early gestation • (girl inside, boy outside)
Male Pseudohermaphrodite (XY) • Testes present, external genitalia are female • Due to androgen insensitivity (testicular feminization) • (boy inside, girl outside)	Double Y Males (XYY) • Phenotypically normal • Severe acne, high risk of anti-social behavior, very tall

Sex Hormone Disorder Labs

Disorder	Testosterone Levels	LH Levels	Description
Primary Hypogonadotropic	↓	↑	No testosterone = no negative feedback = ↑ LH
Defective Androgen Receptor	↑	↑	Can't see the androgens = no negative feedback = ↑ LH ↑ Testosterone
Testosterone Secreting Tumor	↑	↓	↑ Testosterone therefore do have negative feedback = ↓ LH
Exogenous Steroid Use	↑	↓	↑ Testosterone therefore do have negative feedback = ↓ LH
Hypogonadotropic, Hypogonadism	↓	↓	

Aromatase Pathologies
(Aromatase: think estrogen)

Aromatase Deficiency (affect females) Insufficient production of aromatase so **can't convert androgens to estrogens.** Masculinization of females (virilization), **normal female internal genitalia, clitoromegaly** (due to high androgen). SX: Primary amenorrhea, normal blood pressure, tall (because no estrogen, estrogen closes the epiphyseal growth plates). Risk: Predisposed to **osteoporosis** (no estrogen) and polycystic ovaries. Labs: **Increased LH and FSH** (out looking for the estrogen).	**↑ Aromatase production = ↑↑ estrogen** Affects both sexes. In males = gynecomastia, feminized appearance, hypogonadism, oligozoospermia (low sperm count), micropenis. In females = precocious puberty and short stature because estrogen closes epiphyseal plates early, excessively large breast (estrogen is required for breast development), enlarged uterus, menstrual irregularities. Labs: ↑ DHEA-S TX: **Aromatase inhibitors**
5α Reductase Deficiency (46 XY) • Males only • Deficiency in the male chromosome 46XY • 5α Reductase is required to **convert testosterone to DHT** (DHT is responsible for male **external genitalia**) • Male has no external genitalia (virilization at birth – or female genitalia) (DHT: 5α dihydrotestosterone) • Males have internal sex organs: testicles and Wolffian structures • Affects only genetic males (those with a Y chromosome) **Pseudo-hermaphroditism** When an individual is born with the primary genetic sex characteristics of one sex but develops secondary sex characteristics. Ex: If a female is born with testes = male pseudohermaphrodite, if a male is born with ovaries = female pseudohermaphrodite	**Androgen Insensitivity (46 XY)** (Androgens: think testosterone) • Males only (but the patient will present as a female (physiologically) • Mutation in the androgen receptor gene so there is no response to androgens (testosterone), **the receptor "can't see the testosterone".** • This individual is actually a male but develops female characteristics • 1° amenorrhea • Bilateral inguinal masses (testes), these MUST be removed due to ↑ chance of testicular cancer • **Breast development (testosterone is still converted to estrogen. Estrogen = breast)** • **No pubic or axillary hair development (no adrenal hormones (axillary) and no pituitary hormones (pubic)** • No mullerian structures (Testes are present so Sertoli cells do produce MIF (Mullerian Inhibitory Factor) so no uterus or fallopian tubes or upper 1/3 of vagina • Does have blind vaginal pouch • **Watch for a teenage patient that has never had a period but presents normally with breast and genitalia but does not have any pubic or axillary hair.**

Testosterone Deficiency

- MC **Pituitary adenoma**
- SX: Decreased libido, gynecomastia, small testicles, erectile dysfunction, decreased early morning erections, decreased sperm count, hot flashes, osteoporosis
- DX: MRI of pituitary
- TX: **Bromocryptine** (Dopaminergic agonist)

Precocious Puberty Causes

Precocious Pseudo-Puberty (adrenal cause)	**Precocious Puberty (central cause – Pituitary)**
• Most common in boys • Excessive sex steroids • Course pubic and **axillary hair** (**tip**: "**A**"xillary hair due to "**A**"drenal problems) • Significant growth acceleration • Severe cystic acne • Small testicles, large penis • Gonadotropin independent • **Causes:** CAH (21 Hydroxylase), Adrenal tumor, Ovarian cyst, McCune Albright, leydig or germ cell tumors	• Most common in girls • Premature activation of hypothalamus of pituitary – gonad axis • Less dramatic presentation • Testicular and penis enlargement • **Pubic hair** (**tip**: "**P**"ubic hair due to "**P**"ituitary problems) • Premature maturation • Growth spurt • **Causes:** Idiopathic, CNS tumors, Hypothyroid

McCune Albright	**Kallmann's Syndrome**
• Genetic disorder of bones, skin pigmentation and premature puberty • Precocious puberty due to endocrine hormone excess • Unilateral café au lait spots • Polystotic fibrosis (bone fibrosis) 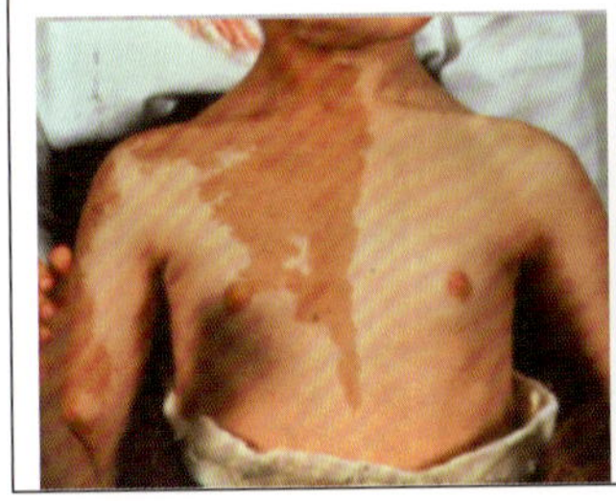 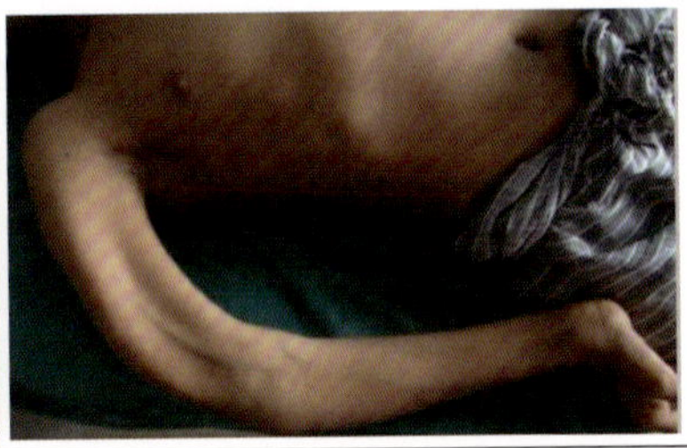	• Failure to start puberty or failure to complete puberty • Occurs in males and females • Hypogonadism and infertility • **Anosmia (reduced or no sense of smell)** **Note: This is the Olfactory Never (CN I). Remember, CN I is the only cranial nerve that does not go to the Thalamus but goes directly to the sensory cortex.** • Cause: **Hypothalamic neurons** responsible for releasing GnRH **fail to migrate** into the hypothalamus during embryonic development

Contraception, Abortive 's, Tocolysis, HRT (hormone replacement therapy)

DRUG GENERIC name Trade name	Clinical Use	Mechanism of Action and Resistance	Toxicity and Notes
Contraception			
OCP (oral contraception)	Contraception **Combined (estrogen/progestin** ↓ **risk of ovarian and endometrial cancer and ectopic pregnancy.** They also ↓ bleeding and cramps. They do **NOT** change the risk of breast cancer.	Inhibits LH/FSH → **no estrogen → no LH surge → no ovulation → no pregnancy.** Various forms containing various levels of estrogen and progestin. MC: Combo of estrogen and progesterone. Unit contains: 21 pills and 7 placebos. Menses occurs during the 7 days of placebo pills. Progestins: Thicken cervical mucus → ↓ access of sperm. Progestin's also inhibit increase in spiral arteries in the endometrium so ↓ implantation. **NOTE:** Estrogen containing OCP's provide a **continual level of negative feedback** to the pituitary, which stabilizes FSH and LH which **prevents the LH surge** which inhibits ovulation.	**Do NOT use in women >35 if they are smokers** (↑ cardiovascular events). **↑ risk for hypercoagulability →** ↑ blood clots so **avoid in anyone with history of blood clotting disorders.** Can cause **hepatocellular adenomas** (benign) (AKA: **Hepatic Adenoma**): discontinue OCP's. **Does NOT cause weight gain. Can cause hypertension.** Note: in any situation where there is a ↓ in estrogen = infertility (ie: Anorexia nervosa) Note: if taken during pregnancy, do NOT increase miscarriage or birth defect risk. Do NOT use in estrogen-positive breast cancer.
Estrogen	Ovarian failure, HRT in postmenopausal women, menstrual abnormalities, men with androgen-dependent prostate cancer.	Binds estrogen receptors.	**↑ risk of endometrial cancer (AKA: endometrial hyperplasia) (any bleeding in a postmenopausal woman is considered endometrial carcinoma until proven otherwise).** **↑ risk for blood clots.** **Prematurely closes epiphyseal plates.** Contraindicated in: Pregnancy, DVT, Smoker > 35 yrs old, acute liver disease, chronic HTN, Diabetes, Depression, Migraines, hyperlipidemia.
Progestin	↑ vascularization of endometrium to prepare the uterus for implantation. (**tip**: PROgestin is PRO pregnancy). Treats: abnormal/ **dysfunctional/** irregular uterine bleeding. "Morning after pill"	Binds progesterone receptors.	Does not ↑ risk of blood clots. Can be used by breastfeeding moms b/c they do not affect milk production. Contraindicated in: Pregnancy, DVT, Smoker > 35 yrs old, acute liver disease, chronic HTN, Diabetes, Depression, Migraines, hyperlipidemia.

Hormone Replacement Therapy (HRT) (estrogen replacement)	Prevention of menopausal symptoms: hot flashes, vaginal atrophy, dyspareunia.	Estrogen replacement	Note: Must add progesterone b/c estrogen only will ↑ risk of endometrial carcinoma in postmenopausal women. Contraindicated in: Estrogen sensitive breast or endometrial cancer, DVT, unexplained vaginal bleeding, liver dz. Additional benefits: ↓ risk of osteoporosis (when there is estrogen there is ↓ osteoclast activity) but is **NOT a treatment for osteoporosis**. ↓ risk of colorectal cancer.
Condoms: Female and Male	Contraception, Protection against STD's.	.	Note: **Be careful of latex allergies**. Other barrier methods: condoms, cervical caps, diaphragms, contraceptive sponges, spermicides.
Tubal ligation (AKA: sterilization)	Contraception	Surgical procedure in which the fallopian tubes are ligated/tied for permanent contraception.	Most effective: 99% effective. Failures most often result in ectopic pregnancy.
IUD (Intrauterine devices)	**Contraception**	**Copper or levonorgestrel device is placed inside the uterus so that ↓ implantation and makes the environment in the uterus non-conducive for pregnancy.**	**Can ↑ risk of PID (pelvic inflammatory dz) and ↑ risk of miscarriages.** **Copper IUD's = ↑ bleeding and cramps.** **Hormonal IUD's = ↓ menstrual bleeding and even stop periods.** **Contraindicated in: Hx of ectopic pregnancy, abnormal uterus shape/size, Abnormal pap smears.**
Diaphragm	**Contraception**	**Circular ring with contraceptive jelly that covers cervical canal. Placed over cervix at least 6 hours before intercourse and left until 6 hours after intercourse.**	**Must be fitted properly, requires advance preparation, improper placement can ↓ efficacy.**
Vaginal Ring	**Contraception**	**Vaginal ring that releases estrogen and progesterone. Stays in the vagina for 3 weeks.**	**Withdrawal bleeding occurs when ring is removed.**
Transdermal Patch	**Contraception**	**Skin patch with combo of estrogen and progesterone. Stays on skin for 7 days and then replaced. 3 weeks of patches with 4th week of no patch.**	
Nexplanon Implanon (Implantable contraception)	**Contraception. Progesterone only.**	**Contraception: subdermal tube that is implanted under the skin in the upper arm and releases hormones.**	**Considered to be the most effective form of birth control. Must replace every 3 years.** **Lighter periods, can be used during breastfeeding, ↓ PMS symptoms.** **Side effects: Weight gain, moodiness, sore breast, lethargy, irregular bleeding first 6 – 12 months.**

Birth Control, cont'd

Depo Provera	**Contraception. Progesterone only.**	**Injection that provides 3 months of contraceptive protection.**	
Vasectomy	**Male contraception.**	**Surgical procedure in which the vas deferens is ligated/ties for permanent contraception**	**Must use protection for up to 6 months after the vasectomy (or 2 negative sperm analysis).**
Levonorgestrel Norgestrel Antiprogestin Mifepristone (AKA: Morning after pills")	**Emergency contraception. (ECP's)** **Progestin only.**	**Delays or disrupts ovulation or fertilization. Contain high doses of estrogens, progestin's or both.**	**Nausea, vomiting, abdominal pain, fatigue, headache, breast tenderness, dizziness.**

Infertility

- A couple is not considered infertile until after **ONE YEAR** of trying to become pregnant.
- 1st Step: Always rule out the male first with a semen analysis. MCC of infertility is due to the male.
  Causes: ↓ sperm motility, abnormal sperm morphology, ↓ sperm count, azoospermia.
  TX: In vitro fertilization, intrauterine insemination. Azoospermia: Artificial insemination.
- Normal semen analysis → anovulation reasons.
  Causes: Hypothyroidism, low progesterone or estrogen, hyperprolactinemia, anorexia.
  TX: Check TSH (treat underlying cause), Induce ovulation (pulsatile) with **Clomiphene citrate**.
- If ovulation is occurring then check for physical causes such as obstructions. (PID due to Chlamydia or Gonorrhea, tubal damage.
  DX: Hysterosalpingogram (HSG) and/or laparoscopy.
  TX: Repair damage or open blockage.

In Vitro Fertilization (IVF)

- Process where multiple eggs are fertilized by the sperm outside the body. (in vitro = "in glass").
- Eggs are aspirated from the ovarian follicles.
- Fertilized eggs are transferred into the uterus with the intention of one of the eggs implanting to establish pregnancy.

Pregnancy

Fertilization

Developmental age: # days from fertilization.
Gestational age: # days since last menstrual period. (2 weeks longer than conception/developmental age).

Due Date Calculation:
"Nägele rule: Date of last menstrual period (LMP), add 1 year, subtract 3 months and add 1 week (7 days).
Ex: LMP = Feb. 12, 2015, estimated delivery date = Feb. 12 plus 1 year = Feb. 12, 2016. Feb. 12, 2016 minus 3 months = Nov. 12, 2015 plus 7 days = Nov. 19, 2015.

Timing/Age Terminology

Gestation: Carrying of embryo/fetus.
Gestation period: Embryonic (fetal age) plus two weeks. Begins at fertilization until birth.

Embryo: Fertilization until 8 weeks.
Fetus: 8 weeks to birth.
Neonate: Birth to 28 days.
Infant: 29 days to one year old.

First trimester: Fertilization till 12 wks (developmental age).
Second trimester: 12 weeks till 24 weeks (developmental age).
Third trimester: 24 weeks till delivery (Developmental age)

Pre-viable: fetus born before 24 wks.
Preterm: fetus born between 25 – 37 wks.
Term: fetus born between 38 – 42 wks.
Post term: fetus born after 42 wks.

34 weeks: Lungs are considered mature. L/S ration (surfactant) is 2:1.

Gravidity – Parity

Gravidity: # times the uterus has been pregnant.
Parity: # of births with gestational age > 24 wks (4 values)

(**tip**: F – PAL)
#1 = F # **F**ull term births.
#2 = P # **P**reterm births.
#3 = A # **A**bortions/miscarriages
#4 = L # **L**iving children

CONDITION	FIVE-DIGIT SYSTEM A B C D E
Jane is pregnant for the first time.	1 – 0 – 0 – 0 – 0
She carries the pregnancy to term and the neonate survives.	1 – 1 – 0 – 0 – 1
She is pregnant again.	2 – 1 – 0 – 0 – 1
Her second pregnancy ends in abortion.	2 – 1 – 0 – 1 – 1
During her third pregnancy, she delivers viable twins.	3 – 2 – 0 – 1 – 3

LEGEND:
A — Times uterus has been pregnant.
B — Number of deliveries.
C — Number of premature deliveries.
D — Number of abortions (spontaneous or therapeutic).
E — Number of living children.

Terminology for Signs	Diagnosis of Pregnancy	Normal Physiologic Changes in Pregnancy
Goodell Sign: 1st sign of pregnancy on physical exam. Softening of the cervix due to ↑ vascularization. At 4 wks. **Chadwick's Sign:** Bluish discoloration of the cervix, vagina, labia due to ↑ blood flow. 6 – 8 wks after conception. **Linea Nigra:** dark vertical line on the abdomen from pubis to umbilicus. Due to ↑ melanocyte-stimulating hormone by the placenta. Can also cause darkened nipples. 2nd trimester. **Ladin Sign**: Softening of the midline of the uterus. At 6 wks. **Chloasma**: "Mask of pregnancy". Hyperpigmentation of the face. 16 wks. **Quickening:** First time the mother feels the fetus move.	• Egg implants: 6 – 8 days after ovulation. • β-HCG (**beta subunit**) picked up at 1 week in serum. • **β-HCG (beta subunit) picked up at 2 weeks in urine.** • **β-HCG doubles every 48 hours for first 4 weeks, peaks at 10 weeks and declines about 16 weeks.** • β-HCG levels are 1000 – 1500 IU/mL at 5 weeks. • β-HCG levels are >6500 IU/mL at 6 weeks. • Vaginal ultrasound: detects pregnancy at 5 weeks. • Abdominal ultrasound detects pregnancy at 6 weeks. • Ultrasound confirms intrauterine pregnancy at 5 weeks by presence of a gestational sac. • Ultrasound detects fetal heart motion. • Fetal movements detected at approximately 20 weeks. **β-HCG** (from trophoblastic tissue) High levels β-HCG at 16 wks indicates multiple gestations, molar pregnancy, possible choriocarcinoma. β-HCG maintains the corpus luteum allowing it to secrete progesterone during the first trimester.	• ↑ Thyroglobulin levels = ↑ T4 levels and **normal TSH.** (if patient is hypothyroid on levothyroxine = must ↑ dose. • ↑ GFR and ↓ BUN/creatine • 50% increase in plasma volume. • ↑ Cardiac output (↑ preload, **S3**) and ↑ HR • Hypercoagulable state. • ↓ motility in large intestine = ↑ risk constipation • ↑ reflux, heartburn (Can be severe enough to damage and cause scarring (strictures) in the esophagus. • ↑ risk of gallstones

Pregnancy Testing

Trisomy Quad Screen Labs

Trisomy	afp	estriol	β HCG	A Inhibin	PAPP
Trisomy 21, Downs Syndrome	↓	↓	↑	↑	↓
Trisomy 18, Edwards Syndrome	↓	↓	↓	normal	↓
Trisomy 13, Patau's Syndrome			↓	↓	

(**tip**: Trisomy 13 quad screen: little vowel's (a and e) are little so they are down. The big letters β and A are up)

AFP: Alpha Fetal Protein: Plasma protein encoded by the AFP gene on chromosome 4. Produced by the yolk sac and liver during fetal development. Levels begin decreasing after the first trimester. Levels <2.2MoM = Normal. Levels >2.2 MoM = abnormally elevated.

Estriol (AKA: E3): Type of estrogen made during pregnancy. Made by the placenta by 16-hydroxydehydroepiandrosterone sulfate (16-OH DHEAS), an androgen steroid made in the fetal liver and adrenal glands.

β HCG (Human chorionic gonadotropin): β HCG is a hormone (glycoprotein) produced by the syncytiotrophoblast after implantation. It is heterodimeric-containing subunits of: alpha (which is identical to the subunits in LH, FSH, TSH) and Beta (unique to hCG). The Beta subunit is used to detect pregnancy because on the Beta subunit is specific for pregnancy.

A Inhibin: Hormone made by the placenta during pregnancy, remaining constant through the 18th week of pregnancy. It inhibits FSH production.

PAPP (Pregnancy-associated plasma protein): Protein encoded by the PAPPA gene. Encodes a metalloproteinase, which cleaves insulin-like growth factor binding proteins that are involved with wound healing and bone remodeling. Low levels can result in IUGR, preeclampsia, placental abruption, premature birth and fetal death.

Amniocentesis

- Sampling of the amniotic fluid for chromosomal/genetic abnormalities, sex determination, fetal infections
- **Do not do prior to 15 weeks gestation**
- Risk of procedure: Amniotic fluid embolism, sudden respiratory failure, cardio shock, seizures, DIC, severe hypotension, miscarriage
- Must be prepared to intubate and ventilate

Chorionic Villus Sampling (CVS)

- Sampling of the chorionic villus (placental tissue) for chromosomal or genetic disorders in the fetus
- **Done between 10 – 12 weeks, preferred at 15 weeks**
- Risk: miscarriage, leakage of amniotic fluid leading to infection or oligohydramnios
- **Do not do before 9 weeks due to risk of limb defects**

Timeline for Testing, Treatment in Pregnancy

- For women planning a pregnancy: Discontinue OCP's **and start folic acid 1 month** before pregnancy.
- For women that are vegetarians: Must supplement Vitamin B-12

(* Indicate test that are needed only for special situations)

Week	Test	Test For	Notes
1st Appointment	CBC	Anemia	↓ Hb, ↓ MCV: Iron deficiency. Give ferrous sulfate. ↓ Hb, ↑ MCV, ↑ RDW: Give folate. NOTE: Caused by ↑ hepcidin (inhibits iron transport). Iron needs are increased during pregnancy and hepcidin stops the absorption of iron.
	Type and Screen, Direct/Indirect Coombs	Blood type, Rh Antibodies	Rh-negative moms, Rh positive fetus. 28 weeks: give RhoGAM to Rh-negative moms after insuring absence of anti-D antibodies.
	Urinalysis	UTI	Do **not give TMP/SMX** for UTI's, Safe to use: **PO: Nitrofurantoin, Cephalosporins or Amoxicillin**
	PAP Smear	HPV, cervical dysplasia	
	Rubella antibodies	Lack of Rubella IgG antibodies = risk of rubella	Do not vaccinate for Rubella during pregnancy. However, if someone is vaccinated b/c they not aware they were pregnant – it IS OK- reassure mom. The **#1 preventive measure** to ↓ **congenital rubella** infections is to vaccinate all women of childbearing age.
	HEP B surface antigen	HBsAg = risk for transmission of HBV from mom to baby	If HBsAg is found with HBeAg = highly infective.
	VDRL, RPR	Syphilis	Confirm with FTA-ABS. Transmitted through the placenta so C-section will not prevent. TX: Penicillin IM. If penicillin allergy: must desensitize and then treat. NOTE: Order HIV test for any patient testing positive for any STD.
	ELISA	HIV	Confirm with Western Blot. If HIV positive: start HAART therapy (do not wait until post-delivery). NOTE: C-section must be done if the mother's viral load > 1000 at the time of delivery. Newborn baby must be treated with AZT for 6 weeks. (gp120 crosses placenta to fetus)
	Cervical culture. NAAT (Nuclear acid amplification)	Gonorrhea, Chlamydia, Trichomonas	Gonorrhea, Chlamydia: **Ceftriaxone PO, Azithromycin IM.** Trichomonas: **Metronidazole PO.** NOTE: Order HIV test for any patient testing positive for any STD.
5 weeks	Ultrasound	Verify pregnancy, gestational sac.	
Throughout			Urinalysis are monitored each visit to check for UTI's.
*12 – 16 wks	Chorionic villus sampling (optional)	Used: Karyotyping, Advanced maternal age, genetic dz in parents, karyotype.	**Do NOT perform under 9 weeks** due to potential of fetal injury: damaged limbs. Also risk of: miscarriage, infection.
*14 – 24 weeks	Cervical cerclage	Closure of incompetent cervix.	
*15 – 20 wks	Amniocentesis (Optional)	Karyotyping, Chromosomal problems, genetic DZ, neural tube defects	**Do NOT perform under 9 weeks** due to potential of fetal injury: damaged limbs. Also risk of: miscarriage, infection.

*15 – 20 wks	Quad or Triple Screen. AFP, β-HCG, Estriol, Inhibin A.	Genetic, congenital problems.	(See chart above)
16 – 20 wks	Quickening	First time mom feels baby move.	Occurs sooner on subsequent births
*20 wks	Percutaneous Umbilical Blood Sample (AKA: Fetal Blood Sampling)	Diagnostic: karyotype, IgG and IgM antibodies and blood gases. Therapeutic: if fetus is anemic, intrauterine transfusions can be administered.	Aspiration of fetal blood from the umbilical vein.
*20 wks	Fetoscopy	Biopsy or laser occlusion of abnormal blood vessels, TX of spina bifida or biopsy.	Allows access to the fetus, umbilical cord, placenta and amniotic cavity.
28 wks	**Glucose Tolerance Test**	Gestational diabetes	**1 hour 50 g OGTT glucose test** given. (Sensitive test: catches all patients that may have the disease). If > 160, patient is considered to have gestational diabetes. If > 140 then patient must take a **3 hour 100 g OGTT glucose test**. (Specific test: catches all people that actually have the disease). If results are >140 Dx patient is considered to have gestational diabetes.
*28 wks	**For Rh Negative Moms**		Give Rh (D) immunoglobulin. **RhoGAM**. For "unsensitized" mothers: Must give RhoGAM to mothers: after miscarriage/abortion, ectopic pregnancy, when doing amniocentesis, chorionic villus sampling, with heavy vaginal bleeding, within 72 hours of delivery.
28 wks	CBC	Check for anemia. Hb < 10 g/dL = anemia	Give iron supplements.
34 wks			Babies lungs are considered to be mature. L/S ration > 2:1. Prior to 34 weeks: **Betamethasone** (steroids) may be administered to ↑ surfactant.
36 wks	**GBS Test**	Group B Strep (rectum and vaginal)	**If positive: Ampicillin IV is given intrapartum** (during labor).
* At delivery.	For Rh Negative Moms		Give Rh (D) Immunoglobulin (**RhoGAM**)
RhoGAM NOTE: Must give RhoGAM in Rh negative, sensitized moms (meaning antibody titer levels > 1:4) at 28 weeks, with any heavy vaginal bleeding, during chorionic villus sampling (CVS), during amniocentesis, after miscarriage or abortion, with 72 hours of delivery. If mother's antibody titers are < 1:16, she is unsensitized (no anti-Rh antibodies are present), no treatment is necessary.			

Pregnancy Pathologies

Hydatidiform Mole (Molar pregnancies)
AKA: Gestational Trophoblastic Disease (GTN)

- Common in the Philippines and Taiwan.
- Other risk factors: Maternal age < 20 and > 35 years old, folate deficiency.
- SX: presents with bleeding <16 weeks of gestation. Also: HTN, hyperemesis gravidarum, hyperthyroidism.
- No fetal heart tones.
- CXR to rule out lung metastasis (lung is the MC location of metastasis).
- Baseline β-HCG. You must follow the levels of β-HCG to track the recurrence so it is important to keep patient on contraceptives so that β-HCG levels are not confused.
- D & C (Dilation and Curettage).

Molar Pregnancies cont'd

	Complete Mole	**Partial Mole**
B HCG	↑↑↑	↑
Karyotype	**46** (46XX, 46XY) Dizygotic ploidy (diploid)	**69** (69XXX, 69XXY, 69XYY) triploidy
Presence of fetal parts	**"Completely"** GONE (none)	Yes, **PARTS** of a fetus
Germ Cells Involved	Sperm and egg	2 sperm and 1 egg
Imaging	**"snowstorm"** on ultrasound or cluster of grapes	Fetal parts will be seen on ultrasound.
Complications	15 – 20% malignant trophoblastic disease, 2% convert to choriocarcinoma	Low risk
	Caution: If the question presents with a patient that presents with pregnancy complications and it sounds like a complete molar pregnancy and you are told the ultrasound shows nothing- - beware it is NOT a complete molar pregnancy because you would not see "nothing" on an ultrasound, you would see a "snowstorm" appearance. 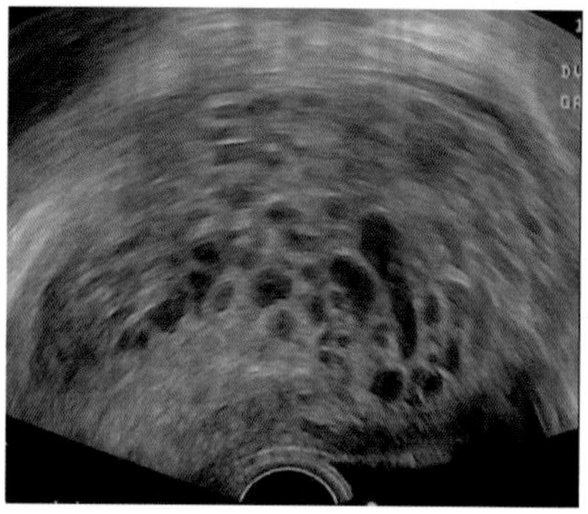	Ultrasound shows **"products of conception"**

Abortions/Miscarriages

- Miscarriage/Spontaneous abortion: natural death (expulsion) of embryo/fetus < 20 weeks from gestation or < 500 gm. SX: vaginal bleeding with/without tissue or clot and pain/cramping. MC complication of early pregnancy. MCC: Chromosome abnormalities. ↑ risk: maternal smoking, advanced maternal age, previous spontaneous abortion, Lupus autoantibodies: Anticardiolipin and Antiphospholipid.
- Fetal demise (AKA: Stillbirth): Fetal death > 20 weeks. SX: lack of fetal movement. MCC: Idiopathic. ↑ risk: trauma, antiphospholipid syndrome, maternal diabetes, fetal infection.
- Complication of prolonged fetal demise > 2 weeks in duration: DIC due to **tissue thromboplastin factor III (coagulation factor)** from deteriorating fetal organs. Check for D-dimers, fibrinogen, PT, PTT. Requires immediate delivery/D & C.
- **First time stillbirth**: important to obtain autopsy of fetus and placenta in order to determine if there were any genetic causes which would impede additional pregnancies.

Type of Abortion	Findings	Treatment
Threatened abortion	**NO dilation** of cervix, intrauterine bleeding before 20 wks, fetus intact, no passage of fetal parts, fetal heart is active.	Bed and pelvic rest
Inevitable abortion	**Dilation** of cervix, intrauterine/vaginal bleeding, fluid discharge, lower abdominal cramps, products of conception can be seen, ultrasound may show rupture or collapse of gestational sac, no fetal heartbeat.	D & C (Dilation and curettage)
Complete abortion	**Cervix closed**, empty uterus (**no products of conception**), abdominal pain, cramping, passage of tissue. Whole conceptus has passed through the cervix (pain and contractions subside once passed)	Follow B-hCG
Missed abortion (< 20 wks) Spontaneous abortion	**Fetus intact** but dead	**Required procedures** **1- Doppler to check for fetal heartbeat** **2- Transvaginal ultrasound for confirm the absence of fetal heartbeat** **TX: D & C to remove products of conceptions or medications to abort: Misoprostol or Mifeprisone**
Fetal demise (> 20 wks) Stillbirth	Fetal demise in utero. Loss of pregnancy symptoms, no increase in the size of the uterus. Retained fetus and placenta. No fetal heartbeat.	
Partial molar pregnancy	**Some fetal parts** (AKA: products of conception) 46 XX, 46 XY	D & C
Complete molar pregnancy	**No fetal parts** found (AKA: products of conception) 69 XXX,69 XXY, 69 XYY	Follow up
Septic Abortion	Infection of uterus. SX: Fever, chills, abdominal pain, bloody purulent vaginal discharge	**TX: Cervical and blood cultures.** **IV Levofloxacin and Metronidazole.** **Gentle suction curettage (do not do vigorous due to possible perforation of uterus), D & C.**

Intrauterine Fetal Demise (IUFD) and Stillbirths

- **Fetal demise or stillbirth is > 20 weeks.**
- **Required procedures**
  1- Doppler to check for fetal heartbeat
  2- Transvaginal ultrasound for confirm the absence of fetal heartbeat
- **TX: D & C to remove products of conceptions or medications to abort: Misoprostol or Mifeprisone**
- **Important: 1st episode: autopsy of fetus and placenta to find cause to try and prevent reoccurrence in future pregnancies.**
- **Must obtain parental permission**

Adolescent Pregnancy

- **Maternal Risk: ↑ perinatal mortality, ↑ preterm delivery**
- **Infant risk: ↑ premature and low birth weight, immaturity due to socio-economic situations, future risk of cognitive disorders**
- **There is NOT an ↑ risk for congenital malformations**

IUGR

Poor fetal growth. Fetal weight is estimated to be < 10th percentile of its gestational age that result in low birth weight.

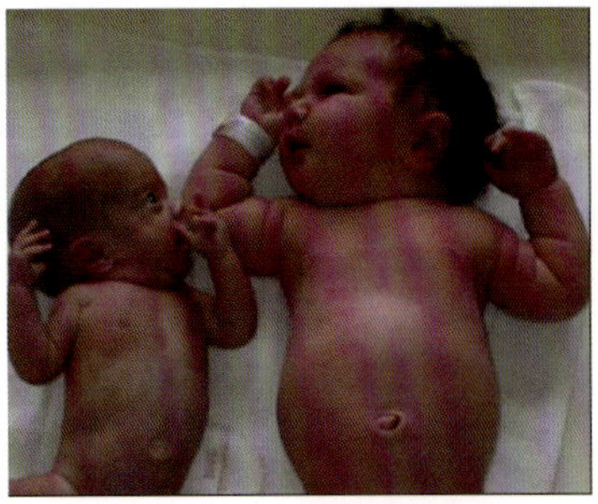

IGUR Normal

Asymmetrical IUGR (most common 70%)	Symmetrical IUGR
Restriction of weight followed by length. Head grows normally but body is thin, out of proportion to head. Exam shows normal head measurement but ↓ abdominal measurements.	Overall growth restriction indicating that the fetus has grown slowly since the beginning. The head and body are proportional. Exam shows all measurements are ↓.
Causes occurred > 28 weeks (MC: **due to maternal causes)** Extrinsic factors. ↓ perfusion to the placenta.	Occurs occurred < 28 wks (MC: **congenital causes**) Intrinsic factors. ↓ growth.
HTN, smoking, hypoxia (causing: polycythemia due to stimulation of erythropoietin and hypoglycemia due to decrease in glycogen and adipose stores), pre-eclampsia, malnutrition, vascular DZ, malnutrition, infarction of placenta, alcohol, drugs, SLE, twin-twin transfusion.	TORCH infections, chromosome problems, structural abnormalities (NTD, congenital heart diseases), aneuploidy, anemia

Complications in Pregnancy, Labor and Delivery

Morning Sickness	Hyperemesis Gravidarum
Metabolic alkalosis. (Loss of H+ and K) ↑ pH, ↑ CO2, ↑ HCO3 **Hyperemesis Gravidarum** (4 – 10 weeks) **Severe vomiting** = wt loss, ketonuria Medication that can be given safely to ↓ nausea and vomiting in first trimester: **Doxylamine, Ondansetron, Promethazine, Metoclopramide, Pyridoxine (B6).**	Causes: severe vomiting in pregnancy between 4 – 10 weeks. Severe vomiting (vomiting out **HCL**) = loss of H+ (↓ Protons) and Chloride (hypochloremia). Loss of weight, ketonuria. Due to hypochloremia, kidneys will be reabsorbing Chloride from the urine. (Bicarb HCO3) is being reabsorbed with Chloride = **metabolic alkalosis.** Labs: Normal BP with ↓ **urine Chloride** (Normal chloride: 20 – 250 mEq/L) **Must check β-HCG for gestational trophoblast disease (hydatidiform molar pregnancy or choriocarcinoma): these can cause severe vomiting. If ↑ β-HCG, perform an ultrasound.** Medication that can be given safely to ↓ nausea and vomiting in first trimester: **Doxylamine, Ondansetron, Promethazine, Metoclopramide, Pyridoxine (B6)**

Gestational - Maternal Diabetes

High risk for **macrosomia babies** (large babies > 5000 gm) causing trouble at delivery: **shoulder dystocia** /shoulder dislocation (**Erb palsy**: upper brachial plexus injuries) or **Klumpke paralysis** (pulling out on the arm) (lower brachial plexus injury).
May require cesarean section.
NOTE: HbA1c > 8.5 in the first trimester are associated with neural tube defects and other congenital malformations.

Induce labor at 39 – 40 weeks if baby is <4500 gm.
If baby is >4500 gm in a diabetic mother or >5000 g in a nondiabetic mother: schedule C-section (macrosomia baby ↑ risk of shoulder dystocia).

Pregnant women are given a **glucose tolerance test b/t 26 and 28 weeks** to check for maternal diabetes.
Monitor HbA1c in each trimester.

1 hour 50 g OGTT glucose test given. (Sensitive test: catches all patients that may have the disease). If > 160, patient is considered to have gestational diabetes.
If > 140 then patient must take a **3 hour 100 g OGTT glucose test**. (Specific test: catches all people that actually have the disease).
If results are >140 Dx patient is considered to have gestational diabetes.

Glucose levels: 2 hour postprandial should be < 120

Timeline Monitor:
HbA1c each trimester.
Triple screen at 16-18 weeks for neural tube defects.
Monthly biophysical profile and sonograms to check for IUGR and macrosomia.

Maternal Diabetes cont'd

26 weeks: Weekly nonstress (NST) and Amniotic Fluid Index (AFI) if there is poor glycemic control.
32 weeks: Weekly nonstress test (NST) and Amniotic Fluid Index (AFI) if baby shows macrosomia or mother is on insulin, had previous stillbirth or has HTN.
Postpartum: 2 hour 75 g OGTT glucose test between 6 – 12 weeks to see if diabetes has resolved.

TX: NPH Insulin (intermediate dose). If NPH is not enough add either Regular or Lispro.
Do not use long acting medications (ie: Glargine)

During Labor: Keep blood glucose between 80 – 100 mg/dL with 5% dextrose in water and insulin drip.
Discontinue insulin after delivery.

Gestational Diabetes Affect on the Infant

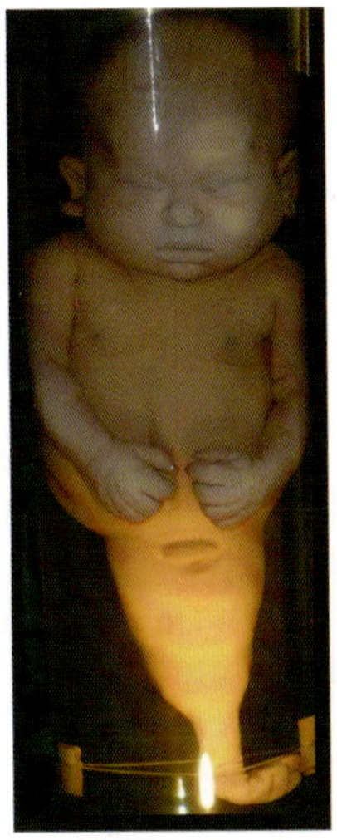

Caudal Regression

- **Macrosomia** (big baby)
  Big baby = more weight = difficulty breathing = RDS
  ↑ risk of shoulder dystocia (anterior shoulder of the infant can't be delivered without
  ↑ manipulation)
- Surfactant decreased
- **Hypoglycemia (after birth)**
- Respiratory Distress = EPO = Polycythemia
- Heart issues (ASD, VSD, **truncus arteriosus**)
- Hypocalcemia
- Polyhydramnios
- Physiologic jaundice (Hyperbilirubinemia)
- IUGR
- Hypocalcemia
- Hypomagnesemia
- Polycythemia
- Abdominal distension (small left colon syndrome).
- ↑ risk of childhood obesity
- ↑risk of developing diabetes
- **Caudal Regression**
- **NOTE:** HbA1c > 8.5 in the first trimester are associated with neural tube defects and other congenital malformations.

Pre-eclampsia

Mild: **BP > 140/90**, **Proteinuria**
> 300 mg, edema in face, hands, feet.
Severe: **BP > 160/110**, Proteinuria >**5 gms** on a 24 hr urine or 3-4 on a dipstick, oliguria, pulmonary and generalized edema, mental status, headache, upper abdominal pain and vision changes, liver dysfunction, DIC.
HELLP Syndrome.
HELLP Syndrome = **H**emolysis, **E**levated **L**iver enzymes, **L**ow **P**latelet count.

Labs: Thrombocytopenia, elevated liver enzymes.

HTN Cause: Abnormal placental spiral arteries = maternal endothelial vasoconstriction, hyperreflexia.
Complications: **Placental abruption**, renal failure, eclampsia, coagulopathy, uteroplacental insufficiency

TX: Mild:
HTN: **Methyldopa (α-agonist) or Labetalol.** **(2nd line: Nifedipine)** If mom at term: induce delivery.

Mild: If preterm: **Betamethasone** to mature fetus lungs and **Magnesium sulfate** as prophylaxis for seizures.

TX: Severe: IV Hydralazine (control BP). Deliver at 34 weeks if severe,
Deliver at 37 weeks if mild
IV Magnesium Sulfate to prevent seizures.
(Overdose of Mg = hyporeflexia).
If Mg Sulfate toxicity: change to **Calcium Gluconate**
If term: induce delivery.
If preterm: **Betamethasone** to mature lungs.

Eclampsia	**Braxton Hicks**
Tonic-clonic (Grand Mal) seizure in patients with history of pre-eclampsia. TX: Stabilize mom and deliver baby immediately. TX: **Magnesium sulfate** to prevent seizures, **Hydralazine** to control BP	(False contractions) Irregular contractions that go away when change positions or movements. There is NO cervical dilation. The rate of contractions can increase closer to the end of pregnancy. MCC: Dehydration
Hypertension **Chronic HTN**: BP > 140/90 before < 20 weeks of the pregnancy. TX: **Methyldopa, Labetalol, Nifedipine.** Transient HTN: Send half of the pregnancy or in labor and delivery when the protein does not exceed 300 mg/24 hrs. If protein exceeds 300 mg/24 hurs it is considered pre-eclampsia. Gestational HTN: BP > 140/90 that starts AFTER 20 weeks of gestation. There is NO proteinuria or edema. TX: **Methyldopa, Hydralazine, Labetalol, Nifedipine.** **Do NOT use these HTN medications during pregnancy:** **ACE inhibitors, ARB's, Thiazide's or renin inhibitors.** **It is ok to use: β-blockers, loops diuretics, and nitrates.**	**HELLP Syndrome** H = hemolysis EL = Elevated Liver enzymes LP = Low platelets MCC: Severe preeclampsia, but can occur without HTN TX: Stabilize mom and **deliver baby immediately** (only definitive cure). TX: **IV Magnesium sulfate** ($MgSO4$) to prevent seizures, **IV Hydralazine** to control BP, and IV Dexamethasone (IV corticosteroid). TX: Give platelet transfusion if platelet count <50,000mm^3
Gestational Thrombocytopenia Don't get this confused with HELLP. This condition only has low platelets, it does not have any other symptoms associated with it. MC cause of thrombocytopenia during pregnancy. Platelet counts are > 70,000. MC during the 3rd trimester.	**Lumbar Lordosis** Presents in the last trimester. Relaxation of ligaments of **sacroiliac joints** (pelvic girdle) (**Tip:** "Lordy, Lordy, I'm pregnant) Also during last trimester: low back pain and ankle edema (better in the mornings and worse at nights)

Rh Incompatibility

Mother: Rh negative (**tip**: **M**om is a **M**inus (-)
Fetus: Rh positive
Dad: Rh positive
(if the mother is Rh negative and the father is Rh positive, there is a ↑ chance the baby will have Rh positive blood = sensitization).
If both parents have Rh-negative blood, the baby will have Rh-negative blood = no sensitization).

Occurs in pregnancies after the first baby. Blood is able to cross from the fetus to the mother's blood various ways: delivery, amniocentesis, placental abruption, abortion, and trauma.

In the first delivery, the baby's Rh-positive blood crosses the placenta into the mother's bloodstream. The mom then makes antibodies against this Rh-positive blood. On subsequent pregnancies the mom's antibodies attach the Rh-positive blood cells of the fetus causing hemolysis of its red blood cells (AKA: **Hemolytic disease of the newborn**).

Rh antibody screening is done on the mother's initial prenatal visit. Rh antibody titer's are done on patients that are Rh negative.
Unsensitized mom: If patient has no Rh antibodies =

unsensitized (which is good – we don't want antibodies to attach the fetus's blood).
Sensitized mom: If a patient does have Rh antibodies they are "sensitized", it means they already have antibodies to the baby's Rh-positive blood. A patient is considered sensitized if she has a **titer level > 1:4**. If the titer **is < 1:16**, no treatment is needed. Sensitized moms must receive RhoGAM prophylaxis at 28 weeks gestation and at birth.

To insure that the patient stays "unsensitized" **RhoGAM** (anti-D Rh immunoglobulin) is given at 28 weeks and during: 72 hours of delivery, vaginal bleeding, abortion/miscarriage, amniocentesis, ectopic pregnancies, placental abruption.

If mother is no "Sensitized" or has a **low titer level of > 1:4** she must receive **RhoGAM**.
If titers levels are **≤ 1:16 RhoGAM is not required**.

Rh Incompatibility cont'd

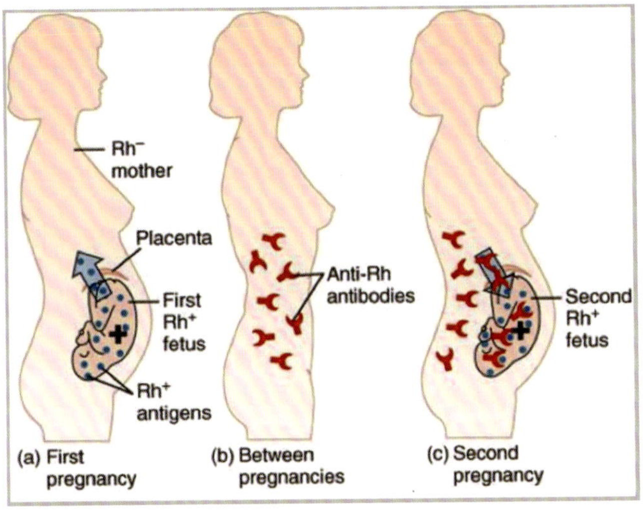

mother \ father	D	D
d	Dd	Dd
d	Dd	Dd

100% Rh+ children

mother \ father	D	d
d	Dd	dd
d	Dd	dd

50% Rh+ children

Management of Fetus Well Being
If Rh antibody levels are ≥ 1:16: amniocentesis at 16-20 weeks to evaluate bilirubin levels.
Results:
Low bilirubin levels: repeat amniocentesis in 3 weeks.
Medium bilirubin levels: repeat amniocentesis in 2 weeks.
High bilirubin levels: Take umbilical blood sample to obtain fetal hematocrit. (Determines if there is anemia. Ie: hemolysis). If hematocrit is low: give intrauterine transfusion.

Premature Rupture of Membranes (PROM)

Rupture of membranes before onset of labor. ↑ risk if infection ascends from the lower genital tract.

DX: Confirmation of amniotic fluid:
Fluid shows **"ferning pattern"** when put on a slide, fluid turns nitrazine paper blue (+ nitrazine test), fluid is in posterior fornix. Common in oligohydramnios.

Complications: Placental abruption, chorioamnionitis, preterm labor, cord prolapse.

Chorioamnionitis: Bacterial infection of fetal membrane MC due to prolonged labor. SX: fever, foul odor, tachycardia (mom or fetus), ↑ WBC in mom, tender uterus.
TX: Culture, IV antibiotics, delivery.

TX: Bedrest if <24 weeks gestation.
Preterm fetus (24-33 wks): Beclomethasone to mature the lungs. ↓ contractions with Tocolytics, antibiotics (**Ampicillin and Azithromycin**) to ↓ chorioamnionitis.
Term fetus (>34 wks): Delivery.

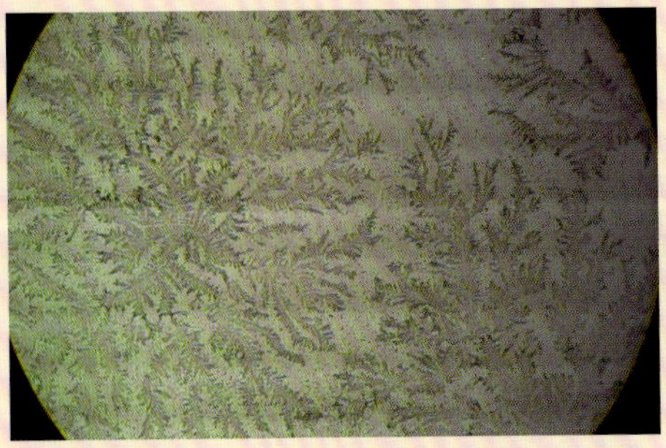

"Ferning" (amniotic fluid)
(Test for premature rupture of membranes)

Cervix Insufficiency

Inability of cervix to stay closed throughout pregnancy.

Causes: **LEEP**, OB trauma, **multiple gestations**, pre-term birth, 2nd trimester pregnancy loss, mullerian anomalies.

Evaluate cervix with transvaginal ultrasound. Cervix length should be > 25 mm at 24 weeks. If < 10% of that measurement = short cervix or if < 25mm at 28 weeks.

TX: Cervical cerclage (stitching cervix shut)

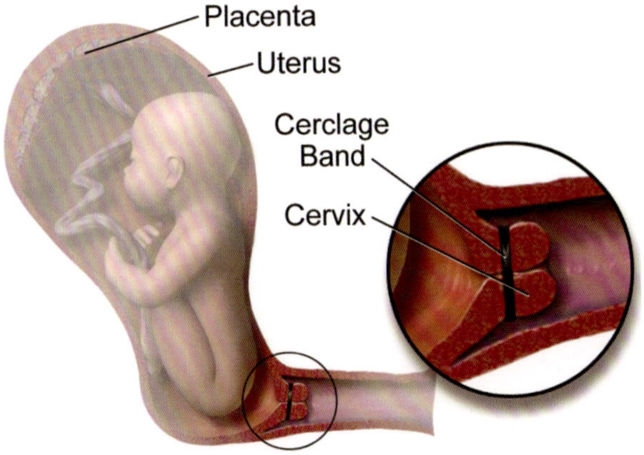

Cerclage Correction of the Cervix

Oligohydramnios	Polyhydramnios
Oligohydramnios Risk: Potter's sequence, hypoplasia of the lungs. <0.5 L of amniotic fluid Fetus is unable to urinate. Causes: Bilateral **renal agenesis, posterior urethral valves in males.**	**Polyhydramnios** 1.5 – 2 L of amniotic fluid Fetus is unable to swallow amniotic fluid. Causes: Duodenal atresia, anencephaly, esophageal atresia. Risk: Multiple gestations, maternal diabetes
Premature (preterm) Labor Combination of contractions with cervical dilation. Premature fetus born before 37 weeks (< 2500 gm). Risk factors for preterm labor: previous preterm labor, multiple gestations, problems with the uterus, placental abruption, cervix or placenta, infections (chorioamnionitis), smoking, drugs (cocaine), anemia, polyhydramnios, preeclampsia, fetal birth defect, little or no prenatal care, less than 6 months since last pregnancy, diabetes, high blood pressure, short cervical length, fetal fibronectin (glue-like substance between the fetal sac and lining of the uterus), uterine anatomical abnormalities (ie; bicornate uterus), intraabdominal surgery. Complications for baby: RDS, low birth weight, breathing difficulties (immature lungs), underdeveloped organs, vision problems, higher risk of learning disabilities and behavior problems, intraventricular hemorrhage, sepsis, necrotizing enterocolitis, kernicterus. TX: **Tocolytics and bed rest with goal to reach 34 to 36 weeks.** Decrease contractions in order to slow the progression of cervical dilation. TX: **Terbutaline** (β-2 adrenergic receptor), **Magnesium sulfate*.** **Calcium channel blockers.** TX: for fetus: If fetus is < 34 weeks or < 2500 gms: **Betamethasone** to mature lungs. (**tip**: "B"etamethasone for "B"abies) ***Mg toxicity: ↑ risk of cardiac arrest or respiratory depression.** **SX: ↓ deep tendon reflexes** **When preterm labor should NOT be stopped:** **Cervical dilation > 4cm, hemorrhage, fetal death, pre-eclampsia/eclampsia, maternal cardiac dz, chorioamnionitis**	**Ectopic Pregnancy** MC in ampulla of fallopian tube. SX: Less than expected rise in β-hCG, sudden lower unilateral abdominal pain, vaginal bleeding. SX if ruptured: ↓ BP, Tachycardia Risk Factors: **PID (Pelvic Inflammatory Dz), IUD** (Intrauterine devices), **Highest risk: previous ectopic pregnancies**, history of infertility, prior tubal surgery **DX: Transvaginal Ultrasound to locate the site.** **(caution: do not confuse with appendicitis) .** **Perform when the β-HCG is between 1500 – 6500.** **TX: Admit and terminate.** **Treatment Options:** **Ruptured:** **If Ruptured and stable = surgery.** **If Ruptured and unstable = IV fluids → surgery.** **Not ruptured:** **Not ruptured and ectopic > 3.5 cm → surgery.** **Not ruptured and patient is immunodeficient → surgery.** **Not ruptured and < 3.5 cm and competent, β-hCG < 6000 mIU/ml, absence of fetal heart beat → Methotrexate.** **Follow patient's β-HCG levels for 4 – 7 days.** **After 7 days reevaluate:** **β-HCG < 15% = one more shot MTX.** **β-HCG same or greater → surgery.**

Cardiac Pathologies

Normal changes in the heart and blood vessels during pregnancy:

- Increase of 40 – 50% in blood volume during the first trimester.
- Increase of 30 – 40% in cardiac output due to ↑ blood volume.
- Increase of 10 – 15 BPM in heart rate.
- Decrease in BP by 10mmHG due to hormone changes and more blood is directed to the uterus.
- Normal SX: fatigue, shortness of breath and light-headedness.

Sudden Death: Pregnancy is contradictory with these high risk pre-existing heart conditions because it can lead to sudden death: Eisenmenger syndrome, severe valve disorders, pulmonary hypertension, prior postpartum cardiomyopathy.

Peripartum Cardiomyopathy
Develops between the 9th month and 5 months postpartum.
Risk factors: multiple gestations, preeclampsia, over 30 years of age.

Mitral or Aortic Stenosis
Repaired by balloon valvuloplasty.

Regurgitation Pathologies
No treatment needed.

Hypercoagulable Pathologies

DVT or Pulmonary Embolism (MCC maternal death)
TX: Anticoagulation with **(LMWH) Heparin (do NOT use warfarin during pregnancy).**

Anticoagulate with **Low Molecular Weight Heparin** these conditions:
PE or DVT, A-Fib if there is also an underlying heart disease, Eisenmenger syndrome, Factor V Leiden, Antithrombin III deficiency, Antiphospholipid/Anticardiolipin syndrome, an ejection fraction is < 30%, Prothrombin gene mutation, or with Hyperhomocysteinemia.

Hyperthyroidism
Causes: IUGR and stillbirth.
TX: β-blockers.

Graves Disease
Complications: Maternal thyroid-stimulating and blocking Ig's can cross over to the placenta causing IUGR, goiter and fetal tachycardia.
TX: 1st trimester: **Propylthiouracil (PTU)**.
TX: 2nd and 3rd trimester: **Methimazole**.
PTU crosses the placenta so may cause hypothyroidism and goiter in the fetus so must switch to **Methimazole** in the 2nd and 3rd trimesters.
PTU and Methimazole are Class D drugs. They can harm the fetus by inhibiting thyroperoxidase (inhibits T3 and T4).

Hypothyroidism
Complications: Miscarriages, mental retardation.
Labs: ↑ T4 with a normal TSH. (Due to the ↑ of the TBG – thyroid binding globulins).
TX: **Levothyroxine**. **The dose of levothyroxine must be increased 25-30% during pregnancy due to the increase in TBG's.**

Placenta previa
Painless bleeding any trimester (but is MC in first trimester)

Placenta covers part or all of cervix.
Risk: Multiparty, prior C-section
TX:
Vaginal delivery if ≥ 36 wks and placenta is > 2 cm from the internal os.
C-section if placenta is < 2cm or covering the internal os.

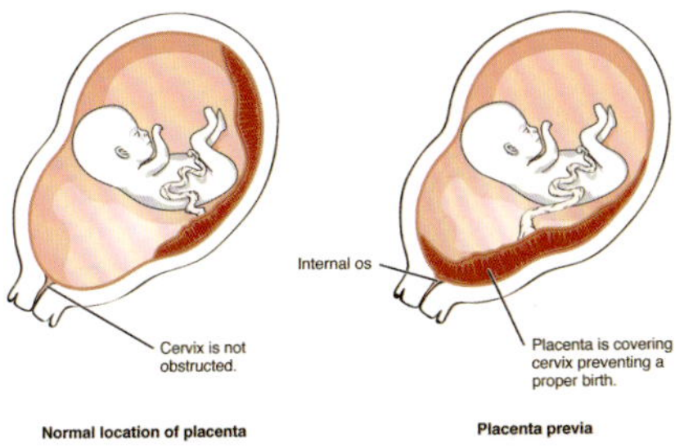

Types of placenta previa
Low-lying: placenta implanted low in the uterus but does not cover the os. <2 cm from the os.
Partial: placenta partially covers the os.
Marginal: placenta is on the edge of the os.
Vasa previa: fetal vessel is over the os.

Placental Abruption
(AKA: abruption placentae)

Occurs: 3rd trimester
Causes: **trauma (MVA, fall)**, smoking, HTN, **cocaine,** preeclampsia, diabetes, SLE, previous abruption, short umbilical cord, folate deficiency, placenta percreta, uterine myomectomy.

SX: **Abrupt, painful dark red 3rd trimester bleeding,** ↑ uterine tone, uterine hyperactivity, uterine tenderness regression of fetus, no uterine contractions, abnormal bump noted on abdomen.
↑ Risk: DIC, Sheehan's Syndrome (postpartum hypopituitarism), fetal hypoxia, fetal death.

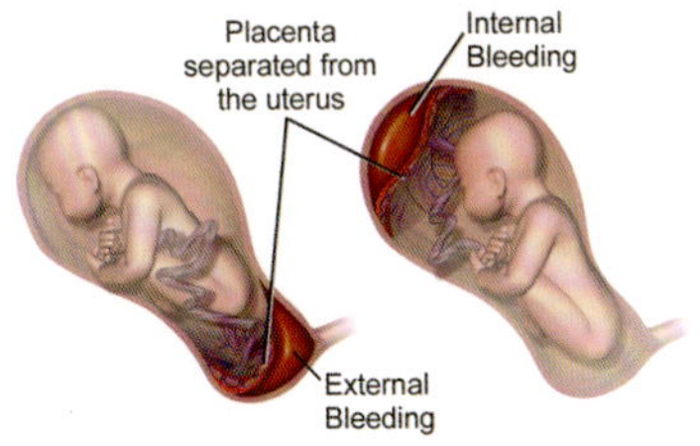

Abruptio Placenta (Placental Abruption)

Types: Concealed: Blood is within uterine cavity.
External: Blood drains through the cervix.

TX: If fetal instability: emergent C-section.
Stable and ≥ 36 wks: vaginal delivery.
Admit and observe < 34 wks.

Uterine Rupture **During delivery** SX: ↑↑ Abdominal pain with ↑ vaginal bleeding, regression of fetal stage, can **palpate (or see) fetal limbs/parts on the mother's abdomen.** (AKA: Abnormal "bump", irregular contours on mother's abdomen), **no uterine contractions, regression of** fetus (fetus was moving downward to delivery but is now withdrawn back up. Loss of fetal station), hypovolemia and shock, agitation, fetal HR abnormal. Tachycardia, ↑ RR, ↓ BP. MCC: **previous C-section**, trauma, uterine overly distended (polyhydramnios, multiple gestations), placenta percreta, fibroids, excessive oxytocin. Complication: Hysterectomy due to excessive bleeding. TX: Immediate C-section	**Placenta Accreta/Increta/Percreta** Occurs: **After delivery**, at delivery of placenta Accreta = Placenta attaches to myometrium – NO penetration. Increta = Placenta penetrates into the myometrium. Percreta = Placenta perforates through the myometrium (can attach to bladder or rectum) (**tip**: "P" for perforates) SX: ↑ Postpartum bleeding Complications: hysterectomy (**Tip**: the placenta is "creeping" into the uterus) 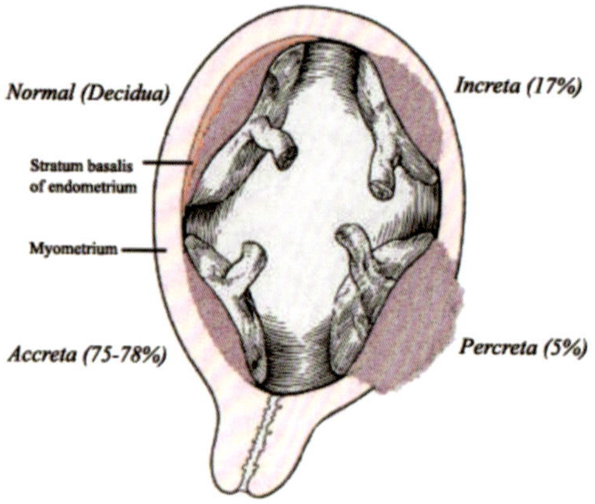
Vasa Previa During ROM (rupture of membranes) the fetal umbilical vein is ruptured = severe bleeding (fetus bleeding). Can be more common with multiple gestations. SX: Severe bleeding after ROM, fetus tachycardia and then bradycardia. No affect on the mother. Perform "APT" (Alkali Denaturation Test) test to determine if the blood is from fetus or mother. *(Vasa Previa cont'd)* 75% fetal mortality Fetus SX: Tachycardia → bradycardia Tx: Emergency C-section	**Benign Edema of Pregnancy** Leg cramps that worsen at night. Bilateral edema. No HTN and No proteinuria, no pre-eclampsia. TX: Reassure and follow up
Urinary Tract Infection (UTI) **All patients with > 100,000 organisms.** **MCC: E. coli** **Complication if not treated:** **Pyelonephritis → septicemia → preterm labor and low weight baby** **Asymptomatic bacteriuria SX: no fever, no urgency, no burning, no frequency.**	**Amniotic Fluid Embolism** SX: Sudden respiratory failure, cardiogenic shock, seizures, DIC TX: Respiratory support, intubation and mechanical ventilation.

UTI cont'd

Labs: + urine culture.

Symptomatic Acute Cystitis SX: No fever, urgency, burning, frequency.
Labs: + urine culture.

Pyelonephritis (hospitalize):
SX: Flank pain (costovertebral tenderness), fever, urgency, burning, frequency.
Labs: + urine culture.

TX: DO NOT give TMP/SMX during pregnancy.

Asymptomatic and Symptomatic Outpatient TX: Nitrofurantoin, Amoxicillin, Ampicillin or 1st generation Cephalosporin (Cephalexin) for 7 days.
(Note: if a pregnant patient has symptoms of a UTI, treatment should be started immediately)

Pyelonephritis TX: Hospitalize.
IV Cephalosporins or IV Gentamicin and tocolysis.

Postpartum Fever

PP Day 0: Atelectasis. Follows general anesthesia, patient's pain inhibits deep breaths. Mild fever. TX: Incentive spirometry and ambulation.
PP Day 1: UTI. Follows vaginal exams during labor and catheterizations. High fever, CVA tenderness. TX: IV antibiotics.
PP Day 2-3: Endometritis. Follows retained products of conception or prolonged rupture of membranes. Moderate-high fever. TX: IV **Gentamycin and Clindamycin**.
PP Day 4-5: Wound infection. Follows C-section incision or episiotomy. Spiking fevers, wound erythema. TX: IV antibiotics, wound care.
PP Day 5-6: Septic thrombophlebitis. Follows a prolonged labor. Fever swings. TX: IV **Heparin** for 7 – 10 days.
PP Day 7 and over: Mastitis. Follows cracking of the nipple after breastfeeding. Fever, breast erythema and tenderness. TX: IV **Nafcillin**.

Post Partum Hemorrhage

TX: Fundal/bimanual massage, IV Access, Crystalloid infusion (Keep SBP > 90mm), notify blood bank for PRBC (blood transfusion)

Administer one: **Oxytocin, Methylergonovine or Carboprost**.

MCC of uterine atony.

Uterine Atony

MC cause of excessive postpartum bleeding.

Causes: Postpartum hemorrhage, multiple gestations, uterine distention, polyhydramnios, prolonged labor

TX:
Uterine massage.
Uterotonic agents: **Oxytocin, Methylergonovine, Carboprost**

Pregnancy Pruritis

Can occur on the scalp, anus, vulva, abdomen.

TX: Topical steroids, antihistamines, oatmeal baths emollients, UVB

Herpes Gestationis

AKA: Pemphigoid Gestationis

Benign Autoimmune disease of pregnancy.

SX: Vesicles and papules around the umbilicus.

TX: Topical mild corticosteroids (**Triamcinolone**)

Herpes Management

If no exposure or background of herpes: no test required.
If background or outbreak of herpes during pregnancy: TX: **Acyclovir** at 36 weeks.
If outbreak of herpes at delivery: C-section.
If no background but patient is exposed to herpes during pregnancy:
TX: Herpes Simplex Virus IgG Antibody screen. If positive: **Acyclovir** at 36 weeks.
If negative: no treatment.

If active lesions at the time of delivery = must do C-section.

Pregnancy Acne

Do NOT use: Class C or Class D drugs:
No retinoids: topical or systemic (Class C). Severe teratogen.
Other category Class C: Benzoyl peroxide, sodium sulfacetamide.
Class D: Tetracycline, Doxycycline, Minocycline

Ok to use Class B drugs:
TX: Topical **azelaic acid, topical clindamycin, topical erythromycin** (Class B).

Bacterial Vaginosis **AKA: Gardnerella** SX: Amine odor, Clue Cells on KOH prep, Vaginal pH ≥ 4.5, Vaginal discharge. Complications of no treatment: Risk of preterm birth, STD's, premature rupture of membranes, spontaneous abortion. TX; Oral **Metronidazole, Clindamycin**	**Bipolar and Depression** **TX: ECT (Electro Convulsive Therapy)** **(Note:** watch the vignette that indicates a bipolar woman presents at > 12 weeks gestation on Lithium or Valproic Acid. The answer is NOT to discontinue or change medications despite the fact that these are teratogenic. Leave her on the medications, she needs the treatment and any damage that would have been done has **already been done**. It is past 8 weeks).
Group B Strep (GBS) Cervical culture at 37 weeks to check for active GBS (norma flora). Rectum and vagina. If positive = TX: **IV ampicillin prophylaxis peripartum (during delivery)**	**Lacerations** Vaginal or perineal tears due to delivery. 1st degree tears (Superficial): involves skin of the perineum and tissue around opening of the vagina – does not involve muscles. 2nd degree tears: deeper, involving the muscles. Each layer must be sutured. TX: Suture
Uterine Inversion Placenta does not detach from the uterus when it exits which pulls out the uterus and turns it inside out. Potentially fatal. TX: Uterine replacement, IV Oxytocin **Normal Lochia (post-partum)** Lochia Rubra: 1 – 3 days: bloody discharge with clots with leukocytosis, low-grade fever is normal. Lochia Serosa: 3 – 4 days: serous pale discharge. Lochia Alba: 3 – 4 days: White or yellow discharge. Foul smelling lochia indicates endometritis. **Urinary Retention (hypotonic bladder)** Residual volume (normal < 50 mL) is > 250 mL. TX: **Bethanechol**. If meds do not work: catheterize.	**Endometritis** (AKA: Retained placental tissue, retained products of conception). Post partum polymicrobial infection (gram positives and negatives and anaerobic bacteria). MCC: Polymicrobial Infection. Other causes: Prolonged ROM > 24 hrs, C-section, prolonged labor > 12 hours, intrauterine catheter, fetal scalp electrodes, forceps delivery SX: 2 – 3 days of fever (fever usually > 100.4° within 24 hours of deliver) and chills, uterine tenderness, lower abdominal pain, abnormal bleeding or discharge, leukocytosis, and foul smelling lochia. **Lochia: vaginal discharge during postpartum period. Consisting of blood, tissue shed from lining of uterus and bacteria. Lochia is normal after birth and should decrease daily and end approximately 10 days after birth. But if bleeding increases or foul smell to lochia = ↑ risk of endometritis)** Risk: C-section, prolonged rupture of membranes, long labor with multiple vaginal exams. TX: **IV Clindamycin and Gentamicin**

Intrahepatic Cholestasis of Pregnancy	Acute Fatty Liver
(ICP) MC in 3rd trimester. Associated with multiple pregnancies. SX: ↑↑ **pruritis** (especially in the palms and soles at night), ↑ bile acids, ↑ ALT, ↑ AST, ↑ Alk Phos, jaundice. DX: ↑↑ in serum bile acids (from 10 to 100 times the normal level) TX: Ursodeoxycholic Acid	SX; Nausea, malaise, headache, abdominal pain, pre-eclampsia (can lead to renal failure), ↑ PT, ↑ AST.
Misc **Bloody show**: blood tinge from the release of the mucus plug. **Lightening**: Fetal descent into the pelvis. **Amniotomy** ("Break the water"): Puncture of the amniotic sac. **Beware:** rule out a prolapsed umbilical cord before puncturing. **Episiotomy** (AKA: perineotomy): incision of the perineum and posterior vaginal wall during 2nd stage of labor to make the opening larger for the passage of the baby. Complication: damage to anal sphincter or rectum causing fecal incontinence, scar tissues can make sexual intercourse painful, difficulty in defecating. **Sitz bath:** Warm shallow bath that patients sit in to help relieve discomfort/pain from the stitches of episiotomy.	**Postpartum Depression** 10- 15% incidence Starts within **4 weeks** of delivery and last **from 2 weeks to 1 year.** SX: **Anxiety**, poor concentration, depression, **worried.** TX: **SSRI**, psychotherapy
Postpartum Blues 50 – 80% incidence Starts **2 – 3 days** post delivery and ends within **10 days**. SX: **Tearful, fatigue**, depressed. Tx: Supportive	**Postpartum Psychosis** 0.1 – 0.2 % Incidence Last from a few days – 2 months SX: **Delusions, hallucinations**, confusion, possible **suicidal or homicidal** ideas or attempts. TX: Inpatient hospitalization, antipsychotics, antidepressants. **Assess child safety.**

Breastfeeding

Contraindications to Breastfeeding	Safe to Breastfeed
• HIV • Illicit (street) drugs • Active, untreated tuberculosis • Active lesion of Herpes simplex on breast, boils, impetigo • Avoid for 2 hours after drinking alcohol • Untreated varicella • Medications: radioactive isotopes, chemotherapy, antimetabolites, thyrotoxic agents, Methotrexate, Cyclosporine • HTLV-1: Human T-cell leukemia virus Type I or Type II • Infants with galactosemia • Maternal lead levels > 40 micrograms/dL • Women undergoing radiologic procedures	• Hepatitis A, B and C • Mastitis • Women who have received vaccines (live or killed) • Women who have had breast surgery • Women who have pierced nipples • Most medications are safe • Women that smoke

Breast Pathologies in Pregnancy and Post Partum

Breast Engorgement: 24 – 72 hrs post partum. SX: Both breasts: tense, warm, tender, fullness. Peaks 3 – 5 days. Improves spontaneously. TX: Cool compresses, **Acetaminophen, NSAIDS**	**Mastitis** SX: Unilateral, pain, firm, tenderness, erythema, fever, swelling MCC: S. aureus TX: Continued breast feeding on infected side, **heat packs, Dicloxacillin, Cephalexin**
Breast Abscess: Similar to mastitis but has a palpable, fluctuant mass. Fever, unilateral, pain, firm, tenderness, erythema. TX: Drainage, **Dicloxacillin, Cephalexin**	**Plugged Ducts** Similar to mastitis but **NO fever and NO systemic symptoms.** TX: Improve the quality of breast-feeding. For persistent plugged ducts indicates a galactocele (retention cyst containing milk in the mammary glands). TX: Aspiration
Superficial Vein Thrombosis of the Breast (Mondor's Disease) Painful, cord-like lesion, local redness. Self-limiting.	**No Milk Production** SX: Breast are full and tender, warm. TX: No medications. Use tight bras, avoid nipple stimulation, ice packs, analgesics.
Sheehan's Syndrome (AKA: Postpartum hypopituitarism) Cause: Ischemic infarction in pituitary following heavy postpartum blood loss and hypovolemic shock. SX: Inability to breastfeed: No lactation postpartum (agalactorrhoea), amenorrhea/oligomenorrhea, cold intolerance, constipation, weight gain, hypoglycemia, hyponatremia.	

Labor and Delivery

Fetal Testing helps determine the well being of the fetus.

Test	Description	Results
Non-Stress Test (NST)	Measure fetal heart rate during normal activity. Measures fetal HR and movements.	**Reactive (assuring)** results: The fetus is doing well. Requires: detection of 2 fetal movements and ↑fetal HR > 15 bpm lasting 15 – 20 seconds > 20 minutes. **Nonreassuring** Test results: 1st step (baby could be sleeping): vibroacoustic stimulation to wake the fetus. 2nd step: if the test is still nonreassuring: proceed to the Biophysical Profile Test (BPP)
Biophysical Profile (BPP)	Measures 5 categories worth 2 points each. 1) NST 2) 2) Fetal chest expansions/breathing movements (normal is ≥ 1 in 30 minutes). 3) Fetal movements (normal: ≥ 3 in 30 minutes). 4) Fetal muscle tone (fetus flexes an extremity) 5) Amniotic fluid index	BPP Score: 8 – 10: Normal 4 – 8: Inconclusive For normal and inconclusive test: fetus must be rechecked weekly. < 4: Abnormal: Immediate delivery.
Kick Count	Measures number of fetal movements over a certain period. < 28: fetal movement can be felt 3 – 4 times a day. ➢ 28 weeks, movements can be tracked by mom. Should feel 10-15 movements in 24 hrs. ➢	Immediate concern if no fetal movements or less than 10 detected within a 12-hour period.
Amniotic Fluid Index (AFI)	Estimate of the amount of amniotic fluid.	Normal AFI: 8 – 18 cm Oligohydramnios: AFI < 5 – 6 cm Polyhydramnios: AFI: > 20 – 24 cm

False Labor verses True Labor

False Labor	True Labor
Irregular contractions. Interval of contraction do not shorten. Contractions do not ↑ in intensity. No progression/no cervical changes. Can last 4 – 8 weeks. Contractions and pain are in the low abdomen. Pain is relieved by sedation. TX: Reassure and send home.	Contractions at regular intervals. Contractions are progressive, there is cervical change. Contraction intervals shorten (grow closer). Contractions ↑ in intensity. Contractions and pain in upper abdomen and back. Pain is not relieved by sedation.

Labor Inducers and Labor Abortives

Induction of Labor

When it is necessary to deliver the baby before the due date.

- Cervical ripening: Administer Prostaglandin E_2 (Do not give prostaglandins to patients with breathing problems: asthma, COPD, etc., because it may provoke bronchiospasm).
- ROM (Rupture of Membranes/Break the water)
- Stimulate uterine contractions: Oxytocin

↑ Uterine Tone: Labor Inducers and Abortives			
Mifepristone	Termination of pregnancy.	Competitive inhibitor of progestin at the progesterone receptors. ↑ uterine tone = ↑ contractions.	Abdominal pain, nausea, cramping, heavy bleeding, ↓ appetite. Note: Given with **misoprostol (PGEi) or Methotrexate** for abortions. Misoprostol: (PGEi) prevents NSAID induced ulcers (inhibits adenylate cyclase → ↓ cAMP → ↓ proton pump activity → ↓ gastric acid).
Methotrexate	Termination of pregnancy.	Folate antagonist. Folate necessary for synthesis of **thymidine** (Pathway to making purines/DNA).	Methotrexate used when: No fetal heart detected, B-hCG <6,000 mIU, fetal tissue is <3.5 cm in diameter and mother has not taken folate.
Dinoprostone	Stimulates labor. Used in vaginal inserts for contraceptions.	PGE2. Prostaglandin E2. Softens cervix and causes uterine contractions.	**NOTE: Do not give** prostaglandin's to asthmatic's, COPD or any patient with breathing difficulties because it may provoke a bronchospasm.
Oxytocin Pitocin	**IV to induce labor.** **↓ postpartum hemorrhage.**	↑ uterine tone. Given IV or by nasal spray b/c it is destroyed in the GI tract. Nasal administration crosses the blood brain barrier.	↑ heart rate, ↓ blood pressure, cardiac arrhythmias, ↑ fetal blood flow, Subarachnoid hemorrhage
↓ Uterine Tone: Slow/Stop Labor (Tocolysis)			
Terbutaline	**Tocolytic**: ↓ uterine tone (stops contractions in premature labor).	Greatest effects on **β-2 receptors**. **Relaxes uterine smooth muscle.**	Tachycardia, anxiety, tremors, headaches, hyperglycemia, hypotension, hypokalemia.

Fetal Readings and Monitoring

Heart Rate

- Normal: 110 – 160 bpm
- Tachycardia: > 160 bpm
- Bradycardia: < 110 bpm

Cardiotocography

Monitoring fetal heartbeat and uterine contractions during labor

- **External: Pressure gauge on the abdomen that monitors fetal HR and contractions**
- **Internal: Electrode placed on fetus's scalp to monitor HR. Catheter in the uterus monitors contractions.**

Accelerations

Abrupt ↑ fetal heart rate (FHR). Reassuring (normal): The rate must increase from the baseline (onset of acceleration) to the peak in ≤ 30 seconds and the peak must be ≥ 15 bpm and last ≥ 15 seconds from the onset to return to baseline. This should occur at least twice in 20 minutes.

Decelerations

Decreases in fetal heart rate (FHR) due to contractions.

Fetal Heart Rate Classifications

- **Category 1: Normal – reassuring pattern.**
  - **Baseline rate 110 – 160 bpm**
  - **Moderate variability**
  - **Absence of late, or variable decelerations**
  - **Early decelerations may/may not be present**
- **Category II: Indeterminate (continue monitoring and reevaluate) – nonreassuring pattern.**
  - **Bradycardia or tachycardia**
  - **Minimal or marked baseline variability of FHR**
  - **Periodic/recurrent decelerations longer than 2 min and shorter than 10 min.**
  - **Variable decelerations that have a slow return to base**
- **Category III: Abnormal (Abnormal fetal acid-base status) - nonreassuring pattern.**
  - **Absence of baseline variability with recurrent late or variable decelerations or bradycardia**
  - **Sinusoidal FHR**

Nonreassuring Pattern Causes to Evaluate/Identify

- **Non hypoxic causes (MC medicine causes: β agonist, β antagonist, oxytocin), discontinue meds**
- **Provide IV normal saline fluids and high-flow oxygen**
- **Put mother in left lateral position**
- **Vaginal exam to check for prolapsed umbilical cord**
- **Stimulate fetus's scalp and observe for accelerations/reassuring patterns**
- **Check pH of fetal scalp (normal pH 7.20)**
- **If none of these measures restores a reassuring pattern: emergency cesarean delivery**

Deceleration	**Result**	**Cause**
Early Decelerations	↓ in FHR occurring WITH contractions. The onset, nadir and recovery coincide with the beginning, peak and end of the contraction.	Head compression
Late Decelerations	↓ in FHR AFTER contraction has started and does NOT return to baseline until AFTER contraction ends. The nadir occurs after the peak of the contraction.	Fetal hypoxia, uteroplacental insufficiency (uterine perfusion). **EMERGENCY**: Cesarean delivery
Variable Decelerations	↓ and ↑ in FHR (onset and return to baseline) that vary, without any relationship to the contraction. **Absence** of variability is a nonreassuring pattern. Severe variables are nonreassuring patterns = **fetal acidosis.**	Umbilical cord compression. (**tip**: umbilical cords VARY in length)
Prolonged Deceleration	↓ in FHR from baseline ≥ 15 bpm lasting ≥ 2 minutes and ≤ 10 minutes.	

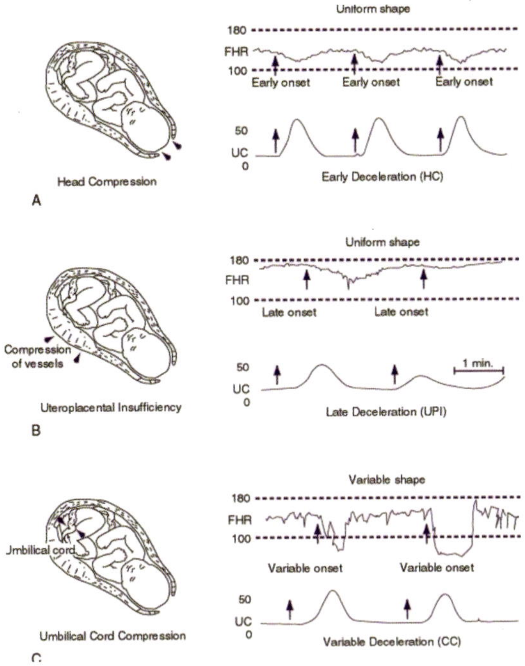

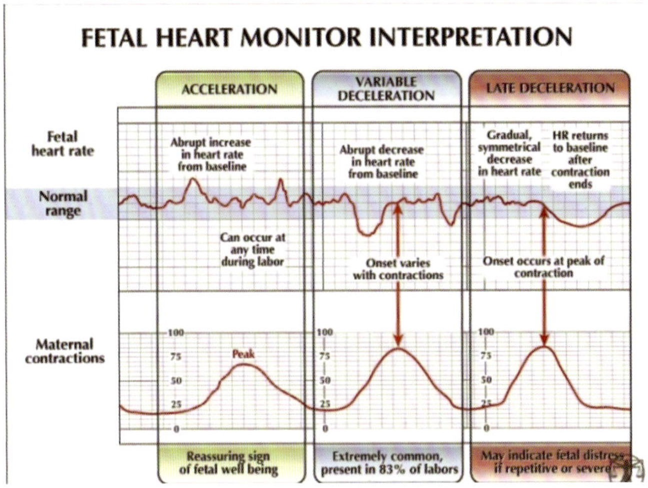

Stages of Labor

Stage	Description	Duration	Notes
Stage 1	Onset of labor ➔ full dilation of cervix (10cm)	Primipara: can last up to 20 hours. Multipara: can be very quick: < 14 hours.	
Stage 1 Latent stage	Onset until 4 cm dilated. **Cervical Effacement.**	Primipara (1st baby): < 20 hours. Multipara: < 14 hrs.	Abnormal: < 3cm cervical dilation or no cervical change in 20 hrs (primipara) or 14 hrs (multipara) TX: rest and hydration.
Stage 1 Active phase	From 4 cm until 10 cm dilated. **Dilation.**	Primipara: 1.2 cm/hour. Multipara: 1.5 cm/hour.	**Abnormal:** Prolongation or arrest. **Based on the 3 "P"s: P**ower (strength and frequency of uterine contractions), **P**assenger (size and position of fetus) and **P**assage (is passenger to large for the pelvis). No cervical change in ≥ 2hours. **Causes**: fetus to large, abnormal presentation of fetus, too small pelvis or dysfunctional contractions. (AKA: The 3 "P's") **TX**: Weak contractions: **IV oxytocin** To strong of contractions: morphine to sedate Adequate contractions (something else is wrong): emergency cesarean delivery.
Stage 2	Begins 10 cm till delivery of baby. Descent	Primipara: several hours, usually < 2 hrs. Multipara: can be very quick, usually < 1 hr. Epidural will slow This stage down.	Abnormal: Prolonged stage. Causes: Fetus head is not engaged ➔ emergency cesarean delivery. Fetal head is engaged ➔ forceps or vacuum delivery. **Normal delivery:** Engagement (fetal head enters pelvis) ➔ Descent ➔ Flexion of head ➔ Internal rotation when fetus reaches **I**schial spines and sagittal sutures are forward ➔ Extension so head can pass through the vagina ➔ External rotation (head rotates so shoulders can descend) ➔ Anterior shoulder delivery (downward pressure on fetal head will deliver the shoulder) ➔ Posterior shoulder delivery (upward pressure on fetal head will deliver the shoulder) ➔ body of fetus will follow shoulder deliveries.
Stage 3	Delivery of placenta. Repair of lacerations. Expulsion.	< 30 minutes	Abnormal: Prolonged stage. Causes: Placenta accrete/increta/percreta. Initial TX: Oxytocin IV. If this does not work: try manual removal, last resort hysterectomy.

Fetal Stations

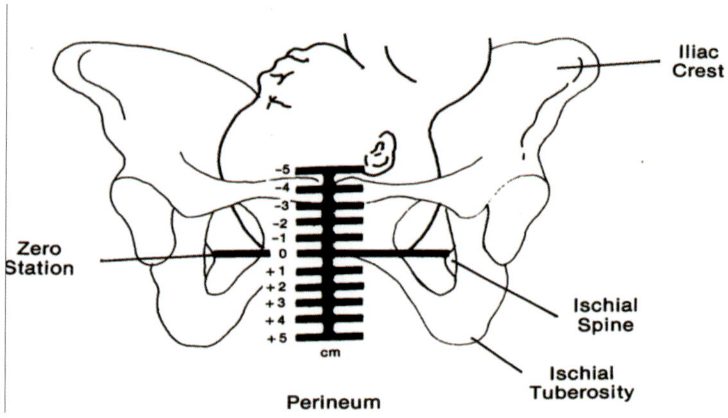

Cephalic Vertex and Abnormal Birth Presentations

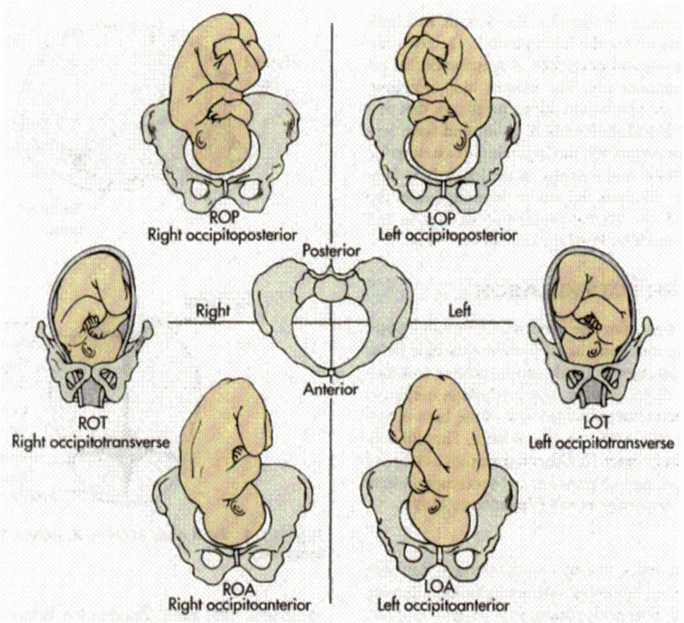

(**tip**: Right: ATP Left: ATP)

Delivery Complications

Breech Presentations (legs or bottom first)

- Normal presentation: Cephalic (head first)
- Frank Breech: fetus hips flexed with knees extended bilaterally (folded in half).
- Complete Breech: Fetus hips and knees flexed bilaterally.
- Footling Breech: Fetus feet are first.
  Single footling: one leg down.
  Double footling: two legs down.

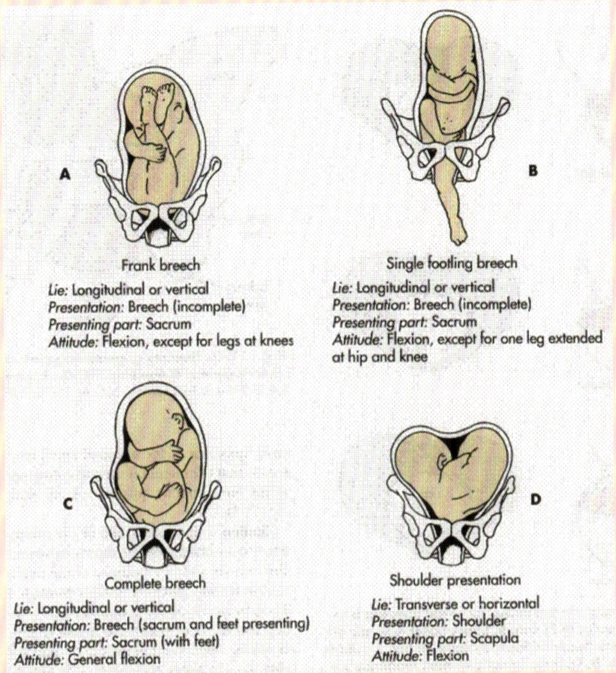

Malpresentation can be determined by:

Physical exam: Leopold maneuvers.
4 actions to help determine the position of the fetus: Fundal grip, Lateral grip, Pawlik's grip, Pelvic grip.

Vaginal exam:
If exam reveals a soft mass: malpresentation.
If exam reveals a hard surface: skull (normal cephalic)

Treatment of Breech:

- Most fetus's will rotate into a cephalic position on their own after 36 weeks
- External Cephalic Version. Performed after 37 weeks. Attempt to rotate the fetus is done externally on the abdomen. (Internal Cephalic Version is done internally through the cervix).

Cesarean Delivery

Delivery done by either low transverse incision (most common) or classic vertical incision in cases involving: Fetal distress (non-reassuring EFM reading), active genital herpes infection in the mother, HIV-positive mother with a high viral load, placenta previa, breech (preterm and on frank) or transverse position, failure of progression, arrest of labor, previous classic C-section, prolapsed cord, risk of uterine rupture or previous uterine rupture, failed instrumental delivery (forceps), macrosomia, vasa previa, instability of mother, high risk fetus, pre-eclampsia, bicornuate uterus, posthumous birth after death of the mother.

Patients with a previous low transverse C-section are usually able to have a normal vaginal birth in subsequent deliveries.

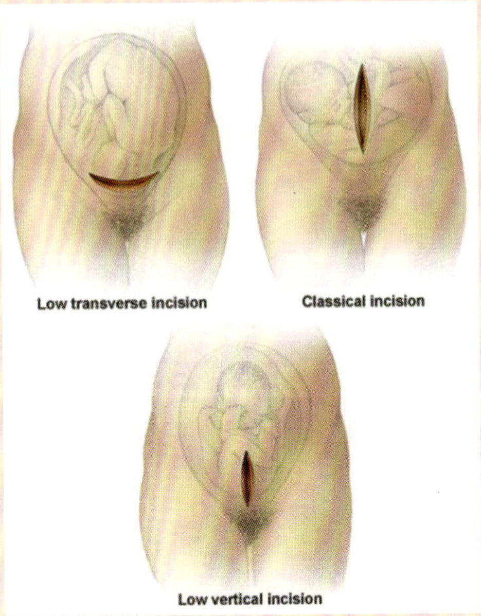

Shoulder Dystocia Anterior shoulder will not deliver; it is stuck behind the pubic symphysis. Causes: Fetal macrosomia (maternal diabetes), post term pregnancy, prior history of shoulder dystocia. Complication: Erb Palsy: damage to the upper brachial plexus. **TX: 1st line: McRoberts Maneuver** Mother flexes knees to chest in order to create a larger opening angle in the pelvis. 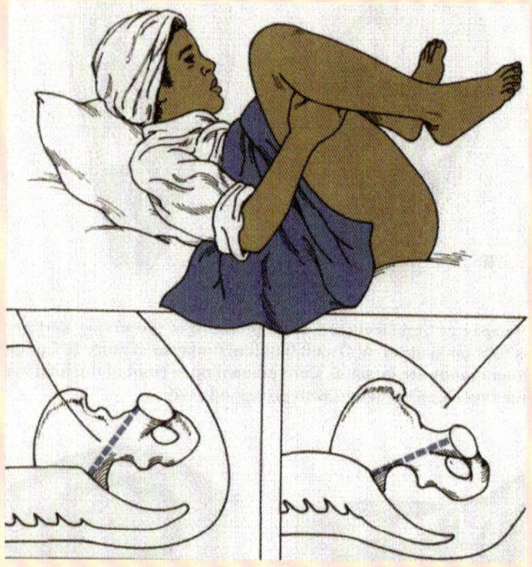 Additional Maneuvers: Woods and Rubin Maneuvers: Delivery of posterior shoulder. Zavanelli Maneuver: push fetus head back into uterus and perform cesarean delivery.	**Postpartum Hemorrhage** More than 500 mL after delivery. Complication: Sheehan syndrome. (see above for more details) Early postpartum bleeding: Within 24 hrs of delivery. Late postpartum bleeding: ≥ 24 hrs to 6 weeks. **Postpartum Infection and Fever. Endometritis.** Retained products of conception after delivery. (see above for more details) TX: **Gentamycin and Clindamycin** **UTI** Causes: catheterizations and vaginal exams. Wound Infection: Causes: Cesarean incision, stitches from lacerations. **Mastitis** Cause: **S. aureus** infects cracked nipples. SX: Unilateral breast erythema, tenderness. Must continue breast-feeding during treatments. TX: **Dicloxacillin** **Septic Thrombophlebitis** Cause: Prolonged labor. TX: **Heparin** **Fecal Incontinence** Causes: Midline episiotomy that goes into the anal sphincter and rectum, prolonged childbirth, forceps delivery.
Umbilical Cord Prolapse Emergency C-section. MC: prolapse occurs after rupture of membranes before the head is engaged. Compressed cord causes hypoxemia in the fetus, ↓↓ oxygen supply. SX: Severe bradycardia and variable accelerations present on fetal monitor. TX: Do not try and put the cord back in. Place mother in knee-chest position with vaginal area elevated. IV **Terbutaline** (B-2 agonist that decreases uterine tone by ↑ cAMP) to decrease contractions.	**Vacuum or Forceps Assisted Delivery** **Appropriate** to use in cases of: Nonreassuring pattern during absence of other contraindications. If mother has cardiac, pulmonary or other issues which could become dangerous during pushing. MC: Prolonged 2nd stage of labor. **Inappropriate** to use in cases of: The mother's pelvis is too small. Cervix is not fully dilated. Fetal head is not engaged. Orientation of the head is not clear. Membranes have not ruptured.

Fetal Growth and Maturity

Pre Term Infant	Post Term Infant
< 37 weeks gestation, < 2500 gm Few creases in the feet, they are smooth. Covered in lanugo "Peach fuzz", ↓ fat causes hypothermia, thin skin so veins are visible, ↓ cartilage in the ears, hypoglycemia, ↓ temperature stability. Risk: immature lungs, RDS, ↑ infections	> 42 weeks gestation, peeling skin, long fingernails. Risk: meconium aspiration

Postpartum Contraception

Breastfeeding Mothers

- **Breastfeeding causes anovulation so can temporarily be utilized for contraception, but is not assured. Recommended using an additional method of contraception.**
- **Progestin (OCP's, Depo-Provera, Implanon) can be used immediately after delivery and is safe during breastfeeding. Progesterone only OCP's: Do not affect the milk or the baby and there is no DVT risk.**
- **IUD or Diaphragm: May be used after 6-week postpartum check up.**

Non-breastfeeding Mothers

- **Estrogen-progestin (OCP's, vaginal ring, patch) can't be started > 3 weeks postpartum due to risk of DVT's. Do not use in breastfeeding mothers due to ↓ lactation.**
  Estrogen and Progesterone OCP will ↓ milk production and will pass on to the baby
- **IUD or Diaphragm: May be used after 6-week postpartum check up.**

Gynecologic Pathologies and Conditions

Pelvic Pain Differentials in Gynecology

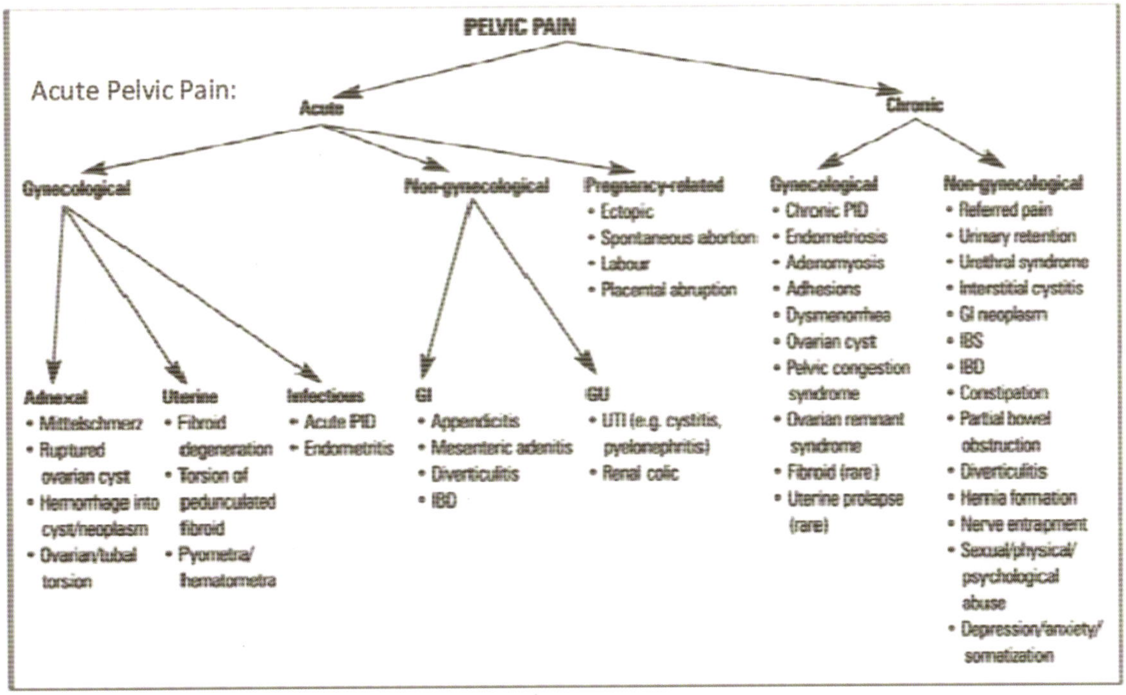

Endometriosis	Adenomyosis	Polycystic Ovarian Syndrome (PCOS)
Endometrial tissue (cells that line the womb) that is growing outside of the uterus. MC sites for ectopic tissue: ovaries (Adnexa mass = ovarian endometriosis). Other locations: Cul-de-sac, Uterosacral ligament, Broad ligament, oviducts. SX: **Classic triad**: Dysmenorrhea, dysuria and dyspareunia. Pelvic pain **during** periods, **dysmenorrhea** (painful cramps, chronic pain worse in the premenstrual period), **dyspareunia** (pain with intercourse), recto-vaginal tenderness (tenderness on any movement of the uterus), **dysuria** (urinary urgency/frequency), **dyschezia** (pain with defecation), **infertility**, pelvic pain, tender pelvic lymph nodes, fixed retroverted uterus, the uterus is NOT enlarged. ↑ risk of infertility. If ectopic tissue is on the ovary = endometrioma/ endometrioid cyst that is filled with blood (AKA: "**Chocolate cyst**") Pelvic exam: normal size uterus, retroverted uterus, uterosacral nodularity. Tenderness on rectovaginal exam. CA-125 marker may be elevated. Biopsy shows: **Proliferative endometrial tissue inside a cyst**. DX: **Laparoscopy is the only way to DX.** TX: Combination of estrogen and progestin OCP pills. GnRH analog: **Danazol** (antiestrogen) **, Leuprolide.** (GnRH agonist that down regulate the pituitary gland), progestins, **NSAIDS (Naproxen).** **Surgical TX: Adenolysis for fertility.** **Complete pain relief: Radical TAH-BSO.** Asymptomatic: no treatment needed	Ectopic endometrial tissue inside the **myometrium** caused by hyperplasia of the glands in the basalis layer of the endometrium (myometrium). MC: Women in 4th and 5th decades. SX: Painful, severe dysmenorrhea, menorrhagia (heavy periods). Exam: Large, **boggy**, soft, **symmetrically diffuse,** enlarged, **tender** uterus with cystic areas in the myometrium. Does not change with hormones. Associated with daughter's who's mother's were exposed to DES, tubal ligation, pregnancy termination, history of endometriosis, caesarean section, uterine fibroids.. **DX: Biopsy to rule out endometrial cancer. Ultrasound and MRI.** **TX: Hysterectomy is the only cure. No medical treatment.** **(Note: if it is a fibroid or leiomyoma, the uterus will be an irregular shape).**	Hormone imbalance. MCC of infertility in women. Suspected that it is a genetic disease. Polycystic ovaries produce excessive amounts of androgens (male hormones – testosterone). Aromatase converts free testosterone to estrogen. (↑ risk in obese women because adipose tissue also contains aromatase, which makes additional estrogen). This patient has no estrogen receptors in the hypothalamus it does not "see" the estrogen so GnRH, LH and FSH are all increased. SX: **hirsutism, infertility**, irregular periods, acne, pelvic pain, **obesity (> 30 BMI),** oligomenorrhea/amenorrhea. Associated with: Metabolic syndrome (central obesity), insulin resistance, increased homocysteine levels. **Labs: ↑ androgen levels, ↑ GnRH, ↑ LH, ↑ FSH.** (LH:FSH ratio: 3:1 normal LH:FSH is 1.5:1). DX: Ultrasound shows bilateral enlarged ovaries. TX: **Weight reduction**, OCP's to ↓ amount of free testosterone, **Spironolactone** (antiandrogen), **Clomiphene** (SERM inhibits negative feedback of estrogen on GnRH which ↓ LH and FSH causing a pulsatile cycle) and Metformin to ↑ insulin sensitivity → ↓ testosterone → LH surge. **Idiopathic Hirsutism** MC cause of hirsutism. Hirsutism in the presence of all normal labs and no virilization. TX: DOC: **Spironolactone**. **Eflornithine** (*Vaniqa*) for topical treatment of unwanted facial hair.

Pelvic Inflammatory Disease (PID)
AKA: Cervicitis
Cause: Chlamydia trachomatis and Neisseria gonorrhoeae.
MC bacterial STD in the USA.
MCC of infertility in women <30 with normal periods.

SX: **Cervical motion tenderness** (Chandelier sign), **purulent (mico-purulent discharge), infertility,** endometritis, tubo-ovarian abscess, **salpingitis** (inflammation of fallopian tube), hydrosalpinx (blocked fallopian tube with serous or clear fluid), fever, leukocytosis (↑ WBC), adnexal tenderness, lower abdominal pain.

Complications:
Hugh-Curtis Syndrome: infection of liver capsule leading to adhesions (AKA: Violin string adhesions).
If no treatment: may develop abscesses, peritonitis, sepsis.

Risk Factors: Adhesions can cause intestinal **obstruction** (air/fluid levels on abdominal x-ray), **infertility**, **ectopic pregnancy**

Pelvic Inflammatory Disease
Continued

TX: Must start TX immediately, do now wait for results of cultures.
Outpatient TX: one dose IM Ceftriaxone *(Rocephin)* (for Gonorrhea) **and oral Doxycycline or oral Azithromycin** (for Chlamydia).
YOU MUST TREAT FOR BOTH ORGANISMS.

CAUTION: watch the vignette: if the patient has been throwing up: you must hospitalize her to use IV meds (she will not keep the oral meds down). This goes for ANY situation in which a patient must receive medication but is throwing up.
In Patient TX: IV Cefoxitin or Cefotetan and Doxycycline OR Clindamycin and Gentamycin.

Initial test: β-hCG, cervical culture
Accurate test: Laparoscopy

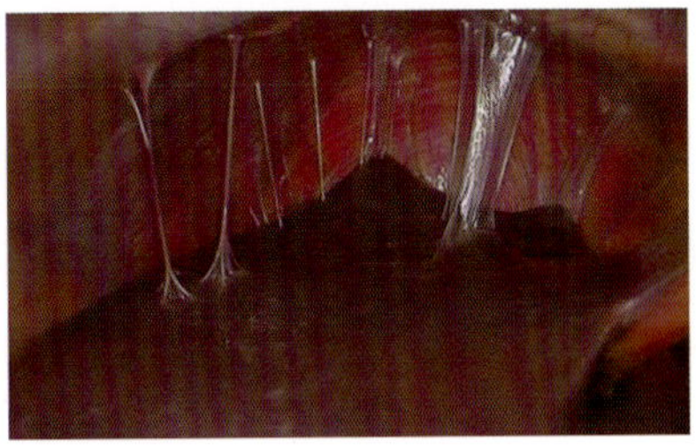

Fitz Hugh-Curtis Syndrome (complication of PID)
("Violin string" adhesions can cause intestinal obstruction)

Pelvic Inflammatory Disease
Continued

Chronic Pelvic Inflammatory Disease
Patient has past history of STD (PID) as well as abnormal vaginal bleeding and/or ectopic pregnancies.

SX: Infertility and/or dyspareunia, bilateral lower abdominal-pelvic pain. No fever, no adnexal mass, no discharge.

DX: Cervical cultures and labs will be normal.
Ultrasound shows bilateral hydrosalpinges (cystic pelvic masses).
Laparoscope will diagnose adhesions.

TX: Adenolysis (lysis) of tubal adhesions for infertility,
Analgesia (temporary treatment for pain),
Pelvic clean-out: TAH-BSO to eradicate pain. Do not give antibiotics: this is not an infection.

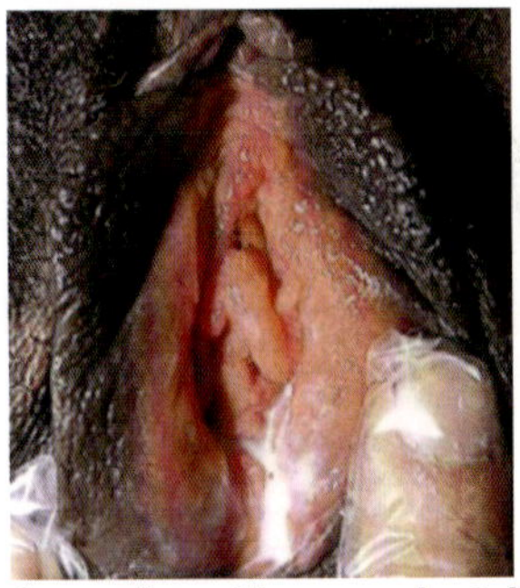

Gonorrhea: Mucopurulent discharge

Bacterial Vaginosis
(aka: Gardnerella Vaginosis, BV)
Gm variable
Is **NOT an STD** but is associated with sex

SX: **Gray vaginal discharge, fishy smell,** is NOT painful, **NO redness or inflammation.**

DX: **Clue cells (squamous epithelial cells covered with adherent bacteria** due to an overgrowth of anaerobic bacteria in the vagina).
pH 5 – 6.

TX: **Metronidazole**
Nursing moms: discontinue nursing while taking meds and then resume once meds have stopped

Candida albicans
(aka: Yeast infection) Dimorphic yeast.
Pseudohyphae and budding yeast at 20° C
Germ tubes at 37°C
NO β 1-3 Glucan in the walls
↓ Glucan = osmotic instability

Vaginal Candidiasis: Not sexually transmitted (due to overgrowth of Candida, normally because of antibiotic use).
Local infections: T cells.
Systemic Infections: ↑ in neutropenic patients.
DX: **Germ Tube test. pH: 4 – 5.**

Vulvovaginitis (Vaginitis/yeast): due to antibiotic use (esp. in diabetics).
Antibiotics, steroids, diabetes, OCP's, immunocompromised allow for the **decrease in the normal flora bacteria Lactobacilli**, which allows for the **overgrowth of Candida**.
SX: White **"cottage cheese"** coating.
TX: **topical "azole" cream, Nystatin, Fluconazole, Miconazole**

Trichomonas vaginalis
(aka: Vaginitis)
Protozoan

Source: **STD**

SX: Vaginal **pruritis and burning. Red vaginal mucosa** (AKA: Strawberry cervix), dyspareunia (pain with sex). Inflammation of vagina and vulva.

High risk for: preterm labor, premature rupture of membranes (ROM).

DX: Motile Trophozoites on wet mount in pear shape with flagella.
Vaginal ph of 6 - 7 (alkalotic)

TX: **Metronidazole**
MUST treat partner also. (**tip**: "trichy dicky").

Nursing mothers: Must stop nursing for a few days while on the medicine and then resume.

Premature Ovarian Failure (premature menopause) Loss of function of ovaries, loss of eggs (lack of viable oocytes), surgical removal of ovaries before the **age of 40**. Causes: genetic, autoimmune, Turn Syndrome, Fragile X syndrome, smoking, enzyme defects, radiation/chemotherapy. Labs: ↑ **FSH**, ↑ LH, ↓ estrogen **An ↑ FSH is the identifying lab to confirm menopause.** **TX: In vitro fertilization with donor oocytes.**	**Ovarian Torsion** Acute/sudden lower unilateral abdominal pain with adnexal mass. Negative β-hCG. DX: Laparotomy TX: Detorsioning of the ovaries. If there is necrosis: oophorectomy is performed. If blood supply is intact a cystectomy is performed. Differentials: Pain for weeks or days: PID, Ectopic pregnancy, appendicitis (if RLQ pain), Diverticulitis (if LLQ pain).	**Tubo-ovarian Abscess (TOA)** Complication of PID (Pelvic Inflammatory Disease). Encapsulated pocket of pus that forms on the ovary and/or fallopian tube as a result of an upper genital tract infection. The TOA can also occur without a preceding problem of PID or sexual activity. SX: Fever, ↑ WBC and ESR count, lower abdominal pain, low back pain, rectal pain, vaginal discharge, nausea, vomiting. DX: Ultrasound, MRI, laparoscope, X-ray show a unilateral abscess (mass). Culdocentesis shows pus. Blood cultures show anaerobic organisms. TX: Inpatient treatment: Cefoxitin and Doxycycline.
Lichen Sclerosus (Post menopausal) SX: Vulvar pruritis, white, polygonal macules, atropic, thin **"cigarette or parchment paper -like" covering over the vulva and anus**, scarring. Obliteration or **atrophy** of the labia minora and clitoris, ↓ diameter of the vaginal opening (introitus: entrance into a hollow organ). ↑ risk of squamous cell carcinoma. **DX: Vulvar punch biopsy** **TX: Topical corticosteroids** 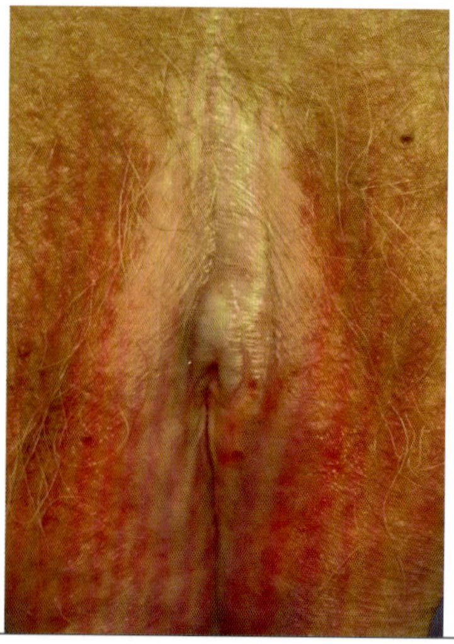	**Normal: Physiologic Discharge** Physiologic leukorrhea. Copious (mucoid) discharge: white or yellow. No odor, no other symptoms. Squamous cells with few PMN's. All other discharges = pathologic	**First Menses: Normal** Periods in young girls: First 2 years may have irregular cycles because of the immature hypo-pituitary axis is not producing enough hormones (FSH and LH) which is needed for ovulation. Without ovulation, period will lack regularity. **Premenarchal Vaginal Bleeding** Bleeding before menarche. MCC: Foreign body in the vagina. Other causes: Sarcoma botryoides (cancer), pituitary tumor, adrenal tumor or ovarian tumor, sexual abuse. DX: Pelvic exam under sedation. Imaging: CT or MRI to look for tumor. If all test are negative: Idiopathic precocious puberty.

Dysfunctional Uterine Bleeding (DUB)
Heavy bleeding without structural or organic problems/disease.
Occurs because anovulation. With no progesterone to signal cycle to begin sloughing (menses). Estrogen stabilized the endometrium.

MCC: Anovulation
↑ Risk with HTN, > 35 age, Diabetes, obesity.

In adolescents:
If mild: Add iron supplements
If moderate with no active bleeding: Add progestin (Medroxyprogesterone) and iron supplements.

If moderate with active bleeding or severe bleeding: High dose IV estrogen therapy. Combo OCP with high estrogen promotes hemostasis (estrogen followed by progesterone). Severe bleeding despite treatment may require a D & C.

In women >35 or other high risk patients (obese, diabetics, chronic HTN): Endometrial biopsy (rule out hyperplasia and carcinoma).
If biopsy is negative: TX: Cyclic progestins. If progestin fails → ablation or hysterectomy.

Primary Dysmenorrhea

SX: ↑ cramps, colicky pain, lower abdominal pain that radiates to thighs and back before the period – usually occurs within 2 years after the start of menarche. Causes: nausea, vomiting, diarrhea, headaches.

DX: History and PE. Pelvic exams are normal.

Cause: PG mediated. ↑ levels of prostaglandins due to breakdown of the endometrium.

TX: NSAIDS, PG inhibitors, OCP's.

Secondary Dysmenorrhea

SX: Cramping pain arising in the mid-reproductive years. Can show: infertility, dyspareunia, dyschezia, vaginal bleeding.

DX: Ultrasound for Adenomyosis, liomyoma. Laparoscopy: Endometriosis, adhesions.

Cause: Organic lesions: endometriosis, adhesions, adenomyosis, liomyoma, cervical stenosis.

TX: treat underlying condition.

Sexual Assault

Prophylaxis:
HIV **HAART therapy** (Tenofovir, Emtricitabine, Raltegravir, Efavirenz)

Hep B and Hep B Ig. (If patient has already been vaccinated against HEP B they do not need the Ig)

Azithromycin for Chlamydia
Ceftriaxone for Gonorrhea
Metronidazole for Trichomonas Vaginalis.

Premenstrual Syndrome (PMS)

Physical and emotional symptoms that occur 1 – 2 weeks prior to a woman's menses (luteal phase). Believed to be caused by the changes of hormones during this time period.

SX: Bloating, acne, tender breasts, cramps, irritability, mood swings, fatigue, constipation/diarrhea, low back pain, food cravings.
Symptoms do not occur during pregnancy or menopause. Most symptoms resolve when bleeding starts.

Symptoms can be worsened by a diet high in caffeine, salt or alcohol and increase exercise.

TX: **SSRI's: Fluoxetine, Sertraline** (Increase serotonin). To help relieve pain: 800 mg **Ibuprofen** three times a day, beginning 10 days prior to period.

Primary Amenorrhea
AKA: Anovulation
No period by the age of 14 without secondary sexual development or by the age of 16 with secondary sexual development.

MCC: Pregnancy
(**Beware**: questions will appear to lead you to a pathology when a woman has missed a period or is late **– it is pregnancy in most all cases!**)

Signs of pregnancy:
Cervix, vagina and labia have a "blue" tinge color (AKA: Chadwick's Sign) due to the increased blood flow.
Missed/late/unusual period, tender and enlarged breast, nausea and vomiting, frequent urination, fatigue, strange cravings, skin changes. **NOTE:** Pregnancy can occur prior to the first menses.

DX: **#1: Rule out pregnancy with β HCG**, then check TSH, Prolactin, FSH.

Other reasons for Amenorrhea or Anovulation:

Physical Causes: Imperforate hymen, anorexia nervosa, excessive exercise, vaginal septum.

Ovarian Causes: PCOS (due to ↑ testosterone (androgens), ovarian failure (AKA: menopause. labs show ↑ FSH).

Hypothalamic Causes: Stress, Cancer, GnRH deficiency (Kallmann's Syndrome: no smell/anosmia = No GnRH, ↓ FSH, ↓ LH).
Genetic Causes: (**Turners 45XO or 54X**: (No ovaries = ↑ FSH. Absence of one X chromosome).

Pituitary Causes: Prolactinoma (labs: prolactinemia), Empty sella.

Premenstrual Dysphoric Disorder (PMDD) Severe and disabling form of premenstrual syndrome (PMS) causing difficulty in day to day functions and relationships. Symptoms are cyclic (like PMS) during the luteal phase of the menstrual cycle. SX: Hostility, irritability, depression, anxiety, difficulty concentrating, fatigue, bloating, breast tenderness, headache, aches, excess tension. Complication: Associated with lifetime depression, mood and anxiety disorders. TX: SSRI: **Fluoxitine** and Cognitive Behavioral Therapy (CBT).	*Primary Amenorrhea cont'd* **NOTE:** If breasts are present, this indicates that estrogen is being produced. **Secondary Amenorrhea** **When normal periods are absent for >3 months or irregular menses is absent for >6 months.** **Due to estrogen deficiency** because of ↓ LH and GnRH Common with elite female athletes. **Other problems** due to ↓ estrogen: Osteopenia, osteoporosis, infertility, vaginal atrophy breatst atrophy, amenorrhea. **MOA of amenorrhea:** If no ovulation occurs, the corpus luteum (site of initial progesterone synthesis) does not form. If this does not form there is no progesterone spike and decline, which results in amenorrhea (no menses).	*Amenorrhea/Anovulation cont'd* **Endocrine Causes**: Hypo/Hyper-Thyroidism (Hypothyroidism = ↑ TSH = ↑ prolactin), Diabetes, Adrenal disorders (Androgen insensitivity: no pubic or axillary hair, ultrasound shows testes in the low abdomen and karyotype shows male genotype). **Uterine Causes:** Asherman Syndrome (uterine/endometrium fibrosis and adhesions due to dilation and curettage (D & C), IUD or miscarriage). **Embryo Causes:** Müllerian Agenesis (internal sex organs are absent: ovaries, fallopian tubes, uterus, cervix and upper 2/3 of vagina. PE: shows blind vagina (AKA: foreshortened vagina). Menopause: ↑ FSH is seen in labs. (LH is also high, but ↑ FSH is pathognomonic). **NOTE:** **Leuprolide** (GnRH analog) when used continuously will inhibit FSH and LH secretion, which inhibits menstrual cycles and puts women in a "state" of menopause. This is beneficial in endometriosis and fibroids (or other disease states that are stimulated by the menstrual cycle). If the drug is used in a pulsatile manor it stimulates the release of FSH and LH causing the menstrual cycle/ovulation.

Amenorrhea not due to Pregnancy

- Central Causes: Due to Hypothalamic/Pituitary. Labs will show ↓ FSH = check pituitary by MRI
- Peripheral Causes: Due to gonadal issues. Labs will show ↑ FSH = check karyotyping
- Primary amenorrhea with 2° sexual characteristics: normal up to 16 years old.
- If 2° traits are absent, perform ultrasound at 14 years old
- **If only pubic hair present = due to GnRH issues**
- **If both pubic and axillary hair present = due to adrenal issues**
- **Estrogen is required for breast development**. If no estrogen = no breast. If there is no breast development check FSH levels. FSH will be ↑ and estrogen will be absent.
- Breast development: seen "breast buds" in Tanner Stage 2. Breast buds = estrogen
- Hypothyroidism: Has elevated TSH leading to elevated prolactin causing amenorrhea. TX: hypothyroidism.
- If prolactin is up (without hypothyroidism): review medications (antidepressants and antipsychotics) due to anti dopamine side effects which will increase prolactin. If no meds: Rule out pituitary tumor with CT. If pituitary tumor treat with Bromocriptine (dopamine agonist). If tumor is large (>1 cm: remove tumor with transsphenoidal surgery).
- **Estrogen-Progesterone Challenge Test (EPCT): 3 weeks of oral estrogen followed by 1 week progesterone. Positive test (has withdrawal bleeding) = lack/decreased estrogen. Check FSH level: ↑FSH = premature ovarian failure or no ovaries (Turners).**
  ↓ FSH = hypothalamic-pituitary deficiency. Rule out tumor with a brain CT/MRI.
  Negative test (no withdrawal bleeding): Indicates a potential outflow obstruction or scarring/adhesions. Identify lesions with a hysterosalpingogram.
- **Progesterone Challenge Test (PCT): 7 – 10 days of progesterone. Positive test: If withdrawal bleeding occurs = anovulation. TX: Clomiphene for cyclic stimulation. Negative test: No withdrawal bleeding indicates a potential outfox obstruction or scarring/adhesion or lack of estrogen. Identify lesions with a hysterosalpingogram.**

Ultrasound Results:

Uterus Present	Check FSH	If ↑ FSH = check karyotype for Turner's If ↓ FSH = check brain with MRI
Uterus Absent	Check Karyotype and Serum Testosterone	If Karyotype is 46XX, normal female and testosterone level = problem is due to abnormal mullerian development. If Karyotype is 46XY, normal male and testosterone level = problem is due to androgen insensitivity.

Differentials in Hormones for GYN Pathologies and Conditions

Pathology	**LH/FSH**	**Testosterone**	**DHEAS**	**17-hydroxyprogesterone (17-OH)**	**Diagnosis**
Adrenal tumor	NL	↑	↑	NL	US/CT adrenals
Congenital Adrenal Hyperplasia	NL	NL to ↑	NL - ↑	↑	ACTH stimulation test
Ovarian Tumor	NL	↑	NL	NL	US/CT ovaries
Polycystic Ovarian Syndrome	↑LH, ↓FSH	↑	NL - ↑	NL	US abdomen
Menopause	↑FSH, ↑LH	NL - ↓	NL - ↓	**NL - ↓**	FSH levels

Menopause

- **12 months of amenorrhea with elevation of FSH and LH.**
- Mean age 51 years. Smokers can present in menopause 2 years earlier.
- **DX: ↑ FSH** (LH will also be increased but the definitive dx is increased FSH)
- Hirsutism after menopause is due to increased androgen production.
- Menopause: failure of the anterior pituitary to secrete gonadotropins.
- **Premature Ovarian Failure:** When menopause occurs **before age 40**. DX: ↑ FSH.
- Menopause symptoms (due to lack of estrogen)
  Note: Remember: adipose tissue continues to make estrogen by converting androgens to estrone, so women that are overweight have less severe symptoms and decreased risk of osteoporosis.
  - Hot flashes
  - Amenorrhea
  - ↑ risk of osteoporosis
  - Vaginally: Vaginal atrophy, ↓ lubrication, ↑ vaginal pH, ↑ vaginal infections
  - Urinary: Urgency, frequency, urge incontinence, nocturia
  - After menopause women have the same risk for cardiovascular DZ as men. It is the MCC mortality in postmenopausal women.
  - ↓ sleep, emotional, ↑ risk of depression

Hormone Replacement Therapy (HRT)

Treatments for HRT	**Benefits of HRT**	**Conditions not for HRT**	**Side Effects/Risk of HRT**
Helps to reduce the vasomotor symptoms of menopause. Hot flashes and night sweats (AKA: vasomotor symptoms) due to hormonal fluctuations. Vaginal atrophy. Dyspareunia. **NOTE:** Do not use HRT >4 years. Treat for shortest time possible and at lowest dose.	Decreases risk of fractures and colorectal cancer.	Estrogen-sensitive breast of endometrial cancer. Osteoporosis. Current or history of blood clots. Unexplained vaginal bleeding. Liver disease.	Increased risk of blood clots. Increased risk of breast cancer if used > 4 years. Increased risk of heart attack.

Gynecologic Tumors and Cancers

- **Gynecology Epidemiology**
  - Incidence: #1) Endometrial, #2) Ovarian, #3) Cervical
  - Mortality: #1) Ovarian, #2) Cervical, #3) Endometrial
  - **CAUTION:** Be **VERY** careful to read exactly what epidemiology fact they are asking for on the exam! Be sure its not the "general" public (male/female) incidence or mortality. Just because they say it's a woman in the vignette, do not assume they want GYN. If they want GYN, be careful to note if it is incidence or mortality!
- Screening: PAP smears (cytology) begin at 21 and continue every 3 years until 65 unless the patient is immunocompromised. For the immunocompromised, PAP smears should begin after their first sexual encounter. If >30 years old, screening can be done every 5 years if the PAP is also done with HPV testing. (See more details in the screening chapter).
- Endometrial carcinoma: ↑ risk with longer exposure to estrogen
- Ovarian cancers: ↑ risk with PCOS, endometriosis, advanced age, BRCA-1 or BRCA-2, family history.
  ↓ Risk: OCP's, pregnancy, breastfeeding (decreased exposure to estrogen).
- Tumor Marker for Ovarian Cancer: CA-125 (used to follow reoccurrence, not used for screening).

Human Papilloma Virus (HPV)
No Envelope
Double stranded, circular

Causes:
HPV 1, 2, 6, 11, CIN (Cervical Intraepithelial Neoplasia), Cervical Cancer (CIN associate with HPV 16, 18),
Anal cancer in men, genital warts

Transmission: Sexual activity
High risk: MC: due to higher number of sexual partners. Also: Early age of intercourse, immunosuppression, cigarette smoking. Condoms do NOT totally protect against HPV because areas around genitals and thighs are not covered.

Prevention: Gardasil (HPV vaccine) **given to all females from 13 – 26. Gardasil is also indicated for males 9 – 26 years of age to prevent genital warts due to HPV.**
Protects against: HPV 6, 11, 16, 18.
Do not vaccinate pregnant, lactating women and do not vaccinate the immunosuppressed.

HPV warts, associated with HPV 6, 11
Condylomata acuminate. (Benign).

SX: Heaped up, white, flesh, transparent colored. (Resembles cauliflower)

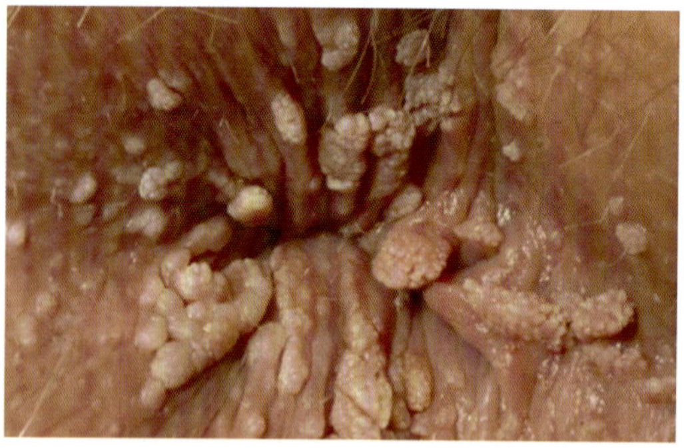

TX: **Cryotherapy with liquid nitrogen, laser removal, trichloroacetic acid, podophyllin** (melts them away, but is potentially teratogenic, causes tissue damage. Do NOT use during pregnancy),
Imiquimod (sloughs off wart **without any damage to surrounding tissues** and causes no pain).
(**tip**: I in Imiquimod for "I" for Ideal to use)

CIN (Cervical Intraepithelial Neoplasia)

Location: **"Transitional zone": squamocolumnar junction**.

CIN 1, CIN 2, CIN3 (carcinoma in situ) is the extent of the dysplasia.
PAP smear classifications:

- **ASCUS: Atypical squamous cells of undetermined significance. (MC: due to early HPV infection). On first occurance: repeat PAP in 3-6 months along with HPV DNA typing. If second PAP smears indicate ASCUS or HPV 16 or 18, must do colposcopy (magnifies the cervix 12x) and ectocervical biopsy. Must have 2 consecutive negative PAP smears.**
  (If patient is unlikely to follow up in 3 – 6 months for a second PAP, perform the colposcopy and ectocervical biopsy after the first ASCUS result).
  Ectocervical biopsy is done for abnormal lesions (ECC).
  Cone Biopsy is done if abnormal cells are found on ECC and/or colposcopy. NOTE: Cone biopsies can result in an incompetent cervix or cervical stenosis.
- **CIN 1: Low-grade squamous intraepithelial lesion (mild dysplasia). CIN 2, CIN 3: High-grade squamous intraepithelial lesion (moderate to severe dysplasia).**
  CIN 2, CIN 3: Requires a LEEP (loop electrosurgical excision procedure) or Cold-knife conization (excision of tissue from the cervix). Note: these can result in an incompetent cervix or cervical stenosis.
  If recurrent CIN 2 or CIN 3 or biopsy confirms cancer: treatment: hysterectomy.
- **Cancer: Invasive.**
  MC: Squamous cell carcinoma.
  TX: Hysterectomy.
  Adjuvant therapy (radiation and chemotherapy) is used if: the cancer has metastasized to the lymph nodes, is poorly differentiated, tumor is >4 cm or is recurrent.
- **Pregnant Patients: Managed the same way a nonpregnant patient is except that no ECC (Endocervical curettage) or LEEP procedure is preformed due to the high vascular condition of the cervix during pregnancy. Colposcopy and biopsy are ok to do.**
  Invasive cancer in pregnancy: Diagnosis <24 weeks: radical hysterectomy or radiation. Diagnosis >24 weeks: C-section at 32-34 weeks.

Cancers due to HPV

- 90% of cervical cancer
- 90% of anal cancer in males.
- 70% of the cancer of the oropharynx (base of the tongue and tonsils, and back of throat). 30% due to smoking and alcohol.
- 70% of cancer of the vulva, vagina
- 60% of cancer of the penis

Associated with: **HPV 16 and HPV 18**
MOA: **HPV 16 and 18 produce the E6 and E7 gene** products.
E6 inhibits **p53** suppressor gene. (**tip**: E**6** is next to p5**3**)
E7 inhibits **RB** suppressor gene.

Risk: #1 Multiple sex partners, smoking, early sexual intercourse, HIV

Early dysplasia:
Koilocytes (squamous epithelia cell) that has undergone structural changes due to HPV. Shows **enlarged dark, wrinkled (like a raison) nucleus** (2 – 3 x normal size) with **halo around nucleus (perinuclear halo)** and irregular nuclear membrane;

Dysplasia on a PAP smear are preneoplastic cells: Koilocytes and atypical cells

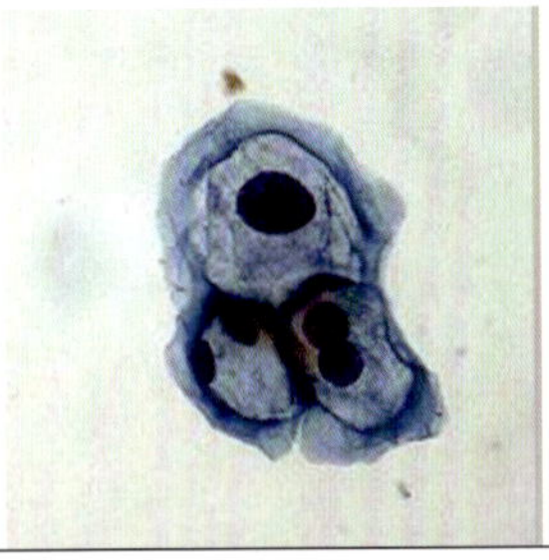

HPV Screening Guidelines (PAP Smears)

- **Normal healthy patients: Begin PAP's at age 21 until 65 every 3 years**
- You **MUST** also test for Chlamydia in sexual active women
- In **immunocompromised** patients (HIV, SLE, transplants) do PAP at time of **1st sexual activity**, twice in 1st year and then every year.
- No screening required if no risk and no DES exposure (ie: hysterectomy with cervix removed)
- If cytological abnormality occurs on a PAP smear:
  1) Colposcopy is performed. Acetic acid is applied to cervix at the **squamocolumnar junction (transformation zone**). Areas that turn white or have an abnormal vascular pattern are **biopsied**.
  2) If biopsy shows **dysplasia** then a **LEEP** (loop electrical excision procedure) procedure is done. (End of cervix is removed using a wire loop with an electric current. Future risk of LEEP is **cervical incompetence** during pregnancy (cervix is tied shut until term) and increased potential of spontaneous abortion.

PAP Smear Results

- **Both low and high-grade dysplasia must have colposcopy and biopsy.**
- **Low Grade Squamous Intraepithelial Lesion (LGSIL)**
  Shows atypical squamous cells in the cervix
  DX: Colposcopy and biopsy to confirm
  Monitor patient, most LGSIL is self-resolving. If progression the same steps as used in HGSIL are taken.
- **High Grade Squamous Intraepithelial Lesion (HGSIL)**
  Indicates moderate to severe cervical dysplasia that if untreated can lead to cervical cancer.
  DX: Colposcopy with biopsy to confirm.
  TX: LEEP (Loop Electrosurgical Excision Procedure
  Other treatment options: Cryotherapy, Conization (cone biopsy), laser therapy.
  Regular follow up with PAP smears and colposcopies to monitor for reoccurrence.

Endometrial Carcinoma

MC gynecologic malignancy.

ANY postmenopausal bleeding is considered to be endometrial carcinoma until proven otherwise.

Initial presentation: **Endometrial hyperplasia**.
Presents with vaginal bleeding.

Risk factors: **Prolonged exposure to estrogen (unopposed estrogen)** without progestin's (**anything** that allows estrogen to be present longer: early menses, late menopause, few/no children (nulliparity), OCP's), obesity, diabetes, HTN, granulosa cell tumor (produces estrogen), HRT (hormone replacement therapy), PCOS, Tamoxifen use, chronic anovulation (ie: PCOS).
NOTE: In women with chronic anovulation give progestins to prevent endometrial hyperplasia, which leads to cancer.

(**Remember: women being treated with Tamoxifen have an increased risk for Endometrial hyperplasia/Endometrial carcinoma**).

DX: Endometrial biopsy.
Negative results: Biopsy shows atrophy and no cancer cells: no additional work up necessary.
Positive results: Adenocarcinoma. Surgery and staging of cancer.

TX:
Radiation therapy if: >50% of myometrium is involved, biopsy was poorly differentiated, or metastasis to the lymph nodes.
Chemotherapy is: the cancer has metastasized.

Squamous Cell Carcinoma of the Vulva
MC vulvar cancer.

Risk factors: Increasing age (average age 65), exposure to HPV, smoking, HIV, skin conditions that involve the vulva (ie: Lichen sclerosus), history of precancerous conditions of the vulva.

SX: Itching (pruritis) that does not go away; bleeding that is not from menstruation, ulcers (small to larger, cauliflower-like lesions), pain, tenderness, skin changes (color and thickening).

DX: Biopsy
TX: Surgical resection and reconstructive surgery. Can include radiation and chemotherapy.

Vulvar melanoma: Cancer that begins in the pigment producing cells in the vulva.

Vulvar Cancer Stages (Squamous Cell)

- Stage 0: Carcinoma in situ
- Stage I: Small tumor confined to the vulva or limited to the vaginal wall. <2 cm in size.
- Stage II: Tumor has grown to include nearby structures (ie: lower urethra, vagina, anus. Still limited to the vulva or perineum, but is >2 cm.
- Stage III: Cancer has spread to lymph nodes.
- Stage IVA: Cancer has spread to other areas: bladder, rectum, pelvic bone, bilateral lymph nodes.
- Stage IVB: Cancer has metastasized to distant parts of the body.

Paget's Disease of the Vulva
AKA: Extramammary Paget Disease
Noninvasive intraepithelial (in the skin) adenocarcinoma.
MC: Postmenopausal Caucasian women.
Can often be associated with other cancers in the urethra, rectum or Bartholin glands.

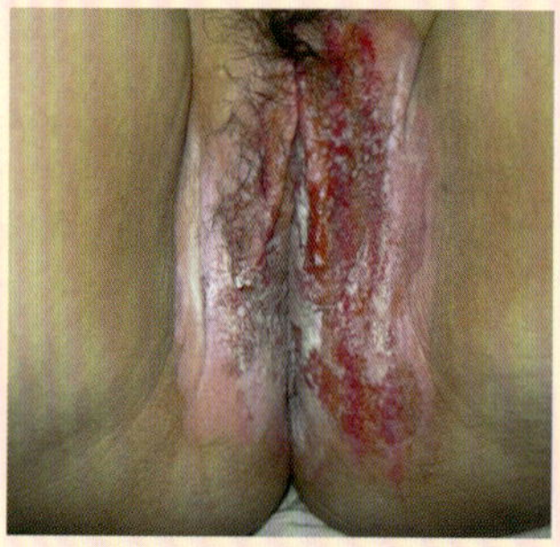

SX: Itching, burning, soreness. Presents as a erythemic skin lesion with a white coating (can be mistaken for eczema).

DX: Biopsy.
TX: Surgical excision.

Leiomyoma
(AKA: Uterine Fibroid)

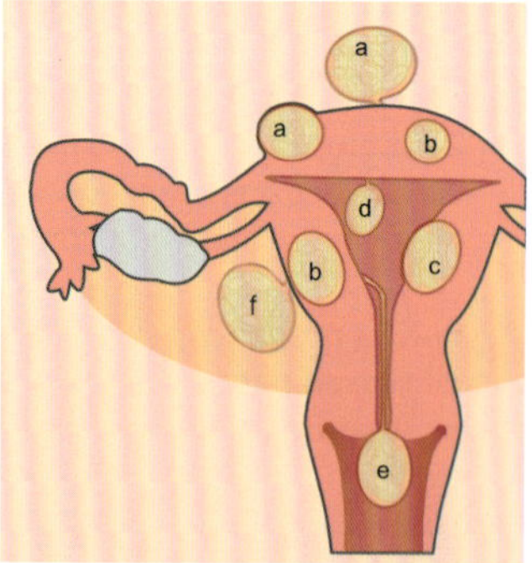

MC benign smooth muscle (myometrium) tumor in women.
Estrogen dependent: ↑ size with OCP use or during pregnancy and ↓ size in menopause.
(Myometrium: inner layer of the uterus made up of smooth muscle composed of actin and myosin).
Types: Intramural, subserous, submucosa.
MC: African American women.

SX: Estrogen sensitive = increases in size with periods and pregnancy and decreases in size with menopause, heavy periods (menorrhagia), dysmenorrhea. Uterus is firm, **asymmetric**, **nontender**, enlarged.
Lab: β-hCG is negative.

DX: Hysteroscopy for submucosa fibroid. Ultrasound and MRI for intramural or submucosa.

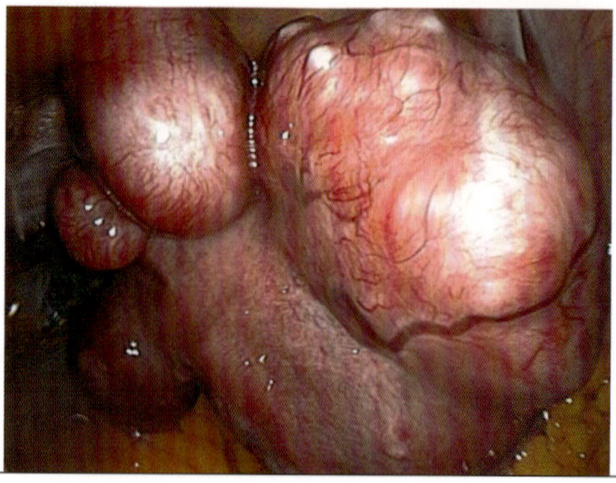

Complications: Infertility (difficult for implantation of the embryo), menorrhagia (excessive menstrual bleeding), anemia (if ↑ chronic bleeding), acute abdominal pain in pregnant women because of the degeneration of the tumor due to lace of blood supply, can compress the ureter/bladder or rectum.

Histology: **Whorled**/ball of smooth muscle bundles.

TX: Asymptomatic: no treatment.
Symptomatic: Embolization. Surgery: Hysteroscopic resection or hysterectomy.

Ovarian Cysts

Luteal or Follicular Cyst:
MC cyst during reproductive years. Asymptomatic, Negative β-hCG, ultrasound shows simple, fluid filled cyst.
DX: Transvaginal or abdominal ultrasound. If asymptomatic no additional follow up.
Removal of cyst by laparoscope if cyst is >7 cm in diameter or there has been a previous steroid contraception that did not resolve the cyst.

Corpus Luteum Ovarian Cyst
Ovarian cyst that ruptures at menstruation once egg has been released from follicle. Ceases after menopause.

Follicular Ovarian Cyst
MC ovarian cyst in young woman.
Cyst occurs when the follicle does not rupture to release the egg and becomes a cyst. Has thin walls, lined by granulosa cells with clear fluid.

Endometrioid Ovarian Cyst
Associated with endometriosis. Cyst forms on the ovary and is filled with blood ("chocolate cyst")

Hemorrhagic Ovarian Cyst
Develops when a blood vessel inside of an ovarian cyst ruptures. Blood filled cyst expands causing abdominal pain. Blood clots can form restricting the blood flow and causing damage to the ovaries. Usually self-limiting.

Ovarian Cysts continued

Theca-lutein Ovarian Cyst
Bilateral ovarian cyst filled with clear fluid. Cyst occur when there is an abnormal level of β-HCG. Associated with multiple gestations or molar pregnancies. Cyst resides when β-HCG levels decrease. Can increase risk of choriocarcinoma.

Dermoid Ovarian Cyst
Benign **teratoma** (germ cell tumor) that contains mature, solid tissues: skin, bone, teeth, thyroid tissue (produces TSH so can cause hyperthyroidism), cartilage, blood, hair.
MC in women during reproductive years: Ages teens to forties).

TX: Laparotomy to remove the tumor or oophorectomy.

Dermoid/Teratoma Cyst/Tumor

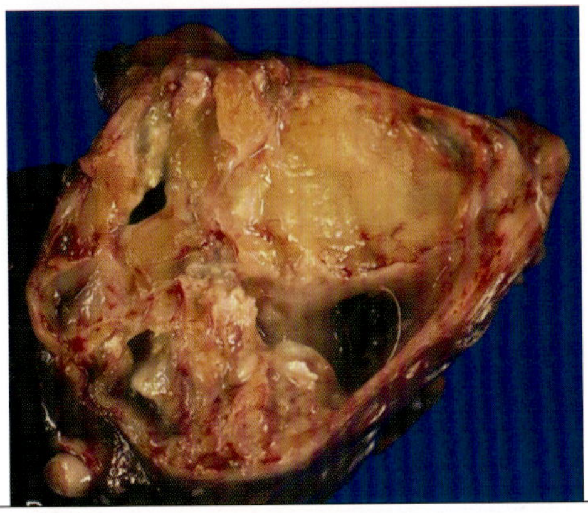

Ovarian Benign Tumors

Brenner Ovarian Tumor
Unilateral, benign. Surface epithelial stromal tumor.
Histology: Nest of **transitional** epithelial (bladder) cells that is yellow/tan in color.
Stain shows: "Coffee bean" shaped nuclei.

Fibroma Ovarian Tumor
Benign sex cord-stromal tumor (tumor derived from stromal components of the ovary and testis).
Occurs during perimenopause and Postmenopause.
Histology: Bundles of **spindle cells** producing **collagen**.

Endometrioma Ovarian Tumor
Associated with endometriosis. Cyst forms on the ovary and is filled with blood ("chocolate cyst")

Mature Cystic Ovarian Teratoma
(AKA: **Dermoid cyst**)
Benign teratoma that contains mature, solid tissues: skin, bone, teeth, **thyroid tissue (can produce TSH)**, cartilage, blood, hair.

NOTE: All ovarian masses must be evaluated by:
An ultrasound, β-hCG, Laparotomy if the tumor is complex and/or >7 cm.

Immature Teratoma
Germ cell tumor.
Malignant, immature teratoma. Like the mature teratoma/dermoid, it contains hair, bone, teeth, etc., but also contains primitive neuroepithelium (embryonic tissue).
MC in girls and young women up to their early twenties.
Labs: Increased HCG and AFP.

Ovarian Malignant Neoplasms

- SX: MC in women > 50, weight loss, enlarging abdomen.
- **CA-125 marker** is used to follow the response to treatment and progression of cancer.
  NOTE: CA-125 can be also be elevated with pancreatitis, cirrhosis, endometriosis, peritonitis.
- **DX: Sonogram for premenopausal. CT for postmenopausal women.**
  Biopsy. Check for tumor markers.

Ovarian Mutations
NOTE: **K-RAS and BRAF** (downstream mediator of K-RAS) are associated in serous tumors of the ovary (ovarian teratoma).
C-KIT mutations are associated with dysgerminomas (ovarian counterpart of a seminoma: MC type of malignant ovarian germ cell tumors.

Additional Ovarian Benign Tumors

Mucinous Cystadenoma Ovarian Tumor
Benign cystic tumor lined by mucus secreting epithelium.

Ovarian Serous Cystadenoma Tumor
MC type of benign ovarian tumor.
Histology: Unilocular cysts that containing clear fluid. The cyst is lined with simple ciliated epithelium.

Thecoma Ovarian Tumor
Benign sex cord-stromal ovarian tumor composed of theca cells. They are able to produce estrogen. Cause postmenopausal bleeding.
Histology: Consist of ovarian cortex with cells having abundant lipid-filled cytoplasm.

- **TX: Surgical debulking of the visible tumor. Premenopausal: Salpingo-oophorectomy. Postmenopausal: Total abdominal hysterectomy (TAH).**

Choriocarcinoma
Germ cell tumor (testes/ovary). Malignancy of trophoblastic tissue (cytotrophoblasts, syncytiotrophoblasts). No placental chorionic villi. Can occur during or after pregnancy.
Labs: Abnormal ↑ β-HCG.
Early hematogenous spread to lungs.
SX: During pregnancy: hydatidiform mole, spontaneous abortion, ectopic pregnancy, hyperemesis gravidarum.

Dysgerminoma
Malignant germ cell tumor. (Germ cells give rise to the gametes: sperm and egg).
(Equivalent to the male seminoma). MC: in adolescence and young adults.
Associated with ↑ serum lactic dehydrogenase (LDH).
Tumor markers: LDH, β-HCG, AFP.
Histology: Smooth, knobby external surface. Uniform cells resembling primordial germ cells. Stroma contains granulomas and lymphocytes.
Ultrasound shows cystic mass.
Metastasis to lymph nodes.

Ovarian Malignant Neoplasms

Krukenberg Ovarian Tumor
Malignant metastasis from stomach adenocarcinoma.
Histology: shows mucus producing **signet ring cells.** (Cells filled with mucus that pushes nucleus to the cell periphery).
Tumor marker: CEA

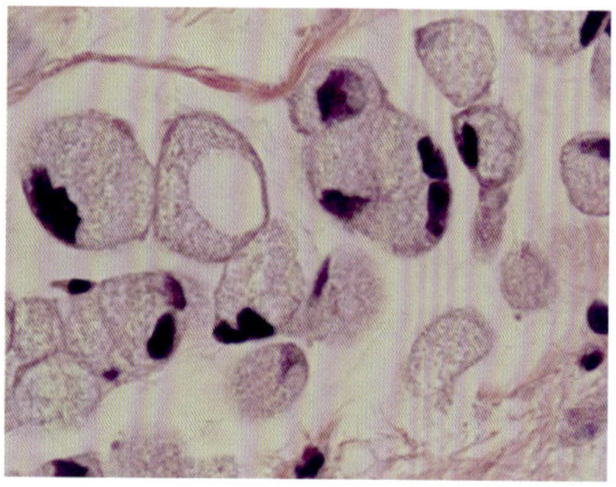

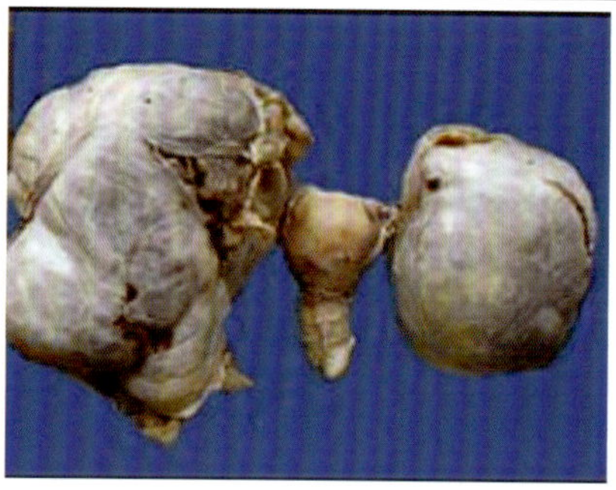

Granulosa-theca Cell Tumor627
MC Sex cord-stromal tumor.
Malignant. Arises from granulosa cells.
MC: presents in the 50's.
Tumor marker: Inhibin, Estrogen

Produces ↑ estrogen and/or progesterone, which cause endometrial hyperplasia. Presents with abnormal uterine bleeding in postmenopausal women. Women of reproductive age present with menometrorrhagia (irregular and more frequent periods), uterus myohyperplasia and absence of postmenopausal signs and in children can present with precocious puberty.
Removal of the tumor will cause regression of all precocious signs.

Histology: "call-Exner" bodies (primordial follicles)

Yolk Sac Ovarian Tumor
(AKA: Endodermal sinus tumor)
Malignant germ cell tumor. MC tumor in male infants.
Histology: endodermal cells that secret alpha-fetoprotein (AFP), Schiller-Duval bodies (resemble a glomerulus: mesodermal core with central capillary) with cytoplasm containing **AFP and A1AT**.

Mucinous Cystadenocarcinoma
Malignant ovarian epithelial tumor. Tumors are multilocular with multiple smooth, thin walled cyst. Cyst contain hemorrhagic and/or cellular debris.

Papillary Serous Cystadenocarcinoma
AKA: Epithelial-stromal ovarian tumor or Ovarian Adenocarcinoma.
MC malignant ovarian cancer in postmenopausal women.
Bilateral.
Histology: Psammoma bodies. Tall, columnar ciliated epithelial cells filled with clear serous fluid.
Tumor markers: CA-125, CEA

Sertoli-Leydig Cell (stromal tumor).
Ovarian tumor that secretes testosterone.
Woman presents with masculine symptoms: hirsutism, clitoral enlargement, balding.
Tumor markers: Testosterone.

Vaginal Tumors

Sarcoma Botryoides
(AKA: Embryonal Rhabdomyosarcoma)
Presents on mucosal surface of the wall of the vagina in girls < 8 years old, onset by age of 3.

Microscopy shows rhabdomyoblasts that contain cross-striations.

SX: "bunch of grapes" protruding from vagina and vaginal bleeding.
Histology: Spindle shaped tumor cells with cross striations.
Desmin +.

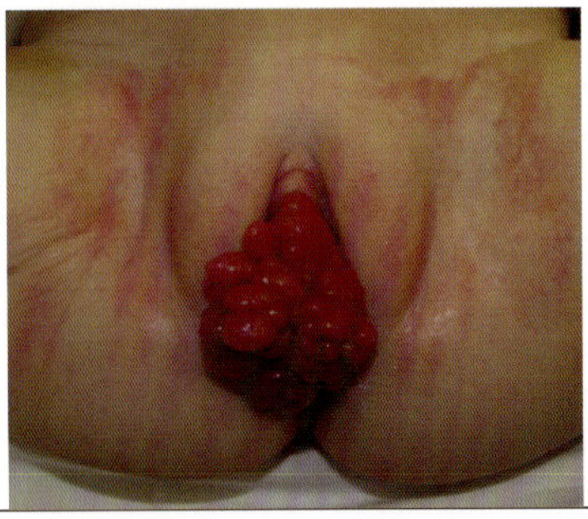

Vaginal Tumors

Clear Cell Adenocarcinoma
Associated with daughters of mothers who took DES (diethylstilbestrol- drug believed to prevent miscarriages 1938 – 1971)) while pregnant.
DES also increases risk of adenomyosis.

Vaginal Tumors

Squamous Cell Carcinoma of the Vagina
Found in women > 60 with multiple medical issues.
Arises from the squamous cells that line the vagina.
Radiation TX is excellent for poor surgical candidates.
Stage 1 and II or < 2 cm = surgical removal.

Pregnancy Tumor

Luteoma of Pregnancy
Benign tumor (stromal cell) that occurs in the ovaries during pregnancy due to an increase of progesterone and testosterone (sex hormones).
Bilateral, multi-nodule, solid masses on both ovaries.
B-HCG influences stromal cells to replace normal ovarian tissue.
↑ risk in pregnant Afro-Caribbean > 30, PCOS, previous luteoma, multiple pregnancies, advance maternal age.

SX: Masculinization of mother and sometimes the fetus. Sudden onset of hirsutism, acne, temporal balding, clitoromegaly.

TX: Self-limiting.

(Note: most all solid tumors indicate malignancy, but not with luteoma of pregnancy)

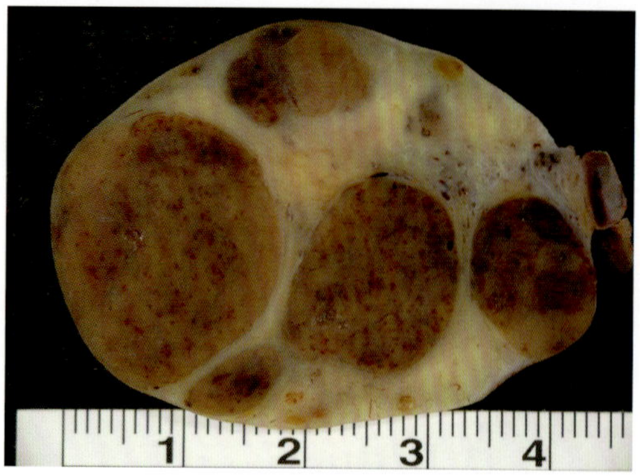

Differentials For Sudden Onset Hirsutism and Virilization (clitoromegaly) During Pregnancy
- **Ultrasound (US) to study ovaries**

US Results and differentials	**No Ovarian Masses.** **Must to abdominal CT to rule out adrenal mass.**	**Bilateral Cystic.** **Theca Lutein Cyst. Check for ↑ HCG**	**Bilateral and Solid.** **Rule out pregnancy or Luteoma**	**Unilateral Solid.** **Perform laparotomy to rule out malignancy**

Management for Asymptomatic Post Menopausal Pelvic Masses
- **Transvaginal ultrasound**
- **CA-125 level. Any ↑ in CA-125 indicated ovarian cancer**
- **If ultrasound shows a simple cyst and negative CA-125 and the mass < 10 cm: follow and monitor the mass**

GYN Cancer Risk

Cancer	**Risk Factors**
Squamous Cell Carcinoma of Cervix or Vagina	HPV (↑ number of sex partners)
Endometrial Adenocarcinoma	HTN, Tamoxifen, Diabetes, Obesity, Nulliparity, unopposed estrogen
Ovarian Cancer	Nulliparity, Lack of OCP use, early menses, late menopause, Family Hx. (**Anything** that allows more time of exposure to estrogen)

GYN Cancer Markers

Cancer	**Marker/Notes**
Granulosa Cell or Theca Cell Tumor	↑ Estrogen. Cuboidal cells with ↑ lipids (acidophilic: Exner Bodies). Solid ovarian mass that causes vaginal bleeding older postmenopausal women.
Ovarian Carcinoma	↑ AFP. Also see this with liver cancer and non-seminoma testicular cancer.
Ovarian Cancer	CA-125 marker. This marker is monitored for the reoccurrence of the cancer.

Breast Pathologies , Tumors and Cancers

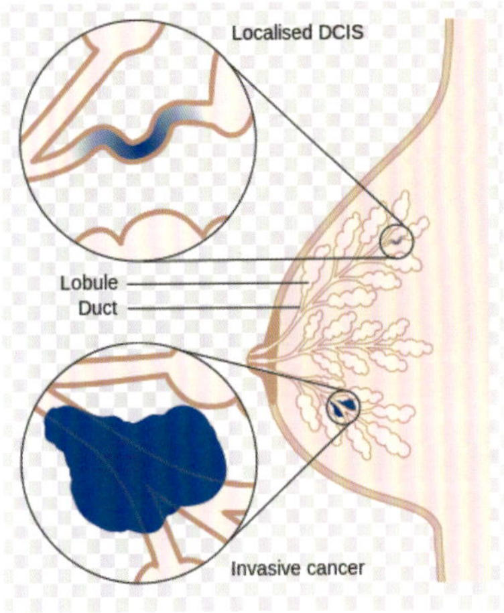

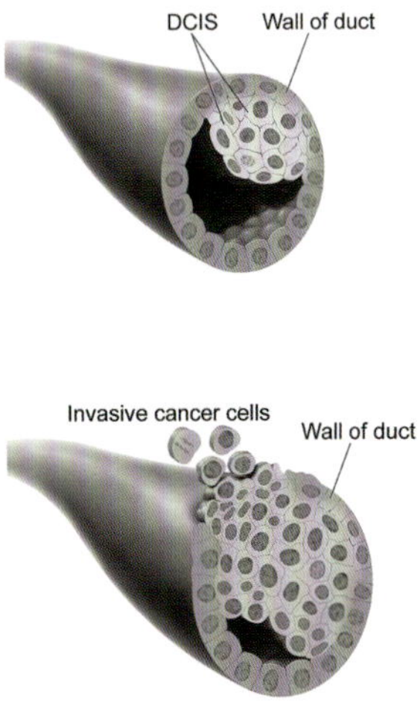

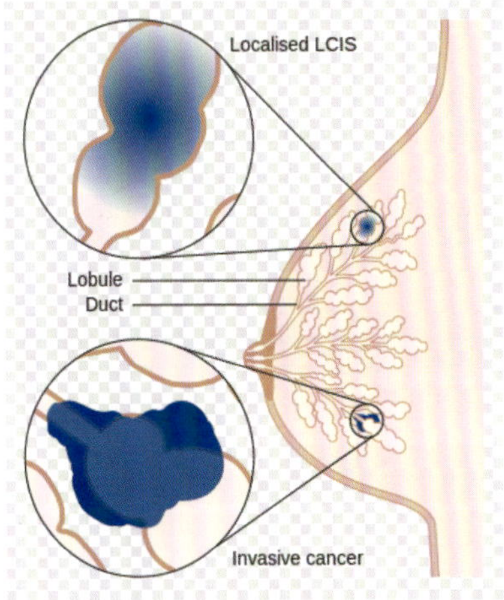

Breast Cancer and Breast Cancer Characteristics

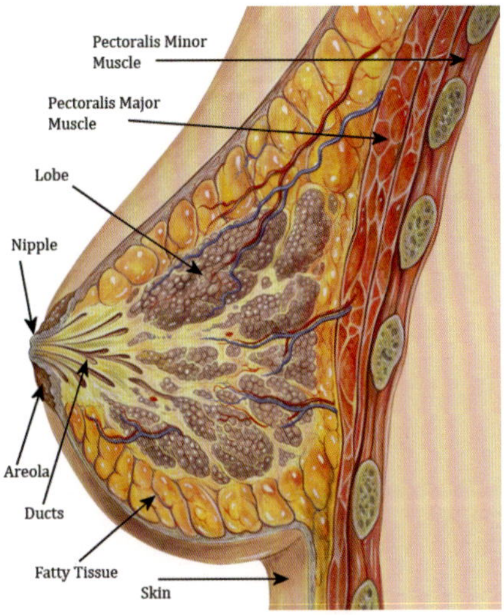

- **Risk factors:** previous breast cancer, age, sex, nulliparous, late menopause, early menarche, obesity, first degree-relative with breast cancer, high-fat diets.
- Most important prognosis: **TMN staging (Axillary lymph node involvement)**
- Breast cancer metastasizes to: **lung, brain, liver, bone**
- Malignant breast cancer is MC in women > 45: mobile mass in the upper outer quadrant, irregular boarders, no calcifications. Initial Test: FNB (Fine needle biopsy)
- Early detection is critical
- **Screening:** Mammography begins at **50 years old** and then every 2 years until the age of 75.
- NOTE: MC bilateral nipple milky discharge is a prolactinoma. Check prolactin and TSH levels.
- If family history of breast cancer, screening should begin 5 years before the age of the family member was diagnosed.
- Infiltrating Ductal and Lobular Carcinomas have the worse prognosis. Medullary and Mucinous have intermediate and Tubular and Cribriform have the most favorable prognosis.
- Anatomy: 10 – 15 lobes in each breast.

- **DX Options:**
  - **Ultrasound: if the mass is painful or varies in size during menses. It will also show if the mass is solid or cystic.**
  - **Biopsy: Abnormal mammogram requires a biopsy to rule in or rule out cancer and to test for the presence of estrogen and progesterone receptors. If cancer is ruled in, an axillary lymph node is dissected (open biopsy during surgery) and then a sentinel node (first group of lymph nodes that drain a cancer) biopsy is performed to see if the cancer has metastasized.**
  - **Pet Scan: Used to evaluate lymph nodes that cannot be reached by biopsy. If there is cancer, there will be an increased uptake on the PET scan.**
- TX: Lumpectomy and radiation.
  Tamoxifen: Preventive therapy in patients that have more than one first-degree relative that has breast cancer and when there are positive receptors found for estrogen and/or progesterone. If axillary nodes are positive or the cancer is > 1 cm in size, add adjuvant chemotherapy with the Tamoxifen.
  Adjuvant chemotherapy used if: Cancer is > 1 cm or is located in the axilla.
  Trastuzumab (monoclonal antibody) to treat HER-2/NEU. It decreases risk of the cancer reoccurring.
- **Infiltrating Ductal and Lobular Carcinomas have the worse prognosis. Medullary and Mucinous have intermediate and Tubular and Cribriform have the most favorable prognosis.**
- Anatomy: 10 – 15 lobes in each breast.

Benign	Malignant
• Freely **mobile** mass, round, not attached to surrounding tissue • Movable mass that **change** in size with **menstrual cycle** • **Well circumscribed** • Wider than deep • **Smooth** and round with surrounding fibrous capsule • Cells multiple slowly • Tumor grows by expanding and pushing away and against surrounding tissue • Never metastasizes • Easy to remove and does not reoccur • **Foamy macrophages** • **Course calcifications** • Bilateral discharge that is clear, milky, yellow or green (nonbloody). • Bloody discharge (intraductal papilloma: benign)	• **Fixed** or ulcerating, or nodular mass • **Irregular** shaped with no capsule • Cells multiple rapidly. Irregular size/shape of cell and nucleus • Chromatin clump irregularly • Nucleoli are large, irregular, prominent • Tumor grows by invading and destroying surrounding tissue • Mass is fixed. Attached or deeply fixed to surrounding tissue • Metastasizes if not removed/destroyed • Difficult to remove and can reoccur • **Microcalcifications** • Unilateral discharge • Bloody, serous (watery), sticky, brown, black discharge • **Dimpling** of skin • Osteoblastic bone metastasis (Osteoblastic: deposition of new bone. Osteolytic: destruction of normal bone.)
Benign Pathologies	**Malignant Pathologies**
Fibroadenoma **Fibrocystic change** Fat necrosis (due to trauma to breast tissue) Mastitis (breastfeeding moms) Intraductal papilloma Prolactinoma (due to pituitary tumor)	DCIS (Ductal Carcinoma In Situ) LCIS (Lobular Carcinoma In Situ) Paget's disease of the breast Inflammatory breast cancer Invasive ductal carcinoma Invasive lobular carcinoma

Breast Cancer Definitions

- HER2- positive
  - 20 - 25% of breast cancers.
  - Abnormal estrogen receptor.
  - Aggressive, fast growing.
  - Cancer cells have more of the protein, which cause these cells to grow and spread faster than the cells with the normal level of the HER2 protein.
  - DX test: FISH or IHC test
  - **Trastuzumab** (Herceptin) decreases risk of cancer reoccurring.

- Endocrine receptor-positive (estrogen or progesterone receptors)
  - 80% of all breast cancers are estrogen-positive (ER): cancer cells grow in response to estrogen.
  - 65% of all breast cancers are progesterone-positive (PR): cancer cells grow in response to progesterone.
  - ER/PR – positive cancers respond better to hormone therapy than ER/PR – negative.
  - **SERM's: Tamoxifen, Raloxifene**: inhibits cancer from coming back by blocking hormone receptors, preventing hormones from binding to them. (Tamoxifen: pre and postmenopausal women. Raloxifene (postmenopausal women)
    Aromatase Inhibitors: Anastrozole, Exemestane: stops estrogen production (only for postmenopausal).

- BRCA1 and BRCA
  - ↑ risk of ovarian and breast cancer.
  - BRCA mutations also increase the risk of pancreatic, colon, stomach, gallbladder, uterine or melanoma cancers.
  - Men who test positive for BRCA run a risk for breast, pancreatic, testicular and prostate cancer.
  - 20 - 25% of inherited cancers: breast and ovarian.
  - 10% of all breast cancers and 15% of all cervical cancers. 20 - 25% of inherited cancers: breast and ovarian.
  - Can be inherited from a person's mother or father.
  - Child of a parent with the BRAC1 or BRAC2 mutation has a 50% of inheriting the mutation.
  - Human genes that produce tumor suppressor proteins. (Tumor suppressors repair damaged DNA). If either BRAC1 or BRAC2 are mutated then it can't protect against DNA damage, leading to a higher risk of cancer.
  - Screen for the BRCA mutation: If a family member has breast or ovarian cancer.
    ↑ Risk of the BRCA mutation if ≥ 2 or more close relatives had breast cancer before age 50, a male relative has breast cancer, a female relative has both breast and ovarian cancer, 2 relatives have ovarian cancer or you are of Ashkenazi Jewish ancestry and a close relative has breast or ovarian cancer.
    Low risk of having a BRCA mutation if: No relatives had breast cancer before age 50, no relatives with ovarian cancer and no male relatives that had breast cancer.
  - Prophylactic treatment: mastectomy and/or oophorectomy

Diagnosing Breast Cancer

- Ultrasound and/or Mammogram: **MUST be done before a biopsy.**
  Mammography and biopsy if woman >50 years old. (Biopsy can be done alone on women <40).
- Mammography is performed when these SX present:
  Bloody nipple discharge, blood fluid upon aspiration of a cyst, if a cyst recurs > twice within 4-6 weeks, skin edema with erythema, or the mass does not disappear completely during a FNB.
- **Biopsy Types**
  - **BIT: Fine needle biopsy (FNA).**
  - **Core Biopsy. Takes more breast tissue than FNA. Will test for estrogen (ER) and progesterone (PR) and HER 2/NEU.**
    Core biopsy is superior to FNA.
  - **MAT: Sentinel Lymph Node Biopsy. Performed during mastectomy/lumpectomy surgery. Sentinel node biopsy (sentinel nodes are the first group of lymph nodes draining the cancer) is used to stage the cancer, to see if the cancer has metastasized. If the sentinel node is negative then axillary lymph node dissection is not necessary.**

Breast Cancer Grading and Staging

Grades

Indicates the severity of the mutation and the likelihood that it will spread.
How closely the cells resemble healthy cells.
The shape and size of the nuclei.
How rapidly the cells divide and multiply.
Grades determine the best treatment plan.
The lower the grade the better chance of full recoveries at every stage (including aggressive ones)

- Low grade (1): well differentiated
- Intermediate grade (2): moderately differentiated
- High grade (3): Poorly differentiated

Staging: TNM

"T" Tumor size = the size of the tumor and the number of lymph nodes affected.
"N" Nodes = the nearest lymph nodes are the axillary (under the arm)
"M" Metastases = Signs of metastases in other organs (bones, liver, lungs, brain)

- Stage 0,1: Earliest detection. Cells confined to limited area
- Stage 2, 2A: Early stages but beginning to spread. Responds well to treatment
- Stage 3 A, B, C: Advanced, evidence of invasion of surrounding tissues near the breast (lymph nodes/muscle)
- Stage 4: Cancer has metastasized (brain, bones, lungs, liver)

Breast Cancer Epidemiology

- Steady increase in the incidence of breast cancer as women age. Highest rates are in postmenopausal women ≥ 50 years old.
- Family History: Relative risk in a woman with breast cancer in a first degree relative (mother, sister, daughter) ranges 1.5 – 2.5
- Reproductive factors: The younger a woman's age at menarche, the higher her risk of breast cancer. For each 2 yrs delay in onset of menses, the risk is reduced by 10%
- The earlier a woman has her first birth, the lower her lifetime risk for breast cancer. Women who have their first birth after the age of 30 have an increased risk. A nulliparous woman has an increased risk.
- The later a woman's age at menopause, the higher her risk of breast cancer. Women who have menopause after 55 yrs. Have twice the risk of those who had menopause before 45.
- Women who have had breast cancer have a 10 fold increased risk in developing a second primary breast cancer
- Breast cancer is more common in Western industrialized countries than in developing countries
- Additional risk factors: hormone therapy, obesity (BMI ≥ 30), higher socioeconomic status, history of breast cancer, exposure to ionizing radiation, BRCA1/BRCA2 carrier, benign breast disease.

Breast Cancer Treatments

- Invasive cancer when the tumor is <5 cm: Lumpectomy (breast conserving) and radiotherapy. Chemotherapy (adjuvant) can also be added.
- Chemotherapy is added to therapy when tumor is >1cm and/or if the cancer is lymph node positive.
- Hormone therapy (adjuvant): for all hormone receptor-positive tumors (ER+ and PR+ receptors).
  Tamoxifen (binds estrogen receptors) for 5 years. For pre and postmenopausal women.
  LHRH analogs (**Goserelin**): can be used separately or with **Tamoxifen**. For premenopausal women.
  Oophorectomy can be done separately or with Tamoxifen.
  Aromatase Inhibitors (**Anastrozole, Letrozole, Exemestane**) block peripheral production of estrogen. For postmenopausal women.
- Trastuzumab (monoclonal antibody against the HER2/neu receptor) is used for: HR-positive, premenopausal women, HR-negative, pre- or postmenopausal women, and HR-positive, postmenopausal women.
- Inflammatory cancer when the tumor is >5 cm: systemic therapy.
- Sentinel node biopsy (preferred) or axillary node dissection.

Benign Breast Pathologies

Acute Mastitis	Fat Necrosis
Breast abscess during breast-feeding caused by milk stasis or a bacterial infection. Infection cause: MCC: **S. aureus** (enters through cracks in the nipple). (Also by: S. epidermidis or streptococci) SX: pain, swelling, erythema, warmth, fever, chills. An abscess is also possible. TX: Heat packs, antibiotics, and patient **MUST** continue nursing. (The baby will not get infection) **Dicloxacillin. Cephalexin** (Abscess: will need incision and drainage)	Benign painless lump that develops after an injury to the breast (sports, accidents, seat belt, surgery, needle biopsy, spouse abuse). It does not increase chances of breast cancer. SX: Hard lump, usually painless but can have pain around the necrosis, possible drainage from the nipple (if near the bruised area), dimpled/retracted skin around the damage. Oil cyst: oily fluid that the necrosis contains. Mammogram: Shows necrotic fat cells. TX: Self -limiting. If it develops an oil cyst, drainage may be necessary.
Gynecomastia Development of breast tissue in males due to ↑ estrogen as compared to androgens. **Normal in infants** (estrogen produced by the placenta) **and in puberty** development in males. Also normal to be seen in older males due to ↓ in testosterone and increase of fatty tissue (fat synthesizes estrogen). (**Caution**: this question will generally show a concerned mother bringing her son in because he is embarrassed in the locker room at school. He will be 14 – 17 yrs old. If all else (tanner scale corresponds to puberty), simply reassure the mother. This is normal and he will grow out of it). **Other causes**: Klinefelter dz, kidney failure (damage to testicles/testosterone synthesis due to ↑ urea), Leydig or Sertoli cell tumors. Drugs: **anti-androgen therapy (flutamide, spironolactone) 5-alpha-reductase inhibitors (finasteride), ketoconazole, cimetidine, GnRH analogues, Verapamil, Amlodipine, anabolic steroids, alcohol, omeprazole, opiods, digitalis, estrogen, marijuana, heroin, Dopamine antagonist.**	Gynecomastia 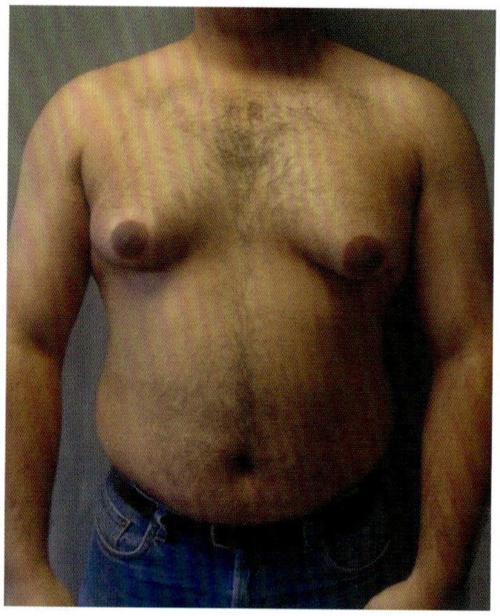

Benign Breast Tumors

Fibroadenoma	Fibrocystic Breast Disease
Benign tumor of glandular and fibrous tissue (stromal and epithelial cells). MC benign tumor of women **under 35** years old. SX: 1 lesion, can be painless or tender, **mobile**, clear defined **sharp edges**. Hormone dependent: **Changes size with menstrual cycles**, or ↑ estrogen (pregnancy). Subside after menopause. Histology: **Foam** cells (macrophages), FNB shows: epithelium and **stromal** cells. Nodular and encapsulated. TX: None	Benign breast lumps common in women of childbearing ages. SX: Bilateral, tender breast lumps ("cobblestone" texture) that changes with menstrual cycles. Lumps peak before periods. MC in upper, outer sections of breast (armpit region). Subsides after menopause. Histology: Cystic mass filled with clear fluid. Little risk of progression to cancer unless family hx. TX: Initial: Mammography to determine if lump is a cyst. If a cyst: FNB. If fluid is bloody or foul smelling → cytology If fluid is clear: no treatment, follow up in 6 weeks.

Intraductal Papilloma	Phyllodes Tumor
Benign "wart like" tumor that develops in the lactiferous ducts near or under the nipple/areola that can puncture a duct causing a discharge. MCC of clear or bloody nipple discharge in women 20 – 40 yrs. Increased risk for breast cancer. 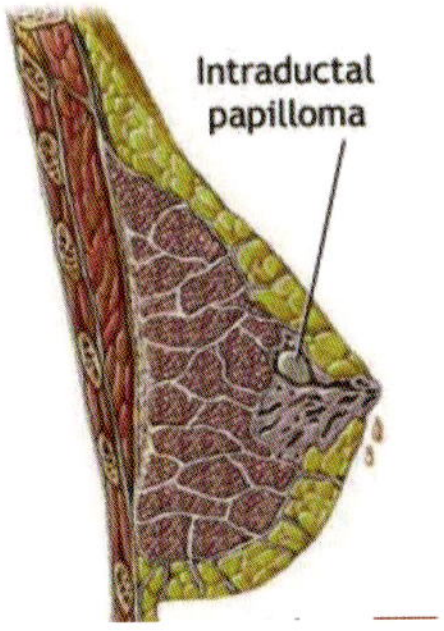 	Normally benign but can progress to malignant. MC: older women 40 – 50 yrs. (but can be found in any age) SX: Large and fast growing mass (increases in size in just a few weeks). Histology: Epithelial, glandular (lobule and duct), stromal (connective) tissue. Grows in a "leaf like" (Phyllodes – leaflike). TX: Surgical removal. (Phyllodes tumors can reoccur after removal).

Malignant Breast Tumors

Non-invasive Malignant Breast Tumors

Ductal Carcinoma in situ (DCIS)	Comedocarcinoma
(**"in situ"** = "in place" – not having moved out of the duct. It has not "YET" become invasive = **has not crossed basement membrane to invade surrounding tissues**). (**tip**: cancer is still "In Side" the tube) Pre-cancerous/non-invasive lesion. Stage 0. MC in women in their 50's. SX: Lump in breast or under the arm, nipple discharge, tenderness, warmth, and erythema. Histology: abnormal cells lining the ducts and lobules of the mammary gland. Microcalcifications (calcium deposits) found on mammogram. DX: Mammogram TX: Surgical removal with clear margins (lumpectomy), Radiation and **Tamoxifen** for 5 years to decrease risk of progressing into invasive breast cancer. **Lobular Carcinoma in situ (LCIS)** MC: Premenopausal women. TX: **Tamoxifen** for 5 years to decrease risk of developing breast cancer.	Non-invasive, intraductal tumor involving multiple ducts. Type of Ductal Carcinoma in situ. (Early stage of breast cancer). Increased risk for breast cancer. Histology: Tissue showing areas of black or white-to-pale yellow **necrosis** surrounded by large pleomorphic cancer cells with irregular nuclei. Mammograms show a branching pattern along with calcifications. 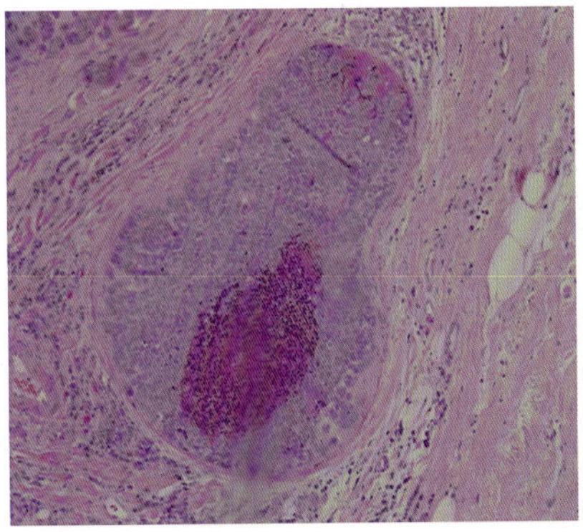

Paget Disease of the Breast/Nipple

Lesion that affects the nipple and areola.

SX: **Eczema-like rash** on the skin of the nipple and areola (does not heal). Red, itchy, scaly, flaky, inflammation. Burning sensation. Bloody or yellow **discharge**. Nipple can be inverted.

Histology: Infiltration of Paget cells (large neoplastic cells with abundant **clear or pale cytoplasm ("halo")** with eccentric, hyperchromic nuclei and prominent nucleoli). Cells stain **positive for mucin.**

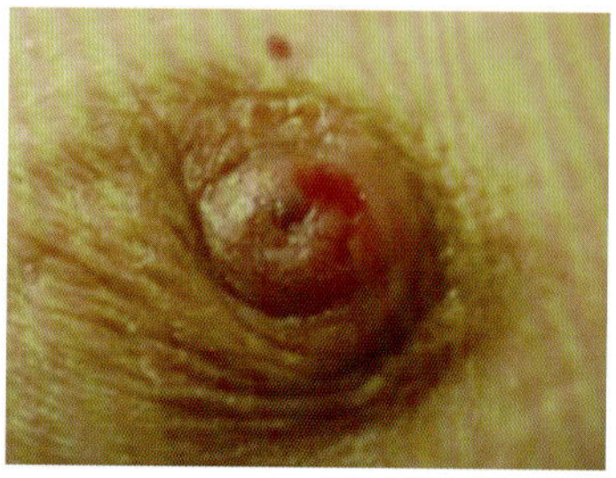

DX: Mammogram and FNB. Surgical removal.

Increased risk of breast cancer.

Cribriform/Micropapillary Carcinoma

Histology: Growth patterns form papillary structures with small fenestrations. Tumor cells are smaller and more uniform as compared to Comedocarcinoma. There is also **NO necrosis.**

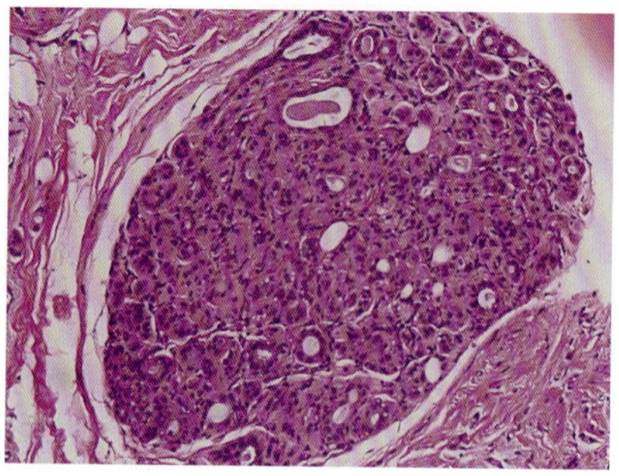

Cribriform/Micropapillary Carcinoma

Invasive Malignant Breast Tumors

Invasive Ductal Carcinoma

(AKA: Infiltrating Ductal Carcinoma)
MC: Invasive breast cancer.

SX: Unilateral. Hard, bumpy, irregularly shaped lump with sharp margins beneath the areola or central area of the breast. Nipple retraction.

Cancer begins in the ducts (the tubes that carry milk from the milk-producing lobules to the nipple). It attaches to surrounding structures and can cause dimpling of the skin and nipple retraction (due to traction on the suspensory ligaments).
MC type of breast cancer and MC in women 55 or older. Is the most common type of breast cancer that affects men.

Histology: Cancer cells have invaded into surrounding breast tissue. **Microcalcifications** and debris blocking the duct. Cells are small, **glandular** with irregular margins with **stellate infiltration**. Show yellow, chalky streaks. Malignant cells are infiltrating/invading the duct wall.
Express: e-cadherin.
Estrogen sensitive.

Metastasizes to #1) lymph nodes, then into bones, lung, liver, brain.

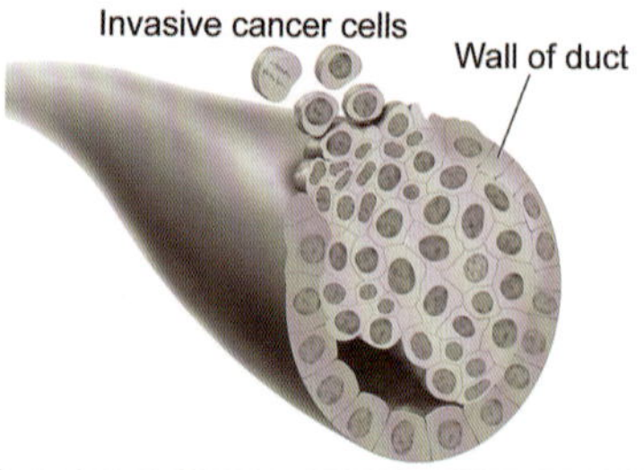

Invasive Lobular Carcinoma

(AKA: Infiltrating Lobular Carcinoma)
2nd MCC of invasive breast cancer.

SX: Can be bilateral with most being unilateral. Hardening/thickening in the breast, rather than a lump. It cannot normally be palpated. It is usually a coincidental finding. Swelling of the breast, breast and nipple pain, erythema, nipple discharge (other than breast milk).

Cancer begins in the milk-producing lobules (these empty into the ducts that carry milk to the nipple). Cancer cells have invaded into surrounding breast tissue.
MC in women in their 60's.

Histology: Cells are small and uniform with a round to oval nuclei and moderate pale cytoplasm. Cells infiltrate in **orderly rows** ("Indian file") and are larger than ductal carcinoma cells.
Estrogen sensitive.

DX: Mammography, ultrasound, Fine Needle/Core Needle biopsy.

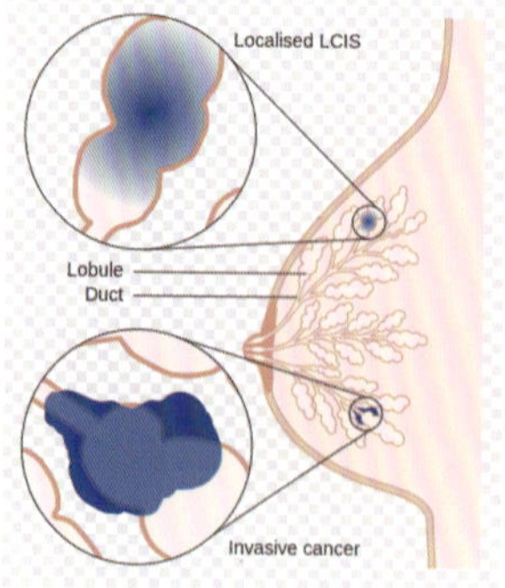

Medullary Carcinoma

Form of Invasive Duct Carcinoma.
Well-circumscribed mass. Soft, fleshy with areas of **necrosis and hemorrhage**.

SX: Feels more like a spongy area of breast tissue rather than a lump. May also feel smooth-sided (similar to a breast cyst)

Histology: Solid sheets of cells forming a **syncytium** (multinucleate mass of cytoplasm that is not separated into cells) with large pleomorphic nuclei, prominent nucleoli and a high mitotic rate. There is little fibrous stroma.
↑ lymphocytes and plasma cells around the sheets of tumor cells.

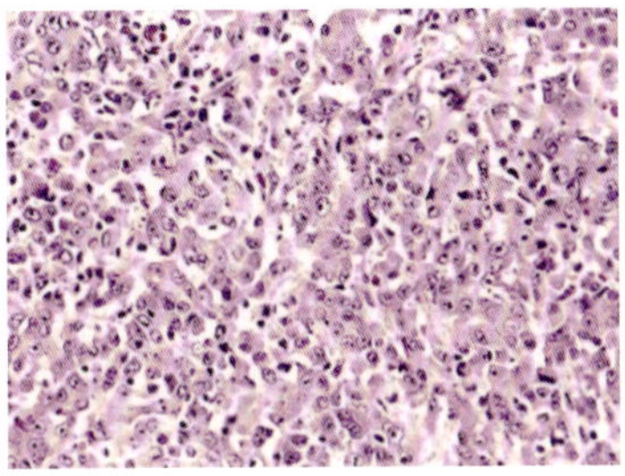

Mucinous Carcinoma
(AKA: Colloid Carcinoma)

Form of Invasive Duct Carcinoma.
MC in women in their 60's and 70's.
Less likely to spread than other types of breast cancer.

Histology: Sharply circumscribed, lacks fibrous stroma. Soft and gelatinous. Has a shinny surface when cut.
Majority of tumor is **mucinous** composed of isolated tumor cells floating in pools of extracellular mucin.

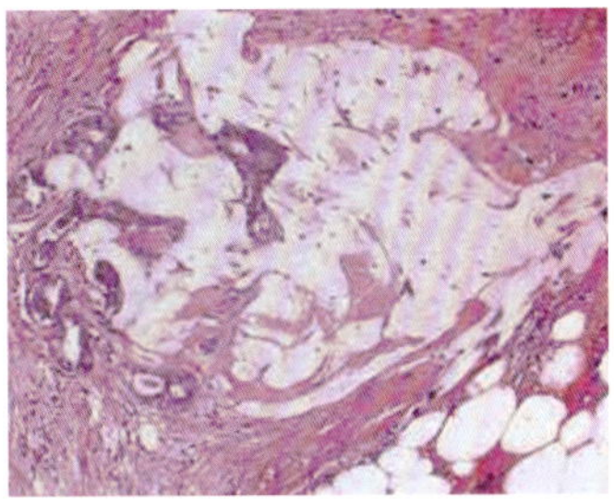

Tubular Carcinomas
Type of Invasive Ductal Carcinoma

Histology: Small glands (tubules) of varied shapes. Distribution is haphazard with single layers of cells lining each gland.
Calcifications on mammogram.
Estrogen receptor positive.

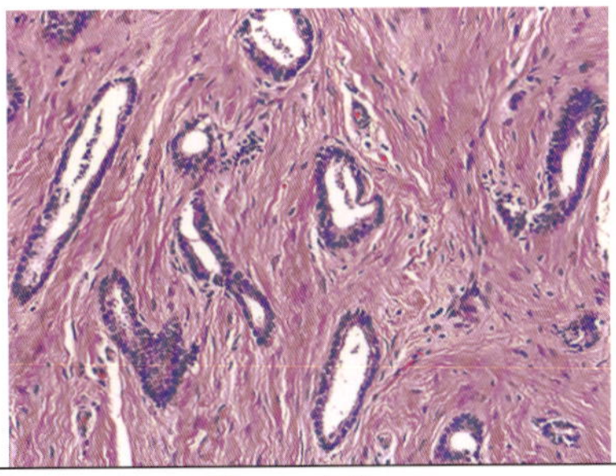

Cribriform Carcinoma
Type of Invasive Ductal Carcinoma

Cancer cells invade the stroma (connective tissue) in nest like formations between the ducts and lobules. Uniform, sharply outlined tumor cells are embedded in fibrous stroma within glandular spaces so that it looks like holes. (looks like Swiss cheese)

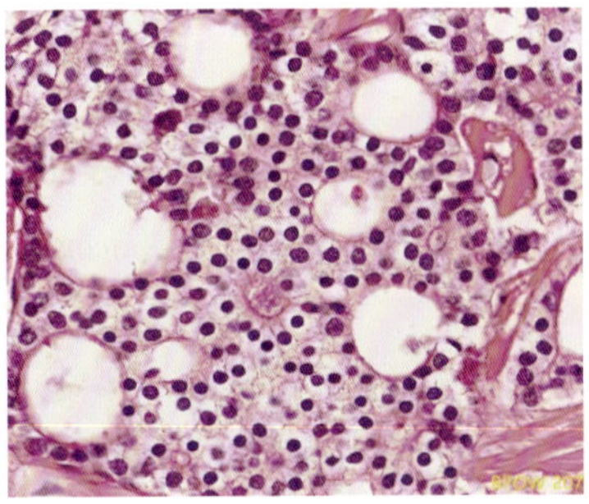

Inflammatory Breast Cancer

Aggressive breast cancer. Rapid and metastasizes early.
Occurs in woman of any age, MC between 40 – 60 yrs.
Difficult to detect by mammography or ultrasound.

SX: Skin changes, **dimpling of the skin (Peau d'orange),** nipple retraction, rapid increase in breast size, erythema, pruritis, skin is hot to touch (resembles mastitis), breast is harder/firmer/swollen.

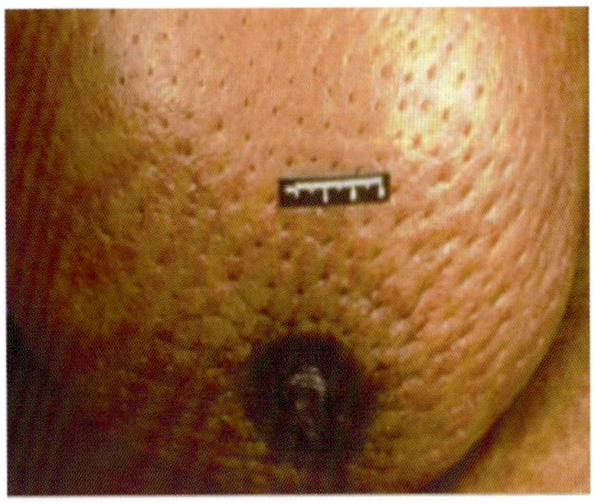

Peau d'orange: (**Dimpling of the skin** is caused by the **suspensory ligaments: Cooper's ligaments**). Cooper's ligaments connect mammary glands to the dermis of the overlying skin.

Cancer cells **invade the local lymph ducts causing** edematous swelling of the breast. (Lymph cannot drain).

Overexpression of **E-cadherin** and caveolin

DX: Biopsy

Breast Cancer in Men

Male breast cancer accounts for 1% of all breast cancers.

Increased risk: ↑ estrogen (due to genetics, drugs, alcohol, cirrhosis), radiation exposure (usually treatment for Hodgkin's lymphoma), family history of breast cancer, diseases of the testicles (mumps/orchitis), testicular injury, undescended testicle, genetic (Klinefelter's), breast cancer in close female relative.

MC: Infiltrating (Invasive) Ductal Carcinoma

SX: Non-painful mass **beneath the nipple**. Can be asymptomatic or can show skin changes: ulceration of the skin, puckering/dimpling of the skin, erythema, scaling, itching, retraction of the nipple, bloody or opaque discharge. Most are unilateral, 1% can be bilateral.
Malaise, weakness, unintentional weight loss. Symptoms in other organs that it may have metastasized to.

Prognosis: TMN Staging (same as for women)

DX: Biopsy, MRI, Ultrasound

TX: Surgery/mastectomy, Chemotherapy, Radiation therapy

Remember: It is normal for a baby boy to have "nodules" under his nipples and it is normal for a teenage boy to have gynecomastia.
It is NOT normal for a grown man to have a nodule under his nipple.

Breast Cancer Test

- **HER2: FISH (Fluorescence In Situ Hybridization) or IHC (Immunohistochemistry)**
- **P53: Gel Electrophoresis**
- **S Phase: Flow cytometry (↑proliferation = poor prognosis)**

Management of Palpable Breast Masses

- **If patient is < 30: perform an ultrasound**
  If US shows a simple cyst → needle aspirate (patient option)
  If US shows a complex cyst (solid) → core needle biopsy
- **If patient is > 30: perform an US and mammogram → suspicious results → core biopsy**

Recurrence of Breast Cancer

- Radical mastectomy (when involves **axillary lymph nodes**) → chronic lymphedema → Angiosarcoma (AKA: Steward Treves Syndrome) shows nodules in the arm.
- The only treatment for the lymphedema in the arm is **compression sleeves**

Prostate, Penis and Testicular Pathologies and Tumors

Benign Prostatic Hyperplasia (BPH)

Hyperplasia of the prostate gland.
MC in men > 50 years.

Digital exam: **Smooth, firm/rubbery enlargement** of the prostate gland.
Affects the **center** of the prostate where the urethra runs through. (Where as prostate cancer affects the periphery of the prostate).

SX: Gradual **change in urinary habits**. Difficulty starting and stopping the flow of urine, dribbling, dysuria, frequency, nocturia.

Complications: Inability to empty bladder may cause back up of urine = hydronephrosis, UTI's.
Stasis of urine can lead to urinary bladder stones.

NOTE: PSA levels can rise after digital exams of the prostate. PSA reading may not be accurate for several months.

TX: **α-1 antagonist: Doxazosin, Tamsulosin, Terazosin (relaxes smooth muscle), Finasteride (5α-reductase).**

TX: Surgical repair: **TURP** (Transurethral resection of the prostate). Side effects: **Retrograde ejaculate, AKA: dry ejaculate** (the prostate is responsible for adding semen to sperm).

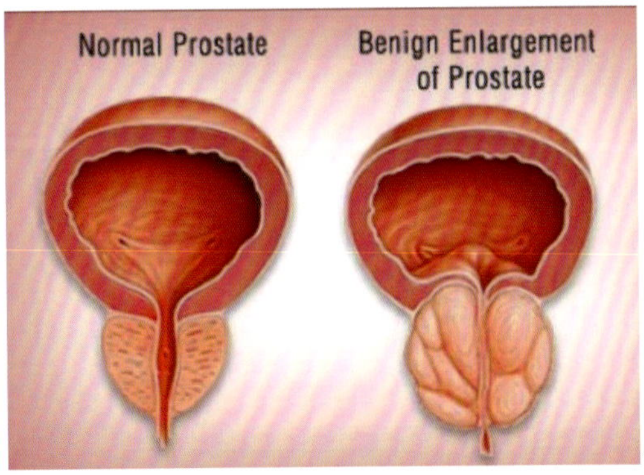

Acute Prostatitis

Acute inflammation of the prostate gland usually due to a bacterial infection. MC: **E. coli** (E. coli also the cause of UTI's and urethritis).

SX: (male UTI). Tender, boggy prostate, dysuria, urgency, frequency, supra-pubic pain and/or low back pain, tenderness in the perianal area and testicles, possible blood in the semen, high fever, chills, cloudy urine, urgency, dribble, frequency.

Caution: **Do not do massage the prostate** (will spread the bacteria)

DX: Urinalysis, urine cultures.

TX: 1st line: **Quinolones, Ciprofloxacin or Levofloxacin**.
2nd line: **TMP/SMX**

Chronic Prostatitis

Non-bacterial, > 20 leukocytes.
TX: Sitz baths and **anti-inflammatory's**

Epididymitis (AKA: Epididymo-orchitis)

(Orchitis: Inflammation of the testicle/s, but has same MOA, causes, treatment as Epididymitis)
(Epididymitis: where sperm mature and are stored)

SX: Pain of the epididymis, inflammation, erythema, warmth and swelling in the scrotum. Dysuria, urethral discharge.
Cremasteric reflex is intact (in testicular torsion, the reflex is absent).

Cause: In sexually active men <35: #1: Chlamydia and #2: Gonorrhea. In men > 35: E. coli.

TX: **Azithromycin and Ceftriaxone** for Chlamydia and gonorrhea. **Doxycyline** can be used instead of Azithromycin.
Ofloxacin, Levofloxacin for E. coli

Varicocele

Due to the backing up of blood draining the left testicle via the left gonadal vein, high pressure causes the veins in the **pampiniform plexus** to become **dilated** causing the scrotum to swell. (AKA: Bag of worms appearance)
(**Remember** most varicoceles occur on the **left side**: the left testicle must drain **via the left gonadal vein** (AKA: testicular vein) **into the left renal vein** at a 90° angle **and then into the IVC** while the right testicle drains via the right gonadal vein (AKA: right testicular vein) which drains directly into the IVC.

SX: Will not transilluminate, aching pain, feeling of heaviness in the testicle, "bag of works" disappears when lying down.
Complication: Infertility due to ↑ temperature in scrotum.
TX: Surgery

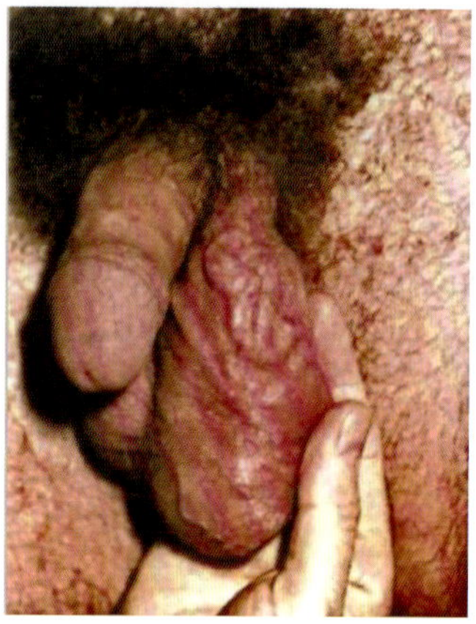

Hydrocele

Accumulation of clear fluid in the **tunica vaginalis** because the **processus vaginalis** in the embryonic development did not obliterate, it is still patent. (Tunica vaginalis is the membrane covering the testicle and epididymis).

SX: Painless, **swollen scrotum**. Can appear in boys or girls (Boys: swollen scrotum. Girls: swollen labia)
Transilluminates.

Causes: trauma, infection, tumor.

TX: Surgery

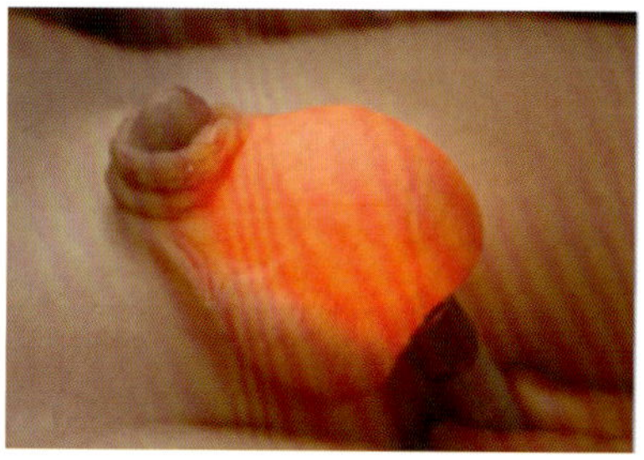

Illumination of a hydrocele

Cryptorchidism
Undescended Testis (one or both).
(This is NOT monarchism: having only one testicle)

Testes should descend within the **first few months** of life. If they have not descended, treatments **MUST** be done between 1 year and 2 years of age.
Treatments: β-hCG or testosterone hormone injections or surgery (orchiopexy).

Spermatogenesis requires cooler temperatures (<37°C). Testes that do not descend remain in the abdomen (too warm).

Complications if they do ascend: Infertility (↑ temperatures), increased risk of germ cell tumors.

Labs: If unilateral: LH, FSH, Inhibin are normal.
If bilateral: ↑FSH, ↑ LG, ↓ Inhibin.
(↑ temperatures = no Sertoli cells = no sperm)

Hypospadias (pictured below)
- **No fusion of urethral folds**
- Urethra opens on ventral (inferior) side of penis
- Risk of UTI's if not repaired
- In the female, no fusion of urethral folds = vagina

Epispadias
- Faulty positioning of genital tubercle
- Urethra opens on dorsal (superior) side of penis
- Associated with exstrophy (AKA: Ectopia vesicae) of the bladder (bladder outside of abdomen). Exstrophy of bladder: due to failure of caudal fold closure

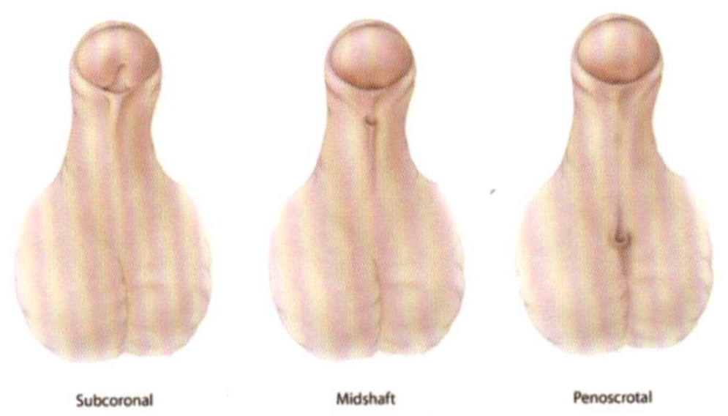

Testicular Torsion

When the **spermatic cord twists** (testicle is suspended from the spermatic cord). When it twist it cuts off blood supply to the testicle = ischemia.

SX: Acute, severe testicular pain, nausea, vomiting, testis is higher than its normal position, swelling. **Loss or decrease of cremasteric reflex** (stroking the inside of the thigh normally causes the testicles to be pulled up, but this reflex is lost in testicular torsion).

Note:
Cremasteric reflex is elicited via nerve roots **L1 and L2**. The Genitofemoral nerve mediates Cremasteric reflex.

DX: Ultrasound.

TX: Surgical emergency.

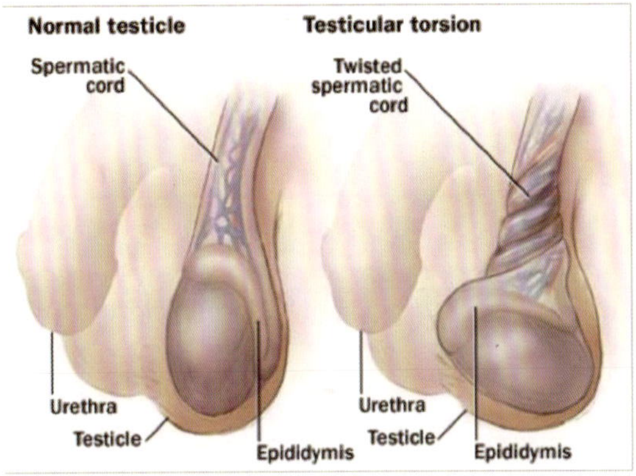

Priapism

Painful, sustained erection without the presence of physical or psychological stimulation. Blood stays to long in the penis causing ischemia to the penis.
If it is not restored timely, disfigurement of the penis, erectile dysfunction or penile gangrene can occur.

TX: Initial: Ice packs and **α-agonist (epinephrine or phenylephrine)**
Erection should not go **beyond 4 hours**.
Medical emergency.

Associated with: Sickle Cell, Fabry's Dz, Leukemia, neurologic disorders, trauma, **cocaine, heroin, alcohol**, black widow spider bites, **anticoagulants, anti-convulsants** (**Valproate**), **anti-depressants** (**Trazodone**), anti-psychotics (**Chlorpromazine, Clozapine**), **Phosphodiesterase Inhibitors, α-Blockers**.

Peyronie's Disease

Connective tissue disorder in which scar tissue forms in the tunica albuginea (thick sheath of tissue surrounding the corpora cavernosa). "Broken penis".

SX: pain, abnormal curvature, erectile dysfunction.

Cause: Trauma/injury to the penis usually through sexual activity. In particularly when positions are used cause the penis to hit in a straighter path (ie: woman on top).

Erectile Dysfunction	Premature Ejaculation
Consistent/recurrent inability to acquire or sustain an erection for sexual intercourse. Causes: Psychological stress, diabetes, alcohol, metabolic syndrome, substance abuse, advancing age, neurological conditions, injury, smoking, cardiovascular disease, medications. Determination if physiological/neurological or psychological: **Ask: If patient is having night time or early morning erections.** If he is: psychological. If he is not: neurological/physiological. TX: If psychological, in addition to lifestyle changes, counseling, managing medicines: add **phosphodiesterase inhibitor (PDE-5): Sildenafil (Viagra)*** *Caution: **PDE-5 inhibitors can NOT be given with nitroglycerin (nitrates)** = potentially fatal hypotension. *Caution: Emergency medical attention needed for erections **lasting > 4 hours**. (Priapism: see above)	Male ejaculates soon after sexual activity with minimal penile stimulation. Defined: within one minute. (Average ejaculatory latency: 4 to 8 minutes) Non pharmacology TX: • Kegel exercises to strengthen the pelvic floor muscles. • Masters and Johnsons "squeeze technique": Just before the "point of no return" the man signals their partner to squeeze the head of the penis between the thumb and index finger to suppress the ejaculatory reflex. • Masters and Johnsons "stop-start" technique: during intercourse when the man feels he is approaching climax, both partners stop moving, remaining still until the feels of ejaculatory subside, the resume activity. TX: **SSRI** (increase serotonin signals in the brain slows ejaculation). **Paroxetine, Dapoxetine, Clomipramine**. Analgesic: **Tramadol**

Scrotum Trauma	Male Urethral Injuries
Mild: Minimal swelling, normal PE, bed rest, Ice packs, supportive briefs, NSAID's, Follow up in 48 hours or sooner if needed. **Moderate:** Moderate pain and swelling. Check ultrasound. If normal US: Follow up in 48 hours or sooner if needed. If abnormal: surgery consult. **Severe:** Severe pain and swelling or abnormal ultrasound exam: Surgical consult.	**Anterior Urethra**: "Saddle injury" Blunt trauma to the perineum or instrumentation of the urethra. SX: Normal prostate, bleeding from urethra, **able to urinate.** **Posterior Urethra:** Fractured pelvis. Major trauma. SX: Supra pubic pain, bleeding at urethra meatus, high ride prostate, scrotal hematoma, is **NOT able to urinate**. TX: Retrograde Urethrogram BEFORE placing Foley.
Hematomas **Scrotal Hematoma** Testicle rupture ➔ ultrasound **Penile Shaft Hematoma** **Trauma to erect penis (fracture to corpus cavernosus)** **SX: Large hematoma midshaft.** **Normal arterial inflow without venous outflow**	

Erectile Dysfunction (AKA: ↓ libido) Differentials

Can show gynecomastia and testicular atrophy

Lab Results	What to check (cause)
If ↓ Testosterone with normal FSH and LH	Check serum prolactin
If ↑ Prolactin	Check MRI for Pituitary prolactinoma
If Prolactin and MRI is normal	Give testosterone therapy

Hernias

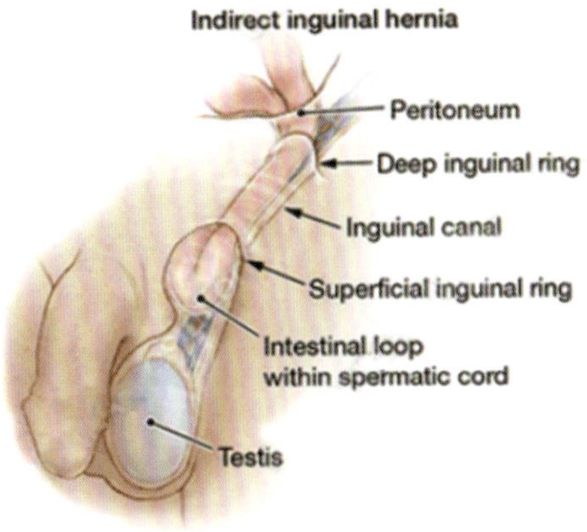

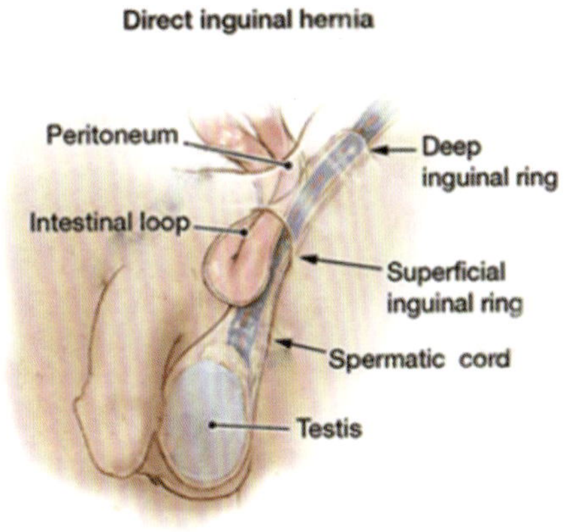

Direct Hernia

- Loop of intestine protrudes through **Hesselbach's triangle** in the abdominal wall through the superficial inguinal ring
- **Medial to inferior epigastric vessels**
- MC in older men due to weakness in abdominal wall: breakdown of the **transversus abdominalis aponeurosis and transversalis fascia.**
- MC acquired.

Hesselbach Triangle boarders:
Medial boarder: Lateral margin of rectus sheath.
Superolateral boarder: Inferior epigastric vessels.
Inferior boarder: Inguinal ligament (AKA: Poupart's ligament)

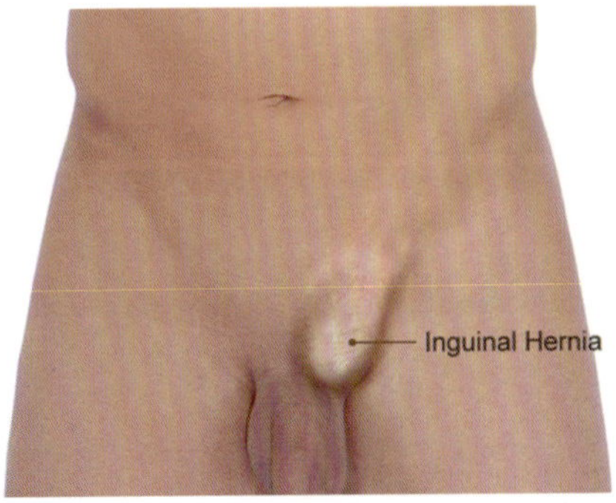

Indirect Hernia

- Loop of intestine extends through the deep (internal) inguinal ring, the superficial (external) inguinal ring and into the scrotum. (same path as the decent of the testes)
- Lateral to the inferior epigastric vessels
- MC in infants and children due to failure of closure of process vaginalis (can cause hydrocele).
- Infant ↑ risk due to a **patent processus vaginalis.**
- MC congenital.

(**tip**: Indirect ➔ lateral to vessels: you go **IN**to the **LAT**rine to pee)
(**tip**: "IN"direct = "IN"fant)

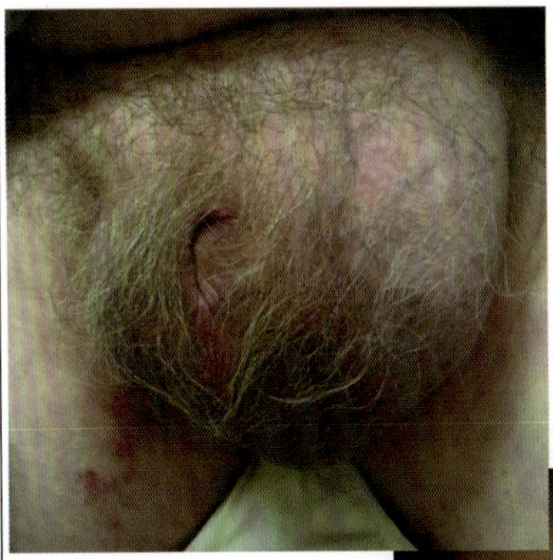

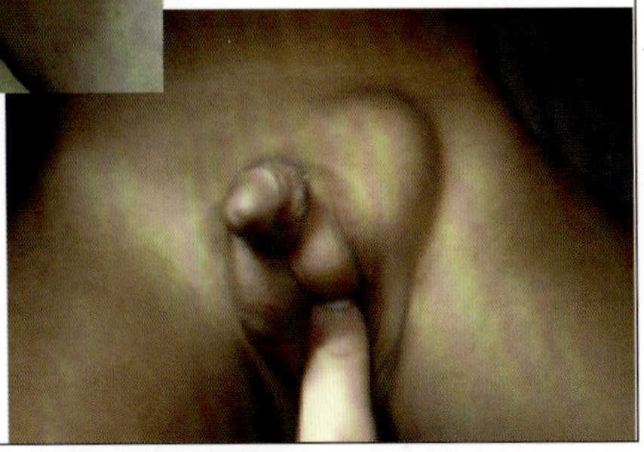

Hernia Surgery Layers

Skin ➔ Superficial fascia (contains 3 fascia: Camper's, Scarpa's) ➔ Camper fascia (adipose tissue) ➔ Scarpa fascia (fibrous tissue that helps form the fundiform ligament of the penis and contains 3 fascias: Colles: posterior perineum; Dartos: scrotum/labia majora; Deep superficial fascia: penis/clitoris) ➔ **External oblique** (inguinal ligament, superficial inguinal ring, external spermatic cord, anterior rectus sheath) ➔ **Internal Oblique** (cremasteric and muscle fascia, medial rectus sheath) ➔ **Transverse abdominis** (conjoining tendon, posterior rectus sheath) ➔ **Transversalis fascia** (deep inguinal ring, internal spermatic fascia, posterior rectus sheath, femoral sheath (femoral canal: femoral artery, vein) ➔ **Extraperitoneal layer** (testes) ➔ **Parietal Peritoneum**

Penis, Prostate and Testicular Tumors/Cancer

Prostate Cancer
(AKA: Prostatic Adenocarcinoma)

Occurs on the **peripheral** sides of the prostate gland (whereas BPH occurs centrally).

SX: Digital exam shows **hard, nodular, asymmetrical** prostate. Presents similar to BPH (obstructive symptoms: difficult to stop/start). Many are asymptomatic.

Labs: **↑ PSA, ↑ AFP** (PSA is useful to follow the reoccurrence of the cancer, but it is not used for screening. But if the patient requests a PSA screening, do the screen).

Metastasis to the **bone**, in particularly the lower back = Osteoblastic.

Prognosis: Metastasis and Gleason score (Grade of the differentiation/abnormality of the cells. Grades of < 6 have a good prognosis and grades of ≥ 8 have a poor prognosis and are aggressive.

Drug TX: 1st: **Flutamide** (anti-androgen),
2nd: **Leuprolide** (GnRH agonist: will raise testosterone levels initially), Ketoconazole.
Prostate cancer hormone drugs help to slow the progression, not prevent reoccurrences.

TX: Surgical repair (Prostatectomy): **TURP** (Transurethral resection of the prostate).
Side effects: **Retrograde ejaculate, AKA: dry ejaculate** (the prostate is responsible for adding semen to sperm), erectile dysfunction, urinary incontinence.

HPV Anal Cancer

Human Papilloma Virus
No Envelope
Double stranded, circular

Causes:
HPV 1, 2, 6, 11, CIN (Cervical Intraepithelial Neoplasia), Cervical Cancer (HPV 16, 18),
Anal cancer in men, genital warts

Transmission: Sexual activity
High risk: Homosexual males due to anal intercourse.
Condoms do NOT totally protect against HPV because areas around genitals and thighs are not covered.

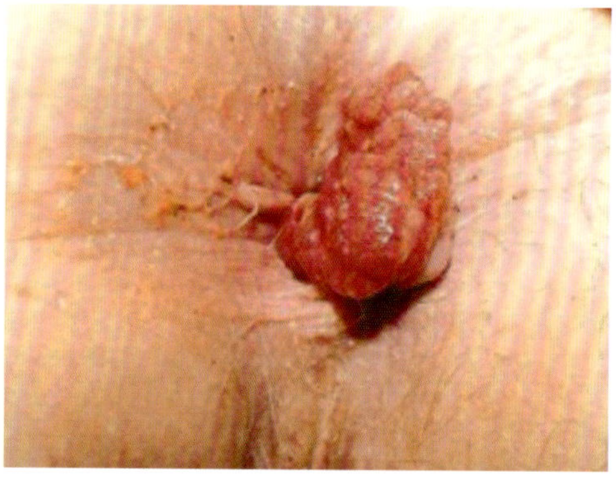

Penile Squamous Cell Carcinoma

SX: Erythema, rash, foul smelling discharge, sore that doesn't heal, bleeding from penis or foreskin,
Phimosis (foreskin can't be retracted over the glans).

Risk: HIV, HPV, genital warts, poor hygiene, trauma, smoking, chewing tobacco, UV light

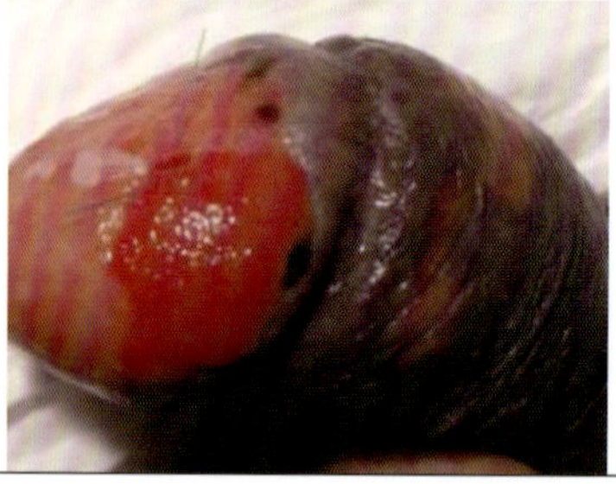

TURP (Transurethral Resection of the Prostate)

Repair of BPH if α-blockers do not work or removal of the prostate gland in prostate cancer.

Complications: **Retrograde ejaculation (AKA: Dry ejaculate)**. Sperm flows back into the bladder because the bladder neck fails to close.

Hyponatremia because of ↑↑ flushing solutions.
SX: Twitching, nausea, disorientation.

Testicular Germ Cell Tumors

- Germ Cell Tumors: Seminoma's and Nonseminomas.
- MC in young men (<35)
- SX: Painless mass in the scrotum
- 95 % of all testicular tumors
- Tumors will not transilluminate
- Do not biopsy the tumor.
- Labs: AFP (Alpha fetoprotein) is **only** secreted by **Nonseminomas**; HCG is elevated in both seminomas and nonseminoma.
- Prognosis: CT of pelvis and abdomen.
- DX: Do not biopsy.
  TX: Inguinal orchiectomy (removal of affected testicle/s and spermatic cord/s).
  Localized: radiation
  Metastasis: Chemotherapy
  Seminoma (chemo and radiation);Non-seminoma (chemo)
- Risk Factors: Klinefelter syndrome, cryptorchidism

Choriocarcinoma Malignant, solid tumor, derived from syncytiotrophoblastic and cytotrophoblastic origins. Nonseminomatous germ cell tumor. SX: Painful, progressive swelling. Metastasizes hematogenously to lungs, liver and brain. If they bleed in the brain, leads to a stroke. Labs ↑ **β-HCG** (↑ β-HCG is a TSH and LH analog) so can cause hyperthyroid symptoms and gynecomastia) TX: Radical orchiectomy	**Embryonal Carcinoma** Malignant. SX: Palpable testicular mass, asymmetric testicular enlargement, low back pain, dyspnea, hemoptysis, hematemesis, neurologic problems. Histology: Pale grey tumor with **hemorrhage and necrosis**. Labs: **↑ hCG, normal AFP**
Teratoma, Mature (AKA: Dermoid) Malignant. (Teratoma 's in women are benign) On-seminomatous germ-cell tumor. Histology: Cystic and multiloculated. Contains: cartilage, nerve, various types of epithelium. DX: Contain **well differentiate tissues** from all three embryonal layers (ectoderm, mesoderm, endoderm) Labs: **↑ hCG, ↑ AFP** Hematogenous spread to lungs, brain, bone, liver. TX: Orchidectomy **Immature Teratoma** Histology: Areas of immature tissue (stroma, epithelial, neural).	**Yolk Sac Tumor** **(AKA: Endodermal Sinus Tumor)** **Malignant Germ Cell Tumor.** **(Correlates to the Yolk sac tumor in females)** MC tumor in males < 3 yrs. Histology: endodermal cells that secret alpha-fetoprotein (AFP), **Schiller-Duval bodies** (resemble a **glomerulus**: mesodermal core with central capillary) with cytoplasm containing **AFP and A1AT**.

Seminoma	Teratocarcinoma
Germ cell tumor of the testicle and can be in the mediastinum (chest) MC: Men between 15 and 35 yrs. (Corresponds to the dysgerminoma in the ovaries). MC germ cell tumor. Two types: Classical and Spermatocytic. Histology: Solid, homogenous, light well, sharply circumscribed areas of necrosis. Tumor cells are uniform, large, round, abundant clear cytoplasm and large central nucleus with 1 or 2 prominent nucleoli. Malignant. Originates in the germinal epithelium of the seminiferous tubules. SX: Painless, testicular enlargement. MC: men in their 30's. Histology: Large cells in lobules and watery cytoplasm. Labs: **↑ AFP, ↑ LDH**	Mix of adult teratoma and embryonal carcinoma. Histology: Multicystic areas of adult teratoma and solid with **hemorrhagic and necrotic areas** of embryonal carcinoma.

Testicular Non-Germ Cell Tumors

- 5 % of all testicular tumors
- Tumors will not transilluminate
- Risk Factors: Klinefelter syndrome, cryptorchidism

Leydig Cell Tumor	Sertoli Cell Tumor
Sex cord-stromal tumor arising from Leydig cells. MC in young adults. SX: **Precocious puberty** in boys due to excess **testosterone**, **gynecomastia**. Palpable testicular mass (approx.: 5 cm). Females can have. Due to ↑ testosterone they present with masculinization, anovulation, acne, hirsutism, clitoromegaly, amenorrhea. Immunohistochemical shows: inhibin, calretinin, melan-A. Histology: **Rinke crystals** (rod-like cytoplasmic inclusion). Cells: polygonal with round/oval nucleus and acidophilic granular cytoplasm.	Sex cord-stromal tumor arising from Sertoli cells. Produces excess estrogen: males present with feminization. Histology: Solid, well-circumscribed, white/yellow, firm with focal cystic areas. Tubular formations lined by elongated cells having appearance of Sertoli cells.
Testicular Lymphoma MC **Secondary** cancer in older men > 50 yrs. Extra nodal presentation of **non-Hodgkin lymphoma**. Arises from lymphoma metastases to testes. Prognosis depends on type and stage of lymphoma. TX: Surgical removal.	

Differentials for Germ Cell Tumors

Tumor	BHCG	AFP	LH & FSH	Estradiol	Testosterone	Notes
Non-seminoma germ cell tumor	↑	↑				
Seminoma	↑	none				Markers usually normal. See syncytiotrophoblast giant cells.
Hepatocellular Carcinoma	none	↑				
Choriocarcinoma (germ cell tumor)	↑↑	none				
Ledig Cell Tumor (sex cord tumor)			↓	↑↑	↑↑	Gynecomastia, Precocious puberty
Teratoma	↑	↑				
Yolk Sac (germ cell tumor)		↑				endodermal sinus tumor

REPRODUCTIVE PHARMACOLOGY

Contraception, Abortives, Tocolysis

DRUG GENERIC name Trade name	Clinical Use	Mechanism of Action and Resistance	Toxicity and Notes
OCP (oral contraception)	Contraception **Combined (estrogen/progestin ↓ risk of ovarian and endometrial cancer.** They also ↓ bleeding and cramps. They do **NOT** change the risk of breast cancer. **Protective** against: Ovarian cyst and ovarian cancer, endometrial cancer, benign breast disease, dysmenorrhea.	Inhibits LH/FSH ➔**no estrogen ➔ no LH surge ➔ no ovulation ➔ no pregnancy.** Various forms containing various levels of estrogen and progestin. Progestin's: Thicken cervical mucus ➔ ↓ access of sperm. Progestin's also inhibit increase in spiral arteries in the endometrium so ↓ implantation.	**Do NOT use in women >35 if they are smokers** (↑ cardiovascular events). **↑ risk for hypercoagulability ➔** ↑ blood clots so **avoid in anyone with history of blood clotting disorders.** **Does NOT cause weight gain.** Associated **with HTN, increase in triglycerides.** Note: in any situation where there is a ↓ in estrogen = infertility (ie: Anorexia nervosa) Note: if taken during pregnancy, do NOT increase miscarriage or birth defect risk. Do NOT use in estrogen-positive breast cancer. Note: OCP's can cause a **hepatic adenoma.** OCP's should be discontinued if this occurs and the cyst will go away.
Estrogen	Ovarian failure, HRT in postmenopausal women, menstrual abnormalities, men with androgen-dependent prostate cancer.	Binds estrogen receptors.	**↑ risk of endometrial cancer (any bleeding in a postmenopausal woman is considered endometrial carcinoma until proven otherwise).** **↑ risk for blood clots.** **Prematurely closes epiphyseal plates.** Contraindicated in: Pregnancy, DVT, Smoker > 35 yrs old, acute liver disease, chronic HTN, Diabetes, Depression, Migraines, hyperlipidemia.
Progestin	↑ vascularization of endometrium to prepare the uterus for implantation. (**tip**: PROgestin is PRO pregnancy). Treats: abnormal/ **dysfunctional**/ irregular uterine bleeding. "Morning after pill"	Binds progesterone receptors.	Does not ↑ risk of blood clots. Can be used by breastfeeding moms b/c they do not affect milk production. Contraindicated in: Pregnancy, DVT, Smoker > 35 yrs old, acute liver disease, chronic HTN, Diabetes, Depression, Migraines, hyperlipidemia.

Hormone Replacement Therapy (HRT) (estrogen replacement)	Prevention of menopausal symptoms: hot flashes, vaginal atrophy. ↓ risk of osteoporosis (when there is estrogen there is ↓ osteoclast activity).	Estrogen replacement	Note: Must add progesterone b/c estrogen only will ↑ risk of endometrial carcinoma in postmenopausal women.
Condoms: Female and Male	Contraception, Protection against STD's.	.	Note: **Be careful of latex allergies.** Other barrier methods: condoms, cervical caps, diaphragms, contraceptive sponges, spermicides.
Tubal ligation (AKA: sterilization)	Contraception		Most effective: 99% effective. Failures most often result in ectopic pregnancy.
IUD (Intrauterine devices)	Contraception	Copper IUD: causes inflammation, which prevents fertilization and implantation.	Can ↑ risk of PID (pelvic inflammatory dz) Copper IUD's = ↑ bleeding and cramps, PID. Hormonal IUD's = ↓ menstrual bleeding and even stop periods. Contraindicated in: Hx of ectopic pregnancy, abnormal uterus shape/size, Abnormal pap smears.
Nexplanon Implanon (Implantable contraception)	Contraception. Progesterone only.	Contraception: tube is implanted under the skin in the upper arm and releases hormones. Last 3 years.	Lighter periods, can be used during breastfeeding, ↓ PMS symptoms. Side effects: Weight gain, moodiness, sore breast, lethargy, irregular bleeding first 6 – 12 months.
Depo Provera	Contraception. Progesterone only.	Injection that provides 3 months of contraceptive protection.	
Levonorgestrel Norgestrel Antiprogestin Mifepristone (AKA: Morning after pills")	Emergency contraception. (ECP's) up to 120 hours. Progestin only.	Delays or disrupts ovulation or fertilization. Contain high doses of estrogens, progestin's or both.	Nausea, vomiting, abdominal pain, fatigue, headache, breast tenderness, dizziness.
Medroxy-progesterone	IM once every 3 months for birth control		
DES (Diethylstilbestrol)	To ↓ risk of miscarriage. Estrogen replacement therapy for estrogen deficiency.		**WITHDRAWN from market in 1971.** **Clear cell carcinoma (vaginal tumor) and adenomyosis in daughters of mother's who used DES.** Sons of mothers who took DES had ↑ risk of testicular cancer and infertility.
Mifepristone	Termination of pregnancy.	Competitive inhibitor of progestin at the progesterone receptors. ↑ uterine tone = ↑ contractions.	Abdominal pain, nausea, cramping, heavy bleeding, ↓ appetite. Note: Given with misoprostol (PGEI) or Methotrexate for abortions. Misoprostol: (PGEI) prevents NSAID induced ulcers (inhibits adenylate cyclase → ↓ cAMP → ↓ proton pump activity → ↓ gastric acid).
Dinoprostone	Stimulates labor. Used in vaginal inserts for contraception's.	PGE2. Prostaglandin E2. Softens cervix and causes uterine contractions.	
Terbutaline Ritodrine	**Tocolytic**: ↓ uterine tone (stops contractions in premature labor).	**β-2 receptor agonist.** **Relaxes uterine smooth muscle.**	Tachycardia, anxiety, tremors, headaches, hyperglycemia, hypotension, hypokalemia.

Oxytocin Pitocin	**IV to induce labor.** **↓ postpartum hemorrhage.**	↑ uterine tone. Given IV or by nasal spray b/c it is destroyed in the GI tract. Nasal administration crosses the blood brain barrier.	↑ heart rate, ↓ blood pressure, cardiac arrhythmias, ↑ fetal blood flow, Subarachnoid hemorrhage

Phosphodiesterase Inhibitors (PDE5)

DRUG GENERIC name Trade name	Clinical Use	Mechanism of Action and Resistance	Toxicity and Notes
The "fil's" **Sildenafil** *Viagra* **Vardenafil** *Levitra* **Tadalafil** *Cialis* **Avanafil** *Stendra*	Erectile dysfunction (**tip**: Fils the penis)	Inhibits phosphodiesterase 5. **↑ cGMP causes smooth muscle relaxation** (stops the degradation of cGMP) in the corpus cavernosum → ↑ blood in the dorsal artery → erection.	**Do NOT give within 4 hours of patients on nitrates due to dangerous hypotension affects that can cause death.** Flushing, headache, color vision changes.

Pharmacology Sexual Side Effects

Drug Family	Dysfunction/Action
α-1 Blockers	↓ ejaculation
β - Blockers	Erectile dysfunction (esp. in African Americans)
Dopamine Agonist	↑ libido
Neuroleptics	Erectile dysfunction
SSRI's	Anorgasmia
Trazodone	Priapism

Antiandrogens

DRUG GENERIC name Trade name	Clinical Use	Mechanism of Action and Resistance	Toxicity and Notes
Finasteride	**BPH** (↓ DHT), Hirsutism, Male pattern baldness	**Inhibits 5 α-reductase** so that the conversion of testosterone to DHT is decreased. Antiandrogen properties.	↑ risk of prostate cancer (treating BPH lowers PSA which mask the development of prostate cancer).
Minoxidil *Rogaine*	Androgenic alopecia, Refractory HTN.	Antihypertensive vasodilator that also slows hair loss and promotes regrowth.	Irritation of the eyes and treated areas, unwanted hair growth on other areas of the body, temporary hair loss.
Flutamide	**Prostate cancer.** PCOS (Polycystic ovarian syndrome), hirsutism. Treats excess androgens in women.	Antagonist at the testosterone receptors. If no testosterone = no DHT. Inhibits entire axis: No GnRH = No LH = No FSH.	Gynecomastia, GI symptoms, mild hepatotoxicity

Ketoconazole	PCOS, hirsutism (also: fungal infection drug)	**Inhibits 17, 20 Desmolase** (enzyme that converts cholesterol to the steroid hormones testosterone and cortisol). No testosterone = no DHT.	**P-450 Inhibitor** Gynecomastia, amenorrhea
Spironolactone	PCOS, hirsutism (also: K sparing renal drug. Also: one of 4 main drugs that ↓ mortality)	**Inhibits both 17,20 Desmolase and 17α-hydroxylase** (enzyme that converts cholesterol to the steroid hormones testosterone and cortisol). No testosterone = no DHT.	Gynecomastia, amenorrhea

Androgen Agonist

DRUG GENERIC name Trade name	Clinical Use	Mechanism of Action and Resistance	Toxicity and Notes
Danazol	Endometriosis. Hereditary angioedema.	Synthetic androgen that acts at the androgen receptors. ↓ estrogen so tones down estrogen effects.	Weight gain, hepatotoxicity, hirsutism, acne, ↓ HDL
Testosterone **Methyltestosterone**	Promotes development of 2° sex characteristics, hypogonadism, promotes healing after burns/injuries.	Agonist at androgen receptors.	Masculinization in females, premature closure of epiphyseal plates, inhibits LH → ↓ testosterone → testicular atrophy.

GnRH Pharmacology

DRUG GENERIC name Trade name	Clinical Use	Mechanism of Action and Resistance	Toxicity and Notes
Leuprolide	Prostate cancer (continuous use), Uterine fibroids (continuous use), Precocious puberty (continuous use). Infertility (pulsatile use), Endometriosis.	GnRH analog has agonist properties in pulsatile use. When used for antagonist properties with continuous use, GnRH is down regulated so that FSH/LH are ↓.	Impotence, hot flashes, antiandrogen effects, nausea, vomiting. Note: Prostate cancer treatment: there is an ↑ in testosterone for the **first dose** and then testosterone will ↓. **NOTE**: **Leuprolide** when used continuously will inhibit FSH and LH secretion, which inhibits menstrual cycles and puts a women in a "state" of menopause. This is beneficial in endometriosis and fibroids (or other disease states that are stimulated by the menstrual cycle). If the drug is used in a pulsatile manor it stimulates the release of FSH and LH causing the menstrual cycle/ovulation.

α-1 Antagonist

Tamsulosin *Flomax*	**BPH**	α1-antagonist. Relaxes smooth muscle so less resistance to urinary flow. Prostate has $\alpha 1_A$ receptors and vessels have $\alpha 1_B$ receptors.	Sulfa allergies. Hypotension.

Selective Estrogen Receptor Medulators (SERMs)

DRUG GENERIC name Trade name	Clinical Use	Mechanism of Action and Resistance	Toxicity and Notes
Clomiphene	Infertility due to anovulation (PCOS)	Antagonist at estrogen receptors in the hypothalamus preventing normal negative feedback. ↑ release of LH and FSH from pituitary which stimulates ovulation. Imitates natural estrogen.	Hot flashes, multiple pregnancies, visual disturbances.
Tamoxifen	**Breast cancer** (estrogen receptor- positive), Infertility in anovulatory disorders, prevent estrogen-related gynecomastia.	Acts as **antagonist at breast tissue** (anti-estrogen) and an **agonist at the uterus (endometrium) and bone.** In breast (antagonist): inhibits estrogen sensitive breast cancer. In bones (agonist): inhibits osteoclasts and prevents osteoporosis. In uterus: agonist → ↑ estrogen → endometrial cancer (↑ or longer exposure to estrogen = ↑ risk of endometrial and cervical cancers)	**Endometrial cancer (AKA: Endometrial hyperplasia),** ↑ risk of blood clots (thromboembolism), hot flashes, ↑ triglycerides, memory impairment. Good for bones and breast. Bad for uterus. **Do NOT use**: if patient is an active smoker, has had previous blood clots or is a high risk for blood clots (thromboembolism).
Raloxifene	**Breast Cancer** (estrogen receptor- positive)	Acts as an **antagonist at uterus** and an **agonist at the bone.** Antagonist at the uterus → ↓ estrogen so no ↑ risk for endometrial carcinoma. Agonist at the bone → ↓ osteoclast activity (↓ bone resorption) so ↓ osteoporosis and bone fractures.	Hot flashes, leg cramps, blood clots., pulmonary embolism. Teratogen. Must stop Raloxifene 4 weeks prior to any surgery due to ↑ risk of thrombosis. Good for bones, breast and uterus. (**tip**: RELAX (ralox) your bones are fine)

SSRI's (Selective Serotonin Reuptake Inhibitor)

SSRI's are the drug of choice for: Depression, Bulimia nervosa, anxiety, PTSD, OCD, Panic Disorder, Social Phobia, Premature ejaculation.

DRUG GENERIC name Trade name	Clinical Use	Mechanism of Action	Toxicity
CITALOPRAM *Celexa* **FLUOXETINE** *Prozac* **PAROXETINE*** *Paxil* **SERTRALINE** *Zoloft*	**Post Partum Depression, panic disorder, OCD, eating disorders (bulimia), anxiety disorders, social phobia, PTSD.** **TX: Premature ejaculations**	5-HT (Serotonin) reuptake inhibitors	**Sexual dysfunction**: ↓ libido, anorgasmia, GI SX **Serotonin Syndrome*** Avoid use with: SNRI, MOA's, TCA's, St John's Wart, Meperidine, Dextromethorphan, Triptans (Migraines). *Paroxetine **is NOT safe in pregnancy**. All other SSRI's are safe in pregnancy.

ENDOCRINOLOGY

Properties

- Made in gland(s) or cells
- Made in advance and stored (in most cases)
- Transported by blood
- Distant target tissue receptors
- Exert effects at very low concentrations
- Half-life indicates length of activity

Functions

- Control of rates of enzymatic
- Control of transport of ions or molecules across cell membranes
- Gene expression and protein synthesis

Glands

- **Ap**ocrine "smelly" (**tip**: like an **Ap**e) = breast, axilla, genital
  In issues of **precocious puberty** this helps to identify the origin of the problem between hypothalamus/pituitary and adrenal. If axillary hair (underarm) NOT present and there is pubic hair, the problem is in the hypothalamic/pituitary axis. If there is axillary hair and no pubic, the problem is in the adrenal glands.
- Holocrine = Sebaceous glands (this involves the entire (HOLE) cell)
- Merocrine = Sweat glands. Sweat glands bring ↑ Na and Cl to skin (affected in cystic fibrosis)
- Paracrine – like endocrine = Diffuses to target cells

Hormone Classifications

- Peptide or protein hormones (linked amino acids)
- Steroid hormones (all derived from cholesterol)
- Amine hormones (derived from tryptophan or tyrosine)

Hormone interactions

- Synergism (multiple stimuli, more than additive)
- Permissiveness (needs a second drug to get full expression). (**tip**: the 2nd drug gives it "permission" to work better)
- Antagonism (opposes. Ie: glucagon opposes insulin)

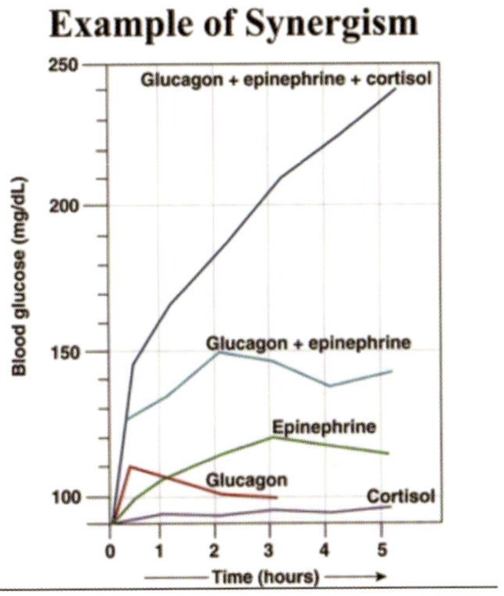

Signaling Pathways of Endocrine Hormones

Signal	Hormones	Notes
cAMP	HCG, PTH, Calcitonin, Glucagon, ADH (V2 receptors), FSH, LH, ACTH, TSH, CRY, GHRH,	Adenylate cyclase
cGMP	NO, ANP	Vasodilation
IP3	ADH (V1 receptor), Oxytocin, GnRH, TRH, Histamine (H1 receptor), Angiotensin II, Gastrin	Phospholipase C
Steroid Receptor (lipophilic) Circulate bound to globulins which increase solubility. **Intranuclear**	**T3/T4**, Testosterone, Estrogen, Vit D, Cortisol, Aldosterone, Progesterone	These receptors are **intracytoplasmic, nuclear receptors** and go directly to gene expression. They are NOT on the cell surface. Associated with **Chaperones (heat shock proteins hsp90 and hsp 56)** Chaperones assist in folding/unfolding, assembly/disassembly of proteins. **SHBG (Steroid Hormone Binding Globulin)** ↑ SHBG lowers free testosterone = gynecomastia ↓ SHBG raises free testosterone = hirsutism ↑ SHBG raises with OCP's and Pregnancy
Tyrosine Kinase (AKA: **RTKs** = receptor tyrosine kinase) (**Cell surface** receptor. Extracellular **ligand-binding** domain, **transmembrane-spanning protein (7 spans)**	**Insulin** **Growth Factors**: IGF-1, FGF (fibroblast), PDGF, EGF	**MAP kinase pathway**. (**RAS/MAP** Kinase pathway) Transfers a phosphate group from ATP to a tyrosine residue (phosphorylation) - **downstream**. Regulate cells growth, signal PMN's, proliferation, differentiation, adhesion, migration, apoptosis and regulate the immune system.
Tyrosine Kinase (Intrinsic) (AKA: nRTK's = non-receptor tyrosine kinase) **Cytoplasmic**, No surface receptors, no transmembrane domains). Do not bind to a ligand.	**Cytokines**: IL-2, IL-6, IL-8, IFN, Prolactin, EPO, TCR (T cell receptors), BR (B cell receptors), **Growth Hormones**: Acidophils (organisms that thrive under acidic situations)	**JAK/STAT pathway.** Triggers a **cascade** of events through phosphorylation that **transmits the extracellular signal** to the nucleus causing changes in gene expression. Associated with cancers. **LACK:** extracellular ligand-binding domain, transmembrane-spanning. Regulation: Tyrosine phosphorylation

Tyrosine kinases receptors verses G protein receptors: Tyrosine kinases do not require the use of a 2nd messenger, G protein receptors do require a 2nd messenger.

TIP to help determine 1°, 2° and tertiary causes for TSH, PTH and Cortisol problems.

- Think of the system as you would jobs in a company. In a company you have the employee (1°, the gland: thyroid, parathyroid, or adrenal), the supervisor (2°: pituitary or kidney/Vit D) of the employee and the CEO (tertiary: hypothalamus or an ectopic site) of the entire company.
  Meaning: When things are working normal, every person in the company does what their boss tells them to: Example: If the gland (worker) would happen to make more hormone than it was instructed, the manager would see this overproduction and tell the worker to decrease production (he sends this message to decrease production by decreasing his levels/orders). If everything is working properly, when the manager sends this order to decrease production, the worker (gland) should do as told and decrease production.
- Remember that none of these "employees" come out to "work" (to increase or decrease levels) unless:
  1) they see their employee not producing properly (making to much or to little hormone) or
  2) if this employee is defective themselves and does their own thing (over producing or not producing hormones) without any regard to their normal job function and they will ignore all orders given to them by their boss.

- **Thyroid Examples: (Worker: gland (T3, T4), Manager: (TSH in Pituitary): CEO: (Hypothalamus, ectopic site)**
  Example for 1° hyperthyroidism: If the manager (TSH/pituitary) sees that the hormone production by their employee/gland is high (🡅 T3, T4) they will instruct he employee (gland) to make less (they do this by coming out "low" = 🡇 TSH). If all is normal, the employee/gland will do as told and decrease production. However, if the gland ignores the instructions to produce less and continues to produce without regard to instructions, this is the fault of the gland = 1° pathology.

  Example for 2° hyperthyroidism (pituitary: The problem is going to be with the manager (TSH/pituitary) not the worker/gland. The worker/gland will be producing high hormones (🡅 T3, T4). In a normal situation the manager would see the high production and tell the workers to decrease production (by lowering its levels = 🡇 TSH) and the worker/gland would obey and make less T3 and T4. But in this case the manager (TSH) ignores the high production by his workers/gland tells his workers/gland to keep on making the high level of hormones, ignoring the fact they are already making too much.

- **Parathyroid Examples**: (Think of the PTH/parathyroid gland as the manager in this case and the serum calcium levels as the "employee").
  PTH levels from the gland respond to the levels of Calcium. Serum calcium and phosphate levels are always opposite in normal functioning. PTH normal function: When serum calcium is low it is the manager's job (parathyroid) to recognize this and release instructions (🡅 PTH) to increase calcium levels through various means such as: resorption of bone or 🡅 reabsorption of Ca in the gut.

  Example for 1° Hyperparathyroidism: Serum calcium levels will be high (causes: cancer, excess Vit D). In the normal situation the manager (Parathyroid/PTH) would see the high levels of calcium and send out instructions (🡇 PTH) so that no more calcium is resorbed so that calcium levels drop, but the problem is with the manager (Parathyroid/PTH), the manager is ignoring the high serum calcium levels and continues to to release high levels of PTH. Because the calcium level (employee) is responding to the instructions, the level of calcium remains high. So you will see both 🡅 PTH and 🡅 Ca.

  Example for 2° Hyperparathyroidism: In this case there will be low serum calcium levels (due to either kidney problems causing the lack/decrease of production of calciferol (active Vit D) so 🡇 reabsorption of calcium in the gut or lack of Vitamin D). In normal function the manager would see this low calcium and send a message (🡅 PTH) so that the calcium (employee) increases. But in this case the calcium (employee) ignores the order to increase and stays low. So you will see 🡅 PTH and 🡇 Ca.

Adrenal Gland

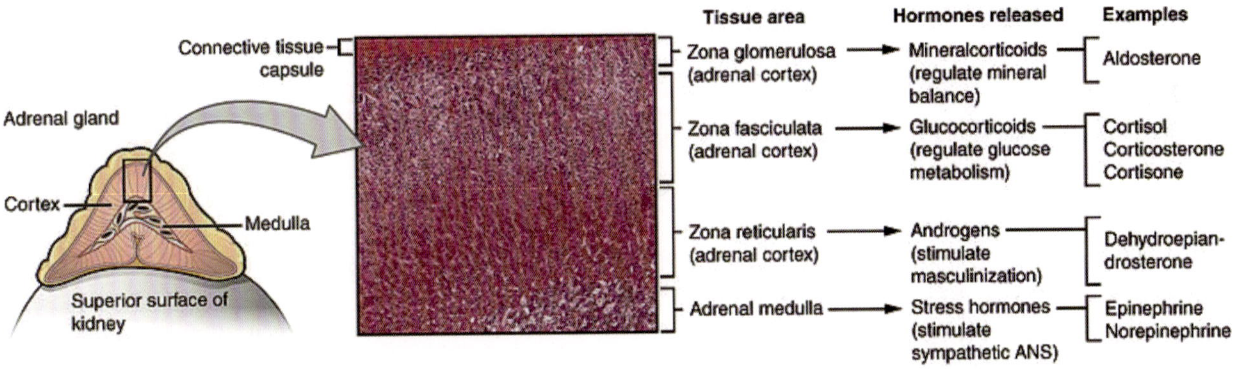

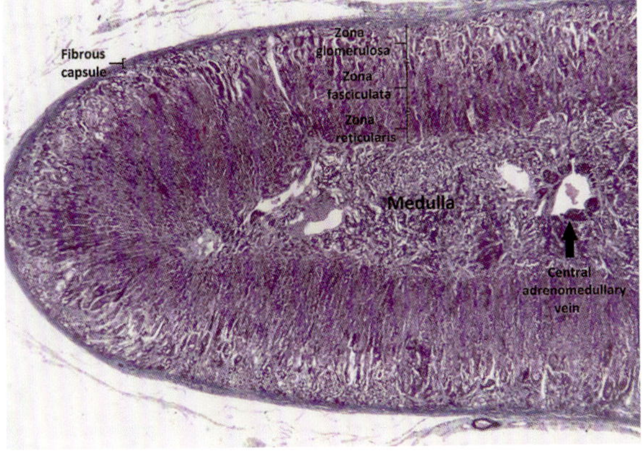

Adrenal gland drainage
Right adrenal gland ➔ right adrenal vein ➔ IVC (Direct route to IVC)
Left adrenal gland ➔ left adrenal vein ➔ left renal vein ➔ IVC (Indirect route to IVC via left renal vein)

Cortex: Adrenal Gland Layers
"GFR" (**tip**: sweeter as you go deeper)
G = zona glomerulosa (Salt)
F = Fasciculata (Sugar)
R = Reticularis (Sex)

Medulla: Adrenal Gland Layer
Chromaffin Cells: Catecholamines

Cortex (zona glomerulosa) ➔ Mineralocorticoids ➔ Aldosterone

Aldosterone

- Synthesized from **cholesterol via 11β hydroxylase**
- Central role of regulating blood pressure (holds Na and excretes K)
- **Acts on DCT and collecting ducts** of nephron by activating the basolateral Na/K pumps (pumps 3 Na out of the cell into the interstitial fluid and 2 K ions into the cell from the interstitial fluid creating a concentration gradient which results in reabsorption of Na and water into the blood and secretes K ions)
- Increases retention of Na to ↑ reabsorption of water = ↑ blood pressure and blood volume
- Increases the secretion of K
- Activated by the renin-angiotensin system (stimulated by angiotensin II)
- Aldosterone synthesis stimulated by:
  ↑ angiotensin II, ↑ K levels, ↑ ACTH levels
  (Angiotensin II is regulated by angiotensin I which is regulated by renin)
  (K levels are the most sensitive stimulators of aldosterone)
- In response to low blood pressure, stretch receptors in the atria stimulate the adrenal gland to release aldosterone

Exchanges to keep in mind (when one goes out, the other stays in = visa versa). Know your teams!

- **K and H stay together. They both go out or stay in together. So when anything talks about one, know that the other is right with it**
- **Na and Cl and HCO3 stay together. They all go out or stay in together. So when anything talks about one, know that the other 2 are right with it**
- When K and H go one direction, then Na, Cl and HCO3 go the opposite. If you retain K and H, then you will lose (excrete) Na, Cl, and HCO3
- The AKA's of H = acid, proton
- H (acid) and HCO3 (base) are opposite. If H goes out, it leaves more room for HCO3 to increase = alkalosis
  If HCO3 goes out, it leaves for room for H to increase = acidosis
- **If you vomit or have diarrhea** = means that H and K are leaving making you more alkalotic and hypokalemic
- Symptoms of ↓ K (hypokalemia) = paresthesias, tetany, muscle spasms, rhabdomyolysis

Potassium Pathology

- Potassium levels are **critical**, their normal range is narrow and normal levels must be maintained. Levels to high or to low can cause **fatal arrhythmias**. Increased extracellular potassium causes depolarization of the membrane potential of the cells and opens the voltage-gated sodium channels, never generating an action potential. This causes the potassium channels to open so that the cells become refractory (causing electrically excitable cells). This leads to cardiac impairment leading to ventricular fibrillation or asystole.
- **Arrhythmias can occur once potassium levels reach > 6 mmol/L. This is an emergency situation.**
- When a vignette shows any labs: you should immediately look to two lab values first: 1) Potassium and 2) Creatinine. **If the potassium is abnormal – STOP – do an EKG (1st step) and treat the potassium disorder first BEFORE you do anything else. Beware: This includes giving fluids in severe hypovolemia from whatever cause: accidents, hemorrhage, etc.** They may have a heart attack before you can even give fluids. **Treat the potassium FIRST and FOREMOST**.
- 95% of the bodies' potassium is located inside the cells.
- **Normal Potassium levels: 3.5 – 5.0 mEq/L**

Hyperkalemia = to much potassium is outside the cells, it must be sent back into the cells or excreted.

- **Arrhythmias can occur once potassium levels reach > 6 mmol/L. This is an emergency situation.**
- IV Potassium chloride is the final of the three drugs administered in capital punishment. It is what stops the action potential in the heart causing it to stop beating. Oral potassium chloride does not cause this reaction.
- **Hyperkalemia causes:**
  Hemolysis, cell death, tumor lysis syndrome, decrease in insulin (insulin drives potassium into the cell), burns, tissue necrosis, rhabdomyolysis, Addison's DZ (lack of aldosterone causes loss of sodium and retention of potassium), Aldosterone deficiency, forms of Congenital Adrenal Hyperplasia, massive blood transfusion, excessive intake of potassium, Acidosis, Renal insufficiency, Box jellyfish venom, **Drugs:** ACE inhibitors/ARB's; Aldosterone inhibitors: Spironolactone and Eplerenone; Potassium sparing diuretics: Amiloride, Triamterene; NSAID's: Ibuprofen, Celecoxib, Naproxen; Trimethoprim, Pentamidine, Renal Tubular Acidosis, Sodium/Potassium pump inhibitors: Beta blockers, digoxin, Heparin.
- **Hyperkalemia = Acidosis** (Cells bring in hydrogen ions/protons into the cell releasing potassium out of the cell).
- Symptoms: Muscle weakness, paralysis of muscles, including GI muscles (ileus), cardiac arrhythmias. It does NOT cause seizures.
  EKG shows: Peaked T waves, Wide QRS complexes, PR interval prolongation.
- **Treatment for hyperkalemia: forces extracellular potassium back into the cell.**
  - **IV Calcium gluconate** or Calcium chloride (Increases threshold potential) Used **in abnormal EKG's**.
  - IV Insulin injection of 10 – 15 units of regular insulin along with 50 ml of 50% dextrose (to prevent hypoglycemia) (insulin shifts the potassium into the cells and increases the sodium-potassium ATPase pump)
  - Hemodialysis in severe cases
  - Kayexalate (Sodium polystyrene sulfonate with sorbitol) binds potassium in the GI tract and will cause potassium to be excreted in the stool but this takes to long. **Beware: Never** choose this answer, it takes several days to be effective).
  - Loop diuretics and fludrocortisone can increase potassium excretion in patients with good kidney function.
  - Salbutamol, Albuterol (β2 selective agonist) by nebulizer.

Hypokalemia = decreased extracellular potassium because potassium has shifted inside the cells

- **Hypokalemia = Alkalosis** (hydrogen ions/protons come out of the cell in exchange for potassium going into the cell)
- **Hypokalemia causes:**
  Loop diuretics, hypomagnesemia (if magnesium is low, the magnesium-potassium channels open and lose potassium into the urine. **Low Mg = Low K**), Conn's syndrome (AKA: Hyperaldosteronism), anything that increases aldosterone (aldosterone keeps sodium and gets rid of potassium), Bartter syndrome, anything that shifts potassium into the cells: insulin, β2 agonist (stimulates the sodium/potassium ATPase pumps), **alkalosis, vomiting, diarrhea, laxative abuse**, licorice.
  NOTE: If a patient is vomiting or has diarrhea (or both) you must think: they are getting rid of potassium. The electrolyte balance will be abnormal.
- Symptoms: Similar to hyperkalemia. Potassium affects muscles and the heart. Paralysis and weakness of the muscles, **loss of reflexes**.
  EKG shows: U waves, inverted or flattened T waves, ST depression, PVC's
- **Treatment for hypokalemia**: Replace the potassium. Oral or IV potassium replacement.
  Note: If IV potassium is replaced to fast it can result in a fatal arrhythmia. The potassium must equilibrate before it shifts out of the cells. Oral potassium replacement is safe, there is no limit on time frame to administer.

Aldosterone Pathologies

Hyperaldosteronism (AKA: Conn's Syndrome)

Primary Cause: Adrenal hyperplasia or Aldosterone-secreting adrenal adenoma. Presents: High BP and hypokalemia. Low risk of malignancy. Can be bilateral or unilateral. **Secondary Cause:** Renin secreting tumor or overactive renin system due to low intravascular volume (low BP). Ie: renal artery stenosis, CHF, cirrhosis, nephrotic syndrome. SX: Both causes have HTN (aldosterone is holding in Na which is retaining water and ↑ BP), HTN. DX: Confirm with CT after biochemical testing shows: High aldosterone (even with a high-salt diet), low potassium and low plasma renin levels) **RENIN level** will determine what the cause is: an Aldosterone tumor or a renin tumor. TX: tumor removal **Spironolactone**	**Aldosterone-secreting Tumor.** Tumors secrete aldosterone so Na is retained, K and H (AKA: proton, acid) are lost. Loss of K = Weakness and paraesthesia. Loss of H means that ↑ HCO3 = metabolic alkalosis **If Conn's is due to a mineralocorticoid excess** (**aldosterone secreting tumor**) there will be **HTN but ↓ Renin, ↑ Aldosterone, ↓ K.** Renin activates if there is low BP. Since there is ↑ BP (HTN) renin should not be active. **If Conn's is due to a renin tumor**, there will be **HTN and ↑ Renin, ↓ K.** **Renin should not be on with HTN, it should only activate when there** is low BP, which means there is a tumor secreting renin at will. TX: tumor removal **Spironolactone**
	"Aldosterone Escape" Mechanism by which the body counteracts to much aldosterone in an attempt to ↓ BP. The natriuretic peptide **ANP is released** from the atria of the heart (to much stretch is detected b/c ↑ fluid volume). ANP causes renin to be shut down and Na to be excreted so that fluid is decreased and therefore ↓ in BP. (ANP generates sodium loss). (**Note**: both BNP (from ventricles) and ANP causes a ↓ systemic vascular resistance, ↓ central venous pressure, ↓ preload because of the ↓ in blood volume from the natriuresis and diuresis).

Hyperaldosteronism/Conn's Disease

Type	Renin	Aldosterone	Potassium	HTN	Causes
Primary 1°	↓	↑	↓	↑	Adrenal Hyperplasia TX: surgery, **Spironolactone, Eplerenone**
Secondary	↑	↑	↓	↑	Diuretics, CHF, Cirrhosis, Coarctation, Renal HTN, Renal Tumor, Malignant HTN
Other Causes	↓	↓	↑	↓	CAH, Cortisol resistance, hyperaldosteronism, Cushing's

Cortex (zona fasciculata) ➔ Glucocorticoids ➔ Cortisol

Cortisol

- Release of cortisol is controlled by the hypothalamus (CRH) which triggers the anterior pituitary to release ACTH (adrenocorticotropic hormone) into the blood which then goes to the adrenal cortex.
- ACTH stimulates synthesis of cortisol, glucocorticoids, mineralocorticoids and DHEA (dehydroepiandrosterone) DHEA functions in the biosynthesis of androgen and estrogen sex steroids
- Synthesized by cholesterol via 11 β hydroxysteroid dehydrogenase
- Steroid hormone
- Released in response to stress and low blood glucose
- Works along with glucagon and norepinephrine (fasting state)
- Counteracts insulin. It inhibits the peripheral utilization of insulin (AKA: insulin resistance) by decreasing GLUT4 transporters
- Increases blood sugar through gluconeogenesis
- Increases glycogenesis in the liver (unknown mechanism)
- Suppresses the immune system: inhibits IL-12, INFγ, TNFα, TH1 cells (T cells, cell mediated responses)
- Upregulates TH2, IL-4, IL-10, IL-13 so creates an immune response (humoral, antibodies)
- Activates anti-stress and anti-inflammatory pathways
- Stimulates copper enzymes to increase copper availability for immune purposes (copper is co-factor for lysyl oxidase in cross linking for collagen and elastin)
- Stimulates superoxide dismutase for the making of the oxidative burst to kill bacteria
- Aids in metabolism of fat, protein, and carbohydrates
- Excess levels can lead to proteolysis (breakdown of proteins) and cause muscle wasting
- Decreases bone formation = ↑ osteoporosis (progressive bone disease, loss of bone matrix)
- Transports K out of the cell = hyperkalemia
- ↓ Calcium absorption in the gut
- ↓ collagen synthesis = ↑ free amino acids leaving less available for uptake by muscle = ↓ protein synthesis
- Inhibits IgA and IgM, but does not inhibit IgG
- ↑ wound healing time
- Acts as a diuretic = ↑ GFR and RPF (renal plasma flow)
- Also can cause Na retention and K excretion
- Stimulates gastric acid secretion
- Long term exposure damages the hippocampus = impaired learning and memory retrieval
- Cortisol levels peak in the early morning (8 am) and are lowest from midnight till 4 am
- ACTH levels affect cortisol levels. Abnormal levels are associated with depression, psychological stress, hypoglycemia, fear, pain, etc.
- ↑ production in the fetus between 30 and 32 weeks stimulates surfactant production

Cortisol Production Disorders

Primary Causes

- ↓ Cortisol production (hypocortisolism): Addison's disease, Nelson's syndrome
- ↑ Cortisol production (hypercortisolism): Cushing's syndrome

Secondary Causes

- ↓ Cortisol production: Pituitary tumor, Sheehan's syndrome
- ↑ Cortisol production: Pituitary tumor, ectopic tumor (Small Cell lung cancer), Cushing's disease, Pseudo-Cushing's syndrome

Cortisol Levels

Normal blood plasma cortisol levels: 9 am: 140 nmol/L to 700 nmol/L
Normal blood plasma cortisol levels: Midnight: 80 nmol/L to 350 nmol/L

Factors to Increase Cortisol Levels	Factors to Decrease Cortisol Levels
Caffeine	Omega 3 Fatty Acids: suppresses IL-1 and IL-6, enhancing IL-2 (promotes CRH release) (Omega 6 has an inverse effect)
Sleep deprivation	Massage therapy
Prolonged aerobic exercise (↑ gluconeogenesis to maintain blood glucose levels)	Laughing
Severe calorie restriction	Music (peaceful)
Trauma, stressful events	
Anorexia nervosa	
Smoking marijuana	
Viral infections via activation of cytokines	

Cortisol Pathologies

Addison's Disease (AKA: Adrenal insufficiency, Hypoadrenalism)

Affects products of both levels of the cortex: CORTISOL and ALDOSTERONE

(**tip** "ADD"isons = is the "ADD"ing of two layers for this pathology)

Adrenal glands do not produce enough steroid hormones: **BOTH** mineralocorticoids (aldosterone) and glucocorticoids (cortisol) due to adrenal atrophy or destruction due to disease.

1° Primary causes of Adrenal Insufficiency:
Chronic Causes: **Atrophy** or destruction of gland by autoimmune diseases or administration of iatrogenic steroids in developed countries and TB in developing countries.
Acute Causes: Sudden onset due to hemorrhage: Waterhouse-Friderichsen syndrome (due to Neisseria meningitides).

↓ Aldosterone, ↓ Cortisol, ↓ Na, ↑ K, ↓ sex hormones, ↓ BP (hypotension), **↑ ACTH, ↑ MSH (hyperpigmentation),** ↑ Renin. **Includes ALL 3** of the cortex layers (GFR), it spares the medulla.

2° Secondary cause of Adrenal Insufficiency: Due to other **disease process.**
MCC: TB of adrenal glands, autoimmune destruction, metastasis.
See: Calcification of adrenal glands.

↓ Aldosterone, ↓ Cortisol, ↓ Na, ↑ K, ↓ sex hormones, ↓ BP (hypotension), **↓ ACTH, ↓ MSH (NO hyperpigmentation),** ↑ Renin, non-ion gap metabolic acidosis, eosinophil's.

SX: Nausea, vomiting, **hypotension, hyponatremia, hyperkalemia**, weakness, fatigue, confusion/altered mental status, hyperpigmentation, hypoglycemia, metabolic acidosis, high BUN, eosinophilia, anorexia, weight loss.

TX: Steroid replacement: (**Fludrocortisone, Hydrocortisone**).
For stable patients (non hypotensive): **Prednisone**

Primary adrenal insufficiency:
SX: Abdominal pain and weakness, ↓ BP (due to excretion of Na), Hyperkalemia (retention of K), acidosis (retention of H), skin/mucosal **hyperpigmentation** (due to MSH – Melanocyte stimulating hormone). (MSH and ACTH share the same precursor molecule (POMC – pro-opiomelanocortin). ACTH is ↑ because of the low cortisol levels. **If ACTH is ↑ then MSH is ↑.**
Adrenal atrophy and no hormone production.

MCC is due to iatrogenic administration of steroids.

2° Secondary adrenal insufficiency:
SX: Weight loss, fever, cough with sputum production, abdominal pain, dizziness, nausea, non-ion gap acidosis, eosinophil's.
↓ BP (due to excretion of Na), Hyperkalemia (retention of K), acidosis (retention of H), **no hyperpigmentation (MSH) and ↓ ACTH.**
Calcification of adrenal glands.

DX: Cosyntropin Stimulation test.
Adrenal Insufficiency:
24-hour urine cortisol (more specific than overnight dexamethasone test).
Give ACTH and cosyntropin (synthetic ACTH).
If ↑ cortisol > 20 after 30 – 60 min after giving cosyntropin, this rules OUT Addison's.
If minimal or no rise in cortisol = confirms 1° adrenal insufficiency.

Note: ↑ ACTH = primary adrenal insufficiency.
↓ ACTH = hypothalamic or pituitary dysfunction.

Incidental Finding of a Tumor on the Adrenal Gland

An incidental finding of an asymptomatic tumor on the adrenal gland. (4% incidence).
Evaluate the test below to determine if this tumor is what is causing the actual symptoms.

Overnight dexamethasone suppression test.
Renin and aldosterone levels to exclude hyperaldosteronism.
Metanephrines in blood or urine to rule out pheochromocytoma.

Cosyntropin Stimulation Test
Most specific test of adrenal function.
Cosyntropin (synthetic ACTH).
Cortisol is measured before and after the administration of Cosyntropin. If the gland is normally functioning, there will be a rise in cortisol levels after giving Cosyntropin.

If hypoadrenalism is due to insufficiency/failure of the adrenal gland: **ACTH levels will be ↑ and aldosterone levels will be ↓** = 1° Adrenal Insufficiency.

If hypoadrenalism is due to pituitary failure: **ACTH level will be ↓, aldosterone will be ↑** = 2° Adrenal Insufficiency.

Cortisol Negative Feedback Loop

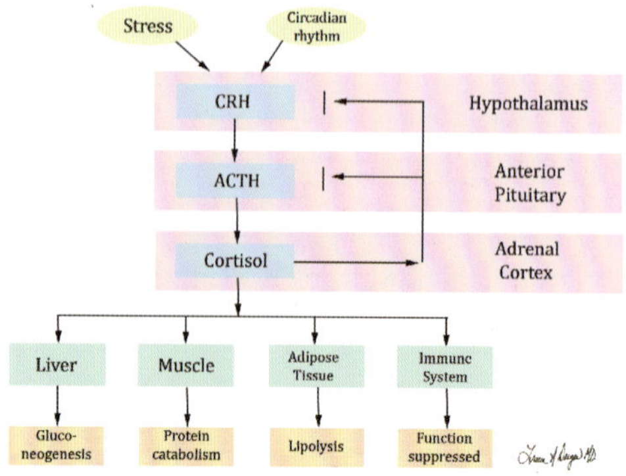

Cortisol Feedback

Cushing's syndrome and Cushing's disease (aka: **hyperadrenocorticism**)

- Cortisol is in the Zona Fasciculata in the adrenal cortex
- Cushing's syndrome is due to high cortisol
- Cushing's syndrome: same as "hypercortisolism". (Ectopic production of ACTH from cancer or carcinoid, overproduction of cortisol in adrenal gland, use of prednisone or other glucocorticoids).
  The MC cause is exogenous administration of steroids.
  TEST for Cushing's syndrome: 24-hour urine cortisol or 1 mg overnight dexamethasone test.
  To determine source of Cushing's syndrome: Look at the ACTH level: High ACTH: Pituitary or ectopic. Low ACTH: Adrenals.
- Cushing's disease: **pituitary overproduction of ACTH.** MC due to pituitary adenoma.
- Cortisol is anti-insulin.
- **↓ ACTH levels = adrenal source of problem**
- **↑ ACTH levels = either pituitary cause (cortisol is suppressed with high dose dexamethasone) or an ectopic cause located in the lung cancer or carcinoid (cortisol is not suppressed with high dose dexamethasone).**
- **Hypercortisolism Effects**:
  Hyperglycemia, Hyperlipidemia (fat distribution), Leukocytosis (from demargination of WBC), easy bruising, striae (due to ↓ in fibroblast activity), hypertension, hirsutism, muscle wasting, ↑ insulin resistance, ↑ gluconeogenesis, lipolysis and proteolysis, ↓ osteoblast activity (↓ bone formation), ↓ immune and inflammatory response by inhibiting or decreasing IL-2 production, histamine release, leukotrienes, prostaglandins, eosinophils, WBC adhesion. (see full list below)
- **Cortisol stimulates gluconeogenesis to increase blood glucose levels**. It breaks proteins down (ie: bones, and skin) so they can be made into sugar, which causes the symptoms of osteoporosis (due to cortisol induced bone breakdown), central obesity (cortisol induced hyperglycemia leads to fat deposition), bruising, striae (due to central obesity and fragile capillaries that rupture) and muscle wasting. Excess cortisol also causes hypertension (due to mineralocorticoid affects at the kidney),

Cushing's Syndrome Causes:

1) Excessive cortisol-like medications (ie: steroids: prednisone) MCC: **exogenous corticosteroids.**
2) **Tumor** that is producing excessive cortisol in either the **adrenal glands, the pituitary or ectopic cancer** (paraneoplastic, carcinoid) ie: Small Cell lung or carcinoid)

Cushing's disease = is in the pituitary and ↑ ACTH
Cancers = High dose does not suppress and ↑↑ ACTH

TX: Surgical removal of the source (pituitary or adrenal).

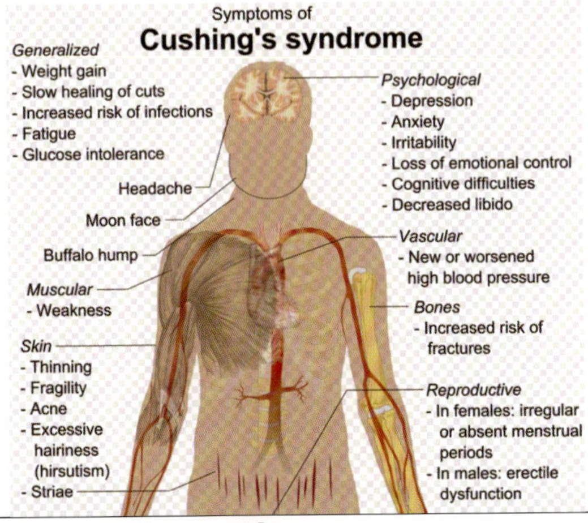

SX: **(Metabolic Syndrome)** Rapid weight gain (esp. in face and trunk: ie: **Central/Truncal obesity (fat redistribution)**: it is measured by **waist to hip ratio**), fat redistribution: **"buffalo hump"** (**pads of fat on the back of the neck**), **hypokalemia**, **metabolic acidosis**, increased abdominal fat, fat face ("moon face") red cheeks, ↑ sweating, dilation of capillaries = thinning of skin and bruising), red/purple **striae** (stretch marks on the skin due to weight gain), **hirsutism** (due to increased androgen levels), baldness, brittle hair, thin arms and legs, muscle wasting, hypocalcemia, insomnia, decreased libido or **impotence**, amenorrhea, infertility (elevated androgens), erectile dysfunction, depression, anxiety, memory dysfunction, insulin resistance (**↑ risk of diabetes**), polyuria (from hyperglycemia and increased free water clearance), polydipsia, HTN (b/c epinephrine is constantly stimulated = vasoconstrictive), GI disturbances, impaired wound healing, muscle and bone weakness (**osteoporosis**), hypercholesterolemia, hypertension (due to fluid and sodium retention), hyperglycemia, **leukocytosis** (from demargination of WBC).

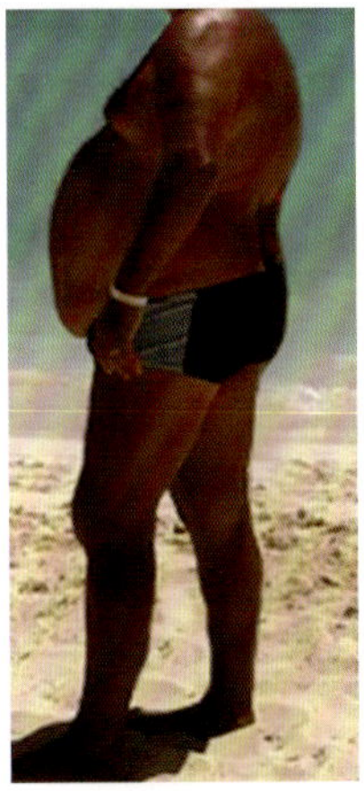

Acanthosis nigricans and skin tags in the axilla and around neck.

Exogenous corticosteroids MC Cause of Cushing's. ↓ ACTH, bilateral adrenal atrophy	**1° Primary Adrenal Adenoma** Due to either hyperplasia or cancer ↓ ACTH, atrophy of the uninvolved adrenal gland
ACTH Secreting Pituitary Adenoma (AKA: Cushing's disease) **↑ ACTH**	**Ectopic (paraneoplastic) ACTH secreting tumor** MC: **Small Cell Cancer or bronchial cancer** in the lungs ↑ ACTH

Screening Test: 24 hr Free Cortisol Urine Test
Used to diagnose Cushing's syndrome.
Cortisol levels rise in the early morning (highest 8 am). Patients are given glucocorticoids so **should have** suppressed cortisol in the morning if they are normal (due to negative feedback. Their system says they have cortisol so no need to make any more. But in Cushing's syndrome the Cortisol is made irregardless, so it is higher than normal in the morning)

↑ 24 hour urinary excretion of cortisol = Cushing's syndrome/adrenal tumor.

False positive test can be caused by**:** Alcoholism, depression, stress (emotional or physical).

NOTE: Cortisol causes hyperglycemia by stimulating gluconeogenesis. Protein breakdown releases amino acids which act as precursors to gluconeogenesis to stimulate lipolysis. When lipolysis occurs, free fatty acids are released and act as the energy source for gluconeogenesis.

Dexamethasone Suppression Test
(suppression test: given to see if the hormone levels can be suppressed)

A low dose of Dexamethasone is administered and if the **cortisol levels decreases = normal, no disease**.
This is due to negative feedback. Dexamethasone will indicate to ACTH in the pituitary that there is increased cortisol, so ACTH levels (manager) will decrease (↓ ACTH) to tell the adrenal to decrease/suppress production of cortisol, thereby causing cortisol levels to be suppressed. This indicates everything is working properly and the cause of increased cortisol is due to other "normal" problems.
(**Normal problems** being: obesity, depression, depression, alcoholism, emotional or physical stress can cause ↑ cortisol levels).

But if low dose Dexamethasone is administered and the cortisol levels do **not suppress** after the ↓ ACTH levels tell it to decrease = **Cushing's Syndrome = adrenal tumor**. Remove tumor.

If ACTH levels can't be suppressed then high doses of dexamethasone are given to find the source.

If a high dose of Dexamethasone **suppresses the ACTH** level and cortisol levels decrease = **Cushing's Disease (pituitary adenoma).** This means that the excess levels of cortisol (dexamethasone) got the attention of the pituitary (manager/ACTH) and it realized that there was too much cortisol, so the pituitary finally does its job by ↓ ACTH to tell the adrenals (employee) to decrease cortisol production. Confirm the pituitary adenoma with an MRI and remove tumor.

If a high dose of dexamethasone does **NOT suppress ACTH** levels (they continue to be high) and cortisol levels are **not suppressed** = it means that the cause is the production of ACTH in an **ectopic site**: MC: **Small Cell Lung cancer**. Scan chest for a tumor.

Dexamethasone Test Summary:
Low dose Dexamethasone test:
If a low dose of dexamethasone causes ↓ **ACTH levels** and cortisol levels from the adrenal **are suppressed** = **No disease**.
If a low dose of dexamethasone causes ↓ **ACTH levels** and cortisol levels are **not suppressed** (they stay high) = **Cushing's syndrome/Adrenal tumor**. It means that there is a tumor in the adrenal secreting cortisol. The tumor is causing the adrenal gland to ignore the instructions from the pituitary (ACTH) to decrease the production of cortisol.

High dose Dexamethasone test:
If a high dose of dexamethasone causes suppression of **ACTH and cortisol level suppress (decrease) = there is a pituitary tumor = Cushing's disease**.
If a high dose Dexamethasone does not suppress **ACTH and cortisol levels do not suppress** (they stay high) then the ACTH production is coming from an ectopic site.
MC: **Small Cell lung cancer**, carcinoid.

Small Cell Cancer of the lungs (Paraneoplastic cancer)
Centrally located and associated with smoking.
Produces ACTH-rP and ADH-rP.
ACTH-rP causes Cushing's syndrome and ADH-rP causes SIADH (syndrome of inappropriate antidiuretic hormone)

Tip: **CAREFUL on hormones from ectopic sites:** On all hormone secreting paraneoplastic cancers in the lungs (Small cell and Squamous: these hormones are peptide LIKE, not the real hormone. If the exam wants to be trick, the questions will clearly indicate there is a "mass in the lung" so you know the cancer is secreting one of the hormones (PTH, ACTH, or ADH). If they have BOTH hormones in the answer choices: PTH and PTH-rP, you MUST pick the hormone with the "rP" because it is the "related" peptide. Do NOT pick the straight PTH hormone. However, in most cases they will just put one of these in the answer choices in which case pick the PTH.

Lab Test in Cushing's

- BIT: 24-hour urine cortisol and 1 mg overnight dexamethasone suppression test. These test are used to diagnose Cushing's syndrome.
- The ACTH level determines the origin (location) of Cushing's syndrome.
  - If the ACTH is ↑ then the source is either an ectopic site (Small Cell lung cancer) or a Pituitary adenoma.

	Pituitary Tumor Cushing's Disease	**Ectopic ACTH (Small cell or Carcinoid)**	**Adrenal Adenoma Cushing's Syndrome**	**No Disease**
Low Dose Dexamethasone Administration			↓ ACTH and Cortisol does not suppress	↓ ACTH and Cortisol suppresses
High Dose Dexamethasone Administration	Both ACTH and Cortisol suppresses	ACTH and Cortisol do not suppress		
Test to Perform	MRI, Petrosal vein sample (Petrosal sinus)	CT chest and abdomen for cancer	CT adrenal glands	Look for underlying cause:
Treatment	Surgical removal. Access through: Trans-sphenoid.	Surgical removal.	Surgical Removal.	Treat underlying cause.

Additional Test and Pathologies

DIAGNOSIS	**CRH Levels**	**ACTH Levels**	**Cortisol Levels**
Tumor in adrenal gland cortex: Primary hypersecretion	↓	↓	↑
Tumor in anterior pituitary: Secondary hypersecretion	↓	↑	↑
Damage to adrenal gland		↑	↓
Hypopituitary adrenal insufficiency		↓	↓
Hypothalamus Pathology: Secondary hypersecretion	↑	↑	↑

Cortex (zona reticularis) ➔ Sex Steroids

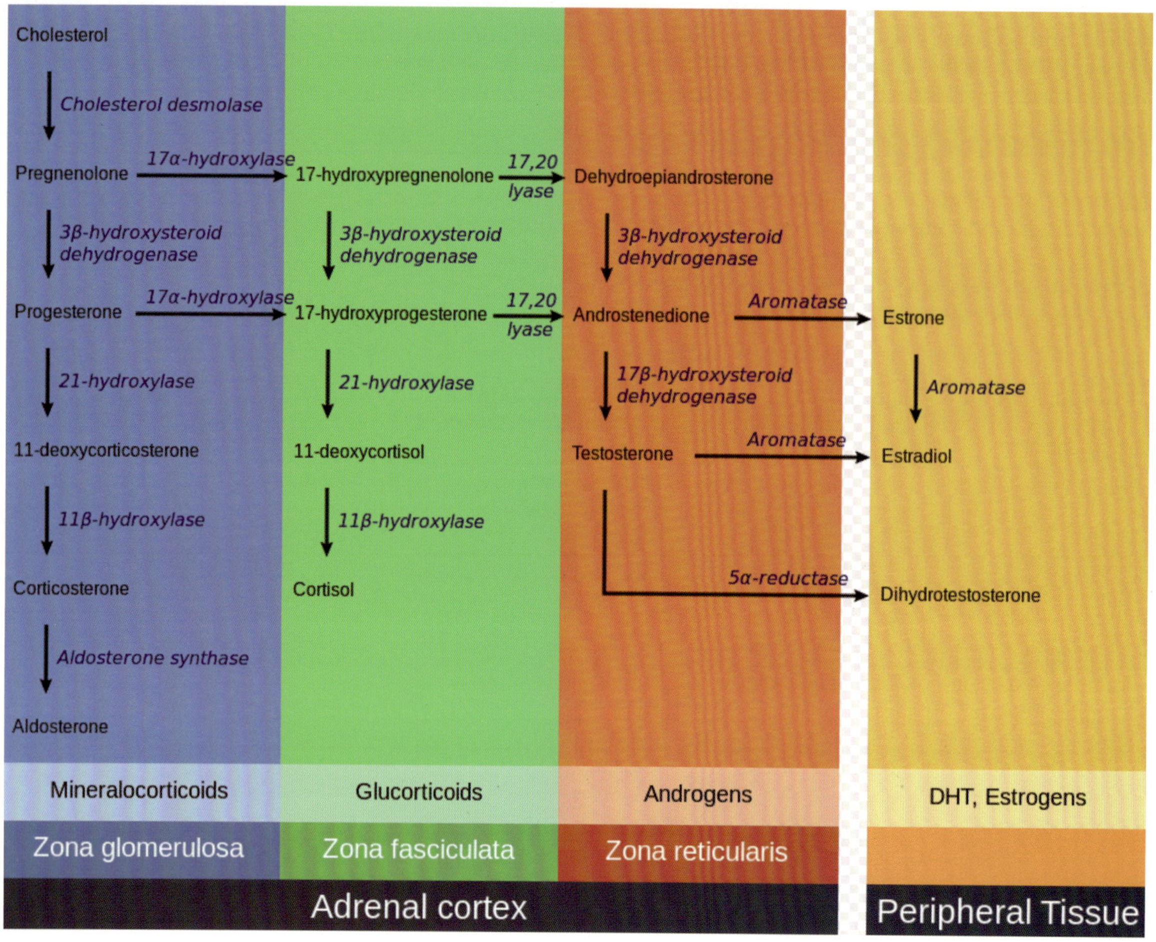

Sex Steroid General Rules

- If no cortisol = 🡅 androgen production b/c ACTH is activated which 🡅 androgens
- Androgens (Testosterone) is converted to estrogen via aromatase
- Testosterone is converted to DHT
- Cholesterol is the precursor in the synthesis of the adrenal cortex hormones
- ACTH activates the enzyme Cholesterol desmolase for Cholesterol to proceed, Ketoconazole inhibits Cholesterol desmolase
- DHEA –S is marker for Adrenal tumors
- Adrenal glands are enlarged in all forms of Congenital Adrenal Hyperplasia (CAH) because of 🡅 ACTH. ACTH is increased because of low levels of cortisol.

Sex Steroid Pathologies

Congenital Adrenal Hyperplasia's (CAH)

Enzyme Deficiency	**Aldosterone** (Mineralocorticoid) Zona Glomerulosa. Cortex of Adrenals.	**Cortisol** (Glucocorticoid) Zona Fasciculata. Cortex of Adrenals.	**Sex Hormones** (Androgens) Zona Reticularis. Cortex of the Adrenals.	**Labs**	**Notes**
21 Hydroxylase MOST COMMON	↓ Aldosterone which causes salt wasting.	↓ Cortisol (so will see an increase in ACTH)	↑androgen excess (lack of 21 hydroxylase will shunt pathway to androgen synthesis)	↓Na, ↓ Cl, **Hypotension and dehydration (due to salt wasting)**, ↑ renin, ↑ testosterone, hypoglycemia, ↑ ACTH, **↑K (Hyper-kalemia)**	**Build up of 17α Hydroxylase.** **Inability to covert progesterone to deoxy-corticosterone so production of corticosterone is decreased.** **Females have ambiguous genitalia** (masculinization). Boys present with precocious puberty at 2 – 4 years old. Hirsutism due to ↑ adrenal androgens. **See:** adrenal hyperplasia. **TX: If salt wasting: Fludrocortisone, If there is salt wasting: Hydrocortisone (Prednisone = inhibits pituitary). Corrective surgery for females.**
17α Hydroxylase	↑	↓	↓	**HTN**, ↑ Na, ↓ DHT, **↓testosterone** low renin, ↑ ACTH, ↓ andro-stenedione, **↓K (hypo-kalemia)**	**ALL babies show female phenotype.** (Males show pseudo-hermaphroditism, ambiguous genitalia, undescended testes. Females lack 2° sexual development)
11β Hydroxylase	↓	↓	↑	**HTN**, ↓ renin, ↓Na, **↑testosterone** ↑ ACTH, **↓ K (hypo-kalemia)**	**Build up of 11 deoxy-corticosterone which causes the HTN.** Ambiguous genitalia in females. Males normal at birth. Hirsutism due to ↑ adrenal androgens.
3β Hydroxysteroid dehydrogenase				**↑DHEA**	

Aromatase Pathologies

When you think of the word aromatase: think estrogen.

Aromatase Deficiency (affect females) Insufficient production of aromatase so **can't convert androgens to estrogens.** Masculinization of females (virilization), **normal female internal genitalia, clitoromegaly** (due to high androgen). SX: Primary amenorrhea, normal blood pressure, tall (because no estrogen, estrogen closes the epiphyseal growth plates). Risk: Predisposed to **osteoporosis** (no estrogen) and polycystic ovaries. Labs: **Increased LH and FSH** (out looking for the estrogen).	**↑ Aromatase production = ↑↑ estrogen** Affects both sexes. In males = gynecomastia, feminized appearance, hypogonadism, oligozoospermia (low sperm count), micropenis. In females = precocious puberty and short stature because estrogen closes epiphyseal plates early, excessively large breast (estrogen is required for breast development), enlarged uterus, menstrual irregularities. Labs: ↑ DHEA-S TX: Aromatase inhibitors

5α Reductase Deficiency (46 XY)	**Androgen Insensitivity (46 XY)**
• Affects males only • Deficiency in the male chromosome 46XY • 5α Reductase is required to convert testosterone to DHT (DHT is responsible for male external genitalia) • Male has no external genitalia (virilization at birth – or female genitalia) (DHT: 5α dihydrotestosterone) • Males have internal sex organs: testicles and Wolffian structures • Affects only genetic males (those with a Y chromosome)	**When you think of the word androgen: think testosterone.** • AKA: Testosterone insensitivity (receptors don't "see" testosterone) • Affects males only • Mutation in the androgen receptor gene so there is no response to androgens (testosterone), the receptor "can't see the testosterone". • This individual is actually a male but develops female characteristics • 1° amenorrhea • Bilateral inguinal masses (testes), these MUST be removed due to ↑ chance of testicular cancer • Breast development (testosterone is still converted to estrogen. Estrogen = breast) • No pubic or axillary hair development (no adrenal hormones (axillary) and no pituitary hormones (pubic) • No mullerian structures (Testes are present so Sertoli cells do produce MIF (Mullerian Inhibitory Factor) so no uterus or **fallopian tubes or upper 1/3 of vagina** • Does have **blind vaginal pouch**
Pseudo-hermaphroditism When an individual is born with the primary genetic sex characteristics of one sex but develops secondary sex characteristics. Ex: If a female is born with testes = male pseudohermaphrodite, if a male is born with ovaries = female pseudohermaphrodite	**Testosterone Deficiency** • MC Pituitary adenoma • SX: Decreased libido, gynecomastia, small testicles, erectile dysfunction, decreased early morning erections, decreased sperm count, hot flashes, osteoporosis • DX: MRI of pituitary • TX: **Bromocryptine** (Dopaminergic agonist)

Amenorrhea

#1 MCC amenorrhea: Pregnancy

Primary amenorrhea

- Cause: Genetic defect
    - **Turner's Syndrome**, 45 XO (no ovaries, no estrogen), ↑ FSH, ↑ LH
    - Testicular feminization. No testosterone receptors. (Has no penis, scrotum, and prostate). Genetically male but looks and feels like a woman, but does not have menses. Patient presents as a female with breast but no ovaries, cervix or top third of the vagina (blind vaginal pouch).
- Secondary amenorrhea
    - Pregnancy, hyperprolactinemia, extreme weight loss, anorexia nervosa, extreme exercise.
    - Polycystic ovary syndrome (PCOS): Hirsutism, obesity (↑ BMI), amenorrhea, cystic ovaries, ↑ adrenal androgens.

Hypogonadism

- **Klinefelter's Syndrome**, **47 XXY, or XXY** (no testosterone), **↑ FSH**, ↑ LH
- **Kallmann's Syndrome** (Hypothalamus pathology), **Anosmia (lack of smell, Cranial nerve I = Olfactory)**, ↓ GnRH, ↓ FSH, ↓ LH

Precocious Puberty Causes

Pathology Tip for precocious puberty: Development of hair is a good tip as to where the pathology is from. If only pubic hair is developed: then look to the pituitary ("P"ubic = "P"ituitary). If there is axillary hair: then look at the adrenal's ("A"xillary = "A"drenals).

Precocious Pseudo-Puberty (adrenal cause)	Precocious Puberty (central cause – Pituitary)
• Most common in boys • Excessive sex steroids • Course pubic and **axillary hair** (**tip**: "A"xillary = "A"drenal problem) • Significant growth acceleration • Severe cystic acne • Small testicles, large penis • Gonadotropin independent • **Causes:** CAH (21 Hydroxylase), Adrenal tumor, Ovarian cyst, McCune Albright, Leydig or germ cell tumors	• Most common in girls • Premature activation of hypothalamus of pituitary – gonad axis • Less dramatic presentation • Testicular and penis enlargement • **Pubic hair** (**tip**: "P"ubic hair = "P"ituitary problem) • Premature maturation • Growth spurt • **Causes:** Idiopathic, CNS tumors, Hypothyroid

McCune Albright

- Genetic disorder of bones, skin pigmentation and premature puberty
- Precocious puberty due to endocrine hormone excess
- Unilateral café au lait spots
- Polystotic fibrosis (bone fibrosis)

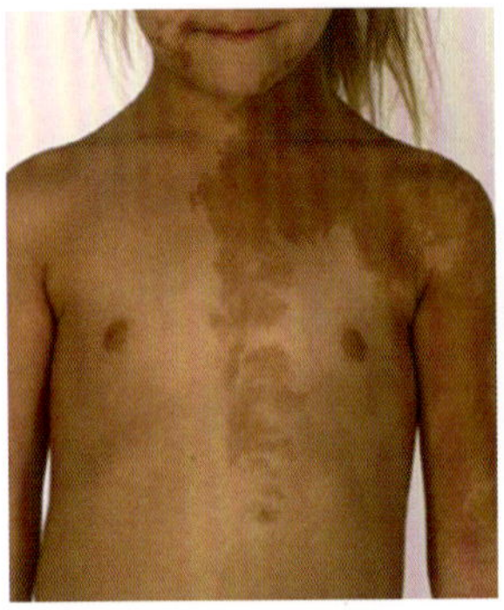

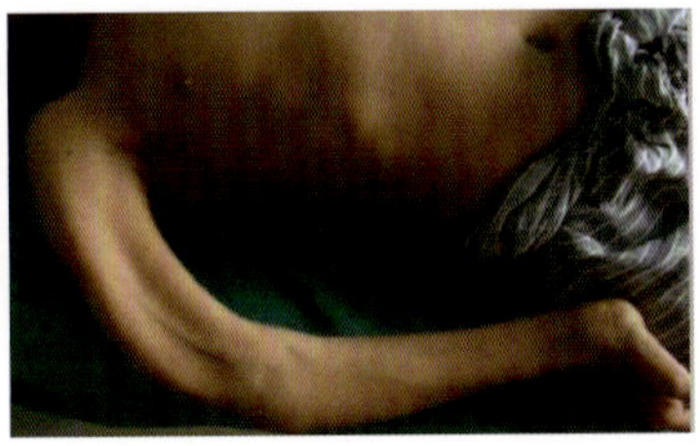

Kallmann's Syndrome

- Failure to start puberty or failure to complete puberty
- Occurs in males and females
- Hypogonadism and infertility
- **Anosmia (reduced or no sense of smell)**
- Cause: **Hypothalamic neurons** responsible for releasing GnRH **fail to migrate** into the hypothalamus during embryonic development
- Labs: ↓ GnRH, ↓ FSH, ↓ LH

Adrenal Medulla → Chromaffin Cells → Catecholamine's (Norepinephrine and Epinephrine)

- Pre-ganglionic sympathetic fibers
- Nicotinic Receptor and ACh neurotransmitter (cholinergic fibers)
- Chromaffin Cells release catecholamine's
- Chromaffin cells are neuroendocrine cells
- Norepinephrine (AKA: noradrenaline) and epinephrine (AKA: Adrenaline)
- **Norepinephrine is a neurotransmitter and epinephrine is a hormone**
- Neural crest origin
- Innervated by the splanchnic nerves
- Secrete catecholamine's when stimulated by sympathetic nervous system
- Associated with pheochromocytoma (MEN IIA and MEN IIB, RET oncogene)
- Epinephrine is a "back up" to glucagon, along with cortisol in order to maintain blood glucose levels
- Low insulin levels will stimulate epinephrine and cortisol, which will then stimulate glycogenolysis, gluconeogenesis, lipolysis and proteolysis.
- Epinephrine (catecholamines) and cortisol will activate lipolysis by acting on G protein β-adrenergic receptors to stimulate adenylate cyclase which ↑ cAMP, which stimulates PKA. PKA stimulates lipolysis by activating hormone sensitive lipase (HSL) intracellularly in the adipose tissues which hydrolyzes triglycerides to release free fatty acids (FFA) and glycerol.

Adrenal Pathologies

Pheochromocytoma	Adrenal Crisis
• (MEN IIA, MEN IIB), RET gene • Derived from neural crest cells • Catecholamine's released from the chromaffin cells in the adrenal medulla • Secretes norepinephrine, epinephrine and dopamine • **DX in urine**: VMA (breakdown product of norepinephrine and epinephrine) and plasma-free metanephrine. High plasma and urinary catecholamine levels. Plasma-free metanephrine and VMA levels. CT or MRI of adrenal glands. • Episodic ↑↑ HTN (Episodic: AKA: Comes and goes, you have been treated before, spells, relapsing) • TX: Surgical removal, **but MUST treat patient with α-antagonist (phenoxybenzamine) FIRST before treating with beta blockers (Propranolol).** If treated with beta blockers first it leaves the alpha receptors unrestrained and will cause a hypertensive crisis. (**tip**: A comes before B)	• Medical emergency – insufficient level of cortisol • Due to Addison's, Waterhouse-Frederickson, sudden stoppage of exogenous steroids, pituitary disorders (Sheehan's, pituitary adenoma), congenital adrenal hyperplasia (CAH) • In the case of sudden stoppage of exogenous steroids, **Watch for patients on chronic steroids.** Exogenous steroids shut down the entire hypo-pituitary axis so that no cortisol is produced naturally. The body relies on the exogenous steroids. Cortisol is a stress hormone, meant to be released when the body is under stress When patients are admitted to the hospital, all home meds are discontinued If a patient experiences stress in the hospital (usually after surgery) and they are dependent on the exogenous steroid, they are not able to produce any cortisol so throws them into an adrenal crisis • SX: Confusion, psychosis, convulsions, hyperkalemia, hypercalcemia, hypoglycemia, hyponatremia, hypotension, hypothyroid, severe vomiting and diarrhea • TX: **Injectable steroids and fluids**

Waterhouse-Friderichsen Syndrome	Neuroblastoma
• Adrenal insufficiency due to adrenal hemorrhage associated with overwhelming bacterial infection by **Neisseria meningitides** (Meningococcus) • SX: organ failure, coma, widespread purpura, DIC, endotoxic shock, septicemia, death 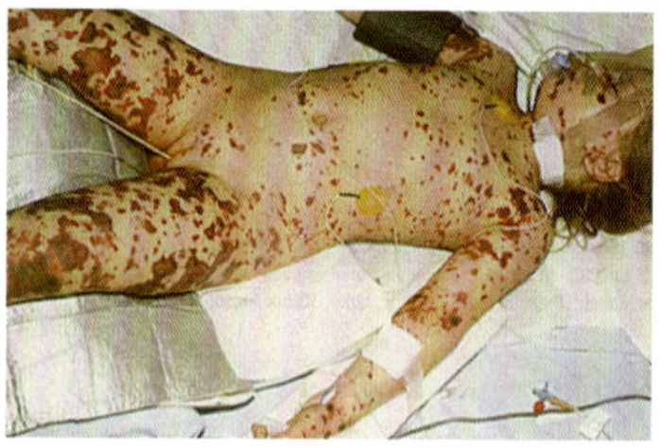	• MC extracranial solid cancer (tumor) in children, most occurring in children under 2 • Neuroendocrine tumor arising from **neural crest cells** (sympathetic nervous system). AKA: Ganglioneuroblastoma. • Originates in adrenal glands or in nerve tissues in the chest, abdomen, neck, pelvis • MC is in the adrenal glands • Histology: small, round/blue, rosette patterns (Homer-Wright rosettes) • DX **Urine or blood: Increased levels of catecholamines: HVA** (homovanillic acid), **VMA** (vanilmandelic acid), dopamine. • Associated with the **N-myc** (N=Neuro) • SX: Abdominal distension, firm/irregular mass that **can cross the midline** (verses Wilms tumor (cancer of the kidneys): does **not** cross the midline and is smooth and unilateral). Can also develop in the pelvis (pressing on the spine causing inability to crawl/walk), in the chest (causing difficulty in breathing), in the bones (causing anemia).

Pituitary

- Anterior pituitary is derived from Rathke's pouch. Rathke's pouch is a depression in the roof of the embryonic mouth. (AKA: diverticulum of the roof of the embryonic mouth/oral cavity).
- Posterior pituitary is derived from a ventral outgrowth of the primitive hypothalamus.
- Located in the sella turcica.

Hypothalamus Endocrine Control (3 levels)

- Hypothalamic stimulation from CNS
- Pituitary stimulation from hypothalamic trophi hormones
- Endocrine gland stimulation from pituitary trophic hormones

Hypothalamus

- Located below the thalamus, just above the brainstem
- Part of the limbic system
- Ventral part of the diencephalon
- Controls: hunger, thirst, body temperature, sleep, circadian rhythms
- Synthesizes and secretes neuro hormones (AKA: releasing hormones, hypothalamic hormones) to stimulate or inhibit pituitary hormones

Anterior Secreted Hormones RH= releasing hormone IH = inhibitory hormone	Abbreviation	Produced By	Released By	Effect and Notes	End Result
Thyrotropin RH	TRH	Parvocellular Neurosecretory cells Of Paraventricular Nucleus	Reach anterior Pituitary by Hypophyseal **Portal System**	Stimulates TSH release in pituitary. TSH is synthesized by Thyrotrophs. Note: Stimulated by TRH. Note: Inhibited by T3. Note: **TRH also stimulates prolactin.**	TSH stimulates Thyroid gland to release **thyroid hormones** (TH) (thyroxine). T3 and T4. Target organ: Thyroid. Regulation of **metabolism**. Note: Deficiency leads to hypothyroidism. Note: Excess leads to hyperthyroidism.
Prolactin RH	PRH PRH is inhibited by PIH (dopamine)	Parvocellular Neurosecretory cells of Paraventricular Nucleus	Reach anterior Pituitary by Hypophyseal **Portal System**	Stimulates prolactin release in pituitary. Pituitary prolactinoma = Amenorrhea, osteoporosis. Prolactin synthesized by Lactotrophs. Note: Stimulated by: PRH and TRH. Note: Inhibited by dopamine (PIH).	Prolactin release (lactation) for milk production and promotes growth of the reproductive organs. Target organ: **Mammary glands** and reproductive organs. Note: Deficiency leads to failure of lactation postpartum (aka: hypoprolactinemia). Note: Excess leads to amenorrhea, galactorrhea, infertility in females, impotence and decreased libido in males. It does not cause galactorrhea in males. (aka: hyperprolactinemia). Note: Suckling of the baby stimulates release of prolactin to allow for lactation. This can inhibit the release of GnRH, causing anovulation (infertility), acting as a natural birth control. (patient should not rely on this as a birth control).

Hormones	Abbreviation	Produced By	Released By	Effect and Notes	End Result
Dopamine (PIH) (Prolactin IH)	DA	Dopamine neurons of Arcuate nucleus	Reach anterior Pituitary by Hypophyseal **Portal System**	Inhibit release of Prolactin (PRH) in pituitary. Antipsychotic meds (dopamine antagonist) Causes galactorrhea.	
Corticotropin RH	CRH	Parvocellular Neurosecretory cells Of paraventricular Nucleus	Reach anterior Pituitary by Hypophyseal **Portal System**	Stimulates ACTH release in pituitary. ACTH is produced by Corticotrophs. 🡻 in chronic exogenous steroid use. Note: Stimulated by CRH. Note: Inhibited by glucocorticoids (steroids).	ACTH stimulates adrenal cortex to release glucocorticoids (cortisol) and androgens. **Target organ: Adrenal cortex.** Note: Deficiency leads to decrease in cortisol and androgens (aka: Adrenocortical insufficiency). Note: Excess leads to Cushing's disease (increased cortisol and androgens).
Growth Hormone RH	GHRH GHRH is inhibited by GHIH (somatostatin)	Neuroendocrine neurons Of Arcuate nucleus	Reach anterior Pituitary by Hypophyseal **Portal System**	Stimulates GH release From pituitary to produced IGF-1 in the liver and opposes insulin. GH is synthesized by Somatotrophs. Note: Stimulated by GHRH. Note Inhibited by IGF-1.	GH stimulates the liver to release insulin-like growth factors. GH stimulates **body growth** and a higher metabolic rate. **Target organ**: **Liver**, bones, muscles Note: Deficiency leads to dwarfism in children or GH deficiency syndrome in adults. Note: Excess leads to gigantism in children and acromegaly in adults.
Gonadotropin RH	GnRH	Neuroendocrine cells of Preoptic area	Reach anterior Pituitary by Hypophyseal **Portal System**	Stimulate FSH and LH release from pituitary. LH and FSH are produced by Gonadotrophs. Regulated by prolactin. Tonic GnRH suppresses HPA axis.	Note: LH stimulates the production of sex hormones: Estrogen and Progesterone in the female and androgens in the male. FSH stimulates the production of sperm and eggs. Target organs: **reproductive organs** Note: Deficiency leads to decrease in sex steroids (aka: gonadal insufficiency). Note: Excess leads to infertility. Note: Stimulated by GnRH, sex steroids. Note: Inhibited by prolactin, sex steroids. Note: Pulsatile GnRH = puberty and fertility.
Somatostatin GHIH (Growth hormone IH)	SS	Neuroendocrine cells of Periventricular nucleus	Reach anterior Pituitary by Hypophyseal **Portal System**	Inhibits GH and TSH from pituitary. Analogs treat: acromegaly, VIPomas, gastrinomas.	
Melanocyte-stimulating hormone.	MSH	Synthesized by Corticotrophs.			Melanin synthesis. **Target organs: Melanocytes** in the skin.
Beta endorphin		Synthesized by Corticotrophs.			Pain control.

Posterior Secreted Hormones	Abbreviation	Produced By	Released	Effect and Notes	End Result
Oxytocin	OXY	Magnocellular Neurosecretory cells of **Paraventricular nucleus** (**tip**: have a PARA ovaries)	Stored & released into blood by **Capillary plexus**	Lactation (milk let down reflex) and uterine contractions (smooth muscle contraction) during childbirth. Note: Stimulated by estrogen and stretch receptors in the nipples and cervix. Note: Inhibited by stress.	Target organ: mammary glands and **uterus.**
Vasopressin (antidiuretic hormone)	ADH	Magnocellular Neurosecretory cells of **Supraoptic nucleus**	Stored & released into blood by **capillary plexus**	↑ permeability to water to cells of distal tubule and collecting duct in kidney. (water reabsorbed by Aquaporin proteins on the apical membranes of the epithelial cells in the collecting ducts). Note: Stimulated by ↑ OSM and ↓ low blood volume. Note: Inhibited by low OSM.	Target organ: **Kidney,** sweat glands, circulatory system

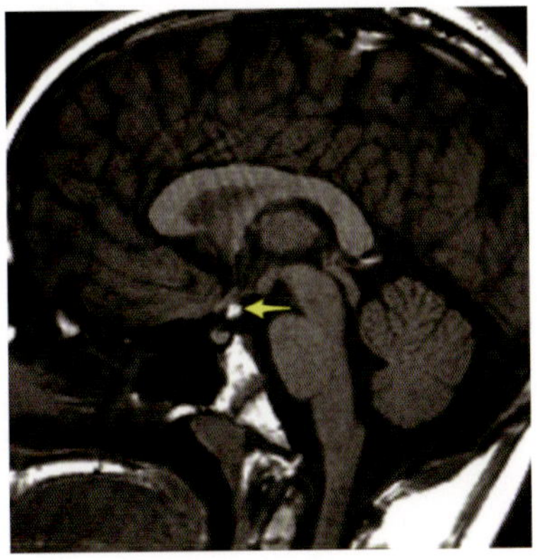

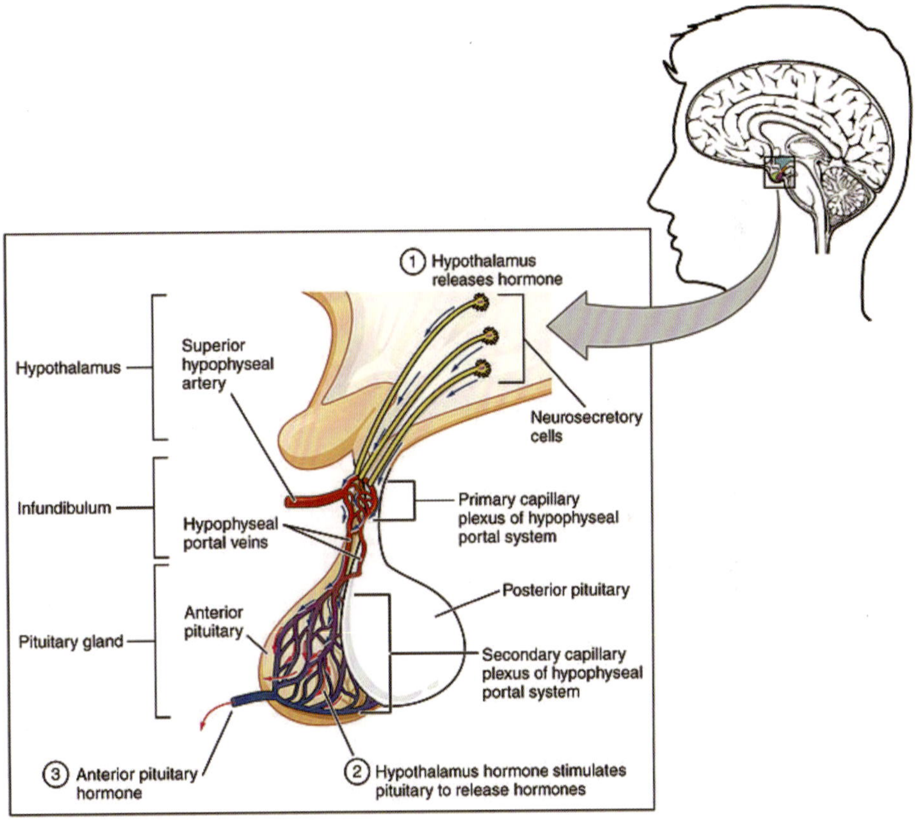

Anterior pituitary (AKA: adenohypophysis)

- Secretes: FSH, LH, ACTH, TSH, PRL, GH

Posterior pituitary (AKA: Neurohypophysis)

- Stores and releases oxytocin and ADH

Pituitary Hormone Pathologies

Anti-diuretic Hormone (ADH) = Water balance of the body.
With ADH = body is able to retain water.
Without ADH = body is in need of water = polydipsia, polyuria. (Diuretics can also cause this reaction).

Made in Magnocellular Neurosecretory cells of **Supraoptic nucleus.** Stored and released from the **posterior pituitary** by **capillary plexus**. **↑ permeability to water to cells of distal tubule and collecting duct in kidney. Inability to concentrate urine is due to lack of ADH.** Water is reabsorbed by **Aquaporin** proteins on the apical membranes of the epithelial cells in the collecting ducts. Angiotensin II plays a major part in regulation of ADH: If body needs more fluid (dehydration, low BP, low volume) the RAAS (renin) will kick in. Angiotensin II stimulates ADH to hold in more water, stimulates aldosterone to retain more Na which retains more water and vasoconstricts to increase blood going back to heart. If the body has too much fluid (hyponatremia), levels of aldosterone will decrease fluid. BNP/ANP stretch receptors in the brain will also pick up to much fluid and stop RASS and diureses.	**Diabetes Insipidus** (ADH is not working – **getting rid of to much water**) **Caused by osmotic diuresis:** due to high blood sugar leaking into the urine and taking excess water with it. **Causes:** **Central DI** = deficiency of arginine vasopressin (↓ADH) from the **CNS.** Shows ↑ serum OSM. MCC: Pituitary tumor, autoimmune, trauma, surgery. (**tip**: if **DDAVP/Desmopressin** test given and there is a **C**hange in osmolality = **C**entral DI. **C = C**) (**Desmopressin** is also used to treat nocturnal enuresis (bedwetting) **Nephrogenic DI** = kidney dysfunction due to an insensitivity of the **receptors** in the kidney to ADH. There is normal release of ADH from posterior pituitary. Dilute urine and ↑ serum osmolality. ↑Ca, ↓K. MCC: Hereditary, **lithium demeclocycline**, ↑ Ca. **Psychogenic Polydipsia** = intake of excessive amounts of water. **BOTH** urine and plasma osmolality will be diluted. Sodium will be normal – it does not have to correct. Misc: = GI, alcohol, drug abuse	SX: **Polyuria**: Excessive urination (especially at night), **Polydipsia**: excessive thirst (esp. for ice), dehydration. DX: **Desmopressin test** (**DDAVP**) or water deprivation = differentiates between central, nephrogenic, polygenic. Test results: If the osmolality **CHANGES** after the test, the cause is **CENTRAL**. (**Tip**: **C**hange = **C**entral). Serum OSM will ↓ and urine specific gravity > 1. 0 TX: **Desmopressin (DDAVP)** If the OSM **stays the same** or only slight change = **nephrogenic**. Shows a urine specific gravity or < 1.0 TX: **Hydrochlorothiazide, amiloride, indomethacin** To determine if it is **polygenic** it will correct – look at the **Na levels** – they will be **NORMAL**. Both central and nephrogenic Na levels will take a while to correct/adjust.

SIADH (Syndrome of Inappropriate Anti-diuretic Hormone) **Excessive water retention.** Serum is watered down. **Hyponatremia** (normal Sodium: 136 – 145 mEq/L) Urine OSM > serum OSM	**SIADH Causes:** **Ectopic ADH-rP** in **Small Cell lung cancer** (**TIP**: if the exam is referring to the ADH associated with small cell lung cancer, look at the answer choices. If they list BOTH ADH and ADH-rP you must pick ADH-rP. If only one of these choices is given in the answers, then pick that one. ADH from small cell lung cancer is not the "real" ADH, it is a related peptide: ADH-rP) Drugs (ie: **cyclophosphamide**) Head trauma CNS disorders Pulmonary disease TX: Na levels 115 – 125 = **water restriction** Na levels < 155 = **demeclocycline, IV hypertonic saline**	**Central Pontine Myelinolysis (CPM)** (AKA: Osmotic demyelination syndrome) Severe damage of the myelin sheath of the nerve cells in the pons in the brainstem. When Na serum levels get too low (hyponatremia) cerebral edema can occur causing **seizures.** **These low Na levels MUST be brought back to normal SLOWLY**. If they are corrected to quickly = CPM **TX rate: No more correction than 10 mmol/L of sodium per day or 0.5 mmol/L of sodium per hour.**

Prolactinoma
MCC: Pituitary adenoma

SX: Galactorrhea, amenorrhea
↓ LH, ↓ FSH (because prolactin inhibits GNRH = no LH and no FSH).

SX: Females = no cycles = amenorrhea and galactorrhea. Inhibits lactation after childbirth.
(**tip**: "Pro" lactin = "Pro" lactation).
SX: Males = gynecomastia, headaches and visual disturbances.

Labs: Very high prolactin levels > 200.

Neuro: **Dopamine Tubero Pathway**:
⃠ Dopamine = ↑ Prolactin.

TX: **Bromocriptine, Cabergoline** (dopamine agonist)
Surgery: **Trans-sphenoidal** Pituitary Surgery

Add'l SX: **Bitemporal hemianopia**, headache, hypopituitarism, decreased libido, infertility, acromegaly

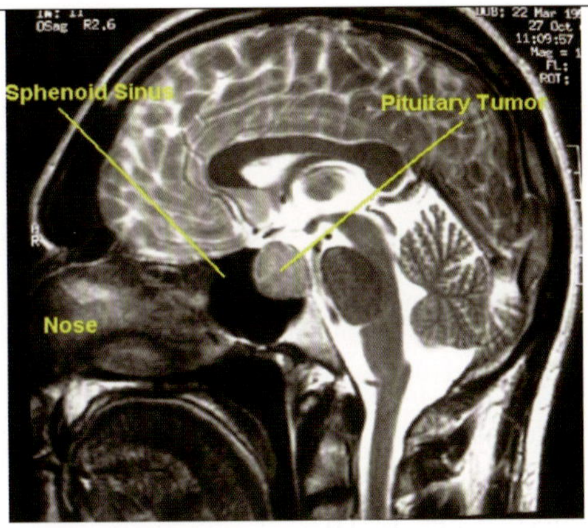

Pituitary adenoma
(removed by transsphenoidal surgery)

Absence of Pituitary
The absence of the pituitary can be due to trauma, congenital (the pituitary normally develops in embryo during the 3rd week), surgical removal, infections, radiation, stroke/infarction (Sheehan's). So all end products of the different hormones released from the pituitary will be affected. This requires hormone replacement therapy. There can be additional complications due to some types of hormone replacements. Example: If a male has had a pituitary adenoma removed by transsphenoidal surgery and he is put on hCG replacement. **hCG has the same alpha unit as LH, FSH and TSH.** By increasing the hCG this will increase the LH, which will increase the testosterone in the Leydig cells, which makes **more estradiol** via aromatase in the adipose tissue and testis leading to gynecomastia.

Prolactinemia
Physiologic causes (other than Pituitary adenoma)

Prolactin can be co-secreted with GH. Hypothyroidism can cause hyperprolactinemia because extremely **high TRH levels stimulate prolactin** secretion.

Pregnancy, renal insufficiency (kidney DZ ↑ prolactin), liver disease (liver DZ ↑ prolactin), intense exercise, stimulation of nipples (chest), cutting of pituitary stalk (motor vehicle accident) stops dopamine from going to the anterior pituitary (dopamine inhibits prolactin release).
Medications: Antipsychotic, Verapamil, Methyldopa, Metoclopramide, Opioids, TCA antidepressants.

SX: **Women** present with galactorrhea and infertility.
Men present with erectile dysfunction, ↓ libido, headache, visual disturbances. Gynecomastia and galactorrhea can also present, but are uncommon.

DX:
1st test: β-HCG to rule out pregnancy.
TSH, BUN/creatinine (kidney dz ↑ prolactin levels), LFT's (liver dz ↑ prolactin levels) and review all medications patient is taking.

If ALL of the above are negative, then do an MRI.
TX: **Dopamine agonist. Bromocriptine, Cabergoline.**
Removal: **Transsphenoidal surgery**

Growth Hormone - GH

From GHRH from the Neuroendocrine neurons of the Arcuate nucleus in the hypothalamus.
Reaches the anterior Pituitary by Hypophyseal Portal System.

GH is mediated by IGF-1. Induces targets to produce insulin-like growth factors (IGF) . IGF stimulates metabolism and body growth. Maximum secretion is in the middle of the night.

Promotes anabolic actions on bone and skeletal muscle, stimulates gluconeogenesis, stimulates lipolysis.
GH is stimulated by stress, sleep and hypoglycemia.

GH is an antagonist against the actions of insulin. It is inhibited by glucose, IGF-1 and Somatostatin.

IGF-1 growth hormone from liver and stimulates cartilage in the bone cells.

Uses **Tyrosine Kinase** (AKA: **RTKs** = receptor tyrosine kinase)
(**Cell surface** receptor.
Extracellular **ligand-binding** domain, **transmembrane-spanning. (7 spans). Ras/Map Kinase pathway.**

Tyrosine kinase growth factors = ↑ growth proliferation and differentiation.

GH is suppressed by glucose.
GH is anti-insulin.
GH ↑ glucose (GH is a stress hormone. ↑ stress = ↑ cortisol).

A **pituitary tumor** can cause an increase in GH.
NOTE: If this occurs prior to fusion of the epiphyseal plates it will cause gigantism. If it occurs after the closure of the epiphyseal plates it will cause acromegaly.

Acromegaly
(**tip**: A for Adults)

↑ GH in adults. Happens after epiphyseal plates close.
MCC: Excess GH in adults due to pituitary adenoma

SX:
Large hands and feet, course facial features, large tongue, insulin resistance (**Patient will mention that their hat, shoes, and rings do not fit anymore**), ↑↑ sweating (odor) due to enlarged (hypertrophied) sweat glands. **Carpal tunnel**, Joint abnormalities (growth of articular cartilage), colonic polyps, skin tag, HTN , macroglossia, large jaw (macrognathia), deep voice, organomegaly, cardiomegaly, amenorrhea (**GH ↑ prolactin**), cardiomegaly, central obesity, ↑ LDL and cholesterol, **diabetes (GH is anti-insulin).**

Abuse of GH presents the same as acromegaly.

DX:
BIT: **↑ serum IGF-1 (insulin-like growth factors) in the liver.**
MAT: Supression of GH by administering glucose excludes acromegaly. (Normal: GH should be suppressed by glucose).
MRI: shows pituitary tumor,
GH fails to suppress after oral glucose.
If glucose levels are ↑, then GH should ↓.
Supression of GH by giving oral glucose excludes acromegaly.

The exam prefers: the most inexpensive and non-invasive routes of diagnosis and treatments.
To DX Acromegaly = have patient bring in a younger picture of themselves.

TX:
Surgery to remove pituitary tumor (transsphenoidal removal).
Med: **Octreotide** (Somatostatin analog), **Pegvisomant** (GH receptor antagonist), **Bromocriptine, Cabergoline** (Dopamine agonist inhibit growth hormone release)

Gigantism
(**tip**: all kids like the jolly great GIANT)

↑ GH in children which increases linear bone growth. Happens before epiphyseal plate closure.

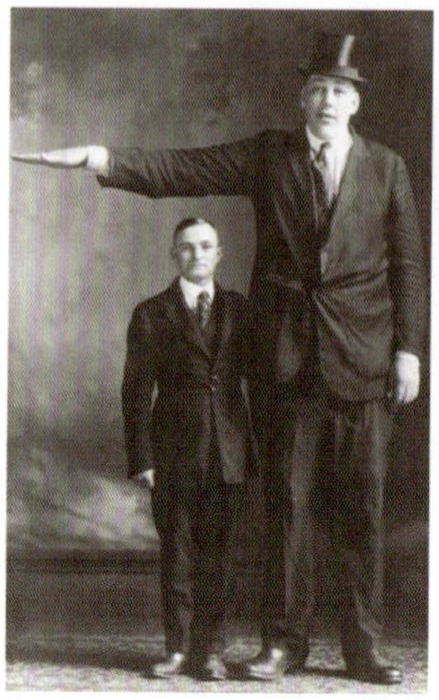

Dwarfism
Due to defective growth hormone receptors so that ↓ linear growth occurs.
↓ IGF-1 levels in liver.

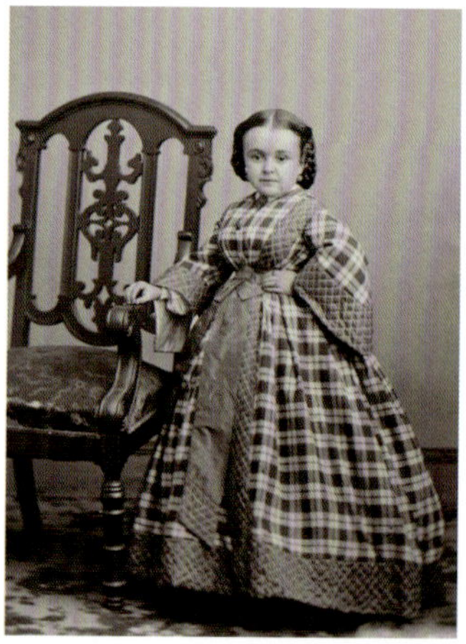

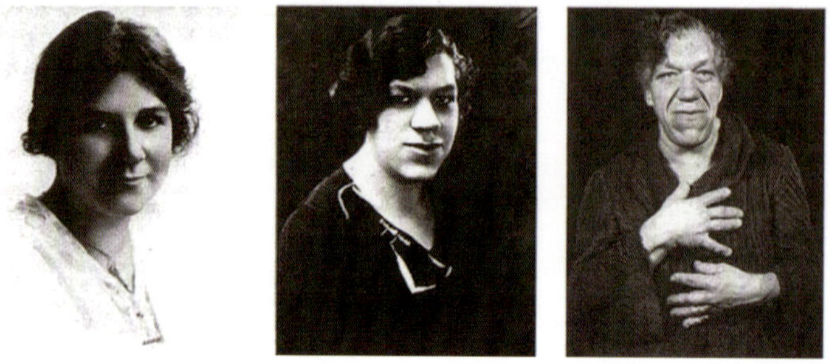

Picture sequence of acromegaly

GnRH

LH and FSH Deficiency	Kallmann Syndrome	
LH and FSH stimulate the female gonads to release estrogen and progesterone. Causes anovulation, amenorrhea, decreased libido. LH and FSH stimulate the male gonads to release androgens. Causes lack of testosterone, inability to make sperm, decreased libido, erectile dysfunction, decreased axillary and pubic hair, decreased muscle mass.	• Failure to start puberty or failure to complete puberty • Occurs in males and females • Hypogonadism and infertility • **Anosmia (reduced or no sense of smell)** • Cause: **Hypothalamic neurons** responsible for releasing GnRH **fail to migrate** into the hypothalamus during embryonic development • Labs: ↓ GnRH, ↓ FSH, ↓ LH	

Additional Pituitary Pathologies

Empty Stella Syndrome (ESS)	Sheehan's Syndrome
The pituitary gland shrinks or is flattened. The sella turcica (a depression located in the sphenoid bone that holds the pituitary gland. It is held in the hypophyseal fossa area). This area becomes filled with CSF instead of the pituitary gland. Causes: Primary: Increased pressure in the sella turcica, which causes the gland to flatten (high blood pressure, obesity, intracranial HTN). Secondary: Due to the gland regressing because of trauma, surgery or radiation therapy. Increased risk for precocious puberty, pituitary tumors, growth hormone deficiency, pituitary gland dysfunction, low testosterone and/or hypogonadism in men.	Postpartum pituitary gland infarction/necrosis due to ischemia because of severe blood loss during or after childbirth. SX: Inability to lactate after childbirth (agalactorrhoea), hypopituitarism (intolerance to cold, weight gain, constipation, bradycardia, low blood pressure). Gonadotropin deficiency (↓ LH and FSH) may cause amenorrhea, hot flashes, decreased libido. Adrenal insufficiency (↓ ACTH) may cause hypoglycemia, anemia, hyponatremia (SIADH).

Pancreas

- Performs both endocrine (acinar and duct cells) and exocrine rolls.
- Produces: Insulin, glucagon, somatostatin, pancreatic polypeptides.
- Secretes digestive enzymes to help digest and absorb nutrients in the small intestine:
  Bicarb from centroacinar cells stimulated by secretin.
  Digestive enzymes from basophilic cells stimulated by CCK.
- Digestive enzymes:
  Trypsinogen and Chymotrypsinogen (**Enteropeptidase (enterokinase) cleaves trypsinogen to form trypsin**).
  (**tip**: when you go on a **TRYP** (trip) you rent from **Enterp**rise)
  Pancreatic Lipase
  Pancreatic Amylase
  Phospholipase A2, lysophospholipase
  Cholesterol esterase
- Blood supply:
  Splenic artery supplies the neck, body and tail.
  Superior and inferior pancreaticoduodenal artery supply the anterior and posterior surfaces and head
  Drainage of the body and neck into the splenic vein
  Drainage of the head into the superior mesenteric and portal veins
- Make up:
  Islets of Langerhans composed of:
  α (alpha) cells on periphery secrete glucagon
  β (Beta) cells in the central secrete insulin (**tip**: INsulin is on the INside)
  δ (Delta) cells interspersed secrete somatostatin
  F cell secrete pancreatic polypeptide
- NOTE: Extremely high glucose levels artificially drops sodium levels

Pancreatic Cell

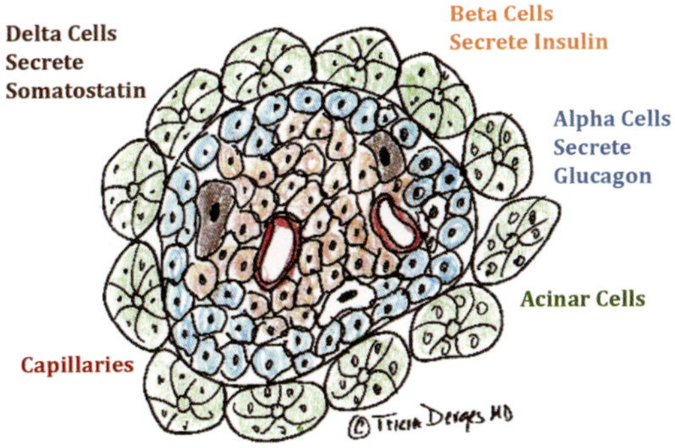

Insulin

- Peptide hormone produced by **Beta cells**
- Regulates metabolism of carbs and fats by promoting absorption of glucose from the **skeletal muscles and fat tissues** through **GLUT-4** receptors
- Preproinsulin is synthesized in RER ➔ proinsulin (**secretory granules**) ➔exocytosis of insulin and **C-peptide**
- **C-Peptide** is present if the body has made its OWN insulin. **If C-peptide is not present then the insulin was taken exogenously**
- **Well fed state = glycolysis and insulin is on and glucagon is off**
- Insulin opposes glucagon
- **Tyrosine Kinase** (AKA: **RTKs** = receptor tyrosine kinase) (**Cell surface** receptor. Extracellularly **ligand-binding** domain, **transmembrane-spanning**
- Insulin does **not cross the placenta**

Physiological effects of Insulin

- ↑ glycogen synthesis, liver
- ↑ lipid synthesis. Forces fat cells to take in blood lipids which are converted to triglycerides
- ↑ esterification of fatty acids. Makes adipose tissues make fats from fatty acid esters
- ↑ amino acid uptake in cells
- ↑ DNA replication and protein synthesis
- ↑ serum potassium uptake into cells
- ↑ HCL by parietal cells
- ↓ proteolysis (protein b/d)
- ↓ lipolysis, causes reduction in conversion lipid stores into blood fatty acids
- ↓ gluconeogenesis, causes decrease in production of glucose from nonsugar sources
- ↑ arterial muscle tone by forcing arterial muscle walls to relax = ↑ blood flow
- ↑ GnRH = ↑ fertility
- ↑ Na retention
- ↓ glucagon release

Insulin Dependent Glucose Transporters (must have GLUT receptors to bring glucose into the cell)

GLUT-1: Brain, RBC's, cornea
GLUT-2: β islet cells, kidney, liver, small intestine
GLUT-4: Skeletal muscle, adipose tissue
GLUT-5: Spermatocytes (need fructose for their "trip"), GI tract

Organ insulin utilization
Brain: Highest use of glucose, uses ketone bodies during starvation..

Heart: Glucose and fatty acids

RBC's: Use glucose because they must rely on anaerobic metabolism due to lack of mitochondria

Insulin-independent glucose uptake. These organs can bring in glucose **without** the help of insulin: Brain, RBC's, Intestine, Cornea, Kidney, Liver
(**Tip**: BRICK L)

Insulin Regulation

- Glucose regulates insulin release
- GH = insulin resistance = ↑ insulin
- β 2 agonist = ↑ insulin
- Glucagon, cortisol, epinephrine, norepinephrine, TNFα, catecholamine's = stop insulin
- Parasympathetic (Cholinergic/ ACh) releases insulin (Digest)
- Sympathetic can stimulate either ↑ or ↓ in insulin
- Epinephrine binds both α and β receptors. So if an α blocker is given, epinephrine will still stimulate β therefore releases insulin. If you block α receptors, β is still working

Insulin Secretion (Beta Cells)

- Glucose enters Beta cells through **GLUT-2**
- Glucose ➔ glycolysis to ↑ **ATP:ADP** ration in the cell
- ↑ATP/ADP ratio **closes K** channels to prevent K from leaving the cell by facilitated diffusion so ↑ K ions making the cell more positive, leaving to depolarization
- On depolarization, voltage gated **Ca channels open** to allow Ca to move **into (influx)** the cell by facilitated diffusion
- ↑ Ca concentration ➔ activates **IRS** and **phospholipase C that makes IP3 and DAG.**
- Phospholipase C inhibits fructose 1,6 biphosphate and gluconeogenesis promoting glycolysis
- IP3 binds to receptors on the endoplasmic reticulum to allow the release of Ca from the ER through IP3 gated channels, ↑ Ca concentration even more
- **↑↑ Ca causes release (exocytosis) of insulin in secretory vesicles into the blood stream**

Glucose Uptake in Muscle/Adipose

- Insulin binds receptors in dimeric form and activates the receptor tyrosine-kinase domain
- **Tyrosine Kinase** (AKA: **RTKs** = receptor tyrosine kinase) (**Cell surface** receptor. Extracellular **ligand-binding** domain, **transmembrane-spanning**
- The tyrosine receptor **phosphorylates IRS-1** (Insulin Receptor Substrate) which stimulates **PIP3** a (phosphoinositide-3) and **RAS/MAP** kinase pathway (RAS/MAP continue on to promote cell growth and DNA synthesis).
- **PI3K** (Phosphatidylinositol 3 Kinase) stimulates the **GLUT-4** receptor to be expressed on the plasma membrane
- **GLUT-4** brings in glucose via facilitated diffusion to move down a concentration gradient into the muscle and fat cells
- Once glucose is inside the cells it is phosphorylated by glucokinase (liver) or hexokinase (other tissues) to form G6P, which enters glycolysis. G6P can't diffuse back out of cells
- Muscle contraction ↑ surface GLUT-4 receptors due to ↑ need for energy. Especially important in cardiac muscle

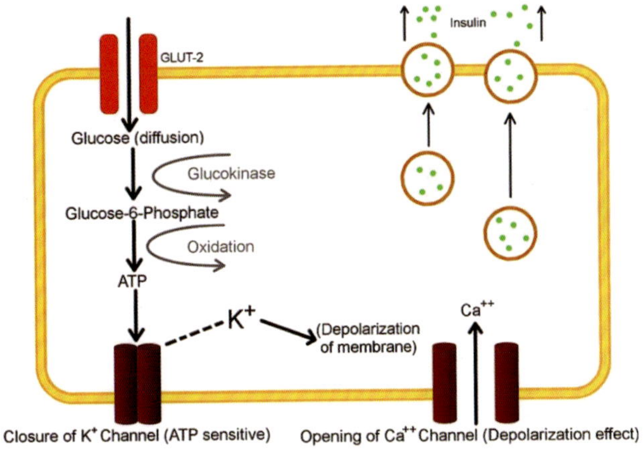

Insulin Release

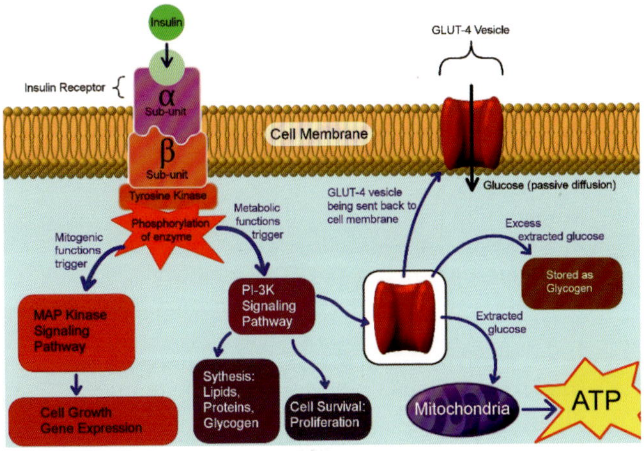

Insulin Signal Pathway

Insulin and Diabetes mellitus

Diabetes Type 1	Diabetes Type 2	
• **Autoimmune** destruction of the insulin producing beta cells in the pancreas.. • Once 90% of the beta cells are destroyed the blood glucose levels will rise. • Usually presents first time as DKA. • DKA • Weight loss • Younger <30 • Destruction of beta cells is by T lymphocytes. • **Histology: Islet leukocytic infiltrates** • HLA-DR3, HLA-DR4 • Not uncommon to have other autoimmune diseases	(AKA: Metabolic syndrome) • **↑ Resistance to insulin** • Initial stage is due to insulin resistance and hyperinsulinemia. • Later stage is caused by beta cell dysfunction and impaired insulin secretion. • Insulin resistance = weight gain • Histology: **Amyloid (amylin)** polypeptide (IAPP) deposits in the Islet cells • Hyperosmolar DKA • Older > 40 **NOTE: Patients with Acanthosis nigricans should be tested for diabetes (hyperinsulinemia).**	SX: **Polydipsia, polyuria, polyphagia,** blurry vision (reoccurring), recurrent infections. **Diagnosis of Diabetes** **Fasting Glucose ≥ 126 mg/dl** **Random Glucose with symptoms ≥ 200 mg/dl** **Abnormal 2 hour Glucose Tolerance Test.** **HbA1c > 6.4** **(normal: 4.8 – 5.6** **pre-diabetic: 5.7 – 6.4)** HbA1c: can give you average glucose levels of patient: **HbA1c x 20** = average glucose reading over the past 90 days. **Equivalents:** **DM = CAD = PAD** **Annual checkups required for diabetics:** Ophthalmologist, Podiatrist, Nephrologist

Type 1 DKA Diabetic Ketoacidosis	Type 2 DKA Hyperosmolar Hyperglycemic	Diabetic Eye Pathologies (nonenzymatic glycosylation)
• SX: **Kussmaul breathing** (hyperventilation = **rapid/deep = respiratory alkalosis**), urine and serum **ketones**, confusion, **fruity breath (acetone)** odor (exhaled acetone), **polydipsia, polyuria,** dehydration, delirium, psychosis, **abdominal pain**, nausea, coffee grounds vomiting • Can be brought on by any type of stress or infection • Labs: **Anion Gap Metabolic Acidosis** Na – (HCO3 + Cl) Normal: < 15 > 15 = Anion Gap Metabolic acidosis • **Acid/Base: Anion Gap (> 12) Metabolic Acidosis with compensation Respiratory alkalosis** (Kussmaul breathing) • **Labs: ↓pH, ↓ HCO3, ↓ CO2, ↑ K, hyperglycemia. (tip: Hyperkalemia = Acidosis. Hypokalemia = Alkalosis)** • **↑ levels: Acetone, Acetoacetate, Beta Hydroxybutyrate** • Finger stick glucose: high > 250. (can be as high as 600+) • **Hyperkalemia** ↑ K, because there is no insulin. K is extracellular, out in the serum and not inside the cell because it is exchanged for hydrogen ions going into the cell trying to compensate for the metabolic acidosis. (K must be trapped in the cell to release insulin. **Insulin drives potassium into the cell with glucose**) • **Acidosis = hyperkalemia.** **Alkalosis = hypokalemia.** • TX: **IV Fluids (normal saline), IV Insulin, Replace K** once potassium levels come down towards a normal level (to replace intracellular stores), and **glucose** to prevent hypoglycemia. **Follow improvement by monitoring the anion gap and/or arterial pH**	• Extreme high blood sugars cause severe dehydration because of ↑ in OSM • **NO ketones in the urine** • **Glucose levels > 600 (can reach > 1200)** • Hyperviscosity • **↓↓K, Hypokalemia** due to high urinary output • Hypercoagulability • **Serum OSM >320** • Substantial polydipsia due to severe dehydration • Usually due to an infection, MI, stroke, illness • TX: **IV Fluids** (must correct over a 24 hour period) with normal saline, **replace K** (rate of 10 mEq per hour). **IV insulin** is **not started** until K levels have stabilized. Insulin moves K into the cells and patient is already ↓↓ K due to urination. If patient's K levels are low, do not start insulin as it will make the serum K levels even lower.	**Diabetes Retinopathy** Takes 10 years to develop Is the first damage due to DM 2 stages: **1st stage** **Non-proliferative** diabetic retinopathy. No symptoms, eyesight 20/20. DX: **Microaneurysms** (bulges in the artery walls). Blocked retinal blood vessels due to ischemia (lack of blood flow) **Macular edema** causes retinal thickening (blood vessels leak) = blurred vision and darkened images. **2nd stage** **Proliferative** diabetic retinopathy. **Neovascularization** – formation of abnormal NEW blood vessels that burst and bleed (vitreous hemorrhage) and blur vision and causes **"floaters"** (specks of blood/spots floating in the visual field). Hemorrhages increase causing larger spots of bleeding = **"Cotton Wool Spots" (flame hemorrhages)** **Osmotic Damage** Due to **accumulation of sorbitol** in organs with **aldose reductase** or ↓ in sorbitol dehydrogenase. Causes: **Cataracts** Neuropathies 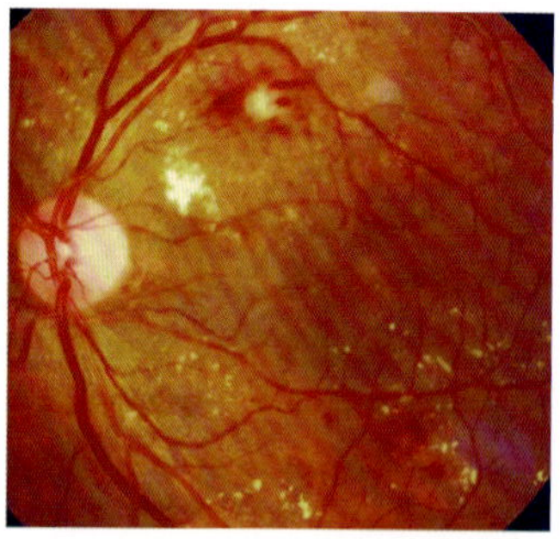

Diabetic Nephropathy	**Neuropathies**	**Hypoglycemia**
(Nonenzymatic glycosylation) Nephrotic Syndrome Progressive kidney disease, taking 5 – 10 years to occur. Damages the capillaries in the glomeruli, scarring the glomeruli. SX: **Progressive proteinuria**, chronic renal failure Histology: **Kimmelstiel-Wilson nodules** **Progression monitored by urine microalbumin.** Micro (tiny) bits of protein will start to show in the urine due to loss of negative charge in the basement membrane of the glomerulus. So a ↓ of filtration is needed so more damage/larger holes are not made. **Ace Inhibitors** dilate the efferent arterioles so that the filtration fraction is decreased. Monitor GFR (eGFR). (Hyaline: shows pink with stained with H & E). TX: **Ace Inhibitors (or ARB's) are a MUST** to **slow down the progression** of diabetic nephropathy in patients that have **normal** kidney function. 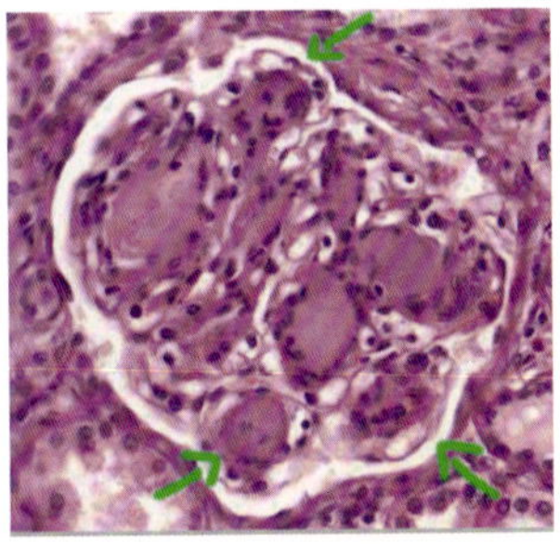	Diabetics can suffer from neuropathies in various organs. **Feet:** ↓ sensation makes patients unable to feel anything in their feet so sores or injuries go untreated and can lead to ulcers which can become **gangrene and require amputation.** **TX: Gabapentin** *(Neurontin),* **Pregabalin** *(Lyrica)* Penis: **Erectile dysfunction** Bladder: **Overflow incontinence**. They are unable to feel when their bladder is full or whether or not they have emptied it when urinating so the urine will overflow when the bladder fills and causes dribbling. **Gastroparesis:** Diabetics can't sense stretch in stomach (stretch is what stimulates gastric motility) so ↓ motility/emptying of stomach contents (Succussion splash noted in abdomen) and SX of bloating, **constipation**, fullness, diarrhea. TX: **Metoclopramide, Erythromycin** (increase gastric motility) **Constipation:** This is due to the **dysfunction of the Pelvic Splanchnic Nerves.** Cardiovascular: Equivalent to CAD. Increased risk of stroke, CHF.	Condition where there is ↑↑ insulin (insulin is taking to much glucose out of the blood) SX: Loss of consciousness, confusion, blurred vision, tremors, sweating, coma, death **Causes:** **Insulinoma** (insulin secreting tumor in the pancreas). **Exogenous** insulin injection. **Sulfonylurea** overdose. **To determine cause:** (Remember the exam likes inexpensive and non-invasive procedures) 1st: Check urine for drugs (**Sulfonylurea**). This patient is usually a health professional wanting attention. They are admitted into the hospital, their condition is stabilized but become hypoglycemic again) 2nd: If urine is drug free. Take a blood sample. **Check for C-Peptide.** If there is C-Peptide then do an ultrasound and look for a tumor. TX: **Octreotide** 3rd: If there is no C-Peptide then insulin has been injected.

Dawn Phenomenon (Dawn Effect)

Early morning (between 2 and 8 am) **increase in blood sugar** (glucose) due to decreasing insulin and a growth hormone surge. (Growth hormone antagonizes insulin)

TX: Avoid carb intake at bedtime,
Adjust the dose of insulin meds, or administer extra insulin in the early morning.
TX needs to leave more insulin in the body. Glucose is rising because there is no insulin left to pull it out. If you eat less before bed (↓ carb) then your insulin won't be used up on this and more will stay in the body. If you add more insulin to your evening dose, more will last until the morning.

Somogyi Effect

Elevated blood sugar in the morning due to a **rebound (reflex)** of the body in response to a low blood sugar.

TX: The rebound will not happen if enough glucose is left in the body. So you need to insure more glucose is available through the night. Eat a snack before bedtime or reduce the amount of the evening dose of insulin.

Diabetics are ↑ risk for:	Health Care for Diabetics	KETONES:
Infections from pseudomonas, mucormycosis (AKA: Rhizopus, Zygomycosis, Absidia, Mucor, Cunninghamella). **Diabetes is the equivalent to Coronary Artery Disease.**	Annual eye exam (check for neovascularization/proliferative retinopathy). Annual screening for nephropathy. (UA is checked for **microalbuminuria**: levels of urine albumin 30 – 300 mg/24 hrs. Positive UA for proten is > 300 mg/24 hrs). All **vaccines** required for immunocompromised patients (annual influenza, pneumococcal). **ACE inhibitors/ARB's** for to slow progression of kidney failure. ACE inhibitors/ARB's to control BP below 130/80 (this ↓ risk of MI). **Aspirin** (all Diabetic patients > 30 years). **Statins** if the LDL is > 100 mg/dL. Annual foot exam (check for ulcers and nephropathy).	Fuel used when glucose is gone. **Organs that can use ketones:** Skeletal, Cardiac, Renal, Brain **Organs that can't use ketones:** RBC (no mitochondria) Liver (no **thiophorase**) (**Note**: Remember from bio chem that anything that inhibits the beta-oxidation pathway inhibits ketones from being made).

Condition	Fasting Glucose Level	2 Hour Glucose Level	AbA1c
Normal	< 110 mg/dl	< 140 mg/dl	< 6.0
Diabetes mellitus DX	≥ 126 mg/dl	≥ 200 mg/dl	≥ 6.5

Anion Gap Acidosis and DKA

- Insulin is needed to bring glucose into cells to use as fuel for energy.
- Absence of insulin means no glucose comes into the cell so there is no fuel to use to make energy.
- The cells then use free fatty acids and ketones for fuel instead.
- The acid base is now acidic because the negatively charged ketones decrease the levels of HCO3 (bicarb)
- Formula for Anion Gap: Sodium minus (HCO3 + Cl). If total is > 14 = DKA.
- Other Anion Gap causes: MUDPILES
  Methanol, Uremia, DKA, Paraldehyde, Iron/INH, Lactic acidosis, Ethylene glycol, Salicylates (aspirin)

Management of Diabetes

- Lipid goal in a diabetic without CAD: LDL goal < 100.
- **Lipid goal in a diabetic with CAD: LDL goal < 70**. (Diabetes = CAD) (TX: **Statin**)
- **Blood Pressure goal** < 130/80 mm Hg.
- **Slow progression of renal disease**. Monitor urine microalbumin. Use of **ACE inhibitors**.
- Annual eye exam to monitor for **proliferative retinopathy**. TX with **VEGF inhibitors: Ranibizumab, Bevacizumab**.
- Annual **foot exams by a podiatrist** to monitor for neuropathies. TX neuropathy with **Gabapentin or Pregabalin**.
- Monitor other **neuropathies:** Gastroparesis (TX: **Metoclopramide, Erythromycin**), bladder incontinence (TX: overflow with **Oxybutynin**), erectile dysfunction (TX: **Sildenafil**).
- Overall drug TX: Statin, Ace Inhibitor, Neuropathies as indicated.

Treatment Management for Diabetes Type 2

- Lifestyle changes: Diet (↓ calories), exercise = weight loss.
- Initial drug therapy: Metformin (blocks gluconeogenesis). Side effects: lactic acidosis, do not use if renal failure, must stop Metformin if surgery, do not use contrast dyes.
- If DM 2 still not controlled, add a second drug to Metformin: Sulfonylurea (increases release of insulin): Glipizide, Glyburide. Side effects: SIADH, Hypoglycemia.
- If DM 2 is still not controlled after 2-drug regimen add insulin, sub Q.

Maternal (Gestational) and Fetus Diabetes Pathology

Maternal Diabetes	Diabetes in Fetus and Neonate
High risk for **macrosomia babies** (large babies > 5000 gm) causing trouble at delivery: **shoulder dystocia** /shoulder dislocation (upper brachial plexus injuries) or **Klumpke paralysis** (pulling out on the arm) (lower brachial plexus injury). Pregnant women are given a **glucose tolerance test at 28 weeks** to check for maternal diabetes.	• **Macrosomia** (big baby) Big baby = more weight = difficulty breathing = RDS • Surfactant decreased • **Hypoglycemia** • Respiratory Distress = EPO = Polycythemia • Heart issues: Transposition of Great Arteries • Hypocalcemia • **Caudal Regression** • Polyhydramnios • Physiologic jaundice • IUGR

Additional Pancreatic Hormone Pathologies

- Note: Pancreatic hormones are required to help absorb Vit. B12. After eating Vitamin B12 it binds to the **R-protein** (AKA: Transcobalamin I, Haptocorrin, Cobalophilin) in the stomach before it goes to the small intestine to be absorbed. Pancreatic enzymes unbind Vit B 12 from the R-protein so that B-12 can then bind with Intrinsic Factor to be absorbed.

Insulinoma	**Glucagonoma**
Tumor of Pancreatic Beta Cells, Spontaneous hypoglycemia. ↑↑ Insulin = hypoglycemia. Labs: Low blood glucose and **C-Peptide will be present** (body produced) SX: Palpitations, confusion, sweating, loss of consciousness, no pain, HTN (↑ blood pressure) DX: Fasting insulin and glucose levels TX: **Octreotide**, surgical resection	Tumor of the Pancreatic Alpha Cells. ↑↑ glucagon production. Labs: Blood serum glucagon > 1000 pg/mL (normal 50 – 200 pg/mL) Glucagon ↑ blood glucose via gluconeogenesis and lipolysis = hyperglucagonemia and ↓ amino acids, anemia, diarrhea, weight loss. TX: **Octreotide**, surgical resection
VIPomas Endocrine tumor originating from **non-Beta islet cells in the pancreas**. Produces ↑↑ vasoactive intestinal peptide (VIP) **Highly associated with MEN I** SX: **Severe watery diarrhea (up to 3 liters/day)**, dehydration, hypokalemia, achlorhydria (↓ HCL production in the stomach), flushing, hypotension, hypercalcemia, hyperglycemia. DX: Fasting VIP plasma level TX: **Octreotide**, surgical resection	**Gastrinoma** **Zollinger-Ellison Syndrome** (Associated together) Tumor in the pancreas or duodenum in **non-beta islet cells** that secretes ↑↑ gastrin (parietal cells) causing multiple ulcers in the stomach, duodenum, small intestine. **Highly assocated with MEN I** SX: Hypergastrinemia, multiple recurrent ulcers, severe diarrhea, steatorrhea, vomiting blood (stomach ulcers), weight loss, malabsorption issues, abdominal pain DX: Fasting serum gastrin TX: **Octreotide, PPI,** surgery resection

Parathyroid

- Parathyroid and Thyroid are in control of **calcium regulation.**
- PTH is secreted from the parathyroid chief cells. It raises the level of calcium. It is a polypeptide of 84 amino acids.
- Calcitonin is secreted from the Thyroid parafollicular cells. (**tip**: calci "tone" in, "tones" down calcium when its too high)
- **Calcium forms: Ionized, bound to albumin, and bound to anions.**
  When calcium is bound to albumin it is not active = ↓ calcium levels. ↑ in pH it causes calcium to bind to albumin (aka: the negative charge increases the affinity of albumin to calcium), resulting in ↓ calcium.
- Calcium is needed for teeth, bones, transmission of signals in nerve cells and muscle contraction.
- Parathyroid function is to **maintain calcium (raise calcium levels) and phosphate levels** so that nerves and muscles function properly via Parathyroid Hormone (**PTH**).
- The serum-ionized calcium via negative feedback determines PTH secretion.
- PTH uses the Gq G-protein path: phospholipase C. When there are high levels of extracellular calcium: Phospholipase C hydrolyzes PIP2 (phosphatidylinositol 4,5-bisphosphate) to IP3 and DAG (diacylglycerol) to cause calcium to be released from intracellular stores into the cytoplasm, raising the extracellular concentration of calcium. This increase of extracellular calcium inhibits PTH.
- **PTH is stimulated** by: ↓ serum calcium, ↓ serum magnesium, ↑ serum phosphate (decreases calcium sensitive receptors).
- **PTH is inhibited by**: ↑ serum calcium, ↓↓ serum magnesium, calcitriol (Vitamin D3).
- PTH raises **blood calcium levels by stimulating osteoclast** to break down bone and release calcium (resorption) and increasing the amount of calcium reabsorbed in the small intestine. **Rank-L** (secreted by osteoblast and osteoclast) **and M-CSF** mediate this.
- PTH can stimulate the reabsorption of calcium in the distal tubules and renal collecting ducts in the kidney.
- PTH **inhibits the reabsorption of phosphate** from the lumen of the renal tubules in the PCT (phosphate is excreted in the urine), which causes a decrease in the plasma phosphate concentrations which increase the amount of calcium that is ionized.
- PTH upregulates 1-alpha hydroxylase to **convert vitamin D to its active form** (converts 25-hydroxy vitamin D to 1,25-dihydroxy vitamin D). The active form of vitamin D (Calciferol) goes to the intestine to increase the reabsorption of calcium and phosphate by **calbindin** (calcium binding proteins).
- PTH **raises GI calcium absorption by activation vitamin D** and conserving (reabsorption) of calcium in the kidneys.
- PTH regulates phosphate in the kidneys. It stops the PCT reabsorption of **phosphorus so that it is excreted**
- In the **normal** physio of calcium and phosphate in the serum = **Calcium and phosphate are opposite** (ie: if Ca ↑ then Phosphorus ↓).
- Magnesium is similar to calcium in its effects on PTH. Hypomagnesemia inhibits PTH secretion, resulting in hypoparathyroidism. Administration of magnesium can reverse this effect.
- Low calcium levels can cause paresthesias, pain, cramps, carpopedal spasms (spasmodic contractions of the muscles of the hands, feet, wrists, ankles).
- 4 Parathyroid glands located on the thyroid gland. **Superior glands arise from the fourth brachial pouch and the inferior glands arise from the third brachial pouch.**
- Blood supply correspond to the thyroid gland: Superior parathyroids = **inferior thyroid artery** which is off the subclavian. The inferior parathyroids have various blood supplies.
- Histology: **Chief cells**: synthesize and release PTH.
- **Thyroid** is in charge of decreasing the calcium levels – **Calcitonin** is from the **parafollicular cells (C Cells)**
  Calcitonin inhibits osteoclast. (**tip**: Calcit "tone" in = "tones" down calcium).
  Highly associated with MEN 2A and 2B (Medullary Thyroid Cancer = ↑ Calcitonin)

Regulation of Calcium

Serum Levels	PTH Response
↓ Calcium	↑ PTH
↑ PO4	↑ PTH
↓ Mg	↓ PTH
↓↓ Mg	↓ PTH

Parathyroid Pathologies

Hyperparathyroidism

Release of too much PTH = ↑ calcium because of Breakdown of bone.
Normal Ca level: 9 – 10.5 mg/dL
High Ca levels of > 10.5 – 12 = pathology
↑↑ Ca levels of ≥ 13 is indicative of cancer

Breakdown of bone by PTH:
Macrophage colony stimulating factor (**M-CSF**) (in bone marrow progenitor cells) and **RANK-L** (receptor activator of NF-κB ligand) secreted by osteoblast bind the RANK receptor on osteoclast and stimulate them to breakdown bone in order to ↑ Calcium.

↑ in PTH will ↑ serum Ca and will then ↑ serum 1, 25 Dihydroxyvitamin D, and will ↓ serum phosphorus (with good renal function. Remember: poor renal function increases phosphorus).

PTH-rP
(PTH related peptide)

Released from an ectopic site. MC: Squamous cell carcinoma in the lungs.
(**TIP**: if the exam is referring to the PTH associated with squamous cell lung cancer, look at the answer choices. If they list BOTH PTH and PTH-rP you must pick PTH-rP. If only one of these choices are given in the answers, then pick that one. PTH from squamous cell lung cancer is not the "real" PTH, it is a related peptide: PTH-rP)

Primary Hyperparathyroidism
Problem is with the parathyroid gland itself.
MCC: Hypercalcemia.

DX: **↑ PTH with hypercalcemia**.

LABS: ↑ Calcium, ↑ PTH, ↓ Phosphate
(Ca is up because the adenoma is doing its own thing and continually producing PTH, despite what the serum calcium level is. As long as PTH is being secreted the body will continue to break down bones to get the calcium that the PTH is demanding)

Causes:
MCC: Adenoma = benign proliferation of chief cells (hyperplasia).
Additional causes of hypercalcemia: Defective calcium receptors on the parathyroid glands, Malignancy, granulomatous disease (granulomas release stimulate Vitamin D), Vitamin D toxicity, Thiazide diuretics (↑ reabsorption of calcium), Berylliosis, Histoplasmosis.

Complications of hypercalcemia:
Constipation, kidney **stones**, Acute tubular necrosis, renal insufficiency, polyuria, polydipsia (DI), **short QT** on EKG, abdominal pain, **confusion**, fractures, **osteoporosis**, osteomalacia.

TX: **Furosemide** (excretes calcium), **Bisphosphonate (Pamidronate),** insure hydration, **Calcitonin** (if Furosemide is not working), **Steroids** with granulomatous disease.

Secondary hyperparathyroidism
Due to a disease that lowers calcium levels, forcing the parathyroid glands to overwork to compensate for the loss of calcium.

LABS: Normal to ↓ Calcium, ↑ PTH, ↑ Phosphate
(Because Calcium is low, PTH is at work trying to raise the level. Phosphate is high because the kidneys are not excreting it, so its building up)

Causes:
MCC: Chronic **renal disease = less active vitamin D is converted = ↓ Ca =** parathyroid compensates and works harder (hypertrophy) to release more PTH trying to find more calcium. Failing kidneys also do not excrete phosphate so it is retained. This causes calcium phosphate to form in the body and remove calcium from the circulation = hypocalcemia.
(Remember: Calcium is reabsorbed in the DCT)

Can also result from any malabsorption problem.
Severe Vitamin D deficiency.
Severe Calcium deficiency.

If the secondary cause is not corrected it will continue on to Tertiary Hyperparathyroidism

Tertiary hyperparathyroidism	**SX of Secondary Hyperparathyroidism:**
Occurs when the secondary cause becomes chronic which causes the body to be unresponsive to blood calcium levels = PTH is continually released. Labs will show **everything is up**. ↑ Ca, ↑↑ PTH, and ↑ Phosphate (normally phosphate is opposite of Ca) **Hyperparathyroidism Associations:** MEN I and MEN 2A Post menopausal women Radiation treatment that exposed the neck Severe deficiency in Vitamin D or Calcium People on lithium **Familial hypocalciuric hypercalcemia (FHH)** Family history. Defective Ca receptor on parathyroid cells. PTH is not suppress by ↑ Ca = mild hypercalcemia with normal to ↑ PTH Don't forget: **Hydrochlorothiazide's retain Ca**	Fragile bones = osteoporosis, osteomalacia, kidney stones (excess calcium in the blood = excess calcium in the urine), abdominal pain, weakness, tiring easy, depression, HTN, forgetfulness, bone and joint pain, nausea, vomiting, anorexia, CONSTIPATION Neonatal hypoparathyroidism: severe hyperparathyroidism in pregnant women may cause dangerously low levels of calcium in newborns **Screening for bone density**: **DEXA scan** (duel-energy x-ray absorptiometry) Screening: Women at age 65 and every two years. **Calcium** Recommendations: Girls 9 – 18: 1300 IU/day (International units) Women 19 – 50: 1000 IU/day Women over 50: 1200 IU/day **Vitamin D** Recommendations: Most: 200 IU – 600 IU/day > 70: 600 IU – 800 IU/day

Hyperparathyroidism and Hypercalcemia

Causes of Hypercalcemia	Complications of Hypercalcemia	Treatment
Parathyroid adenoma Hyperplasia of glands Vitamin D Intoxication Granulomatous Diseases (ie: Sarcoidosis. Granulomas make Vitamin D) Malignancy (look for a very high Ca level > 13) Tuberculosis Berylliosis Histoplasmosis Thiazide Diuretics (Ca is reabsorbed in the DCT)	Constipation Peptic ulcers (calcium stimulates gastrin) Lethargy/slow Abdominal pain Nausea, vomiting Anorexia Kidney stones (Nephrolithiasis) Muscle weakness Confusion Fractures **Osteoporosis/Osteomalacia** Acute Tubular Necrosis (renal insufficiency) Short QT Syndrome Dehydration/volume depletion (↑ Ca inhibits ADH at collecting duct = nephrogenic diabetes insipidus).	IV Normal Saline **Bisphosphonates** (slow) **Furosemide** to ↑ renal Ca excretion **Calcitonin** (works faster than Bisphosphonates. **Steroids** used in granulomatous dz. Surgery: Remove parathyroid gland (s). Bone screening: **DEXA test** for bone density.

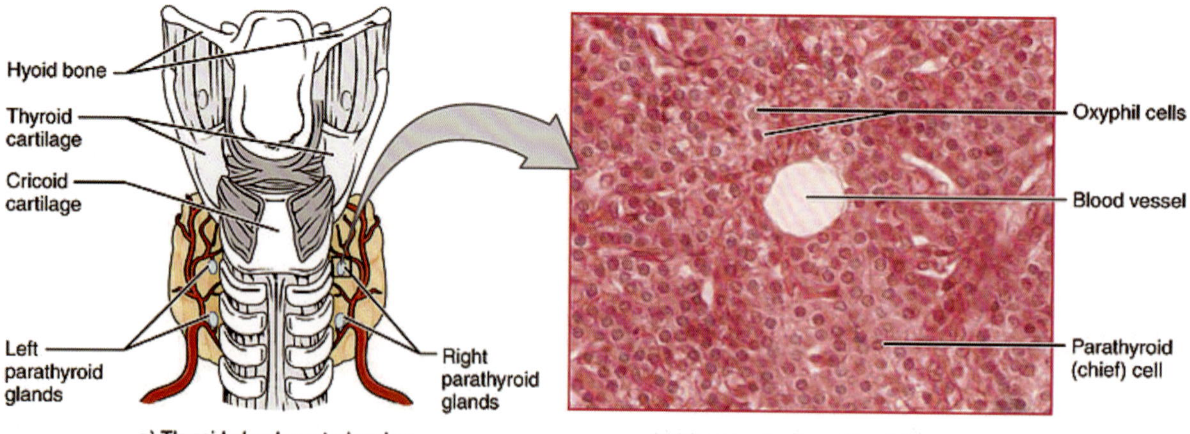

a) Thyroid gland, posterior view

b) Micrograph of parathyroid tissue

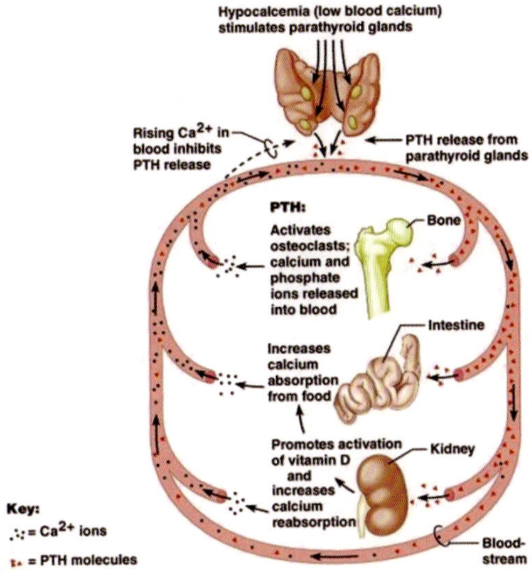

Calcium Pathologies

	Serum Calcium	Serum PO4	Serum PTH	Alkaline Phosphatase	Urine Calcium	Urine PO4	Vitamin D (25 vs 1,25)
Primary Hyperparathyroidism	↑	↓	↑	↑ or NL	↑	↑	
Secondary Hyperparathyroidism	↓ or NL	↑ to NL	↑	↑ or NL	↓	↓	
Tertiary Hyperparathyroidism	↑	↑	↑↑	↑ or NL			
Hyperparathyroidism	↑	↓	↑				25: NL 1,25: ↑
Vitamin D Toxicity	↑	↑	↓				25: ↑ 1,25: NL to ↑
Hypoparathyroidism	↓	↑	↓				25: NL 1,25: ↓
Vitamin D Deficiency	↓	↓	↑				25: ↓ 1,25: NL

Relationship between Mg and Calcium

- Mg can stimulate PTH similarly to Calcium
- Acute decrease in Mg stimulates PTH and an acute increase in Mg decreases secretion
- Severe hypermagnesemia can cause hypoparathyroidism
- ↑ Mg will cause ↓ deep tendon reflexes (DTR)
- ↓ Mg can be caused by: diuretics, diarrhea, alcohol abuse, aminoglycosides

Calcium and albumin relationship

- **Calcium is either bound to albumin or is in its free form (ionized). Ionized Ca is the active form. Calcium bound to albumin is inactive. The concern is for the active form (ionized).**
- **When albumin is low = lower total calcium due to less albumin. Total calcium = ionized calcium + calcium bound to albumin (Lab results are given for Total Calcium)**
- **Calcium is + charged and albumin is – charged = attraction**
- **Calcium correction for hypoalbuminemia:**
  Corrected Ca = {0.8 x (normal albumin – patient's albumin)} + serum Ca level
- **(AKA: Corrected Ca = serum total calcium + 0.8 (4 – serum albumin)**
  (normal albumin = 4 mg/dL or 40 g/L)
- **Gives estimate of what the total Ca level would be if the albumin were a normal level. The corrected calcium level is higher than the total calcium.**
- **Alkalosis can also cause hypocalcemia. When serum is alkalotic, hydrogen ions bound to negatively charged albumin are released. This opens binding spots up for ionized calcium to bind, which reduces the amount of active calcium. This still shows a normal (unchanged) total serum calcium because the ionized just shift spots (unbound to bound), so the total serum calcium is the total of all unbound and bound.**

Vitamin D Metabolism, Names, Pathologies

- Ingested from the diets and supplements
  D3 (derived from ultraviolet **sunlight**, saltwater fish, fish liver oil)) = Cholecalciferol
  D2 (derived from plants, milk, dairy, juices) = Ergocalciferol
- Liver: 25-hydroxy = **Calcidiol**
- Kidney: 1,25 Dihydroxycholecalciferol = Active form Vitamin D = **Calcitriol** (absorbs calcium and phosphorus in the gut)
  Requires calcium for 25 – hydroxyl to be converted to active form 1, 25 via **1α hydroxylase**
- Activated Vit D 1,25 then goes to the small intestine to reabsorb Calcium and Phosphorus
- **Rickets (children), Osteomalacia (adults)**
  Vitamin D-deficient rickets: lack of vitamin D in diet.
  Vitamin D-dependent rickets: inability to convert 25-OH to 1,25 OH (active form).
  Must supplement Vit D.
  X-linked hypophosphatemic rickets: Kidney failure causes inability to retain phosphate so bones become weak (soft) due to poor bone mineralization.
  Can also cause pectus carinatum (aka: pigeon chest) in children (Rickets) due to increased deposition of unmineralized **osteoid** causing an outward protrusion of the sternum.

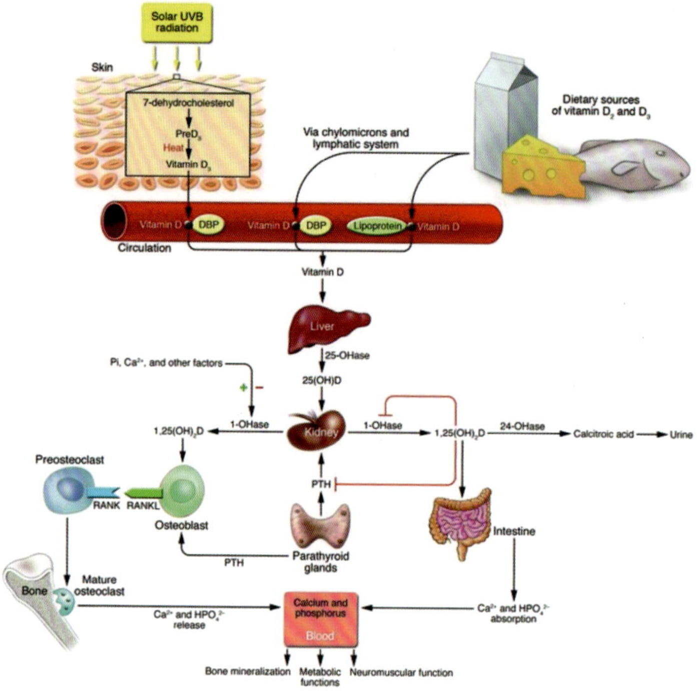

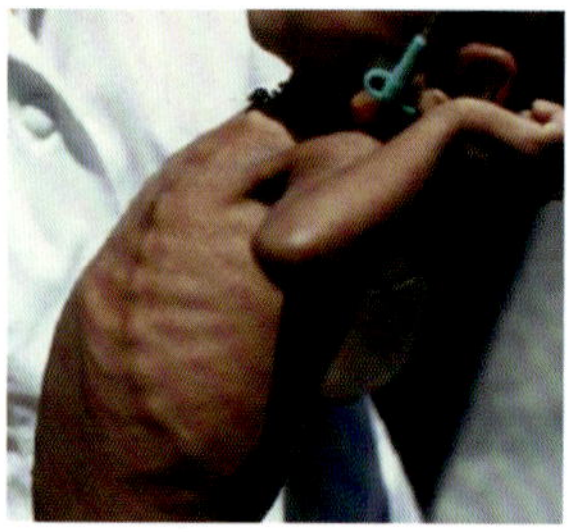

Rachitic Rosary in Rickets

Associated with a mutation in the PHEX gene sequence, which deregulates the fibroblast growth factor 23.
NOTE: Infants that are strictly breastfed must be given vitamin D supplements beginning at 2 months old.
SX: Lateral bowing of the legs. (AKA: Bowlegs)
DX: CXR shows rachitic rosary (beading of the ribs): knobs of the bone at the costochondral joints.
TX: Replacement of Vitamin D, phosphate and calcium

Differentials in Vitamin D Pathologies

Vitamin D Pathology	25 OH	1,25 OH	Calcium	Phosphate	Cause
Vitamin D-Deficient	↓	↓	↓ to NL	↓	Lack of Vit D in diet
Vitamin D-dependent	NL	↓	↓	NL	Inability to make active Vit D
X-Linked Hypophosphatemia	NL	NL	NL	↓	Inability of kidney to retain phosphate

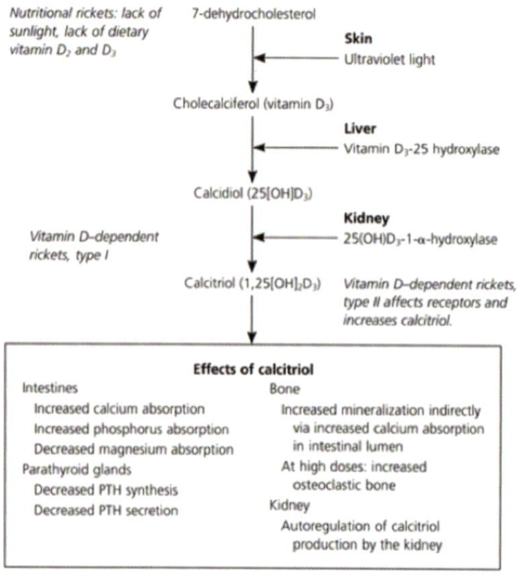

Hypoparathyroidism

Hypocalcemia
↓ Calcium in the blood.
Affects normal muscle contraction and nerve conduction.

Labs: ↓Ca, ↓ PTH, ↑ Phosphate

EKG shows prolonged QT.

TX: Replace calcium and give Vitamin D (oral)

Causes

- **MCC: #1: accidental removal during thyroid surgery.**
- Autoimmune destruction.
- Hemochromatosis.
- **DiGeorge syndrome.**
- **Magnesium deficiency** (Mg and Ca are closely related): **Magnesium is required for PTH to be released from the gland.** Low magnesium levels also lead to ↑ urinary flow of calcium.
- Defect in the calcium receptor.
- **Renal failure**: Kidney converts 25 hydroxy-D to the active 1-25 hydroxy-D.
- Genetic disorders.
- Fat Malabsorption
- Low albumin (for every point decrease in albumin, the calcium level decreases by 0.8), but the calcium levels are normal.
- Acute hyperphosphatemia (Phosphate binds with calcium and lowers it).

SX: Cramping, twitching of muscles (AKA: **tetany** = involuntary muscle contraction), paresthesia, fatigue, headaches, bone pain, insomnia, seizures, irregular heart beats, spasm of the upper airways (bronchi), perioral numbness, mental irritability, carpopedal spasm (involuntary, sudden, violent contraction of muscles of the wrist, hands, thumb, fingers, feet, toes).

Chvostek's sign (tapping on the facial muscles (facial nerve) = twitching, tetany

Trousseau sign: Occlusion of the brachial artery with BP cuff = carpal spasm = ↓ calcium.

Pseudohypoparathyroidism, AD
(AKA: Albright hereditary Osteodystrophy)

Resistance to PTH = ↓ Ca
Due to a dysfunctional G Proteins

Labs: ↓ Ca, ↑ PTH ↑ Phosphate

SX: Short stature, rounded faces, shortened 4th/5th metacarpals, tetany, muscle spasms, calcification of the basal ganglia in the white matter of the brain

Associated with TSH resistance

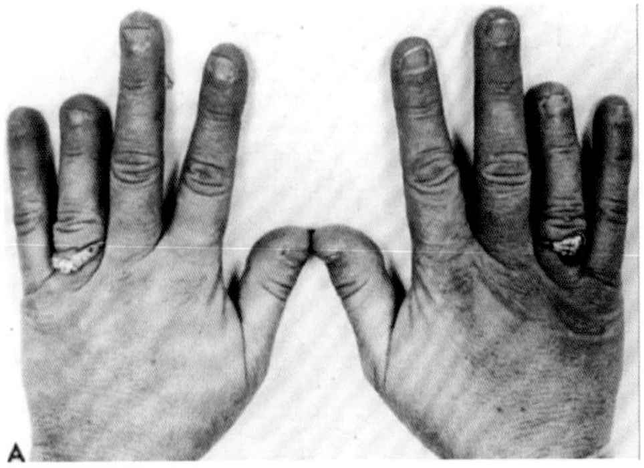

Pseudohypoparathyroidism

Calcium Tip:

- High calcium: lethargic and slow
  High calcium: volume depletion (↑ Ca inhibits ADH at collecting duct = nephrogenic diabetes insipidus).
- Low calcium: twitching (Chvostek's sign, Trousseau's sign) and hyperexcitable, seizures, prolonged QT

PTH and Ca^{2+} Pathologies

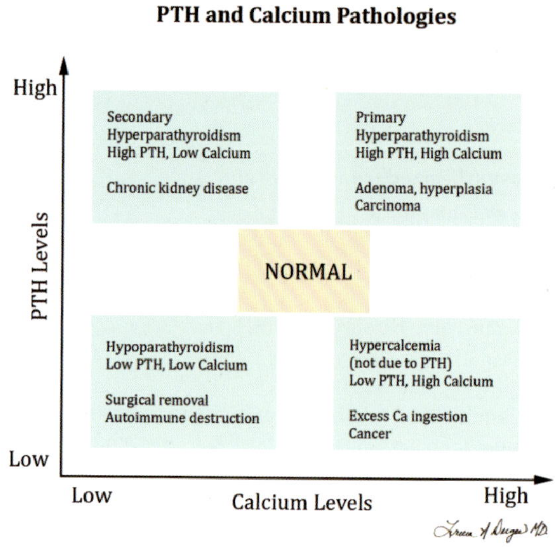

Hypercalcemia

High Calcium (hypercalcemia) **If PTH is normal to high**	**High Calcium** **If PTH is ↓, then check Vit D**	**Effects of ↑ Calcium**
1° hyperparathyroidism Parathyroid adenoma Parathyroid hyperplasia Parathyroid carcinoma Family History Lithium	Vitamin D excess Vitamin A excess Immobilization Granuloma Dz Hyperthyroidism Thiazides Theophylline **↑↑↑ Calcium > 13 = malignancy**	Fragile bones = osteoporosis, osteomalacia, kidney stones (excess calcium in the blood = excess calcium in the urine), abdominal pain, Lethargy/slowness, weakness/tiring easy, depression, forgetfulness, bone and joint pain, nausea, vomiting, anorexia, **CONSTIPATION** HTN, arthritis, acute pancreatitis, increase of 1,25 Dihydroxyvitamin D.

Hypocalcemia

↓ Calcium (hypocalcemia)	**Signs of ↓ Calcium**	**Effects of ↓ Calcium**
Hypoparathyroidism Vitamin D Deficiency Chronic Kidney Dz Genetic Dz Eating disorders Fat malabsorption Prolonged vomiting Chelation therapy (removes heavy metals from body) Bisphosphonates Calcitonin Tumor lysis syndrome Alkalosis Neonatal hypocalcemia Low albumin	**Chvostek's sign** (tapping on the facial muscles (facial nerve) = twitching, tetany **Trousseau sign:** Occlusion of the brachial artery with BP cuff = carpal spasm	Tetany (AKA: **Trousseau's sign**): twitching, contraction of muscles, AKA: hyperexcitability of muscles. Cardiac arrhythmias Laryngospasm Positive chronotropic = ↑ HR Negative inotropic = ↓ Contractility **QT prolongation** Oral, perioral paresthesias,(numbness), petechiae, purpura Convulsions/Seizures, Mental irritability, Carpopedal spasm (spasm of feet/hands), **Chvostek's sign** (tapping on the facial muscles (facial nerve).

Thyroid

Thyroid Hormone Synthesis

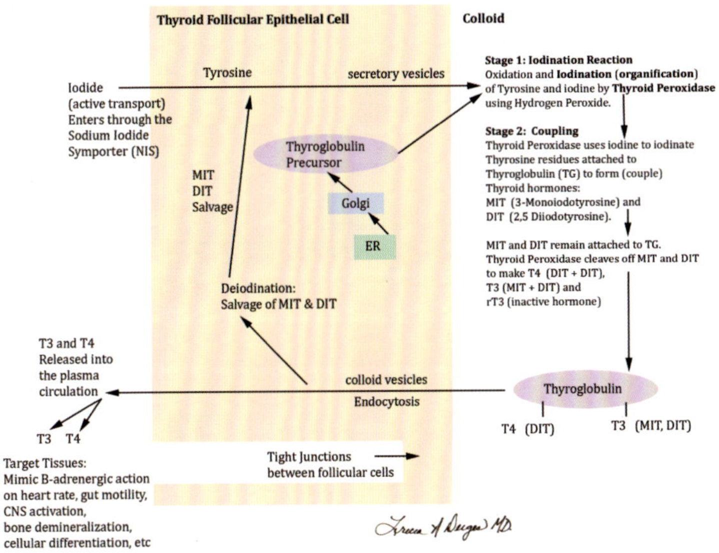

- Controls how fast the body uses energy (metabolic rate), makes proteins and its sensitivity to other hormones
- Produces thyroid hormones T3 (triiodothyronine) and T4 (thyroxine), synthesized from iodine and tyrosine
- Produces calcitonin
- Thyroid hormone output is controlled by TSH (thyroid-stimulating hormone) produced by the anterior pituitary and regulated by TRH (thyrotropin-releasing hormone)
- Follicular cells (Thyroid epithelial cells) secreted T3 and T4
- Parafollicular cells (AKA: "C cells" secrete calcitonin). **Calcitonin decreases the level of calcium** in the serum when it gets to high. (**tip**: calci"tone"in = "tones" down calcium). Reduces calcium uptake in the intestines and kidneys. Stimulates calcium deposition in the bones.
- **β HCG mimics TSH** (same α subunit)
- **TSH (T3 and T4) are steroid hormones = intranuclear receptor.**
  T3 binding activates DNA binding activity in an intracellular receptor.
- **LABS:**
  TSH: Thyroid-Stimulating hormone: TSH is ↑ in hypothyroidism, ↓ in hyperthyroidism.
  Thyroxine (AKA: T4)
  Free T4 is T4 that is not bound to a protein in the blood. Most T4 is bound.
  Total T4 test: Measures BOTH kinds of T4 (free T4 and bound T4). Total T4 is ↑ in hyperthyroidism, ↓ in hypothyroidism.
  Free T4 test: Measures only Free T4.
  Total T3 (triiodothyronine). Total T3 is ↑ in hyperthyroidism, ↓ in hypothyroidism.
  Free T3 (triiodothyronine). Total T3 is ↑ in hyperthyroidism, ↓ in hypothyroidism.
  Thyroxine-binding globulin (TBG): An ↑ in TBG results in an ↑ in total thyroxine (T4) and triiodothyronine (T3) without an ↑ in thyroid hormones. Unsaturated TBG ↑ when thyroid hormones are ↓.
  Pregnancy causes an ↑ TBG which causes an ↑ in T4 production, TSH levels remain normal.
  Thyroid hormone uptake: measures unbound (unsaturated) serum TBG.

  Example: In hyperthyroidism, labs would show: ↓ TSH, ↑ T3, ↑ T4, ↑ Total Thyroxine (T4), ↑ Free Thyroxine (T4), and Normal TBG.

Thyroid Hormone T3 Function

- Controls metabolism
- ↑ β1 receptors = ↑ HR, CO, SV, contractility.
- ↑ base metabolic rate by ↑ Na/K ATPase activity = ↑ O2 use, RR, body temperature.
  Location: Cell membrane.
- ↑ gluconeogenesis, glycogenolysis, lipolysis so ↑ metabolism (energy production).
  Location: Nucleus.
- Normal development of the CNS and the skeleton.
  Location: in the neonatal cells.
- ↑ heat production.
  Location: Mitochondria.

Thyroid Hormone Production Pathway (T3 and T4)

- T4 synthesized in the **follicular cells** from free tyrosine
- Iodine is brought into the cell for **organification and oxidation by thyroid peroxidase**
- Once organified is coupled into **MIT** (monoiodotyrosine) and **DIT** (diiodotyrosine)
- One MIT and one DIT = **T3**
- Two DIT's = **T4**
- T3 and T4 are released into the blood
- **Thyroxin-binding globulin (TBG)** binds and carries both T3 and T4 in the blood. Only free hormone is active
- **TBG is synthesized in the liver**
- **TBG Deficiency:** There is a ↓ in serum T4 concentration and a normal serum TSH. The venous blood will show normal free T4 concentrations.

Thyroid Hormone Synthesis Cont'd

- T4 (inactive) is converted to T3 (active) in the peripheral tissues by **5'-deiodinase** (**tip**: (t) 3… (t) 4…..5")
- RT3: (AKA: Reverse Triiodothyronine (isomer of T3), reverse T3). RT3 levels increase in cases of: euthyroid sick syndrome, physical or biological stress, after surgery, trauma, diabetes, extreme cold exposure, because its clearance decreases but production remains the same. Comes from the conversion of T4.
- T4= 90% of serum thyroid hormones; T3 = 9% of serum thyroid hormones; fT3 = 1 % of serum thyroid hormones

	Hyperthyroidism (Overactive Thyroid Gland)	Hypothyroidism (Underactive Thyroid Gland)
General	Increased Appetite	Normal Appetite
	Weight Loss	Mild Weight Gain (~3 kg)
	Heat intolerance	Cold intolerance
		Feeling Run Down
Nervous System	Increased Nervousness	Calmness or indifference
	Sleeplessness	Drowsy or sleepy
	Mental competence (ok / Normal)	Dull or Confused
	Hand Tremors	No tremors
	Anxiety	Depression
Circulatory System	Palpitations (pounding Heart beats)	None unless (thyroiditis)
	Very Fast Pulse (Tachycardia)	Slow Pulse Rate
	Increased Blood Pressure (Gen; Systolic)	Hypertension (Often diastolic as well)
	No Fluid retention (No swelling/Odema)	Puffiness and Odema (swelling present)
Digestive system	Fast transit of Food (Stool frequency)	Indigestion
	Frequent Bowel Movements	Constipation
Skin	Warm and smooth skin	Cold & dry Skin with increased pigments
	Increased Perspiration	Decreased sweating
	Increased Nail Growth	Brittle Nails
Muscle	Weakness (due to muscle loss)	Cramps & Aches
Blood	Low cholesterol levels	High Cholesterol Levels
		Anemia (Low RBC count)

TSH

- Released from thyrotrope cells in the anterior pituitary from stimulation by TRH from the hypothalamus.
- TSH receptor is located on the follicular cells of the thyroid.
- Stimulates the thyroid to produce thyroid hormones: Thyroxine (T4) and Triiodothyronine (T3).
- Somatostatin, made in the hypothalamus, can inhibit or decrease the release of TSH.
- TSH is responsible for metabolism in the body. T3 and T4 regulate the release of TSH.
- **TSH shares the same alpha subunit as LH, FSH and hCG. This alpha subunit** (92 amino acids long) **also stimulates adenylate cyclase and cAMP and PKA.**
- TSH helps with energy homeostasis by stimulating lipolysis. **TSH stimulates hormone sensitive lipase (HSL).**
    - Epinephrine is a "back up" to glucagon, along with cortisol in order to maintain blood glucose level.
    - Low insulin levels suppress lipolysis by ↓ cAMP and PKA. Low insulin levels will also stimulate epinephrine and cortisol, which will then stimulate glycogenolysis, gluconeogenesis, lipolysis and proteolysis.
    - Epinephrine (catecholamines) and cortisol will activate lipolysis by acting on G protein β-adrenergic receptors to stimulate adenylate cyclase which ↑ cAMP, which stimulates PKA. PKA stimulates lipolysis by activating hormone sensitive lipase (HSL) intracellularly in the adipose tissues, which hydrolyzes triglycerides to release free fatty acids (FFA) and glycerol.
    - TSH raises the metabolism rate (by any of these catabolic pathways) and therefore causes a higher rate of metabolites, which in turn can cause acidosis.
- **TSH receptors are located on the heart.** T3 increases heart rate and contractility, thereby increasing cardiac output via β-adrenergic receptors. This increase in heart rate and contractility create a wide pulse pressure (aka: bounding pulse). This can cause the cardiac symptoms seen in a thyroid storm.

Hyperthyroidism

- MCC Graves in the developed world
- 2nd MCC: Toxic multinodular goiter in the developed world
- MCC in the undeveloped world: iodine deficiency
- **Labs:**
  If **primary** hyperthyroidism: ↑ total T3 and T4 and ↓ TSH, ↓ cholesterolemia (b/c ↑ LDL receptor expression)
  If **primary** hypothyroidism: ↓ total T3 and T4 and ↑ TSH, ↑ cholesterolemia (b/c ↓ LDL receptor expression)
- **Only pituitary adenomas have a high TSH level.** In all other forms, the pituitary release of TSH is inhibited.

Additional causes of hyperthyroidism

- Thyroiditis
- Levothyroxine overdose
- Iodine reduced

Hypothyroidism (TSH levels are markedly increased if the thyroid gland has failed)

- Failure of thyroid gland
- Dietary deficiency of iodine
- Amiodarone

Hyperthyroid Pathologies

Graves Disease

MCC of hyperthyroidism **(Autoimmune** Dz of Thyroid TSH receptor antibodies HLA DR3 Anti-TSH receptor **Labs: ↓ TSH, ↑ T3 and T4** IgG pretends its TSH = ↑T3, T4 IgG against **TSH receptors**. SX: (triad: goiter, ophthalmopathy, dermopathy). Hyperthyroidism **Exophthalmos** (AKA: proptosis, extraocular, muscle swelling). **Pretibial myxedema** (anterior shin nodules) **Diffuse goiter (**swelling of the neck or larynx due to an enlarged, dysfunctioning thyroid gland (thyromegaly) (Graves DZ cont'd) DX: RAIU (Radioiodine) (radioactive iodine) shows ↑ diffuse uptake throughout gland. TX: Radioiodine ablation (shrinks the thyroid, destroying the gland) Meds: **Propylthiouracil (PTU)** (inhibits BOTH peroxidase and 5"-deiodinase) Use **PTU** during first trimester of pregnancy then switch to Methimazole. (**tip**: PTU = **P** for **P**regnancy and for "**P**air" (both MOA's) **Methimazole** inhibits peroxidase only.	**Graves Exophthalmos** **Antibodies against fibroblast of the eye muscles** causing differentiation into fat (adipose) cells. These muscle cells become inflamed and swell → compressing veins → veins won't drain = edema around the eyes. TX: **Prednisone**	**Graves Pretibial Myxedema** Waxy, discolored induration of the skin (peau d'orange appearance) on the anterior aspect of the lower legs/feet, non-pitting edema of the skin. Cause: factors in the serum that **stimulate fibroblasts** to ↑ synthesis of glycosaminoglycans (long, unbranched polysaccharides consisting of a repeating disaccharide unit. Polar and attract water) Untreated hyperthyroidism can lead to **osteoporosis** due to accelerated bone resorption (osteoclast)
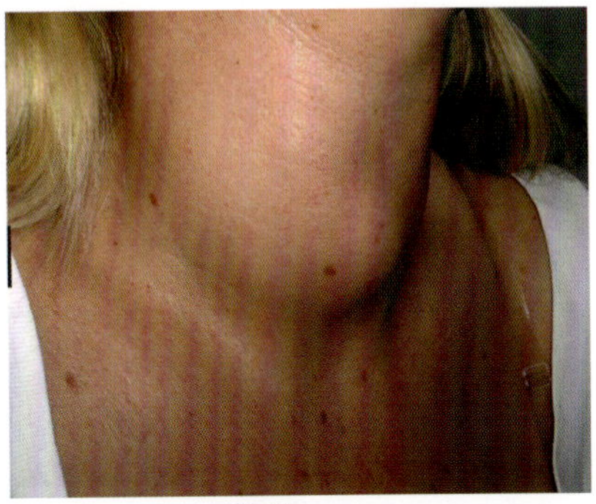 Goiter	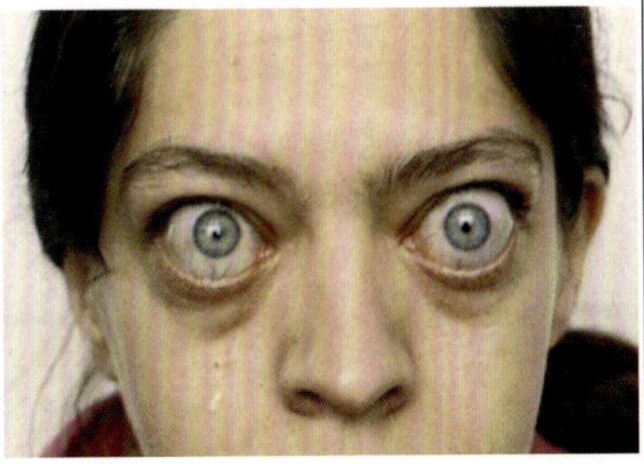 Exophthalmos	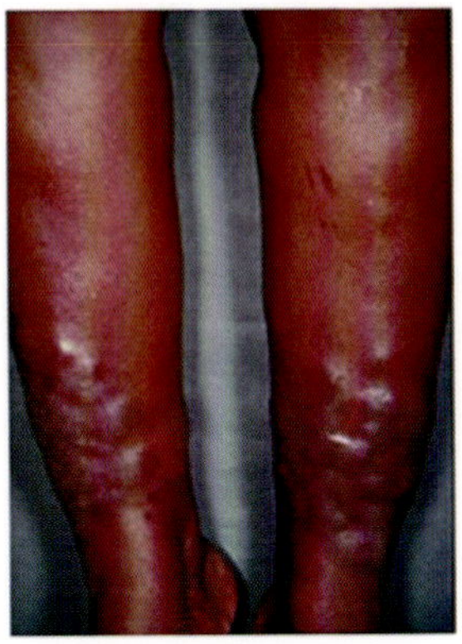 Pretibial Myxedema

Thyroid Storm (AKA: Thyrotoxicosis) Stress induced catecholamine surge Emergency SX: Tachycardia, agitation, delirium, coma, ↑↑ fever 106°, hypermetabolic, hyperadrenergic, CHF TX: "Triangle of Treatment" **Propranolol** = ↓ sympathetic outflow (AKA: increase parasympathetic affect) and blocks actions on target organs. **PTU** = (blocks production of thyroxine) ↓ Thyroid hormone synthesis and release and ↓ conversion from T4 to T3 so thyroid action is ↓ on tissues. **Methimazole**: Blocks production of thyroxine. **Dexamethasone**: Blocks peripheral conversion of T3 and T4. **Iodine**: Blocks uptake of iodine into the thyroid gland.	**Toxic Multinodular Goiter** AKA: Toxoid nodular goiter, Plummer syndrome Hyperthyroidism Excess production of thyroid hormones from thyroid nodules in the follicular cells which do not require stimulation of TSH due to a **mutation in the TSH receptor** Risk factors: female and individuals > 60 SX: Similar to Graves hyperthyroidism but **does NOT** have the exophthalmos (proptosis) ophthalmologic problems that Graves does. Additional SX include: osteoporosis, non-painful goiter, tachycardia, irritability, muscle weakening/wasting, tremor, fatigue, A-fib, other cardiac problems. DX: ↑ Focal uptake of radioactive iodine = in one or a few hot nodules. Hot nodules are seldom malignant.	**Factitious Thyrotoxicosis (AKA: Exogenous, Thyrotoxicosis factitia)** Intentional or accidental ingestion of large amounts of thyroid hormones. Labs show hyperthyroid: ↑ T3, ↑ T4, ↓ TSH and **atrophied** thyroid gland. SX: Weight loss. Looks like Graves but no symptoms except palpitations and sweat. Gland is not palpable. **↓ Radioiodine uptake (RAIU)** throughout the thyroid. **Exogenous use has the same labs as hyperthyroidism.** To determine the difference, look at the RUAI uptake. If it is due to the thyroid, the RUAI will be increased (thyroid is taking up iodine in order to make thyroid hormones). If it is exogenous the RUAI will be low because the gland is not making the thyroid hormone and does not need the iodine. Results from a radioiodine uptake test: If ↓ or no uptake = exogenous/factitious If ↑ uptake = Graves (actual thyroid dz)
Hyperthyroidism can lead to A-Fib ↑T3 and T4 stimulate the beta 1 receptors on the heart → g protein = ↑ sympathetic → palpitations Untreated Hyperthyroid → Bone loss → ↑ osteoclast activity → ↑ serum Calcium → cardiac arrhythmia A-Fib Tx: **Propanolol**	**Sick Euthyroid Syndrome** (AKA: "Low 3 Syndrome") Occurs with a patient with acute or severe illness or starvation Labs: ↓ T3, NL T4 and NL TSH After the patient recovers all returns to normal Recheck every 8 weeks. If T4 is ↓ = bad prognosis	**Struma Ovarii** **Ovarian teratoma** tumor that makes thyroid hormones causing hyperthyroidism **↓ Radioiodine uptake (RAIU)** throughout the thyroid.

Silent Thyroiditis **(AKA: Painless Thyroiditis)** Brief hyperthyroid phase. Spontaneous recovery. SX: Small non-tender goiter. Normal exam. Labs: ↑ T4, ↓ TSH Histology: Lymphocytic infiltrate Low radioiodine uptake (↓ RAIU)	**Subacute Thyroiditis** (AKA: de Quervain's thyroiditis) Can cause **both** thyrotoxicosis and hypothyroidism. Causes: **After a viral or flu-like illness (URI).** Self-limiting Releases preformed thyroid hormones Histology: Mixed cell infiltrate (lymphocytes, PMN, histocytes) with multi-nucleated giant cells. **Granulomatous** inflammation. Labs: **↑ ESR, ↑ CRP,** **↓ Radioiodine uptake (RAIU)** throughout the thyroid. SX: very painful upon palpation. Jaw pain. **Thyroid SX: Tender and painful thyroid goiter** **TX: NSAIDS, Propanolol**	**Pituitary Adenoma** **Labs: ↑ TSH, ↑ T3, ↑ T4** **TX: Surgery** (transsphenoidal) **Drugs causing hyperthyroidism** **Amiodarone** **Lithium** **Non-thyroid pathologies that can cause hyperthyroidism:** **Dermoid Cyst** (teratoma): due to thyroid tissue within the dermoid.
Iodine-induced Hyperthyroidism (aka: Jodbasedow effect) Iodine overload stimulates nodules to hypersecrete thyroid hormone. **↓ Radioiodine uptake (RAIU)** throughout the thyroid. SX: Usually presents as thyrotoxicosis after patient has been administered radioiodine contrast and iodinated drugs (ie: Amiodarone).	**Trophoblastic tumors** Malignant trophoblastic tissue that secretes human chorionic gonadotropin that stimulates the TSH receptor. Causes by: Choriocarcinoma, hydatidiform moles, embryonal carcinoma of the testis. **↓ Radioiodine uptake (RAIU)** throughout the thyroid.	

Radioiodine Uptake Results on Nodules (RAIU)
Nodule Management: Fine Needle Biopsy (FNB) nodule if thyroid function test are normal.
Hot Nodules

- Benign. DX hyperthyroidism = Hyperfunctioning and show ↑ uptake
  Hot Nodule = Adenoma
- ↑ radioiodine uptake occurs when high levels of thyroid hormone are being made
- Radio uptake = toxic nodule

Cold Nodules

- Malignant (**tip**: **C**old = **C**ancer) = hypofunctioning.
  Must do a FNB (Fine needle biopsy)
- ↓ radioiodine uptake
- ↓ uptake if thyroid is not making any thyroid hormones
- Surgical removal of nodule

Hyperthyroid Differentials

Condition	T3	T4	TRH	TSH	RAIU	Notes	Treatment
Primary Hyperthyroidism	$\uparrow$	$\uparrow$	$\downarrow$	$\downarrow$	$\uparrow$	Graves	Radioactive iodine
Secondary Hyperthyroidism	$\uparrow$	$\uparrow$	$\downarrow$	$\uparrow$		Pituitary adenoma, α sub unit	
Tertiary	$\uparrow$	$\uparrow$	$\uparrow$	$\uparrow$		Hypothalamic tumor	
Thyrotoxicosis	$\uparrow$	$\uparrow$		$\uparrow$			
Pregnancy	$\uparrow$	$\uparrow\uparrow$		NL		Due to $\uparrow$ TBG	
Familial Hyperthyroid	NL	$\uparrow$		NL			
Sick Euthroid Syndrome	$\downarrow$	NL		NL		Acute/severe illness – returns to normal after recover	
Subacute Thyroiditis				$\downarrow$	$\downarrow$	Tender thyroid	Aspirin
Factitious Thyrotoxicosis				$\downarrow$	$\downarrow$	Non-palpable thyroid gland	
Pituitary Adenoma				$\uparrow$		Dx: MRI of head	Transsphenoidal surgery to remove pituitary adenoma.

Hypothyroid Pathologies

Hashimoto Thyroiditis
Autoimmune
Anti-microsomal
Anti-TPO (anti-thyroid peroxidase)
Anti-Thyroid Peroxidase Antibodies
Antithyroglobulin
HLA-DR5
Chronic lymphocytic infiltration

Histology: Hürthle cells
AKA: lymphoid aggregate with **germinal centers**
AKA: granular cytoplasm
AKA: mononuclear infiltrate germinal centers

SX: (See hypothyroid SX in above table) and $\uparrow$ LDL, bradycardia, delayed reflexes and knee jerk, amenorrhea, $\uparrow$ triglycerides, periorbital puffiness, **"Tinsels Sign" (tapping on the wrist) produces carpel tunnel.** Note: hyperthyroidism is initially seen followed by hypothyroidism.

Thyroid SX: is rubbery and non-tender and diffusely enlarged

DX: If patient raises arms and see face plethora (rounded, ruddy/red face) and/or neck vein distension

Highly associated with Pernicious Anemia and other autoimmune DZ: SLE, Celiac, Addison's, DMI, Non-Hodgkins lymphoma.

Congenital Hypothyroidism
(AKA: Cretinism)

Causes: maternal hypothyroidism, iodine deficiency, thyroid agenesis, thyroid dysgenesis, genetic defects in the synthesis of thyroid hormones (AKA: dyshormonogenic goiter)

SX:
Large, protruding tongue, umbilical hernia, puffy face, poor brain development

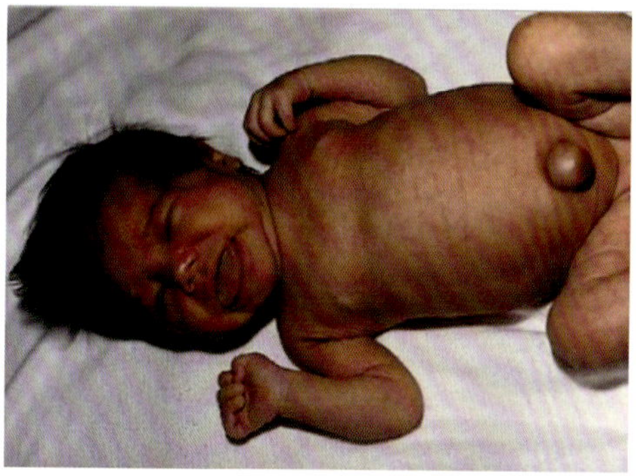

Riedel Thyroiditis

Thyroid replaced by **fibrous** tissue

Labs:
Antibodies against peroxidase

Thyroid SX:
Hard (rock hard), painless and fixed

Subacute Thyroiditis (AKA: de Quervain) Can cause both thyrotoxicosis and hypothyroidism. Causes: **After a viral or flu-like illness** Self-limiting Releases preformed thyroid hormones Histology: Mixed cell infiltrate (lymphocytes, PMN, histocytes) with multi-nucleated giant cells. **Granulomatous** inflammation. Labs: **🡅 ESR, 🡅 CRP, 🡇 Radioiodine uptake (RAIU)** SX: jaw pain **Thyroid SX: Tender and painful thyroid goiter** **TX: NSAIDS, Propanolol**	**Wolff-Chaikoff Effect** 🡇 in thyroid hormones due to excess ingestion of iodine. This **stops the iodine pumps** and **stops the organification** which causes the 🡅 of circulating iodine in serum Effect last approximately 10 days. Used to be used as a treatment against hyperthyroidism before meds **Thyroid SX: Painless**	**Myxedema Coma** Extreme Hypothyroidism Patient same labs as a hypothyroid state but any stressful event (MI, stroke, infection, sickness) causes a coma state SX: altered mental status, low blood sugar, low blood pressure, low body temp, hyponatremia, hypercapnia, hypoxia, bradycardia
Prolactin and TSH Hypothyroid = 🡇 T3, 🡅T4, 🡅 TSH 🡅 TRH = 🡅 Prolactin (Feedback: 🡅 TSH, 🡅 TRH = 🡅 Prolactin)	**Hypothyroid and Dementia** On ALL elderly presenting with potential dementia, **TSH and B12 levels must be checked**. Deficiency of either an cause a patient to present signs like dementia.	**Hypothyroid and Carpel Tunnel** Hypothyroidism causes weight gain. Weight gain can cause compression on the median nerve causing carpel tunnel.

Hypothyroid Differentials

Condition	T3	T4	TSH	Notes
1° Primary Hypothyroid	🡇	🡇	🡅	Problem in the thyroid gland
2° Secondary Hypothyroid	🡇	🡇	NL	Problem in the pituitary
Subclinical	NL	NL	Mildly 🡅	
General Resistance	🡅	🡅	Mildly 🡅	

Causes of Hypothyroidism

Primary Hypothyroidism (the gland is the problem)

- Idiopathic hypothyroidism, **Hashimoto's Thyroiditis**, Surgical removal of the thyroid, Fibrous Thyroiditis, Iodine Deficiency, Drug Therapy (Lithium, Interferon), Infiltrative Diseases (Sarcoidosis, Amyloidosis, Scleroderma, Hemochromatosis)

Secondary Hypothyroidism (No TSH is stimulating)

- Pituitary or hypothalamic neoplasms, Congenital hypopituitarism, Pituitary necrosis (Sheehan's syndrome)

Tertiary Hypothyroidism: No TRH. Hypothalamic disease (ie: Sarcoidosis is destroying TRH)

Pregnancy and the Thyroid

Pregnancy and Normal Affects on the Thyroid	Pregnancy and Hyperthyroidism
Thyroid hormone blood levels are ↑ during pregnancy due to hCG and estrogen. hCG is similar to TSH → stimulates thyroid to produce more thyroid hormone. It is possible for the TSH to show a slight increase because of the hCG. ↑ estrogen causes more TBG (thyroid-binding globulin) to be made in the liver. 1st trimester the fetus depends on maternal thyroid hormone. The fetus makes its own thyroid hormone at 12 weeks. **Normal pregnancy labs**: ↑ T3, ↑↑ T4, Normal TSH	MCC: Graves Must be monitored throughout pregnancy Uncontrolled hyperthyroidism can cause: CHF, Preeclampsia, Thyroid storm, Miscarriage, Premature birth, Low birth weight TSI (Thyroid-stimulating immunoglobulin) can cross the placenta and stimulate the fetal thyroid which can lead problems with the infant: ↑ heart rate, early closure of the soft spots, poor weight gain, irritability, enlarged thyroid that presses on the trachea and interferes with breathing. If the mother is on antithyroid medications, the baby is less likely to develop hyperthyroidism because the meds cross the placenta. Hypothyroidism is a preventable cause of mental retardation.
Pregnancy and Hypothyroidism	**Postpartum Thyroiditis**
MCC: Hashimoto's Hypothyroidism can cause: CHF, Preeclampsia, Anemia, Miscarriage, Stillbirth, Low birth weight Uncontrolled hypothyroidism during the first semester can affect the growth and brain development of the fetus. TX: **Levothyroxine** Women with pre-existing hypothyroidism **must ↑ their dose during pregnancy** to maintain normal thyroid function. Synthetic thyroxine is safe for the mother and fetus during pregnancy.	Inflammation of the thyroid that presents during the first year after giving birth (Thyroiditis). This causes stored thyroid hormone to leak out of the inflamed thyroid and raise the hormone levels in the blood. Autoimmune condition causes mild hyperthyroidism lasting 1 – 2 months then experience hypothyroidism for 6 – 12 months before the thyroid returns to normal function. If the thyroid is too damaged, the hypothyroidism becomes permanent requiring lifelong Levothyroxine. Postpartum Thyroiditis tends to recur with future pregnancies. Postpartum Thyroiditis is often confused with post-partum blues.

Thyroid Differentials

Etiology	Goiter	TBG	RAIU Radio Uptake	Symptoms
Graves	Yes	↑	↑ (taking iodine in to make T3, T4)	Exophthalmos, pretibial edema, diffuse hyperplasia
Subacute, De Quervain's	Yes	↑	↓	Painful, fever
Painless	+/-		↓	Short hypothyroid and returns to hyperthyroid
Hashimoto's	+/-		NL	
1° Follicular Cancer		↑	NL	
Toxic Nodular			↑ in the nodule only	Single nodule. Palpable thyroid nodule
Toxic Multi Nodular	Yes	↓	NL to ↑	Gradual onset: cough, dysphagia, dyspnea
TSH Secreting Adenoma	Yes		↑	All high: ↑T3, T4, TSH
Iatrogenic/factitious	No	↓	↓	NL T3, ↑ T4, ↓ TSH

Thyroid Cancer

Follicular Carcinoma
(AKA: Follicular Thyroid Cancer)

Thyroglobulin (Tg) = tumor marker.
Follicular cells make thyroid hormones.
Invades the thyroid **capsule**,
Invades vessels.

Histology: **Uniform** follicles.

Metastasizes to: lung and bone via blood.
Good prognosis (5 yr = 91%, 10 yr = 85%)

TX: Thyroidectomy followed by radioiodine

Colloid Nodular Goiter
AKA: Colloid Nodule

Benign, overgrowths of thyroid tissue.
Asymptomatic
Small nodules found on physical exam

MC: Adolescent girls with normal thyroid test

DX: Gelatinous mass of colloid both surrounding and contained within follicular cells.

Papillary Carcinoma
(AKA: Papillary Thyroid Cancer)

Most common thyroid cancer

Asymptomatic thyroid nodule (neck mass).
Thyroglobulin (Tg) = tumor marker

Histology: "Orphan Annie eyes" (nuclei that appear empty),
AKA: Ground glass nucleus.
AKA: Follicular hyperplasia with tall epithelial cells.
Psammoma bodies, NO capsule, local infiltrate
Mitochondria, ↑ RER, apical microvilli

Metastasizes through lymph to lung.

Risk: RET and BRAF mutations

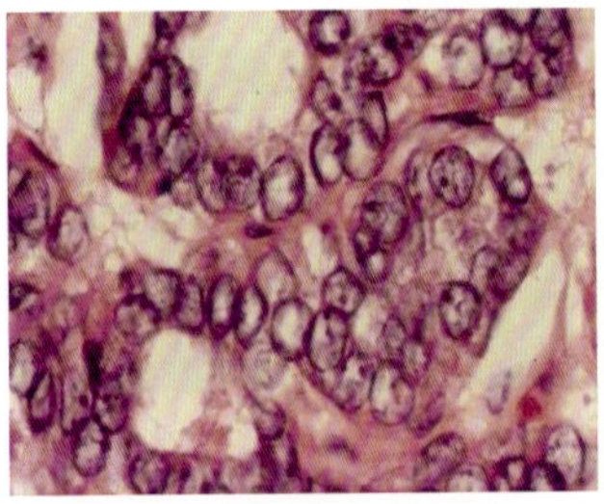

"Orphan Annie Eye"

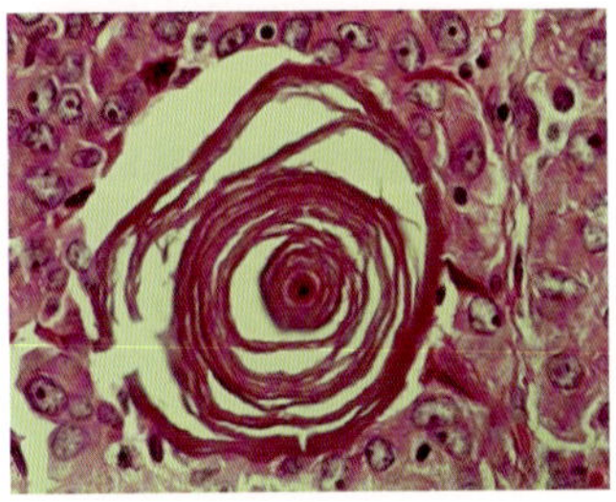

Psammoma Bodies

Medullary Carcinoma
(AKA: Medullary Thyroid Cancer)

Originates from **Parafollicular Cells** (C Cells) that produce calcitonin.

MC: RET proto-oncogene with **MEN 2A and 2B**
MC sites: lymph nodes in the neck, mediastinum, liver, lung, bone.

Histology:
Polygonal cells with **amyloid deposits shown on Congo Red stain**.
AKA: Sheets of cells in an amyloid stroma

SX: Diarrhea and flushing, pruritis (similar to Carcinoid) are caused by ↑ levels of calcitonin, enlarged cervical lymph nodes. (The symptoms in **Carcinoid** are caused by ↑ levels of serotonin).

DX: ↑ **5-HIAA in** urine (5-hydroxyindoleacetic acid), ↑ Calcitonin.

Metastasizes to the liver

Multiple Endocrine Neoplasia, MEN Syndrome

- **Autosomal Dominant, so watch for ANY family history in the question (male or female, parents, siblings) that has had thyroid "issues" (neck surgery), low calcium problems, or blood pressure "issues". It does NOT have to be the patient that has had them.** The patient may have just ONE pathology but the question will mention a family member with history of one of these issues.
- Tumors of endocrine glands
- If parathyroid tumors are involved: watch for ↑ **calcium levels.**
- If thyroid tumor is involved: watch for ↑ **calcitonin levels.**
- If pancreatic tumors are involved: watch for ↑ **gastrin.**
- If pituitary tumor is involved: watch for ↑ **prolactin.**
- If adrenals are involved: watch for ↑ **urinary metanephrines.**

MEN I (Wermer Syndrome)	MEN 2A (Sipple Syndrome)	MEN 2B
Menin Gene **The 3 "P's"** Pituitary tumors Parathyroid tumors Pancreatic tumors Gastrinoma (Zollinger Ellison) VIPomas, Glucagonoma, Insulinoma	**Ret Gene (proto-oncogene)** **The 2 P's and 1M** Medullary Thyroid Cancer Spindle shape cells secrete **Calcitonin** (C Cells/Parafollicular) Parathyroid tumors Pheochromocytoma	**Ret Gene (proto-oncogene)** **The 2 M's and 1 P** Medullary Thyroid Cancer Pheochromocytoma Oral/intestinal mucosal neuromas/ulcers Marfanoid characteristics.

Multiple Endocrine Neoplasia (MEN)

Autosomal Dominant

MEN 1	**MEN 2A**	**MEN 2B**
MENIN Gene	RET Gene	RET Gene
Pituitary adenoma (high prolactin)	Medullary thyroid cancer (high calcitonin)	Medullary thyroid cancer (high calcitonin)
Parathyroid hyperplasia (high calcium)	Parathyroid hyperplasia (high calcium)	Mucosal neuromas
Pancreatic tumors (VIP, Gastrinoma) (high gastrin)	Pheochromo-cytoma (high urinary metanephrines)	Pheochromo-cytoma (high urinary metanephrines)
		Marfanoid body habitus
3 P's	2 P's, 1 M	2 M's, 1 P

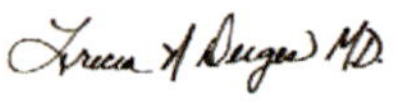

ENDOCRINE PHARMACOLOGY

Diabetic Pharmacology

Diabetes Mellitus Treatment Goal

- Type 1 Diabetes: Insulin replacement, low-carbohydrate diet.
- Type 2 Diabetes: Weight loss (decreased calories), dietary modifications, exercise and lifestyle changes. If these lifestyle changes do not work then oral diabetes medication and/or insulin replacement. (**Note**: if the answer choice give both: weight loss and exercise, choose weight loss (decrease in calories) and not exercise. Exercise does not necessarily mean weight is being lost. If someone exercises but continues to eat high calories they will not lose weight).
- Gestational Diabetes: Dietary modifications, exercise. If these lifestyle changes do not work then insulin replacement.
- Hemochromatosis, amyloidosis: watch for an older patient that is newly diagnosed as a diabetic. The deposits in their pancreas have damaged their beta cells so ↓ in insulin.

DRUG **GENERIC name** **Trade name**	**Clinical Use**	**Mechanism of Action and Resistance**	**Toxicity and Notes**
TYPE 1 Diabetes Mellitus			
Insulin: **RAPID acting** **Aspart** **Glulisine** **Lispro**	Diabetes Mellitus, DM1, DM2 Given at mealtime, last 2 hours.	Binds insulin cell membrane receptor: **Tyrosine Kinase Receptor**. Actions: Liver: ↑ Glucose so it can be stored as glycogen. Muscle: ↑ Glycogen, protein synthesis, ↑ K uptake (presence of ADP required and K must be trapped inside the cell for insulin to be released). Adipose: ↑ Triglyceride storage.	Hypoglycemia. Is usually seen with fictitious use (most with medical personnel for attention). If insulin is fictitiously injected there will be no C peptide. Insulin made by the body will always have C peptide. In cases of hyperkalemia. Giving glucose and insulin can drive K into the cell to help reduce levels of K. Given along with **Calcium Gluconate.**
Insulin: **SHORT acting** **Regular**	Same Given at meal time, last 6 hours.	Same	**Drug of choice for DM Type 1**
Insulin: **Intermediate acting** **NPH** *(Twice a day)*	Same	Same	
Insulin, **LONG acting** **Detemir** **Glargine** *(Lantus: Once a day)*	Same	Same	Glargine can be added to other insulin drugs

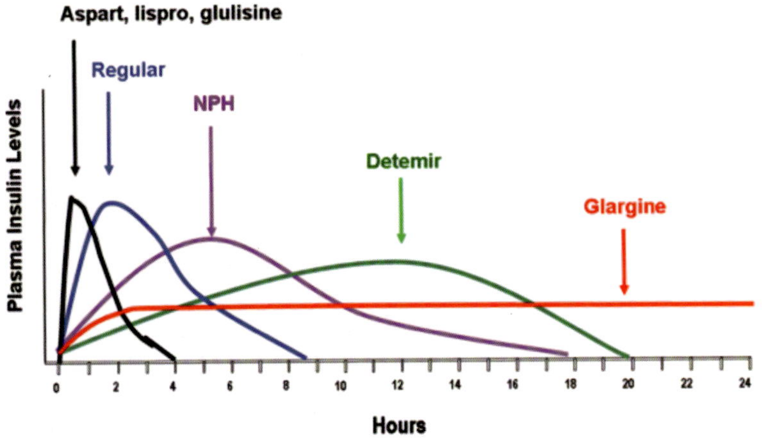

DRUG GENERIC name Trade name	Clinical Use	Mechanism of Action and Resistance	Toxicity and Notes
TYPE II Diabetes Mellitus			
Biguanides **Metformin**	First line therapy for DM Type II and pre-diabetics. PCOS for weight loss.	Unknown. It is thought to ↓ gluconeogenesis	**Lactic Acidosis** (**do not use in renal disease/insufficiency**), GI disturbances (diarrhea). Metformin is contraindicated in use with contrast dyes or surgery as it may lead to acute renal failure. **Metformin blocks B12 absorption.** **MUST stop** Metformin before any surgery or any use of contrast dyes. Does not cause weight gain. (**tip**: Metformin is the **BIG** one)
Sulfonylureas **1st Generation:** **Chlorpropamide** **Tolbutamide** **2nd Generation:** **Glimepiride** **Glipizide** **Glyburide**	DMII	Stimulates the release of endogenous insulin from the pancreas (brings insulin to the surface) **Closes K channels in the beta cell membrane → depolarization → insulin increase due to ↑ Ca influx.** (**tip**: think of "Sulfonylurea" as "surfing". You surf on the surface. So it causes the insulin to rise to the surface)	**1st Generation: Disulfiram-like effects.** 2nd Generation: **Hypoglycemia**, SIADH, Sulfa allergies. Sulfonylureas brings ↑ glucose intracellularly = ↑ obesity. Hypoglycemia: Is usually seen with fictitious use (mostly with medical personnel for attention). If insulin is fictitiously injected there will be no C peptide. Insulin made by the body will always have C peptide. DX: **Check urine for Sulfonylureas.**
Secretagogues Nateglinide Repaglinide	DMII	Simulates the release of insulin from the pancreas (similar MOA to Sulfonylureas).	Hypoglycemia. Do not contain sulfa.

Glitazones Thiazolidine-diones **Pioglitazone** **Rosiglitazone**	DM II	↑ insulin sensitivity in peripheral tissue. Binds **PPAR-Y nuclear transcription regulator** which ↑ insulin sensitivity and levels of adiponectin. (PPAR-Y regulates glucose metabolism and storage of fatty acids).	**Hepatotoxicity,** **Weight gain,** Edema, hepatotoxicity, heart failure. **Do not use with CHF** (may worsen the condition). Rosiglitazone: contraindicated with CHF due to ↑ fluid overload. (**tip**: Its **PARR** for the course that **GLITZ**y stones are **heavy on your liver**)
α - Glucosidase Inhibitors **Acarbose** **Miglitol**	Postprandial hyperglycemia	**Inhibits/delays carbohydrate (sugar) absorption** in the intestine by inhibiting intestinal brush-border α-glucosidases.	**GI disturbances.** Flatus, abdominal pain, diarrhea, bloating. (**tip:** a Caboose is at the end of the train, this med is for the end of dinner. And a MIG (jet fighter plane) is also always after the enemy).
Meglitinides Nateglinide Repaglinide	Postprandial insulin release in DM II	Binds the K channels on the βeta cell membranes.	Weight gain, hypoglycemia
GLP-1 Analogs Exenatide Liraglutide	DM II	↑ Insulin, ↓ Glucagon release. Lowers glucose, ↓ gastric emptying.	GI disturbances, slow gastric emptying, and weight loss. **Exenatide: acute pancreatitis**

DPP-4 Inhibitors (Dipeptidyl Peptidase) Linagliptin Saxagliptin Sitagliptin	DM II. Used as a 2nd agent to Metformin.	↑ Insulin release, ↓ Glucagon release. ↑ incretin levels (GLP-1 and GIP) which inhibits glucagon causing an increase in insulin secretion. ↓ gastric emptying.	UTI, URI. Slow gastric emptying.
Amylin Analog	DMI, DMII	↓ Glucagon release, ↓ gastric emptying	GI disturbances, hypoglycemia
SGLT-2 Inhibitors (Sodium-glucose co-transporter 2) Canagliflozin Dapagliflozin Empaglifozin	DMII	Blocks reaborption of glucose in PCT	UTI, Glucosuria, Vaginal yeast infection, Hyperkalemia.
Pramlintide		↑ Insulin, ↓ Glucagon, ↓ appetite Analog of amylin (protein secreted by the pancreas along with insulin)	

Thyroid Pharmacology

DRUG GENERIC name Trade name	Clinical Use	Mechanism of Action and Resistance	Toxicity and Notes
Levothyroxine (T4) **Triiodothyronine (T3)**	**Hypothyroid**, myxedema	Replaces thyroid hormones	Heat intolerance, arrhythmias, tachycardia, and tremors. **During pregnancy, the dose of Levothyroxine must be increased.** (**tip**: think of "Levo" as Levitate – if you levitate something, it rises)
Thioamide **Propylthiouracil (PTU)**	**Hyperthyroidism.** **Hyperthyroidism in pregnancy.**	Inhibits **organification** (coupling, the making of MIT, DIT) by blocking **thyroid peroxidase** with stops thyroid hormone synthesis (T3 and T4, AKA: MIT, DIT). AND It also blocks peripheral conversion of T4 to T3 by blocking **5' deiodinase**. (**tip**: 3 → 4 → 5)	**Agranulocytosis,** aplastic anemia, hepatotoxicity, skin rash. (**tip**: P in PTU is for Pregnancy and P for "pair" (2): it works in 2 places)
Thioamide **Methimazole**	**Hyperthyroidism**	Inhibits **organification** (coupling, the making of MIT, DIT) by blocking **thyroid peroxidase** with stops thyroid hormone synthesis (T3 and T4, AKA: MIT, DIT).	**Teratogen** (aplastic cutis/Curis aplasia = congenital absence of the epidermis). (**tip**: M for Mono (one) = only works in 1 place. PTU works in 2 places)

Parathyroid Pharmacology

DRUG GENERIC name Trade name	Clinical Use	Mechanism of Action and Resistance	Toxicity and Notes
Cinacalcet	Hyperparathyroidism (AKA: Hypercalcemia)	Mimics the action of calcium on the tissues by activating the calcium receptors in the parathyroids → ↓ PTH levels → ↓ serum calcium levels.	Hypothyroidism

Hypothalmamic/Pituitary Pharmacology

DRUG GENERIC name Trade name	Clinical Use	Mechanism of Action and Resistance	Toxicity and Notes
Octreotide (AKA: Somatostatin)	**Gastrinoma** **Carcinoid Syndrome** **Acromegaly** **Glucagonoma** **VIPomas**	**Somatostatin analog**	
Oxytocin **Pitocin**	**Stimulates uterine contractions, milk let down, controlling uterine hemorrhage following delivery.**		
ADH Antagonist Conivaptan Tolvaptan	**SIADH**	Blocks ADH at the **V2 receptors** in the kidney	
Demeclocycline	**SIADH**	**ADH antagonist.** Used with serum Na drops to ≤ 115 mEq/L) (normal 135 – 145 mEq/L)	Tetracycline family: Do not use in pregnancy due damage to teeth and bones. Photosensitivity, nephrogenic DI.
Desmopressin acetate	Central DI		
Growth Hormone	GH deficiency, Turner's syndrome		

Glucocorticoids (Steroids) Pharmacology

DRUG GENERIC name Trade name	Clinical Use	Mechanism of Action and Resistance	Toxicity and Notes
Beclomethasone Dexamethasone Hydrocortisone Cortisone Prednisone Triamcinolone Fludrocortisone Methyl-Prednisolone Betamethasone Deoxy-corticosterone Methylprednisolone	Hyperparathyroidism (AKA: Hypercalcemia) Beclomethasone: *asthma* Dexamethasone: *Adrenal insufficiency, dexamethasone suppression test, increase surfactant* Hydrocortisone: *Anti-inflammatory* Prednisone: *autoimmune diseases, allergic reactions, immunosuppressant Anti-inflammatory* Cortisone: *anti-inflammatory, joint injections* Triamcinolone: *musculoskeletal problems, topical for skin rashes: poison ivy* Fludrocortisone: *1° adrenal insufficiency.* Methyl-Prednisolone: *asthma, breathing exacerbation.* Betamethasone: *increase surfactant, skin diseases, rheumatic disorders* Deoxy-corticosterone Methylprednisolone: *COPD exacerbation, respiratory diseases, acute bronchitis, arthritis*	Inhibits Phospholipase A2 in the Arachidonic Acid Pathway stopping both the leukotriene and cyclooxygenase pathways. (Shuts down entire ACTH axis). Inhibits transcription factors NF-κB. Inhibiting the Arachidonic Pathway decreases inflammation and immunity.	Side effects: Cushing's syndrome: truncal obesity (increased hip to waist ration), muscle wasting, **osteoporosis** (treat with bisphosphonates), avascular necrosis, peptic ulcers, skin atrophy and thinning (decreased dermal collagen), easy bruising (ecchymosis), telangiectasia. Chronic use: Individuals are considered immunocompromised. Adrenal insufficiency (AKA: Adrenal crisis) can result if steroids are abruptly stopped (not tapered if used for more than one week). WATCH for the patient that is admitted for surgery (or other inpatient procedure) and goes into adrenal insufficiency due to stress but the body is not able to supply cortisol (stress hormone) to deal with their stress because their entire ACTH axis has been shut down due to chronic steroid use. Steroids must be continued in hospitalized patients in order to avoid this emergency.

NEUROLOGY

NEURAL DEVELOPMENT

- Notochord differentiates into neuroectoderm and forms neural plate
- Neural plate forms neural tube and neural crest
- **Notochord** becomes **nucleus pulposus** in the intervertebral disk

Fetal Layers

Endoderm layer becomes:

- Digestive system, Liver, Pancreas, Lungs (inner layers)
  (GI and tube above the pectinate line, liver, lungs, pancreas, thymus, thyroid follicular cells, parathyroid, bladder, urethra, serous linings of body cavity)

Mesoderm layer becomes:

- Circulatory system, Lungs (epithelial layers), Skeletal system, Muscular system
  (muscles, connective tissue, bone, cartilage, blood, lymph, spleen (from foregut), adrenal cortex, kidney and ureter, skin, INTERNAL genitalia: ovaries, testes, vagina)

Ectoderm layer becomes

3 Layers of Ectoderm

- **Surface**
  Anterior Pituitary (AKA: Adenohypophysis from Rathke's Pouch (roof of mouth). Location of Craniopharyngioma with cholesterol crystals), lens, sensory of smell and hearing, glands: sweat, mammary, salivary, anal below pectinate line

- **Neural Tube**
  CNS and brain, **posterior pituitary (AKA: Neurohypophysis),** retina, CNS neurons, oligodendrocytes, astrocytes, spinal cord. Anterior horn motor neurons are derived from the **basal plate**.

- **Neural Crest**
  ANS, cranial nerves, melanocytes, chromaffin cells of adrenal medulla, parafollicular cells of the thyroid, melanocytes, larynx, Schwann cells, pia and arachnoid skull, odontoblast, aorticopulmonary septum (SPIRALING: Transposition of Great Vessels, TET of Fellow, Truncus Arteriosis and Migration: Hirschsprung's)

The Neuro Crest Queen

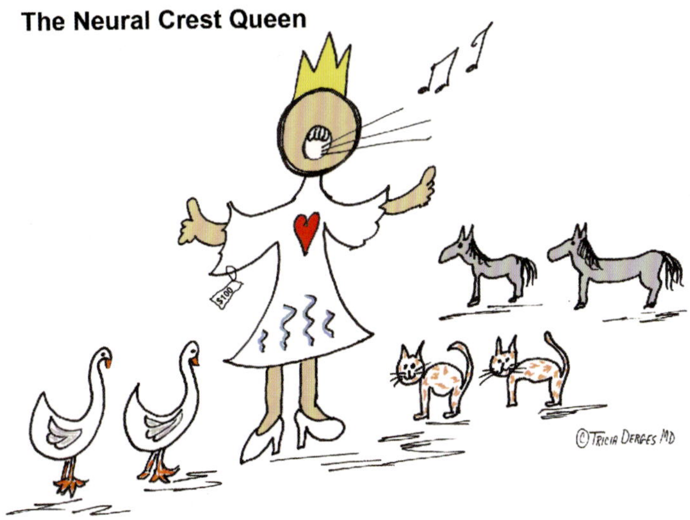

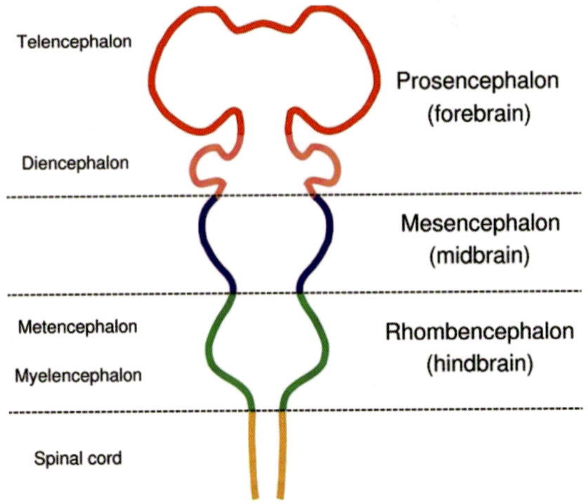

Tongue Development

- Anterior 2/3: 1st and 2nd brachial arches
- Posterior 1/3: 3rd and 4th brachial arches

Taste Development: From the **Solitary Nucleus** (**tip:** I have a **taste** for just one **Solitary** thing)

- **Anterior 2/3: CN VII (AKA: Chorda tympani, Facial nerve)**
- Posterior 1/3: CN IX
- Very Back (extreme posterior): CNX

Sensory Development (pain sensation)

- Anterior 2/3: CN V3
- Posterior 1/3: CN IX
  Pain sensation for the **posterior pharynx is by CN IX**
- Very Back (extreme posterior): CNX

Motor Development

- CN XII
- Muscles are from the occipital myotomes

Sweet vs Bitter

- Sweet taste receptors are controlled by CN VII on the anterior 2/3 of the tongue
- Bitter taste receptors are controlled by CN IX and X on the posterior of the tongue
  (This is why there is a bitter taste in the mouth in the morning when one suffers from GERD)

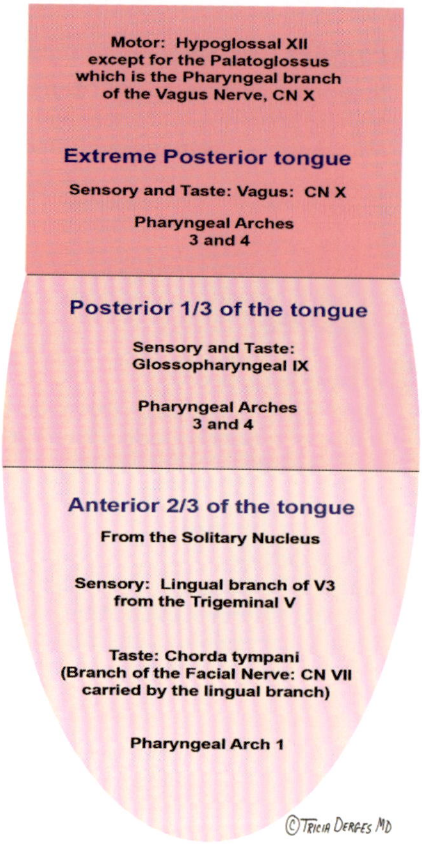

Primitive Reflexes

- Normal reflexes in an infant (More reflexes in the Child Development Chapter)
- Disappear within first year of life. Normal frontal lobe development inhibits the reflexes.
- Can reappear in adults due to lesions involving the frontal lobe (AKA: loss of inhibition)

Reflex	Description
Galant Reflex	Infant face down: stroking down one side of the spine causes lateral flexion of lower body toward the stroked side
Moro Reflex	Infant abducts and extends limbs when startled
Palmar Reflex	Stoking infants palm causes the fingers to curl
Plantar Reflex	Babinski sign (normal for infant, abnormal in an adult = UMN lesion) Stroking the bottom of an infants foot causes dorsiflexion of big toe and fanning out of other toes
Rooting Reflex	If the side of the cheek or mouth is stroked on an infant they will turn their head toward the side (position to nurse)
Suckling Reflex	If the roof of the mouth is touched on an infant they will begin to suck (nurse)

Neural Pathologies

Forebrain Pathologies

Anencephaly

- Malformation of anterior neural tube = no forebrain
- High AFP
- Polyhydramnios due to absence of swallowing center of brain
- Higher risk with maternal diabetes type I
  Decrease risk by supplementing folate

Holoprosencephaly

- Failure of brain hemispheres to separate
- Mutations of hedgehog gene
- SX: Cleft lip, cleft palate or cyclopia (one eye)

Posterior Fossa Malformations
Arnold-Chiari Malformation (AKA: Chiari II)

- **Herniation** of cerebellar vermis and tonsils through foramen magnum
- Aqueduct stenosis
- Hydrocephalus
- Myelomeningocele and paralysis

Dandy Walker

- Agenesis of cerebellar vermis
- **Enlargement of 4th ventricle**
- Hydrocephalus and spina bifida
- (**tip:** have a large ventricle to WALK around in)

Neural Tube Defects: Increased Alpha Fetal Protein (AFP) and ACK **(Failure to Fuse)**

- **#1 Cause of high AFP: DATING ERROR or multiple gestations**
- Gastroschisis (intestines NOT covered by peritoneum) (**tip**: "gast"ly)
- Omphalocele (intestines covered by peritoneum)
- Spina Bifida Occulta: No herniation: failure of bony spinal canal to close (tuft of hair)
- Meningocele: Meninges herniates through spinal canal
- Meningomyelocele: Meninges and spinal cord herniated
- Anencephaly: Absence of part of the brain or skull

Neural Crest Migration Failure

- **Hirschsprung**
- 12th week: **Ganglion cells do not migrate to rectum**
- **No Meissner (sub mucosal), no Auerbach** (bowel wall)
- Biopsy shows no ganglion cells
- Higher risk in Downs Syndrome
- Transposition of the Great Vessels: No **SPIRALING of aorticopulmonary septum (AKA: Failure of septation)**

DERIVATIVES of the PHARYNGEAL ARCHES

ARCH	BRANCHIAL POUCH (Endoderm)	SKELETAL (Mesoderm and Neural Crest)	AORTIC ARCH (Mesoderm)	MUSCLES (Mesoderm)	CRANIAL NERVE (Neural Tube)	Cleft
1 Mandibular	Ear (Middle ear, Eustachian tube)	Incus, malleus, mandible, maxilla, temporal bone, spheno-mandibular ligament, spheno-malleolar ligament (**Meckel's** cartilage), zygomaticum	**Maxillary branch** of the carotid artery	Jaw muscles, floor of mouth, soft palate, Muscles of the ear. **Muscles of mastication**. Tensor palatine muscles, **anterior** belly of digastric, mylohyoid, tympani	5	External acoustic meatus
2 Hyoid	Palatine Tonsil	**Stapes** bone of middle ear, **styloid process** of temporal bone, stapedius, hyoid bone of neck, (**Reichert's** cartilage)	Cortico-tympanic artery (adult), **stapedial** artery (embryo), arteries to the ear	Muscles of facial expression, jaw and upper neck muscles, stapedius, Stylohyoid, **posterior** belly of digastric muscle	7	Cervical sinus
3	Thymus, **Inferior** Parathyroids	Lower rim and greater horns of the hyoid bone	**Common carotids, Internal carotid**	Stylopharyngeus (elevates pharynx)	9	Cervical sinus
4	**Superior** Parathyroids, C Cells of Thyroid	Laryngeal cartilages	Arch of the Aorta, Right **Subclavian** Artery	Constrictors of pharynx and vocal cords, larynx, striated muscle of the esophagus	10 **Superior laryngeal** branch of Vagus nerve	Cervical sinus
6		Laryngeal cartilages	**Pulmonary Artery**, Ductus Arteriosus	Intrinsic muscles of the larynx, pharynx, striated muscle of the esophagus, Sternocleidomastoid, Trapezius	10 - XI **Recurrent laryngeal** branch of Vagus nerve, Spinal Acc'ry	

Brain Anatomy

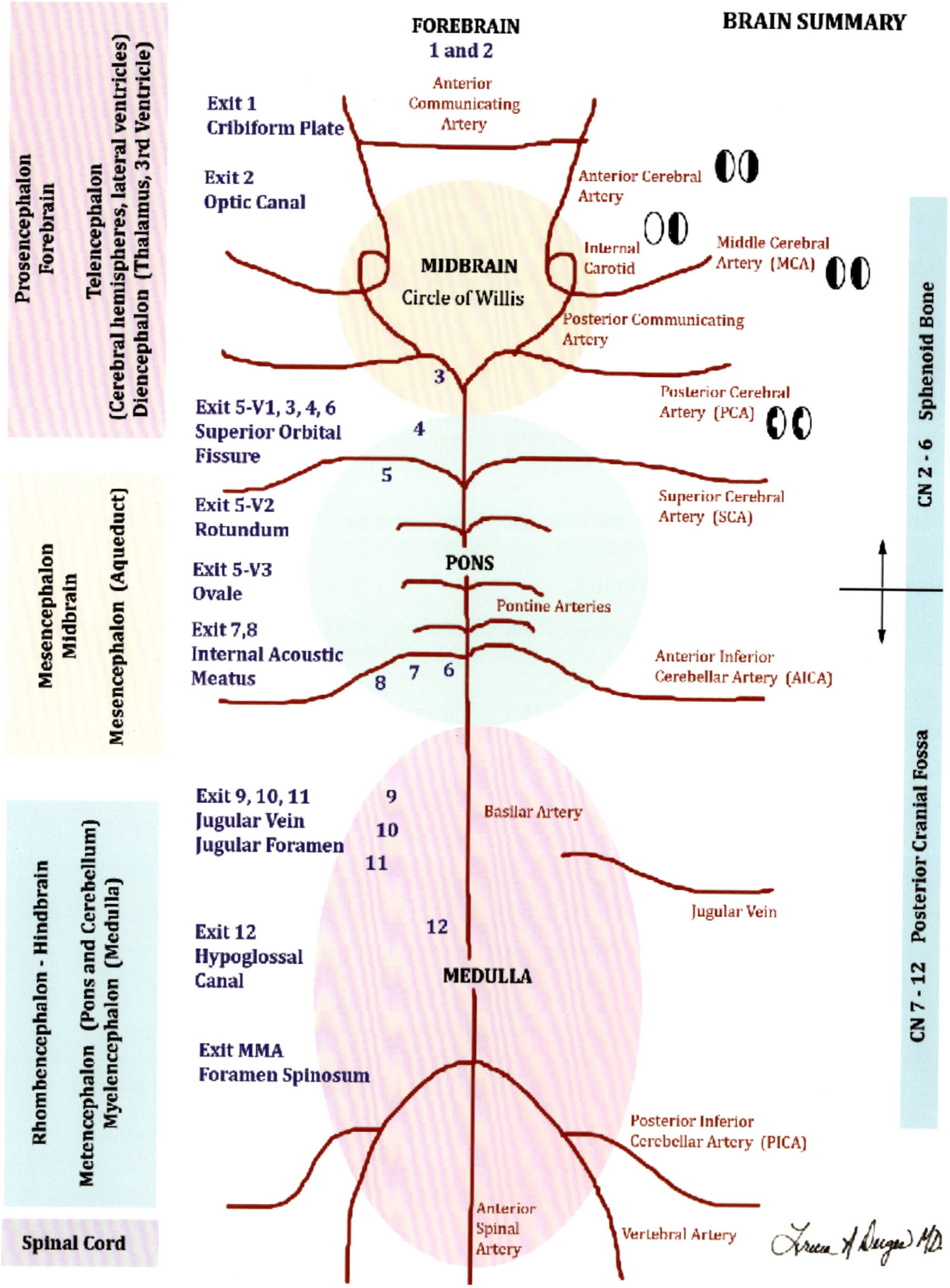

Brain Stem: Sagittal plane

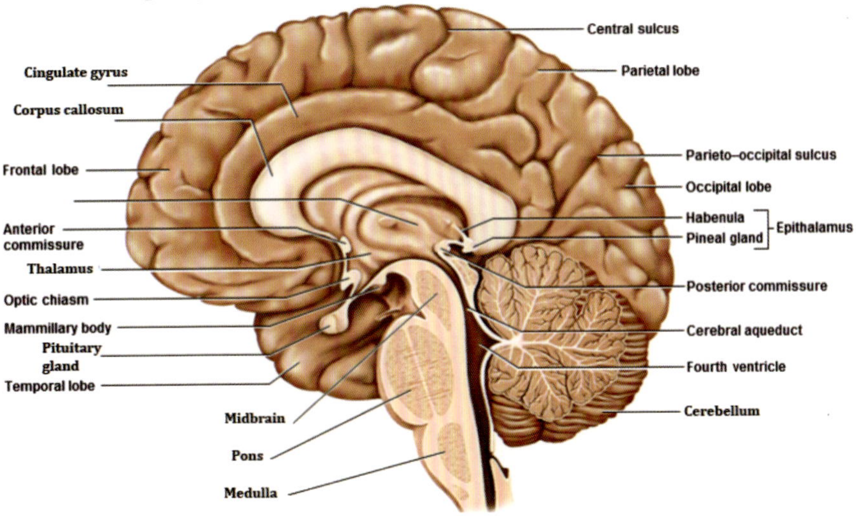

Brain: Coronal

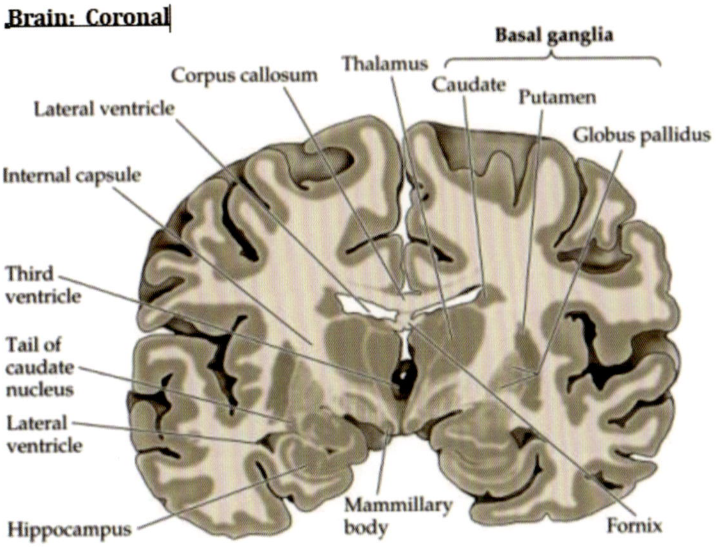

Twelve Cranial Nerves

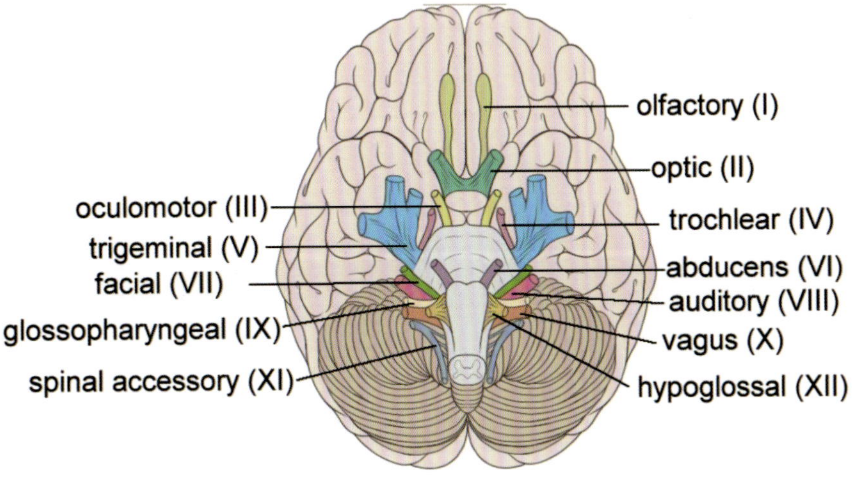

Cranial Nerves

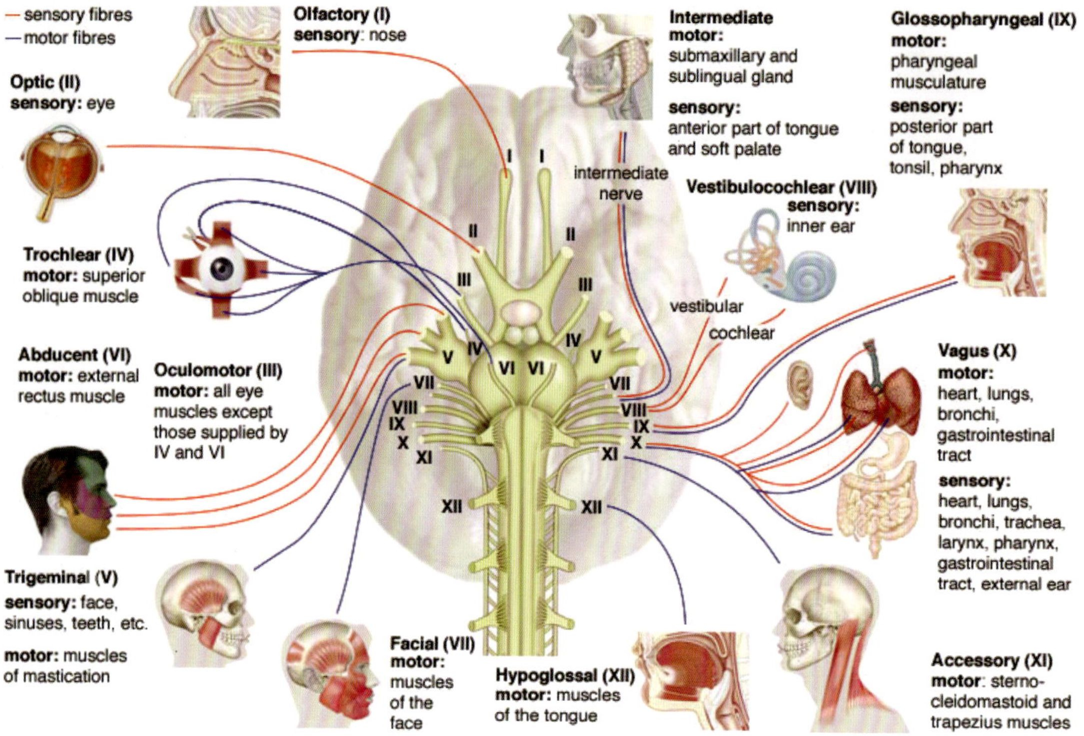

Cranial Nerve	Fibers	Origin	Brainstem Nucleus	Exit	Function	Neuropathy
CN1 – Olfactory	S: Olfactory epithelium	Temporal lobe	--------	Cribriform Plate	Olfaction (smell)	↓Smell, Taste
CN II – Optic	S: Retina	Only CN from CNS	--------	Optic Canal	Vision	Visual dysfunction
CN III – Oculomotor	M: Superior/middle/inferior rectus; inferior oblique, levator palpebrae. PNS: Pupillary constrictor, ciliary muscle of eye: both by ciliary ganglion.	Midbrain	Oculomotor Nucleus	Superior Orbital Fissure	Movement of eyeball. Pupillary constriction and accommodation.	"Down & Out" Syndrome, Mydriasis, Ptosis, Diplopia, lost accommodation, light reflexes.
CN IV – Trochlear	M: Superior oblique	Only CN from dorsal brainstem	Trochlear nucleus	Superior Orbital Fissure	Movement of eyeball.	Vertical diplopia
CN V – Trigeminal (V1, 2, 3)	S: Face, scalp, cornea, nasal, oral cavities, cranial dura mater M: Muscles mastication, Tensor Tympani muscle	Supero-lateral Pons	S: Trigeminal sensory nucleus. M: Trigeminal motor nucleus.		General sensation. Opening/closing mouth. Tension of tympanic membrane.	↓ corneal reflex, Herpes Zoster (V1>V2>V3)
V1 - Opthalmic	S: Forehead, nose, eye, frontal sinus, ↑ eyelid.	Pons	S: Trigeminal sensory nucleus	Superior Orbital Fissure	General sensation	Most affected by Herpes
V2 – Maxillary	S: Cheek, ↑ teeth, ↓ eyelid, maxillary sinus	Pons	S: Trigeminal sensory nucleus	Foramen Rotundum	General sensation	Tic douloureux
V3 – Mandibular	S: lower face, ↓ teeth, anterior 2/3 tongue, temple, TMJ, lingual gingiva. M: Mastication, Tensor Tympani, Tensor Veli Palatini, Mylohyoid, Anterior Digastric Belly.	Pons	S: Trigeminal sensory nucleus. M: Trigeminal motor nucleus.	Foramen Ovale	Sensation and motor	Tic douloureux, Abnormal chewing.

CN - VI Abducens	M: Lateral rectus	Ventral brainstem thru cavernous sinus	Abducens nucleus	Superior Orbital Fissure	Movement of eyeball	Cavernous sinus syndrome, medial eye deviation, diplopia.
CN – VII Facial	S: Anterior 2/3 tongue (Chorda Tympani), soft palate. M: Facial expression, Stapedius muscle, Posterior Digastric Belly, Stylohyoid. PNS: Submandibular/sublingual/lacrimal glands	Ventral brainstem (lateral to VI)	S: Nucleus Solitarius M: Facial Motor Nucleus PNS: Superior Salivatory Nucleus	Internal Acoustic Meatus	S: Taste M: Facial Movement, tension of ossicles PNS: Salivation and lacrimation	Bell's Palsy, Unilateral facial paralysis, lower motor nerve palsy.
CN – VIII Vestibulocochlear	S: Cochlea (sound), Vestibular apparatus (balance)	Ventral brainstem. Petrous Ridge of Temporal bone	Cochlea: Cochlear Nucleus Vestibular: Vestibular Nucleus	Internal Acoustic Meatus	Hearing, Proprioception of head and balance.	Hearing, balance loss. Vertigo.
CN – IX Glossopharyngeal	S: Taste & sense of posterior 1/3 of tongue, tonsil, pharynx, middle ear, carotid sinus, Eustachian tube. M: Stylopharyngeus PNS: Parotid gland	Lateral Medulla (inferior to VIII)	General sensation, Chemo/Baroreceptors: Trigeminal Sensory Nucleus. Taste, swallowing, salivation: Nucleus Solitarius.	Jugular Foramen	General sensation, Chemo & Baroreceptors, taste, swallowing, salivation	↓ taste and salivation, syncope (messenger in carotid massage)
CN – X Vagus	S: Pharynx, larynx, external ear, Aortic bodies, Aortic arch, Thoracic and abdominal viscera, oesophagus. M: Soft Palate, larynx, pharynx, upper oesophagus. PNS: Cardiovascular, respiratory, GI system.	Lateral Medulla (inferior to IX)	General sensation, Chemo/Baroreceptors: Trigeminal Sensory Nucleus. Visceral sensation: Nucleus Solitarius. Speech, swallowing: Nucleus Ambiguus. PNS: Control of systems: Dorsal Motor Nucleus of Vagus.	Jugular Foramen	General sensation, Chemo-Baroreceptors, taste, visceral sensation, speech, swallowing, control of systems.	Dysphagia, hoarseness, stridor.
CN – XI Accessory	M: Sternomastoid (SCM), trapezius, laryngeal, Pharyngeal	Spinal roots enter magnum, joining medullary roots to form IX.	Nucleus Ambiguus, Cranial nerves	Foramen Magnum and Jugular Foramen	Movement of head and shoulders	Paralysis of SCM and Trapezius (drop shoulder, torticollis)
CN – XII Hypoglossal	M: Tongue (intrinsic & extrinsic)	Medulla (b/t pyramids & olive)	Hypoglossal Nucleus	Hypo-glossal Canal	Movement of tongue	Tongue deviates towards lesion

Cranial Nerve Nuclei Locations

- Lateral nuclei are sensory
- Medical nuclei are motor
- Cranial nerve III, IV = Midbrain
- Cranial nerve V, VI, VII, VIII = Pons
- Cranial nerve IX, X, XII = Medulla
- Cranial nerve XI = Spinal cord

Olfactory Nerve

- **Only sensory nerve to go directly to the sensory cortex and not the Thalamus.**
- Olfactory nerve synapses in the Pyriform Cortex.

Cranial Nerve Reflexes

Reflex	Afferent	Efferent	Notes
Corneal (close eyelids)	V1 Opthalmic	VII Temporal branch	Foreign object causes orbicularis oculi To close eyelids
Carotid sinus	IX	X	Mechanical means to decrease HR
Gag	IX	X	1st reflex lost in **botulism** (**descending paralysis**), Stroke pharynx
Cough		X (via the superior laryngeal branch)	
Jaw jerk	V3 Mandibular - Sensory (masseter)	V3 Mandibular –Motor	Stretch reflex for masseter
Lacrimation	V1 Opthalmic	VII	
Pupillary	II	III	Pupil constricts to responding light
Vestibulo-ocular	VIII	III, IV, VI	Head/eye compensatory movements To stay on a target when head/body moves

Cranial Nerve X (Vagus) Nuclei

Nuclei	Innervation	Cranial Nerves
Nucleus a**M**biguus	**M**otor: pharynx, larynx, upper esophagus. Palate elevation, swallowing. Efferent.	IX, X, XI
Nucleus **S**olitarius	**S**ensory: baroreceptors, taste (tongue), distention of gut. (**tip**: I have **taste** for only one **SOLITARY** thing: steak!). Afferent.	VII, IX, X
Doral Motor Nucleus	Parasympathetic fibers to heat, lungs, upper GI	X

Cranial Nerve Lesions

- If the question is wanting where the lesion is at, look at all the symptoms and identify which cranial nerve belongs with each symptom. The lesion will be at the highest cranial nerve.
  (ie: Patient can't hear (CN VIII), patient can't smell (CN I), patient can't swallow (CN IX), patient is looking "down and out" (CN III), the highest cranial nerve lesion out of the CN VIII, CN I, CN IX, CN III is cranial nerve IX. So cranial nerve IX is where the lesion is.

Cranial Nerve Lesion	Lesion Description
Cranial Nerve V	Jaw deviates **toward** side with lesion b/c unopposed force of opposite pterygoid muscle
Cranial Nerve VII	Bells Palsy (entire ½ of face): Face droop, tearing, decrease in taste, can't close eyelid. All facial expressions.
Cranial Nerve X	Uvula deviates **away** from side with lesion
Cranial Nerve XI	Weakness turning head contralateral side of lesion (sternocleidomastoid) so causes shoulder droop on side of lesion (trapezius)
Cranial Nerve XII (LMN)	Tongue deviates **toward** side of lesion b/c weak tongue muscles on affected side (**tip**: lick your wounds). So lesion on the right side would cause tongue to deviate to the right. Nerve damage: CNXII (hypoglossal- retracts tongue) and genioglossus.

Nerves

Nerve	Function
Neuron	**Permanent** Cells – **stays in G0 phase**, have no stem cells. If in CNS: Nissl substance. Can't regenerate. In PNS: Injury to axon (Wallerian degeneration) axon can regenerate over time.
Microglia	**CNS macrophages** = phagocytosis. Responds to damage in the CNS
Astrocytes	Derived from the neuroectoderm. Removes excess neurotransmitters, foot process in the blood-brain barrier. Causes **reactive gliosis** in the repair of CNS damage (**Glial Scar**). Repairs K metabolism. **GFAP = marker.**
Myelin	Wraps and insulates axons in the CNS (oligodendrocytes) and PNS (Schwann cells). Increases conduction speed. Conducts through saltatory conduction between **Nodes of Ranvier**.
Oligodendrocytes	**Myelinates** multiple axons of the **neurons in the CNS**. Majority of cell in the white matter. Associated pathologies: Lesions in **Multiple Sclerosis** are due to demyelination of the oligodendrocytes. Lesions in PML (multifocal leukoencephalopathy). Lesions in Leukodystrophies. Derived from neuroectoderm.
Schwann Cells	Myelinates a **single PNS** axon. Increases conduction speed. Conducts through saltatory conduction between **Nodes of Ranvier**. Associated pathologies: **Guillain-Barre, NF2 acoustic meatus (CN VIII).**

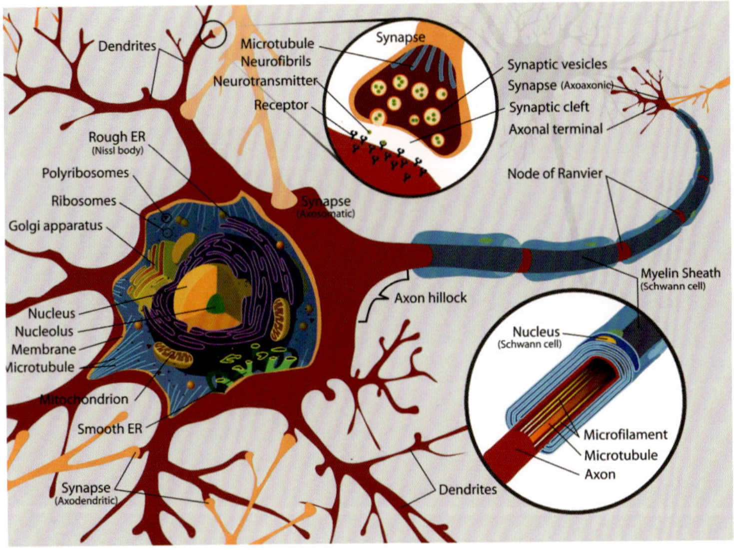

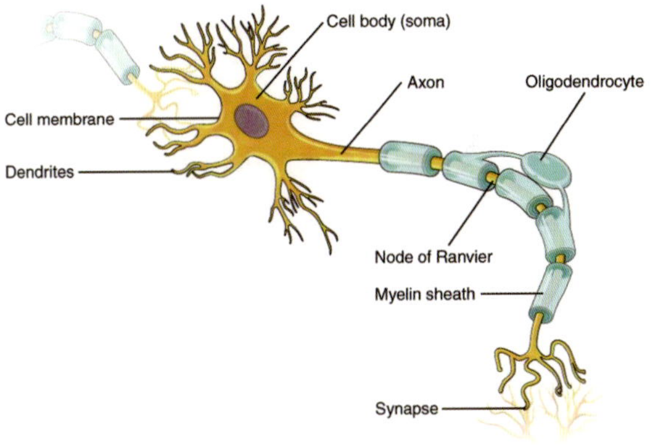

Sensory Receptors

Mechanoreceptors: sensory receptor that responds to pressure or distortion

Receptor Type	Nerve Description	Location	Senses
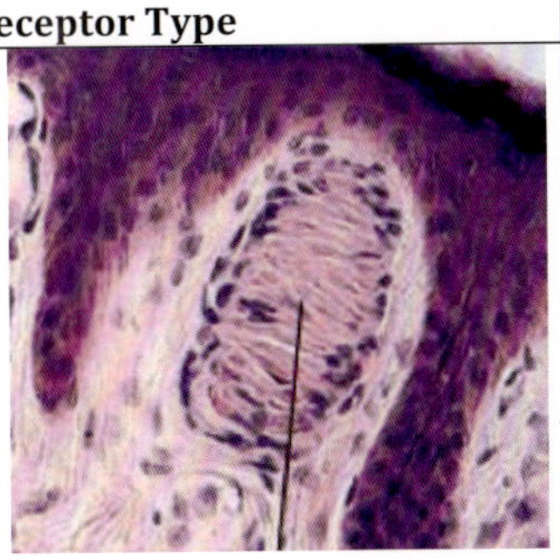 **Meissner Corpuscles** Mechanoreceptor. AKA: Tactile corpuscle.	Myelinated fibers –rapidly adapting	On hairless, glabrous skin and finger pads under the epidermis layer	**Fine touch, light touch,** position, sense (**tip**: mighty Fine tornado)

Pacinian Corpuscles Mechanoreceptor. AKA: Lamellar receptor. 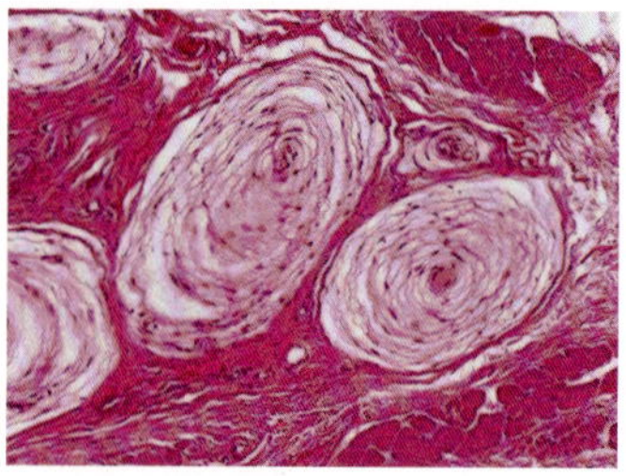	Myelinated fibers – rapidly adapting	Deep skin, joints, ligaments, Pancreas	**Vibration and pressure**, grasping/releasing object. Looks like a thumb print.
Merkel Disc Mechanoreceptor	Myelinated fibers, adapt slowly	Hair follicles, basal epidermis	Pressure, **deep touch**, position and sense (shapes) and edges)/ **These receptors are lost in burns**.
Ruffini Endings Mechanoreceptor AKA: Bulbous receptor	Enlarged dendritic endings with capsules	Subcutaneous tissues. Spindle shape	Skin stretch, finger position and control, grip objects.
Nociceptors Pain Fibers Free nerve endings (FNE). Perception of pain.	**Type I Fibers:** **C Fibers = slow conduction, unmyelinated,** small diameter fibers. Prolonged depolarization transmits slow, dull, aching, burning pain. Glutamate is the neurotransmitter in the dorsal horn along with Substance P. **Type II Fibers: A Delta δ Type = fast conduction, myelinated,** medium diameter fibers. Glutamate in the dorsal horn transmits sharp, fast pain by acting on ligand gated ion channels. Afferent nerve ending = brings info from the bodies periphery to the brain. (**tip**: 2 legs makes you fast)	Skin, epidermis, viscera	Pain (AKA: nociception), temperature, mechanical stimuli (**tip**: on **II legs** you can run **fast**. Myelinated nerves are always faster)

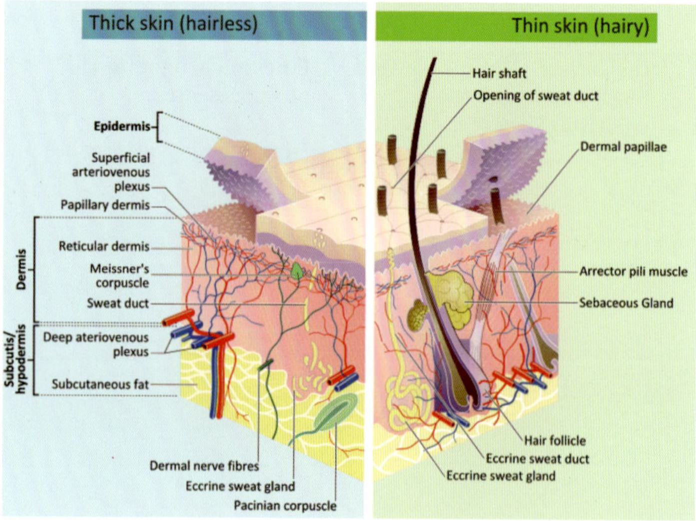

Dermatomes

- C4 = Collarbone
- C6 = Thumb/1st finger (**tip**: curve thumb to 1st finger and it makes a "6")
- C8 = Pinkie
- T4 = Nipple
- T10 = Umbilicus (initial appendicitis pain point) (**tip**: Belly But TEN)
- L4 = Knee
- S1 – S2 = Foot (**tip**: you have 2 feet)
- S3 – S4 = Anal/Penile
- Referred Pain: Right shoulder pain from gallbladder pain via phrenic nerve.
  Left shoulder pain from stomach via phrenic nerve.

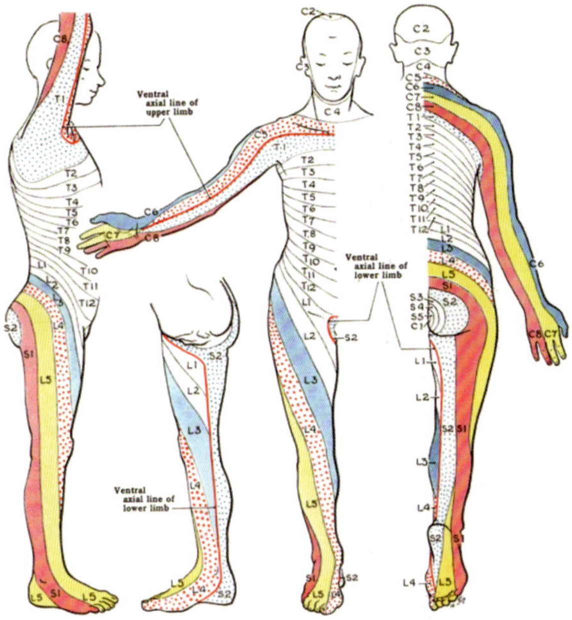

Reflexes

- Biceps = C5 nerve root
- Brachioradialis = C6 nerve root
- Triceps = C7 nerve root
- Patella = L4 nerve root
- Achilles = S1 nerve root
- Cremaster = L1, L2
- Anal = S3, S4

Layers a needle goes through during a lumbar puncture (spinal tap)

- Skin ➔ Fascia ➔ Supraspinous ligament ➔ Interspinous ligament ➔ Ligamentum flavum ➔ Epidural space ➔Dura mater ➔ Subarachnoid space

Vertebra Anatomy

Note: When gaining access to the spinal cord (neural canal) the **point of entry is through the lamina** because the lamina does not lie directly on a nerve or the spinal cord.

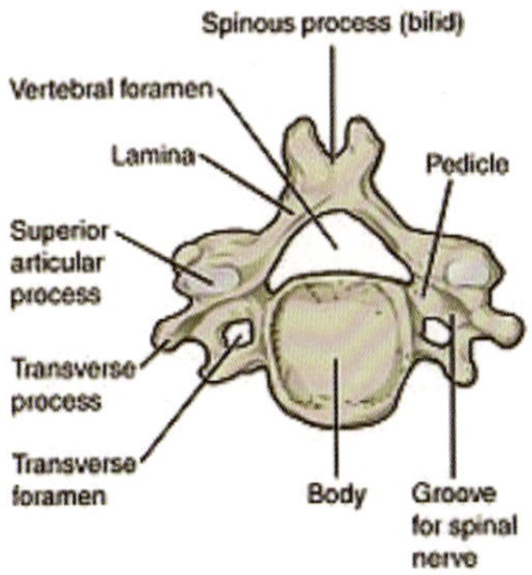

Neurotransmitters

Neurotransmitter	Nucleus (Synthesis)	Pathologies
5-HT Serotonin	Raphe nucleus	↑ Parkinson's (Substantia Nigra) ↓ Anxiety and Depression
ACh Acetylcholine	Basal nucleus of Meynert	↑ Parkinson's (Substantia Nigra) ↓ Alzheimer's ↓ Huntington's (Caudate Nucleus)
Dopamine	SNc in midbrain (substantia nigra pars compacta), Ventral tegmentum	↓ Parkinson's ↑ Huntington's (Caudate Nucleus) ↓ Depression
GABA	Nucleus Accumbens	**Inhibitory** neurotransmitter ↓ Huntington's (Caudate Nucleus) ↓ Anxiety Cells in the Striatum, Pallidum and Substantial Nigra use GABA.
Glutamate	**Subthalamic Nucleus**	**Excitatory** neurotransmitter. Released by cortical cells in the Primary Motor Cortex. Glutamate stimulates cells in the striatum creating 2 pathways: The "Direct" (causing movement) and "Indirect" (preventing movement) pathway in the Basal Ganglia. Cells in the Cortex, Thalamus and STN = glutamatergic. **Associated: Hemiballismus**

Dopamine Pathways/Tracts

Dopamine Pathways

Active Dopamine Pathways (Dopamine is on)

Tubero Pathway	Nigro Pathway	Mesolimbic Pathway
Inhibits Prolactin	Creates movement (ie: tics)	Euphoria of drug use. Delusions, schizophrenia. Increased visions and feelings

Inactive Dopamine Pathways (Dopamine is off)

Tubero Pathway	Nigro Pathway	Mesolimbic Pathway
Prolactin is on Prolactinoma Galactorrhea	Increase in EPS symptoms. Increase in Parkinsons.	Gives theraputic effects of anti-psych meds. Slows down schizophrenia.

Brain Structures and Functions

Brain Anatomy	Function
Anterior Pituitary	AKA: Adenohypophysis: Releases hormones: TSH, GnRH, MSH, ACTH, GH, FSH, LH, Prolactin (PRL), Endorphins
Area Postrema	Area in the medulla by the floor of the 4th ventricle that controls vomiting. Detects toxins in the blood.
Basal Ganglia	Base of the forebrain. Postural adjustments, voluntary movements, procedural learning, routine behaviors (habits), cognition, emotion, **controls eye movements**. **Components: Striatum** (AKA: **Internal Capsule = Caudate nucleus (cognitive) and putamen (motor)** = Huntington's), **Lentiform = globus pallidus/pallidum (GPe: externus, GPi: internus) and Putamen,** nucleus accumbens, **subthalamic nucleus (STN): Associated with Hemiballismus), Substantia nigra** pars compacta **(SNc) associated with Parkinson's.** Associated pathologies: Huntington's, Parkinson's, Tourette Syndrome, Hemiballismus, OCD, and Dystonia. Glutamate (excitatory neurotransmitter): Released by cortical cells in the Primary Motor Cortex. Glutamate stimulates cells in the striatum creating 2 pathways: The "Direct" (causing movement) and "Indirect" (preventing movement) pathway in the Basal Ganglia. **Direct Pathway** (Creates movement) AKA: **Dopamine D-1** Pathway – Excitatory. **(GABA released) which disinhibits the thalamus = ↑ movement.** **Path:** Cortex (stimulates → Striatum (inhibits) → SNr-GPi complex (disinhibits thalamus) → **Thalamus (stimulates) →** Cortex (stimulates) → Muscles → **Increases movement (hyperkinetic)** **Indirect Pathway** (Decreases movement) AKA: **Dopamine D-2** Pathway – Inhibitory. **Path:** Cortex (stimulates) → Striatum (inhibits) → GPe (disinhibition of STN) → STN (stimulates) → SNr-GPi complex (inhibits) → **Thalamus (inhibited)** → Cortex (inhibited) → Muscles → **Decreases movements (hypokinetic)**
Blood Brain Barrier	Selective permeability that separates circulating blood from the CNS/CFS. Endothelial cells connected by **tight junctions**. (Note: tight junctions also located in scrotum). Allows **passive diffusion** of: gases, **small (lipid, non-polar) molecules**, **water**, amino acids and **glucose**. **Astrocytes** create the BBB.
Cerebellum	Coordination and balance. All cerebellum lesions are ipsilateral. Lateral lesions: involve voluntary movement of extremities. Medial/midline lesions: involve ataxia, nystagmus, head tilting. Input nerves: Middle and Inferior cerebellar peduncle via **mossy fibers** (**tip**: IN = Inferior). Output nerves: Superior cerebellar peduncle via Superior cerebellar peduncle via **Purkinje fibers**. Injury: Intention tremor, ataxia, loss of balance. Ipsilateral deficits (falls toward side of lesion) TX: **Romberg Test** (test neurological function and drunk driving. Test proprioception (ability to know where the body is in space), vestibular function (ability to know head position in space), and vision. Patient stands with feet together with hands at side. Closes eyes for one minute. If patient sways or falls = positive test.

Cerebral Cortex	Cerebrum (brain) outer layer. Functions in attention, perception, thought, language, consciousness, memory, awareness. Gray matter with **astrocytes being the most abundant cell** type. Note: If a movement is planned but is not carried out, the premotor cortex will increase in its activity. **Contains: Brodmann's areas.** **Brodmann areas:** 1, 2, 3 = primary somatosensory cortex, area 4 = primary motor cortex, area 17 = primary visual cortex, **areas 22 (Wernicke's area)**, areas 41, 42 = primary auditory cortex, **areas 44, 45 = speech and language (Broca's areas).** The **Arcuate fasciculus** connects Broca's area (in the inferior frontal gyrus) and Wernicke's area (posterior superior temporal gyrus).
	Broca's Area: **"Broca's Aphasia"** (frustrated patient): **(Speech production).** Can hear and understand but is unable to say what they want to. It does not come out the way intended. **Posterior, Inferior frontal lobe, dominant left side, areas 44, 45.** **Wernicke's Area: (Speech comprehension). Posterior region of the superior temporal lobe. "Fluent Aphasia"** The patient is able to fluently connect words but the words totally lack meaning. **Brodmann's area 22.** Associated with **Wernicke-Korsakoff Syndrome**. (Vitamin B-1 deficiency in alcoholics) (**tip**: if you have trouble remembering which one goes with which lobe: keep it alphabetical: "B"roca's is closest to "F"rontal. Were "W"ernicke's is closer to "T"emporal lobe). **Conduction Aphasia**: Damage to the **arcuate fasciculus** (thick band of fibers that connects Broca's and Wernicke's areas). **Unable to repeat words.**
Colliculi	Inferior and Superior Colliculi lie just inferior to pineal gland. (**Tip**: Your eyes are above (vision - superior) to your ears (auditory – inferior) Inferior Colliculi: **Auditory** Superior Colliculi: Conjugate vertical **gaze center**. (In Parinaud syndrome, the conjugate vertical gaze is paralyzed due to pressure from a pinealoma)

Cerebral Cortex and its Functions

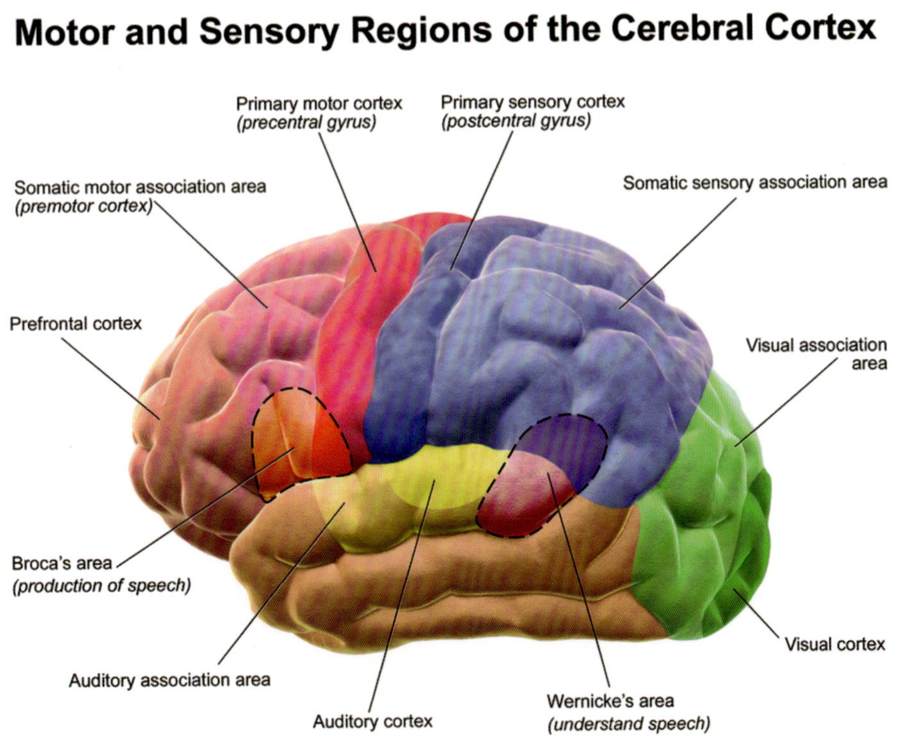

Frontal Lobe	A major lobe of the cerebral cortex. **Separated from parietal lobe by the central sulcus** and the **temporal lobe by the lateral sulcus** (AKA: Sylvian fissure). Precentral gyrus forms posterior border, containing the primary motor cortex. Contains most of the dopamine-sensitive neurons in the cortex. Executive decisions, personality, reward, attention, planning, motivation, mood. Injury: Disinhibition, decreased concentration, judgement, aggression.
Hypothalamus	Adenohypophysis: regulates anterior pituitary. Neurohypophysis: regulates posterior pituitary. Regulates: hunger, temperature, sexual urges, osmolality, area postrema, autonomics, water. **Paraventricular nucleus**: makes oxytocin (**tip**: you have a PARA ovaries) **Supraoptic nucleus**: makes ADH **Anterior** Hypothalamus: Regulates **cooling** (**tip**: **A**ir conditioning = cools) = p**A**rasympathetic. Dysfunction causes heat stroke. (Note: heat exhaustion is due to dehydration). **Posterior** Hypothalamus: Regulates **heating** = sympathetic. **Lateral** Hypothalamus: Regulates **hunger** (makes us eat). **Inhibited by leptin**. Lesions cause failure to thrive in infants and anorexia. **Ventromedial** Hypothalamus: Controls **satiety** (tells you are full so you stop eating). Lesions cause hyperphagia = weight gain. **Stimulated by leptin**. (**tip**: lesions to Medial makes you grow medially). **Suprachiasmatic** Nucleus: **Circadian rhythm.**
Limbic system	**Hippocampus:** In the medial temporal lobe under the cerebral cortex. Consolidates short-term memory to long term memory. REM sleep processes long term memory. **First area in the brain that is damaged when there is hypoxia.** Injury: Anterograde amnesia (unable to make new memories) **Amygdala**: Deep and medially in temporal lobes. Functions in emotions, reactions, decision making, reward center and memory. Left amygdala is assocated with negative emotions. Right amygdala is assocated with memories that can be consciously recalled. This area is associated with damage in **Klüver-Bucy syndrome** (hypersexuality, disinhibition). **Fornix:** Nerve fibers that carries info from the hippocampus to the mammillary bodies to the anterior thalamus, associated with recall memory. **Mammillary Bodies:** Located by the anterior arches of the Fornix. Associated with recollective memory. **This is the area damaged in Wernicke-Korsakoff syndrome**: impaired memory causes the "fill in" of memories = confabulation. **Cingulate Gyrus:** Located medially in the cerebral cortex above the corpus callosum. Links behaviors to motivation.
Pineal Gland	Circadian rhythms and melatonin secretion **Parinaud Syndrome: A Pinealoma** causes pressure to superior colliculi (conjugate vertical gaze center), which causes paralysis of conjugate vertical gaze.
Posterior Pituitary	AKA: Neurohypophysis: Receives and releases ADH and oxytocin from hypothalamus
Reticular Activating System	In the midbrain. Controls consciousness. ↓ levels of wakefulness = coma

<table>
<tr>
<td>Thalamus</td>
<td>

SENSORY. Sensory relay for all ascending tracts, except olfactory.
If a stroke is purely sensory, the lesion is in the thalamus.

VPL Nucleus (Ventral posterolateral): Receives info from: **Spinothalamic and Dorsal Columns (AKA: medial lemniscus) and projects them to the postcentral gyrus (Brodmann's Areas 1, 2, 3) in the cortex. Pain and temperature, vibration, proprioception**, touch, pressure. (Brodmann's areas 1, 2 and 3 make up the somatosensory cortex).

VPM Nucleus (Ventral posteromedial): Receives info from: Trigeminal tract and gustatory (taste) from the solitary tract and the trigeminal nerve and projects it to the postcentral gyrus in the cortex. **Face sensation and taste**.

LGN Nucleus (lateral geniculate): CN II – Vision. Receives input from the retina. Connects the optic nerve to the occipital lobe. Goes to the superior colliculus (AKA: Calcarine sulcus).

MGN (medial geniculate): Auditory (hearing). Relays info between the inferior colliculus and auditory cortex in the temporal lobe.

VL (Ventral lateral): Receives input from basal ganglia (nuclei) = substantial nigra, globus pallidus, cerebellum. Sends output to the primary motor and premotor cortex. Coordinates movement.

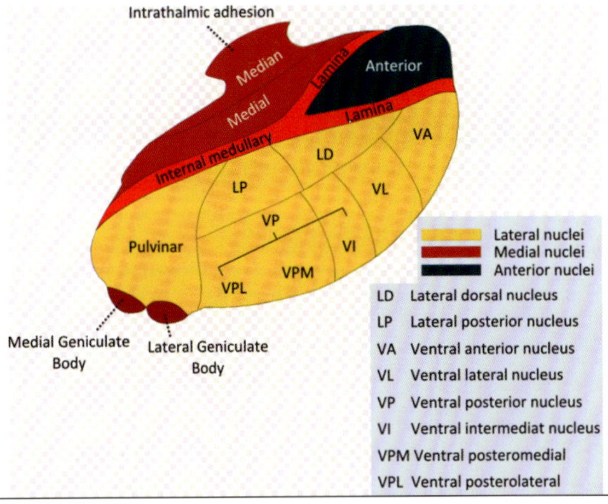

</td>
</tr>
</table>

Dominant and Non-Dominant Brain
Dominate – Left Parietal – Temporal Cortex

- Left side: majority
- Verbal and language processing
- Analytic processing
- Critical thinking
- Reasoning and logic
- **Writing** ability (damage causes: Agraphia)
- **Mathematics**: adding, subtracting, multiplying (damage causes: acalculia)
- Ability to name, distinguish and **recognize the fingers** (Damage causes: Finger agnosia)
- (**tip**: Count (math) on the fingers)
- Left-right orientation

Non-Dominant – Right Parietal-Temporal Cortex

- Right side of the brain
- Able to recognize the left side of the world (**Damage causes: left side neglect (AKA: Spatial Neglect** Syndrome, Hemineglect, Hemispatial Neglect: Is agnosia of the contralateral side of the world. Meaning the patient is unable to see the left side of themselves, the left side of their plate, etc. They will shave only their right side of their face or think there is only food on the right side of their plate)
- Interprets body language and facial expressions
- Identifies **shapes**, sizes, contours, sounds, melodies, color
- Emotions, creativity, intuition
- **Position** relative to other things/others
- Depth and breadth

Note: Inability to read (alexia) with preservation of the ability to write (agraphia): indication lesion is in the left occipital cortex and splenium of the cerebral cortex.

Lesions to the Dominant and Non-Dominant Lobes

Dominant Lobes	Nondominant Lobes
Lesion to the Left Dominant Parietal Lobe (AKA: Gerstmann Syndrome) • Inability to do mathematics - Acalculia • Inability to name fingers • Inability to write - Agraphia • Inability to identify left or right sides	**Lesion to the Right Non-Dominant Parietal Lobe** • Inabilty to do construction (copy an object) - Apraxia • Inability to dress (Dressing Apraxia) • Confusion
Lesion to the Left Dominant Temporal Lobe • Visual: Homonymous Superior Quadrantanopia • Aphasia, no speech • Wernicke's (word salad) • No comprehension of the spoken or written language • Unable to express thoughts	**Lesion to the Right Non-Dominant Temporal Lobe** • Visual: Homonymous Superior Quadrantanopia • Inability to perceive complex sounds

Brain Sulcus and Gyrus

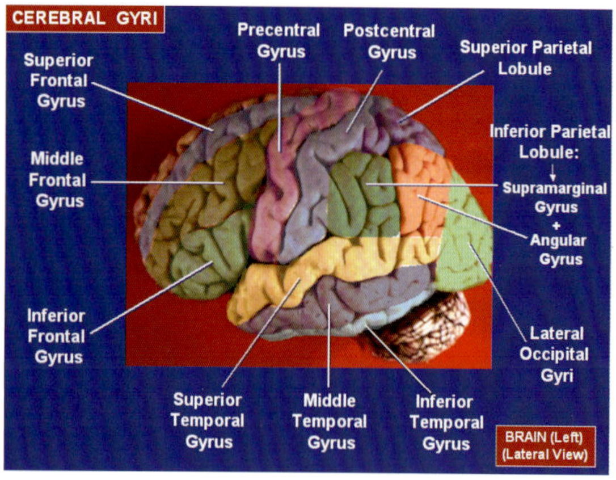

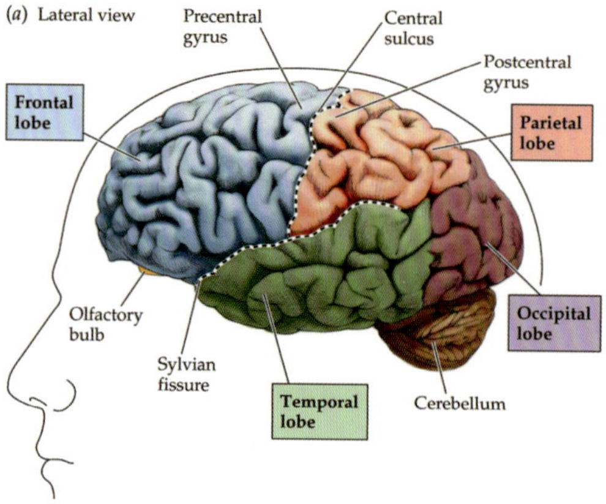

Brain Sinuses

Venous channels that run through the dura that drain blood from cerebral veins and receive CSF from arachnoid granules. These empty into the internal jugular vein and return to the heart. **Internal jugular vein** is the location that central lines are inserted to deliver medicines to the heart.
(**tip**: Meds need to go **IN**to the heart via the **IN**ternal jugular vein)

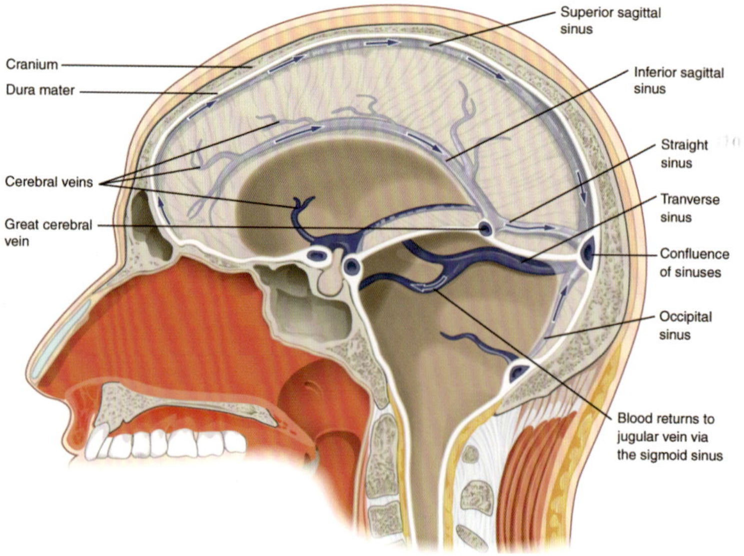

Ventricles and CSF

- CSF made by **choroid plexus** of the ventricles
- Produced by **ependymal cells in the choroid plexus**. Secrete sodium into the lateral ventricles = osmotic pressure which draws water into the CSF. Negative chloride binds with the positive sodium = neutral charge.
- Ependymal cells secrete Na into the ventricles creating osmotic pressure drawing water into the CSF space. The positive charge of the Na draws in the negative charged Cl creating a neutral charge. This causes CSF to have a higher concentration of Na and Cl than plasma.
- CSF contains higher levels of Na and Cl than plasma, but contains lower levels of Ca, glucose, K and protein than plasma.
- Cushion for the cortex
- Immunological protection to the brain
- Autoregulation of cerebral blood flow
- CSF occupies the subarachnoid space (between the arachnoid mater and pia mater) and the ventricle system
- Produces 500 mL of CSF per day
- **CSF circulation**: Produced in the lateral ventricles ➔ 3rd ventricle via foramen of Monro ➔ 4th ventricle via Aqueduct of Sylvius (AKA: Cerebral aqueduct) ➔ subarachnoid space via Foramen of Luschka (lateral) and Foramen of Magna (AKA: Magendie (medial) ➔ reabsorbed by **arachnoid granulations (AKA: Villi)** ➔ drains into the dural venous sinuses.

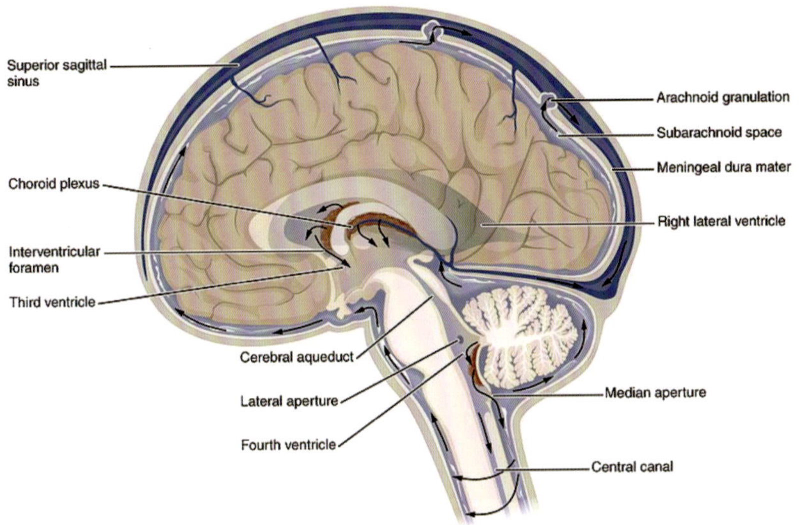

CSF Pathologies

Non-Communicating Hydrocephalus	**Communicating Hydrocephalus**	**Enlarged Ventricles**
Cause: **Blockage of CSF exiting the ventricles**. Usually due to stenosis of the aqueduct of Sylvius. CSF backs up causing swelling of the ventricles and hydrocephalus. **Dandy-Walker Syndrome** Congenital brain malformation of the cerebellum. Absence of the cerebellar vermis blocks drainage of the 4th ventricle enlarging it. SX: ↑ ICP, vomiting, convulsions, vomiting.	Cause: CSF is produced and **exits the ventricles** but is **not reabsorbed by the arachnoid granules (villi)** causing ↑ ICP, papilledema and herniation. (**tip**: If you can't get outside (ventricles), you can't communicate with anyone. If you can get outside (ventricles) you can communicate)	Other pathologies that will show enlarged ventricles: **AIDS/HIV** Gaucher's Disease **Excess Vitamin A (Retinol)** Excess Vitamin A can cause idiopathic intracranial hypertension

Hydrocephalus ex vacuo

Atrophy of the brain due to injury: stroke, trauma. The ventricles are not enlarged, they look enlarged **due to the atrophy of the brain** (neuronal atrophy).
There is more than normal amounts of CSF but there is **NO increase in pressure**.

Normal Pressure Hydrocephalus

Normal aging.

Decreased absorption of CSF due to normal aging.
SX: **Gait disturbances/stumbling (wobbly), urinary incontinence/dribbling (wet) and forgetful/dementia (wacky).**

Caused by increase in ICP due to abnormal accumulation of CSF in the ventricles.

TX: Shunt placement

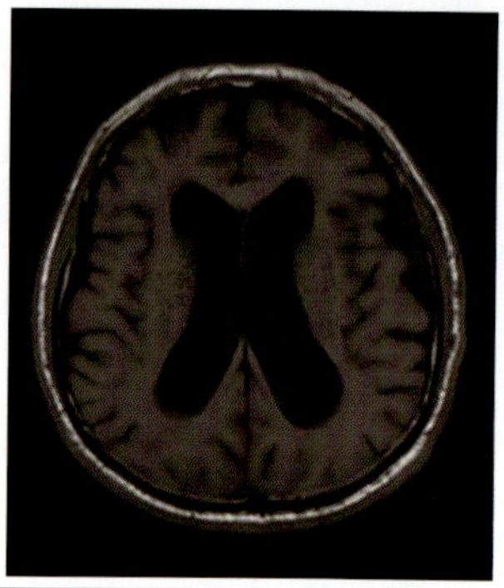

CSF Findings in Diseases (Lumbar punctures)

Disease	PMN's	Glucose	Lymphocytes	Protein	Pressure	RBC	Other
NORMAL	0 – 5	45 – 80		18 – 58		0	
Bacterial Meningitis	**↑↑ >1000**	**↓ <40**		> 400	↑		
Fungal Meningitis		**↓**	**↑↑**	↑	↑		
Viral Meningitis (AKA: Aseptic Meningitis)		**NORMAL**	**↑↑ > 90%**	Normal	↑		Note: there is an ↑ in WBC over the normal ratio of WBC and RBC in meningitis. In a subarachnoid hemorrhage the WBC is ↑ but the ratio is normal. **Normal ratio:** 1 WBC to every 500-1000 RBC
TB Meningitis	5 – 1000	**↓↓ <10**		↑↑ >400			
Lyme, Cryptococcus, Rickettsia		↓	↑↑	↑			
Guillain Barre	Normal	Normal		**↑↑ 45 - 1000**			
Tertiary Syphilis							**Positive VDRL**
Pseudo Tumor Cerebri					**↑↑**		
Multiple Sclerosis				**↑↑**			
Subarachnoid Hemorrhage (SAH)						**↑**	**Xanthochromia** Note: there is an ↑ in WBC but the WBC and RBC ratio is **normal**. In meningitis the WBC is ↑ than the normal ratio. **Normal ratio:** 1 WBC to every 500-1000 RBC.
Injury/improper stick technique						↑↑	
Herpes			**↑↑ > 90%**	↑	↑	**↑↑**	**(RBC with viral profile)**
HIV Toxoplasmosis							**EBV DNA**
Creutzfeldt-Jakob Disease				14-3-3 Protein			
Normal Pressure Hydrocephalus (NPH)				Normal			
Subacute Sclerosing Panencephalitis (SSPE)							Antibodies to the measles virus

Lumbar Puncture Rules

- **BEFORE performing an LP, a CT of the head must be obtained if the patient has ANY of these signs:**
  Papilledema (Indicates increased intracranial pressure), confusion, focal neurological abnormalities or having/had seizures
- **Do any cultures BEFORE starting antibiotics**
- **If no LP can be performed start antibiotics immediately**
- **LP (or spinal anesthesia)_ Anatomy: Landmark: Iliac crest for L3 to L4**
  Layers to penetrate (in order): Skin, fascia, supraspinous ligament, interspinous ligament, ligamentum flavum, epidural space, dura mater, subarachnoid space.
- **Normal WBC to RBC ratio in CSF: 1 WBC to every 500 – 1000 RBC.**
  Note: In SAH: there is a higher WBC's count but the ratio to RBC is still normal.
  In meningitis: there is a higher WBC count but that count is higher than the normal WBC:RBC ratio (abnormal).

Movement Disorder Differentials

Movement	Description	Pathology	Notes
Akathisia	Restlessness, constant tapping of leg, arm, etc.	Side effect of anti-psych meds	
Athetosis	Basal ganglia. **Slow, writhing** movements In the hands	Huntington's, Rett Syndrome	
Bradykinesia	**Slow** movements, difficult to start movements	**Parkinson Disease**	Patient has a hard time starting to move, but once started can't stop
Chorea	Basal ganglia. Sudden, purposeless movements	**Huntington's,** **Rheumatic Fever**	
Dystonia	**Sustained**, involuntary muscle contractions. Neck is sustained to one side.	Blepharospasm (eyelid twitch), Side effect anti-psych meds	
Essential Tremor (AKA: Postural tremor, Shaky Hand Syndrome, Kinetic tremor)	Tremor with **intentional (voluntary)** movement such as eating, writing, pointing.		AD inheritance. **Improves with alcohol.** TX: **Propanolol**
Flapping tremor (AKA: Asterixis)	Tremor of the hand when wrist is extended. Jerking movements of outstretched hands.	Liver damage, **Hepatic encephalopathy**: damage to brain cells due to build up of ammonia in the brain because liver is not metabolizing ammonia to urea.	TX: **Lactulose**
Hemiballismus	**Subthalamic nucleus** in basal ganglia. **Sudden, uncontrolled flailing of an arm or leg**	Lacunar stroke, damage to the Putamen or Caudate Nucleus	Dopamine D-1 pathway (disinhibits thalamus = ↑ movement)
Intention tremor	**Zigzag** motion when pointing or extending hands	**Cerebellar dysfunction**	
Myoclonus	Sudden, uncontrolled **muscle contraction**. Hiccups, jerks, twitches		
Myotonia	**Prolonged contraction** of skeletal muscles after voluntary contraction.	Myotonic muscular dystrophy, Malignant hyperthermia	
Resting tremor	**Tremor at rest.** Tremor is better when intentionally using hands.	**Parkinson Disease**	
Tardive dyskinesia	**Repetitive oral (tongue),** facial movements	Irreversible side effect of anti-psych meds	

Gait Differentials

Gait	Description
Parkinson	Shuffling, narrow base, fenestrating, no arm swing
Distal Motor Neuron	Steppage gait
Spastic Paraparesis or Stroke	Scissoring gait
Cerebellar Ataxia	"Drunken Sailor"
Senile Gait	"walking on ice" or "expecting to fall", precautious gait
Trendelenburg Gait	Polio (Sup. Gluteal Nerve, Gluteus Maximus, Medius)
Tabes Dorsalis Gait	Walks w/legs wide apart due to ↓ proprioception. Feet are lifted higher than normal causing a slapping sound on the floor
Muscular Dystrophy Gait	Waddle gait because of weak gluteal muscles
Normal Pressure Hydrocephalus Gait	Slow, broad based shuffling gait due to ↓ CSF absorption
Cerebellar Tumor	Ipsilateral ataxia. Wide base with erratic staggering. Difficult to maintain balance = ↑ falls
UMN	Spastic gait. Damage to Corticospinal tract
Vestibular Ataxia	Staggering gait due to ↓ movement of head
Dystonic Gait	Involuntary, sustained. Must twist to move limb or trunk
Foot Drop Gait	Can't dorsiflex foot due to peripheral neuropathy. Damage to spinal nerves L4 – S2, Common Peroneal nerve.
Tarsel Tunnel Gait	Antalgic gait (limp – favors foot) to avoid weight bearing on foot. Due to damage of the Tibial Nerve. Plantar surface of foot is numb.

Movement and Degenerative Pathologies

Huntington's

Autosomal Dominant
Trinucleotide repeat of CAG on chromosome 4
(AKA: **Hypermethylation** of histone gene)
(Methylation = stops)
Basal ganglia lesion

↓ GABA, ↓ ACh, ↑ Dopamine

Neuronal death via NMDA-R binding.
Glutamate toxicity.

Location: **Caudate Nucleus**

Anticipation (future generations are affected at earlier ages)
Presents between 20 – 50 years

SX: Cognitive and physical decline, **aggression, violence, changes in personality** (frontal lobe), psychotic problems, high risk of **suicide.**

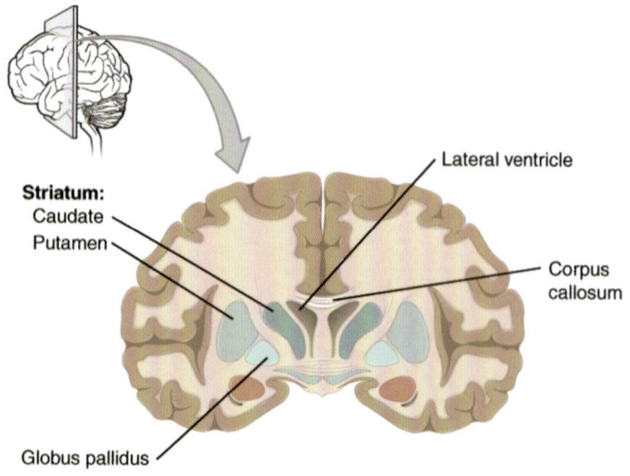

Frontal section

Parkinson Disease

Degenerative disorder of CNS
Location: **Substantia Nigra**
Cause: Loss of **Dopaminergic neurons in Substantia Nigra** causing **depigmentation** (paleness).
Loss of myelination.

↑ ACh,
↓ Dopamine

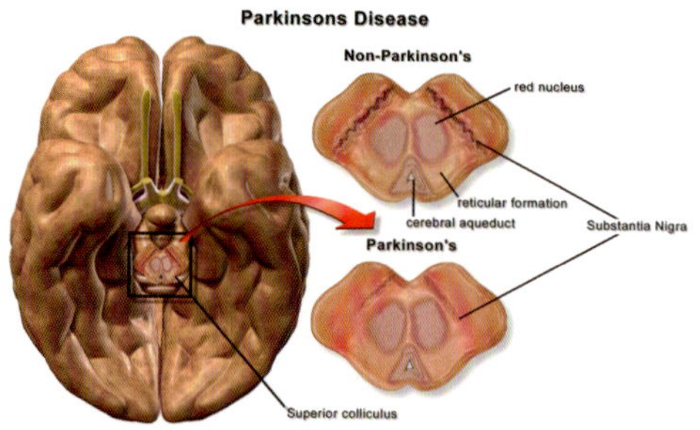

SX: **Triad: Resting tremor, rigidity, bradykinesia.** (AKA: Akinesia): slow movements. Once get started can't get stopped. **Resting tremor** (tremor stops with intentional movements), **cogwheel rigidity** (oscillating movement), **postural instability** ("lead pipe" movements – stiff, uniform moves), **shuffling gate**, **hypomimia** ("mask" faces = ↓ face expressions, **flat effect**), frequent falls, **hypophonia** (soft speech), **micrographia** (tiny handwriting), **Asymmetrical resting tremors**: tremors start in 1 hand and then generalizes and spreads to other side of the body.

DX: **Handwriting will show micrographia**
DX: **Lewy Bodies, made of α-synuclein**
(AKA: intracytoplasmic eosinophillic inclusion bodies)
DX: **Handwriting will show micrographia**
TX: Levodopa (L-Dopa), Carbidopa (increases bioavailability).
Dopamine Agonists: Bormocriptine, Pergolide, Pramipexole, Ropinirole, Piribedil, Cabergoline, Apomorphine, Lisuride.
MAO Inhibitors: Selegiline, Rasagiline
Add Quetiapine for psychosis.
Add Modafinil for daytime sleepiness.

Poliomyelitis (Polio) **Caused by the poliovirus.** Infection and destruction of the **anterior horn** of the spinal cord (LMN) and the brainstem. Transmission: **Fecal/Oral (fecal contamination of water).** **Method of spread**: Oropharynx (and small intestine) spread via blood (hematogenous) to the CNS. SX: **LMN lesion**: **Fasciculations,** flaccid paralysis, hyporeflexia, muscle pain, atrophy and weakness, hypotonia, fever, headache, nausea DX: CSF shows **viral panel**: ↑ WBC and ↑ Protein, normal glucose. Virus found: stool or throat Vaccines: Live (Sabin) and Killed (Salk) **Trendelenburg gate:** Weakness of abductor muscles: **gluteus medius and gluteus minimus and superior gluteal nerve**. Are not able to abduct the thigh at the hip.	**Friedreich Ataxia** Reduced expression of the **mitochondrial** protein **Frataxin.** **Trinucleotide repeat GAA** on chromosome 9 that encodes the Frataxin gene Degeneration of spinal cord tracts. SX: **Ataxia**, **HCM (Hypertrophic Cardiomyopathy),** kyphoscoliosis, nystagmus, hammer toes, vision and hearing impairment, high plantar arches
Amyotrophic Lateral Sclerosis (ALS) AKA: Lou Gehrig's Disease Death of motor neurons and muscular atrophy. Scarring (sclerosis) of the lateral regions of the spinal cord. **Glutamate** is not reabsorbed by the astrocytes so toxic levels build up in the tissues. Combined **LMN and UMN lesions** (strictly motor defects). Motor: muscle twitching and weakness, difficulty speaking, dysphagia. **No sensory or intellectual defects.** Defect is on Chromosome 21, which codes for **superoxide dismutase**. Mutant SOD1 gene. Degeneration of both corticospinal tracts and atrophy of the ventral roots. SX: Both UMN (hyperreflexia, positive Babinski) and LMN (**Fasciculations**, **flaccid paralysis**, muscle atrophy), tripping/falling, difficulty speaking, swallowing, breathing, death 3 – 5 years from onset. TX: **Riluzole** (↓ presynaptic glutamate release)	**Shy-Drager Syndrome** AKA: Multiple System Atrophy Damage due to cell loss and proliferation of astrocytes in the CNS. This area of damage forms glial scars. SX: Presents similar to Parkinson's dz. (muscle rigidity, tremors, slow movements), autonomic dysfunction (incontinence, ↓ BP, regulation = orthostatic HTN, impotence), poor coordination (ataxia). (triad: Parkinson's SX, erectile dysfunction or incontinence, orthostatic HTN) DX: Abundant glial cytoplasmic inclusions in the CNS. Little improvement with Parkinson's drugs. Progresses faster than Parkinson's with no remission. Average lifespan after onset of symptoms: < 8 years.
Creutzfeldt-Jakob Disease (CJD) AKA: **Spongiform** encephalopathy, BSE, Mad Cow Dz., Prion Dz. Caused by prions (misfolded proteins). Build up of amyloids. Degenerates brain tissue rapidly. Mutation in the gene for **PrP, PRNP**. CSF shows **14-3-3 protein**. Incurable and fatal. SX: Rapidly progressive dementia, **sharp waves on EEG**, personality changes, hallucinations, ataxia, myoclonus (muscle twitches), gait changes, seizures. Transmitted by contaminated brain products.	**Cerebral Palsy** Permanent movement disorders that appear in early childhood. Due to damage occurring to the developing brain. MC: occurs during pregnancy or within the first month of life. Causes: Multifactorial: Intrauterine developmental problems (IUGR, exposure to radiation, infection), **hypoxia of the brain** during labor and delivery, premature babies. SX: Spastic, hyperreflexia, hypotonic, persistence of primitive reflexes, positive Babinski sign, stiff and weak muscles, abnormal muscle tone, difficulty swallowing, joint and bone deformities, speaking, hearing, contractures (tight muscles/joints). Milestones of sitting, crawling and walking are delayed. Difficulty with reasoning, learning disabilities. May also have seizures. TX: Therapy for the specific areas of need, botulinum toxin injections (to ↓ spastic muscles), surgery, orthotics.

Restless Leg Syndrome
Neurological disorder that causes an **irresistible urge** to kick or move one's extremities (MC: legs) to stop or relieve odd or uncomfortable sensations.
Partners of the patient may complain of being kicked during the night. Occurs during any period of relaxation (sleep, study, watching TV, sitting and relaxing).

Potential causes: MC: low iron levels < 50 μg/L. Other causes: caffeine, fibromyalgia, diabetes, thyroid dz, Mg or folate deficiency, varicose veins or valve insufficiency, peripheral neuropathies, Parkinson's.
TX: **Pramipexole** (Dopamine agonists), **Levodopa.**

Hemiballismus
Repetitive, **involuntary flailing, ballistic** movements of the proximal limbs.
AKA: Chorea

Caused by a decrease in the activity of the **subthalamic nucleus** in the basal ganglia. (The subthalamic nucleus stimulates the globus pallidus).

The hemiballismus movements are always on the **contralateral** side of the lesions.

Locations of Brain Lesions/Pathologies

Pathology	Location
Hemiballism Lacunar Strokes	Subthalamic Nuclei
Huntington's	Caudate Nucleus
Parkinson's	Substantia Nigra
Wilsons (Hepatolenticular degeneration)	Lentiform Nucleus (Globus Pallidus and Putamen)
Kluver-Bucy Syndrome	Amygdala

Spinal Cord Lesions

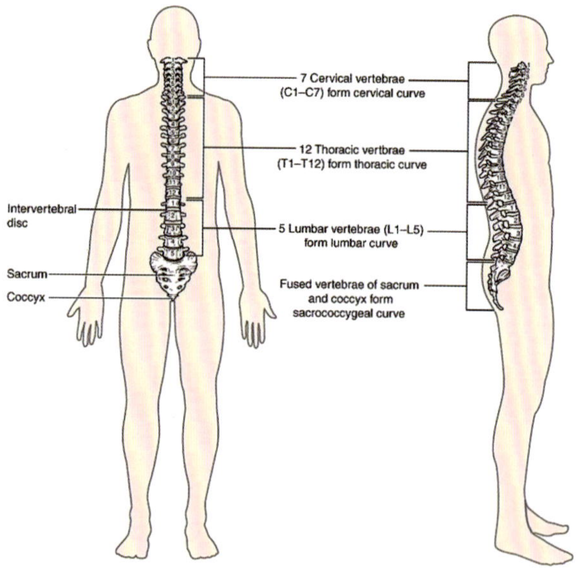

- **Lesions between C1 and C5**
  Upper motor neuron signs present in both upper and lower limbs.
- **Lesions between C6 and T2**
  Upper motor neuron signs present in the lower limbs and lower motor neuron signs are present in the upper limbs.
- **Lesions between T3 and L3**
  Upper motor neuron signs are present in the lower limbs. The upper limbs are normal.
- **Lesions between L4 and S2**
  Lower motor neuron signs are present in the lower limbs. Upper limbs are normal.

Back and Spine Pathologies

Nerve Root Innervation

Nerve Root	Reflex Lost	Motor Deficit	Sensory Deficit
C5	Biceps	Deltoid weakness	Shoulder
C6	Brachioradialis	Biceps, wrist extensors	Lateral arm and thumb
C7	Triceps	3rd finger (middle finger)	3rd finger
C8	5th finger	Hand dysfunction (innervates small muscles to hand	Medial hand
L4	Knee Jerk	Dorsiflexion of foot	Medial calf
L5	None	Dorsiflexion foot and big toe	Dorsal foot
S1	Ankle Jerk	Weakness of gastrocnemius, eversion of foot	Lateral foot

Back/Spine Pathologies

- Diagnostic Test: Imaging is required for: ankylosing spondylitis, epidural abscess, Cauda equine, and cord compressions
- **BIT is plain flat film x-ray** for fractures, infection, cancer with compression
- **MAT is an MRI** unless contradiction to an MRI (ie: pacemaker, metal plates) then use a CT
- **DO NOT do imaging** in patients with low back strain or without focal neurological abnormalities
- **Treatment for back with WITHOUT neurological defects: No bed rest. Stay active.**
    - **Conservative TX for 4 – 6 weeks: Early mobilization (NO bedrest), no exercise program, muscle relaxants and NSAIDS**
    - **SX: Acute onset pain with positive straight leg test = possible herniated disc if no neurological defects**
    - **Rule out cauda equina (perianal area is functional)**
    - **If rapidly progressing neurological defects (foot drop, weak leg, perianal dysfunction) = emergent surgical decompression**

Disk Herniation **AKA: Sciatica**	**Spinal Cord Compression**	**Spinal Epidural Abscess**
Herniation at the **L4/5 and L5/S1**. SX: **Acute pain** radiating down the thigh into the leg and foot. Pain and numbness of medial calf and/or foot. Pain is worse when sitting. DX for disc herniation: **Straight Leg Raise Test** (SLR). Patient lies flat and the leg is raised straight upward to 70°. If pain radiates into the buttocks and **below the knee into the foot** = **positive test**. If patient claims pain radiates in the low back or hamstrings: negative test = patient faking. Imaging: No imaging for low back pain and a positive SLR test unless neurological deficits are present (numbness, weakness, paralysis, bowel or bladder incontinence, erectile dysfunction). TX: **NSAID's**, **Continue ordinary activity**. **NO bed rest**, it will delay healing. Steroid injection into the epidural space if no improvement with conservative mgmt.. **Caution:** If the question says that the pain goes "to the knee", the nerve involved is the femoral, not the sciatic. The sciatic must go to the foot.	**MCC: Cancer** Metastasis from: non-small cell type lung cancers, breast cancer, prostate cancer, renal cell carcinoma, thyroid cancer, lymphoma, multiple myeloma. Medical emergency. DX: MRI SX: **Pain worse at night. Wakes patient up.** Vertebral tenderness, hyperreflexia, ↓ sensation to pin prick/touch, ↑ tendon reflex, positive Babinski. TX: **Glucocorticoid (Dexamethasone)** to ↓ pain and ↓ swelling. Give **radiation** to decrease pain. Give chemotherapy (lymphoma) or radiation for cancers (solid tumors). Surgical decompression if steroids and radiation/chemotherapy are not effective or if neurological symptoms are present. (S3 and S4 issues causes: numbness, weakness, paralysis, bowel or bladder incontinence, erectile dysfunction).	Collection of pus or inflammatory granulation between dura mater and the vertebral column. Causes: **Hematogenous spread** of infection elsewhere in the body (ie: UTI, cellulitis), IV drug use, IC states (Diabetes, HIV, alcoholic), from injections (epidural anesthesia, steroids). SX: Similar to spinal cord compression symptoms. Vertebral tenderness over lumbar spinal area with constant back pain, hyperreflexia, fever, ↓ sensation to pin prick/touch, ↑ tendon reflex, positive Babinski. **Triad: Fever**, focal spine pain, and neurological defects. Can progress to: Motor/sensory defects, bowel/bladder dysfunction, paralysis. Labs: ↑ ESR DX: MRI TX: Surgical drainage for large abscesses. Empiric treatment until cultures return. Empiric TX: **Vancomycin or Linezolid and Gentamicin.** Upon return of culture/sensitivity: Staph sensitive: **Oxacillin, Nafcillin, and Cefazolin.**

Cauda Equina Syndrome (CES) Medical Emergency Loss of function of the lumbar plexus (nerve roots) below the conus medullaris of the spinal cord. **CES is a lower motor neuron lesion**. Involves the **spinal nerve roots**. Involves the lower end of the spine. SX: **Asymmetrical** weakness, radiates pain, Severe back pain, **saddle anesthesia** ("pens and needles"). Involves the **S3 – S5** dermatomes (includes perineum, external genitalia, anus), absent bilateral Achilles (ankle) reflex, bladder and bowel dysfunction/incontinence, affects the anus/bladder sphincters. **Hyporeflexia.** TX: Emergency surgical decompression.	**Lumbar Spinal Stenosis** MC: Persons over 60. Degenerative change. **SX**: Back pain that radiates bilaterally into the buttocks and thighs when walking. **Pain is worse when walking downhill** (upon extension), pain continues when standing. Pain is **better walking uphill, sitting, cycling and leaning forward** (upon flexion). (can present similar to peripheral artery disease). (Presents similar to PAD but in PAD there are poor pulses and pain is better when standing). Spinal stenosis can simulate peripheral arterial disease., but ankle/brachial index is normal. DX: MRI. Pulses are normal. TX: Weight loss, NSAID's, steroid injections into lumbar epidural space if standard pain medications do not control the pain. Physical therapy. Surgical decompression to dilate the spinal canal.	**Ankylosing Spondylitis** Chronic Inflammatory disease of **sacroiliac joints** (axial skeleton) in the pelvis and spine. **Fusion** of joints in spine. Onset between < 40 years of age. SX: **Stiff in the mornings or with rest** and **improves throughout the day with activity**, **uveitis** (inflammation in anterior chamber of the eye, redness and floaters), inflammation of the prostate and aorta, **aortic valve insufficiency**. Pain is worse at night. Leaning forward relieves pain. Peripheral arthritis of the hips, shoulders, knees. Complications: **Kyphosis** (Flattening of the normal lumbar curvature), ↓ chest expansion, disorder of tendon attachment of the Achilles tendon, AV block. DX: BIT: Flat film XR of **sacroiliac joint** in the pelvis. MAT: MRI is more sensitive than flat film. MRI detects abnormalities years before x-rays. XR shows "bamboo spine" (fused vertebral joints) Associated with **HLA-B27** Negative for RF. Labs: **↑ CRP and ESR** TX: Best: Exercise and **NSAIDS.** **Can also use: Infliximab, Sulfasalazine.** **Do not use Steroids – they do not work.**
Anterior Spinal Artery Infarction All sensation lost. Position and vibratory senses preserved. No TX	**Brown-Sequard Syndrome** MC: Knife wound injury to the spine.. SX: Loss of ipsilateral vibratory and position senses and loss of contralateral pain and temperature.	**Conus Medullaris** **UMN and LMN lesion.** **SX: Symmetrical** weakness. Involves **L1 and L2**. Involves the higher end of the spine. **Hyperreflexia**
Vertebral Osteomyelitis AKA: Spinal osteomyelitis) Infection and inflammation of the bone and bone marrow. Occurs: IV drug use, Sickle Cell, Immunocompromised, S. aureus, or distant infections that spread (ie: UTI, cellulitis). SX: Pain and tenderness over vertebra. Pain is not relieved with rest. Fever, swelling at the infection site, night sweats, difficulty moving from a standing to a sitting position, muscle spasms. DX: MRI, ↑ ESR, ↑ WBC TX: IV antibiotics, surgery (depends upon the severity).	**Lumbo-sacral pain** Pain after physical exertion (lifting). SX: No radiation, No weakness, No sensory changes, No neurological defects. Local tenderness to the paraspinal muscles. DX: Normal leg raise test. TX: NSAID's continued activity, Do NOT advise bed rest.	**Compression Fracture** **Pathologic fracture** MC: **Osteoporosis**, Ankylosing spondylitis, multiple myeloma, Osteomalacia. Things that predispose to this condition: Post menopause, senile osteoarthritis, and steroid use. Caused by demineralization (↓ bone density). Microarchitecture is disrupted. SX: Acute intense pain in vertebra, spine tenderness. Pain does NOT stop when lying down or resting, ↑ pain on strain or cough. **NOTE:** There will be ↓ ankle reflexes in the elderly but this IS **NORMAL AGING.** **NOTE:** If pain is due to a ligamentous sprain, the pain will ↑ with movement but get better with rest.

Spondylolisthesis	Back Pain Recommendations
Forward displacement/slip of a vertebra. MC: L5 slips to S1 ("Step off") between 6 and 16 years old. Can also be due to degenerative DZ due to joint arthritis and ligamentum flavum weakness. SX: Constant back pain, general stiffening of the back, tightened hamstrings, change in gait, atrophy of the gluteal muscles, paresthesias, neurological dysfunction (ie: bed wetting).	• When lifting: Keep back straight and bend knees • Regular exercise (strength support for the back and abdominal muscles) • Good sleeping position, do not sleep on stomach • Warm up before activities/sports • Avoid exercise with repetitive twist and bending

Epilepsy/Seizures

- Seizure disorder: ≥2 unprovoked seizures occur > 24 hours apart.
- ↑ Risk: Family history, initial seizure before 9 months old, preexisting neurological disorder, atypical seizures, abnormal development.
- Anti-seizure medications are often assocated with bone loss and osteoporosis.
- Causes of seizures: medication/drug side effects, renal failure, liver failure, brain tumors, brain abscesses/infections, meningitis, trauma, alcohol withdrawal, drug abuse, epilepsy, hypoglycemia, stroke, brain injury/congenital brain defect, electrolyte imbalance (abnormal potassium levels do not causes seizures, they cause heart arrhythmias), choking, electric shock, fever, very high blood pressure, family history.
- Symptoms: blackouts, loss of consciousness, confusion, muscle spasms, drooling, falling, sudden/rapid eye movements, making unusual noises (grunting), sudden mood changes, loss of bladder or bowel control, clenching of the teeth, feeling of fear or anxiousness, nausea, dizziness, vision changes, strange taste in the mouth
- DX: BIT: Head CT, Check electrolyte levels, urine toxicology, renal function, liver function
  If all BIT test are normal then do an EEG (Electroencephalogram)
- TX: If this is the first seizure, antiepileptic medicine is not required unless:
  Abnormal EEG, status epilepticus, family history of seizures, causes that are not treatable (ie: tumor in the brain).
  Medicines may be discontinued after 2 years with no seizures.
- **Posterior shoulder dislocation: MC dislocation due to seizures.**
- **Driving and Seizures:** A physician can never make the decision to take away a driver's license or to keep someone from driving regarding a seizure. But as long as the patient is well controlled on their medications (no seizures) they are able to drive.

Partial Seizure – Simple	Partial Seizure – Complex
• **No loss of conscience** • Has memory of seizure • EEG Findings: **"Spike and Sharp" waves**, multifocal spikes. • SX: Jerking, stiffening of part of the body. Weakness, speech can be affected. Can have an aura (smell or taste things), hear ringing, illusions or hallucinations, changes in heart rate, sweating. • 1st line: **Carbamazepine.** 2nd line: **Valproic acid**, **Phyenytoin**	• **Loss of conscience or "out of touch/unaware"**, automations such as: biting, **lip-smacking, chewing, hand wringing**, fidgeting, picking, biting (mouth injuries), urination, moving their mouth, pick at the air or their clothing, or perform other purposeless actions. Person can wander, lose bladder control, have an aura (warning) prior to seizure (smell, sound or taste), feeling of anxiety. Very lethargic after the seizure. • Does not have any memory of seizure • Last 30 seconds to 2 minutes • EEG Findings: **Sharp waves, focal spikes** in anterior temporal lobe. • 1st line: **Valproic Acid, Phenytoin**

Tonic-Clonic Seizures (Formerly known as Grand Mal Seizures) • Generalized seizure that affects both hemispheres of the brain. • MC associated with epilepsy. • These seizures are what is produced in ECT therapy • Tonic phase: loss of consciousness and skeletal muscles becoming rigid. • Clonic phase: Convulsions, cyanosis in the lips or extremities, incontinence. • Seizure is followed (postictal) by confusion, drowsiness, headache, nausea, disorientation.	**Absence Seizures** (AKA: Petit-Mal) • Resembles "day dreaming". Person **stares into space** < 10 seconds, lapses of awareness. Begins and ends abruptly. • MC in children 4 – 14 • EEG Findings: "**3 second spike**" • 1st line: **Ethosuximide**. 2nd line: **Valproic Acid.**
Status Epilepticus • When a seizure lasts **too long** (> 5minutes) or too close together and patient **doesn't recover** between the seizures, patient is having repeated seizures for 30 minutes or longer, if patient goes into a 2nd seizure without recovering consciousness from the 1st seizure. • Medical emergency • 1st line: **Benzodiazepine** (**Diazepam, Lorazepam**). (**tip**: to drive a "Benz" is status) 2nd line **Phenytoin.** **If seizures continue add Fosphenytoin.** **If seizures still continue add Phenobarbital.** **If seizures still continue must put under anesthesia**	**Myoclonic Seizure** • Jerking or twitching of a muscle, hiccups • Person is awake, no altered mental status • EEG Findings: **Irregular "spike and wave"** pattern • 1st Line: **Valproic Acid.** 2nd line: **Lamotrigine**
Infantile Spasms (West Syndrome) • **Infant seizures during first 12 months** • **Clusters of spasms lasting for minutes with brief intervals in between each spasm.** • **MC: Downs Syndrome, others: underlying CNS disorder.** • **EEG Findings: High voltage, slow waves. Irregular spokes and sharp waves.** **1st line: ACTH, prednisone, B6 (Pyridoxine), Vigabatrin**	**Unprovoked Seizure Management** If all other test are negative: Labs, EKG, UA, cervical spine image then: Must do a CT without contract to look for bleeds and any head injury obtained in a fall. If the CT is negative: then perform an EEG
Febrile Seizures • Seizure caused by a high fever. • MC in children 3 months to 6 years. • Risk increased with family history of febrile seizures. • Children that have their first febrile seizure before their first birthday, half will have at least one more. • Cannot be prevented by cool clothes, acetaminophen, ibuprofen, lukewarm baths. • Seizure should not last more than 5 minutes, if so go to ED/911 TX: Self limiting, reassure family	

Seizures verses Syncope

Situation	**Seizure**	**Syncope**
Causes	Sleep loss, emotions, alcohol withdrawal, flashing lights	Emotions, vasovagal response, heat, crowds, standing still in one spot
Symptoms	Aura, hallucinations, chewing, twitching, biting the tongue, rapid/strong pulse, unusual body position, Can occur when sleeping or sitting	Light headedness, unlikely to occur in sleep or when sitting unless cardiac causes, pallor, sweating, nausea, weak/slow pulse, seldom any shaking
Post Symptoms	Delay in returning to baseline, sleepy, confused, lethargic, disoriented	Immediate spontaneous return to baseline.

Cerebral Blood Supply

Circle of Willis

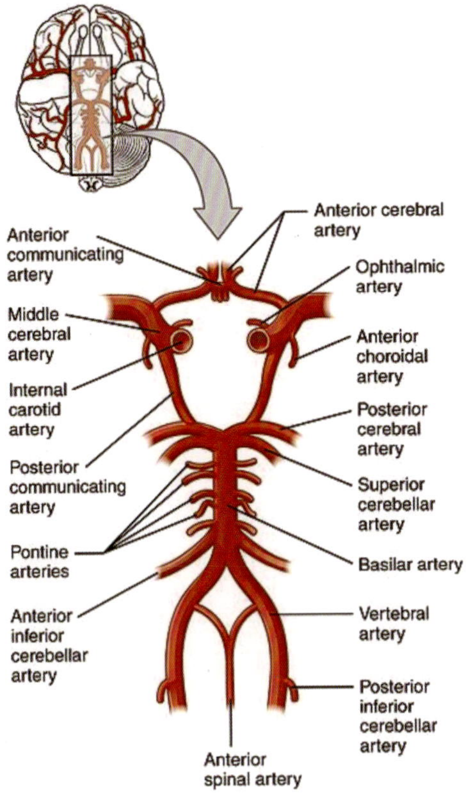

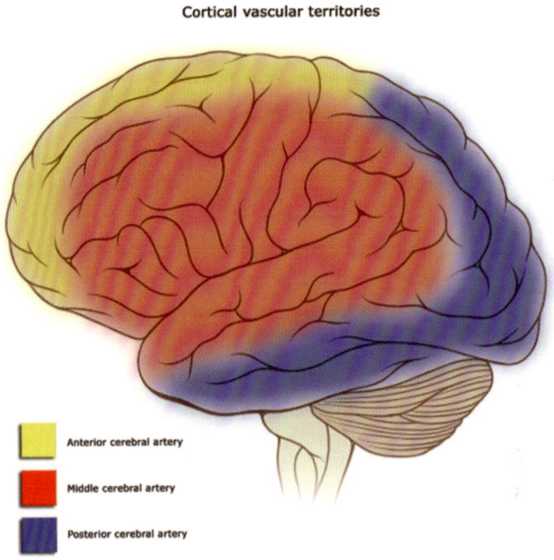

Cerebral Perfusion Control

- **Regulated by PCO2**
- ↑ CO2 (hypoventilation = ANYTHING that decreases oxygen that causes hypoxia: **COPD**
- ↑ CO2 **vasodilates vessels** in the brain (surrounded by skull that does not give) = ↑ ICP
- ↑ ICP = papilledema, headaches
  (First sign of carbon dioxide poisoning = headaches)
- Hyperventilation = ↓ CO2 therefore ↓ ICP by vasoconstriction
- TX: **Mannitol**

Strokes

- Irreversible damage begins after **5 minutes** of hypoxia
- **First area to show damage: hippocampus**
- Stroke Imaging:
  Dark image with no contrast = ischemic stroke
  Bright image with no contrast = hemorrhagic stroke (**do NOT give TPA**)
- DX: MRI/MRA for the brainstem
- Evaluation for all strokes:
  ECHO for source of clots (A-Fib: TX: Warfarin, Endocarditis or Myxoma : TX: surgery)
  Carotid Doppler/Duplex (TX: Endarterectomy for > 70% stenosis, but not 100%)
  Holter monitor if EKG is normal.
- **Hemorrhagic strokes**: Intra-cerebral bleeding
  MC Sites: Basal ganglia
  MCC: HTN, anticoagulation, cancer
- **Symptoms last ≥ 24 hours (TIA's last < 24 hours)**
- **Permanent neurologic deficits**
- Strokes do not affect the forehead (no loss of wrinkles) only the bottom half of the face, whereas Bells Palsy affects the entire unilateral/bilateral side of the face (bottom part of face and forehead).
- **Ischemic stroke: Disruption of blood flow leads to ischemia and liquefactive necrosis. Caused by emboli or from a thrombosis.**
  Embolic stroke: embolus from another part of the body: Either cardiac or carotid artery. Emboli present with more sudden symptoms.
  Thrombotic stroke: Due to atherosclerotic plaque (MC: MCA)
  Hypoxic: Due to hypoperfusion or hypoxemia = affects watershed areas (MCA – ACA)
- TIA (Transient Ischemic Attack): See below.
- Younger patients < 50 years: etiology of a stroke is more commonly due to a hypercoagulable state, vasculitis, Diabetes, or HTN: Check for DX: VDRL/RPR, Protein C and Protein S deficiency, Factor V Leiden mutation, Antiphospholipid syndrome, ANA, Double-stranded DNA, ESR rate
- **Treatment of Ischemic strokes:**
  Must be < 4 hours of onset of stroke and **must RULE OUT a hemorrhagic stroke before thrombolytics by doing a CT without contrast of the head first**.
  < 4 hours = give **TPA's** as long as there are **NO** other contraindications for TPA's (see contradictions below)
- Hemiparesis = weak one side
- Hemiplegia = paralysis one side

Contraindications for Thrombolytics

- Previous stroke within past 1 year
- History of a hemorrhagic stroke
- Brain surgery or trauma within past 6 months
- Chest compressions (CPR) within past 3 weeks
- Hypertensive urgency
- Active bleeding
- Major surgery within past 6 weeks
- Presence of intracranial mass/neoplasm
- Any bleeding disorder
- Concern of an aortic dissection
- Patient on anticoagulation
- Bleeding ulcer
- TIA

Diagnostic Test for Strokes

- Head CT, no contrast: Most sensitive for blood. It will take > 3 days to identify a nonhemorrhagic stroke.
- MRI: Most sensitive for nonhemorrhagic stroke (within 24 hours).
- Magnetic Resonance Angiogram (MRA) Most accurate for brain stem images.

Transient Ischemic Attacks (TIA)

- Present same as strokes, but neurologic dysfunction returns back to normal **within 24 hours** (Strokes last > 24 hours).
- Symptoms resolve completely.
- Can present with **Amaurosis fugax** (transient loss of vision in one eye) due to emboli in the ophthalmic artery.
- TIA's are caused by thrombosis or emboli, never hemorrhage.
- Do not give thrombolytics for TIA's.

Stroke and TIA Treatments

- Echocardiogram (evaluate heart pathologies that would throw emboli).
- Carotid Doppler/Duplex to evaluate for atherosclerosis emboli (Endarterectomy for > 70% and < 100% stenosis).
- Head CT to determine if stroke was hemorrhagic and MRI to determine if stroke was ischemic
- EKG (to check for arrhythmias). If **A-Fib**: TX: **Warfarin, Rivaroxaban or Dabigatran**
- Holter monitor if EKG is normal.
- In young patients without history of HTN or diabetes: Test for clotting disorders: Factor V Leiden, Protein C and S Deficiency, Antiphospholipid syndrome.
- **No thrombolytics for TIA's**
- **Thrombolytics** only for strokes if < 4 hours from onset as long as there are no contraindications for administering thrombolytics.
- Paradoxical emboli's due to a patent foramen ovale: closure of ovale.
- Note: In the case of A-fib, clots or endocarditis: add **Warfarin**
- If patient has a history of diabetes, HTN or hyperlipidemia: Must control levels:
  Diabetes: < 100
  HTN: < 130/80
  Hyperlipidemia: LDL < 100
- Anti-platelet medicines (**aspirin or clopidogrel**)
- **Statin's** for nonhemorrhagic strokes.

Brain Infarct Repair Timeline

Timeline	Cell Reaction	Description
12 – 48 hours	**Red Nuclei (red neuron)**	Eosinophilic cytoplasm, pyknotic nuclei, **loss Nissl substance**
24 – 72 hours	Neutrophil infiltration	Necrosis
3 – 5 days	Macrophage **(Microglia)** infiltration	Phagocytosis by microglia
1 – 2 weeks	**Astrocytes "Reactive gliosis"**	Vascular proliferation, **liquefactive necrosis**
> 2 weeks	**Astrocytes "Glial Scar"**	Cystic area surrounded by **gliosis, astrocytes proliferate forming Glial scar**

Strokes and Bleeds

Artery	Location	Symptoms
ACA Anterior Cerebral Artery	Motor and Sensory Cortex affects **lower limbs**	CONTRA Paralysis and loss of sensation of **lower limb**, urinary incontinence, personality changes
MCA Middle Cerebral Artery	Motor and Sensory Cortex of upper limb and face. Temporal lobe (Wernicke area) Frontal Lobe (Broca area)	CONTRA Paralysis and loss of sensation of **upper limb and face.** Aphasia if dominant side affected (left). Left sided "neglect syndrome" if non-dominant side affected (right). Eyes deviate to the side of the lesion (ipsilateral)
Lenticulostriate (AKA: **Lacunar Stroke/Infarct**)	Basal Ganglia, Striatum, Internal Capsule **Purely Motor Stroke** **Lenticulostriate arteries** arise from MCA	CONTRA Hemiparesis/hemiplegia, ataxia, Parkinsonian signs MCC: **uncontrolled HTN, Diabetes**
ASA Anterior Spinal Artery	Lateral Corticospinal tract Medial lemniscus. Caudal medulla (hypoglossal nerve) **CN 12** STROKE: Medial Medullary Syndrome	CONTRA Hemiparesis of upper and lower limbs, 🡻 proprioception. IPSI **Hypoglossal** dysfunction (**tongue deviates** IPSI)

PICA Posterior Inferior Cerebellar Artery	Lateral medulla, lateral Spinothalamic, Inferior cerebellar peduncle **CN IX, X** **Lateral Medullary Syndrome (AKA: Wallenberg Syndrome)**	IPSI: Face = **Horner's** (Horner's is always IPSI) **CONTRA**: Body = dysphagia, **hoarseness,** ↓ gag reflex Ataxia, dysmetria, vomiting, vertigo, nystagmus.
AICA Anterior Inferior Cerebellar Artery	Lateral pons. Middle and inferior cerebellar peduncles **CN VII** **Lateral pontine syndrome**	IPSI: Face = Horner's Paralysis of face, ↓ **taste** (2/3 tongue), ↓ lacrimation/salivation, ↓ pain and temp face Ataxia, dysmetria (coordination of movement: over or undershoot of intended position), vomiting, vertigo, nystagmus
PCA Posterior Cerebral Artery	Occipital cortex = visual	CONTRA Hemianopia with **macular sparing,** Prosopagnosia (inability to recognize faces)
Basal Artery	Pons, medulla, lower midbrain, corticospinal, corticobulbar, pontine reticular formation	"Locked in Syndrome" Preserved consciousness, blinking. Quadriplegia, loss of movements: facial, mouth.

VBI Vertebrobasilar Artery	Posterior circulation of the brain: supplies: medulla, cerebellum pons, midbrain, thalamus, occipital cortex (vision) (Note: Anterior circulation of the brain involves the Carotid arteries).	Vertigo, Vertical nystagmus, ataxia, dysarthria, dystonia, nausea, vomiting, diplopia. Patient may complain of feeling like their knees are buckling due3 to weakened quadriceps (AKA: drop attack).
Anterior Communicating	MC Saccular aneurysm (AKA: Berry, AKA: **Sub-arachnoid**) - NOT a stroke	Visual defects
Posterior Communicating	Saccular aneurysm (AKA: Berry, AKA: **Sub-arachnoid**) - NOT a stroke	**CN III Palsy (Down and Out, ptosis, pupil dilation) (aka: Oculomotor Nerve Palsy)**
Opthalmic Artery		**Amaurosis fugax**

Moyamoya Syndrome	**Stenosis/obstruction (clots) of arteries in the brain**. MC: Internal carotid, MCA and ACA. Collateral circulation develops but **leaks blood** due to increased pressure causing a "puff of smoke" (Japanese for moyamoya) appearance on angiography. Congenital (chromosome 17) or can be acquired. ↑ risk in Downs Syndrome, NF 1, and head trauma. SX: TIA's, strokes, numbness/paralysis of extremities), convulsions, migraine-like headaches.	**Not** due to atherosclerosis (damage to walls of arteries). This is due to the inner layer of the carotid proliferating into the lumen. The blood clots inside the artery can cause strokes.
Thalamus	**Purely Sensory Stroke**	
Cranial Nerve Lesions	To determine where lesion is located if all lesions in question pertain **ONLY** to cranial nerve deficits (no spinal tracts), look at each lesion description and identify the highest cranial nerve that is responsible for that lesion and that is the CN that is the lesion. (Example: Patient can't smell (CN II), they can't feel their face (CN VII) and they can't move their tongue (CN XII) = the lesion is at CN XII)	

Stroke Lesions

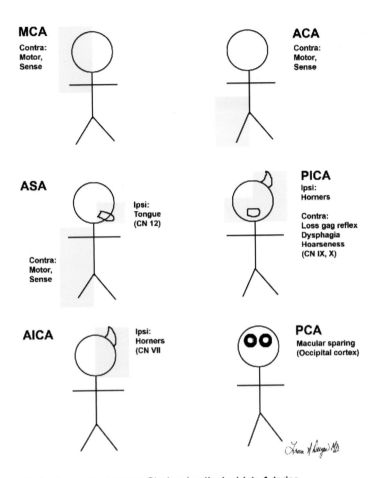

Motor loss only: Lacunar Stroke: Lenticulostriate Arteries
Sensory loss only: Thalamus

Elevated Intracranial Pressure

- Goal of treatment is to maintain brain perfusion (not ↓ ICP)
- Emergency
- SX: headaches, unequal pupil sizes, ↓ response to light
- Beware of signs of end organ damage: papilledema
- TX: Elevate head, no fluid overload, hyperventilation, hypothermia lowers oxygen demand, sedation lowers oxygen demand
- Mannitol, Furosemide
- Caution: Must get a head CT before performing a lumbar puncture to rule out ICP. If there is ICP and an LP is performed it may cause the brain to herniate

Head Trauma and Intracranial Hemorrhage

- All head trauma causing altered mental status or loss of consciousness requires a head CT without contrast.
- Do not use skull X-rays for head trauma.

Injury	Location	Symptoms
Epidural Hematoma	**Rupture Middle Meningeal artery, which** is a branch off of the **maxillary artery**, which is off of the **external carotid**. 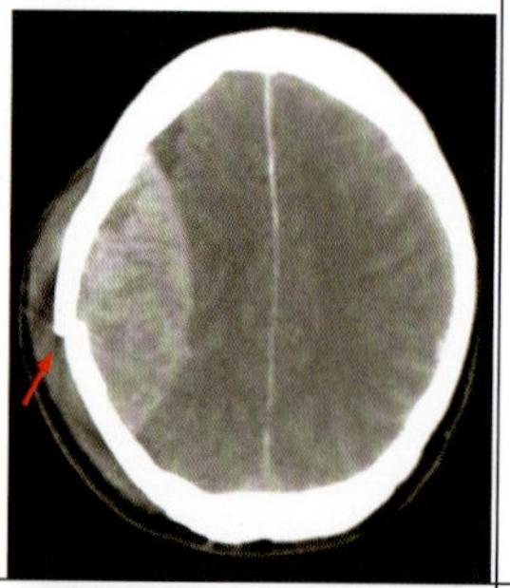	Due to skull **fracture of temporal bone (trauma),** can have **"Lucid" intervals** (2nd loss of consciousness following the 1st LOC within minutes to hours), **sudden loss of consciousness, CN III Palsy.** **CT: shows biconvex** (lentiform) Does not cross suture lines TX: Emergency craniotomy Note: Lucid interval is considered the time between the 1st LOC and 2nd LOC.
Subdural Hematoma	**Rupture of bridging veins.** MC Chronic: Older people. Brain atrophy causes **bridging veins** to stretch and break (esp. with falls) (AKA: Vessel fragility) (**tip**: "Sub" dural is shaped like a "sub"marine) 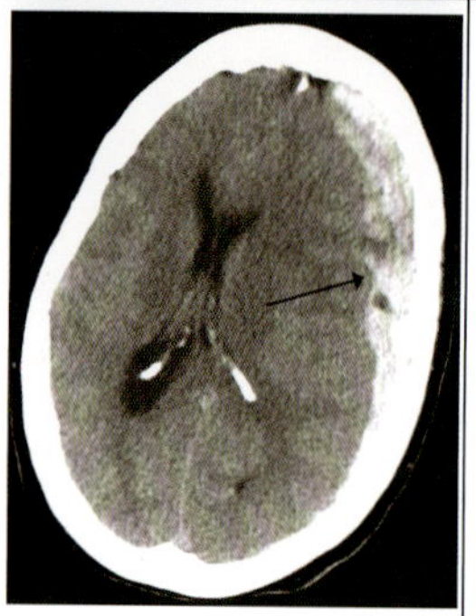 Acute: trauma, shaken baby, alcoholics	Acute: due to head trauma and fluctuating consciousness. Chronic: Venous bleeding that **develops over time**. Can cross suture lines. **Can also have "Lucid" intervals** (2nd loss of consciousness following the 1st LOC within minutes to hours**).** DX: CT
Subarachnoid Hemorrhage	MC sites: **Anterior Communicating Artery**, Anterior Cerebral, **Posterior Communicating Artery** 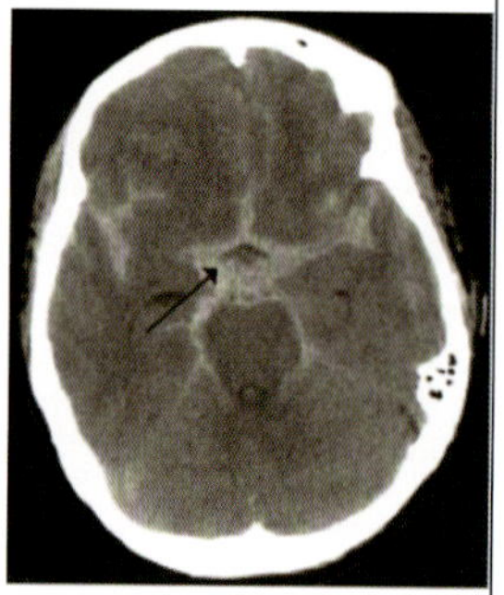 Risk: ADPKD, Marfan's, HTN, smoking, sudden $\uparrow$ BP, Ehlers-Danlos, smoking, African Americans, hyperlipidemia.	**Sudden, severe headache**. Bi-temporal hemianopia via compression of optic nerve. Photophobia, stiff neck, can also have loss of consciousness. DX: **RBC and xanthochromia** (yellow spinal tap due to discoloration from breakdown of RBC's) in CSF and increased WBC count but the ration of WBC to RBC will be **NORMAL.** Note: In meningitis the WBC will still be increased but the ratio of WBC to RBC will be increased, **not normal.** **NORMAL** CSF WBC to RBC Ratio: 1 WBC for every 500 to 1000 RBC. Complications: Rebleed in 24 hours. 3 – 10 days **vasospasm** = TX: **Nimodipine**
Cerebral Contusion (Bruising)	Bruising of the brain tissue due to a blow to the head. Head CT shows ecchymosis due to small vessels bleeding in to the brain. 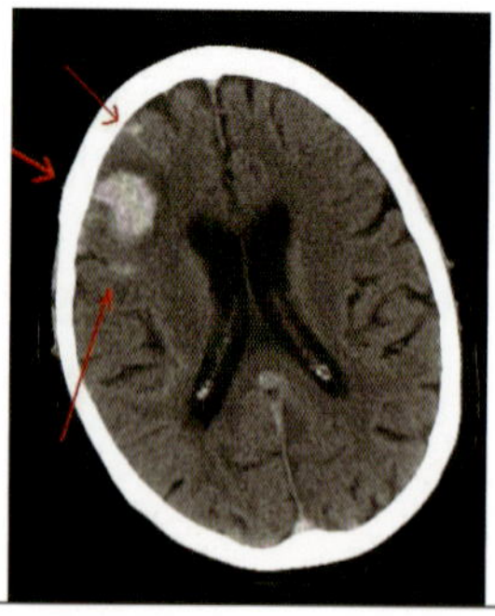	Depends upon the location in the brain and the severity of the bleed: Headache, difficulty focusing attention, edema, confusion, dizziness, sleepiness, loss of consciousness, nausea and vomiting, seizures, loss of coordination, difficulty in memory, speech, hearing, vision. Injury can cause a decline in mental function in the long term. Acutely can cause brain herniation due to $\uparrow$ ICP. TX: $\downarrow$ swelling of the brain. Observe in the hospital to monitor for any signs of ICP.

Concussion (AKA: MTBI: Mild Traumatic Brain Injury)	MC type of traumatic brain injury (TBI). Head injury with temporary loss of brain function. MCC sports injuries, bicycle and car accidents, falls, nearby explosions, acceleration forces without a direct impact. The brain is shaken hard enough to bounce against the skull. No focal defects. Normal head CT	Must exclude neck injuries and skull fractures. Physical and cognitive rest, light activity, non-contact sports, no drug or alcohol use, close follow up. Must wait 24 hours before returning to activities. TX: Observe at home for new symptoms, lucid intervals.
Diffuse Axonal Injury	Acceleration-deceleration injuries to the head. SX: unconsciousness	MC: Automobile accidents
Brain Abscesses	Collection of infected material in the brain that come from local or remote infections (contiguous infection from: dental abscesses, sinus, ear or mastoid infections), head trauma, skull fractures, surgical procedures, HIV infections.	Cause ↑ intracranial pressure because they are space-occupying lesions. Symptoms: headaches, nausea, confusion, seizures, coma. DX: CT with contrast shows a ring-enhancing lesion. MAT: Brain biopsy (the only way to distinguish an abscess from cancer). TX: IV antibiotics.

Skull Fractures and Affected Arteries

Artery	Fracture Location
Maxillary Artery (gives off the Middle Meningeal Artery)	Where the frontal, temporal and parietal lob meet
Occipital Artery	Posterior scalp
Opthalmic	Eyes and nose
MCA off of the Internal Carotid	Parietal and Temporal lobes. Subarachnoid and intracranial hemorrhage
Facial Artery off of the External Carotid	Mouth and cheeks

Spinal Tracts General Concepts

- Tracts: bundle of nerves in the CNS
- **Dorsal (posterior) = sensory**
  Dorsal root ramus: Skin on the back and dorsal neck and deep intrinsic back
- **Ventral (anterior) = motor**
  Skin on the anterolateral trunk, limbs and skeletal muscle of the anterolateral trunk and limbs
- Dorsal root ganglia: location of ALL cell bodies of primary sensory neurons.
  Dorsal root ganglia are of Neural Crest origin.
  Dorsal root is outside of the spinal cord
- Spinal nerves: Peripheral nerves that carry sensory info and motor commands out of the spinal cord.
  31 pairs spinal nerves made of roots.
  Contained mixture of dorsal and ventral roots.
  Cervical nerves exit above the vertebra.
  Cervical nerves: C1 – C8, Thoracic nerves: T1 – T12, Lumbar nerves: L1 – L5, Sacral nerves S1 – S5, Coccygeal nerve.
- Spinal nerves: ALL spinal nerves have LMN on the same side of the spinal cord as the muscle innervated.
  (EX: Right radial nerve leaves the ventral horn on the right side)
- Somatic Nerves: Part of the peripheral nervous system that controls all voluntary muscle systems in the body and controls the involuntary **reflex arcs**.
- Reflex arc: Reflex actions that are activated by spinal motor neurons so the reflex can happen immediately without having to send the message all the way to the brain (ie: patellar reflex: knee jerk)
- Cauda equine: roots of: lumbar, sacral, coccygeal spinal nerves
- White matter in the spinal cord: contain tracts of axons (AKA: fasciculi)
  Surrounds great matter
- Grey matter in the spinal cord: contains the dorsal, ventral nerve and Lateral (Intermediate zone: preganglionic sympathetic nerves located between T1 – L2, S2 – S4
- Voluntary skeletal contraction: UMN → LMN (Brodmann 4 and 6)
- Axon is what goes out to the muscle (runs in a nerve)
- Decussation: Spinal tracts cross over (in spinal cord or medulla) to the other side of the body (contra)

Upper Motor Neurons (UMN)	Lower Motor Neurons (LMN)
UMN: Cell body is in the motor cortex in the precentral gyrus of the cerebral hemisphere of the brain. UMN: Is inhibitory of the Muscle Stretch Reflex. UMN= Contra to LMN (opposite side of the body) UMN are in tracts	LMN: Cell body is in the α-neuron in the ventral horn. Its axon goes out to the spinal nerve directly to the muscle. LMN: are not in tracts, they extent out of the spinal cord to innervate the muscle.
UMN Signs **+ Babinski** (toes go up and fan out when sole stroked) **Spastic paralysis** Clasp Knife spasticity Increased reflexes Increased tone	**LMN Signs** **Fasciculations** Atrophy **Flaccid paralysis** Decreased tone Decreased reflexes

Spinal Tracts

Ascending Tracts – ALL SENSORY TRACTS (ends in Sensory Cortex)

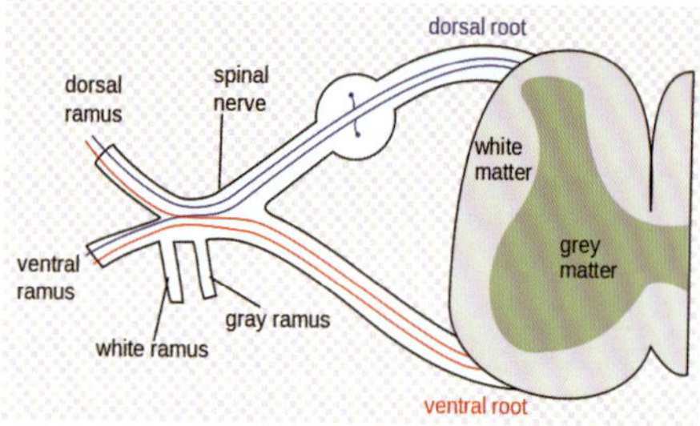

- Dorsal Columns (**Medial Lemniscus**, Posterior Column): Vibration, proprioception, pressure, fine touch.
  - Fasciculus **gracilis**: Relays information from the legs and lower thorax (T7 and below).
    (tip: Gracilis = Gastrocnemius).
  - Fasciculus **cuneatus**: Relays information from the upper thorax (C2 – T6) and the arms. It is lateral to the Fasciculus gracilis.
  - **NOTE:** Syphilis (Tabes dorsalis: demyelination of the dorsal columns).
    NOTE: Vitamin B12 deficiency (Subacute Combined Degeneration SCD) causes demyelination of the dorsal columns.

  Vitamin B12 vs Vitamin E
  NOTE: Deficiency of Vitamin E can sound **exactly** like a deficiency of Vitamin B12. Both can show ataxic gait and other neuro symptoms.
  If the question stem wants B12, it will have to associate it with one or more of: MCV >100, hypersegmented neutrophils, homocysteine, methionine, methylmalonic acid, macrocytic or macrocytosis anemia.
  If the question stem wants Vitamin E, it will have to associate it with one or more of: Malabsorption (Vitamin E is a fat soluble vitamin: so ANY pathology that involves malabsorption of Vitamin E: Cystic fibrosis (due to decrease in pancreatic hormones), antioxidant (protects RBC from hemolysis and oxidative stress), hemolytic anemia, (destruction of RBC's), or fatty stools. Vitamin E can be used in the treatment of abetalipoproteinemia (helps restore and produce lipoproteins), atherosclerosis (inhibits the oxidation of LDL) and some cancers.

- Spinothalamic tract: Pain and Temperature = Lateral. Crude touch and pressure = Anterior.
  (**tip**: spino**T**halamic = **T**emp)

- Spinocerebellar Tract: limb and joint position (proprioception).
  Always IPSI.
  The Golgi tendon organs and muscle spindle fibers obtain proprioceptive information.

  Golgi Tendon Organs: Senses changes in muscle tension. It is a proprioceptive sensory receptor located at the origins and insertions of skeletal muscles fibers into the tendons of skeletal muscles.
  Function: Monitors the stretch (force) being exerted by muscles. This feedback generates spinal reflexes that control muscle contraction.

  Muscle Spindle Fibers: Sensory receptors within a skeletal muscle that detect change in the length of the muscle.

Descending Tract – MOTOR TRACT (starts in Motor Cortex)

- Corticospinal tract: Voluntary movement of contralateral limbs
  (**tip**: corti**GO**spinal)

Spinal Tracts: Neurons and Synapses

Tract	1st Order Neuron	1st Synapse	2nd Order Neuron	2nd Synapse	3rd Order Neuron
ASCENDING SENSORY					
Dorsal Column **At T6 and below it uses the gracilis. Above T6 uses the cuneatus.**	**Dorsal Root Ganglion** outside the spine. Then enters Spine	Ascends IPSI side up the spinal cord. **Fasciculus gracilis** (legs) **and Fasciculus cuneatus** (arms)	Medulla (Medullary pyramids) **Decussates in Medulla and axons now become "medial lemniscus" and goes to the VPL.**	VPL Thalamus Thalamus sends to Sensory Cortex	Sensory Cortex
Spinothalamic	**Dorsal Root Ganglion** outside the spine. Then enters Spine. **Pain and Temp Type II Fibers:** **A delta (δ) fibers** = sharp pain and cold. Fast fiber. Afferent. (**tip**: 2 legs makes you fast) **Type I Fibers:** **C Fibers** = dull, aching pain and warmth. Slow Fibers. Unmyelinated.	IPSI grey matter of spinal cord	Decussates in the **Ventral White Commissure** (white Matter) in the spinal cord (Lumbar region) and then ascends IPSI to VPL. **In the Spinal Cord:** Dorsal ganglion is located 2 levels up from the site of the lesion. Lesion is always on contra Side. Therefore, the lesion will always be 2 levels down from the Dorsal root ganglion and on the contra side. (**Example**: Lesion is at T4 on the right. The Dorsal root ganglion will be located at T2 on the left side. If the Dorsal root ganglion is located at C5 on the left side, the lesion will be located at C7 on the right side) **Lissauer's Tract:** Is the "tract" the nerves take in this "journey" of going up or down between the lesion and dorsal root ganglion.	VPL Thalamus Thalamus sends to Sensory Cortex	Sensory Cortex
Spinocerebellar – Dorsal (posterior) tract	Dorsal Root Ganglion Muscle spindle, Golgi tendon organs	Clarke's nucleus (Between T1 – L3)	Dorsal horn, Ascend IPSI to the cerebellum via inferior cerebellar peduncle on mossy fibers		Cerebellum
Spinocerebellar – Anterior tract	Dorsal Root Ganglion Golgi tendon organs	Clarke's Nucleus (Between T1 – L3)	Dorsal horn, Ascend IPSI to the cerebellum via inferior cerebellar peduncle on mossy fibers		Cerebellum

DESCENDING MOTOR					
Corticospinal	Is **UMN at this point** until it leaves the spinal cord to an extremity. Motor Cortex then descends IPSI to the Medulla and decussates (Medullary pyramidal decussation) and then descends Contra.	Ventral horn of the spinal cord (AKA: Anterior)	Is the point it leaves the spinal cord and goes out to the extremity/muscle. **At this point it is now a LMN.**	NMJ Nicotinic Receptor, ACh	

Spinal Tracts

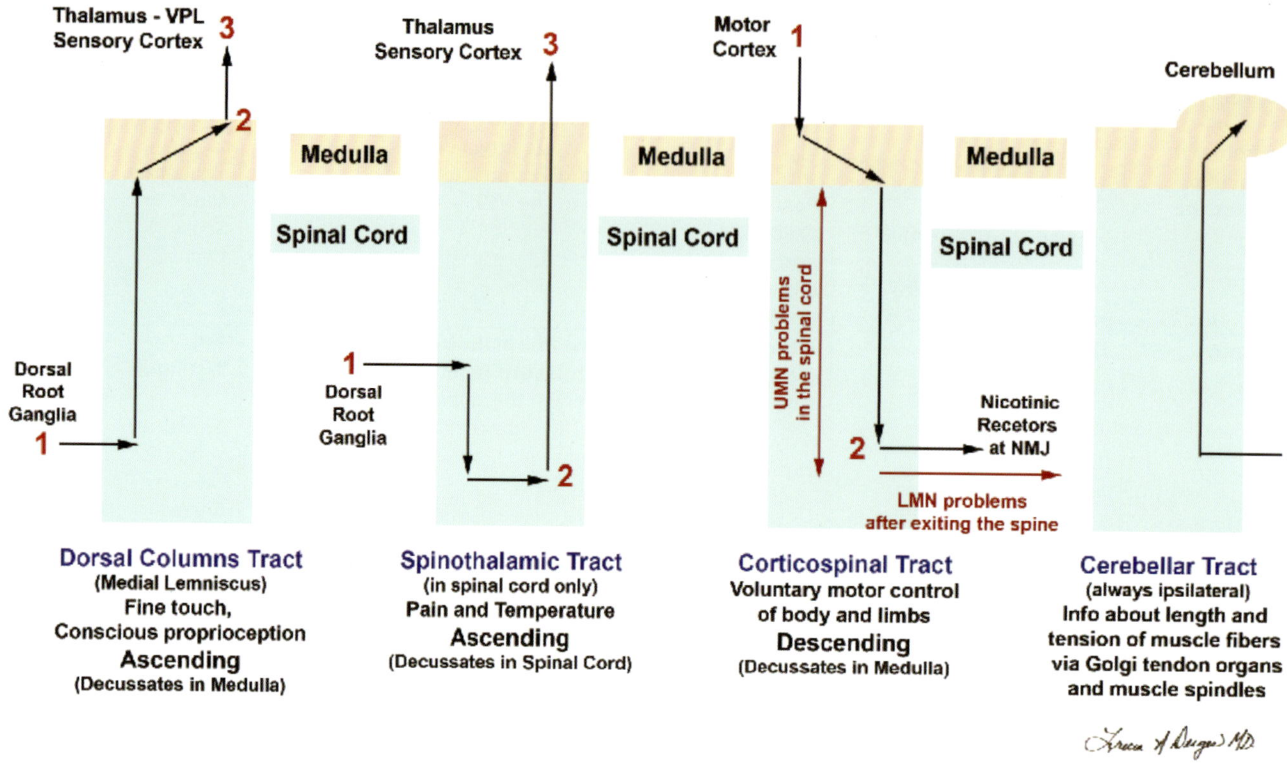

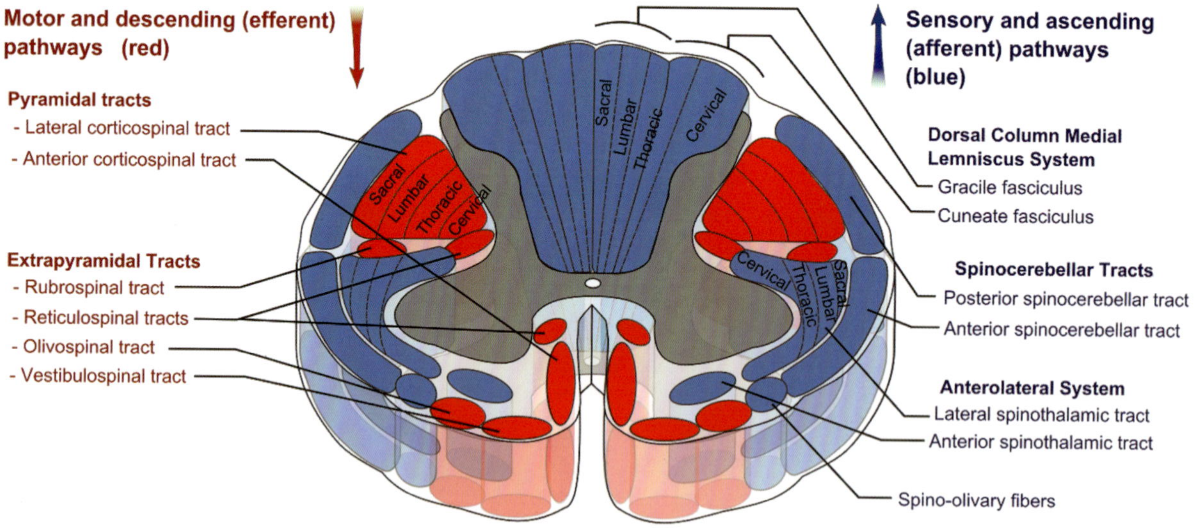

Dorsal (Posterior) Column Spinal Tract and Spinothalamic Tract

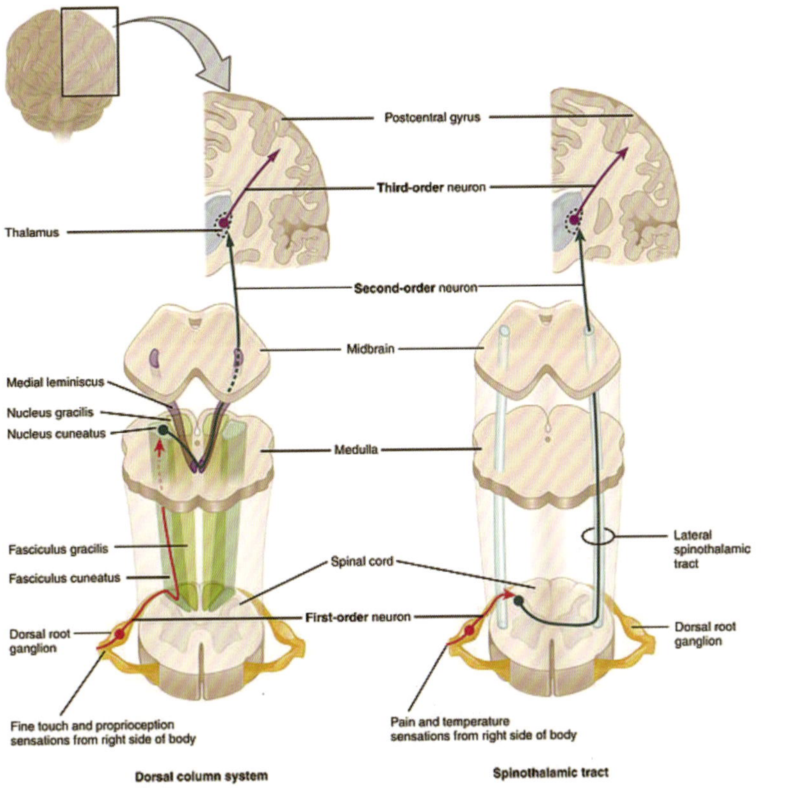

Corticospinal Tract

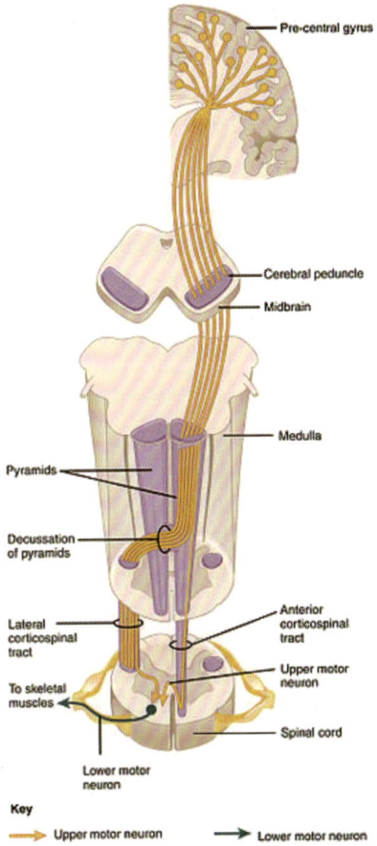

Spinocerebellar Tract

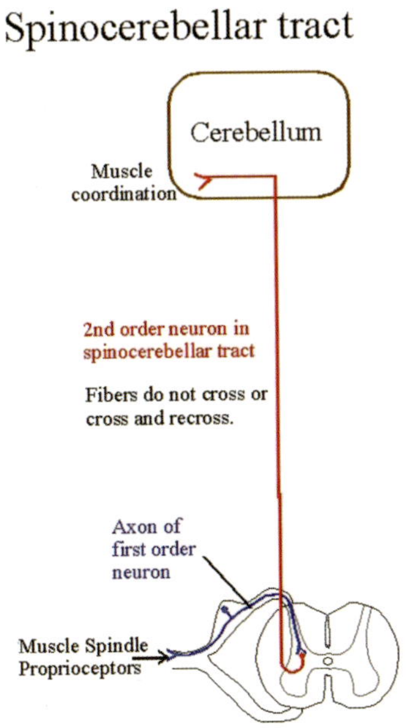

Golgi Tendon Organs (Proprioceptor)

- Function to protect the muscle and connective tissue from injury.
- Capsular structure located in muscle tendons.
- Connected in **series** to extrafusal skeletal muscle fibers.
- Detects changes/tension within **muscle tendons**.
- Reflex activity: **Tendon Reflex**.
- The Golgi tendon organ also mediates the inverse myotactic reflex (reflex that protects against excessive loads).
- They are stimulated with excessive tension during muscle shortening or when the muscle is stretched passively.
- Causes a reflex inhibition of the muscle which causes the muscle to relax and drop the load (weight).
- Stretch: Inhibits contraction of agonist and facilitates antagonist contraction.

Muscle Spindle Fibers (Proprioceptor)

- 3 – 12 (or more) intrafusal fibers (fusiform shaped)
- **Parallel** attachment to sheaths of extrafusal skeletal muscle fibers.
- Reflex activity: **Stretch Reflex.**
- Imbedded in the perimysium between muscle fascicles.
- Detects stretch of skeletal muscle (changing length of a muscle). Monitors **muscle length**.

Reflex Arc of the Golgi Tendon Organ and Muscle Spindle Fibers

An increase in muscle tension activates receptors (Golgi tendon organ) in the tendon and fires ➔ Afferent input from the sensory neurons of the muscle spindle fiber go to the spinal cord (dorsal root) ➔ these sensory neurons synapse with inhibitory interneurons that then synapse with the Alpha Motor Neurons ➔ the Alpha motor neuron sends output to the regular skeletal-muscle fiber and stretch reflex pathway (ventral root) ➔ the Gamma motor-neuron sends output to the contractile end portions of the spindle fiber ➔ the descending pathways coactivates alpha and gamma motor neurons ➔ the inhibition of the Alpha Motor Neurons causes muscle relaxation, relieving the tension that had been applied to the tendon ➔ the load (weight) is dropped.

Joint Kinesthetic Receptor (Proprioceptor)

- Sensory nerve endings within the joint capsules

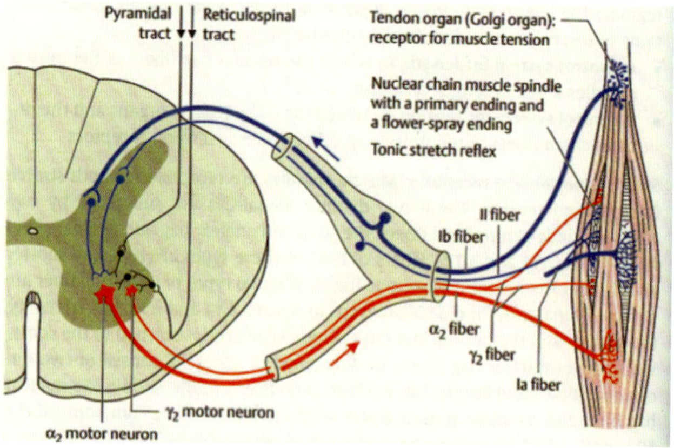

Spindle and Golgi Tendon Organ Feedback System

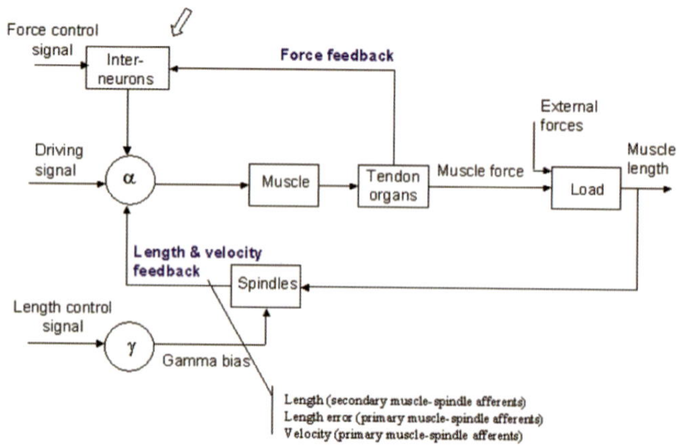

Levels of the Spinal Cord

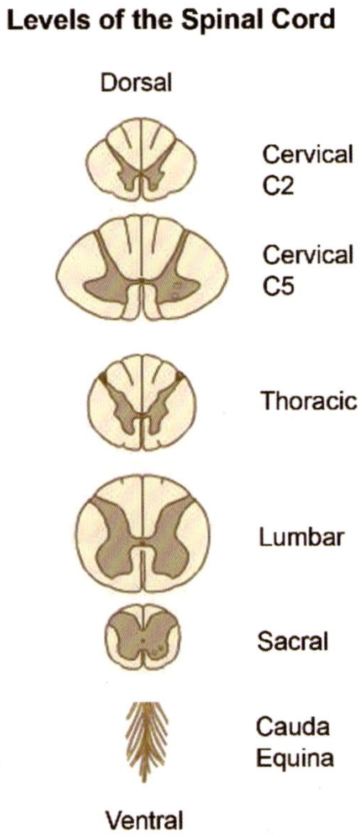

HOMUNCULUS

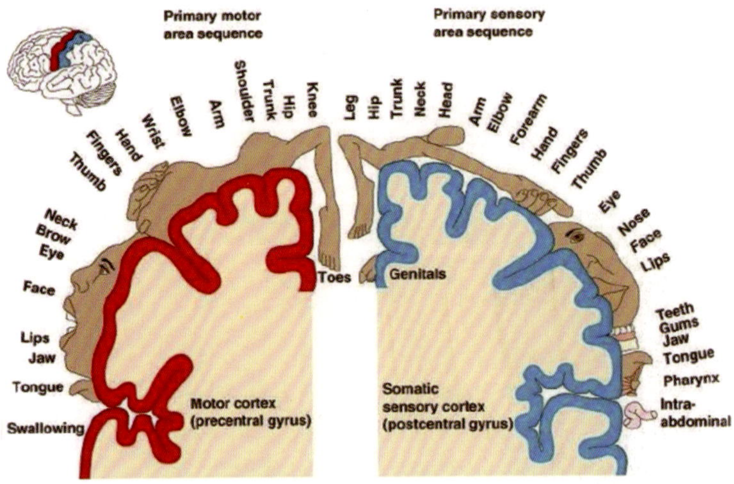

Cerebral Lobe Functions

Lobe	Function
Dominant Lobe	Handwriting, reading, spelling, mathematics, talk, understand
Non-dominant Lobe	Skilled moves, dressing, orientation (steadiness)
Frontal Lobe	Personality, behavior, executive function, reasoning, judgment
Parietal Lobe	Sense, touch, pain, temperature, interpretation
Temporal Lobe	Memory, hearing, sequencing, organization,
Occipital Lobe	Vision: color, light, movement

Lobe Lesions

- Global aphasia: Not able to talk or understand
- Conduction aphasia: Poor repetition but understands ok

Lobe	Lesion
Right Parietal **(non-dominant)**	Hemi-neglect to everything on the left side
Left Temporal **(dominant)**	**Wernicke/Brodmann's Area 22** **Broca (Inferior, Posterior frontal lobe)** Can understand language but is frustrated because **they can't say what they want to** (AKA: **Expressive aphasia**). Comprehension is fine. No fluent speech. Difficulty in production of speech, word finding and repetition. **Wernicke (superior temporal lobe)** Can't understand written/spoken language. Is able to still speak fluently but it makes no sense. Patient is unable to repeat words. (AKA: **Receptive aphasia**). No comprehension, things are meaningless. **Not able to interpret or understand.**
Occipital Lobe	Visual disturbances: color, light, movement
Frontal Lobe	Hemiparesis

Facial Nerve Lesions

Bells Palsy (AKA: Facial Nerve Palsy)	Central Nerve Palsy (stroke)
Due to CN VII and is a LMN lesion **Ipsilateral** (peripheral) facial paralysis (face stiffness). Loss of forehead and brow expression lines, inability to close eye, drooping eye lid, loss of nasal folds and lateral side of lower lip droops = all one side of the face. (AKA: the **entire length, upper and lower,** half of the face is paralyzed), hyperacusis (loud sounds due to CN VII not innervating the stapedius muscle), taste dysfunction (due to CN VII not supplying taste to the anterior 2/3 of the tongue). Associated with: **Lyme DZ** (Lyme DZ can cause bilateral facial palsy), herpes (simplex or zoster), diabetes, CREST, HIV, sarcoidosis, tumors. TX: Self-resolving, Because the eyelid is not able to close, **MUST keep lubricating drops in the eye to keep it from drying out and tape the eye shut (especially at night)** to avoid corneal ulcerations/abrasions. (tip: **B**ells = **B**oth sides: top and bottom) 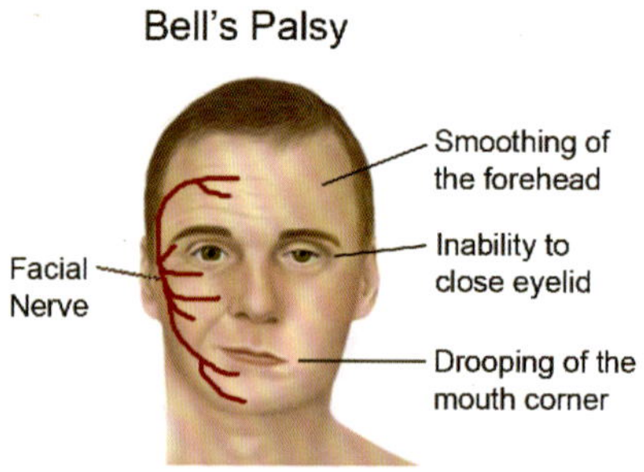	**Due to an UMN lesion** **Contralateral** paralysis of lower face (loss of nasal folds and the lateral side of the lower lip droops), **but no loss of forehead or brow expression.** 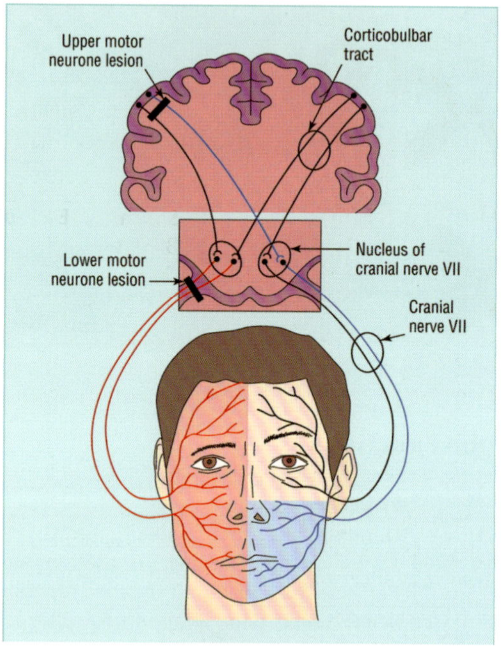

Brown-Séquard Syndrome

Hemisection of spinal cord

Damage to half of the spinal cord.	
MC: stabbing injury, gun shot wound Loss of motor function (hemiparaplegia) (**Lateral corticospinal tracts**) Loss of proprioception, two-point discrimination, vibration, pressure on **ipsilateral** side to lesion. (**Dorsal column-medial lemniscus tract**) Loss of pain and temperature and crude touch **contralateral** to lesion. (**Spinothalamic tract**) DX: MRI	

Herniations

- **Uncal** herniation: (Uncus) Compresses **CN III Palsy** ("Down and Out" gaze)
- **Cerebellar tonsillar** herniation: into foramen magnum = coma and **death** due to compression on brain stem = inhibits **respiration.**
  Associated with Chiari malformation (AKA: Arnold-Chiari malformation)
- Cingulate (Subfalcine) herniation under falx cerebri compresses the anterior cerebral artery
- Transtentorial (central) herniation

CNS Tumors

- MC brain cancer: Metastasis
- Metastasis location: **Grey/white matter junction**
- Treatment:
  Single lesion = **S**urgery
  Multiple lesions = Radiation, Chemo

MC METS to the Brain	**Solitary METS to Brain Lesion**	**Multiple METS Brain Lesion**
1) Lung 2) Breast, kidney 3) Kidney, prostate (female and male urogenital neoplasms **4) Melanoma** 5) Colon	Breast Colon	Lung Melanoma
Rare METS to Brain Esophagus Liver Non-melanoma	**MC METS to Brain – Non-Smokers** Breast	**MC METS to Brain – Smoker** Lung

Metastasis to Brain

Multiple lesions at **gray – white matter border**.
(Primary tumor is a single lesion).

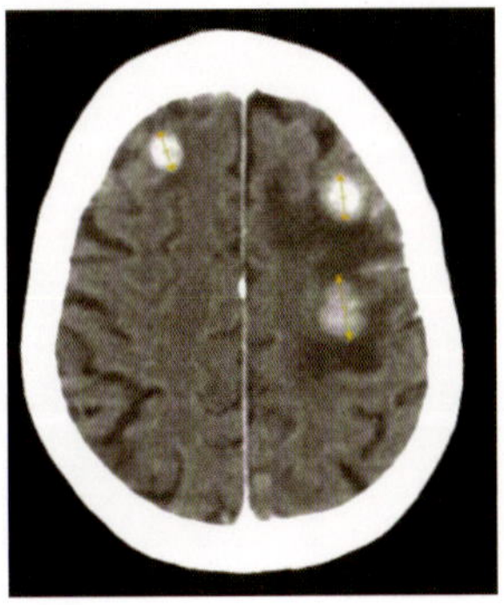

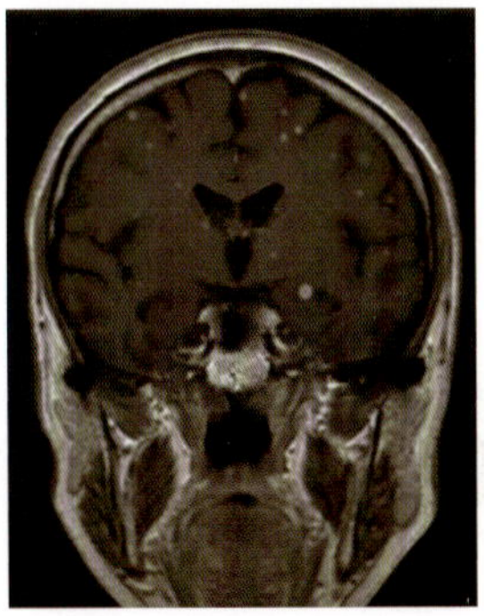

Primary Mass verses Metastasis

Primary Mass	**Metastasis**
Poorly circumcised (can't see where it stops and starts because it is part of the brain) Single mass Varies in its locations	Well circumcised (pushes brain out) Multiple masses Grey white matter junction

Prognosis – Based on:

- Location
- Infiltrative behavior
- **GRADE**
  How abnormal the tumor cells and the tumor tissue look under a microscope.
  Grades 1, 2, 3, 4
  1 = Well differentiated, low grade
  4 = Poorly differentiated, high grade

Adult Tumors

Oligodendroglioma
Malignant – oligodendrocytes
40 – 50 yrs
+ GFAP

Frontal Lobe: personality changes, seizures.

Histology: **Spherical nuclei** with **perinuclear halos**, (AKA: "fried egg" appearance, AKA: round nuclei with clear cytoplasm), **capillaries look like chicken wire** with **granular** chromatin (AKA: **eosinophilic** cytoplasm), **Calcifications**

Meningioma
#2 MC Adult Tumor
Benign
Arises: Arachnoid cells.
Attached to the dura (has "tails" on both sides where it attaches)

Histology: **Spindle cells, psammoma** bodies (**whorled** pattern) and **calcification**.

SX: Personality changes, new onset tumor

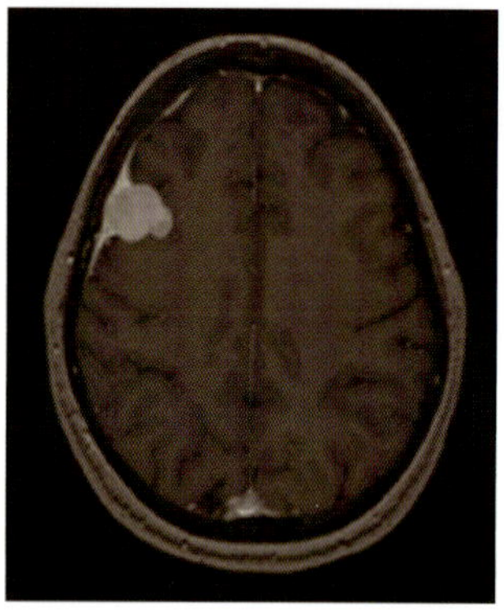

Hemangioblastoma

Cerebellar
Associated: VHL (von Hippel-Lindau)

Produces **erythropoietin** (causes 2° polycythemia)
EPO stimulates growth cells in tumor.
Histology: Foamy cells (foamy blood), highly vascular.

SX: Retinal angiomas

Glioblastoma Multiforme
(AKA: Grade IV Astrocytoma)

#1 MC Adult Tumor
Malignant – 1 year survival
+ for GFAP (Glial Fibrillary Acidic Protein)
P53 is mutated

Histology: Pseudopalisading cells
Boarder: central areas of **necrosis and hemorrhage.**
AKA: Microvascular proliferation and **necrosis**
"butterfly" appearance that can cross midline.
Loss of heterozygosity on
Chrom 10.
SX: Papilledema, nausea, vomiting, **headaches** that worsen with change of positions or pressure (coughing, sneezing), **personality change**, strange behaviors.
TX: Nitrosoureas

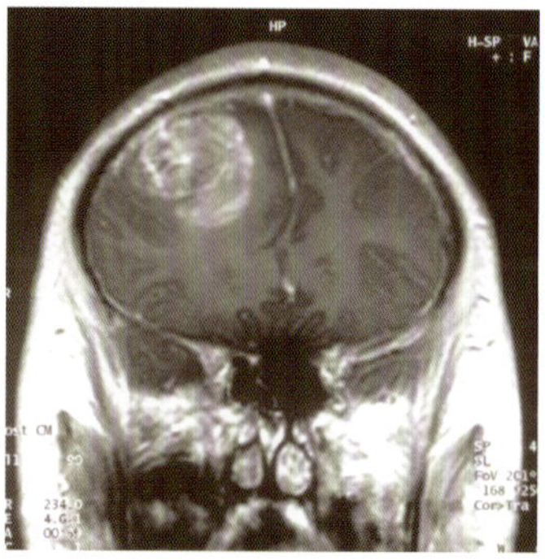

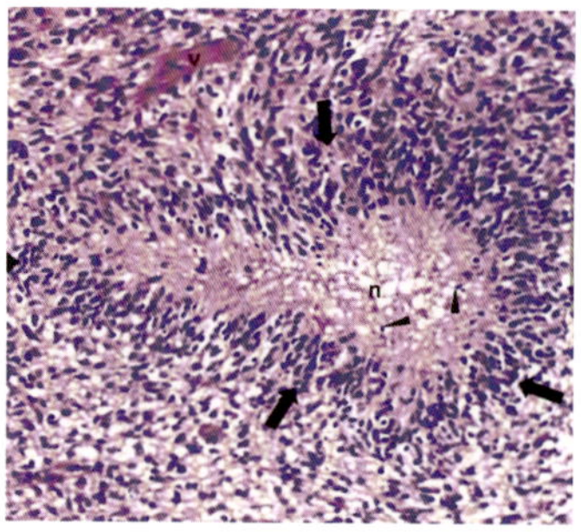

Pseudopalisading Cells

Schwannoma
Benign nerve sheath tumor.

Cerebellopontine angle.
Neural Crest origin.
+ S-100

Associated with **NF-2: CN VIII Acoustic schwannoma** (AKA: Acoustic neuroma)

Histology: **Oval nuclei, spindle shape**

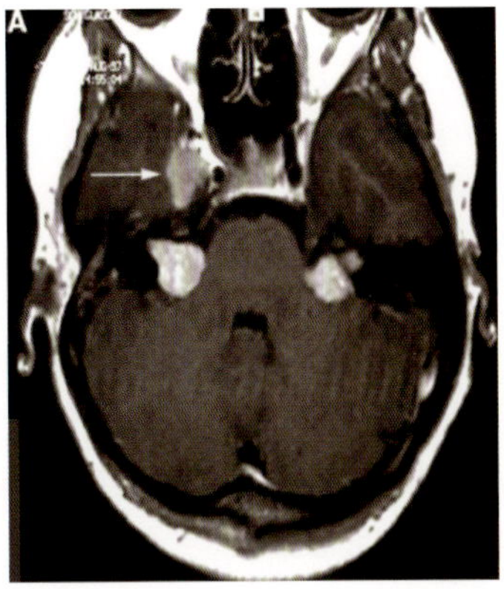

Empty Sella Syndrome
AKA: Sella Turcica

Pituitary gland shrinks or becomes flattened.

Primary: Pressure is increased in the sella turcica cavity from an anatomical defect above the pituitary. This compresses and flattens the pituitary.
MCC: Obesity and HTN in women.
Can also be a sign of idiopathic intercranial HTN (Psudotumor cerebri)

Secondary: Pituitary gland is destroyed because of an injury, surgery or radiation. See ↓of all functions associated with the pituitary gland.

DX: MRI

Pituitary Adenoma
Is NOT a cancer
MC: **Prolactinoma**

SX: Galactorrhea, amenorrhea
↓ LH, ↓ FSH
(Females = no cycles)
(Males = gynecomastia)

Bitemporal hemianopia = pressure on optic chiasm.

Neuro: Dopamine Tubero Pathway (Tuberoinfundibular Pathway: dopamine neurons in the arcuate nucleus in the tuberal region of the mediobasal hypothalamus):
⊘ Dopamine = ↑ Prolactin

Surgery: **Trans-sphenoidal** Pituitary Surgery

TX: **Bromocriptine, Cabergoline** (dopamine agonist)

Add 'l SX: Bitemporal hemianopia, headache, hypopituitarism, decreased libido, infertility, acromegaly, galactorrhea.

↑ ACTH = ↑ cortisone = Cushing's.
↑ LH/FSH = hypogonadism
↑ GH = Gigantism or Acromegaly.
NOTE: If this occurs prior to fusion of the epiphyseal plates it will cause gigantism. If it occurs after the closure of the epiphyseal plates it will cause acromegaly.
↑ **Prolactin** = infertility, galactorrhea, amenorrhea.
↑ ADH = SIADH
↑ TSH = ↑ T3, T4
↑ MSH = hyperpigmentation

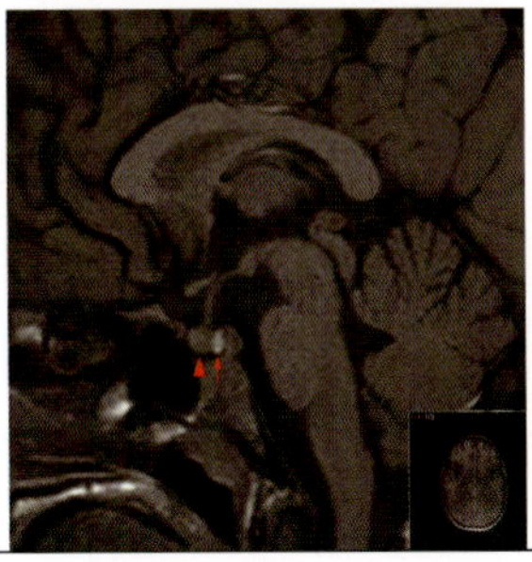

Children's Tumors

Pilocystic Astrocytoma
MC in child and young adult
Cerebellum, below the tentorium.
Benign
(Pilo = hair)
+ GFAP
Cystic mass with mural (wall) nodules.

(Is both cystic and solid)
Associated with NF-1

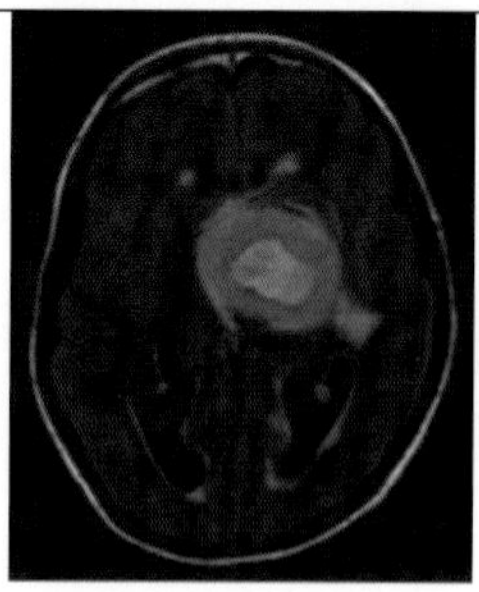

Histology:
Astrocytes (spindle cells) have bipolar processes (look like long hairs: **Rosenthal fibers**)
(AKA: Rosenthal fibers (corkscrew)**:** **eosinophilic** structures)

PNET (Primitive Neuroectoderm Tumor)
1) Medulloblastoma
2) Retinoblastoma (retina, Rb gene)

Medulloblastoma
Malignant, aggressive
Neuro ectoderm tumor.
Vermis of the cerebellum.
Arises in midline of cerebellum.
(Catch early = good prognosis. Catch late = spread in CSF and seeds everywhere)

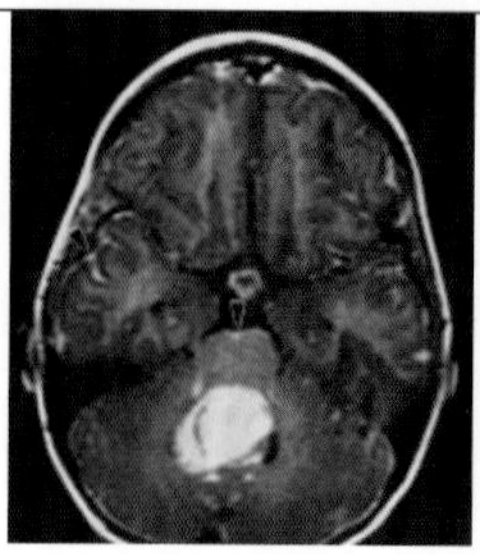

Histology:
+ PNET
Scant cytoplasm, **Homer-Write rosettes** (cells line up around a space). Solid tumor with **sheets of small blue cells.** (AKA: Dark tumor cells surrounding pale neurofibrils)
SX: Diplopia, CN VI lesion, falls, ataxia, gate dysfunction, vomiting
TX: Surgery, radiation

Ependymoma
Tumor in the **4th ventricle** = obstructs CSF = hydrocephalus.
+ GFAP
Poor prognosis

Histology: Perivascular pseudorosettes around vessels, rod shaped blepharoplasty (basil ciliary bodies)

Risk: Syringomyelia

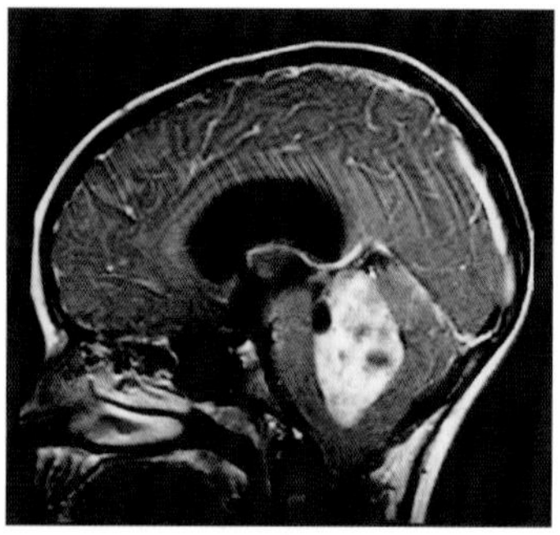

Craniopharyngioma (AK: Sella tumor. Suprasellar)
Benign
MC: supra tentorial tumor

Remnant of **Rathke pouch** (Anterior pituitary), roof of mouth.
Compresses optic chiasm: bitemporal hemianopsia, ↑ ICP, headaches, hypopituitary

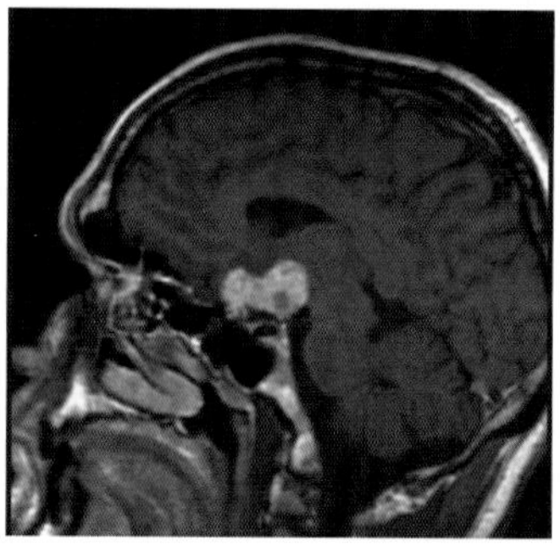

Histology: **Calcified** multiple **cystic** masses, keratin pearls, **tooth enamel, cholesterol crystals** (yellow brown fluid), stratified squamous spongy stroma, gliosis, nesting squamous epithelium

Kids: retarded growth
Adults: Sexual dysfunction (↓ libido), amenorrhea
DX: MRI or CT

Pineal Gland Tumor (AKA: Pinealoma)
Dorsal midbrain
Germinoma: secretes βHCG = **precocious puberty** in males

Parinaud Syndrome = Due to Pinealoma or Germinomas.
Impaired upward gaze, bilateral papilledema, vertical gaze paralysis, ataxia, nystagmus, loss pupil reaction, retraction of eyelid. Affects CN III. Also has deep voice and facial hair due to BHCG secretion and Leydig cell stimulation.

Obstructive hydrocephalus (due to compression of tumor on ventricles). CT will show **enlarged ventricles.**

Extracranial Neural Tumors

Paraganglioma Tumor by the Carotid Body or Aortic Arch, head, Neck, thorax, abdomen Neuro granules: **Chromogranin** Enolase **Synaptophysin** protein (stains positive on tumor cells in CNS.	**Neuroblastoma** MC Extracranial tumor **Adrenal Medulla** Neural Crest derivative + S-100 Histology: Solid tumor. Solid sheets **of small round blue cells.** **N-myc** on chromosome 2 Labs: High urinary **HVA or VMA** SX: Abdominal mass, can cross the midline, Myotonia, non-rhythmic eye movements (dancing eyes), myoclonus (involuntary muscle jerk), hypotonia. **NOTE**: Do NOT confuse this with nephroblastoma.
Beckwith-Wiedemann Syndrome (BWS) Overgrowth disorder that increases the risk of childhood cancer. MC cancers that develop: Wilms tumor (nephroblastoma), pancreatoblastoma and hepatoblastoma. Neuroblastoma, rhabdomyosarcoma. SX: Macrosomia, macroglossia, visceromegaly (large liver and kidneys), neonatal hypoglycemia, hyperinsulinemia, prominent occiput and eyes, abdominal wall defects: umbilical hernia and/or omphalocele, hearing loss, musculoskeletal abnormalities. **Caution**: Do not confuse BWS with Congenital hypothyroidism. Congenital hypothyroidism has umbilical hernias but not omphalocele. It also does not have hypoglycemia or hyperinsulinemia.	

Horner Syndrome

- Associated with **Pancoast Tumor**, Brown-Séquard Syndrome, syringomyelia
- SX: (Sympathetic) Ptosis (drooping of eyelid), Anhidrosis (no sweating), and Miosis (pupil constriction)
- Deficiency of sympathetic activity
- Compression of sympathetic chains = cervical or thoracic cancer

Demyelinating Pathologies

Multiple Sclerosis

Sclerosis = scars (plaques/lesions)

MC autoimmune disorder affecting the CNS.
Demyelination and loss of oligodendrocytes. (Cells responsible for creating and maintaining myelin sheaths that help carry action potentials)
2:1 occurance in women verses men
5 – 10 years lower life expectancy than normal

Relapsing (comes and goes/waxes and wanes) disease

Initial presentation are normally **visual issues**: Nystagmus (involuntary eye movement), diplopia (double vision), optic neuritis (inflammation of optic nerve that can lead to complete or partial loss of vision) or **MLF** (Medial longitudinal fasciculus: When the eyes look laterally, **CN III** of the eye that follows (must move medially) **does not get the message from CN VI to turn**. So the initial eye (that only needs a message to turn laterally CN VI) is looking to the side, but the other eye is still looking straight ahead)
Then other symptoms: **paresthesias**, muscle spasms, depression, loss of sensitivity, lethargy, pain, bladder incontinence, difficulty swallowing, **scanning speech** will follow.
These symptoms will improve and then relapse on a continually declining scale.
Inflammation occurs with the demyelination caused by **T cells that attack the myelin** (seen as foreign).

DX: CSF studies = ↑ **IgG Protein. (AKA: IgG oligoclonal bands)**
Increase in astrocytes (due to destruction of nearby neurons)

(Multiple Sclerosis cont'd)

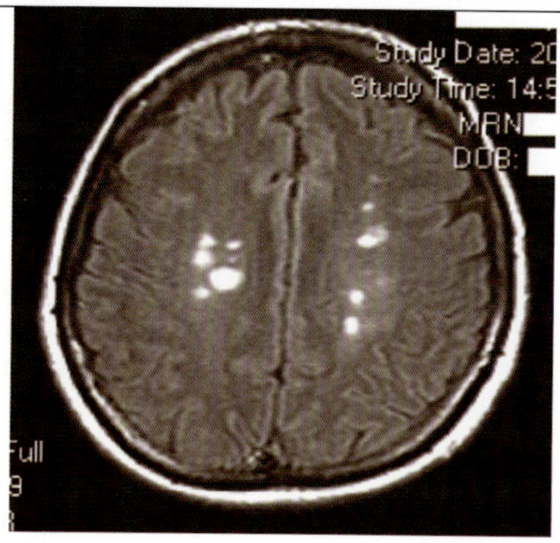

MRI = **Periventricular plaques** in the white matter (areas of oligodendrocytes have been lost and reactive gliosis has occurred).

Test: **Length-Space Constant Test**: Measures how far an axon travels.
↓ Myelin = ↓ Space Constant (AKA: myelin is not thick, takes up less space)
↓ Myelin = ↓ Length Constant (AKA: length of the action potential is less, it can't go as far. Myelin is what insulates the nerve and allows the impulse (action potential) to travel longer distances)

TX: **INF β and Steroids**
(β = Brain)

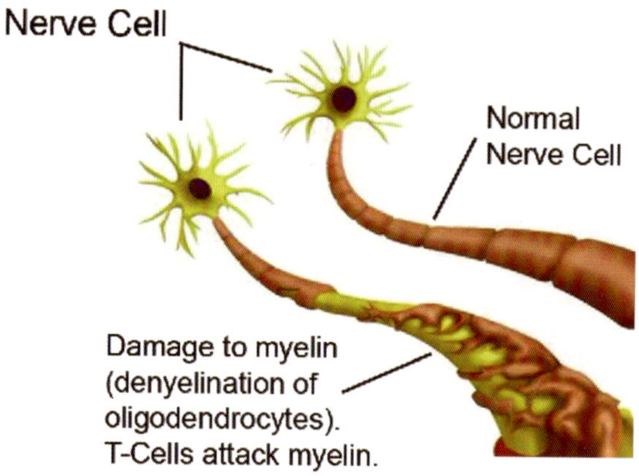

NOTE: Remember that **any** use of steroids puts the individual at risk for all side effects of steroids: avascular necrosis, osteoporosis, atrophied adrenal gland, Cushing's symptoms, etc.
Many treatments add **steroids** as an adjunctive therapy's:
Lupus and Rheumatoid Arthritis (Methotrexate and Steroids), PCP (TMP/SMX and Steroids), Multiple Sclerosis (INF-β and Steroids).

Guillain-Barré Syndrome

Autoimmune.
Body is attacking peripheral nerves causing **demyelination** and damage to motor fibers.
No sensory loss.
↓ Neuron firing.

Rapid onset: 1 day to 2 weeks. Usually follows a gastrointestinal infection or URI.
MCC: **Campylobacter**, CMV (in immunocompromised)

SX: **Symmetrical, ascending** weakness and paralysis.

Risk: Involvement of **diaphragm muscle (Phrenic Nerve)** = causes respiratory failure.
Must be prepared to **ventilate/intubate**.
(AKA: what to watch for in this disease: ↓ chest expansion (breathing)

DX: CSF studies show: ↑ **protein**

TX: Self resolving
Do **NOT** use **steroids** = worsens condition

Charcot-Marie-Tooth Disease

Inherited disorder of the peripheral nervous system. Loss of muscle tissue and touch sensation over the body. Subtype of muscular dystrophy.

Caused by mutation that affects the myelin sheath and/or the nerve axon that leads to continual demyelination and remyelination.

SX: Foot drop, hammer toes (curled toes), wasting of muscles in the legs ("stork leg"), high/flat arched feet, pain, scoliosis, difficulties in chewing and speaking.

DX: Nerve conduction studies and biopsy of the nerve.
TX: Physical therapy and orthotic footwear.

Note: Vincristine is contradicted in patients with Charcot-Marie.

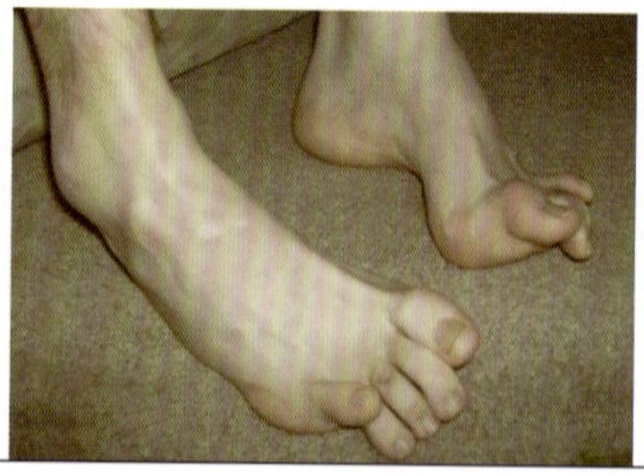

	Krabbe Disease **Lysosomal Storage Disease** (AR) Deficiency of **Galactocerebrosidase and build up of galactocerebroside.** Dysfunctional metabolism of **sphingolipids**. Myelin sheath is destroyed SX: **Renal** involvement, developmental delays, peripheral neuropathy, optic atrophy, **multinucleated globoid cells**
Subacute Sclerosing Panencephalitis (SSPE) Associated with infection of the **measles virus** prior to the age of 2. Asymptomatic for 6 to 15 years. SX: Gradual and progressive psychoneurological deterioration: personality changes, seizures, ataxia, photosensitivity, myoclonia, coma, visual changes. DX: Due to antibodies against the measles virus in the CSF. Brain biopsy will show RNA virus with hemagglutinin encapsulated in brain tissue **Central Pontine Myelinolysis** **(AKA: Locked In Syndrome)** Severe **axonal demyelination** in the nerve cells in the **pons**. AKA: Destruction of the myelin sheath. Cause: **Correcting hyponatremia to quickly** or in withdrawal from chronic **alcoholism**. SX: Acute paralysis, dysphagia, dysarthria (difficulty speaking), quadriparesis, loss of consciousness Maximum correction: **Rate not exceeding** 10 mmol/L/24 hours or 0.5 mEq/L/hour. Add vitamins for alcoholics. TX: Correction of sodium levels, Sodium levels 115 – 125 = **withhold/restrict water** Sodium levels < 115 = **Demeclocycline**	**Metachromatic Leukodystrophy** **Lysosomal Storage Disease** (AR) Deficiency of **arylsulfatase A** and build up of sulfatides. **Impaired production** of myelin sheaths. SX: Peripheral and central demyelination with ataxia and dementia **Progressive Multifocal Leukoencephalopathy (PML)** **AKA: JC Virus** **Demyelination** and **destruction of oligodendrocytes** (white matter of the brain) caused by **JC Virus (polyomavirus)**. Similar to MS but is much more rapidly progressing. SX: Rapidly progressive, fatal (6 months). Hemiparesis, speech disturbances, vision problems, gate problems, **non-ring enhancing lesions** in the cortical white matter. Labs: Positive for TOXO with CD4 < 100, but *(PML cont'd)* **be careful** to be sure it says "ring enhancing" and not **NON-RING enhancing lesions** (TOXO **has** ring enhancing lesions. CNS lymphoma also has ring-enhancing lesions). Risk: **HIV** and other immunocompromised patients Associated with: use of **Natalizumab** (drug has been withdrawn from use)

Acute Disseminated Encephalomyelitis (ADEM)
Autoimmune that attacks and inflames the brain and spinal cord. The inflammation attacks the myelin sheaths and destroys the white matter.

Cause: **Viral infections** (measles, flu, rubella, varicella, EBV, herpes, etc.) and **vaccinations (rabies)**
SX: **Abrupt onset** 1 – 3 weeks after infection, fever, headache, confusion, vision impairment, seizure, coma

(Caution: do not mix this up with **Subacute Sclerosing Panencephalitis (SSPE)** due to the **measles virus**.
SSPE has a history of **measles prior to the age of 2** followed by 6 – 15 asymptomatic years.
Gradual and progressive psychoneurological deterioration: personality changes, seizures, ataxia, photosensitivity, myoclonia, coma.

Early TX: INF, Ribavirin Late: Palliative care.

Encephalitis and Abscess Pathologies

Encephalitis:

- Acute inflammation of the brain
- SX: Fever combined with confusion

<table>
<tr>
<td>
Herpes Encephalitis
Retrograde transmission of HSV virus in the temporal lobe in the CNS.
Virus lies dormant in the trigeminal ganglion.
Rapidly progressing. Fever, confusion, change in personality. Can present in as short of time as a few hours.

BIT: CT/MRI shows changes in the temporal lobe.
MAT: PCR: Lumbar puncture shows a viral CSF presentation.

TX: IV Acyclovir. Treat immediately; do not wait for the results of the CSF test. If resistant to Acyclovir: use Foscarnet.
</td>
<td>
Viral Encephalitis
Acute or latent infections caused by:
HSV, Rabies, HPV, Poliovirus, measles, arbovirus (St. Louis encephalitis, West Nile encephalitis), bunyavirus (La Crosse), arenavirus (lymphocytic choriomeningitis), Reovirus (Colorado tick virus).

Bacterial, Protozoal, Parasitic Encephalitis
Acute or latent infections caused by:
Toxoplasmosis, malaria, Lyme disease, Bartonella henselae, Mycoplasma, amoeba (Naegleria fowleri)

SX of encephalitis:
Confusion, hallucinations, seizures, ataxia, irritability, fever, stiff neck.
DX: MRI, EEG, Lumbar puncture, blood test, urinalysis.

TX:
Viral causes: antiviral meds.
Bacterial causes: Antibiotics.
Steroids to reduce brain swelling.
Sedatives for restlessness.
Acetaminophen for fever.
</td>
</tr>
<tr>
<td>
Brain Abscess
Collection of infected material in the brain that come from local or remote infections (contiguous infection from: dental abscesses, sinus, ear or mastoid infections), head trauma, skull fractures, surgical procedures, HIV infections.

SX: Rapidly progressing. Fever, headache, neurological problems (hemiparesis, aphasia), ↑ ICP, confusion, drowsiness, seizures, coma.

DX: BIT: CT with contrast shows ring-enhancing lesion. (Ring-enhancing lesion indicates: infection or cancer).
If HIV is negative perform brain biopsy.
MAT: Brain biopsy. (The only way to distinguish between an abscess and cancer).
Do not do lumbar puncture (alters the ICP which can cause brain herniation).

TX: ↓ ICP, IV antibiotics if indicated by culture).
If HIV is positive: TX: TMP/pyrimethamine
</td>
<td>
Toxoplasmosis
Intracellular, parasitic protozoan

Source: Ingestion of oocysts (sporozoites). Cat feces, deli meats, skins of raw vegetables (peel vegetables). Pregnant women must avoid these things – oocysts cross the placenta and infect the fetus.

Highest risk: HIV

SX: Brain CT shows Ring Enhancing Lesions
Triad of: Chorioretinitis (cotton like- white/yellow lesions in the eyes), hydrocephalus, intracranial calcifications.
(Tip: tOxOplasmosis: the “O”s make a RING)

DX: Blood sample showing tachyzoites

TX: Sulfadiazine and pyrimethamine
(If the TX of Sulfadiazine and pyrimethamine does not work then the differential DX is Primary CNS Lymphoma
</td>
</tr>
</table>

Naegleria fowleri AKA: Naegleriasis Protozoan Fatal primary amoebic meningoencephalitis Enters brain through cribriform plate. Source: **Warm freshwater** ponds, lakes, rivers, hot springs, poorly chlorinated swimming pools, warm water discharges from industrial plants (is not found in salt water) DX: Amoebas in spinal fluid TX: **Amp B**	**Cysticercosis or Neurocysticercosis** Caused by: Taenia solium (Pork tapeworm) Worm lives in the intestine and infections are asymptomatic unless infection occurs during the larval stage causing Cysticercosis or Neurocysticercosis (**Very common in Mexico**). Source: Ingestion of larvae in **uncooked or undercooked pork**, eggs, undercooked vegetables SX: Seizures, **Cysticercosis** (tissue infection), **neurocysticercosis** (brain infection causing seizures) DX: **Eosinophils in the CSF, CT/MRI of brain shows multiple cysts that will calcify over time.** **TX:** **Praziquantel** for Cysticercosis **Albendazole** for Neurocysticercosis if uncalcified.

Dementia

Normal Aging

- This patient **is concerned** and **aware** of their memory loss
- This patient **does not have** impairment of daily functions
  (**Caution**: Normal again and Alzheimer's will sound exactly alike in the question. Look to see if the patients is aware and worried about their memory loss and/or if they are still able to do daily task, if they are it is NORMAL aging)

Mini Mental Status Exam

- ≥ 25 normal again
- ≤ 10 severe impairment
- 11 – 18 moderate impairment
- 19 – 24 mild impairment (mild Alzheimer's)

Required Test For All Patients With Memory Loss (abnormal test in these areas can mimic dementia)

- **TSH**
- **B12 levels**
- Head CT
- VDRL/RPR

Pick's Disease Dementia AKA: Frontotemporal Dementia Frontal temporal atrophy (frontal and temporal lobes) SX: **Change in personality and behavior**, compulsive, **Klüver-Bucy Syndrome** (inappropriate behavior, use of dirty language, hypersexual, hyperorality, hyperphagia), strange eating habits. No problems with movement. DX: **Pick bodies** (**tau protein aggregates**), atrophy of frontal and temporal lobes. Degeneration of cortical and basal forebrain neurons. Silver stain shows: Zebra bodies (AKA: inclusion bodies).	**B-12 and Hypothyroidism Dementia** Patient shows all the signs of dementia but it is due to one of these two issues. Before you ever diagnose anyone with dementia, **ALWAYS** run a **TSH test** and check their **B-12 levels**. Do not condemn someone to a diagnosis of dementia when it is something that can be easily fixed.

Alzheimer Dementia

MCC: Elderly and Downs Syndrome
Downs Syndrome (early onset at 40) due to APP protein on chromosome 21.
Elderly (late onset) due to **ApoE4 protein** on chromosome 19.
(Apo-E2 on chromosome 19 is protective)

DX:
↓ ACh, ↓ Glutamate at the NMDA receptors, Aβ Proteins (made from precursor protein APP),
Tau protein, senile plaques (β amyloid core), neurofibrillary tangles. No focal defects.

Stages of Alzheimer's
Note: **Patients are not concerned** it is the family that will bring them in.
Alzheimer's is slow onset and slow progression.
Stage 1: Subtle memory loss (↓ memory loss for recent events and conversations), difficulty in language (hard to find the words they want), **loss of ability to perform task** that they had always been able to do. (Ie: pay bills = bills piling up), can **become lost** in familiar areas (walk or drive), ↓ ability to operate appliances, los of interest in social activity, forgets appointments, mood swings, confusion and irritability, trouble with language, long term memory difficulty, can remember RECENT events.
IT IS NOT: misplacing things or minor short-term memory loss.
Stage 2: Impaired judgement and **personality changes**
Stage 3: **Late** in the disease: psychotic features **(hallucinations)**

DX: MMSE (mini mental status exam) score ≤ 24
Always check: Head CT, **B12, TSH**, and VDRL or RPR. If these levels are abnormal, they can cause symptoms of Alzheimer's.

TX: Donepezil, Galantamine, Rivastigmine, Memantine
(**tip**: I am DONE with Alzheimer's).

Lewy Body Dementia

(**Caution:** Lewy Body and Alzheimer's can be presented to sound alike. If the patient falls (stumbles, falls, trips, or is unstable for any reason) or if the patient has hallucinations and either (or both) these symptoms appear EARLY on, the dementia is Lewy Body. Hallucinations do not appear until the last stages in Alzheimer's and Alzheimer's doesn't have movement problems). Lewy Body Demential is basically dementia plus Parkinson's.

DX: **α-synuclein deficiency** (structural component of the Lewy Bodies). **Lewy Bodies (AKA: eosinophilic** inclusion bodies). AKA: Clumps of Alpha Synuclein.

SX: **↑ EPS movements, falls, hallucinations, fluctuating or periodic impairment** (variations in attention and alertness daily). **Have motor features of Parkinson's** (shuffling gait, ↓ arm swings, stiff movements).

TX: **Rivastigmine** (ACh inhibitor)
Does **NOT** respond to dopamine (Parkinson's drugs) and worsens with epileptic drugs

Neuro Syphilis Dementia

Final stage of syphilis. (Tertiary)
Slow and progressive destructive infection of the brain and spinal cord.

SX: tremors in fingers and lips, irritable, ↓ concentration, dysarthria (not able to articulate – difficulty in saying words), memory loss, personality changes, poor judgment, hallucinations, paranoia

DX: **Positive RPR**, history of STD's

TX: **penicillin**

Pseudo-Dementia

Severely **depressed** elderly with memory loss. Patient is very concerned and **aware of memory loss**.

Drug Induced Dementia

Memory loss due to medications. Dementia can be reversed if the offending drug is stopped.

Lenticular Nucleus Atrophy = Wilson's

Caudate Nucleus Atrophy = Huntington's

Vitamin B-12 Dementia: Dementia with megaloblastic anemia and dorsal column symptoms (ataxia).
MCC: Pernicious anemia

Multi-Infarct Dementia (AKA: Vascular Dementia)

2nd MC cause of dementia in the elderly due to series of minor strokes. History of **HTN and TIA's**.

SX: **Sudden** forgetfulness and deterioration in functioning ability. Mood, behavior changes, cognitive changes, possible weakness and aphasia.

DX: MRI shows numerous old infarctions

Klüver-Bucy Syndrome

Syndrome caused by lesions in the temporal lobe or amygdaloid nucleus.

SX: **Hypersexuality** (saying inappropriate sexual comments, seeking sexual stimulation from inappropriate objects), **hyperorality** (examine everything by mouth), hyperphagia, amnesia, and agnosia (inability to recognize familiar people or things).

Klüver-Bucy Syndrome is associated with several diseases and pathologies: tumors, herpes simplex encephalitis, subcortical gliosis, stroke, carbon monoxide poisoning, Alzheimer's Disease, **Pick's Disease** and Rett Syndrome.

Normal Pressure Hydrocephalus	
Normal aging. Decreased absorption of CSF due to normal aging. SX: Wide based **gait disturbances**/stumbling/ataxia (**wobbly**), **urinary incontinence**/dribbling (**wet**) and **forgetful/dementia (wacky).** Caused by increase in ICP due to abnormal accumulation of CSF in the ventricles. DX: Head CT shows enlarged ventricles without brain atrophy. Lumbar puncture shows normal pressure. TX: Shunt placement (**tip:** the best way to approach this question is that if you see "normal pressure hydrocephalus" in the answer choices, go pick out anything that would represent: wet, wobbly, wacky. The question will do an excellent job of casually hiding these three symptoms and it will be highly likely you will fall for a distractor. If you do not find all three of these hidden symptoms it is not normal pressure hydrocephalus).	

Delirium verses Dementia

Delirium	Dementia
• **Acute onset (few days)** • ↑ elderly with medical issues • **Hospital or nursing home setting** • Causes: medications, dehydration, B-12, electrolyte disturbances, hyperglycemia, UTI, infections, Parkinson's, prior stroke • SX: Symptoms fluctuates, can fluctuate in/out consciousness, **hallucinations**, talks to people not there, delusions, wanders around, disoriented, agitated, anxiety • Important to check BMP and CBC to see if there are **electrolyte issues** • **Haloperidol** is used to treat aggression	• **Slow, progressive** • Elderly • Home or office setting • Gradual memory loss • Problems planning and carrying out task: balancing a check book, writing a letter • Depression is common • Not keeping up with persona grooming

Mini Mental Status Exam

Category	Possible Points	Description
Orientation to time	5	Begins at broad time reference and ending in a very specific, narrow point
Orientation to place	5	Begins at broad time reference and ending in a very specific, narrow place
Registration	3	Repeating named prompts
Attention and calculation	5	Serial sevens, spelling words backwards, counting backwards by 3's
Recall	3	Registration recall
Language	2	Naming items (ie: pen, clock)
Repetition	1	Repeating back a phrase
Complex commands	6	Drawing a figure shown
Results		≥ 25 normal aging, 19 – 24 mild impairment, 11 – 18 moderate impairment, ≤ 10 severe impairment

Prion Diseases

Creutzfeldt-Jakob Disease (CJD)	Kuru Disease	Mad Cow Disease
(AKA: **Spongiform** Encephalopathy) Rapidly progressing to dementia with myoclonus and death. DX: **Prions PrP** (misfolded β-pleated sheet protein, changes from an α helical to a β pleated sheet), brain shows cyst (multiple vacuoles) in the grey area, brain takes on the look of a "sponge". **EEG shows Sharp waves.** MAT: Brain biopsy. CSF shows a **14-3-3 Protein**. If protein is present, biopsy is unnecessary. SX: Patient younger than in Alzheimer's. Personality changes, memory loss, hallucinations, **myoclonus (involuntary muscle twitching),** psychosis, speech impairment, nystagmus, positive plantar reflex, ataxia, seizures, death **Note**: Prions can **not be destroyed** like other bacteria/spores/viruses using the 120° pressure/steam for > 15 min. Prions can only be killed with bleach or by autoclave (steam/pressure) at 270° for 15 minutes.	**Cannibalism** (Papua New Guinea tribes) Transmission of prions via eating of the brains of people that were infected with the disease.	(AKA: Bovine Spongiform Encephalopathy) BSE Transmission: humans eating **contaminated cows** (brain, spinal cord or digestive tract) (Variant of Creutzfeldt-Jakob)

Neurocutaneous Diseases

Neurofibromatosis Type I (AKA: Von Recklinghausen Disease), AD	Neurofibromatosis Type II, AD
Tumor disorder caused by **microdeletion on the NF1 gene on chromosome 17 that encodes for the protein neurofibromin** SX: **Lisch nodules** in the iris, flat pigmented skin lesions (**café au lait spots**), **freckling of the axillae** and/or inguinal areas, dermal neurofibromas (single/multiple firm rubbery bumps) on the skin, scoliosis, kyphosis, ADHD, **neurofibromas (derived from Schwann cells** or fibroblasts). Neurofibromatosis café au lait spots 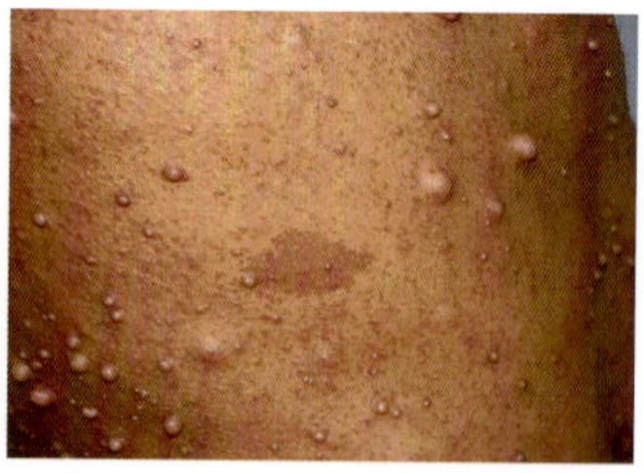 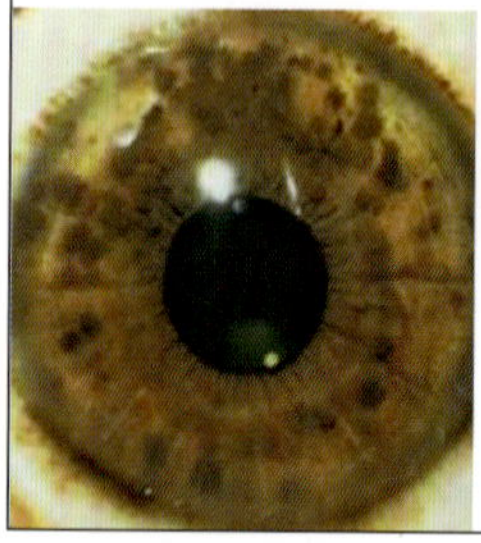 Lisch Nodules	Mutation of the **Merlin** gene (influences the form and movement of cells) **Microdeletion of the NF2 gene located at chromosome 22** **SX: Bilateral acoustic neuromas (Schwannomas)** Schwannomas, meningioma's, ependymomas, Symmetric, non-malignant brain tumors in the **region of cranial nerve VIII** by the internal auditory meatus. Schwannomas are **neural crest** derivatives. Marker: **S-100** 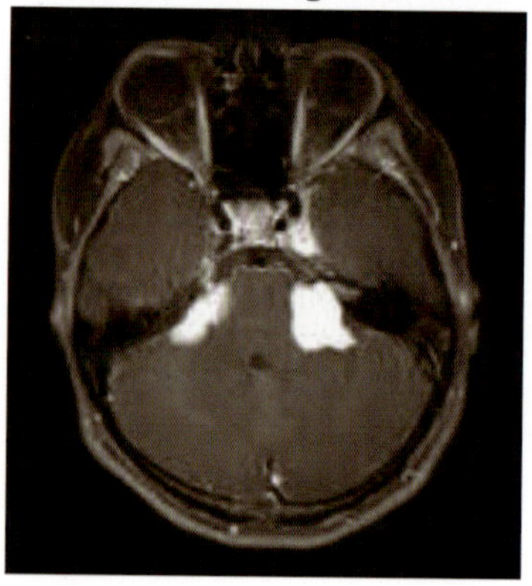

Sturge-Weber Syndrome

Mutation of **GNAQ gene.**
Affects capillary (small) blood vessels.
Neural crest derivative. Errors in mesodermal and ectodermal development.

SX: **"Port wine stain" in V_1 and V_2 distribution on face**, cerebral malformation and tumors with abnormal blood vessels on the brain surface (ipsilateral leptomeningeal angioma), seizures, mental retardation, glaucoma.

DX: CT shows bilateral tram track **calcifications**

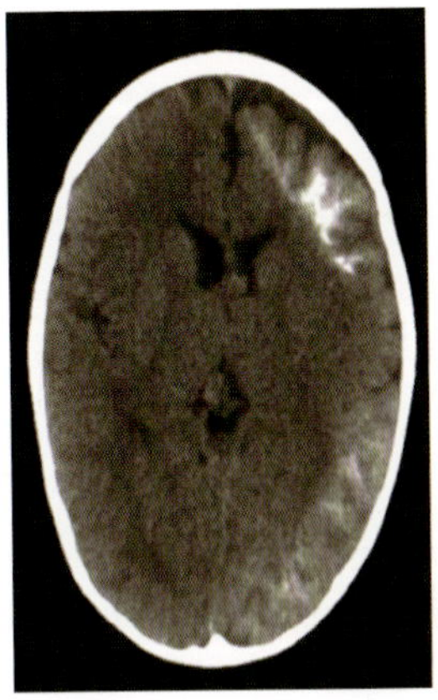

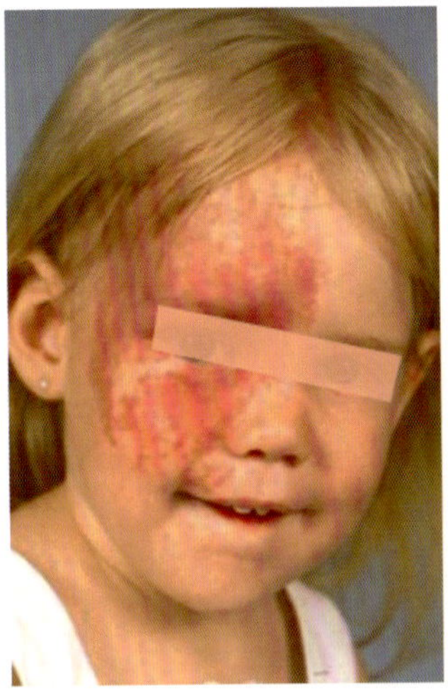

Tuberous Sclerosis (TSC)

Autosomal Dominant disease of benign tumors (**Hamartomas)** in the brain and other organs (heart, kidneys, eyes, lungs, skin)

Mutation of **TSC1 and TSC2** that code for the **Hamartin and Tuberin** proteins (normally act as tumor growth suppressors). TSC1 and TSC2 are tumor growth suppressors.
Intracranial subependymal nodules and cortical/subcortical tubers. These subependymal nodules (swollen glial cells) can transform into a subependymal giant cell astrocytoma close to the foramen of Monro causing a non-communicating hydrocephalus which can cause papilledema.

SX: **Rhabdomyoma (heart),** angiomyolipomas (kidney), **angiofibromas (skin), "ash leaf" spots** (light patches of skin due to lack of melanin), **Shagreen patches** (thick leathery skin dimpled like an orange), **Koenen's tumors** (fleshy **tumors under fingernails** or toenails), seizures, **Coloboma** of the Iris, **Subependymal tumors** and **Cortical tubers** (brain).

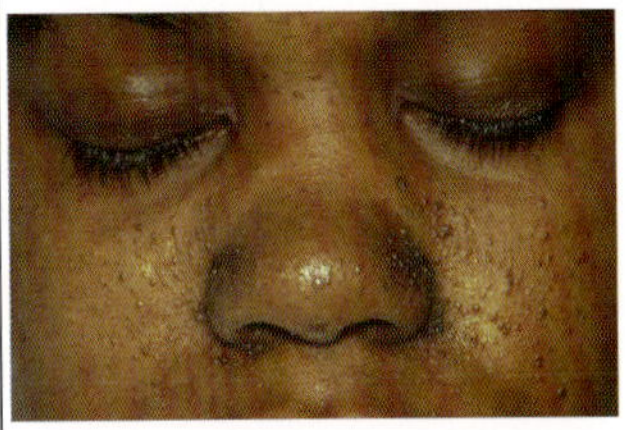

Tuberous Sclerosis (angiofibromas)

Tuberous Sclerosis (Koenen's tumors)

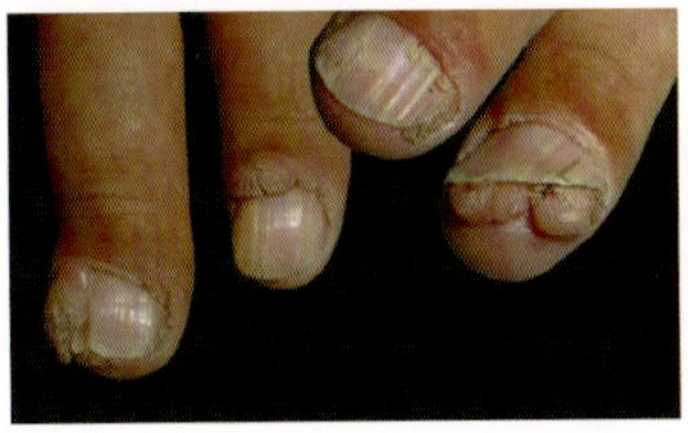

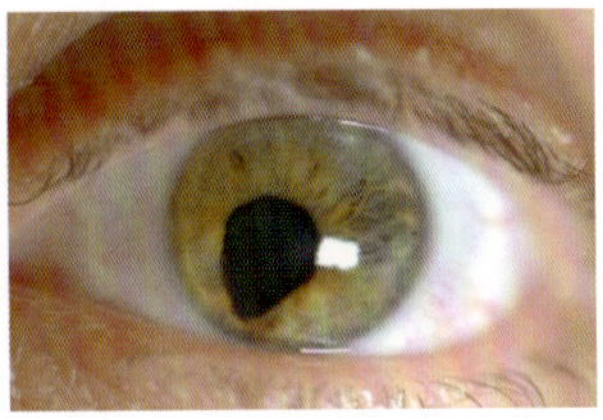

Coloboma of the Iris

Headaches and Face Pain

Headache	Description	Treatment
Cluster	**Episodic/repetitive**, occur in clusters. **Unilateral.** **Severe pain behind the eye**. (stabbing/knifelike pain) Eye watering, nasal congestion (rhinorrhea), eye redness. No aura. **↑ in men.** Can last up to 3 hours. Can be triggered by alcohol, so can occur while drinking. MC: in spring and fall.	**100% oxygen**, **Sumatriptan, Ergonovine, Steroids** **Prophylactic TX: Verapamil**

(**Caution**: Cluster headaches can sound similar to trigeminal neuralgia, temporal arteritis (Giant Cell) and TMJ.
Trigeminal neuralgia: sharp, repetitive shooting pains involving CN V with pain lasting < 1 minute.
Temporal arteritis: Pain is at the temple and there is tenderness on the scalp. It can also have jaw and tongue claudication, tinnitus and is associated with polymyalgia rheumatic.)
TMJ: Joint pain in the jaw accompanied by popping/clicking sound of joint.

Migraine	Pulsating, sensitive to light, sound, aura of smell and/or sound, nausea, vomiting. Can be unilateral or bilateral. Patient wants to stay in a dark room. Can last from 4 – 72 hours. Due to neurons in the trigeminal nucleus (CN V). Triggers: OCP's, menses, caffeine	**Sumatriptan (Serotonin 5-HT agonist)** (Triptans vasoconstrict vessels: can provoke ischemia), **NSAIDS (ibuprofen)** Prophylactic and Recurrent migraines: **Propanolol, Botox (Botulism) injections, Calcium Channel Blockers**
Migraines in Children	MCC of acute headaches in children. SX: Unilateral, bifrontal pain, photophobia, nausea, vomiting, aura, visual dark spots. Occipital headaches are rare. Must see a doctor.	**1st line: Acetaminophen, NSAID's, Ibuprofen.** Lie in a dark room with cool rag on head. **2nd line: Triptans**
Tension	Tension, "band like", squeezing, steady pain. No focal findings, no stiff neck, no aura, no seizures. Can last up to 4 – 6 hours. Associated with stress.	**NSAIDS, Acetaminophen**
Pseudotumor Cerebri	**Morning headaches**, **papilledema**, double vision, pulsatile tinnitus, visual field loss, Sixth nerve palsy. **Overweight female (↑ BMI).** Possible ↑ use of Vitamin A (Vitamin A is needed to make CSF). DX: **CSF: shows ↑ opening pressure**. CT/MRI are normal.	Weight loss. **Acetazolamide.** Surgery.
Subarachnoid	Acute onset, severe, MC in occipital region. Can be accompanies by nuchal rigidity (neck stiffness/pain due to irritation of the meninges), CN III problems, vision changes, stroke signs, neurological signs (paralysis, tingling in extremities). Medical emergency.	CT scans. If SAH, **Nimodipine** given to prevent vasospasms. DO NOT take aspirin or NSAID's if suspected due to potential bleed.
Coital Cephalalgia (AKA: Sexual headaches, Pre/Post Coital Headaches)	Headache that occurs in the skull and neck during sexual activity (organism, masturbation). Begins as a dull headache and increases with sexual excitement, becoming intense at orgasm. It can suddenly begin at orgasm. Pain can last from 1 minute to 72 hours. Occurance is unpredictable. MC in men.	Sudden and severe pain must be evaluated for intracranial hemorrhage. Indomethacin, β-Blockers
Hangover Headache	Occurs after drinking.	

Face Pain

Temporal Arteritis	Inflammation of the blood vessels in the head (branches of the external carotid artery). Sharp pains on the side of head (temple area) with **tenderness to the scalp.** **DX: Biopsy the temporal artery.** (See full details in vascular disease section)	TX: **Steroids** (must start treatment immediately due to risk of blindness, do not wait until biopsy results come back).
TMJ (Temporomandibular Joint Disorder)	Dysfunction of the muscles of mastication and the temporomandibular joints. **Audible clicks** when opening/closing jaw, **referred** pain to ear, pain with chewing, teeth grinding.	TX: Nighttime teeth guard to prevent bruxism, surgery.
Trigeminal Neuralgia	**Sharp shooting pains** from the side of the face originating from the trigeminal nerve (MC: V2 and V3 divisions). Can be a trigger area on the face.	TX: **Carbamazepine, Oxcarbazepine**

Headache Sources and Symptoms

- Primary headaches are recurrent
- Secondary headache causes are sudden and severe

Location	Description of symptoms accompanying headache
Meningitis	Nuchal rigidity and fever. DX with CT
Inter-hemorrhage	SAH, "worst headache of my life" DX with CT, nuchal rigidity, vision/neuro changes
Tumor	Deep, dull ache, wakes you up from sleep. DX with CT
Posterior Fossa Tumor	Vomit proceeds headache by weeks. Headache worsens if one bends, lifts, coughs. DX with CT
Temporal Arteritis	Unilateral pounding pain, head tenderness, visual changes, ↑ ESR. DX with biopsy

Latent Herpes Virus

Postherpetic Neuralgia: (AKA: Nerve Pain is burning)

- Herpes Virus I: Lies dormant in the **trigeminal ganglia**
- Herpes Virus II: Lies dormant in the **sacral root ganglia**
- Herpes Zoster (AKA: Shingles, Varicella Zoster): Lies dormant in the **dorsal root ganglia**
  TX: **Acyclovir, Famciclovir, Valganciclovir**
  Prophylaxis Vaccine: Shingles: Patients ≥ 60 years old.
- Nerve pain TX: **Gabapentin** *(Neurontin)*, **Pregabalin** *(Lyrica)*, **Carbamazepine, Amitriptyline, topical Capsaicin.**

Vertigo/Dizziness

Vertigo	Description
Benign Paroxysmal Positional Vertigo	Patient feels like they are **moving/spinning/swaying** when they are not. **Sudden onset. Positional in onset – can only be induced by change in position.** **Short** in duration (paroxysmal) Caused by changes in the position of the head. SX: **No tinnitus or hearing loss**. MC: occurs when moving from lying position to standing. Eyes: Range from a mild horizontal nystagmus to severe vertical nystagmus, nausea. Cause: **calcium crystals** in the labyrinth dislodge and get trapped in the **semicircular canal**. TX: Epley maneuver (AKA: repositioning maneuver) the head is tilted to free the calcium from the semicircular canals.
Central Vertigo	Due to brain stem or cerebellar lesions (stroke, CNS injuries)
Ménière's Disease	Inner ear disorder that affects hearing and balance. SX: Hearing loss, **tinnitus**, and dizziness. Cause: build up of **endolymph** in the inner ear. (AKA: excess fluid in the inner ear) Can last minutes to 24 hours. TX: **Meclizine (↓ endolymph)**, Sodium restriction and diuretics. ↓ intake of caffeine, alcohol, nicotine, chocolate, bright lights, noise.
Labyrinthitis	Inflammation of the labyrinth of the inner ear that controls balance. Sudden hearing loss, **tinnitus** due to a recent viral or bacterial infection, head injury or reaction to medication. Self-limiting.
Perilymph Fistula	Hearing loss with history of trauma
Vestibular Neuritis	Inflammation of the vestibular nerve (CN VIII) in the inner ear causing vertigo. MC causes are a viral upper respiratory infection. It is not related to a change in position as in benign positional vertigo.

Heat Stroke verses Heat Exhaustion (Hyperthermia, thermogenesis)

Heat Stroke (AKA: Exertional)	Heat Exhaustion
Healthy person doing heavy work in direct sun SX: **Temp > 105° (40° C), Dry skin** (they can't sweat), Nosebleeds, altered mental status, rhabdomyolysis, **myoglobin** in urine (dipstick test shows no RBC's), because extreme heat is breaking down proteins. Labs: ↑ CPK and K Cause: **Failure of the thermoregulator** (**anterior hypothalamus malfunction**). Body is getting hot but the sensor is broken. TX: **Evaporation cooling**. Spray/mist lukewarm water on naked patient and use circulating fans (**convection** over water). Ice baths or ice packs may also be used. DO NOT infuse iced/cold saline into the body, this can stop the heart. **NOTE**: The **fastest form of cooling is convection** (**moving air**) verses conduction (molecules must pass heat/cold from one to another). It provides a mist over the skin so that moving air-cools it down. (AKA: **Evaporation**)	Healthy person doing heavy work in the heat but is not staying **hydrated = ↑ dehydration** Cause: **inadequate sodium and fluid replacement.** SX: **Normal body temp,** excessive **sweating**, NO altered mental status, NO delirium. Can lead to renal failure. Labs: Normal: no rise in CPK and K TX: Move patient into cool environment, normal IV saline and electrolytes.

Other forms of Hyperthermia (thermogenesis)

- **Malignant hyperthermia** due to anesthetics (Halothane)
- **Neuroleptic malignant syndrome** due to antipsychotic medications
- **Malignant hyperthermia** due to the uncoupling of the electron transport chain in the inner mitochondrial membrane, which dissipates the proton gradient before it can be used for oxidative phosphorylation. This energy is now used to generate heat instead of producing ATP. (Salicylic acid, brown fat, 2,4-dinitrophenol (DNP: antiseptic, pesticide, sulfur dyes, wood preservatives).
- TX: **Dantrolene**

Fevers

Fever Defined as: • Temperatures > 38°C/100.4°F rectally in children < 3 years old lasting < 1 week • Temperatures > in an adult. • Causes of concern for fevers in children: meningitis and pneumonia due to group B Streptococcus, E. coli, Listeria	**Fever of Unknown Origin (FUO)** Patient has a fever but no explanation for the fever can be found. Criteria: Fever > 101° on various occasions or a fever that persist without any diagnosis. 3 outpatient visits or 3 days in the hospital without finding a cause.
Treatment for fevers in children with suspected meningitis • SX: Lethargy, poor feeding, irritability • Blood cultures and lumbar puncture (Note: If signs of ICP do not do a lumbar puncture: bulging fontanelles, paralysis of visual gazes) • Do NOT wait until test result return to begin empiric treatment: **Vancomycin plus Cefotaxime or Ceftriaxone**. • Treat for specific organism once test results return: N. meningitis: **Penicillin** for 5 – 7 days. S. pneumonia: **Penicillin or 3rd generation Cephalosporin** for 10 – 14 days. HiB: Ampicillin for 7 – 10 days. E. coli: 3rd generation Cephalosporin for 3 weeks. • **Rifampin** for prophylaxis for all close contacts in cases involving HiB or N. meningitis	

Tremors

Tremor	Description	Association and Notes
Essential Tremor	Continuous, Coarse. No tremor at rest, only when use of hands.	Cerebellum, Basal ganglion. TX: **Propanolol**. Alcohol improves tremor. Autosomal dominant.
Intention Tremor	Irregular, Coarse. Gets worse when approaching target.	Cerebellum, brain stem.
Resting Tremor	Slow, "pill rolling", improves/disappears with purposeful movement. Only occurs at rest.	Parkinson's. Basal ganglion.
Postural Tremor	Action tremor present while voluntarily maintaining a position against gravity.	
Flapping Tremor (AKA: Asterixis)	Tremor, flapping motion, of the hand when the wrist is extended.	Associated metabolic encephalopathy, liver or kidney failure, hepatic encephalopathy, Wilson's dz, CO2 toxicity, phenytoin

Brain Death Criteria

- **No respiratory drive for 10 – 20 minutes**
- **Body temp < 34°**
- **Irreversible absence of all cerebral and brainstem reflexes and no spontaneous breaths**
- **EEG isoelectric for 30 minutes**
- **No cerebral circulation by Doppler or angiography**
- **Minimum of 24 hour observance in adults with anoxic-ischemic brain damage with a negative drug screen**
- **NOTE: Is is normal to see spinal reflexes or limbs move/twitch after death (AKA: Lazarus sign/Lazarus reflex): causes false hope for family members.**

Inhaled Anesthetics

- ↑ Cerebral blood flow = ↑ ICP
- Myocardial depression = ↓ CO
- Hypotension
- Respiratory depression = ↓ TV
- ↓ Renal function
- **Reversal** of anesthetics: **Naloxone or Naloxone with Flumazenil**
- **Malignant Hyperthermia** caused by anesthetics (fever and severe muscle contractions/rigid: same MOA as neuroleptic malignant syndrome and ETC uncoupling): TX: **Dantrolene** (blocks Ryanodine receptors to stop release of Ca from sarcoplasmic reticulum)
- ↑ MAC = ↓ Potency = Low volume of distribution = low solubility in the blood = fast onset (ie: nitrous oxide)
- ↓ MAC = ↑ Potency = High volume of distribution = high solubility in the blood = slow onset = greater gradient in the tissues

(MAC: Minimum Alveolar Concentration: **tip**: Notice the Volume of Distribution and Solubility both follow the direction of Potency)

Local Anesthetics (nerve blocks)

- Blocks Na channels
- If given with epinephrine = vasoconstriction to stop bleeding.
  Do not use epinephrine on extremities, fingers, toes, penis: vasoconstriction = ischemia
- **Order of loss: pain → temperature → touch → pressure**
- Order of nerve blockade: small diameter fibers > large diameter fibers
  Myelinated fibers > unmyelinated fibers
  small myelinated fibers > small unmyelinated fibers > large myelinated fibers > large unmyelinated fibers

Nerves and Anesthetics

- Anesthetic block (AKA: pudendal block, saddle block) injected near the **ischial spine** in the pelvis blocks the **pudendal nerve.**
  MC used in obstetrics to block pain in the perineum, vulva and vagina. (MC: Lidocaine or Chloroprocaine).
  Injected into the pudendal canal where the pudendal nerve is located.

OPHTHALMOLOGY

Eye Anatomy

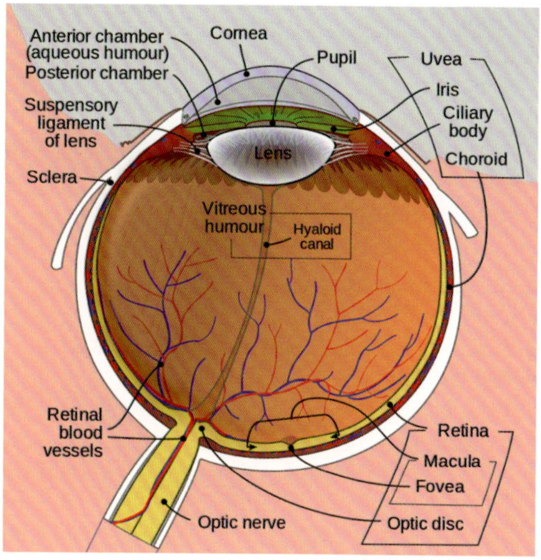

- Optic Nerve: (AKA: CN II) transmits visual information from the retina to the brain via the route: retina (optic disc) → optic nerve → optic chiasm → optic tract → lateral geniculate nucleus (LGN) → optic radiations → occipital cortex (visual cortex).
  Develops from the optic stalks in the 7th week of embryonic development and is composed of retinal ganglion and glial cells
- Retina: Inner light-sensitive coat of the eye. The cornea and lens create an image on the retina via chemical and electrical events that lead to nerve impulses via the optic nerve to the brain
- Choroid: Vascular layer of the eye between the retina and sclera. Provides oxygen and nutrients to the retina.
- Blood supply: Two circulations: Retinal and uveal, both are supplied by posterior ciliary arteries which come off the ophthalmic artery.
  Ophthalmic Artery branches off into the Central Retinal Artery travels, which travels with the optic nerve and enters the eye.
  Central retinal artery and vein are the sole source of blood supply and drainage to the retina. Blockages can cause damage to the retina as well as blindness due to ischemia and edema.
  Uveal Circulation: Supplied by branches directly off the ophthalmic artery. Supplies uvea and outer and middle layers of the retina.
  Retinal Circulation: Supplies by the Central retinal artery (branch of the Ophthalmic artery). Central retinal artery supplies nutrients to the inner retina and surface of the optic nerve.

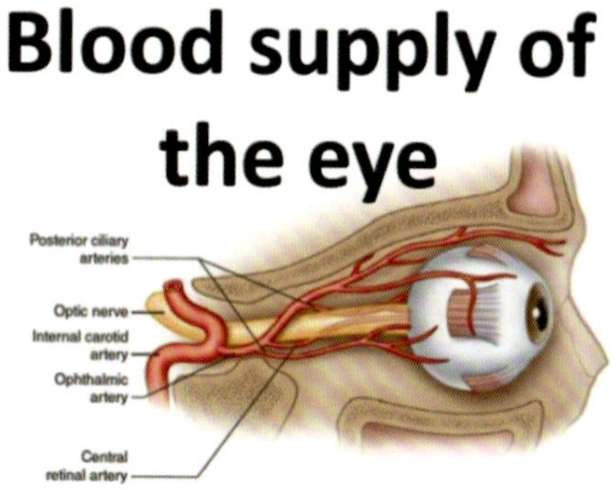

- Macula of the Retina: (AKA: Macula lutea): Pigmented area near the center of the retina containing the largest concentration of cone cells. It is responsible for central, high-resolution vision
- Cone Cells: Photoreceptor cells in the retina responsible for **color vision** and function best in bright light
- Rod Cells: Photoreceptor cells in the retina responsible for **peripheral vision** and do not require bright light
- Sclera: The "white of the eye". Outer layer of the eye consisting of collagen and elastic fibers
- Iris: Controls the diameter and size of the pupil and the amount of light reaching the retina
  This is the structure that gives our eyes their "color" (blue eyes, green eyes, brown eyes)
  (The iris and pupil work like a camera with the pupil being the aperture and the iris the diaphragm)
- Pupil: A black hole in the center of the iris that allows light through to strike the retina
- Lens: Biconvex structure in the eye. The lens can change shape to allow it to focus on objects so that a sharp image of this object can be formed on the retina. It works with the cornea to refract light.
- Cornea: Clear front surface of the eye that covers the iris, pupil and anterior chamber. Works with the lens to refract light (change the direction of a wave of light).
- Anterior chamber: Fluid (aqueous humor) filled space inside the eye between the iris and cornea.
  This area is pathologic for glaucoma (blockage of the canal of Schlemm = increased intraocular pressure) and for Hyphema (blood collecting in the anterior chamber)
- Aqueous Humour: Gelatinous fluid secreted from the ciliary epithelium (structure supporting the lens). It functions to maintain intraocular pressure, provide nutrition, has immunoglobulins and provides protection against dust and pollen.
- Canal of Schlemm: Channel in the eye that collects aqueous humor from the anterior chamber and sends it to the blood stream via anterior ciliary veins.. If the channel is blocked = ocular HTN
- Ciliary Muscle: Ring of smooth muscle that controls accommodation (viewing objects at varying distances) by changing the shape of the lens
- **Sphincter Pupillae Muscle: Circular muscle in the iris, circling the pupil, that functions to constrict the pupil**
- **Sphincter Pupillae Muscle: Parasympathetic**
- **Radial Dilator Muscle: Dilates the pupil.**
- **Radial Dilator Muscle: Sympathetic**
- Suspensory Ligament: Fibrous strands connecting the ciliary body to the lens
- Vitreous Humor/Body: Clear viscous gel that fills the space between the lens and retina. It is composed of phagocytes to remove cellular debris in the visual field.
- Uvea: Contains vascular structures, iris, ciliary body and choroid. Pigmented layer that is between the retina and the sclera

Pupillary Controls

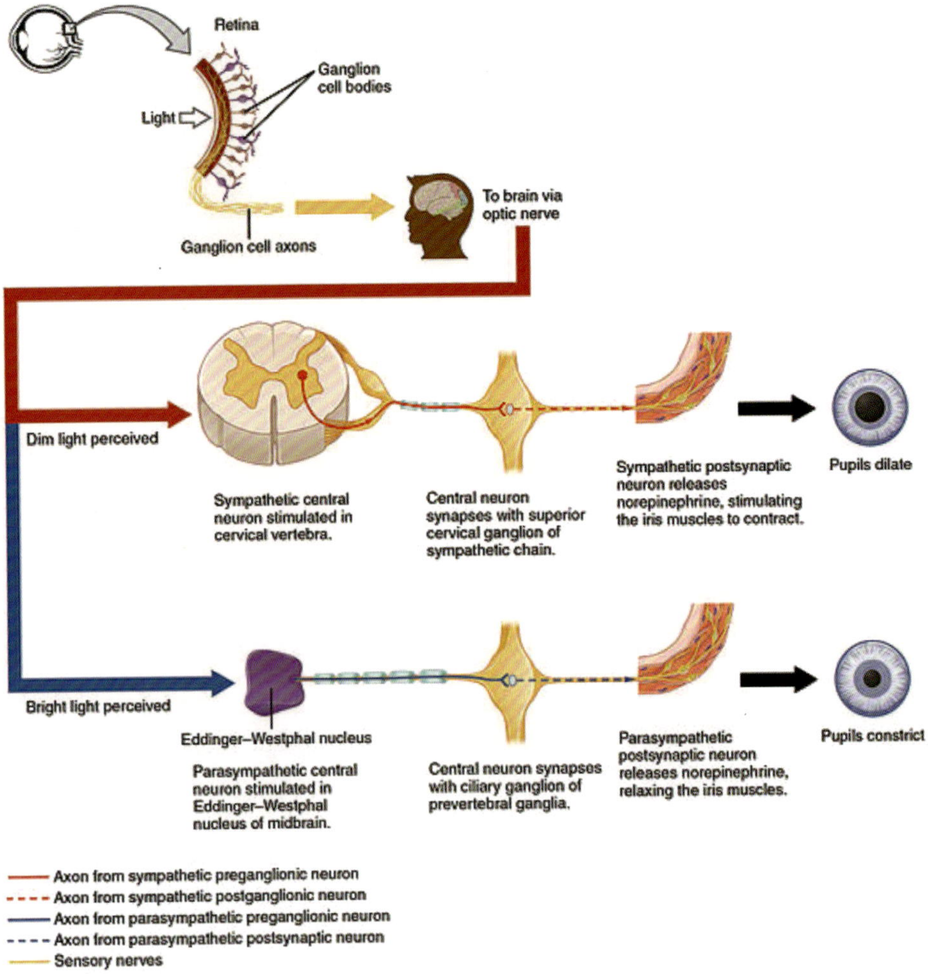

Pupillary Control: Sympathetic vs Parasympathetic

Sympathetic and Parasympathetic Control

Mydriasis
- Sympathetic
- Dilates iris
- **Radial muscles constrict ➔ dilation**
- (**tip**: my**D**riasis = **D**ilated)

Miosis
- Parasympathetic
- **Sphincter (Circular) muscle constricts ➔ contraction** (**tip**: "**C**"ircular = "**C**"onstricts)
- Controlled by CN III
- Damage to CN III = lose consensual response
- **Damage to CN III = CN III Palsy ("Down and Out")**

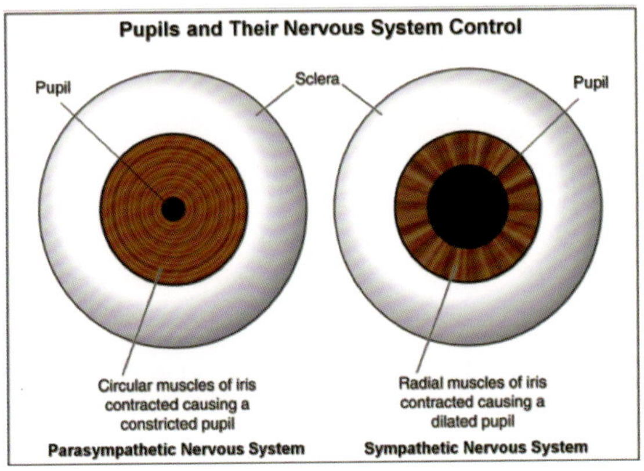

Refractive Errors (Cornea or lens isn't evenly curved so light rays aren't bent (refracted) properly)

Myopia (Nearsightedness: Objects near to you are clear but object further away are blurry)

- **Convex, ciliary muscles contract = lens relaxes/curves**
- Eye is too long or the **lens is curved** too much so light is focused in front of the retina
- **NOTE**: Be aware the eyesight in a patient with myopia can **temporarily improve as they age**. As they age, the lens will begin to relax. During the time it has relaxed to the curve of a normal eye, the patient's vision will improve. As they continue to age and the lens continues to flatten, their vision quality will decrease and they will experience hyperopia.

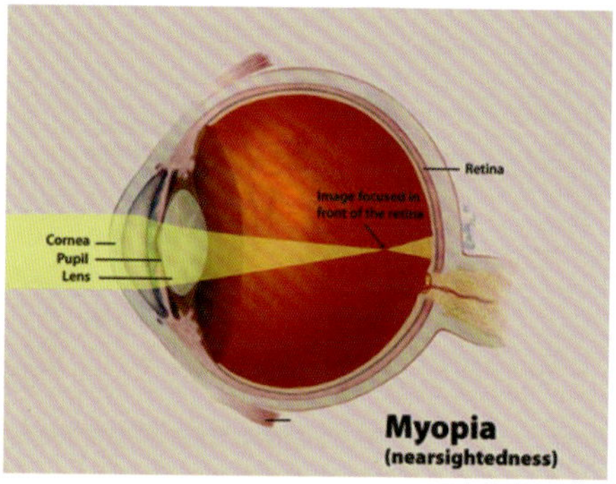

Hyperopia (Farsightedness: Objects far from you are clear but objects close are blurry)

- **Ciliary muscles relax** = **lens flattens**. Loss of elasticity.
- Eye is too short so light is focused behind retina

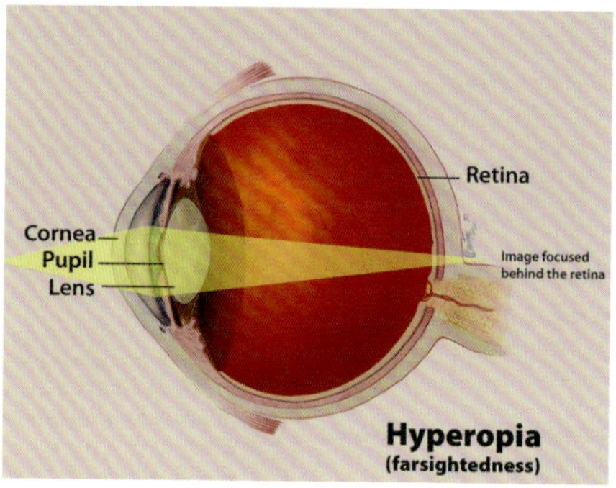

Astigmatism

- Cornea or lens is curved too steeply in one direction, blurring the vision

Presbyopia – Age related

- **Normal aging** due to ↓ **elasticity in the lens.**
- Difficulty ready things up close. Can't read fine print, must hold things far to read.
- Begins occurring in the 40's
- TX: Reading glasses

Corneal Reflexes

- Afferent arm: CN V
- Efferent arm: CN VII

Cranial Nerves and the Eye

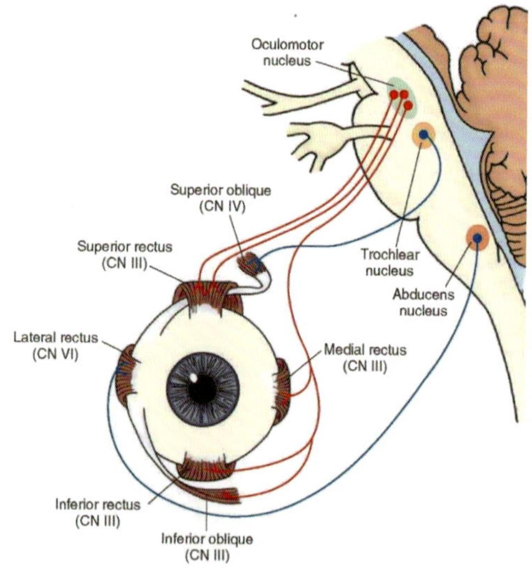

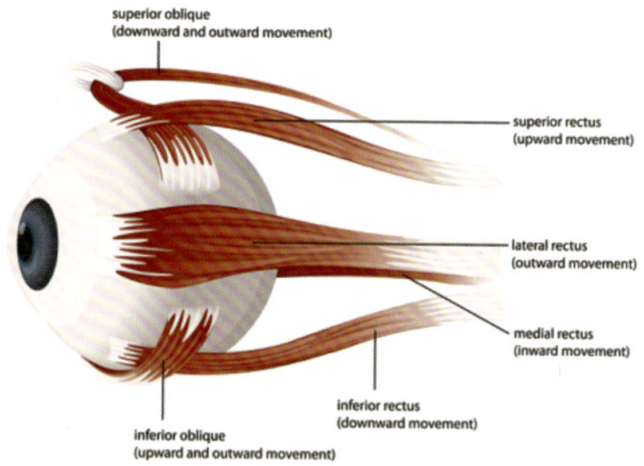

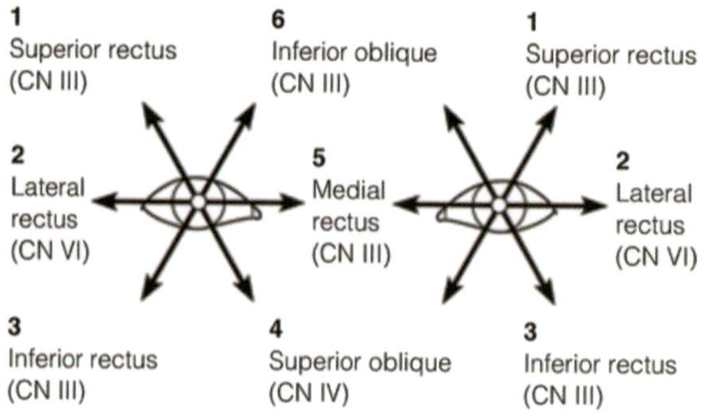

Eye Muscles, Innervation, Lesions

Cranial Nerve	Muscle and Function	Lesion
CN III MC site of intracranial Aneurysm (PCA)	Superior Rectus: Adduct Medial Rectus: Depress Inferior Rectus: Elevate Inferior Oblique: Externally rotate Levator Palpebrae: Elevating upper eyelid	**"Down and Out" causing: ptosis, pupil dilation and loss of accommodation**. **Cranial Nerve III Palsy (aka: Oculomotor Nerve Palsy)** (SR) Eyes down and lateral (MR) Diagonal diplopia (IR) Dilation of pupil (IO) Loss of accommodation (LP) Ptosis
CN IV	**Superior Oblique**: Internally rotate, depress, abduction. Elevates eye in the abducted position.	Vertical and horizontal diplopia, Eyes deviate up. Unable to look down (can't read paper or go down steps).
CN VI	**Lateral Rectus**: Abduct	Horizontal diplopia, Eye deviates medially. Unable to look medial, only to center.
Optic Nerve		Blindness – ipsilateral side
Optic Chiasm		Bitemporal hemianopia
Optic Tract		Contra homonymous hemianopia
Frontal Lobe Destruction		Ipsilateral deviation of eye
MLF (Medical Longitudinal Fasciculus) (AKA: Medial Rectus Palsy)	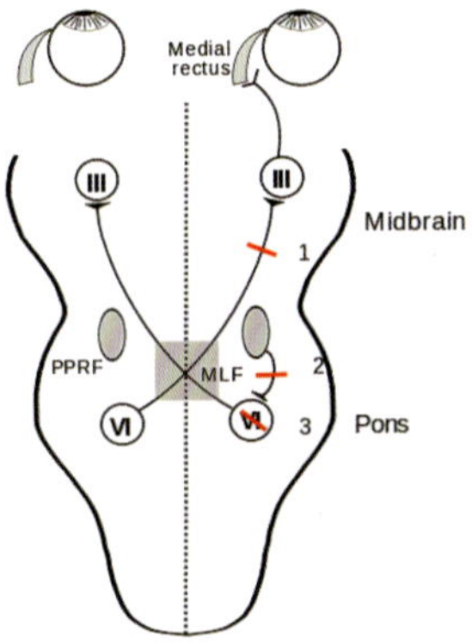 CN VI is not able to signal CN III.	Demyelination **(Multiple Sclerosis):** abducts one eye and the other stays straight with nystagmus. Neither eye can look medially.

Eye Pathologies and Injuries

Central Retinal Artery Occlusion	Central Retinal Vein Occlusion
Blood flow from the Central Retinal Artery is blocked. Central retinal artery provides oxygen and nutrients to the retina. Ischemia to inner retina = ↓ blood flow. MCC: carotid artery atherosclerosis SX: Monocular **Sudden**, acute, **PAINLESS** loss of monocular vision (vision loss in one eye). Funduscope exam shows: **red lesion ("cherry red spot")** with **pale (halo)** color of the retina surrounding it and dark macula. Paleness is due to ischemia from blocked vessel. Associated with transient Amaurosis Fugax. ↑ risk from: CAD, endocarditis, long bone fractures, valvular disease, hypercoagulability, vasculitis, myxoma. TX: **100% oxygen, Acetazolamide**, ocular massage	Milder form of Central Retinal Artery Occlusion (same causes), Monocular loss of vision. SX: **Very bloody, sudden painless** loss of monocular vision. (**tip**: central Vein = V for Very bloody). Due to the extravasation of blood into the retina. Tortuous veins, retinal hemorrhage, cotton wool spots, pallor of the optic disc. Associated with HTN. The Central retinal artery and vein are the sole source of blood supply and drainage to the retina. Blockages can cause damage to the retina as well as blindness due to ischemia and edema. TX: **Ranibizumab**

Diabetic Retinopathy
Retinal damage due to diabetes. Persistent hyperglycemia causes microvascular retinal changes.

Non-proliferative: Initial stage. Most patients do not notice any change in their vision. Early changes are reversible. Damaged capillaries can leak lipids and blood into the retina causing retinal swelling (macular edema).

Proliferative: **Neo-vascularization** (blood vessels proliferate). The fragile new vessels hemorrhage and destroy the retina. These hemorrhages show up as white spots (AKA: microvascular changes) on the retina ("**Cotton wool spots**")

TX: Laser photocoagulation (cauterize ocular blood vessels). VEGF has also been injected into the vitreous chamber every 1 – 2 months to control neovascularization (ie: Ranibizumab, Aflibercept or Bevacizumab). .

All diabetics must see an ophthalmologist and podiatrist once a year.

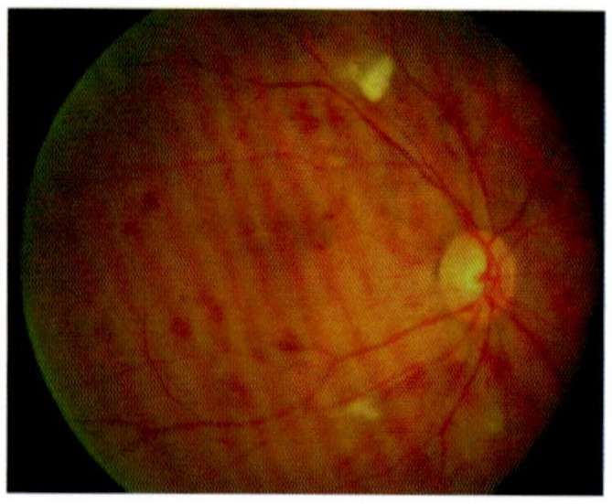

Vitreous Hemorrhage
MC: seen with Proliferative Diabetic Retinopathy. This occurs when a diabetic loses sight.

SX: Sudden loss of vision, **floaters**, fundus is hard to see, dark red glow.
TX: Sleep upright. Vitrectomy can remove a vitreal hemorrhage that is obstructing the vision.

Uveitis
Inflammation of the uvea.
MC: Seen with autoimmune diseases.
3 Classifications:

Anterior Uveitis: MC: 90% of Uveitis cases.
Inflammation of **anterior chamber**, iris and ciliary body.
SX: Redness (red conjunctiva), **eye pain**, blurred vision, floaters (dark spots floating in visual field), irregular pupil, **keratic precipitates (mutton fat)** on the cornea, dilated ciliary vessels, **photophobia, hypopyon** (sterile pus), iris nodules.
Associated with: **HLA-B27, arthritis diseases**

Intermediate Uveitis: Affects one eye.
SX: Floaters, blurred vision.
No pain or photophobia

DX: Slit lamp exam
TX: **Topical steriods**

Posterior Uveitis: Inflammation of back of eye.
SX: Floaters, Blurred vision, photopsia, seeing flashing lights, NO pain, ↓ visual acuity.

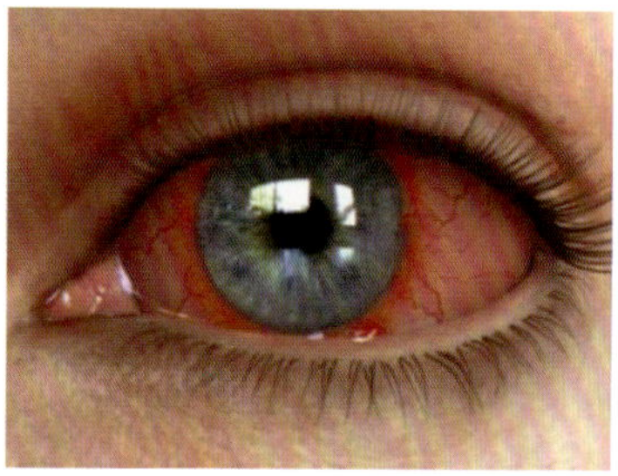

Optic Neuritis

Inflammation of the optic nerve because of the swelling and **destruction of the myelin sheath** covering the **optic nerve**.

MCC: Multiple sclerosis in females from 20 – 45 years old.

SX: Sudden loss of vision (partial or complete), sudden blurred vision, pain on movement of affected eye. . Color vision can appear "washed out", difficulty in judging depth and vision worsens with increased body temperature., swollen optic disc, central scotoma, afferent pupillary defect.

Visual function spontaneously improves over several months.

Postoperative Endophthalmitis

Inflammation of the vitreous humor in the anterior and posterior segments of the eye following cataract surgery due to perioperative introduction of the microbial organisms into the eye from the patients normal flora or contaminated instruments.
Usually occurs within 6 weeks post surgery.

SX: ↓ vision, dull ache, swollen eyelid, red conjunctiva, corneal edema.

TX: **IV Vancomycin and Cefuroxime**

Retinitis
(AKA: Retinitis Pigmentosa)
Inflammation of the retina of the eye.

SX: Necrosis and edema causing scarring and blindness.

Causes: CMV, Candida, Toxoplasmosis, Herpes

CMV Retinitis **MC of blindness in HIV**.
Candida spreads through bloodstream causing abscesses in the retina.

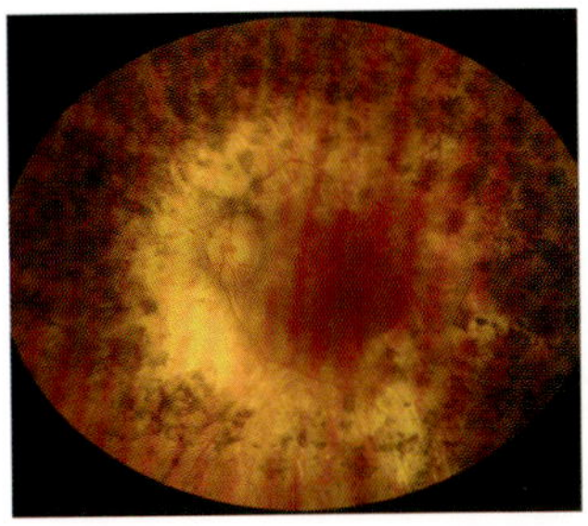

Papilledema

Optic disc swelling due to ↑ **ICP.**

Papilledema is the sign for **end organ damage** in cases of hypertensive emergencies. It is also a key factor that must be present in Pseudotumor Cerebri.

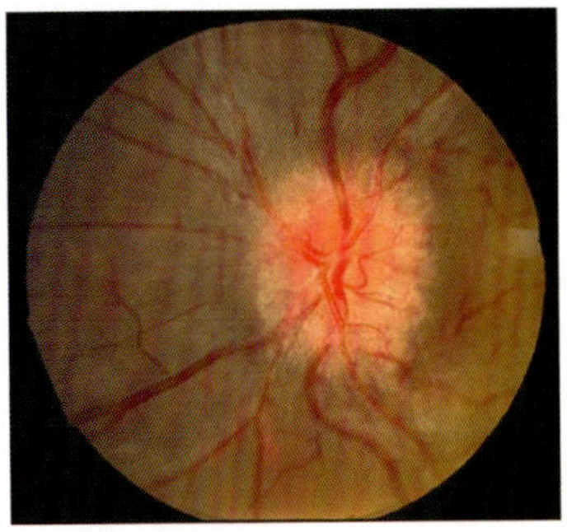

Glaucoma
Eye disorders that result in optic nerve damage due to increased intraocular pressure.
Two categories: Open-angle and Closed-angle

Open-angle (AKA: Chronic Glaucoma)
SX: Slow to develop, painless, asymptomatic
DX: tonometry (measures "tone" of t intraocular pressure (IOP)
TX: **Pilocarpine**, topical beta blockers: **Timolol**

Closed-angle - Emergency
SX: **Sudden, severe pain**, redness, nausea, vomiting, **rock-hard eyes** (↑↑ IOP), **halos** around lights, ↑ IOP pushes iris forward, **fixed and dilated midpoint pupil** (does not react to light)

Caution: do NOT give epinephrine due to mydriatic action

TX: IV Mannitol or Acetazolamide

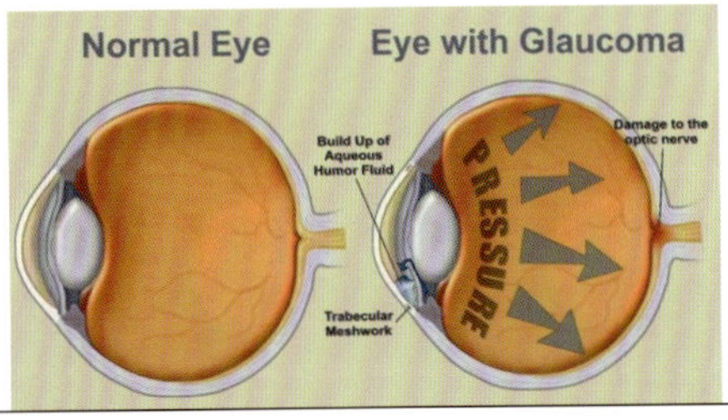

Cataract

Opacification (clouding) and thickening of the lens resulting in ↓ vision affecting one or both eyes.

Risk: MCC: ↑ **age**.
Build up of sorbitol (aldolase reductase).
Smoking, trauma, diabetes, alcohol, **chronic steroid use**, prolonged exposure to sunlight (ultraviolet light), congenital, galactosemia (Aldolase Reductase)

SX: **faded colors**, blurry vision, halos around light, difficulty seeing at night.
(Note: don't forget the bio chem connection with sorbitol and aldolase reductase).

TX: Surgery to remove lens.

Complication: **Postoperative Endophthalmitis**
(see above)

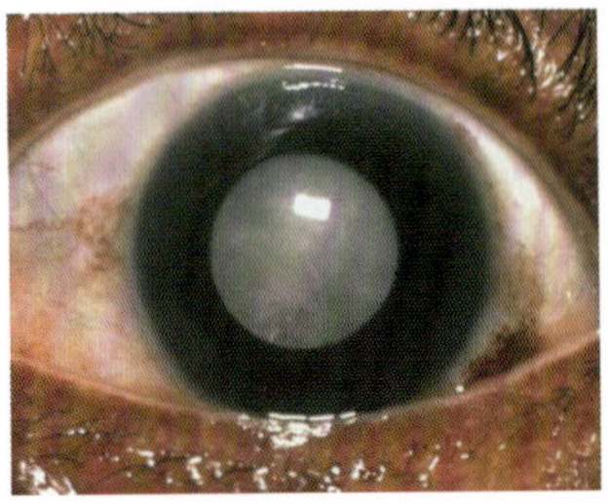

Closed Angle Glaucoma	Macular Degeneration
Closed Angle Glaucoma **Emergency** **If not treated within 2 – 5 hours = blindness.** SX: **Sudden, unilateral severe pain**, **red eye**, nausea, vomiting, **rock-hard eyes** (↑↑ IOP), **halos** around lights, ↑ intraocular pressure (IOP) pushes iris forward, **fixed and dilated midpoint pupil** (does not react to light). DX: Tonometry **BIT:** **Pilocarpine drops** (to constrict the pupil), **IV Mannitol or Acetazolamide** **(helps open up the angle)** and Acetazolamide ↓ production aqueous humor. Others drugs: **Latanoprost, Travoprost** (Prostaglandin analogs), **Timolol** (topical beta blocker). **Do NOT use epinephrine in closed angle glaucoma.**	**Macular Degeneration** MCC blindness in elderly in the USA Two types: Atrophic (dry) and Neovascular (wet). Wet type is the cause of 90% of the blindness. SX: Bilateral **loss of central vision.** Atrophic: Accumulation of drusen (cellular debris) between the retina and the choroid. No therapy. Neovascular (wet) is MCC of permanent blindness from macular degeneration TX: **VEGF inhibitor**: **Ranibizumab, Bevacizumab, Aflibercept** 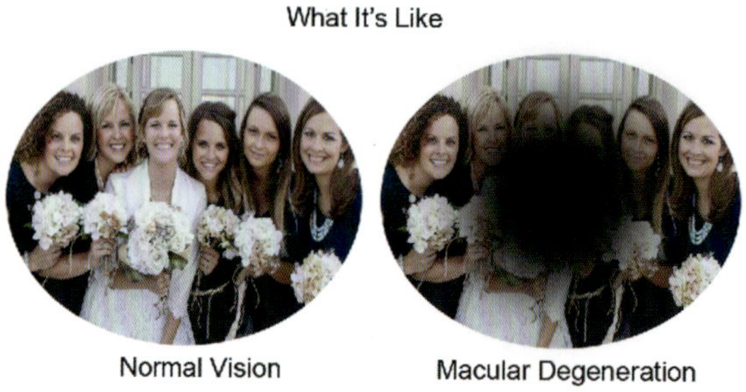 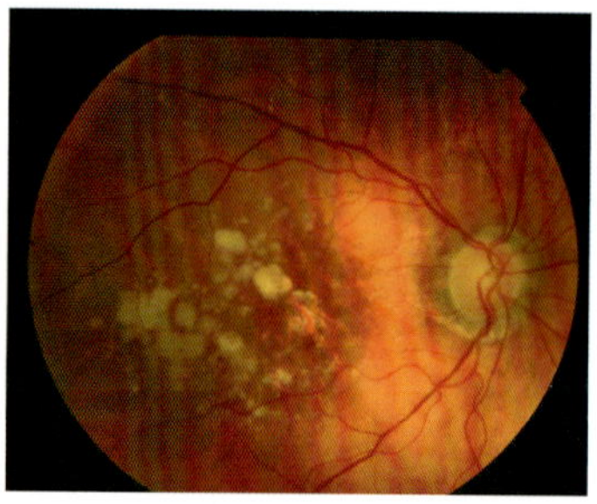
Open Angle Glaucoma **Gradual loss of peripheral vision (tunnel vision).** Common in African Americans	

Amaurosis Fugax	
Amaurosis Fugax **Painless**, transient monocular visual loss normally due to **emboli** from an atherosclerotic **carotid artery**, cardiac emboli, atrial myxoma, vasospasm, Temporal Arteritis. Can present as a TIA. SX: Monocular vision loss that appears as a **"curtain coming down"** into the field of vision, dimming, blurring. Vision loss last from a few seconds to hours. TX: Diagnostic work up to treat underlying cause. **Carotid Doppler and an ECHO** to look for the source of the emboli. **WARNING: This is a sign for an impending stroke.**	

Abrasions

Scratch to the cornea due to trauma or contact lenses.

SX: Feels like sand in the eyes
DX: Fluorescein stain drops. Blue light is shined on the eye; the dye makes the cornea appear green so that it shows any abrasions or scratches.
No treatment. Refer to ophthalmologist. Do not patch abrasions caused by contact lenses.

Fluorescein stain (drops) under blue light.

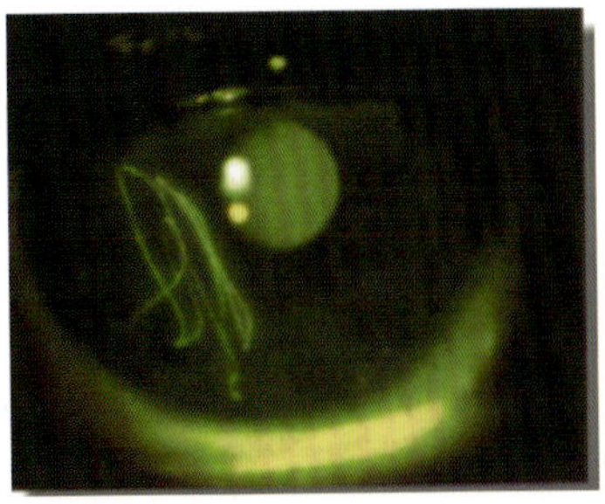

Corneal abrasion after fluorescein drops

Retinal Detachment – Emergency

Retina pulls away from its underlying support tissue. Separation of the layers of the retina.

Risk: Trauma. Anything that pulls on the retina, diabetic retinopathy, severe myopia (nearsightedness).

SX: Sudden, **painless, unilateral loss of vision** described as **"curtain coming down"** photopsia (flashes of light), increase in floaters. Retina has grey appearance.

Without immediate treatment it can lead to blindness.
TX: Various methods: laser, injectable gas, cryotherapy, surgery.

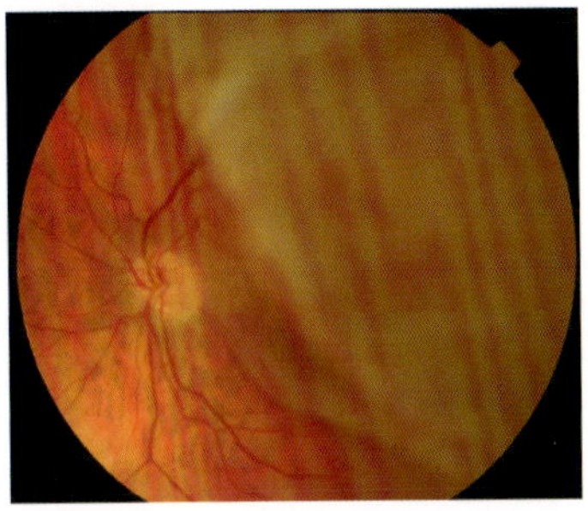

Eye Injuries

High Velocity (drilling or grinding)
Foreign body sensation, photophobia, excess lacrimation

DX: Fluorescein Exam. Woods lamp.

Low Velocity
↑ possibility of globe penetration.
Interocular foreign body formation.

Spared Eye Injury

Immune mediated inflammation of one eye after a penetrating injury to the other because it uncovers **hidden antigens**.

SX: Floating spots, blurred vision, redness.

Aniridia
Absence of the iris.
Associated with **Wilm's Tumor**

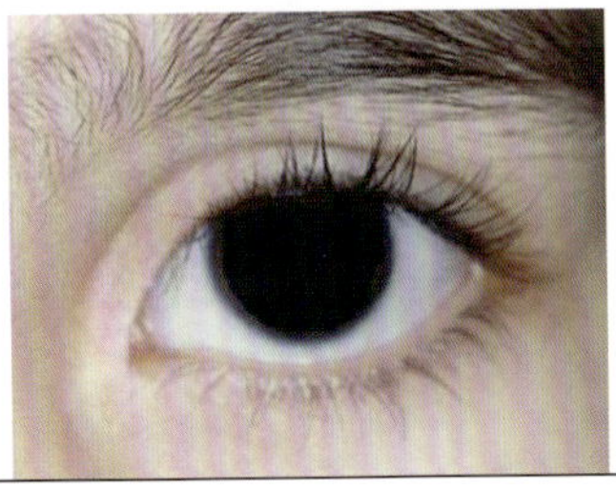

Coloboma of the Iris
A hole in one of the structures of the eye (iris, chorioid, retina or optic disc) that is present from birth. Occurs when a gap (chorioid fissure) fails to close. MC occurrence is in the iris.

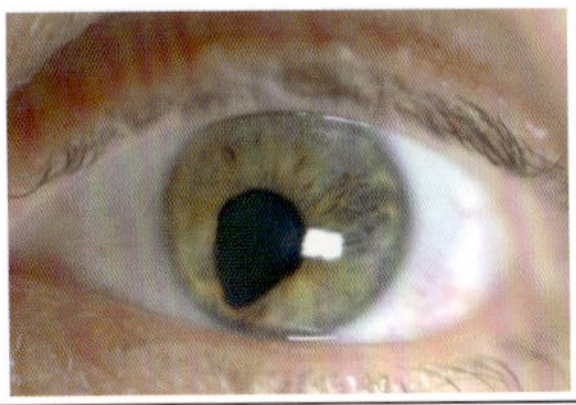

Eye Infections

Orbital Cellulitis
Pre-Orbital and Orbital SX:
Eyelid edema, erythema, tenderness,
Fever, leukocytosis.

Orbital Cellulitis (dangerous), caused by Bacterial Sinusitis:

Additional SX: (above Sx) **plus**:
Ophthalmoplegia (weak eye muscles), pain with ocular movement, proptosis (forward push of eyeball).
Complication: blindness, intracranial abscess, sinus venous thrombosis
TX: **IV antibiotics: Vancomycin + Ampicillin/Sulbactrum**

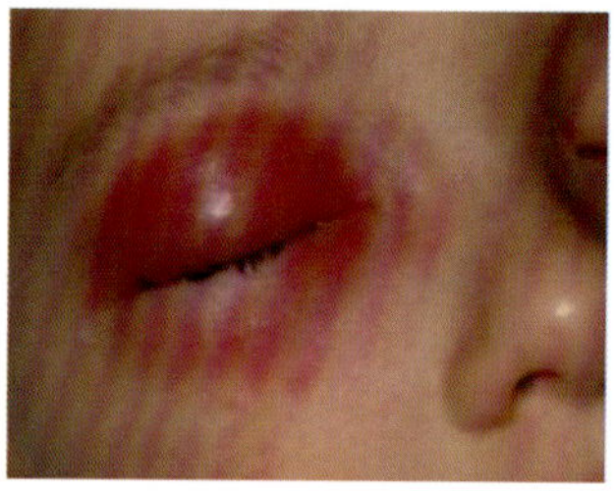

Bacterial conjunctivitis
(AKA: Keratitis)

SX: Unilateral infection,
Mucopurulent discharge, not itchy, swelling of eyelid,
No adenopathy (swollen lymph nodes), low level contagious

TX: topical antibiotics: Erythromycin, Gentamicin, Bacitracin

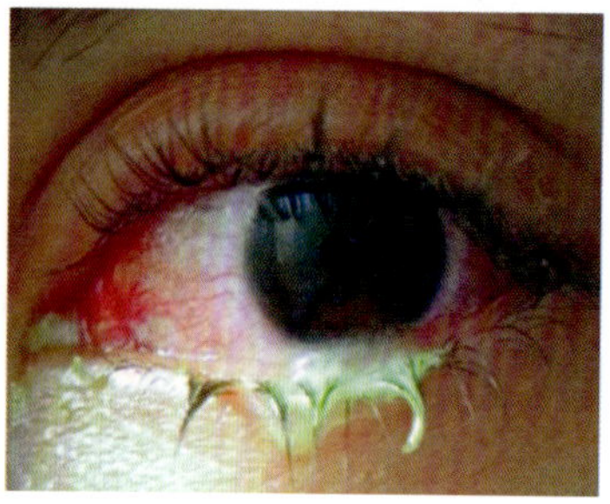

Pink Eye (Conjunctivitis)
Adenovirus, No Envelope, Double stranded, linear

Inflammation of the conjunctiva (outermost layer of the eye and inner surface of the eyelid)
Can affect one or both eyes.
Highly contagious

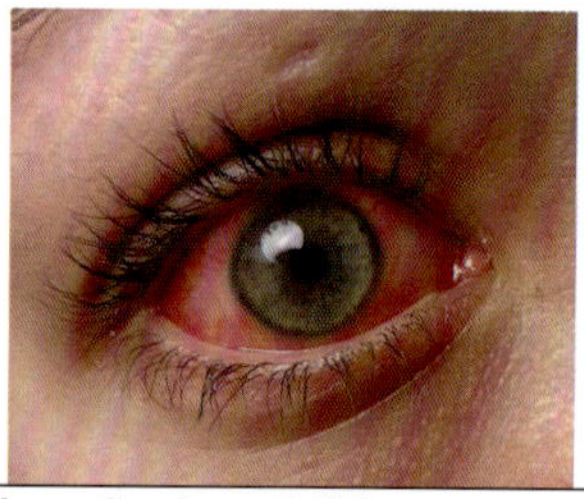

Viral Conjunctivitis
1 or both eyes
Discharge of fluid: red and crusty
Assoc. with common cold, URI, sore throat

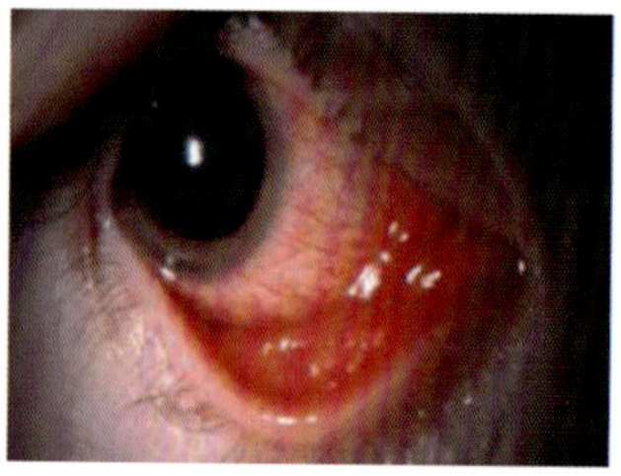

Allergies - Conjunctivitis
Both eyes
Bilateral itching and redness
Nasal congestion (pale, boggy mucosa)
Increased tearing (lacrimation)
Cobblestone appearance of conjunctiva
SX due to histamine from mast cells

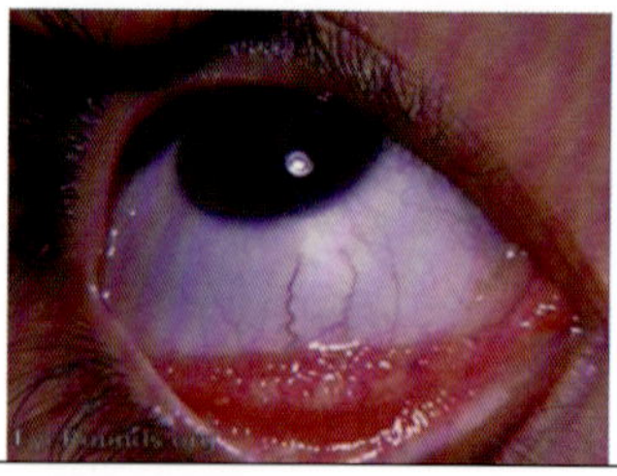

Chalazion (AKA: Meibomian gland lipogranuloma)	**Hordeolum (AKA: Stye)**
Cyst in the eyelid due to inflammation of a blocked **meibomian gland.** MC: upper eyelid SX: Subacute and **painless nodule** on the inside of the lid verses on the lid margin, swelling of eyelid, increased tearing, heaviness of eyelid, sensitivity to darkness. Chronic inflammation and will not resolve without intervention. TX: Antibiotic **eye drops: chloramphenicol, fusidic acid** 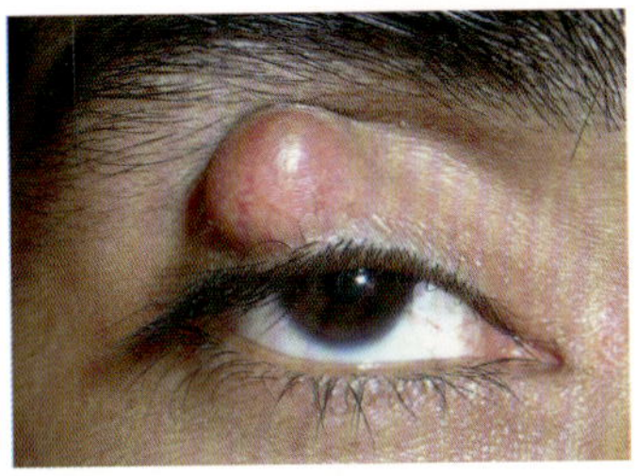	Infection of the **sebaceous glands** of Zeis at the base of the eyelashes or an infection of the apocrine sweat glands of Moll. They can be external or internal styes. External: form on the outside of the lids. Internal: due to infections of the meibomian sebaceous glands on the inside of the eyelid. MCC: **S. aureus** Acute onset and shorter in duration than chalazion's. SX: **Painful, contain water and pus**, crusting of eyelid margins, burning in the eye, redness, itching, discomfort when blinking, sensation of foreign body in eye, tearing, mucous discharge Complication: progression to a chalazion, eye cellulitis TX: Self-resolving in 7 – 10 days without treatment. Good hygiene: proper hand washing, warm washcloths in the morning to remove residue from oil glands around the eyes preventing blockage. No sharing of cosmetics. Med TX: Ophthalmic **erythromycin ointment** 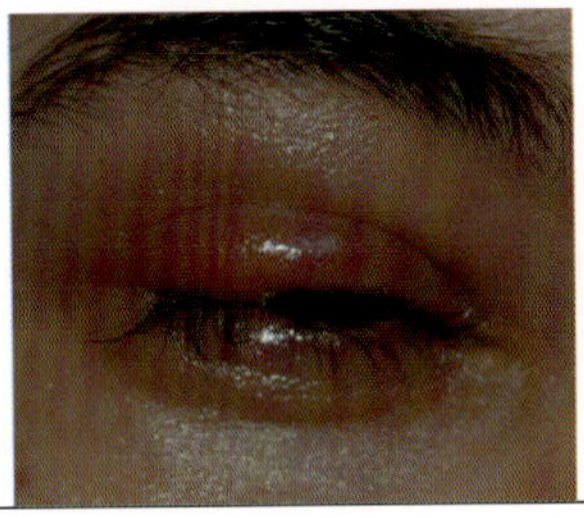

Differentials in Conjunctivitis

Bacterial Conjunctivitis	**Viral Conjunctivitis**
Purulent, pus, thick discharge	Watery discharge
Not itchy	Itchy
Difficult to transmit	Easy to transmit
Unilateral	Bilateral
No lymph node swelling	Preauricular lymph node swelling

Eye Pathologies Related to HIV and other Communicable Diseases

Herpes and Varicella Retinitis (VZV)
(Acute Retinal Necrosis)

- Eye pain.
- Central necrosis of the retina.
- Whitening of the retina with marked blood vessel closure. No hemorrhages.
- Maculopapular-vesicular rash preceded by pain with trigeminal distribution (forehead and eye)
- Fever, malaise, burning, itching
- Dendriform corneal ulcers.
- Keratitis of the eye.
- Peripheral retinal lesions.
- Rapid peripheral vision loss.
- Conjunctivitis
- Due to the reactivation of a latent infection by Varicella Zoster in the dorsal root of the trigeminal nerve ganglion.
- Complications: Optic neuritis, Retinal detachment.
- TX: **Acyclovir**

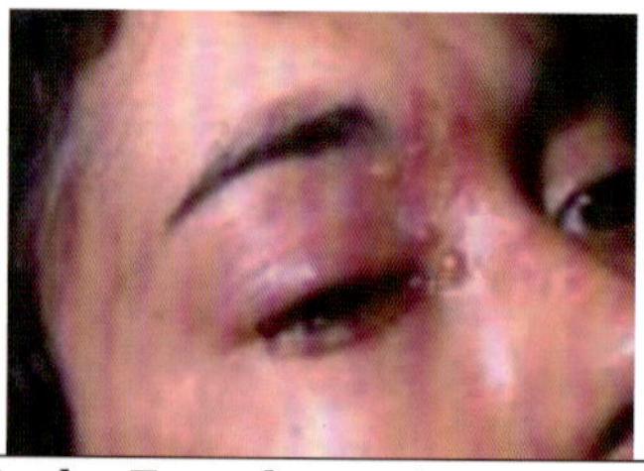
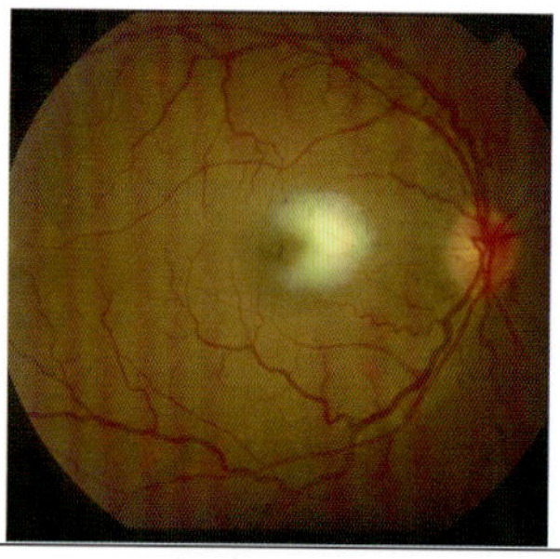

CMV Retinitis

- MC ocular opportunistic infection in HIV
- Painless. Floaters, flashing lights, mild, blurred vision.
- Fluffy, granular lesions by hemorrhages of the retinal vessels.
- Yellow-white patches (retinal opification): "Cotton Wool Spots"
- No keratitis.
- No Conjunctivitis.
- TX: **Gancyclovir, Foscarnet**

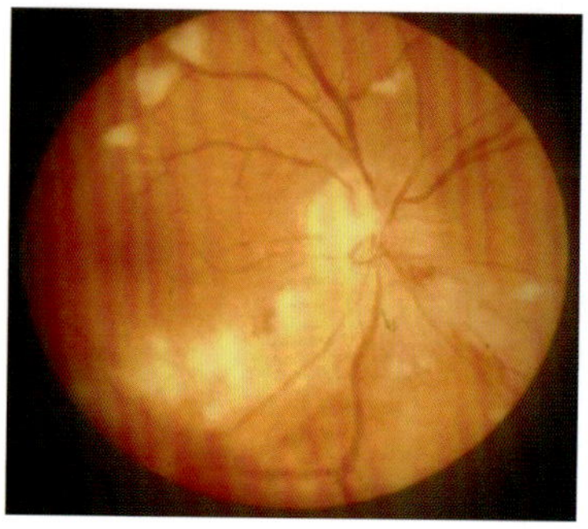

Ocular Toxoplasmosis
(Toxoplasma Retinochoroiditis)

- Necrotizing retinochoroiditis (posterior pole) of the inner layers of the retina
- White fluffy lesions surrounded by retinal edema

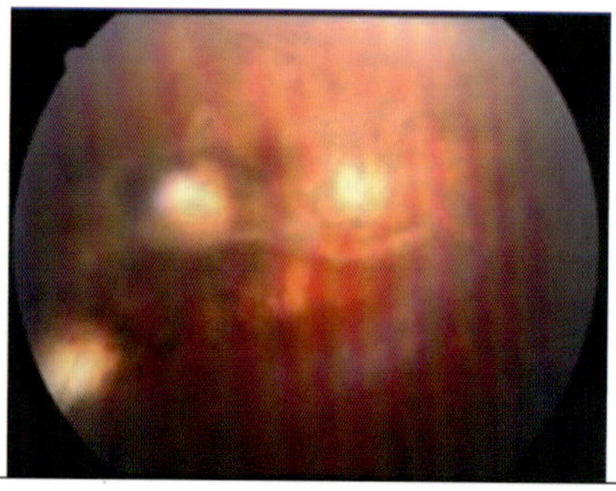

HIV Retinopathy

- **MC non-infectious complication of HIV individuals**
- **Oncotic lesions in the retinal nerve fiber layer**

Cotton Wood Spots, intraretinal hemorrhages, impaired color vision and contrast sensitivity that worsens with age.

Kaposi Sarcoma of the Eye

- Vascular neoplasm
- Non-tender nodule on the eyelid or conjunctiva. Normally only involves the skin but can progress to the GI tract or CNS.
- TX: Radiotherapy, cryotherapy, chemotherapy

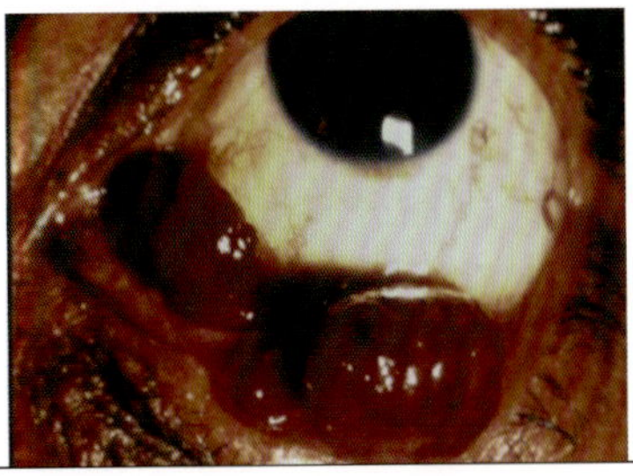

Squamous Cell Carcinoma of the Eye

- 3rd MC neoplasm associated with HIV
- Pink, gelatinous growth in the interpalpebral area
- Engorged blood vessels can be seen feeding the tumor
- TX: Local excision, cryotherapy
- Deep invasion and metastasis are rare

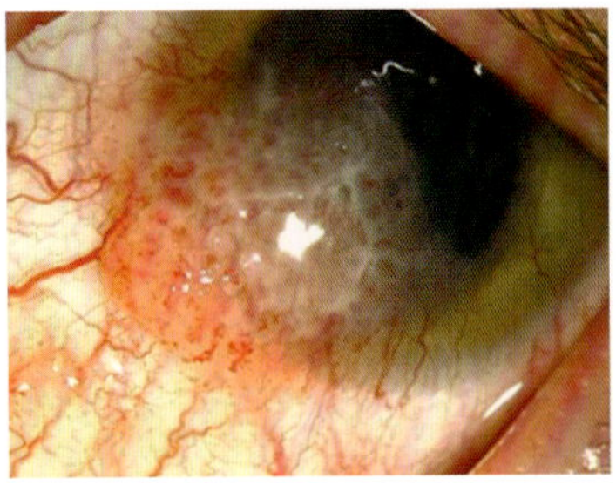

Trichomegaly
(AKA: Hypertrichosis)

Exaggerated growth of the eye lashes. Occurs in the later stages of HIV.

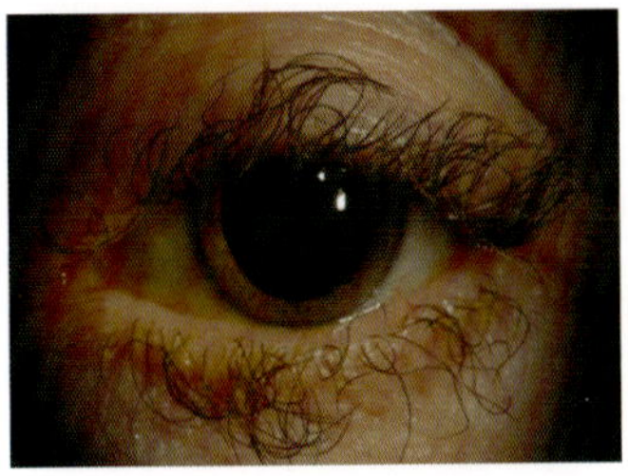

Sicca Syndrome
(Dry eye)

- Burning, uncomfortable red eyes
- Can be due to infection from blepharitis or destruction of the lacrimal glands.
- Can be associated with Sjogren's dz.
- TX: tear supplements

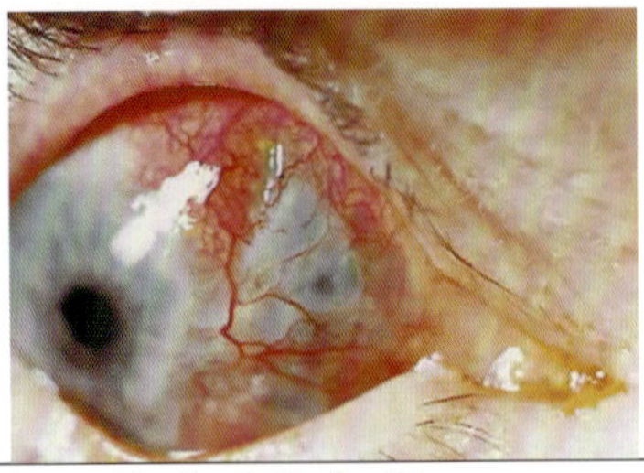

Syphilis Retinitis
AKA: Retinitis Pigmentosa, Syphilitic Chorioretinitis

- Uveitis, optic neuritis, nonnecrotizing retinitis
- Dermatologic and CNS symptoms may accompany
- Unilateral or bilateral pale yellow retinal lesions that involve the macula.
- Retinal detachment.
- **TX: Penicillin G**

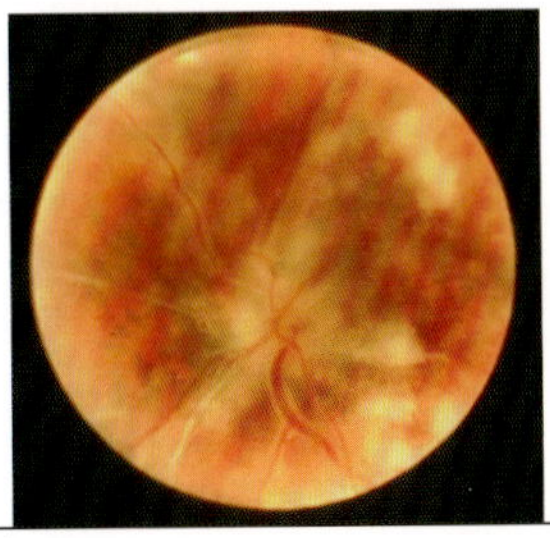

Candida Albicans Endophthalmitis

- History of IV drug use or indwelling central lines
- Floaters, whitish "puff-balls", vitreous strands. Infiltrates in the choroid and retina.
- **TX: Amp B and Fluconazole**

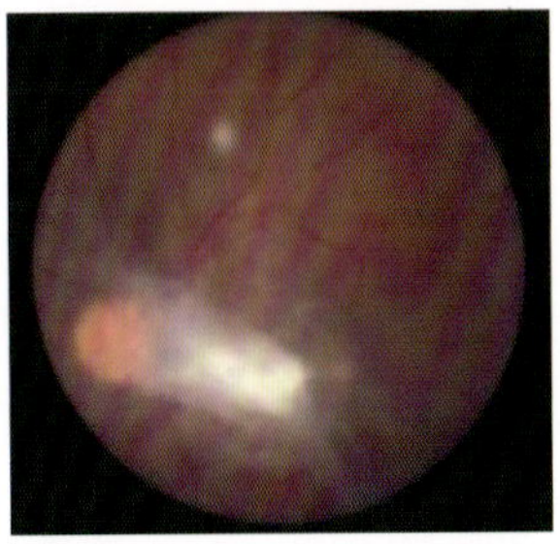

Herpes Keratitis
(AKA: Keratitis)

Infection of the cornea caused by the Herpes simplex virus

SX: Unilateral redness, swelling of conjunctiva and eyelids, small white itchy lesions on the cornea.

Complications: can lead to dendritic ulcers

DX: Fluorescein staining confirms dendritic pattern

EX: Oral Acyclovir, Famciclovir, Valacyclovir

Eye Tracts and Lesions

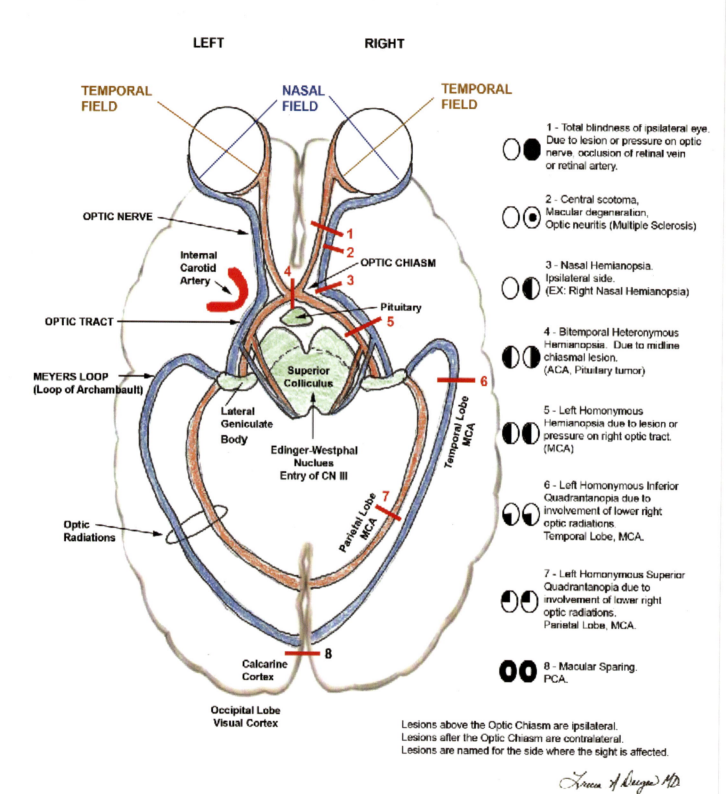

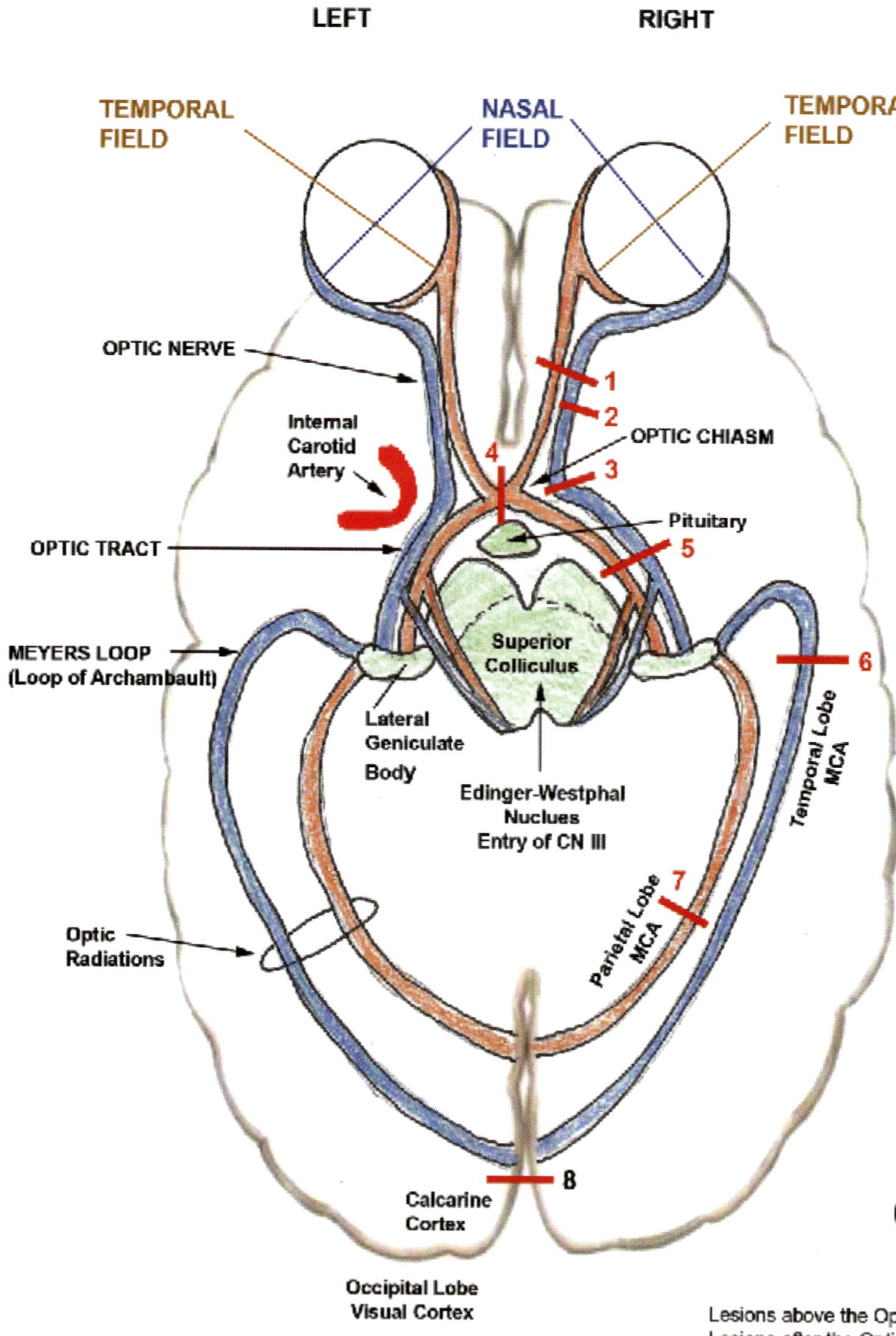

1 - Total blindness of ipsilateral eye. Due to lesion or pressure on optic nerve, occlusion of retinal vein or retinal artery.

2 - Central scotoma, Macular degeneration, Optic neuritis (Multiple Sclerosis)

3 - Nasal Hemianopsia. Ipsilateral side. (EX: Right Nasal Hemianopsia)

4 - Bitemporal Heteronymous Hemianopsia. Due to midline chiasmal lesion. (ACA, Pituitary tumor)

5 - Left Homonymous Hemianopsia due to lesion or pressure on right optic tract. (MCA)

6 - Left Homonymous Inferior Quadrantanopia due to involvement of lower right optic radiations. Temporal Lobe, MCA.

7 - Left Homonymous Superior Quadrantanopia due to involvement of lower right optic radiations. Parietal Lobe, MCA.

8 - Macular Sparing. PCA.

Lesions above the Optic Chiasm are ipsilateral.
Lesions after the Optic Chiasm are contralateral.
Lesions are named for the side where the sight is affected.

Eye Lesions

- Lesions that occur before the optic chiasm are ipsilateral effects
- Lesions that occur after the optic chiasm are contralateral effects
- Lesion Names: Are named for the side that the eye sight is affected.
  Example: If the lesion is **after** the optic chiasm (it becomes contra). So if the lesion occurred on the right side, it is named "left" to correspond to where the loss of vision actually takes place.
- Hemianopia = Hemi = half. This means that half of the eye/visual field is affected
- Homonymous = Homo = same. This means the same half/quarter of both eyes/visual fields are effected
- Quadrantic = quarter ("Pie in the sky" or "Pie down low")
- Bi = involves both left and right visual fields
- Anopia = blindness
- **Outer superior loop = temporal lobe** (don't forget, **Herpes** loves the temporal lobe)
- **Inferior loop = parietal lobe**
- Nasal retina = nasal field (inside/medial view). Information **crosses over** to the contralateral brain.
- Temporal retina = temporal field (outside/lateral view). Information does **not cross** over to the contralateral brain, it stays ipsilateral.

Structure Lesioned	Lesion Name	Associated Artery	Notes
Optic Nerve with both nasal and temporal Tracts lesioned	Anopia of the ipsilateral eye	Retinal Artery or Retinal Vein	Ipsilateral
Temporal tract lesioned	Macular Degeneration (Central sight) (AKA: Optic Neuritis, Central Scotoma) on the Temporal, ipsilateral side		Ipsilateral
Nasal tract	Binasal (nasal) Hemianopia. The nasal tract is lesioned so the nasal (medial) visual field is gone. The patient can still see fine out of both of their lateral views (temporal field).	Internal Carotid Artery	
Optic Chiasm	**Bitemporal Hemianopsia**. The temporal (lateral) visual field is gone in both eyes. MCC: Pituitary tumor	Anterior Comm. Artery	
Optic Tract	Homonymous Hemianopia (named left or right based on side vision loss) Vision loss is contra to lesion.	Middle Cerebral Artery	Contra
Optic Tract	If the visual blindness is on the left sides of both eyes this is called **left hemi-neglect** and is due to lesion in the **non-dominant (right)** side of the brain.	Middle Cerebral Artery	Contra
Superior Loop of Meyer's Loop	Upper quadrantic anopia. Visual blindness will be in the upper quarter (same side) of both eyes (named left or right based on the side of vision loss). Vision loss is contra to lesion. (**tip**: "pie" in the sky)	Middle Cerebral Artery	**Temporal lobe – Herpes Goes to the temporal lobe.** Contra
Inferior Loop of Baum's Loop	Lower quadrantic anopia. Visual blindness will be in the lower quarter (same side) of both eyes. ("Pie" in the bottom)	Middle Cerebral Artery	Parietal Lobe. Dorsal optic.
Occipital Cortex	Hemianopia with Macular Sparing (named right or left based on the side of vision loss). Vision loss is contra to the lesion.	Posterior Cerebral Artery	Occipital Lobe Contra

AUDIOLOGY

Sound

- **High frequency** sounds ➔ **oval** and round window ➔ **base of the cochlea**
- **Low frequency** sounds ➔ Apex of cochlea ➔ **helicotrema** (hair cells in this area detect low frequency sound)
- **Prolonged loud noise** damages the ciliated hairs of the Organ of Corti
- Organ of Corti: sensory epithelium on the basilar membrane that allows for transduction of auditory signals into action potentials. Vibrations move cochlear fluid and hair cells in the organ of Corti in order to produce electrochemical signals. Located in the cochlea.
- Semicircular Canal: Filled with endolymph in order to maintain balance of the body
- Tympanic Membrane (AKA: eardrum): Separates external ear from middle ear. Transmits sound from the air through the middle ear to the oval window.
- Auditory canal (AKA: ear canal, external auditory meatus): Extends from the pinna (ear outside of the head) to the eardrum
- Eustachian tube: Links the nasopharynx to the middle ear
- **Auditory Pathway**: Spiral ganglion ➔ CN VIII ➔ dorsal/ventral cochlear nuclei of the medulla ➔ superior olivary nuclei ➔ lateral lemniscus ➔ inferior colliculus of the midbrain ➔ medial geniculate body of the thalamus ➔ auditory cortex.
- Recurrent ear infections can be due to 2nd hand smoke causing damage to the cilia.

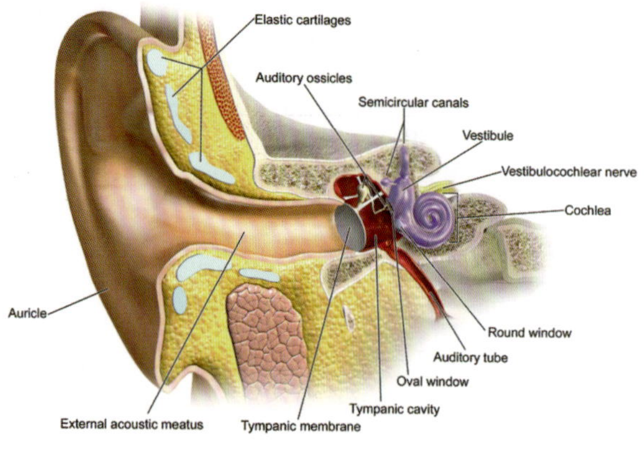

The Anatomy of the Ear

Innervation, Blood Supply and Anatomy of the Ear

- Outer Ear: Outer visible ear (AKA: pinna, auricle), ear canal, ear drum (outer layer of the tympanic membrane). Sensation to the outer ear, skin of the ear and ear cavity supplied mainly by facial nerve (CN VII).
- Blood supply: Anterior and posterior auricular arteries (branches of superficial temporal artery, external carotid artery and branches of the occipital artery.
- Middle Ear: Air filled cavity behind the tympanic membrane, 3 bones (ossicles): malleus (hammer), Incus (anvil), Stapes (Stirrup), oval window, round window, connects to the upper throat via the Eustachian tube.
  Innervated by CN VII (facial).
  Blood supply: Branches of the occipital, posterior auricular arteries, middle meningeal artery, and internal carotid.
- Inner Ear: Consist of bony and membranous labyrinths. Contains sensory organs for motion and balance: Vestibules and Semicircular canals, Cochlea.
  Bony labyrinth: bone matrix that transmits vibrations into endolymph in the membranous labyrinth. This then transmits the vibrations into the cochlea.
  Blood supply: branch of the tympanic branch of the maxillary artery, stylomastoid branch of posterior auricular artery, branch of middle meningeal artery, basilar artery, anterior inferior cerebellar artery.

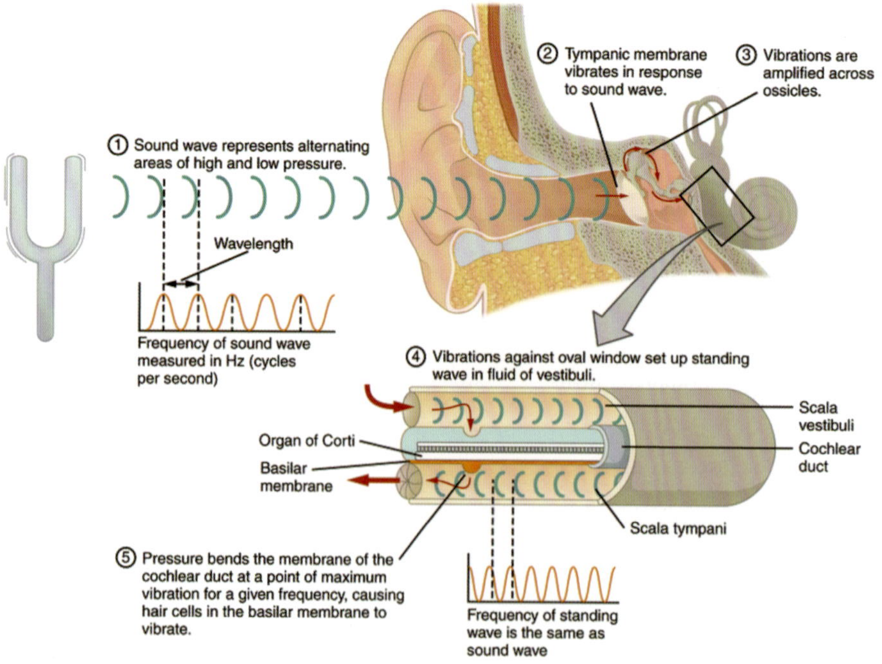

Hearing Test

- MCC conductive hearing loss in younger adults: Otosclerosis
- Ototoxic antibiotics = sensorineural loss

Weber Test (tuning fork on top of the head) If sound is equal in both ears = normal test. If sound is louder in one ear than the other = abnormal. The affected ear "hears" the vibration the most. **Conductive hearing loss** = causes lateralization to the **affected ear** because noise in the room so the person "feels" the vibrations better. **Sensorial hearing loss** = causes lateralization to the **unaffected ear** because unaffected ear "senses" vibration better.	**Rhine Test** Tuning fork is placed on the mastoid bone. Normal if air sounds better (sense) than vibration on the bone (conduction). (air > bone) If the vibration on the bone is last less than the sound heard in the air = normal test. (air > bone) If the vibration on the bone last longer than the sound heard in the air = abnormal = Conductive hearing loss in the affected ear. (bone > air) **Abnormal Rhine Test** Conductive hearing loss = causes lateralization to the **affected ear** when bone vibration is greater than air. **Normal Rhine Test** Sensory hearing loss = causes lateralization to the **unaffected ear** when the air vibration is greater than the bone.

Hearing Loss

- 2 types: due to an intense noise incident (gunfire, fireworks, explosion, drums) or gradually over time due to constant exposure to noise (music, workplace machinery, concerts, nightclubs, personal media players).
- Long-term exposure to sound levels over 80 dB can cause permanent hearing loss.
- Other factors affecting hearing: smoking (damages cilia), ototoxic chemicals or drugs, exposure to heavy metals, high viscosity of the blood (polycythemia), Type 2 diabetes
- Conductive hearing loss: MC causes: (due to middle ear issues): impacted earwax, fixed/missing ossicles (bones), holes in the tympanic membrane, middle ear inflammation.
- Deafness as a result of injury/damage to outer ear: conductive deafness.
- Deafness as a result of injury/damage to inner ear, brain or vestibulocochlear nerve: sensorineural deafness.

Ear Pathologies

Ménière's Disease **(tip:** Meniere's = My Ears) Inner ear disorder that affects hearing and balance. SX: Hearing loss, **tinnitus**, dizziness. Cause: build up of **endolymph** in the inner ear. (AKA: excess fluid in the inner ear) Can last minutes to 24 hours. TX: **Meclizine (↓ endolymph)**, Sodium restriction and diuretics. ↓ intake of caffeine, alcohol, nicotine	**Otosclerosis** Inherited abnormal growth of bone near the middle ear that can result in hearing loss. Causes conductive and sensorineural hearing loss. TX: Surgery
Labyrinthitis (AKA: Otitis Interna) Sudden hearing loss due to a recent viral illness, bacterial infection, head injury, stress, medication, allergy, pressure changes from flying or scuba diving SX: hearing loss, **tinnitus**, severe **vertigo**, **nystagmus** TX: Self-limiting	**Cholesteatoma** Growth of keratinizing squamous epithelium in the middle ear and/or mastoid process. They can spread through the base of the skull, through the middle ear bones (malleus, incus and stapes) or cause chronically draining ears. SX: Ear discharge and/or hearing loss, vertigo, bleeding from the ear, tinnitus, headaches, imbalance

Perilymph Fistula (AKA: Labyrinthine Fistula)	Otitis Media (children)
Abnormal opening in the bony capsule of the inner ear causing leakage of perilymph from the semicircular canals. SX: Dizziness, imbalance, hearing loss	MC: 6 – 36 months old SX: **Bulging**, erythematous, **non-mobile tympanic membrane**. Fever, irritable, ear drainage, fluid in middle ear, decreased hearing, pain. **High Risk**: **2° smoke** (smoke damages cilia), allergies, formula, facial deformities) Healing: Takes up to 2 months. Tympanic membrane may continue to be swollen, but no other SX. Reassure patient. **TX: Amoxicillin plus clavonic acid**
Acute External Otitis Media (Otitis Externa) (AKA: **Swimmers Ear**) Infection by bacteria due to water remaining inside the ear after swimming (showers). Complication: Untreated Otitis Media can lead to Mastoiditis. TX: **Ciprofloxacin w/dexamethasone otic drops**	**Otitis Externa** (adults – not connected with swimming) (Different than Otitis Media) MC: Pseudomonas **Granulation tissue** (fibrous tissue) deposits inside ear canal SX: **NORMAL** tympanic membrane, **purulent drainage, severe pain**

Neurofibromatosis Type II , AD
(Acoustic Neuroma)
Autosomal Dominant

Mutation of the **Merlin** gene (influences the form and movement of cells)
Microdeletion of the NF2 gene located at chromosome 22

Bilateral acoustic neuromas (Schwannomas)
in the **region of cranial nerve VIII** by the internal auditory meatus
Schwannomas are **neural crest** derivatives.
S-100 marker.

Acoustic Neuroma (NF2)

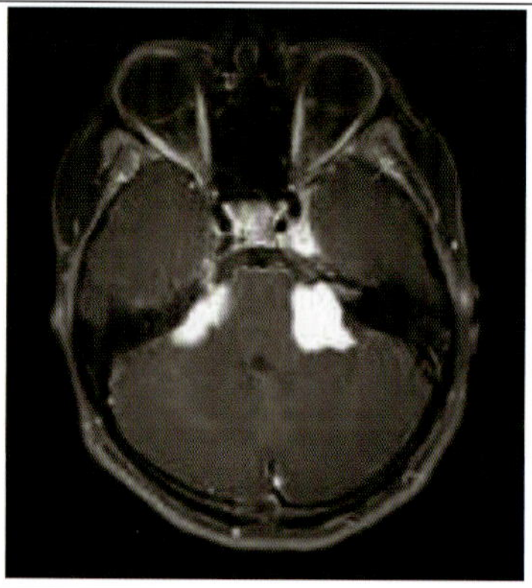

Mastoiditis	
Inflammation of the mucosal lining of the mastoid antrum and mastoid air cells inside the mastoid process (area of the temporal bone that is behind the ear). Emergency MCC: Untreated acute otitis media. Complications: Deafness, vertigo, facial-nerve palsy, meningitis, brain abscess, dural venous thrombophlebitis, epidural abscess. SX: Ear pain (otalgia), tenderness, swelling in the mastoid area. Fever, headaches, irritability, possible drainage (see brown discharge on bedding upon waking). TX: IV Ceftriaxone.	

Vertigo/Dizziness

Vertigo	Description
Benign Paroxysmal Positional Vertigo	Patient feels like they are **moving/spinning/swaying** when they are not. **Sudden onset. Positional in onset – can only be induced by change in position.** **Short** in duration (paroxysmal) Caused by changes in the position of the head. SX: **No tinnitus or hearing loss, vertigo**. MC: occurs when moving from lying position to standing. Eyes: Range from a mild horizontal nystagmus to severe vertical nystagmus, nausea. Cause: **calcium crystals** in the labyrinth dislodge and get trapped in the **semicircular canal**. Test: Infusion of warm water in the affected ear when the patient is supine will cause the top of the eye to rotate toward the affected ear (rotatory nystagmus). TX: Epley maneuver (AKA: repositioning maneuver) the head is tilted to free the calcium from the semicircular canals.
Central Vertigo	Due to brain stem or cerebellar lesions (stroke, CNS injuries)
Ménière's Disease	Inner ear disorder that affects hearing and balance. SX: Hearing loss, **tinnitus**, dizziness. Cause: build up of **endolymph** in the inner ear. (AKA: excess fluid in the inner ear) Can last minutes to 24 hours. TX: **Meclizine (↓ endolymph)**, Sodium restriction and diuretics. ↓ intake of caffeine, alcohol, nicotine
Labyrinthitis	Acute/Sudden hearing loss, tinnitus due to a recent viral or bacterial illness. Infection affecting both branches of the vestibule-cochlear nerve. Self Limited.
Perilymph Fistula	Hearing loss with history of trauma
Vestibular Neuritis	Vertigo that occurs without any change in position and does not affect hearing. Inflammation of the vestibular nerve associated with balance resulting in dizziness/vertigo. TX: **Meclizine**.

SPEECH

- Sound requires 3 things: lungs (produces airflow and pressure to vibrate vocal folds), the vocal cords/folds within the larynx (muscles of the larynx adjust length and tension of vocal cords to create pitch and tone), and articulators (tongue, palate, lips, cheeks).
- Vocal Cords (AKA: Vocal folds): folds of mucus membranes across the larynx that vibrate (due to the air flow expelled from the lungs) to allow phonation.
- Vocal cords are controlled by the vagus nerve, are located at the top of the larynx, and are part of the glottis.
- Vocal cords are attached anteriorly to the thyroid cartilage
- **Epiglottis** (flap) that closes off the larynx during swallowing so that food enters the esophagus and not the trachea. If food or liquid contact the vocal cords a cough reflex is triggered to prevent aspiration. Inflammation of the epiglottis is due to **Haemophilus influenza**. Epiglottitis is a medical emergency. TX: **Racemic epinephrine** (sympathomimetic bronchodilator via aerosol) and antibiotics. Possible need for tracheal intubation.
- Vocal cords = true vocal cords/folds.
- **False vocal cords**/folds (AKA: vestibular folds). Thick folds of mucus membrane above the true vocal cords/folds as protection.
- Vocal polyps/nodules: nodules that form on the vocal cords due to repeated abuse of the vocal cords. (SX: hoarseness or breathiness > 2 weeks. TX: speech-language therapy, surgery).
- Important: If a child is showing language delay the first thing to have evaluated is the hearing. (by age 3, children should have a vocabulary of 900 words)

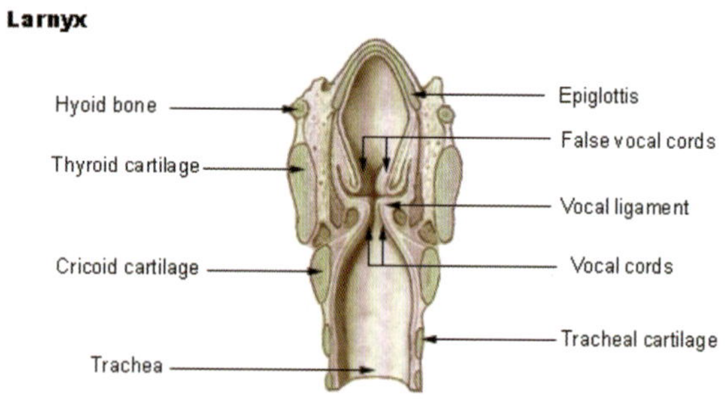

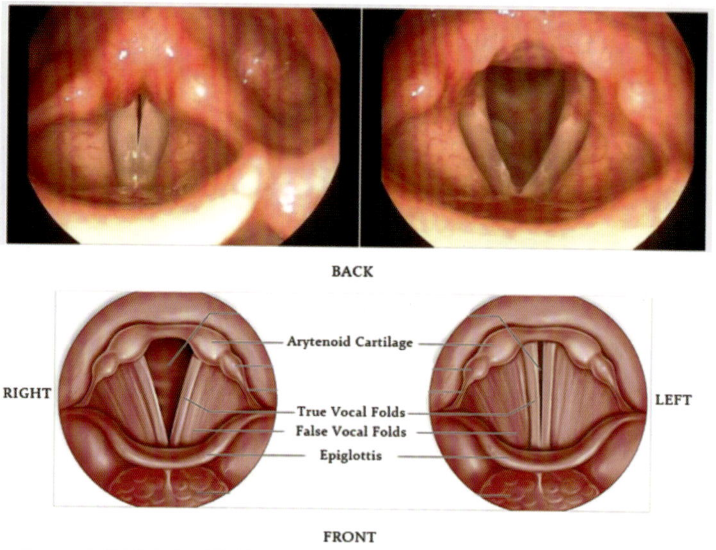

True and False Vocal Cords

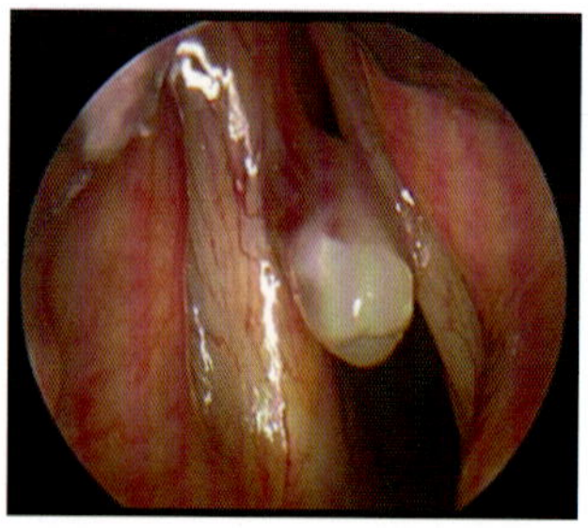

Vocal Polyp

NEUROLOGY PHARMACOLOGY

Epilepsy Pharmacology

Partial Seizure – Simple

- **No loss of conscience**
- Has memory of seizure

Partial Seizure – Complex

- **Loss of conscience**, biting, **lip-smacking**, chewing, hand wringing, **picking**, injury to mouth/teeth, loss of bladder or bowel control, may have an aura prior to seizure (smell, sound, taste, visual), feel of anxiety,
- Does not have any memory of seizure
- Last 30 seconds to 2 minutes

Absence Seizures

- Resembles "**day dreaming**". Person stares into space < 10 seconds
- MC in children 4 – 14

Status Epilepticus

- When a seizure **lasts too long** (> 5minutes) or to close together and person doesn't recover between the seizures or person is having repeated seizures for 30 minutes or longer
- Medical emergency

Myoclonic Seizure

- Jerking or twitching of a muscle, hiccups

DRUG GENERIC name Trade name	**Clinical Use**	**Mechanism of Action**	**Toxicity** (Anti-epileptic meds can lead to osteoporosis)
CARBAMAZEPINE *Tegretol*	**1st Line: Trigeminal neuralgia (CN V)** Also: partial simple, partial complex seizures, mood stabilizer, mania	**Inhibits** voltage gated **Na channels** in neurons (AKA: ↑ Na channel inactivation, ↓ Na current)	**Agranulocytosis, aplastic anemia, induces cytochrome P-450, liver toxicity, teratogenesis, Stevens-Johnson, SIADH, diplopia.**
Oxcarbazepine	Epilepsy, aniety, mood disorders, benign motor tics	Derivative of Carbamazepine.	Hyponatremia, diplopia, headaches, dizziness.
BENZODIAZEPINE (IV Diazepam, Lorazepam, Clonazepam)	**1st Line**: Status Epilepticus. **2nd line** for eclampsia (1st line is $MgSO_4$)	**↑ GABA action** (Main inhibitory neurotransmitter in the CNS. It reduces neuronal excitability)	Sedation**, respiratory depression**, dependence, tolerance. (**tip**: It is **STATUS** to drive a Benz)
ETHOSUXIMIDE *Emeside, Zarontin*	**1st Line**: Absence Seizures.	**Blocks** T-type **Ca channels** = stops action potentials	Steven-Johnson, fatigue, GI symptoms, urticaria (hives) (**tip**: Ethyl is always **ABSENT**)
VALPROIC ACID *Depakote, Convulex*	**1st Line: Myoclonic seizures. 2nd Line: Absence Seizures** Also: Mood stabilizer, mania, bipolar.	**Inhibits** voltage gated **Na channels** in neurons. (AKA: ↑ Na channel inactivation, ↓ Na current). **↑ GABA** by **inhibiting GABA transaminase.** Stops post transcription. Inhibits histone deacetylase.	**Teratogen** (neural tube defects), **severe liver toxicity** (must follow LFT's), GI SX.
PHENYTOIN *Dilantin*	Partial seizures: Simple and Complex. 2nd line: Status Epilepticus.	**Inhibits** voltage gated **Na channels** in neurons (AKA: ↑ Na channel inactivation, ↓ Na current) **ZERO ORDER kinetics.**	**Gingival hyperplasia**, **SLE-like** symptoms, **Induces cytochrome P-450**, **Acute Intermittent Porphyria**, Stevens-Johnson Syndrome, hirsutism, megaloblastic anemia, teratogenic, nystagmus, diplopia
FOSPHENYTOIN	Parenteral use		
GABAPENTIN *Neurontin*	Peripheral, **Diabetic, postherpetic** Neuralgia. **Restless leg** syndrome. Bipolar, migraine prophylaxis.	**Inhibits** voltage **Ca Channels** GABA analog.	Sedation, ataxia

PHENOBARBITAL	1st Line in neonates.	↑ **GABA**	Confusion, lethargy, induces **cytochrome P-450**, sedation. **PRIMIDONE is metabolized to Phenobarbitol.**
LAMOTRIGINE *Lamictal*	**1st Line: Mood disorder in pregnancy**. 2nd Line: Myoclonic seizure.	**Inhibits** voltage gated **Na channels** in neurons. (AKA: ↑ Na channel inactivation, ↓ Na current).	**Stevens-Johnson** Syndrome
TOPIRAMATE *Topamax*	Seizures in adults, children. Prophylaxis for **migraines**. Addictions.	**Inhibits** voltage gated **Na channels** in neurons. (AKA: ↑ Na channel inactivation, ↓ Na current). ↑ **GABA** by **inhibiting GABA transaminase.**	**Kidney stones**, sedation, weight loss
TIAGABINE *Gabitril*	Partial seizures in ages >12. Anxiety, fibromyalgia	↑ GABA by inhibiting re-uptake	Confusion, difficulty speaking, sedation, paresthesia
VIGABATRIN *Sabril*	Partial seizures	↑ **GABA** by **inhibiting GABA transaminase.**	Sedation, headaches, depression, vertigo, diplopia, confusion
ZONISAMIDE	Partial seizures, infantile spasms, myoclonic seizures, resting tremors of Parkinson's dz, Tardive dyskinesia	Sulfonamide. Blocks Na and T-type Calcium channels.	Depression, anorexia, somnolence

Opioid Analgesics

Opiates bind to mu, kappa, delta receptors.

DRUG GENERIC name **Trade name**	**Clinical Use**	**Mechanism of Action**	**Toxicity**
HEROIN **MORPHINE** **OXYCODONE** **DEMEROL** **PENTAZOCINE** **FENTANYL** **CODEINE**	**Analgesic**	**Opioid receptor mu agonist. Opens K channels, closes Ca channels = ↓ synaptic transmission (action potential).** (stops transmission of pain by **hyperpolarizing** the cell). Inhibits release of **Substance P** (pain), ACh, Norepinephrine, 5-HT, glutamate. Note: Morphine, when **chronically** used will metabolize itself and become stronger. **However**, in a patient that does not use opioids chronically, the risk of becoming addicted to morphine (when needed due to pain control for injury or surgery) is **extremely low**.	Addiction, **miosis (pinpoint pupils/constricted pupils), respiratory depression.** **Overdose SX: Miosis,** ↓ respiratory rate, confusion, **cold/clammy skin**, weak, drowsy, coma. **OD Toxicity TX: Naloxone, Naltrexone (opiod receptor antagonist)** **Note:** Opioids cause **constipation** (look for this common side effect in a patient following surgery).
LOPERAMIDE *Imodium*	Diarrhea, IBD	**Opioid receptor mu agonist in the myenteric plexus of large intestine.**	**Must not be used in children <2 due to potential fatal paralytic ileus.** Not to be used if blood in the stool.

DIPHENOXYLATE *Diocalm*	Diarrhea, IBD	**Opioid receptor mu agonist.** ↓ peristalsis so body has time to remove water from the intestine.	Does NOT cause addition.
METHADONE *Dolophine*	Detox program for opiod/heroin addicts	Synthetic opioid.	
DEXTROMETHORPHAN (DXM or DM) *Robitussin, NyQuil, Vicks, Dimetapp, TheraFlu, Dimetapp*	Antitussive (cough suppressant)	Serotonin reuptake inhibitor. (Dextrorphan is NMDA receptor antagonist)	Sedative, GI SX, nervousness. Recreationally used in excessive dosages → Hallucinations, dissociation, diplopia, sweating, HTN, euphoria, paresthesia.
MEPERIDINE	Use for pain in **acute pancreatitis** because it does not cause Sphincter of Oddi to contract=pain. (**Fentanyl** is also used for acute pancreatitis)	Synthetic opioid.	**Do not use with MAO inhibitors → Serotonin Syndrome**
PENTAZOCINE	Pain	Synthetic agonist-antagonist opioid.	**Can cause opioid withdrawal in patients dependent on opioids**
BUTORPHANOL *Stadol*	Migraines, Labor	Synthetic mu-opioid receptor agonist.	↑ perspiration can cause opioid withdrawal in patients dependent on opioids. Not easily reversed by Naloxone.
TRAMADOL *Ultram*	Chronic Pain. Fibromyalgia. Is not as strong as full strength opioids so can use during daily activities.	**Weak opioid receptor mu agonist. Inhibits serotonin and norepinephrine.**	Increases the risk of **seizures**. Serotonin Syndrome

Amphetamines

DRUG **GENERIC name** **Trade name**	**Clinical Use**	**Mechanism of Action**	**Toxicity**
Dextroamphetamine *Adderall, Adderall XR, Vyvanse* **Phentermine** *Qsymia, Vites, Adipex* Amphetamine type stimulants: Cannabis, Cocaine, Ecstasy, Opioids.	ADHD, Narcolepsy, Obesity, cognitive and performance enhancer, recreationally as an aphrodisiac, euphoria. Phentermine: appetite suppression in treatment of obesity.	CNS Stimulant. Increases excitatory neurotransmitters dopamine, norepinephrine and serotonin in the brain. Phentermine: substitute amphetamine	Avoid in patients with history of drug abuse, glaucoma, anxiety, heart disease, HTN, hyperthyroidism, BPH, pregnancy, epilepsy, peptic ulcers, MAOI's HTN or hypotension (vasovagal response), tachycardia, Raynaud's (due to reduced blood flow to extremities), dry mouth, nasal congestion, decreased seizure threshold, weight loss, erectile dysfunction or priapism, bruxism,

Barbiturates

DRUG GENERIC name Trade name	Clinical Use	Mechanism of Action	Toxicity
PHENOBARBITAL PENTOBARBITAL SECOBARBITAL	CNS depressant: sedation, anesthesia, anxiolytics, anticonvulsants, analgesic.	Keeps **Chloride channels open LONGER** so that neuron firing ↓ (AKA: ↑ **duration** of the opening) (**tip**: BARB talks a really **LONG** time, or BARB wants it longer)	↓↓ **respiratory depression**, bradycardia. **Induces cytochrome P-450**, ↑ risk for addiction, CNS depression, ↑ toxicity when combined with alcohol. OD TX: Supportive treatment = monitor respiration (be ready to intubate).
THIOPENTAL	Induction of anesthesia	.	

Benzodiazepine

DRUG GENERIC name Trade name	Clinical Use	Mechanism of Action	Toxicity
Short Acting: **ALPRAZOLAM** **TRIAZOLAM** **OXAZEPAM** **MIDAZOLAM** **(tip: ATOM is very small)** **Long Acting:** **CHLORDIAZEPOXIDE** **CLONAZEPAM** **DIAZAPAM** **FLURAZEPAM** **Intermediate Acting:** **LORAZAPAM** **TEMAZEPAM**	Status epilepticus, Anxiety, night terrors, DT's related to alcohol withdrawal, anesthesia, insomnia (sleeping aid). Alprazolam + Botox treats resting tremor of Parkinson's.	↑ **Frequency** of the opening of **Chloride channels** so that neuron firing is decreased and GABA ↑. (AKA: Allosterically binds GABA = ↑ GABA) (**tip**: BEN wants it more often)	CNS depression when combined with alcohol, dependence. OD TX: **Flumazenil*** (GABA receptor antagonist) (***must not be used** in patients that are benzodiazepine dependent. It also stops the action of benzodiazepine that the patient is on, causing withdrawal and seizures).

Non-benzodiazepine Hypnotics (Sleep aids)

DRUG GENERIC name Trade name	Clinical Use	Mechanism of Action	Toxicity
ZOLPIDEM Ambien **ZALEPLON** **ESZOPICLONE** (**tip**: Sleep = ZZZ's)	Insomnia	Inhibitory neurotransmitter that binds GABA receptors	Confusion, headaches. Reversal by **Flumazenil*** (GABA receptor antagonist) (***must not be used** in patients that are benzodiazepine dependent. It also stops the action of benzodiazepine that the patient is on, causing withdrawal and seizures).

Neuromuscular Blocking Drugs

- Used to relax/paralyze muscles before induction of general anesthesia or tracheal intubation.
- Works at the nicotinic receptor (ACh)

Depolarizing Neuromuscular Drugs

DRUG GENERIC name Trade name	Clinical Use	Mechanism of Action	Toxicity
SUCCINYLCHOLINE	Muscle relaxer, Induction of muscle relaxation/short term paralysis	Nicotinic ACh receptor agonist. Causes **persistent depolarization** of the motor end plate. Reversal of Action: **Neostigmine** (cholinesterase inhibitor = stops the breakdown of ACh in synapses)	Prolonged depolarization = ↑↑ Ca (hypercalcemia). Repolarization blocked = ↑↑ K (hyperkalemia = TX: **Calcium gluconate**) ↑↑ K = Lengthens QRS, Peak T Waves.

Non-depolarizing Neuromuscular Drugs

DRUG GENERIC name Trade name	Clinical Use	Mechanism of Action	Toxicity
CURAIRE (Poison arrows made from plant extracts in Central and South America) (Tubocurarine, Calabash, Atracurium, Vecuronium)	Poison: Causes weakness of skeletal muscles → death by paralysis of diaphragm.	Reversibly **inhibiting nicotinic ACh receptors** at the neuromuscular junction. This causes inhibition of action potential.	Death due to paralysis of diaphragm. TX: **Neostigmine or Pyridostigmine** (cholinesterase inhibitor). Must be given with **Atropine**. Atropine prevents **muscarinic** effects)

Muscle Relaxant

DRUG GENERIC name Trade name	Clinical Use	Mechanism of Action	Toxicity
DANTROLENE	Muscle relaxant that ↓ contraction in muscles in Neuroleptic **Malignant Syndrome** (Antipsychotic drugs) and **Malignant Hyperthermia** (anesthetics and ETC uncoupling)	**Inhibits Calcium** release from the sarcoplasmic reticulum by **blocking (antagonizing) the ryanodine receptors.** **D2 agonist.**	GI symptoms.

Anesthetics

Local Anesthetics

- To decrease bleeding, epinephrine can be combined with local anesthetics. MOA: Vasoconstriction.
  Do not use local anesthetics with epinephrine on extremities or penis = ischemia
- Order of loss of pain: 1st = pain, 2nd = temperature, 3rd = touch, 4th = pressure
- Order of nerve blockade: Myelinated fibers > unmyelinated fibers. Small-diameter fibers > large diameter fibers

DRUG **GENERIC name** **Trade name**	**Clinical Use**	**Mechanism of Action**	**Toxicity**
Amides: **LIDOCAINE** **BUPIVACAINE** MEPIVACAINE **Esters:** PROCAINE **COCAINE** TETRACAINE	Spinal anesthesia, minor surgeries/suturing.	Block Na channels → action potential	Bupivacaine can cause cardiotoxicity. Cocaine can cause arrhythmias (diffuse ST elevations). HTN, hypotension. Do not use Bupivacaine IV. It is for nerve blocks: carpal tunnel. Epinephrine can be added to vasoconstrict so that bleeding ↓.

IV Anesthetics

DRUG **GENERIC name** **Trade name**	**Clinical Use**	**Mechanism of Action**	**Toxicity**
THIOPENTAL (aka: Sodium Thiopental) (barbiturate)	Induce anesthesia. High potency because it has high lipid solubility. Status epilepticus.	Rapid onset in the brain. Rapid distribution in skeletal muscles and adipose tissue. Milky white in the blood.	Cardiovascular and respiratory depression. Hypotension, apnea, airway obstruction. Note: has been replaced by propofol.
KETAMINE (Aryl-cyclohexylamines)	Anesthesia	Blocks NMDA receptors. (Glutamate)	Hallucinations, bad dreams, ↑ cerebral blood flow.
Propofol	Sedation, Fast induction anesthesia. (less nausea than Thiopental)	↑ GABA.	
MIDAZOLAM (Benzodiazepine)	Anesthesia. MC used in endoscopy.		Respiratory depression, ↓ BP, anterograde amnesia. TX: Overdose: Flumazenil
MORPHINE FENTANYL (Opioids)	Sedative, pain.		

Inhaled Anesthetics

- ↑ Cerebral blood flow → ↑ ICP
  Myocardial depression → ↓ CO
  Hypotension
  Respiratory depression → ↓ TV
  ↓ Renal function
- Reversal of anesthetics:
  IV: Naloxone for opioids
  Oral: Naloxone with Flumazenil, Midazolam
- Tissues = Greater the gradient = slower the onset of action
- MAC = Minimal Alveolar Concentration = amount of anesthetic required to prevent 50% of the patients from feeling stimulus (ie: incision)
- **Lipid soluble drugs = cross the blood brain barrier**
- **↑ MAC = ↓ Potency = Faster onset of action = ↓ volume of distribution = ↓ solubility in the blood (does not have to saturate all of the blood before it goes to the brain – goes straight to the brain = fast. Ie: Nitrous Oxide) = rapid recovery**
- **↓ MAC = ↑ Potency = Slower onset of action = ↑ volume of distribution = ↑ solubility in blood (has to saturate all of the blood before it gets into the brain = takes longer/slower)**
- **Onset of gas anesthetic depend upon solubility in the blood**

DRUG GENERIC name Trade name	**Clinical Use**	**Mechanism of Action**	**Toxicity**
HALOTHANE **NITROUS OXIDE** ISOFLURANE ENFLURANE SEVOFLURANE METHOXYFLURANE	Anesthesia.	Rapid onset in the brain. Rapid distribution in skeletal muscles and adipose tissue. Milky white in the blood.	Respiratory depression, Myocardial depression. **Halothane**: Fulminant liver disease (severe **hepatotoxicity** = death) – not used in the USA. **↑↑ LFT's, ↑ PT** (like Reye syndrome) Methoxyflurane: nephrotoxicity, Enflurane: ↑ Seizure risk Malignant hyperthermia (hereditary). Is not caused by nitrous oxide or succinylcholine. TX: **Dantrolene**

Neurology Pathology Pharmacology

Glaucoma

DRUG GENERIC name Trade name	**Clinical Use**	**Mechanism of Action**	**Toxicity**
EPINEPHRINE	Glaucoma	α–agonists ↓ aqueous humor synthesis	**DO NOT USE in closed-angle glaucoma.** Foreign body sensation, blurry vision, mydriasis (epinephrine is sympathetic)
TIMOLOL CARTEOLOL BETAXOLOL	Glaucoma	**B-blocker** ↓ aqueous humor synthesis	
ACETAZOLAMIDE	Glaucoma	↓ aqueous humor synthesis by inhibition of carbonic anhydrase = ↓ HCO_3.	
PILOCARPINE, CARBACHOL	Glaucoma	Direct Cholinomimetic. ↑ outflow aqueous humor by contraction of ciliary muscles. Opens canal of Schlemm	Contracts ciliary muscle = miosis and cyclospasm (false nearsightedness). Eye can't keep a clear vision of objects at a distance due to eye muscle spasms). MCC: eye fatigue.
PHYSOSTIGMINE, ECHOTHIOPHATE	Glaucoma	Indirect Cholinomimetic. ↑ outflow aqueous humor by contraction of ciliary muscles. Opens canal of Schlemm	Contracts ciliary muscle = miosis and cyclospasm (false nearsightedness). Eye can't keep a clear vision of objects at a distance due to eye muscle spasms). MCC: eye fatigue.
Latanoprost (PGF_2)	Glaucoma	Prostaglandin. ↑ outflow aqueous humor	Darkens color of iris

Headaches

DRUG GENERIC name Trade name	Clinical Use	Mechanism of Action	Toxicity
SUMATRIPTAN	Acute migraines, Cluster headaches (1st line for Cluster headaches = 100% O_2)	**Serotonin agonist**. 5-HT agonist that stimulates postsynaptic receptors. Inhibits trigeminal nerve. Induces vasoconstriction.	Do not use in patients with coronary vasospasms: Prinzmetal angina, CAD

Essential Tremors

DRUG GENERIC name Trade name	Clinical Use	Mechanism of Action	Toxicity
PROPANOLOL	↓ **Essential tremors** (hand tremors that worsen with intentional use)	B-Blocker	(Note: Essential tremors improve with alcohol. BUT DO NOT tell a patient is ok to drink).

Alzheimer's

DRUG GENERIC name Trade name	Clinical Use	Mechanism of Action	Toxicity
DONEPEZIL GALANTAMINE RIVASTIGMINE TACRINE	Alzheimer's (due to ↓ ACh)	**AChE inhibitor.**	Insomnia, dizziness, nausea. Use with caution in patients with heart diseases, COPD and arrhythmias. (**tip**: I am **DONE** with Alzheimer's)
MEMANTINE	Alzheimer's (due to ↓ ACh)	NMDA receptor antagonist (Glutamate). ↓ excitotoxicity. Mediated by Calcium.	Hallucinations, confusion, dizziness, drowsiness, agitation.

Huntington's

DRUG GENERIC name Trade name	Clinical Use	Mechanism of Action	Toxicity
TETRABENAZINE, RESERPINE	Huntington's (Due to ↑ dopamine, ↓ ACh, ↓ GABA)	Inhibits VMAT (monoamine transporter) so ↓ release of dopamine.	
HALOPERIDOL	Huntington's (Due to ↑ dopamine, ↓ ACh, ↓ GABA)	Dopamine receptor antagonist (inhibits dopamine)	

Parkinson Disease

DRUG GENERIC name Trade name	Clinical Use	Mechanism of Action	Toxicity
BROMOCRIPTINE	TX: **Prolactinoma** (pituitary tumor) Parkinson's (Due to ↓dopamine, ↑ ACh, ↑ 5-HT)	**Dopamine agonist**	**Parkinson's Drugs can cause Hallucinations and confusion**.
PRAMIPEXOLE, ROPINIROLE, CABERGOLINE	Parkinson's (Due to ↓dopamine, ↑ ACh, ↑ 5-HT)	Dopamine agonist	Note: Dopamine agonist has fewer adverse side effects than Levodopa/Carbidopa but are less effective.
AMANTADINE	Resting tremor in Parkinson's (Due to ↓dopamine, ↑ ACh, ↑ 5-HT) TX: Influenza A. TX: Rubella	↑ Dopamine release, ↓ reuptake	CNS side effects (due to dopaminergic and adrenergic effects), livedo reticularis, Stevens-Johnson syndrome, suicidal ideation. Note: Better treatment in Parkinson's in patients > 60. ↓ side effects than anticholinergic agents.
SELEGILINE RASAGILINE	Parkinson's (Due to ↓dopamine, ↑ ACh, ↑ 5-HT)	**MAO Inhibitor**. Stops breakdown of dopamine. Inhibits conversion of dopamine into DOPAC by inhibiting MAO-B.	
ENTACAPONE, TOLCAPONE	Entacapone = ↑ quality of L-dopa entering the brain. Tolcapone = ↑ L-dopa available to the brain.	**COMT inhibitor**. Prevent L-dopa degradation = ↑ dopamine availability to the brain by inhibiting conversion of dopamine into 3-OMD (3-O-methyldopa) by inhibiting COMT. (AKA: Block the metabolism of dopamine) and extend the effect of dopamine-based meds). (**tip**: If you have "Capone's", your dinner is COMT (comp your meal)	(**tip**: If you eat **CAPON**'s for dinner they will **COMT** your meal). (A capon is a Cornish hen)
L-DOPA (AKA: LEVODOPA)	Parkinson's (Due to ↓dopamine, ↑ ACh, ↑ 5-HT) Greatest efficacy for Parkinson's.	**↑ Level of dopamine in the brain**. L-dopa crosses blood brain barrier (tight junctions) and is converted to **dopamine by dopa decarboxylase**.	**DO NOT give vitamin B-6** with L-dopa. It will ↑ conversion and ↓ effects and ↓ motion. Psychosis caused by Levodopa: Add **quetiapine.** Anxiety, agitation, dyskinesia, arrhythmias due to ↑ formation of catecholamines.
CARBIDOPA	Parkinson's (Due to ↓dopamine, ↑ ACh, ↑ 5-HT)	Peripheral **decarboxylase inhibitor**. Given with L-dopa to ↑ **bioavailability of L-dopa** to the brain.	
BENZTROPINE HYDROXYZINE	Parkinson's (Due to ↓dopamine, ↑ ACh, ↑ 5-HT)	Anticholinergic. Antimuscarinic.	Most commonly used in patients < 60. Anticholinergic drugs can decrease the memory in Parkinson's. Side effects: urinary retention, constipation, and glaucoma.

HEMATOLOGY

- **Fetal Erythropoiesis**
  3 – 8 weeks: Yolk Sac; 6 – 30 weeks: liver (main) and spleen (secondary):
  28 weeks to birth: bone marrow
- **Fetal Blood Hb**: 2 alpha, 2 gamma (adult: 2 alpha, 2 beta)
  Hb F = Higher affinity for O2 than mother
  Hb F = Left shift in Oxy Hb curve
  Hb F = Decreased 2,3 BPG (2,3 BPG loves to give oxygen away to mothers tissues)
  Hydroxyurea: given to **sickle cell patients to increase Hb F**
  SE: Pulmonary Fibrosis and bone marrow suppression
- Adult Hb: 2 alpha, 2 beta
- Hemoglobin: Iron-containing substance in RBC's, each transporting 4 molecules of oxygen. Each RBC holds 250 million hemoglobin molecules, so each RBC carries 1 billion molecules of oxygen. There are approximately 25 trillion RBC in the 5 liters of blood in the human body.
- Erythropoiesis is the process that produces new RBC (7 days) from stem cells. 2 million RBC's are produced per second in the red bone marrow of large bones in healthy adults.
- Hematocrit: proportion, by volume, of the blood that consist of RBC
- **Primary hemostasis**: formation of the platelet plug.
  Secondary hemostasis: activation of the coagulation cascade and formation of the fibrin plug.
- RBC Shape: Biconcave in order to give it more surface area and flexibility as it squeezes through narrow passages and then returns to its original shape. Their diameter is 7 – 8 μm
- RBC last 120 days. The mature RBC's are anucleate (lack a nucleus) so are unable to perform glycolysis/aerobic respiration. They are able to generate 2 ATP in anaerobic respiration.
- Anisocytosis: RBC's are not the same size. Typical finding in anemias.
- Poikilocytosis: RBC's with abnormal shapes (note the variety of shapes in the table below)
- MCV = Mean corpuscular volume: average volume of a RBC. Indicates the size of the RBC's.
- MCH (Mean Corpuscular Hemoglobin: average mass of Hb per RBC in a sample of blood) and MCHC (Mean Corpuscular Hemoglobin Concentration: concentration of Hb in a given volume of packed RBC) reflect the Hb content of RBC's.
- MCV measurements differentiate anemias.
- ↓ MCV: Microcytic: Smaller than normal RBC's. Anemia with MCV < 80. (Iron deficiency, thalassemia, sideroblastic, blood loss, chronic disease, inflammation).
- Normocytic: Anemia with normal MCV values (prosthetic heart valves, sepsis, tumor, aplastic anemia, deficiency of erythropoietin, chronic disease, sudden blood loss)
- ↑ MCV: Macrocytic: Larger than normal RBC's. Anemia with MCV > 100. (B-12 or folate deficiency, pernicious anemia, alcoholism, chemotherapy).
- RDW: Red blood cell width distribution
- Hypochromic anemia: RBC's that are more pale than normal: area of central pallor is increased, ↓ HB concentration and ↓ MCH.
- Hyperchromic anemia: RBC's with ↑ concentration of Hb and ↑ MCH. (Celiac, alcoholism).
- Pure Red Cell Aplasia: Bone marrow ceases to produce RBC's.
- Aplastic Anemia: Deficiency of all three blood cell types (pancytopenia): RBC's (anemia), WBC's (leukopenia), and platelets (thrombocytopenia).
- Pancytopenia: Reduction in the number of RBC, WBC and platelets
- Leukopenia: Reduction in the number of WBC's
- Thrombocytopenia: Reduction in the number of platelets
- Neutropenia: Low concentration of neutrophils (majority of WBC's that are the primary defense against infections by destroying bacteria and immunoglobulin bound viruses in the blood).

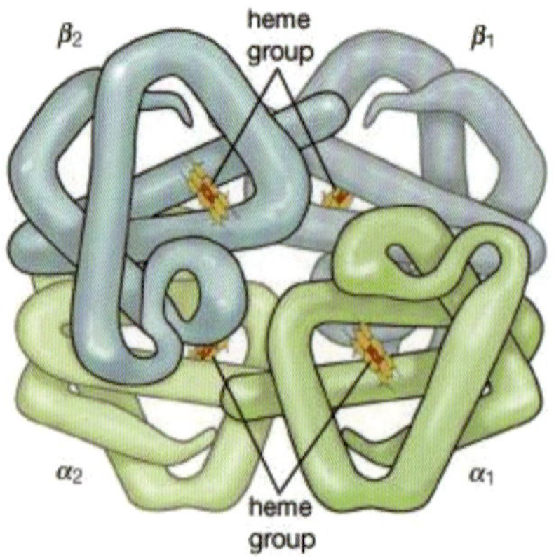

Structure of Hemoglobin

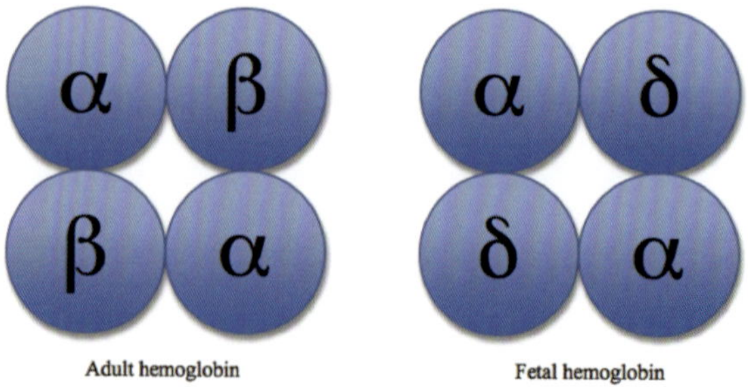

Hematopoietic Precursors

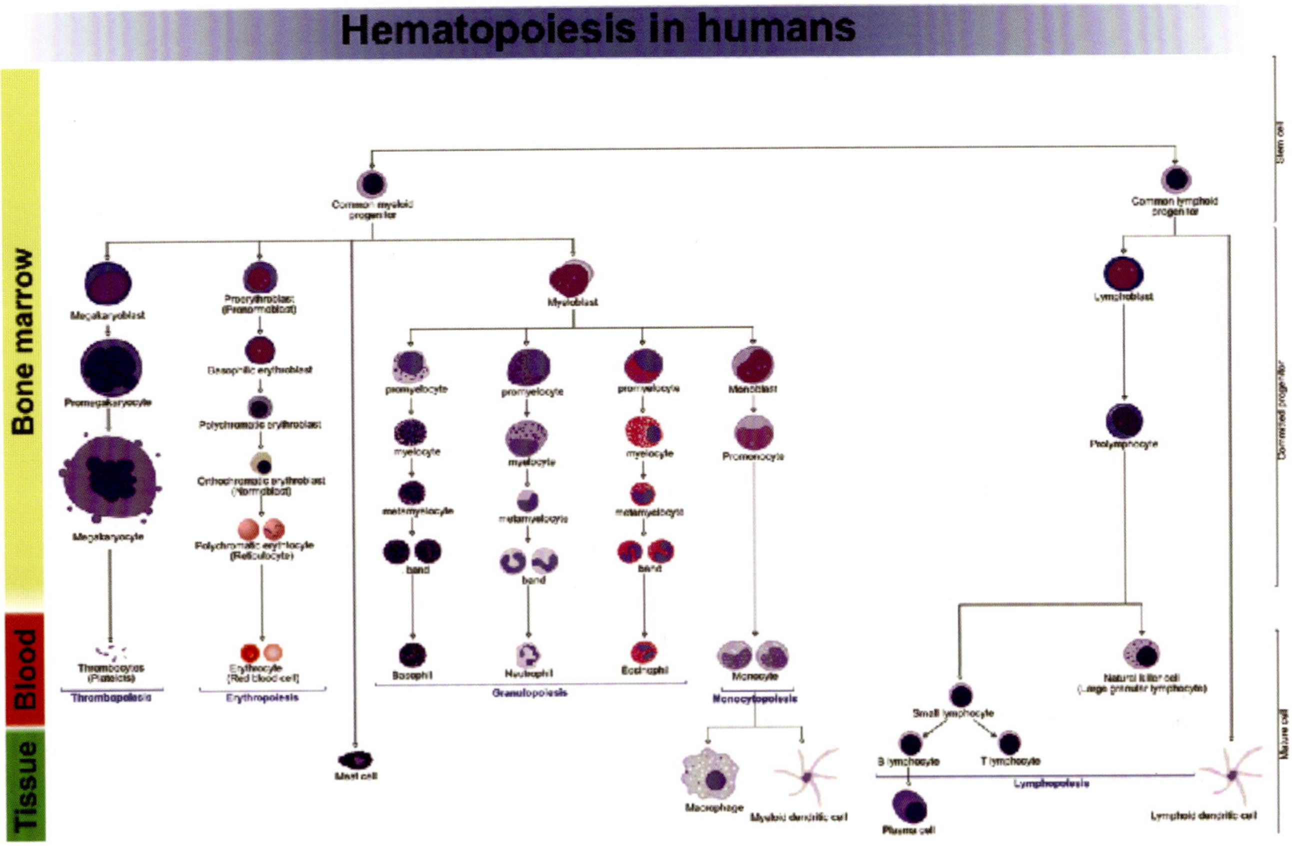

- Blood cells that give rise to all other blood cells
- Derived from the mesoderm
- Located in the red bone marrow. MC: pelvis, femur and sternum, umbilical cord
- Extramedullary hematopoiesis: hematopoiesis occurring outside of the main bone marrow (liver, spleen or other bones not normally used hematopoiesis.
  This occurs due to increased need of RBC production (Thalassemia major, Sickle Cell) or in pathologies of fibrosis taking up the bone marrow causing the hematopoietic cells to be squeezed out (Myelofibrosis).
- Myeloid lines: monocytes, macrophages, basophils, eosinophils, neutrophils, erythrocytes, dendritic cells, megakaryocytes (AKA: platelets)
- Granulocytes (**tip**: BEN): basophils, eosinophils, erythrocytes
- Lymphoid lines: T cells, B cells, and natural killer cells.

Cell Types

- Leukocytes: **ALL** white blood cells
- Lymphocytes: B cells, T cells, Natural Killers, Macrophages
- Basophils: (AKA: Granulocytes): (**tip**: BEN) Basophils, Eosinophil's, Monocytes
- WBC Normal Labs (Leukocytes)
  Neutrophils (PMS's): 60 – 70%
  Lymphocytes: 20 – 30%
  Monocytes: 3-7%
  Eosinophil's: 1 – 3%
  Basophils: 0 – 1%

Macrophages "Names" in Different Tissues

Tissue	Macrophage Name
Blood/Bone Marrow	Monocyte
Bone	Osteoclasts
CNS	Microglia
Connective Tissue	Histocyte, Giant Cell
Granuloma	Epithelioid Cells
Kidney	Mesangial Cells
Liver	Kupffer Cells
Lymph Node	Sinus histocytes
Placenta	Hofbauer Cells
Pulmonary/lungs	Alveolar Macrophage, Dust Cells
Skin/Mucosa	Langerhans Cells
Spleen (Red pulp)	Sinusoidal Cells, RES

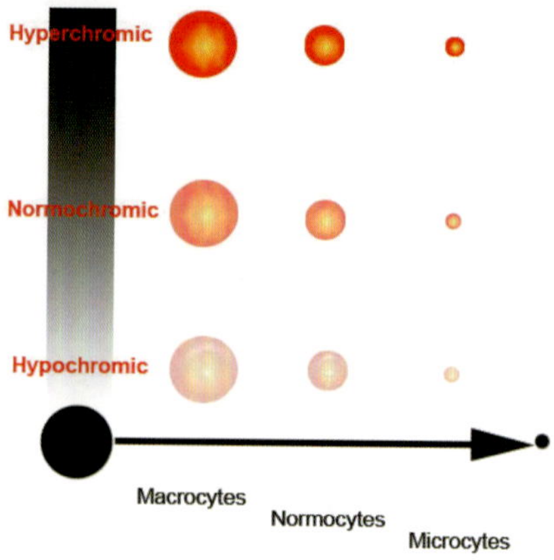

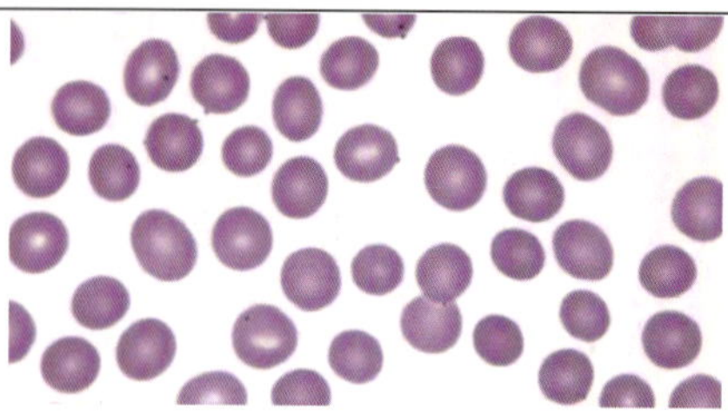

Erythrocyte (RBC)

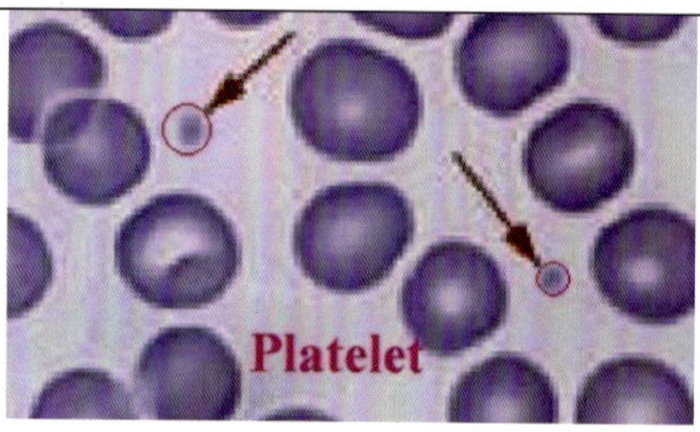

Thrombocyte (platelet)

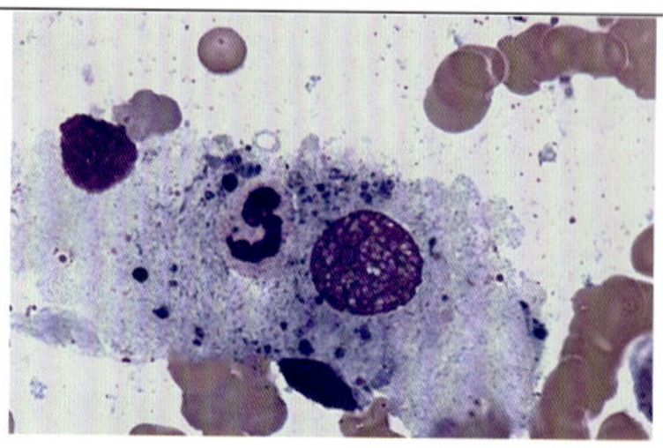

Macrophage

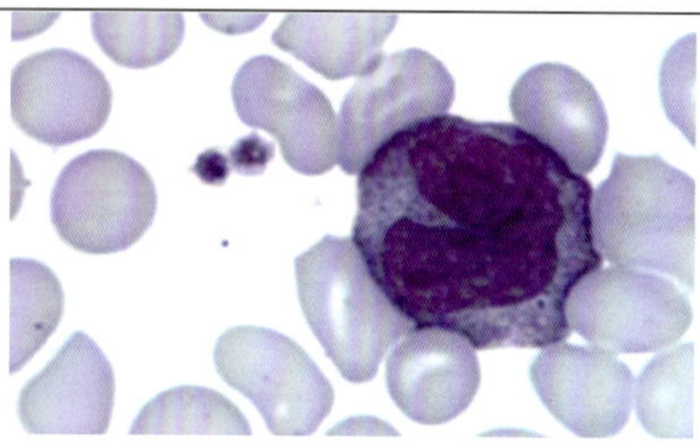

Monocyte

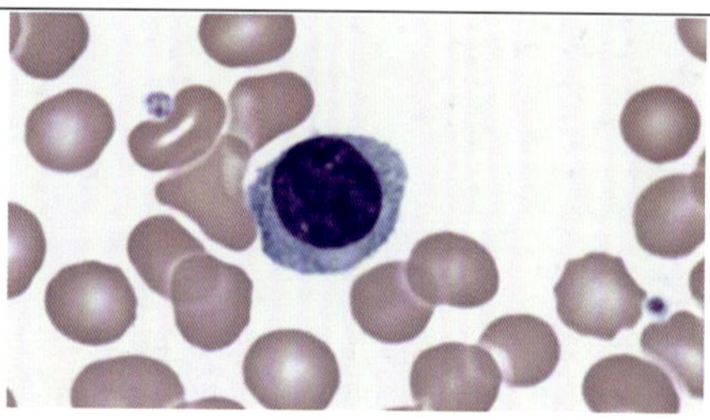

Lymphocyte

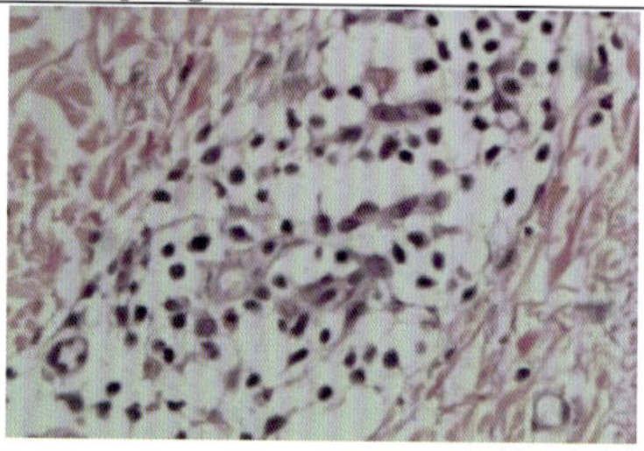

Infiltration of lymphocytes

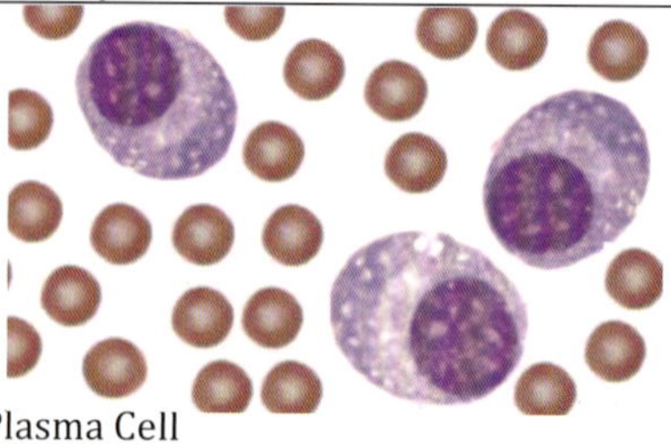

Plasma Cell

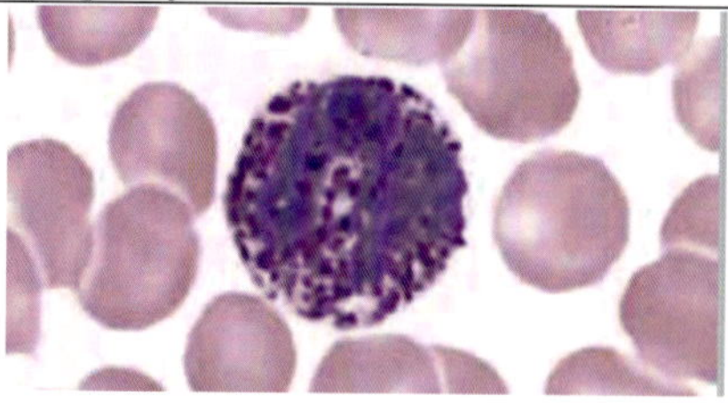

Basophil

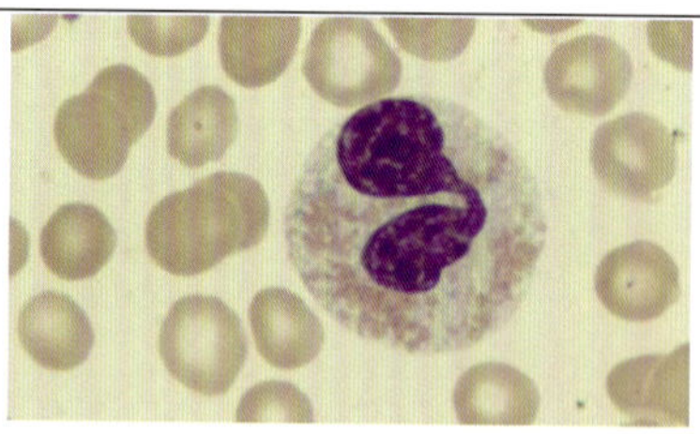

Eosinophil

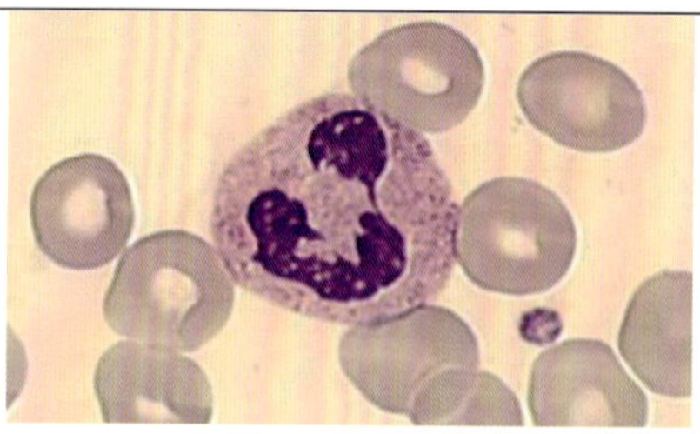

Neutrophil

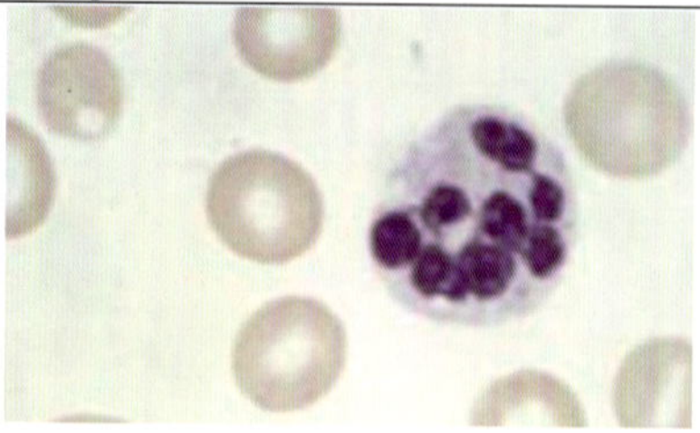

Hypersegmented Neutrophil

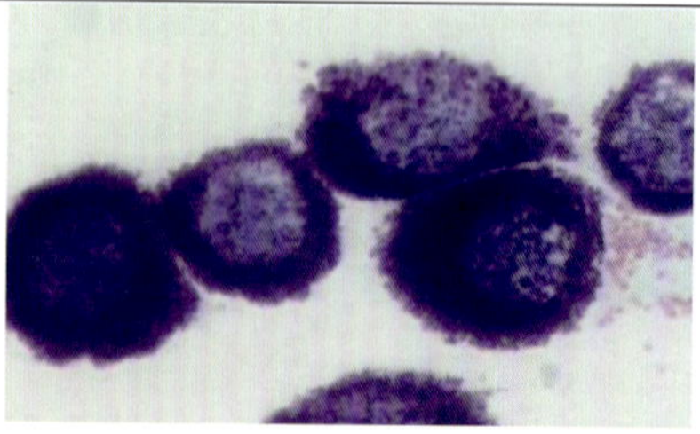

Mast Cell

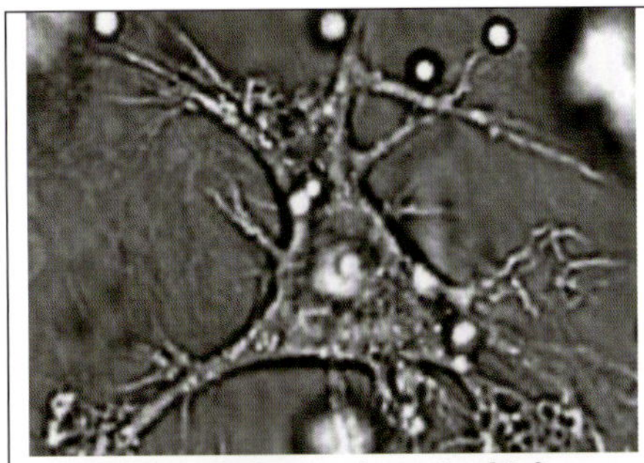

Dendritic Cell (Langerhans in skin)

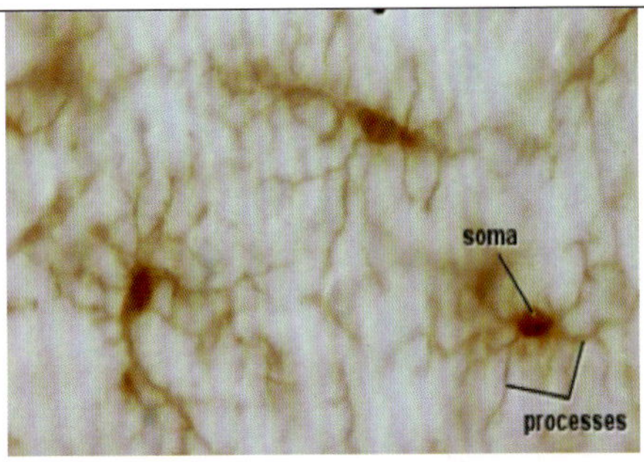

Microglia Cells

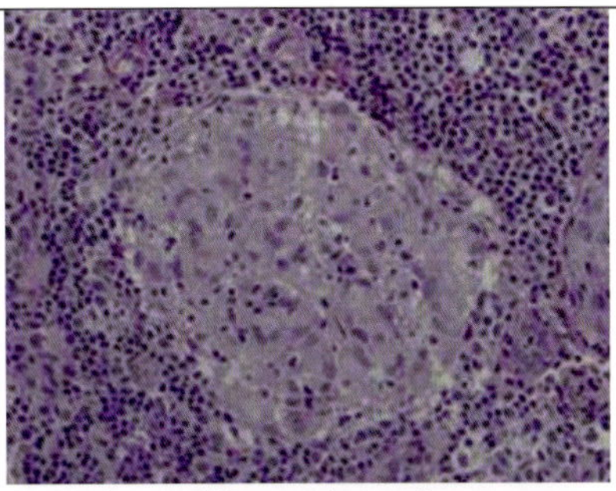

Granuloma (Macrophages)

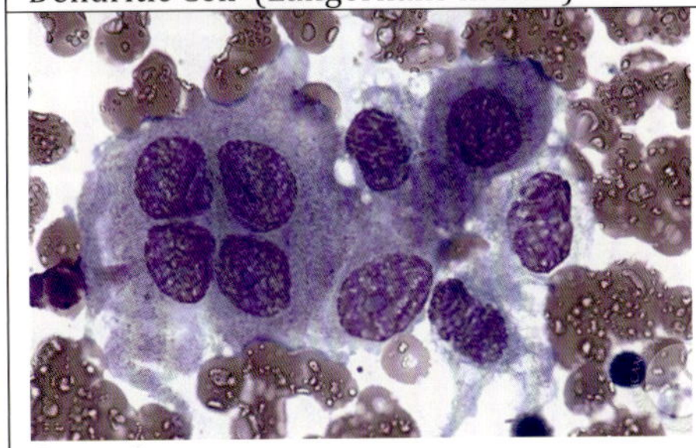

Osteoclast

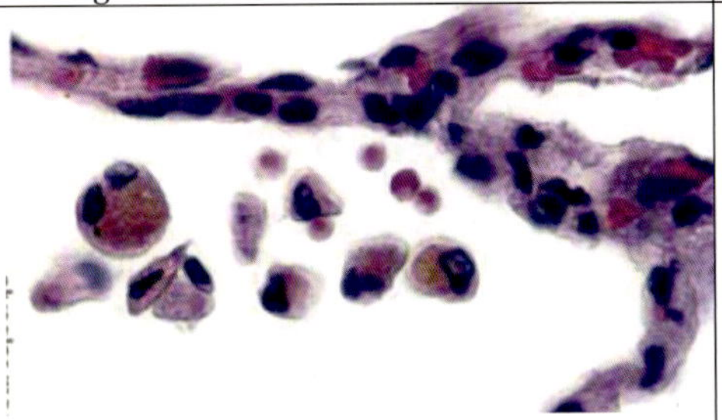

Aveolar Macrophage (Dust Cell)

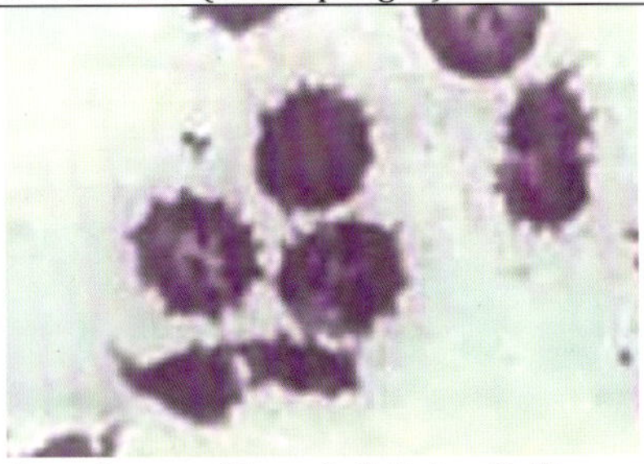

Acanthocyte (Spur Cell, Spiny Cell)
Abetalipoproteinemia (B48, B100)

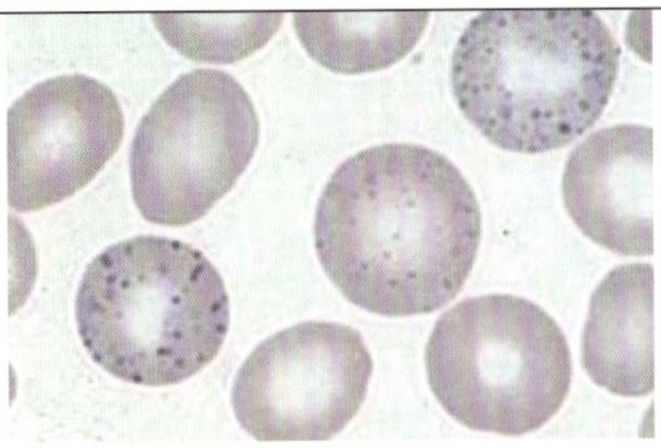

Basophillic Stippling
Lead poisoning, alcohol use, TTP,
Arsenic poisoning, Thalassemia,
Chronic Disease

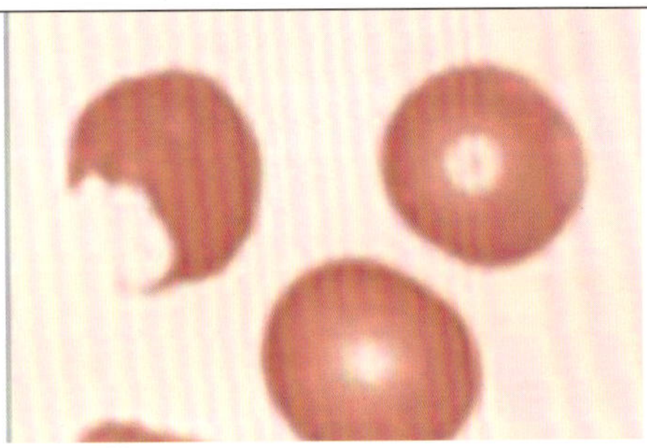

Bite Cell
(AKA: Degmacytes)
G6PD
RBC that spleenic macrophage was trying to remove

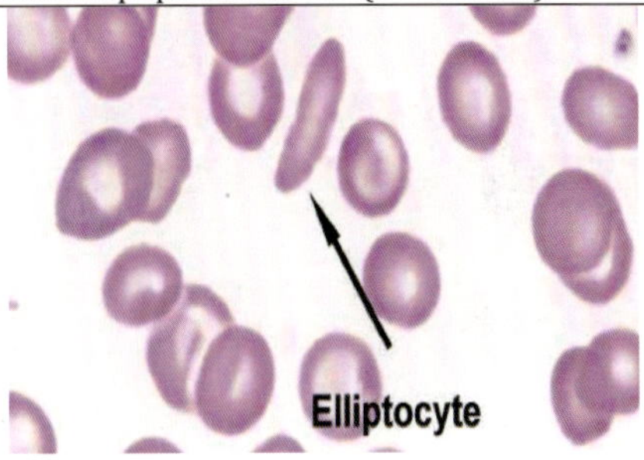

Elliptocyte
(AKA: Ovalocytes)
Hereditary elliptocytosis

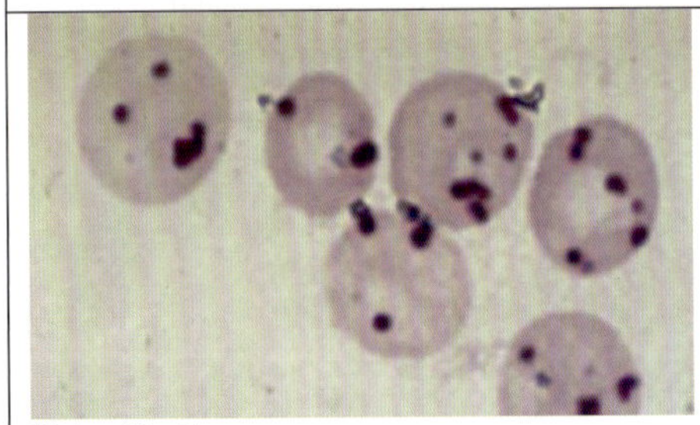

Heinz Bodies
Oxydation of Hb
G6PD deficiency
α-thalassemia

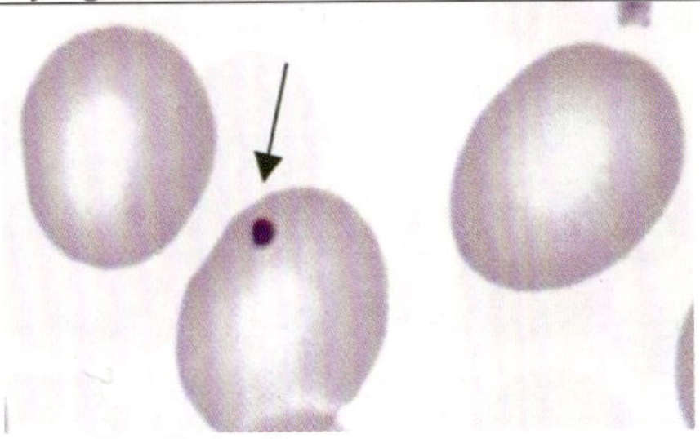

Howell-Jolly bodies
Nuclear remnants
Asplenia, hypospenia

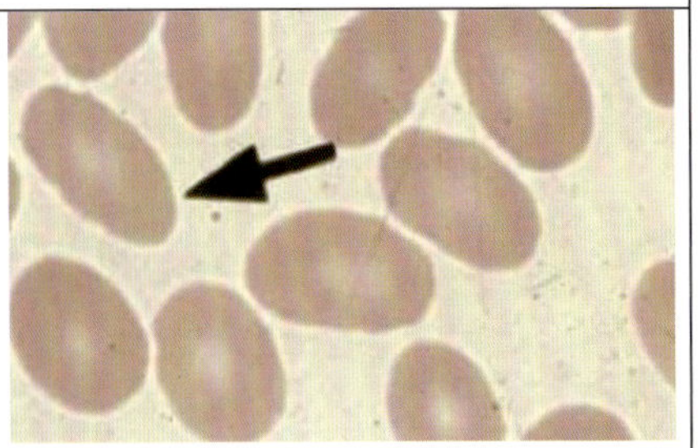

Ovalocyte (Macro)

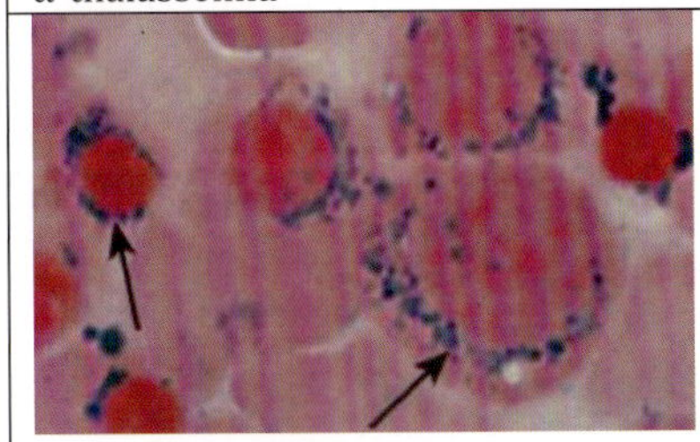

Ringed Sideroblast
Iron overload

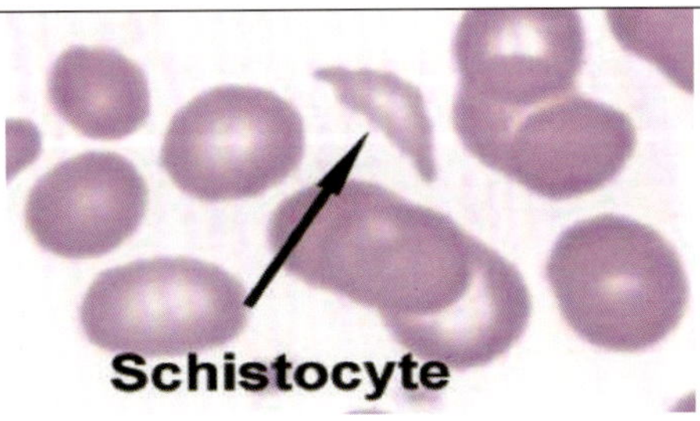

Schistocyte
Indicates hemolysis

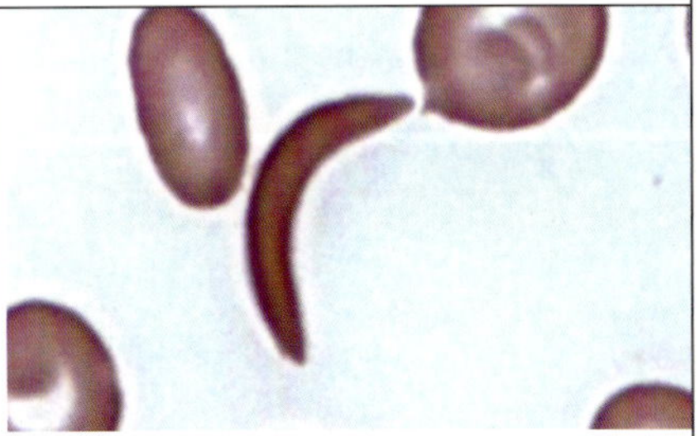

Sickle Cell
(AKA: Drepanocytes)

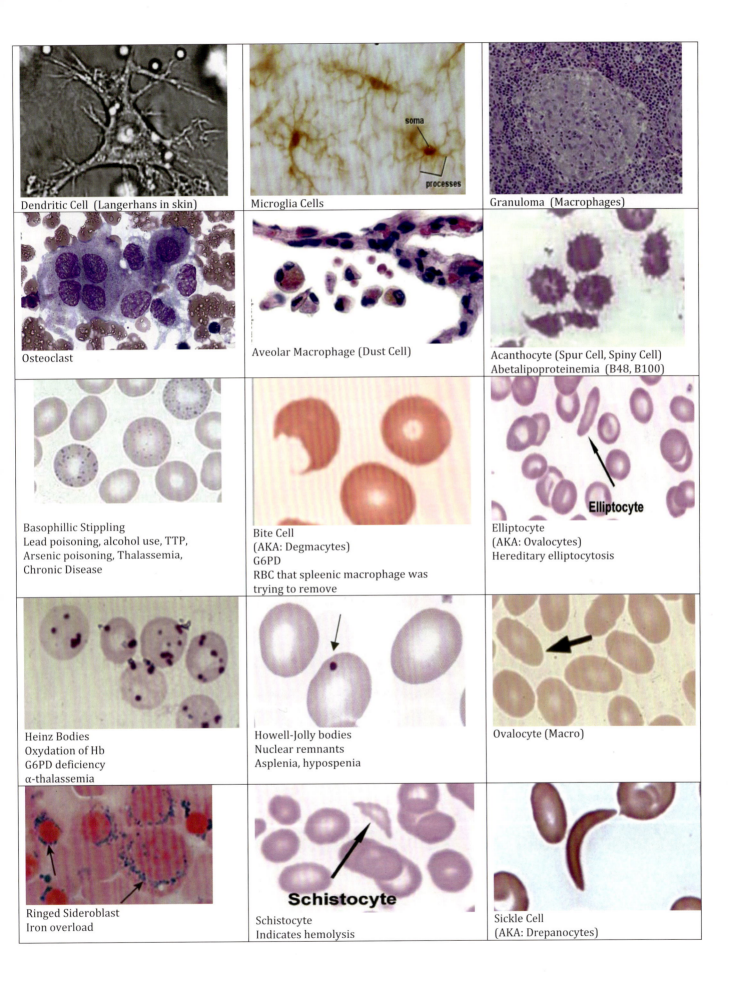

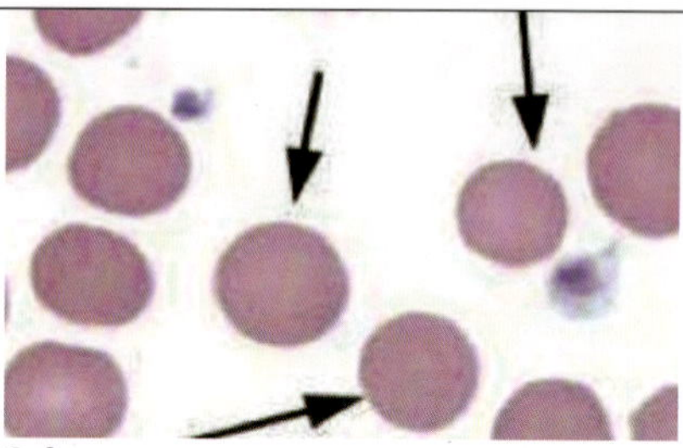

Spherocyte
Hereditary Spherocytos
(Osmotic fragility)

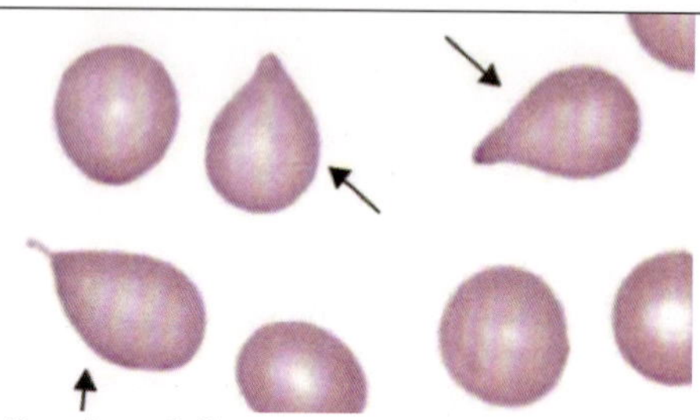

Teardrop Cell
(AKA: Dacrocytes)
Bone Marrow Fibrosis (Myelofibrosis)

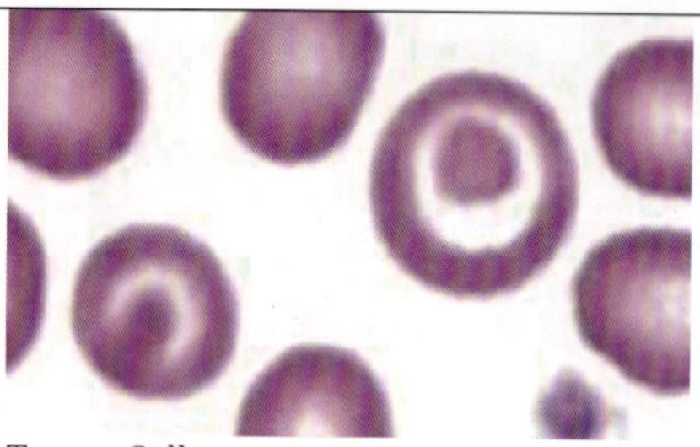

Target Cell
(AKA: Codocytes)
Thalassemia

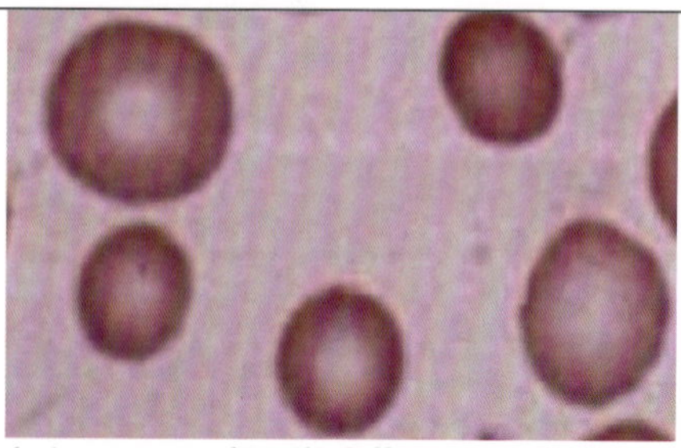

Anisocytosis (RBC's different sizes)

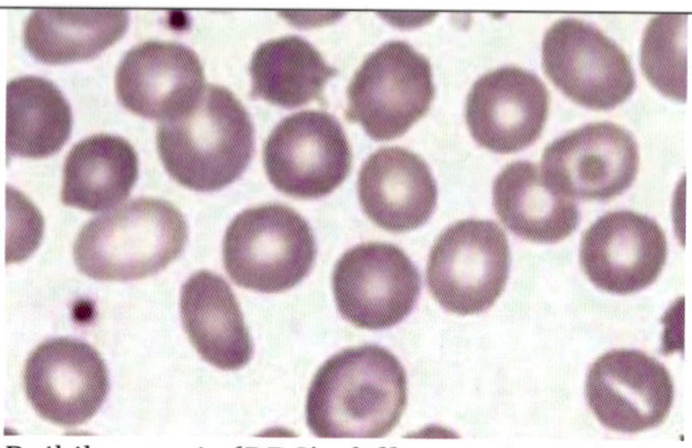

Poikilocytosis (RBC's different shapes)

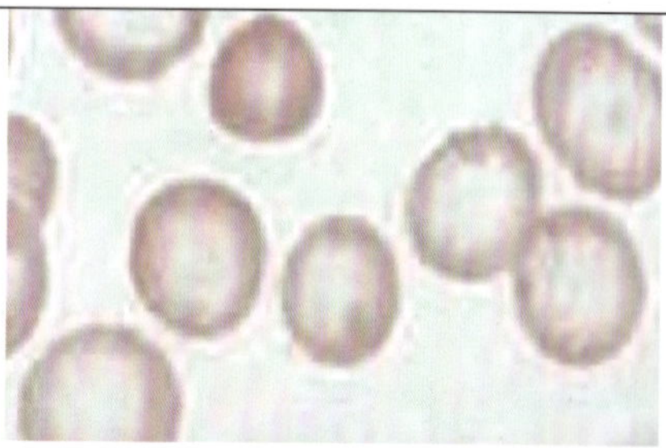

Hypochromic RBC's

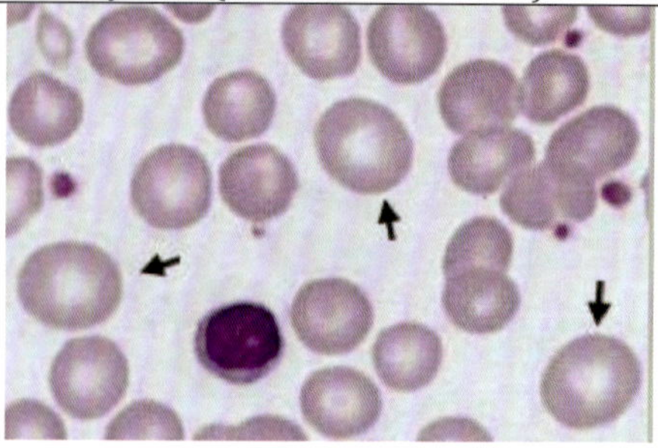

Macrocytic RBC's (Larger)

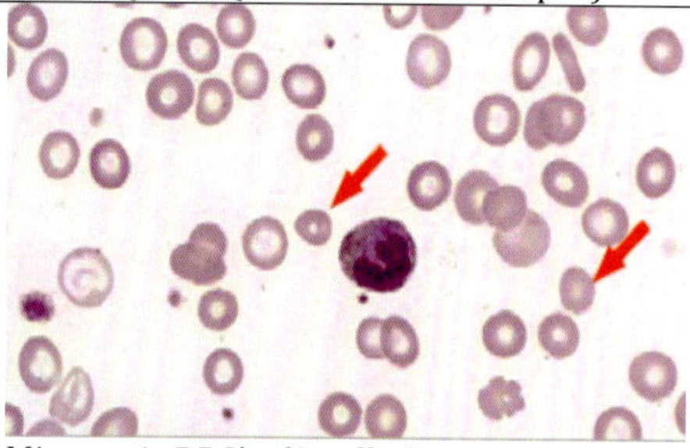

Microcytic RBC's (Smaller)

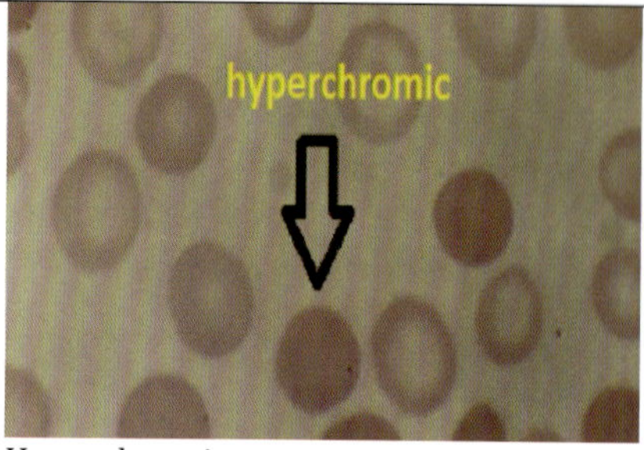

Hyperchromic

Blood Types

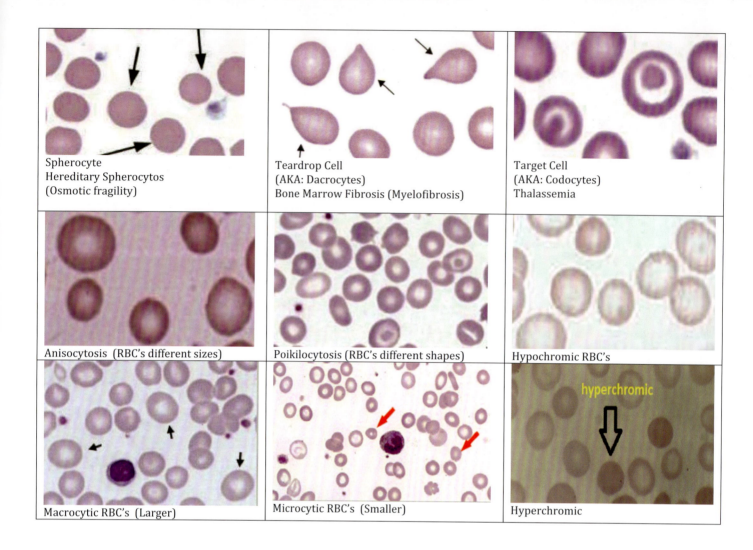

Blood type	RBC Surface Antigen: Donor/Recipient	Notes
A	A Antigen on RBC, Anti B in plasma (Attacks B)	
B	B Antigen on RBC, Anti A in plasma (Attacks A)	
AB	A, B Antigens on RBC. No antibodies in plasma	Universal Recipient of RBC's. Universal Donor of Plasma.
O	No A, B Antigens. A, B antibodies In plasma	Universal Donor of RBC's. Universal Recipient of Plasma.
Rh	Rh antigen on RBC. Rh – mother, Rh + fetus. (**tip**: **M**om is "**M**" for **M**inus (-) In first birth, mother is exposed to infant's blood causing her blood to make antibodies against Rh+ blood for all subsequent births. In subsequent pregnancies with Rh+ fetuses, mother IgG antibodies (anti-Rh IgG) cross the placenta and attacks the fetus's blood causing hemolytic disease of the newborn. (AKA: erythroblast fetalis).	**RhoGAM (Rho (D) immune globulin** is given to mother at 28 weeks. (Passive immunity). If mother is alloimmune: no vaccine needed.

Oxygen Capacity Comparisons

Pathology	Hb	PO_2 (Dissolved O2 in blood)	O_2 Sat on Hb	Total O2 (O_2 Sat + PO_2)
CO	NL	NL	↓	↓
Anemia	↓	NL	NL	↓
Polycythemia	↑	NL	NL	↑

BLOOD TRANSFUSION REACTIONS

Reaction	Timeline	Pathology	Signs	Treatment	Prevention
Allergic-Urticaria	2 – 3 hrs	Donor anti-leukocyte antibodies Lung infiltrates, **IgE Mast** Cells, Type I hypersensitivity	Wheezing, flushing, pruritis, angioedema, pulmonary edema, fever	Antihistamines	
Anaphylactic	**Seconds** to Minutes	**Anti-IgA Antibodies**. Patient is IgA deficient	Dyspnea, hypotension, bronchospasm, urticaria, respiratory arrest, tachycardia, angioedema.	1- **STOP** transfusion 2- IM Epinephrine	Wash RBC, or give blood that has no IgA
Delayed Hemolytic	2 – 10 days	+ Coombs, Hemolytic anemia antibody response	Mild Fever		
Febrile	1 – 6 hrs	**Host antibodies against donor HLA antigens** and WBC's (Leukocytes). Caused by cytokine accumulation in **blood storage. Type II Hypersensitivity**	**Chills, low grade fever**, flushing. No hemolysis.	**Wash/filter RBC** and decrease WBC (Leukocyte antigen)	
Hyperacute Hemolytic	Within 1 hour	**ABO group incompatibility. Extravascular hemolysis. Hemolytic Disease of the Newborn. Host antibodies against foreign antigen on donor RBC.** **+ Coombs**. Due to mismatched blood type. **Antigen/Antibody complex. Type II hypersensitivity. RH incompatible activates compliment which activates MAC = lysis of RBC. DIC** (Compliment mediated cell lysis)	Fever, flank pain, chills, dark urine, **jaundice** = extravascular **hemolysis**, hypotension, hemoglobinemia= intravascular, tachycardia. **Urinalysis shows Hb**, ↑ LDH, ↑ Bilirubin, ↓ Haptoglobin.	1- **STOP** transfusion 2- Hydrate with normal saline	Careful cross and match

Additional Transfusion Information

TRALI: Transfusion-related acute lung injury. AKA: Leukoagglutination reaction.	1 hr	Antibodies in the donor blood against **recipient WBC.**	Acute onset of non-cardiogenic pulmonary edema. Shortness of breath, flank/back pain, fever, chills, hematuria, CXR shows transient pulmonary infiltrates.	Supportive, diuretics, resolves spontaneously.
Minor Blood Group Incompatibility	Days	Blood incompatibility to antigens (Lewis, Kell, Duffy, Kidd) or Rh.	Jaundice after several days, otherwise asymptomatic. No rise in Hct after transfusion.	No treatment.
Fluid Overload		After transfusion of large numbers of RBC's the patient becomes short of breath and rhonchi and crackles are heard.		
Elderly patients with ↓↓ HCT		Must resuscitate with Red Blood Cells		
Platelet Transfusion		1 Unit raises platelet count 5000. If after administration the platelet count rises only a small amount or none at all check patient for antibodies against platelets.		
Jehovah Witness		(Adults) Do not accept blood. In situation of hypovolemia give IV fluids and vasopressors.		

Blood Product Replacements

- **When to transfuse:**
  - **HCT < 25 in the elderly or those with heart disease**
  - **Symptomatic patient**
- **Transfuse packed red blood cells (PRBC's) (Concentrated whole blood = HCT 80%. It is usually double the normal HCT because a percentage of plasma has been removed). Each unit of PRBC should raise HCT 3 points.**

Packed Red Blood Cells (PRBC's) Transfusions for anemia. Concentrated whole blood = HCT 80%. It is usually double the normal HCT because a percentage of plasma has been removed. Each unit of PRBC should raise **HCT 3 points**. Transfusions for anemia • HCT < 25 in the elderly or those with heart disease • Symptomatic patients (lightheaded, dizzy, confused, hypotensive, angina, shortness of breath, tachycardia) • No need to transfuse young and/or asymptomatic patients	**Fresh Frozen Plasma (FFP)** Replaces clotting factors for active bleeding in patients due to **Warfarin toxicity (↑↑ PT/INR).**
Cryoprecipitate Replaces fibrinogen to ↑ clotting. Contains clotting factors, VWF and Factor VIII.	**Plasmapheresis** Removal, treatment and return of blood and blood plasma from the circulation. The filtered plasma is discarded (removing antibodies) and the RBC's with donor plasma (or albumin) are returned to the patient. The patient's plasma can also be returned if the antibodies or other undesired macromolecules are removed. **TX** used in many diseases, in particularly autoimmune. Guillain-Barre, Myasthenia gravis, TTP, Goodpasture syndrome, HUS, Lambert-Eaton, SLE, hyperviscosity.

Heme Pathway

Glycine and succinyl-CoA to d-aminolevulinic acid (d-ALA) via ***d-aminolevulinic acid synthase**
(rate limiting step) with cofactor B6
d-ALA to Porphobilinogen via ****ALA dehydratase**
Porphobilinogen to Hydroxymethylbilane via *****Porphobilinogen deaminase**
Hydroxymethylbilane to Uroporphyrinogen
Uroporphyrinogen to Coproporphyrinogen III via ******Uroporphyrinogen decarboxylase**
Coproporphyrinogen III to Protoporphyrin to Heme via ****Ferrochelatase** with cofactor Fe

Decrease in heme = increase in ALA synthase
Increase in heme = decrease in ALA synthase

(**tip**: to help remember the beginning substances and the enzymes in order for the heme path: Guys (Glycine) suck (succinyl) ALA and tell Poor Bill (Porphobilinogen) that Yur (Uro) a good Fello (ferro).

Heme Pathway Pathologies

****Lead Poisoning**

- Lead stops heme synthesis by inhibiting **ferrochelatase** (causing Protoporphyrin to accumulate) and **ALA dehydratase** (causing δ-ALAs to accumulate).
- Deficiency or absence of **ALA dehydratase and accumulation of d-ALA**; **OR**
- Deficiency of absence of **Ferrochelatase and accumulation of Protoporphyrin**
- Stops heme synthesis
- Higher rates with low socio-economic status
- Lead Exposure Risk: House paint in houses pre 1978, painted children's **toys from China**, plumbers, miners, auto mechanics (batteries), **battery** factory workers, paper hangers, hunters (lead bullets), **ammunitio**n factory workers, imported toys, crayons, vehicle exhaust, old claw foot bathtubs or cosmetics.
- PICA: **eating unusual things** (ie: ice, paper, dirt)
- Pregnancy: miscarriages and still births
- SX: **Abdominal pain**, **Spoon nails**, headache, **constipation**, insomnia, irritability, **learning difficulties**, joint/muscle aches, confusion (**mental lethargy**), **basophilic stippling** of RBC's (aggregates of rRNA retained in the RBC's), **aggressive**, anemia, miscarriage, stillbirth, **behavior problems (hyperactivity)**, ↓ libido, HTN, kidney failure, behavior problems, fatigue, seizures, mental deterioration, constipation, hemolytic anemia, coma, death.
- Initial testing of iron blood levels at 12 and 24 months old. . Levels should be ≤ 5 mcg/dL.
- DX: X-Ray shows **lead lines** (lighter lines: Burton Lines) on gingivae and metaphyses of long bones.
  Labs: Microcytic, hypochromic anemia, basophilic stippling, ↑ FEP (Free erythrocyte porphyrins).

  TX: (Chelation therapy) **Dimercaprol, EDTA. Succimer** for children. Begin chelation for lead levels ≥ 45 mcg/dL.

  Blood Lead levels ≤ 10 μg/dL = no risk
  Blood Lead levels < 45 μg/dL = remove child from house and retest in one month.
  Blood Lead levels > 45 μg/dL = Chelation Therapy
  Blood Lead levels 45 – 69 μg/dL = DMSA SX: abdominal pain, constipation.
  Blood Lead levels >70 μg/dL = EDTA SX: hemolytic anemia, cognitive, behavior disorders.
- **Report to Dept of Health when lead levels > 15 mcg/dL.**

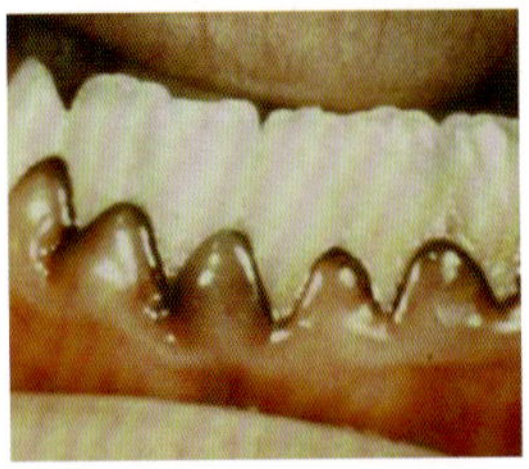

Gingival Lead Lines

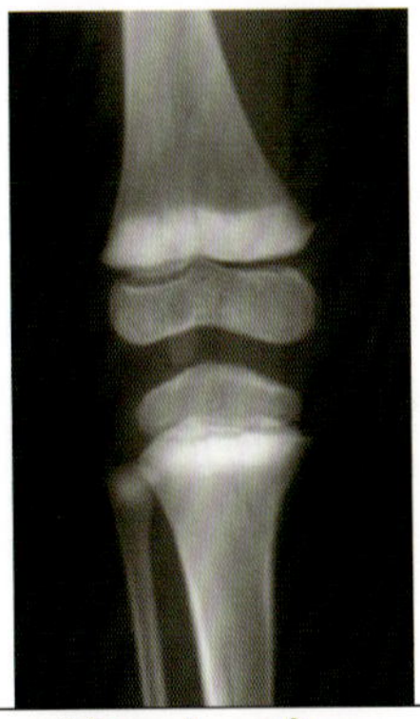

Lead Lines on bones

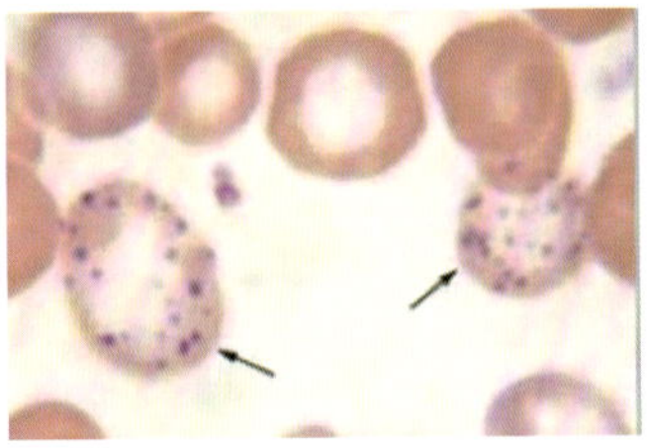

Basophilic Stippling

*****Acute intermittent porphyria (AD, Autosomal Dominant)**

- Deficiency or absence of **Porphobilinogen deaminase and accumulation of ALA and Porphobilinogen**
- See Coporphobilinogen in the urine
- Precipitated by stress, drugs, alcohol, starvation
- SX: **Severe abdominal pain**, **urine turns dark**, **psychological** problems, seizures, anxiety, electrolyte disturbances and paranoia
- TX: Glucose and heme

******Porphyria cutanea tarda, AD**

- Deficiency or absence of **Uroporphyrinogen decarboxylase and accumulation of Uroporphyrin**
- Blistering reaction to sun exposure due to high porphyrin accumulation in the body.
- See Uroporphyrin in urine = tea color urine
- Labs: Increased 24-hour urinary uroporphyrins.
- Associated with Hepatitis C, alcoholism, liver disease (hepatitis, hemochromatosis), diabetes.
- Precipitated by estrogen and OCP's
- **Photosensitive** (only come out at night)
- SX: **Blistering on sun-exposed skin** (painless blisters), excessive hair growth on the face (Werewolf syndrome, hypertrichosis).
- TX: No estrogen or alcohol, avoid the sun or use high SPF sunscreen, phlebotomy (or **Deferoxamine**) if due to hemochromatosis

Anemias

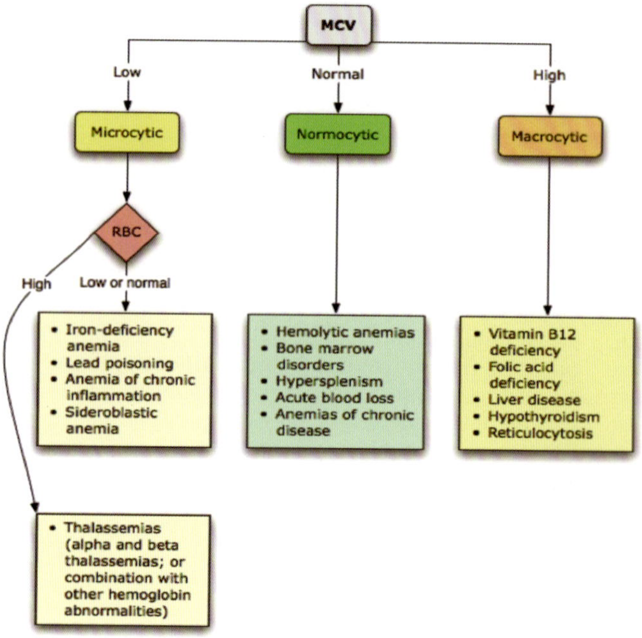

- Anisocytosis: RBC's are not the same size. Typical finding in anemias.
- Poikilocytosis: RBC's with abnormal shapes (note the variety of shapes in the table below)
- MCV = Mean corpuscular volume: average volume of a RBC. Indicates the size of the RBC's.
- MCH (Mean Corpuscular Hemoglobin: average mass of Hb per RBC in a sample of blood) and MCHC (Mean Corpuscular Hemoglobin Concentration: concentration of Hb in a given volume of packed RBC) reflect the Hb content of RBC's.
- RBC measurements diagnose the types of anemia.
- Microcytic Anemia: Smaller than normal RBC's. Anemia with MCV < 80, ↓ MCH. (iron deficiency, thalassemia, sideroblastic, blood loss, chronic disease, inflammation).
- Normocytic: Anemia with normal MCV values (prosthetic heart valves, sepsis, tumor, aplastic anemia, deficiency of erythropoietin, chronic disease, sudden blood loss)
- Macrocytic: Larger than normal RBC's. Anemia with MCV > 100. (B-12 or folate deficiency, pernicious anemia, alcoholism, chemotherapy).
- Hypochromic anemia: RBC's that are more pale than normal: area of central pallor is increased,
↓ HB concentration and ↓ MCH.
- Hyperchromic anemia: RBC's with ↑ concentration of Hb and ↑ MCH. (Celiac, alcoholism)
- Aplastic Anemia: Deficiency of all three blood cell types (pancytopenia): RBC's (anemia), WBC's (leukopenia), and platelets (thrombocytopenia).
- Normal Labs: **Hb** (**Low Hb = anemia**)
Male: 13.5 – 17.5 g/dL; Female: 12.0 – 16.0 g/dL
- Normal Labs: **HCT** (proportion, by volume, of the blood that consist of RBC).
Male: 41 – 53%; Female: 36% - 46%
Example: 36% means there are 36 mL of RBC in 100 mL of blood.
Low Hct = **anemia**. High Hct = **polycythemia, dehydration, EPO use**.
- DX: BIT: CBC (Complete Blood Count) to evaluate the anemia (specifically the **MCV/MCHC**)
MCV: differentiates microcytic from normocytic from macrocytic.
MCHC: indicates problems with synthesis of hemoglobin, which will differentiate between hypochromic, normal chromic and hyperchromic.
- **Labs to help differentiate between anemias: B12, Folate levels (macrocytic), iron studies (microcytic – iron deficiency), Bilirubin (direct and total), Reticulocyte count, Haptoglobin, LDH.**
- SX: Fatigue, pallor, pale conjunctiva, jaundice, scleral icterus (yellow eyes), **pica (craving for ice, dirt, or other odd substance)**, systolic murmur (AKA: flow murmur).

Anemia and Symptoms (Normal HCT: Male 41- 53%; Female 36 – 46%)

Hematocrit	**Symptoms**
> 30%	No symptoms
25 – 30%	Shortness of breath, fatigue
20 – 25%	Lightheadedness, angina
< 20%	Syncope, angina

Note: CBC is best test to indicate anemia.
Note: MCV (Mean Corpuscular Volume) is the best test to differentiate between anemia's/causes.
Note: ↓ oxygen delivery = ischemia = cyanosis = tissue death.
Note:: Ischemia to cardiac tissue = angina = death.
Note: Ischemia (↓ oxygen) can be caused by anemia, carbon monoxide, hypoxia, coronary artery disease.

Microcytic Anemia
(MCV <80, hypochromic)

AKA: Microcytes, Microcytosis

- ↓ MCV < 80, ↓ MCH
- Cell proliferation is faster than hemoglobin synthesis, which causes smaller cells to be produced.
- Due to production problems = ↓ reticulocyte count (except for alpha thalassemia with 3 genes deleted has ↑ reticulocytes).
- All are **hypochromic** and can show target cells on a blood smear.
- BIT: Iron studies

Iron Deficiency Anemia
MCC of microcytic anemia
MCC in adults = chronic blood loss due to colon cancer

↓ in RBC (Hb) because ↓ in iron.

SX: Microcytosis (AKA: Microcythemia) = small RBC, fatigue, **blood loss** (MC: upper or lower **GI bleed, colon cancer, parasites**), weakness, pallor of mucus membranes and/or skin), pale conjunctiva, **hypochromia** (central pallor of the RBC – pale/colorless RBC), poikilocytosis (various shapes of RBC's), anisocytosis (various sizes of RBC's), **PICA** (desire to eat odd food: dirt, paper, ice), **glossitis** (shinny, smooth, red tongue), **koilonychias (spoon shaped nails)**, depression, **Restless Leg Syndrome** (irresistible urge to move legs/body to stop odd, crawling f or uncomfortable sensations), **occult blood** (hidden blood in the stool), **Plummer-Vinson** syndrome (triad: iron deficiency, glossitis, esophageal webs).

Labs: MCV < 80
Iron Labs: ↓ Serum iron (Fe sat), ↑ TIBC,
↓ Ferritin (ferritin is the most sensitive test), **↑ RDW, ↓ Reticulocytes, ↓ Hb, ↓ Platelets.**

MAT: Bone marrow biopsy

Causes: chronic blood loss, malabsorption (iron is absorbed in the duodenum with the help of Vit. C), breastfed infants (supplemented in formulas), poor diet in children, heavy periods, bleeding ulcers, pregnancy, colon polyps in elderly, helminthes infections (hookworm, tapeworm, fluke, roundworms, Yersinia, other invading bacteria, malaria, Vitamin A deficiency.

TX: Oral **Ferrous Sulfate,** adding **Vitamin C** (ascorbic acid) to aid in absorption. Do not take with dairy products.
If dietary cause: ↑ intake of iron rich foods: lentils, red meat, beans, dark green leafy vegetables.

NOTE: Early stages of Anemia of Chronic Dz and Iron deficiency can present as normocytic anemia and then as bleeding continues (chronic) will be come microcytic.
NOTE: Mononucleosis (EBV) can present with mild anemia due to antibodies attacking virus and RBC (RBC look similar to the virus). No treatment needed. Transient.

Iron deficiency in infants:
Iron stores in newborns last 4 – 6 months. Normal iron levels in infants: 9 – 11mg/dL by 12 weeks. Breast milk has low iron but is better absorbed in the babies intestinal tract than formula. May need to supplement with **Ferrous Sulfate**.
Watch for iron deficiency in children >1 year old due to drinking cows milk (verses breast milk or formula) as **cows milk is low in iron**. Milk also decreases the absorption of milk in the gut.

Beta Thalassemia Major: (homozygote)
(AKA: Cooley Anemia)
All B chains absent.

Point mutation (aka: missense) in **splice sites on the mRNA** which **↓ β-Globin beta chain synthesis or absence, which causes shortened** genes.
Splice sites: AKA's: **Spliceosome, introns, exons, snRNAs** (small nuclear RNA), **defect in processing mRNA.=, defective translation of β-globin on mRNA protein.**
B-thalassemia disrupts the normal splicing by the creation of a new 3' splice site.

SX: microcytic/hypochromic anemia, severe **bone deformities (frontal bossing, "chipmunk" faces)** due to bone marrow expansion, **extramedullary hematopoiesis** (hematopoiesis occurring outside the medulla of the bones of the skull and face), nucleated RBC's may be seen (reticulocytes), hepatosplenomegaly, cardiac decompensation (when the Hb < 4 mg/dL).

DX: MAT: **Hb electrophoresis shows: ↑ HbA2 and**

↑ HbF with normal Alpha genes.
↓↓ MCV < 80, Target cells. Normal Iron Studies.
X-rays show "**crew cut**" appearance due to bone marrow expansion from ↑ erythropoiesis, **target cells, normal iron studies** (thalassemia has **nothing to do with iron**), severe anemia, ↓ LDH, ↓ haptoglobin, ↑ indirect bilirubin, ↓ reticulocytes.

MAT: Hemoglobin electrophoresis.

Risk: ↑ risk aplastic crisis by Parvo B-19.

TX: **lifelong blood transfusions** causing **2° hemochromatosis** (iron overload) which requires regular phlebotomy. Splenectomy (note: any Asplenic person is at increased risk for infection from encapsulated organisms). **Deferoxamine** (chelation therapy) and vitamin C for toxicity. Bone Marrow transplant.

Folate and penicillin prophylaxis daily. Immunization: Give all standard immunization vaccines but should add pneumococcal, influenza, meningococcal, Hepatitis B, growth hormone (excess iron may cause deficiency in growth hormone).

(NOTE: ANY Asplenic person must receive Pneumococcal vaccine to protect against infection from encapsulated organisms).

Iron Deficiency Anemia   Cont'd

Iron Needs:
4 mg/day absorbed in the duodenum (assisted with Vit. C).
Average daily requirement: 1 – 2 mg/day.
Pregnancy 5 – 6 mg/day.
Menses 2 – 3 mg/day.
Iron deficiency: can occur with 5 mL (1 tsp) blood loss/day.

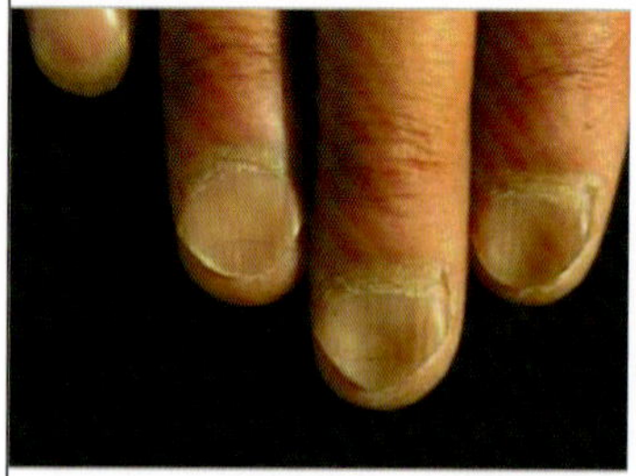

Spoon shaped nails

Glossitis

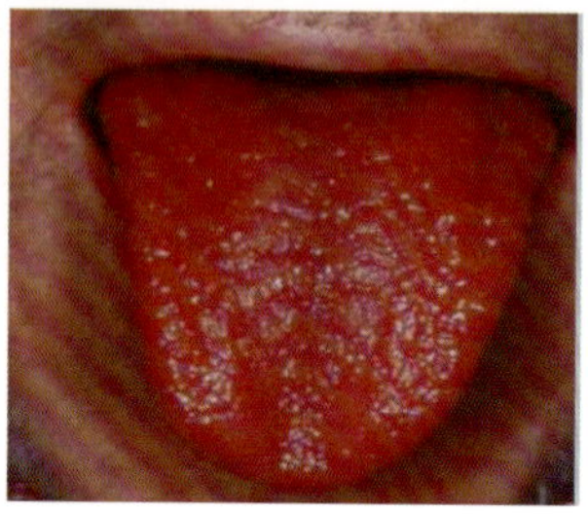

β-thalassemia Minor   Cont'd

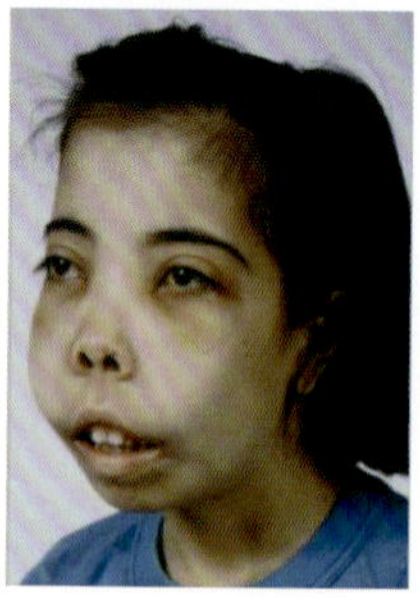

Chipmunk Face

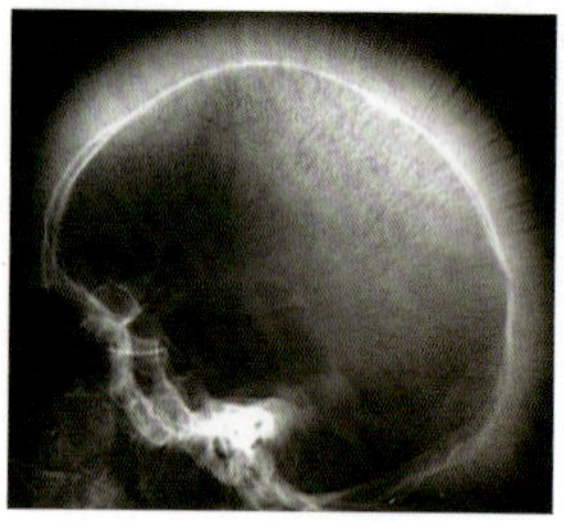

Crew Cut Skull

β-thalassemia Minor: (heterozygote)
SX: asymptomatic, β chain is underproduced.
Only 1 bad β gene.
DX: ↑ **HbA2 (>3.5%)**
TX: No treatment = reassure.

A-thalassemia

Gene **deletion** of the α globin gene. (HBA1, HBA2) =
↓ alpha-globin production so that there are excess β globin chains.

Pathology:
Normal adult Hb = 2α, 2β
1 alpha gene (alleles) deleted = silent carrier = no affect.
2 alpha genes deleted = alpha thalassemia minor.
3 alpha genes deleted = HbH disease (Hemoglobin H disease).
4 alpha genes deleted = HBH = **Hemoglobin Barts** (hydrops fetalis) = baby can't survive. No alpha Hb made so there is excess γ so it binds all oxygen so that no oxygen goes to fetus.

SX: **Target cells**, microcytic/hypochromic anemia),
Heinz bodies, hepatosplenomegaly.

DX: DNA analysis

Labs: MCV < 80, normal RDW
3 Gene Deletion (HbH) shows ↑ reticulocyte count.

MAT: Genetic studies, DNA sequencing.

.

Sideroblastic Anemia

Bone marrow produces ringed **sideroblast** instead of normal RBC's. Abnormal iron builds up in the mitochondria.

MCC: alcohol. (Suppresses bone marrow)
Other causes: genetic (X-link defect in δ-ALA synthase gene in the heme synthesis pathway), copper deficiency, Vitamin B6 deficiency, myelodysplastic syndrome (ineffective production of all blood cell lines), lead poisoning, **Isoniazid**.

Histology:
MAT: Prussian blue staining is positive for **ringed sideroblasts**. Bone marrow shows **iron granules** forming a "ring" inside the **mitochondria**.
AKA: Atypical, abnormal nucleated erythroblasts with granules of iron accumulated in the mitochondria.

Labs: ↑ iron, normal TIBC, ↑ ferritin, MCV < 80,
↓ reticulocyte count, ↑ RDW (RBC volume).

Sideroblastic Anemia can be either microcytic or macrocytic (macrocytic due to myelodysplasia (preleukemic syndrome).

TX: **Pyridoxine (B_6).** (B_6 = cofactor for δ-ALA synthase)
TX for iron overload: Oral iron chelator: **Deferasirox, Deferiprone.**
Remove source of exposure.
Parenteral iron chelator: **Deferoxamine.**

Chronic Anemia - later stage Cancer, chronic infection/disease or internal bleeding. (Rheumatoid arthritis). If chronic DZ is renal failure, **must give erythropoietin**. **↓ TIBC, ALL else is NORMAL to ↓ serum iron (Fe sat), ↑ ferritin, ↓ iron** Ferritin (stored iron) is "locked away" in storage or inside macrophages so that the offending organisms are not able to get to the iron and use it for themselves. TX: Treat underlying cause.	

Thalassemia Differentials

Differential	Alpha Thalassemia	Beta Thalassemia
Cause	**Gene deletion on the α globin gene**	**Point mutation** (aka: missense) in **splice sites on the mRNA**
Hemoglobin	If deletion of 3 genes: Presence of HbH and ↑ reticulocytes	**Increased HbF and HbA2**
Diagnosis	DNA analysis	Hb electrophoresis

Iron

- Ferritin: Iron storage protein. Iron in storage. (**tip**: ferrit**IN** = iron **IN** storage. It is like a bank vault for iron). Storage is inside of the macrophages.
- Ferrous: Iron in the F2 state. Iron that we can use. (**tip**: ferro**US** is the iron that all of **US** use)
- **Haptoglobin**: Binds to free Hb (Hb that has been released from dead/dying RBC's) so that it can escort it to the spleen to be recycled in the bone marrow) (**tip**: I just **HAPTIN** to be going along and picked up a Hb)
- Hepcidin: From liver. Regulates iron metabolism. Binds and inhibits Ferroportin so iron is not exported outside the cells so that it is sequestered inside enterocytes, hepatocytes and macrophages causing ↓ in plasma iron levels. Assist in keeping iron "hidden" in storage (Ferritin) so that antigens do not use the iron for themselves. Helps "lock" it inside the vault.
- Ferroportin: transmembrane protein that transports iron from inside of the enterocytes (basolateral surface) in the gut to the outside of the cell/gut.
- Transferrin: Glycoprotein mainly synthesized in the liver and controls iron concentrations in the serum. Part of the innate immune system found in the mucosa. Binds iron in order to control free iron levels low so that antigens/bacteria can't use it for themselves.
  Transferrin saturation = Iron divided by TIBC.
  Delivers (transports iron in the blood) iron to tissues from the macrophages and enterocytes in the duodenum (vaults where the iron is stored).
  Each transferrin carries 2 iron in the F^3, ferric state.
  Transferrin is ↑ in pregnancy and OCP use.
- Serum Iron (Iron saturation): the amount of iron that is in the serum
- **TIBC (AKA: Transferrin): (Total Iron Binding Capacity):** This is the "guy" who's job is to go out and find iron when it is low/gone from the serum and the storage vault (ferritin). The ONLY time it is working (above normal) is if there is little or no iron left anywhere. (Storage or serum). If it can "see" any iron, it does not increase. So if there is no iron in the serum but it does see iron "hidden away" inside the iron vault (ferritin) it does not care if it is being held hostage (sequestered to keep it from antigens), it only knows it "see's iron so will not go to work.
  (**Note**: so in the questions, always look to see if there is ANY iron, ANYWHERE in the body: serum or storage. If there is ANY iron, TIBC will always be normal because it "sees" iron so has no reason to work).
  Note: TIBC is a measure of unbound/open sites on transferrin. When ↑ open sites on transferrin = ↑ unbound (capacity) sites.

Microcytic Anemia Iron Studies

	Serum Iron (Iron O_2 Sat) (circulating iron)	TIBC	**Ferritin (storage)**	**MCV**	**Transferrin (TIBC & Iron O_2 sat)**	**HCT**	**Notes**
Iron Deficiency Anemia	↓	↑	↓	↓	↓	<30	↑ RDW ↑ Platelets
Thalassemia (genetic) **Only one with normal iron studies**	↑	↓	↑	↓↓↓	↑↑	>30, t Target cells, ↑ HbA2	
Chronic Disease	↓	↓	NL to ↓	NL to ↓	NL - ↓		
Sideroblastic	↑	NL					
Hemochromatosis	↑	↓	↑		↑↑		
Pregnancy, OCP		↑			↓		

GI Blood Loss Source

- Blood loss of > 30% can present with a systolic blood pressure < 100 or heart rate > 100
- Most critical step in severe GI bleed is fluid resuscitation (bolus of 9% normal saline, AKA: Lactate ringers)
- Stool color indicates location of bleed
  Heme positive stool can occur from as little as 5 – 10 mL of blood loss.
  - Red, bright red: From the left side (descending colon, sigmoid, rectum), lower GI bleeds.
  - Maroon, burgundy: From the right side (ascending colon), lower GI bleeds.
    Lower GI bleeds due to: Cancer, Ischemic colitis, polyps, inflammatory bowel disease, Angiodysplasia, Diverticular disease.
  - Black, tarry: **Upper GI bleeds**
    Upper GI considered proximal to the **ligament of Treitz** (where the duodenum and jejunum meet).
    Coffee ground emesis (vomited blood: Bleeding from the duodenum, stomach or esophagus. This can occur with as little as 5 – 10 mL of blood loss.
    Upper GI bleeds: due to: Ulcer disease, cancer, varices, esophagitis, gastritis, duodenitis
- Test: Stood Guaiac Card (AKA: Hemoccult, Occult)
  - Only the iron in Hb or myoglobin will make the Guaiac card positive.

Normocytic Anemia (MCV 80 – 100, normochromic)

- Hemolytic and Nonhemolytic
- Hemolytic anemias are either intravascular (inside vessels) or extravascular (inside spleen: AKA: Reticuloendothelial system). Macrophages (AKA: sinusoidal or RES cells) are the phagocytic cells in the spleen.
- Antigens enter spleen and are phagocytized by dendritic cells in the white matter (Germinal Centers = B Cells)

Hemolytic Normocytic Anemia

Intravascular (inside vessels)	**Extravascular (inside spleen)**
• High RBC destruction: ↑LDH, ↓ **Haptoglobin**, **schistocytes**, ↑ reticulocytes, ↓ Hb, ↑ bilirubin, urobilinogen in urine • Causes: ATN (Acute tubular necrosis: Hb and myoglobin, dark urine) seen in TTP (Thrombotic thrombocytopenic purpura) and PNH (Paroxysmal Nocturnal Hemoglobinuria), prosthetic aortic value (valve replacement for aortic stenosis)	• Normal Haptoglobin (Macrophages can't remove RBC's so they are not broken down so no haptoglobin is needed), ↑ LDH, spherocytes, ↑ unconjugated bilirubin (jaundice). • Causes: Hereditary spherocytosis, sickle cell, G6PD, autoimmune hemolysis, bilirubin gallstones, skin ulcers (S. aureus), osteomyelitis (Salmonella), aseptic necrosis of femoral head

Markers of Hemolysis

- ↑ indirect (non-conjugated) bilirubin
- Bilirubin gallstones if hemolysis becomes chronic (due to ↑ bilirubin)
- ↑ LDH
- ↓ Haptoglobin (**tip**: I just "Haptin" to be going by. The haptoglobin binds to the free Hb that was released from the dying RBC's) and then this complex is then removed by the spleen (reticuloendothelial system). So when haptoglobin counts go down this means that they are being bound up and used – meaning a lot of RBC's are dying (lysis).
- ↑ nucleated RBC's (RBC's being kicked out of the marrow before they totally mature because of such critical need of RBC's in circulation).
- ↑ Reticulocytes
- Hyperkalemia due to ↑ cell breakdown.
- Folate deficiency due to ↑ cell production.
- No hyperuricemia because RBC's do not have nuclei.
- Sudden ↓ in HCT
- Slight ↑ MCV. Reticulocytes are larger than normal cells.
- Hepatosplenomegaly
- Anemia
- Cardiac decompensation: failure of the heart to maintain adequate blood circulation.
- If severe: may see **"crew cut"** appearance of skull on x-ray due to extramedullary hematopoiesis (the main bone marrow can't keep up with RBC production so other bones not normally used to produce RBC's are now having to help in production).
- **Note:** Acute substantial hemolysis or blood loss/hemorrhage will drop HCT quickly, but the MCV will not change as quickly to reflect the change to microcytic anemia (showing iron deficiency). Chronic loss will stimulate the ↑ in reticulocytes which will then ↑ MCV (reticulocytes are larger than normal RBC's).

Non-hemolytic Normocytic Anemia

Anemia of Chronic Disease (early in the disease)	**Aplastic Anemia**
MOA: inflammation. Inflammation causes acute phase reactants to be released from liver. One of the reactants, Hepcidin binds ferroports in macrophages and in the enterocytes (in gut) to inhibit iron release/transport so that it is kept away from the invading organisms. Labs: ↓serum iron, ↑ ferritin, ↓ TIBC (TIBC is not out working because it "sees" iron in storage) Causes: RA, heart disease, infections, RA, acute inflammation, autoimmune disease, diabetes As diseases become chronic, this normocytic anemia will become iron deficiency anemia.	Pancytopenia. Failure or destruction of all myeloid stem cells in the bone marrow causing pancytopenia: RBC (anemia), WBC (leukopenia), platelets (thrombocytopenia). The bone marrow is replaced by fat (AKA: hypocellular bone marrow with fatty infiltration). Labs: **↓ WBC, ↓ RBC, ↓ Platelets (thrombocytopenia), ↓ HCT, ↓ Hb, ↑ MCV, ↑ bleeding (due to thrombocytopenia).** SX: Anemia, pallor, hemorrhage, bruising, petechiae, reticulocytopenia (immature RBC's), infection* (*Infection: due to the lack of defense cells, **even the slightest fever** must be considered an emergency). Labs: Pancytopenia. DX: MAT: Bone marrow biopsy. Causes: MCC: Fanconi's Anemia (see below), Exposure to chemicals, viruses (esp: **Parvo B19**), radiation, B12 and/or folate deficiency, SLE, HIV, PNH, CMV, EBV, Hepatitis, toxins (benzene, insecticides). Drugs: **Carbamazepine, Chloramphenicol, Alcohol, PTU, Methimazole, Phenytoin, Sulfa drugs, chemotherapy drugs.** **TX: Blood transfusions for anemia.** **Antibiotics for infections,** **Cyclosporine** (inhibits T cells) **or Tacrolimus.** **Packed platelets for bleeding.** **Allogenic bone marrow transplant. If unable to do bone transplant: Cyclosporine.**

Chronic Kidney Disease	
Chronic Kidney Disease All kidney functions are decreased or nonfunctional in chronic kidney dz. ↓ EPO = ↓ hematopoiesis TX: Give EPO exogenously. Must also supplement iron replacement in IV iron prep: **Dextran**.	

Normocytic Anemia – Intrinsic Hemolytic Anemia – Extravascular and Intravascular

- ↑ reticulocyte count due to hemolysis and/or blood loss

Sickle Cell Disease
(AKA: Sickle Cell Anemia (HbS)

HbS point mutation (aka: missense) in the β chain. Substitution of a single amino acid: glutamic acid with valine at position 6.
Valine is hydrophobic.
Autosomal recessive.
Homozygous for HbS.
HbA = 0%, HbS = 85 – 90%, HbF <2%
Extravascular

Complication: Vaso-occlusive crisis (disease): sickling of cells which causes them to be unable to bend/curve in vessels or to get caught at bifurcation of vessels thereby blocking flow of blood = ischemia, necrosis = severe pain.
Newborns: asymptomatic due to ↑ HbF (high affinity for oxygen)
(AKA: polymerization of Hb with hypoxic situations due to the substitution of amino acids.
AKA: aggregates on the unloading of oxygen)

Additional complications: **Avascular necrosis of the femoral head,** lower extremity skin ulcers (erythema nodosum), stroke, bilirubin gallstones (due to chronically ↑ bilirubin), infections from **encapsulated organisms**, **Osteomyelitis** (MC from Salmonella if they are asplenic, S. aureus if they have not become Asplenic yet <4 yrs old), Enlarged heart (hyperdynamic due to anemia), Retinopathy. Kidney problems (due to chronic kidney damage), macrocytic anemia (due to folate deficiency), dactylitis, Aplastic crisis.

Causes that precipitate a vaso-occlusive crisis (sickling crisis): **dehydration**, stress, infections, **low oxygen** situations, acidosis, changes in weather, cold temperatures, sickness, **Aplastic crisis (MCC: Parvo B19:** Parvo B-19 affects the bone marrow and cell production. First signs of a Parvo infection is a sudden ↓ in the reticulocyte count. **MAT for Parvo B-19 is a PCR for DNA).**

SX: Dactylitis (swelling of hands), severe pain, Acute chest syndrome (MCC death), avascular necrosis, stroke, priapism,
Splenomegaly in children and atrophy/absence of spleen in adults.

Autosplenectomy: (AKA: spleen sequestration): Howell-jolly bodies and target cells in blood smear. **Due to infarctions**. Normally occurs by the time a child reaches 5

Additional Sickle Cell Disease Complications

↑ Risk of infections by encapsulated organisms, malaria and babesiosis.
(MC: SHiN: Strep pneumo, H. influenza, N. meningitis)
All encapsulated: S. pneumo, Klebsiella, H. influenza, Salmonella, Pseudomonas, N. meningitis, Cryptococcus neoformans (**tip**: **S**ome **K**illers **H**ave **S**ome **P**retty **N**ice **C**rypts)

Osteomyelitis (infection/inflammation of the bone or bone marrow).
If it occurs before autosplenectomy: due to **S. aureus** because spleen is clearing organisms.
If it occurs after autosplenectomy: due to **Salmonella** because spleen no longer clearing encapsulated organisms.

Aplastic Crisis due to virus **Parvo B19** (Smallest, only SS non-enveloped DNA virus). Labs: ↓ reticulocyte count < .5, ↓ Hb.

Autosplenectomy: (AKA: spleen sequestration): Howell-Jolly bodies and target cells in blood smear. **Due to many micro-infarctions**. Occurs between 5 and 7 years old. Spleen will be atrophied.

Avascular Necrosis of the femoral head. (**Circumflex artery**).
SX: Hip pain with gradual restriction of movement.

Renal papillary necrosis due to low oxygen in papilla.

↑ Risk of strokes: MC: Broca's area because of occlusion and sludge of cerebral arteries. Common in children.
TX: Exchange transfusion to ↓ sickle cells in blood.

Macrocytic anemia due to **folate deficiency**. (↑ RBC breakdown = ↑ consumption of folate in bone marrow)
TX: Daily supplements of **folic acid**.

Dactylitis (AKA: sausage digits), presents between 6 and 9 months old.

Sickle Cell cont'd

years old. Spleen will be atrophied.
Complications: Patient is at increased risk for **encapsulated organisms** ongoing. (In particularly: **SHiN** (S. aureus, H. influenza and Neisseria), sepsis, acute chest syndrome, acute **splenic sequestration** (intrasplenic sickling prevents blood from leaving the spleen causing engorgement of the spleen which leads to drop in hemoglobin, thrombocytopenia, reticulocytosis, painful splenomegaly, fever, leukocytosis, splenic rupture and death).

NOTE: If a young sickle cell child gets osteomyelitis (before the age of becoming Asplenic) the cause is Staph aureus because the spleen is still able to remove encapsulated organisms. If the child is > 4/5 years old, they are Asplenic, so the cause would then be due to Salmonella. So be aware of the age if both answers are in the choices).

X-ray shows "crew cut" on skull due to bone marrow expansion due to ↑ erythropoiesis.
LABS: **Sickle cells, target cells, ↑ reticulocytes, Howell Jolly bodies (indicate no spleen: remnants of nuclear material).**

DX:
BIT: Blood smear for sickled cells. (Sickle cell trait does not have sickled cells).
MAT: Hemoglobin electrophoresis. On HbS electrophoresis, HbS moves the slowest due to loss of glutamate.
Prenatal DX: Chorionic villus sampling (**not** before 9 weeks) or amniocentesis (best at 16 weeks).

TX: **Hydroxyurea** (↑ HbF = ↑ affinity for oxygen)
Must vaccinate: **Pneumococcal, H. influenza B, influenza, Meningococcal.**
Antibiotics in case of infections.
Transfusion in the case of shortness of breath or chest pain.
Exchange transfusion to ↓ sickle cells in blood = used to ↓ risk of strokes, acute chest syndrome and used in high-risk surgeries. Is used anytime a patient presents in a sickle cell crisis with any comorbidities such as Acute Chest Syndrome, stroke, retinal infarction (visual problems), and priapism.
Bone marrow transplant is the only definitive treatment.
TX for children: **Penicillin prophylaxis: 3 months until 5 years old; Folate daily; Immunization: Give all standard immunization vaccines but should add pneumococcal (2 months), influenza (6 months), meningococcal (at 2 years old).**
(NOTE: ANY Asplenic person must receive Pneumococcal vaccine to protect against infection from encapsulated organisms).

TX: Vaso-occlusive crisis: Oxygen, IV fluids, blood transfusion, analgesics, and hospitalize.
(Must give pneumococcal vaccine, hydroxyurea and folate upon discharge).
If fever or ↑ WBC start antibiotics immediately (do not wait for lab results): Ceftriaxone, Levofloxacin, Moxifloxacin.

Dactylitis

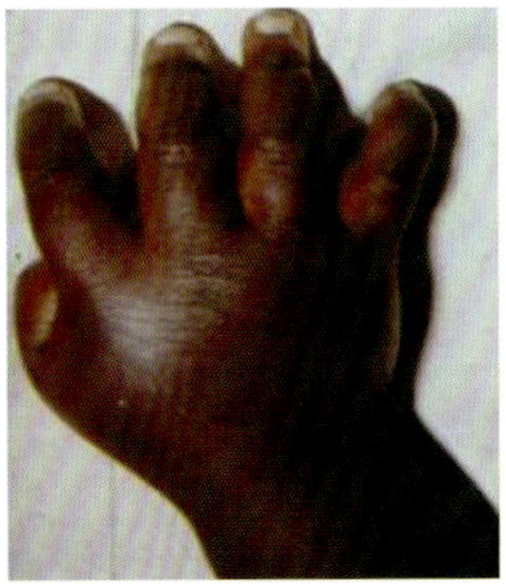

"Crew Cut" skull x-ray

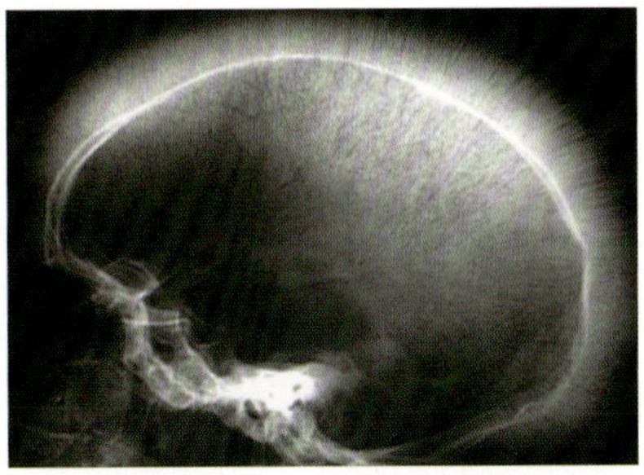

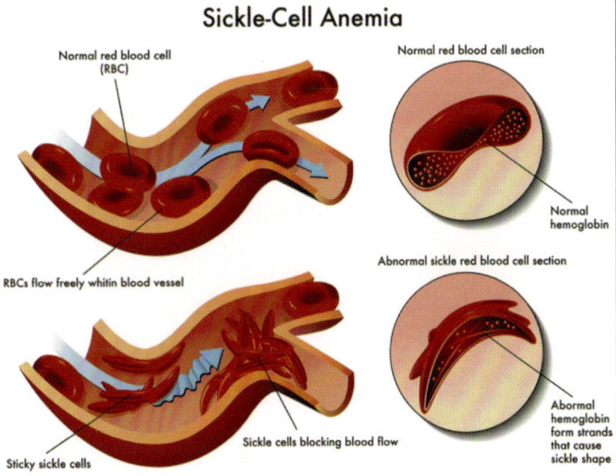

Sickle Cell cont'd
Folic acid replacement, Hydroxyurea (↑ HbF).
TX: If due to Parvo B-19: IVIG.

MCC death in children with Sickle Cell Anemia:
- Infection from encapsulated bacteria due to autosplenectomy (by age 5)
- Splenic sequestration (6 months to 3 years old)
- Acute Chest Syndrome
- Sepsis
- Stroke

Sickle Cell Trait (HbSC, hemoglobin C)
Heterozygous for the sickle gene. Person has one abnormal and one normal allele of the β gene.
HbA = 50 – 60%, HbS = 35 – 40%, HbF <2%.
Extravascular
Missense mutation. Amino acid substitution of **Glutamate for Lysine** in the β Chain at position 6.

Advantage: Resistant to malaria. (P. falciparum)

SX: MC problems are all urinary = hematuria (sickled cells in renal medulla), ↑ UTI's, Isosthenuria (urine whose specific gravity is the same as protein-free plasma because **no ability to concentrate the urine**), fewer and less severe vaso-occlusive crisis. Cramping in physical activity/exertion, body aches,

TX: Gradual acclamation, ↑ hydration, ↑ recovery time.
No medical treatment

Hereditary Spherocytosis
Autosomal Dominant
Extravascular
Hereditary anemia in the white pulp. Defect in RBC cyto-skeleton proteins **ankyrin and spectrin**. Causes the RBC's to be spherical rather than a biconcave shape. The cells are destroyed in the spleen causing a hemolytic anemia.
Hereditary anemia in the **white pulp**.
Extravascular (spleen) hemolysis.

SX: Splenomegaly, intermittent jaundice, recurrent hemolysis, bilirubin gallstones, family history.

Labs: ↑ **MCHC** (>36%), ↑ RDW, ↓ MCV, positive **osmotic fragility** test (↑ RBC fragility), ↑ reticulocyte count, ↑ bilirubin, **negative coombs test**, ↓ or loss of **central pallor,** swelling of RBC's (**osmotic** changes), **hypertrophy of macrophages** in the spleen (taking out damaged RBC).

DX: MAT: **Osmotic fragility test**. (Cells placed in a hypotonic solution → ↑ swelling of cells → hemolysis. (AKA: **Fragile RBC's**)

Complications: ↓ K and water due to dehydration. Hemolysis can lead to pigmented bilirubin gal stones (calcium bilirubinate stones) = acute cholelithiasis (SX: RUQ pain).

Associated with Autoimmune hemolysis.

TX: Splenectomy (NOTE: if splenectomy: must give pneumococcal vaccine to protect against **encapsulated organisms**).
Folic acid replacement.

Glucose-6-Phosphate Dehydrogenase Deficiency
G6PD Deficiency
X-Link
Intravascular and Extravascular
Unable to generate **glutathione reductase** to protect RBC from oxidative stress (MC stress: infection).

Deficiency in G6PD = ↓ glutathione = RBC are not protected against free radicals so there is hemolysis.
Glutathione is formed when cysteine and glutamate are converted to ϒ-glutamylcysteine via γ-glutamylcysteine synthetase. Glutathione protects the RBC against oxidative stress.
Glutathione (ϒ-glutamyl-cysteinyl-glycine) is the main **intracellular antioxidant.**

SX: Males with sudden jaundice (↑↑ cell breakdown) and anemia without splenomegaly after using one of the drugs that cause hemolysis with G6PD or have a current infection.

Labs: Hemosiderin in urine.
DX: BIT: Positive Prussian blue (methylene blue) stains for Heinz Bodies/Bite Cells.
MAT: G6PD level test 1 – 2 months after a hemolysis episode.
- Highest in Africans and Mediterranean decent
- **Protective against malaria**
- **XL condition that predisposes to hemolytic anemia and jaundice in oxidative stress**
- Neonatal jaundice can lead to kernicterus due to large numbers of RBC sequestered (taken out of circulation) in the spleen
- **MCC: Infections**. Other causes: Fava beans (broad beans), drugs (esp. sulfa drugs, anti-malarial drugs, INH, aspirin, sulfa diuretics, dapsone), illness

Pyruvate Kinase Deficiency (AKA: Erythrocyte Pyruvate Kinase Deficiency)	**Paroxysmal Nocturnal Hemoglobinuria (PNH)**
• Extravascular • RBC's can only use Glycolysis to manufacture ATP. They have no mitochondria. • Causes **LACTIC ACIDOSIS** • Common in alcoholics due to Vit B-1 deficiency • Requires a ketogenic diet: **Leucine and Lysine** • Pyruvate Kinase is required to make Pyruvate. Without pyruvate = no ATP • Without ATP, RBC will shrink/deform into echinocytes (burr cells) = cell death • Causes increase in 2,3 BPG = right shift in Oxy Hb curve • **RBC lysis leads to hemolytic anemia in the newborn = jaundice from increased bilirubin** • TX: Blood transfusion or removal of spleen	• Intravascular • Destruction of RBC by complement = **hemolysis** • **DAF** (Decay-Accelerating Factor) protects RBC's, displays cell markers: **CD55 and CD59** • AKA: **GPI anchored** enzyme deficiency • Mutation in the **PIG A gene (leads to absence of GPI anchors on cell membrane)** • Without GPI anchor on membrane **complement** lyse the RBC's • SX: red discoloration of the urine due to presence of Hemoglobin and hemosiderin from breakdown of RBC's, seen mostly in the morning from concentrating overnight. • Labs: hemolytic anemia, **↓ Hb**, **↑ LDH** (Lactate dehydrogenase), **↑ bilirubin**, ↑ Reticulocytes, **↓ haptoglobin**, increased reticulocytes • DX: positive **HAM test** (RBC become fragile when placed in mild acid) or can also be tested using flow cytometry. **Flow cytometry** will show ↓ levels of CD55/CD59. Negative Coombs test. (**tip**: a "PIG" gene is a HAM)

Normocytic Anemia – Extrinsic Hemolytic Anemia

Autoimmune Hemolytic Anemia
Acquired.
Antibodies attack a person's own RBC's = lyse.
MAT: Coombs test + (detects IgG antibody on surface of RBC's).
Associated with Hereditary Spherocytosis.

Classifications:
Warm agglutinin (IgG) (**tip**: warm is **G**ood) or **Cold agglutinin** (IgM) (**tip**: cold is **M**iserable).
Drug induced causes: a=methyldopa, penicillin.
Warm agglutinin (IgG) causes: CLL, lymphoma, SLE, RA, Scleroderma, Ulcerative colitis.
IgG binds Fc receptor of phagocytic cells. Occurs in the **spleen**.
Blood smear: Microspherocytes but does not show-fragmented cells because RBC destruction occurs extravascular in the spleen or liver.
Recurrent episodes: Splenectomy.
Acute hemolysis unable to be controlled by steroids: IVIG.

TX: **Corticosteroids (Prednisolone), Rituximab, Danazol, TNF inhibitors**.

Cold agglutinin (IgM) causes: Mycoplasma pneumonia, infectious **EBV** mononucleosis, viral pneumonias, Waldenström macroglobulinemia.
IgM activates the classical complement pathway = **complement mediated** lysis of RBC's. Occurs in **Kupffer cells.**

DX: Direct Coombs test is only **positive for compliment**. Blood smear is normal.
MAT: Cold agglutinin titer.

SX: Symptoms, mottling and numbness, in cooler parts of the body: ears, fingers, toes, nose.

TX: Staying warm, symptoms resolve when body parts are warmed.
No use of steroids (Prednisone) in Cold agglutinin. **RBC transfusion. Rituximab** and removal of underlying cause.
Cyclophosphamide, Cyclosporine, plasmapheresis.

NOTE: Do NOT confuse Cold agglutinins IgM with Cryoglobulinemia. Cryoglobulinemia is associated with HEP C, Membranous Glomerulonephritis, and arthralgia.

Microangiopathic Hemolytic Anemia	Macroangiopathic Hemolytic Anemia
Intravascular hemolysis. Destruction of RBC's, and formation of schistocytes due to passing over damaged endothelial surfaces (sharp microthrombi) lining small vessels. Labs: **Schistocytes** (helmet cells): fragments of RBC's resulting from the shearing/cutting by the fibrin mesh that results from the aggregation of platelets and fibrin. Seen in: DIC, HUS, SLE, Malignant HTN, TTP, cancer	RBC's are damaged in systemic circulation due to force (turbulent) from large vessels or heart. Associated with: mechanical heart valves, calcified/stenotic heart valve, aortic coarctation, bicuspid aortic valve. Labs: **Schistocytes** (helmet cells), burr cells (echinocytes), ↓ Hb, ↓ haptoglobin, ↑ LDH, ↑ unconjugated bilirubin, ↑ reticulocyte count, normal platelet count TX: Chronic blood transfusions, repair/replacement of valve

Macrocytic Anemia (MCV >100)
AKA: Megaloblastic, Macrocytosis, Megalocytes, Megaloblast

- ↑ MCV
- All show a ↓ reticulocyte count

Macrocytic Anemias

B12 Deficiency
Vitamin B12 is from animal products.= and is stored in the liver. Stores last for 5 – 7 years. B12 stores will be depleted by 5 years for people on vegan diets.

Peripheral smear shows **hypersegmented neutrophils.** (Hypersegmented neutrophils will differentiate B12 from Vit E deficiency. Vit E deficiency does not have macrocytic anemia or hypersegmented PMN's).

Causes of B12 Deficiency:
Malabsorption problems (IBD, Crohn's, Ulcerative Colitis, Celiac Dz, Tropical sprue, Cystic Fibrosis), Pancreatic insufficiency (**Pancreatic enzymes** are required to absorb B12. They **remove B12 from being bound to the R-protein** so it can bind with intrinsic factor.), **pernicious anemia** (confirmed with **anti-parietal or anti-intrinsic factor antibodies**), dietary deficiency (Vit B12 is from animal products and is stored in the liver), gastric bypass, gastrectomy, HIV, Diphyllobothrium latum.
Medications: **PPI's, H2 Blockers, Metformin, Colchicine**.
Metformin blocks B12 absorption.

SX: Ataxia, **presents with neurological symptoms** (MC: peripheral) and/or hematological symptoms, ↓ position and vibratory sensation (damage to posterior columns), **hypokalemia** (when there is pancytopenia, the bone marrow is trying to rapidly make new cells so it takes up all the potassium).

DX: 1st step after seeing ↑ MCV is blood smear to differentiate the cause of the macrocytic anemia by presence of hypersegmented PMN's.

Labs: **Megaloblastic anemia, ↑ LDH, ↑ indirect bilirubin, ↓ reticulocyte count** (RBC's are destroyed as they leave the bone marrow), **↑ homocysteine levels, ↑ Methylmalonic acid levels. Hypokalemia.**
Blood smear: Hypersegmented neutrophils, Macro-ovalocytes

TX: **Replace vitamin B12 and Folate. Replace potassium** if needed, **K can decrease during treatment for B12 deficiency**. B12 replacement will correct the neurologic problems and folate will correct the hematologic problems.
Must supplement B12 for people on vegan diets (B12 supply in the liver last from 3 – 5 years. Vegan's will deplete their supply).

Note: B12 is associated with **↑ Methylmalonic acid** in the homocysteine pathway. Without B12, Methylmalonic acid and Homocystine levels build up. **ONLY B12** is associated with ↑ Methylmalonic acid (MMA) levels. (Note: Homocysteine levels go up in BOTH B12 and folate deficiency).

Note: B12 deficiency (and hypothyroidism) can cause demential-like symptoms. On ALL cases of possible dementia, **you must check B12 and TSH levels.**

Folate Deficiency (Vit B9)
Folate is needed for RBC's to form and grow.
Folate is from green leafy vegetables, liver, citrus fruits.

Peripheral smear shows **hypersegmented neutrophils.**

Causes of Folate (Folic acid) Deficiency:
Dietary deficiency (goat's milk has no folate, must supplement. Goats milk only has iron and B12), Psoriasis (due to skin turnover), drugs (**sulfa drugs, anticonvulsants (Phenytoin, Valproic Acid), Reverse transcriptase Inhibitors, Cholestyramine, OPC's**), chronic alcoholism, hemolytic anemia, malnutrition, eating overcooked foods, Sickle Cell Dz, pregnancy.

NOTE: Any **chemo drug, or Methotrexate** use will require supplementation with folate due to high cell turnover.
Remember: **Methotrexate** is used with many diseases (RA, SLE), so without folate supplementation, any of these diseases could cause folate deficiency.

SX: **Does NOT present with neurological problems.**
(**tip**: "**F**"olate is "**F**"ree from neuro problems).
Hematological symptoms. Loss of appetitive, weight loss, headaches, irritability, behavior disorders, pallor, sore mouth and tongue, fatigue, gray hair, swollen tongue, poor growth.
Note: Folate is absorbed in the small intestine (Jejunum) so any malabsorption pathology will affect the absorption of folate.
Note: ↑ Folate intake is needed with: malabsorption problems, smoking and alcohol consumption, kidney or liver disease, pregnancy (to prevent neural tube defects) and lactation.

DX: 1st step after a CBC confirms ↑ MCV is a blood smear to differentiate the cause of the macrocytic anemia by presence of hypersegmented PMN's.

Labs: **Megaloblastic anemia, ↑ LDH, ↑ indirect bilirubin, ↓ reticulocyte count** (RBC's are destroyed as they leave the bone marrow), **↑ cysteine** levels, Hypokalemia.
Blood smear: Hypersegmented neutrophils, Macro-ovalocytes

TX: **Vitamin B12 and Folate. Replace potassium** if needed. B12 replacement will correct the neurologic problems and folate will correct the hematologic problems.

Pregnancy folate requirement: 400 mcg/day prior to pregnancy through the first trimester. (Overdose levels > 1000 mcg/day)

NOTE: Folate is associated with **↑ cysteine** level in the homocysteine pathway. (Note: Homocysteine levels go up in BOTH B12 and folate deficiency).

"Tea and Toast" diet.
MC seen in the elderly. They do not eat properly.
SX: Fatigue and macrocytic anemia.
TX: Folic Acid

Medications – Non-megaloblastic Anemia
No hypersegmented neutrophils.

Methotrexate, Hydroxyurea, Cyclophosphamide, Busulfan, Zidovudine, 6-MP, Acyclovir, Danorubicin, Adriamycin, Fluorouracil, Benzine

Other causes of macrocytic anemia
No hypersegmented neutrophils.
Alcoholism (can also cause neurologic problems)
Hypothyroidism
Liver Dz
Sideroblastic anemia

Additional Anemia's

Diamond-Blackfan Anemia
AKA: Inherited Pure Red Cell Aplasia

Congenital hypoplastic anemia.
Macrocytic or normocytic anemia with ↓ erythroid progenitors in the bone marrow.

Labs: **↓ reticulocytes**, **↑ fetal hemoglobin**, adenosine deaminase. Macrocytic with no hypersegmented neutrophils. **Pure red blood cell aplasia** (no RBC's in the bone marrow), neutropenia.

SX: Congenital anomalies. web neck, cleft lip, shielded chest, **triphalangeal thumbs**, cleft palate, urogenital malformations, cardiac defects.

DX: Blood count, bone marrow biopsy.

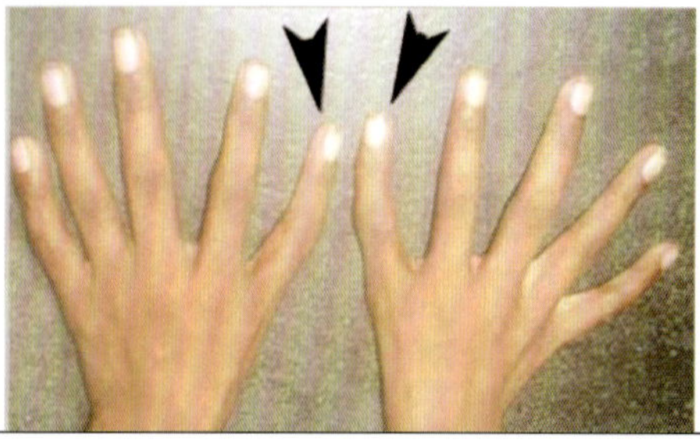

Fanconi Anemia
Genetic DZ with ↑ frequency in Ashkenazi Jews and Africans. Genetic defect in the proteins responsible for DNA repair leading to cancer. MC: AML (Acute Myelogenous Leukemia).
Bone marrow failure.

SX: Congenital defects, short stature, development disabilities, low set ears, endocrine problems, **partially detached, absent, additional thumbs**, small head (microcephaly), pounding in ear, freckles, aplastic anemia, chronic infections, café au lait spots (skin pigmentation), small eyes (microphthalmia), short stature, horseshoe kidney.

Labs: ↓ platelets, ↑ MCV

TX: Bone marrow transplant

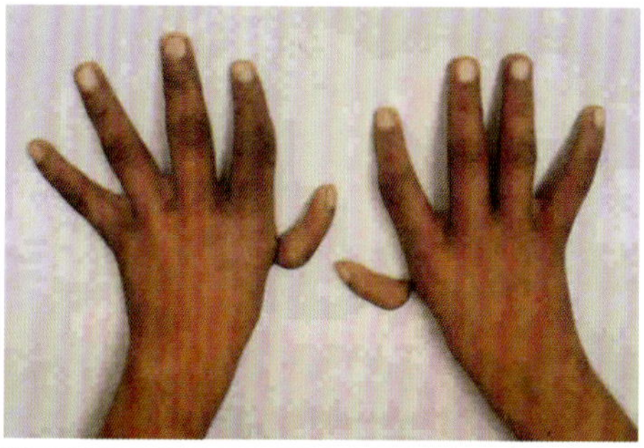

Hemolytic Anemia (hemolysis)

- **Intravascular Hemolysis**
  Breakdown/destruction of RBC's in the blood vessels.
  SX: Schistocytes
  MC: Prosthetic valves, HUS, PNH, TTP
- **Extravascular Hemolysis**
  Breakdown/destruction of RBC's elsewhere in the body (MC: Spleen = Reticuloendothelial system)
- Intrinsic: Hereditary (inherited) Causes
  Defects of RBC membrane production (ie: Hereditary spherocytosis, hereditary elliptocytosis)
  Defects in Hb production (ie: Thalassemia, Sickle-cell disease)
  Defective RBC metabolism (ie: G6PD, Pyruvate kinase deficiency)
- Extrinsic: Acquired Causes
  Immune-mediated (ie: transient Mycoplasma pneumonia, autoimmune hemolytic anemia, SLE, RA, Hodgkins, CLL)
  Paroxysmal nocturnal hemoglobinuria
  Hypersplenism (ie: portal HTN)
  Burns (acquired hemolytic anemia)
  Lead poisoning (non-immune hemolytic anemia)
  Prosthetic heart valves

Pure Red Blood Cell Aplasia

- An anemia only affecting red blood cells. The bone marrow stops producing red blood cells.
  - Diamond-Blackfan anemia
  - Parvo B19
  - Thymoma
  - Lymphocytic leukemia

Pernicious Anemia

- Associated with
    - **B12 deficiency**: due lack of dietary intake (B12 is from animal products) due to **vegans or "tea and toast" diet** (common in elderly), **Diphyllobothrium latum**. B12 deficiency will show as megaloblastic anemia. B12 is essential for the development of RBC's.
      Low B12 levels can lead to nerve damage (loss of balance, depression, confusion, numbness, tingling in hands and feet), false positives on PAP smears (deficiency affects the way epithelial cells look in the cervix), megaloblastic anemia (fatigue, pallor, shortness of breath, low RBC, blood counts), swollen red tongue, bleeding gums, loss of appetite (anorexia).
      Labs will show MCV >100, low B12, high MMA (methylmalonic acid), low RBC count, high LDH (tissue damage: blood cells, heart, liver, kidney, muscles, brain, lungs), high reticulocyte count.
    - **Malabsorption** problems in the terminal ileum. Any malabsorption problems can inhibit the absorption of B12 and intrinsic factor. Most common problems: Pancreatic exocrine insufficiency.
    - It is common for patients with one **autoimmune** diseases to have other autoimmune diseases. The most common autoimmune association with pernicious anemia is **Hashimoto's Thyroiditis**. But others can include: Graves DZ, Addison DZ, Type 1 Diabetes, Vitiligo, Myasthenia gravis, Hypopituitarism, Hypoparathyroidism.
    - **Deficiency of intrinsic factor**. Intrinsic factor is produced in the parietal cells in the stomach and is required for the absorption of Vitamin B12 in the ileum. Anything that effects this production will create an intrinsic factor shortage, this includes pathologies in the stomach that can also affect function of the parietal cells. Examples: Bariatric surgery, excessive consumption of alcohol, gastric ulcers, gastric tumors, autoantibodies against parietal cells or autoantibodies against intrinsic factor, atrophic gastritis.
      Mutation of the GIF gene (gene that encodes for the intrinsic factor protein)
    - Hereditary (aka: Congenital pernicious anemia). These individuals do not make enough intrinsic factor or cannot properly absorb vitamin B12 in the ileum. Higher risk in Northern European or Scandinavian individuals.
    - Mutations in **Haptocorrin** (AKA: **R Protein**, Transcobalamin I, TCN I). Glycoprotein secreted by the salivary glands: Binds to B12 to safely transport it through the acidic environment of the stomach into the duodenum, which then allows it to bind to intrinsic factor and be absorbed in the ileum. (**tip**: intrinsic and B12 the R train to the ileum)
    - Pernicious anemia raises the risk of gastric cancer and gastric carcinoid tumors.
    - Schilling test: Determines if the body is absorbing Vitamin B12 normally. Seldom used today.
      Test consist of several steps:
      Step 1- Patient given oral B12 and intramuscular B12 (this insures the patient's liver is saturated with B12). Normal patients will spill over the B12 saturation into the urine. Presence in the urine is a normal test. If little or no B12 is found in the urine = step 2.
      Step 2 – Step 1 is repeated and oral intrinsic factor is added. If the urine is normal, this verifies that intrinsic factor is not being produced: This defines diagnoses of pernicious anemia. If the B12 level is low again (abnormal test) this indicates the problem is due to a malabsorption problem.
      If problem is due to bacteria: antibiotics and vitamin B12 are administered: verified by a normal urine test.
      If problem is due to lack of pancreatic enzymes: pancreatic enzymes and vitamin B12 are administered: verified by a normal urine test.

Step 1 Test Result	Step 2 Test Result	Diagnosis
Normal		Vitamin B12 deficiency
Low	Normal	Pernicious anemia (intrinsic factor deficiency)
Low	Low	Malabsorption in the terminal ileum

Blood Poisons

Carbon Monoxide Poisoning
Colorless, odorless, nonirritating gas.
Binds to Hb to form carboxyhemoglobin which ↓ oxygen carrying capacity. Binds with a higher affinity to Hb than oxygen. Competes with oxygen for binding sites with 200 times the affinity..

Shifts the oxy-Hb dissociation curve to the left (impairing oxygen release to the tissues).

Uncouples Complex IV of the ETC.

Causes: car exhaust, working in an underground parking garage, smoking indoors, inside wood/propane/charcoal, wood, kerosene or natural gas stove, portable generators, fireplaces.

SX: First sign: headaches. Note: always ask the patient if others in the household also have headaches.
Cherry-red lips, skin and nail beds.

DX: Carboxyhemoglobin
Labs: **O2 saturation is NORMAL on pulse oximeter and normal PaO2.**
TX: **100% pure oxygen**

Cyanide Poisoning
Poison gas that inhibits cellular respiration by inhibiting **Cytochrome C Oxidase in Complex IV of the ETC**.

Shifts the oxy-Hb dissociation curve to the left (impairing oxygen release to the tissues).

Causes: fires when synthetic/natural products burn and are inhaled, plastic manufacturing, artificial nail remover, pesticides.

SX: Headache, HTN, confusion, syncope, seizures, coma, dyspnea, death, skin can be cherry red, breath smells like bitter almonds.

Labs: ↑ Venous O2

Cyanide TX options:
Thiosulfate, Met Blue, Hydroxocobalamin.

Hydroxocobalamin combines with cyanide to form cyanocobalamin (Vitamin B-12), which is excreted.

Sodium nitrate induces methemoglobin in RBC's, which combines with the cyanide. Methemoglobinemia is then treated with Methylene Blue. Methylene blue inhibits Monoamine Oxidase. This changes the iron form Ferric (F^3 iron form) to Ferrous (F^4 iron form). Vitamin C can also assist in treating methemoglobinemia.

Sodium thiosulfate transforms cyanide (donates a sulfur atom) to thiocyanate by rhodanese, which is then excreted.

TX: Nitrites.
Nitrites oxidize Hb to methemoglobin. Methemoglobin binds cyanide. Thiosulfate (sulfur) binds cyanide to form thiocyanate which is then excreted

Methemoglobinemia
Form of Hb that contains the **ferric (Fe3) iron (oxidized state)** instead of the ferrous (Fe2) iron so that there is ↓ in total oxygen carrying capacity.

Shifts the oxy-Hb dissociation curve to the left (impairing oxygen release to the tissues).

Causes: Exposure to drugs: amyl nitrate, **nitroprusside**, dapsone, nitroglycerin, topical anesthetic drugs (lidocaine, bupivacaine, tetracaine).

SX: **Brown blood**, syncope, and dyspnea.
Labs: **Normal O2 saturation. Must obtain ABG.**
TX: Methylene blue.

Coagulation Pathway - Clotting

The three pathways that makeup the classical blood coagulation pathway

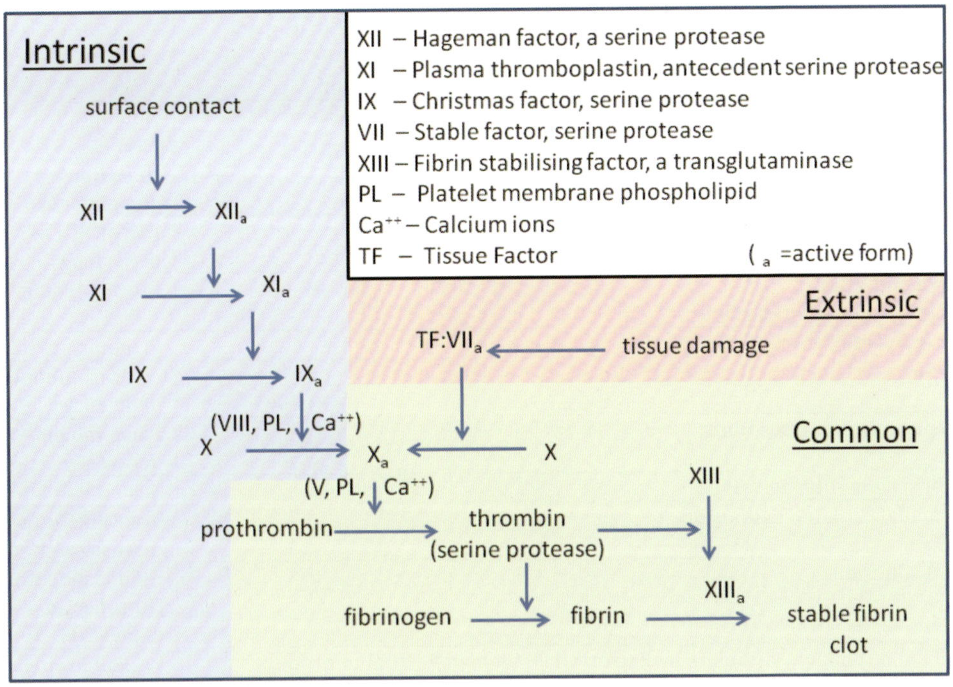

Coagulation Terminology

Factor#	Factor Name	Function	Pathologies
I	Fibrinogen	Thrombin ➔ Fibrinogen ➔ Fibrin ➔clots. Fibrinogen forms bridges between platelets by binding to their GpIIB/IIIa surface receptors. 90-hour half-life.	
	Fibrin	Fibrin combines with platelets to form hemostatic platelet plug over damaged endothelium.	
II	Prothrombin **Longest half-life.**	Activates: I, V, VII, VIII, XI, X!!!, Protein C, platelets. Prothrombin ➔Thrombin ➔Fibrinogen➔ Fibrin = clot **NOTE:** Factor II has a long half life (**65 hours**), all other clotting factors are from 6 – 24 hours. **Heparin is given with Warfarin for several days so that the propagation of the clot is prevented due to the long half-life of Factor II. This is the Heparin "bridge".** Bridging the time over until all clotting factors are totally gone so the DVT will not continue to grow. **Clotting factor:** Needs Vitamin K for synthesis and Calcium for activation.	Thrombophilia
III	Thromboplastin (Tissue Factor)	Cofactor VIIa	
	Thrombin	X activates Prothrombin ➔ Thrombin. Thrombin converts Factor XI to XIa, VIII to VIIIa, XIII to XIIIa, V to Va, Fibrinogen to Fibrin = clots. Thrombin is inactivated by Antithrombin (ATIII). (ATIII is what Heparin acts on)	
IV	Calcium	Required for coagulation factors to bind phospholipids	
V	Factor V	Cofactor for X to form prothrombinase complex. Factor V allows Factor X to activate thrombin = clot. 15-hour half-life.	Factor V Leiden
VII	Factor VII (aka: **proconvertin**) **Shortest half life**	Activates IX, X **Note: This is the first clotting factor to degrade by 50% after Warfarin is administered. It has the shortest half-life (5 hours).** **Clotting factor:** Needs Vitamin K for synthesis and Calcium for activation.	Factor VII deficiency

VIII	Antihemophiliac Factor A	Cofactor of IX. The only clotting factor that is not a protease, it is a transglutaminase.	Hemophilia A
IX	Anti-hemophilia Factor B	Activates X 25-hour half-life. **Clotting factor:** Needs Vitamin K for synthesis and Calcium for activation.	Hemophilia B
X	Factor X	Forms Prothrombinase with Factor V. Activates thrombin. 40-hour half-life. **Clotting factor:** Needs Vitamin K for synthesis and Calcium for activation.	Factor X deficiency
XI	Plasma Thromboplastin	Activates IX 45-hour half-life.	Hemophilia C
XII	Hageman Factor	Activates XI, VII, prekallikrein	Hereditary angioedema
XIII	Fibrin Stabilizing Factor	Crosslinks fibrin. 200-hour half-life.	Factor XIII deficiency
	Protein C	Inactivates Va and VIIIa. Inhibitor of the coagulation cascade.	Protein C deficiency
	Protein S	Cofactor for activated Protein C	Protein S deficiency
ATIII	Antithrombin III	Inhibits IIa, Xa	Antithrombin III deficiency
	Plasminogen	Converts to plasmin and lyses fibrin	Plasminogen deficiency
	Plasmin	Degrades fibrin clots (fibrinolysis)	
	von Willebrand Factor	Binds VIII, mediates platelet adhesion.	Von Willebrand disease
	Fibronectin	Mediates cell adhesion	Glomerulopathy (fibronectin deposits)
	Prekallikrein (Fletcher Factor) (Prekallikrein cont'd)	Precursor of kallikrein. It is stimulate by Factor XII (Hageman Factor) to produce Kallikrein, which activates kinins. Deficiency can be acquired due to angioedema, DIC, Sickle-cell dz. Kallikreins function in coordination of semen liquefaction, blood pressure and skin desquamation. **NOTE:** Kallikrein (kinin-kallikrein system) is the precursor to bradykinin (inflammatory mediator). It is converted to Bradykinin by the enzyme Kallikrein. It is a vasodilator that causes a ↓ in blood pressure, contraction of smooth muscle in the bronchus and gut, ↑ vascular permeability and causes natriuresis (which drops blood pressure even more). Bradykinin is broken down naturally by Angiotensin-converting enzyme (ACE) in the lungs. **ACE inhibitors** increase/over activate bradykinin (inhibits its degradation), which can lead to **angioedema** (vasodilation) and **dry cough** (bronchoconstriction).	Prekallikrein Factor deficiency
	Tissue Plasminogen Activator (tPA)	Activates plasminogen	Thrombophilia and hyperfibrinolysis
	Urokinase	Activates plasminogen	Quebec platelet disorder
	Cancer procoagulant	Activates Factor X = thrombosis in cancer	

Clotting Factors and Platelets

- Platelet disorders: Superficial bleeding
  Involves: Skin, epistaxis, gingiva, purpura, gums, petechia, mucosal, vaginal (menorrhagia)
- Clotting disorders: Deep
  Involve: Joints and Muscles
- Clotting: Extrinsic Pathway (Factor VII), **Warfarin** followed by **PT** (ProTime)
  Clotting: Intrinsic Pathway (Factors: XII, XI, IX, VIII)), **Heparin** followed by **PTT** (Partial thromboplastin time)
  (**tip**: think in 3's for Intrinsic pathway: HEP, PTT, vWF)

Types of Bleeding

- Petechiae <5mm
- Purpura 5mm – 1 cm (red/purple spots on skin that do not blanch.
- Ecchymosis > 1 cm

Normal Labs

- PT/INR: 11 – 15 seconds
- PTT: 25 – 40 seconds
- Bleeding time: 2 – 7 minutes

Bruising (AKA: ecchymosis)

- Caused by trauma to capillaries/veins that causes blood to hemorrhage (seep, extravasate) into surrounding tissues.
- Bruise color: **Heme oxidase** (coverts heme to bilirubin) causes the green color of bruises

Virchow's Triad

- Hemodynamic alterations
  - Stasis (no movement: sitting long periods: flights, truck driver)
  - Turbulence (A-fib, myxoma)
- Endothelial dysfunction
  - Atherosclerosis (hardening of the arteries)
- Hypercoagulability (increase of activation of clotting factors)
  - Factor V, increased homocysteine levels, nephrotic syndromes, anti-phospholipid syndrome, protein C and S deficiency, antithrombin III deficiency

Coagulation

Vitamin K and Clotting

- **Vitamin K is required for carboxylation (gamma-carboxylation = activate) the clotting factors: II, VII, IX, X, Proteins C and S. Needed to synthesize the clotting factors. Note: Factor VII is aka: Proconvertin.**
  Calcium is needed to activate the clotting factors.
- **Epoxide reductase** is required to reduce vitamin K after it has been oxidized in the carboxylation of glutamic acid. Inhibition of this enzyme will stop the gamma carboxylation of the clotting factors = no clotting (action of Warfarin)
- Vitamin K (K-2, menaquinone) is produced by the intestinal flora
- **Newborn babies do not have gut flora so can't produce vitamin K. Babies born in hospitals are automatically given a vitamin K shot at birth. Babies born at home that do not receive a vitamin K shot are at risk for hemorrhagic disease of the newborn.**
- **Vitamin K is a fat-soluble vitamin**.
  - Any **malabsorption** problem will ↓ absorption of vitamin K and can affect clotting
  - Foods containing Vitamin K must be ↓ or discontinued if on warfarin (will decrease the actions of warfarin and cause clotting): Green leafy vegetables (spinach, kale), dried basil, pickles, soybeans, olive oil, dried fruit (blueberries, prunes, pears, peaches, figs, currants), lettuce, cabbage, broccoli, asparagus, okra, Brussels sprouts. Drinks can also ↑ bleeding when on warfarin: alcohol, cranberry juice, green tea
- **Warfarin: Inhibits Vitamin K Epoxide reductase (which stops the reduction of Vit K) so that clotting factors are not activated.**
  - **Warfarin followed by PT and INR** (Prothrombin time: normal: 12 – 13 seconds, normal International Normalized Ration: 0.8 – 1.2).
    PT measures factors I (fibrinogen), II (prothrombin), V, VII, X.
    PT/INR levels for people on warfarin for blood clots and A-fib: target 2.5.
    PT/INR levels for people with prosthetic valves: target 3.5.
  - **HIGHLY AFFECTED by P-450 drugs.**
    P-450 activators will clear warfarin faster, ↓ PT = ↑ clots.
    P-450 inhibitors will build up warfarin, ↑ PT = bleeding
  - **Active bleeding antidote: Fresh Frozen Plasma**
    PT levels up to 5: decrease dosage
    PT levels higher: Administer vitamin K
  - **For patients that: PT levels drop (non-therapeutic), undergoing a surgical procedure (abdominal, pelvic, hip, knee), anti-phospholipid syndrome, treatment of DVT to ↓ the risk of clotting subcutaneous injection of low molecular weight heparin can be taken: Enoxaparin (Lovenox).**
  - **Heparin → Warfarin** Bridge Therapy for DVT and PE's
    Warfarin inhibits vitamin K dependent clotting factors II, VII, IX, and X and Protein C and S. Protein C and S are anticoagulants and have a shorter half life so can initially cause coagulation so Heparin is given along with Warfarin for a few days until Warfarin has time to work, then the Heparin is discontinued.
  - **The first clotting factor to degrade by 50% after the administration of Warfarin is Factor VII because it has the fastest half-life of only 5 hours.**
  - **Heparin must be given along with Warfarin because Factor II will not degrade for 65 hours. It has the longest half-life.**

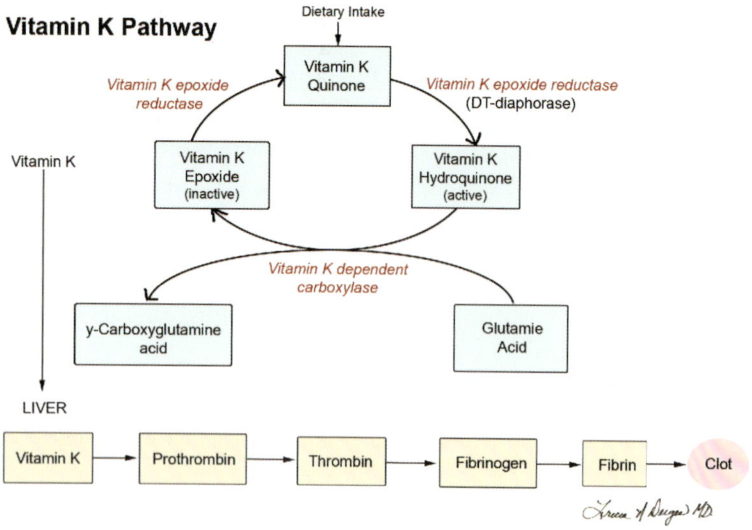

Coagulation – Factor V

- Factor V is homologous to factor VIII and is synthesized in the liver
- Factor V is activated by thrombin and binds activated platelets. Its two chains are bound by Calcium.
- **Factor V is a cofactor of the prothrombinase complex (Factor Xa and Factor V). Factor V allows Factor X to activate thrombin. This prothrombinase complex converts prothrombin (Factor II) to thrombin (Factor IIa) that cleaves fibrinogen to fibrin, which forms the meshwork with platelets that forms clots.**
- In the presence of Thrombomodulin, a cofactor for thrombin, (membrane protein on the surface of endothelial cells), thrombin activates Protein C to decrease clotting (anticoagulation)
- **Factor V is inactivated by Protein C by preventing it from binding to Factor Xa**
- **Point mutation in Factor V (Factor V Leiden) causes hypercoagulability**

Hypercoagulability Pathologies

Factor V Leiden **MCC Autosomal dominant** inherited disorder of hypercoagulability in Caucasians. Point mutation in Factor V gene. **Factor V can't be turned off by Protein C, it is resistant to it.** Incomplete dominance: Homozygous (worst) or heterozygous (milder). Missense mutation (AKA: Point mutation): replacement of **arginine with glutamine**. **Factor V can't be inactivated by Protein C ➔ so Factor V is free to cause clotting.** Labs: **Normal PT and PTT**. (This is because Factor V works fine in the coagulation pathway making fibrin at the normal rate. But later when the body tries to turn off Factor V (with Protein C) it does not turn off and continues to make fibrin = clots) SX: ↑ abortions/miscarriages, pulmonary embolisms, DVT's, strokes, TIA's DX: Russell's viper venom time (**snake venom**)	**Antithrombin III deficiency (ATIII deficiency)** Majority: Autosomal dominant inherited disorder causing recurrent DVT's and PE's. ↑ risk in kidney failure (**Nephrotic Syndromes**): ATIII is lost in the urine allowing Factor II and Factor X and Factor V to form clots. **(Normal action of ATIII: binds to thrombin to form the thrombin-anti thrombin complex ➔ anticoagulation.** **Heparin binds ATIII in order to activate this pathway ➔ no clots)**
Prothrombin G20210A Mutation (Factor II mutation) Genetic mutation which replaces guanine with adenine where the poly-A tail on the pre-mRNA causing elevated prothrombin levels. ↑ prothrombin = ↑ thrombin = ↑ clots.	**Protein C and Protein S Deficiency** Protein C (anticoagulant) inhibits factors V and VIII. Without Protein C Factors V and VIII are able to clot. Protein C deficiency ↑ risk of skin necrosis while on **Warfarin**. (The skin necrosis looks like HIT, but appears **after** the start of Warfarin. If dark skin necrosis occurs after the start of Heparin, but before Warfarin is started, then it is due to **Heparin**).

Increased Plasma Homocysteine Levels (AKA: Hyperhomocysteinemia)
(Homocysteine: amino acid produced by the body that alters adenosine. Homocysteine can't come from diet, it can only be produced by methionine (amino acid). Methionine can be derived from diet: fish, meat, dairy. Production of homocysteine also requires cofactors of B6 (pyridoxine), B12 and folic acid.)

Elevated plasma levels of homocysteine are associated with increased risk of thrombosis and atherosclerosis (stroke and heart attack).

Nephrotic Syndromes

🡅 risk in kidney failure (**Nephrotic Syndromes**): **ATIII is lost in the urine allowing Factor V and Factor X to form clots** (it does not able to inactivate Factor V and Factor X).

Note: Antithrombin III's job is to stop the path of Factor V from occurring, therefore inhibiting clots.
Antithrombin III /// Factor V ➔Prothrombin ➔ Thrombin ➔ Fibrinogen ➔ Fibrin ➔ Clot.

Risk factors
- Stasis: situations which slow blood flow: sitting long periods (plane, driving, bed ridden, wheelchair)
- Turbulent blood flow: A-fib, damage to endothelia surfaces, Myxoma tumor (left atrium)
- Post surgery, hospitalization (prolonged bed rest)
- Overweight, obesity
- Broken bones
- Increased homocysteine levels
- Diabetes, Metabolic syndrome
- Nephrotic syndromes
- Peripheral artery disease, Vasculitis, Atherosclerosis
- Polycythemia (thickened, slow blood)

Risk factors
- OPC's, Hormone Replacement Therapy (HRT)
- Pregnancy
- Smoking
- Cancer
- Heart failure
- Hereditary, Congenital
- HIV and HIV treatments
- Dehydration
- Organ transplants, implanted devices
- Antiphospholipid Antibody Syndrome (APS)
- Autoimmune disorders: Rheumatic disorders (Rheumatic = joints, bones, muscles)
- Bone marrow disorders
- DIC, TTP
- Thrombocythemia

Antiphospholipid Syndrome (APL)

IgG or IgM antibodies against negatively charged phospholipids. (Phospholipid antibodies)
Can be associated with Lupus.

Anti-cardiolipin antibodies associated with spontaneous abortions/miscarriages.
Lupus anticoagulant associated with 🡅 PTT (clotting).
Anti- β2 glycoprotein, Anti-phospholipids.

SX: **Thrombosis** (clotting) of veins and arteries, recurrent **spontaneous abortions/**miscarriages, stillbirths, preterm delivery, preeclampsia, IUGR, thrombocytopenia, livedo reticularis.

Labs: 🡅 PTT, normal PT/INR.

False positives with VDRL/RPR (Syphilis) and normal FTA.

DX:
BIT: Mixing study: Mixing patients plasma with normal plasma. If APL antibody present the PTT level in the mixture will stay elevated.
MAT: Russell Viper Venom Test (RVVT): RVVT is prolonged if APL antibodies are present.

NOTE: APL is important to test for in the case of the first clot for the individual. If APL is the reason for the first clot, they will require lifelong Warfarin.

TX: Check patient for APL antibodies if ≥ 2 first-trimester or 1 second trimester abortion/miscarriage occurs.
Prophylaxis to prevent reoccurrence: Heparin and aspirin.
Caution: do not use Warfarin during pregnancy.

DVT's and Arterial Clots

DVT (veins)	Arterial Clots
Causes: **Virchow's Triad**: Venous stasis (↓ blood flow), hypercoagulability, endothelial wall damage. Stasis: sitting long periods, long drives, long airplane flights, bed ridden, wheel chair, post surgical immobilization, trauma. Hypercoagulability: polycythemia, pregnancy, cancer, antiphospholipid syndrome, OCP's, blood disorders, ↑ homocysteine levels. Blood clot in the veins. MC in the calves in the popliteal vein. Others: Thigh in the femoral or iliofemoral vein. **The higher up and larger the vein the more dangerous and more likely to embolize** (part of the clot breaks off and goes to the lungs = pulmonary embolism) SX: Progressive. Swelling, erythema, warmth, **pain on dorsiflexion of foot (+ Homans sign)** Complications: **Pulmonary embolism** (clot in the lungs). PE signs: acute shortness of breath, clear chest x-ray, low O2 saturation (low 90's). See pulmonary chapter for more details on PE's) Complications if there is a patent foramen ovale (ASD: hole between the right and left atrium, allowing the clot to bypass the lungs and go into the left side of the heart and be ejected = stroke, TIA, arterial embolism) DX: Doppler/ultrasound (veins will not compress) Labs: ↑ D- Dimer TX: **Heparin bridge to warfarin**. Heparin must be given along with Warfarin for several days due to the **long half life of Factor II,** which takes approximately 65 hours to degrade. This prevents the clot from growing. First clot: Warfarin 6 months. Additional clots: Lifelong warfarin therapy. Warfarin PT/INR: 2.5 TX: for patients that can't be anti-coagulated: **IVC filter**. Any patient that is ↑ risk for bleeding: bleeding ulcers, past hemorrhagic stroke, recent major surgery, bleeding disorder. **DVT Prophylaxis (for surgery)** **Low Molecular Weight Heparin (LMWH) or Fondaparinux**: Start on admission and not 12 hours prior to surgery. Restart after surgery. Continue for 10 – 35 days after surgery.	Cause: Emboli that is ejected from the left side of the heart into the arterial system causing ischemia, infarction, necrosis and/or gangrene. Emboli can go to the extremities (arms, legs), kidneys (renal arteries), any other peripheral arteries or emboli can go to the brain and cause a stroke. SX: Acute. Immediate severe pain, hypoxia, discoloration of extremity, no swelling, cold leg, no pulse, numbness, tingling, pallor, muscle spasm, possible paralysis, MI. Echo of the heart must be performed to identify the source for thrombus. Causes for thrombus: A-Fib, Myxoma, Endocarditis, other arrhythmias, mitral stenosis, atherosclerosis, recent surgery, bone fracture (fat embolism), IV therapy (air embolism), cancer, diving (air emboli) Atherosclerosis can cause a thromboembolism and/or a cholesterol embolism. **Types of Arterial Embolisms:** • Thromboembolism: From thrombus/blood clot. • Fat Embolism: From bone fracture. • Air Embolism: (gas emboli): From air bubbles (IV or nitrous (scuba divers rising to the surface to quickly). • Cholesterol Embolism: From cholesterol from atherosclerotic plaque. • Septic Embolism: From pus containing bacteria. • Cancer Embolism • Amniotic Fluid Embolism: From amniotic fluid. Stroke/TIA's emboli can also come from atherosclerosis in the carotid artery. **Anytime there is an ischemic stroke, both the heart (ECHO) and carotid (carotid angiogram)** must be performed to locate the source of the emboli. **(if >70% blockage in the carotid: Carotid endarterectomy must be performed)**

Thrombophlebitis (AKA: Trousseau's Syndrome (Superficial Clots). Superficial Thrombophlebitis) Variant of a DVT. Episodes of **superficial vessel** inflammation that reoccur in various locations. SX: Clot is located just under the skin. It **feels like a "cord"**, extremely painful, swelling over the clot with erythema. Complications: the superficial clot can migrate down the perforating veins into the femoral vein and become a DVT in up to 10% of patients. TX: Hot packs. NSAIDS for pain. Compression stockings. Self Resolving. **Trousseau's Sign of Malignancy**: Recurrent clots in uncommon sites (chest wall, arms). This is associated with pancreatic, gastric or lung cancer. DX: Perform appropriate CT's to rule out cancer.	**Venous Insufficiency (Valve Insufficiency)** Increased swelling of the lower legs/feet at the end of the day causing **pitting edema**. Cause: Due to **venous stasis** caused by **varicose veins**, tortuous veins, incompetent valves. TX: **Compression stockings, elevate legs** above heart level, exercise. Complications: **Venous ulcers** due to the ↑ fluid. **Note:** To determine the difference between CHF and Venous stasis (both cause pitting edema). Pitting edema due to venous stasis will ↓ in the mornings, whereas, pitting edema due to CHF will still be present in the mornings.

Anticoagulation – Protein C, Protein S

- Protein C (zymogen: inactive enzyme precursor is a vitamin K dependent glycoprotein in the plasma) is activated when it irreversibly binds and inactivates Factor V and Factor VIII. Factor V is then unable to bind with prothrombin or Factor Xa, thereby inhibiting thrombin and clotting.
- Protein S is the cofactor for Protein C in the inactivation of Factors Va and Factor VIIIa.

Anticoagulation – Plasminogen

- Plasminogen is converted to Plasmin by the enzyme Tissue Plasminogen Activator (tPA). Plasmin degrades fibrin clots (fibrinolysis).
- tPA is also used to treat embolic or thrombotic strokes that are <3 hours from onset. After 3 hours the fibrin mesh is unable to be broken down by plasmin.

Anticoagulation Pathologies (Non-clotting)

Hemophilia A or Hemophilia B **X-Link** recessive (males and homozygous females). Hemophilia A: genetic deficiency in **Factor VIII** Hemophilia B (AKA: Christmas disease): genetic deficiency in **Factor IX** **No prothrombin → no thrombin → no clotting.** SX: Superficial: Prolonged bleeding, bruising, hematomas. (Common for prolonged bleeding in dental procedures/lacerations/surgery or epistaxis) Deep bleeds: Bleeding into joints (hemarthrosis), muscles, brain, GI. Joints show: **hemosiderin deposits** and fibrosis. Labs: **↑PTT, normal PT, normal bleed time** **DX: MAT: Factor VIII or IX assay.** TX: Hemophilia A: **Recombinant Factor VIII** OR **Thrombin** for major bleeds into the joints or muscles. Minor bleeds: TX: **Desmopressin (DDAVP)** – it ↑ vWF release from endothelial cells. TX: Hemophilia B: **FACTOR IX**	**Vitamin K Deficiency** Due to: malabsorption (Vitamin K is synthesized by colonic bacteria), **Warfarin, Coumadin** Causes ↓ synthesis of clotting factors: II, VII, IX, X, Protein C and S. Labs: ↑PTT, ↑PT, Normal bleed time **Newborns** colonic bacteria are not established for the first 5 – 7 days of life leading to ↑ risk of hemorrhagic disease of the newborn. Vitamin K shots are administered in delivery rooms to newborns. **Babies born at home** are at increased risk. SX: Petechiae, bruising, hematomas, bleeding, ↑ bleeding after surgical procedures.
Factor XII Deficiency AKA: Hageman Factor (plasma protein) Autosomal Recessive Factor XII activates Factor XI and prekallikrein. (Start of the intrinsic pathway). **Does NOT cause bleeding**. It is also activated by endotoxins (Lipid A). Labs: **↑ PTT, no bleeding**. No treatment.	

Platelets

Platelet Plug Formation

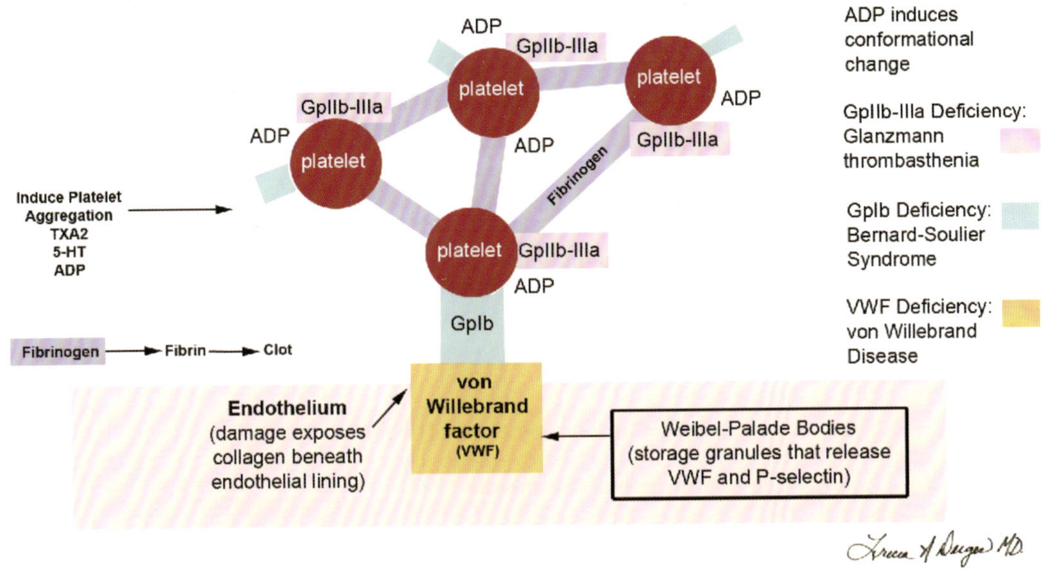

Platelet Plug Formation Pathway

- Endothelial damage exposes collagen
- **Weibel-Palade Bodies** (granules in **endothelial cells** in the inner lining of blood vessels and heart) release **vWF** (coagulation) and **P-selectin** (inflammation).
  (**tip**: Weibel-Palade bodies are the glue factor, vWF is the glue)
- VWF binds platelets at the GpIb receptor
- Platelets release calcium and ADP so the coagulation pathway can be activated
- ADP binds its receptor stimulating GpIIb/IIIa expression
- Fibrinogen then binds GpIIb/IIIa to connect platelets together to form the platelet plug = stops bleeding

Platelet Aggregation Balance

- Thromboxane A2 (TXA2): (Arachidonic pathway) produced by activated platelets.
  ↑ Platelet aggregation, vasoconstrictor, Prothrombotic
- ADP: Released from activated platelets to expose fibrinogen binding sites, ↑ platelet aggregation,
  ↑ mobilization of intracellular calcium. Inhibits adenylyl cyclase from prostaglandins.
- 5-HT: Secreted from enterochromaffin cells into the blood where it is taken up by platelets for storage. Activated platelets release serotonin for vasoconstriction.
- Nitrous Oxide (NO). (AKA: EDRF: Endothelium-derived relaxing factor): Released to promote smooth muscle relaxation (vessels) for vasodilation = increased blood flow = ↓ platelet aggregation.
- PGI2: (Arachidonic pathway): Vasodilator that inhibits platelet activation.

Pro-aggregation	Anti-aggregation
ADP, TXA_2, 5-HT released by platelets to ↓ blood flow so ↑ platelet aggregation	NO and PGI_2 released by endothelial cells ↑ blood flow so ↓ platelet aggregation

Platelet Transfusion:
Transfuse packed platelets when < 10,000 platelets.
1 unit raises platelet count 5000.
If there is little or no rise in platelets after transfusion = antibodies against platelets.

Platelet Pathologies

Bernard-Soulier Syndrome Deficiency of **Glycoprotein Ib (GpIb)** (receptor for vWF) which ↓ the aggregation of platelets = ↑ bleeding. (**tip**: **1** Soldier) SX: Easy bruising, excessive bleeding, epistaxis (nosebleeds), gingival bleeding, post operative/postpartum bleeding, menorrhagia. Labs: ↑ **bleeding time,** ↓ **Platelet count,** Normal PT, PTT	**Glanzmann Thrombasthenia** Deficiency of Glycoprotein IIb/IIIa (GpIIb/IIIa) (receptor for fibrinogen). Without the bridging of fibrinogen no platelet aggregation can occur. SX: Easy bruising, excessive bleeding, epistaxis (nosebleeds), gingival bleeding, post operative/postpartum bleeding, menorrhagia. Labs: ↑ **Bleeding time, normal platelet count**, Normal PT, PTT. Platelet aggregation is normal in Ristocetin assay.
Idiopathic Thrombocytopenia Purpura (ITP) (AKA: Immune Thrombocytopenic purpura) Autoimmune: antibody destruction of platelets. **Anti-GIIb/IIIa antibodies.** **IgG coats platelets** to be removed by splenic macrophages and Kupffer cells (liver macrophages). SX: **Minor**: bruising (ecchymosis), petechiae, bleeding from gums, menorrhagia, petechial, bleeding from gums, nose bleeds (epistaxis). **US show normal size spleen.** DX: Peripheral smears to rule out TTP and HUS. Peripheral smear shows normal RBC's. Bone marrow smear shows hyperplasia of mature megakaryocytes. Labs: ↑ **Bleed time,** ↓ **Platelet count,** ↑ **Megakaryocytes,** can see antiplatelet antibodies. (**Isolated thrombocytopenia**). **Normal PT, PTT, normal HCT, normal WBC.** TX: **1st line best therapy if platelet counts are > 20,000 and < 50,000: Prednisone** (Start therapy before determining diagnosis). **2nd line Therapy if platelet counts are < 20,000:** IVIG or RhoGAM (IVIG is the fastest way to raise platelet count because it stops the macrophages from destroying the platelets. No transfusions (unless life-threatening bleeding). Platelet counts return to normal in approximately 6 months. If ITP continues to occur = splenectomy Chronic ITP after splenectomy: **Eltrombopag or Romiplostim** (stimulate megakaryocytes). . **If platelet count is < 20,000** and the patient present with serious co-morbidities (**life threatening bleeds** in the brain/bowel), **DO NOT** transfuse platelets, it will make the problem much worse, treat with **IVIG or RhoGAM**.	**Thrombotic Thrombocytopenic Purpura (TTP)** Inhibition or deficiency of **ADAMTS 13** (**metalloprotease** responsible for cleaving vWF into smaller units. **Zinc** is what the metalloprotease uses to cleave.) Without ADAMTS 13 vWF can't be cleaved = ↑ platelet adhesion causing ↑↑ **microscopic clots (thrombosis**). RBC are destroyed as they pass over these clots = **microangiopathic hemolytic anemia**. Associated with SLE, HIV, Cyclosporine, Clopidogrel, Ticlopidine. More common in adults. (**TTP is a close pathology** and MOA to **HUS** caused by deficiency in **ADAMTS**13. TTP causes more CNS problems and is more common in adults; HUS causes more renal problems and is more common in children). SX: Microangiopathic hemolytic anemia, **intravascular hemolysis**, neurologic sx (hallucinations, altered mental status/neurological (confusion, seizures), behavior change, strokes), **kidney failure**, bruising, purpura, **thrombocytopenia.** Labs: ↑ **Bleeding time,** ↓ **Platelet count (thrombocytopenia),** ↓ **RBC, Normal PT, PTT.** **Schistocytes,** ↑ **LDH,** ↓ **Hb,** negative Coombs test. TX: Plasmapheresis, Plasma Exchange. **DO NOT** transfuses platelets into TTP (or HUS) → worsens.

Thrombocytopenia
Disorder with ↓ platelets.

Causes: ↓ platelet production, ↑ platelet destruction, diseases, medications (**Myelosuppression caused by: Valproic acid, Isotretinoin (Vit A), PPI, H2 Blockers, Methotrexate, Interferon, Carboplatin**)

Normal platelet count: 150,000 – 450,000.
Platelet transfusions required with < 50,000 platelets.
Platelet Transfusion:
1 unit raises platelet count 5000.
If there is little or no rise in platelets after transfusion = **antibodies against platelets**.

SX: epistaxis, bleeding gums, bruising, purpura, petechia

Labs: ↑ Bleeding time, ↓ Platelet count, Normal PT, PTT.

Heparin-induced Thrombocytopenia (HIT)

Development of thrombocytopenia due to **autoantibodies against Platelet Factor IV (PF4)** when administering **Heparin (MC: unfractionated heparin)**, causing thrombosis in either venous or arterial vessels. HIT does not cause bleeding b/c platelets are precipitated out. IgG antibodies form a complex with PF4 and Heparin.

DX: ELISA is positive for platelet factor 4 (PF-4) antibodies.

SX: Skin rash, fever, chills, HTN, tachycardia, shortness of breath, chest pain, necrotic lesions at injections site.

TX: 1st: STOP Heparin. Change Heparin to a direct thrombin inhibitor: Lepirudin, Argatroban, Danaparoid, Fondaparinux, Bivalirudin. (Do NOT change to a low molecular weight heparin)
Once platelets rise to 150,000, **warfarin** can be started.

Do NOT transfuse platelets in HIT, it will worsen condition.

Warfarin Induced Skin Necrosis (due to Protein C deficiency)

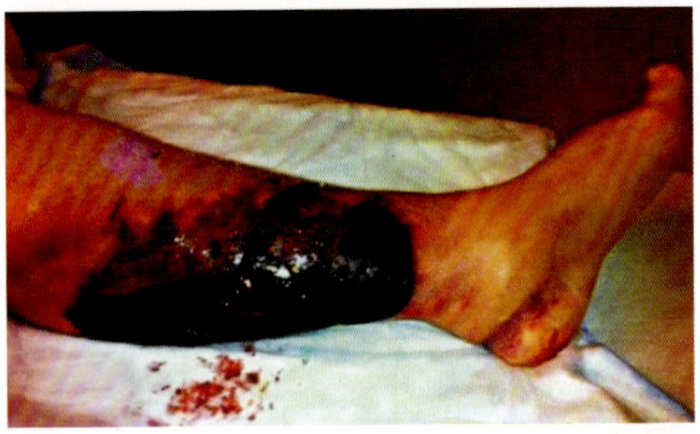

Wiskott-Aldrich Syndrome (WAS)
X-Link recessive.

- **↓ IgM and ↓ platelets (thrombocytopenia)** (**tip**: remember to turn the "W" in Wiskott upside down to an "M")
- ↑ IgE and IgA
- Mutation in **WAS gene**
- High risk of infections by encapsulated organisms (polysaccharide capsules)
- SX: Thrombocytopenic purpura, eczema (rash), recurrent infections, bruising, epistaxis, bloody diarrhea

Essential Thrombocytosis (too many platelets)

↑↑ Platelet count > 1 million → bleeding and thrombosis. MC due to **mutation in JAK 2.**

SX: Bleeding, thrombosis, vision problems, headaches, hand pain. Can be difficult to distinguish from ↑ platelets due to infections, iron deficiency or cancers. **Erythromelalgia** (red, painful hands).

TX: **Hydroxyurea** (can cause suppression of RBC. If RBC suppression, treat with **Anagrelide**).
TX for erythromelalgia: **Aspirin**

Uremia-Induced Platelet Dysfunction
Uremia impairs adhesion, aggregation, and degranulation in platelets.

MC: Dialysis patients. (AKA: Renal failure)

Labs: ↑ bleed time, Normal PT/PTT, **Normal platelet count**.
Ristocetin test is normal. VWF level is normal.

TX: **DDAVP (Desmopressin)**, dialysis

Mixed Coagulation and Platelet Pathologies

Von Willebrand Disease	Disseminated Intravascular Coagulation (DIC)
MC hereditary coagulation disorder. Due to a deficiency in vWF. vWF synthesized by **endothelial cells** in **Weibel-Palade** Bodies (AKA: **Seidel Lewis** Bodies) Intrinsic pathway defect. vWF (carrier protein) is required to bind Factor VIII. Without vWF, Factor VIII breaks down. SX: ↑ bleeding tendencies: nosebleeds (epistaxis), easy bruising, bleeding gums, mucus membrane bleeding, **heavy menstrual periods (menorrhagia)**, ↑ blood loss during childbirth, ↑ post-operative bleeding, petechiae. VWF worsens after the use of aspirin. DX: MAT: **Ristocetin** assay (RIPA) (The antibiotic causes platelet agglutination (clumping) in the presence of vWF). Other test: Factor VIII activity. Labs: **↑PTT, Normal PT, Normal to ↑ bleed time, thrombocytopenia, ↓ VIII, ↓ IX.** TX: Minor bleed: Desmopressin **(DDAVP)** MOA: it ↑ vWF release from endothelial cells. **If DDAVP is not successful: Replace Factor VIII or give VWF concentrate.** Major bleed: vWF from plasma with Factor VIII. Cryoprecipitate (frozen blood product prepared from plasma: contains: fibrinogen, Factor VIII, vWF, Factor XIII)	Widespread activation of the clotting cascade in small vessels throughout the body = ↑↑ bleeds from various sites. Consumptive coagulopathy. ↑ risk of death. Due to underlying causes: Sepsis (MC: by E. coli), endotoxic shock, cancers, pregnancy complications (pre-eclampsia, eclampsia, amniotic fluid embolism), severe trauma, snake bites, transfusion reactions (ABO incompatibility), TTP, HUS, trauma, pancreatitis, burns, cancer. SX: ↑ bleeding from several sites including IV lines. Labs: **↑ PT and PTT, ↑ Bleeding time, ↑ D-Dimers (fibrin split products), ↓ platelet count, ↓ Plasma Fibrinogen (it has been consumed), ↓ Factor V and VIII, schistocytes.** **TX: Platelets < 50,000: Replace platelets and replace clotting factors by giving FFP. Cryoprecipitate to replace fibrinogen (if FFP is not able to control the bleeding).**

Differential Labs in Bleeding and Clotting Disorders

(NL = normal)

Disease/Drug	PT	PTT	Bleed Time	Platelet Count	RBC	D-Dimer
DIC	↑	↑	↑	↓	NL	↑ (↓ Fibrinogen)
Hemophilia A/B	NL	↑	NL	NL	NL	NL
Factor V Leiden	NL	NL	NL	NL	NL	NL
vWF	NL	↑	↑	NL to ↓	NL	NL
ITP	NL	NL	↑	↓	NL	NL
TTP	NL	NL	↑	↓	↓	NL
HUS	NL	NL	↑	↓	↓	NL
Thrombocytopenia	NL	NL	↑	↓	NL	NL
Bernard-Soulier	NL	NL	↑	↓	NL	NL
Glanzmann	NL	NL	↑	NL	NL	NL
Vitamin K Deficiency	↑	NL	NL	NL	NL	NL
End Stage Liver Dz	↑	↑	↑	↓	NL	↑ (↓ Fibrinogen)
Uremia	NL	NL	↑	NL	NL	NL
Heparin	NL	↑	NL	NL	NL	NL
Warfarin	↑	NL	NL	NL	NL	NL
Aspirin	NL	NL	↑	NL	NL	NL

Platelet Pathology Differentials

	HUS	**Henoch-Schönlein purpura**	**TTP**	**ITP (healthy person)**
Platelet Count	↓	↑	↓	↓
Diarrhea	Bloody	No	No	No
Renal Involvement	Yes (Uremia)	Yes (hematuria, IgA)	Yes	No
Abdominal Pain	Yes	Yes	No	No
Fever	Yes	No	Yes	No
Neuro Signs	No	No	Yes (fluctuating)	No
Schistocytes	Yes	No	Yes	No
Microangiopathic Hemolytic Anemia	Yes	No	Yes	No
Joint Pain	No	Yes	No	No

Thrombocytopenia Causes

Pathologies due to ↓ production	**↑ Destruction**	**Misc**
Viral: HIV, HEP C, EBV Chemotherapy Mylodysplasia > 60 years old Alcohol Fanconi's Vit B-12 deficiency Folate deficiency	SLE Medications (ie: Heparin) ITP DIC TTP HUS Anti-phospholipids	Dilution from RBC infusion Splenic sequestration

Misc Heme Notes

- Vitamin B-12 deficiency stops erythroid lines in the bone marrow = ↓ erythropoiesis = anemia and ↑ indirect bilirubin
- Splenic Sequestration: Splenic pooling of RBC = ↑↑ reticulocytes because of ↑ hemolysis
- Jehovah's Witness: No blood transfusions. **For hypovolemia** (↓ BP) give IV fluids and vasopressors (norepinephrine or dopamine). Children < 18, give blood transfusions. Doctors can overrule parents.
- Splenectomy: **Prior to a splenectomy these vaccines must be given:** **Pneumococcus, Haemophilus influenza, Neisseria meningitis**

HEME PHARMACOLOGY

DRUG GENERIC name Trade name	Clinical Use	Mechanism of Action and Resistance	Toxicity and Notes
Heparin	Anticoagulation for DVT, PE, MI, acute coronary syndrome. Pregnancy use: does NOT cross into placenta like warfarin does.	Activates and binds antithrombin III so that IX and X are not activated. This ↓ thrombin and Factor Xa. **Follow PTT.** Creates a "Bridge" to insure the clot does not grow. Protein C & S are the first of the clotting factors (shortest half life and are anti-thrombin III natural anti-coagulants) to be released ahead of II, VII, IX, X. Their purpose is to stop clotting and then quickly disappear leaving II, VII, IX, X free to clot. Heparin is also given with Warfarin because of the long half-life of Factor II, 65 hours. This insures that the proliferation of the clot is inhibited until **Factor II** is degraded.	**Do not use Warfarin in pregnancy, use Heparin.** **HIT** (Heparin Induced Thrombocytopenia). Bleeding, thrombocytopenia. HIT is due to IgG antibodies against Platelet Factor IV. **Overdose: Protamine sulfate** positive charged molecule that binds negatively charged heparin).
Argatroban Bivalirudin Lepirudin Hirudin	Use in HIT patients for anticoagulation. (use instead of heparin)	Does not require antithrombin III. It inhibits thrombin directly.	**(tip:** its RUDe to HIT for the "rudin's")
Apixaban Rivaroxaban Edoxaban Dabigatran	DVT and prophylaxis of DVT, PE, treat A-Fib to prevent strokes.	Directly inhibits Factor Xa. Does not require monitoring of PTT	Bleeding. No reversible agent.
Low Molecular Weight Heparins (LMWH)			
Enoxaparin *Lovenox* **Dalteparin**	Anticoagulation and prophylaxis for DVT, PE, MI, acute coronary syndrome.	Acts on factor Xa. Does not require following PTT.	Difficult to reverse.

Warfarin

DRUG GENERIC name Trade name	Clinical Use	Mechanism of Action and Resistance	Toxicity and Notes
Warfarin **Coumadin**	DVT and prophylaxis of DVT, PE, treat A-Fib to prevent strokes, use after STEMI for anticoagulation.	Inhibits **gamma carboxylation** (aka: carboxylation) of clotting factors II, VII, XX, X and protein C and S. Inhibits **Vitamin K Epoxide Reductase**. **Must follow PT/INR** Normal PT/INR is 1.0 PT/INR with DVT or A-Fib is 2.0 – 3.0 (average of 2.5 is ideal). PT/INR with prosthetic valve is above 3.0 with 3.5 being ideal.	**CAUTION: Interactions with P-450's** **Do not use Warfarin in pregnancy, Must use Heparin.** **Overdose: Fresh Frozen Plasma for active bleeding.** **PT/INR <5: hold warfarin for 1 – 2 days.** **PT/INR 5 - 9: Hold warfarin till INR is stable. Add low dose oral vitamin K (1 – 2.5 mg).** **PT/INR >9 Hold and add high does oral vitamin K (2.5 – 5mg).** Active bleed: **Hold warfarin and FFP.** **Deficiency of Vitamin K**: Bleeding in newborn (no flora in gut) and in those on NPO and antibiotics (kills natural flora). **Warfarin Necrosis**: due to **Protein C deficiency**. Skin necrosis (like HIT).

Thrombolytics (TPA: Tissue Plasminogen Activator)

DRUG GENERIC name Trade name	Clinical Use	Mechanism of Action and Resistance	Toxicity and Notes
Streptokinase Alteplase Tenecteplase Reteplase	Ischemic stroke (must be giving within 3 – 4 hours of stroke onset and MUST do CT first to insure it is not a hemorrhagic stroke). Early, MI, thrombolysis of PE.	Activates plasminogen to convert to plasmin. Plasmin cleaves thrombin and fibrin clots. (After 3 – 4 hours the fibrin and thrombin have become stable and cannot be broken down). (**tip**: Plasmin makes blood like Plasma again) **TPA can only bind plasminogen in the presence of fibrin.** ↑ PT and PTT. No affect on platelets.	**CAUTION: Do NOT use in any patient with active or recent bleeding (hemorrhagic stroke, recent surgery, bleeding disorders, severe HTN > 185 systolic or > 110 diastolic, INR > 1.7, platelet count < 100,000, stroke or head trauma within 3 months, cancer, recent trauma, cancer, etc).**

Platelet Pharmacology

DRUG GENERIC name Trade name	Clinical Use	Mechanism of Action and Resistance	Toxicity and Notes
Aspirin (Salicylic acid)	Antiplatelet to ↓ platelet aggregation. Antipyretic, analgesic, anti-inflammatory. Daily use (81 mg) to ↓ risk of MI. In case of MI, most critical drug to give (regular strength, sublingual) on the way to the hospital to ↓ mortality.	Irreversibly inhibits cyclooxygenase (COX-1 and COX-2) so inhibits platelet aggregation.	**NOTE: Aspirin is one of the 4 drugs that ↓ morality rates! (Aspirin, β-Blocker, Ace Inhibitor, Spironolactone).** **Toxicity: First sign: Tinnitus (CN VIII), mixed acid/base disorder (respiratory alkalosis and metabolic alkalosis = anion gap metabolic acidosis), Constricts afferent arteriole (inhibits prostaglandins), interstitial nephritis, gastric ulcers. Reyes syndrome (given in viral illness to children)**
ADP Receptor Inhibitors			
Clopidogrel Ticlopidine Ticagrelor **Prasugrel**	Antiplatelet. **Better than aspirin in PCI** (Percutaneous coronary intervention/Balloon/ Stent) , unstable angina, ↓ ischemic /thrombolytic stroke.	Inhibits platelets by irreversibly **blocking ADP receptors**. This **inhibits Glycoprotein IIb/IIIa from binding to fibrinogen.** (Fibrinogen is the linking cross bridge that allows platelets to bind).	Ticlopidine causes neutropenia. TTP, HUS, hemorrhage.
GP IIb/IIIa Inhibitors			
Abciximab Eptifibatide TIrofiban	Percutaneous MI, Transluminal Coronary Angioplasty, unstable angina	Binds **Receptor GP IIb/IIIa** on platelets to inhibit aggregation.	Abciximab (MAB: monoclonal antibody) (**tip**: think of Michael Jackson's song: **ABC**.....1, **2, 3**)
Phosphodiesterase III Inhibitors			
Cilostazol **Dipyridamole**	**Claudication in PAD** (peripheral artery disease), prevention of stroke or TIA's, prevention of angina, coronary vasodilation.	**Inhibits platelets and vasodilates.** Inhibits platelet aggregation by inhibiting phosphodiesterase III to ↑ cAMP in platelets → ↓ aggregation. Directly targets arterioles.	Note: Superior to aspirin in treating arterial disease (due to vasodilation). Facial flushing, hypotension, abdominal pain, headache, nausea.

Platelet Treatment Levels

Platelet Presentation	Treatment
Platelet count > 50,000	No treatment
Platelet count < 50,000 with minor bleeding	Prednisone
Platelet count < 20,000 with major bleeding	IVIG or RhoGAM
Continual reoccurring drops in platelet count	Splenectomy
Continued drop in platelet count after splenectomy	Romiplostim, Eltrombopag

BLOOD and LYMPH ONCOLOGY/PATHOLOGY

Leukemia and Lymphoma

Leukemia

- Cancer that begins in the bone marrow with ↑ abnormal, immature WBC's (Blast, lymphoblasts) with ↓ RBC
- Tumor cells are found in the blood
- Causes: Inherited or environmental
  Smoking, ionizing radiation (x-rays, microwaves, radio waves), chemicals (benzene: crude oil/gasoline), chemotherapy, Downs Syndrome
- Types of Leukemia:
  Acute Lymphoblastic Leukemia (ALL)
  Acute Myeloid Leukemia (AML)
  Chronic Lymphocytic Leukemia (CLL)
  Chronic Myeloid Leukemia (CML)
  Hairy Cell Leukemia (HCL)
- SX: bleeding, bruising, petechiae (↓ platelets), fatigue, ↑ risk of infections, anemia (due to ↓ RBC's = pallor), night sweats
- DX: Bone marrow biopsy, blood test
- TX: Bone marrow transplant, chemotherapy, radiation therapy

Lymphoma

- Blood cell tumor that develops from lymph nodes: Neoplasm of the lymphatic tissues.
- Cancer of lymphocytes (WBC that belongs to both lymph and blood)
- Abnormal proliferation of lymphocytes (B and T cells) into monoclonal lymphocytosis.
- Types of Lymphoma's
  Hodgkin's Lymphoma (HL)
  Non-Hodgkin Lymphoma (NHL)
  Multiple Myeloma
  Immuno-proliferative Diseases (Follicular Lymphoma, B-cell Lymphoma, T-cell Lymphoma, Waldenstrom's Macroglobulinemia, Wiskott-Aldrich Syndrome, Post transplant disorder)
- Immuno-proliferative diseases are due to abnormal proliferation of lymphocytes (B and T cells) into monoclonal lymphocytosis.
- SX: B symptoms (Fever, night sweats, weight loss), anorexia, fatigue, pruritis, lymphadenopathy, dyspnea
- DX: Lymph node biopsy.
- DX to determine type of lymphoma:
  Flow cytometry (used in blood cancers: cell study)
  Immuno-phenotyping (proteins expressed)
  Fluorescence (FISH) (DNA chromosome sequence)
- TX: Chemotherapy, radiation therapy

Leukemia and Lymphoma Chromosomal Translocations

Disease	Translocation
ALL	12:21
AML, Type MC	15:17
Burkitt's Lymphoma (c-myc)	8:14
CML (BCR-ABL)	9:22 Philadelphia chromosome
Follicular Lymphoma (bcl-2)	14:18
Mantle Cell Lymphoma	11:14

Transplants

- Autologous: Your own cells back to you
- Allogenic: Someone else's cells. Must be <50 years old
- Stem Cells: No rejection (no graft verses host)

"B" Symptoms of Lymphoma

- Night sweats
- Weight loss
- Fever

Leukemia

Acute Lymphoblastic Leukemia (ALL)
WBC Cancer with **> 20% Blast/lymphoblasts** (immature WBC)
Translocation **12:21 is most common = good prognosis**, 4:11 most common children < 1 year old = poor prognosis.
Acute begins in the bone marrow.

MC in children 2 – 5 years old.
Types: B Cell and T Cell.
Most common: B Cell. Worst prognosis: T Cell.
B Cell: Most common. Markers **CD10**, CD19
T Cell: Markers **CD2, 3, 4, 5, 6, 7 , 8** (will also have throat issues: anterior mediastinum widening (mass), compression on esophagus, trachea, dysphagia, inspiratory stridor, superior vena cava syndrome)
(**tip**: B Cell: ≥ CD 10, T Cell: < CD9 plus **T** cell = **T**hroat issues)

Markers: **CALLA +, + PAS, TdT** (marker of pre-T and Pre-B cells)
↑ Risk: **Downs Syndrome**.

SX: Rubbery, non-tender lymph nodes, bone pain at night (bones grow at night) hepatosplenomegaly, petechiae (↓ platelets), abdominal pain.
CXR shows: wide mediastinum (enlarged lymph nodes due to leukemic infiltration of the thymus))

Labs: ↑ leukocytes, ↑↑ lymphoblasts, tear drop RBC's (bone has cancer)

DX: BIT: Blood smear showing blasts.
MAT: Flow cytometry
Confirm: Bone marrow biopsy

Prognosis: determined by cytogenetics (assessing chromosome characteristics).
Good cytogenetic = ↓ relapse = continue chemotherapy.
Poor cytogenetics = ↑ relapse = Bone marrow transplant.

TX: **Methotrexate (prevents relapse of ALL in the CNS), Filgrastim.**
Rasburicase (inhibits tumor lysis syndrome by ↓ uric acid).

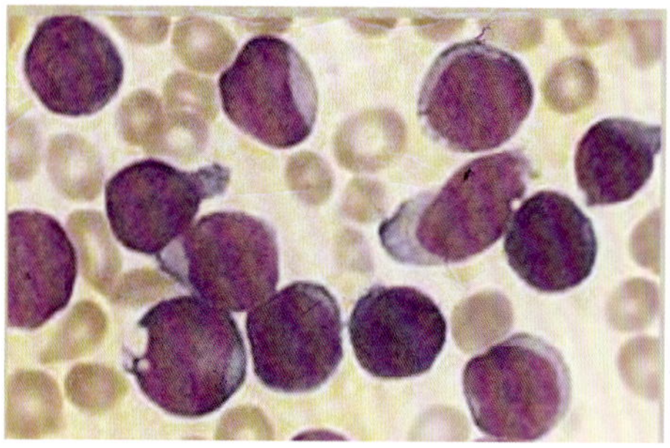

Acute Lymphoblastic Leukemia

Chronic Lymphocytic Leukemia (CLL)
(AKA: CLL is a stage of Small Lymphocytic Lymphoma SLL)
MC leukemia in adults.
B Cell Cancer, affecting **mature B cell lymphocytes** (antibody producing cells) with ↑↑ lymphocytes.
Monoclonal proliferation of mature lymphocytes (old, mature cells).

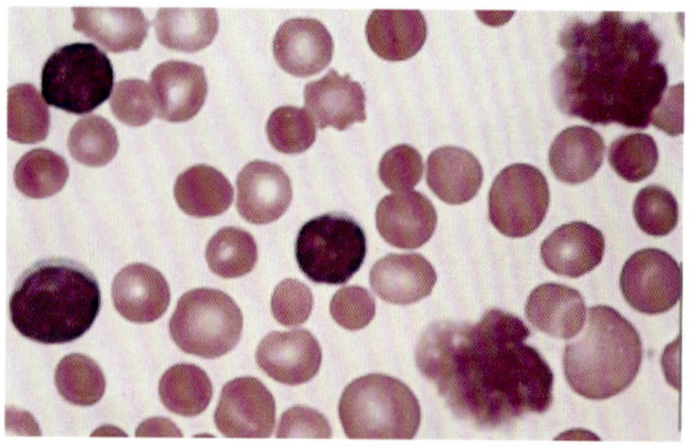

MC in men > 50 years old.
Average age: 71
Chronic: Years to develop, usually found on routine blood work.
Chronic begins in the periphery. No bone pain.
CLL cells attack normal RBC and platelets = anemia and thrombocytopenia.

Markers: **CD5, CD20, CD23**

SX: Fever, **fatigue**, productive cough, lower lob infiltrates, painless lymphadenopathy, early satiety, anemia, hepatosplenomegaly (enlarged spleen compresses stomach causing early satiety), ↑ infections because ↓ function of lymphocytes.

Labs: **↑↑ WBC of 50,000 – 200,000 with > 50% lymphocytes.**
Blood smear shows: **"Fragile" leukocytes ("Smudge/Smear** cells caused by the slide cover crushing them), cells show **hyper condensed nuclear chromatin. Hypogammaglobulinemia,** anemia, thrombocytopenia (due to IgG warm antibodies).

Signaling: **STAT signaling, Tyrosine (Kinase) Phosphatase** activity.

4 stages of CLL: 0) ↑ WBC, 1) Lymphadenopathy, 2) hepatosplenomegaly, 3) anemia, 4) thrombocytopenia
Staging:
Lymphocytes only: good
Thrombocytopenia: poor

DX: Bone marrow biopsy.
Confirmatory test: Flow cytometry of peripheral blood.

DX: **Kappa and Lambda ratio is abnormal (uneven).** There is not a normal distribution of B-lymphocytes, the ratio is abnormal, this indicates a B cell malignancy.

TX: No treatment for Stages 0 and 1.
Stage II and III: Fludarabine.
Stage IV: **Fludarabine with Rituximab**
Mild cases: **Chlorambucil** (alkylating agent)
Autoimmune thrombocytopenia or hemolysis: Prednisone,
Refractory cases: **Cyclophosphamide**

Acute Myeloid Leukemia (AML)

Cancer of the myeloid line of blood cells. (Myeloid line: granulocytes, monocytes, erythrocytes, platelets).
Leukemic cells replace the bone marrow causing drop in RBC's and platelets.
Affects older adults, average age is 67.
CML, myelodysplastic and myeloproliferative diseases can evolve into AML.

MC subtype M3: Acute Promyelocytic Leukemia (APL) subtype of AML
Abnormal accumulation of immature granulocytes (promyelocytes). Associated with **DIC**.
Translocation: 15:17. Translocation of retinoic acid receptor **RAR gene** on chromosome 17. (Retinoic acid receptor is defective).

M5 subtype is associated with **gingival hyperplasia**.

SX: Similar to the flu. Weight loss, anorexia, shortness of breath, petechiae, joint pain, frequent infections.

DX: **Sudan Black stain shows: Auer Rods (AKA: Peroxidase + cytoplasmic inclusions, azurophilic granules, giant cytoplasmic peroxidase granules)**.
DX: BIT: Blood smear showing blasts.
MAT: Flow **cytometry**
Confirm: Bone marrow biopsy

Prognosis: determined by cytogenetics (assessing chromosome characteristics).
Good cytogenetic = ↓ relapse = continue chemotherapy.
Poor cytogenetics = ↑ relapse = Bone marrow transplant.

↑ Risk of DIC

TX: All-trans Retinoic Acid (Vitamin A). (Retinoic is a precursor to vitamin A). **Rasburicase** (inhibits tumor lysis syndrome by ↓ uric acid).
MOA: Retinoic acid causes blast cells to ↑ their cell differentiation so they mature. (They let the cells grow up).

Note: Retinol is converted to retinal, which is oxidized to retinoic acid, the form of Vitamin A that regulates gene transcription. (AKA: retinoids: retinol, retinal, retinoic acid). B-Carotene is converted into retinol (aka: provitamin A). Vitamin a is an essential fat-soluble molecule, stored in satellite cells in the liver in the form of retinyl esters (retinyl palmitate). All-trans-retinol is formed when these esters are hydrolyzed.
All-trans retinoic acid and Retinoic acid (9-cis-RA) act as hormones to affect gene expression. They are transported into the nucleus by retinoic acid binding proteins (CRABP). There they bind to the **RAR** and RXR retinoic acid receptors to affect gene transcription and expression. **Retinoic acid (Retinol) inhibits Histone acetylation so that gene transcription is inhibited.**

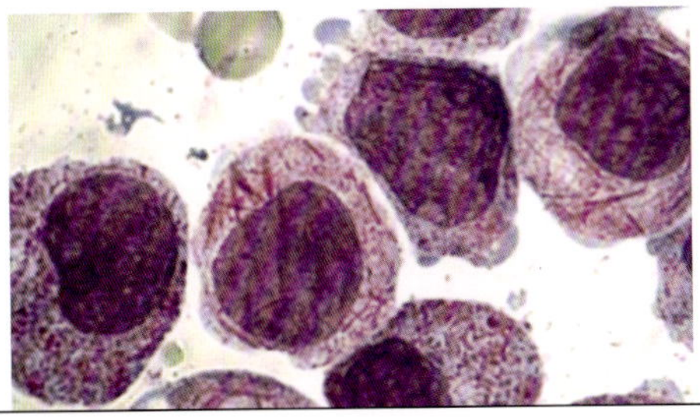

Acute Myeloid Leukemia - Auer rods

Chronic Myeloid Leukemia (CML)

Proliferation of myeloid cells in the bone marrow that accumulate in the blood. (Myeloid line: granulocytes, monocytes, erythrocytes, platelets). ↑↑ production of mature granulocytes (BEN: basophils, eosinophils, neutrophils). (is NOT WBC's/lymphocytic)
MC in middle age to older adults, average age 64.

Translocation: 9:22 "Philadelphia Chromosome", BCR-ABL

SX: Night sweats, pruritus after hot showers/baths (due to release of histamine), fever, ↓ appetite, weight loss, bone pain, early satiety, fatigue, anemia, LUQ pain**, splenomegaly** (enlarged spleen compresses stomach causing early satiety).

Labs: **↑↑ PMS's of 50,000 – 100,000 with ↑ WBC's**, ↑ mature granulocytes, **↓ Leukocyte alkaline phosphatase (LAP)** (due to a low mature granulocytes. LAP is ↑ in Leukemoid Reaction), ↓ Hb, ↓ Hct, ↑ bands > 35%, ↑ segmented PMN's > 25%. CML can present with ↑ WBC on routine exam. Shift to the left with blasts, eosinophilia.
(**tip**: "L"AP is "L"ow in CML)

BIT: Leukocyte alkaline phosphatase (LAP)
DX: MAT: Philadelphia chromosome: BCR-ABL by **PCR or FISH**.

Complication: Progression to Blast crisis and AML = death. (CML Blast crisis: ↓ Alk Phos and Philadelphia chromosome. 9:22) Leukemoid reaction has no Philadelphia chromosome 9:22 and ↑ Alk Phos)

Signaling: **JAK/STAT< Tyrosine Kinase activity**

TX: Cure: bone marrow transplant.
TX: **Imatinib (inhibitor of tyrosine kinase)** (**Gleevec**)

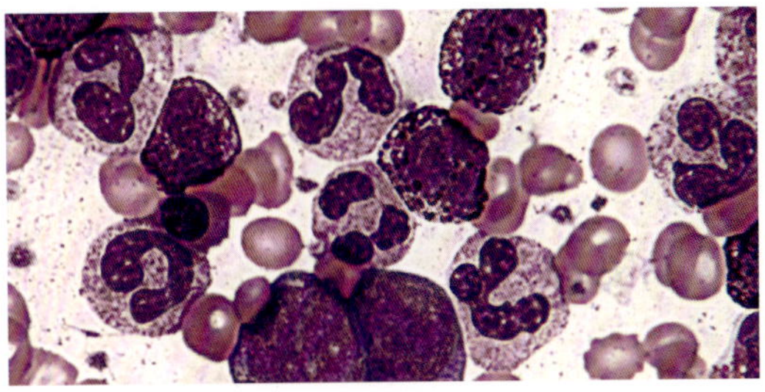

Hairy Cell Leukemia (HCL) Mature B-cell tumor due to accumulation of abnormal B-lymphocytes. Causes fibrotic bone marrow. (Subtype of CLL) MC: middle aged men Associated with **HIV**. SX: ↑ bleeds (due to ↓ platelets), **Dry bone marrow taps** (aspiration) due to fibrotic bone marrow, anemia (↓ RBC), **↑ Splenomegaly.** Markers: **CD11c, is no CD25 expression**, ↓ P53 Labs: (pancytopenia) ↓ platelets, ↓ WBC Stains: **TRAP (tartrate-resistant acid phosphatase)** show "hairy cells" (AKA: hair-like projections, **filamentous projections**, spikes) Hairy cells produce and live on TNFα (stimulated by IL-2) DX: Flow **cytometry** TX: **Cladribine** (2CDA) **(inhibits adenosine deaminase)** Side affects: Neuro and renal symptoms. **Pentostatin, Fludarabine with Rituximab.** 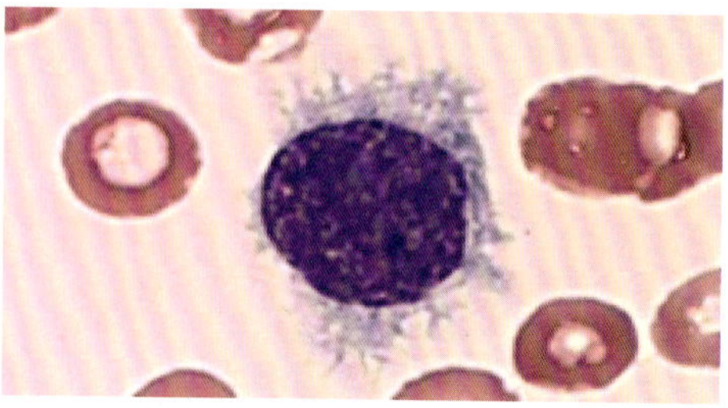 Hairy Cell Leukemia	**Leukemoid Reaction** AKA: Leukostasis Reaction Leukocytosis (↑ WBC) due to an **acute** infection, stress or drugs (**Dapsone, Sulfa drugs, glucocorticoids, All-trans retinoic acid**). **NO Philadelphia chromosome (9:22), ↑ Alk Phos, no anemia, shift to the left (Dohle bodies).** (CML blast crisis has the Philadelphia chromosome 9:22 and ↓ Alk Phos), **↑ Leukocyte alkaline phosphatase (LAP).** **Cause:** ↓ oxygen delivery to tissues because there are so many WBC that the RBC can't get through to the tissues. Labs: > 100,000 WBC (90% PMN's), ↑ Alk Phos. Shows abnormal leukocyte aggregate and clumping. SX: Clogs brain, lungs and vessels causing hypoxia, hemorrhage, ↓ perfusion, shortness of breath, blurred vision, headache, TIA, strokes. TX: **Leukapheresis** (centrifuge to remove excess WBC's) and hydration to ↓ number of leukocytes and break up aggregation. **Hydroxyurea** will ↓ the cells but leukapheresis works much faster. **Differential between CML and a Leukemoid reaction**: CML is ↓ Leukocyte alkaline phosphatase (LAP) and a Leukemoid reaction has ↑ Leukocyte alkaline phosphatase (LAP). **NOTE:** If the vignette does not give you LAP levels, look at the time frame the patient has been sick. **A leukemoid reaction is acute – fast onset** due to an infection or other stress. Look for a patient that presents sick (fever, chills, etc).

Lymphoma

- "B" Symptoms: Night sweats, fever, weight loss

Hodgkin Lymphoma (HL)

Cancer originating from lymphocytes (B Cells, T Cells, NK).
Enlarged lymph nodes, starts centrally in the cervical neck region and spreads outward.

Single group of nodes, localized. MC: Cervical area.
Contiguous spread.
Cell markers: CD30, CD15 (**tip**: 15 x 2 = 30)
Disease occurs in 2 age groups: young adults (15 – 35 yrs) and adults (> 55 yrs).
Hodgkin's can **reoccur** in 20 years as 2° malignancy in the lungs. Radiation therapy can also damage the heart and cause **concentric heart disease** (calcified ring around the heart, pericardial knock).

SX: MC in young adults. Constitutional "B" SX: (Night sweats, fever, weight loss), pruritis, **firm-rubbery painless lymphadenopathy** of one or more nodes (MC: mediastinum or supraclavicular nodes), hepatosplenomegaly, back pain, pain in nodes after alcohol intake, **nodular nodes**.

Stain shows Reed-Sternberg Cells (AKA: "Owl's Eyes", Lacunar cells). Giant binucleate/bilobed cells.
(**tip**: think of a "hodge" as a lodge. A lodge is in the woods and owls live in the woods)

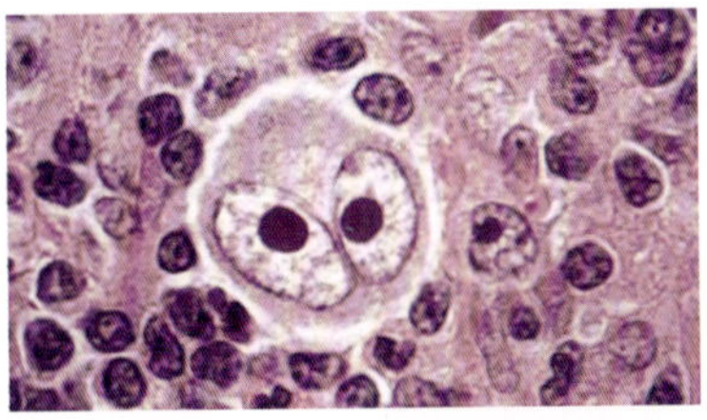

DX: BIT: Excisional lymph node biopsy. Lung biopsy shows large binucleated cells (Reed-Sternberg cells) with granulocytes, histocytes and lymphocytes.

TX: Chemotherapy or Radiation

Staging
80 - 90% of patients present in stages 1 and 2.
Stage 1: One lymph node involved
Stage 2: Two nodes on SAME side of diaphragm
Stage 3: Involves one node on both sides of diaphragm
Stage 4: Organ involvement
TX:
Radiation for local (Stages 1 and 2)
Chemotherapy for wide spread (Stages 3 and 4)
Recurrence: Bone Marrow Transplant.
MOPP or ABVD Chemotherapy
MOPP:
Mechlorethamine, Oncovin (Vincristine), Procarbazine, Prednisone.
ABVD:
Adriamycin (Doxorubicin), Bleomycin, Vinblastine, Dacarbazine

Non-Hodgkin Lymphoma (NHL)

Group of cancers derived from lymphocytes that include any lymphoma **except** Hodgkin's.
Enlarged lymph nodes, widespread.

Multiple peripheral nodes involved.
Noncontiguous spread. Disseminated.
Painless lymphadenopathy: **not tender, no warmth, redness.**
(Infection makes nodes tender, warm, red).
Cell markers: CD20
MC: B Cells
SX: **"B" Symptoms**: night sweats, fever, weight loss.
Disease occurs MC in adults 20 – 40 years old.
80 – 90% of patients present in Stage 3 and 4.

Labs: No Reed-Sternberg cells, ↑ LDH, normal CBC.

DX: BIT: Excisional lymph node biopsy. (**Do NOT do a FNB** (needle aspiration) because the individual nodes will appear normal.

Staging
80 - 90% of patients present in stages 1 and 2.
Stage 1: One lymph node involved
Stage 2: Two nodes on SAME side of diaphragm
Stage 3: Involves one node on both sides of diaphragm
Stage 4: Organ involvement

TX: Stage 1, 2: radiation and ↓ chemotherapy.
Stage 3, 4, or "B" symptoms: Chemotherapy with CHOP and Rituximab.
Rituximab (targets only CD20)
CHOP therapy: Cyclophosphamide, Hydroxydaunorubicin (Adriamycin), Oncovin (Vincristine) Prednisone.

Nodular Sclerosing Hodgkins Lymphoma
MC: Hodgkin's lymphoma in developed countries: MC in girls: adolescents and young adults.

SX: Enlarged lymph **nodes in the neck**, armpits ad chest, mediastinal mass, night sweats, pruritis, anemia, bone pain

Histology: **No Reed Sternberg cells**, Necrotizing granulomatous inflammation

DX: Lymph node biopsy.

TX: Chemo and radiation.

Burkitt Lymphoma (Non-Hodgkin)
MC: children, young adults.

Translocation: 8:14. Translocation of c-myc on 8 and Ig heavy chain on 14.
(**c-myc is a transcription activator/regulator**)
Associated with EBV

Shows high Ki-67 (high mitotic index)

Histology shows: **Macrophages with abundant clear cytoplasm mingled among sheets of lymphocytes**. ("Starry sky" appearance)

TX: **Vinca Alkaloids**

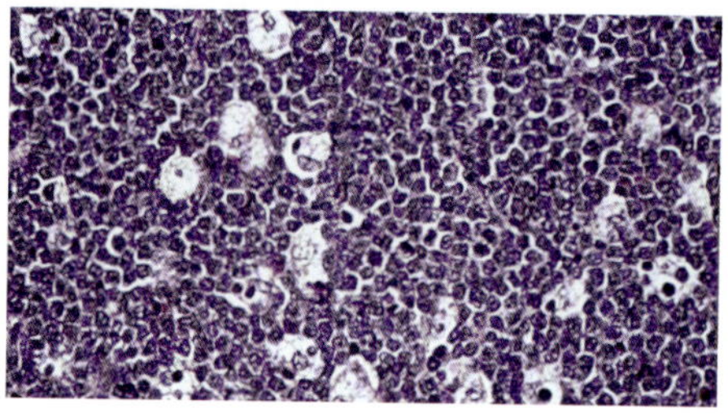

Endemic form (African variant) Burkitt's Lymphoma.
MC: Africa, Brazil, New Guinea (↑ malaria regions).
Associated with EBV.
SX: **Jaw lesions** (ulcerated/draining), abdominal pain, weight loss.

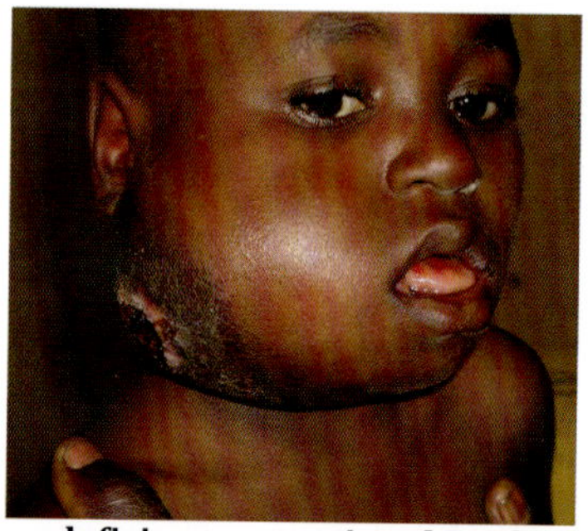

Immunodeficiency-associated Burkitt's
Associated with HIV, post-transplant patients on immunosuppressive drugs.

TX: **Rituximab**

Follicular Lymphoma (Non-Hodgkin)
Lymphoma of follicle center B cells.

Markers: CD10, 19, 22, 20. **Does NOT express CD5**.
Translocation: 14:18. Translocation of Ig heavy-chain on 14 and **bcl-2 on 18.**

Overexpression of bcl-2 (anti-apoptotic gene = does not allow cell to die. This is not good in cancer cells)

SX: Painless/painful, enlarged nodes. The lymphadenopathy comes and goes (AKA: episodic, wax and waning)

TX: **Rituximab**

Mantle Cell Lymphoma (Non-Hodgkin)
B-cell lymphoma in the pre germinal B-cell center in the mantle zone.

Translocation: 11:14. Translocation of cyclin D1 on 11 and Ig heavy chain on 14.

Express **CD5 and over express cyclin D1**.

TX: **Rituximab with CHOP therapy**

Diffuse Large B-Cell Lymphoma (Non-Hodgkin) MC type of non-Hodgkins in adults. **Translocation 14:18** **Aggressive**, fast growing, can arise in lymph nodes outside lymphatic system: GI, testes, thyroid, skin, breast, bone, brain. SX: Painless, rapid swelling in neck, armpit, groin. TX: **CHOP therapy**	**Adult T-Cell Lymphoma (non-Hodgkin)** Associated with **IV drug use**, blood transfusions. Caused by **HTLV-1 (retrovirus)** SX: Lytic bone lesions (RANKL/nuclear factor-κB ligand), hypercalcemia. MC: Japan, Caribbean, South America, Africa.
Mucosal Associated Lymphoid Tissue (MALT) Lymphoma, originating from B Cells in the marginal zone, MC in the **stomach** due to **Helicobacter pylori**. (Can be at any other mucosal location). DX: Endoscopy biopsy shows expansion of the **marginal zone** with sheets of neoplastic small lymphoid cells. TX: H. pylori. **Clarithromycin, Amoxicillin**.	**Sézary Disease** **Cutaneous lymphoma** (late stage of **mycosis fungoides**) Histology: Neoplastic CD4 + lymphocytes. SX: **Pautrier's microabscesses (collection of mycosis cells** in the epidermis), erythroderma (scaling erythremic skin), **Sézary cells (atypical lymphocytes**), lymphadenopathy.

Blood Cancers with Monoclonal Antibody Spikes

Multiple Myeloma Monoclonal **plasma cell** cancer. (Plasma cells produce antibodies). MC tumor arising from the bone in the elderly (> 70 yrs). **Signs/Symptoms** • **Serum protein electrophoresis (SPEP) shows an IgG or IgA Monoclonal M Spike > 3g/dL** • **DX: MAT: Bone marrow biopsy confirms > 10% plasma cells.** • > 30% plasma cells in bone marrow • Plasma cells produce ↑ IgG (55%) and IgA (25%) • ↑ ESR > 100 • **Bence Jones Proteins in** urine (Urine dipstick does NOT pick up Bence Jones Proteins, it is only picked up by urine protein **electrophoresis.** **AKA: Ig light chains in urine** **AKA: Amyloid infiltration** AKA: Gel electrophoresis of proteins in urine AKA: **PARA proteins** AKA: Tamm Horsfall Proteins AKA: VkCk in urine • **↓ anion gap because IgG is cationic.** (Cationic substances ↑ Cl and HCO3 which ↓ anion gap) • MC Death: Renal failure, infection • **Bence Jones proteins** absorbed in tubules can precipitate and form **eosinophilic cast** that cause **obstruction** (PARA proteins obstruct renal tubes/glomeruli) and is toxic to kidney tubules. • **AL Amyloidosis** that show apple green birefringence on **Congo Red stain** → tubular necrosis → renal failure • **Rouleaux** formation seen on peripheral blood smear (RBC stacked due to the **IgG protein** on the RBC which causes them to stick together) • Histology: **Plasma cells with "clock face" chromatin** and intracytoplasmic inclusion containing	**Monoclonal Gammopathy of Undetermined Significance (MGUS)** Resembles Multiple Myeloma but antibody levels and number of plasma cells in the bones are lower. Asymptomatic precursor to multiple myeloma at rate of 1 – 2%/year. Asymptomatic ↑ **IgG** on serum protein electrophoresis. Serum shows **monoclonal M spike < 3 g/dL** (Multiple myeloma shows > 3g/dL spike) **< 10% plasma cells** in the bone marrow. No treatment. **Waldenström's Macroglobulinemia** (AKA: Lymphoplasmacytic Lymphoma) Cancer of uncontrolled **overproduction of IgM** from B cells in the bone marrow and lymph nodes causing **hyperviscosity.** SX: anemia (increase WBC crowd out the RBC's), weakness, vertigo, vision defects (**enlarged vessels** in the eye due to hyperviscosity) fatigue, **bleeding** from gums and/or nose or other mucosal surfaces, **hyperviscosity,** Raynaud's, anemia. **NO** lytic bone lesions, confusion, headache. DX: **Monoclonal IgM spike**. (**tip**: Remember to turn the "W" in Waldenstrom's to an "M" for IgM) BIT: Elevated serum viscosity levels and IgM levels. Labs: B cells produce ↑↑IgM TX: Plasmapheresis (removes IgM and ↓ viscosity), **Lenalidomide, Bortezomib, Fludarabine, Chlorambucil.**

Multiple Myeloma cont'd

- immunoglobulins
  AKA: Plasma cells with large **eccentric nuclei**
- **↑ calcium levels due to Osteolytic lesions by osteoclast regulated by RANKL.**
- Overexpression of **RANKL gene**. Binds receptor at nuclear Kappa B ligand
- RANKL = hypercalcemia (breaking bone down)
- **Lytic lesions** in bones (back bone, skull)
- **↑ BUN/Creatinine**
- ↑ Total protein with normal albumin
- **Hypercalcemia** (due to high plasma cell turnover = ↑ INF, IL-1, constipation
- **Hyperuricemia is toxic to kidney tubules.**
- **↑ Bone resorption** (break down) = **Hypercalcemia**
- ↑ Bone issues (fractures/weakness) of back and skull
- Pathologic fractures = bone pain due to **Osteoclast Activating Factor (OAF) attacking the bone**
- **Anemia:** massive numbers of **plasma cells** in the bone marrow **crowd out** the other cell lines (RBC)
- Radionuclide bone scans will be normal b/c lytic lesions do not pick up the nuclear isotope
- MC in men and in African Americans
- DX: Skeletal survey shows punched out lytic lesions (shows ↑ calcium).
  Serum protein electrophoresis shows ↑ levels IgG monoclonal antibody.
  Urine protein electrophoresis shows Bence-Jones proteins.
  Peripheral smear shows rouleaux formation of RBC's.
  MAT: **Bone marrow biopsy** shows > 10% plasma cells.

- TX: **Bisphosphonates** (to ↓ bone fractures), **Dexamethasone with Lenalidomide or Bortezomib** (reverses renal function).
  Erythropoietin for anemia.
  Autologous stem cell bone marrow transplant.

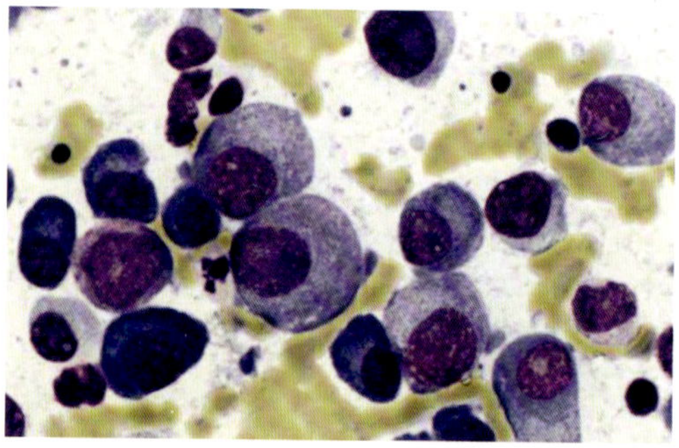

Misc Bone Marrow Proliferation Pathologies

Myelodysplasia
(AKA: Myelodysplastic Syndrome), Preleukemic disorder.

Disorder/dysplasia of hematopoietic stem cells (ineffective hematopoiesis of all blood cells) in the myeloid lineage due to a 5q deletion. (Patients with 5q = better prognosis). Onset >65 years.

SX: Weight loss, fatigue, infection, severe anemia (↓RBC, Hb) and progression to cytopenia due to bone marrow failure, neutropenia (↑ risk of infections), thrombocytopenia (↑ bleeding, ecchymosis, hemorrhage, petechiae), splenomegaly.

Complications: ↑ risk of transformation into AML.. Infection and fatal hemorrhaging before leukemia develops.

Causes: Environmental exposures (radiation, benzene), chemotherapy.

Labs: **Bilobed nucleus** (**Pelger-Huet cells**), anemia with ↑ MCV, ↓ blast, pancytopenia, ↓ reticulocyte count, large/oval RBC's (Macro ovalocytes), nucleated RBC's, hypercellular marrow.
Prussian blue stain is positive for ringed sideroblasts, normal B12.

Prognosis: Based on Blasts percentage.

TX: **Erythropoietin.**
Transfusion (For those patients with **5q deletion,** must add either **Azacitidine or Lenalidomide** to help decrease the need for transfusion).

Pelger-Huet Anomaly
Congenital:
Autosomal Dominant disorder caused by mutations in genes encoding proteins for the **nuclear lamina** (fibrillar network inside the nucleus composed of intermediate filaments). Associated with the **lamin B receptor**.

Histology: PMN that has a hyposegmented /bilobed nucleus.

Acquired: Pseudo-Pelger-Huët Anomaly
Occurs after chemotherapy, vitamin B12/folate deficiency, malaria, muscular dystrophy or during the course of AML, CML or myelodysplasia.

Histology: PMN's with **bilobed nuclei** that have two nuclear masses connected with a thin filament of chromatin.

Langerhans Cell Histiocytosis
(AKA: Hand-Schüller-Christian disease)
Clonal proliferation of **dendritic (Langerhans cells**, AKA: monocyte, histocytes) in the bone marrow that migrate from the skin to lymph nodes.

SX: Painful bone swelling, fever, erythematous scaly rash, anemia, pancytopenia, lytic lesions = fractures, lesions erupting on the scalp and ear canal.

DX: Expression of **S-100**, peanut agglutinin expressing, MHC II, CD1a.
Histology: **Birbeck granules** ("tennis rackets"). Birbeck granules are formed by the protein Langerin (CD207).

Note: Langerhans are APC (Antigen presenting cells).
(**tip**: I play tennis in Burbank, CA)

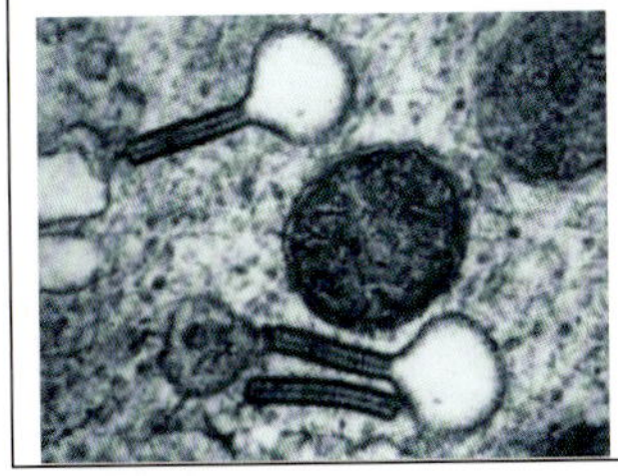

Bone Marrow Transplants

- Both **bone marrow transplants** and **liver transplants** are most at risk for **graft-verses-host** rejection.
- Autologous transplantation (transplant is from the same person) has no rejection (including graft-verses-host).
- Autologous transplantation can be done up to 70 years old.
- Allogeneic transplantation (transplant is from donor, other than self, from the same species) can be done up to 50 years old.
- Allogeneic transplantation are at risk for graft-verses-host rejection.

Myeloproliferative Pathologies

Polycythemia

Polycythemia Vera	Polycythemia Appropriate Absolute
Polycythemia Vera Neoplasm in which the bone marrow overproduces all blood cell lines, with RBC being the most predominant. Mutation in **JAK2 gene (Janus Kinase, JAK/STAT)) a non-receptor tyrosine kinase**. (Protein that regulates bone marrow production). (AKA: Jak2 mutation). SX: **Intense pruritis after hot shower** (due to **histamine** release from ↑ basophils), plethoric face (swollen), ruddiness (rosy/red color), **thrombosis** (due to hyperviscosity), headache, fatigue, splenomegaly, ↑ blood clots (due to thick blood), peptic ulcers (due to ↑ histamine release = stimulates gastric acid), **gout/gouty arthritis** (due to ↑ cell turnover and uric acid (purines), bleeding (due to enlarged blood vessels). **↑ Risk Budd Chari**: (due to hypercoagulable state → clotting in hepatic vein = back up = ascites, abdominal pain, hepatomegaly) Labs: **↑↑ RBC production/mass, ↓ ESR, ↑ ALP, ↑ HCT** > **50%, ↑ Hb = ↑ oxygen content** (oxygen plus oxygen bound to Hb), **↓ EPO levels, ↑ plasma volume, ↓ MCV, ↑ LAP, ↑ WBC, ↑ Platelets, ↓ iron levels** (iron used up to make new RBC's), **↑ B12 levels.** **DX: MAT: JAK2 mutation.** TX: **Phlebotomy and aspirin**: Keeping Hct < 45 (↓ risk of thrombosis). **Antihistamines, Allopurinol or Rasburicase** (↓ uric acid), **Hydroxyurea** (↓ cell count).	**Polycythemia Appropriate Absolute** Polycythemia due to chronic hypoxic conditions. **Hypoxic conditions stimulate EPO (erythropoietin is produced by peritubular cells in the renal cortex)**. EPO binds erythrocyte precursors in the bone marrow (CFU-e/colony forming units) = ↑ RBC production. **ANY chronic hypoxic condition** stimulates EPO: High altitude, RDS, COPD In renal failure/Chronic kidney disease = no EPO production = anemia. Must give exogenous EPO. **Labs: ↑ RBC production, ↑ EPO, ↓ O2 saturation, ↑ HCT** 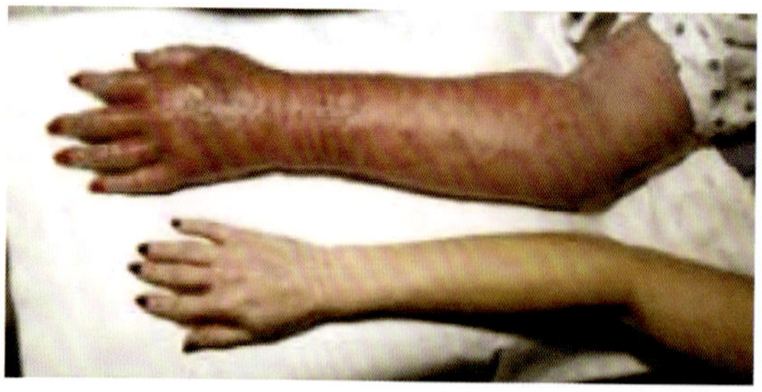 Polycythemia Vera

Polycythemia Inappropriate Absolute (2° Polycythemia)	Polycythemia Relative
Polycythemia 2° due to another pathology. EPO producing tumor, tumors/cancer in the kidney (Wilms, Renal Cell Carcinoma). Labs: ↑ **RBC production/mass**, ↑ **EPO**, ↑ **HCT > 60%, normal O2 saturation.**	Polycythemia due to ↓ plasma volume. Causes: Dehydration, diuresis, burns Labs: ↑ **RBC production/mass**, ↑ **HCT, normal O2 saturation**

Polycythemia Differentials

Polycythemia	RBC Mass	EPO Level	Plasma Volume	O2 Sat	Notes
Polycythemia Vera	↑↑	↓	↑		Mutation in Jak2
Polycythemia Appropriate	↑	↑		↓	Chronic Hypoxia
Polycythemia Inappropriate	↑	↑			2° Pathology
Polycythemia Relative			↓		Dehydration, diuresis, burns

Myeloproliferative Pathologies cont'd

Essential Thrombocytosis	Myelofibrosis
Overproduction of **platelets** leading to thrombosis. **Jak2 mutation.** SX: Erythromelalgia (burning sensation and redness in the extremities that resolve with aspirin and/or cooling), ↑ bleeding, thrombosis, headache, visual disturbance. Histology: Bone marrow contains enlarged megakaryocytes Labs: **↑↑ platelets, all cell lines are ↑** TX: Daily low dose **Aspirin**. Extremely high platelet counts: TX: **Hydroxyurea** (cyto reducing agent: reduction of cells, ↓ platelet count)	Proliferative clonal neoplasm of the hematopoietic stem cells in the bone marrow results in **collagen fibrosis** (replacement of the marrow with **scar tissue**). (AKA: **Fibroblast replace marrow with collagen**) Note: presents similar to Hairy Cell Leukemia. Causes: Mutations to JAK2 (Janus Kinases = non-receptor tyrosine kinase). Change of valine to phenylalanine at 617 position. Labs: **Teardrop RBC** (being "squeezed" out of the marrow), nucleated RBC's, ↑ megakaryocytes, **pancytopenia** (↓ production of all cells in the bone marrow), **↓ reticulocyte count.** **Normal TRAP level.** SX: Hepatosplenomegaly, pancytopenia, ↑ Extramedullary hematopoiesis in the spleen (marked splenomegaly with multiple splenic infarcts), cachexia (loss of appetite/weight loss/fatigue), easy bruising (↓ platelets), bone pain, pallor and shortness of breath (anemia). TX: allogeneic stem cell transplantation

ONCOLOGY - METASTASIS

General Cancer Categories
Please see individual chapters for details on individual types of cancers.

MORTALITY and INCIDENCE RATES: DEATH and CANCER

MCC Death: Heart Disease

MCC Death in a smoker: Lung cancer
MCC Death in a non-smoker: Colon cancer
Mammograms lower the mortality more than any other cancer-screening test.

Cancer Mortality

MC in MEN	MC in Women
Lung Prostate Colon	Lung Breast Colon

Cancer Incidence

MC in MEN	MC in Women
Prostate	Breast

GYN Cancers

Caution: Be careful to read very carefully what type of cancer they want when they are asking about mortality/incidence with women: there is a big difference between GYN cancers and cancers in general in women. **Note: breast cancer is NOT considered GYN cancer!**

MC GYN Mortality	MC GYN Incidence
Ovarian Endometrial Cervical	Endometrial Ovarian Cervical

Tumor Definitions

- Benign: Tumor is well differentiated. It has no metastasis, low mitotic activity (cell proliferation) and no necrosis.
- Malignant: Tumor is poorly differentiated, metastasis, local invasion. (Has high telomerase activity. This inhibits the shortening of the chromosomes and cell death.
- Carcinoma: Cancer that is derived from epithelial cells (epithelial tissues line cavities and the surfaces of organs and blood vessels). Epithelial cells: squamous, cuboidal and columnar. These cells do not contain blood vessels so must get their nourishment from substances that diffuse through the basement membrane. Occur due to damaged DNA: the cell can become malignant.
  Carcinomas spread MC by the lymphatics (except for: Renal cell carcinoma, hepatocellular carcinoma, follicular thyroid carcinoma, choriocarcinoma).
  EX: Breast, colon, lung cancer, adenocarcinoma, squamous cell carcinoma, small cell carcinoma.
- Sarcoma: Cancer that is derived from mesenchymal origin (cartilage, fat, muscle, hematopoietic tissue, vascular tissue).
  Sarcomas spread MC hematogenously (blood).
  EX: Liposarcoma, chondrosarcoma, osteosarcoma, Kaposi's, desmoid, angiosarcoma). Sarcomas are assessed by their grade (low, intermediate or high).

Carcinoma Epithelium Cell Type	Benign	Malignant
	Adenoma Papilloma	Adenocarcinoma Papillary carcinoma

Sarcoma Mesenchymal Cell Type	Benign	Malignant
Blood cells		Leukemia Lymphoma
Blood vessels	**Hemangioma** (Strawberry: children Cherry: adults) (tip: children play with strawberry shortcake)	Angiosarcoma
Bone	Osteoma	Osteosarcoma
Connective tissue	Fibroma	Fibrosarcoma
Fat	Lipoma	Liposarcoma
Melanocyte	Nevus, Mole	**Melanoma**
Smooth muscle	Leiomyoma	Leiomyosarcoma
Striated muscle	Rhabdomyoma **Myxoma**	Rhabdomyosarcoma

Cancer: General

- Most common cancer: metastasis
- Names: Metastasis is named for the original cancer (Example: A metastasis breast cancer that spreads to the lungs is called metastatic breast cancer, not lung cancer).
- **MC places of metastasis: Bone, Liver, Lungs**
- Primary cancer: single lesion
- Metastases: multiple lesions
- **Metalloproteinase** (enzyme requires zinc) causes **invasion leading to metastasis in cancers**
- **Unintentional weight loss, especially in an older person**
- **Benign:** Well differentiated cells. Low mitotic activity. No metastasis.
- **Malignant:** Poorly differentiated, invasive, unorganized/erratic growth, may metastasize.
- **Cachexia:** Muscle atrophy, weight loss, fatigue associated with serious disease. **Weight loss due to cytokine effects of TNF-α and IL-1**.
- **Autophagic degradation (vacuoles) by the autophagy-lysosome system contribute to muscle wasting (cachexia) in cancer.** Autophagy is the process that degrades cellular components leading to organelle damage and it stimulates proteolysis, which breaks down muscle.

Metastatic calcification

- (**tip**: "**M**" etastatic = "**M**"etastases)
- Deposits of calcium in otherwise normal tissue
- Increased absorption or decreased excretion of calcium due to diseases (ie: hyperparathyroidism)
- Labs: Increased calcium levels (hypercalcemia)
  Normal calcium labs: 8.5 – 10.2 mg/dL
  High calcium: > 10.2 indicates a disease process
  Very high calcium: > 13 indicates cancer (mc: PTHrp from Squamous Cell lung cancer)
- Note: Dystrophic calcification: calcification due to tissue damage in necrotic tissue (**tip**: "**D**"ystrophic = "**D**"amage), it is not due to cancer

Mass effect: cancer in the body due to the local presence of cancer cells. The mass effect is due to the growing mass that results in secondary pathologies because of the pressure on or displacement of surrounding tissues.
Example: tumors in the pharyngeal area can lead to dysphagia/hoarseness/stridor, intracerebral hemorrhage (hematoma).

Paraneoplastic syndrome: cancer in the body due to the secretion of peptides (hormones or cytokines) by the tumor cells or by an immune response (antibodies) against the tumor.
Examples: Small Cell lung cancer (Cushing syndrome, SAIDH, Lambert-Eaton), pancreatic carcinoma (Carcinoid. Dermatomyositis, Trousseau sign), neural tumors, thymoma, Insulinoma (hypoglycemia), Adrenal adenoma/Conn's syndrome (hyperaldosteronism), Non-Hodgkin lymphoma, gastric carcinoma (Acanthosis nigricans), bronchogenic carcinoma (Dermatomyositis), renal carcinoma (Polycythemia), thymic neoplasms (anemia).

Tumor Lysis Syndrome: Complication during the treatment of cancer due to large amounts of cell death occur causing abnormalities in metabolites and electrolytes such as: Hyperkalemia, hypocalcemia, hyperuricemia, hyperphosphatemia and high BUN. This condition can cause serious side effects: kidney failure, seizures, arrhythmias, high uric acid and death. MC in leukemias and lymphomas.
TX: Allopurinol, IV hydration to maintain urine output.

Grading and Staging

Staging: TNM

"T" Tumor size = The size of the tumor and the number of lymph nodes affected.
"N" Nodes = The nearest lymph nodes are the axillary (under the arm)
"M" Metastases = Signs of metastases in other organs (bones, liver, lungs, brain)

- Stage 0,1: Earliest detection. Cells confined to limited area
- Stage 2, 2A: Early stages but beginning to spread. Responds well to treatment
- Stage 3 A, B, C: Advanced, evidence of invasion of surrounding tissues near the breast (lymph nodes/muscle)
- Stage 4: Cancer has metastasized (brain, bones, lungs, liver)

Grades

Most common prognosis used in brain cancer
Indicates the severity of the mutation, mitotic activity, differentiation and the likelihood that it will spread.
How closely the cells resemble healthy cells.
The shape and size of nuclei.
How rapidly the cells divide and multiply.
Grades determine the best treatment plan.
TX: Low grade: radiation or chemotherapy.
TX: Intermediate or High: surgery, chemotherapy, radiation.
The lower the grade the better chance of full recoveries at every stage (including aggressive ones)

- Low grade (1): well differentiated
- Intermediate grade (2): moderately differentiated
- High grade (3): Poorly differentiated and likely to metastasize

Cancer Cells vs Non Cancer Cells

- Monoclonal = cancer. Mono (one). One cell produces all the cancer cells.
- Polyclonal = cells from two or more cell lines.

Reversible Cell Plasia

Hyperplasia	Increase in numbers of cells
Metaplasia	One cell type is replaced by another cell type. (Ex: Barrett's esophagus)
Dysplasia	Abnormal growth. Change in cell shape and size. Unorganized.

Irreversible Cell Plasia

Anaplasia	Loss of differentiation and function of cells. (ex: Giant cells with large or multiple nuclei)
Desmoplasia	Fibrous tissue formation due to neoplasm (ie: linitis plastica in stomach cancer)
Neoplasia	Uncontrolled clonal proliferation of cells. Can be benign or malignant.
Differentiation	How closely a malignant tumor resembles the tissue of its origin. Poorly differentiated: is not like the original tissue. Well differentiated: is still similar to the original tissue.

Path of Adenoma to Carcinoma

APC ➔ Methylation ➔ Cox 2 overexpression ➔ K-RAS ➔ Rb ➔ P53

Main Sites of Metastasis

- Brain includes: neural tissue (parenchyma), arachnoid and pia mater, meninges, space containing CSF
- Lung includes: main lung tissue (parenchyma), pleura (membrane covering the lungs and lining chest cavity

Cancer Type	Main Sites of Metastasis	MC Risk Factors
Bladder	Bone, liver, lung	**Smoking.** Other ↑ risk factors: aniline dyes, aging, male, Caucasian, chronic cystitis, family Hx, taking **Pioglitazone** >1 yr (diabetes med), **Cyclophosphamide**
Breast	Bone, brain, liver, lung	Female, aging, family Hx, personal Hx, radiation exposure, obesity, longer exposure to estrogen (beginning period early, late menopause), having first child at older age, never being pregnant, HRT therapy, alcohol, genetics.
Colorectal	Liver, lung peritoneum	Aging, African American, Inflammatory intestinal conditions, family Hx, low fiber/high fat diet, sedentary lifestyle, diabetes, obesity, smoking, alcohol, radiation
Esophageal	Celiac lymph nodes, liver, lungs	**(Alcohol, smoking for upper esophagus: squamous).** (**Achalasia, reflux, GERD** for **lower Barrett's Esophagus**). Other risk: Drinking very hot liquids, obesity, radiation.
Kidney	Adrenal gland, bone, brain, liver, lung	Smoking, aging, obesity, HTN, long term dialysis, family Hx, ↑ risk with diseases: VHL, tuberous sclerosis, familial papillary renal cell carcinoma
Liver	Adrenal gland, bone, brain, liver, lung	Alcohol, smoking, steroids, aflatoxins, arsenic, vinyl chloride (chemical in plastic mfg., cirrhosis, HEP B or HEP C, obesity, aging, male, Asian, diabetes
Lung	Adrenal glad, bone, brain, liver, other lung	**Smoking**, second hand smoke, radon (natural gas from dirt and rocks that gets trapped in houses), asbestos, arsenic, diesel exhaust, silica, chromium, family Hx, radiation therapy to the chest, diet
Melanoma, Skin Most common cancer in the USA	Bone, brain, liver, lung, skin, muscle	**Exposure to UV rays**, fair skin, Hx of sunburns, moles, family Hx, weakened immune system, radiation, arsenic
Ovary	Liver, lung, peritoneum	Aging, smoking, inherited gene mutation, HRT, longer exposure to estrogen (beginning period early, late menopause), fertility TX, IUD, PCOS
Pancreas	Liver, lung, peritoneum	**Smoking**, African American, obesity, diabetes, chronic pancreatitis, family Hx
Prostate	Adrenal gland, bone, liver, lung	Aging, African American, family Hx, genetics, diet, obesity
Stomach	Liver, lung, peritoneum, ovary (Krukenberg tumor)	**Diet** (high in salty and smoked foods/nitrosamines), diet low in fruits and vegetables, **smoking**, aflatoxin fungus, family Hx, **H. pylori**, long term stomach inflammation, pernicious anemia, stomach polys
Thyroid	Bone, liver, lung	Female, radiation, genetics
Uterus (Endometrial)	Bone, liver, lung, peritoneum, vagina	Aging, hormonal changes, longer exposure to estrogen (beginning period early, late menopause), obesity, hormone TX for breast cancer (**Tamoxifen**), HNPCC (colon cancer), never having been pregnant

Most Common Metastasis Sites

Site of Metastases	MC Location of Primary Tumor	Notes
Bone	MC from: Prostate or Breast Others: Lung, thyroid, kidney	
Brain	MC from Lung > Breast > Prostate > Melanoma > GI	MC form of brain cancer is metastasis. Metastasis in the brain is located at the "gray-white" matter junction. TX: If there is a "**S**"ingle lesion = "**S**"urgery. If there are multiple lesions = radiation.
Liver	MC from colon > stomach, pancreas	

Metastasis: Shows multiple lesions

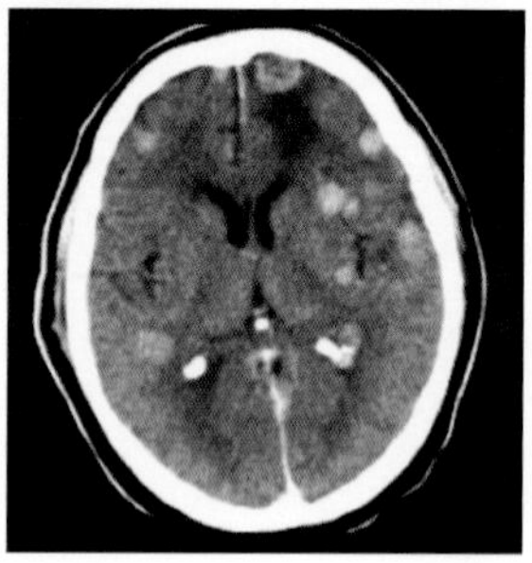

Brain

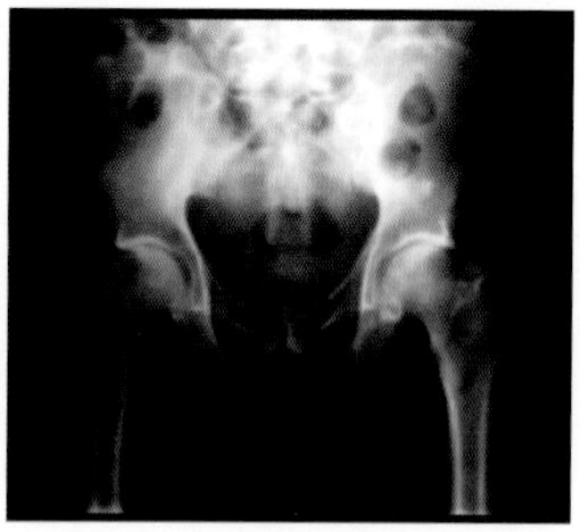

Bone

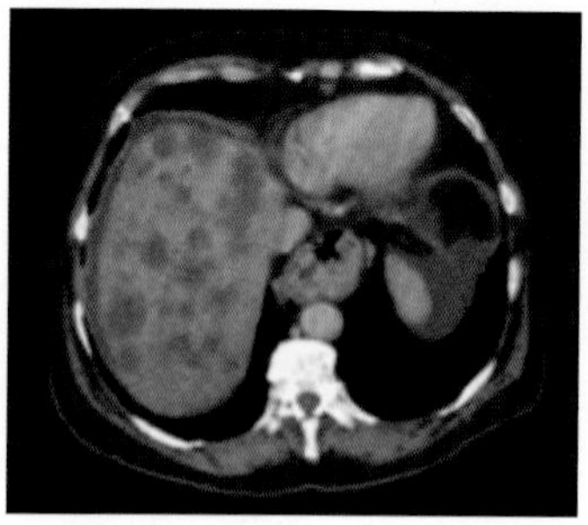

Liver

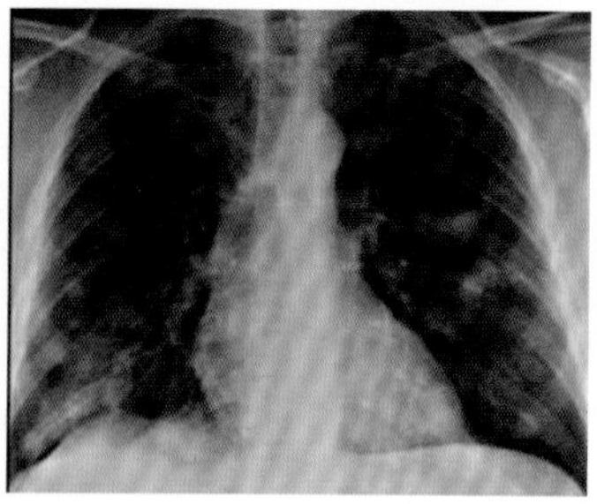

Lungs

Types of Metastasis

Metastasis	Description
Local invasion	Cancer cells invade nearby normal tissue
Intravasation	Cancer cells invade and move through the walls of nearby lymph or blood vessels
Circulation	Cancer cells move through the lymphatic system and bloodstream to other parts of body
Arrest and extravasation	Cancer cells arrest (stop moving) in capillaries at a distant location. Then invade the walls of the capillaries and migrate into the surrounding tissue (extravasation)
Proliferation	Cancer cells multiply at the distant location to form micrometastases (small tumors)
Angiogenesis	Micrometastases stimulate growth of new blood vessels to obtain a blood supply for oxygen and nutrients needed for continued tumor growth

TUMOR SUPPRESSOR GENES

"Anti-oncogenes" **"LOSS of FUNCTION"** (Stops cell proliferation). Inactivation causes tumor development.
Both alleles must be damaged/lost in order for development of disease.
(AKA: **Two hits are required for loss of function**).

GENE	TUMOR	GENE PRODUCT
BRCA1	Breast cancer Ovarian cancer	DNA repair protein
BRCA2	Breast cancer Ovarian cancer	DNA repair protein
PTEN	Breast cancer Prostate cancer Endometrial cancer	
CPD4 SMAD4	Pancreatic cancer	DPC – deleted in pancreatic cancer
DCC	Colon cancer	DCC – deleted in colon cancer
APC	Colorectal cancer	
Menin MEN1	MEN 1	
P53	Li-Fraumeni Syndrome	Transcription factor
P16	Melanoma	Cyclin dependent kinase
NF1	Neurofibromatosis 1	RAS GTPase protein
NF2	Neurofibromatosis 2	Schwannoma protein (Merlin)
TSC1	Tuberous Sclerosis	Hamartin protein
TSC2	Tuberous Sclerosis	Tuberin protein
Rb	Retinoblastoma Osteosarcoma	Inhibits E2F
VHL	Von Hippel-Lindau DZ	Inhibits factor 1a
WT1	Wilms Tumor (nephroblastoma)	
WT2	Wilms Tumor (nephroblastoma)	

ONCOGENES

"Proto-oncogenes" Pro Tumor/stimulates cell proliferation. Over **expression (amplification)** = ↑↑ growth.
"GAIN of FUNCTION" (Turns on tumor development)
One allele is already lost so there only needs to be damage/loss to the last remaining allele to develop the disease.

GENE	TUMOR	GENE PRODUCT
HER2/neu **c-erbB2**	Breast Ovarian	Tyrosine kinase
L-myc	Lung	Transcription factor
N-myc	Neuroblastoma	Transcription factor
c-myc	Burkett lymphoma	Transcription factor
BCR-ABL	CML AML	Tyrosine kinase
bcl-2	Follicular lymphoma	Anti-apoptotic
ras	Colon cancer Pancreatic cancer lung cancer	GTPase
c-kit	GIST tumor (Gastrointestinal stromal tumor)	Cytokine receptor
ret	MEN 2A, MEN 2B	Tyrosine kinase
BRAF	Melanoma	Serine-threonine kinase

TUMOR MARKERS

MARKER	TUMOR
α-fetoprotein	Yolk Sac tumor Testicular cancer Hepatocellular carcinoma Hepatoblastoma Mixed Germ Cell (secreted with β-hCG)
Alkaline phosphatase (ALP)	Paget's DZ Bone metastases Seminoma
β-hCG	Hydatidiform moles Choriocarcinomas (Gestational trophoblastic dz) Testicular cancer
CA-15-3 CA-27-29	Breast cancer
CA-19-9	Pancreatic cancer
CA-125	Ovarian cancer
Calcitonin	Medullary thyroid carcinoma (MEN)
CEA (Carcinoembryonic Antigen)	Colorectal cancer
PSA (Prostate Specific Antigen)	Prostate cancer (Can be elevated in BPH, prostatitis and after massaging the prostate in a prostate exam)
S-100	Melanomas (Neural Crest origin) Schwannomas Langerhans cells
TRAP (Tartrate Resistant Acid Phosphatase)	Hairy cell leukemia

Cancer Tumor Markers

Type of Cancer	Origin	Marker	Notes
Carcinoma	Ectoderm. Epithelial origin.	Cytokeratin	Lymph, glands. Lining of cavities and surfaces of structures. Spreads lymphatically. Exceptions that spread hematogenously: Hepatocellular (hepatic vein), Follicular (thyroid), Renal Cell Carcinoma (renal vein), Choriocarcinoma.
Sarcoma	Mesoderm. Mesenchymal origin.	Vimentin	Connective tissue. Spreads hematogenously.
Lymphoma		CD45	

Cancers Associated with Microbes

EBV	Burkitt Lymphoma, Nasopharyngeal carcinoma, CNS lymphoma
Hepatitis B, C	Hepatocellular carcinoma
HSV-8	Kaposi sarcoma
HPV	Cervical carcinoma (CIN, HPV 16, 18), Anal carcinoma (homosexual males), penile carcinoma
H. pylori	MALT lymphoma, Gastric adenocarcinoma
HTLV-1	Adult T-cell leukemia, lymphoma
Liver fluke	Cholangiocarcinoma (Clonorchis sinensis)
Schistosoma haematobium	Bladder cancer

Cancers Associated with Paraneoplastic Syndromes

Hormone	Cancer	Syndrome/Symptoms
Ectopic ACTH and ACTH-like	Small Cell Lung Carcinoma, Pancreatic carcinoma, Thymoma	Cushing Syndrome. ↑ ACTH.
ADH	Small Cell Lung Carcinoma	SAIDH. Hyponatremia, ↑ ADH.
Aldosterone	Adrenal adenoma (Conn's), Ovarian carcinoma, Non-Hodgkin's lymphoma	Hyperaldosteronism, ↑ Na, ↑ HCO3, ↓ K, ↓ H (protons) = hypertension, metabolic alkalosis.
Antibodies against presynaptic Ca channels at NMJ	Small Cell Lung Carcinoma	Lambert-Eaton. Gets stronger through the day, no eye involvement.
Antibodies against postsynaptic ACh receptors at the neuro-muscular junction	Thymoma	Myasthenia gravis. Gets weaker through the day, eye involvement (ptosis).
Serotonin, Bradykinin	Pancreatic carcinoma, Gastric carcinoma	Carcinoid Syndrome. Flushing, diarrhea, cardiomyopathy, 5-HIAA (5-hydroxyindoleacetic acid) in the urine.
Calcitriol (1,25 Vit D)	Hodgkins lymphoma	Hypercalcemia. ↑ Ca
Erythropoietin	Renal Cell Carcinoma, Hepatocellular carcinoma, Thymoma, Pheochromocytoma	Polycythemia. Labs: ↑↑ Hct
Insulin, Insulin-Like	Insulinoma, Hepatocellular carcinoma	
PTH rp	Squamous Cell Lung carcinoma, Renal Cell carcinoma, Ovarian carcinoma, Multiple myeloma, Breast carcinoma	Hypercalcemia. ↑ Ca
Antibodies against NMDA receptor	Ovarian teratoma	Memory and psychiatric problems, seizures, dyskinesias.
	Pancreatic	Trousseau Syndrome (migratory superficial thrombophlebitis)
	Gastric adenocarcinoma Visceral cancers	Acanthosis nigricans
	Pure red blood cell aplasia	Thymoma. Anemia with low reticulocytes.

Cancers Associated with Paraneoplastic Syndromes cont'd

	Neuroblastoma	Bone lesions in the legs and hips (difficulty standing/walking), tumor in the bones around the eyes (bruising/swelling around the eyes) = "Dancing feet and dancing eyes".
	Pancreatic	Nonbacterial thrombotic endocarditis. (deposits of sterile platelets and fibrin (thrombi) on the heart valves.

Cancers Associated with Diseases

Disease	Cancer
Acanthosis nigricans	Stomach and other visceral cancers (also associated with diabetes)
Actinic keratosis	Squamous cell carcinoma of the skin
AIDS	Kaposi, CNS Lymphoma (think of CNS lymphoma when patient is being treated from Toxoplasmosis and the treatment does not work (ring-enhancing lesions).
Atrophic gastritis, Chronic	Gastric adenocarcinoma
Barrett Esophagus	Esophageal adenocarcinoma (lower 1/3 of esophagus)
Pernicious anemia	Gastric adenocarcinoma
Cirrhosis	Hepatocellular carcinoma
Crohn's	Colon Adenocarcinoma
Cushing Syndrome	Small Cell Lung Cancer (ACTH)
Dermatomyositis	Lung cancer
Down's Syndrome	ALL
Dysplastic nevus	Melanoma
Hashimoto Thyroiditis	Lymphoma (also associated with pernicious anemia)
Hypercalcemia	Squamous Cell Lung Cancer (PTH)
Lambert-Eaton	Small Cell Lung Cancer
Myasthenia Gravis	Thymoma
Paget Disease of the Bone	Osteosarcoma, Fibrosarcoma
Plummer-Vinson Syndrome	Squamous Cell Carcinoma of the Esophagus
Polycythemia	Renal Cell Carcinoma, Hepatocellular Carcinoma
Pure RBC Aplasia	Thymoma
Radiation exposure	Leukemia, Breast cancer, Papillary Thyroid cancer
SIADH	Small Cell Lung Cancer (ADH)
SLE	Lymphoma
Tuberous Sclerosis	Cardiac Rhabdomyoma
Ulcerative colitis	Colon Adenocarcinoma
Xeroderma pigmentosum	Melanoma, Basal Cell Carcinoma, Squamous Cell Carcinoma of the Skin

Carcinogens

Toxin	Cancer	Organ Affected	Notes
Aflatoxins: Aspergillus	Hepatocellular carcinoma	Liver	Dust from peanuts
Alkylating drugs	Leukemia, Lymphoma	Blood	Cyclophosphamide, Carmustine, Busulfan, Cisplatin, Streptozocin, Chlorambucil
Amine Dies	Bladder cancer	Bladder	
Arsenic	Lung, Liver, Skin	Lungs, Liver, Skin	
Asbestos	Bronchogenic carcinoma, Mesothelioma	Lung	For it to be Mesothelioma: must affect the pleura, must be at least 20 years from exposure, ferruginous bodies
Carbon Tetrachloride	Centrilobular necrosis/liver cancer	Liver	Upholstery, insecticide, refrigerant, cleaning agent, used in fire extinguishers
Cigarettes	Transitional Cell, Squamous Cell carcinoma/adenocarcinoma, Renal Cell carcinoma, Pancreatic adenocarcinoma, Small Cell Carcinoma	Bladder, Pancreas, Lung, Esophagus, Kidney, Larynx Cancers	
Ethanol	Hepatocellular carcinoma	Liver	

Carcinogens cont'd

Ionizing Radiation	Papillary Thyroid Carcinoma	Thyroid	
Nitrosamines (smoked foods)	Gastric cancer	Stomach	MC: Japanese diets
Radon	Lung cancer	Lung	Colorless, odorless, radioactive gas. Found in soil and rocks: moves in the air and into underground and surface waters.
Vinyl Chloride	Angiosarcoma	Liver	Used in PVC plastics

Cancer Treatments

- **Additions to cancer treatments:**
  Allopurinol to avoid tumor lysis syndrome/gout.
  Ondansetron: 5HT antagonist (nausea)
  Folic Acid (AKA: Folate, B9) to aid with rapid cell division and growth
- **Salvage: Extended radiation treatment when the first type of cancer treatment failed. Only provides long-term control.**
- **Adjuvant: Treatment in addition to the standard treatment (given together). Ex: Radiation given at the same time chemo**
- **Consolidation: Multi-drug regiment given after induction treatment to further reduce the tumor. Ex: Multi drugs given after induction for cancer.**
- **Induction: Initial dose to rapidly kill tumor cells and send the patient into remission. Ex: Chemo for acute leukemia.**
- **Maintenance: Given after induction and consolidation (or initial) to keep patient in remission. Ex: Daily androgens to treat prostate cancer.**
- **Neo Adjunctive: Treatment given before standard therapy. Ex: Radiation before tumor removal.**

Pain Management in Terminal Cancer

3 Key Principals

- **Try non-narcotics first (unless patient is in severe pain)**
- **Do not be afraid to give narcotics**
- **Prescribe adequate amounts of narcotics**

For patients that have never used narcotics:

- **Try short acting morphine (titrate as needed). Once titrated can then be switched to long acting**

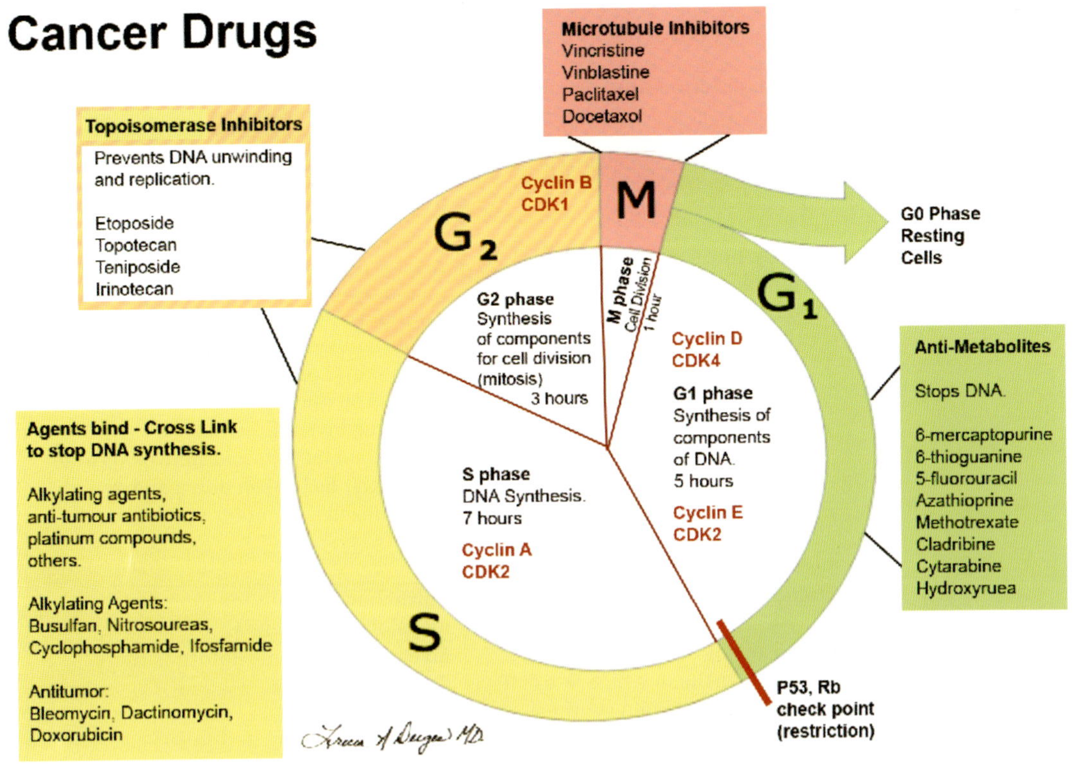

Microtube Inhibitors

DRUG GENERIC name Trade name	Clinical Use	Mechanism of Action and Resistance	Toxicity and Notes
Vincristine **Vinblastine** Vinorelbine	Leukemia's, Lymphomas, solid tumors.	Vinca alkaloids bind β-tubulin, which inhibit the formation of the microtubules (mitotic spindles) in the M-phase of the cell cycle. (AKA: inhibit microtubules in β tubules) (**tip:** all M's = **M** phase, **M**icrotubules, **M**itotic spindle) **Do not allow the microtubule to form or grown.** (**tip**: "VINe" is not able to grow)	**Vincristine: Neurologic toxicities.** **Vinblastine: Bone marrow suppression.** (**tip**: vin**BLAST**ine **BLAST** the **B**one)
Paclitaxel	Breast cancer. Ovarian cancer.	Will not allow microtubules (mitotic spindle) to **break down** so that cell cycle can't progress. Does not allow the microtubule to breakdown.	Myelosuppression, alopecia, hypersensitivity. (**tip**: can't put your back **PAC DOWN**)
Ixabepilone	Breast cancer.	Stabilize microtubules. Used in cancers that are insensitive to paclitaxel.	Peripheral neuropathy.

Antimetabolites

- Stop DNA and RNA synthesis. So always occurs in **"S" phase**. (S phase is where DNA is synthesized)
- Without DNA = ↓ purine, ↓ protein synthesis
- **Must give Allopurinol with cancer drugs** to ↓ risk of gout due to ↑ cell death. **Except with Azathioprine and 6-MP**: both need **xanthine oxidase** to be metabolized (broken down). (**Allopurinol inhibits xanthine oxidase**) so you must use another chronic gout drug instead.
- All drugs that treat cancer and stop DNA will affect bone marrow.

DRUG GENERIC name Trade name	Clinical Use	Mechanism of Action and Resistance	Toxicity and Notes
Azathioprine **6-mercapto-purine (6-MP)** **6-thioguanine (6-TG)**	SLE (Azathioprine), RA, Leukemia, AML, IBD (6-MP, 6-TG), **prevents organ rejection**.	Purine analog. ↓ purine synthesis. Activated by HGPRT. Blocks nucleotide synthesis which Inhibits lymphocyte proliferation.	Bone marrow suppression (anemia), hepatotoxic, GI symptoms, thrombocytopenia, leukopenia. Azathioprine and 6-MP: require xanthine oxidase to be metabolized (broken down) so **do NOT use** **Allopurinol** or **Febuxostat** with these drugs. You must use another chronic gout drug instead. Allopurinol inhibits xanthine oxidase so 6-MP can't be broken down and metabolized so it builds up → toxic.
Cytarabine	Leukemias, Lymphomas	Pyrimidine analog. Inhibits DNA polymerase.	Thrombocytopenia, leukopenia, megaloblastic anemia.
5-Fluorouracil (5-FU)	Colon cancer, intestine, pancreatic cancer, basal cell carcinoma	Pyrimidine analog. **Inhibits thymidylate synthase** which ↓ dTMP to inhibit DNA and protein synthesis.	Myelosuppression, photosensitivity, diarrhea Overdose of 5-FU: **Uridine** (also the treatment for orotic aciduria)
Methotrexate (MTX)	Leukemias, Lymphomas, Choriocarcinoma, Sarcomas. Non cancer uses: Abortion in ectopic pregnancies, rheumatoid arthritis, SLE, psoriasis, IBD	Folic acid analog. **Inhibits dihydrofolate reductase → ↓ dTMP** → inhibits DNA and protein synthesis. By inhibiting dihydrofolate reductase, **thymidylate synthase** is inhibited which **inhibits the conversion of DHF → THF.**	**Pulmonary fibrosis**, myelosuppression, fatty liver, hepatotoxic, stomatitis (mouth ulcers), teratogenic. Myelosuppression can be reversed/rescued with **Leucovorin** (folinic acid). (**tip**: Leucovorin to the rescue)

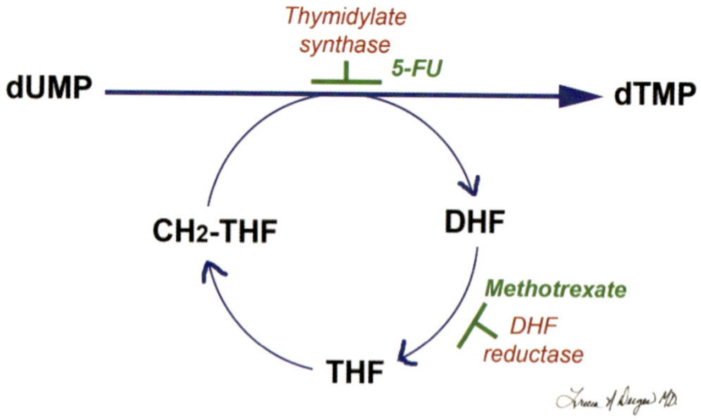

Antitumor Antibiotics

- **Breaks or Intercalates in DNA, stops cross linking**

DRUG **GENERIC name** **Trade name**	**Clinical Use**	**Mechanism of Action and Resistance**	**Toxicity and Notes**
Bleomycin	Testicular cancer. Hodgkin Lymphoma.	Inhibits **G2 phase by intercalating** in DNA to cause **breaks in the DNA**. Form free radicals.	**Pulmonary fibrosis**, skin discoloration, Mild myelosuppression. (**tip**: Bleo the clown blows up your balls and your lungs)
Dactinomycin **Actinomycin D**	Children's tumors: Wilms, Ewing, Rhabdomyosarcoma (**tip**: children with tumors "**ACT**"inomycin **out**)	Stops DNA. Intercalates in DNA.	**Myelosuppression**
Doxorubicin *Adriamycin* **Daunorubicin** *Cerubidine* **Epirubicin** **Idarubicin**	Leukemia's, Lymphomas, Solid tumors	Inhibits **G2 phase by intercalating** in DNA to cause **breaks in the DNA**. Form free radicals.	**Dilated cardiomyopathy**, alopecia, myelosuppression. (**tip:** the "Rubicin" brothers dilate your heart) Prevent cardiomyopathy with **Dexrazoxane** (iron chelating agent)

Alkylating Agents

- Alkylating agents add an alkyl group to DNA. It attaches the alkyl group to the **guanine base** of DNA at the number 7 **nitrogen** atom of the imidazole ring. This inhibits DNA replication by forming intrastrand DNA crosslinks.
- AKA: **Cross links/intercalates in DNA (AKA: terminates DNA)**
- AKA: Alkylates DNA
- AKA: Methylate's (stops) DNA
- Process requires **bioactivation by the liver (first pass metabolism)**

DRUG **GENERIC name** **Trade name**	**Clinical Use**	**Mechanism of Action and Resistance**	**Toxicity and Notes**
Busulfan	CML. Ablates bone marrow before bone marrow transplantation.	Cross-links DNA. Requires bioactivation by liver.	**Pulmonary fibrosis**, skin discoloration, Mild myelosuppression.
Cyclophosphamide Ifosfamide	Leukemia, Lymphoma, brain tumors	Cross-links DNA Requires bioactivation by liver.	**Hemorrhagic cystitis, bladder cancer,** myelosuppression. Partial **prevention of hemorrhagic cystitis** with **Mesna**. Mesna binds the toxic metabolites, **acrolein** in the urine and excretes it.
Nitrosoureas **Carmustine** **Streptozocin** Lomustine Semustine	Glioblastoma multiforme and other brain tumors Streptozocin: pancreatic cancer	Crosses blood-brain barrier. Requires bioactivation by liver. Cross-links DNA	CNS symptoms: seizures, dizziness, confusion, ataxia, headaches, **Pulmonary fibrosis** Streptozocin: insulin dependent diabetes. (**tip**: Mustangs are wild and can cross over barriers)

Selective Estrogen Receptor Medulators (SERMs)

DRUG GENERIC name Trade name	Clinical Use	Mechanism of Action and Resistance	Toxicity and Notes
Tamoxifen	**Breast cancer** (estrogen receptor- positive), Infertility in anovulatory disorders, prevent estrogen-related gynecomastia.	Acts as **antagonist at breast tissue** (anti-estrogen) and an **agonist at the uterus (endometrium) and bone.** In breast (antagonist): inhibits estrogen sensitive breast cancer. In bones (agonist): inhibits osteoclasts and prevents osteoporosis. In uterus: agonist ➔ 🡅 estrogen ➔ endometrial cancer (🡅 or longer exposure to estrogen = 🡅 risk of endometrial and cervical cancers)	**Endometrial cancer (AKA: Endometrial hyperplasia),** 🡅 risk of blood clots (thromboembolism), hot flashes, 🡅 triglycerides, memory impairment. Good for bones and breast. Bad for uterus. **Do NOT use**: if patient is an active smoker, has had previous blood clots or is a high risk for blood clots (thromboembolism).
Raloxifene	**Breast Cancer** (estrogen receptor- positive)	Acts as an **antagonist at uterus** and an **agonist at the bone.** Antagonist at the uterus ➔ 🡇 estrogen so no 🡅 risk for endometrial carcinoma. Agonist at the bone ➔ 🡇 osteoclast activity (🡇 bone resorption) so 🡇 osteoporosis and bone fractures.	Hot flashes, leg cramps, blood clots, pulmonary embolism. Teratogen. Must stop Raloxifene 4 weeks prior to any surgery due to 🡅 risk of thrombosis. Good for bones, breast and uterus. (**tip**: RELAX ("ralox") your bones are fine)

Antiandrogens

DRUG GENERIC name Trade name	Clinical Use	Mechanism of Action and Resistance	Toxicity and Notes
Flutamide	**Prostate cancer.** PCOS (Polycystic ovarian syndrome), hirsutism. Treats excess androgens in women.	Antagonist at the testosterone receptors. If no testosterone = no DHT. Inhibits entire axis: No GnRH = No LH = No FSH.	Gynecomastia, GI symptoms, mild hepatotoxicity

GnRH Pharmacology

DRUG GENERIC name Trade name	Clinical Use	Mechanism of Action and Resistance	Toxicity and Notes
Leuprolide	**Prostate cancer** (continuous use), Uterine fibroids (continuous use), Precocious puberty (continuous use). Infertility (pulsatile use), Endometriosis.	GnRH analog has agonist properties in pulsatile use. When used for antagonist properties with continuous use, GnRH is down regulated so that FSH/LH are 🡇.	Impotence, hot flashes, antiandrogen effects, nausea, vomiting. Note: Prostrate cancer treatment: there is an 🡅 in testosterone for the **first dose** and then testosterone will 🡇. **NOTE**: Leuprolide when used continuously will inhibit FSH and LH secretion which inhibits menstrual cycles and puts a women in a "state" of menopause. This is beneficial in endometriosis and fibroids (or other disease states that are stimulated by the menstrual cycle). If the drug is used in a pulsatile manor it stimulates the release of FSH and LH causing the menstrual cycle/ovulation.

Misc Cancer Pharmacology

DRUG GENERIC name Trade name	Clinical Use	Mechanism of Action and Resistance	Toxicity and Notes
Asparaginase *Elspar*	Leukemia	Converts L-asparagine to aspartic acid and ammonia, which keeps the leukemia cells from asparagine causing cell death.	Bone marrow suppression, hypersensitivity
Bevacizumab	Colorectal cancer, Renal cell carcinoma	Inhibits angiogenesis. Monoclonal antibody against VEGF.	Hemorrhage, slow wound healing
Cetuximab	Colorectal cancer (Late stages)	Monoclonal antibody against EGFR	Hepatotoxic, diarrhea, rash
Cisplatin **Carboplatin** **"the Platin's"**	Testicular cancer, Bladder, ovarian, lung cancer.	Cross links DNA	**Nephrotoxicity, ototoxic** (Do not use with aminoglycosides or cephalosporins), neurotoxicity, hemolytic anemia (hemolysis), Hypomagnesia, hypokalemia, hypocalcemia. **Nephrotoxicity prevented** with **Amifostine.** Amifostine scavenges **free radicals.**
Erlotinib	Non-small cell lung carcinoma.	EGFR tyrosine kinase inhibitor	rash
Etoposide Teniposide	Small Cell lung cancer, Testicular cancer.	Inhibits the G2 phase by **inhibiting topoisomerase II** leading **to DNA apoptosis** (degradation).	Alopecia, vomiting, nausea, myelosuppression
Irinotecan Topotecan	Irinotecan: Colon cancer. Topotecan: small cell and ovarian cancer.	Inhibits DNA unwinding by inhibiting **topoisomerase I.**	Myelosuppression, GI symptoms
Filgrastim	Increases the production of leukocytes (neutrophils). Neutropenia is usually due to chemotherapy and bone marrow transplantation.	G-CSF Granulocyte colony-stimulation factor analog that stimulates the proliferation and differentiation of granulocytes (leukocytes/neutrophils).	Mild bone pain, rash, wheezing, ARDS, hemoptysis.
Hydroxyurea	Sickle cell disease, CML, Melanoma	Cancer treatment MOA: Inhibits DNA synthesis in S phase by inhibiting ribonucleotide reductase in the pyrimidine pathway. Sickle cell MOA: ↑ HbF so there is more affinity for oxygen.	**Pulmonary fibrosis**, bone marrow suppression
Imatinib Gleevec	**CML** GIST (GI stromal tumor),	**Tyrosine kinase inhibitor** of **BCR-ABL** (Philadelphia chromosome 9:22 in CML, JAK/STAT pathway) and in **c-Kit** (GIST tumors).	Edema
Prednisone Prednisolone	Higher doses treat cancer: CLL, Non-Hodgkins lymphoma, immunosuppressant. Lower doses treat: inflammatory diseases, allergic reactions	Synthetic corticosteroid. Promotes apoptosis.	Cushing's type symptoms: central obesity (↑ waist to hip ratio), weight gain. Osteoporosis, HTN, hyperglycemia, edema, mental confusion, joint pain, cataracts, acne. ↑ cortisol levels (can cause damage to adenyl glands). Sudden withdrawal can cause **adrenal crisis. (adrenal insufficiency) and death.** A stressor (such as surgery or hospitalization) can require the need for cortisol (stress hormone) and it is not available → adrenal crisis. Withdrawal must be tapered if on the drug > 1 week.

DRUG GENERIC name Trade name	Clinical Use	Mechanism of Action and Resistance	Toxicity and Notes
Rituximab	Non-Hodgkin lymphoma (B cell neoplasm), Rheumatoid arthritis (with MTX)	Monoclonal antibody against CD20 (B cell).	Possible progression to PML (Progressive multifocal leukoencephalopathy)
Sorafenib	Renal cell carcinoma. Hepatocellular carcinoma.	Targets serine/threonine and tyrosine kinase in tumor cells. Stopping tyrosine kinase stops angiogenesis.	HTN, hemorrhage, hypophosphatemia, alopecia, pruritus, GI symptoms
Trastuzumab Herceptin	**HER-2** positive breast cancer, gastric cancer	Monoclonal antibody against the **tyrosine kinase receptor HER-2** (erbB2). Kills cancer cells that overexpress HER-2 by cytotoxicity (CD 8).	Cardiotoxicity (**tip**: get a TRAING bra for HER-too (2)
Vemurafenib	Melanoma	Inhibits B-Raf kinase enzyme (VEGF, PDGFR) in the B-Raf/MEK/ERK pathway to cause apoptosis in melanoma cells lines.	Arthralgia, photosensitivity, skin rash

Antiemetic for Chemotherapy Pharmacology

DRUG GENERIC name Trade name	Clinical Use	Mechanism of Action and Resistance	Toxicity and Notes
Ondansetron *Zofran*	Antiemetic (stops nausea and vomiting) for chemotherapy. postoperative and Gastroenteritis.	**5-HT (Serotonin) receptor antagonist.**	Constipation, dizziness, headaches. **Torsades de pointes**.
Aprepitant	Antiemetic (stops nausea and vomiting) for chemotherapy. postoperative and Gastroenteritis.	Substance P antagonists. Transmembrane G-protein coupled receptor in the Gq path (PKC, IP3, DAG). (NK1 receptor antagonist)	

Chemotherapy Drug Side Effects

Chemotherapy Drug	Side Effect
Actinomycin D	Myelosuppression
Adriamycin	Cardiomyopathy
Bleomycin	Pulmonary Fibrosis
Busulfan	Pulmonary Fibrosis
Cisplatin	Ototoxicity, Renal toxicity
Cyclophosphamide	Hemorrhagic cystitis
Daunorubicin	Cardiomyopathy
Dactinomycin	Myelosuppression
Doxorubicin	Cardiomyopathy
Etoposide	Myelosuppression, Alopecia
Hydroxyurea	Pulmonary Fibrosis
Methotrexate	Pulmonary Fibrosis, Hepatotoxic
Paclitaxel	Myelosuppression, Alopecia
Prednisone	Cushing's type syndrome, Osteoporosis, Weight gain
Raloxifene	Hot flashes, thrombosis
Tamoxifen	Endometrial carcinoma
Trastuzumab	Cardiotoxicity
Vinblastine	Bone Marrow Suppression
Vincristine	Neuropathy

MUSCULOSKELETAL - ANATOMY

Head, Neck, Chest

Muscles of Mastication (4)	Action and Notes
All are innervated by mandibular division of **Trigeminal V3.** All are derived from the 1st **pharyngeal arch**.	
Temporalis	Elevates and retracts mandible. Backward movement of jaw during chewing.
Masseter	Elevates mandible
Medial Pterygoid	Closes mouth, chews, pulls mandible up/forward/medial
Lateral Pterygoid	**Opens mouth** protrudes and **lowers** jaw. (**tip**: L for Lowers)

Muscle	Action and Notes
Orbicularis oris	Encircles the mouth. Closes and puckers lips
Buccinator	Walls of the cheeks. Holds food in contact with teeth when chewing and assists in blowing air out of the mouth. Area hurt when hit on the side of the face. Innervated by **CN VII.**
Mentalis	Protrudes the lower lip.
Zygomaticus Major	Raises corner of mouth to **smile**.
Geniohyoid	Pulls hyoid bone anteriorly for swallowing. Innervated by the **ansa cervicalis**
Levator Palatini	Elevates soft palate. Innervated by CN X.
Cricothyroid	Only laryngeal muscle that is innervated by the Superior Laryngeal nerve.
Sternocleidomastoid	Flexes and rotates head laterally.
Scalenes (anterior, middle, posterior)	Elevates ribs 1-2, flexes and rotates neck.
Pectoralis minor	Depresses and downwardly rotates scapula.
External intercostals	Elevates rib cage.

Bone	Notes
Orbital Bone	Bone that encircles the eye and is **MC broken** during fights or accidents.
Zygomatic bone (AKA: Cheek bone)	**Forms floor of orbit.** Boarders: orbit, maxilla, temporal bone, masseter.
Maxillary and medical nasal processes	**Failure to fuse causes: cleft lip**

Sinuses	Notes
Sphenoid Sinus	Point of entry to **remove pituitary tumor**. **NOTE: Point of entry** of an infection that leads to a Cavernous Sinus Thrombosis in the Cavernous Sinus.
Cavernous Sinus	Superior opthalmic vein drains into the Cavernous sinus. Facial vein drains into the Cavernous sinus. **NOTE:** Location of a **Cavernous Sinus Thrombosis** due to a spreading infection of the nose, ears, sinus, or teeth **through the sphenoid sinus.** SX: Loss of vision, bulging eyes, inability to abduct the eye.
Sigmoid Sinus	Drains into the Internal Jugular vein
Petrosal Sinus	Is the posterior continuation of the Cavernous Sinus

Nerves	
Posterior pharyngeal area sensation (pain)	CN IX
Posterior tonsillar fossa	CN IX
Soft Palate Innervation	CN X
Uvula deviation	CN X lesion
Superior Laryngeal nerve (internal branch)	Innervates laryngeal mucosa above vocal folds. Only nerve to innervate the laryngeal muscle cricothyroid
Left Recurrent Laryngeal nerve	Innervates laryngeal mucosa below vocal folds. Innervates all of the laryngeal muscles except the cricothyroid.
Superior Laryngeal nerve (external branch)	Cricothyroid

Vessels	
Facial Vein	Drains into the Cavernous sinus
Azygos Vein	Drains the thoracic wall
Superior Laryngeal Artery	Accompanies by the Internal branch of the Superior Laryngeal nerve

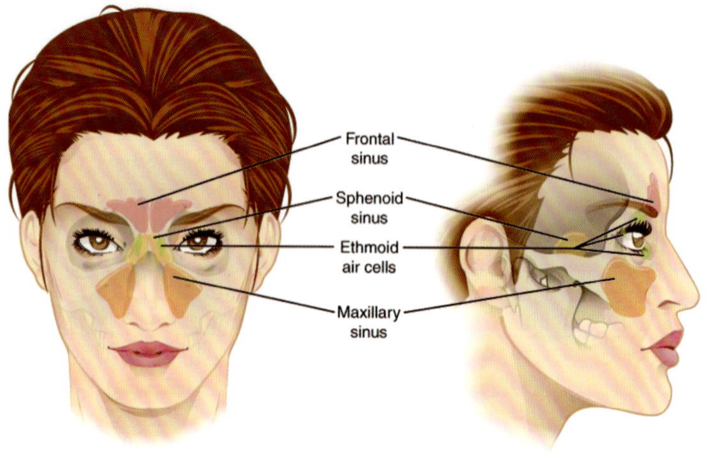

Salivary Glands	Notes
• Chorda tympani controls salivation from the sublingual and submandibular glands • Parotid gland is innervated by the glossopharyngeal nerve (CN IX) • Exocrine glands with ducts that produce saliva and amylase (enzyme that breaks down starch into maltose. First step in digestion). • Parasympathetic innervation via cranial nerves. • Sympathetic innervation via preganglionic nerves that synapse in the superior cervical ganglion. • BOTH parasympathetic and sympathetic innervation increases saliva.	
Parotid Glands	Largest salivary gland. Located on the side of the face over the buccinator muscle. Enters oral cavity via the parotid duct (AKA: Stensen duct). Associated with inflammation during **mumps and bulimia.** **Facial Nerve (CN VII) runs through the parotid gland.** **Parasympathetic innervation**: CN IX via otic ganglion. (IP3 and DAG pathway. Release: ACh and Substance P). **Sympathetic:** Preganglionic nerves that synapse in the **superior cervical ganglion**. Release norepinephrine, ↑ cAMP = ↑ saliva.
Submandibular Glands	Located beneath the lower jaws, superior to the digastric muscles. Enters the oral cavity via the submandibular duct (AKA: Wharton duct). Produce the majority of the saliva. **Parasympathetic innervation:** CN VII via submandibular ganglion. (IP3 and DAG pathway. Release: ACh and Substance P). **Sympathetic:** Preganglionic nerves that synapse in the superior cervical ganglion. Release norepinephrine, ↑ cAMP = ↑ saliva.

Sublingual Glands	Located inferior to the tongue and anterior to the submandibular glands. **Parasympathetic innervation**: CN VII via submandibular ganglion. (IP3 and DAG pathway. Release: ACh and Substance P). **Sympathetic**: Preganglionic nerves that synapse in the superior cervical ganglion. Release norepinephrine, ↑ cAMP = ↑ saliva.

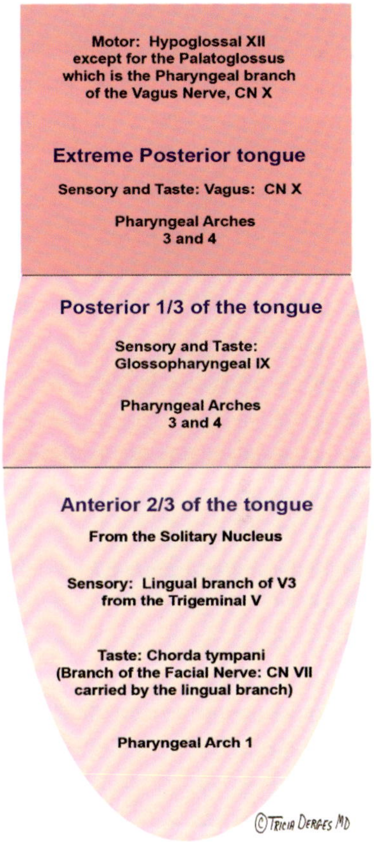

Tongue Development

- Anterior 2/3: 1st and 2nd brachial arches
- Posterior 1/3: 3rd and 4th brachial arches

Taste Development: From the **Solitary Nucleus**
(**tip**: you have a favorite taste for just one SOLITARY thing)

- **Anterior 2/3: CN VII (AKA: Chorda tympani, Facial nerve)**
- Posterior 1/3: CN IX
- Very Back (extreme posterior): CNX

Sensory Development (pain sensation)

- Anterior 2/3: CN Trigeminal, V3 branch
- Posterior 1/3: CN IX
  Pain sensation for the **posterior pharynx is by CN IX**
- Very Back (extreme posterior): CNX

Motor Development

- CN XII
- Muscles are from the occipital myotomes

Facial Nerves

- **Nerves: Facial Nerve (VII) supplies the muscles of facial expression. Ophthalmic, maxillary and mandibular branches of the trigeminal nerve supply the sensation to the skin of the face.**
- **Injuries**
  - Hit in the side of the face with a baseball: Injury to the **Buccal nerve**
  - Break in the side of the jaw (broken jaw): Injury to the **Inferior alveolar nerve**
  - Injury to the chin: **Mental nerve**
  - Loss of any facial expression: **Facial Nerve (VII)**

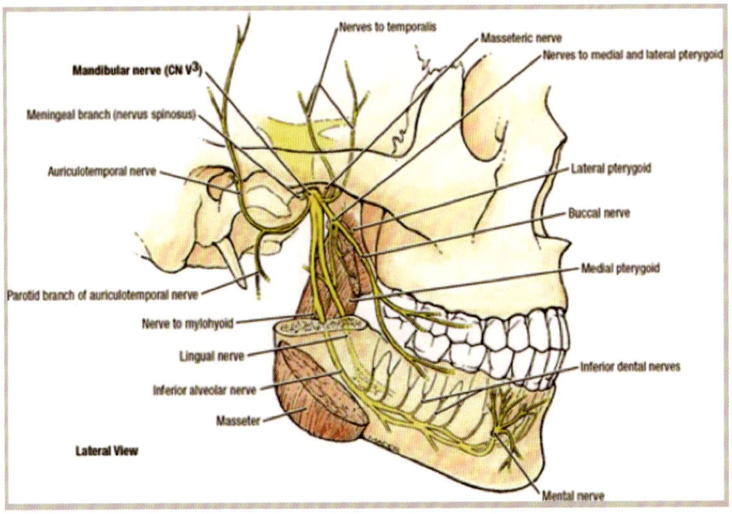

Facial Blood Supply

- **Blood supply: Branches of the external carotid artery supply blood to the face.**
- **Injuries**
  - MC location of a broken bone on the face is on the inferior boarder **zygomatic arch** (cheek bone). The **Infraorbital artery** is in danger of being damaged. (MC: injuries: assault, automobile accidents, falls, sporting accidents). The temporalis muscle passes medial to the arch and inserts into the coronoid process of the mandible.
  - Mandible fractures due to blunt facial trauma. The maxillary artery (branch off of the external carotid) is at risk for damage.

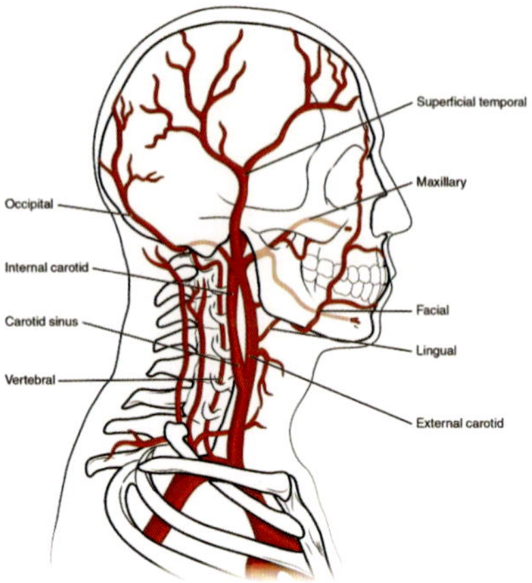

Facial Bones

- Upper face: Frontal and frontal sinus.
- Midface: Nasal, ethmoid, zygomatic, maxillary.
- Lower face: mandible.

Jaw Disorders

Bruxism (teeth grinding, clinching teeth)

- Occurs during the period of sleep.
- Increased tension in the masseter muscle.
- SX can be reduced by massage of the masseter muscle.

Temporomandibular Disorder (aka: TMJ)

- Temporomandibular joint is a hinge that connects the jaw to the temporal bone (front of the ears). Allows the jaw to be moved up and down and side to side.
- Due to problems with the muscles of the jaw or the joint. MC: arthritis, genetics, jaw injury, bruxism.
- Popping or clicking and pain of the jaw joint.
- TX: NSAIDS, TCA's, muscle relaxants, mouth guards, counseling, surgery.

Retroperitoneal Organs (SAD PUCKER)

- Suprarenal (adrenal) gland
- Aorta and IVC
- Duodenum (2nd, 3rd parts)
- Pancreas (head), NOT tail
- Ureters
- Colon (ascending and descending)
- Kidneys
- Esophagus, lower 2/3
- Rectum

GI Ligaments

GI Ligament	Connects	Structures Contained	Additional Anatomy
Falciform	**Liver to anterior (ventral) abdominal wall**	**Ligamentum teres (derivative of fetal umbilical vein).** Derivative of the embryonic ventral mesentery.	
Gastrocolic	Greater curvature of stomach and transverse colon	Gastroepiploic arteries	Part of greater omentum
Gastrohepatic	Lesser curvature of stomach to liver	Gastric arteries	**Left gastric involved in esophageal varices (left gastric is off the Azygos)**
Gastrosplenic	Greater curvature of stomach and spleen	Short gastrics, left gastroepiploic vessels	
Hepatoduodenal	Duodenum to liver	**Portal triad:** Proper Hepatic Artery, Portal Vein, Common Bile Duct	Location in ligament: Posterior: Portal Vein. Right side: Common bile duct. Left side: Hepatic artery.
Splenorenal	Spleen to abdominal wall	Splenic artery and vein, tail of pancreas. Splenic artery runs beneath the stomach.	Concerns of **stomach ulcers eroding into the splenic artery**

Upper Extremities: Shoulder, Arm, Hand Anatomy and Pathologies

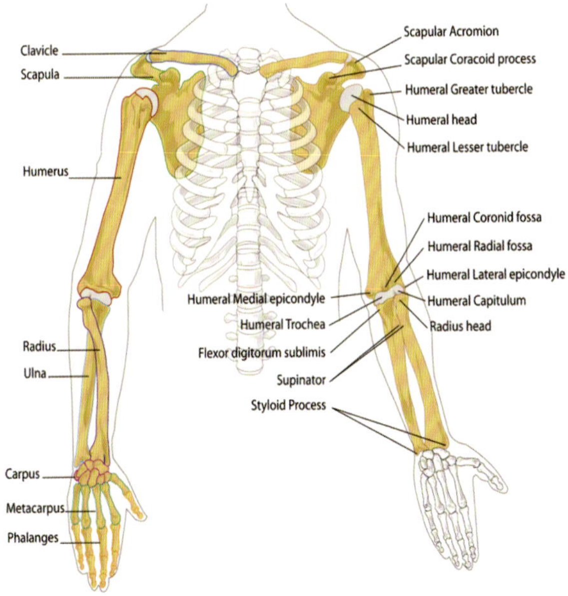

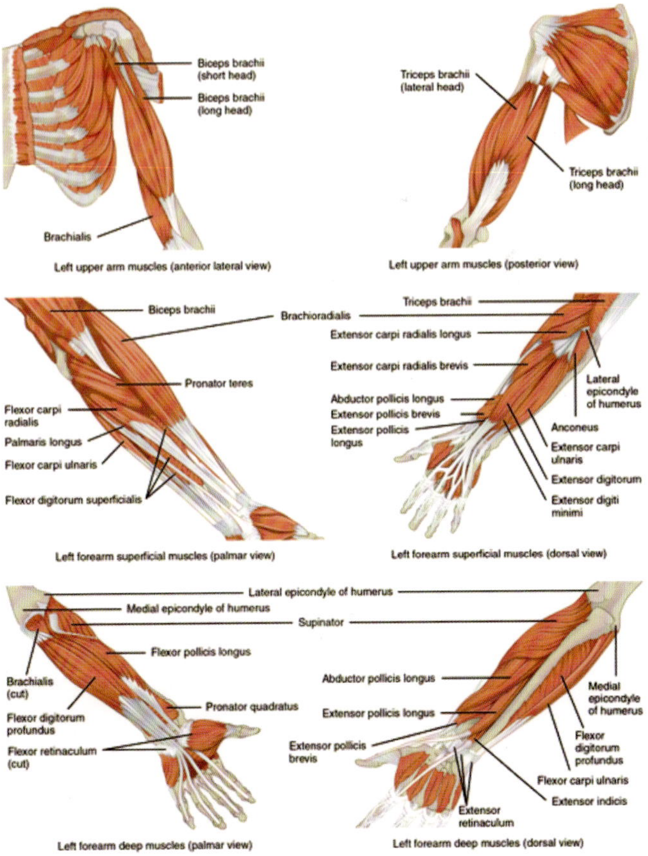

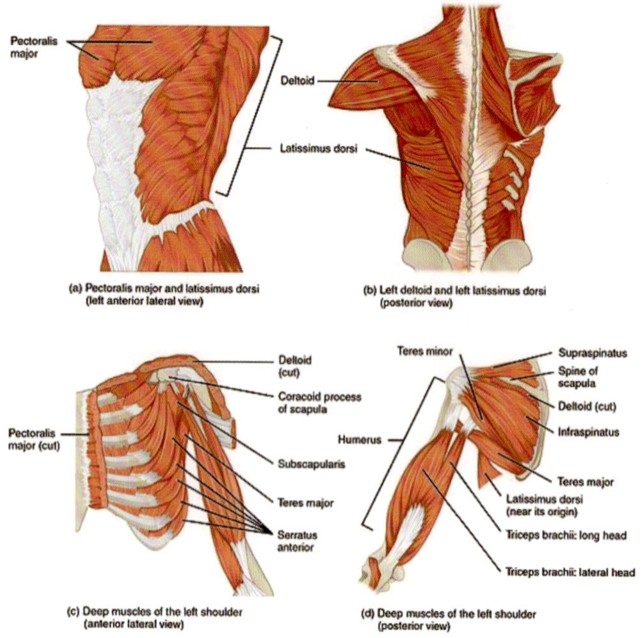
Pectoralis major
Deltoid
Latissimus dorsi
(a) Pectoralis major and latissimus dorsi (left anterior lateral view)
(b) Left deltoid and left latissimus dorsi (posterior view)
Deltoid (cut)
Coracoid process of scapula
Pectoralis major (cut)
Subscapularis
Teres major
Serratus anterior
Teres minor
Supraspinatus
Spine of scapula
Deltoid (cut)
Humerus
Infraspinatus
Teres major
Latissimus dorsi (near its origin)
Triceps brachii: long head
Triceps brachii: lateral head
(c) Deep muscles of the left shoulder (anterior lateral view)
(d) Deep muscles of the left shoulder (posterior view)

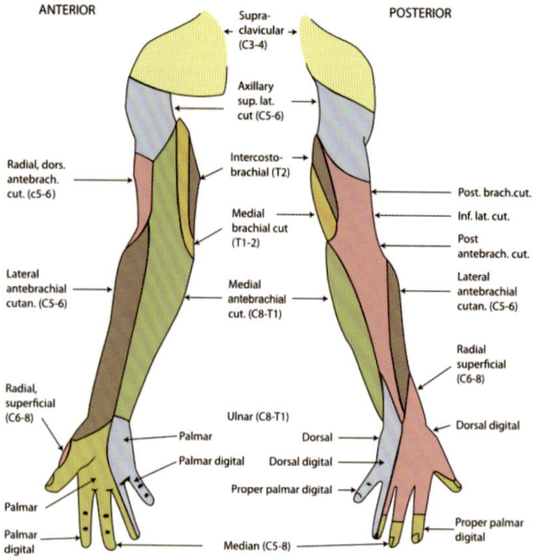
ANTERIOR
POSTERIOR
Supra-clavicular (C3-4)
Axillary sup. lat. cut (C5-6)
Intercosto-brachial (T2)
Radial, dors. antebrach. cut. (c5-6)
Medial brachial cut (T1-2)
Post. brach.cut.
Inf. lat. cut.
Post antebrach. cut.
Lateral antebrachial cutan. (C5-6)
Medial antebrachial cut. (C8-T1)
Lateral antebrachial cutan. (C5-6)
Radial superficial (C6-8)
Radial, superficial (C6-8)
Ulnar (C8-T1)
Palmar
Dorsal
Dorsal digital
Palmar digital
Dorsal digital
Proper palmar digital
Palmar
Palmar digital
Median (C5-8)
Proper palmar digital

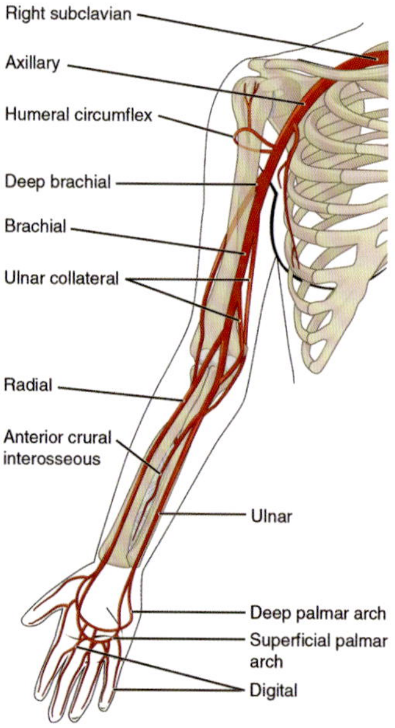
Right subclavian
Axillary
Humeral circumflex
Deep brachial
Brachial
Ulnar collateral
Radial
Anterior crural interosseous
Ulnar
Deep palmar arch
Superficial palmar arch
Digital

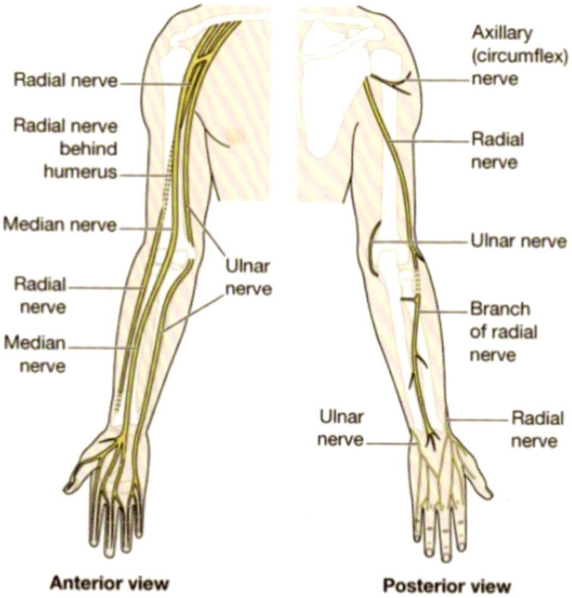
Radial nerve
Radial nerve behind humerus
Median nerve
Radial nerve
Median nerve
Ulnar nerve
Axillary (circumflex) nerve
Radial nerve
Ulnar nerve
Branch of radial nerve
Ulnar nerve
Radial nerve
Anterior view
Posterior view

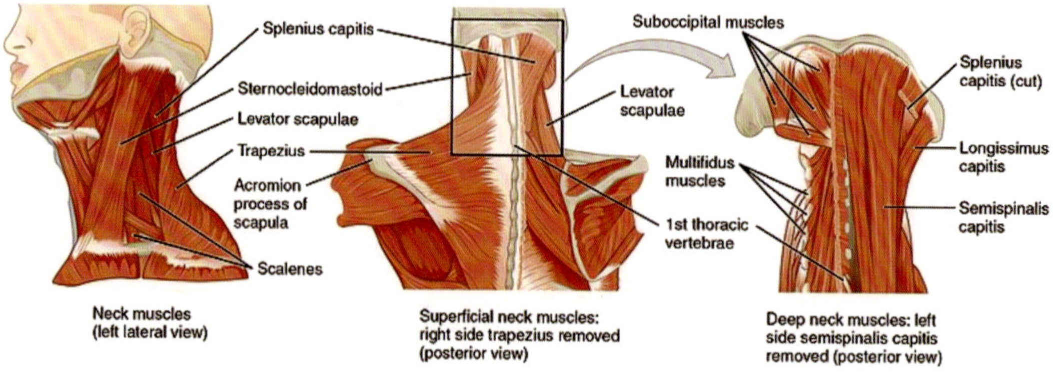
Splenius capitis
Sternocleidomastoid
Levator scapulae
Trapezius
Acromion process of scapula
Scalenes
Suboccipital muscles
Levator scapulae
Multifidus muscles
1st thoracic vertebrae
Splenius capitis (cut)
Longissimus capitis
Semispinalis capitis
Neck muscles (left lateral view)
Superficial neck muscles: right side trapezius removed (posterior view)
Deep neck muscles: left side semispinalis capitis removed (posterior view)

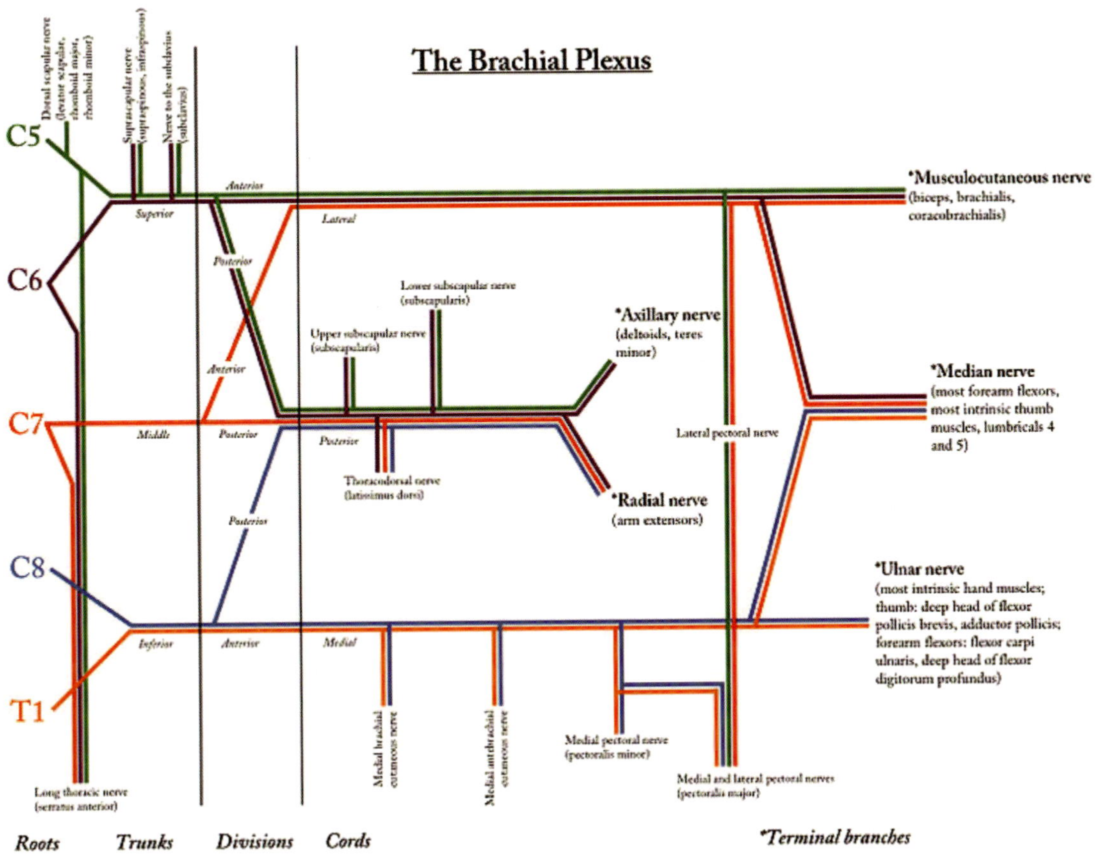

Brachial Plexus and Upper Extremity Injuries/Pathologies

Nerve, Muscle, Vessel	Cause	Nerve-Location	Muscle - Action	Notes	Appearance
Winged Scapula	**Mastectomy**, stab wounds	**Long Thoracic**	**Serratus anterior** Scapula won't anchor to thoracic cage. No **Abduction** of arm horizontally. **Lateral Thoracic Artery runs with Long Thoracic Nerve.**		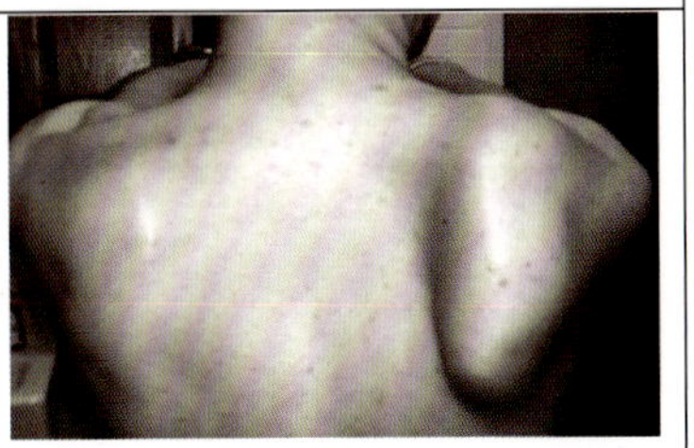
Erb Palsy **"Waiters Tip"** **AKA** **Shoulder Dystocia**	Difficulty Delivering infants head and anterior shoulder causing damage to upper brachial plexus and possibly fracture of clavicle or humerus. Compression ➔Phrenic Nerve injury ➔ diaphragmatic injury	**Upper Plexus: C5, C6**	Deltoid and supraspinatus: **No abduction** of arm (hangs by side). Infraspinatus: arm is **medially rotated** (Can't laterally rotate). Biceps brachii: no flexion of arm (arm is extended and pronated). ⬇Moro and biceps reflex	(**tip**: $5 or $6 is a good tip)	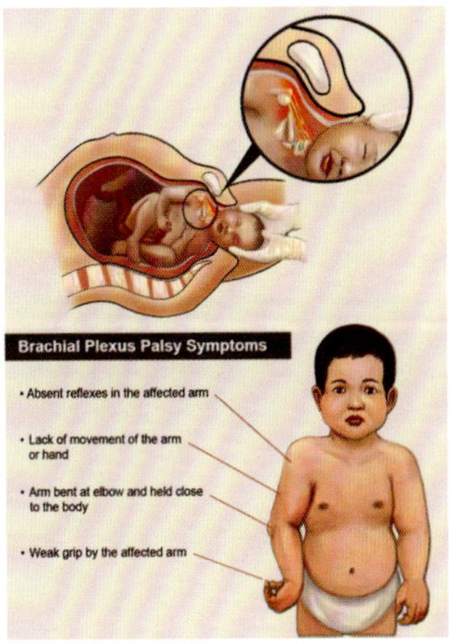

Klumpke's Palsy	Infants: upward pull of arm during delivery. Adults: grabbing, hanging from branch to break fall.	**Lower Plexus: C8 – T1**	**Claw hand,** can't extend fingers. Intrinsic hand : Lumbricals, interossei, **Thenar, Hypothenar**		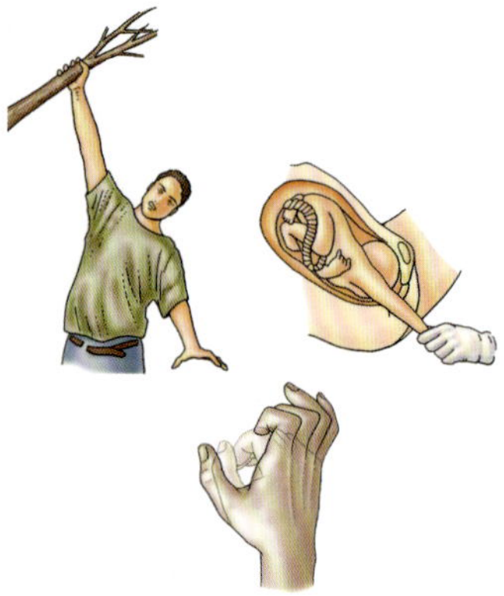
Thoracic Outlet Syndrome	**Pancoast tumor** Cervical rib Injury.	Lower Plexus C8 – T1	Compression of lower plexus and subclavian vessels. **Hoarseness** (due to Left recurrent Laryngeal nerve compression). Muscles: same as Klumpke's	Vascular Compression Causes: **Atrophy** of Intrinsic hand muscles, Ischemia, pain, edema	
Superior Vena Cava Syndrome	**Obstruction of SVC. MC: Bronchogenic Carcinoma.**			Facial edema, Dyspnea, Dysphagia, Stridor, headache	
Clavicle Injury	Fracture of Collar bone	**MC Type of Fracture: Midshaft** X-ray shows: *Medial end* is pulled up due to the sternocleidomastoid muscle. *Lateral end* is stable due to opposing trapezius pulling up and the deltoid pulling down. *The midshaft area* (area broken) is pulled in two different directions: The medial end of the lateral bone is pulled inferomedially by the pectoralis major and latissimus dorsi so it is shortened. The distal end of the medial bone is pulled upward due to the sternocleidomastoid. *Distal fractures* are stable due to the opposing force of the trapezius and the deltoid muscles.			**Muscle attachments:** Medial (proximal) end: Sternocleidomastoid. Distal (lateral): Trapezius and Deltoid. Midshaft: Subclavius **Clavicle attachment:** Medial end: on sternum by the Sternoclavicular ligaments. Distal end: on the scapula by the Coracoclavicular ligaments. **TX:** **Non-displaced: sling** **Displaced/closed: Figure 8 dressing.** **Open FX, non-union: surgery**
Accessory Nerve		Posterior triangle of neck			
Musculocutaneous Nerve	Upper trunk compression	C5 – C7 Arises from the lateral cord.			Paralysis of biceps, brachialis. Loss of **any elbow** Function. No Forearm flexion or supination at **elbow**. **Sensation** loss over **lateral forearm**.

Axillary Nerve	Fracture of the **surgical neck of the humerus.** Fall on outstretched hand. **Anterior dislocation** of shoulder at glenohumeral joint.	C5 – C6	Innervates the deltoid. Damage: Arm externally rotated. Loss abduction of arm > 15°. (unable to raise arm from the side). **Sensation** loss over **deltoid.**		Most common cause is **anterior shoulder dislocation**. **Axillary comes off of Radial Nerve**. **Posterior Circumflex Artery runs with Axillary Nerve.**
Posterior shoulder Dislocation	Seizures		Adduction of arm, internally rotated.		
Radial Nerve **"Wrist Drop"** **"Saturday Night Palsy"** **"Pope's Blessing"**	**Midshaft fracture of humerus, Radial grove** fracture, compression of **axilla** (crutches pressing on the axilla, sleeping with arm over chair = "Saturday night palsy".	C5 – T1	Innervates the **Extensor** pollicis longus. Damage: **"Wrist Drop" inability to extend**: fingers, wrist, elbow. Inability to extend thumb. "Pope's Blessing" Sensation loss over **posterior** arm, forearm, dorsal hand.		**Deep brachial artery** runs along side the Radial nerve. So must check for pulse and color (refill) to insure blood supply is not damaged. Deep branch of the Radial nerve passes through the Supinator.
Nursemaid's Elbow	Pulling child up by one arm	Radial	**Annular ligament** on the head of the radius		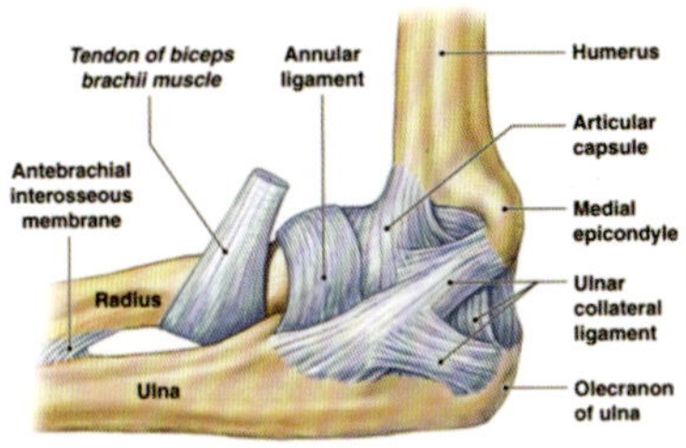
Median Nerve	**Carpal tunnel.** Typist, carpenters, any repetitive action of the wrist. Wrist lacerations (suicide attempts). Supracondylar Fx of humerus. **Other causes**: obesity, hypothyroidism, pregnancy. (Anything that can swell and put pressure on the median nerve).	Median C5 – T1 Formed by lateral and medial cords of brachial plexus.	Abducts, rotates, opposes and flexes the thumb. Innervates the thenar (thumb), Abductor pollicis brevis, Flexor pollicis brevis, Opponens pollicis, 1st two lumbricals, anterior forearm flexors. Sensation over the first 3.5 digits. Damage: Loss of **flexion**: fingers and wrists. Pain in first 3 fingers. "Ape hand". **Loss of thumb (thenar) opposition** (AKA: **Thenar wasting**), (can't hold a piece of paper between thumb and index finger). Sensation loss: first 3 ½ digits =thenar (thumb) and palm.	See wasting of thenar eminence	**(See carpal tunnel under wrist pathologies)** Medial nerve lies between the palmaris longus and flexor carpi radialis on anterior aspect of the forearm. Median nerve passes through the two heads of the Pronator Teres. 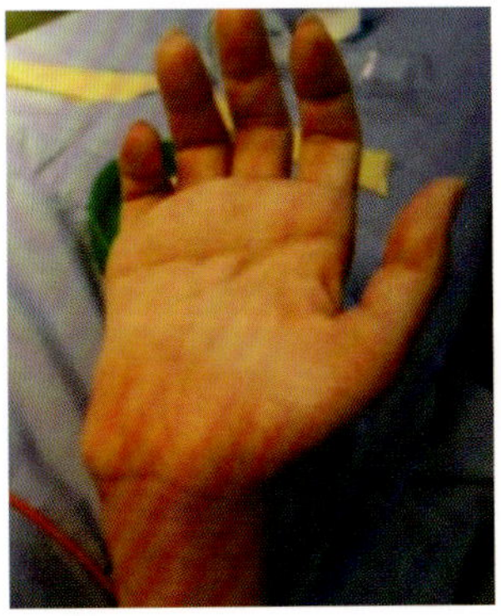

Ulnar Nerve **"Ulnar Claw"**	Fracture/trauma of **medial** epicondyle/ olecranon of humerus (funny bone). Fracture of hamate. **Bikers** putting pressure on the palms of the hand.	Ulnar C8 – T1 Arises from the medial cord.	Adducts the thumb. Innervates the Adductor pollicis. Sensation loss over 4th and 5th fingers and hypothenar eminence. Innervates interossei. Loss of **flexion** of wrist and intrinsic hand. Damage: No abduction or adduction of interossei (fingers). Loss of radial deviation of the hand. Adducts the thumb. Sensation loss and pain in the 4th and 5th fingers and wasting of the hypothenar eminence. Innervates interossei.	(**tip**: **U** are funny! (funny bone and U for **U**lnar).	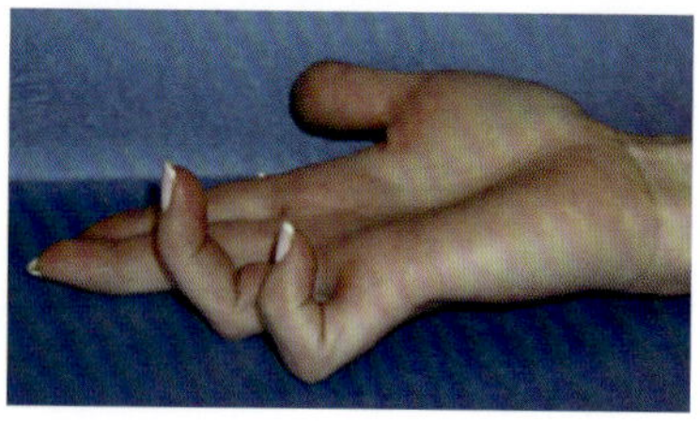 Ulnar nerve passes through the Flexor Carpi Ulnaris.
Recurrent branch Median nerve "Ape hand"	Superficial laceration of palm	Median C5 – T1	Damage: "Ape Hand". Loss of thenar muscle group: opposition, abduction and flexion of thumb. No sensation loss.		
Biceps Rupture "Popeye Sign"	Injury due to heavy lifting. MC: middle age men.		Proximal (at shoulder joint) biceps tendon rupture MC in men > 60. Distal (at elbow joint) biceps tendon rupture MC in middle aged men due to heavy lifting or sports.		**SX: Patient hears or feels a snap in the top of the shoulder followed by sharp pain which normally quickly subsides.** **DX: MRI** 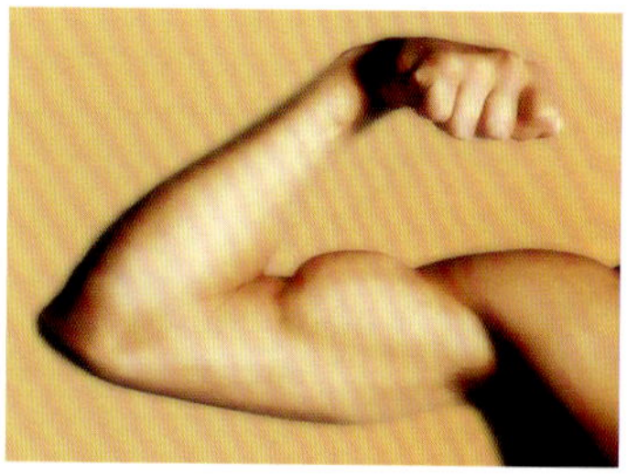

Tennis Elbow	Lateral epicondylitis Overuse of extensors of forearm.		Extensor carpi radialis brevis		(**tip: L** = **L**ove score in tennis) SX: Chronic, nagging pain on lateral epicondyle. 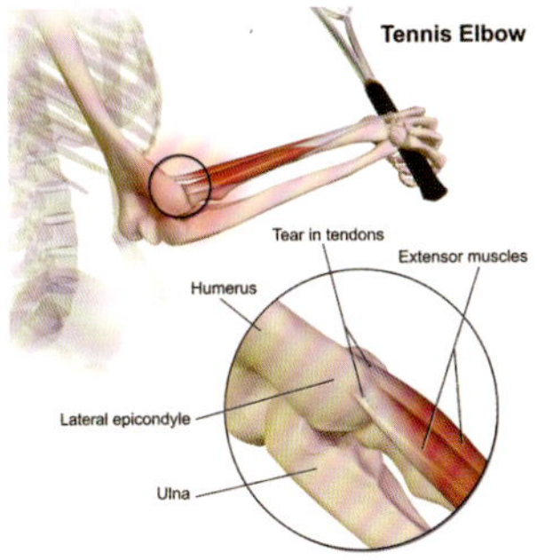
Golfers Elbow	Medial epicondylitis Overuse of Flexors of forearm.		Flexes: Flexor carpi radialis, Flexor carpi ulnaris, Flexor digitorum, Palmaris longus Flexing and pronating wrist.		(tip: I am only a Mediocre golfer) 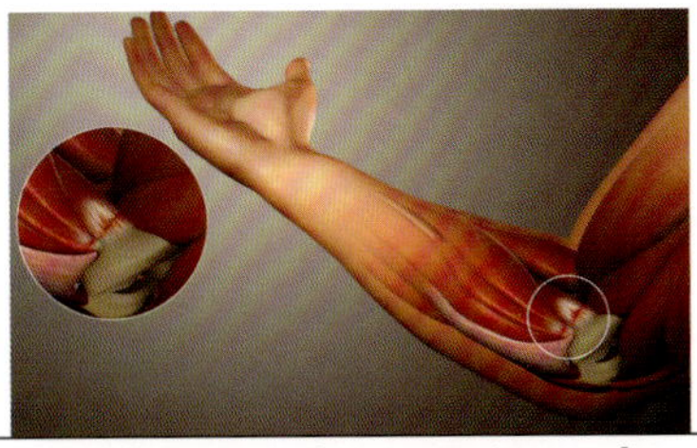
Subacromial Bursitis	Repetitive overhead motions. MC: Tennis		Pain with rotation of shoulder. Worsens when flexing shoulder. There is NO deltoid atrophy.		Bursa between the acromion and supraspinatus.
Olecranon Bursitis "Students elbow"	Injury to the elbow, repeated minor injuries, repeated leaning on the point of the elbow on a hard surface.		Inflammation of the elbow's bursa at the proximal end of the ulna.		SX: Pain, redness and swelling around the olecranon. TX: NSAIDs, RICE. Aspiration of excess bursa fluid. 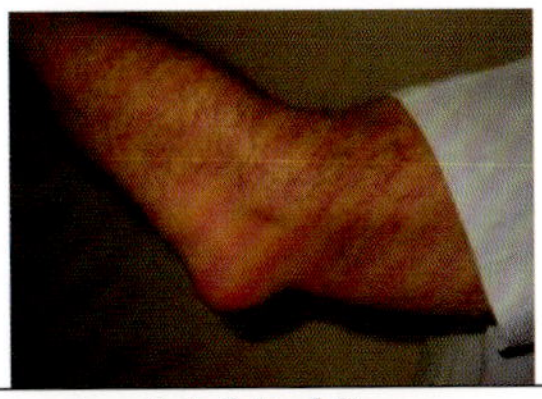
Cubital Fossa	Area on arm where blood is usually drawn.		**Boarders:** Superior: line from medial to lateral epicondyle of humerus. Medial (Ulnar N.): Pronator Teres. Lateral (Radial N.): Brachioradialis muscle. 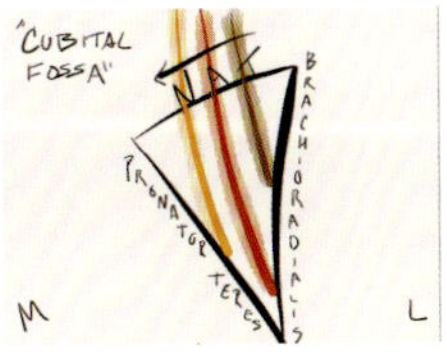		**Contents of Cubital Fossa:** Radial nerve Biceps brachii tendon Brachial artery Median nerve (tip: TAN: T=tendon of Brachioradialis, A=Artery (Brachial) N=Nerve: Median 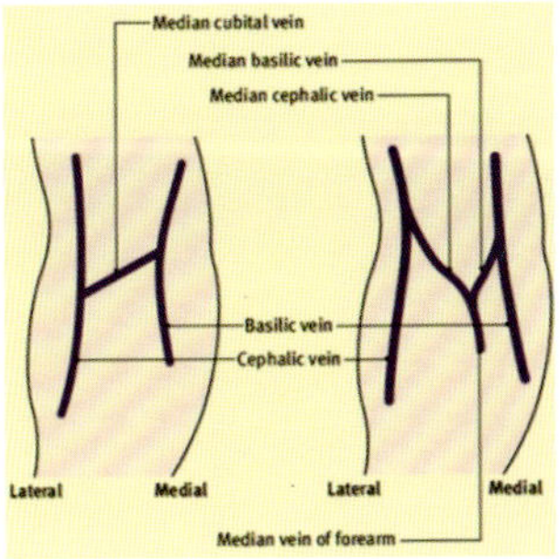

Flexion of the Elbow					3 main muscles that flex the elbow: biceps, brachioradialis, brachialis
Lower Trunk of Brachial Plexus					Formed in the neck and moves independently. It is NOT in the axillary sheath.
Ulna and Radius					Held together by the membranes: Interosseous (big) and Annular (small)

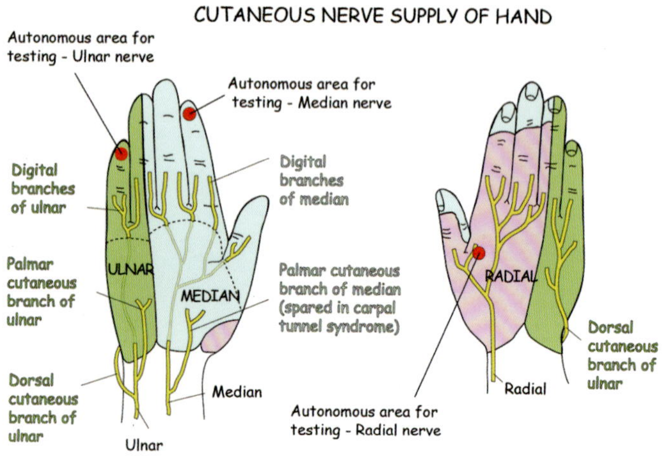

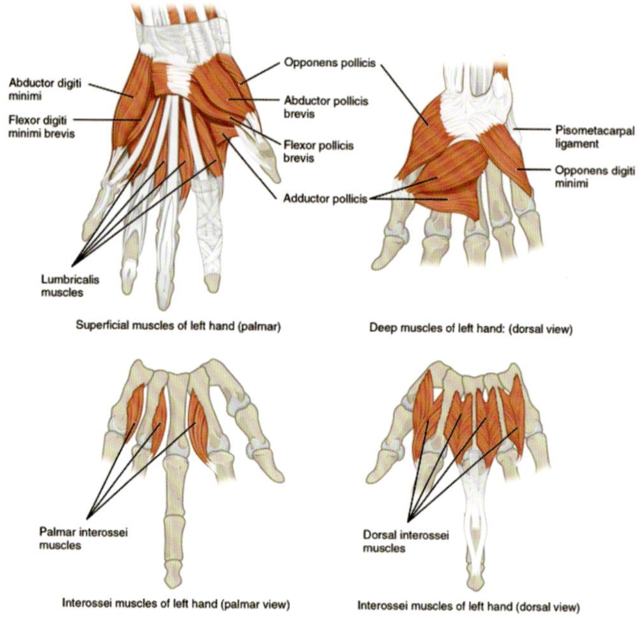

Hand Muscles

Thenar Muscles (Median nerve) (tip: "OAF") Opponens pollicis — **O** = oppose Abductor pollicis brevis — **A** = Abduct Flexor pollicis brevis — **F** = Flex	**Hypothenar Muscles (Ulnar nerve)** (tip: "OAF") Opponens digiti minimi — **O** = oppose Abductor digiti minimi — **A** = Abduct Flexor digiti minimi brevis — **F** = Flex
Interosseous Muscles Dorsal interosseous muscles = abduct fingers Palmar interosseous muscles = adduct fingers (**Tip**: **DAB** = **D**orsal = **AB**ducts) (**Tip**: **PAD** = **P**almar = **AD**ducts)	**Lumbrical muscles:** Flex at MCP joint. Extend at PIP and DIP joints.

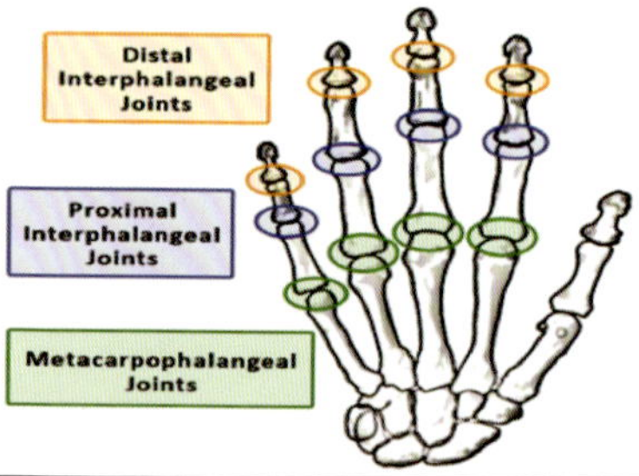

Wrist and Hand Pathologies

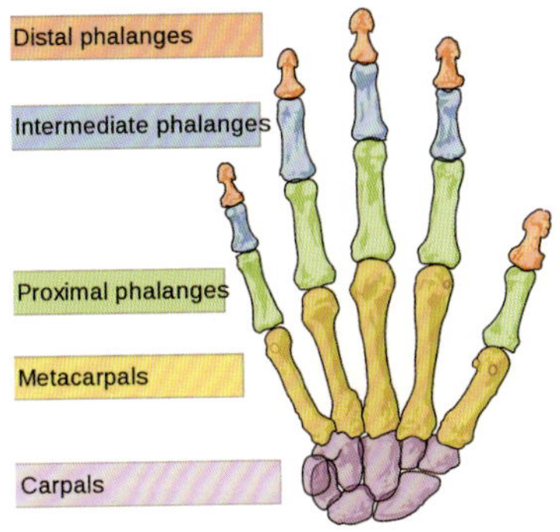

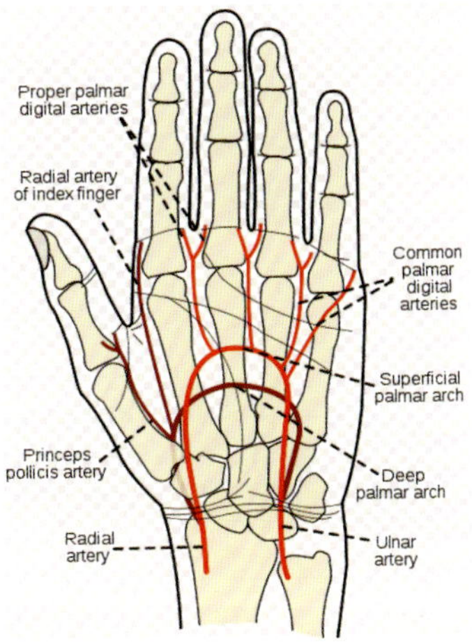

Wrist (Carpal) Bones

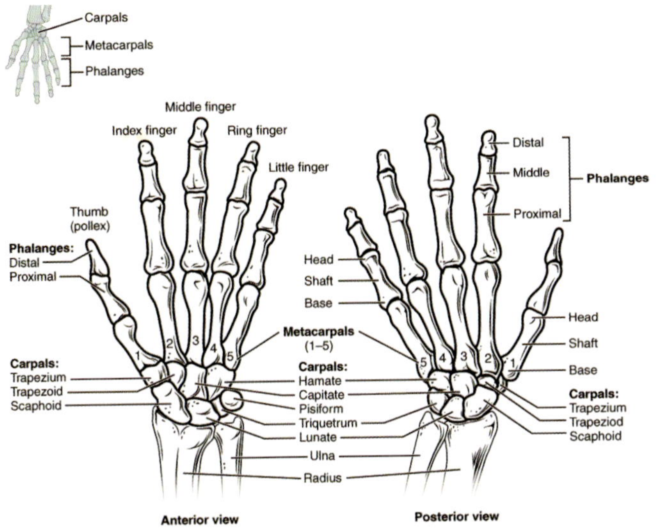

(**tip**: Some Lovers Tri Positions (pinky) That They Can't Handle

Carpal Tunnel

- **Median nerve** (Compression)

  Causes: repetitive movements, pregnancy (↑ fluid = ↑ pressure), hypothyroid (Matrix muco-polysaccharide protein deposit complex), Amyloid (Renal/dialysis), Acromegaly (hyperplasia), Rheumatoid Arthritis (tendons and synovial inflammation), Colles Fracture (compression), dislocation of the lunate
- Flexor digitorum
- **Pain is worse at night.**
- Carpal tunnel test (recreate symptoms)
  Phalen sign = hyper flex wrist.
  Tinel's sign = Tap on median nerve.
  Elevate hand above head.
- **TX: If any of the Carpal Tunnel test are positive = nerve conduction test**
- **TX: Splint wrist for night time only**
  If no improvement = steroid injections
  If no improvement = surgery (last resort)

Scaphoid Fracture

- "Snuff Box" has severe point tenderness. MC fractured carpal bone
- May not show break on first x-ray, must do MRI to insure there is no break
- Danger: **Avascular necrosis**

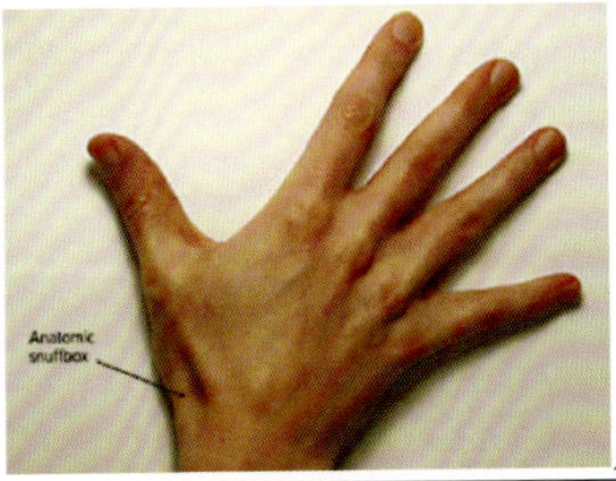

Anatomic snuffbox

Hamate Fracture

- Ulnar nerve injury
- Pain and swelling of hypothenar

	Lunate Fracture • Acute carpal tunnel
	Guyon Canal Syndrome • Ulnar nerve compression at the wrist/hand • MC in cyclist due to pressure exerted on handlebars
De Quervain's Tenosynovitis • MC: Injury to mom's thumb from picking up baby • Inflammation to Polus longus brevis, Abductor pollicis • SX: Tenderness on the radial side when the tendon is stretched	**Boxers Fracture** • 1st and 2nd metacarpal if an experienced fighter. • 5th metacarpal if an inexperienced fighter.
Colles' Fracture • MC: Elderly due to fall on outstretched hand Distal radius	**Amputation of finger/extremity** **Sterile gauge, sterile saline, sterile plastic bag, ice and saline mixed (or sterile water), transport. Do not put bag on just ice, it must be in a saline/water and ice mix.**
Dupuytren Contracture • Hyperplasia (thickening) of the palmar fascia causing contracture of the 4th and 5th fingers. (Unable to extend the fingers). • TX: Joint injections (**Lidocaine, Collagenase, Triamcinolone**), or surgical release.	

Rotator Cuff

- Innervated by C5 and C6
- **Rotator cuff tear:** Due to trauma. Weakness in the shoulder. Lidocaine injections do not improve it. Requires surgery.
- If lateral pain when abducting and externally rotating shoulder = **rotator cuff tendonitis**
  TX: **Lidocaine** injection
- **Rotator cuff tendonitis**: pain when reaching our or lifting arm. Due to repetitive activity, which causes nerve impingement.
- Rotator Cuff injury: Severe tenderness at the insertion of the supraspinatus
- If anterior pain = joint osteoarthritis or biscep tendonitis
- If posterior pain = nerve impingement or cervical disc herniation
- MAT: MRI
- TX: NSAID's, rest, physical therapy, steroid injections for pain. Surgery with complete tears or not responding to therapy

SITS Muscle	Action	Notes
Supraspinatus	**Abducts** (raises) arm first 15° then the deltoid takes over and raises are the rest of the way up.	**Suprascapular nerve.** MC rotator cuff injury
Infraspinatus	**Laterally** rotates arm	**Suprascapular nerve.** Pitching injury
Teres Minor	**ADDucts and laterally** rotates arm (**tip**: "T"eres for "T"wo actions of the arm)	**Axillary nerve**
Subscapularis	**Medially** rotates and ADDucts arm	**Subscapular nerve**

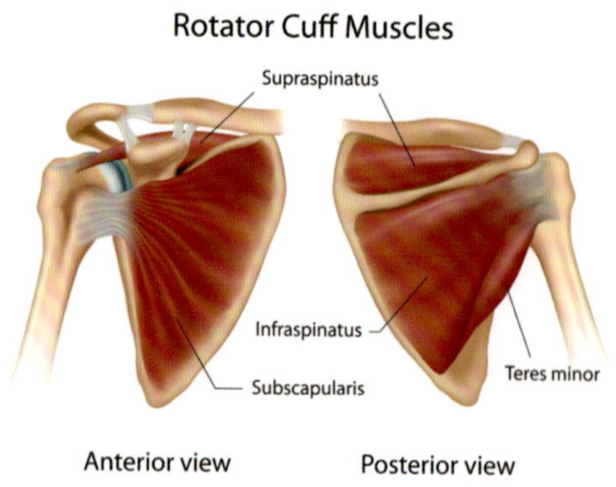

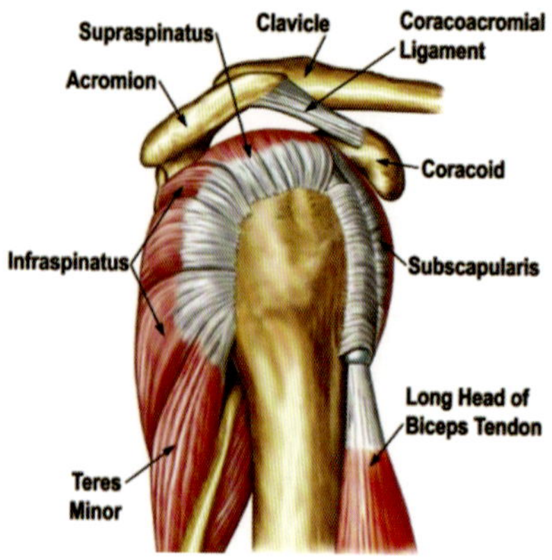

Lower Extremities: Thigh, Leg, Foot Anatomy and Pathologies

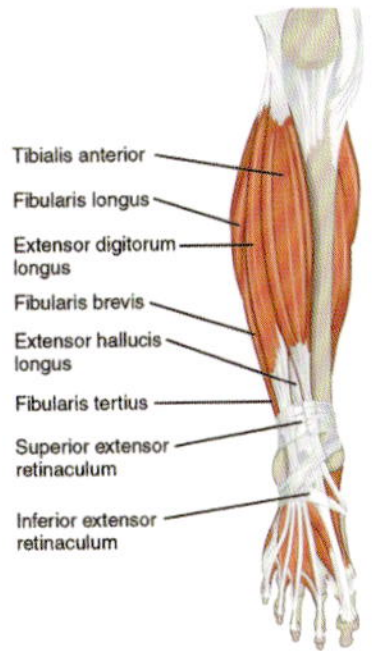

Superficial muscles of the right lower leg (anterior view)

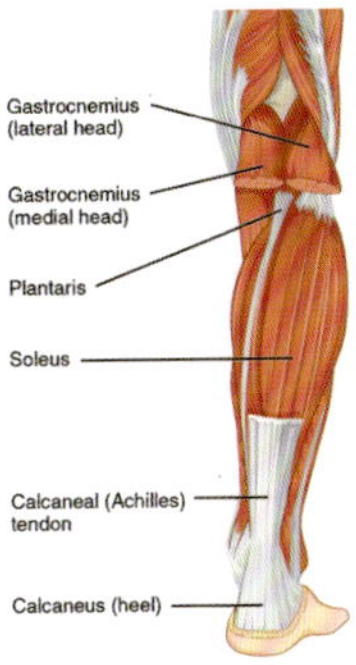

Superficial muscles of the right lower leg (posterior view)

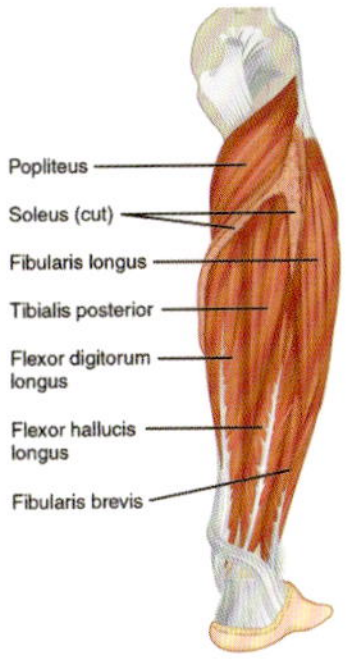

Deep muscles of the right lower leg (posterior view)

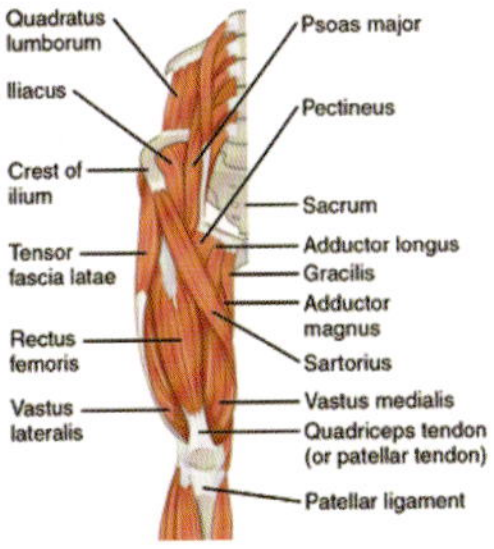

Superficial pelvic and thigh muscles of right leg (anterior view)

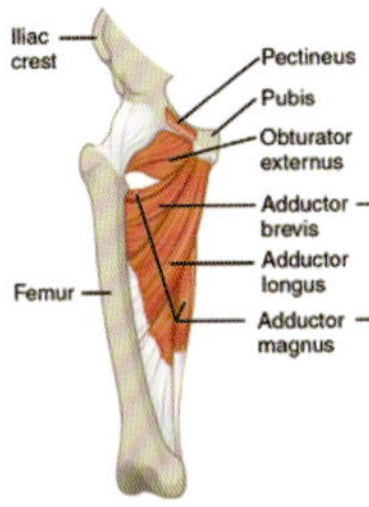

Deep pelvic and thigh muscles of right leg (anterior view)

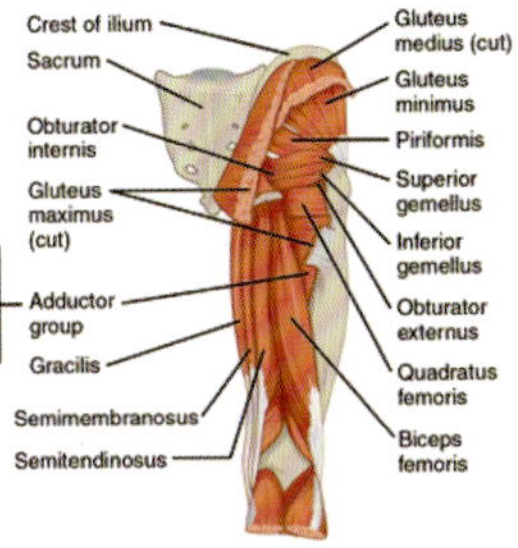

Pelvic and thigh muscles of right leg (posterior view)

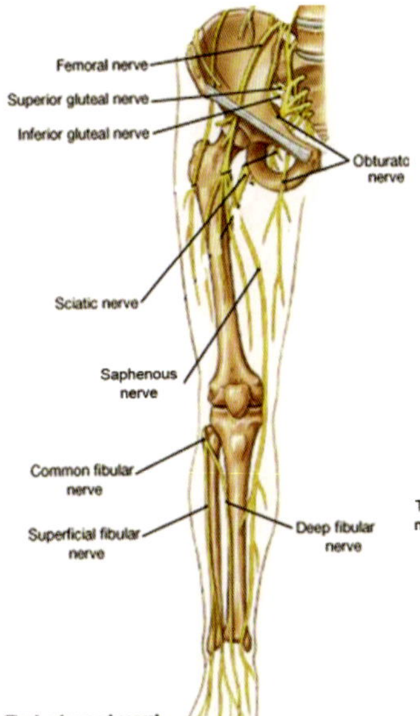

The lumbar and sacral plexuses, anterior view

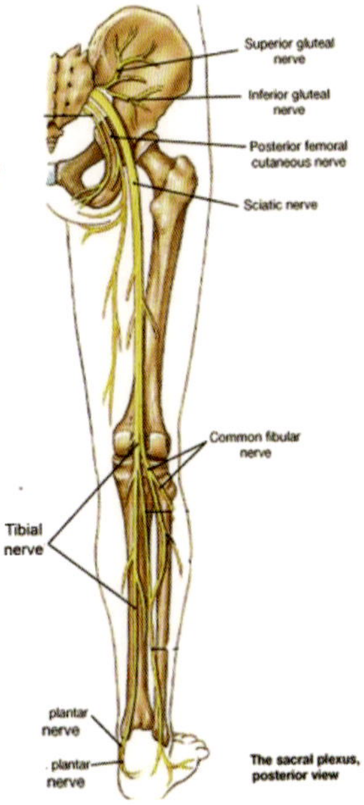

The sacral plexus, posterior view

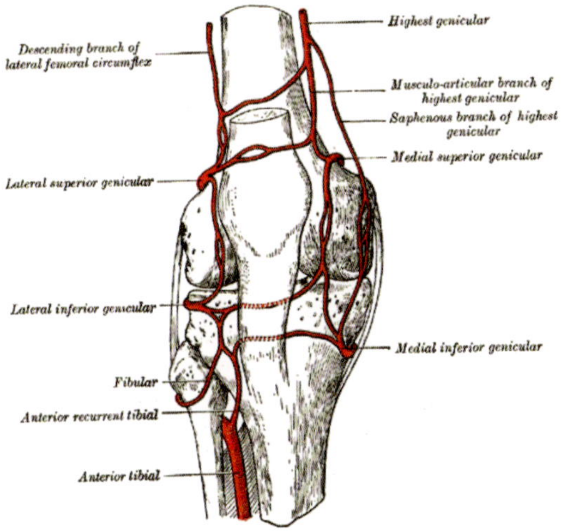

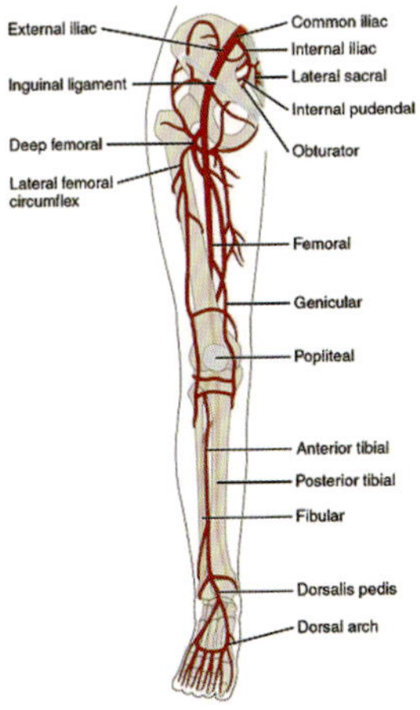

Anterior view

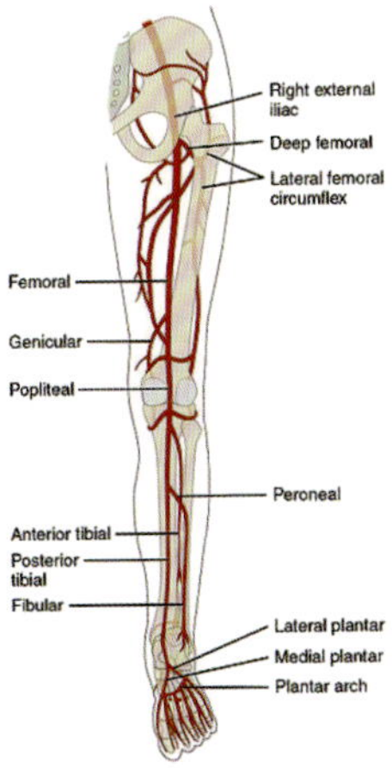

Posterior view

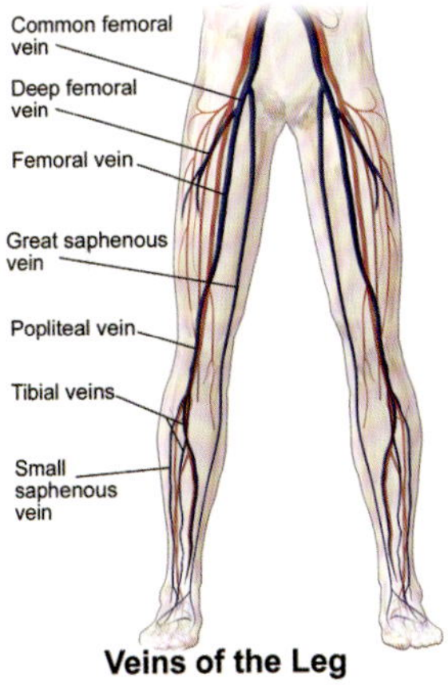

Veins of the Leg

Nerve, Muscle, Vessel	Cause	Nerve	Muscle - Action	Notes	Appearance
Obturator Nerve	Crush injury to pelvis or injury from pelvic surgery	L2-L4	Innervates the **medial compartment** of the thigh (adductors and gracilis). **Damage: No adduction** of thigh. Sensation loss on **medial thigh**		(**tip**: an operator **ADDS** on her calculator)
Lateral Cutaneous Femoral Nerve	Tight jeans or tight belt, obesity, pregnancy, sitting with legs crossed, riding a bike.		Sensation loss or pain on **lateral thigh**		
Femoral Nerve	Crush/fracture of pelvis	L2-L4	Responsible for **knee** extension. Innervates the **anterior compartment** of the thigh. Damage: No thigh flexion (**Knee flexion = knee** will buckle). Sensory loss to a**nterior** thigh.		Note: If KNEE is mentioned, think femoral nerve.
Common Peroneal Nerve	Fibular neck fracture (lateral leg)	L4-S2	Damage: **Foot drop**. No eversion of foot. No dorsiflex of foot. Sensation loss on dorsum (top) of foot. "Steppage gate" (high step gate)		(**Tip**: **PED** = **P=Peroneal** **E=Eversion** **D=Dorsiflex, dorsum**
Tibial Nerve	Knee trauma. Baker's cyst (proximal). **Tarsal Tunnel** syndrome (distal)	L4-S2	Damage: No inversion of foot. No plantarflex of foot. Sensation loss or pain on **sole** (bottom) of foot. Can't curl toes. "Antalgic gait" (Can't put weight on affected foot). Worsens when walking.		(**Tip**: **TIP =** **T=Tibial** **I=Inversion** **P=Plantarflex)**
Superior Gluteal Nerve	**Polio**, Posterior hip dislocation (auto accident, hit from behind)	L4-S1	**Responsible for hip abduction.** **Innervates: Gluteus medius and minimus muscles.** **Damage: "Trendelenburg gait"** No hip abduction-causing pelvis to tilt.		(**tip**: the little gluteus muscles: Gluteus medius and minimus go with the BIG SUPERIOR nerve) (**tip**: "T" in Trendelenburg goes with "T" for two muscles (Gluteus medius and Gluteus minimus). 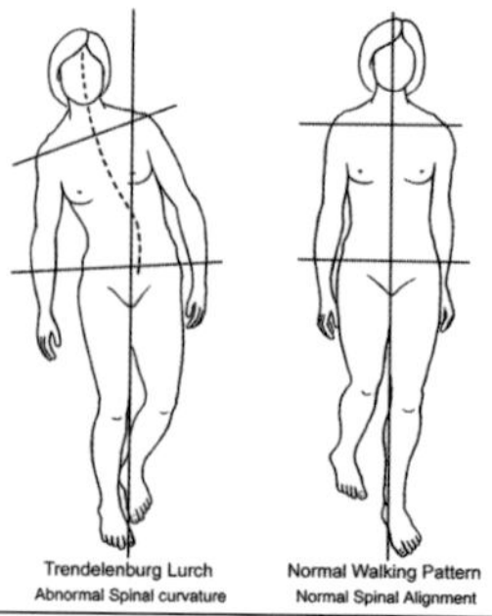

Inferior Gluteal Nerve	Posterior hip dislocation (auto accident, hit from behind)	L5-S2	**Innervates the Gluteus maximus muscle.** Damage: Difficulty climbing stairs, rising from seated position.		(**tip**: the little nerve goes with the BIG muscle)
Saphenous Nerve			Damage: anesthesia of the medial surface of the leg.		
Greater Trochanter					3 muscles that insert into the greater trochanter: gluteus minimus, gluteus medius, piriformis

Pudendal Nerve					Exits pelvis through the Greater Sciatic Foramen just below the piriformis muscle. Anesthesia given at the **ischial spine** blocks the **pudendal nerve** to block pain during delivery. The **Inferior rectal nerve** is a direct branch off of the **Pudendal**.
Psoas Major			**Flexes thigh at the hip**		
Greater Saphenous Vein			Unbranched, runs medially, upward to meet with the femoral vein through the fossa ovalis		
Ankle Sprain	Coming down on foot – inverting ankle, injuring the lateral side of ankle.		Lateral ligament: **Anterior Talo Fibular Ligament.**		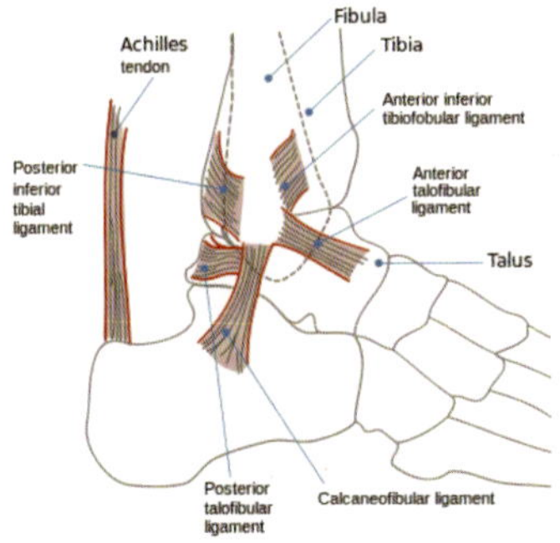
Medial Malleolus					Structures behind the Medial malleolus (from anterior to posterior): Anterior **T**ibialis posterior, flexor **D**igitorum longus, posterior tibial, flexor **H**alluces longus (**tip**: TOM, DICK and HARRY)
Sciatica (Sciatic nerve pain)	Causes: improper hip injection, trauma, lumbar degenerative disc DZ, spinal stenosis, osteophytes, arthritis in the spine.	L3 – S1	Pain, numbness and/or weakness that **extends to the foot**. (it does not stop at the knee. The knee would be due to a femoral nerve problem). Innervates the **posterior compartment** of the thigh.		SX: Patient can have a ↓ knee-jerk or ankle-jerk reflex. May also have foot drop. Sciatic nerve exits the pelvis through the Greater Sciatic Foramen. Be **SURE** the description says the pain **goes to the FOOT (S1 and S2) for sciatica**. If pain only goes to the **KNEE = femoral nerve**.

Osgood Schlatter Disease	MC in adolescent boys and girls ages 9 – 16. MC: males. Coincides with **growth spirts**. Due to repetitive jumping and kneeling.		Episodic knee pain when ascending/ descending stairs, squatting. Occurs at the junction of patellar ligament and tibial tuberosity. Edema and tenderness over the **tibial tubercle** (couple of inches down from kneecap).		DX: Pain reproduced by **extending knee against resistance.** Tenderness at tibial tubercle. Anterior tissue swelling. MC: Traction apophysitis of tibial tubercle. TX: Stretch exercise, **NSAID's**
Patellofemoral Pain Syndrome "Runners knee"	Peripatellar pain in the **patellar ligament** due to contact between the back of the patella and the femur. MC due to sports involving running.		**Anterior** knee pain 2° to trauma or meniscal tear. Pain in front of knee or under patella. **Pain with squatting** and becomes worse after starting to walk after **prolonged sitting** or **climbing stairs.** Pain is worse with activity or prolonged sitting (due to sustained flexion).		DX: Pain on **compressing patella**, crepitus, joint locking, instability. Normal X-rays. Pain **when flexing knee.** Subacute-chronic pain. **Crepitus** with movement of patella. TX: Exercise to strengthen thigh muscles (cycling), physical therapy. Knee braces do not help, no surgery.
Patellar Tendonitis "Jumpers Knee"	**Overuse injury** due to repetitive use of extensor mechanism of the knee causing micro tears. MCC: **Frequent jumping**. MC: athletes (basketball, volleyball, track)		Episodic, anterior, aching knee pain.		DX: Pain at the **inferior patellar**. TX: **RICE (rest, ice, compression, elevation)**
Patellar Tendon Tear/Rupture	Tendon connecting patella to the tibia ruptures.		Anterior knee. Severe pain, unable to bear weight, unable to extend leg, unable to maintain extended knee. Loss of ability to raise the straight leg. Patella sits higher.		DX: Movement of patella further up the quadriceps. Patella moves toward the hip when quads contract. TX: Surgery
Bakers Cyst "Popliteal cyst"	Arises from any arthritis in the knee, meniscus tear, lyme dz.		Posterior herniation of the synovium of the knee. Swelling (bulging into the popliteal space) of **synovial bursa behind the knee.**		TX: Rest and leg elevation. NSAID's for pain. Cyst can be aspirated and injected with corticosteroids. Fluid within the cyst can leak out into inner leg and can form a hematoma over medial malleolus: "crescent sign". MC seen: Osteoarthritis or Rheumatoid Arthritis. NOTE: Presents like a DVT – swollen calf. Must rule out DVT with a Doppler.

Prepatellar Bursa/ Bursitis "Housemaid's Knee"	**Kneeling on knees** (plumbers, roofers, gardeners, carpet layers)		Pain and swelling above the patella (kneecap). Inflammation of the prepatellar bursa.		Presents similar to a DVT. Pain, swelling, inability to flex the knee. Edema and **crepitus** over lower patella. Common in elderly, associated with osteoarthritis
Trochanter Bursitis	Overuse or trauma of the **hip**.		**Pain on lateral hip joint**. Pain when external pressure is applied. Painful to lie on one's side. Inflammation of the Gluteus Medius Bursa.		Located on lateral femur between gluteus medius and gluteus minimus.
Anserine Bursitis (AKA: Not serious)			Sharp pain on the anterior/medial tibia just below the knee.		DX: Valgus stress test does not reproduce pain so there is no damage to the MCL. X-rays are normal. No redness, warmth or swelling noted. TX: RICE
Club Foot **"Metatarsus Adductus"**	Congenital deformity. 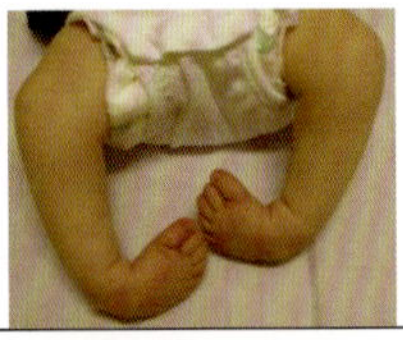		**Internal rotation** of the foot at the ankle. (Junction of the **Calcaneum and Talus**)		**TX:** **Type I: passively overcorrect rotation and reassure patient.** **Type II: correct rotation back to neutral with orthotics (corrective shoes).** **Type III: Rotation is rigid and will not correct requiring a plaster cast.**
Plantar Fasciitis (AKA: Heel spur)	Not clear. Associated with ↑ exercise, obesity, inward rolling of the foot, a lifestyle with ↓ exercise.		Point tenderness/burning pain in the heel and bottom of foot, worse with the first steps at the beginning of the day or after a period of sitting. Disorder at the insertion site of the ligament at the calcaneus.		NOTE: Similar to Tarsal Tunnel Syndrome, but plantar fasciitis **improves with use**. Tarsal Tunnel does not improve with use. TX: Steroid injection, stretching exercises for the foot and calf, arch supports, splinting. NSAID's for pain. Resolves spontaneously over time.
Tarsal Tunnel	Numbness, burning sensations in the foot radiating to the first 3 toes, base of the foot and heel.		Posterior Tibial Neuralgia. **Tibial nerve** is compressed in the tarsal tunnel.		Positive tinel's sign: tingling shock sensation that occurs when the affected nerve is tapped. Pain does **not improve with use** (as it does improve with plantar fasciitis). TX: Avoiding high heels, boots. Steroid injections.
Morton Neuroma AKA: Foot neuroma	Painful, burning, tenderness sensation between the 3rd and 4th metatarsals when weight-bearing pressure is applied. MC: High heels.		Benign neuroma of an intermetatarsal plantar nerve which entraps the affected nerves between the 2, 3 or 4th metatarsals.		TX: Orthotics, corticosteroid injections, sclerosing alcohol injections, Radio frequency ablation.
Stress Fracture AKA: Shin splints	Sharp pain over bony surfaces. MC: shins. Can also occur in arms.		Sudden ↑ in repeat tension without adequate rest.		MC: Runners that suddenly ↑ the intensity of their running (usually training for a race). All x-rays are negative.

Tenosynovitis	Introduction of bacteria into a sheath due to a puncture wound (thorn or needle)		Inflammation of the synovium (fluid-filled sheath) that surrounds the tendon.		Can be associated with infectious arthritis caused by N. gonorrhea. TX: NSAIDs (Naproxen, IBP), cortisone injections.
Pulse: Dorsalis Pedis Artery					Best place to palpate: On the dorsum of the foot, between the tendons of the extensor halluces longus and extensor digitorum longus.
Inguinal Nodes					Lymph from the **medial** side of foot drains into the saphenous vein into the inguinal nodes.
Popliteal Nodes					Lymph from the **lateral** side of the foot drains into the short saphenous vein into the popliteal nodes.

Greater Sciatic Foramen: Contents That Exit the Pelvis

The majority of the Greater Sciatic Foramen space is occupied by the Piriformis muscle.

Location	Vessels	Nerves
Above the Piriformis	Superior Gluteal Vessels	Superior Gluteal Nerve
Below the Piriformis	Inferior Gluteal Vessels. Internal Pudendal Vessels.	Inferior Gluteal Nerve, Pudendal Nerve, Sciatic Nerve, Posterior Femoral Cutaneous Never, Obturator Internus, Quadratus Femoris.

Abnormal Gaits

Gait	Cause	Description
Antalgic Gait	Injury to the tibial nerve.	Limp used so as to avoid pain by not putting any weight on injured side. Unable to bear weight on affect foot/leg. Favors injured side.
Scissors Gait (Spastic)	Cerebral palsy, brain trauma/DZ, Multiple sclerosis, spinal cord tumor, stroke, spastic paraparesis	Legs flexed at hips and knees (like crouching) with the knees and things crossing in a scissor-like movement.
Steppage Gait	**Polio**, herniated lumbar disk, Guillain-Barre, peroneal neuropathy, injuries to the common peroneal nerve, distal motor neuron	"**Foot drop**". The foot hangs with the toes pointing down causing the toes to scrape the ground when walking. It causes the patient to lift the leg higher than normal when walking.
Waddling Gait	Congenital hip dysplasia, myopathies, muscular dystrophy	"Duck-like" walk
Propulsive Gait	CO poisoning, drugs	Stiff posture, stooped with the head and neck bent forward.
Ataxic **Broad Based Gait** "Drunken sailor"	Cerebellar ataxia, alcohol intoxication, cerebellum injury, stroke, drugs, Friedrich's ataxia	Unsteady, uncoordinated walk with a wide base and the feet thrown out, coming down first on the heel and then on the toes with a double step.
Festinating gait, AKA: Shuffling gait, AKA: Parkinsonian gait	**Parkinson's Dz**	Involuntary move with short shuffling steps (AKA: hypokinesia), accelerating steps on tip toes with the trunk flexed forward and the legs flexed stiffly at the hips and knees. It is difficult for patient to get started moving and once he does it is difficult to get stopped so falls/injuries are common.
"Trendelenburg gait"	**Injury to the superior gluteal nerve or gluteus minimus and gluteus medius muscles.**	**No hip abduction-causing pelvis to tilt.** **MCC: Polio,** posterior hip dislocation (auto accident)
Senile Gait	Elderly	"Walking on ice", "expecting to fall", over precautious

Knee Injuries
"Unhappy Triad" = ACL, MCL, Medial Meniscus

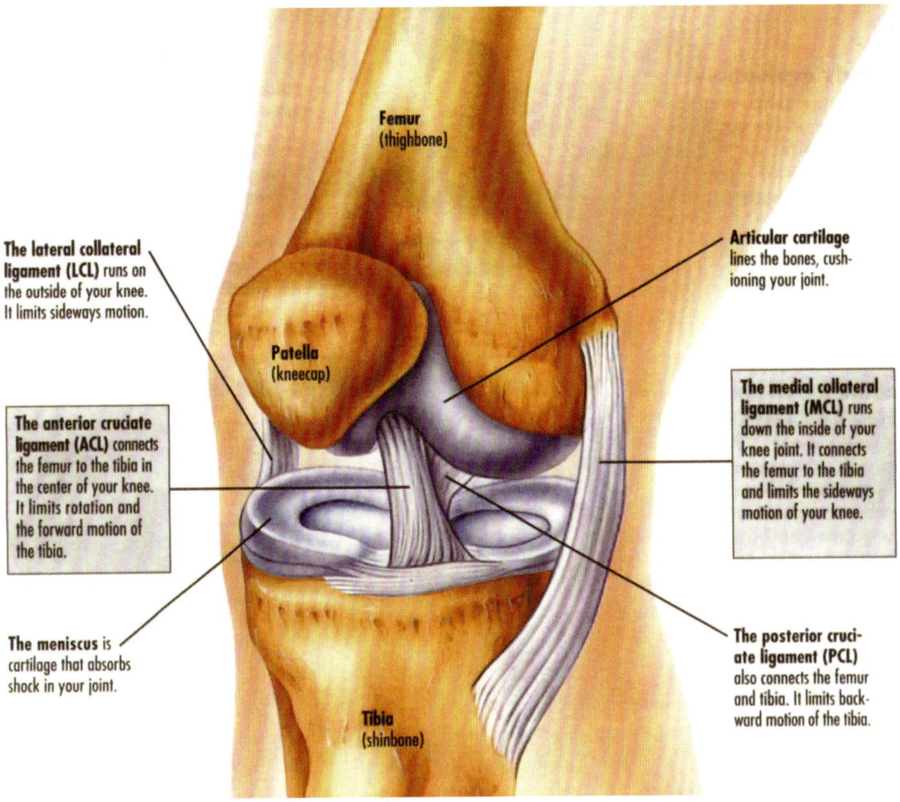

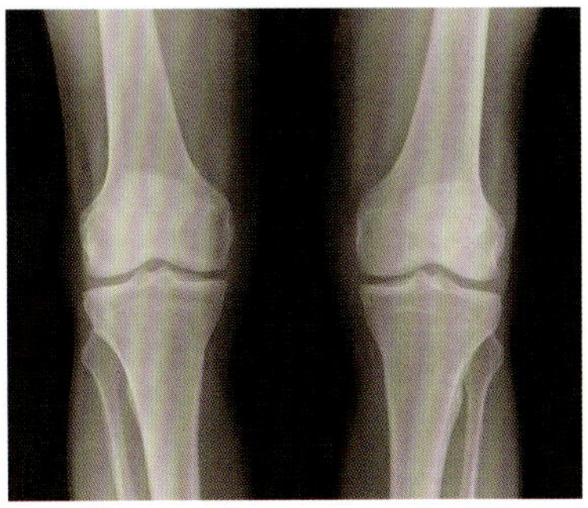

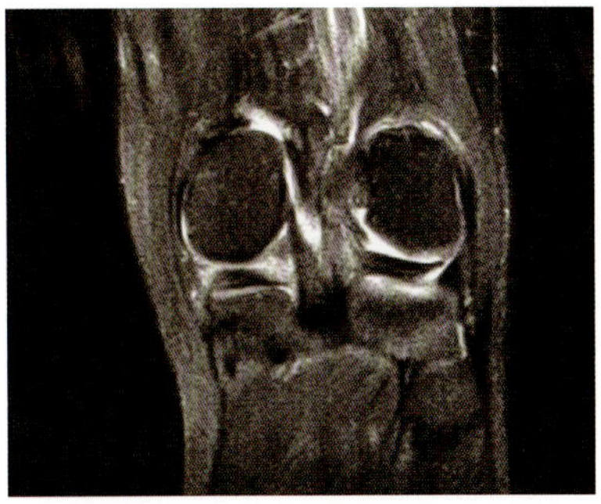

Injury	Cause of Injury	Test	Symptoms and treatments
ACL (Anterior collateral ligament)	Hit/force to the knee during aggressive sports.	DX: **Anterior Drawer** test. (AKA: **Lachman test**) (Anterior site of tibial attachment) (Posterior drawer test = Posterior collateral ligament injury. Posterior site of tibial attachment)	SX: **Rapid, immediate onset**. "Pop", **unable to bear weight**. **Blood in the joint (hemarthrosis).** TX: RICE (rest, ice, compression, elevation), Surgery
MCL (Medial collateral ligament)	**Lateral hit** to the knee causing medial tenderness. MC: skiing or contact sports.	DX: **Valgus Stress Test.** (↑ pain if lateral side of knee is pushed medially while affected let is extended or knee is bent.) Abnormal passive **abduction = MCL**. (**Varus Stress** Test Abnormal passive **adduction = LCL** (Lateral collateral ligament)	SX: ↑ pain if extended knee is rotated. Lower leg abducted when knee is stationary. No blood in the joint **(no hemarthrosis).**
Meniscus	**Twisting force** on the knee. Due to twisting when changing directions when walking/running, twisting on the knee when turning.	**McMurray Test** ↑ pain when knee is bent 90° and lower leg is **externally rotated = medial meniscus.** If lower leg is **internally rotated = lateral meniscus**).	SX: **Slow to develop. "Catching/popping" sensation.**

Additional Nerve Injuries and Anatomy

Nerve	Anatomy	Injury	Notes
Right recurrent laryngeal nerve	Branches off of the vagus nerve just inferior to the right **subclavian artery** (loops under the right subclavian artery). Runs posterior to the thyroid gland. It supplies all intrinsic muscles of the larynx (opens and closes the larynx), but does not supply the cricothyroid muscle. Nerves of the **6th pharyngeal arch.**	Can be injured during thyroid surgery.	Symptoms of injury: hoarseness (weakened or loss of voice).
Left recurrent laryngeal nerve	Branches off the vagus nerve just inferior to the aorta (looping under the **aortic arch**). It supplies all of the intrinsic muscles of the larynx (opens and closes the larynx) but does not supply the cricothyroid muscle. Nerves of the **6th pharyngeal arch.**	Can be injured during thyroid surgery.	Symptoms of injury: hoarseness (weakened or loss of voice).

Hip Injections
- Give intramuscular hip injections in the superior-lateral quadrant of the hip to prevent sciatic nerve injury

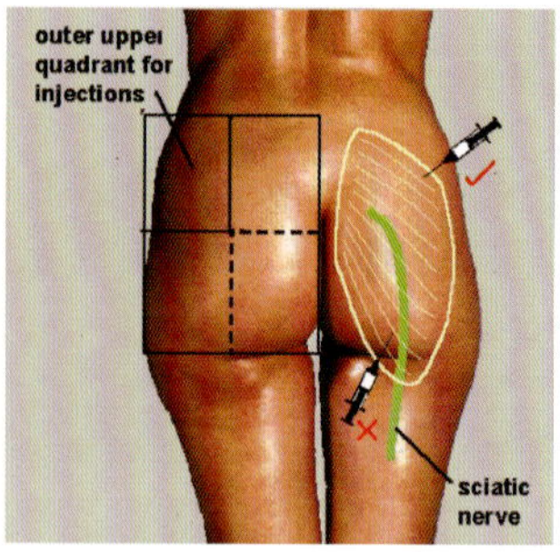

Compartment Syndrome
- SX: Severe pain when limb is moved in any direction – can't get comfortable, pallor (↓ blood flow), pulselessness, paresthesia, paralysis
- Causes: trauma, cast
- TX: **Emergency fasciotomy**

Cartilage, Tendons, Ligaments: Poor healing due to ↓ blood supply.

Neck, Chest, Abdomen Anatomy

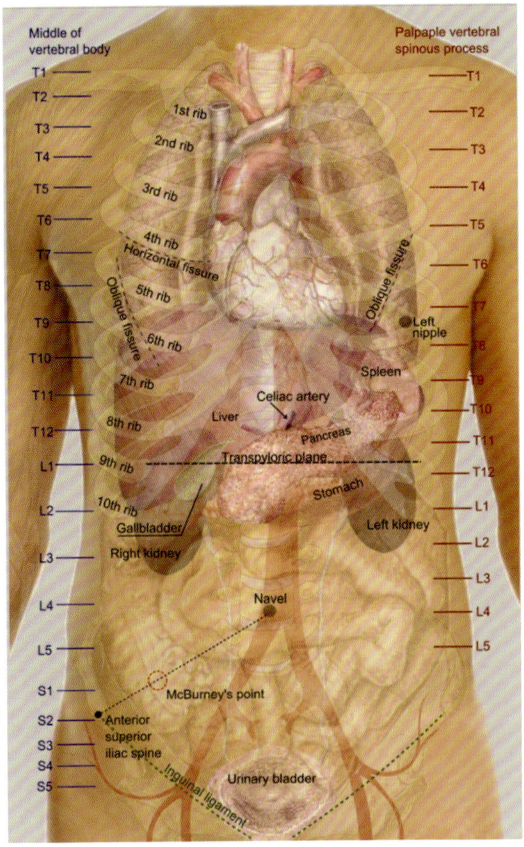

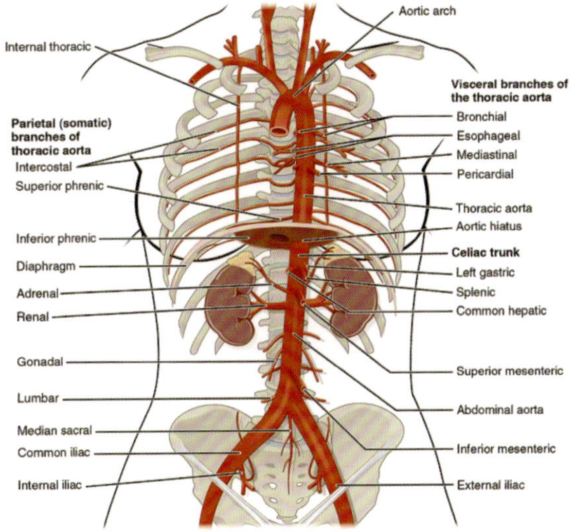

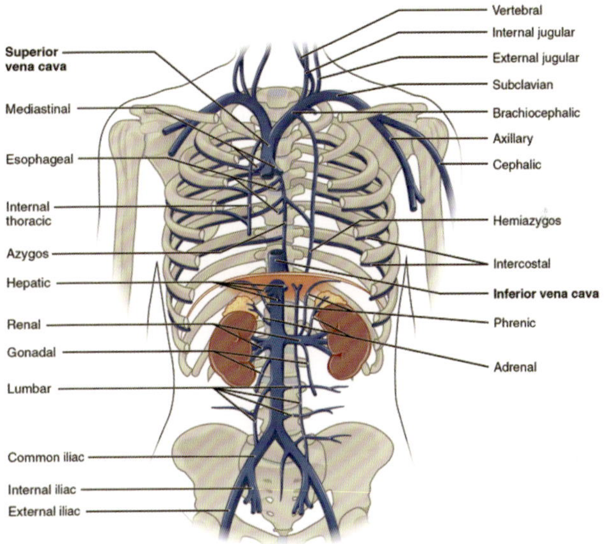

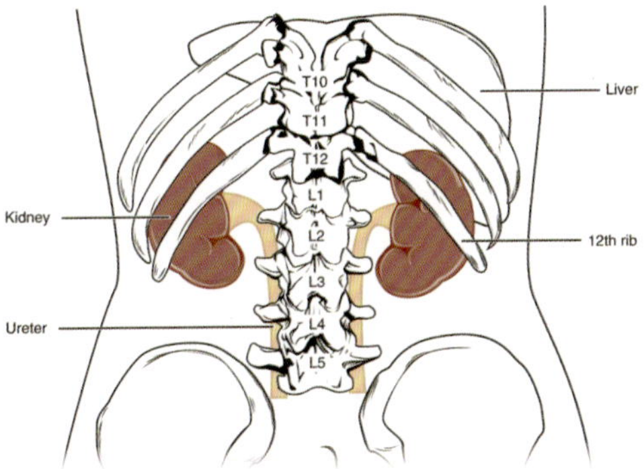

Retroperitoneal Organs

(**tip**: SAD PUCKER)

S = Suprarenal glands (adrenals)
A = Aorta/IVC
D = Duodenum (2nd, 3rd segments)
P = Pancreas (head, neck, body)
U = Ureters
C = Colon (ascending, descending/sigmoid)
K = Kidneys
E = Esophagus
R = Rectum

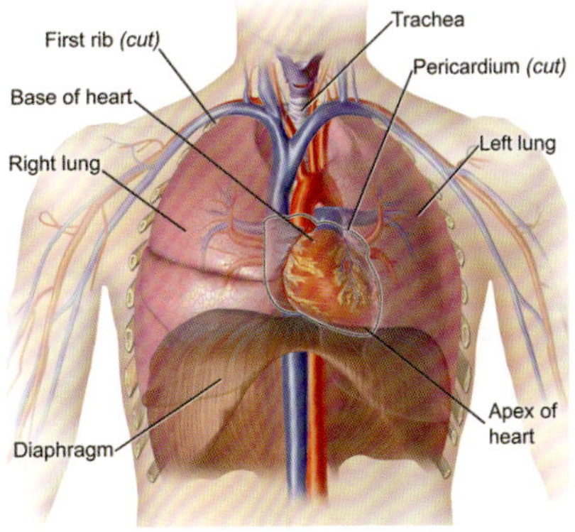

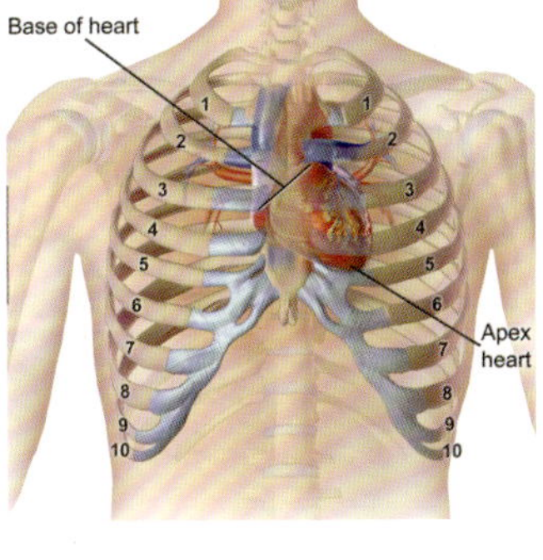

Location for Injuries: Heart, Lung, Neck, Chest

- Ribs 1 – 6 = damage to pleura
- Ribs 8 – 10 (right) = liver
- Ribs 9 – 11 (left) = spleen
- Ribs 11, 12 = floating
- Ribs 12 = Retroperitoneal = kidney injury
- **Stab wound** left **4th intercostal space** immediately lateral to sternal border: Injures right ventricle (Right ventricle extends from right sternal border to 2 inches to the left sternal border at 4th intercostal space, forms anterior sternocostal surface of heart and is medial to left midclavicular line).
- Left ventricle: Forms left boarder and diaphragmatic surface (inferior) of the heart. Also forms the anterior wall of the heart 2 – 3 inches from the left sternal border (midclavicular) from the 5th **intercostal space**.
- Right atrium: Forms right border of the heart. Its anterior surface is on the right sternal border between the 3rd – 6th rib.
- Left atrium is posterior to the left ventricle and forms the base of the heart.
- Apex of lung extends 3 – 4 cm above the first rib into the neck. Base of lung is in contact with the diaphragm. The mediastinal surface of the lungs has a cardiac impression to accommodate the heart.
- Neck: 3 zones.
  Zone 1: Base of neck (2cm above clavicles) (injury: arteriography, esophagogram, bronchoscopy, surgery)
  Zone 2: Midcervical: 2 cm above clavicle to angle of mandible (injury: surgical exploration)
  Zone 3: Angle of mandible to base of skull (injury: arteriography, embolization)

General Pain/Pathology Descriptions for Chest and Abdomen

LOCATION	DESCRIPTION
CHEST	
Pleurisy, pleuritic pain	Sharp pain on inspiration
Costochondritis	Stabbing, dull, aching pain reproduced with palpation
PE	Acute Shortness of breath, clear chest XR, low O_2 Sat
Pneumothorax	Decreased breath sounds
Angina	Pressing, squeezing, tight - radiating
Tamponade	Distant heart sounds
Pericarditis	Sharp, knifelike, feels better when leaning forward
Aortic Dissection	Severe, ripping, tearing pain b/t shoulder blades/back
Esophageal spasms	Severe pressure, squeezing
Reflux esophagitis	Burning, squeezing
ABDOMEN	
Gallbladder	URQ, Pain after eating (Radiates to the right shoulder due to phrenic nerve)
Appendix	LRQ, Pain migrates from umbilicus
Ectopic Pregnancy	LLQ/RLQ severe, sharp pain
Torsion: ovarian, testicular	LLQ/RLQ severe, sharp pain (male = no cremasteric reflex)
Diverticulitis	LLQ, pain (mimics an appendicitis)
Acute Pancreatitis	Severe pain radiating to back
Epigastric Pain	Pain: ulcers, PUD, MI
Ruptured Ulcer (other abdominal organ)	Diffuse, severe abdominal pain, air-fluid levels on x-ray
Intussusception	Colicky pain
PMS	Bloating, cramping
Obstruction	Distended abdomen, air-fluid levels on x-ray
UTI, Cystitis	Suprapubic pain
Pyelonephrosis, Hydronephrosis, Struvite Stone	Costovertebral pain, flank pain
Kidney Stones	Pain radiating to groin
Hypoactive bowel sounds	Blood vessel obstruction, opiates, anesthesia, bowel obstruction, trauma, hypokalemia, mechanical bowel obstruction, peritonitis
Hyperactive bowel sounds	Crohn's Dz, Ulcerative Colitis, diarrhea, infectious enteritis, GI hemorrhage, gastroenteritis, food hypersensitivity, early mechanical bowel obstruction
High-pitched tinkling sounds	Intestinal fluid and air under tension in a dilated bowel.
Bruits	Abdominal: kidneys: renal artery stenosis = HTN Abdominal: Hepatic: carcinoma of liver or alcohol hepatitis
Neuro/Nerve pain	Burning pain

Surgical Injuries

Surgery	Damage
Parotid surgery (cheeks, face)	Facial nerve VII damage, Facial droop/palsy
Mastectomy	**Wing Scapula**: Long thoracic nerve. Serratus anterior muscle.
Submandibular surgery (submandibular salivary gland)	Tongue palsy
Thyroid or Parathyroid surgery	Left recurrent laryngeal (off Vegas nerve) = hoarseness
Thyroid surgery	Loss of parathyroids (hypocalcemia)
Oophorectomy	Ligation of **ureter**

Thoracocentesis – Needle Placement for Pneumothorax or Pleural Effusion

- 7th at mid clavicular line
- 9th at mid axillary line
- 11 at post scapular

Pericardiocentesis – Needle Placement for Cardiac Tamponade

- Parasternal approach: 5th – 6th intercostal space at the left sternal border at the cardiac notch of the left lung.
- Subxiphoid approach: Infrasternal angle. (Lower opening of the thorax at the 12th thoracic vertebra – xiphoid process)

Layers of Chest Wall (Thoracocentesis, Pericardiocentesis)

Chest Wall: Skin ➔ fatty tissue ➔ Intercostal muscle ➔ external intercostal muscle ➔ Innermost intercostal muscle ➔Parietal pleura ➔ Interpleural space ➔ visceral pleura ➔ lung or pericardial sac

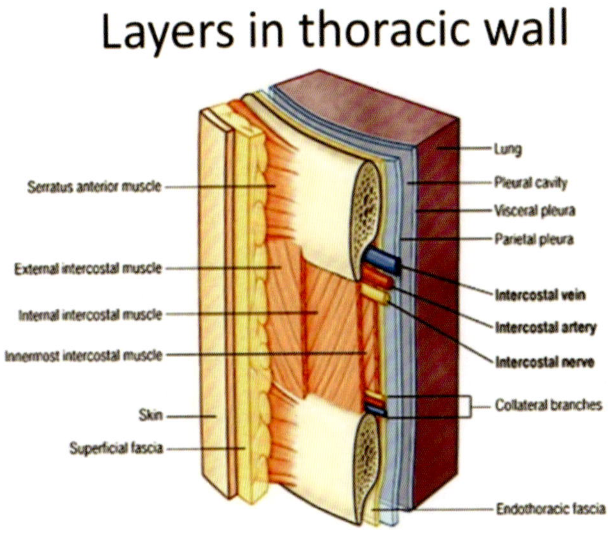

Inguinal Hernia or Abdominal Repair – Layers of abdomen

Abdomen layers: Skin ➔ Camper's Fascia (Superficial fascia) ➔ Scarpa's Fascia (Superficial fascia) ➔ Deep Fascia ➔ Muscular Layers (External oblique, Internal oblique, Transverse) ➔ Transversalis Fascia ➔ Extraperitoneal fat ➔ Parietal peritoneum.

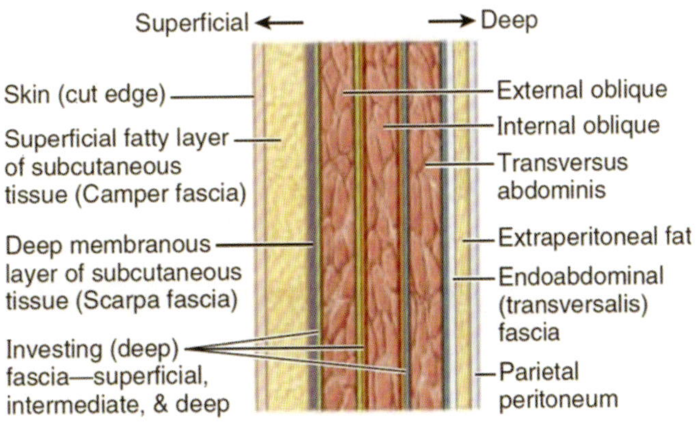

Epidural/Spinal, Lumbar Puncture – Layers

Back layers for Epidural: Skin ➔ Fascia ➔ Supraspinous ligament ➔ Infraspinous Ligament ➔ Ligamentum Flavum ➔ Epidural Space ➔ Dura ➔ Subarachnoid space (contains CSF)

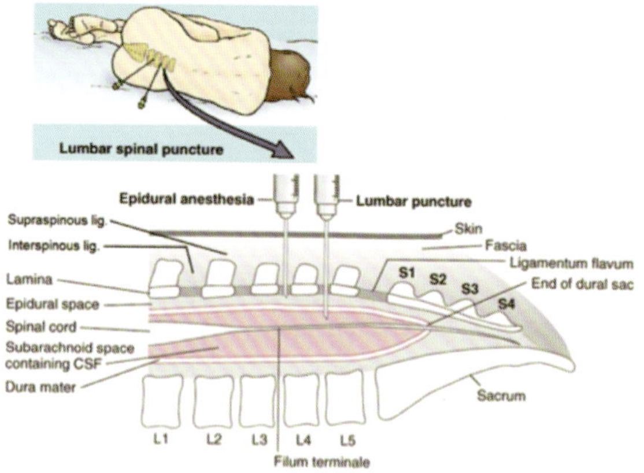

Skull Layers

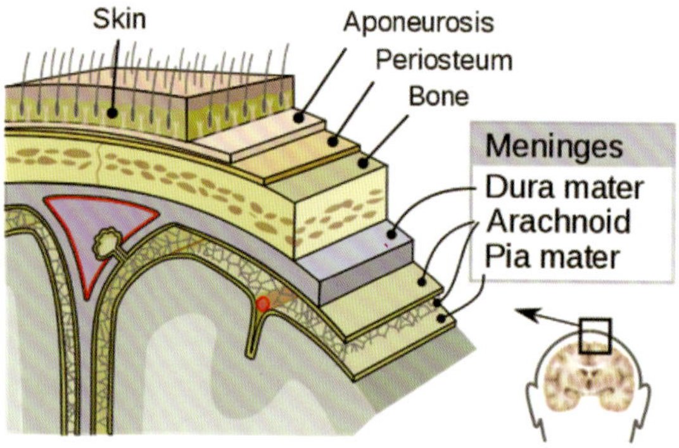

Anatomical Landmarks

Level	Anatomy	Level	Anatomy
C3	Hyoid bone, Bifurcation of Common Carotid Artery	**T9**	Xiphoid process
C4	Superior border of thyroid cartilage	**T10**	Esophagus and Left Gastric Vessels, Vegas Nerve crosses diaphragm
C6	Division of larynx & trachea, Cricoid cartilage	**T12**	Aorta, Thoracic Duct, Azygos vein, Hemi-Azygos vein crosses diaphragm
C6 – T1	Thyroid gland	**L1**	Rib margin (10 cm from midline)
C7	Spinous Process	**L1 – L2**	Renal arteries, Superior Mesenteric Artery, Hilum of kidneys: left kidney is above and right kidney is below, Celiac trunk originates just above
T1	Highest point of apex of lung	**L2**	Thoracic duct begins, Azygos and Hemiazygos begin
T2	Superior border of scapula, Jugular notch	**L3**	Umbilicus, Inferior Mesenteric Artery
T4	Nipples, Azygos vein enters SVC, Arch of aorta begins & ends.	**L4 – L5**	Tubercle of Iliac crest, Bifurcation of the Abdominal Aorta, Union of Common Iliac veins, Inferior Vena Cava formed from Common Iliac veins
T4 and T5	Bifurcation of trachea	**S2**	Posterior Superior Iliac Spine. Middle of sacroiliac joint
T5 – T9	Heart, Body of sternum	**S3**	Posterior Inferior iliac Spine, Pelvic colon ends and rectum begins (landmark in surgery of recto sigmoid carcinoma)
T7	Inferior border of scapula	**S4**	Natal cleft
T8	IVC, Phrenic nerve crosses diaphragm		

LYMPH DRAINAGE

Lymph Node	Drainage
External Iliac Nodes Along the external iliac vessels and drain into common iliac nodes	Leg, buttock, superior uterus **Cervix**: anterior and lateral cervix (drains with uterine arteries and cardinal ligaments at base of broad ligament) and **ultimately drains into the para aortic nodes**
Internal Iliac Nodes Along the internal iliac vessels	All pelvic structures, **upper** anal canal above pectinate line), **vagina, bladder, prostate.** **Cervix:** posterior and lateral cervix (drains with uterine arteries) and **ultimately drains into the para aortic nodes**
Deep Inguinal Lymph Nodes Between the leg and pelvis under cribriform fascia. Affected due to infections of STD's, leg and foot infections	**Penis,** scrotum, **vulva, vagina,** perineum, gluteal region, lower abdominal wall, **lower** anal canal (below the pectinate line)
Superficial Inguinal Nodes Beneath inguinal ligament and **drain into the deep inguinal** lymph nodes	Lower anal canal (below the pectinate line), **scrotum.** **Rectum, vagina, perineum.**
Para-aortic Nodes	**Uterus, ovaries, testes, cervix (from both internal and external iliac nodes)**, kidneys
Lumbar Nodes (AKA: lateral aortic nodes) Between the diaphragm and pelvis along the IVC and aorta. Common iliac drains into the Lumbar nodes and converge to become the **THORACIC DUCT**	Intestinal trunk
Popliteal Nodes Located at back of knees in popliteal fossa of posterior leg	Lower leg and foot
Celiac Nodes	Spleen, stomach, pancreas, upper duodenum, liver
Superior Mesenteric Nodes	Lower duodenum, jejunum, ileum, ascending colon, transverse colon to the splenic flexure
Inferior Mesenteric Nodes	Splenic flexure, sigmoid colon to the upper rectum. **Location of metastasis of cancer of the descending colon.**
Gastroepiploic Nodes	Greater curvature of the stomach
Subpyloric Nodes	Distal stomach, duodenum, pancreas
Axillary Nodes Underarm to the collar bone	**Breast**, upper chest wall, upper limbs
Hilar Nodes Lungs	**Lungs**
Supraclavicular Nodes In the cavity over the clavicle (Right and Left sides).	Lymph from the abdomen and thoracic cavity drain here. **RIGHT NODE:** Drains mediastinum lungs, esophagus. Enlargement: It is a location of metastasis of various malignancies: gastrointestinal, lung, retroperitoneal. Location of: **Virchow's node** (left supraclavicular node with lymph drainage, especially the stomach, passing through the thoracic duct. **LEFT NODE**: Drains thorax, abdomen via thoracic duct. Enlargement: Lymphoma, thoracic or retroperitoneal cancer, bacterial or fungal infection.
Mediastinal Nodes Along the trachea, esophagus, between lungs and diaphragm	Trachea, Esophagus. Location where lymph drains into the **subclavian vein**
Cervical Nodes Over and below the Sternocleidomastoid muscle	Posterior: Scalp and neck, thorax, cervical, auxiliary nodes, thyroid gland, posterior pharynx, tonsils, head, neck. Enlargement: TB, lymphoma, head and neck malignancy.
Sub-Mandibular (AKA: Tonsilar Nodes) Beneath the mandibular angle, base of jaw	Tongue, lips, mouth, molars, submaxillary gland. Enlargement: infections of head, neck sinus, ears, eyes, scalp, pharynx.
Sub-mental Nodes Beneath chin	Lower lip and tip of tongue, floor of mouth, teeth, skin of cheek, submental salivary gland. Enlargement: CMV, Mononucleosis, EBV, Toxoplasmosis, dental periodontitis.
Postauricular Nodes (Posterior) Behind ears	External auditory meatus, pinna, scalp. Enlargement: local infection, **mononucleosis**
Preauricular Nodes (Anterior) In front of ears	Eyelids, conjunctivae, temporal region, pinna. Enlargement: External auditory canal infection, **strep throat.**
Suboccipital Nodes: Between back of head and neck	Scalp and head. Enlargement: Local infection

(**tip:** You have a "**Para**" testes and ovaries, **S**crotum is **S**uperficial and the penis goes **Deep**)

Lymphatic System

- Originates as plasma (fluid portion of blood)
- 2 – 3 liters of lymph is filtered per day
- Lymph (AKA: extracellular fluid: fluid that flows between cells)
- Flows in a continuous loop in one upward direction in its own system, independent of blood
- Upward movement dependent on movement of muscles and joint pumps (lymph has no pump)
- Passes through lymph nodes (afferent vessels) that filter out pathogens, waste products, cancer cells so fluid can be returned to circulatory system
- Lymphocytes (WBC) inside of the lymph node destroy these pathogens
- Damaged or destroyed lymph nodes do not regenerate
- **Thoracic duct (AKA: alimentary duct),** largest lymphatic vessel. Begins at 2nd lumbar vertebra to the neck. **Drains systemic circulation at the left subclavian vein. It drains lymph from most of the body: legs, trunk, left chest (thorax), left arm, left head and neck.**
- **Right lymphatic duct drains the right arm, right chest (thorax), right head and neck. It combines with the right subclavian vein and right internal jugular vein.**
- **Filtered lymph flows into (efferent vessels) the subclavian veins**

Anastomosis

Portal Anastomosis

Portal Anastomosis

Esophageal Varices:
Left Gastric and Esophageal Veins
Increased venous portal pressure dilates left gastric veins. Pathway: left gastrics branch into the esophageal veins which go into the Azygos* veins then into the SVC.

Hemorrhoids:
Superior rectal vein and Middle/Inferior Rectal Veins

Caput:
Paraumbilical and Superior and Inferior Epigastric Veins

***Azygos Vein:** Formed by union of the ascending lumbar veins and right subcostal veins at the 12th thoracic vertebra. It "arches" over the right main bronchus to join the SVC. The "arch of the Azygos Vein" is an anatomic landmark. It drains the posterior intercostal veins on the right side of the body. It connect the systems of the SVC and IVC. **The Azygos Vein provides an alternative path for blood to the right atrium when either of the venae cavae is blocked.** The **hemiazygos vein** is the left-sided equivalent of the Azygos Vein. It drains the posterior intercostal veins on the left side of the body.

Portal Anastomosis

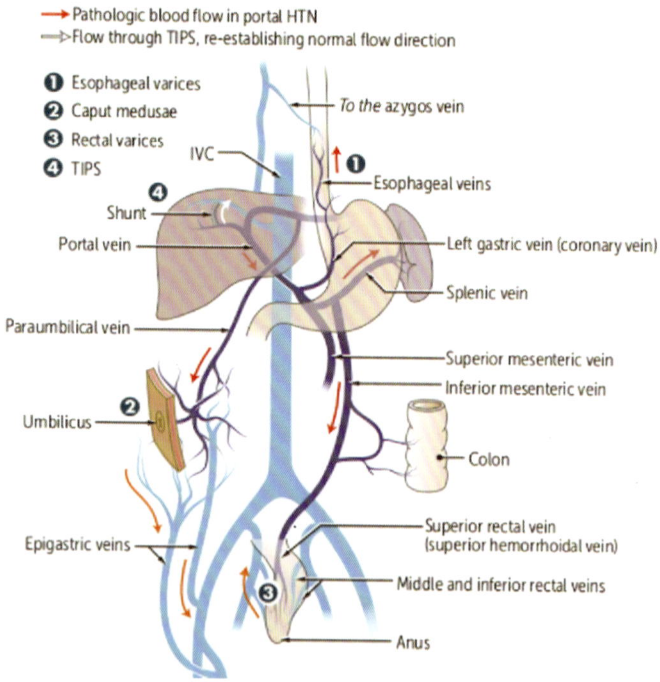

Knee Anastomosis

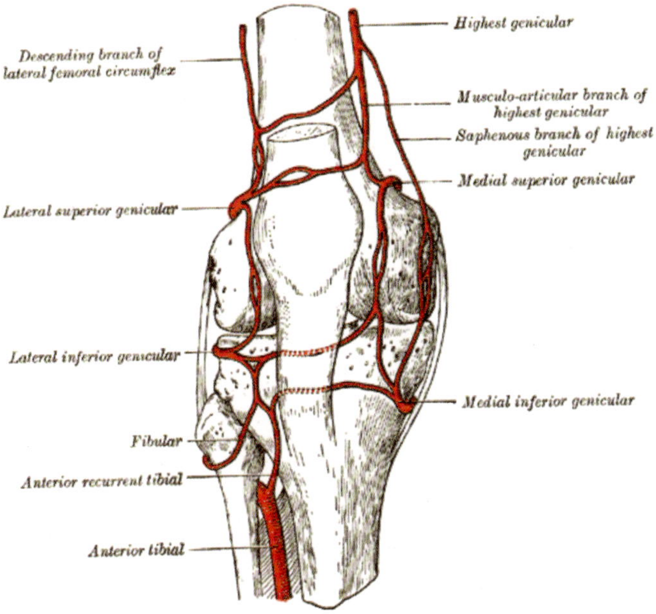

Shoulder Anastomosis

Subscapular artery (branch of the axillary artery) forms an anastomosis with branches of the Subclavian artery.

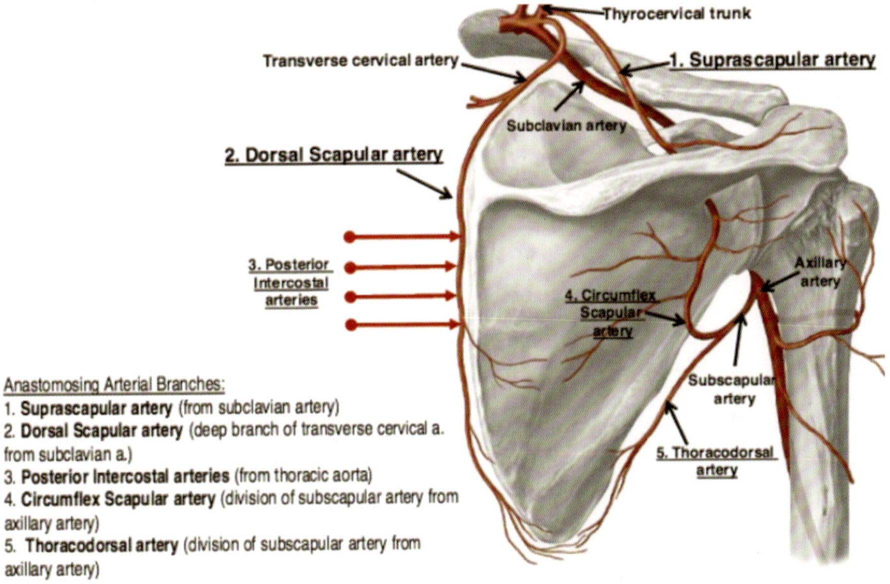

Watershed Areas

Organ	Vessels/Notes
Brain	ACA and MCA (first area of damage: hippocampus)
Splenic Flexure	SMA and IMA
Renal	PCT – Most susceptible to ↓ O2 damage
CNS Neurons	Most susceptible to ↓ O2 damage
Liver- Zone III	Most susceptible to ↓ O2 damage
Heart	Anterior: LAD
Heart	Right lateral side: RCA
Heart	Left lateral side: LCX

Vessel Pathways of the Abdomen

- Celiac Trunk comes off of the abdominal aorta: Splits into the Left gastric, Splenic Artery and the Common Hepatic Artery.
- Common hepatic artery divides into 3 branches: Proper hepatic: supplies the liver, gallbladder and part of the stomach.
  The left and right hepatic arteries supply the right side of the liver. The right hepatic artery supplies the right side of the liver and then branches into the Cystic artery to supply the gallbladder and cystic duct. The left hepatic artery supplies the left side of the liver.
- The venous blood from the GI tract drains into the superior and inferior mesenteric veins; these two vessels are then joined by the splenic vein just posterior to the neck of the pancreas to form the portal vein. This then splits to form the right and left branches, each supplying about half of the liver. The blood then leaves through the hepatic vein, which joins the inferior vena cava, just inferior to the diaphragm and is then returned to the right atrium of the heart.
- Left gastric branches off of the Hepatic Portal Vein and into the esophageal veins (which dilate under increased pressure from the portal system into esophageal varices) which go into the Azygos veins then into the IVC.
- Esophageal veins: main anastomoses that connect the systemic system via the Azygos system; and connects the portal system via the left gastric vein system.
- Azygos system (left and right sides) drain the venous blood of the thorax and some of the venous blood from the abdomen: Right side: Azygos vein. Left side: Hemiazygos and accessory hemiazygos vein.
- Spleen: supplied by the Short gastrics and the splenic artery off of the celiac trunk, which is off of the abdominal aorta.
- Adrenals: Supplies by 3 arteries: Superior suprarenal artery (branch of the inferior phrenic artery), Middle suprarenal artery (branch of the abdominal aorta), Inferior suprarenal artery (branch of the renal artery).
  Venous drainage: Right side drained by the suprarenal vein directly into the IVC. Left side drained by the Left suprarenal vein into the left renal vein and then into the IVC.
- Renal: Order of the arterial supply through the kidneys: Abdominal aorta ➔ the Renal artery ➔ Lobar arteries ➔ Arcuate arteries ➔ Interlobular arteries ➔ Afferent arterioles ➔ Glomerulus.
  Note: the renal artery also branches into the Inferior Suprarenal artery to supply the adrenal glands.
  Order of the venous drainage: Glomerulus ➔ Efferent arteriole ➔ Peritubular capillaries ➔ Interlobular veins ➔ Arcuate veins ➔ Interlobar vein ➔ Renal vein ➔ IVC.
  The efferent arterioles of the juxtamedullary nephron drain into the vasa recta.
- Left gonadal veins (ovarian and testicular) drain into the left renal vein (high pressure here can cause a left varicocele in the testicles: aka: varicose veins of the pampiniform plexus) and the right gonadal veins drain directly into the IVC.
- Head of the Pancreas: Supplied by SMA and the Superior Pancreaticoduodenal Artery.
  Tail and body of the pancreas: Supplied by branches of the splenic artery.
- Stomach: Lessor curvature (lesser omentum) of the stomach is supplied by the left (superior edge) and right (inferior edge) gastrics.
  The greater curvature (greater omentum) is supplies by the right gastro-omental artery inferiorly and the left gastro-omental artery superiorly. The fundus of the stomach, and also the upper portion of the greater curvature, is supplied by the short gastric artery, which arises from the splenic artery.
- Foregut blood supply: Celiac trunk (comes off of the abdominal aorta at T12)
  Midgut: Superior mesenteric artery (comes off of abdominal aorta at L1)
  Hindgut: Inferior mesenteric artery (comes off of the abdominal aorta at L3 – just before the bifurcation into the common iliacs).
- Superior duodenum: Superior Pancreatoduodenal branches from the Gastroduodenal artery (from the Celiac).
  Inferior duodenum: Inferior Pancreatoduodenal branches from the Superior Mesenteric.
- Ascending colon: Right colic artery
  Proximal 2/3 transverse colon: Middle colic and marginal artery.
  Distal 1/3 transverse colon: Marginal and Left colic artery
  Descending colon: Left colic artery
  Sigmoid: Sigmoid artery (Sigmoid becomes the rectum at the S3 vertebral level)
- Rectum: Superior 1/3: Superior rectal branch of the IMA.
  Middle 1/3: Middle rectal branch of the Internal iliac
  Inferior 1/3: Inferior rectal branch of the Internal pudendal

Anatomical Boarders and Contents

Submandibular Triangle (Digastric Triangle) Sup: Mandible, Anterior: Anterior belly of digastric, Posterior: Posterior belly of digastric	**Subclavian Triangle** Sup: Inferior belly of Omohyoideus, Inferior: Clavicle. Base: SCM, Floor: Serratus anterior
Subclavicular Triangle Sup: Inferior belly of Omohyoideus. Inferior: Clavicle, Anterior: SCM	**Occipital Triangle** Anterior: SCM, Posterior: Trapezius. Inferior: Omohyoideus
Subclavian Triangle Sup: Inferior belly of Omohyoideus, Inferior: Clavicle. Base: SCM, Floor: Serratus anterior	**Submental Triangle** Lateral: anterior belly digastric. Inferior: body of hyoid bone, Medical: midline of neck. Floor: Mylohyoid

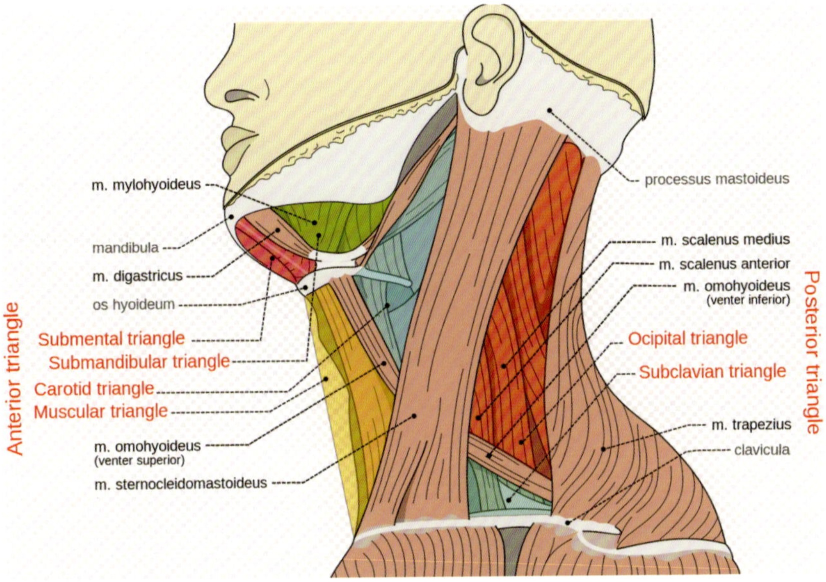

Carotid Triangle Sup: Digastric, Anterior: Omohyoid & hyoid bone, Posterior: SCM	**Carotid Sheath** Ganglion of Vagus nerve, Internal Carotid artery, CN IX, CN X, CN XI, Internal Jugular Vein, Laryngeal nerves (branches off the Vagus Nerve)

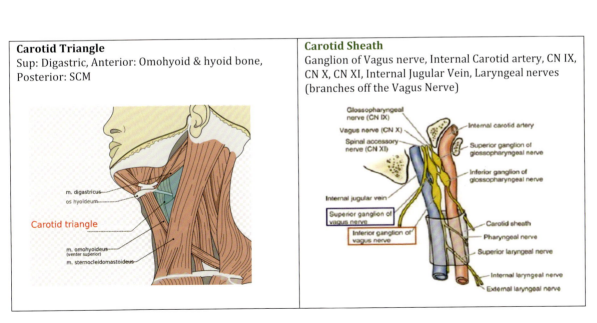

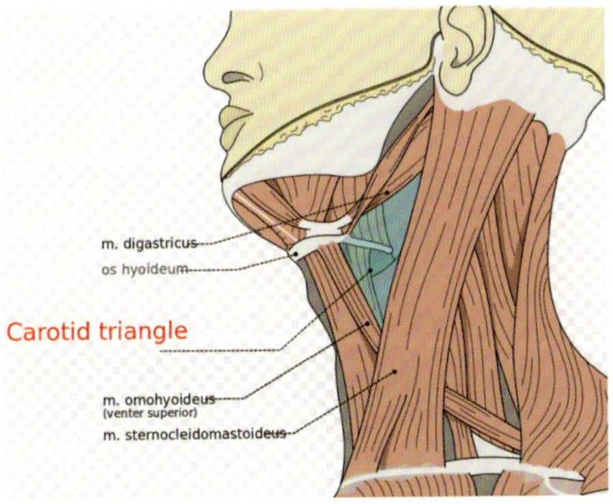

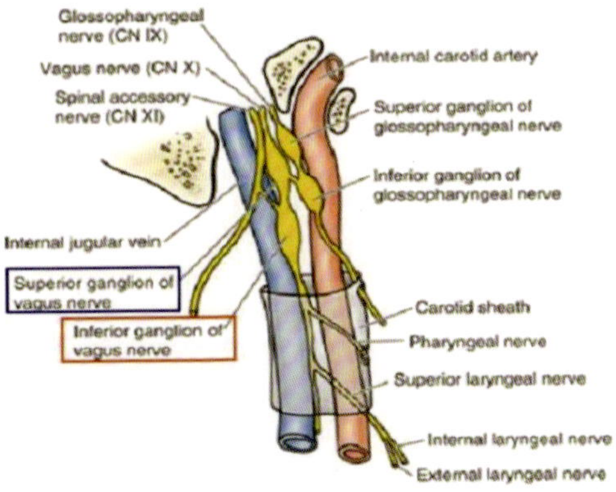

Hesselbach's Triangle

Lateral: Inferior epigastric artery, Medial: Lateral edge of rectus abdominai, Inferior: Inguinal ligament (AKA: **Poupart's ligament**).
Site of Direct Hernia.

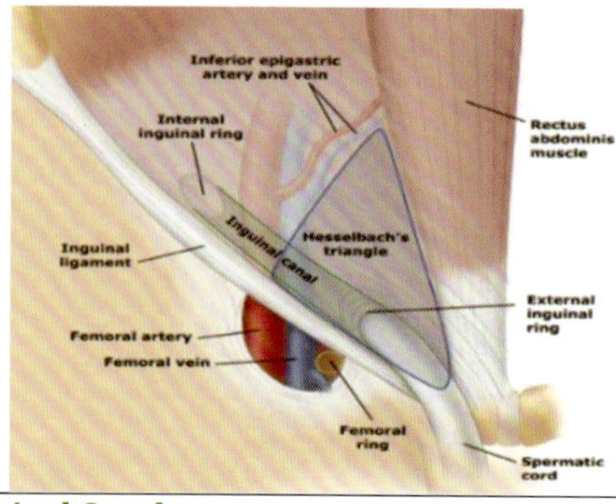

Femoral Triangle

Borders: Sup: Inguinal ligament, Adductor longus, Sartorius.
Contents: (**tip**: NAVeL)
Femoral NERVE, Deep Femoral ARTERY, Femoral VEIN, e = empty, Lymph.

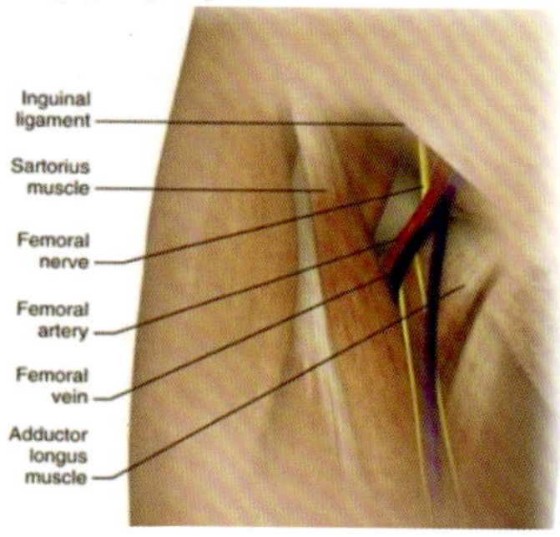

Inguinal Canal

Male: **Spermatic cord, ilioinguinal nerve.**
Female: **Round ligament of the uterus, ilioinguinal nerve**

Spermatic Cord

Arterial blood supply: vas deferens (ductus deferens), testicular artery, cremasteric artery.
Fascia, pampiniform plexus, vas deferens, testicular lymphatic's,
Nerves: genitofemoral, ilioinguinal, sympathetic and visceral afferent fibers.

Hernias

(See the GI chapter for details on hernias)

Indirect Hernia: Lateral to epigastric vessels. Goes into the scrotum. (**tip**: he goes "IN" to the "LAT"trine).

Direct Hernia: Medial to epigastric vessels. Goes through Hesselbach's triangle.

Reflexes

Deep tendon reflexes (DTR)

Grading: 0 = absent, 1= present, 2 = brisk, 3= very brisk, 4 = clonus

- Jaw jerk – lesion above trigeminal motor nucleus – pons
- Supinator: C5 – 6
- Biceps: C5 – 6
- Triceps: C6 – 7
- Knee: L 4 - 5
- Ankle: S 1 – 2

Babinski Reflex (Plantar Reflex)

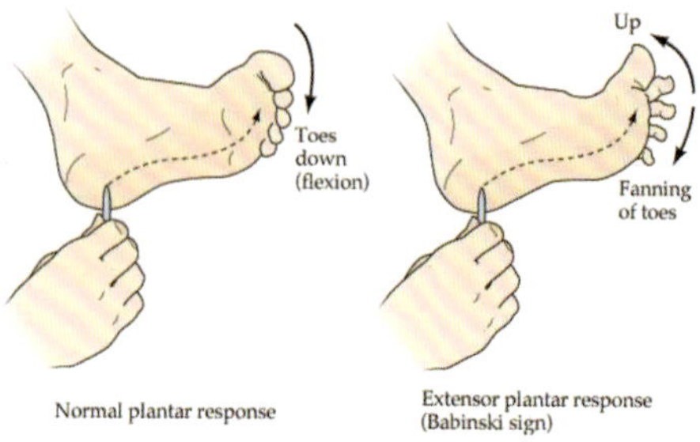

Clinical Diagnostic Test Names

Test	Purpose	Description
Babinski (adult)	Dx upper motor neuron damage	Stroke the bottom of the foot. If the toes flair up and outward, it is a positive test and indicates upper motor neuron damage.
McBurney's Point	Appendicitis	Press in on the LRQ and release. Pain indicates a positive test.
Rovsing's Sign	Appendicitis	Palpation of the LLQ produces pain in the RLQ.
Psoas Sign	Appendicitis	Patient lies on their side with knees extended or the patient can flex their thigh at the hip. This causes the iliopsoas hip flexors to irritate an inflamed appendix. Positive sign = pain. The right iliopsoas lies under the appendix.
Murphy's Sign	Gallbladder, Cholecystitis	Press in on the URQ and release. Pain indicates a positive test.
Romberg's Test	Neuro- balance test (close eyes)	Patient stands with eyes closed, extends arm and try's to maintain balance. Swaying or falling indicates a positive test.
Homans Sign	DVT	Pain on dorsiflexion of the foot.
Chandelier Sign	Cervical motion tenderness (gonorrhea, chlamydia)	When cervix it touched, causes major pain.
Anterior Drawer (Lachman Test)	Anterior cruciate ligament damage (ACL)	Patient supine, hips flexed 45°, knees flexed to 90 °, doctor pulls forward on the tibia just below the knee. Positive test if tibia pulls forward more than normal.
Posterior Drawer	Posterior cruciate ligament damage (PCL)	Patient supine, hips flexed 45°, knees flexed to 90 °, doctor pushes in on the tibia just below the knee. Positive test if tibia moves more than normal.
Straight Leg Test (Lasègue's sign)	Herniated disc (L5)	Patient lies on their back. Keeping one leg straight, the doctor raises the leg. If sciatic pain is experienced between 30 and 70 degrees, it is a positive test and is MC due to a herniated disc.
Obturator Sign	Appendicitis (irritates obturator internus muscle)	Patient lies on their back. The hip and knee are flexed at 90°. Doctor holds patients ankle in one hand and the knee with the other hand. The hip is rotated by moving the patient's ankle away from the body while allowing the knee to only move inward. (Flexion and internal rotation of the hip). This causes appendix to come in contact with the obturator internus muscle causing pain if the appendix is inflamed. Positive sign = pain.
Empty Can Test	Rotator cuff tear (supraspinatus strength)	Patient sits or stands. The shoulder is fully internally rotated, abducted to 90° and placed in 30° of forward flexion (as if emptying a beverage can). The patient try's to hold this position against resistance. Pain or inability to hold the position indicates injury to the supraspinatus muscle.
Drop Arm Sign	Rotator cuff tear	Patient sits or stands. The shoulder is fully abducted by the doctor and released. The patient lowers the arm without support. If the arm falls uncontrollably to the side from a position of 90° of abduction, the test indicates a rotator cuff tear.
Rinne or Weber Hearing Test	Dx conductive or sensory hearing loss	Tuning fork test that compares the duration of perception by bone conduction and by air conduction. Rinne test: The tuning fork is placed on the mastoid bone. In the normal ear the tuning fork vibrations are heard twice as long as by air conduction as by bone conduction. Weber test: The tuning fork is place on the center point of the head. If it is heard better in the affected ear, it is a conductive hearing loss. If it is heard better in the normal ear, it is a sensorineural hearing loss.
Auspitz Sign	Psoriasis	Bleed spots where psoriatic scales have been scraped off.
Excoriation	Intense itching	Picking at the skin or scratching the skin intensely

Muscles

Skeletal Muscle Contraction

- (**Intracellular**) Action potential (ACh synaptic cleft) ➔ **Calcium stored in terminal cisternae** ➔ Ca enters motor end plate via **L type voltage gated calcium channels** ➔**depolarization down T tubules** ➔ bind dihydropyridine (calcium channel) and **ryanodine receptors** ➔ **release of calcium from sarcoplasmic reticulum (AKA: endoplasmic reticulum)**
  ➔ Calcium binds **troponin C** ➔ Conformational change **moves tropomyosin to expose actin heads** ➔ myosin **releases ADP and PO4 to form cross-bridges with actin** ➔ Power Stroke (**contraction**) = **H and I bands shorten between the Z lines, A band stays the same length** ➔ **ATP binds to release the myosin head** ➔ sarco/endoplasmic calcium-ATPase pumps (SERCA) pumps **calcium** out of the cytosol to return back to the terminal cisternae in the sarcoplasmic reticulum.
- If there is no ATP to release the myosin head ➔ Riga mortis.
- Sarcomere is area between two Z lines (Z lines = dark, heavy line)
- H (myosin) and I (actin) banks always shorten
- A = Always stays the same length (actin and myosin) (**tip A = A**lways stays the same)

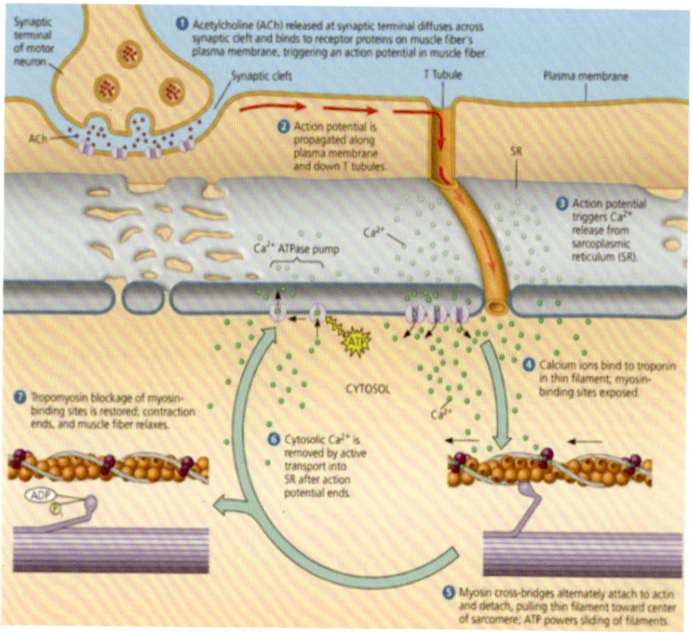

Muscle Fibers

Type 1 (AKA: Slow Twitch)

- Red fibers = ↑ mitochondria and myoglobin
- ↑ Oxidative phosphorylation (aka: making ATP)
- Posture muscles = paraspinal, soleus

Type 2 (AKA: Fast Twitch)

- White fibers = ↓ mitochondria and myoglobin
- ↑ Anaerobic glycolysis
- Biceps, deltoids, pectorals, latissimus (weight training)

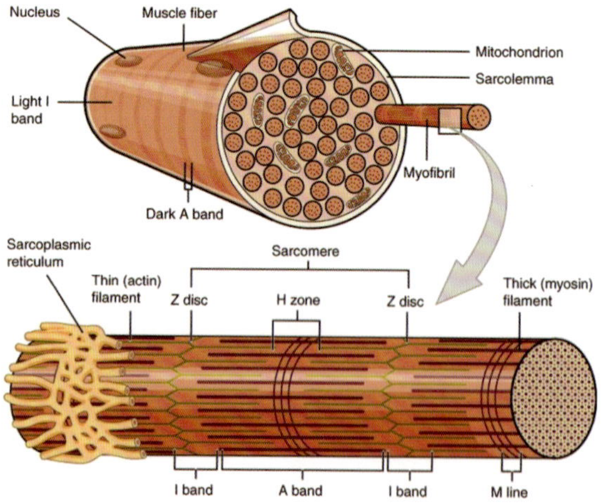

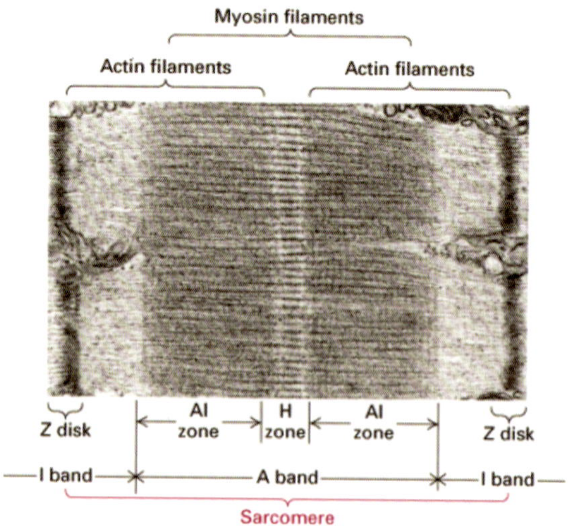

Exercise: Physiologic Effects

- Thought of beginning the exercise automatically increases the HR, acting on β1 adrenergic receptors
- Exercise begins causing INCREASE WORK LOAD ON THE HEART (AKA: increased oxygen demand)
- This increases sympathetic activity:
  1) ↑ Venous return = ↑ EDV, ↑ CO, ↑ SV
  2) Vasodilation is skeletal muscles (so vessels are able to bring more oxygen to the exercising muscles) AND to increase the flow to be able to remove more metabolites (CO_2, K, and H) from the cells.
  3) Vasoconstriction of viscera in GI and skin (this allows more blood to be sent to the muscles and increase the blood flow to the heart.
- Increases the activity of the cells therefore creates more metabolites (waste: CO_2, K and H) – so vasodilation allows for this increase of metabolites to be taken away
- There are more metabolites in venous flow, which ↓ VO_2 because more are made during exercise
- As body temperature increases with exercise, cutaneous arterioles dilate to radiate heat and ↓ body temp
- Aerobics dilates = ↓ TPR
- Isometric (weight lifting) = ↑ TPR, making heart muscles work harder = ↑ BP and ↑ risk of MI
- NO change in arterial content, ONLY venous. Venous content will show ↑ in metabolites (↑ CO_2)
- Exercise = ↑ CO = ↓ TPR
- Cardio exercise also increases blood volume because it stimulates the release of ADH and aldosterone (both cause the kidney to retain water), therefore increasing blood plasma levels
- Exercise also increases the amount of proteins in blood plasma, therefore causing water retention and increased volume

Sore Muscles From Exercise (AKA: DOMS: Delayed Onset Muscle Soreness)

- Note: this is not due to lactic acid
- The damage is caused by ultrastructural disruptions of myofilaments, in particularly the Z-band filaments. (Z-band holds the muscle fibers together).
- The pain is caused by the increased sensitivity of the muscle's nociceptors due to damage to the muscle's connective tissues. The delayed effect of the pain (1 – 2 days after exercising) is due to the time it takes for the inflammatory process to cause the increased sensitivity to the nociceptors. Inflammation to the microscopic muscle tears also causes swelling which can make muscles appear hypertrophied in the days following strenuous exercise or exercise involving muscles that have not been regularly used.
- Methods to minimize muscle soreness after activities are things that will increase the blood flow to the muscles: massage, hot baths, sauna, progressively increase your work outs, low-intensity work outs or continue to do the high intensity exercise/work. By continuing to do the intense work out/movements, the body increases its threshold for pain tolerance (AKA: exercise-induced analgesia).
- Lactic acid, a byproduct of the conversion of glycogen to ATP, is actually used as fuel for exercising muscles. Muscle cells convert glycogen to lactic acid when there is not enough oxygen to allow the conversion to ATP. The mitochondria then use the lactic acid as fuel. Lactic acid allows the body to convert glycogen to energy without the need for oxygen. Lactic acid is then converted to pyruvate and sent into the TCA cycle to be converted to ATP under conditions where there is limited oxygen.
- Endurance training increases the mitochondria in the muscle cells, which aids in the ability to use lactic acid as a fuel. This allows muscles to work harder for longer periods in low oxygen situations.
- Note: Aerobic energy: Conversion of glycogen to ATP. Anaerobic energy: Conversion of glycogen to lactic acid when little oxygen is available.
- VO_2 Max: (amount of O_2 in the venous system) Measure of the maximum capacity of a body to transport and utilize oxygen during exercise. VO_2 decreases during exercise due to increased oxygen drop off/demand in the arterial system and increased metabolites being produced.
- Damage to muscle is measured by blood levels of CPK (Creatine phosphokinase). Enzyme in muscles that is released when muscles are damaged.

Smooth Muscle Contraction

- Action potential ➔ Calcium enters L type voltage gated Calcium channels ➔Calcium-calmodulin complex ➔ **activating myosin=light chain kinase (MLCK)** ➔ Myosin ➔ **cross bridging** ➔ contraction

  Gq pathway: Phospholipase C ➔ IP3 ➔ Extracellular Calcium ➔ Calcium Calmodulin ➔ **MLCK** ➔ Cross bridge

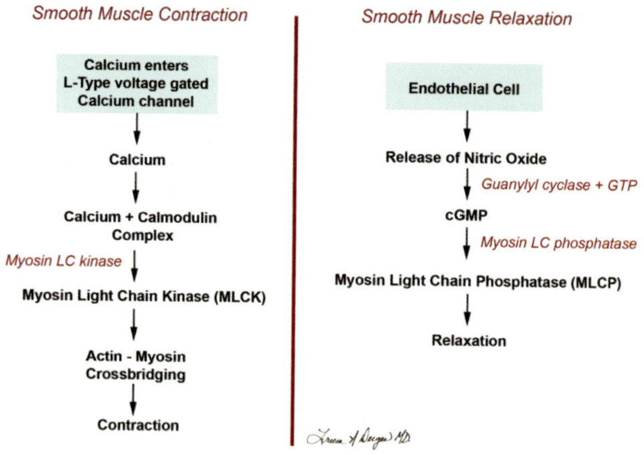

Smooth Muscle Relaxation

- Nitric oxide ➔ **cGMP via Guanylate cyclase ➔ Myosin-light-chain phosphatase (MLCP)** ➔ myosin ➔ relaxation.

Muscle Movements

To rise up from a sitting position.
- Gluteus maximus

To abduct arm. Raise arm from side to over the head.
- Supraspinatus raises the arm the first 30°, then the deltoid raises it the rest of the way up. The muscles that raise the shoulder blade as you are raising your arm are the trapezius and serratus anterior.

To adduct the arm. Lower arm from over the head down to the side.
- Pectoralis major, latissimus dorsi, teres major, teres minor

To Flex the arm. Raise the arm straight forward from the side and then up.
- Anterior deltoid, pectoralis major, long head biceps brachii, short head biceps brachii, coracobrachialis

To Extend the arm. Pull arm straight backwards from the side.
- Posterior deltoid, latissimus dorsi, teres major

To adduct the arm. Lower arm from over the head down to the side.
- Pectoralis major, latissimus dorsi, teres major, teres minor

Lateral rotation of the arm.
- Infraspinatus, teres minor, posterior deltoid

Medial rotation of the arm.
- Subscapularis, latissimus dorsi, teres major, anterior deltoid

To cup the hand.
- The Thenar group makes the cup: Abductor pollicis, flexor pollicis brevis. The hypothenar group: Abductor digiti minimi and flexor digiti minimi brevis.

To shrug the shoulders "scapular elevation"
- Trapezius and Levator Scapulae

To dorsiflex the foot.
- Anterior compartment of the leg. Extensors: Extensor halluces longus, Extensor digitorum longus. Tibialis and peroneus tertius.

To plantarflex the foot.
- Posterior compartment of the leg. Flexors: Flexor halluces longus, Flexor digitorum longus. Tibialis posterior, Gastrocnemius, Soleus, Plantaris.

Pronation of the forearm. Turning the palms from the anatomical position facing anterior to facing posterior.
- Pronator quadratus, pronator teres, brachioradialis

Extension of neck.
- Bilateral sternocleidomastoid muscles (SCM)

Flex the neck (turning it to one side)
- Unilaterally will flex the neck to the same side as the contracting SCM and rotates the neck to the contra lateral side. (Ex: if you rotate the neck to the left, the right SCM is working).

Sit ups. To sit up from a supine position without use of arms.
- Rectus abdominus, external abdominal obliques, iliopsoas muscles (Psoas major, iliacus muscle)

Bone, Joint , Connective Tissue and Muscle Pathologies

Bone

2 types of mineralized osseous tissue.

- Cortical tissue (AKA: compact bone)
  - Supports body, protects organs, aids in movement, stores and releases calcium (and other elements)
  - Forms the cortex (outer shell), dense.
  - 80% of the weight of the skeleton.
  - Functional unit: Osteon.
  - Osteon consist of lamellae (concentric layers of compact bone tissue) that surrounds the Haversian canal
  - Haversian canal contains the bone's nerve and blood supply

- Cancellous tissue (AKA: trabecular bone, spongy bone)
  - Soft, flexible
  - Site of haematopoiesis (production of blood cells)
  - Functional unit: Trabecula.

Endochondral Ossification (long bones) Chondrocytes create a model of the bone with **cartilage**. The cartilage is then converted to woven bone by osteoblasts and osteoclasts. The woven bone is then converted to lamellar bone. Consist of femur, tibia, fibula, humerus, radius, ulna. Contains both red and yellow and fatty bone marrow. Elongation: diaphysis and epiphysis. Longitudinal growth: endochondral ossification at the epiphyseal plate. Bone growth stimulated: growth hormone from the anterior pituitary.	**Membranous Ossification (flat bones)** Woven bone is formed without cartilage when Osteoblasts secrete calcium phosphate to create a bony matrix that is then ossified. The woven bone is then changed to lamellar bone by osteoblasts and osteoclasts. They have only red bone marrow. **NOTE**: The flat bone, ilium in the pelvis, is the main site where erythropoiesis occurs. In pathologies that require heavy replacement of RBC's (ie: Sickle Cell or Beta Thalassemia) additional RBC production sites are required, such as the skull. When this occurs, x-rays will show a "crew cut" appearance around the skull. Consist of skull (calvaria) bones, facial bones, pelvis, sternum, rib cage. Composed of 2 layers of thin compact bone that encloses a layer of trabecular bone (AKA: spongy, cancellous). This trabecular layer contains the red bone marrow (haematopoiesis). Note: in pathologies that
Osteoblast = Builds bone Secretes collagen, **mineralization**. Differentiate from mesenchymal stem cells in periosteum. Live in lacuna.	**Osteoclasts = (AKA: Macrophages)** **Breaks down bone (AKA: resorption)** Secretes acid and **collagenases.** Differentiate from macrophages. **RANK-L, M-CSF stimulates osteoclast**. Live in Lacuna NOTE: Be sure you pay attention if the term is re**SORB** or re**AB**sorb. Resorb means **breaks down** the bone (osteoclasts). Reabsorb means something is bringing things back IN. *Just like in the kidneys.* Re**AB**sorb means things are being brought back out of the tubules and back into the body to reuse. Secrete means that things are being put out of the body and into the tubules to be excreted.
Estrogen Inhibits apoptosis in osteoblast. Induces apoptosis in osteoclast. **Estrogen deficiency leads to osteoporosis.**	**PTH** Parathyroid hormone maintains calcium levels in the body by stimulating osteoclasts to resorb bones.

Periosteum	**Additional bone terminology**
Connective tissue that forms 2 layers on the **outside** surface of bones. Outer layer: Fibrous layer: consist **fibroblasts**. Inner layer: Cambium layer: consist of progenitor cells that develop into **osteoblasts**. Injury to bones: Requires the **periosteum** for repair. Repair: progenitor cells develop into osteoblasts and chondroblasts ➔ healing.	**Endosteum**: Connective tissue that lines the inner surface of bones. **Trabecula**: functional unit of the trabecular bone (AKA: spongy, cancellous). **Osteon**: functional unit of the compact bone (AKA: cortical). **Lacuna**: Sites of osteoblasts and osteoclasts. **Bone marrow**: (AKA: myeloid tissue) found in spongy bone. In children bones are filled with red marrow. Aging: red marrow replaced by yellow or fatty marrow. Red marrow location in adults: pelvic bones, femur, ribs. **Haversian Canals**: microscopic tubes in the cortical bone where the nerves and blood supply to the bone travel. Connect the Volkmann canals. **Volkmann's Canals**: Channels in the cortical bones located inside osteons. Transmit blood from the periosteum into the bone and provide nourishment for the osteons.

Compact Bone & Spongy (Cancellous Bone)

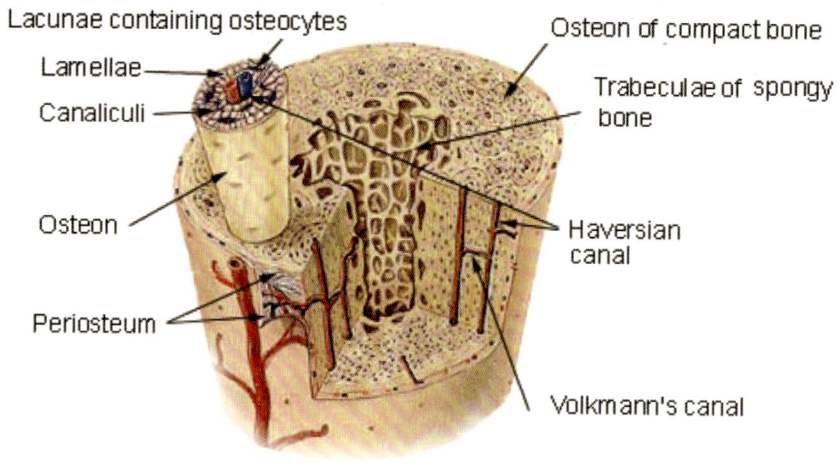

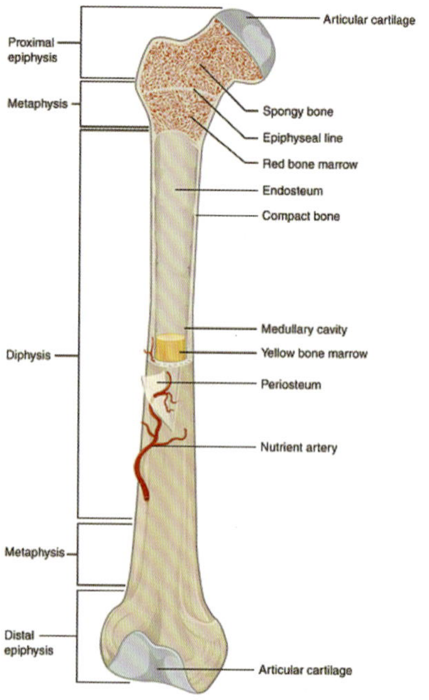

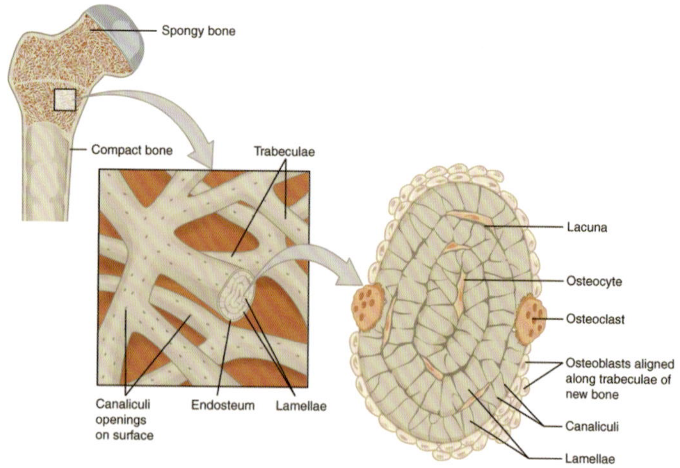

Bone Pathologies

Osteoporosis
Decrease in spongy (AKA: Trabecular) **bone mass.**
Normal bone mineralization.

Cause: **Loss of estrogen**.
Ie: menopause, anorexia, steroids.

Risk: Kyphosis, loss of height, **vertebral compression fracture (collapse)**, **femoral neck fracture** /**avascular necrosis/aseptic necrosis** (**medial circumflex femoral artery).**

NOTE: Cathepsin K is the most potent collagenase (protease). It is secreted by osteoclasts (extracellularly) so that they can break down collagen (the main component of the non-mineral protein matrix of the bone) in bone resorption. This plays a major role in osteoporosis.
(All other Cathepsins are found in the **lysosome and are activated by the low pH**).

MC: Women more than men.
African American women ↓risk due to larger bones.

Labs: **Normal labs** (Ca, PO4, ALP, PTH)

DX: DEXA (Dual Energy X Ray Absorptiometry)
Normal T-score ≥ 1.0
Osteopenia T-score -2.5 to < -1.0
Osteoporosis t-score ≤ - 2.5
(Osteopenia: bone mineral density is lower than normal, precursor to osteoporosis)

TX: **Weight bearing exercise** (non-weight bearing exercises do not increase density: ie: swimming or bicycling). Increase intake of Calcium and Vitamin D.
Additional TX: **Bisphosphonates, Denosumab** (monoclonal antibody against RANK-L), estrogen replacement in postmenopausal women, **Raloxifene** in postmenopausal women (↓ risk of breast cancer and ↓ LDL levels).

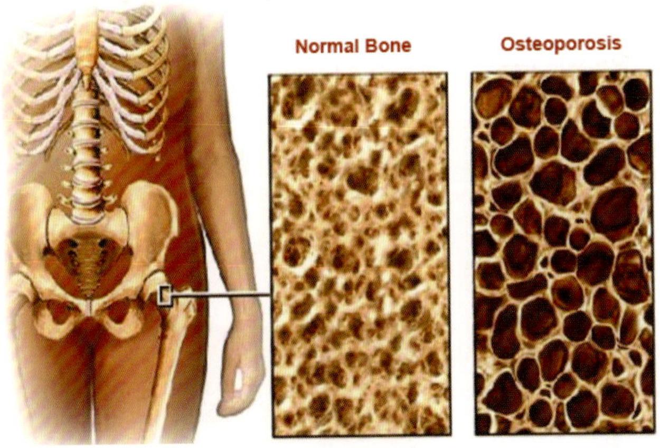

Bone lesions:
Initial findings: Osteolytic lesions that then changes to Osteoblastic lesions.
Osteolytic = Paget's, osteoporosis, multiple myeloma.
Osteoblastic = Metastatic prostate cancer.

Paget Disease of the Bone
(AKA: Osteitis deformans)

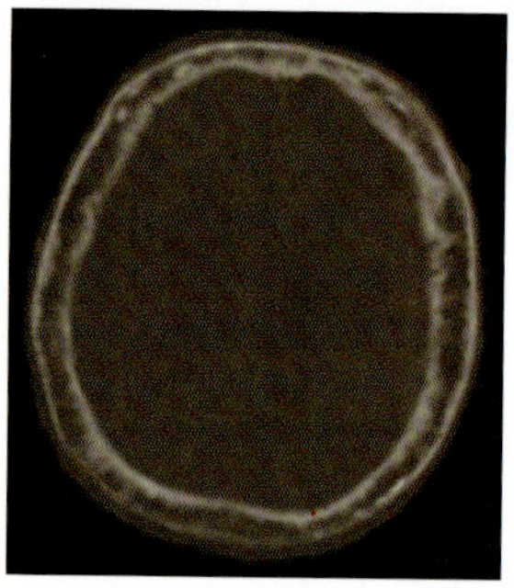

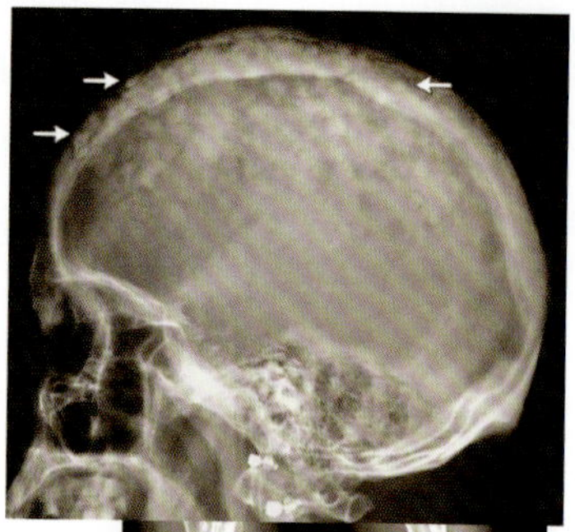

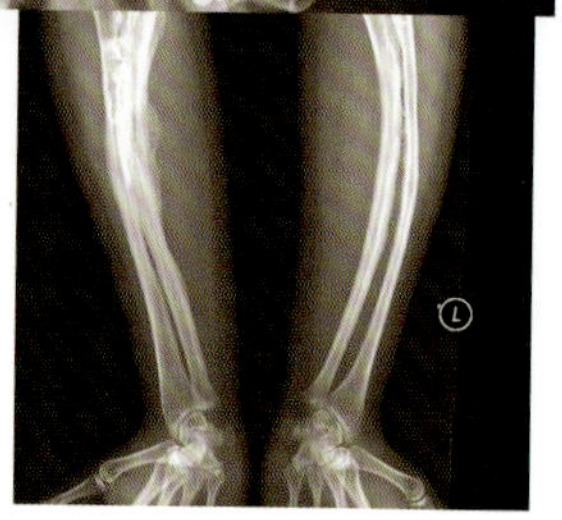

Excessive breakdown and formation of bone due to ↑ in both osteoblast and osteoclast activity resulting in enlarged, misshaped bones.
Abnormal bone architecture.
X-ray shows **thickened skull (calvarium)**

Activated by: **RANK-L** (Kappa Beta Ligand) and **M-CSF** (Macrophage colony stimulating factor)

Localized and affects just a few bones (where Osteoporosis affects all the bones)

Labs:
BIT: ↑ **ALP and normal serum Calcium** and phosphate levels.
MAT: X-ray.

Histology: **Mosaic pattern of lamellar and woven bone** (consist of osteoblast and osteoclast).

SX: **Bone pain, stiffness, fractures**. Loss of hearing or vision if Paget's occurs in the skull.
Can see increase in hat size.

Bone lesions:
Initial findings: Osteolytic lesions that then change to Osteoblastic lesions.
Osteolytic = Paget's, osteoporosis.
Osteoblastic = Metastatic prostate cancer.

TX: **Bisphosphonates, Calcitonin**

Achondroplasia, AD
Defective **fibroblast growth factor receptor 3 (FGFR3) which inhibits chondrocytes**

Endochondral ossification
Chondrocytes

Dwarfism, short limbs, normal head and trunk, normal life span, normal fertility
Affects the **long bones** (longitudinal bone growth).

Note: **Genetics**: Autosomal dominant: If one parent is affected then 50% of the children will be. If both parents are affected then 75% of the children will be.
Note: Higher risk with **advanced paternal age**

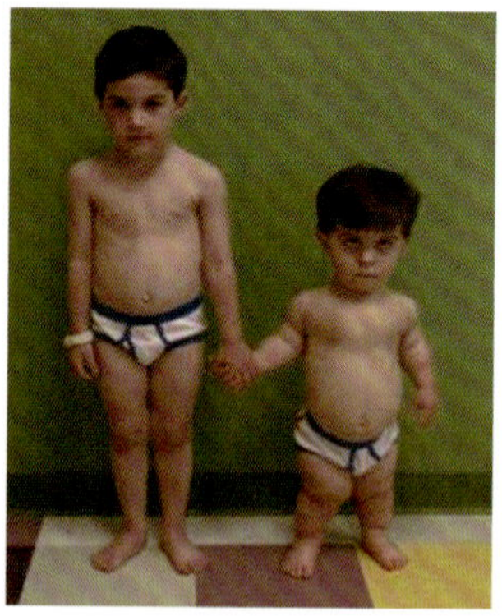

Normal Affected
(twin brothers)

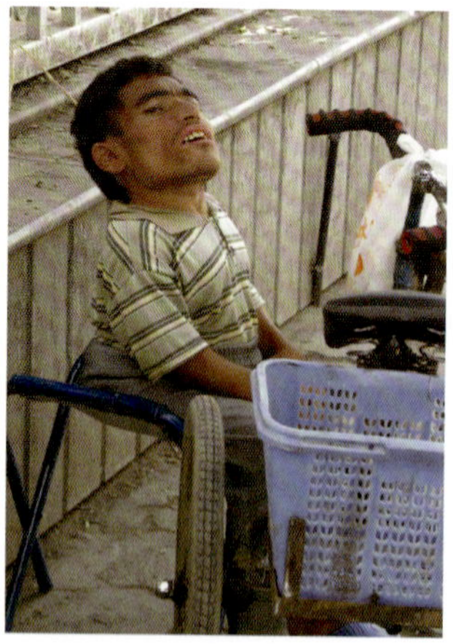

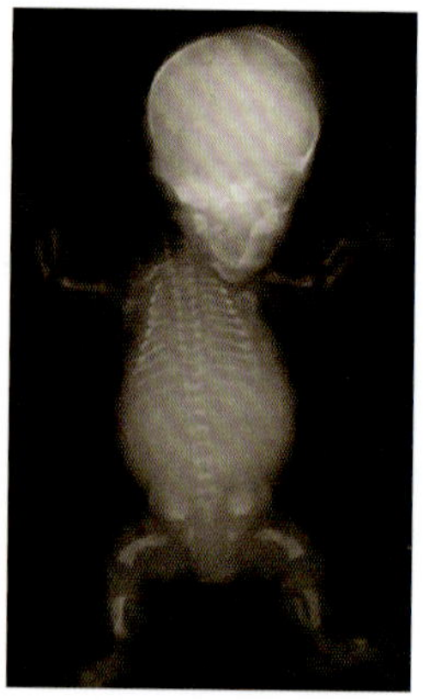

Osteopetrosis
(AKA: Marble Bone Disease)

Thick, dense, brittle bones = ↑ fractures.
Defective osteoclast prevents normal bone resorption.

Bone takes up marrow = pancytopenia, extramedullary hematopoiesis.

Labs: **Normal Labs** (normal to high ALP, Ca, PTH)

DX: XR shows "Erlenmeyer flask"

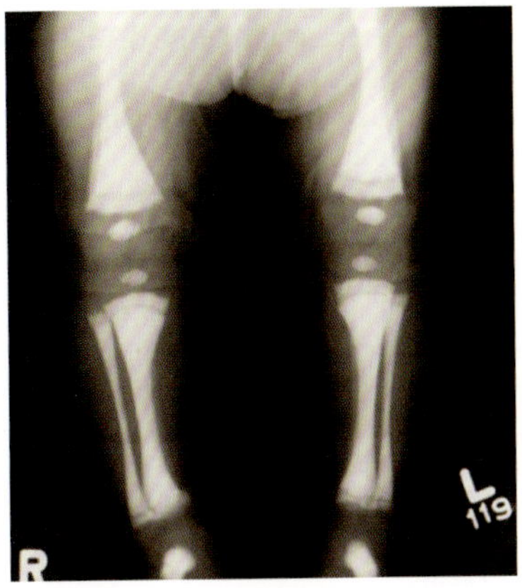

Osteonecrosis
AKA: Avascular Necrosis, bone infarction

Necrosis of the bone due to lack of blood supply. Bone collapses.

MC locations: Head of the femur, neck of the talus (ankle bone), scaphoid.

Blood supply lost:
Femur head: Medial circumflex femoral artery.
Scaphoid: branches of radial artery.

MCC: Chronic steroid use, sickle cell, ↓ or lack of estrogen, alcoholism, Gaucher's Dz.

Osteomalacia (Adults)
Rickets (Children)

Soft bones.
Vitamin D Deficiency.
Defective mineralization ad calcification of osteoid.
Can also cause pectus carinatum (aka: pigeon chest) in children (Rickets) due to increased deposition of unmineralized **osteoid** causing an outward protrusion of the sternum.

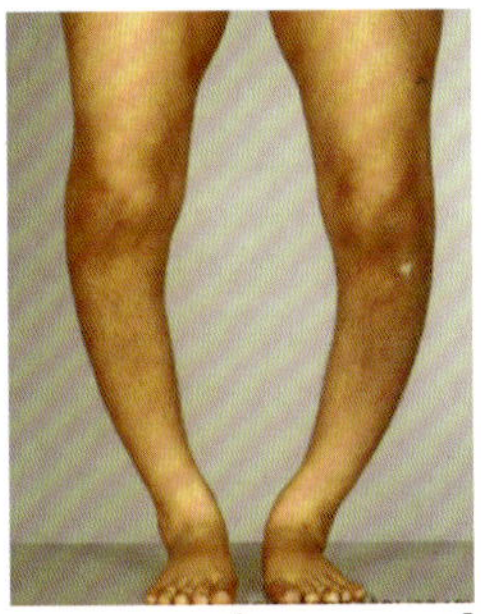

SX: **Lateral bowing** of the legs.
(note: syphilis causes anterior bowing)

Labs: ↑ ALP due to activity of osteoblasts (osteoblast require alkaline environment), ↓ Calcium, ↓ Phosphate, ↑ PTH

↓ Vit D = ↓ serum Calcium = ↑ PTH

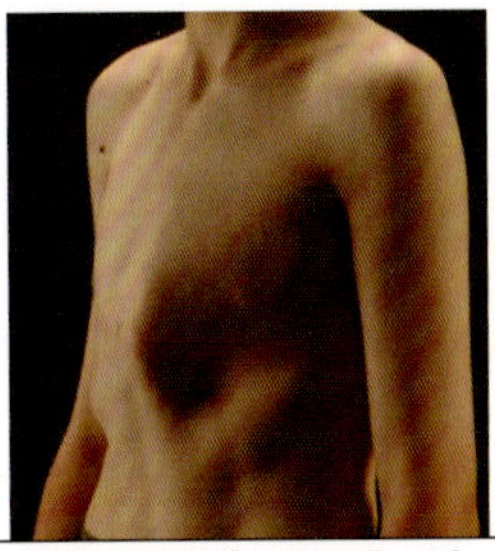

Pectus carinatum

Polyostotic Fibrous Dysplasia (McCune-Albright)

Normal bone is replaced by **fibrous bone**. (AKA: **Fibroblast and collagen**)

SX: Abnormal growth or swelling of the bone, visual deformities of the bone, increased risk of bone fractures, bone pain, **precocious puberty**,
nerve entrapment, **light brown spots** (tumors) on the skin.
(Associated with NF II)

Bony trabeculae are thin and irregular (bony spicules on biopsy)

Labs: ↑ Calcium, ALP and PTH,
↓ Phosphate

Hypervitaminosis D
(AKA: Vitamin D toxicity)

Causes: Excess intake of vitamin D, **granulomatous diseases**.
(MC: **Sarcoidosis)**

SX: Causes **over calcification.**
High levels of calcium (Vit D reabsorbs calcium and PO_4 in the gut), constipation, muscle weakness, metastatic calcification in tissues, fatigue, irritability, HTN.

Osteitis Fibrosa Cystica
(AKA: Von Recklinghausen's Bone Dz)
(this is not related to NF I)

Caused by hyperparathyroidism. PTH stimulates osteoclasts that cause bone weakness and loss.

SX: Areas of loss are replaced with fibrous tissues (peritrabecular fibrosis), brown cyst like tumors in and around the bone, thin bones.

Complications: fractures, kidney stones due to ↑ calcium.

Causes: parathyroid adenoma, genetic, parathyroid carcinoma, renal osteodystrophy.

Labs:
If 1°: ↑ Ca, ↓ PO_4, ↑ ALP, ↑ PTH.
If 2°: ↓ Ca, ↑ PO_4, ↑ ALP, ↑ PTH.

Differentials in Bone Pathology

Pathology	Calcium	Phosphate	Alk Phos	PTH	Notes
Osteopenia	NL	NL	NL	BL	↓ bone mass
Osteopetrosis	NL	NL	↑	NL	Marble bone: thick, dense. Erienmeyer flask look on x-ray
Osteomalacia/Rickets	↓	↓	↑	↑	Soft bones. Lateral bowing of the legs
Osteitis Fibrosa Cystica	↑	↓	↑	↑	Brown, cyst like tumors
Paget's Disease of the bone	NL	NL	Varies	NL	Abnormal bone architecture (mosaic patterns)

Osteomyelitis
Infection of the bone.

MC ↑ risk in: Soft tissue infection, skin ulcers, diabetics (with ulcers), peripheral arterial DZ, trauma, Hx orthopedic surgery.

MCC: **Staph aureus** (MC due to Diabetes or vascular insufficiency).
MC in **Sickle Cell: Salmonella** (unless it is a child under 4 years old before they become asplenic: then MCC S. aureus.
MC in **Pseudomonas** when there is a puncture wound that penetrates through a tennis shoe.

Spread:
Children: through hematogenous spread.
Adults: from contiguous (nearby) infection.

SX: Warmth, redness, swelling of skin/tissue around infection, possibly purulent sinus tract, afebrile.

DX:
BIT: Periosteal elevation on X-ray. If X-ray is normal and suspicion is high, perform an MRI.
MAT: Bone biopsy and culture.
(Bone scan only if MRI is contradicted)

TX: **Based on biopsy to identify organism**:
Gram-positive sensitive: Oxacillin, Cefazolin, Nafcillin, Ceftriaxone.
Gram positive resistant MRSA: IV Vancomycin, Linezolid, Ceftaroline, Daptomycin
Gram negative: Ciprofloxacin.

Charcot Joint
AKA: Neuropathic arthropathy

Progressive degeneration of a weight bearing joint causes bone destruction, bone resorption and deformity.

Loss of sensation and proprioception allows damage to go unnoticed resulting in continued damage that worsens.

MC: Diabetic neuropathy.
Other neuropathies: alcoholic neuropathy, spinal cord injury, syringomyelia (shoulder joints), syphilis (knee joints).
SX: ↓ pain, proprioception, ↑ skin temperature due to inflammation around the joint, deformed joints, large osteophytes, extra bone fragments, degenerative joints, erythema, edema, plantar ulcers.

TX: Orthotic shoes, casting, braces.

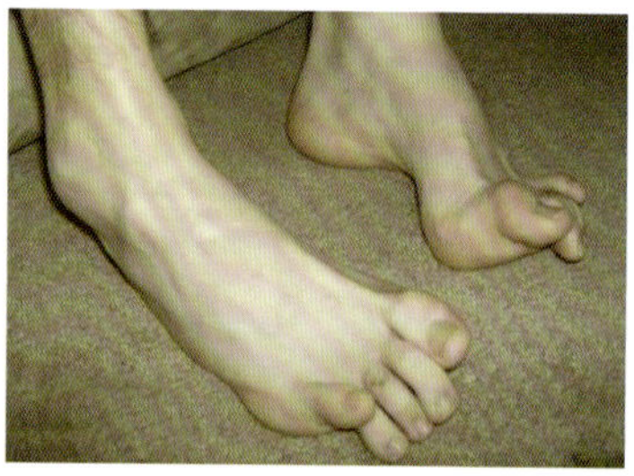

Legg-Calve-Perthes Disease
(AKA: Avascular necrosis of femoral head)

Childhood hip disorder due to a disruption of blood flow to the femoral head causing an idiopathic avascular necrosis and bone death. Even though healing occurs there is a loss of bone mass, which weakens the femoral head causing collapse and deformity.

MC: Boys from 4 – 10 years old.

SX: Slow onset, Antalgic gait (painful), groin pain worsened by leg or hip movement. Chronic hip pain.

DX: Hip X-ray, MRI. Shows joint effusions and joint widening.

TX: Rest, NSAIDS. Removing pressure from the hip: traction, braces, physiotherapy, orthotics.
Surgery: Required on both hips. If there is necrosis of one hip it will eventually involve the other hip.

Growing Pains

MC: Children from 2 – 12 years old.

SX: Night pain, bilaterally in the lower legs, below the knees.
Pain is always gone in the morning.

TX: Reassure, massage, analgesics

Congenital Hip Dysplasia in Infants
(Dislocation of femoral head)

Must check baby's hips at all pediatric visit until 1 year old or walking.

↑ Risk: breech, Caucasian, female, family Hx.
Must diagnose and treat **before 6 months** = best prognosis.
Complications if not treated: limp (Trendelenburg gate), scoliosis, arthritis, avascular necrosis.

SX:
Leg length discrepancy.
Asymmetrical inguinal skin folds

DX: Ultrasound of hips.
Barlow Maneuver: Adduction with posterior pressure on the hip.
Ortolani Maneuver: Abduction with anterior left hip.
Positive test: Palpable "clunk" sound = hip dislocation. TX with Pavlik Harness if < 6 months old. Must refer to orthopedic surgeon.
TX: Pavlik harness

Metatarsus Adductus
Congenital foot deformity that causes toes to point inward when walking.
(AKA: Pigeon toe, clubfoot)

Type 1:
Feet that overcorrect.
Mild, corrects on their own.
TX: Reassurance.

Type II:
Feet that correct to neutral.
TX: Orthopedic shoes

Type III:
Rigid feet
TX: Serial cast

If feet do not correct y 4 years old: orthopedic surgery.

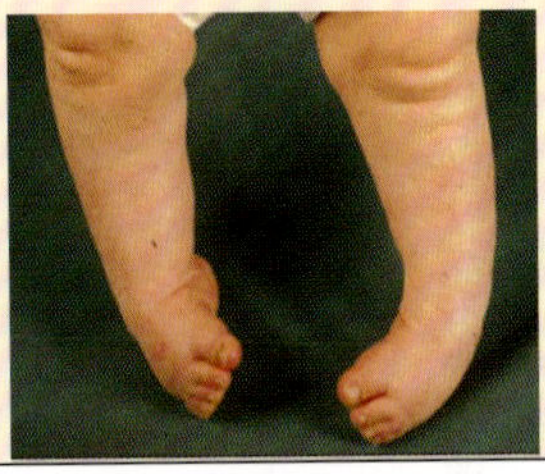

Slipped Cap Femoral Epiphysis
Displacement/fracture through the growth plate due to the slippage of overlying end of the of the femoral cap from the femoral neck (epiphysis).

MC: Obese boys 10 – 16 yrs old.

SX: Dull hip pain, referred knee pain.
Hip externally rotated.

DX: X-ray shows frog leg appearance and widening of joint space.

TX: Immediate surgery. Internal screw fixation to prevent avascular necrosis.

Osteomyelitis

Condition	Infection Cause
Newborns, children, adults	#1 MCC: S. aureus #2: Group A Strep
Sickle Cell	#1 MCC: Salmonella #2: S. aureus (NOTE: check the age. If the child is under 5 and still has function spleen then the #1 MCC is S. aureus. If the child is over 5, they are asplenic and the #1 MCC will be Salmonella)
Potts DZ	M. tuberculosis
Puncture wounds to the foot (particularly through rubber sole of tennis shoes)	Pseudomonas

Rheumatology (Arthritis)

Osteoarthritis
AKA: Degenerative Joint Disease (DJD).
"**Wear and Tear**" destroys **articular cartilage**. (bone on bone).
Non-inflammatory.

SX: **Crepitus**, **subchondral cyst**, **osteophytes (bone spurs), osteophytic changes**, Heberden nodes on **DIP** and Bouchard nodes on **PIP**. **NO MCP** involvement, **narrowed joint spaces**

MC: Pain in weight bearing joints.
Disease progression: Early stage of disease shows and ↑ articular cartilage (with ↑ water content, proteoglycan synthesis, hypertrophic repair of articular cartilage), then as disease progresses there is a loss of articular cartilage and joints become narrowed (wear and tear), short duration of stiffness (as compared to RA). Involves DIP and PIP.
Morning stiffness < 30 minutes

Labs: **Lab test are normal** (ESR, RA, ANA, CBC, RF).
Arthrocentesis: < 2000 leukocytes.

DX: MAT: X-Ray shows: joint space narrowing, **osteophytes**, bone cysts, dense subchondral bone.

TX: **#1: Weight loss.**
NSAIDS (acetominophen),
Intra-articular glucocorticoid injections.
joint replacement if warranted.
(**Note: be careful on the exam** when weight loss is the concept they want you to pick. If they have the choice of exercise or reduce calories in the answer – do NOT select exercise. Reducing calories is **always the best answer** for weight loss. Someone can exercise all day but if they are eating fattening foods in between, they are not going to be losing any weight!)

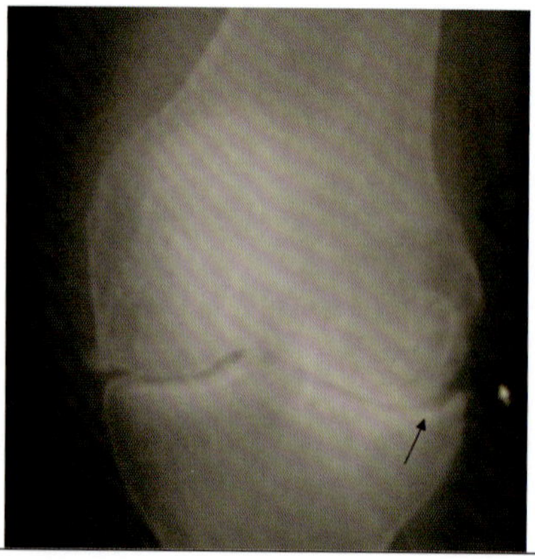

Rheumatoid Arthritis
Autoimmune.
Inflammatory, **bone erosion**, destruction of synovial joints.
(Erosion: Deformity of joints, narrowing of joint space, abnormality of x-rays)
Can occur at any age.

SX: **Morning stiffness > 1 hour for at least 6 weeks. Pannus** formation (**granulation** tissue), **MCP (swelling and pain), PIP involvement, NO DIP involvement**, rheumatoid **nodules** (fibrinoid **necrosis**), **ulnar deviation** of fingers (AKA: Swan neck fingers), Flexion of PIP and hyperextension of the DIP (Boutonniere Deformity), Baker's cyst (mimics a DVT), **C1/C2 cervical spine subluxation (must do cervical spine imaging to verify stability of C1/C2 prior to any surgeries where the patient will be intubated (neck hyperextended) to avoid subluxation (dislocation)**, (reminder: Subluxation is also a common problem in Down's Syndrome), pleural effusions and nodules in the lungs (this pleural effusion shows the lowest glucose level), episcleritis (inflammation of the episcleritis- think tissue between the conjunctiva and the sclera), carpal tunnel syndrome.

Sacroiliac joint is spared in RA.

Note: Remember that **Parvo B-19** can mimic RA because it also has symmetrical joint involvement.

Labs/DX: **Anti-citrullinated antibody (anti-CCP) (most specific for RA),**
RF: Rheumatoid factor (not specific),
Associated with **HLA-DR4**.
Anti-IgG antibody.
MC: IgM to IgG Fc region.
↑ ESR, ↑ CRP (C-reactive protein).
Normocytic, normochromic anemia.
Arthrocentesis: shows 5000 – 50,000 leukocytes..

TX: **Methotrexate (DMARD)** slows down progression of RA, **glucocorticoids (add to Methotrexate in cases of ↑ inflammation, they do not stop progression), TNFα inhibitors**.

NOTE: In cases where the RA patient is being treated with drug (ex: TNFα inhibitors) and the drug initially works but then symptoms return, it is due to **antibodies that were developed against the drug.**

Juvenile Rheumatoid Arthritis
AKA: Adult-onset Still's Disease
AKA: Juvenile idiopathic arthritis.

MC arthritis in children under 17 yrs old.

SX: High **spiking fever > 104°**, persistent **joint pain, swelling, myalgias**, stiffness, often presents with a **salmon color rash** on chest and/or abdomen. Can also present with splenomegaly, **lymphadenopathy**, hepatomegaly, splenomegaly and pericardial effusion. Symptoms last from months to their entire lifetime.

DX: **↑ Ferritin levels** (due to chronic DZ),
↑ LFT's, ANA is normal. May or may not show: leukocytosis, anemia, hypoalbuminemia.

TX: Control pain, improve function and prevent joint damage.

	Rheumatoid Arthritis cont'd **NOTE:** In any pathology where systemic steroids (glucocorticoids) are being used (ie: RA, Lupus) remember that **any of the side effects or signs from steroid use can be seen** in the patient: osteoporosis, atrophied adrenal gland, avascular necrosis. (DMARD: Disease-modifying antirheumatic drug) **Methotrexate** is the best DMARD. **Other DMARD's: Hydroxychloroquine (toxic to the retina), Rituximab (removes CD20 lymphocytes), Sulfasalazine (Bone marrow toxicity, do not use with G6PD), TNF inhibitors (Do PPD to avoid reactivation of TB).** 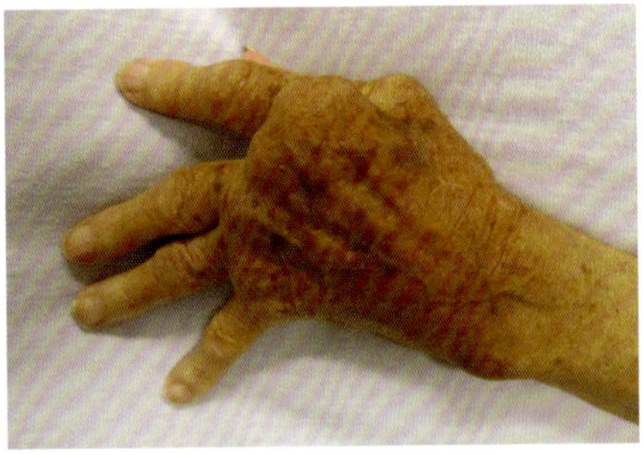	
Caplan Syndrome Combination of rheumatoid arthritis, pneumoconiosis that presents as lung nodules (seen on CXR). MC pneumoconiosis: mining coal dust, asbestos, silica. Smoking is an aggravating factor. SX: Similar to rheumatoid arthritis but must have a **pneumoconiosis and lung nodules.** Can also include: cough, shortness of breath, symptoms of rheumatoid nodules, rales upon auscultation.	**Felty's Syndrome** Combination of rheumatoid arthritis, splenomegaly, neutropenia, low WBC. MC: ages 50 – 70. SX: Similar to rheumatoid arthritis but have a triad of: **splenomegaly, neutropenia, ↓ white blood count and rheumatoid arthritis**. Can also include: fever, weight loss, fatigue, skin discoloration (legs are darker/brown), hepatomegaly, ulcers/sores on lower legs, anemia, thrombocytopenia, vasculitis, and hepatosplenomegaly. Labs: Neutropenia. ↓ WBC, ↓ PMN's	

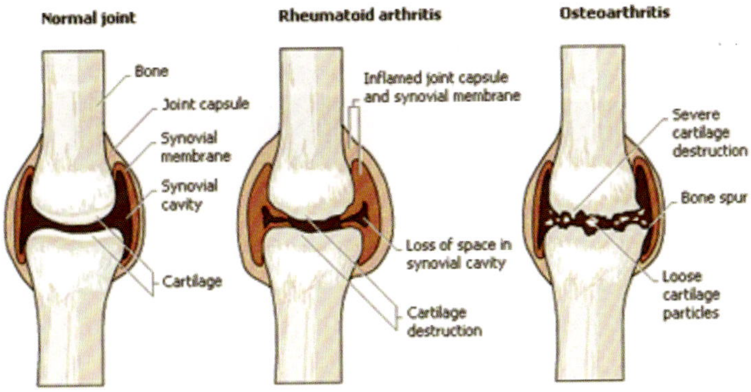

Differentials between Osteoarthritis and Rheumatoid Arthritis

Symptom	Osteoarthritis	Rheumatoid Arthritis
MOA	"Wear and Tear" of articular cartilage	Bone erosion, necrosis, destruction synovial joints
Auto Antibodies	None	Anti-CCP (cyclic citrullinated peptide), RF
DIP	YES	NO
PIP	YES	YES
MCP	NO	YES
Joint WBC/Leukocyte count	< 2000	5,000 – 50,000
Morning stiffness	< 30 minutes	> 1 hour
Inflammation	No	Yes, ↑ ESR, CRP
Treatment	NSAID's, lose weight	Methotrexate
Key Symptoms	Crepitus, osteophytes, subchondral bone cysts, narrowing of joints	Pannus, bone deformity, symmetrical joint involvement, cervical subluxation

Seronegative Spondyloarthropathies

Arthritis negative for RF (Rheumatoid Factor), Not autoimmune

Ankylosing Spondylitis

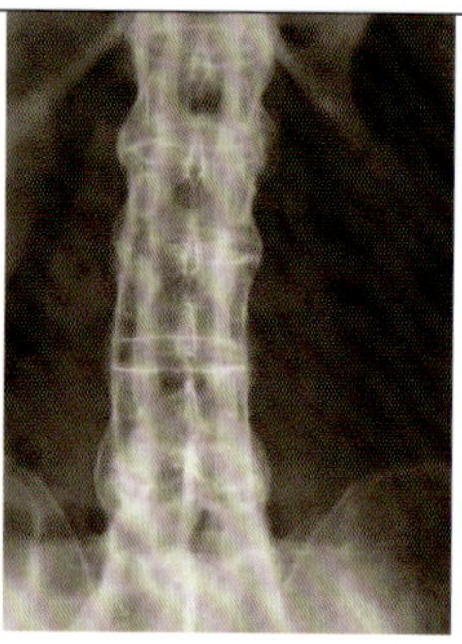

Chronic Inflammatory disease of **sacroiliac joints** (axial skeleton) in the pelvis and spine.
Fusion of joints in spine.

Onset between < 40 years of age.

SX: **Stiff in the mornings or with rest** and **improves throughout the day with activity**, **uveitis** (inflammation in anterior chamber of the eye, redness and floaters), inflammation of the prostate and aorta, **aortic valve insufficiency**. Pain is worse at night. Pain is relieved by leaning forward. Peripheral arthritis of the hips, shoulders, knees.
Complications: **Kyphosis** (Flattening of the normal lumbar curvature), ↓ chest expansion, disorder of tendon attachment of the Achilles tendon, AV block.

DX:
BIT: Flat film XR of **sacroiliac joint** in the pelvis.
MAT: MRI is more sensitive than flat film. MRI detects abnormalities years before x-rays.

X-ray shows "bamboo spine" (fused vertebral joints)
Associated with **HLA-B27**
Negative for RF.

Labs: **↑ CRP and ESR**

TX: Best: Exercise and **NSAIDS.**
Can also use: Infliximab, Sulfasalazine.
Do not use Steroids – they do not work.

Parvo B-19

(AKA: Fifth DZ, Slapped cheek, Erythema infectiosum)

DNA virus: Single stranded, smallest DNA virus.

Seronegative arthritis (negative for RF – rheumatoid factor)

MC in **adults**.
Self-limiting. SX: last 1 – 3 weeks.

Cause: usually transmitted from a child infected with Parvo B-19.
Look for the adult in the vignette to have a job **associated with children** in some way: teacher, daycare, school nurse, etc.

Is the **ONLY** other arthritis that has **symmetrical joint** involvement (Rheumatoid arthritis has symmetrical joint involvement).

NOTE: Pregnant women must not be exposed to Parvo B-19. It can lead to Hydrops Fetalis and fetal death (Hemolytic disease of the newborn).

Psoriatic Arthritis

Inflammatory arthritis that develops in patients with chronic skin psoriasis.

Associated: HLA-B27.
Negative for RF.

SX: **Asymmetrical**, pain, swelling in one or more joints. Involves DIP, **dactylitis ("sausage-like digits), pitting**/lifting/**separation of nails** (onycholysis). (Be careful not to confuse this with onychomycosis), spondylitis or sacroiliitis (sacroiliac joint), pain in the sacrum, **scaly-silver lesions on extensor surfaces** (elbows, knees), Enthesitis (Inflammation of tendinous insertion sites)
Involves the DIP joints.

X-ray shows "pencil in cup" fingers.

TX: NSAIDS (ibuprofen, naproxen), Methotrexate if NSAID's do not work, **sulfasalazine.**
Do not treat with steroids or TNF inhibitors.

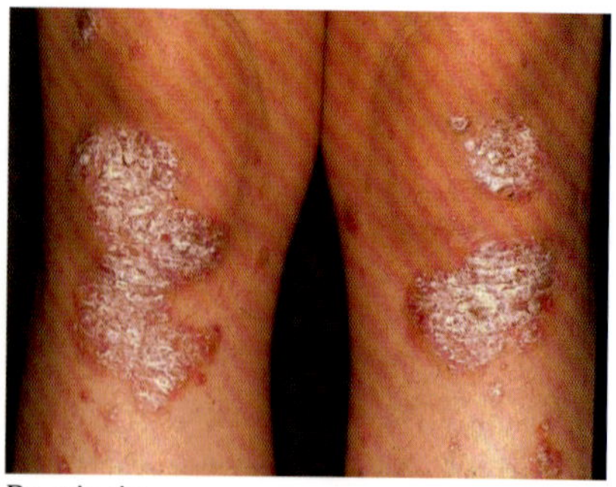

Psoriasis

Psoriatic Arthritis cont'd

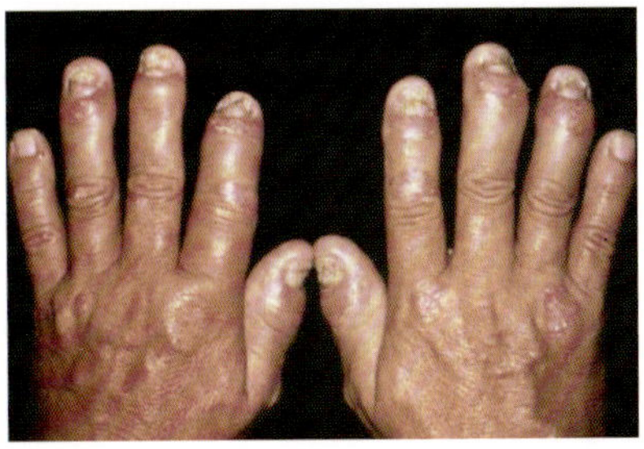

Psoriasis Dactylitis

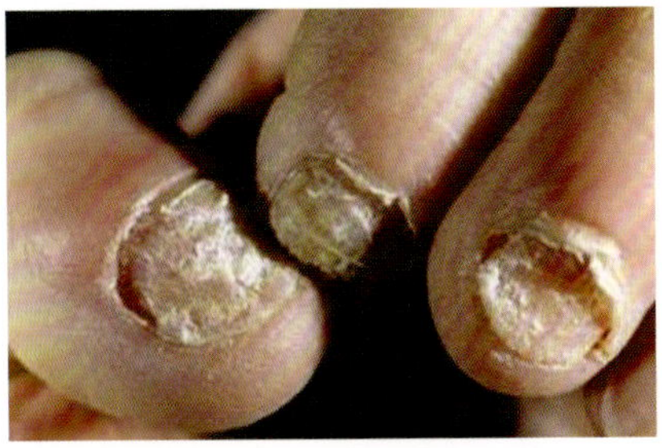

Psoriasis Pitting and separation of nails

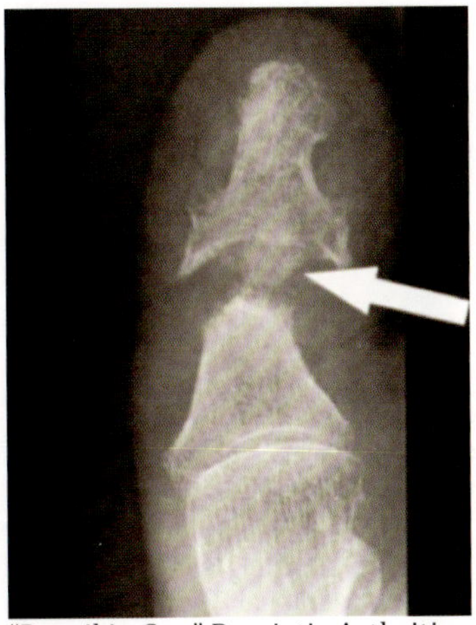

"Pencil in Cup" Psoriatic Arthritis

Lyme Disease Arthritis
Infections disease causes by the Borrelia types of bacteria transmitted via the Ixodes tick.
MC: NE United States)

Lyme arthritis (pain and swelling in the large joints) can occur over a period of several weeks if treatment has not been received. Can result in sporadic bouts of arthritis with neurological issues such as shooting pains, numbness or tingling in the hand and feet and short-term memory problems that worsen from months to years after the infection.

DX: Synovial fluid shows an inflammatory profile: 20% leukocytes (↑ WBC), 50% PMN's, yellow color and negative gram stain.

Confirmatory: Elisa, Western Blot

TX: Doxycycline. If <8 or pregnant: Amoxicillin.

Reactive Arthritis
AKA: **Reiter Syndrome**

Autoimmune condition that develops in response to an infection.
(MC: genitourinary, **Inflammatory bowel** (Ulcerative colitis, Crohn's), **STD**, GI infections, genital lesions (Circinate balanitis: annular dermatitis of the glans penis), urethritis or cervicitis in women, food poisoning, from Salmonella, Shigella or Campylobacter, Yersinia, Chlamydia), **Keratoderma blenorrhagicum** (skin lesions that resemble psoriasis, crusty plaques, found on the palm and soles).
Associated with **HLA-B27**
Negative RF.
SX: Triad of: **Anterior uveitis** (Conjunctivitis – eye pain, redness), Nongonococcal **urethritis (genital abnormalities)**, asymmetric **arthritis**.

(**tip**: Can't pee, see or climb a tree).

TX: **NSAID's,** correct underlying condition. **Sulfasalazine** if NSAID's do not control.

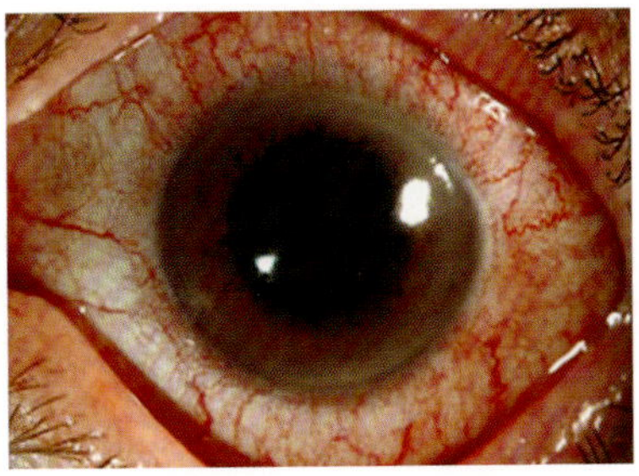

Anterior Uveitis (Conjunctivitis)

Enteropathic Spondylitis
Arthritis associated with **Inflammatory Bowel Disease's**

Ulcerative Colitis
Crohn's Disease

SX: Inflammation of one or more joints that affects either the large weight-bearing joints (knees, hips, shoulders, elbows) or small joints (hands, feet).
Arthritis can involve spine causing ankylosing spondylitis (entire spine) or sacroiliitis (sacroiliac joint).
Painful, warm, swollen, stiff joints

Juvenile Idiopathic Arthritis
AKA: Juvenile Rheumatoid Arthritis (JRA)

Autoimmune, non-infective, Inflammatory.
MCC arthritis in children.
No known cause.
Self-limiting. Last approx.. 6 wks.

SX: ↓ appetite, lethargy, flu-like symptoms, swelling of the joint (MC: knee, ankle, wrist, hands, feet), pain, morning stiffness that improves throughout the day, iridocyclitis (inflammation of the iris).

Septic Arthritis
Gonorrhea/Chlamydia

History of **STD or in sexually active** young persons. MC occurrence during menses.

Septic arthritis (Destroys joints)
SX: Red, swollen, tender joint, immobile, **polyarticular, tenosynovitis** (inflammation of tendon sheaths), **petechial rash.**

DX: Arthrocentesis,

Labs:
WBC (Leukocytosis) 30,000 – 50,000,
↑ **ESR,** turbid synovial fluid.
High risk with arthritic or prosthetic joint.
NOTE: with Gonococcal arthritis cultures must be taken from multiple areas: cervix, rectum, urethra, pharynx.

DX: MAT: arthrocentesis.

TX: **Ceftriaxone, Cefotaxime or Ceftizoxime.**

NOTE: If recurrent gonorrhea infections be sure to check for MAC compliment deficiency.

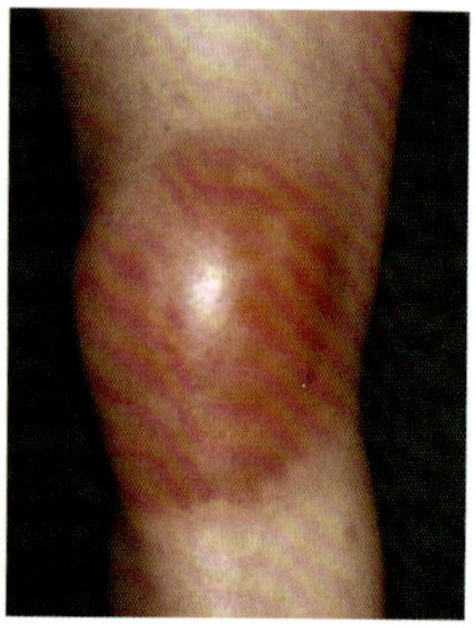

Septic Arthritis
MCC: Staph aureus
MCC: prosthetic joints: S. epidermidis

MCC **Septic Arthritis (destroys joints)**
Bacterial arthritis in **children** and **non-sexually active** adults. MC affects previously damaged joints.

SX: Usually proceeded by cellulitis.
Unilateral (monoarticular) joint, pain, swelling, erythema, immobile joint, chills, fever, unable to bear any weight.

WBC (leukocytosis):
PMN's 50,000 – 100,000,
↑ **ESR,** turbid synovial fluid.

DX: MAT: arthrocentesis.

TX:
Best empiric until culture results: Once culture results return, adjust antibiotics.
Ceftriaxone and Vancomycin.

Sensitive Gram-Positives: **IV Oxacillin, Nafcillin, Cefazolin, Piperacillin with Tazobactam.**

Resistant Gram-Positives: **Linezolid, Daptomycin, Ceftaroline, Tigecycline.**

Gram Negatives: **Fluoroquinolones, Aztreonam, Piperacillin with Tazobactam, Aminoglycosides, and Cefotaxime.**

Penicillin allergy: **Aztreonam, Fluoroquinolone.**

Gouty Arthritis

Gout
Monosodium Urate Crystals

Acute or Chronic. (Acute occurs overnight)
Monoarthritis.
Asymmetric.

Deposits in joint: **Urate crystals due to the crystallization of uric acid (monosodium urate crystals).**

Causes: Binge drinking of **Alcohol**, ↑ **intake of protein (meats)**, **Hyperuricemia** caused by ↑ **production of uric acid** (Lesch-Nyhan, ↑ cell death and turnover (Tumor Lysis Syndrome: ↑↑ cell death due to cancer treatment), ↑ PRPP, von Gierke disease) or **underexcretion of uric acid** (**Thiazide diuretics**, idiopathic), nicotinic acid.

MOA: Alcohol competes for same secretion sites as uric acid in the kidney = ↓ secretion of uric acid = uric acid build up in the blood.

SX: MC: Swollen, red, painful metatarsal-phalangeal joint of **big toe** (1st **podagra**, 1st digit), **Tophus** formation (deposits of uric acid in the joints, bones, cartilage or nodules on the skin. MC: **Achilles tendon**, Pinna of ear (external ear).

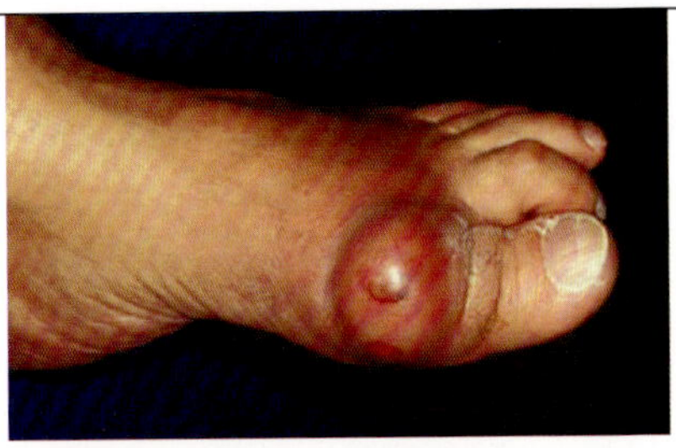
Gout on the big toe (podagra)

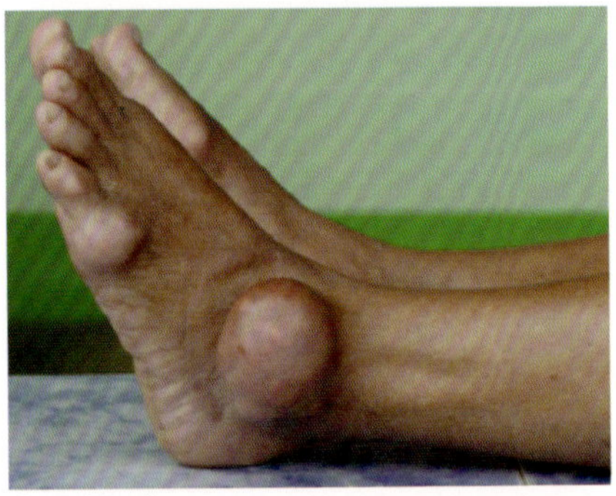
Gout Tophus

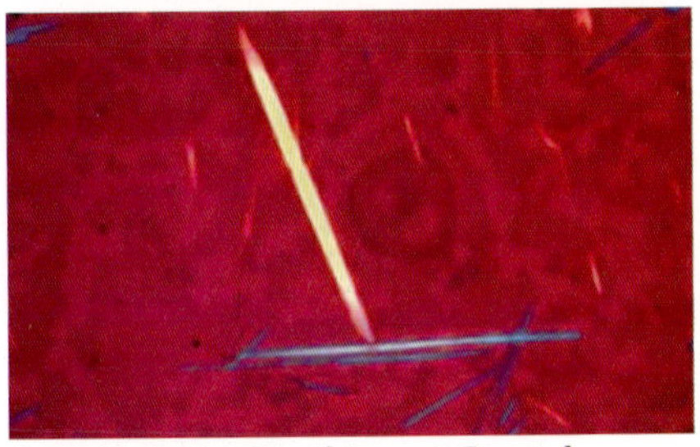
Gout Negative Birefringent Crystals

(**tip**: the crystals in gout look like a negative (-) sign (for negative birefringence), verses the crystals in pseudogout that are rhomboid).

Labs:
MAT: Arthrocentesis (Joint aspiration).
Must tap the joint to make a diagnosis.
Shows: Polarized light shows: **Negative birefringent yellow or blue crystals.**
WBC: 2,000 – 50,000.
X-Ray shows punched-out lesions.

TX:
Acute: #1 =**NSAIDS (indomethacin),**
#2 = colchicine, glucocorticoids.
(Caution: **ALWAYS** pick NSAID's #1 unless patient has a contraindication to NSAID's).

Decrease reoccurrence: Decrease alcohol intake, decrease high protein/purine foods (meat, seafood), no thiazide diuretics.

Chronic or prevention: Allopurinol, Febuxostat (alternative to Allopurinol), Probenecid, Rasburicase, Pegloticase.

Pseudogout
Calcium Pyrophosphate Crystals
(AKA: Chondrocalcinosis)

DX: Deposits in joint: Calcium pyrophosphate crystals

SX: MC: deposits in the larger joints (MC joint: knee. Others: wrist, hip).

Associated with: Hypothyroidism, acromegaly, hemochromatosis, hyperparathyroidism, Hypoparathyroidism, hypophosphatemia, renal osteodystrophy, Wilson's DZ, Osteoarthritis.

Labs:
MAT: Polarized light shows positive birefringent rhomboid crystals.
↑ WBC.

(**tip**: remember: all "P's": Pseudo, Pyrophosphate, Positive crystals)

Associated with: Hypoparathyroidism, Hyperparathyroidism, Hemochromatosis, hypophosphatemia, renal osteodystrophy, Wilson's DZ, Osteoarthritis.

TX:
Acute: #1 =**NSAIDS (indomethacin),**
#2 = colchicine, glucocorticoids.
(Caution: **ALWAYS** pick NSAIDS #1)

Chronic or prevention: Allopurinol, Febuxostat, Probenecid

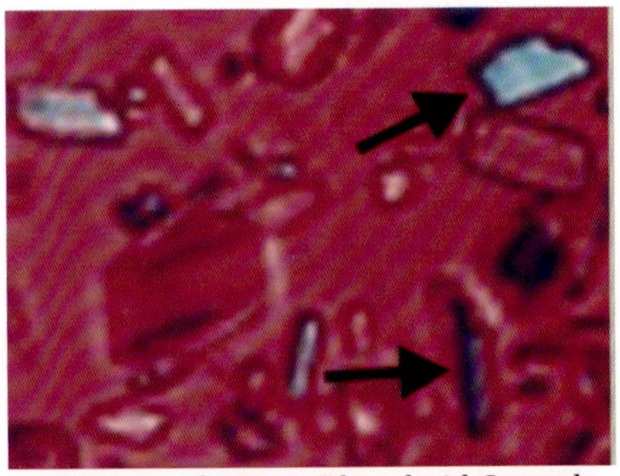
Positive Birefringent Rhomboid Crystals

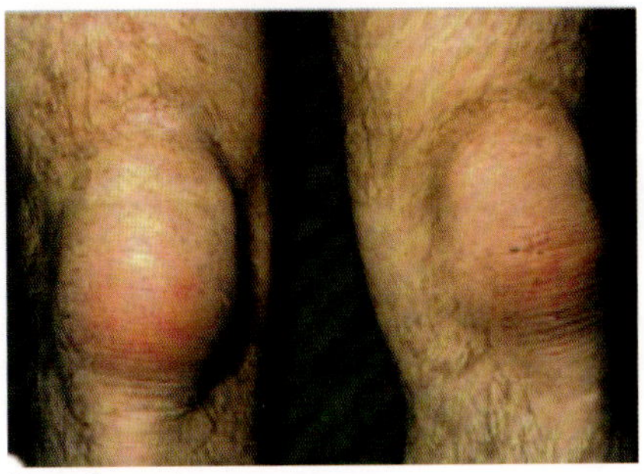
Pseudogout

Back and Spine Pathologies

Nerve Root Innervation

Nerve Root	Reflex Lost	Motor Deficit	Sensory Deficit
C5	Biceps	Deltoid weakness	Shoulder
C6	Brachioradialis	Biceps, wrist extensors	Lateral arm and thumb
C7	Triceps	3rd finger (middle finger)	3rd finger
C8	5th finger	Hand dysfunction (innervates small muscles to hand	Medial hand
L4	Knee Jerk	Dorsiflexion of foot	Medial calf
L5	None	Dorsiflexion foot and big toe	Dorsal foot
S1	Ankle Jerk	Weakness of gastrocnemius, eversion of foot	Lateral foot

Back/Spine Pathologies

- Diagnostic Test: Imaging is required for: ankylosing spondylitis, epidural abscess, Cauda equine, and cord compressions
- **BIT is plain flat film x-ray** for fractures, infection, cancer with compression
- **MAT is an MRI** unless contradiction to an MRI (ie: pacemaker, metal plates) then use a CT
- **DO NOT do imaging** in patients with low back strain or without focal neurological abnormalities
- **Treatment for back with WITHOUT neurological defects: No bed rest. Stay active.**
    - Conservative TX for 4 – 6 weeks: Early mobilization (NO bedrest), no exercise program, muscle relaxants and NSAIDS
    - SX: Acute onset pain with positive straight leg test = possible herniated disc if no neurological defects
    - Rule out cauda equina (perianal area is functional)
    - If rapidly progressing neurological defects (foot drop, weak leg, perianal dysfunction) = emergent surgical decompression

Disk Herniation	Spinal Cord Compression	Spinal Epidural Abscess
AKA: Sciatica Herniation at the **L4/5 and L5/S1**. SX: **Acute pain** radiating down the thigh into the leg and foot. Pain and numbness of medial calf and/or foot. Pain is worse when sitting. DX for disc herniation: **Straight Leg Raise Test** (SLR). Patient lies flat and the leg is raised straight upward to 70°. If pain radiates into the buttocks and **below the knee into the foot = positive test**. If patient claims pain radiates in the low back or hamstrings: negative test = patient faking. Imaging: No imaging for low back pain and a positive SLR test unless neurological deficits are present (numbness, weakness, paralysis, bowel or bladder incontinence, erectile dysfunction). TX: **NSAID's**, **Continue ordinary activity**. **NO bed rest**, it will delay healing. Steroid injection into the epidural space if no improvement with conservative mgmt. **Caution:** If the question says that the pain goes "to the knee", the nerve involved is the femoral, not the sciatic. The sciatic must go to the foot.	**MCC: Cancer** Metastasis from: non-small cell type lung cancers, breast cancer, prostate cancer, renal cell carcinoma, thyroid cancer, lymphoma, multiple myeloma. Medical emergency. DX: MRI SX: **Pain worse at night. Wakes patient up.** Vertebral tenderness, hyperreflexia, ↓ sensation to pin prick/touch, ↑ tendon reflex, positive Babinski. TX: **Must give Glucocorticoid (Dexamethasone) immediately to decrease pressure on the cord. Radiation can be given to help ↓ pain.** Give chemotherapy (lymphoma) or radiation for cancers (solid tumors). Surgical decompression if steroids and radiation/chemotherapy are not effective or if neurological symptoms are present. (S3 and S4 issues causes: numbness, weakness, paralysis, bowel or bladder incontinence, erectile dysfunction).	Collection of pus or inflammatory granulation between dura mater and the vertebral column. Causes: **Hematogenous spread** of infection elsewhere in the body (ie: UTI, cellulitis), IV drug use, IC states (Diabetes, HIV, alcoholic), from injections (epidural anesthesia, steroids). SX: Similar to spinal cord compression symptoms. Vertebral tenderness over lumbar spinal area with constant back pain, hyperreflexia, fever, ↓ sensation to pin prick/touch, ↑ tendon reflex, positive Babinski. **Triad: Fever**, focal spine pain, neurological defects. Can progress to: Motor/sensory defects, bowel/bladder dysfunction, paralysis. Labs: ↑ ESR DX: MRI TX: Surgical drainage for large abscesses. Empiric treatment until cultures return. Empiric TX: **Vancomycin or Linezolid and Gentamicin.** Upon return of culture/sensitivity: Staph sensitive: **Oxacillin, Nafcillin, Cefazolin.**

Cauda Equina Syndrome (CES) Medical Emergency Loss of function of the lumbar plexus (nerve roots) below the conus medullaris of the spinal cord. **CES is a lower motor neuron lesion**. Involves the **spinal nerve roots**. Involves the lower end of the spine. SX: **Asymmetrical** weakness, radiates pain, Severe back pain, **saddle anesthesia** ("pens and needles"). Involves the **S3 – S5** dermatomes (includes perineum, external genitalia, anus), absent bilateral Achilles (ankle) reflex, bladder and bowel dysfunction/incontinence, affects the anus/bladder spincters. **Hyporeflexia.** TX: Emergency surgical decompression.	**Lumbar Spinal Stenosis** MC: Persons over 60. Degenerative change. The **ligamentum flavum** (yellow ligament that connects the laminae of adjacent vertebrae) thickens and compresses the spinal cord in the lumbar vertebra. **SX**: Back pain that radiates bilaterally into the buttocks and thighs when walking. **Pain is worse when walking downhill** (upon extension), pain continues when standing. Pain is **better walking uphill, sitting, cycling and leaning forward** (upon flexion). (can present similar to peripheral artery disease). (Presents similar to PAD but in PAD there are poor pulses and pain is better when standing). Spinal stenosis can simulate peripheral arterial disease (PAD), but ankle/brachial index is normal. **DX:** MRI. Pulses are normal. **TX:** Weight loss, **NSAID's**, steroid injections into lumbar epidural space if standard pain medications do not control the pain. Physical therapy. Surgical decompression to dilate the spinal canal.	**Ankylosing Spondylitis** See Ankylosing Spondylitis above under Seronegative Spondyloarthropathies.
Anterior Spinal Artery Infarction All sensation lost. Position and vibratory senses preserved. No TX	**Brown-Sequard Syndrome** MC: Knife wound injury to the spine.. SX: Loss of ipsilateral vibratory and position senses and loss of contralateral pain and temperature.	**Conus Medullaris** **UMN and LMN lesion.** **SX: Symmetrical** weakness. Involves **L1 and L2**. Involves the higher end of the spine. **Hyperreflexia**

Vertebral Osteomyelitis AKA: Spinal osteomyelitis) Infection and inflammation of the bone and bone marrow. Occurs: IV drug use, Sickle Cell, Immunocompromised, S. aureus, or distant infections that spread (ie: UTI, cellulitis). SX: Pain and tenderness over vertebra. Pain is not relieved with rest. Fever, swelling at the infection site, night sweats, difficulty moving from a standing to a sitting position, muscle spasms. DX: MRI, ↑ ESR, ↑ WBC TX: IV antibiotics, surgery (depends upon the severity).	**Compression Fracture** **Pathologic fracture** MC: **Osteoporosis**, Ankylosing spondylitis, multiple myeloma, Osteomalacia. Things that predispose to this condition: Post menopause, senile osteoarthritis, steroid use. Caused by demineralization (↓ bone density). Microarchitecture is disrupted. SX: Acute intense pain in vertebra, spine tenderness. Pain does NOT stop when lying down or resting, ↑ pain on strain or cough. **NOTE:** There will be ↓ ankle reflexes in the elderly but this IS **NORMAL AGING.** **NOTE:** If pain is due to a ligamentous sprain, the pain will ↑ with movement but get better with rest.	**Lumbo-sacral pain** Pain after physical exertion (lifting). SX: No radiation, No weakness, No sensory changes, No neurological defects. Local tenderness to the paraspinal muscles. DX: Normal leg raise test. TX: **NSAID's** continued activity, NO bed rest.
Spondylolisthesis Forward displacement/slip of a vertebra. MC: L5 slips to S1 ("Step off") between 6 and 16 years old. Can also be due to degenerative DZ due to joint arthritis and ligamentum flavum weakness. SX: Constant back pain, general stiffening of the back, tightened hamstrings, change in gait, atrophy of the gluteal muscles, paresthesias, neurological dysfunction (ie: bed wetting).		

Back Pain Recommendations

- When lifting: Keep back straight and bend knees
- Regular exercise (strength support for the back and abdominal muscles)
- Good sleeping position, do not sleep on stomach
- Warm up before activities/sports
- Avoid exercise with repetitive twist and bending

Back Pain Differentials

Pathology	Symptoms	Physical Exam/Notes
Ankylosing Spondylitis	Stiff in the mornings, improves through the day	"Bamboo spine" on XR, ↓ chest expansion
Cauda Equina	Erectile dysfunction, bladder and/or bowel incontinence	Saddle anesthesia
Compression Fracture	Due to Osteoporosis, demineralization/↓ bone density	Intense pain in vertebra, spine tenderness
Cord Compression	Cancer	Vertebral tenderness, hyperreflexia
Disk Herniation (Sciatica)	Numbness/pain down to the foot and/or medial calf	Positive straight leg test, loss of knee and ankle reflexes
Lumbar Spinal Stenosis	Pain/stiffness walking downhill or standing. Better when going uphill and leaning forward	Pain radiates bilaterally into the buttocks and thighs
Lumbo-Sacral Pain	Pain after exertion (lifting)	Tenderness to the paraspinal muscles, no radiation/weakness or sensory problems.
Spinal Epidural Abscess	↑ ESR, Fever, focal spine pain	Intense pain in vertebra, spine tenderness

Bone Cancer

MC Cancers that metastasis to the bone

- Breast, lung, thyroid, testes, prostate, kidney

Prognosis based on stage

Dull achy pain, worse at night

Osteoblastic	Osteolytic (AKA: Lytic lesions)	Osteoblastic or Osteolytic
Prostate Small Cell Lung Hodgkins **DX: Tech 99 Bone Scan Positive findings on X-Ray**	Multiple Myeloma Non-small cell Non-Hodgkins **DX: X-ray or PET scan, CT (CT or MRI to access Fx risk, MRI to access neuro involvement)**	Breast **DX: PET scan, CT, MRI, Bone scan (CT or MRI to access Fx risk, MRI to access neuro involvement)**

Bone Marrow Transplants

- Rejection: **Graft vs Host** (also seen with liver cancer)
  TX: Steroids
- Leads to ↑ risk of Aspergillus pneumonia (Patchy upper lob infiltrate)

Giant Cell Tumor	Osteochondroma	Osteosarcoma
Benign Tumor Location: Epiphyseal end of long bones. MC: Knee MC: Ages 20 – 40 years old SX: Pain and limited motion, fracture at site of tumor. DX: Biopsy shows Multinucleated giant cells (osteoclast-like cells) X-Ray: **"Soap Bubble" appearance**.	**MC benign tumor of the bone.** MC in children 13 – 15 years old during skeletal growth. X-Ray: **Cartilage-capped bony projection (overgrowth)** located where cartilage forms bone. (AKA: Cartilaginous cap). Pedunculated (stalk) – looks like a cauliflower. TX: Surgery	AKA: Osteogenic Sarcoma Malignant tumor. (#2 MC malignant bone cancer, #1 is Multiple Myeloma) Mesenchymal origin. Presents: 10 – 20 years and again at > 65 years. Cause: Familial: **RB Gene (Retinoblastoma)**, Li-Fraumeni syndrome (P53 mutation), Bone dysplasias: Paget's DZ of the bone, fibrous dysplasia. 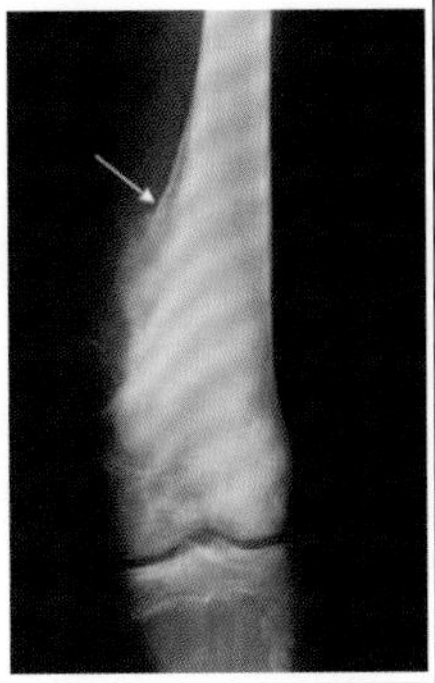 SX: **Pain worse at night.** Pain generally in lower femur, just below knee. Fracture with minor trauma, swelling

Giant Cell Tumor
"Soap Bubble" tumor

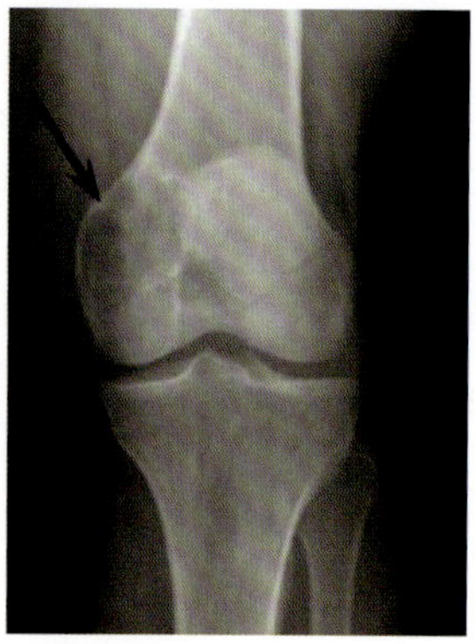

Osteochondroma

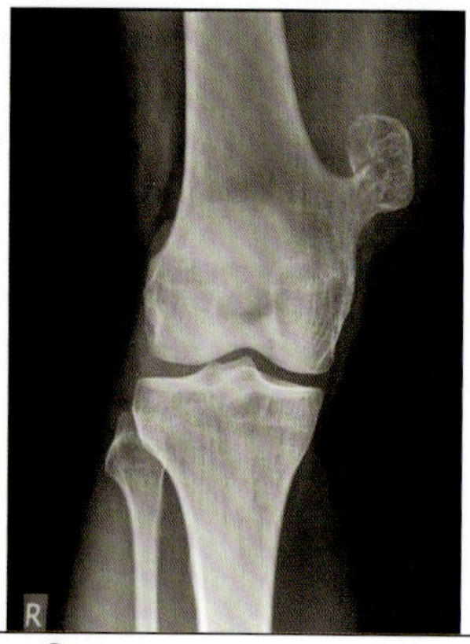

DX: X-ray shows **Codman triangle (elevation of the periosteum)**, AKA: **Sunburst pattern**.

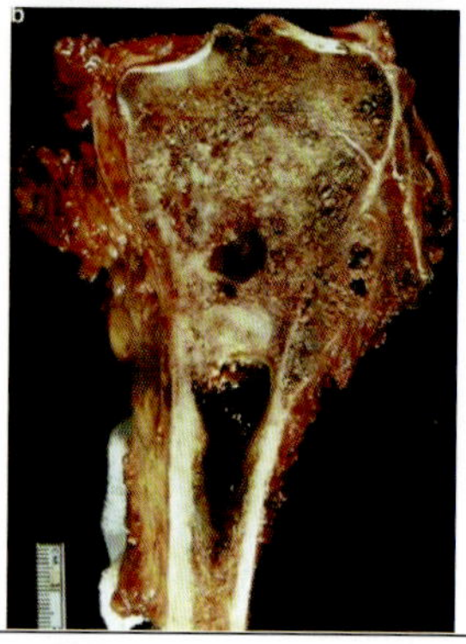

Chondrosarcoma

Malignant, Cartilage tumor.

Presents at all ages.
Affects MC: axial skeleton.

DX: Biopsy, immunohistochemistry (detecting antigens by antibody binding).

DX: **Shinny mass inside the central cavity** of the bone shaft (medullary cavity).

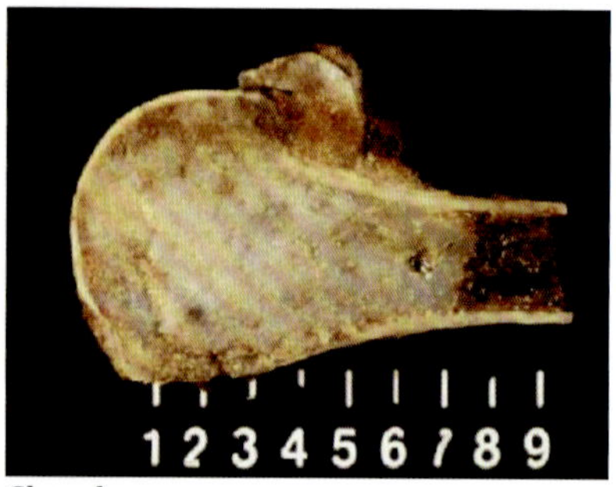

Chondrosarcoma

Ewing Sarcoma
Malignant.

DX: **Small, round, blue cell tumor** with clear cytoplasm (due to glycogen).

MC: teenagers, young adults. MC: pelvis and long bones at growth plate. Other locations: femur, humerus, ribs, clavicle, and scapula).

Associated with **translocation 11:22.**

SX: anemia, fever, pain.

Labs: ↑WBC (leukocytosis), ↑ ESR.

X-Ray: Periosteal reaction (AKA: onion-skin appearance).

TX: Chemotherapy

"Onion-Skin"

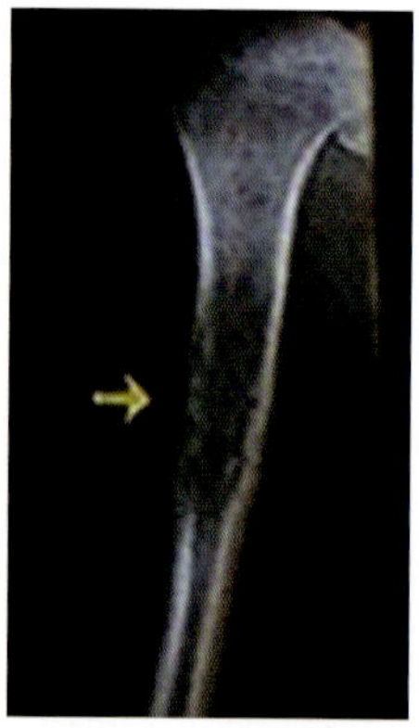

Liposarcoma

Malignant, Fat cell tumor in deep soft tissue (ie: thighs or retroperitoneum). High rate of mitosis.

DX: Biopsy shows **lipoblasts**: Shows small round blue cells or myxoid cells. Clear multi-vacuolated cytoplasm and an eccentric darkly staining nucleus (AKA: Signet ring-type cell). Nucleus and nuclear membrane shows scalloping.
Spindle cells can also be present in variants of the liposarcoma.

Risk Factors: Exposure to herbicides, wood preservatives, radiation. Can be associated with: Neurofibromatosis, Tuberous sclerosis, Retinoblastoma.

SX: Deep mass in the soft tissue (arm, leg, trunk) will show swelling. If located in the chest: cough and SOB. In the abdomen: vomiting, constipation, abdominal pain. In the uterus: bleeding and pelvic pain. Most are slow growing and painless.

TX: Surgery, radiation, chemotherapy

NOTE: A liposarcoma is NOT a lipoma.

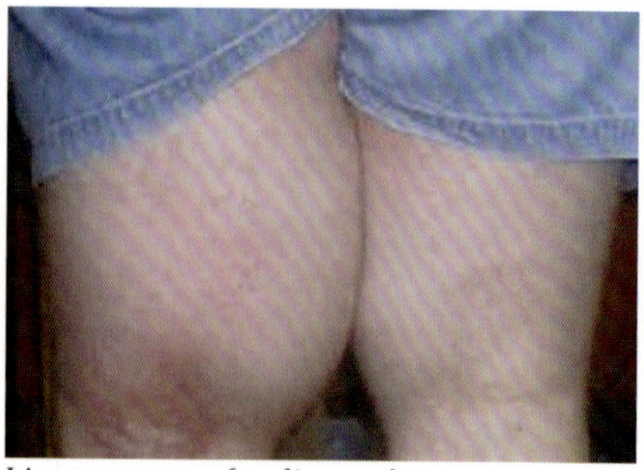

Liposarcoma (malignant)

Lipoma **Lipoma** is a benign tumor composed of **adipose tissue.** MC soft tissue tumor. SX: Soft, mobile and painless. TX: Excision or mesotherapy. 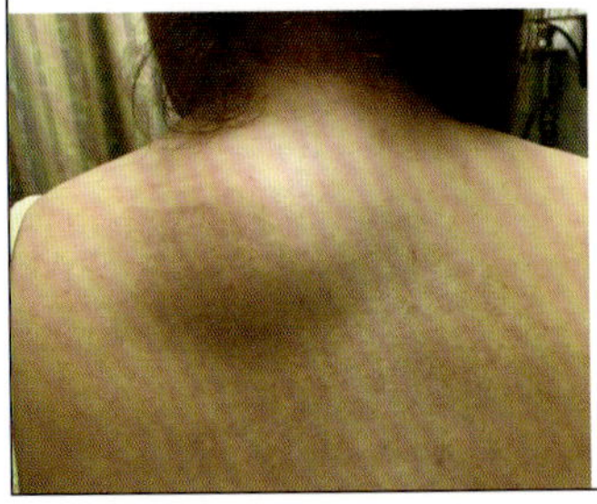 Lipoma (Benign)		

Connective Tissue, Muscle Autoimmune Disorders

The "pathway" to autoimmune disorders: Autoimmune disorders are due to mutation in the FAS protein that occurs during the negative selection process of the T cells in the thymus (Negative selection: when the T cell recognizes itself too much and attacks its own self). **Mutation in the FAS protein** does not allow the activation of the extrinsic pathway in which caspase 8 mediates apoptosis/deletion of that T cell. The mutation allows the Fas protein to bind with the FADD protein and inhibit apoptosis. Thereby allowing the T cell that recognizes itself too much (auto-antibody) to live and be released to attack ones own body.

Note: ALL autoimmune diseases (below and in other chapters) are all due to **mutations in the FAS protein**. It is important to understand all parts of this extrinsic pathway (above and in the immunology chapter) in case the question uses any other part of the pathway, other than a FAS mutation, in their answer choices.

Sarcoidosis
Noncaseating granulomas (macrophages) that form nodules in multiple organs.
Type IV hs.
MC: African American females.

SX: **Erythema nodosum**, **bilateral hilar adenopathy,** uveitis, arthritis, Lupus pernio (raised, hardened purplish lesion on the face), interstitial fibrosis (pulmonary fibrosis, **restrictive lung DZ pattern**: ↓ RV, ↓ TLC, ↓ FVC, ≥ 80% FEV_1/FVC ratio). Cardia shows **restrictive cardiomyopathy**. Neuro affects CN VII. Vision: **Uveitis** that can cause blindness.
Can also include the kidneys and liver.
Lupus pernio (**purple lesions on skin of the face**).

Labs:
HLA-B7, DR15, HLA-DR3
↑ **ACE levels**, ↑ **Calcium** (macrophages release Vit D = ↑ 1α Hydroxylase = ↑ intestinal reabsorption of calcium), ↑ **1,25 Dihydroxycholecalciferol**.

DX:
BIT: CXR show bilateral **hilar adenopathy** (enlarged lymph notes).
MAT: Lung or lymph node **biopsy** showing **noncaseating granulomas**.
Bronchoalveolar lavage shows ↑ helper cells.

TX: **Steroids.**

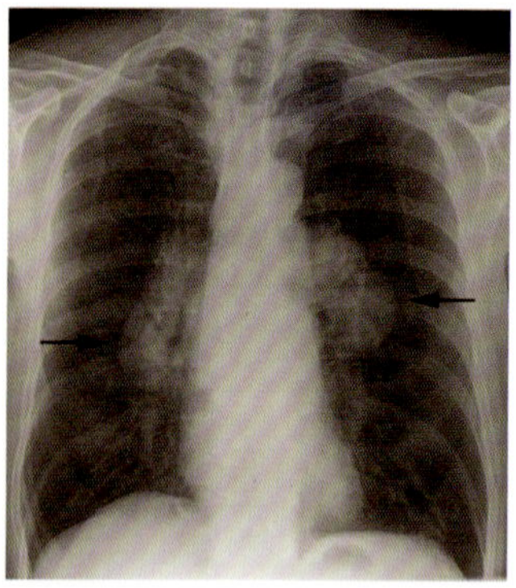

Bilateral Hilar Adenopathy

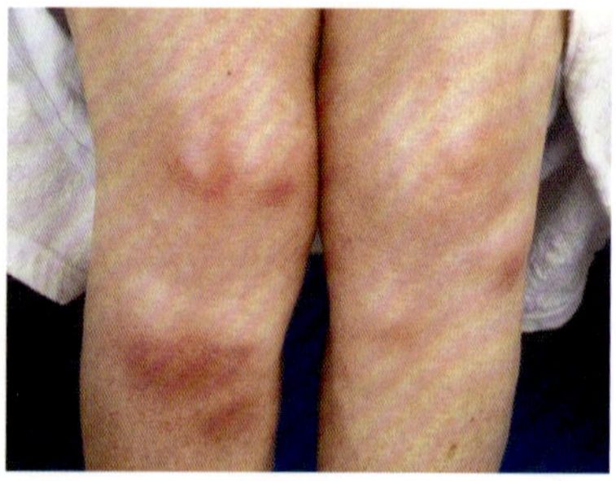

Erythema Nodosum

Scleroderma
AKA: Systemic (Diffuse) Sclerosis
Multi-organ involvement
(AKA: CREST Syndrome plus involvement of the kidney, heart and lungs)
SX: Triad of SX: **Sclerodactyly:** Fibrous **thickening** and tightening of the skin on fingers due to fibroblast overproducing and ↑ collagen deposition in the skin. (MC seen on the face and hands).
Raynaud's: stress or cold temps cause vasoconstriction of arterioles causing cyanosis and pain. Complications: ulcers, gangrene.
Heartburn (GERD, **Esophageal dysmotility** = **dysphagia** from food stuck in esophagus (**↓ UES and LES tone**).
Cardiac: Pulmonary HTN causes right ventricular hypertrophy. Pericarditis, heart block, myocardial fibrosis.
Pulmonary: Pulmonary **fibrosis** (aka: diffuse interstitial fibrosis) and pulmonary HTN.
Renal: Malignant HTN.

Labs: **Scl-70 antibody, ANA, anti-topoisomerase.**

TX: **Methotrexate**.
Renal: **ACE inhibitors**
Esophageal dysmotility: **PPI's**
Raynaud's: **Calcium Channel Blockers**
Pulmonary Fibrosis: **Cyclophosphamide**
Pulmonary HTN: **Bosentan, Sildenafil, Prostacyclin analogs**

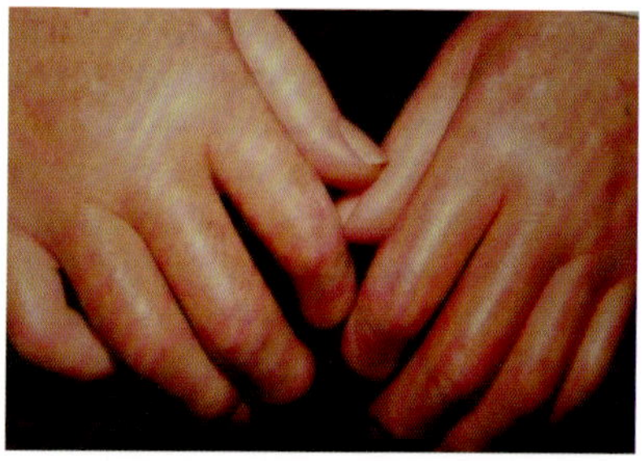

Sclerodactyly

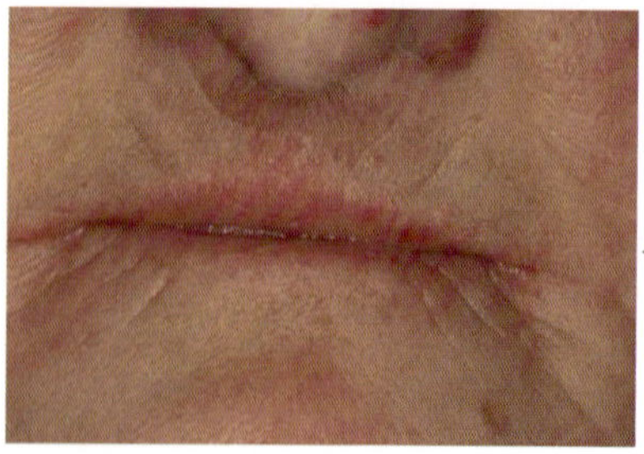

CREST Syndrome
Limited Scleroderma
(AKA: CREST only involves C-R-E-S-T and not kidney, heart and lungs)

SX:
C= ↑ Calcium
R = Reynaud's phenomenon
E = Esophageal dysmotility
S = Sclerodactyly
T = Telangiectasia

DOES **NOT** PRESENT WITH:
Cardiac, Lung, Kidney, or Joint symptoms.
(this is Scleroderma – Diffuse/Systemic)

Labs:
Anticentromere antibodies (specific)
ANA (antinuclear antibodies)
Normal ESR.

Calcium ↑: causes thickening, tightening of skin, calcinosis (calcific nodules).
Reynaud's: stress, cold temps cause vasoconstriction of arterioles causing cyanosis and pain. Complications: ulcers, gangrene and giant capillaries in the nail folds).
Esophageal dysmotility = **dysphagia** from food stuck in esophagus (**↓ UES and LES tone**).
Sclerodactyly: Thickening of the skin on fingers due to fibroblast overproducing and ↑ collagen deposition in the skin.
Telangiectasia: Dilated capillaries. (MC sites: face, palms of hands).
Sclerodactyly: Fibrous thickening and tightening of the skin on fingers due to fibroblast overproducing and ↑ collagen deposition in the skin. MC on the face and hands).

TX: **Methotrexate**.
Esophageal dysmotility: **PPI's**
Raynaud's: **Calcium Channel Blockers**

Dermatomyositis
(Related to Polymyositis)
Perimysial inflammation (the sheath surrounding the muscle fibers).
Mixed B, T , CD4 cell Inflammation of muscles and skin.
(**tip**: "D" in dermatomyositis for "D" for involvement of duel (two) cells = B and T)

Labs:
Anti-Mi2 antibodies
ANA antibodies
Histidine-tRNA autoantibodies.
↑ CPK, ↑ aldolase, ↑ ESR, abnormal electromyogram (EMG) showing spontaneous muscle fibrillation, **RASHES**.

If presence of **anti-Jo-1 antibodies** =
↑ risk of pulmonary fibrosis (interstitial lung DZ)

Complication: Malignancy.
Dermatomyositis is associated with cancers of: lymphoma, GI, lung, ovary.

DX: MAT: **Muscle biopsy**. Biopsy shows shrunken polygonal muscle fibers. Muscle fiber atrophy. Muscle inflammation. (AKA: perivascular infiltrates of inflammatory cells).
Microscopy shows aggregates of mature lymphocytes with small, dark nuclei and scant cytoplasm surrounding vessels. Immunohistochemistry shows B and T cells.

SX: **Gottron papules** (scaly, red patches over the MCP joints, knuckles, knees, elbows), **heliotrope rash** (red, itching, swelling over the upper eyelids or around the eye), periungual telangiectasia's, dysphagia, Mechanic's hand (rough, cracked skin), "Shawl Sign (shoulder and neck erythema), symmetric **proximal (girdle) muscle weakness** and pain, **difficulty in ascending stairs, rising from a chair, combing hair.**
Presents with various skin rashes.
Calcinosis (deposits of calcium) in the skin, joints and tissues.

Note: Statin's have been linked to dermatomyositis/polymyositis but biopsies showed rhabdomyolysis.

TX: **Steroids (Glucocorticoids), Methotrexate, Azathioprine, IVIG, Mycophenolate.**
Hydroxychloroquine for skin lesions.

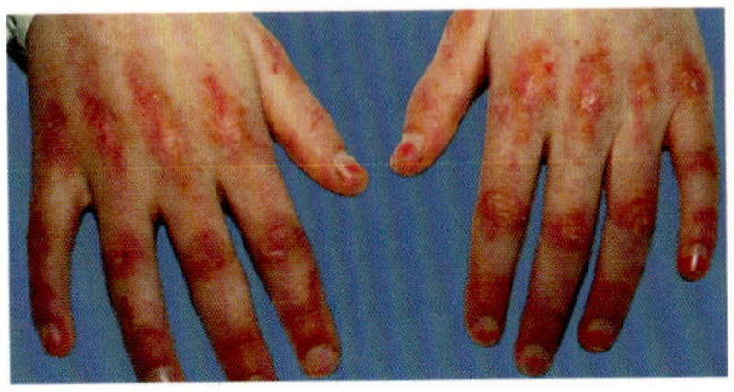

Gottron Papules

Heliotrope Rash

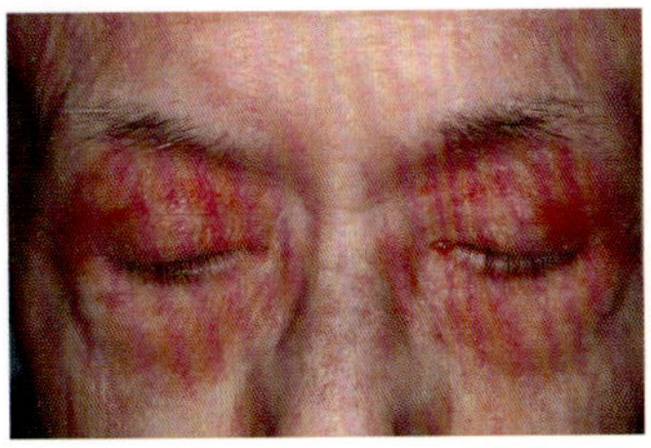

Polymyositis
(Related to Dermatomyositis)
Endomysial inflammation (within the muscle/within the sheath).

Cytotoxic T cells (CD8) Inflammation of muscles.

Labs: Autoantibodies:
ANA antibodies
IFNγ, IL-1, TNFα.
↑ CPK, ↑ aldolase, abnormal electromyogram (EMG). **NO RASHES.**

If presence of **anti-Jo-1 antibodies** =
↑ risk of pulmonary fibrosis (interstitial lung DZ)

Complication: Malignancy.

DX: MAT: Muscle biopsy.

SX: **Proximal (girdle) weakness** and pain with loss of muscle mass. **Difficulty in ascending stairs, rising from a chair, combing hair**, dysphagia (↓ esophageal motility), interstitial lung dz.
Does NOT present with skin rashes.

TX: **Steroids (Glucocorticoids), Methotrexate, Azathioprine, IVIG, Mycophenolate**

Dermatomyositis vs Polymyositis

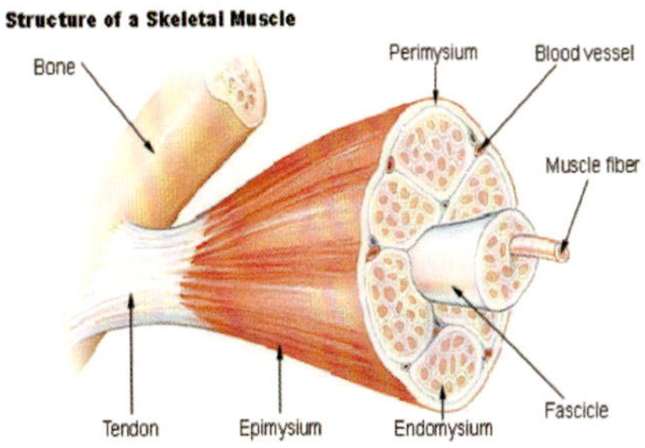

Fibromyalgia

Chronic, widespread pain and response to pressure.

Cause: Unknown. Current theories state that it is due to central sensitization. This lowers threshold for pain because of increased activity of pain nerve cells in the CNS.

SX: Associated with **depression**, anxiety and fatigue. Pain is noted at many locations (hips, back, shoulders). Will also see dysphagia, paresthesias, joint stiffness, fatigue, sleep disturbances, myalgia, **non-refreshing sleep**, muscle spasms, palpitations, bowel disturbances, GU symptoms.

DX: **"Point Tenderness"** upon exam.
AKA: Multiple tender points, Tenderness at trigger points.
All blood test are normal.

TX: **Exercise,**
Best initial medical therapy:
Duloxetine, Pregabalin, Milnacipran, TCA's (Amitriptyline), Anti-seizure meds, weak opioids, trigger point injections.

Polymyalgia Rheumatica (PMR)	Chronic Fatigue Syndrome
SX: Pain and stiffness in the **proximal neck, shoulders** and **hips (pelvic girdle).** Additional symptoms: Weight loss, fatigue, normocytic anemia, no muscle atrophy. **Associated with temporal arteritis.** **MC: > 50 years old.** **Labs: ↑ ESR,** normal CPK, EMG aldolase and muscle biopsy. TX: **Prednisone,** exercise to strengthen weak muscles. **Note**: Do not get this confused with Syringomyelia. Syringomyelia is a cyst (syrinx) inside the spinal cord that results in paralysis and weakness of the back and shoulders ("Cape-like" area). It does NOT Include the hips like Polymyalgia Rheumatica does.	Long term fatigue that it limits person's ability to carry out daily activities **> 6 months.** Cause unknown. SX: Symptoms are sudden onset accompanied by a flu-like illness. Malaise after exertion, non-refreshing strength, arthralgia (joint pain), widespread muscle and joint pain, headaches, chronic mental and physical exhaustion, recurring sore throats, tender lymph nodes, depression, sensitivity to light, dizziness, irritable bowel syndrome, cognition deficits (↓ memory, reaction time, attention), Fibromyalgia type symptoms but **no trigger points.** DX and TX: All test and labs normal. **No** diagnosis or treatments. Must rule out other potential causes of symptoms.

Proximal Weakness Differentials

Proximal weakness means difficulty rising from a chair, ascending steps, brushing hair. These involve the central, postural muscles.

Disease	Differential	Notes
Dermatomyositis	**Perimysial** inflammation. Skin lesions/rashes: Heliotrope rash, Gottron papules. **Anti-Mi-2 antibodies**. Mixed **B & T cell, CD4** inflammation.	
Polymyositis	**Endomysial** inflammation. Cytotoxic **T cell, CD8** inflammation.	No rash involvement.
Polymyalgia Rheumatica (PMR)	Involves neck, shoulders, **hips (pelvis).**	Don't confuse this with Syringomyelia: (cyst/cavity that forms inside the spinal cord): this involves ONLY the neck and shoulders (arms): "Cape like pattern". Loss of feeling with pain, weakness or paralysis. Associated with Temporal Arteritis.
Lambert Eaton	Antibodies against **calcium** channels. Associated with **Small Cell** lung cancer,	Weakness improves through the day.
Myasthenia Gravis	Antibodies against **ACh receptors**. Associated with **Thymoma**.	Becomes weaker through the day.

Systemic Lupus Erythematosus Lupus, SLE	Antiphospholipid Syndrome (APL)	Sjögren Syndrome
Multiorgan: affects heart, kidney, lungs, joints, blood vessels, nerves, skin Type III HS Labs: **BIT: Anti-nuclear (ANA)** **MAT: Anti-dsDNA** **MAT: Anti-smith (anti-Sm)** **Antihistone (drug induced lupus).** **Anti-cardiolipin, Antiphospholipid (hypercoagulability)** **Anti-SSA, Anti-SSB, ↑ clots, emboli, spontaneous miscarriages/abortions).** **Anti-Ro.** **↓ Compliment C3 (always check levels) (tip:** C3 for 3 letters of SLE) **Eosinophilia (in drug induced).** **Thrombocytopenia,** hemolysis, leukopenia. **Can have ↑ ESR** **NOTE: Presence of anti-RO or anti-SSA increases the risk of heart block.** **BIT: ANA** **Most specific test: Anti-DS DNA or Anti-Smith (Anti-Sm).** **Monitoring guidelines: (Must monitor compliment levels to track progression of Lupus) Compliment ↓ in flair ups.** **Anti-DS DNA ↑ in flair ups.** SX: **Any 4 of the following is a diagnosis of Lupus:** (Basically if patient has joint pain, rash, fatigue). Arthralgia (joint pain), fatigue, **malar face rash** (butterfly rash over the nose and cheeks), photosensitive, **oral ulcers, Raynaud's, endocarditis** (Libman-Sacks), pulmonary emboli, pulmonary HTN, **kidney failure (membranous glomerulonephritis: red cell casts, hematuria)**, neurologic/CNS (headaches, seizures, depression, psychosis, stroke, meningitis), **spontaneous abortions** (miscarriage due to **Antiphospholipid** syndrome), fatigue, anemia, mucosal ulcers, emboli, clotting, photosensitivity, serositis (inflammation of the pleura and pericardium = chest pain), Ocular problems (photophobia, retinal lesions/cotton wool spots, blindness), myocarditis. **Endocarditis**: Libman-Sacks (non-bacterial endocarditis). Can also lead to pericarditis, pulmonary HTN and pneumonia.	IgG or IgM antibodies against negatively charged phospholipids. Can be associated with Lupus. **Anticardiolipin antibodies** associated with spontaneous abortions/miscarriages. **Lupus anticoagulant** associated with ↑ PTT (clotting). SX: **Thrombosis** (clotting) of veins and arteries, recurrent **spontaneous abortions/**miscarriages. Labs: ↑ PTT, normal PT/INR. **False positives with VDRL/RPR** (Syphilis) and normal FTA. DX: **BIT: Mixing study: Mixing patients plasma with normal plasma. If APL antibody present the PTT level in the mixture will stay elevated.** **MAT: Russell Viper Venom Test (RVVT): RVVT is prolonged if APL antibodies are present.** **NOTE: APL is important to test for in the case of the first clot for the individual. If APL is the reason for the first clot, they will require lifelong Warfarin.** **TX: Check patient for APL antibodies if ≥ 2 first-trimester or 1 second trimester abortion/miscarriage occurs.** **Prophylaxis to prevent reoccurrence: Heparin and aspirin.** **Caution: do not use Warfarin during pregnancy.**	Associated with Rheumatoid arthritis, SLE, Hashimoto's, Primary biliary cirrhosis, Polymyositis. Autoimmune: WBC **destroys exocrine glands** (salivary and lacrimal). Labs: **Anti-Ro, Anti-La, Anti-SSA, Anti-SSB, RF, ANA (antinuclear antibodies)** **Autoantibodies to snRNP's** (AKA: Ribonucleoprotein antigens, spliceosome, introns and exons). ↑ CSF levels of IL-1. SX: Xerostomia (**dry mouth**), Keratoconjunctivitis sicca (AKA: **dry eyes**, Xerophthalmia. Feels like grains of sand in the eye), Dental **cavities**/caries (no saliva so can't help prevent cavities), polydipsia (due to dry mouth), dyspareunia (due to vaginal dryness), dry skin, fatigue, bilateral parotid enlargement, **dysphagia** (no saliva to help swallow). Complications: **Lymphoma (in 10% of patients – test for), lung DZ, Pancreatitis, Vasculitis, Renal tubular acidosis.** DX: **MAT: Lip or parotid gland biopsy: show lymphoid infiltration.** **Schirmer test: ↓ eye lacrimation (tearing) shows ↓ wetting of filter paper when placed on the eye.** **TX: Must keep eyes and mouth moist.** **Pilocarpine, Cevimeline** (↑ ACh = ↑ secretions) to ↑ secretions and saliva. Artificial tears to ↓ risk of corneal ulcers. **Note:** Remember that Sjogren's and Beta Thalassemia are results of mutations in the snRNP's (spliceosome's).

Systemic Lupus Erythematosus cont'd

Kidney failure: Nephrotic: Membranous glomerulonephritis showing **"wire looping"** and Nephritic symptoms: Diffuse proliferative glomerulonephritis.

False positives for syphilis.

TX: Methotrexate and steroids, NSAIDS, Hydroxychloroquine.
NOTE: In any pathology where systemic steroids (glucocorticoids) are being used (ie: RA, Lupus) remember that **any of the side effects or signs from steroid use can be seen** in the patient: osteoporosis, atrophied adrenal gland, avascular necrosis.

Specific TX:
Joint pain: NSAID's.
Acute flair ups: Prednisone.
Severe DZ: Cyclophosphamide, Belimumab (inhibits B cells), Azathioprine.
Nephritis: Mycophenolate (fore effective than Cyclophosphamide).

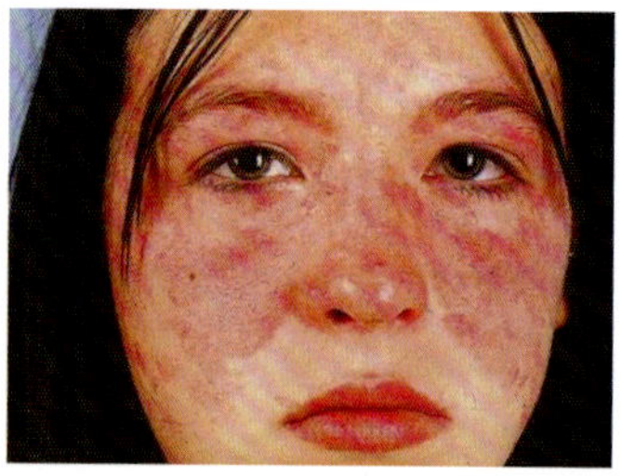

Malar Rash

Drug Induced Lupus

Most common drugs that cause Lupus-like syndrome:
Isoniazid, Procainamide, Hydralazine.

Labs: **anti-Histone antibodies** or Positive ANA

Normal labs: compliment, anti-DS DNA.
No CNS involvement

Lambert - Eaton	Myasthenia Gravis	Felty's Syndrome
Autoantibodies against presynaptic (P/Q type) voltage gated calcium channels, which causes ↓ in release of ACh. Labs: HLA-DR3. Associated with **Small Cell Cancer** of the lung. (Paraneoplastic syndrome: cancer effects not due to cancer cells but hormone/cytokines excreted by the tumor) (**Caution:** Be careful when the questions mention there is a mass seen on X-ray. It could be a thymoma or small cell so carefully read the SX to decide if it is MG or LE). SX: **Proximal weakness** of the arms, legs and trunk. ANS SX: dry mouth, sweating, orthostatic hypotension (blackouts), blurred vision. **Weakness gets better through the day.** As compared to Myasthenia Gravis, Lambert Eaton has more lower extremity weakness and less weakness of the eye muscles = **no ptosis., no eye involvement. Lambert-Eaton also gets better through the day.**	Autoantibodies against postsynaptic **ACh receptor** at the **neuromuscular junction** which ↓ action potential (excitatory effects). Labs: HLA-DR3, HLA-DR1. Type II hs. Associated with **thymoma** (described as **"thymic shadow" on x-ray**) TX: **Diplopia** (double vision), ptosis (weak levator palpebrae superioris), fatigue, weakness, **dysphagia** (esophagus is a muscle = weak ↓ ability to swallow), **dyspnea** (diaphragm is a muscle = respirator arrest). **Gets weaker as the day progresses.** **Complication:** Muscle weakness will eventually affect the diaphragm so in a myasthenia gravis crisis, ventilation may be necessary. DX: Edrophonium test. (seldom used today). (aka: Tensilon Test) **TX: Pyridostigmine (Acetylcholinesterase inhibitor), Atropine.** Thymectomy. **Caution:** Do NOT mix this up with Lambert-Eaton. LE gets better though the day, MG gets weaker. Both LE and MG will show a "mass" on a chest x-ray: LE = Small Cell lung cancer and MG: Thymoma. LE does NOT affect the eye, MG affect the eyes. LE is against channels and MG is against receptors.	Combination of rheumatoid arthritis, splenomegaly and neutropenia. MC: 50 – 70 years old. Labs: HLA-DR4, ↓ WBC, ↓ Platelets SX: Painful, stiff, swollen joints, enlarged spleen, ↓ WBC (neutropenia), fever, fatigue, weight loss, skin pigmentation, ulcers, ↑ bleeding (thrombocytopenia **Caplan Syndrome** Combination of rheumatoid arthritis, Pneumoconiosis (most common: coal mining dust, asbestos, silica) and pulmonary nodules. Labs: HLA-DR4, ↓ WBC, ↓ Platelets SX: Cough, shortness of breath, rales on auscultation, painful joints, morning stiffness, rheumatoid nodules, swollen metacarpophalangeal (MCP) joints DX: LFT's show mixed restrictive and obstructive defects, ↓ TLC. Labs: RF, ANA (antinuclear antibodies)

Eosinophilic Fasciitis
AKA: Shulman's syndrome

Inflammation disease that affects the fascia (connective tissues that surround the muscle, blood vessels, nerves).

Presents with thickened/tightened skin with peau d'orange (orange peel) look similar to sclerodactyly as seen in scleroderma and systemic sclerosis, but there is NO symptoms of:
Raynaud's, Cardiac, Lung or Kidney involvement.

DX: BIT: ↑ eosinophils in the blood.
MAT: Fascia and muscle biopsy.
TX: Corticosteroids, hydroxychloroquine

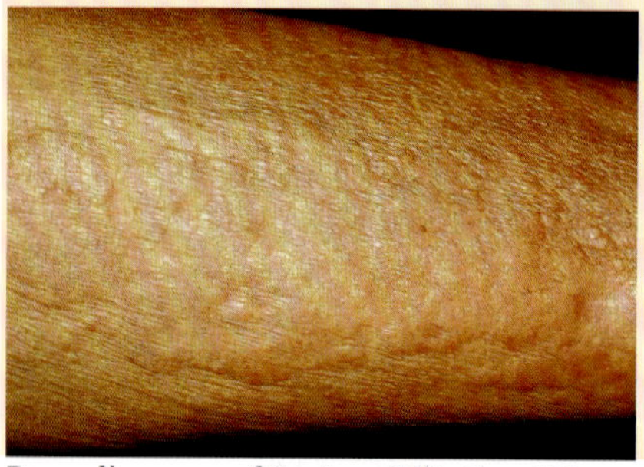

Peau d'orange of Eosinophilic Fasciitis

MUSCULOSKELETAL PHARMACOLOGY

Analgesics, Anti-inflammatory, Antipyretics

DRUG GENERIC name Trade name	Clinical Use	Mechanism of Action and Resistance	Toxicity and Notes
Aspirin (Salicylic acid)	Antipyretic, Analgesic, Anti-inflammatory. MI to inhibit platelet aggregation and ↓ mortality rate. ↓ Platelet aggregation (81 mg/day) and ↓ chance of MI and/or stroke. Antipyretic, Analgesic: 300 – 2400 mg/day. Anti-inflammatory: 2400 – 4000 mg/day.	**Irreversible inhibits COX-1 and COX-2** (Cyclooxygenase path in the Arachidonic Acid pathway). Inhibits platelet aggregation: ↑ bleeding time. (no effect on PT, PTT). ↓ Synthesis of prostaglandins and TXA2 (thromboxane A_2). **Constricts afferent arteriole → ↓ GFR.** (Prostaglandins (PG's) keep the arteriole open/vasodilate)	**NOTE: Aspirin is one of the 4 drugs that ↓ morality rates! (Aspirin, β-Blocker, Ace Inhibitor, Spironolactone).** **Toxicity: First sign: Tinnitus (CN VIII), mixed acid/base disorder (respiratory alkalosis and metabolic alkalosis = anion gap metabolic acidosis),** **Constricts afferent arteriole (inhibits prostaglandins), interstitial nephritis, gastric ulcers.** **Reyes syndrome (given in viral illness to children)** **Do NOT use in patients dependent on ↑ GFR for kidney function.** **Peptic ulcers: Prostaglandins are needed to maintain the mucous lining in the stomach and intestines.**
NSAID's **Diclofenac** **Ibuprofen** **Indomethacin** **Ketorolac** **Naproxen**	Antipyretic, Analgesic, Anti-inflammatory. Indomethacin: Closes PDA's. DOC in acute gout.	**Reversible inhibit COX-1 and COX-2. Inhibit prostaglandin synthesis.** **Constricts afferent arteriole → ↓ GFR.** (Prostaglandins (PG's) keep the arteriole open/vasodilate). The analgesic, anti-inflammatory, anti-pyretic effects are achieved by inhibiting the COX pathway and **reducing prostaglandin production.**	**Do NOT use in patients dependent on ↑ GFR for kidney function.** **Peptic ulcers: Prostaglandins are needed to maintain the mucous lining in the stomach and intestines.** **Indomethacin:** do NOT use with Lithium. It causes ↑ retention of lithium in the kidneys → lithium toxicity. It also ↑ renin and aldosterone levels → ↑ sodium and potassium levels and edema.
Acetaminophen *Tylenol*	Antipyretic, Analgesic. Does **NOT** provide anti-inflammatory benefits.	**Reversible inhibit COX-1 and COX-2. Inhibit prostaglandin synthesis.**	**Use instead of aspirin in children with viral sickness (flu) to avoid Reye's syndrome.** **Overdose causes hepatic necrosis (↑↑↑ ALT and AST):** **N-acetylcysteine. MOA: Regenerates glutathione.**
COX-2 Inhibitor **Celecoxib**	Patients with ulcers. (Stomach protective), Rheumatoid arthritis, Ankylosing spondylitis, osteoarthritis.	Reversibly **inhibits COX-2** (expressed in cells involved in inflammation) It reduces pain and inflammation without adverse GI issues (ulcers).	Sulfa allergies

Gout Pharmacology

DRUG GENERIC name Trade name	Clinical Use	Mechanism of Action and Resistance	Toxicity and Notes
Acute Gout			
NSAID's **Indomethacin** **Naproxen**	DOC in acute gout.	**See above**	**See above** (note: NSAIDS are also the treatment for pericarditis)
Colchicine	Acute gout **(NSAID's are #1 DOC – Colchicine is only used as #1 treatment in acute gout if patient has NSAID allergies)**, Dressler's syndrome (antibody reaction several weeks following an MI)	Inhibits chemotaxis of PMN's (leukocytes) by binding tubulin, which **inhibits microtubule** polymerization.	**GI side effects.** (Note: Colchicine is also the treatment for Dressler's Syndrome)
Chronic Gout			
Allopurinol	Chronic gout, Use with chemotherapy to prevent tumor lysis syndrome.	**Inhibits xanthine oxidase** so that synthesis of uric acid is inhibited. Builds up xanthine and hypoxanthine.	Azathioprine and 6-MP: require xanthine oxidase to be metabolized (broken down) so **do NOT use** **Allopurinol** or **Febuxostat** with these drugs. You must use another chronic gout drug instead. Allopurinol inhibits xanthine oxidase so 6-MP can't be broken down and metabolized so it builds up → toxic.
Febuxostat	Chronic gout	**Same as Allopurinol**	Same as Allopurinol
Benzbromarone	Chronic gout	Non-competitive inhibitor of xanthine oxidase. Used when first line, Allopurinol, does not work.	**P-450 Inhibitor**
Probenecid	Chronic gout	Inhibits **reabsorption** of **uric acid in PCT.** (**tip**: **P**robenecid = **P** for **P**ct)	Requires good renal function when using this drug. Can cause uric acid stones. Can use this drug instead of Allopurinol when using Azathioprine and 6-MP.
Rasburicase **Pegloticase**		Metabolizes uric acid to **allantoin** so that it is easier to excrete.	Immunogenicity (provoke an immune response)

TNF-α Inhibitors

- **MUST check PPD on patients before using TNF-α drugs because of risk of reactivation of latent TB. TNF-α prevents activation of macrophages so ↓ destruction occurs of microbes.**

DRUG GENERIC name Trade name	Clinical Use	Mechanism of Action and Resistance	Toxicity and Notes
Etanercept	Rheumatoid arthritis, ankylosing spondylitis, psoriasis. Used with MTX.	TNF **decoy** receptor. It "pretends" to be the macrophage.	**Check PPD.**
Infliximab **Adalimumab**	Ulcerative colitis, Crohn's, HLA-B27's (Rheumatoid arthritis, psoriatic arthritis, IBD, akylosing spondylitis)	Anti-TNF-α antibody. (MAB = monoclonal antibody)	**Check PPD.** (**tip:** I'm **FIX**in my Crohn's)

Bone Pharmacology

DRUG GENERIC name Trade name	Clinical Use	Mechanism of Action and Resistance	Toxicity and Notes
Bisphosphonates "the dronate's" **Alendronate** *Fosamax* Ibandronate *Boniva*	Prevents loss of bone mass. Osteoporosis, Paget's DZ of bone, hypercalcemia	**Inhibits osteoclast mediated bone resorption** (inhibits RANK-L, M-CSF (Macrophage colony-stimulating factor) by binding hydroxyapatite (mineral form of calcium apatite) in the bone. Pyrophosphate analog.	**Corrosive esophagitis.** Patient must take pill with water and remain upright for 30 minutes so that it does not lodge in the throat and erode through the esophagus.
Teriparatide	Osteoporosis	PTH analog. Increases osteoblast activity.	Potential rare risk of osteosarcoma. Hypercalcemia.
Denosumab	Osteoporosis when Bisphosphonates fail to work.	RANK-L inhibitor. Inhibits osteoclast function.	
Leflunomide *Arava*	Rheumatoid arthritis, psoriatic arthritis	Inhibits pyrimidine synthesis and T-cell proliferation by inhibiting dihydroorotate dehydrogenase.	Hepatotoxic, HTN, teratogenic

Sunscreens

- Protection factor (SPF is the measure of the fraction of sunburn-producing UV rays that will reach the skin).
  Example: SPF 20 means that 1/20th of the burning radiation will reach the skin if the lotion is applied thickly over the skin). So if it takes 20 minutes for your unprotected skin to start turning red, using an SPF 20 prevents reddening 20 times longer – for about 6.5 hours.
- SPF's of 15 or higher do a good job of protecting against UVB rays
- UVA = A for Aging
  UVB = B for Bad
- UVA and UVB both cause DNA damage
- **#1 protection: Wear full clothing**
  Other protection: If you must go out: do not go out between 10 – 3 (highest rays) or wear proper sunscreen.
  Apply sunscreens 30 minutes before sun exposure to allow time to bond to the skin.
  Reapply every two hours and after swimming or sweating.

DRUG GENERIC name Trade name	Protection
PABA (para-aminobenzoic acid) , Salicylates, Cinnamates	Sunscreen, protects against UVB only.
Benzophenone	Sunscreen, protects against short length UVA.
Zinc Oxide, Avobenzone, Ecamsule, Titanium dioxide	Sunscreen, protects against longer UVA rays.

Skin Lesion Removal

DRUG GENERIC name Trade name	Mechanism of Action	Clinical Use and Notes
Podophyllin	Inhibits topoisomerase II	Topical – genital warts . Will damage skin. Do not use during pregnancy.
Liquid Nitrogen (cryotherapy)	Liquid nitrogen	Warts, skin tags, actinic keratosis
Salicylic acid (over the counter)	Acid	Warts
Imiquimod	↑ interferon production. Signals the **toll-like receptor 7** (TLR7) to activate cells to release IFN-α, IL-6 and TNF-α.	Topical – genital warts, basal cell carcinoma, actinic keratosis. **Does NOT cause tissue damage**. **Safe** to use during pregnancy. (**tip**: "I"miquimod for "I" deal)

Acne Treatment

Pustules caused by **Propionibacterium acnes.**

Type of Acne	Treatment	Notes
Mild acne-initial treatment	**Benzoyl peroxide**	
No response to initial treatment	**Topical antibiotics:** Erythromycin, Clindamycin, Sulfacetamide	
More serious acne/no response to topical treatments	**Oral antibiotics:** Tetracycline, Minocycline, Clindamycin	The tetracycline family is **sun sensitive**. So be careful of the teenager that goes on vacation (sun or suntan bed) that breaks out in a rash. The tetracycline family also discolors developing **teeth** and affects **bone growth** in the fetus and discolors permanent teeth in children.
Severe acne	Topical retinoids	
Severe acne, scarring acne and no response to topical retinoids	**Oral retinoic acid** derivative: Isotretinoin, Tretinoin, Tazarotene, Adapalene	**Retinoic acids are severe teratogens. Must check β-hCG for pregnancy** before prescribing and must insure female is on birth control while on the drug.

DERMATOLOGY

Dermatology Lesions

Lesion	Description	Example	
Vesicle	Small blister < 1 cm, fluid filled	Poison Ivy, Herpes, Varicella (chickenpox), Zoster (shingles)	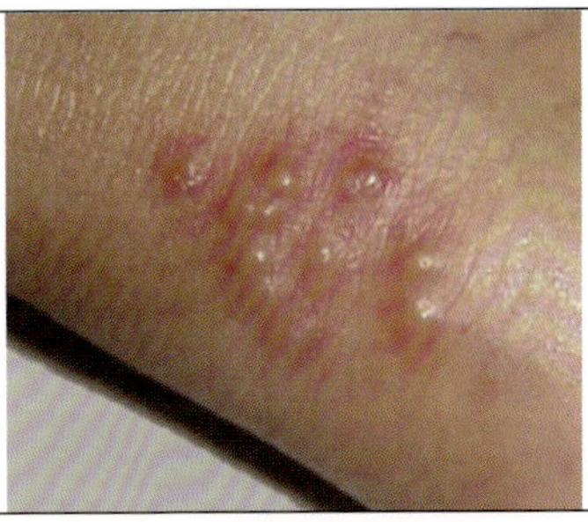
Bulla	Large blister > 1 cm, fluid filled	Bullous pemphigoid (negative Nikolsky's sign), Stevens Johnsons, Toxic Epidermal Necrolysis.	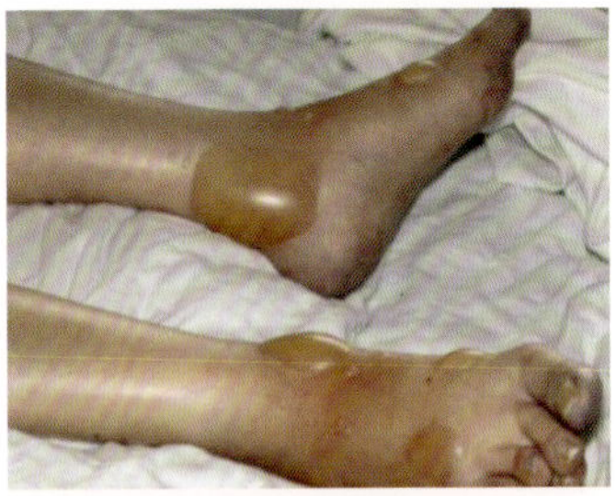
Pustule	Vesicle containing pus	Acne, Pustular psoriasis	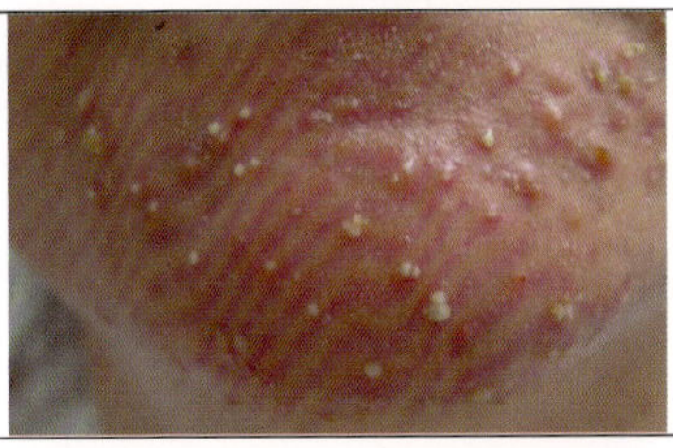
Crust	Dry exudate	Impetigo	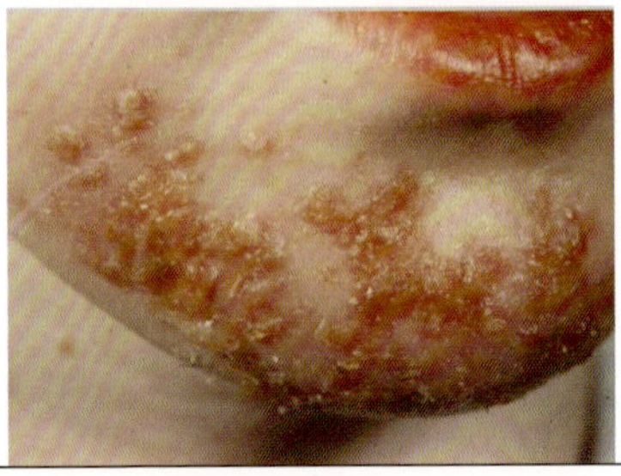
Scale	Flaking	Eczema, Psoriasis	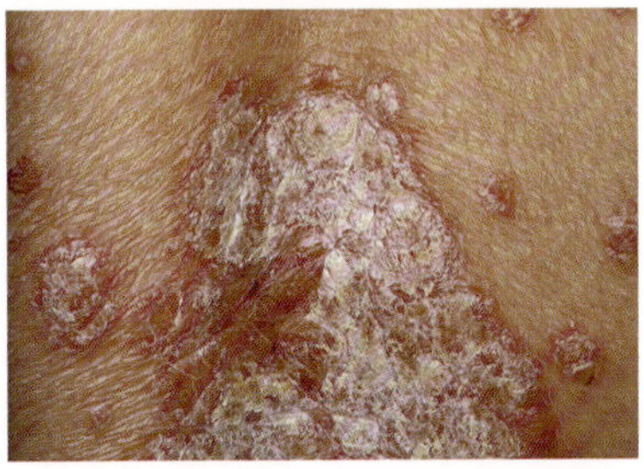

Wheal	Raised, pruritic area of skin	Urticaria (hives)	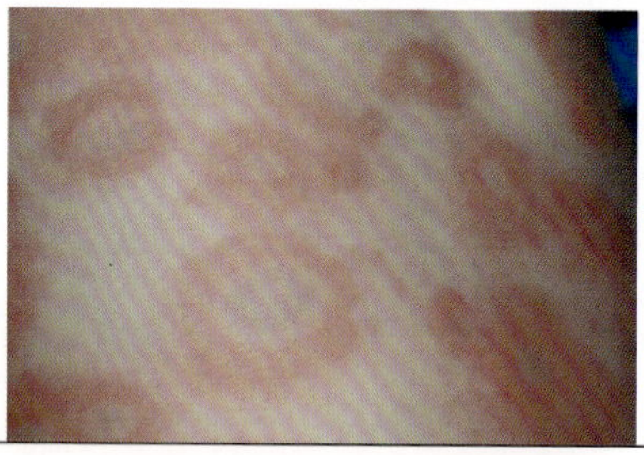
Macule	Flat lesion < 1 cm, different color Than surrounding skin color	Freckle AKA: Ephelis	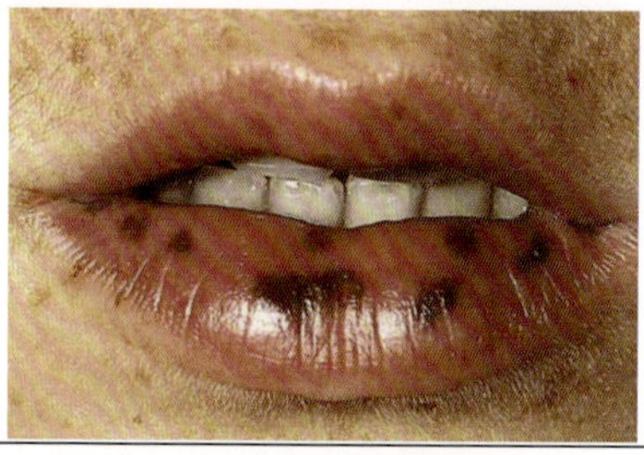
Patch	Macule > 1cm	Birthmark	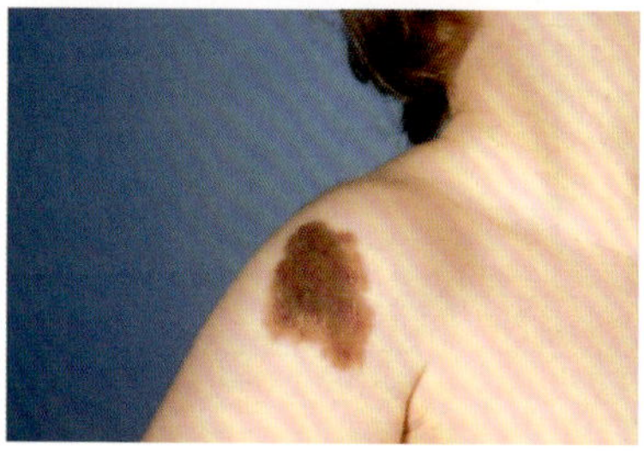
Papule	Elevated solid skin lesions < 1 cm	Nevus (mole)	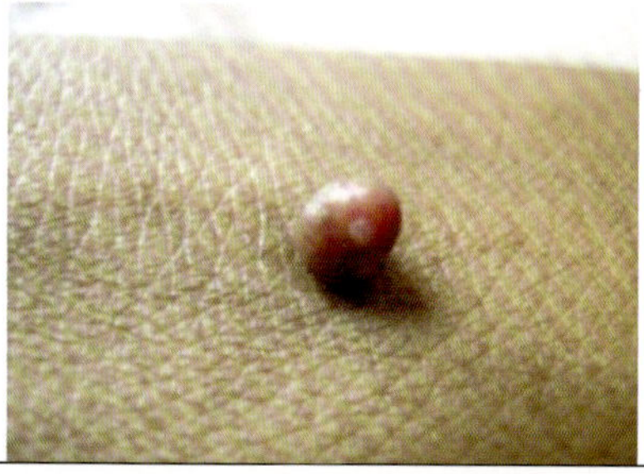
Plaque	Papule > 1 cm	Psoriasis	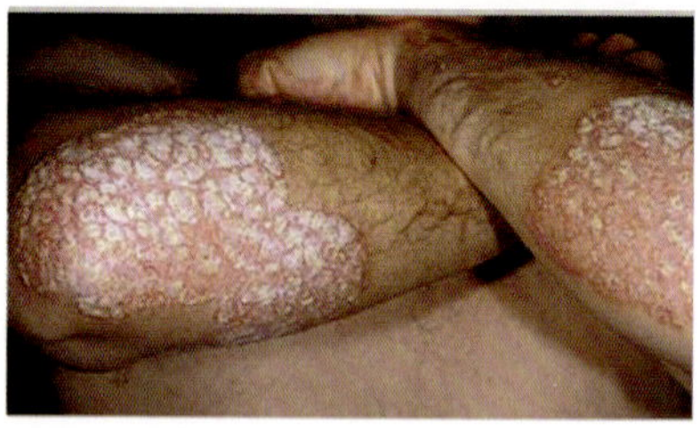

Dermatology Conditions - General Rashes and Lesions

Severity of rashes: Toxic Epidermal Necrolysis > Stevens-Johnson Syndrome > Erythema Multiforme > Morbilliform Rash.

Morbilliform Rash Type of rash seen in the measles. Drug allergies: Penicillins and sulfas. Does not involve mucus membrane. **Blanches** with pressure. TX: **Antihistamines.** 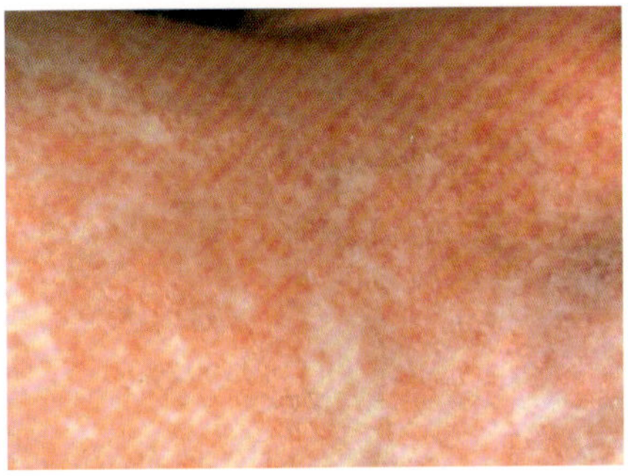	**Erythema Multiforme** Lesions can be various: Papules, macules, vesicles and target lesions. MC: Multiple target lesions with multiple rings that can show center crusting lesions (AKA: epithelial damage). Also common to be seen on the palms and soles. Causes: Sulfa drugs, NSAIDS, Penicillins, Phenytoin, Mycoplasma, Herpes simplex. TX: Antihistamines. 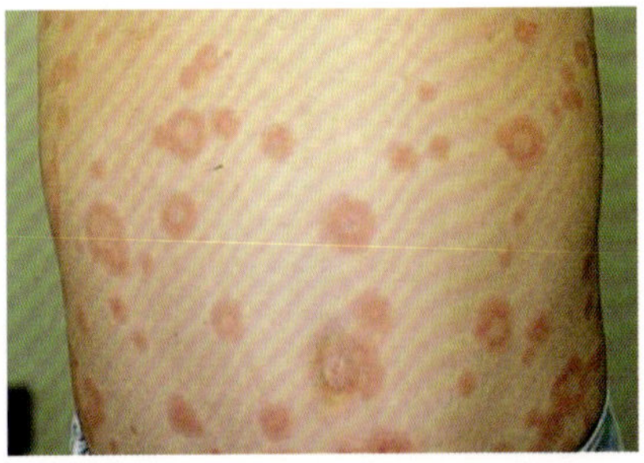	**Xerosis** **AKA: Asteatotic Dermatitis** **Xerosis/dry skin.** **TX: E Emollients** (Vaseline, Mineral Oil, Eucerin, Lubriderm, Aquaphor, Dermasil, Lac-Hydrin), humidifier. 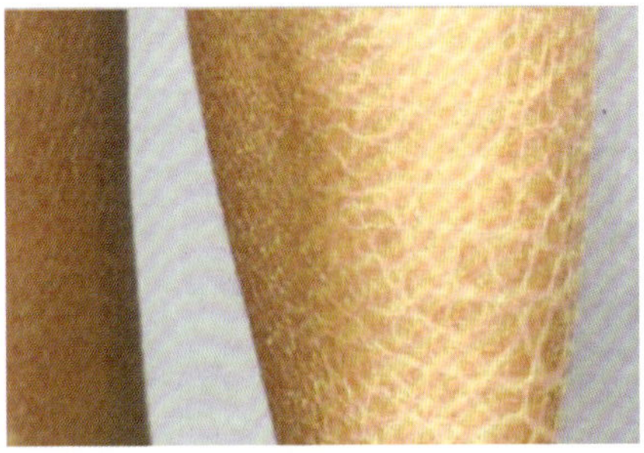
Erythema Nodosum Inflammatory, **erythematous, painful lesions/bumps** of **subcutaneous fat**. It is a secondary inflammation due to current or recent inflammatory conditions. MC seen on **shins** (anterior lower leg). Nodules last 6 weeks. No ulcers. DX: **NOT** by biopsy. MC associated with **Sarcoidosis (DX: by CXR for hilar lymphadenopathy)**. Can also be seen with TB, leprosy, Crohn's, Coccidioidomycosis, Histoplasmosis, Syphilis, Hepatitis, pregnancy. 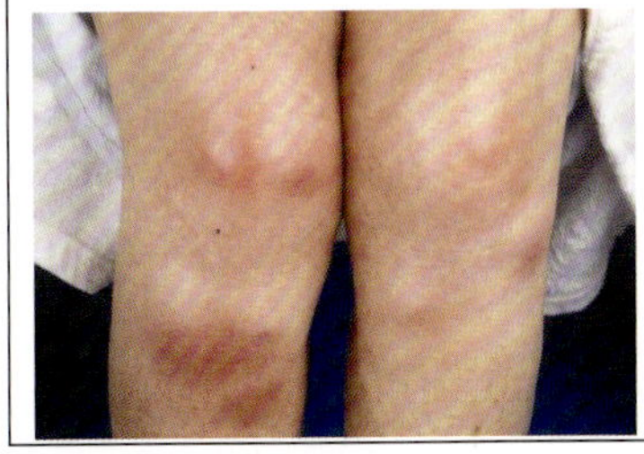	**Urticaria** AKA: Hives. Mediated by **IgE aggregating** to stimulate **mast cells** degranulation causing pruritic **wheals**. MC seen with drug allergies, insect stings/bites. **Hypersensitivity Type I.** (Allergies: foods, insect bites, contact with **latex** (note: this includes **condoms**), medications) TX: **Antihistamines, Prednisone, Danazol, Stanozolol.** 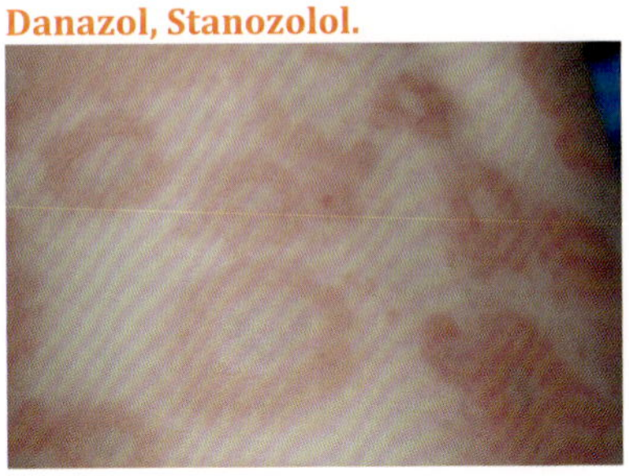	**Ephelis (Freckle)** Macule: Flat lesion < 1 cm, different color than surrounding skin color 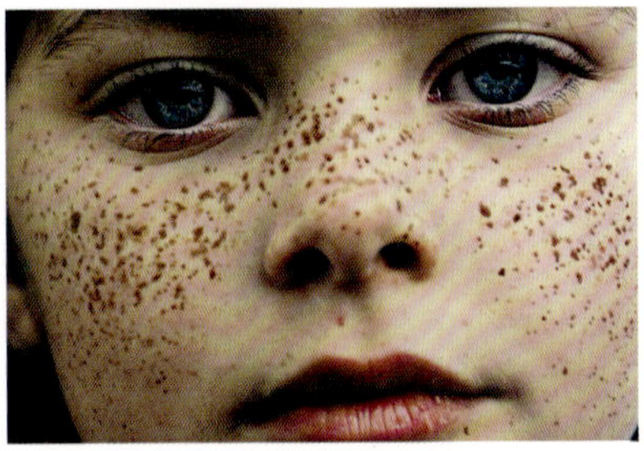

Telangiectasia – spider angioma 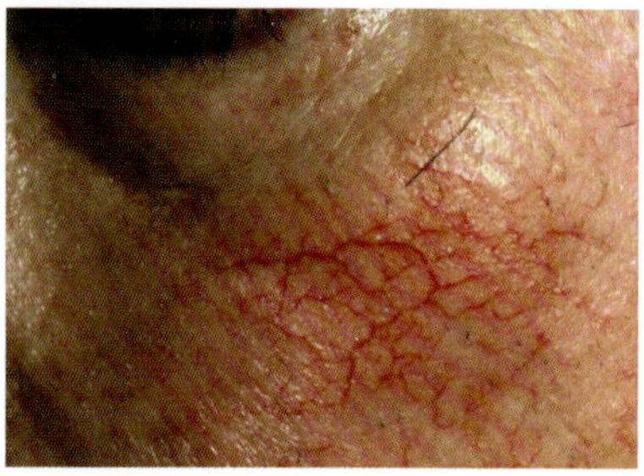	**Skin Tags** 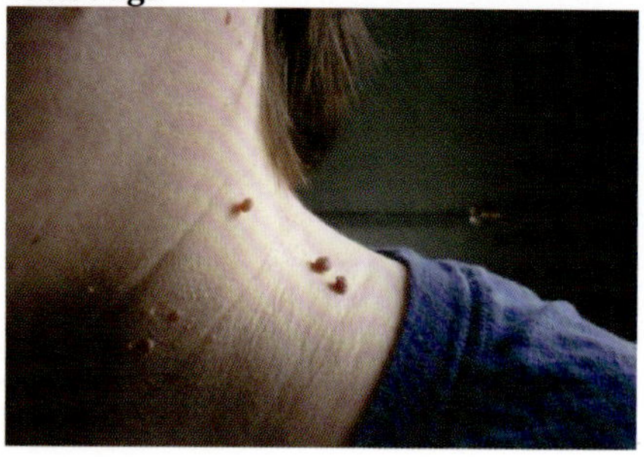	**Bruise** 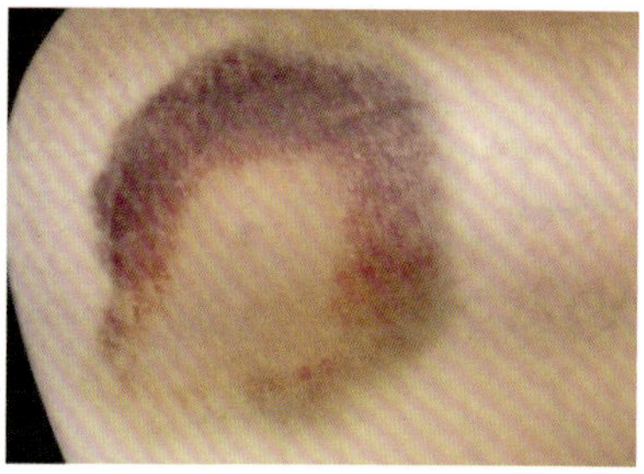
Melanocytic Nevus AKA: Common **mole**. Benign. 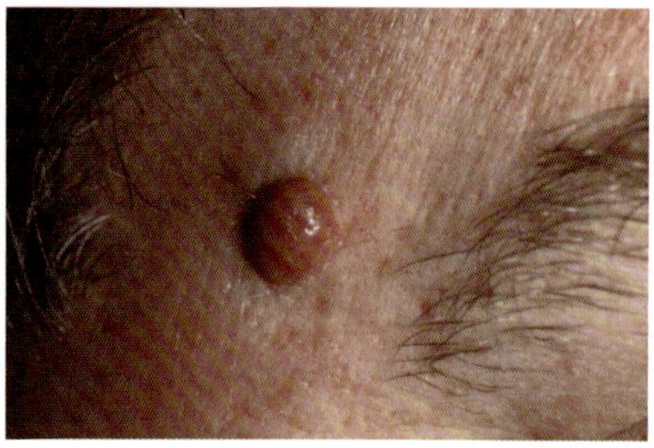 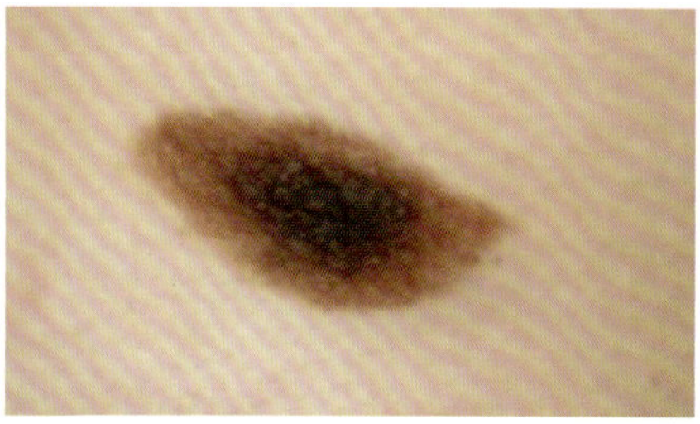	**Livedo reticularis** **Bluish, netlike, arborizing pattern.** 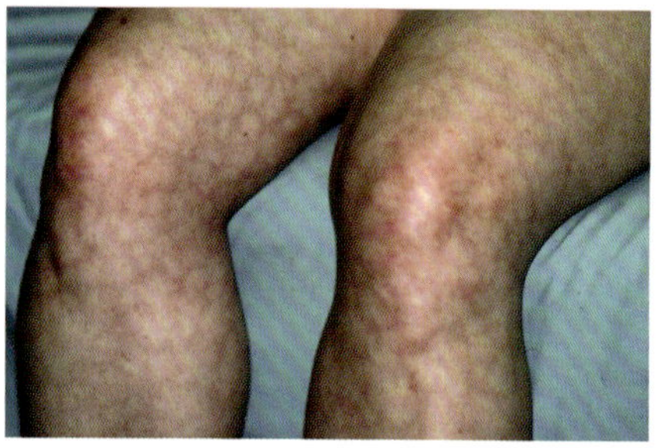	**Mongolian spot** Due to the melanocytes being trapped in the lower dermis due to failure of migration of neural crest cells. MC in Asian's. (Do not confuse with child abuse). 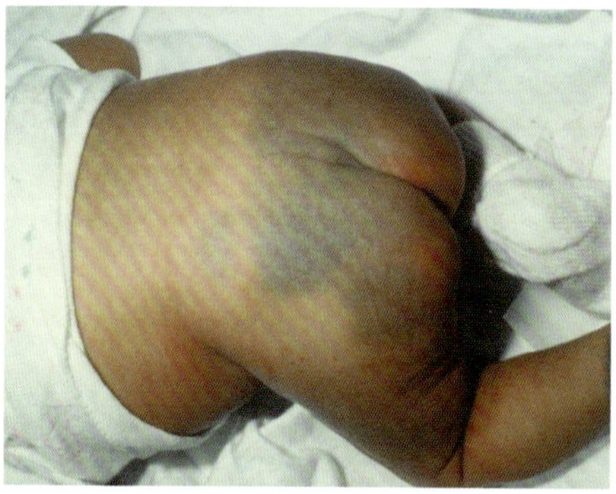
Birth mark 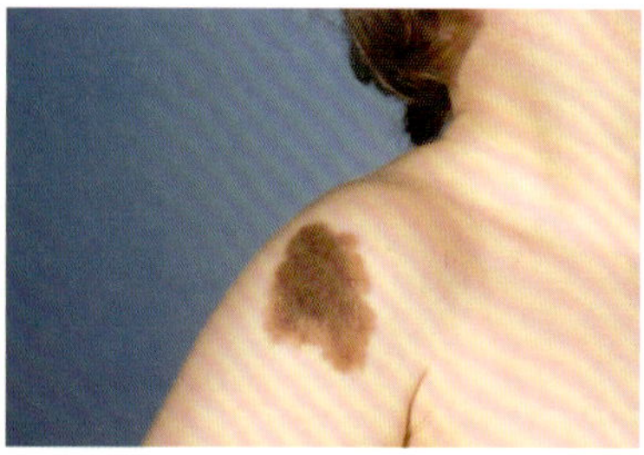	**Pannus** 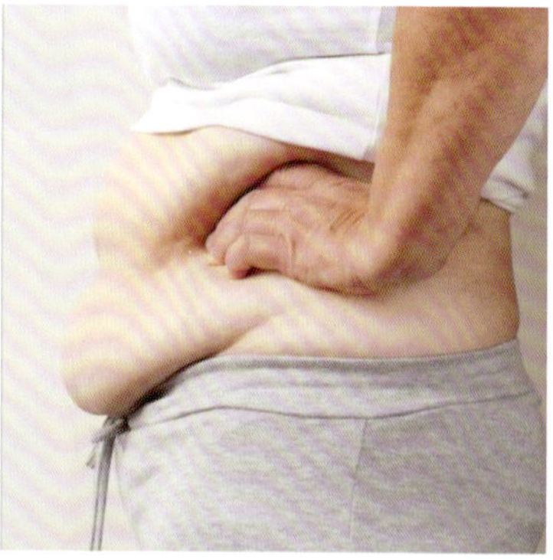	

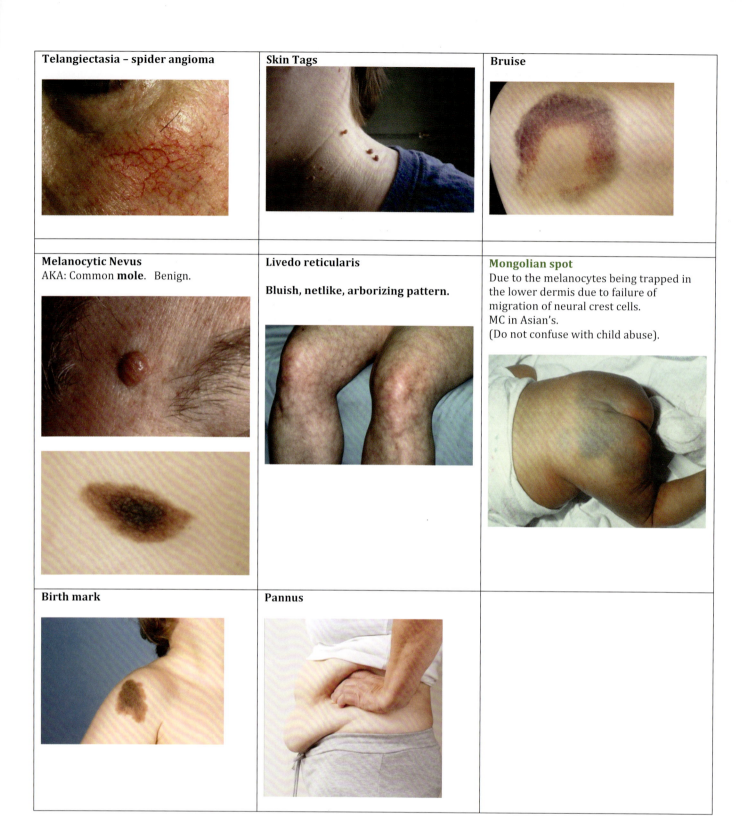

Blanching vs Non-blanching rashes

Blanching Rashes	Non-blanching Rashes
Telangiectasias	Petechiae/purpura rashes (ruptured blood vessels under the skin): Henoch Schonlein Purpura (HSP) Idiopathic Thrombocytopenia (ITP) Hemolytic Uremic Syndrome (HUS) Acute leukemias
Erythema	Ecchymoses
Scarlet fever	Measles (early rash) then becomes non-blanching in 3 – 4 days
Kawasaki disease	Meningococcus
Juvenile rheumatoid arthritis	Rotavirus

Eczema - Atopic Dermatitis
Overactivity of release of histamine from mast cells and immune system.

Combination of **eczema** (erythremic, pruritic rash/plaques on flexor surfaces), **asthma, allergic rhinitis (↑ IgE levels)**.
Seen with: **Churg Straus**.
Seen with **eosinophil's** (allergies).
Family history is common, onset before the age of 5.

SX: Pruritus, erythremic, scaly, rough, thickened skin (**lichenified skin**), MC found on the face, neck and behind knee (flexor surfaces). Pruritus causes scratching which leads to skin infections by Staph aureus.

Preventative TX: Emollients avoid drying soaps and hot water and use cotton clothing. Avoid scratching.

TX: Coal tar, topical steroids, antihistamines.
Moisturize skin and avoid soaps/baths to keep from drying and itching. Wear soft clothes (cotton) so the skin is less irritated.
Doxepin (TCA that treats pruritus).
Tacrolimus, Pimecrolimus (IL-2 inhibitors which inhibits T cells), antihistamines

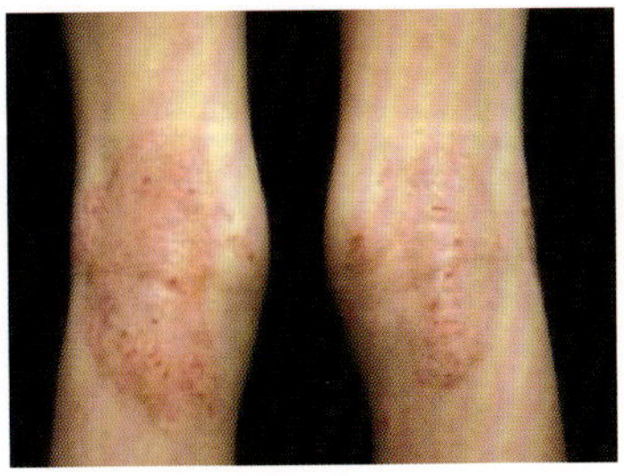

Seborrheic Keratosis
Squamous epithelia proliferation with keratin-filled cysts (AKA: horn cysts or liver spots).
Appears like "**stuck on**" flat, greasy wart-like lesions. Common in elderly.

Leser-Trélat sign: sudden appearance of multiple seborrheic keratoses. Associated with HIV and malignancy.

TX: Removal by cryotherapy, laser or surgery.

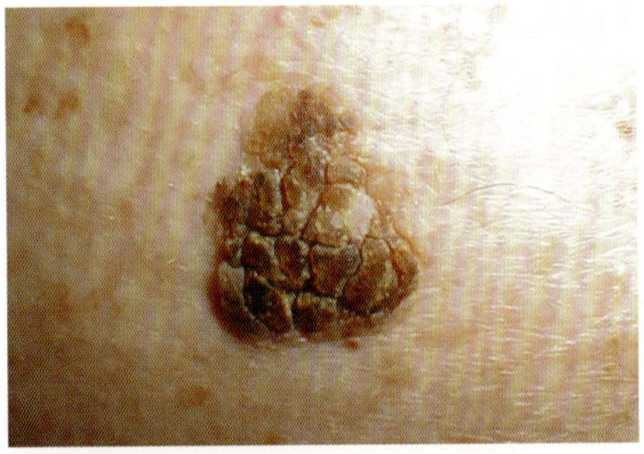

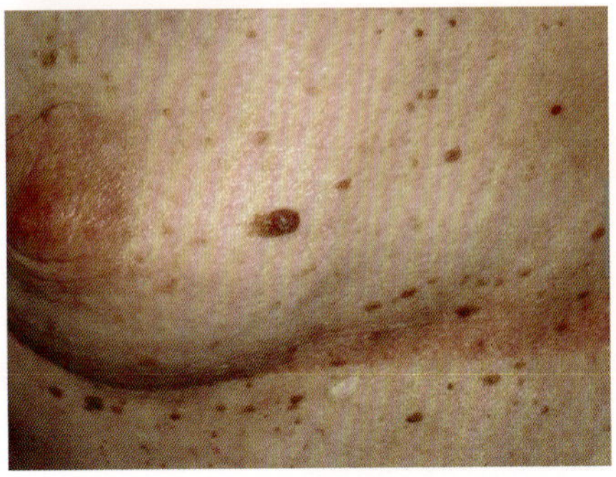

Sebaceous Hyperplasia
Benign.

Sebaceous glands (holocrine glands – sensitive to androgens) become enlarge causing shiny bumps on the forehead, nose and cheeks. Can also occur on the areola, mouth, scrotum, foreskin, vulva, and shaft of penis.

Affects newborns and middle age to elderly adults.

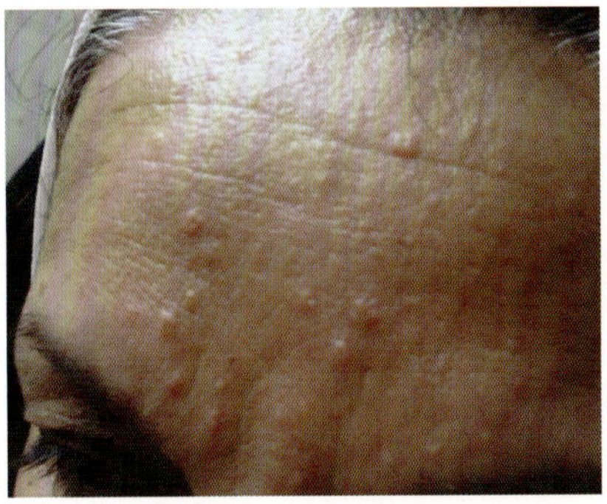

Infants (Congenital, embryonic)

Erythema toxicum
White papules/pustules with a red base that appear on newborns (looks like little white pimples). Benign.

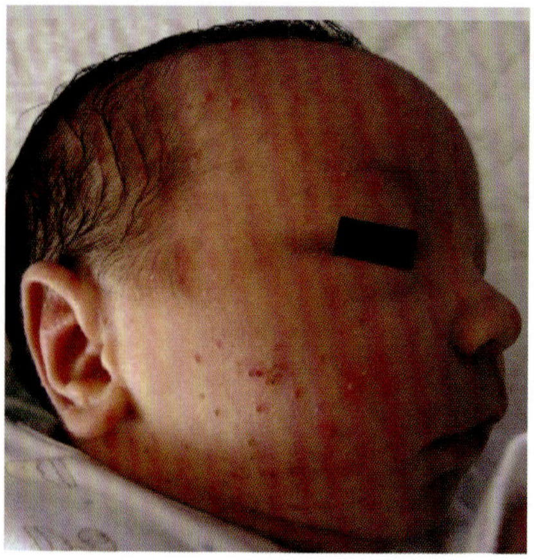

Birth mark

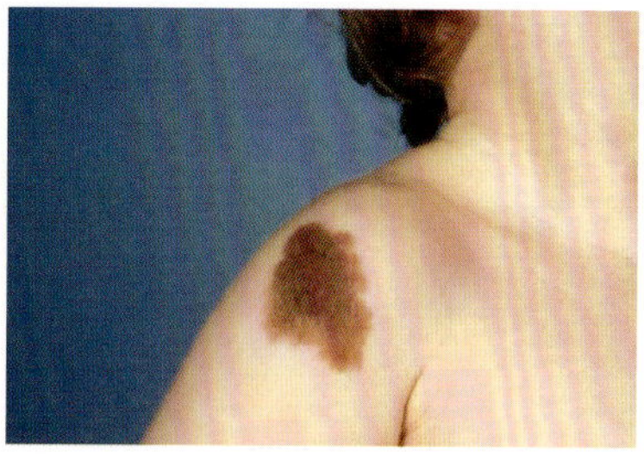

Preauricular tags
(AKA: accessory auricle)
Epithelial mounds of skin that arise near the front of the ear. Thy have no bony, cartilaginous or cystic components. They do not connect to the ear canal or middle ear.
Can be associated with GU abnormalities and/or hearing loss.

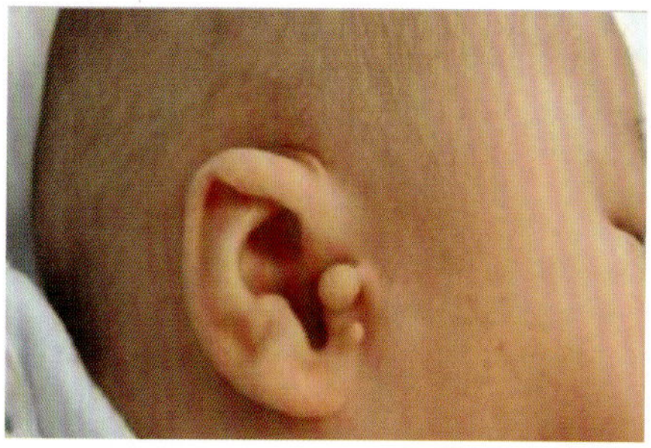

Brachial Cleft Cyst
Mass **LATERAL** to midline.
Congenital epithelial cyst, arises on the lateral neck due to failure of obliteration of the 2nd brachial cleft in embryonic development.

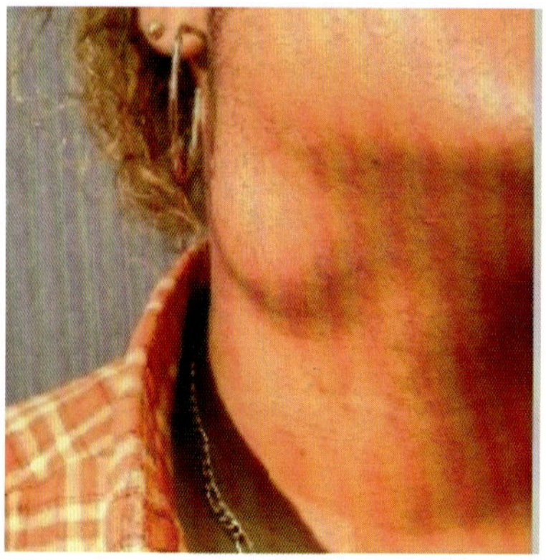

Thyroglossal Duct Cyst
Mass in the midline (**anterior neck**).
Congenital cyst due to anomalous development and **migration of the thyroid** gland during the 4th – 8th week of gestation. Cystic remnant along the thyroglossal duct between the tongue base and thyroid bed in the neck.

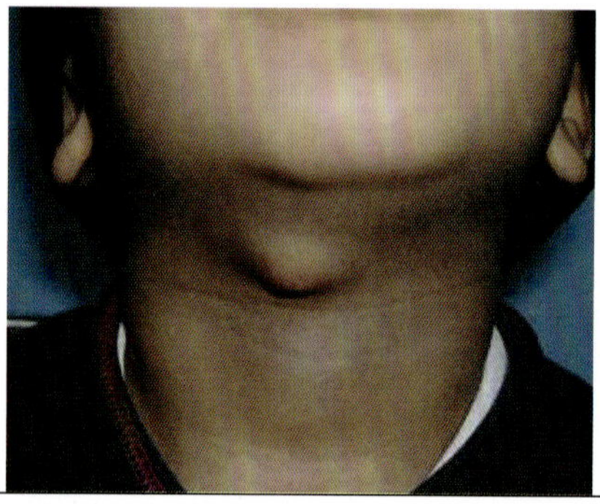

Strawberry hemangioma
Benign growth of endothelia cells (blood vessel). Self-resolving by 10 yrs old.

(**tip** to remember cherry hemangioma verses strawberry hemangioma: Strawberry hemangioma 's are in children: children play with Strawberry Shortcake)

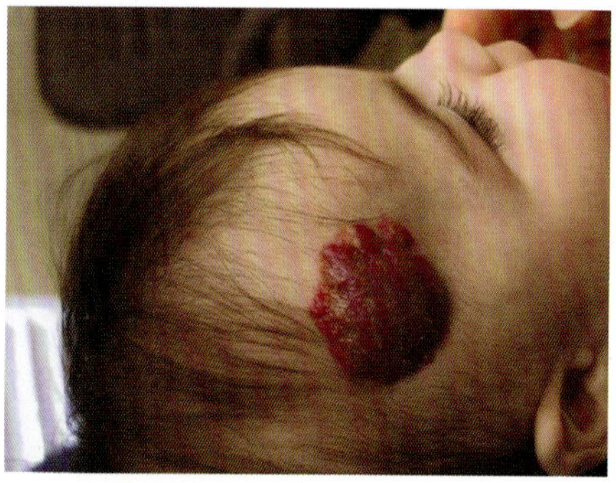

Skin Conditions Due to Drug Reactions, Hypersensitivities.

Urticaria
AKA: Hives.
Mediated by **IgE aggregating** to stimulate **mast cells** degranulation causing pruritic **wheals**.
MC seen with drug allergies, insect stings/bites.
Hypersensitivity Type I. (Allergies: foods, insect bites, contact with **latex**, medications)
TX: **Antihistamines, Prednisone, Danazol, Stanozolol.**

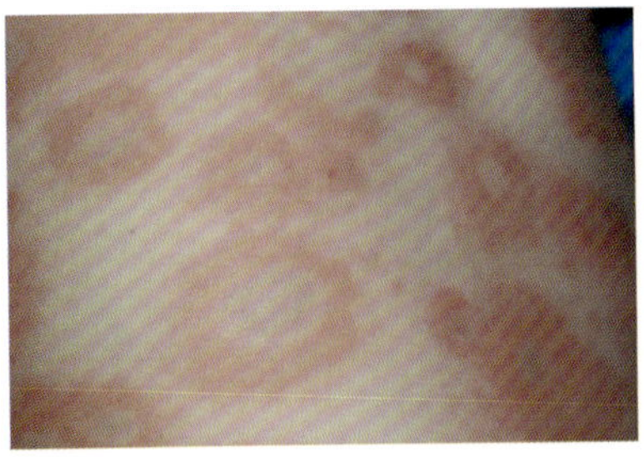

Stevens Johnson Syndrome (SJS)
Target-like lesions: sloughing of skin, bulla formation and necrosis of skin along with fever.
< 30% of the body is involved.
(> 30% of the body = Toxic epidermal necrolysis)

MCC: adverse drug reaction.
(↑ anti-seizure drugs, sulfa drugs, penicillin's, NSAIDS, Phenytoin, Phenobarbital).

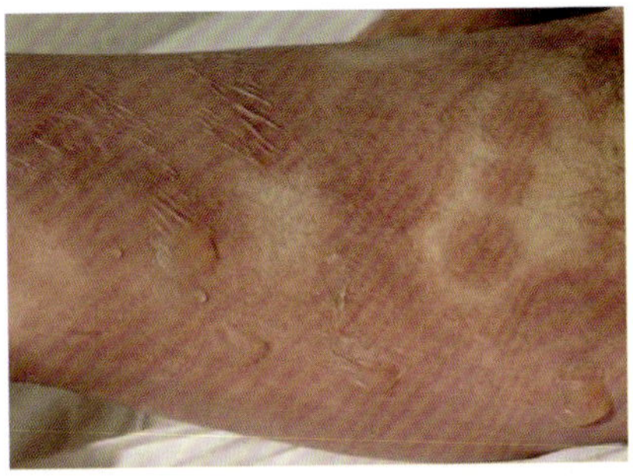

Toxic Epidermal Necrolysis (TEN)
Bulla formation with rapid desquamation.
Sloughing off of sheets of skin due to destruction of epidermal-dermal junctions.
Sloughing off causes skin depigmentation.
Often fatal.
Positive Nikolsky's sign.
>30% of the body involved.
(< 30% of the body = Stevens Johnson)

DX: Skin Biopsy.

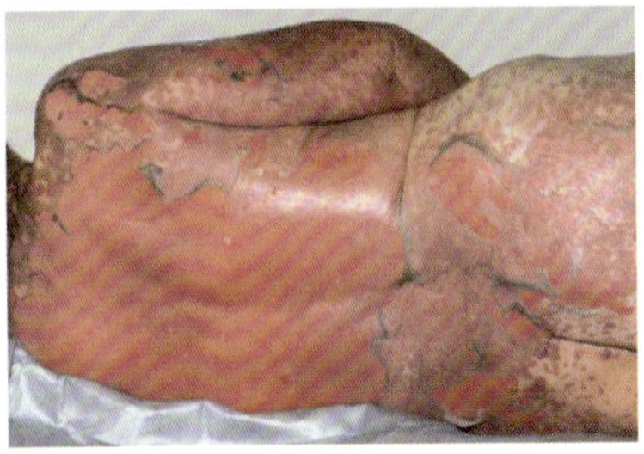

Photosensitivity
Blisters erupt on skin when exposed to sunlight or tanning beds.
Causes: Medications (**tetracycline**: be aware these are used for acne in teens that go to the beach, Porphyria Cutanea Tarda (accumulation of porphyrins),

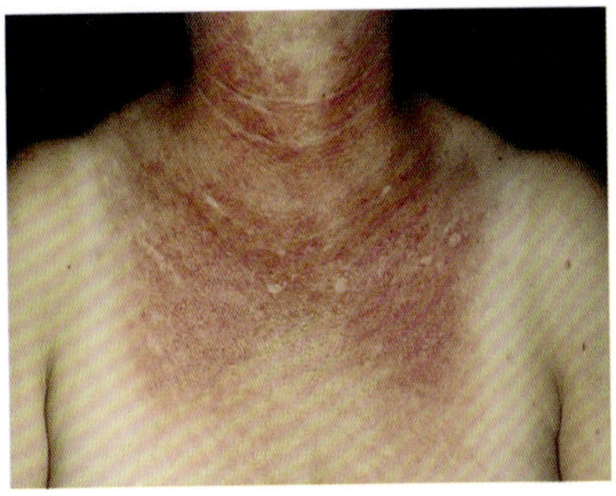

Contact Dermatitis
Hypersensitivity reaction in an area where the skin contacts the specific allergen. The rash usually takes the shape of the allergen or in the area of the allergen was used.
Causes: Jewelry (specifically **nickel**), poison ivy, reaction to soaps, detergents).
Type IV HS mediated by T Cells, Macrophages, CD4.

DX: Specific allergin by patch test.

TX: **Antihistamines, topical steroids.**

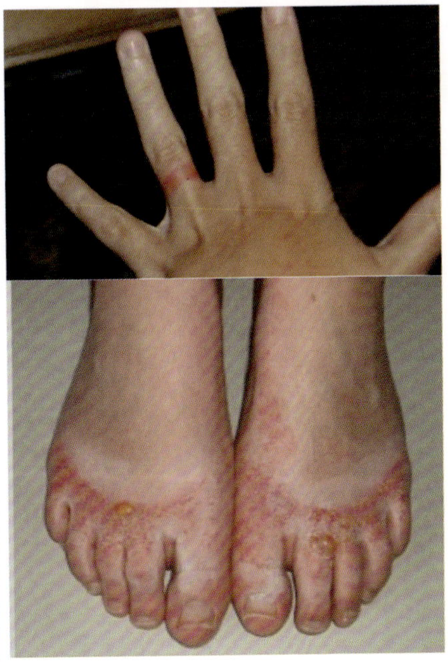

Poison Ivy
Contact Dermatitis.
"Linear vesicular lesion".
HS Type IV. Mediated by T Cells, Macrophages, CD4.

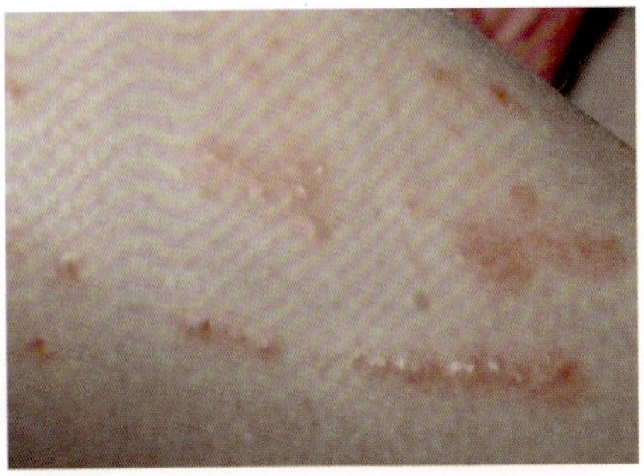

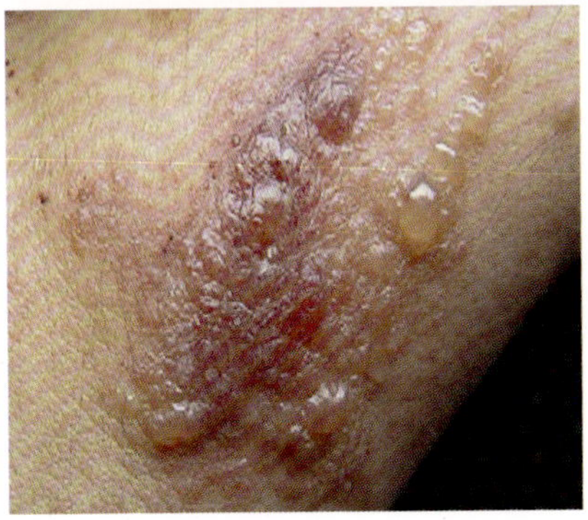

Red Man Syndrome Allergic reaction to **Vancomycin** due to a fast infusion rate. TX: Slow infusion rate and **antihistamines**. 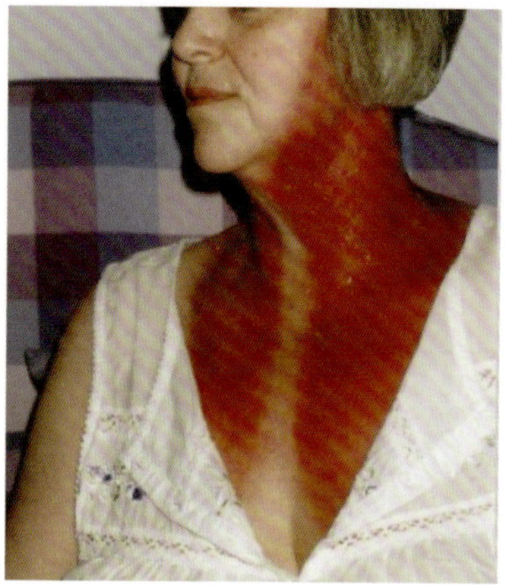	**Acanthosis Nigricans** Velvety **thickening** and hyperplasia of skin. MC seen on neck or axilla. Skin is **hyperpigmented** showing a brown color. Associated with **diabetes**, Cushing's syndrome, obesity and malignancy (MC: **gastric adenocarcinoma**) 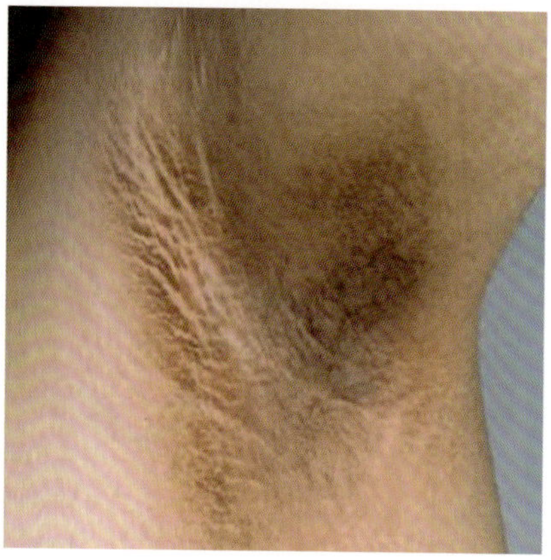	**Heparin Induced Thrombocytopenia (HIT)** (due to antibodies against Platelet Factor IV) **AND** **Warfarin Induced Skin Necrosis** (due to Protein C deficiency) 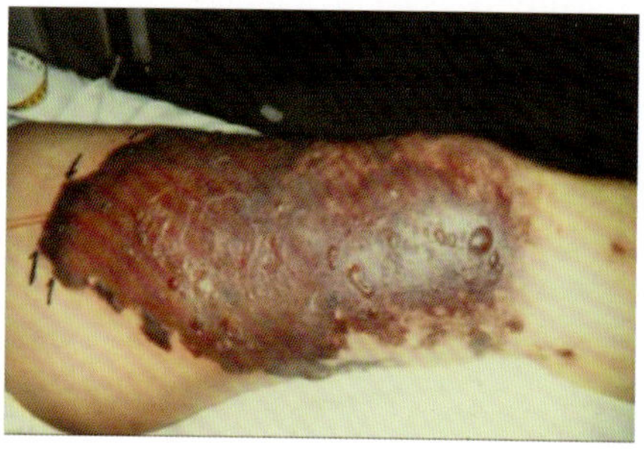

Pigmentation Skin Disorders

Ash Leaf Spots Tuberous sclerosis (associated with hamartomas)  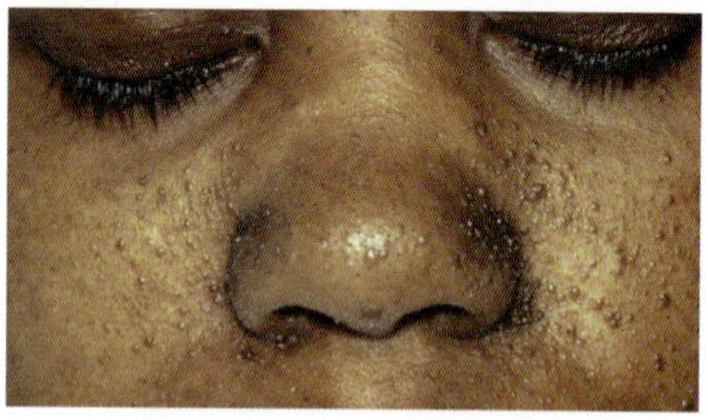	**Café au Lait Spots** (Associated with NF-1 and McCune Albright Syndrome) 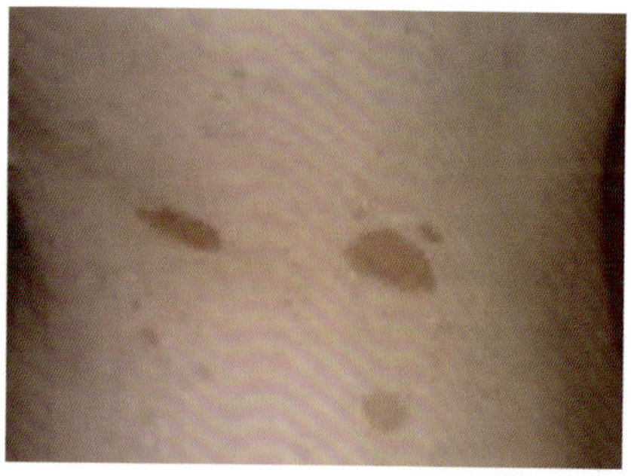	**Albinism** ↓ Melanocyte production due to ↓ **tyrosinase** activity in the dopamine to tyrosine pathway. **Failure of neural crest cell migration**. ↑ risk of skin cancer (Caution: test questions will try and confuse you between PKU, Chediak-Higashi and Albinism – *know your SX*) 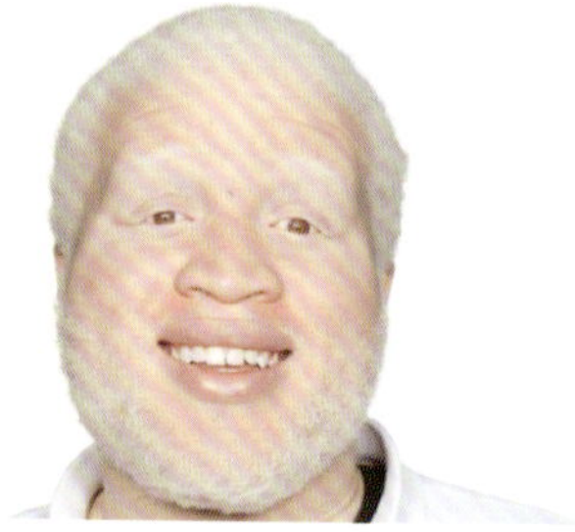

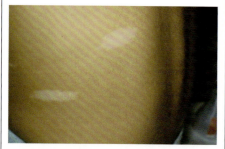

Vitiligo
Autoimmune destruction of melanocytes.
SX: Irregular areas of complete depigmentation.

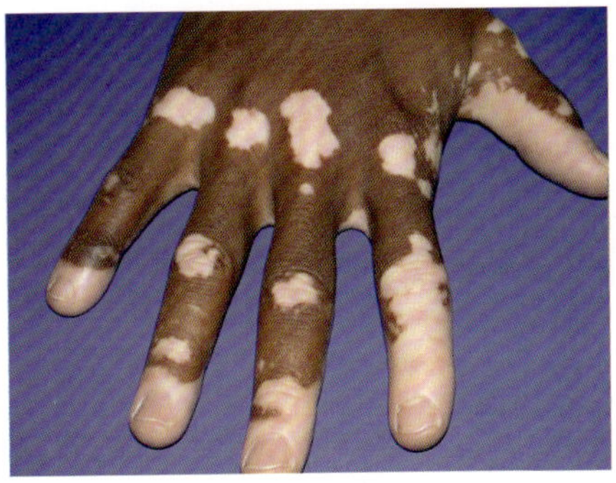

Chloasma (AKA: Melasma)
AKA: Mask of Pregnancy

Hyperpigmentation due to pregnancy or OCP use.

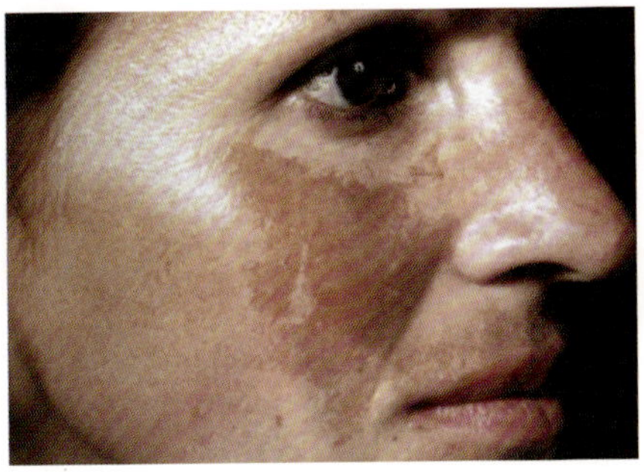

Port Wine Stain
Sturge-Weber
Involves the V1 and/or V2 branch of the trigeminal nerve.

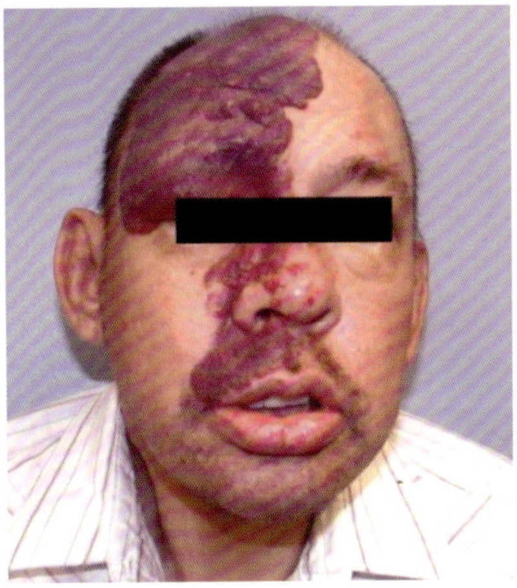

Dermatology Conditions Associated With Blistering, Desquamation

Positive Nikolsky's Sign: The top layers of skin slide away from the lower layers of skin when slightly rubbed.

- Seen in Pemphigus Vulgaris, Toxic Epidermal Necrolysis, Staphylococcal Scalded Skin Syndrome.

Bullous Pemphigoid
Autoimmune. IgG antibodies against **hemidesmosomes** in the **basement membrane** (epidermal-dermal junction).
Does **NOT** involve oral mucosa.
MC in older patients 70's and 80's.

Negative Nikolsky skin.
Immunofluorescence shows **linear pattern at epidermal-dermal junction**.
Bullae filled with serous fluid.

(**tip**: **HE** is a **BULL** and stays in the **basement**)

TX: **Prednisone, Tetracycline, Erythromycin** (combined with **Nicotinamide**).

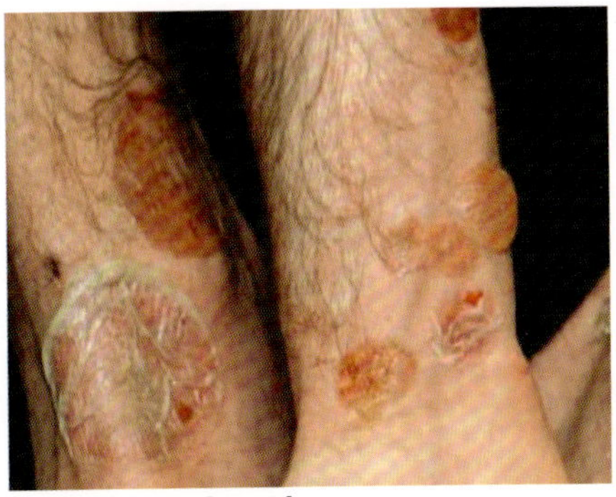

Bullous Pemphigoid

Pemphigus Vulgaris
Autoimmune. IgG **antibodies** against **desmoglein (desmosomes)**.
Ulcers on oral mucosa.

Epidermal cells (keratinocytes) in stratum spinosum are connected by desmosomes.
MC in mid-age patients: 30's and 40's.

Positive Nikolsky sign. (Separation of epidermis when skin stroked).

Drugs can also induce Pemphigus Vulgaris:
Ace Inhibitors, Penicillin, Phenobarbital, Penicillamine.

(**tip**: **Demi** is bad she has a **PIMP** so will have **sores** in her mouth. **P** for Pemphigus and for **P**ositive Nikolsky)

TX: Due to massive infection of the blisters, treatment is critical or Pemphigus **can be fatal**.
High dose Prednisone (systemic), IVIG, Methotrexate, Rituximab, Mycophenolate, Azathioprine, Cyclophosphamide.

Sunburn and Burns
Inflammatory reaction due to UV irradiation. Mutation of **thymine dimers** (DNA mutation).
UVA: aging, tanning beds.
UVB: sunburn
(tip: uvA = A for aging. uvB = Bad)

1st Degree Burn: Damage to epidermis.

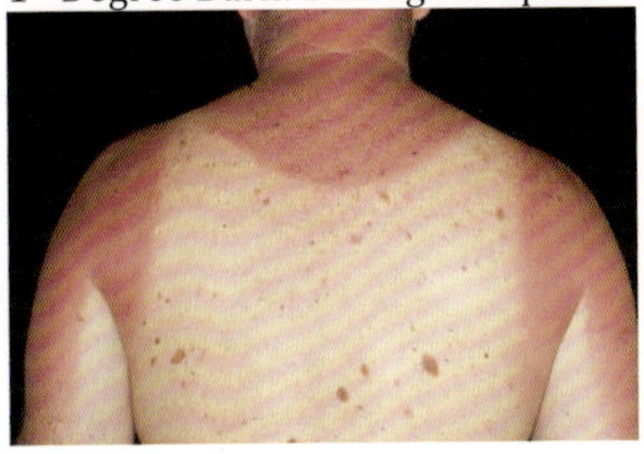

2nd Degree Burn: Destroys epidermis and part of dermis. Fluid-filled **blisters**.
Heals 3 – 4 wks.

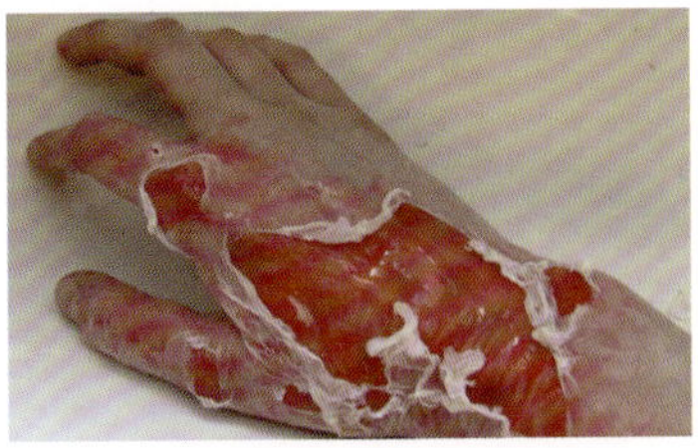

3rd Degree Burn: Destroys epidermis, dermis, and epidermal derivatives. Skin may be black, white, or red. Large amounts of fluids lost. Area is numb due to loss of sensory nerves.

	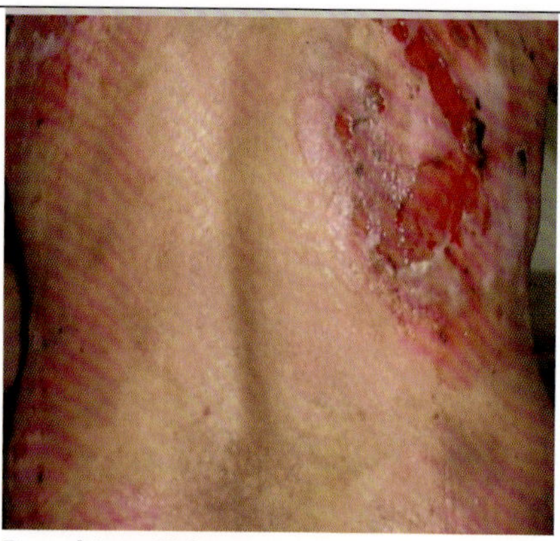 Pemphigus Vulgaris	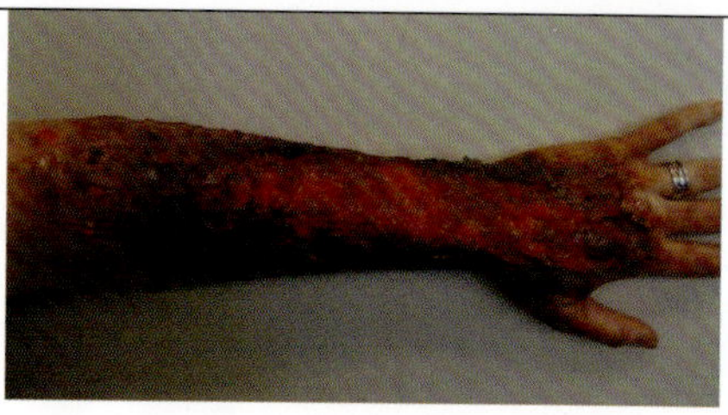 4th Degree Burn: Body parts are partially or completely burned away.
Scalded Skin Syndrome Sloughing off the superficial layers of the epidermis due to exotoxin that destroys the upper layers (stratum granulosum) only. Due to infection by **S. aureus**. Positive Nikolsky sign. MC: newborns and children. TX: IV Nafcillin, Oxacillin, Cefazolin. 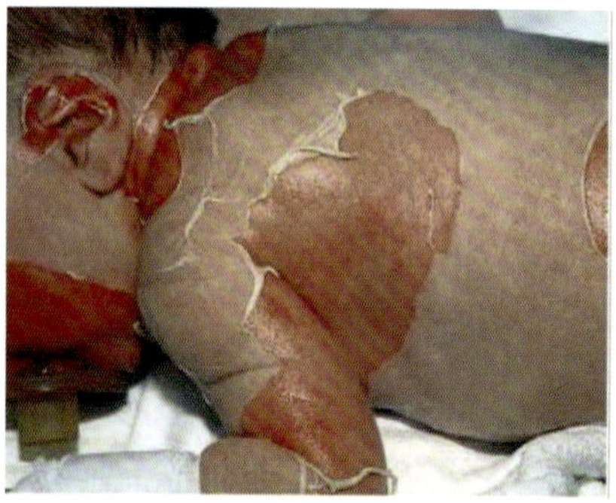	**Kawasaki** Skin desquamation (peeling) 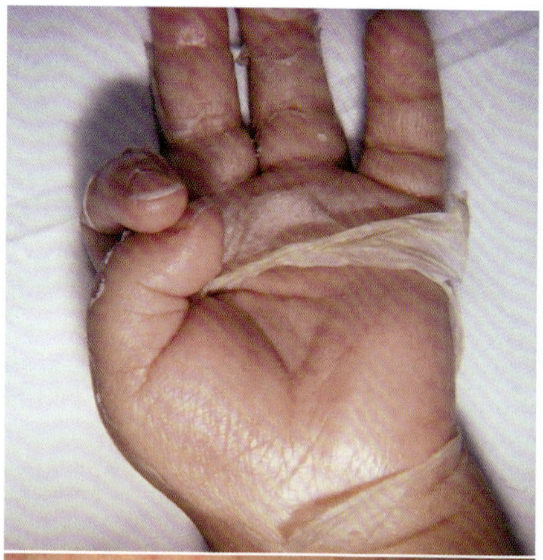 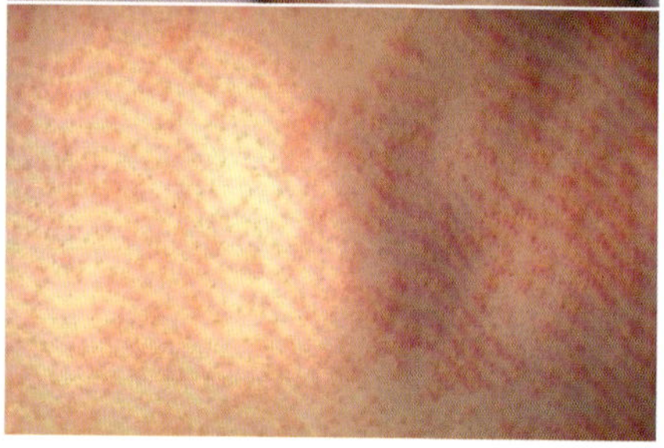	**Lightning Strike: "Ferning"** 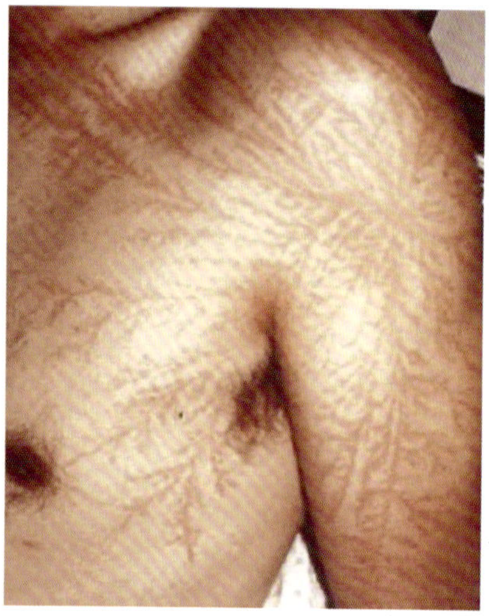

Porphyria Cutanea Tarda

Deficiency of uroporphyrin decarboxylase (heme pathway) causing severe skin damage/blistering when the porphyrins are exposed to sunlight.
SX: Excessive hair growth on the face (Werewolf syndrome, hypertrichosis) blisters on sun-exposed skin.

Exacerbating factors:
Estrogen, Iron overload, alcohol.
Associated with: Hepatitis C.

DX: Increased uroporphyrins in a 24-hour urine collection.

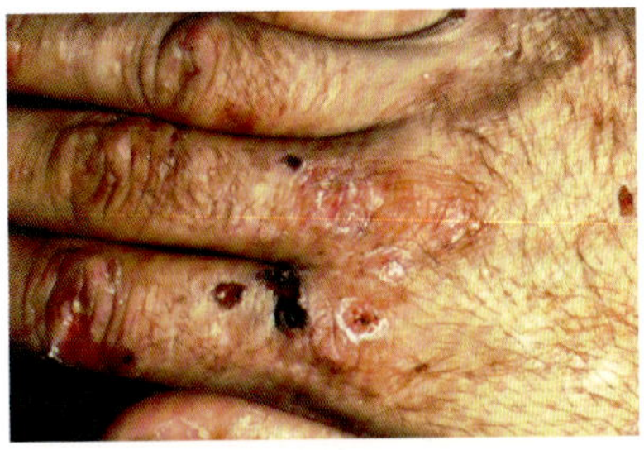

Pemphigus foliaceus
Autoimmune blistering with lesions that are scaly, with crusted over lesions on an erythematous base.
Antibodies block desmoglein 1 from being formed into a desmosome.

MC in river valleys in rural Brazil.
Can also be drug induced due to:
Penicillamine, Captopril, Nifedipine, and NSAIDS.

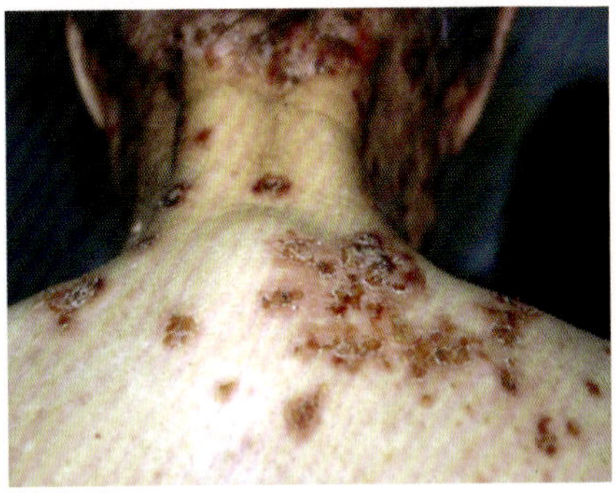

Toxic Shock Syndrome
TSST: caused by S. aureus (enterotoxin).
TSLS: caused by S. pyogenes (exotoxins).
Severe systemic bacterial infection due to a superantigen toxin that allows the binding of MHCII with T cell receptors.

SX: High fever > 102°F, BP < 90 mmHg, desquamation (especially on the hands and soles), involvement of ≥3 organ systems (GI: vomiting/diarrhea), Muscular (myalgia), Kidney failure (↑ serum creatinine), CNS (confusion without any focal neurological features), thrombocytopenia (< 100,000), liver inflammation (↑ LFT's).

TX: ↑ Normal Saline fluids and Dopamine (pressers). Treat for both S. aureus and S. pyogenes. **Vancomycin or Linezolid (for MRSA), Cephalosporins, Penicillins, Oxacillin, Nafcillin, Cefazolin**.

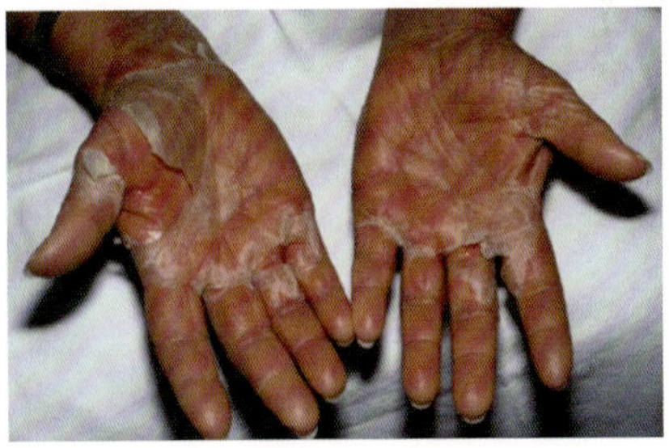

Dermatology Conditions Associated With Bacterial Infections

Cellulitis
Infection of soft subcutaneous tissues and dermis due to **S. aureus** or S. pyogenes. Organisms usually enter through a break in the skin (trauma, athlete's food – cracks between toes, breastfeeding (**mastitis**). Associated with venous stasis.

TX: See skin infection antibiotics below. The answer for treating cellulitis is **never** surgical debridement. (This is only for flesh eating bacteria in necrotizing fasciitis).

Stasis Dermatitis
Edema and hyperpigmentation due to build up of hemosiderin (from microscopic extravasation) in the dermis of the tissues.
Cause: **Venous insufficiency, varicose veins** (venous incompetence) of valves in the lower extremities.
Edema/swelling of legs is ↓ in the mornings after lying down all night, whereas in CHF, the edema is not decreased in the mornings).

TX: **Compression hose, elevation of lower legs.**
Surgical to provide some relief: "Closure Procedure", obliteration of the great saphenous and lesser saphenous veins.

Varicose Veins

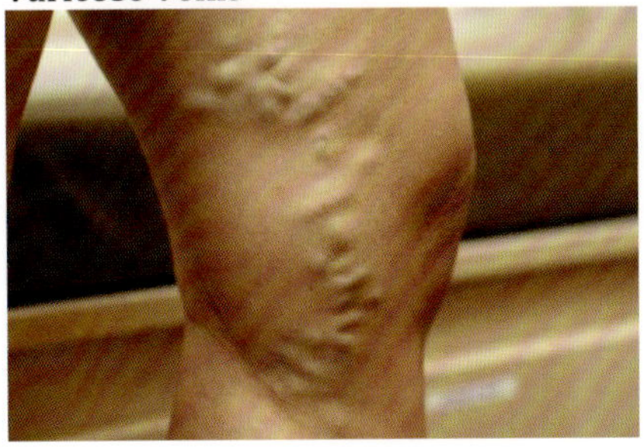

Chronic Venous Insufficiency

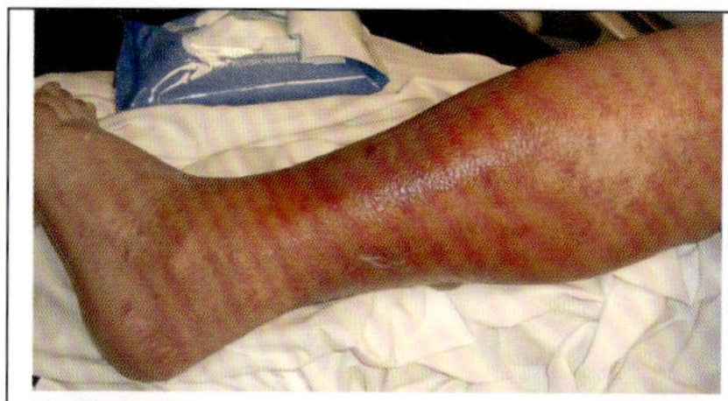

Cellulitis

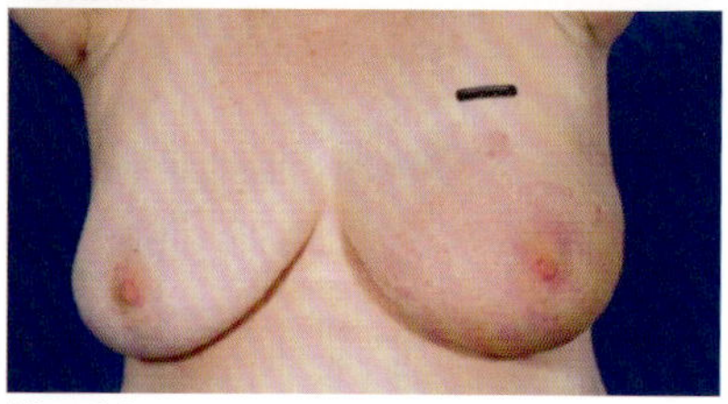

Mastitis

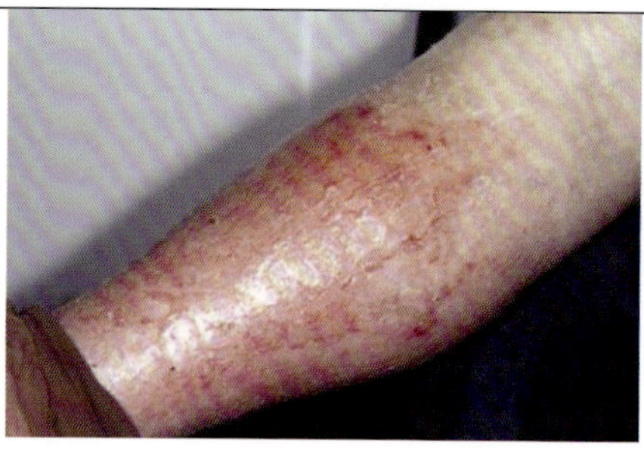

Stasis Dermatitis

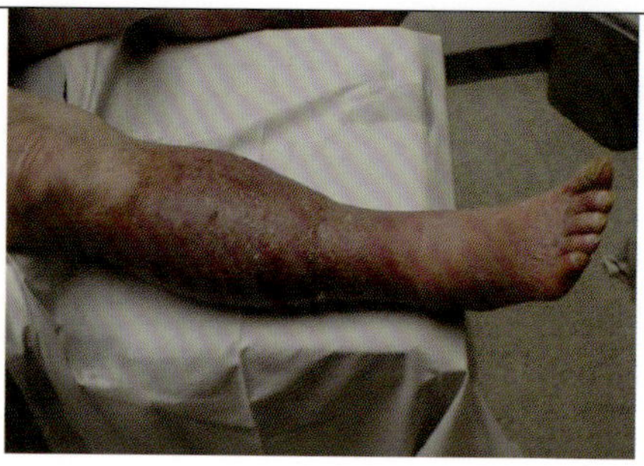

Erysipelas

Inflammation of the dermis and epidermis due to **S. pyogenes** (group A Strep) or Staph aureus.

SX: **Bright red, raised, shinny appearance with marked boarders**. Leukocytosis, bacteremia, fever, chills.

MC on faces, but can be anywhere. (Caution: don't confuse with cellulitis, which is not raised, boarders are difficult to see where they start and are not bright red).

TX: You must **treat for both**: Staph aureus and Strep pyogenes. See treatment for skin infections below. If left untreated, DZ can be fatal.

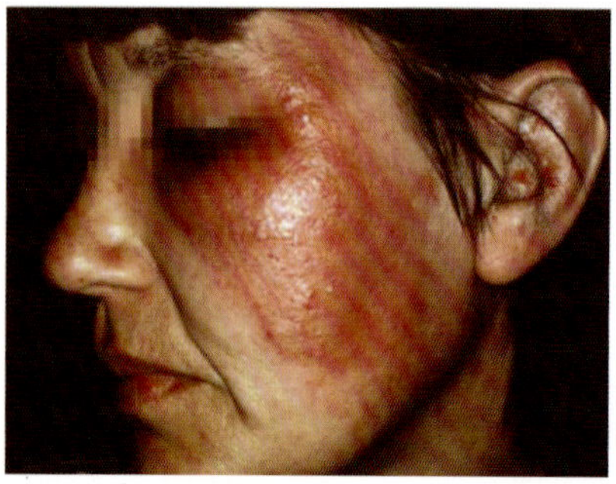

Erysipelas

Folliculitis, Furuncle, Carbuncle (boil), abscess.

Staph infection around a hair follicle. Pseudomonas can cause when source is a poorly sanitized hot tub/whirlpool.

Folliculitis: when infection is superficial around the hair follicle.
TX: **Mupirocin.**

Furuncle: when folliculitis spreads into a small group of these infections and becomes painful.
Carbuncle: Furuncle becomes a skin abscess (boil) that is extremely painful and must be drained.

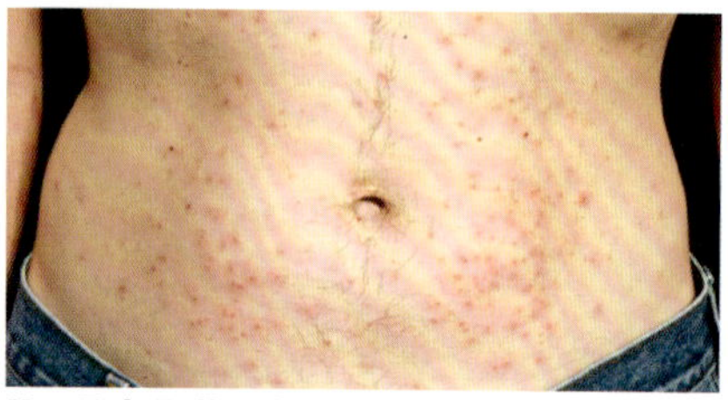

Hot Tub Folliculitis

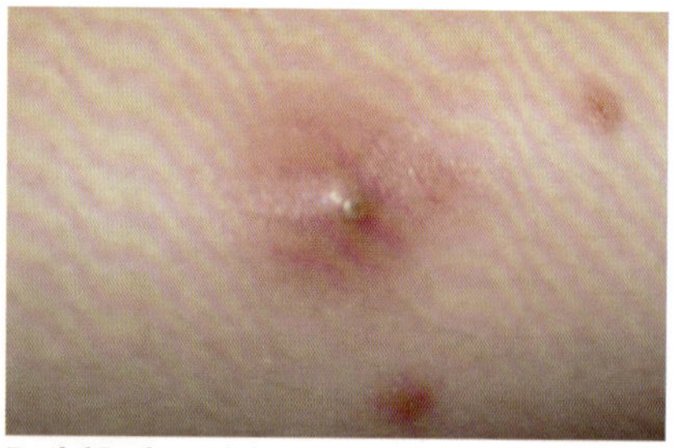

Boil (Carbuncle)

Impetigo

Honey-crusted lesions. MC found face but can be anywhere. Superficial infection caused by S. aureus or S. pyogenes.

TX: **Mupirocin, Bacitracin**

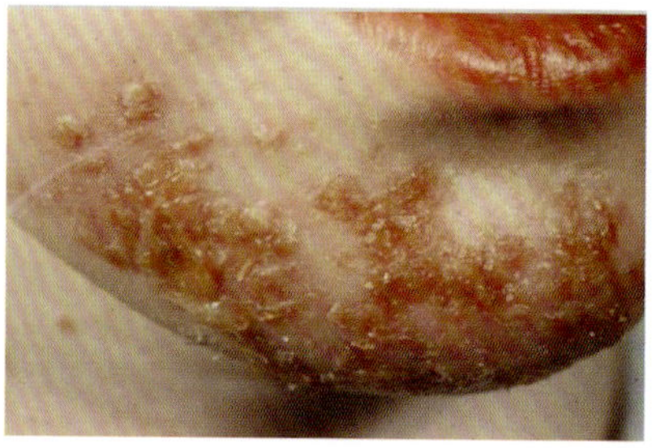

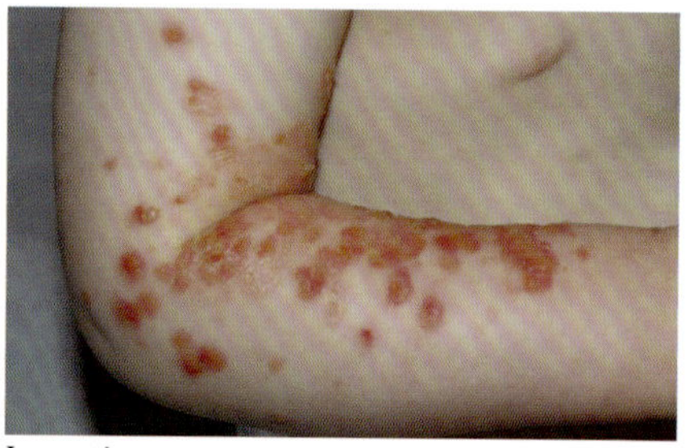

Impetigo

<table>
<tr>
<td>

Necrotizing Fasciitis
"Flesh eating bacteria"
Methane and CO2 gas production causes **crepitus** in the **deep** fascia and muscles due to S. pyogenes.
TX: **Surgery and debridement**.

Causes: **Superficial** flesh eating crepitus due to **C. perfringens**. **Only** infects the **superficial** skin and superficial fascia- NOT deep.
If the infection has affected the **deep tissues and fascia** it is due to **Strep pyogenes.**
Read description of SX carefully in questions.

SX: High fever, pain, **crepitus**.

DX: ↑ CPK. CT, MRI or X-ray shows air in the tissues and/or necrosis. High mortality rate.

TX: Surgical debridement. Ticarcillin-Clavulanate, Piperacillin-Tazobactam, Ampicillin-Sulbactam.
If Strep A: TX: **Penicillin and Clindamycin**.
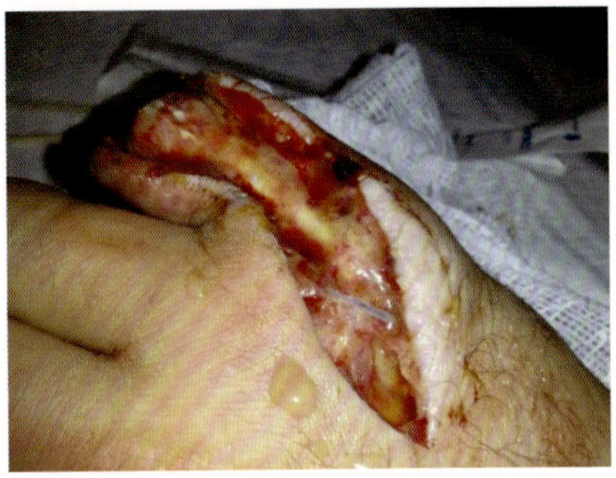
Necrotizing Fasciitis

</td>
<td></td>
<td>

Treatments for Bacterial Skin Infections

Topical: **Mupirocin.**
Mild Infections: **Oral Cephalexin, Dicloxacillin.**
If Penicillin allergies: Mild penicillin allergy: **Erythromycin (Macrolides) , Clindamycin, Clarithromycin, Doxycycline, TMP/SMX.**
Note: Cephalosporins only have a cross over reaction with penicillin in <5% of cases. If reaction to penicillin is mild (rash) it is ok to use Cephalosporins.
If the reaction to the penicillin rash is severe (anaphylactic) then you must use: **IV Vancomycin, Ceftaroline, Tigecycline, and Linezolid.**
MRSA: **TMP/SMX, Clindamycin.**
Severe: (chills, fever)
IV Nafcillin, Penicillin, and Clindamycin.
MRSA: **IV Vancomycin, Linezolid, Daptomycin, and Tigecycline.**

</td>
</tr>
<tr>
<td>

Janeway Lesions
Endocarditis.
Painless.
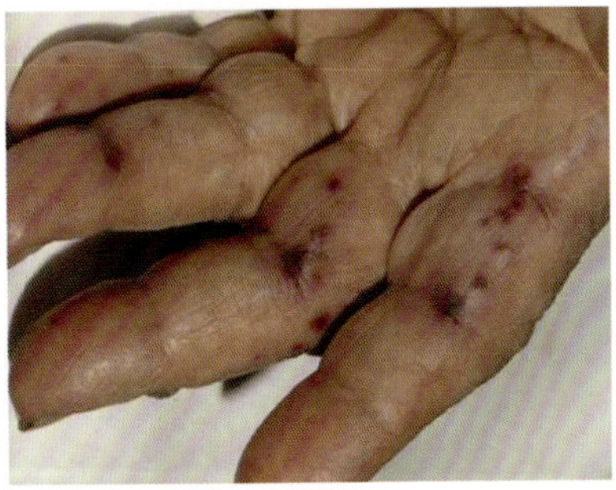

</td>
<td>

Osler Nodes
Endocarditis
Painful. (**tip**: O for Ouch)
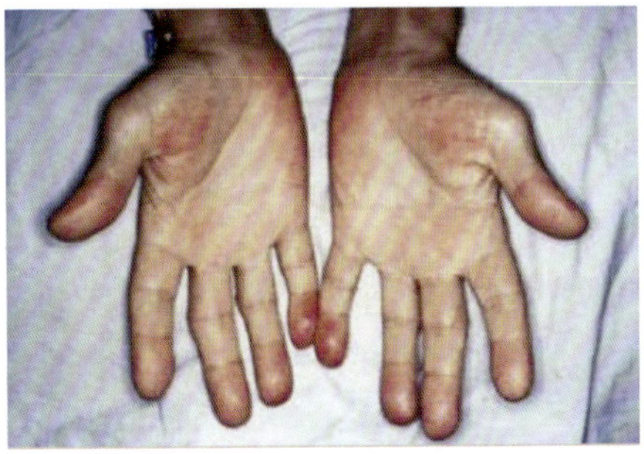

</td>
<td>

Splinter Hemorrhages
Endocarditis
Micro emboli.
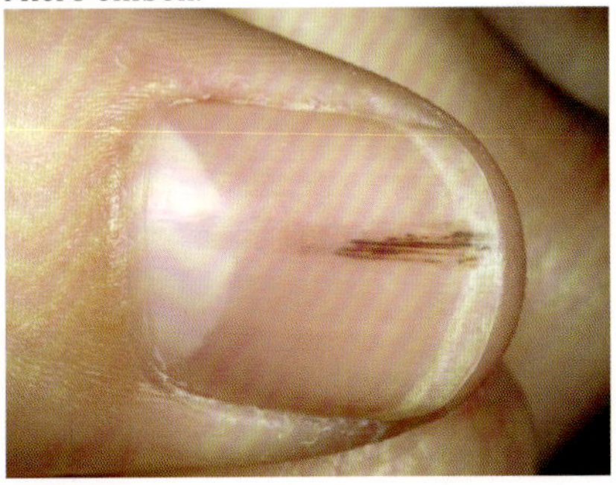

</td>
</tr>
</table>

Acne

Comedone
Blackheads (open to air) and whiteheads (closed over by skin).
Oxidation (open to air) causes the black color.
Cause: Clogged hair follicle (pore) in the skin from keratin and oils (from sebaceous glands). **Stimulation of sebaceous glands by androgens = increase oil (sebum) production.**

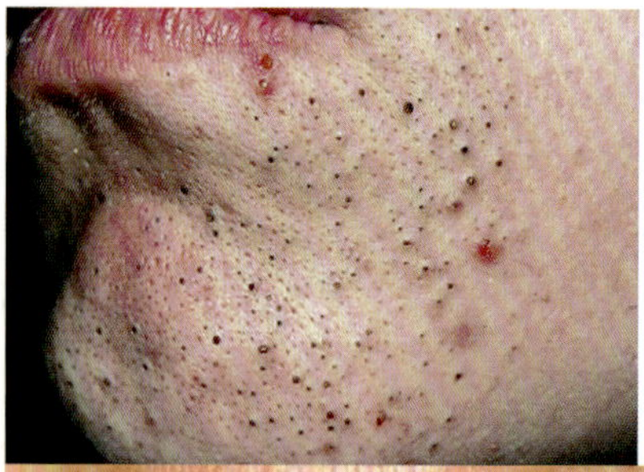

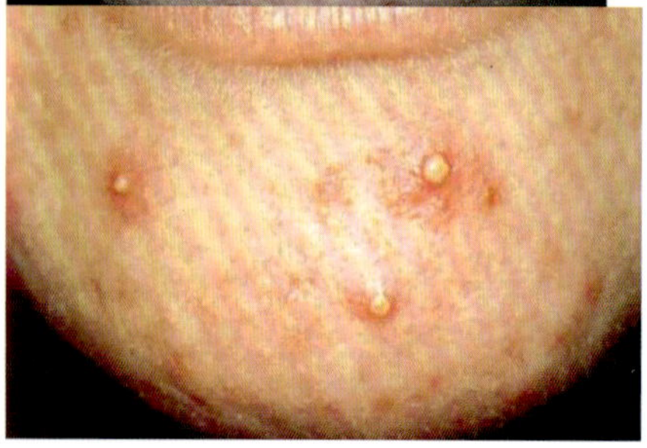

Acne
Pustules caused by **Propionibacterium acnes.**

Initial TX for mild acne: **Benzoyl peroxide.**

2° TX: Topical antibiotics: **Erythromycin, Clindamycin, Sulfacetamide.**

3rd TX: Oral antibiotics: **Tetracycline, Minocycline, Clindamycin.**
(The tetracycline family is **sun sensitive** so watch for the teenager that goes on vacation (**sun or sunbed**) and develops a rash. The tetracycline family also causes **discoloration of developing teeth and poor bone** development in the fetus and discoloration of the teeth in children).

4th TX: Topical retinoids
Last TX or for severe, scarring acne: **Oral retinoic acid derivative: Isotretinoin, Tretinoin, Tazarotene, Adapalene.** **Retinoic acids are severe teratogens. Must check β-hCG for pregnancy** and must insure female is on birth control while on the drug.

Acne Vulgaris

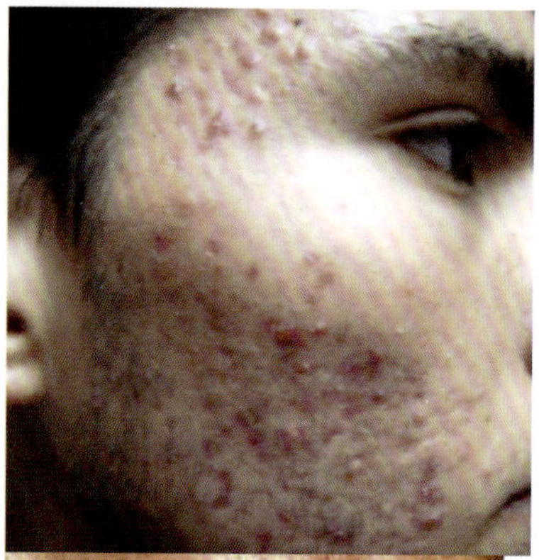

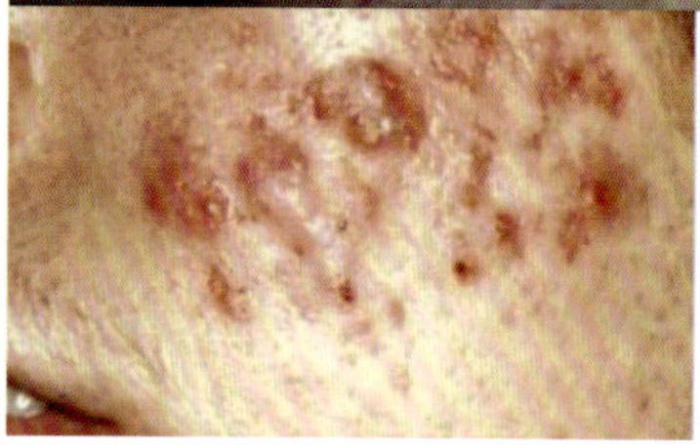

Leprosy
AKA: Hanson's DZ
Mycobacterium
TX: **Dapsone**

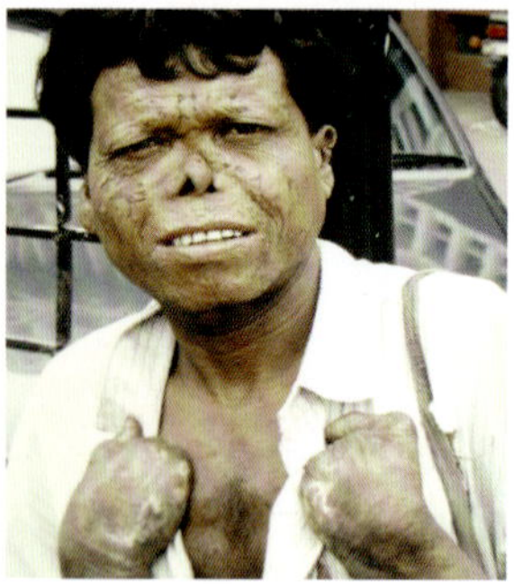

Meningococcemia.
Blood infection from N. meningitides.
Can lead to death.

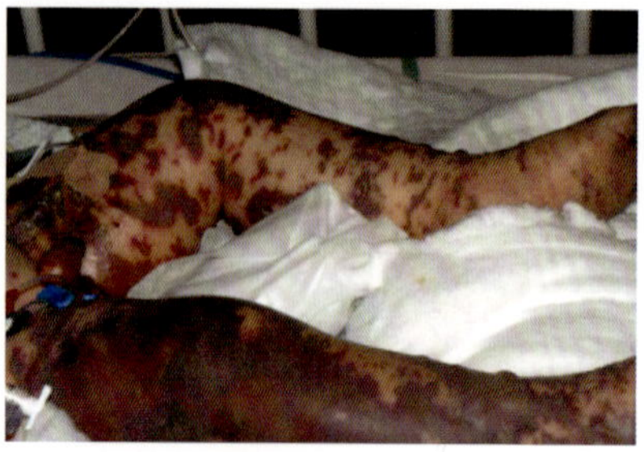

Septic Arthritis
High WBC counts in synovial fluid.
Unilateral joint involvement.

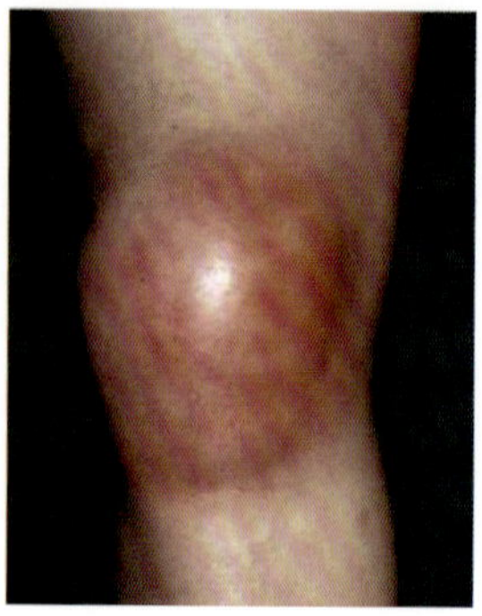

Bacterial Diaper Rash	Scarlet Fever Rash	Bacterial Infections:
Does not go into the folds of the skin. Not as red as a fungal rash. (Fungal Candida rash goes IN to the folds and is much redder) 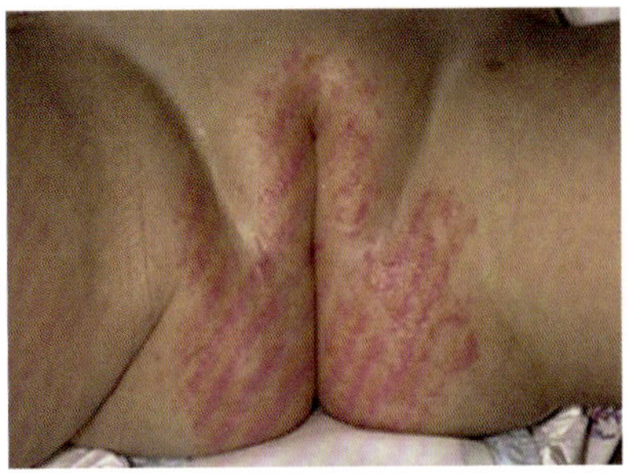	Infection by S. pyogenes (Group A Strep). SX: sore throat, fever, erythematous "Sand paper" (rough) blanching skin rash and bright red tongue ("Strawberry tongue"). 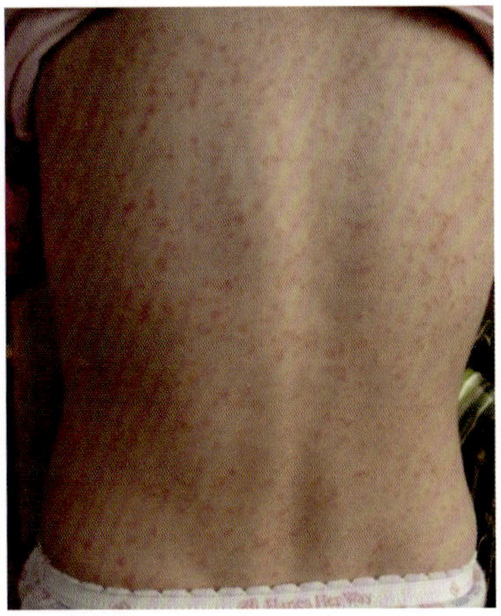 Scarlet Fever rash	Carbuncles, Cellulitis, Erysipelas, Folliculitis, Furuncles, Impetigo, Necrotizing fascitis, Paronychia. TX: **Oral: Cephalexin (Keflex), Cefadroxil (Duricef), Dicloxacillin.** **If organism is Strep: Ampicillin (add β-lactamase inhibitor), Penicillin G.** **Penicillin rash allergy: Use Cephalosporins.** **Penicillin allergies if more than just a rash reaction (anaphylaxis): Macrolides (Erythromycin, Azithromycin, Clarithromycin), Fluoroquinolones (Levofloxacin, Gatifloxacin, Moxifloxacin).** **MRSA resistance: IV Vancomycin.** **Oral: Linezolid, Bactrim.** **IV: Oxacillin, Nafcillin (equivalent to Dicloxacillin. Cefazolin (equivalent of Cefadroxil.**

Dermatology Conditions Associated With Viruses

Erythema infectiosum	Measles	Shingles (Varicella Zoster)
AKA: Slapped Cheek DZ due to Parvo B-19 (AKA: Fifth DZ). 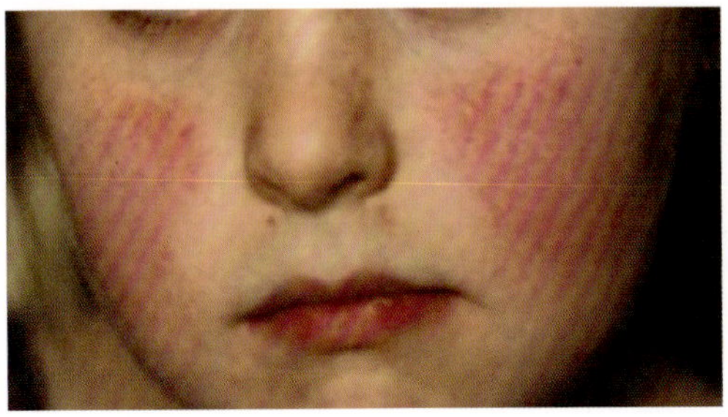	"Morbilliform rash" TX: **Vitamin A** 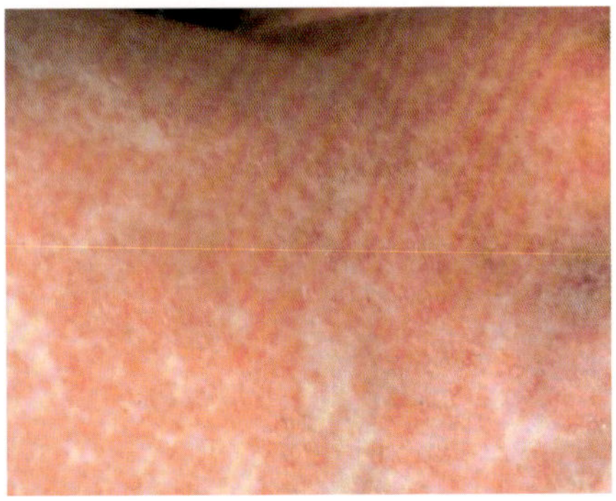	Lies dormant in the dorsal root ganglia. Erupts along dermatome lines. TX: **Famciclovir, Acyclovir, Valacyclovir**. 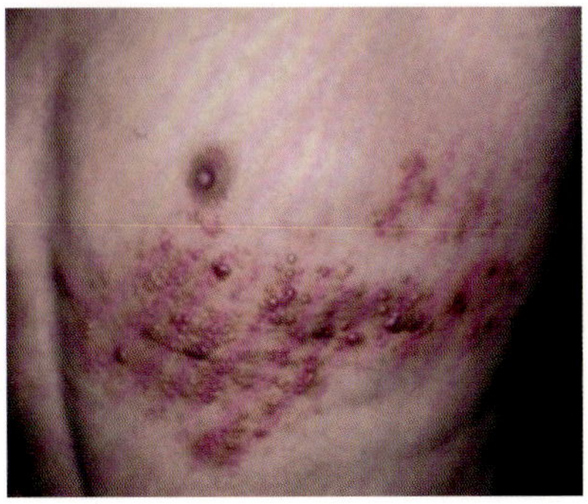

Warts

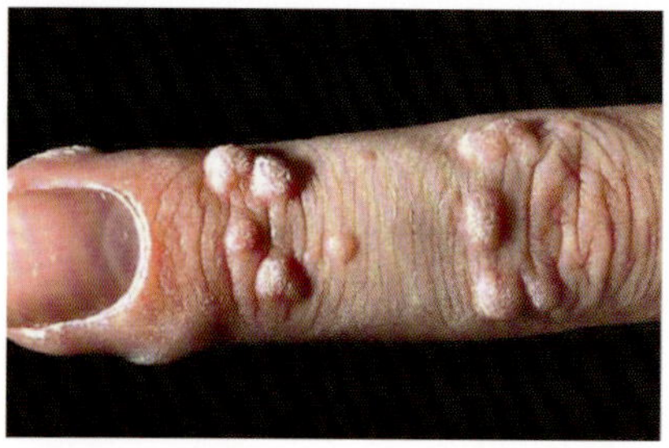

Planters Wart

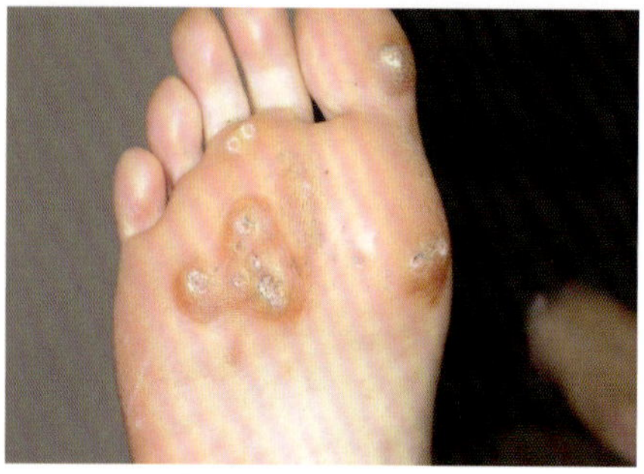

Pityriasis rosea
Erythematous pruritic and pink colored pigmentation. Presents as a single lesion (AKA: "herald patch") then spreads into a generalized rash for several months.
Resembles 2° syphilis but spares the palms and soles. (Has a negative VDRL).
Self-limited.

TX: Ultraviolet light and **steroids.**
Oral antihistamines can also decrease the itching.

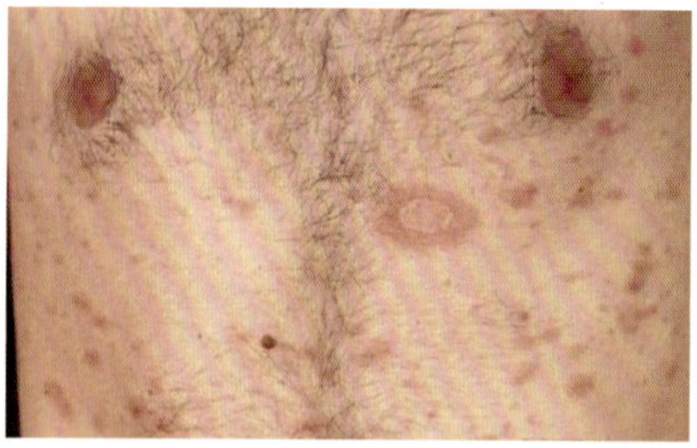

Herpes Simplex
Multiple, painful **vesicles** on the lips/oral mucosa or genitals. (AKA: vesicular rash).
Herpes 1: dormant in trigeminal ganglia.
Herpes 2: dormant in sacral ganglia.
DX: best initial: Tzanck smear.
Most accurate: Viral culture

TX: **Oral Acyclovir, Valacyclovir, Famciclovir.**
Acyclovir resistance: Foscarnet.

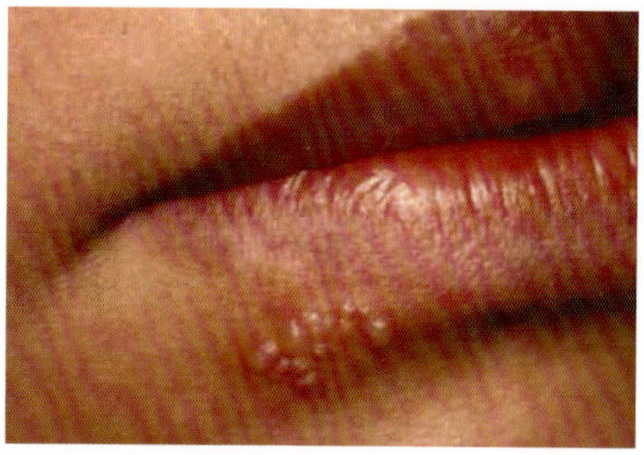

Herpes Simplex I

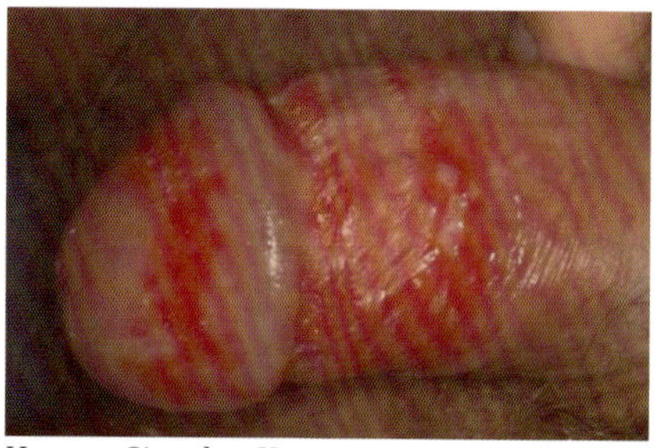

Herpes Simplex II

Herpes Zoster
(AKA: Varicella, Chickenpox, **Shingles**)
Shingles (AKA: Dermatomal Herpes Zoster)

Chickenpox: vesicles in different stages of healing. In children: no treatment.
Adults TX: **Acyclovir, Valacyclovir, Famciclovir.**

Herpes Zoster (Shingles):
Vesicles break normally out along a dermatome but the rash can break out anywhere. Usually due to a stress.
Lies dormant in the **dorsal root ganglia.**
Outbreak is preceded by burning/itching.
(Remember: Herpes 1 lies dormant in the trigeminal ganglia. Herpes 2 lies dormant in the sacral ganglia and Herpes Zoster (Shingles) lies dormant in the dorsal root ganglia).

TX: **Acyclovir, Valacyclovir, Famciclovir.**
IV Acyclovir for ↓ postherpetic neuralgia.
Oral TX for postherpetic neuralgia:
Gabapentin (most effective), TCA's, topical Capsaicin.

Adult exposure to chickenpox: if adult is nonimmune: TX: **Varicella zoster immune globulin** within 96 hours of exposure.

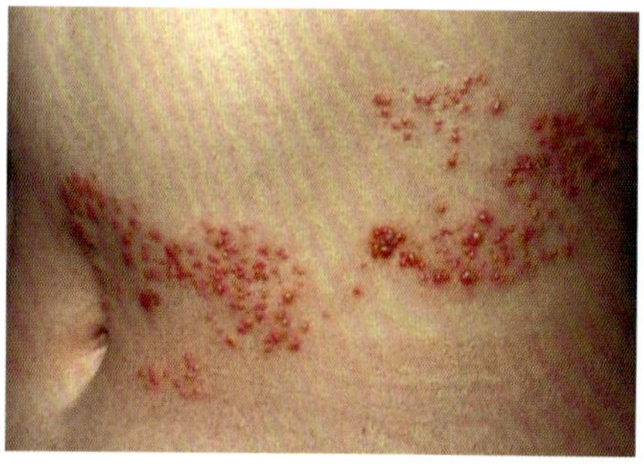

Dermatology Conditions Associated With Fungus/Molds

Tinea pedis 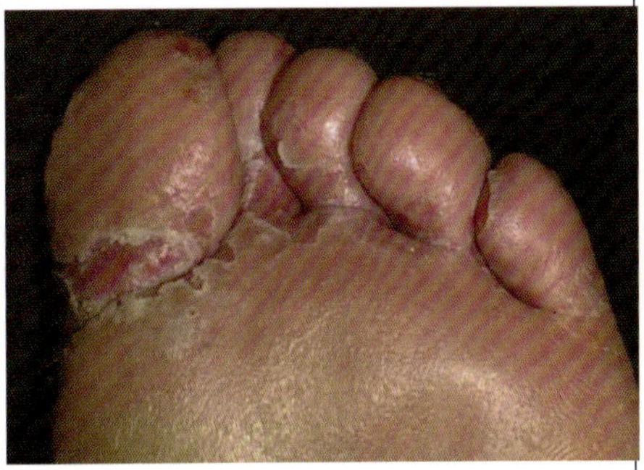	**Tinea cruris** 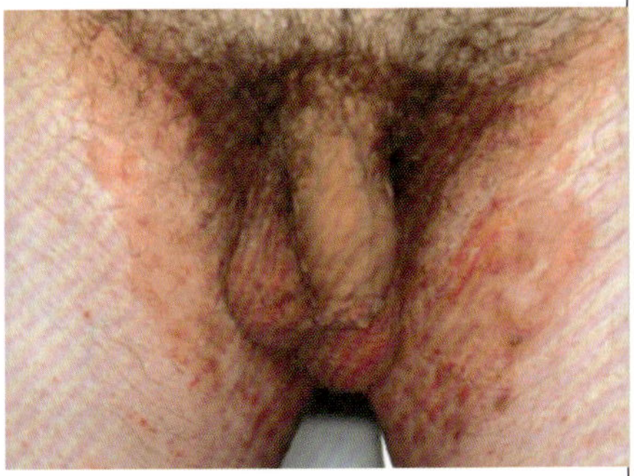	**Tinea corporis** 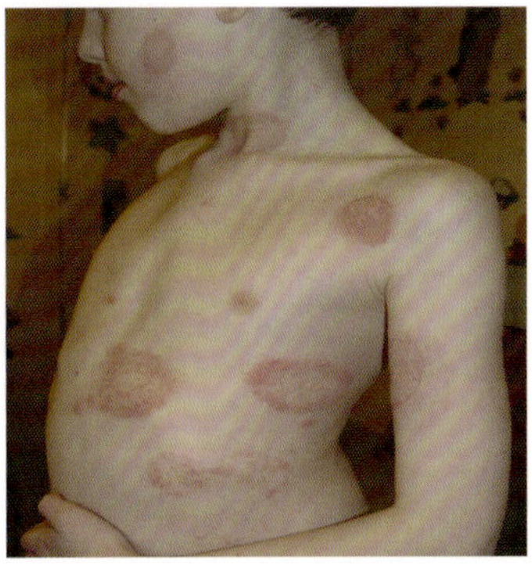
Tinea versicolor **Malassezia furfur** 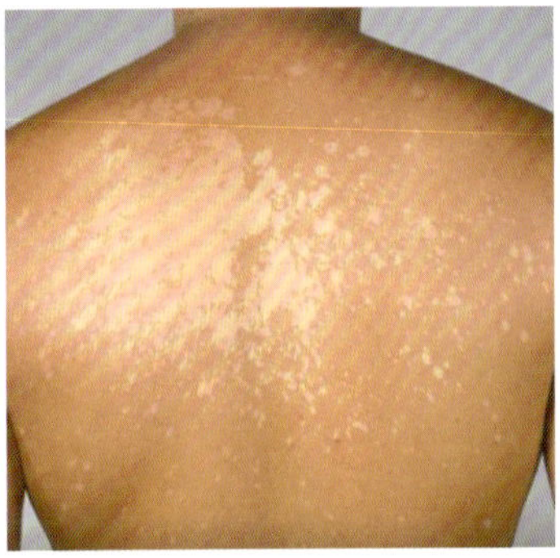	**Tinea capitis** 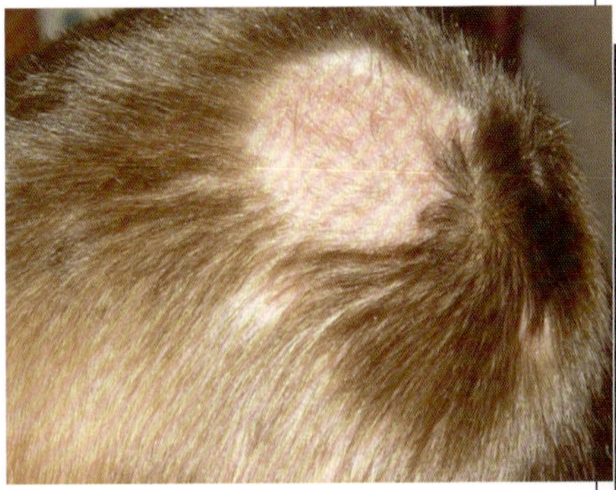	**Onychomycosis** **(AKA: Tinea unguium)** 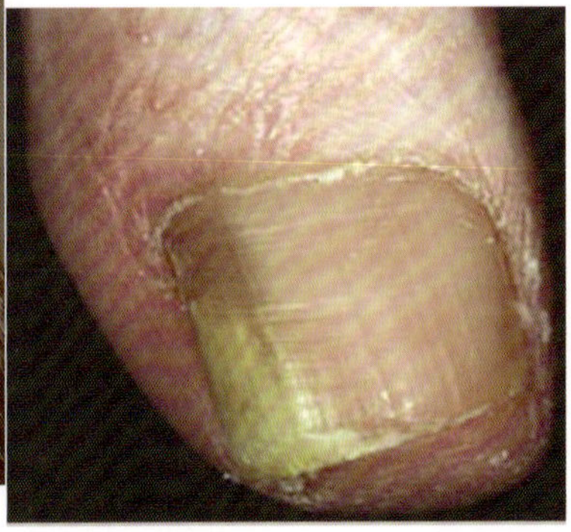
Seborrheic Dermatitis **AKA: Dandruff** **(Infants: AKA: Cradle cap)** Excess secretion of sebaceous glands – inflammatory skin disorder. SX: **Dandruff**. Can occur on the **hair, eyebrows and nasolabial folds.** Flaky skin and scalp or patchy scaling thick crust on the scalp. Can also occur on the face, eyelashes, eyebrows and sides of the nose. Associated with Malassezia furfur. Multifactorial causes. TX: **Zinc pyrithione** as a shampoo, topical antifungal, **Corticosteroids (hydrocortisone), antifungals (ketoconazole), antihistamines.**	**Sporothrix schenckii** "Rose Gardner's DZ" Dimorphic fungus. Subcutaneous nodules/ulcers ascending up the lymphatics. Host tissues: yeast. Outside of body: mold. TX: **Potassium iodide, Itraconazole, Terbinafine, Fluconazole. (Disseminated: Amp B)** 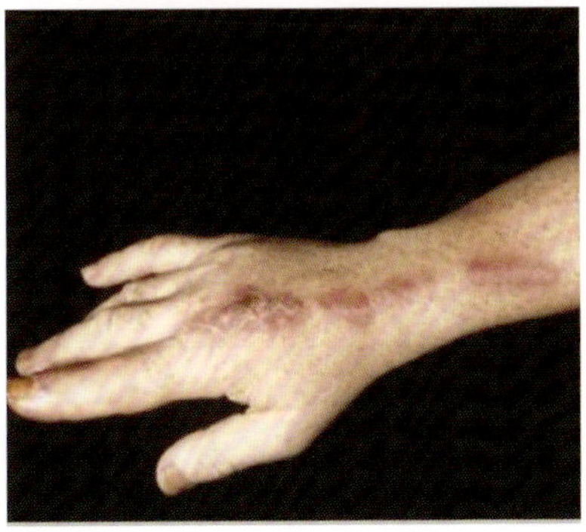	**Cryptococcosis** 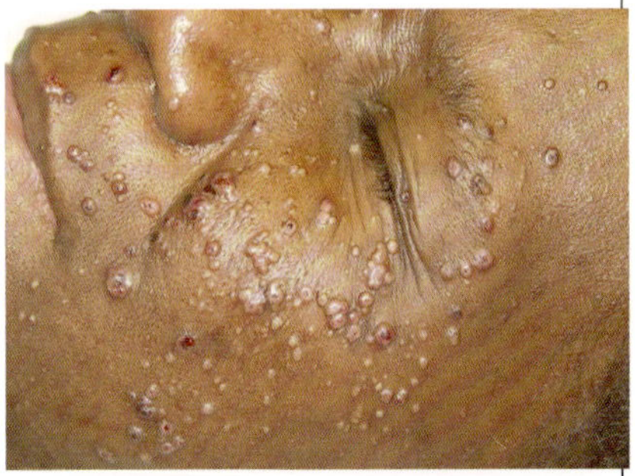 **Coccidioidomycosis** Southwest US. 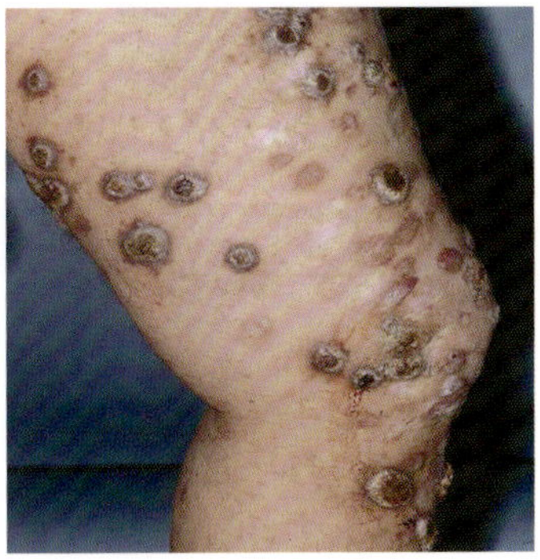

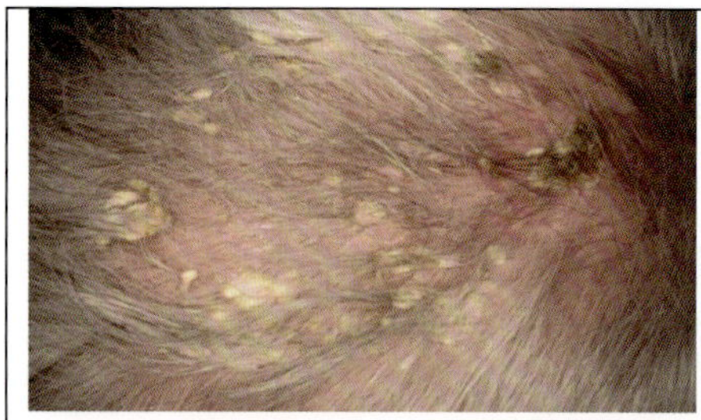

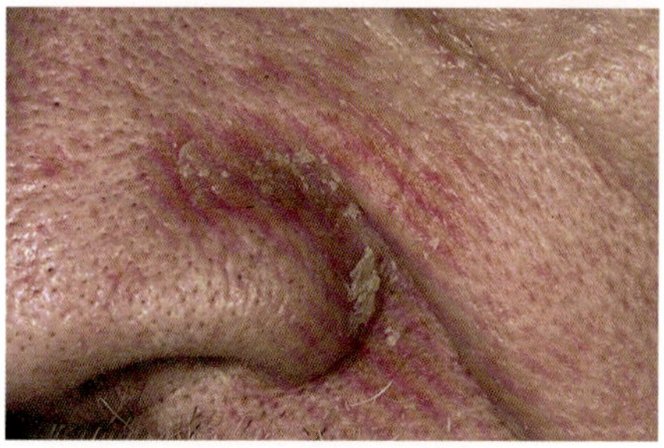

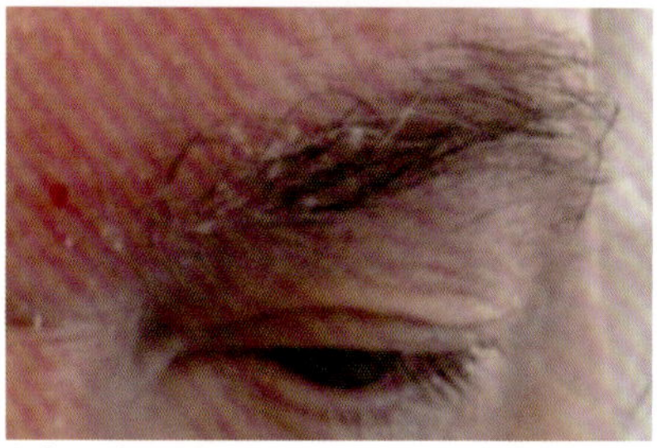

Seborrheic Dermatitis

Blastomycosis
Northeast US.

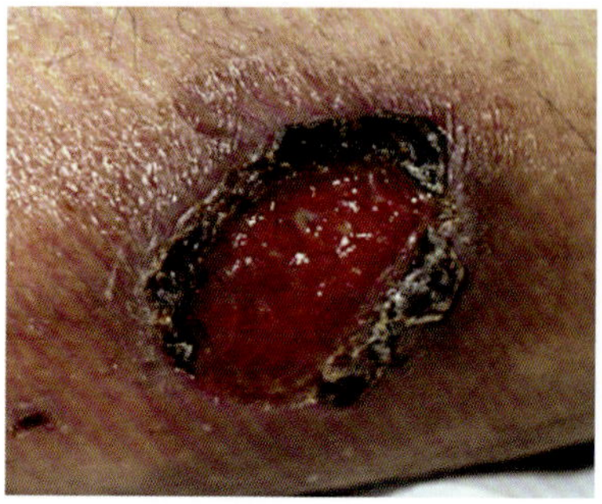

Mucor
AKA: Rhizopus, Absidia, Rhizomucor.
90 degree branching.
Black eschar.
MC: Diabetics. Mucor spores enter through Cribriform palate.
Usually fatal.
TX: **Amp B.**

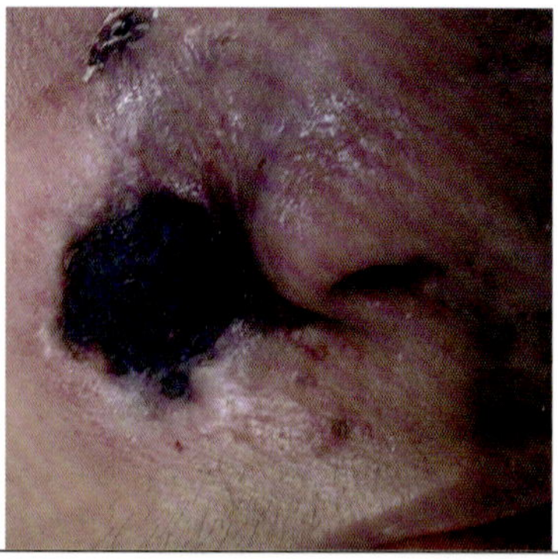

Fungal Diaper Rash.
Diaper rash due to Candida.
Rash goes into the folds of the skin and is bright red.
"candINda" IN the crevices.
(Bacterial diaper rash: lighter red/pink and does NOT go into the folds).

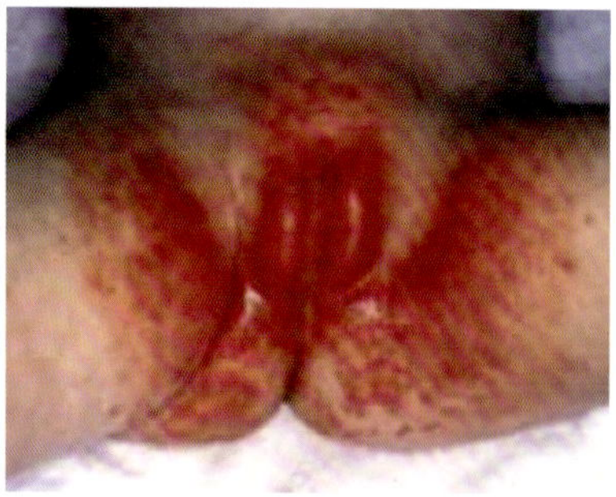

Histoplasmosis

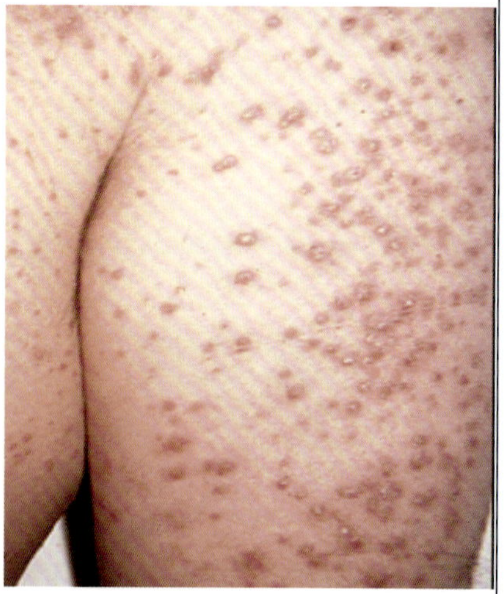

Dermatology Conditions Associated With Parasites and Zoonotics

Lyme DZ

SX: **Target lesion**. (AKA: erythema's lesion with central clearing) appearing 7 – 10 days after bite and is ≥ 5cm in diameter.
Tick: Ixodes tick.
System infection: SX: joint pain/arthritis, cardiac, neurological problems.

TX: Oral doxycycline. If patient I pregnant or under 8 yrs old: use Amoxicillin.

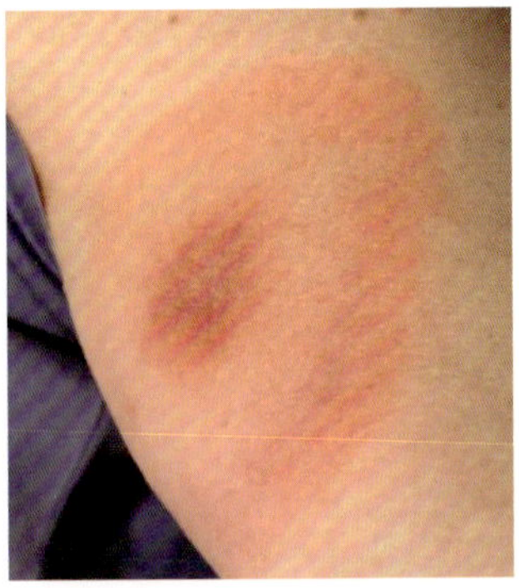

Rocky Mountain Spotted Fever

Rash starts on wrist and spreads to trunk.
Dermacentor tick.

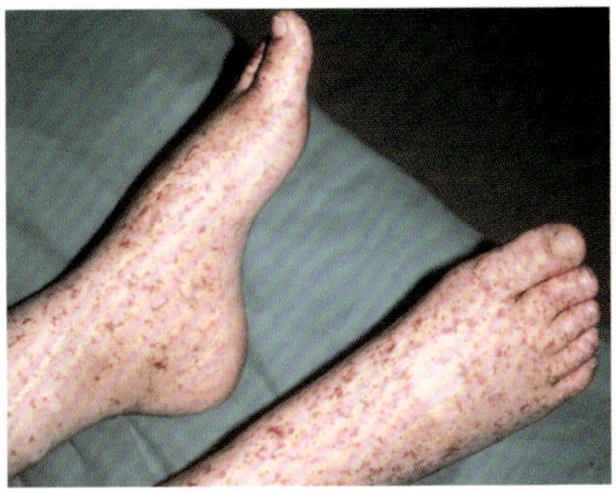

Scabies

Pruritic lesions causes by the organism burrowing in the web spaces between fingers and toes, breast and penis.
SX: "tunnels" in thee webs between the toes/fingers and excoriations (scratch marks due to intense pruritus).
DX: Apply mineral oil over the lesion and scrap out the organism.
TX: Topical **Permethrin, Lindane**.
(Norwegian scabies: form that ↑ with HIV.
TX: **oral Ivermectin**

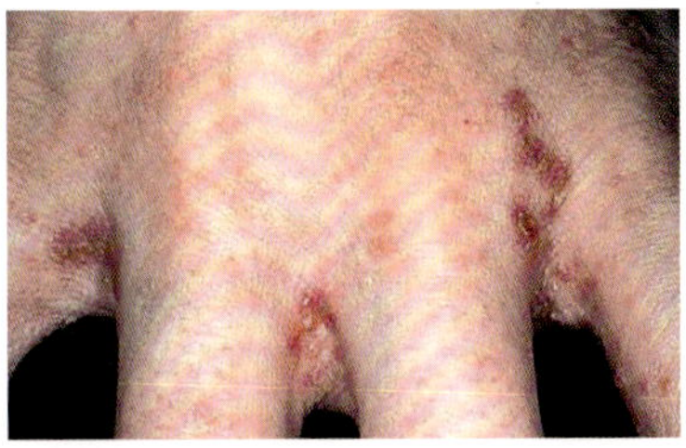

Pediculosis

Lice and Crabs
Organisms that infect areas with hair.
Cause: sharing personal items: hairbrush, hats, and sexual contact.

TX: **Permethrin**.

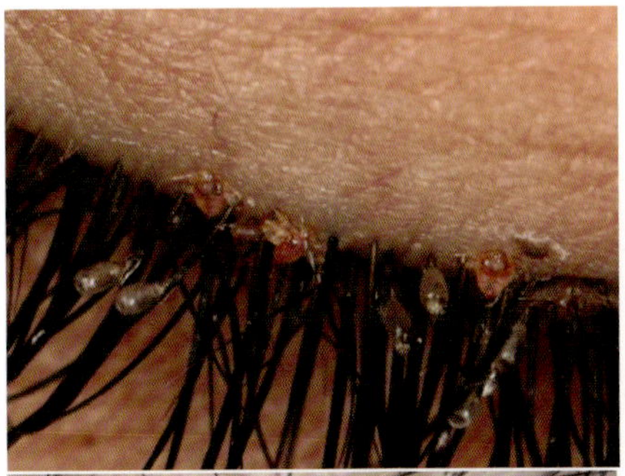

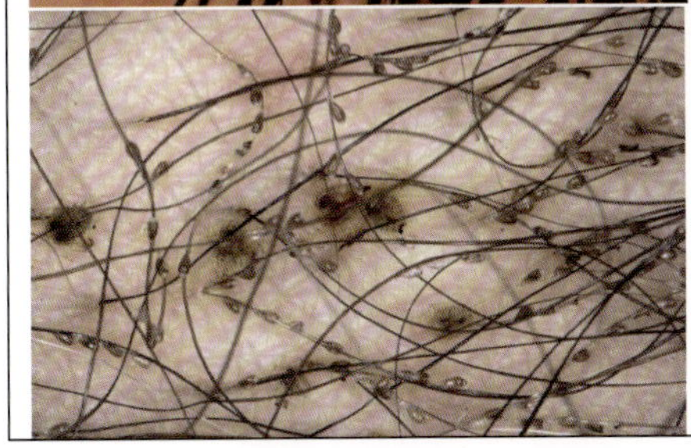

Anthrax: Cutaneous

Cause: contact with animals (sheep, goats, any animal with a coat of hair/wool).
Bioterrorism agent.
SX: Lesion with **central black necrosis**.

DX: Gram stain and culture.

TX: **Ciprofloxacin, Doxycycline.**

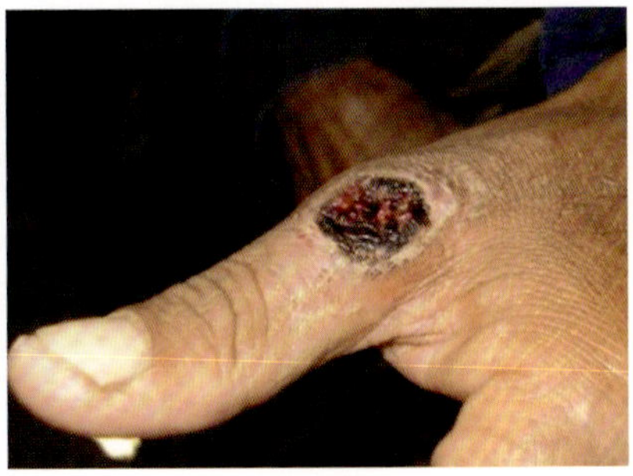

Leishmaniasis

Black Fever via sandfly

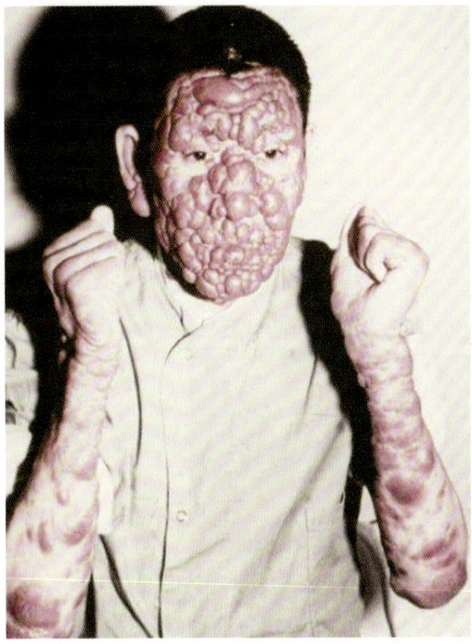

Flea bites

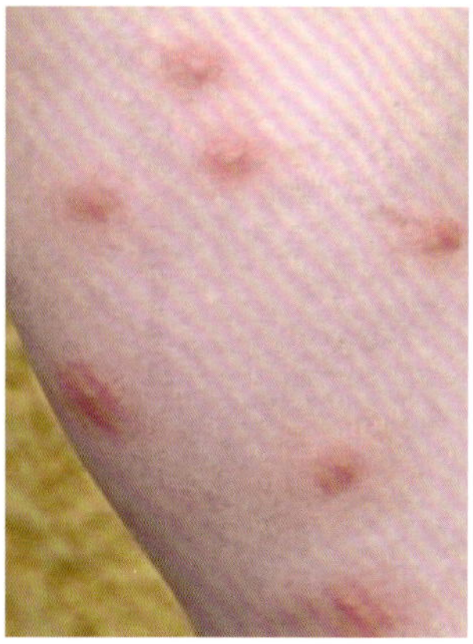

Bed bug bites

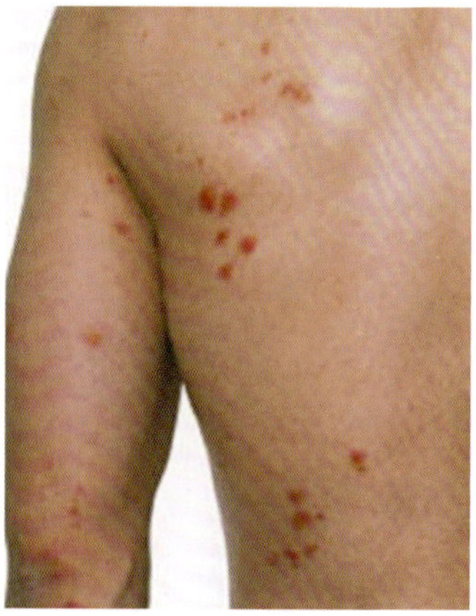

Wuchereria bancrofti
Elephantiasis
Lymphatic's blocked.

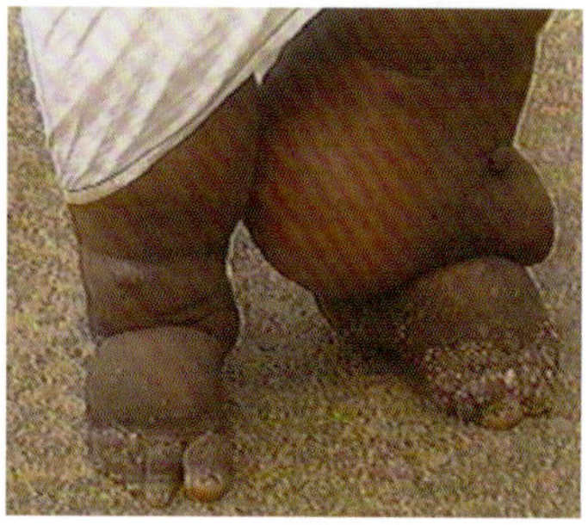

Dermatology Conditions Associated With Chronic or Autoimmune Diseases

Dermatitis Herpetiformis
Pruritic **vesicles** that **mimics a herpes** rash. MC found on elbow or knees.
Due to **IgA deposits** at dermal papillae.
Associated with **Celiac DZ** (blunted villi, grains: rice, barley, rye)

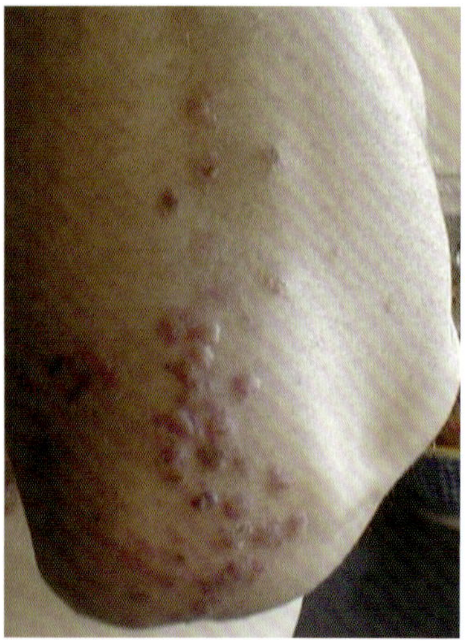

Henoch Schonlein Purpura
Systemic vasculitis: Palpable purpura, joint, abdominal pain shortly following an URI or GI infection.

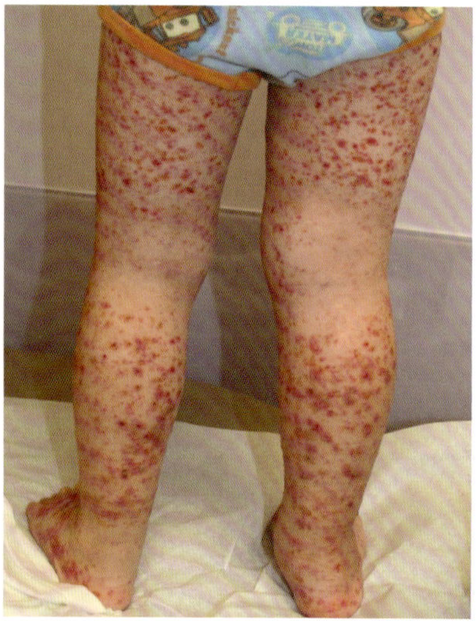

Dermatomyositis
Heliotrope rash.

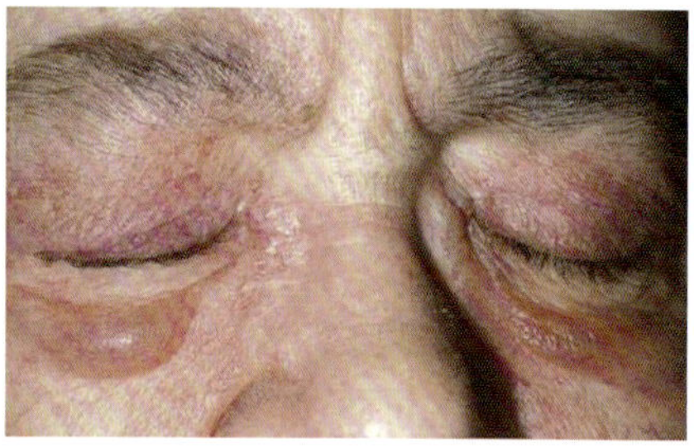

Gottron's Papules
Dermatomyositis

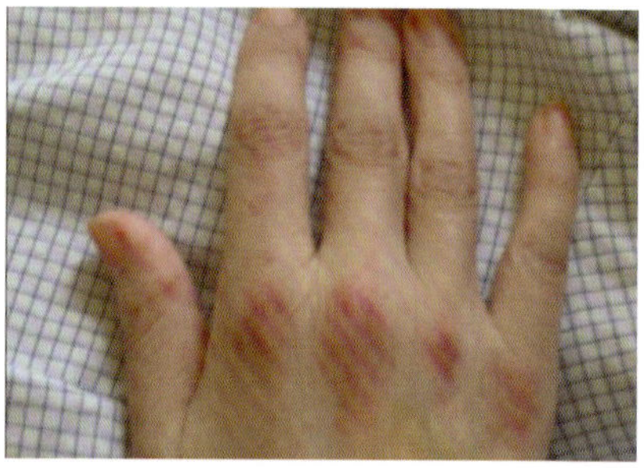

Malar Rash
AKA: Butterfly rash.
Involves cheeks and bridge of the nose but **spares the nasolabial folds.**
SX in: SLE, Pellagra, and Dermatomyositis.

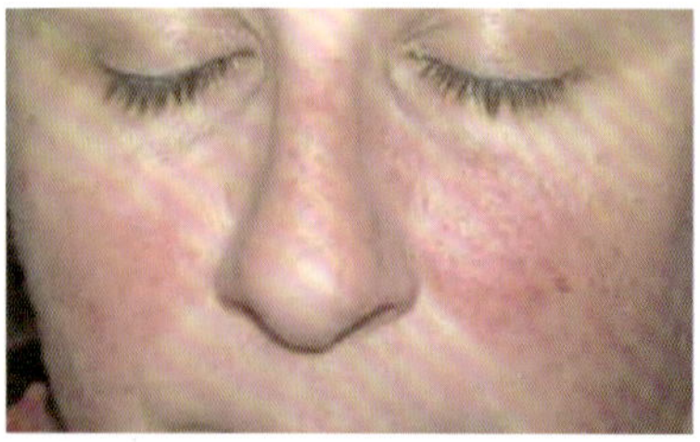

Sclerodactyly
Scleroderma (CREST) syndrome.
Thickening and tightening of the skin on the fingers/and or toes.

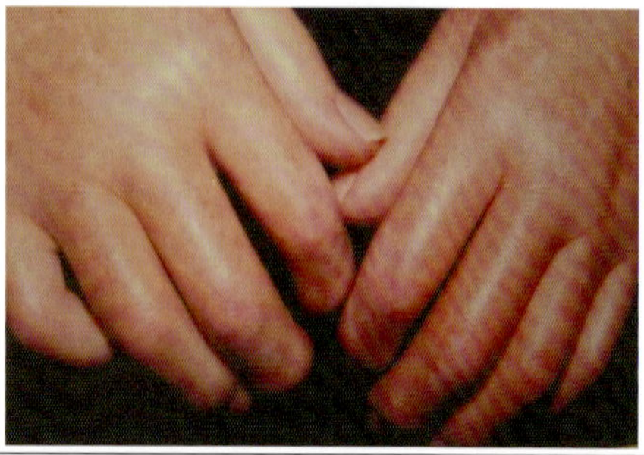

Rosacea
Chronic. Pustules, papules, swelling, erythema, and superficial dilated blood vessels. (Looks like acne, but is not, do not confuse with acne vulgaris).

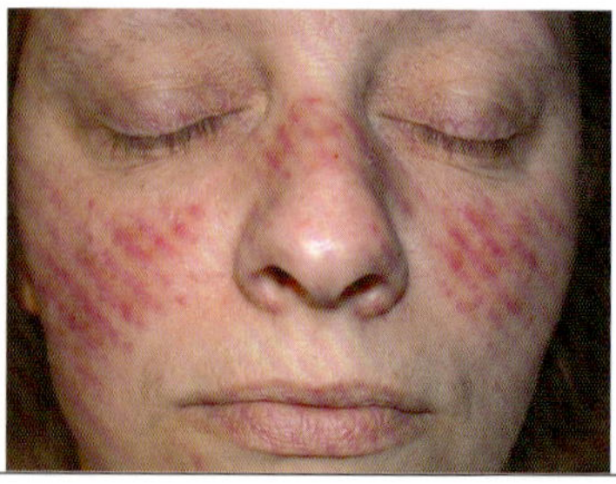

Rheumatoid Arthritis

Specific: anti-CCP (cyclic citrullinated peptide test).
Involves the MCP joints. RA is symmetrical and improves through the day.
TX: **Methotrexate, steroids.**

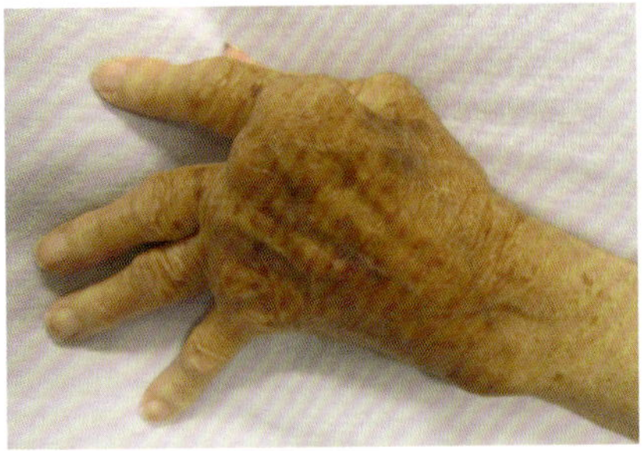

Reynaud's Phenomenon

Decreased blood flow due to cold or stress that results in pale color of hands/fingers.
SX in: CREST syndrome, SLE, RA, Sjogren's, Dermatomyositis.
TX: **Calcium Channel Blockers.**

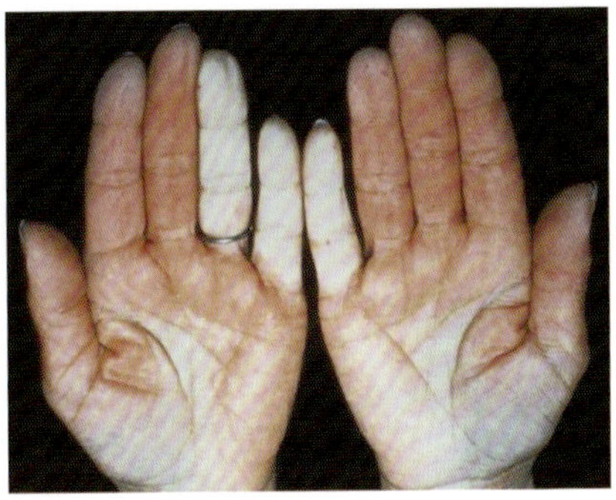

Lichen Planus

Reticular white, pruritic lines/plaque (**looks like lace**) over an area of purple flat papules due to lymphocytes at dermal-epidermal junction.
Associated with Hepatitis C.

Thought to be autoimmune.
No cure, symptomatic relief only.

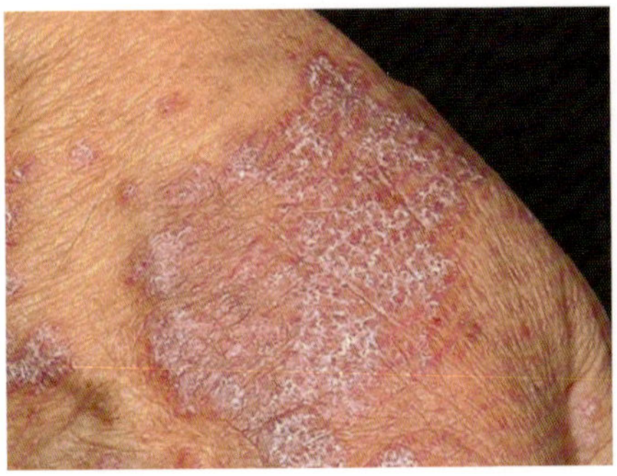

Psoriasis

Silver scaling covering plaques on skin, most common on **extensors**: **knees and elbows**.
Auspitz sign: bleed spots where psoriatic scales are scraped off.

Seen with: **nail splitting or pitting** and psoriatic arthritis.

TX: **Emollients** for all patients (Vaseline, Mineral Oil, petroleum base, Eucerin, Lubriderm, Aquaphor, Dermasil, Lac-Hydrin).
Use **Salicylic acid** to break down scaly build up so medicines can reach the psoriasis.
Localized infection: **topical steroids (fluocinonide, betamethasone, triamcinolone) or steroids containing Vitamin D**.
Coal tar, Anthralin, Topical Vitamin D (Calcipotriene) and Vitamin A (Tazarotene) derivatives.
Extensive infection: **Methotrexate**, TNF Inhibitors: **(Infliximab, Etanercept, Efalizumab, Alefacept),** ultraviolet light.

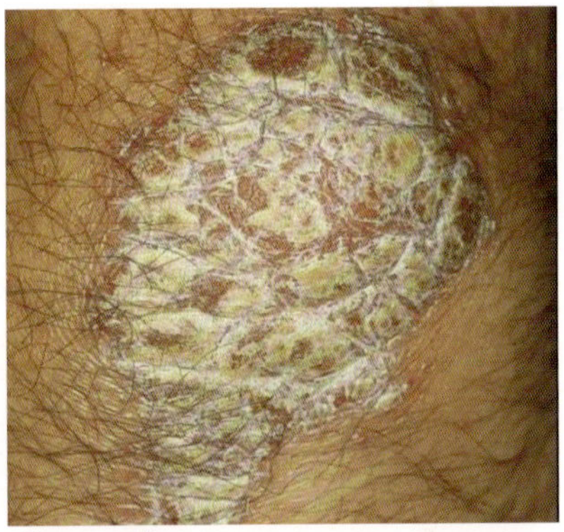

Silver scaling

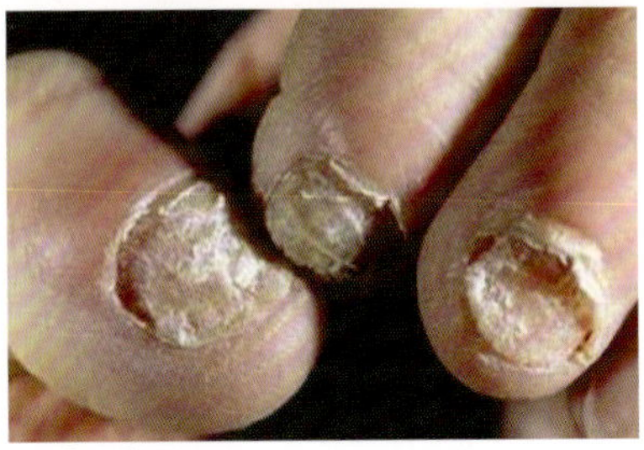

Nail splitting

Dermatology Conditions Associated Tumors, Growths, Moles, Cancer

Actinic Keratosis

Premalignant lesions due to sun exposure.

Small erythematous patch of skin with a rough, scaly scab (flaking) on the surface. Slow to develop.

Lesion can also present as a "horn" (aka: horns of actinic keratosis, Cutaneous horn).

The horn is composed of compacted keratin.

Seen on surfaces of skin with most sun exposures (MC: **top of head**).

🡅 **risk of squamous cell carcinoma** – depends on amount of dysplasia.

TX: **Cryotherapy, Curettage, Topical 5-fluorouracil (5-FU), Imiquimod, Topical retinoic acid.**

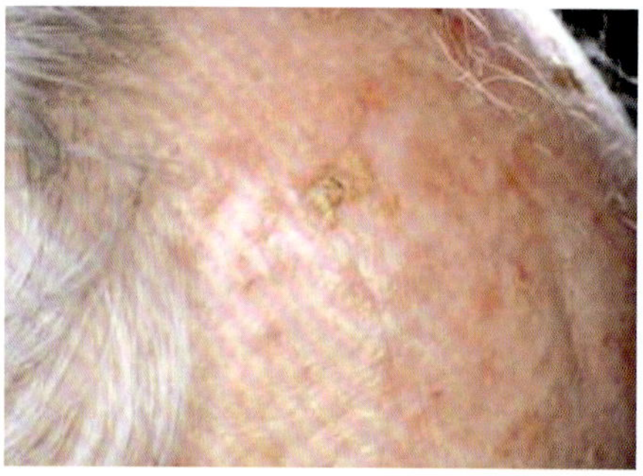

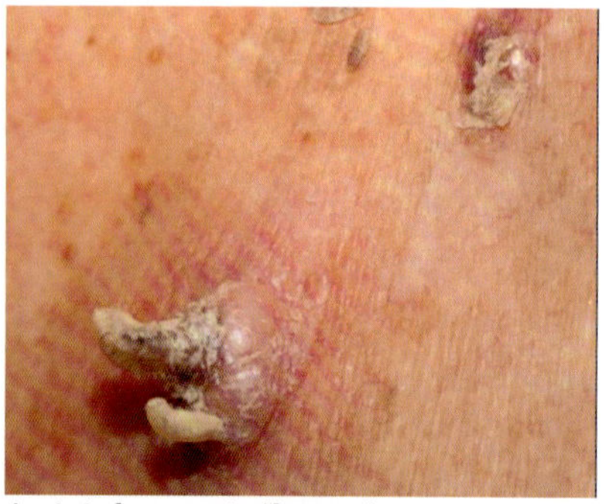

Actinic keratosis "horns" (AKA: Cutaneous horn, The "horns" of actinic keratosis)

Squamous Cell Carcinoma

Second most common skin cancer.

MC: Elderly.

Causes: Associated with: tobacco (smoking and chewing tobacco), alcohol use, exposure to **sunlight**, arsenic exposure, organ transplants, immunocompromised conditions and chronic use of immunosuppressive drugs. The combination of heavy alcohol use and smoking increases the risk of developing oral squamous cell carcinoma 100 fold in women and 38 fold in men.

Locally invasive. MC: lower lip and face. Histology: shows **"keratin pearls**" and ulceration. **Ulceration** does not heal and grows.

Actinic Keratosis is a precursor.

Histology: Squamous epithelial cells arising from the epidermis and **extending into the dermis**. Malignant cells have abundant eosinophilic cytoplasm and a large nucleus. Keratin pearls are also present.

DX: Biopsy, surgical removal.

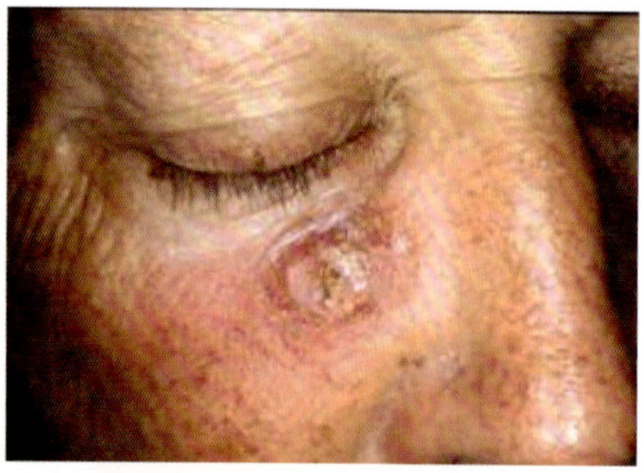

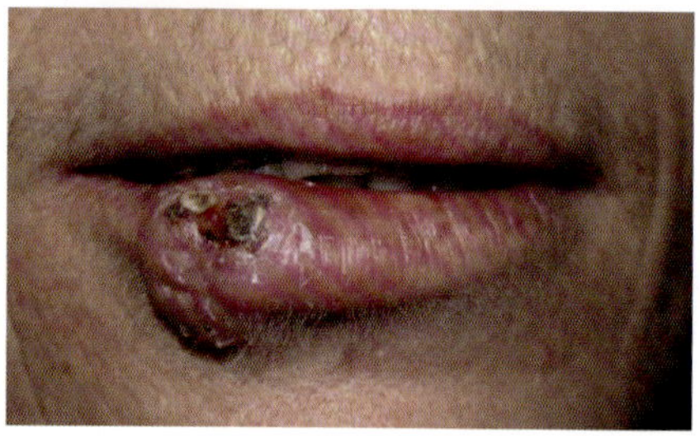

Basal Cell Carcinoma

MC skin cancer.

Located in sun-exposed areas (usually MC in areas from the level of the ear, upper lip and up). Rarely metastasizes.

SX: **Pink, pearly, waxy nodules** (no hyperpigmentation) **with central area of necrosis** (like a volcano). Grows gradually.

Histology shows "palisading" nuclei. Looks similar to molluscum contagiosum but has central area of necrosis with telangiectasis)

DX: Shave or punch biopsy, surgery. No need of wide margin excision.

Mohs surgery (during removal of cancerous lesion, thin layers of the tissue is removed and evaluated by frozen section for cancer cells, this allows for only very small amounts of tissue loss).

TX: Cryotherapy

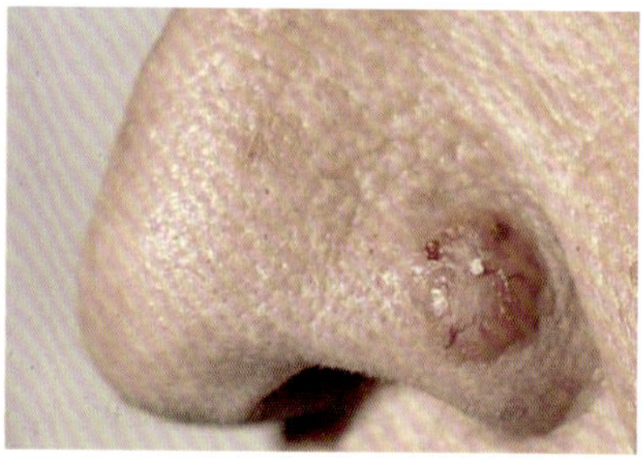

Melanoma	Neurofibromatosis-1	Keratoacanthoma
Malignant skin tumor. MCC excessive exposure to sunlight. Tumor marker: **S-100 (neural crest).** ↑ metastasis to brain. MC: Mutation if **BRAF kinase**. Metastasis depends **on invasion (depth) of tumor. Invasion due to metalloproteinase.** **Xeroderma pigmentosum has increased risk of developing a melanoma.** **Note: Before a melanoma becomes dysplastic, it is a nevocellular nevi.** **DX: Biopsy**: excision with **WIDE margins** and full thickness. Do not do shave biopsy. **Histology:** Melanocytes are located between the epidermis and dermis. Dysplasia of the keratinocytes in the basal layers of the epidermis, dermal **solar elastosis**, buds of atypical epidermis extending toward the papillary dermis, Parakeratosis, thinning of the granular layer. **Prognosis**: If the subcutaneous tissues (aka: hypodermis) are involved, it is a poor prognosis. This is the area beneath the dermis (hypodermis contains: adipose cells, macrophages and fibroblasts). **SX: ABCDE's**: **A**symmetry, **B**oarders are **irregular** (each half is not a mirror of the other half**)**, **C**olor variations in the tumor (brown, black, red), **D**iameter > 6mm, and **E**volution over time. TX: **Vemurafenib** (BRAF kinase inhibitor) 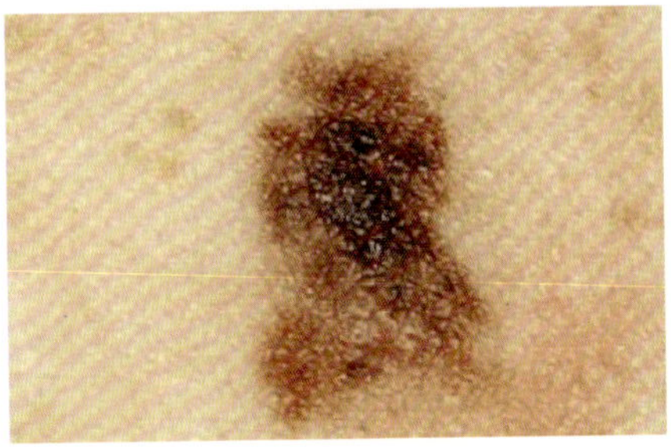 NOTE: **Dysplastic Nevus Syndrome** (AKA: Familial atypical multiple mole-melanoma: FAMMM) is another form of melanoma that runs in families. Caused by a genetic mutation in the CDKN2A gene located on chromosome 9:21.	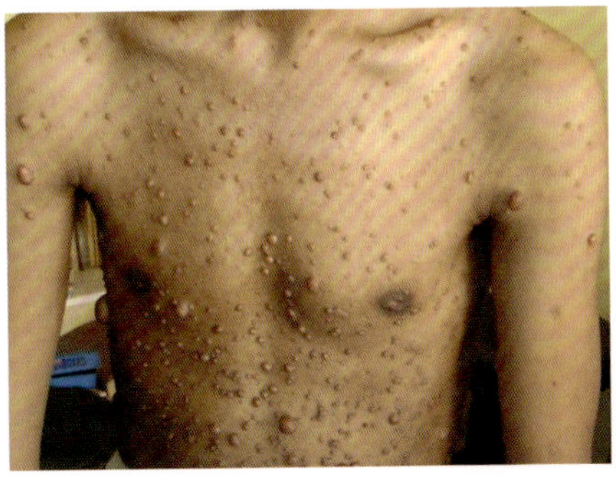	Tumor arising from the hair follicle. SX: Dome shape, symmetrical, smooth wall, topped with ceratin scales. Rapid growth: becomes large within days/weeks. Seldom metalizes and will usually necrose and heal. Don't confuse with squamous cell carcinoma. 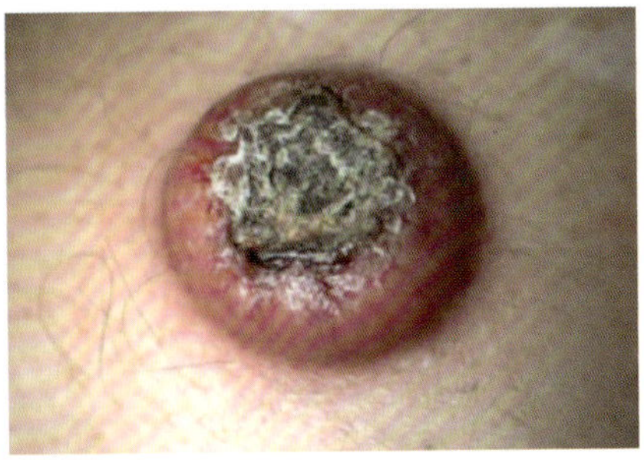

Cherry hemangioma
AKA: Senile angiomas.
Proliferation of blood vessels. Benign. Color: red to purple. Common as one ages.

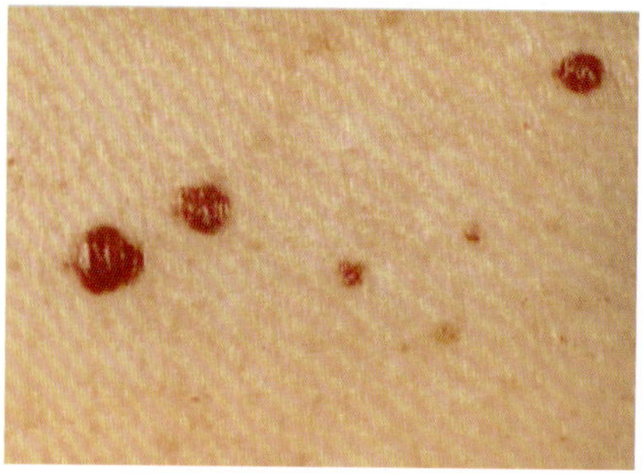

Strawberry hemangioma
Benign growth of endothelia cells (blood vessel). Self-resolving by 10 yrs old.

(**tip** to remember cherry hemangioma verses strawberry hemangioma: Strawberry hemangioma 's are in children: children play with Strawberry Shortcake)

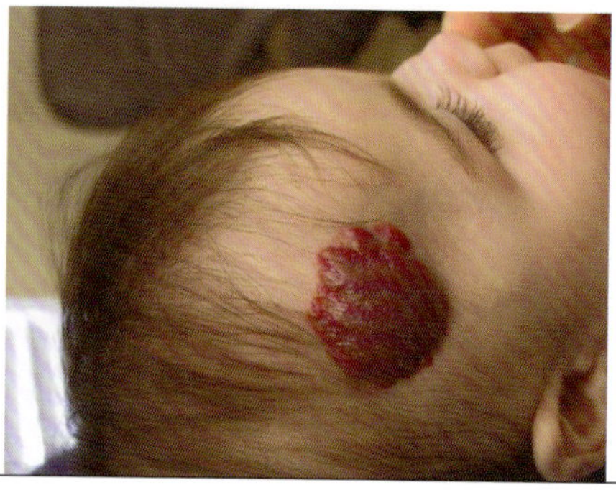

Pyogenic Granuloma
Vascular lesion following minor trauma.

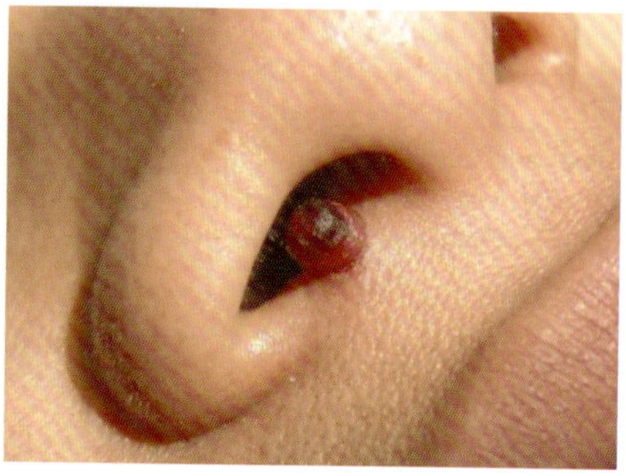

Paget's DZ of the Nipple
Discharge (bloody, yellow), crusting, flaking on the nipple or areola.

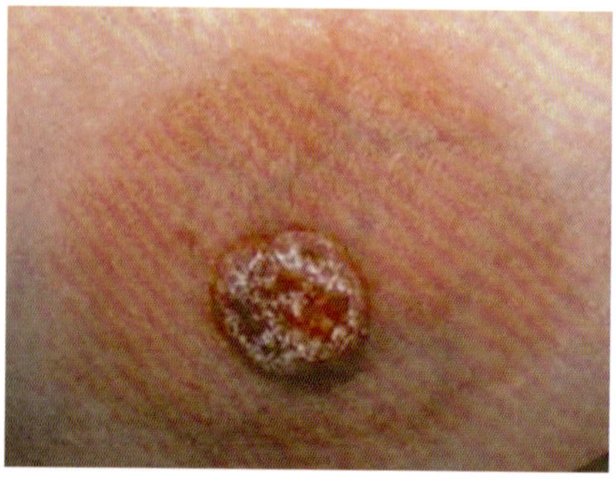

Inflammatory Breast Cancer
"Peau d'orange" Due to blocked lymphatic vessels. "Orange look" is due to **Cooper's ligaments.**

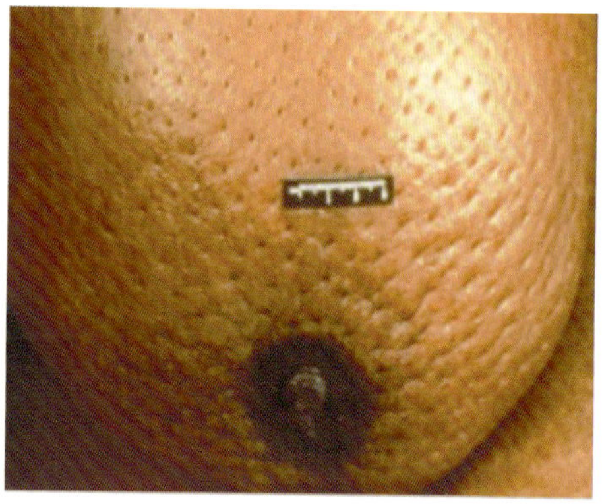

Benign and Malignant Skin Lesion Differentials

Description	**Benign**	**Malignant**
Boarders	Even	Uneven
Symmetry	Same shape/round (sides mirror each other)	Asymmetric
Size	Remains the same	Grows, increases in size
Color	Consistent	Multiple colors

Dermatology Conditions Associated With Genitals or STD's

Genital Lesions

Pathology	Ulcers on genitals	Lymph nodes	Treatment
Syphilis chancre	NOT painful, ulcerated lesions	Not painful lymphadenopathy	Penicillin G (single dose)
Haemophilus ducreyi ("you cry")	Painful ulcers	Not painful lymphadenopathy	Azithromycin (single dose)
Klebsiella inguinale (AKA: Donovanosis, Granuloma inguinale)	NOT painful, Beefy red granulation	NO lymphadenopathy	Doxycycline, Tetracycline
Lymphogranuloma venereum	NOT painful	Painful lymphadenopathy	Doxycycline
Genital herpes	Painful ulcers	Not painful lymphadenopathy	Acyclovir, Famciclovir, Valacyclovir. (Foscarnet for acyclovir resistant)

Condyloma Acuminatum
SX: Cauliflower-like/wart-like lesions on genitals. Associated with **HPV** and koilocytes.

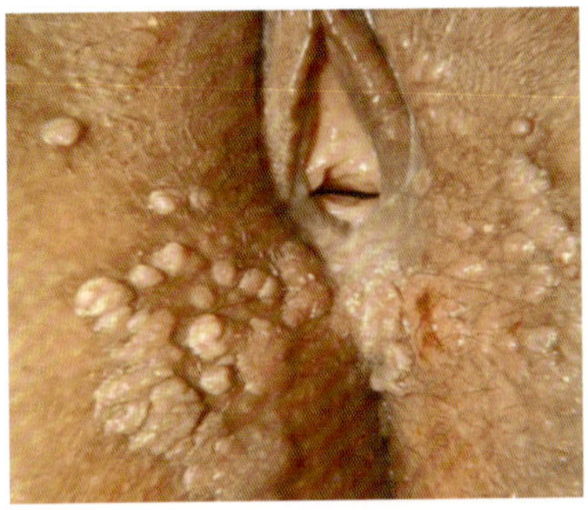

Condylomata Lata
SX: Lesions on genitals associated with secondary **syphilis**.

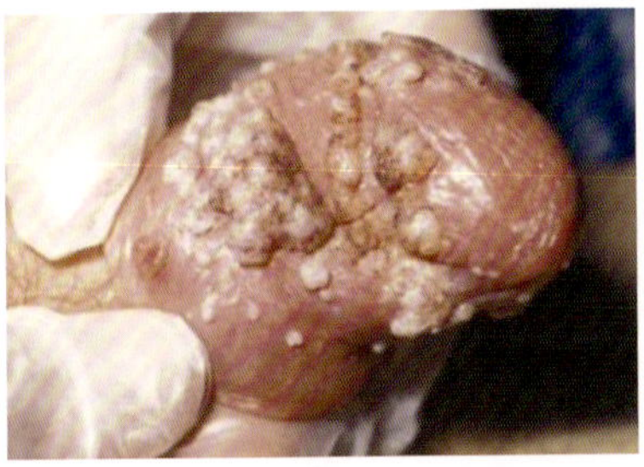

Syphilis Rash
Secondary Syphilis
TX: Penicillin G
(Must **desensitize** if allergic to penicillin, even if pregnant)

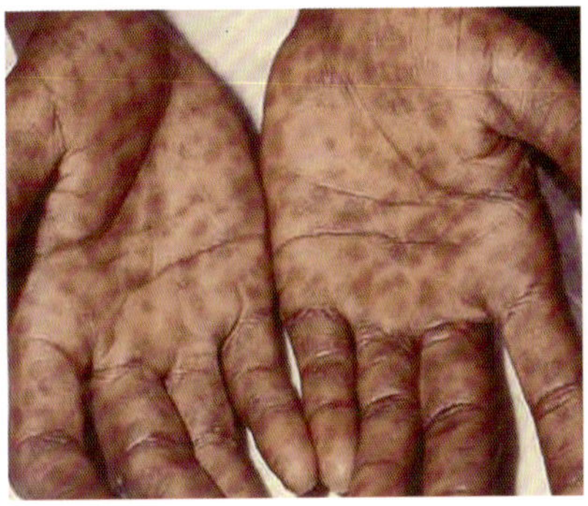

Chancroid
"Punched out" ulcers with indurated boarders.

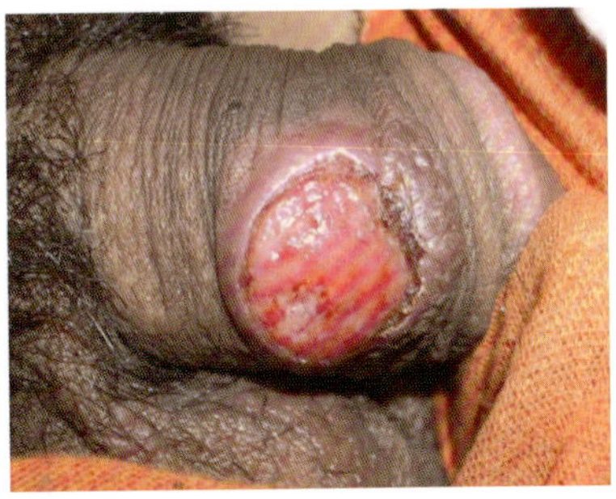

Klebsiella granulomatis
Painless, red, beefy granulation ulcer.
No lymphadenopathy.
Donovan Bodies.

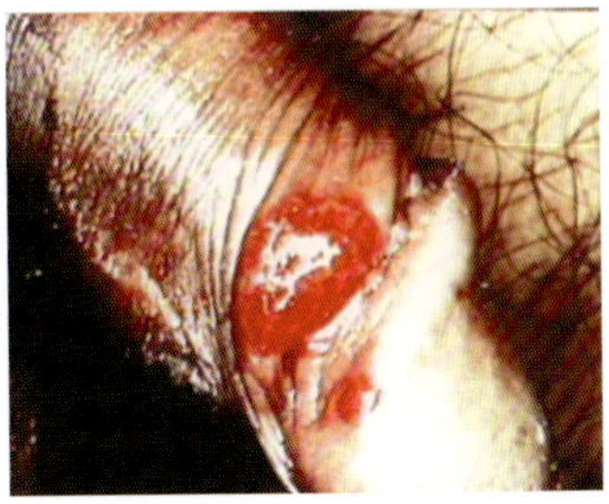

Haemophilus ducreyi
Painful ulcer. Inguinal lymphadenopathy.
Satellite cells (parallel chains).

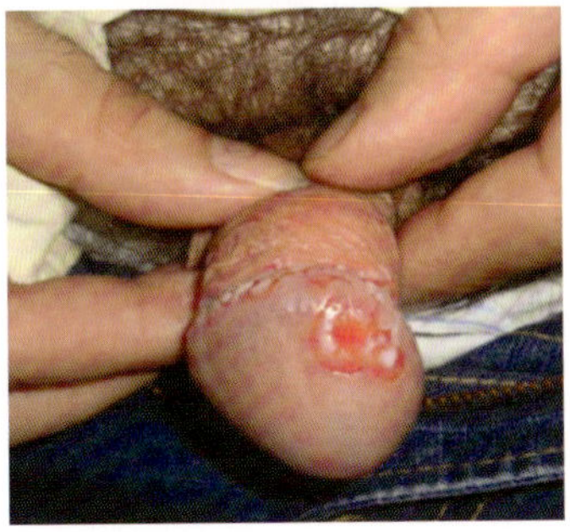

<table>
<tr>
<td>Chlamydia Lymphogranuloma venereum

Painful, swollen inguinal lymph nodes, painless genital ulcers.
TX: Doxycycline
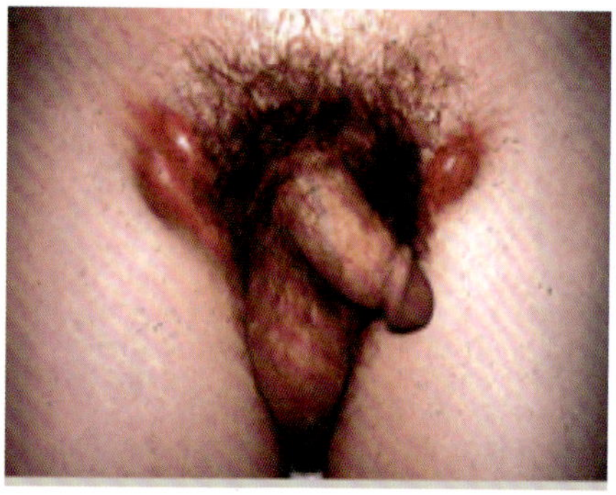</td>
<td>Lichen Sclerosus of the Vulva
MC Post menopausal women. Thinning and atrophy of the vulva covered with white patches (like paper).
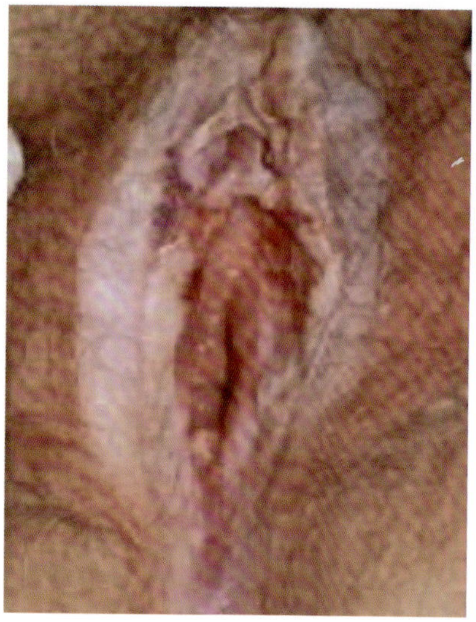</td>
<td>Pearly Penile Papules
AKA: Hirsutoid papillomas, Pearly Penile Papules.
Benign tiny, pearly (flesh color) bumps on the glans of the penis.
(Can also be found on the vulva of the female and confused with HPV).
Normal, no pathology.
TX: CO2 laser vaporizes the papules.
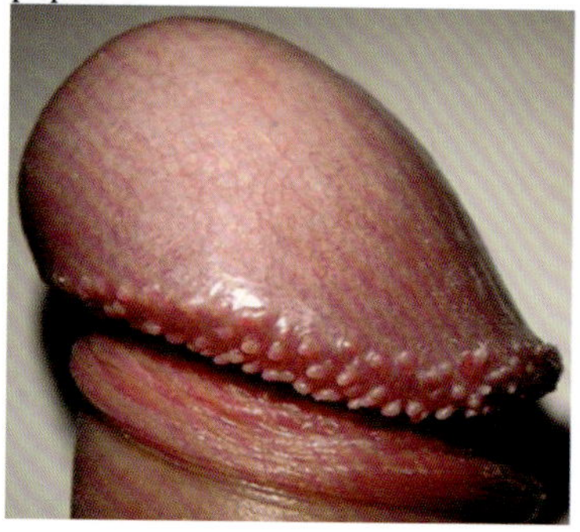</td>
</tr>
</table>

Dermatology Conditions Associated With HIV

<table>
<tr>
<td>Hairy Leukoplakia
White, painless plaques on the lateral SIDE of the tongue that can't be scraped off.
Mediated by EBV and associated with HIV.
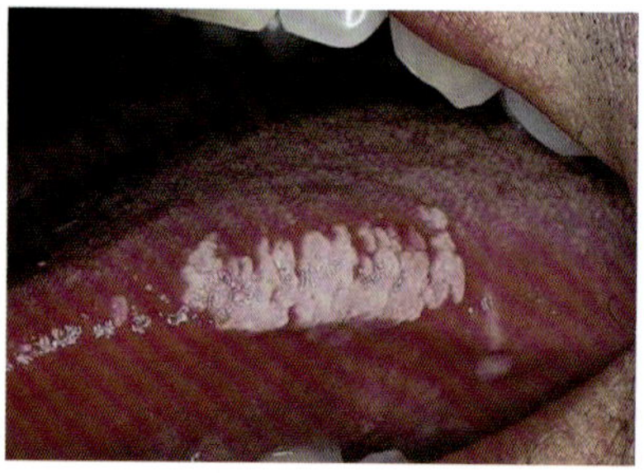</td>
<td>Kaposi's Sarcoma (HSV 8)
Herpes Virus VIII. Purple/red vascular lesions in HIV and other immunocompromised patients with CD4 counts <100.
Lesions can also be found in the lung and GI tract.

TX: HAART (raises CD4 count), Adriamycin, Vinblastine.
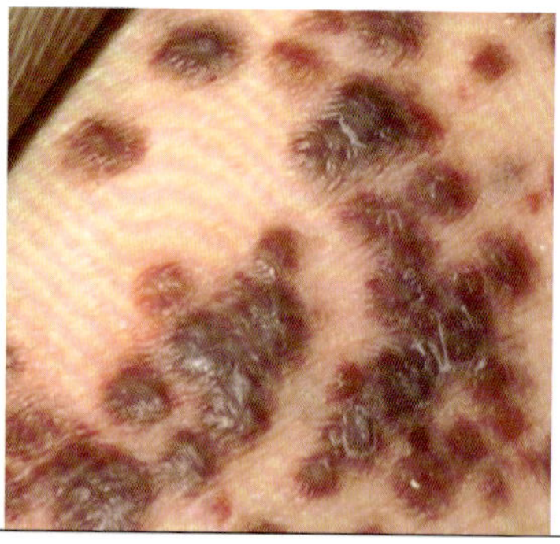</td>
<td>Anal Cancer
Male: HPV from anal sex.
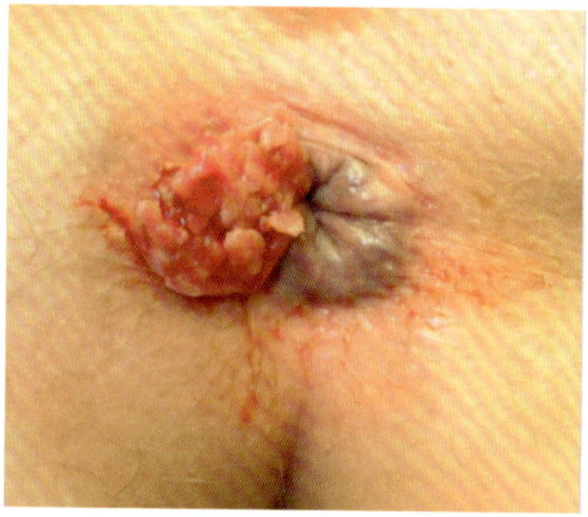</td>
</tr>
</table>

Dermatology Conditions Associated With the Mouth, Neck

Actinomyces
Gm + branching filaments.
Facial/oral abscesses with draining tracts.

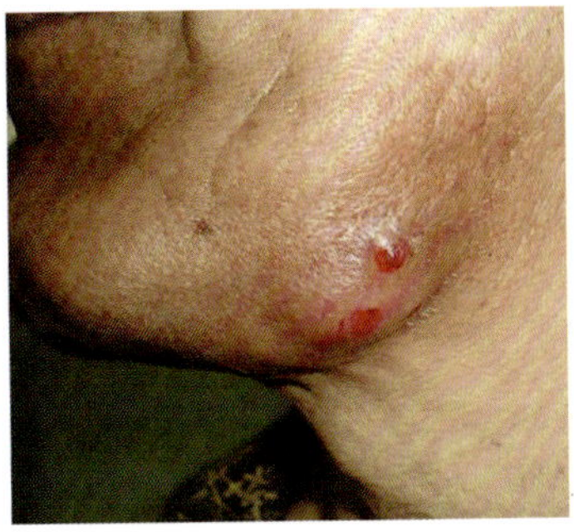

Candida Esophagitis
Associated with HIV. Can scrape off.

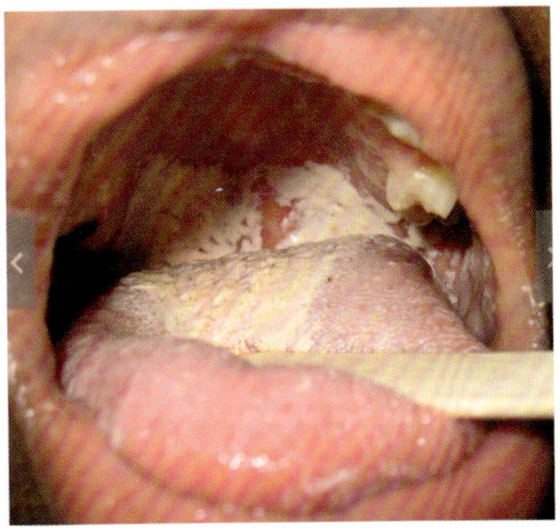

Corynebacterium diphtheria
Do **NOT** scrape off.

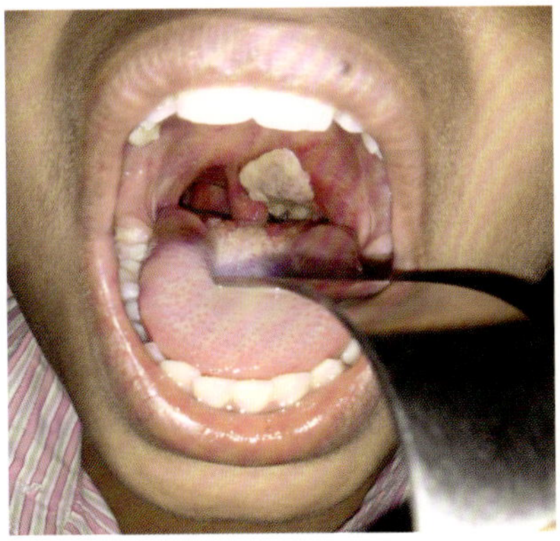

Glossitis
Iron deficiency
Zinc deficiency

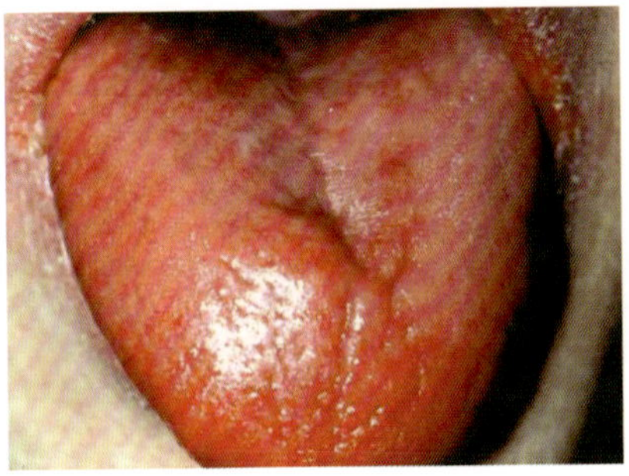

Gingival Hyperplasia
Vitamin C Deficiency, pregnancy, Scurvy, M5 form of AML.
Phenytoin, CCB, Lamotrigine, Ethosuximide, Topiramate.

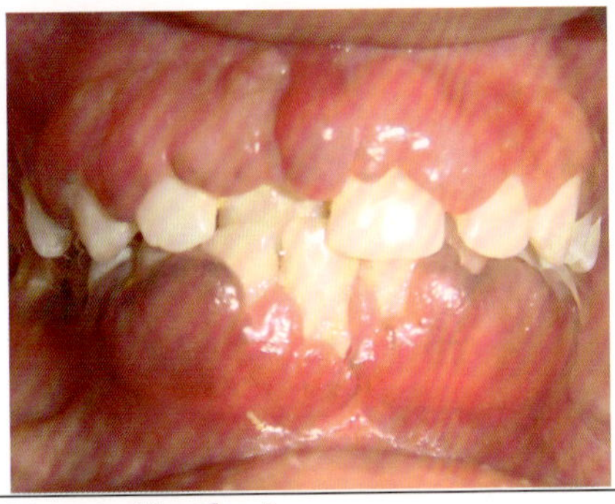

Koplik Spots
Rubeola Measles Virus (on buccal mucosa)

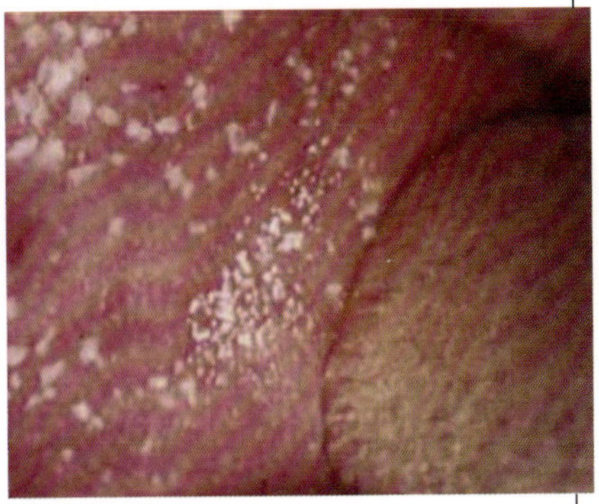

Peutz-Jeghers Syndrome
AD. Benign hamartomatous polyps in GI and hyperpigmented macules (due to increased melanin) on lips and oral mucosa.

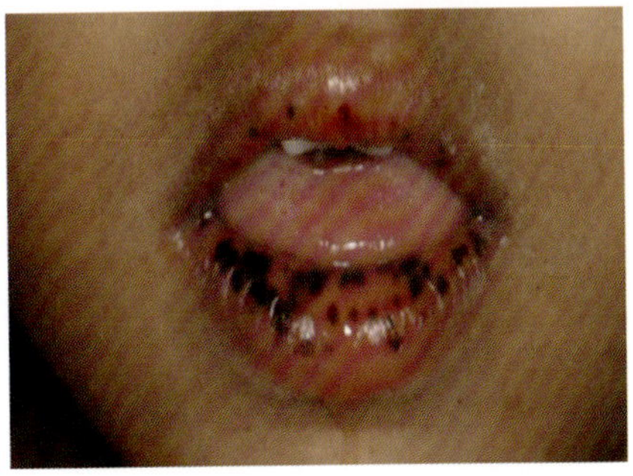

Herpes Simplex I
DS, DNA, Enveloped Virus
Latent in trigeminal ganglia.

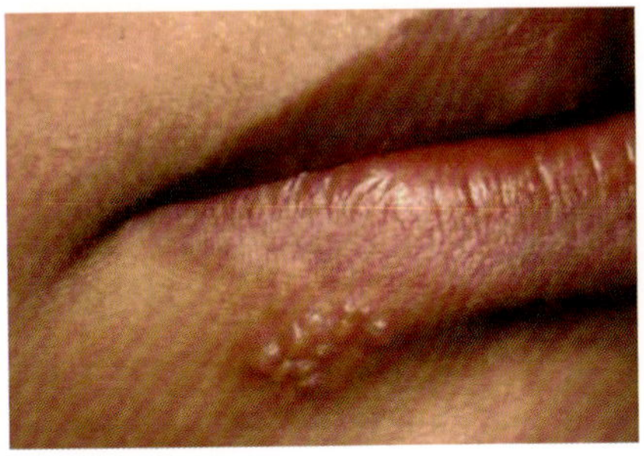

Herpes Simplex I

Scarlet Fever
"Strawberry Tongue"

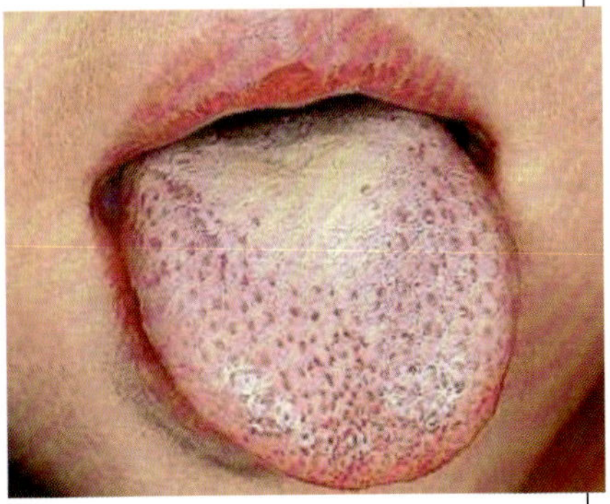

Kawasaki **"Strawberry Tongue"** 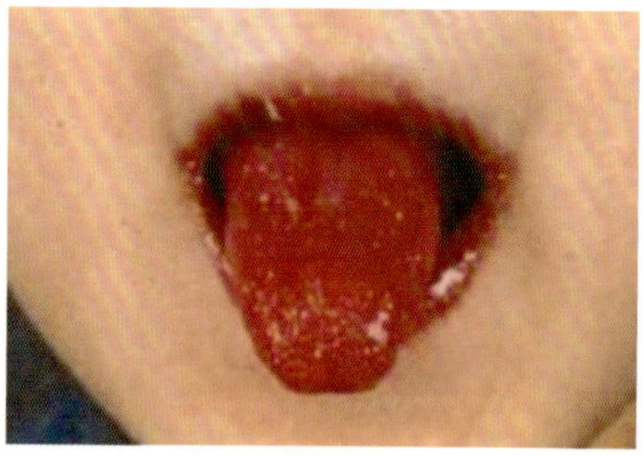		

Dermatology Conditions Associated With the Eyes

Pink Eye Adenovirus Bilateral or unilateral. 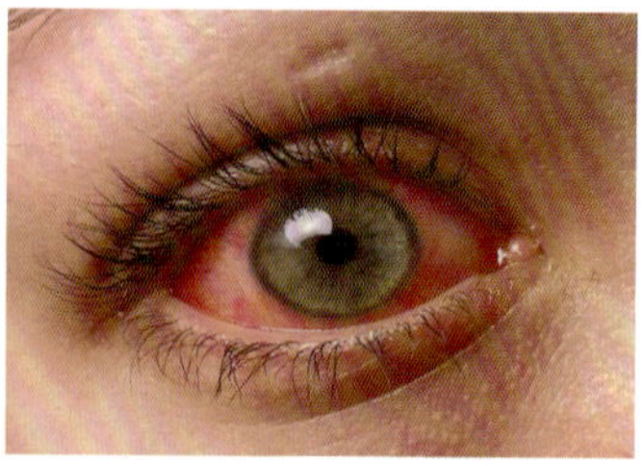	**Bacterial Conjunctivitis** Unilateral. 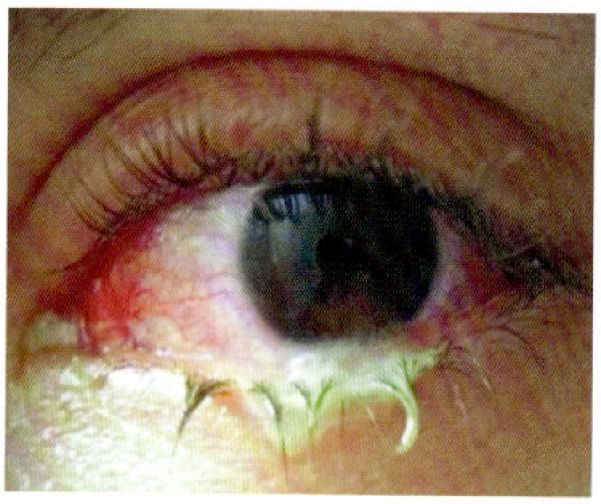	**Viral Conjunctivitis** Bilateral. 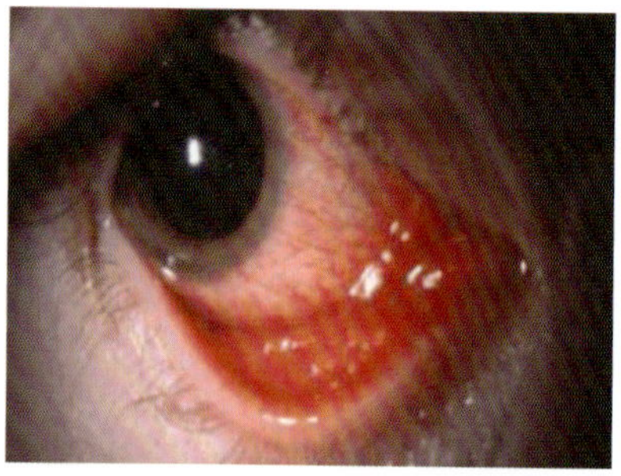
Allergy Conjunctivitis Bilateral. 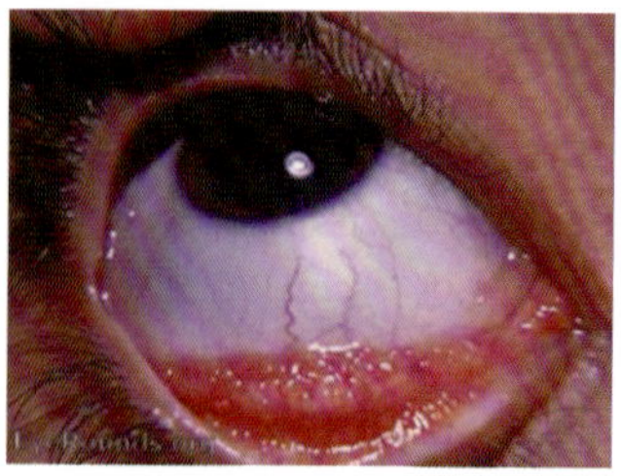	**Anterior Uveitis (Iridocyclitis, Iritis)** Inflammation of the anterior chamber and iris and ciliary body of the uvea. SX: Floaters, blurred vision, photophobia. 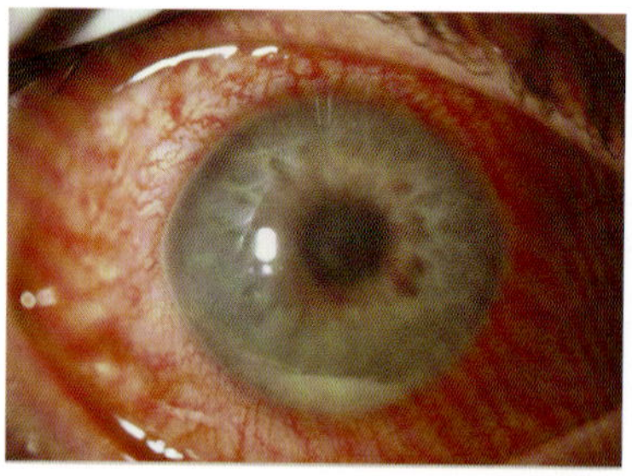	**Chalazion** Inflammation of **blocked** meibomian gland. 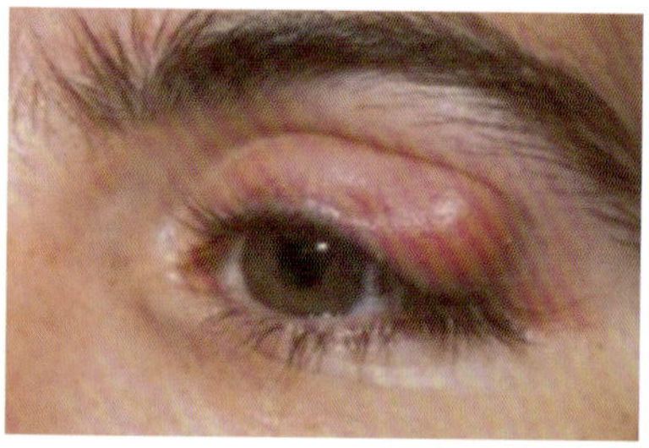

Hordeolum (Stye) **Infection** of glands of Zeis. (**tip**: a wHORe has infections) 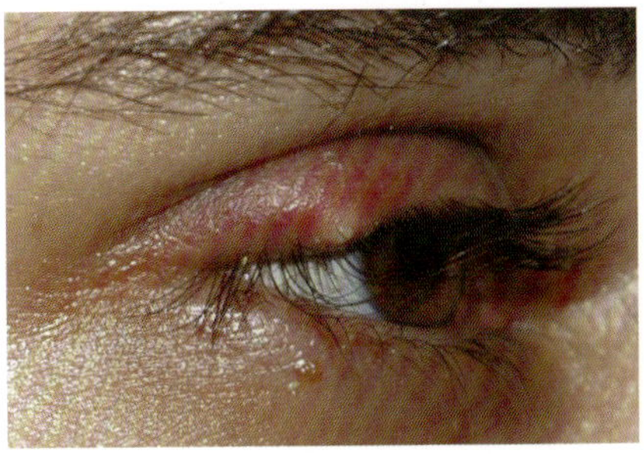	**Orbital Cellulitis** 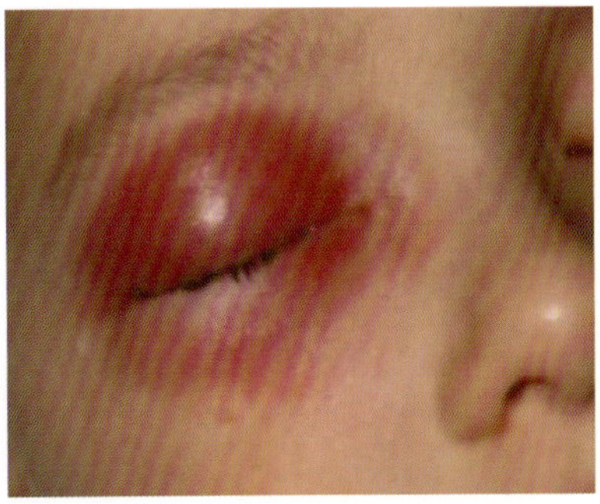	**Bacterial Keratitis** Inflammation of cornea. S. aureus or Pseudomonas can infect **contact lens** that have not been cleaned or worn to long. 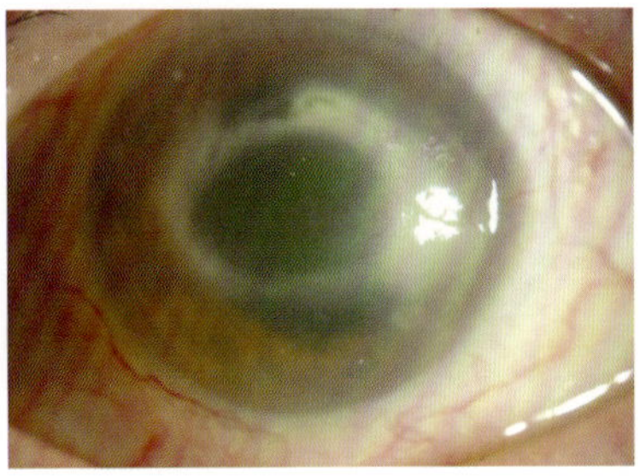
Aniridia Absence of the iris. Associated with **Wilm's Tumor** (AKA: Nephroblastoma) 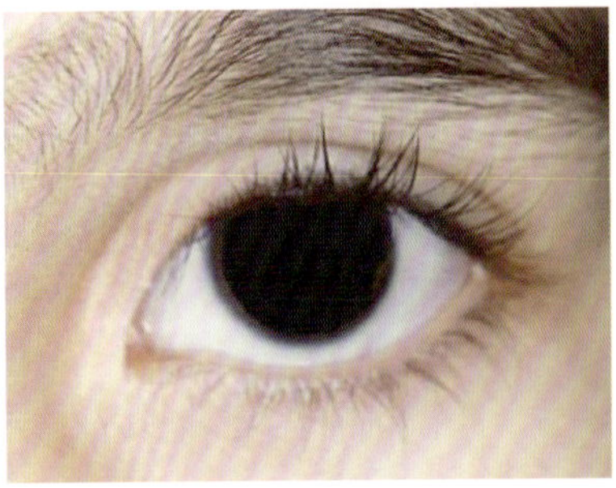	**Coloboma of the Iris** A hole in one of the structures of the eye (iris, chorioid, retina or optic disc) that is present from birth. Occurs when a gap (chorioid fissure) fails to close. MC occurrence is in the iris. Associated with Tuberous Sclerosis. 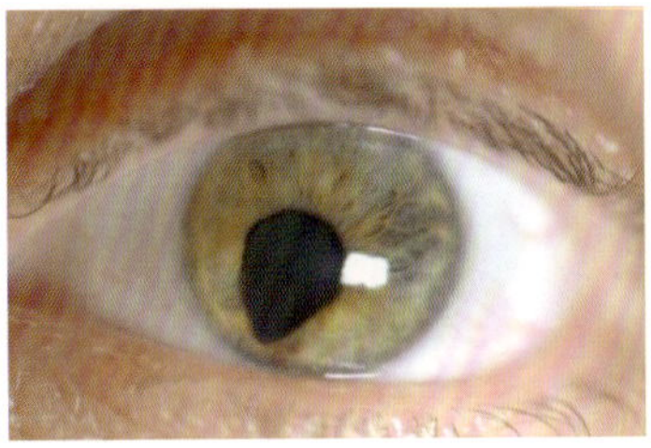	**Abrasions** Scratch to the cornea due to trauma or contact lenses. SX: Feels like sand in the eyes DX: Fluorescein stain drops. Blue light is shined on the eye, the dye makes the cornea appear green so that it shows any abrasions or scratches. No treatment. Refer to ophthalmologist. Do not patch abrasions caused by contact lenses. Fluorescein stain (drops) under blue light. 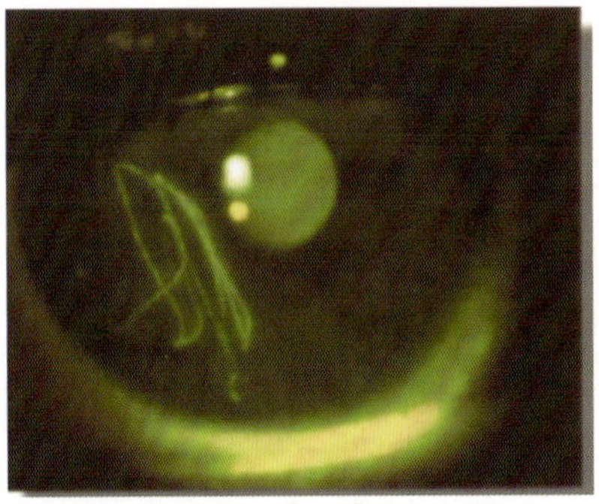 Corneal abrasion after fluorescein drops

Dermatology Conditions Associated With Hair

Male Pattern Baldness **Hereditary.** 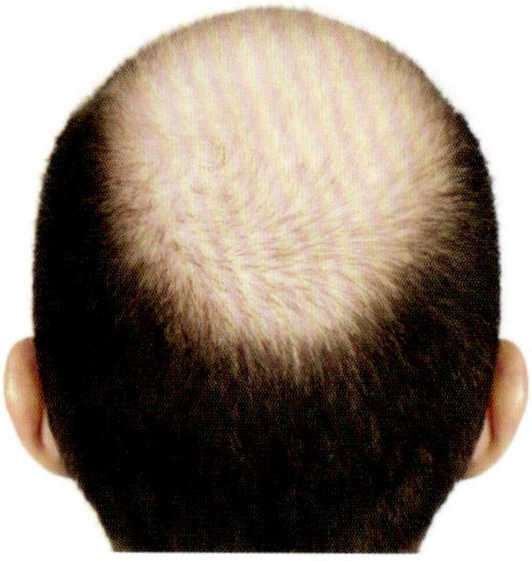	**Alopecia Areata** Autoimmune. 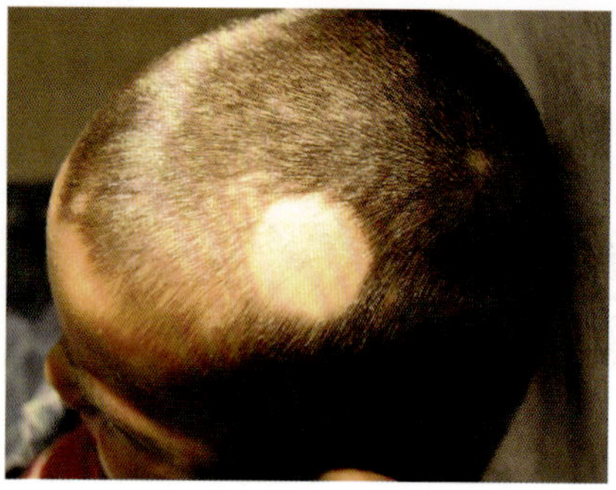	**Trichotillomania** Psychological problem – impulse disorder. (OCD). Compulsive urge to pull out one's hair. SX: broken hair, missing eyelashes/brows. TX: **SSRI** 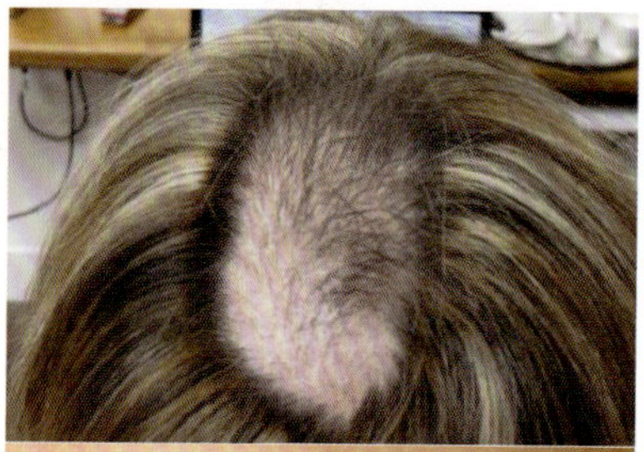 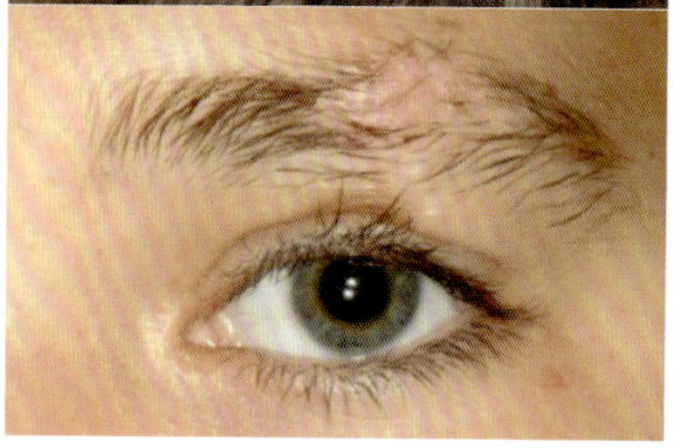
Alopecia Areata Universalis Total loss of hair. 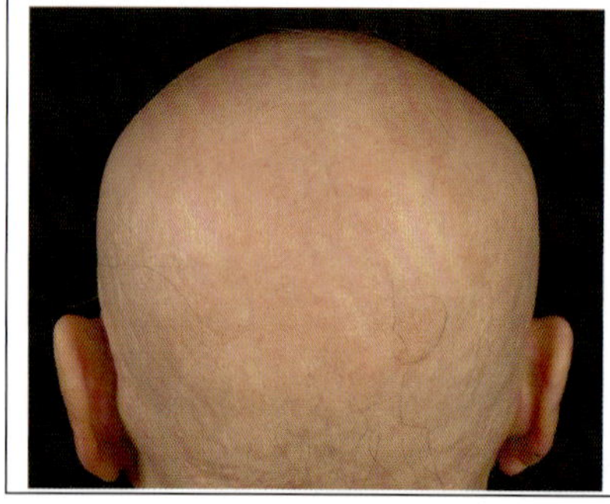	**Hair loss:** Thinning: caused by: poor nutrition (high diets in animal fats = fast food), iron deficiency, hypervitaminosis A. Prescription drugs, chemotherapy, steroids, OCP's, HRT. **TX: Minoxidil (Rogaine), Finasteride, hair transplantation.**	

Dermatology Conditions Associated With Healing

Keloid 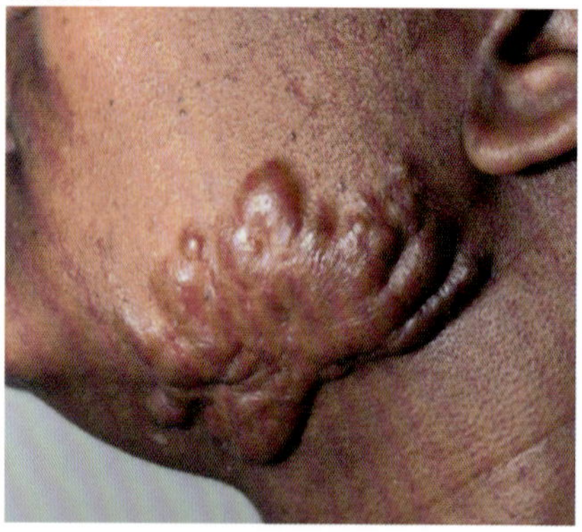	**Contracture** MC: burn healing. 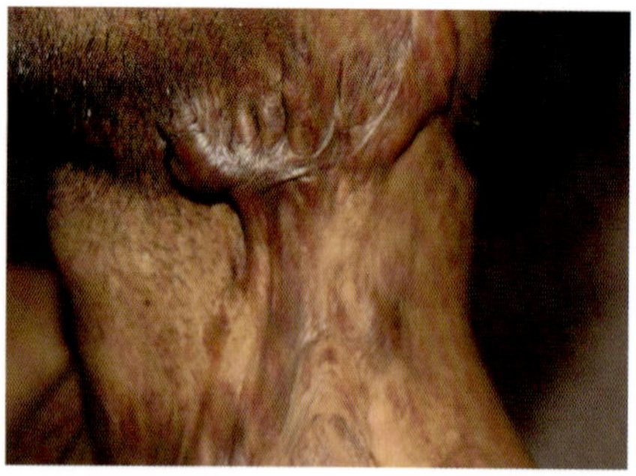	

Dermatology Conditions Associated With Nails

Nail Pitting, Splitting, Fraying.

Psoriasis. Folic acid, protein, Vitamin C deficiencies.

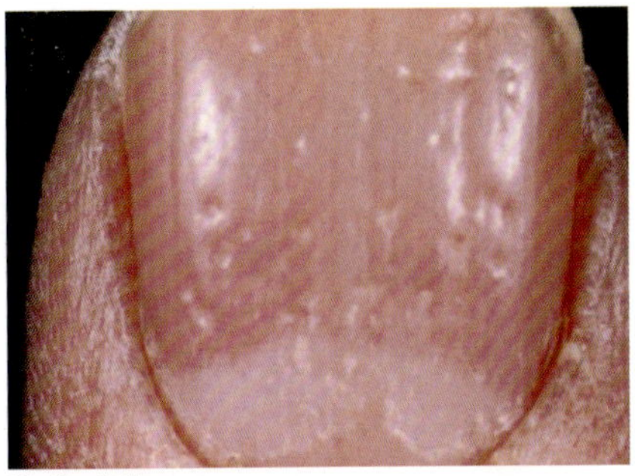

Nail pitting.

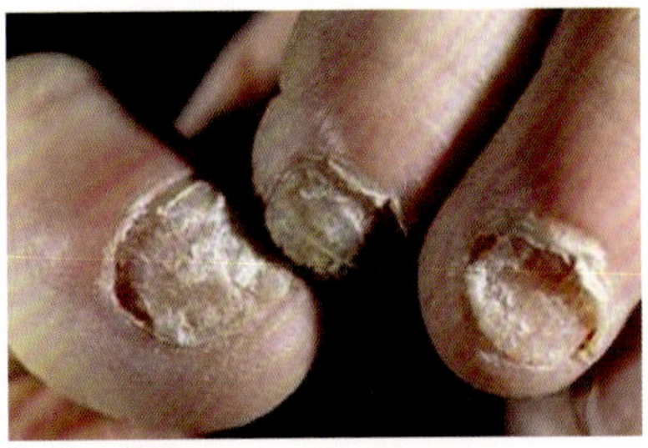

Nail splitting
(Associated with psoriasis)

Clubbing

Indicates a disease. MC: lungs, heart, GI, liver and hypoxia.

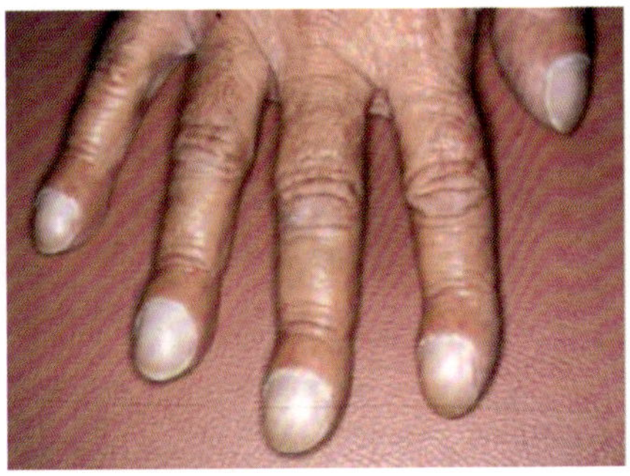

Nail Spooning (Koilonychia)

Iron deficiency.
B_{12} deficiency.

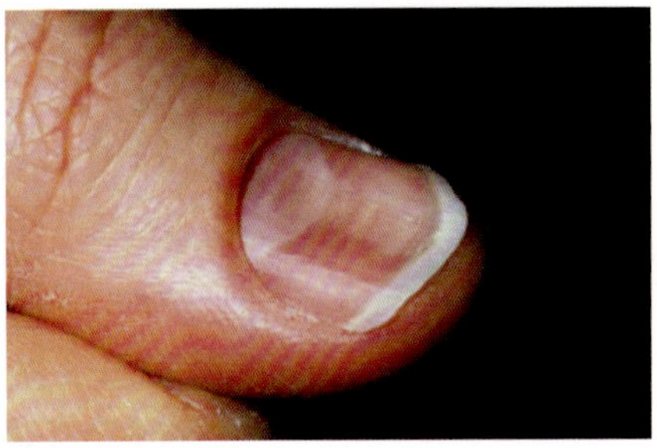

Leukonychia

White discoloration of the nail in the stria that runs parallel to the base of the nail.
MCC injury to the base of the nail.

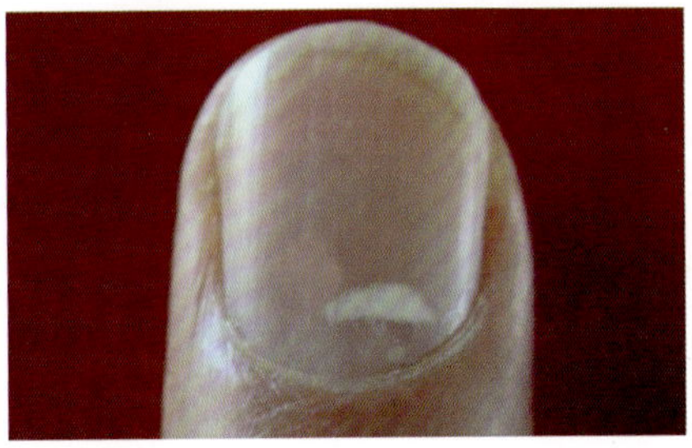

Glomus Tumor

Benign tumor from the glomus body under the fingernail or toenail.
Painful lesion and the pain can be reproduced if placed in cold water.

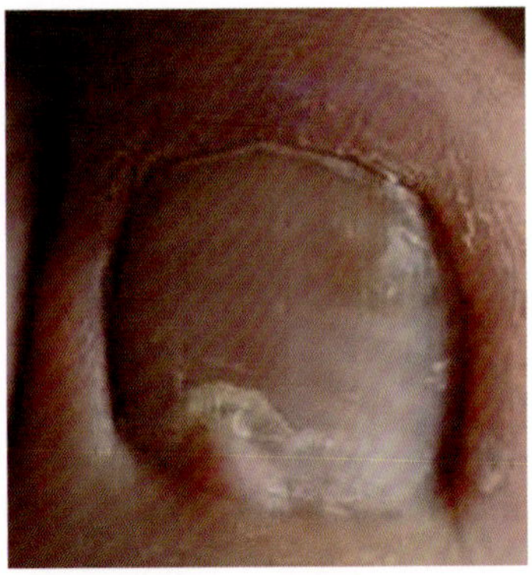

Nail Info/Terminology:

Brittle nails: thyroid problems, iron deficiency, impaired kidney function.
Thick nails: circulation problems.
Yellowing: chronic bronchitis, diabetes, liver dz, lymphatic dz.
Brown/copper color: copper poisoning, fungal infection.
Redness: heart dz.
Dark nails: B_{12} deficiency.
Stains on nail plate (not bed): smoking, henna dyes.
Beau's lines: horizontal ridges.
Mees' lines/Muehrcke's lines: white lines across the nail.

Hangnail

Tiny, torn piece of skin (paronychium) next to the nail. Infected hangnails can cause paronychia, which can lead to an abscess.
TX: hand lotion to prevent.
Trims lose skin with clean nail clipper.

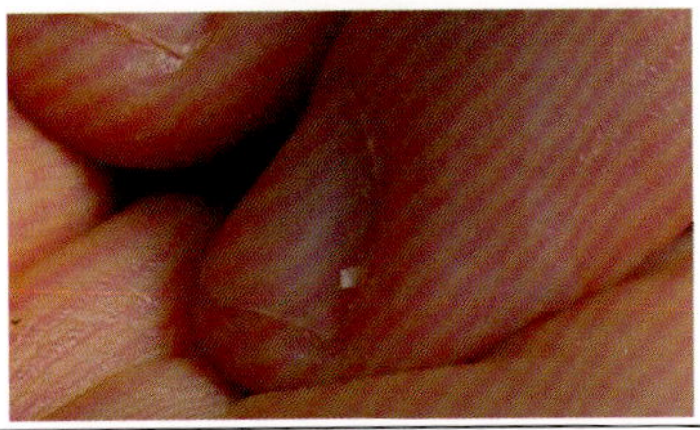

Paronychia

Staff infection of the skin surrounding the nail.
MC: Infection from a hangnail.
TX: I & D (incision and drainage) with antistaphylococcal antibiotics.

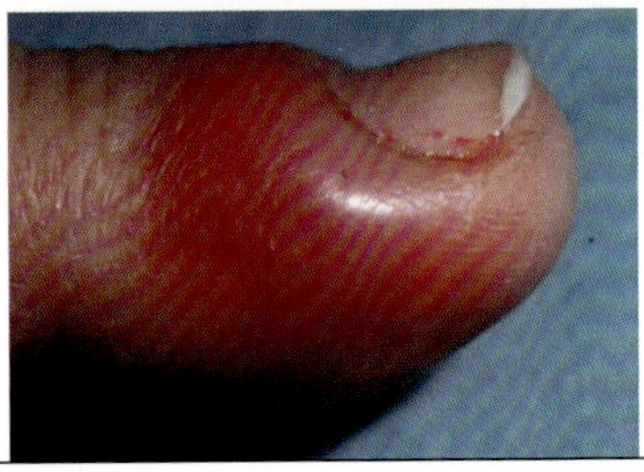

Misc. Dermatology Conditions

Tophaceous Gout

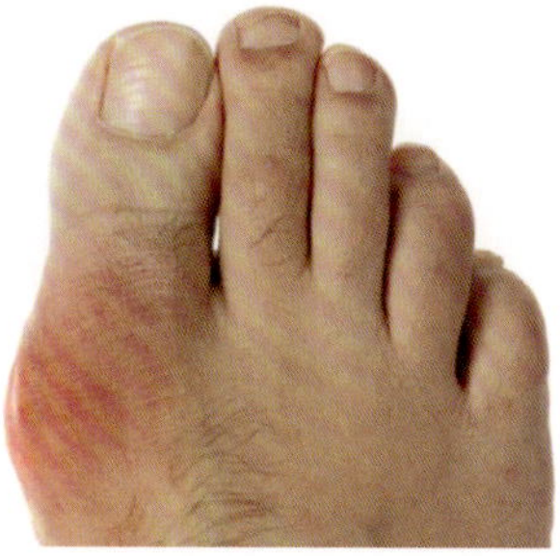

Wet Gangrene

Worst prognosis due to high-risk septicemia.
NC: C. perfringens, B. fusiformis.
TX: Amputation

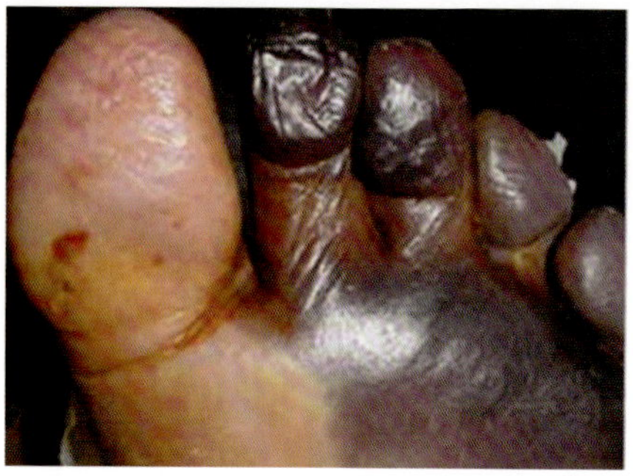

Dry Gangrene

Due to chronic ischemia without infection.
MC: Diabetes, smoking.
TX: Amputation

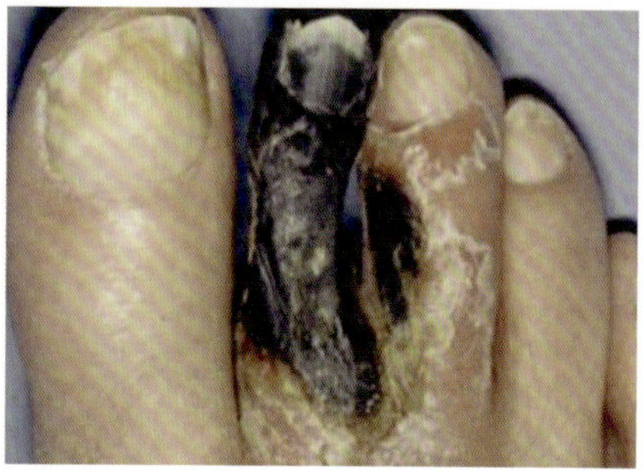

Angioedema

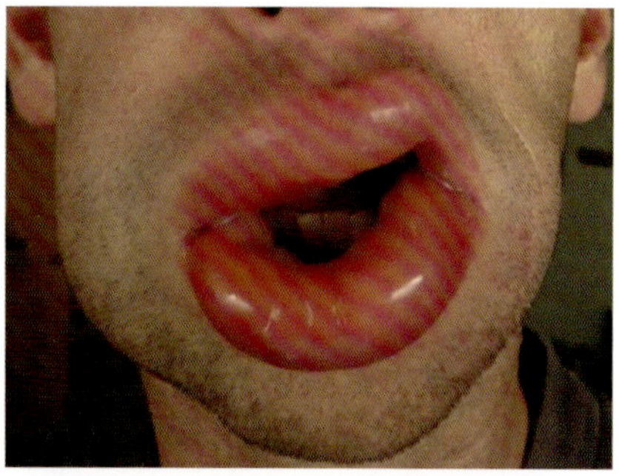

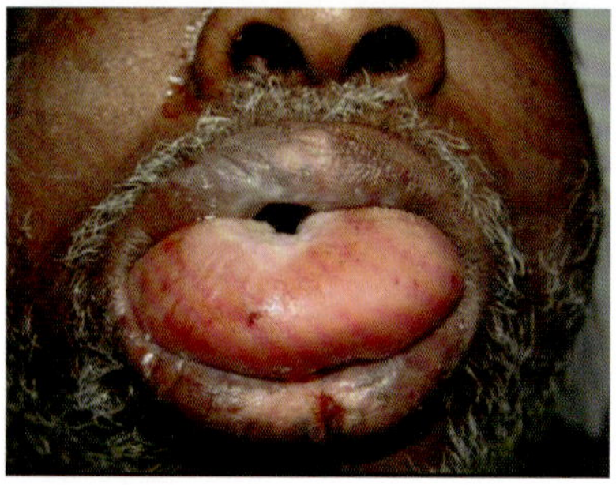

Ichthyosis

"Lizard Skin" or "Fish Skin"
Genetic skin dz.

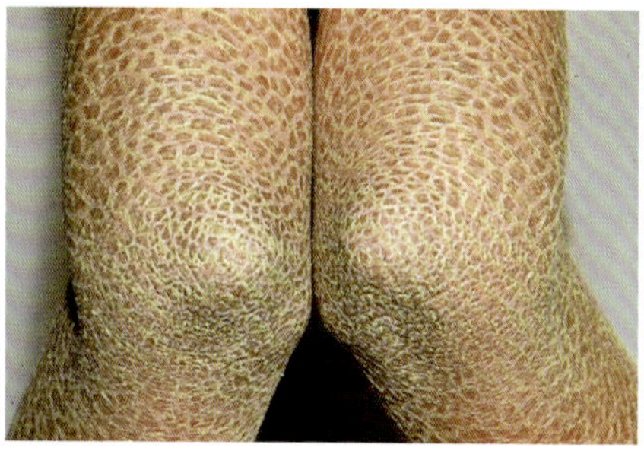

Xanthoma

High levels of cholesterol.

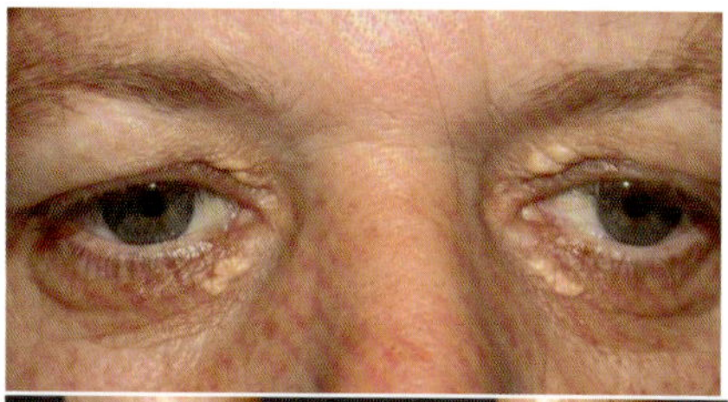

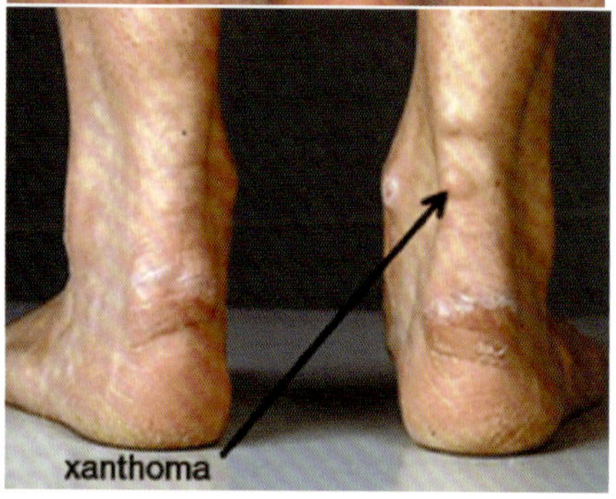

Hirsutism

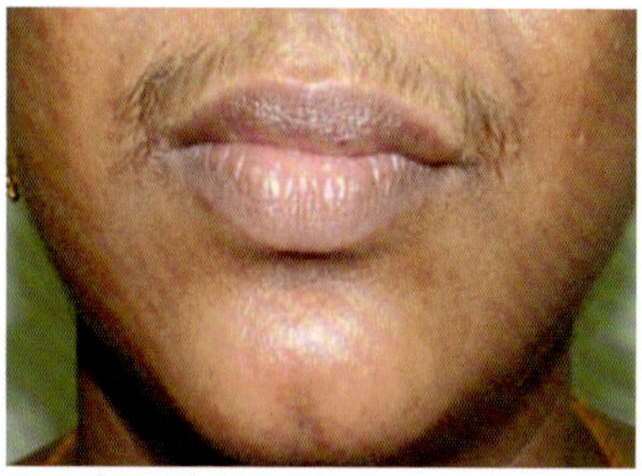

Female with hirsutism

Bells Palsy

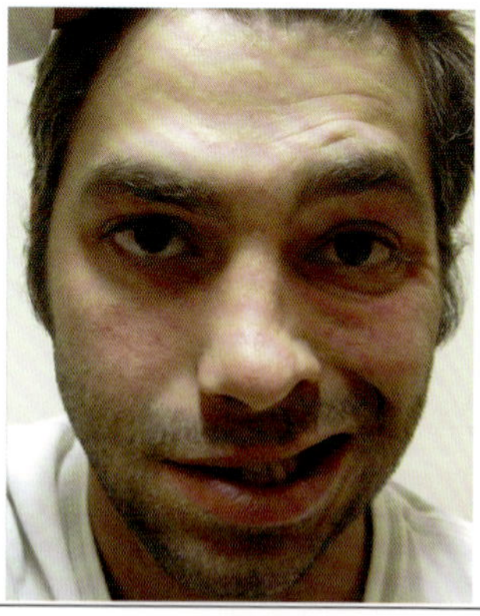

Streaks of Infection

Inflamed lymph vessels due to infection.

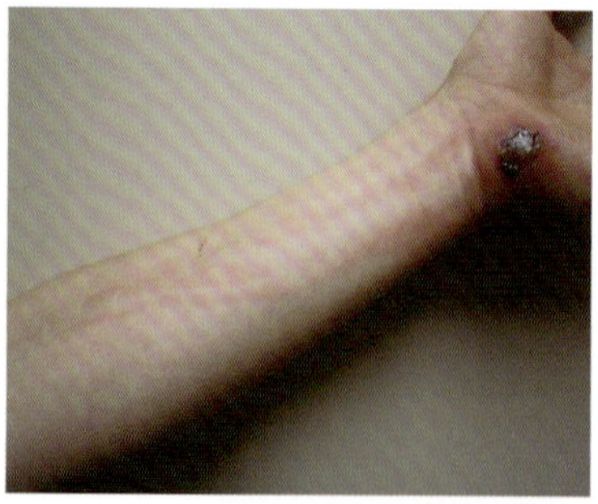

Cushing's Striae 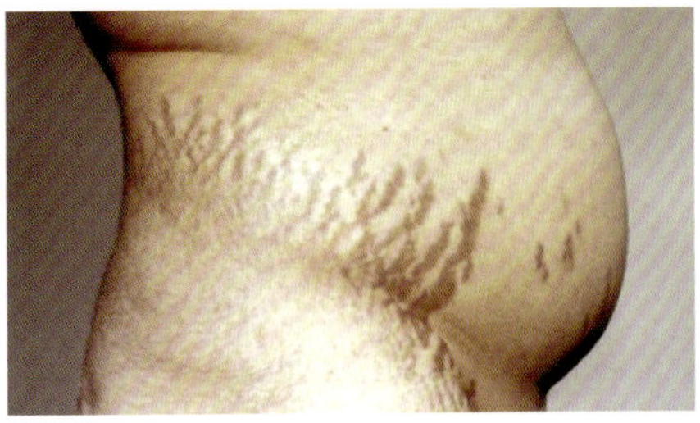	**Caput Medusae** Portal HTN 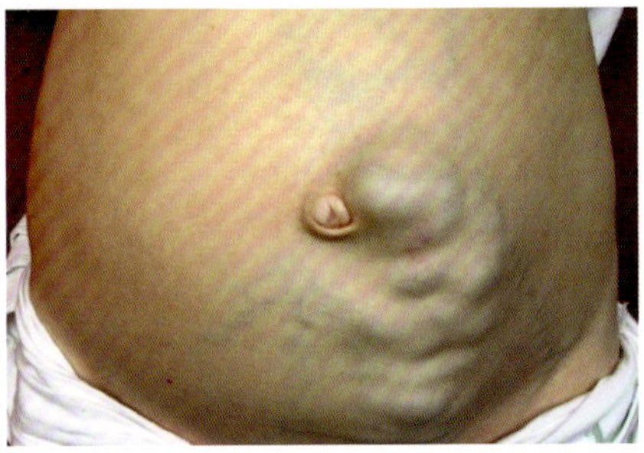	**Stretch Marks** Pregnancy 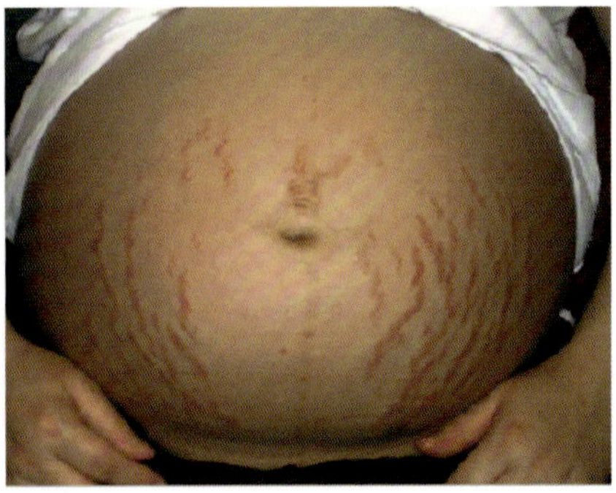
Child abuse 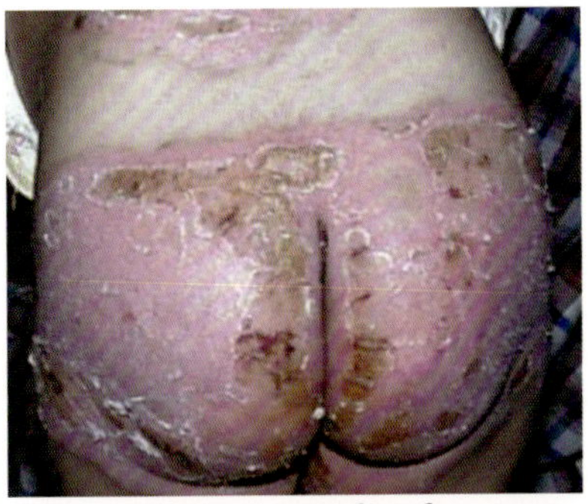 Hot water burns: exact line from water level. 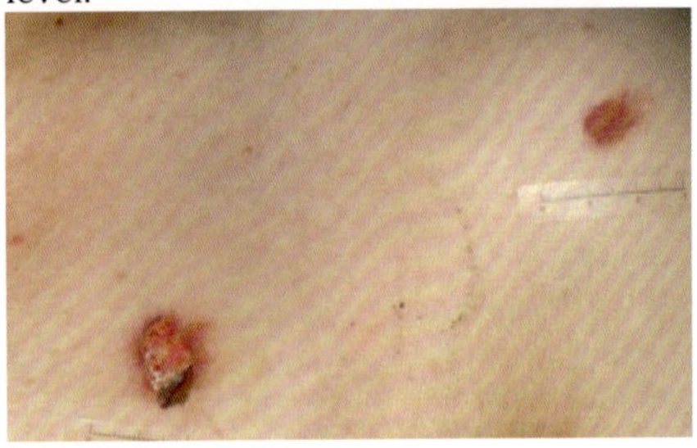 Cigarette burns.	**DIC** Disseminated Intravascular Coagulation 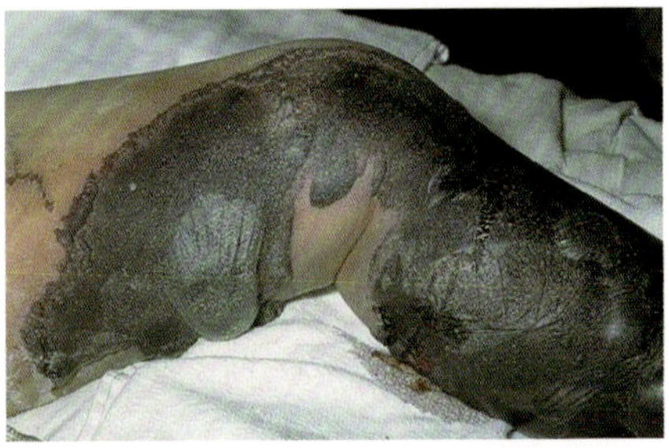	**Cryoglobulinemia** Blood contains high cryoglobulins (immunoglobulin) and become insoluble with < 37° C temperature. It will dissolve again once blood is heated. Insoluble (precipitates) block vessels causing gangrene. IgM against Fc region of IgG. Associated with: Membranous Glomerulonephritis (which is associated with Cancer, HEP C and B). (**tip**: "Member" of the "C" Club: Cancer, HEP C, Cryoglobulinemia) 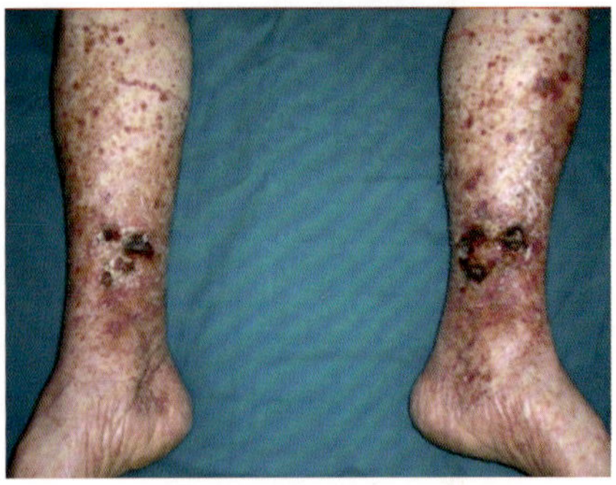

Venomous Bites, Burns, Stings, Trauma Dermatology Conditions

Black Widow Spider Bite

Most victims do not know they were bitten.
Double fang marks can sometimes be seen at the bite location.

SX: Immediate pain (but no tenderness), burning, swelling, erythema, **hypocalcemia**, **severe abdominal pain**, **severe muscle cramps**, nausea.

Labs: Hypocalcemia

TX: **Anti-venom, Calcium, Muscle relaxant, IV Calcium Gluconate**.

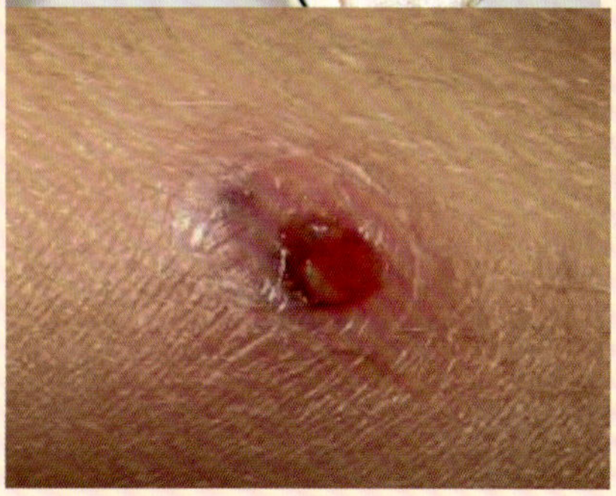

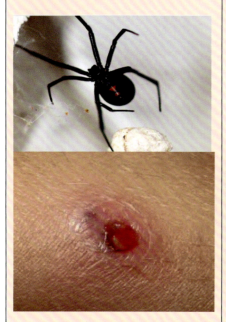

Brown Recluse Bite (AKA: Fiddler spider, Violin spider)

Mild stinging, local erythema. Severe pain within 8 hours. Area around bite can be blue/purple surrounded by a whitish ring and large red outer ring in a "bull's eye" pattern. A fluid-filled blister at the bite site, which sloughs becoming a deep ulcer that turns black. **Necrotic center and ulceration with surrounding erythema.**

SX: Fever, nausea, vomiting, abdominal pain, joint pain, rash, muscle cramping.

TX: Debridement (resect dead skin) and graft, **Dapsone**, steroids.

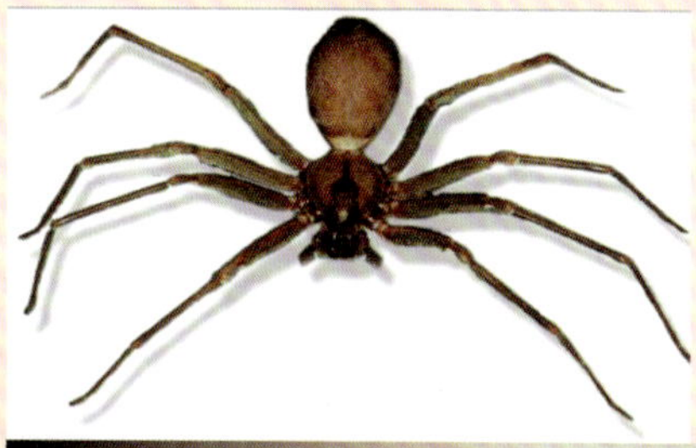

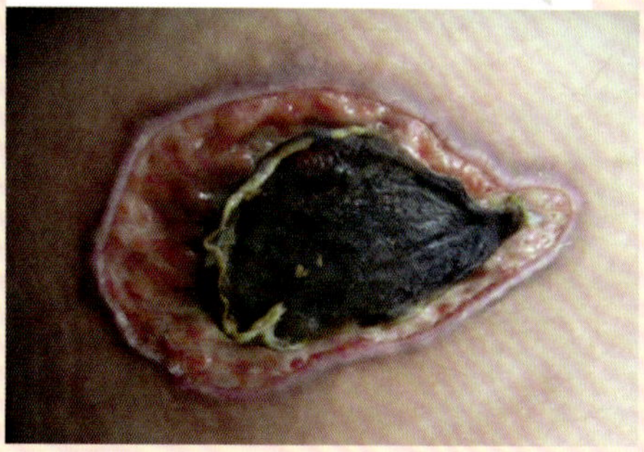

Venomous Snake Bite
Venomous snakes in the USA: copperhead, rattlesnake, cottonmouth (water moccasin), and coral snakes.

SX: a pair of puncture marks at the wound, erythema, severe pain at the site of the bite, nausea, vomiting, labored breathing, disturbed vision, sweating, salivation, numbness/tingling.

TX: Keep wound below heart level, keep patient still. **Anti-venom and Tetanus** prophylaxis.

Venom Toxins:
Cardiotoxins: act on cardiac tissue.
Neurotoxins: act on the nervous system, which can cause respiratory failure.
Cytotoxins: act on the tissue at the site of the bite where the toxin is absorbed.
Hemotoxin: anticoagulate the blood causing internal bleeding.

Anti-venom: (dosed per size of venom not size of patient)
Mild bite: 5 vials.
Extensive bite: 10 vials.
Severe bite: 20 vials.

DO NOT: apply tourniquet, slash wound with a knife, suck out the venom, do not apply ice or immerse in water, do not drink alcohol or caffeinated beverages.

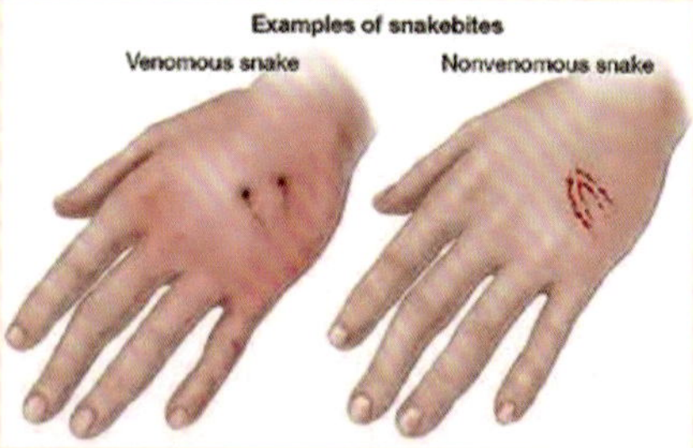

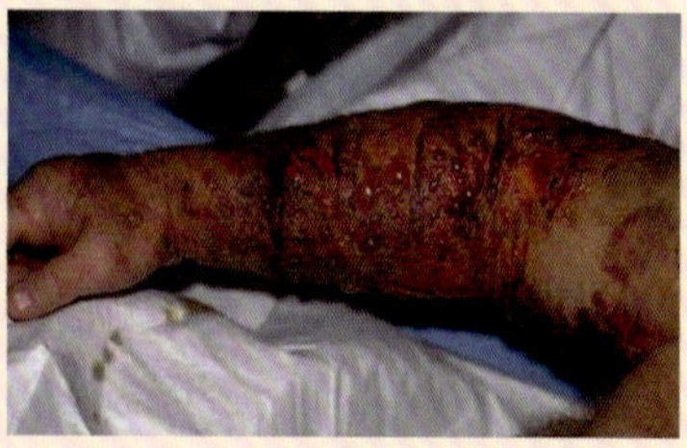

Venomous Snake Bite

Burns	Scorpion Stings	Wasp, Bee, Hornet Stings
MCC death in fires: carbon monoxide. BIT: 100% oxygen MCC death after a fire: infection. TX: Observe for swelling (difficulty breathing, normal saline fluids. **Caution**: if the question indicates that the patient in the ER is feeling fine, no outward burns are noted, but there is hoarseness, erythema (burns) inside the nose or mouth, or SOOT around their mouth – DO NOT send them home. They must be monitored for potential need of intubation due to swelling. (Don't forget the first sign of inflammation is SWELLING). Intubate if: patient exhibits: wheezing, stridor, burns inside the mouth or nose, hoarseness. **See the different types of burns and treatments below.**	Most people present with minor problems: pain, swelling, numbness/tingling at the bite site. Most serious reactions are in children and elderly. TX: Antihistamine, hydrocortisone cream. The "bark" scorpion in the Southwestern US (AZ, NM, CA) can cause more severe symptoms: high blood pressure, tachycardia, weakness, twitching, drooling, vomiting, inconsolable crying in children, unusual head, neck and eye movements. (Lethal scorpions are found in Mexico, South America, Africa, Middle East, India). 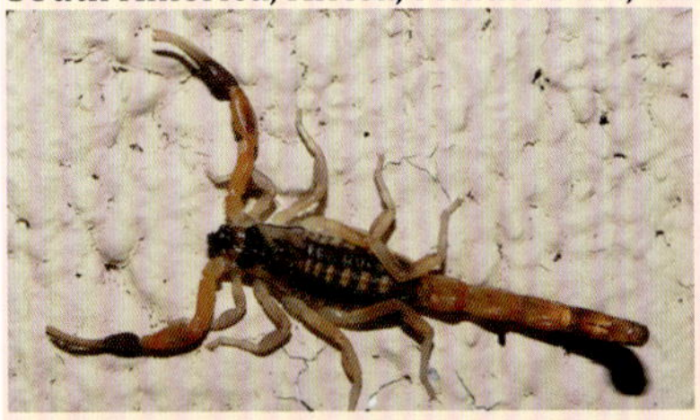 Bark Scorpion 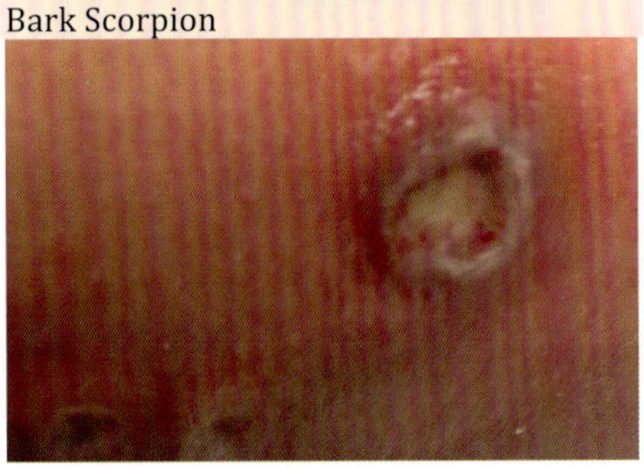	Most people have mild reactions: swelling, itching, pain. TX: remove stinger (scrape off or use tweezers to remove, do not pinch the stinger as it can inject more venom). Ice the area, ibuprofen for pain and antihistamine for itchiness. Soothing measures: calamine lotion, mix of baking soda and water. **Emergency: Anaphylaxis reaction. Type 1 Hypersensitivity** (mediated by T cells, macrophages, CD4). Swollen tongue, hives, difficulty breathing, faintness, tightness in the chest, tachycardia, anxiety, loss of consciousness. **TX: Remove stinger and give Epinephrine IM** 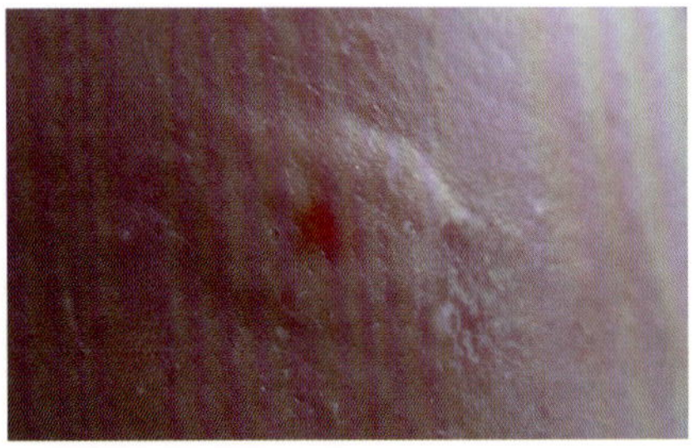

Dog/Cat Bites **Pasteurella multocida**	**Human Bites** Eikenella corrodens	
If bite on hand or any other part of the body, except the face: Rabies prophylaxis: If domestic dog/cat and bite was provoked, dog/cat to be observed by a veterinarian = no treatment required. If domestic bite was not provoked = prophylaxis is required. Bites on the face = require prophylaxis (it is too close to the brain) If bite was from wild animal (and bite was not on the face): kill animal and check brain for Negri bodies. If wild animal bite was on the face: prophylaxis is required. **If bitten but are not able to capture animal: Rabies vaccine and Ig required.** TX: **Amoxicillin/Clavulanate, tetanus booster.** Puncture wounds: Do NOT suture or close. Leave open to drain. Only suture closed lacerations.	Most dangerous type of bites. TX: Surgical debridement and cleaning.	

Burns

Chemical Burns

Burn continues as long as there is contact with chemical.

TX: Get clothes off, mass water irrigation to wash off chemical (1/2 hour to 1 hour shower/water down).

Electrical Burn: High voltage

Most damage is deep and little damage outside.

SX: Myoglobinemia, myoglobinuria, compression vertebral fractures.

TX: Debridement and possible amputation.
Administer high fluids**, diuretics and Mannitol**

Thermal Burns
(House fires, b'que fires, etc)
Burns around mouth and/or nose.
Smoke Inhalation (flames in an enclosed space)
MCC death after a fire: infection.
MCC death in fires: carbon monoxide.

SX: Soot in/around mouth.
Caution: if the question indicates that the patient in the ER is feeling fine, no outward burns are noted, but there is hoarseness, erythema (burns) inside the nose or mouth, stridor, wheezing or SOOT around their mouth – DO NOT send them home. They must be monitored for potential need of intubation due to swelling.
(Don't forget the first sign of inflammation is SWELLING).

DX: Blood gases: Results will tell you how to treat.
Bronchoscopy: Will DX inhalation damage.
Be prepared to intubate and mechanically ventilate.

TX: BIT: 100% oxygen, administer IV fluids (Normal saline or lactated Ringers).
Observe for swelling (difficulty breathing, normal saline fluids.
Intubate if: patient exhibits: wheezing, stridor, burns inside the mouth or nose, hoarseness.

Boiling water/scalding burns

MCC: Child abuse. Report to CPS (Child Protective Services)

Circumferential Burns
Burns that go all the way around a body part.
3rd degree, full-thickness burn.

SX: Leathery, thick skin, swelling, eschar (burnt tissue)

Complication: Limit or cut off blood supply from swelling.

TX: Escharotomy: Cut down both sides of burn tissue to allow expansion of skin and restoration of blood flow.

Burn Guidelines
↑↑ Fluids must be administered.
Amount of fluids needed depend upon size of patient (Kg) and extent of burn (% of body burnt)

% of Body Calculation "Rule of 9's"
Head = 9% (1 head x 9%) = 9%
Each arm = 9% (2 arms x 9%) = 18%
Each leg = 2 parts. 2 parts x 2 legs = 4 parts x 9% = 36%
Trunk = 2 parts front and 2 parts back = 4 parts x 9% = 36%

1st day of therapy:
Weight (kg) x % of total body burned (can't go over 50%) x 4 cc's = amount of electrolyte solution to give in the first 24 hours.
(Over 50% of the body burned = maximum loss of fluid. No more fluid is able to be lost).

First ½ amount is given in the first 8 hours. Second ½ is given in the last 16 hours.
3rd day of therapy:
No more fluids needed. Patient reabsorbs fluid from the tissues → mass diuresis.

Iron Burn
Standard care: 3 weeks
Extensive care: > 3 weeks

TX: Extensive 3rd degree burns in small area.
or Surgical: cut away bad area and graft.

Burn Management

- Tetanus prophylaxis
- Cleaning
- Topical agents:
  Silver sulfadiazine
- If cartilage involved: Mafenide Acetate
- If area around eyes involved: Triple antibiotic
- IV pain medications
- Grafts
- ↑ nutrition support (va gut)
- Rehabilitation: starts on day 1

Trauma Injuries

ABC Assessment First

A = Airway (secure the airway)

- With facial trauma: cricothyroidotomy
- Without facial trauma: intubation with orotracheal tube
- Cervical spine injury: intubation with orotracheal tube using a flexible bronchoscopy

B = Breathing

- Goal to keep oxygen saturation >90%

C = Circulation (fluid)

- IV normal 9% saline (Ringers Lactate) with large-bore needles
-

Crush Injury **SX/Labs: Hyperkalemia, Myoglobinemia, Myoglobinuria.** **TX: Give ↑ fluids, alkalize urine** **Complications:** **Compartment Syndrome** Severe high pressure in a body compartment (arm/leg) that contains muscles and nerves resulting in ↓ blood supply. SX: Severe pain regardless of position, ↓ pulse, ↓ circulation **TX: Emergency Fasciotomy**	**Fat Embolism** Embolism due to fracture of **long bones**, soft tissue trauma and burns. SX: Acute cor pulmonale, respiratory failure, tachycardia, hypoxemia, hypercapnia, ↑ temperature. TX: To ↓ risk, must reduce long bone fractures as soon as possible after the injury and respirator.
Embedded objects Do not remove at the scene of an accident or in the ER. Send to OR. This includes objects inserted into closed body cavities (rectum).	

Rhabdomyolysis

Due to trauma/crush injuries, seizures, venomous bites, prolonged immobility.

SX: red urine (myoglobin)

DX: **You must do an EKG before anything else in rhabdomyolysis because of the hyperkalemia. There is a high risk of fatal arrhythmias.**

IT: Urinalysis shows positive for blood but no RBC's seen on microscopic exam.

MAT: Urine **myoglobin**.

Labs: ↑ CPK, **hyperkalemia** (K is released from dying cells), hypocalcemia (see below: calcium binds damaged muscle), ↓ serum HCO3

TX: Normal 9% saline (NaCl), mannitol to increase excretion (diurese) the myoglobin urine, alkalinize the urine.

Beware of the vignettes that have a patient on a **Statin drug**. They will have "red" urine (myoglobin due to rhabdomyolysis) because of either excessive exercising/running or because a fibrate or niacin has been added to the statin.
In myoglobin no RBC are noted because this is **myoglobin. Myoglobin is very toxic to the kidneys and ↓ serum calcium levels. (causes a left shift to the oxy-heme curve**).

Bullet Damage (gunshot) Mass and velocity are proportional. Faster bullets = ↑ damage. Big guns ≥ 3000 ft/sec = ↑ damage. Small entrance and large exit. Require extensive treatment, possible amputation. Low velocity guns 1000 ft/sec are limited to the trajectory of the bullet.	**Treatment to extremities** If concern for damage to vessels: DX: Doppler. If injury is not near vessels: Clean, send home. If hematoma present or ↓ pulse: surgical repair. If multiple injuries (bleeding, bones, nerves): surgical repair. If it involves extremities (arm/leg) monitor for ischemia and compartment syndrome.

Urological Injuries	Spleen Injury
Blunt trauma: blood in urine. If rib fracture and no pelvic fracture: CT kidneys (renal) If pelvic fracture: Female = bladder injury. Male = Urethra or bladder injury. (Evaluate urethra in male with retrograde urethrogram. If negative then do cystogram (do not start with a cystogram).	MCC: injury from seat belt in an automobile crash. Always try and save the spleen, especially in a child. **If splenectomy is performed: must immunize against encapsulate organisms (SHiN): S. pneumo (Pneumovax Vaccine), H. influenza Vaccine, N. meningitis (Meningococcal vaccine).** **Caution:** The pancreas could also be damaged. If the exam has both in the answer, look at the labs. If only amylase is shown, the answer is the spleen. But if the labs show ANY lipase, even if there is amylase present, the answer is the pancreas. Lipase is specific to the pancreas.

Blunt Abdominal Trauma	Abdominal Trauma
1.5 Liters of blood loss = shock Top 3 locations of high bleeding: Pelvic Fx, Femur Fx, and Abdomen. DX: Pelvic Fx and Femur Fx with X rays. DX: Abdomen imaging is based on the hemodynamic stability of the patient. If stable: CT. If unstable: FAST (Focused Assessment with Sonography for Trauma) Abdominal Sonogram in ER or Diagnostic peritoneal lavage. (FAST: rapid bedside ultrasound performed in the ER to screen for blood around the heart or abdomen after trauma). TX: See management of abdominal bleeding under abdominal trauma.	Gunshot in abdomen: Exploratory lap to repair injuries. A gunshot below the nipple line is considered a chest and abdomen injury. Knife injury: If it enters the peritoneal cavity: must do exploratory lap. If via digital exam appreciates that the wound does not enter the peritoneal cavity, no surgery is required.
Management of abdominal bleeding: 1st: IV fluid resuscitation with normal saline (9% saline, Ringer's Lactate) with large boar needle. In children < 6 years old: Intraosseous access (fluid injection direction into the marrow of the bone (MC proximal tibia). Then exploratory laparotomy if needed. **Hemodynamically unstable patients**: must have an exploratory laparotomy. DX: FAST ultrasound evaluates for intraabdominal bleeding. CT to evaluate retroperitoneal bleeding. Upright CXR and Thoracic X-ray to evaluate for air under the diaphragm for organ (stomach or bowel) perforation. **Bruising and Bleeding location in Abdominal Trauma** Renal trauma: No ecchymosis. Pancreas trauma or acute pancreatitis: Bruising in the flanks (retroperitoneal) due to hemorrhage. Flank bruising: retroperitoneal hemorrhage.	**Signs Associated with Abdominal Trauma** • Seatbelt sign: From seatbelt due to deceleration injury. MC injury: Spleen • Cullen Sign: Bruising around umbilicus due to ruptured abdominal aortic aneurysm or hemorrhagic pancreatitis • Kehr Sign: Pain in left shoulder due to splenic rupture • Grey Turner Sign: Flank bruising due to retroperitoneal hemorrhage • Balance Sign: Dull percussion on the left and shifting dullness on the right due to splenic rupture

Chest/Thoracic Trauma	Pulmonary Failure after Chest Trauma
Blunt trauma to chest due to deceleration injury: Treat obvious injuries. Observe 48 hrs for pulmonary contusion or myocardia damage. Verify that there is not transection of the aorta by CXR of the mediastinum. Mediastinum Evaluation: If it is wide: probable injury. If normal: probable no injury. Follow up with a Spiral CT. If Spiral CT is positive = surgical repair. If Spiral CT is negative but mediastinum was side = do aortogram. If Spiral CT is negative but mediastinum normal = no TX	If multiple rib fractures, or fracture of 1st rib, sternum or scapula = Pulmonary Contusion. If multiple long bone fractures with subsequent pulmonary failure = Fat Embolism
Air Embolism Gas bubble/s in the vascular system. Caused by air getting into the blood accidently during surgery (🡻 risk when head of the bed is lowered during brain surgery or when inserting/removing a central venous catheter), trauma to the lungs, divers holding their breath during ascension, injected into the vein, patients on ventilators, air entering the system from the placenta during birth. TX: Place patient in Trendelenburg position (head down) and on the left lateral decubitus position. Administration of 100% oxygen in hyperbaric therapy. **(Note: Beware of what the diver is doing when he becomes short of breath: if he is just swimming along, it is a PE because of the DVT he developed while flying to where he was going to dive. If he is rising to the surface, it is an air embolism).**	**Subcutaneous Emphysema** AKA: Subthoracic Emphysema Gas or air is trapped in the layer under the skin (subcutaneous). SX: Crepitus (crackling feel), respiratory distress, difficulty swallowing, swelling. DX: Chest X-ray Causes: • Rupture of the esophagus. DX: Endoscopy • Tension Pneumothorax. SX: Shock, distended veins, respiratory distress, displacement of trachea. • Injury to the trachea or bronchus. DX: Fiberoptic bronchoscopy. TX: Intubate and ventilate. • Penetrating trauma (gunshot or stab wounds). • Infection (gas gangrene).

Tension Pneumothorax	Pulmonary Contusions
MCC: Blunt trauma, broken ribs, pleural bleb that burst (COPD). Air going into the chest but not able to escape. SX: Displaced trachea (deviated **away** from injured lung), respiratory distress. Tachycardia, tachypnea (rapid breathing), chest pain, hyperresonance and/or decreased breath sounds. Can lead to cardiac arrest. DX: CXR TX: Emergency needle decompression and chest tube. Needle entry: 2nd intercostal space and insertion of chest tube. Chest tube is connected to a one-way valve system into a water seal. (**Pneumothorax**: Tracheal deviation **toward** lung injury. Hyperresonance and/or decreased breath sounds. DX: CXR. MC: Pleural bleb burst in COPD, Marfan's, lung injury. TX: Chest tube) (**Atelectasis**: CXR shows trachea pulled **toward** the injured lung)	Contusion of the lung caused by blunt chest trauma (rapid deceleration), penetrating trauma, or explosions. Excess fluid from damage (blood, other fluids) causes difficulty with gas exchange. SX: May take hours to a day to appear, 🡻 Oxygen sat, dyspnea, cyanosis, 🡹 RR and HR, rales, coughing up blood, hypotension. DX: CXR and CT TX: Supportive: Fluid restrictions, diuretics, must use crystalloid fluids if fluids are needed, if blood gases 🡻 must use respirator, chest tubes.

Deceleration Injury. If 1st rib, sternum or scapula is broken, it is a very serious deceleration injury. CXR: If widened mediastinum: this indicates transection of the aorta (aortic dissection). Conform with a Spiral CT and do surgical repair.	**Aortic Dissection** SX: **Ripping, tearing pain** to the back, between the shoulder blades. Causes: MCC: **Blunt chest trauma** in an automobile crash. **Falls from 10 feet**.
Hemothorax Blood in the thorax/pleural space. SX: Absent breath sounds and dullness to percussion. DX: CXR shows blunting of costophrenic angle, CT MCC: Most bleeds into the thorax are from the lung. Small amounts of blood (<350 mL): No surgery, self-resolving. TX: Chest tube placed in the base of the lung (pleural base). Do not leave blood in the chest or will result in an empyema (collection of pus). Thoracotomy. Large amounts of blood (1250 mL): requires surgery to stop bleeding.	**Rib Fractures** Cause ↑ pain when breathing, leading to actelectasis and pneumonia. **Pain MUST be controlled and respiratory support must be given**. TX: Topical anesthetic block (nerve block), NSAIDS. Better to not use opiates because of ↓ breathing (respiratory depression) and no not strap chest.
Neck Trauma Penetrating wounds: Injury location: Above the angle of the mandible: DX: Arteriogram (AKA: Angiogram) to determine where the vascular damage is. TX: Embolization of the bleeding vessel. Injury location: Below cricoid cartilage (surgery): DX and TX: Arteriogram (AKA: Angiogram), Esophagram, Esophagoscopy, Bronchoscopy Gunshot wounds require surgery except in cases where the gunshot is above the mandible causing only vascular injury, but no injury to the trachea, esophagus. Bullets cause more damage than knives. If knife injury and patient is asymptomatic: observe. If patient has expanding hematoma or is going into shock = surgery Neck trauma indications for surgery: Rapidly deteriorating vital signs. Expanding hematoma, gunshot wound in the middle area of the neck. Spitting or vomiting of blood. Blunt trauma to neck: Do CT to check for cervical spine or spinal cord injury.	**Brain Bleeds:** There is not enough blood in the brain to cause symptoms of shock. If there are shock symptoms: bleeding is somewhere else. There are no intracranial bleeds responsible for shock. Imaging of brain bleeds: Ruling out bleeds: CT without contrast (blood and contrast look the same so the contrast can cause of false positive). **Epidural hematoma:** MC due to fracture of temporal bone. "Lucid" intervals, sudden loss of consciousness. CN III Palsy. Pupil fixed and dilated, sudden loss of consciousness. Can be quick deterioration, death within hours. Due to rupture of the Middle Meningeal Artery (branch of the Maxillary artery which is a branch of the external carotid artery). Biconvex form. Emergency craniotomy to evacuate hematoma. DX: CT scan with no midline deviation. TX: Emergency craniotomy. **Subdural Hematoma (AKA: Chronic Subdural Hematoma):** MC due to venous bleeding over time. Brain atrophy causes bridging veins to stretch and break. Crescent, semilunar shape. May or may not have midline shift. Fluctuating, gradual loss of consciousness if due to trauma. Other causes: Shaken baby. Elderly and alcoholics (Brain shrinks). DX: CT of head, If midlines shift: surgery, craniotomy to evacuate hematoma. Epidural and Subdural: If no midline shift: Monitor ICP. Fluid restrictions, diuretics (Mannitol, Furosemide), hyperventilation to ↓ ICP, ↓ oxygen demand by sedation or hypothermia.

Skull Fractures: Basal Skull Fracture

SX:
Clear fluid leak from nose (CSF).
"Raccoon eyes" hematoma/ecchymosis behind/around eyes.
Clear fluid leak (CSF) from ear or nose.
Hematoma or ecchymosis behind the ear.

DX: CT of head and neck with no contrast will show a skull fracture).
TX: No treatment for CSF leak, it is self-limiting.
Complication: temporary facial palsy may occur within a few days due to motor and sensory dysfunction of the peripheral nervous system (neurapraxia). Self-limiting in 6 – 8 weeks.

ANY loss of consciousness requires a CT (even if the patient believes they are fine).

Head Trauma

Penetrating injury to the skull: surgery.
Do NOT remove any foreign body in the ER; it must be done in surgery.

Head trauma with loss of consciousness: CT of the head and neck without contrast. If normal CT and neurological exam patient can be sent home and observed for 24 hours. Patient must be awakened often to see if there are any changes in mental status.

Linear skull fractures: Can be assessed and TX in the ER.

Closed skull fracture: No surgery if asymptomatic.

Depressed or commuted (bone fragments) skull fractures: Surgery is required. Bone fragments can be cleaned away from the brain.

NOTE: Intracranial bleeds do not cause hypotension.

Diffuse Axonal Injury
Due to **acceleration-deceleration** injury to the head.
Surgery will not improve.
TX: Keep intracranial pressure down to prevent more injury.
Poor prognosis.

Elevated Intracranial Pressure due to head trauma (ICP)
Emergency
SX: Decreased consciousness after injury → improvement → decline/drowsiness.

DX: Gradual dilation of one pupil due to decrease in responsiveness to light.
Head CT will show midline shift or dilated ventricles.
NOTE: Do not perform lumbar puncture in anyone with high ICP or it will cause the brain to herniate and the patient will die.

TX:
Head elevation.
Hyperventilation causes the decrease of CO2 which causes vasoconstriction in the vessels of the brain → ↓ blood volume → ↓ ICP. Brain perfusion must be maintained.
Caution: do not fluid overload, it will ↑ ICP.
Mannitol (↓ Na and water reabsorption → extracellular fluid). If severe: hypothermia and/or sedation to lower oxygen demand in the brain.

Diaphragmatic Rupture

MCC: Blunt trauma.

DX: X-Ray shows: Loops of bowel in the chest, air fluid levels in the lungs, it is always on the left side because the liver is in the way on the right side so the bowels are not able to go up into the chest.
TX: Nasogastric tube, laparoscopic evaluation, surgical repair.

Hip Fractures
Two locations:
Intrascapular (femoral neck and femoral head)
Extra scapular (Intertrochanteric and subtrochanteric)

Management:
Stabilize, treat pain, DVT prophylaxis.
Must establish the reason the patient fell (ex: MI, stroke)

(Note: Beware of the patient that is bedridden, they do not need to go to surgery).

Pelvic Fractures

Patient can bleed to death and nearby organs can be damaged.

If patient is hemodynamically stable: observe and rule out injuries to nearby organs.

If patient is bleeding into the pelvis and is hemodynamically unstable = shock and not responding to fluids:

- FAST ultrasound to verify if there is a bleed in the abdomen.
- In FAST negative for bleeds = no surgery required.
  Bleeds = surgery.
- Arteriogram.
- External fixation to immobilize broken bones to stop bleeding.

Other organ damage due to pelvic fracture:
Females: Rectum, vagina, bladder (SX: Blood in urine)
Males: Rectum, urethra (perform urethrogram first and then a cystogram), bladder (perform a retrograde cystogram).

Bleeding (Hypovolemic Shock)

MC areas of large volume of bleeding: abdomen, thigh (due to Fx of femur).

SX: ↓↓ BP, cool extremities, cold, clammy skin, oliguria, flat neck veins.
Body is releasing CATS, ATII and ADH to get fluids up.
Body response: Tachycardia (first response to low BP), ↓ CO,
↓ SV, ↓ EF, ↓ preload, ↓ PCWP, ↓ right atrial pressure, ↓ venous saturation (VO2), ↑ TPR (vascular resistance),

TX: Find and repair cause of bleed.

Pericardial Tamponade

SX: Severe hypotension, JVD, distant (muffled) heart sounds, tachycardia, pulsus paradoxus, Kussmaul sign, electrical alternans on EKG, CXR shows clear lungs.
Body response: ↓↓ BP, ↓ CO, ↓ SV, ↓ venous return, equilibrium of diastolic pressure in all 4 chambers, ↓ filling of left ventricle (preload).
MCC: Penetration to the pericardium: broken ribs, bullet or knife puncture wounds.

DX: Echocardiogram

TX: Immediate pericardiocentesis.
Long term TX: Pericardial window.
DO NOT treat with diuretics.

Vasogenic Shock

Causes: Septic Shock and Anaphylactic Shock (due to severe allergy reaction: bee sting, penicillin allergy), spinal anesthesia.

MOA: IgE (allergy, Hypersensitivity type 1) aggregates with another IgE causing the degranulation of mast cells to release histamine. This causes tachycardia, vasodilation, bronchoconstriction and swelling.

SX: Hypotension, tachycardia, extremities are warm.
Body reaction: No adequate filling of ventricles: normal to low PCWP and ↓ EDV, ↑ CO, ↓ TPR.

TX: Vasoconstrictors (Epinephrine) and IV fluids.

Misc Emergencies

Hypothermia

MC: Intoxicated person that fell asleep outside in cold temperatures.
MCC death is cardiac arrhythmias due to the hypothermia.
Hypothermia: the body core temperature is <95.0° F (35.0° C)

SX: **Mild:** Sympathetic system kicks in: shivering, HTN, tachycardia, ↑ respirations, vasoconstriction of vessels. Hyperglycemia (due to ↓ in glucose consumption by the cells and ↓ in insulin release, and ↑ release of glucose from the liver by the sympathetic system). Hypoglycemia can be found in alcoholics.
Moderate: Shivering becomes severe; muscle movements become slow and uncoordinated. Mild confusion begins. Surface blood vessels vasoconstrict even more so that blood is kept closer to the vital organs. Extremities become blue (fingers, toes, lips, ears).
Severe: Systems begin to fail: HR, RR and BP decrease. (ie: at a body core temperature of 82° F, the HR will be at 30 bpm), amnesia, stumbling, walking becomes difficult/impossible, paradoxical undressing (removing clothes), irrational behavior, arrhythmias can occur, organs fail, death.

Causes: extreme cold, conditions that ↓ heat production in the body or ↑ heat loss in the body: alcohol intoxication, low blood sugar, anorexia, elderly.
Heat loss is faster in the water (immersion) than air.

TX: First step: EKG to look for "J-waves of Osborn" or "J wave" or "Osborn wave" (ST elevation-like patterns). Active core rewarming (ACR) if the most effective way to **increase core body temperature**.
Warmed, humidified airway (tube or mask), peritoneal dialysis: (warm fluid cycled through the abdomen, this helps warm the liver which allows it to clear toxins), heated irrigation, diathermy: (ultrasound delivers heat to deeper tissues), extracorporeal: (blood is circulated from the body through a warmer then back into the body's blood stream).

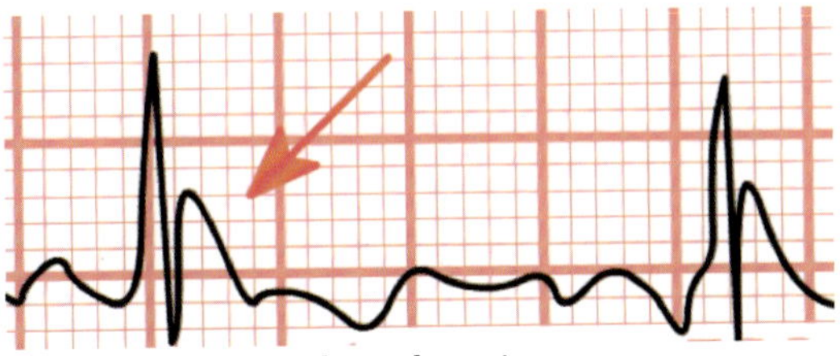

J waves of Osborn - hypothermia

Drowning

(Based on osmosis)

Salt water drowning

Salt water is **hypertonic.** Salt water is inhaled into the lung, it draws water out of the cells so that accumulates in the lungs and causes **thickening of the blood** (causing them to be like CHF), flushing out the surfactant causing **ARDS**. Thicker blood also causes more work on the heart, which can lead to **cardiac arrest** in <10 minutes.

Fresh water drowning

Fresh water is **hypotonic**. Fresh water is inhaled into the alveoli, which are in direct contact with the capillaries. The water is hypotonic so it diffuses into the capillaries and into the RBC's causing **hypervolemia** leading them to **swell and rupture causing hemolysis.** The dilution of the blood will result in an elevation in potassium and depression in sodium, which can cause V-fib causing cardiac arrest in minutes. Hemoglobin from the RBC lysis can cause acute renal failure. If enough cold water moves into the blood stream this can drop the temperature of the heart as the blood moves through causing **cardiac arrest**.

TX: Correction of hypoxemia and acidosis. Give 100% oxygen. Intubation and positive end-expiratory pressure (PEEP) with mechanical ventilation. Monitor for hypothermia for the first 24 hours. Monitor blood glucose and for hypotension. Drowning in warm water has a poor prognosis.

Heat Stroke (AKA: Exertional)	Heat Exhaustion
Healthy person doing heavy work in direct sun SX: **Temp > 105° (40° C), Dry skin** (they can't sweat), Nosebleeds, altered mental status, rhabdomyolysis, **myoglobin** in urine (dipstick test shows no RBC's), because extreme heat is breaking down proteins. Labs: ↑ CPK and K Cause: **Failure of the thermoregulator (anterior hypothalamus malfunction)**. Body is getting hot but the sensor is broken. TX: **Evaporation cooling**. Spray/mist lukewarm water on naked patient and use circulating fans (convection over water). Ice baths or ice packs may also be used. DO NOT infuse iced/cold saline into the body, this can stop the heart. **NOTE**: The **fastest form of cooling is convection (moving air)** verses conduction (molecules must pass heat/cold from one to another). It provides a mist over the skin so that moving air cools it down. (AKA: **Evaporation**)	Healthy person doing heavy work in the heat but is not staying **hydrated = ↑ dehydration** Cause: **inadequate sodium and fluid replacement.** SX: **Normal body temp,** excessive **sweating**, NO altered mental status, NO delirium. Can lead to renal failure. Labs: Normal: no rise in CPK and K TX: Move patient into cool environment, normal IV saline and electrolytes.

Other forms of Hyperthermia (thermogenesis)

- **Malignant hyperthermia** due to anesthetics (Halothane)
- **Neuroleptic malignant syndrome** due to antipsychotic medications
- **Malignant hyperthermia** due to the uncoupling of the electron transport chain in the inner mitochondrial membrane, which dissipates the proton gradient before it, can be used for oxidative phosphorylation. This energy is now used to generate heat instead of producing ATP. (Salicylic acid, brown fat, 2,4-dinitrophenol (DNP: antiseptic, pesticide, sulfur dyes, wood preservatives).
- TX: Dantrolene

Overdose – Poisoning

Gastric Lavage (AKA: Stomach pumping)	Unclear Etiology of ER Presentation
• Eliminates ingested poisons or overdoses from the stomach. • Tube is passed from either the nose or mouth into the stomach. • Saline is administered and suctioned/siphoned out. • Use is limited due to the short time the poisons/pills are actually in the stomach before passing through the pyloric sphincter (30 – 60 minutes). • Only 50% of the substance can be removed at 1 hour from ingestion. • It is of no value after 2 hours from ingestion. At 2 hours only 15% of the substance is able to be removed. • Contradicted if patients have a compromised airway, GI hemorrhage, altered mental status or perforation. Do not use for corrosive/caustic substances (acids and alkali may burn the esophagus and oropharynx), acetaminophen OD, hydrocarbons (organic chemical of carbon and hydrogen) or for poisons/overdoses that have an effective antidote. • DO NOT USE: Syrup of Ipecac, cathartics (sorbitol), forced diuresis (can cause pulmonary edema), whole bowel irrigation (polyethylene glycol). Whole bowel irrigation is only used in large ingested quantities of lithium iron, drug packets (packs of drugs that smugglers keep their drugs stored in).	This is a situation when a patient is brought into the ER in an unconscious state or altered mental status and no information is available to determine the cause of their condition. Certain things are automatically done immediately in order to access what the underlying cause of the patient's condition is. • EKG- 12 lead to access cardiac/circulation issues • Vitals • Airway is secured (pulse oximetry, oxygen) • Finger stick glucose to access blood sugar levels for hypo/hyperglycemia • Administration of Naloxone and dextrose in case of an opiate overdose • Blood work: CBC, OSM, electrolytes, kidney, thyroid, cortisol levels, ammonia, BMP, B12 • ABG, drug/toxicology screen, cardiac enzymes • Cultures: blood and urine • Head CT without contrast to evaluate for stroke

Activated Charcoal	Caustic Poisoning – Acids and Alkalis
• Charcoal is more effective than gastric lavage. • Safe to give in most any toxic drug or chemical overdose. • Is able to remove toxic substances even after they have been absorbed. Repeated doses of charcoal will decrease toxin levels in the blood quickly. • Reduces absorption of poisonous substances up to 60%. • It binds the chemicals so that it reduces their toxicity throughout the GI tract. • It does not bind with: Lithium, iron, lead, iodine, sodium, corrosive/caustic substances (strong acids and bases), alcohols, hydrocarbons, acetaminophen. (charcoal will absorb the drug given to treat an acetaminophen OD). (Polyethylene glycol in whole bowel irrigation will bind lithium and iron).	• Ingestion of acids (battery acid, toilet bowl cleaners, rust removal products) and alkalis (drain cleaner, lye, ammonia) and burn and perforate the pharynx, larynx, esophagus and stomach. • Alkalis damage occurs once the pH > 11.5 • Acidic damage occurs one the pH <2 • Do not induce vomiting or the substance will re burn on the way back up causing further damage. • Patient should ingest high volumes of water. • Evaluate airway: stridor, drooling due to damage causing closed airways.

See respective emergencies in their separate chapters:
Cardiac, Pills (Acetaminophen, aspirin, TCA's), Organophosphate, Atropine, Gases, Digoxin, Metals, Alcohol, Strokes, Head trauma, Pulmonary.

Pharmacology P-450 Interactions

- Note: anytime a question mentions that a patient has been on a drug for a while and has been properly responding, THIS is NEVER the problem. Always look for what is ADDED into the question. THIS is what will be the cause of the new side effects now presenting. If the "new" addition is a drug, check to see if it is a P-450. If a patient is on a statin and the "new" addition is red urine (myoglobin) look for a new strenuous activity the patient has begun (pushing their muscles: ie: training for a marathon, increased weight lifting – anything that is pushing muscles more and then look for the new drug added to be a P-450 inhibitor. (usually a fibrin).
  (If someone has pushed their muscles and myoglobin is presenting, but the patient is not on any medications: remember to check for other clues that could point to McArdle's).
- It is critical to be aware of all drugs a patient is on. A P-450 inhibitor is MCC for toxicity. If a patient is on a P-450 inhibitor, all other drugs will not be cleared normally and will build up. This is especially dangerous if the patient is on a drug that has a narrow therapeutic margin (esp: **warfarin = building up = ↑ bleeding**) or a drug that had major side effects (ie: **statin** = muscle damage).
- If the drug is a P-450 inducer, it means that any other drugs the patient is on is being cleared quickly, so the original drug will not be working as well. The main drugs that this would affect would be: OCP's (patient could become pregnant), warfarin (PT/INR is ↓ so patient can beginning clotting: so look for someone that has A-fib (irregularly irregular rate) and has been well controlled with warfarin to now present with signs of a stroke due to clots now being thrown due to ineffective warfarin. Could also see the improvement for other treatments (antibiotics, etc) simply not working, the condition does not improve.
- Drugs that have a narrow therapeutic window and are affected either way (substrates): if the P-450 is an inhibitor or inducer: Phenytoin (other anti-ecliptics), Warfarin, Theophylline, OCP's.

P-450 Inhibitors: **Causes other drugs to build up = toxicity.**	**P-450 Inducers:** **Clears other drugs so they do not work.**
Acute Alcohol abuse **Fibrates (Gemfibrozil)** Ciprofloxacin Isoniazid Grapefruit Juice Quinidine Amiodarone **Ketoconazole** **Erythromycin (Macrolides)** Sulfonamides **Cimetidine** Ritonavir	Chronic Alcohol Modafinil St. John's wort Phenytoin Phenobarbital Nevirapine Rifampin **Griseofulvin** Carbamazepine

DRUG TOXICITY

ALCOHOL

- Moderate alcohol can raise serum HDL levels.
- Alcohol has anti-platelet affects.
- Low doses of alcohol acts as a vasodilator and reduces peripheral blood pressure.
- Alcohol is a cardio-depressant. Chronic alcohol can cause congestive or dilated cardiomyopathy (dilated chambers of a heart predisposes development of a thrombus)
- Binge alcohol drinking can cause atrial and ventricular arrhythmias in individuals with no previous heart disease. ("Holiday heart")

Intoxication Symptoms	Intoxication TX	Withdrawal Symptoms	Withdrawal TX
Disinhibited, talkative, unstable, disruptive, moody, respiratory depression, **nystagmus**, **ataxia**, amnesia. Wernicke Korsakoff Syndrome. Labs: **AST twice** of ALT value, ↑ GGTP, ↑ LDH Note: Always run UA, blood, breath to look for other drugs.	**IV or IM Thiamine and Mg, B12, Folate. Chlordiazepoxide or Diazepam** to inhibit Alcohol dehydrogenase. Sleep it off. Mechanical ventilation if needed. **Disulfiram (Antabuse)** to help with addiction. Best TX: Alcoholics Anonymous	Tremors, Hallucinations, Seizures, **Delirium tremens. (The DT's)**	**IV or IM Thiamine and Mg, B12, Folate. Chlordiazepoxide or Diazepam (Benzodiazepines)** Do **not** give seizure prophylaxis.

ALCOHOL WITHDRAWL TIMELINE

Initial Withdrawal Symptoms	Hallucinations	Withdrawal Seizure	Delirium Tremens
6 hrs after last drink: SX: **Anxiety,** Diaphoresis, Insomnia, Tremors, Headache TX: **Thiamine, Mg, Folate, Chlordiazepoxide or Diazepam. (Benzodiazepines)**	12 – 24 hrs after last drink: SX: Visual **hallucination** and/or tactile hallucinations (feeling or seeing bugs crawling on their skin).	48 hrs after last drink: SX: Seizures	48 hrs after last drink: Delirium tremens (onset of rapid confusion), Hallucinations, altered mental status, shivering, agitation, sweating, fever, seizures, HTN, death

SUBSTANCE OVERDOSE and WITHDRAWL

- **The most common deaths due to overdose are: Aspirin and Acetaminophen**
- **If the OD was due to a suicide attempt be sure to get psychiatric help for them**

Substance	**Intoxication Symptoms**	**Intoxication TX**	**Withdrawal Symptoms**	**Withdrawal TX**
IV drug use (track marks) be sure to check for HEP B and C, HIV, TB (PPD)				
Amphetamines **Cocaine** Methamphetamines Bath Salts, Coke, Crack, Blow, Rock.	**Sympathetic** activity: autonomic hyperactivity. SX: ↑ HR, ↑ BP, **mydriasis** (dilated pupils), sweating, altered mental status, nausea, sudden headache, flushed skin, **euphoria**, dehydration, hallucinations, headache, palpitations). **Cocaine MI** (AKA: Sudden cardiac death) (**diffuse ST elevations – cardiac vasospasms**), **↑ risk abruptio placenta.**	**Benzodiazepines,** Vitamin C (promotes excretion). **In a cocaine induced MI, do NOT give β-blockers. You must give Calcium Channel Blockers.** (β-Blockers leave α-1 receptors unopposed = HTN emergency).	**↑ appetite (hunger),** paranoia, irritability, agitation, anxiety, **depression**, ↑ risk suicide, headache, **anhedonia** (lack of pleasure), **Hypersomnolence**.	**Antidepressants**
Anabolic Steroids	Aggression, irritability, psychosis, , mania	**Antipsychotics**	Depression, anxiety, concern about physical appearance	**SSRI**
Anticholinergics (TCA's), pesticides (Jimson weed – Atropine poisoning)	Dry skin, flushing, dilated pupils **(mydriasis),** cardiac conduction problems, thirst, urinary retention (sympathetic symptoms)			
Barbiturates	Severe respiratory depression, somnolence, impaired memory, ataxia, inappropriate sexual behavior, anxiety. (High addiction rate, low safety margin as compared to Benzodiazepines)	Respiratory support. **Flumazenil*** *Must **NOT** use Flumazenil if patient is chronically taking Benzodiazepines (or Barbiturates), it will cause them to go into withdrawal.	Delirium. Cardiovascular collapse. Hyperactivity, Seizures Insomnia, Anxiety	Use short-acting benzodiazepines or barbiturates: **Chlordiazepoxide, Phenobarbitol.**
Benzodiazepine (Bennies, Ice, Speed, Uppers, Dexies.	Aggressive behavior, impaired concentration/memory, somnolence, ataxia, inappropriate sexual behavior, anxiety, lessor respiratory depression than Barbiturates.	**Flumazenil*** *Must NOT use Flumazenil if patient is chronically taking Benzodiazepines (or Barbiturates), it will cause them to go into withdrawal.	Hyperactivity, Seizures Insomnia, Anxiety	Use short-acting benzodiazepines or barbiturates: **Chlordiazepoxide, Phenobarbitol.**

Caffeine (Coffee, Tea, Soda, Energy Drinks)	Restlessness, diuretic, muscle twitching, ↑ HR	None	Headache, ↓ ability to concentrate	None
Cannabis (**Marijuana**, THC: tetrahydrocannabinol, Grass, Hash, Pot, Tea, Weed)	**↑ appetite, red conjunctiva (eyes), anxiety**, everything is funny, euphoria, **slow/impaired motor coordination ↓ reaction time** (so rate of accidents increases), ↑ libido, dry mouth, tachycardia.	None	**Irritability, insomnia,** cravings, depression, sweating, sleep disturbances, anxiety, **↓ appetite**/weight loss. Detectible in urine for up to 10 days.	None
Cholinergic Toxicity: Organophosphate poisoning, anti-cholinesterases (more parasympathetic symptoms)	Salivation, vomiting, urination, ↓ heart rate, pupil constriction (**Miosis)**			
Ecstasy (AKA: MDMA: Methylenedioxy-methamphetamine, Molly)	**Hyperthermia, bruxism (teeth grinding).** Euphoria, extreme dehydration (renal failure), hyperthermia, bruxism, insomnia, ↑ HR and BP, agitation, paranoia, hallucinations, convulsions, DIC.			
Flakka (AKA: Gravel)	Paranoia, delusions of superhuman strength, agitation, **bizarre behavior** (ex: biting chunks out of another person) , euphoria, increased awareness, energy, stimulation.			
GHB (Gamma Hydroxybutyric Acid) (AKA: Date rape drug, "meow meow", Club drug)	CNS depressant, psychoactive drug. ↑ sex drive, euphoria. (GABA receptor agonist). Sweating, loss of consciousness, hallucinations, amnesia, nausea, coma. Colorless/odorless and can be added to alcohol.	Hospitalization and supportive.		
Heroin **Opiates** (Opioids, Smack, Stuff, Bug H, Darvon, Codeine, morphine)	**Miosis** (constricted/pinpoint pupil), ↓ gag reflex, **respiratory depression**, apathy, drowsiness, coma, difficulty with memory, slurred speech, death	**Naloxone, Naltrexone** and possible respiratory support. **Note**: Opiates bind to mu, kappa, delta receptors. **Note:** Naltrexone decreases cravings for alcohol.	**Lacrimation (rhinorrhea- runny eyes and nose), yawning, piloerection** (goose bumps), fever, chills, insomnia, **muscle cramps** (flu-like symptoms)	**Methadone, Clonidine, Buprenorphine**
Inhalants **Sniffing glue** (airplane model glue, spray paint cans), gasoline, cleaning fluids.	Belligerence, impaired judgment, blurred vision, apathy, coma	Antipsychotics	None	None

Ketamine	Fast acting: 10 minutes. Dissociative state, sense of detachment from one's physical body, visual and auditory hallucinations. ↑ or ↓ HR and BP, transient erythema, nausea, ↑ salivation, ↑ muscle tone, double vision, tunnel vision, respiratory depression, ↑ ICP.			
LSD (Hallucinogens)	Hallucinations, **flashbacks**, **mydriasis** (dilated pupils), colorful hallucinations, mydriasis, tremors, panic, impaired judgment, distorted perception, lack of coordination.	Supportive. "Talking down".	None	None
Magic Mushrooms (AKA: Psychedelic Mushrooms, Shrooms). Contain psychedelic compounds: psilocybin and psilocin)	Visual enhancement: halos around lights, open/closed eye visual hallucinations, enhanced colors, altered sense of time, spiritual experiences, increased sense of well-being and satisfaction with life.			
Nicotine	Restlessness	None	Irritability, anxiety, cravings.	**Varenicline, Bupropion, Nicotine patch, Nicotine gum**

PCP (Phencyclidine) AKA: Angel Dust	**Aggressiveness**, assaultive, **belligerence**, **vertical and horizontal nystagmus**, **hostility**, HTN, seizures, agitation, impulsiveness, hyper sensitive to sounds, panic, bruxism (grinding teeth), random acts of violence, hyperthermia, rigidity, catatonic. (These are the people that are "superman", they keep coming, even after being shot several times).	"Talking down": Leave in a quiet, dark room to ↓ stimulation. Possible respiratory support.	None	None
Skittles Parties	Varied, depending upon which drugs were ingested. Skittles parties: when all drugs in a home (over the counter and prescription) are dumped into a community bowl and mixed up. Everyone reaches in and takes a handful.			

Pharmacology Toxicities/Overdoses and Antidote

Toxicity	Antidote	Notes
Acetaminophen *Tylenol*	**N-acetylcysteine** (NAC) to replace glutathione. Note: Acetaminophen is metabolized by the P-450 system, which produces N-acetyl-p-benzoquinoneimine (NAPQI). NAPQI is hepatotoxic. It is detoxified by glutathione.	Is also a mucolytic for cystic fibrosis. **Ingestion of 8 – 10 g of Acetaminophen can be toxic. 15 g is fatal.** **If the OD occurred more than 24 hours ago = no TX.** **Draw 4 hr serum acetaminophen concentration to determine hepatotoxicity risk (Rumack-Matthew scale). If the level is below the toxicity level – no TX.** **If the level is above the toxicity risk: administer N-acetylcysteine (NAC).** **NOTE: If they have ingested a bottle: treat them.**
Ammonemia	Lactulose	Binds NH4 in the GI to excrete and ↓ ammonia levels (hepatic encephalopathy)
Amphetamines (basic)	Ammonium Chloride (NH_4Cl) to acidify urine	
Aspirin (Salicylic acid)	Sodium Bicarb ($NaHCO_3$) to alkalinize urine so that the rate of aspirin clearance is increased, dialysis	SX: **Tinnitus, anion gas acidosis, mixed acid base disorder** (**respiratory alkalosis due to hyperventilation progressing to metabolic acidosis due to lactate**), renal toxicity, altered mental status. **Blood gases:** pH is alkalotic, **both** CO2 and HCO3 are **very low** (CO2 is usually in the low 20's (normal 40) and HCO3 will be in the mid teens: 16 (normal 24).
Atropine (antimuscarinic, anticholinergic)	**Physostigmine**	
Benzodiazepine	Flumazenil*	*Caution: If the patient is dependent on benzodiazepines do NOT treat with Flumazenil. This can cause the patient to go into withdrawal.
β-Blocker	**Glucagon**	
Carbon monoxide (competes with Oxygen to bind heme)	100% Oxygen Hyperbaric Oxygen	Inhibits Complex IV of the ETC.
Cisplatin Carboplatin	**Amifostine**	Amifostine (free radical) scavenger prevents nephrotoxicity when using Cisplatin
Copper, arsenic (garlic breath), gold	Penicillamine	(**tip**: PENney's are COPPER)
Cyanide (Almond breath)	Cyanide poisoning is a side effect of nitroprusside and nitric oxide. TX: Thiosulfate, Met Blue, Hydroxocobalamin. Hydroxocobalamin combines with cyanide to form cyanocobalamin (Vitamin B-12), which is excreted. Sodium nitrate induces methemoglobin in RBC's, which combines with the cyanide. Methemoglobinemia is then treated with Methylene Blue. Methylene blue inhibits Monoamine Oxidase. This changes the iron form Ferric (F^3 iron form) to Ferrous (F^4 iron form). Vitamin C can also assist in treating methemoglobinemia. Sodium thiosulfate transforms cyanide (donates a sulfur atom) to thiocyanate by rhodanese, which is then excreted.	HTN emergencies are TX with nitroprusside, which can cause Cyanide poisoning. Methylene blue is then given so that F3 (ferritin) can be converted to F2 (ferrous) and excreted. Inhibits Complex IV of the ETC.

Cyclophosphamide	**Mensa**	Partially prevents hemorrhagic cystitis. Thiol group in **Mesna binds acrolein** in urine.
Digoxin (Digitalis)	Anti-dig Fab, Atropine, Mg	Digitalis "looks" like Potassium so competes for the same receptors, causing digoxin toxicity.
Doxorubicin Daunorubicin Adriamycin	Dexrazoxane	Prevents dilated cardiomyopathy. Iron chelating agent
Ethanol (alcohol)	Ethanol, Fomepizole, dialysis Must: Thiamine B-1, Potassium IV: "Banana Bag"	**Caution**: You MUST give thiamine BEFORE you give glucose.
Heparin	**Protamine sulfate**	Methadone for heroin addition treatments. "Methadone Clinics".
Heroin (Opioid)	**Naloxone**	Acts on Mu receptors
Iron	Deferoxamine	
Nitroprusside (used to TX HTN emergencies)	Sodium Thiosulfate	Treatment with nitroprusside can cause Cyanide poisoning. Methylene blue is then given so that F3 (ferritin) can be converted to F2 (ferrous) and excreted.
Potassium – elevated	**Calcium Gluconate,** loop diuretics, insulin (drives K into the cell), hemodialysis, Kayexalate (polystyrene sulfonate)	**Caution**: if the patient's BP is severely low and his K is to high, the answer is ALWAYS to treat the high K FIRST (Calcium Gluconate). BEFORE fluids. Kayexalate is NEVER the answer; it takes to long to work. High K must come down immediately.
Lead	**Blood Lead levels ≤ 10 μg/dL = no risk.** **Blood Lead levels < 45 μg/dL = remove child from house and retest in one month.** **Blood Lead levels > 45 μg/dL = Chelation Therapy.** **Blood Lead levels 45 – 69 μg/dL = DMSA SX: abdominal pain, constipation.** **Blood Lead levels >70 μg/dL = EDTA SX: hemolytic anemia, cognitive, behavior disorders.**	Lead levels > 45 μg/dL require the child to be removed
Mercury, arsenic (garlic breath), gold	Dimercaprol, succimer	
Methanol, Ethylene ***glycol (antifreeze)	Fomepizole	
Methemoglobinemia	Methylene blue, Vitamin C	
Neuroleptic malignant syndrome	Dantrolene, Bromocriptine	
Norepinephrine	Phentolamine to stop tissue necrosis	Norepinephrine and epinephrine vasoconstrict – blanching out veins which causes ischemia.
Opioids (Heroin)	**Naloxone**	Acts on Mu receptors
Orotic Aciduria	**Uridine**	Inhibits CPS II (Carbamoyl Phosphate Synthetase II) in Pyrimidine pathway
Radioactive isotopes	Potassium Iodide to stop thyroid absorption of isotopes.	
Serotonin Syndrome	**Cyproheptadine** (1st gen histadine)	
TCA's (Amitriptyline)	Sodium Bicarb ($NaHCO_3$) to alkalinize the plasma and protect the heart.	Question will usually present as a patient in the ER that was found with an open bottle of pills, being treated for depression.
tPA, Streptokinase, Urokinase	Aminocaproic acid	
Warfarin	Active bleeding: **Fresh frozen plasma**.	PT/INR levels: ******

Antibiotics Safe in Pregnancy Azithromycin Aztreonam Cephalosporin's Erythromycin Nitrofurantoin (use in UTI's instead of TMP/SMX) Penicillin's	**Unsafe Drugs in Pregnancy** Ace Inhibitors Aminoglycosides (ototoxic) Chloramphenicol (grey baby, no UDP) Clarithromycin (embryotoxic) Cyclin's (Tetracycline, Doxycycline) (bone damage, teeth discoloration) Fluoroquinolones (tendon, cartilage damage) Griseofulvin (teratogen) Lithium (Ebstein's anomaly) Phenytoin Ribavarin (teratogen) Sulfonamides (kernicterus) Valproic Acid (neural tube defects) Vitamin A (Retinol, Isotretinoin) (teratogen)
PERICARDITIS INH Procainamide Phenytoin Hydralazine	**DILATED CARDIOMYOPATHY** Daunorubicin Doxorubicin (Can be prevented with Dexrazoxane)
TORSADES DE POINTES Class 1A antiarrhythmics (quinidine) Class III antiarrhythmics (Sotalol) TCA's Macrolides (Erythromycin) Antipsychotics (Haloperidol) Antiemetics (Ondansetron)	**CORONARY VASOSPASMS** **Cocaine** Sumatriptan Ergot alkaloids (Antimigraine drugs: nonspecific 5-HT agonists: ie: Ergotamine. Vasoconstrictor)
THYROID PROBLEMS (Hypo/hyperthyroidism) Amiodarone Lithium	**ADRENAL INSUFFICIENCY** Withdrawal of steroids (glucocorticoids)
HYPERGLYCEMIA Protease Inhibitors Steroids (Corticosteroids) β-Blockers Hydrochlorothiazide's Tacrolimus Niacin (must increase DM medicine dosage)	**HOT FLASHES** Tamoxifen Clomiphene
ENDOMETRIAL CARCINOMA Tamoxifen	**LIVER DAMAGE** Alcohol INH Metformin Statins Rifampin, Pyrazinamide Fibrates
PANCREATITIS (ACUTE) Didanosine Valproic Acid Fibrates Furosemide, Hydrochlorothiazide Alcohol Azathioprine Steroids (Corticosteroids)	**PSEUDOMEMBRANOUS COLITIS (AKA: Megacolon)** Ampicillin Amoxicillin Cephalosporin's Clindamycin
DIARRHEA Erythromycin Orlistat Excessive Mg intake Colchicine Metformin	**MEGALOBLASTIC ANEMIA** Phenytoin Methotrexate Sulfa Drugs

AGRANULOCYTOSIS Clozapine Carbamazepine Colchicine Propylthiouracil (PPU) Dapsone Ganciclovir	**PURE RED BLOOD CELL APLASIA**
APLASTIC ANEMIA Carbamazepine Methimazole Chloramphenicol NSAID's Propylthiouracil (PTU) Cimetidine Sulfonamides (Gantanol)	**BONE MARROW SUPPRESSION** Hydroxyurea Chemotherapy drugs
G6PD HEMOYSIS Sulfonamides Primaquine Chloroquine INH Aspirin Ibuprofen Dapsone Nitrofurantoin	**DIABETES INSIPIDUS** Lithium Demeclocycline
SLE – LIKE Procainamide Hydralazine, INH Phenytoin Sulfa drugs Quinidine Minocycline Etanercept	**GINGIVAL HYPERPLASIA** Phenytoin Cyclosporine Verapamil Nifedipine
STEVENS JOHNSON SYNDROME Anti-epileptic's: Phenytoin, Carbamazepine, Lamotrigine, Phenobarbital) Allopurinol Penicillin Sulfa Drugs	**TENDON and CARTILAGE DAMAGE** Fluoroquinolones
GOUT (HYPERURICEMIA) Hydrochlorothiazide Furosemide Pyrazinamide Niacin Cyclosporine	**MYOPATHIES** Statins Fibrates Niacin Steroids (glucocorticoids) IFNα Colchicine Penicillamine Hydroxychloroquine
DYSLIPIDEMIA (Fat Redistribution) Protease Inhibitors Steroids (Glucocorticoids)	**TEETH DISCOLORATION and BONE DAMAGE** Tetracyclines

PHOTOSENSITIVITY Cyclins (Tetracycline, Doxycycline) Sulfonamides 5-FU Amiodarone	**FANCONI SYNDROME** Expired Tetracycline
TINNITUS Aspirin	**CINCHONISM** Quinidine Quinine

PARKINSON-LIKE SYNDROME Metoclopramide Reserpine Antipsychotics	**OTOTOXICITY and NEPHROTOXICITY** Do not use Cephalosporin's with Loop Diuretics Cisplatin (prevent with Amifostine) Loop diuretics Aminoglycosides Vancomycin
DYSTONIA and TARDIVE DYSKINESIA Antipsychotics Metoclopramide	**SIADH** SSRI's Carbamazepine Cyclophosphamide
SULFA DRUGS Furosemide Sulfonylureas Sulfasalazine Probenecid Acetazolamide Thiazides Celecoxib Sulfa antibiotics	**HEMORRHAGIC CYSTITIS and Bladder Cancer** Cyclophosphamide (prevent with Mensa)
INTERSTITIAL NEPHRITIS Furosemide NSAID's Methicillin	**PILL INDUCED ESOPHAGITIS** Bisphosphonates, potassium chloride, tetracyclines
DRY COUGH Ace Inhibitors	**ANTIMUSCARINIC** Atropine Tricyclics Antipsychotics H1-Blockers
DISULFIRAM-LIKE SYMPTOMS Metronidazole Griseofulvin 1st Generation Sulfonylureas Specific Cephalosporins Procarbazine	**OTOTOXICITY** Aminoglycosides Vancomycin Loop Diuretics Cisplatin
NEPHROTOXICITY Aminoglycosides Vancomycin Loop Diuretics Cisplatin	**DIABETES INSIPIDUS** Lithium Demeclocycline
CUTANEOUS FLUSING Vancomycin Ca Channel Blockers Niacin, Adenosine Echinocandins	**HEPATIC NECROSIS (AKA: FULMANENT LIVER FAILURE, ACUTE LIVER FAILURE)** Acetaminophen Aspirin, Halothane, Valproic Acid, Amanita phalloides (death cap mushrooms)
PULMONARY FIBROSIS Amiodarone Bleomycin Busulfan Hydroxyurea Methotrexate Carmustine Nitrofurantoin	**GREY BABY SYNDROME** Chloramphenicol
THROMBOCYTOPENIA Heparin	**HYPERCOAGULABILITY** Hormone replacements, OCP's
SEIZURES Tramadol Bupropion Imipenem (Cilastatin) INH (if B6 deficiency) Enflurane	**OSTEOPOROSIS** Steroids (Corticosteroids) Heparin
DISULFIRAM-LIKE REACTION Metronidazole, 1st Generation sulfonylureas Griseofulvin Procarbazine Some of the Cephalosporins	**Odd Taste** Metronidazole (metallic taste)

SURGERY

Patient Assessment: Preoperative valuation of risk factors to decrease perioperative and postoperative complications

- Age
  - ≤40: Labs: Hb, urine screen for pregnancy in women of childbearing age
  - >40 EKG and blood glucose
- Complete history and physical exam
- EKG
  - No need if patient <35 without cardiac Hx
  - Requirements of patients with any history of cardiac disease
    - EKG
    - Stress test (evaluation for ischemia)
    - Echocardiogram (evaluation for heart function, murmurs (valve function) and ejection fraction)

Increased Risk Factors for Surgery

- Sex: Male > 45 years old
- Co-morbidities
  - Hypertension
  - Diabetes: equivalent to coronary artery DZ
  - Thromboembolism risk and anticoagulation management
  - Obesity
  - Infections
  - Immunocompromised
- Cardiac
  - Recent MI ≤6 weeks, unstable angina, decompensated CHF, significant arrhythmias, severe valve disease: Cardiology consultation
  - Previous MI > 6 weeks ago, mild angina, compensated CHF (severe JVD, pitting edema), diabetes: Stress test for high-risk procedures. For patient with low functional capacity perform echocardiogram for left ventricular function.
  - Rhythm other than normal sinus rhythm, abnormal EKG, Hx of stroke, advanced age, functional capacity: Stress test for high-risk procedures or if patient has low functional capacity.
  - Ejection fraction ≤35%
- Pulmonary Evaluation if: Asthma, COPD, cough, dyspnea, smoking
  To improve risk factors: have patient stop smoking 6 – 8 weeks prior to surgery
  - COPD: If severe (FEV_1 <1.5 L) is ↑ risk for postoperative pneumonia. They are unable to clear secretions.
- Renal Function
  All patients must maintain adequate perfusion to the kidneys. BP decreases under anesthesia and if it becomes too low may activate the renin pathway causing a decrease in renal function.
  - All surgeries: IV normal 9% saline before and during surgery
  - Dialysis patients: dialyze 24 hours before surgery
- Hepatic Function: Contraindication to surgery.
  1 risk factor: 40% mortality, ≥3 risk factors: >80% mortality
  - High mortality risk: Prothrombin time: > 16, Bilirubin >2, Albumin <3, encephalopathy (altered mental status)
- Nutritional Risk
  Improve risk with 5 – 10 days of nutritional supplements before surgery.
  - Diabetic coma, serum albumin <3.0, ≥20% loss of body weight over recent few months, serum transferrin <200 mg/dL
  - Nutritional supplements are given thought the gut (not parenteral (TPN): feeding by IV bypassing digestion)

Post Operative Fever Complications

"Five W's" mnemonic Guideline for Post Operative Fever
Fever: 101° F - 103°F

	PO Day	Cause	DX Test	Treatment
WIND	1	Atelectasis	Chest X-Ray	Incentive Spirometry
	3	Pneumonia	CXR, sputum culture	Nosocomial pneumonia antibiotics
WATER	3 - 5	Urinary Tract Infection	Urinalysis and urine culture. UA positive for nitrates and esterase.	Antibiotics
WALKING	5 - 7	DVT's and PE's	Doppler, CT	Anticoagulation with Heparin bridge to Warfarin for 6 months if 1st DVT. If Hx of DVT, Warfarin for life.
WOUND	7 - 9	Wound Infection, cellulitis	Physical exam for erythema, Swelling, pus	Antibiotics, Incision and drainage if abscessed.
WEIRD	9 – 15 days	Deep Abscess, drug fever	CT scan	Percutaneous abscess drainage.

Postoperative Complications

Complication	Symptoms – Possible Causes	Diagnosis and Treatment
Fever - See Above. 101° F - 103°F		
Post operative confusion	Hypoxia, Sepsis	Hypoxia: Check blood gases Sepsis: Block cultures, CBC
Aspiration	Infiltrates on CXR, hypoxia, SOB	Remove gastric contents (lavage), Bronchodilators, Respiratory support if needed.
Delirium Tremors	Altered mental status, hyperthermia, hypertension, tachycardia	Benzodiazepines
Bacteremia	Temp ≥ 104°. Soon after invasive procedures: catheters, instrumentation.	Blood cultures, Empiric antibiotics
Malignant Hyperthermia	Temp ≥ 104°. Soon after administration of anesthetic. MC: Halothane, Succinylcholine. Can also develop myoglobin due to muscle damage (rhabdomyolysis).	IV Dantrolene, 100% O2, cooling blankets, correction of acidosis
Hypoxia		Blood gases. This helps to determine the underlying acid/base to identify causes.
Myocardial Infarction	Caused by hypotension during surgery.	No thrombolytics (due to surgery).
Tension Pneumothorax	Due to positive-pressure breathing. BP ↓and CVP ↑.	Thoracentesis and chest tube placement.
Pulmonary Embolus	MC: End of first week. Acute shortness of breath, hypoxia (clear CXR), ↑ A-a gradient, tachycardia.	CT Heparin. If contradictions to anticoagulation: IVC filter.
Acute Respiratory Distress Syndrome (ARDS)	Atelectasis, Hypoxia and bilateral pulmonary infiltrates. (not CHF)	Positive end-expiratory pressure ventilation (PEEP)

GI Surgery and Non-Surgical Pathologies

Perforation of Abdominal Organ
MCC:
Diverticulitis due to chronic pressure: MCC: constipation and low fiber.
Crohn's disease.
Perforated peptic ulcer (gastric) due to eroding ulcers from NSAID use, H. pylori infections, head injury, burns, trauma, cancer.

SX: Acute/diffuse abdominal pain, rebound tenderness, guarding, abdominal rigidity.
DX: Upright abdominal with thoracic X-ray shows **air under the diaphragm.**

TX: NPO and IV fluids: Normal 9% Saline, NG tube.
Emergency surgery for perforation.
Antibiotics: Metronidazole and Cipro; Cefoxitin, Cefotetan, Ampicillin/Sulbactam, Piperacillin/Tazobactam.
NOTE: Do NOT do colonoscopy or barium enema to dx diverticulitis due to risk of perforation.

Bowel Obstruction
SX: Absence of feces/flatus (gas), high pitched (tinkling) bowel sounds on auscultation, severe colicky pain, nausea, vomiting, pain, fever.

MCC: **Adhesions from previous abdominal surgeries**. Other causes: Fitz-High-Curtis syndrome (PID), Chron disease (fistulas), tumors, hernias, volvulus, carcinoid, intestinal atresia, intussusception, foreign bodies.
NOTE: obstruction can also be due to stool impaction (due to opioids: chronic use or use following pain/surgery). TX: Stool softeners. **Methylnaltrexone** (*Relistor*).

DX:
BIT: Upright abdominal X-ray shows air/fluid levels in the bowel, dilated loops of bowel, absence of gas in the rectum.
If complete obstruction: (volvulus) X-ray shows "birds beak" sign.
MAT: CT with contrast shows change from dilated loops of bowel with contrast to those with no contrast.

Labs: ↑ Lactate (acidosis), CBC and WBC.

TX: NPO, NG (nasogastric) tube, IV fluids (normal saline) if partial obstruction
Complete obstruction: emergency surgery.

Ischemic Bowel and Mesenteric Ischemia
MCC of Ischemic Bowel: Lack of blood flow to the SMA, IMA. (Watershed areas: Splenic flexure, Hepatic flexure).
MCC of Mesenteric Bowel: Acute occlusion of SMA or IMA due to emboli from A-Fib. (**Look for hx of past MI's or strokes**).

Ischemic Bowel Onset: Progressive
Mesenteric Bowel Onset: Acute

Ischemic Bowel SX: Abdominal pain after eating (↑ oxygen need because intestines are "working". Pain subsides after digestion because ↓ in oxygen demand. AKA: same as stable angina), and bloody diarrhea.
Mesenteric Bowel SX: Severe pain that is out of proportion to the physical exam (no guarding, no rebound tenderness, soft abdomen).

Ischemic Bowel DX: BIT: CT of abdomen. MAT: Angiography.
Mesenteric Bowel DX: BIT: Abdominal X-ray. MAT: Angiography.

TX:
Ischemic Bowel TX: Surgery to remove necrotic bowel.
Mesenteric Bowel TX: Emergency surgery to resect necrotic bowel.

Esophageal Perforation

MCC: Iatrogenic due to endoscopy perforation.
Can also be due to drugs that erode through the esophagus (Biphosphates, iron pills, NSAIDS, Doxycycline).

SX: Acute chest or upper abdomen pain, dysphagia, odynophagia (pain on swallowing), air under the skin (subcutaneous emphysema).

DX: Gastrografin contrast esophagram. Do not use barium.

TX: Emergency surgery

Acute Pancreatitis MCC: Alcoholic, Gallstones SX: Severe pain radiating to the back, nausea, vomiting, possible bruising on the back/flank due to retroperitoneal hemorrhage. SX of hemorrhagic pancreatitis: ↑ WBC (>18,000), decreasing Hct, decreased calcium. DX: ↑↑ Serum or urinary amylase and lipase. (Amylase is sensitive, but lipase is specific for pancreatic damage). TX: NPO, IV Normal Saline, NG tube (suction). Complications: **Abscess:** Fevers, chills, ↑ WBC. TX: surgical drainage. **Pseudocyst** (collection of pancreatic fluids, forming thin wall cyst anterior to the pancreas): 4 – 6 weeks afterwards. Pain, palpable, anorexia. DX: CT. TX: If painless: no drainage needed. If painful: Surgical drainage. Chronic Pancreatitis: Diabetes, steatorrhea, malabsorption. TX: Insulin for the diabetes and replace pancreatic enzymes.	**Appendicitis** Acute inflammation of appendix due to **fecalith obstruction** (AKA: Obstruction of lumen by fecalith). **Labs:** Polymicrobial infection (MC: E. coli or B. fragilis). ↑ WBC with left shift. **Perforation** of appendix shows: ↑ WBC (> 18,000) DX: Ultrasound (children): Thickening of appendix walls. Adults: CT. SX: Fever, right lower quadrant pain (beginning initially in the umbilical region and migrating to the RLQ), anorexia, nausea, vomiting. DX signs: **Positive McBurney's Point** (rebound pain in RLQ), **Positive Rovsing's Sign** (palpation of the LLQ produces pain in the RLQ), Obturator Sign: pain with flexing or internal rotation of the right thigh. **Psoas Sign:** pain with extension of the hip. MAT: CT Complications: Ruptured appendix → peritonitis (abscess formation, gangrenous perforation). TX: Appendectomy (Laparoscopic surgery), IV antibiotics: Metronidazole and Cipro, Ampicillin/Sulbactam, Cefoxitin, Cefotetan, Levofloxacin and Clindamycin.
Gallbladder/Gallstones/Bile Duct • **Biliary Colic:** Cystic duct irritation: RUQ colicky pain (positive Murphy's sign), radiates to right shoulder and/or back. MCC: fatty foods. DX: Ultrasound. TX: Cholecystectomy. • **Acute Cholecystitis:** Stones in the cystic duct: Constant pain, fever, ↑ WBC (leukocytosis), RUQ pain (positive Murphy's sign), radiation to right shoulder and/or back. DX; Ultrasound shows gallstones and thick walled gallbladder. TX: NPO, IV fluids, antibiotics, NG tube, cholecystectomy • **Obstructive Jaundice: due to stones.** MC: Obese female (MC: in 40's, but can be any age) SX: ↑ ALP, Ultrasound shows dilated ducts, stones in the gallbladder, ↑ direct bilirubin, recurrent abdominal pain. DX: Ultrasound. Confirm: EUS or MRCP. TX: ERCP, Cholecystectomy • **Obstructive Jaundice: due to tumor.** MCC: Cancer of head of pancreas, ampullae of Vater or common bile duct. SX: Unintentional weight loss, progressive. DX: CT. If CT is negative: MRCP TX: Surgical resection. • **Acute Ascending Cholangitis** Ascending infection and obstruction of the • common bile duct due to obstruction. **NOTE**: Initial presentation is a triad of jaundice, fever and abdominal pain. **BEWARE**: if these symptoms progress to **include shock and altered mental status** (Reynold's Pentad), it can be fatal. SX: ↑ ALP, ↑ WBC, fever, ↑ LFT's, ↑ direct and total bilirubin. TX: IV Antibiotics, ERCP to decompress common bile duct, Cholecystectomy	**Diverticulitis** Inflammation due to fecal (fecalith) impaction into diverticula (pouches) in the bowel wall. SX: Severe LLQ pain, fever, nausea, can be bleeding. DX: CT scan. Do NOT do endoscopy (risk of perforation) TX: Antibiotics: **Metronidazole and Ciprofloxacin.** Recurrent cases or perforation: surgery resection.

Orthopedic Surgical Pathologies (Bone, Ligament)

Orthopedic Repairs

- Closed reduction: simple fractures with no displacement
- Open reduction and internal fixation: severe fractures with displacement or misalignment
- Open fractures: bone has broken the skin, fracture is repaired in surgery

Types of Fractures and Ligament Injuries

Fracture	Description/Notes
Greenstick Fracture	Fracture in young/immature bones. They are soft so the bone bends and breaks. SX: Pain in the injured area. Difficult to see on X-ray.
Stress Fracture AKA: Hairline fracture	Fatigue-induced from repetitive loading (jumping or running) trauma to the bone. MC: Athletes Locations: MC fracture: metatarsals and tibia. SX: Pain with weight bearing that increase with exercise or activity. DX: X-ray does not normally show the fractures. Must use CT or MRI. TX: Rest the limb. Discontinue the exercise that caused it. If necessary, casting or walking boot may be used. Note: Look for an athlete that has **increased the intensity** of his/her training for an upcoming event.
Spiral Fracture AKA: Torsion fracture.	Bone fracture due to a rotating force. This fracture should raise concern about **child abuse** (twisting and jerking of the limbs). NOTE: Do not mix this up with Osteogenesis imperfect (OI). In OI the break will be straight.
Comminuted Fracture	Bone is broken into multiple pieces: splintered or crushed. Common in crush injuries.
Compression Fracture	Collapse of a vertebra. MCC: Complication of osteoporosis (loss of bone mineral density in post menopausal women. Can also be seen in osteogenesis imperfect, metastatic or primary tumors. SX: Severe back pain. DX: Spinal X-rays. Tumors are DX by CT or MRI.
Pathologic Fracture	Fracture caused by a disease that weakened the bone. Fracture occurs from very little trauma. MCC due to metastatic cancers (Multiple myeloma, Paget's DZ, breast, colon). Notes: Colles Fracture (fall on outstretched hand), fractured ribs due to coughing in the elderly. TX: Closed reduction and casting.
Open/Compound Fracture	Broken bone breaks through the skin surface. Note: ↑ Risk of contamination and infection. Note: Beware of gas gangrene developing within a few days due to contamination. SX: Site is swollen, erythematous, painful with **crepitus**. Patient may also show signs of sepsis. TX: Surgery
Traumatic Fracture	Fracture due to sustained trauma. MCC: Falls, automobile accidents, fights.
Periprosthetic Fracture	Fracture at the end of a prosthetic implant.
Closed Fracture	Fractures in which the skin is left intact/unbroken.
Displaced Fracture	Fracture that is not in anatomical alignment. **NOTE: Clavicular fractures (collarbone):** Non-displaced clavicular fractures are put into a sling to stabilize. Surgery is indicated when: open fracture (breaks the skin), distal third of the clavicle is broken, broken in multiple pieces, non union after 3 – 6 months, or nerve or vascular involvement.
Fragmented Fracture	Incomplete: fracture where bone fragments are still partially joined. Complete: fracture where bone fragments are completely separated. Comminuted: fracture where the bone is broken into several pieces.
Facial Fractures	SX: Pain, bruising, swelling, nosebleeds if fracture of the nose, base of the skull or maxilla. Deformity of the nose if a nasal fracture. Mandibular fractures have difficulty opening their mouth with numbness to the lip and/or chin. Be aware of swelling around the face and be prepared to intubate if necessary in case the airway is compromised.
Scaphoid Fracture	SX: Pain in the anatomical "snuffbox" after a fall on an outstretched hand. Complications: Avascular necrosis due to disruption of blood supply from branches off of the radial artery. DX: Initial X-rays do not always show a fracture. Must do an MRI because of the possible complications. TX: Thumb spica cast.
Hamate Fracture	SX: Pain and swelling of the hypothenar. Causes ulnar nerve injury.
Lunate Fracture	SX: Acute carpal tunnel.
Femoral Neck Fracture (Hip Fracture)	SX: Externally rotated and shortened leg. MC: Due to falls by the elderly, **Osteoporosis**. Other: **chronic steroid** use, alcoholism, **Sickle Cell Anemia**, Gaucher's DZ, radiation, chemotherapy. Complication: Blood supply loss at the **Medial Circumflex Femoral Artery**.

Femur Fracture	Caused by major force. TX: Intramedullary rod fixation. **NOTE: ↑ risk for fat emboli.** (Note: ANY bone fracture can be a risk for fat emboli, but the larger bones are more prone).
Shoulder Dislocations	Anterior Dislocation: MCC: Fall on an outstretched hand. SX: Arm is held close to the body and forearm is externally rotated and loss of sensation over the deltoid. (Axillary nerve involvement: Surgical head of the humerus). DX: Postero-anterior (PA) and lateral X-rays. Posterior Dislocation: MCC: Seizures, electrical burns. SX: Arm is held close to the body and forearm is internally rotated. DX: Axillary or scapular X-ray.
Hip Dislocations	Posterior Dislocation: MCC: Head-on automobile crash when knees hit the dashboard. SX: Leg is internally rotated and shortened. TX: Emergency surgery.
Compartment Syndrome	SX: Severe pain when limb is moved in any direction, especially passive extension – can't get comfortable, pallor (↓ blood flow), pulselessness, paresthesia, paralysis. Common causes: **cast (Patient will complain at pain at the site of the cast)**, trauma, crush injuries, prolonged ischemia followed by reperfusion. **NOTE:** Monitor for (6 P's): Pain, Pallor (lack of blood flow), Paresthesia, paralysis, pulselessness, Poikilothermia (cold to touch). If there is pain at the site of the cast, the cast must be removed to evaluate for compartment syndrome. TX: **Emergency fasciotomy.**
De Quervain's Tenosynovitis	SX: Tenderness on the radial side of the hand when the tendon (thumb) is stretched. MCC: mothers picking up their babies (flexed writs and extended thumb). TX: Steroid injections.
Rupture of Achilles Tendon	SX: Sudden popping, pain, swelling, walking severely impaired, unable to stand on the toes, unable to plantarflex (point foot downward). MCC: Sudden or forced plantarflexion or dorsiflexion of the ankle. Usually due to fast acceleration (pushing off at a race or jumping). TX: Casting, possible surgical repair and physical therapy.
Medial Collateral Ligament and Lateral Collateral Ligament	SX: **Pain if extended knee is rotated. No blood in the joints.** Cause: Lateral hit to the knee. MC: Skiing or contact sports. Trauma to the opposite side of the injury. DX: Valgus Stress Test. Abnormal passive abduction = MCL. Abnormal passive adduction = LCL. DX: MRI. TX: Surgical repair.
Anterior Cruciate Ligament Posterior Cruciate Ligament	SX: Severe pain: rapid onset, unable to bear any weight, blood in the joint (hemarthrosis). Causes: Direct hit/force to the knee during aggressive sports. DX: Anterior Drawer (Lachman) Test, Posterior Drawer Test. MRI. TX: Young patients: arthroscopic repair. Older patents: immobilization and rehabilitation.
Meniscus	SX: Slow to develop. "Catching or popping" sensation. Causes: Twisting force on the knee (changing directions quickly). DX: McMurray Test: Pain when knee is externally rotated = medial meniscus. Laterally rotated = lateral meniscus. MRI. TX: Arthroscopic repair.
Carpal Tunnel	SX: Pain, paresthesia (median nerve), loss of opposition of thumb, atrophy of thenar muscle, pain is worse at night. Causes: repetitive movements, pregnancy (↑ fluid = ↑ pressure), hypothyroid (Matrix muco-polysaccharide protein deposit complex), Amyloid (Renal/dialysis), Acromegaly (hyperplasia), Rheumatoid Arthritis (tendons and synovial inflammation), Colles Fracture (compression), dislocation of the lunate. DX: Carpal tunnel test (recreate symptoms), Phalen sign = hyper flex wrist, Tinel's sign = Tap on median nerve or Elevating hand above head causes tingling. TX: NSAID's and splinting.

X-Ray Views for Fractures

- **2 views at 90° to each other**
- **Joints above and below the fracture should be included in the view**
- **Include any other areas of impact that could be affected**

PSYCHIATRY – BEHAVIORAL SCIENCE

Classical Conditioning

- A stimulus that causes a natural response (behavior) to occur. Reward based.
  Example: Pavlov's Dog. A dog is given food every time a bell is rung. So every time the bell rings the dog begins to salivate (natural).
- The natural response (behavior) is **involuntary**.
- Standard time interval.

Random Conditioning

- Response takes longer to extinguish
- Random time interval
- EX: Casino's

Operant Conditioning

- Behavior that is modified because a reward. The response is **voluntary**.
- Extinction
  - When the response (behavior) discontinues because the reward is discontinued.
- Negative Reinforcement
  - When a response (behavior) is required to **stop** a negative stimulus.
    ("When you stop crying I will let you out of the corner")
- Positive Reinforcement
  - When a response (behavior) is **produced** a reward is received.
    ("Stop crying and I'll give you some candy")
- Punishment
  - Negative stimulus is given until the unwanted response (behavior) is stopped.
    ("Sit in the corner until you stop crying")

Simple Learning

- Habituation: repeated stimulus ↓ response
- Sensitization: repeated stimulation ↑ response

Amnesia

- Anterograde: (wipes out new memories). Unable to store new memory but is able to remember old memories
- Retrograde: (wipes out old memories). Loss of old memories but is able to record new memories.
- Korsakov Amnesia: Alcoholic. (Note: In ER must give thiamine before glucose (dextrose) or will cause brain damage.
- Dementia: Memory loss, loss of cognition, **↓ in IQ**
- Normal aging: **IQ is the same** but decrease in memory

Psychiatry Responses/Communication

- **Facilitation:** Doctor facilitates continuing the conversation:
  Example: "Yes....I am listening, please continue". "And then what happened..."
- **Empathy:** Doctor understands what the patient is experiencing because he/she has "walked in their shoes" (it has actually happened to them). Do NOT express "empathy" unless you HAVE been through it and can relate.
  You can express **compassion** to show you feel for their situation.
- **Confrontation:** Last resort. This does NOT provide continued communication. The doctor points out something wrong to the individual.
  Example: "You are upset today, what is wrong?".
- **Reassurance:** This increases compliance. Be truthful.
- **Leading question:** Doctor answers a question with a question. Avoid this because it is helpful for malingering patients. Always have the patient describe the pain, symptoms, etc. Do not give them information to use.
- **Reflection:** Doctor summarizes what the patient has said. Repeat back.
- **Support:** Doctor expresses concern. This is independent of understanding (empathy). The situation has NOT happened to the doctor (as with empathy).

Countertransference verses Transference

- Countertransference: Doctor sees a resemblance in the patient to someone else. (Patient reminds the physician of one of his medical school teachers)
  (**tip**: The **DOCTOR** always stands behind the **COUNTER**)
- Transference: The patient sees a resemblance in the doctor to someone else. (The doctor reminds the patient of their father).

IQ Testing

- Adult > 17 years old. WAIS-R Wechsler (**tip**: w "A" is = "A" for Adult)
- Child 6 – 17 years old. WISC-R Wechsler (**tip**: w "I" is = "I" for infant-child)

Mental Retardation, Mental Illness

Amniocentesis can be preformed on women over 35 to evaluate mental retardation in the fetus.

- IQ < 70.
  85% of mentally retarded are in this category.
  Mild retardation. ↑ difficulty as child gets older.
  MCC: Fetal alcohol syndrome
  Rate: 1.5 to 1 of boys over girls
- IQ 50 – 70
  Mild, is able to achieve 6th grade.
  Able to live independently in the community with minimal supervision. Is able to make their own decisions.
- IQ 35 - 50
  Able to achieve 2nd grade. Is able to work in sheltered workshops. They are not able to live alone, must live in groups.
- IQ 20 – 35
  Severe. Able to be taught basic skills: brush teeth, etc.
- IQ < 20
  Profound. Like babies. Require custodial care.

Phases of Illness in Mental Illness (Depression, Schizophrenia, Bipolar diseases)
Helps to determine medications.
Acute Phase

- **Goal is to achieve remission. (Absence of minimal symptoms with return to pre-morbid wellness)**
- **Response to treatment. Responds to treatment, progressing.**
  If patient attains substantial improvement, there will be a 50% reduction of symptoms.

Continuative Phase

- **The goal is to sustain remission/stabilize remission.**
- **Prevent relapse (the return to the acute phase).**
  Any medications used prior to this phase are continued.

Maintenance Phase

- **Recovery. The episode is over. Patient decides to continue or discontinue therapy.**

Reoccurrence: Has another episode after recovery.

Personality Development

STAGE	YEARS	DEFINITION
Sigmund Freud Theories		
Stage 1 – Oral Stage	Birth – 18 months	Weaning
Stage 2 – Anal Stage	18 mos – 3–4 years	Toilet training. Leads to OCPD, anal retentive, perfectionistic, cheapness in adults.
Stage 3 – Phallic Stage	3-4 years to 5-7 years	Sexual identity. Loves the opposite parent. "Oedipus Complex"
Stage 4 – Latent Stage	5-7 years to puberty	Learning. Super ego, conscious.
Stage 5 – Genital Stage	1-13 to adult	Genital intercourse. True intimacy.
Jean Piaget Theories		
Stage 1	Birth to 2	Learns: Sensory-Motor exploration
Stage 2	2 to 7 years	Learns: Symbols, language, believes they are the center of the universe, death is reversible, blame themselves for everything, inanimate objects are alive, no sense of equal sizes, does not understand the law of conservation.
Stage 3	7 to 11 years	Learns: Death is permanent, understands size difference and the law of conservation.
Stage 4	> 11 years	Learns: Abstract thinking
Erickson's Theories		Believes that personality is developed based on childhood experiences
Stage 1		Learns trust and mistrust
Stage 2	1 – 3 years	Learns: Mastery over environment. Learns to use "no". Autonomy is developed if child is able to make their own decisions. Without autonomy, child learns shame and doubt.
Stage 3	3 – 5 years	Learns Motor and intellectual skills
Stage 4	6 – 11 years	Learns, sets goals, gains sense of accomplishment. If child does not learn this it can cause sense of inferiority, violence and future problems.

Stage 5	11 years to teen	Learns group ID, peer pressure, morality, ethics, sexual experimentation. Without this learning there may be role confusions.
Stage 6	21 years to 40	Early adult. Learns intimacy and about relationships.
Stage 7	40 years to 65	Gains sense of accomplishment. Learns generatively verses stagnation. Without this may experience mid-life crisis and depression.
Stage 8	> 65 years	Has satisfaction with life, is happy and has integrity. Without this there is a risk of suicide and despair.

Sigmund Freud's Psyche

- **Id**
  Present at birth. A person's instincts and drives (aggressive, sexual)
- **Ego**
  Is a defense mechanism present after birth. It is the unconscious (organized, realistic part that mediates between the Id and super-ego. It helps to ward off anxiety by making us not aware.
- **Super-ego: Is conscience. It is ones sense of ethics and duty. It can stop the person from doing things that the Id may want one to do.**

Adolescents/Teens: It is IMPORTANT to understand what determines the probability that an adolescent/teen will be compliant is based on whether their PEERS are doing it.

Psychosis

- Losing contact with reality. Can exhibit: hallucinations, delusions, thought disorder (disorganized thinking, speaking, writing), bizarre behavior, impairment of carrying out daily activities, catatonia (moving a part of one's body and that position is held).
- Causes: Schizophrenia (all categories of schizophrenia), mania/bipolar, PTSD, delusional disorders, grief, sleep deprivation, personality disorders, stress, drugs/medications, postpartum psychosis.

Hallucinations:

- Believing something that is not really there.
  Visual: Seeing something that really is not there.
  Auditory: MC: Schizophrenia.
  Tactile (feeling): MC: Alcohol or cocaine withdrawal causes feelings that bugs are crawling on the skin.
  Olfactory: Smell. Can occur prior to migraines, syncope, epilepsy, brain tumors.
  Gustatory: Taste.
  Hypnagogic: Associated with Narcolepsy. Hallucinations before going to sleep. (tip: hypna**GO**ogic = **GO**ing to sleep).
  Hypnopompic: Associated with Narcolepsy: Hallucinations when waking up.

Delusion

- A false belief (bizarre, untrue, implausible) that one believes with absolute conviction despite evidence to the contrary.
- Individuals with delusions are able to maintain regular function lives.
  (Example: A man has been a cab driver and married for the past 15 years, yet he believes everyday that a space ship will be coming for him one day). These are beliefs that could actually happen but most likely they will never happen.

Narcolepsy (Sleep disorder)

- Loss of the brain's ability to regulate sleep-wake cycles.
  SX: **Excessive daytime sleepiness**, REM immediately after falling asleep, cataplexy
  TX: **Modafinil** or **Amphetamines** and scheduled daytime naps.

Cataplexy

- Symptom of narcolepsy
- Sudden loss of muscle strength/tone.
- Triggered by strong emotions: terror, crying, laughing or loud noises.

Hypnogogic

- Symptom of narcolepsy
- Hallucinations that occur as a patient is going to sleep
- (**tip**: Hypno "GO" ic for "GO" to sleep)

Hypnopompic

- Symptom of narcolepsy
- Hallucinations that occur as a patient is waking up

Sleep Attacks

- Symptom of narcolepsy
- Irresistible sleep. Experiencing REM within 5 minutes of falling asleep.

Sleep Paralysis

- Temporary inability to move or talk upon awakening – lasting seconds to minutes.

Catatonia (Catatonic)

- Stupor: not actively relating to environment, apathetic. Does not react to stimuli.
- Mutism: little speech.
- Loss of motor skills: Waxy Flexibility: patient maintains a position that they are placed in (Example: Put an arm above the head and it is held in that position).
- Echolalia: Mimicking another person's speech.
- Echopraxia: Mimicking another person's movements.
- TX: **Benzodiazepines**

EPS (Extra Pyramidal Symptoms): Side effects to anti-psych meds

Movement Disorder	Symptoms	Notes
Dystonia (Can begin by 4 hours till 4 days)	Muscle spasms, stiffness, or forces sustained contraction of the neck or eyes.	TX: Anti-histamine: **diphenhydramine,** Anti-cholinergic: **Benztropine.**
Akathisia	Restlessness, unable to sit still, repeated leg crossing, stepping in place	TX: Anti-psych meds, β-Blockers
Tardive Dyskinesia	Tongue protrusion, lip smacking, chewing movements, spreading fingers and toes, grunting noises, torticollis, shoulder shrugging, rocking and swaying.	MC caused by typical anti-psychotics. TX: Replace typical anti-psychotics with **Clozapine**.
Parkinsonism (Can begin by day 4 till 4 months)	Symptoms of Parkinson's movements	TX: Anticholinergic: **Benztropine**

Thought and Speech Disorders

- **Circumstantial** Speech (AKA: Circumstantiality)
  Speaker begins at one point, drifts in different directions, but eventually comes back "full circle" to the point. Delay in getting to the point.
- **Tangential** Speech
  Speaker begins on one topic, drifts in different directions and never returns to the original topic.
- Echolalia
  mimicking another person's speech.
- "Flight of Ideas"
  Abrupt leaps from one topic to another. Connects many ideas. Typical of mania in bipolar illness.
- "Pressured speech"
  Rapid speech without pauses.
- Loose Associations: No connections between any thoughts. Seen with psychotic disorders.
- Disorganized speech: "Loose Associations".
  Moving from one subject to another that is totally unrelated.

Suicide Risk

- #1 suicide risk: men > 65 years old.
  #2 suicide risk: teens
- **Most important predictor** of suicide is a history of suicide threats and attempts.
- Signs of suicide risk: **Anhedonia (AKA: No Hope, demoralized)** (no longer able to find pleasure from activities that brought enjoyment),
  depression, alcohol/drug use, no spouse (whether single, divorced or widowed), no social support, no children, sickness/chronic illness, previous attempt, organized plan, family history of suicide, low job satisfaction/unemployment, psych conditions: schizophrenia, borderline, antisocial.
- Anhedonia: is considered the worst of the signs. It is when a person **loses hope**.
- Suicide: **exception to confidentiality**. A person with suicide thoughts must be hospitalized.
- Women attempt suicide more (pills) but men succeed more (guns).
- Caution when giving anti-depressants to persons at risk for suicide. The medication may raise the energy level of the individual just enough to allow them to carry out the suicide.
- Management: Take all threats seriously. Never leave the patient. Hospitalize the patient. Do not identify with the patient. TX: SSRI and psychotherapy. ECT used if in immediate danger.

Substance Abuse (alcohol or drugs: illegal or prescription)

- **Tolerance**: individual requires more of the medicine to achieve the same effect.
- Substance **Dependence**: Individual feels that they need the drug in order to make it through the day.
- Substance **Abuse**: individual uses the drugs so much that it leads to harmful consequences. Relationships are impacted. Failure to fulfill obligations.
- Substance **Addiction**: individual is psychologically and physically dependent on the drug. They will go to any lengths to get the drug. They are unable to hold down a job and may risk illegal activities to obtain the drug. If they discontinue the drug they will suffer withdrawal symptoms.

Stages of Overcoming Substance Addiction

- **Precontemplation**: Individual does **not** recognize there is any problem.
- **Contemplation:** Individual now realizes there is a problem but has **no interest** in changing the behavior. (This usually occurs when a partner leaves.)
- **Preparation**: Individual now realizes they **need/want to change** their behavior. (This usually happens when someone is harmed: emotionally or physically). "I am prepared to change".
- **Action:** Individual is actively taking steps to change their behavior.
- **Maintenance**: Individual is maintaining the change in behavior.
- **Relapse**: Individual stops maintaining behavior changes and returns to old behaviors.

Delivering Bad News

- **Set the stage**
- **Ask/assess the patients comprehension of their problem: "What do you think is going on with your ……"**
- **Warn the patient that you have bad news. Deliver the news straightforward and with compassion/empathy.**

Order of Decision Making Power

This is used when the patient is unable to make decisions for themselves: due to incompetence, unconscious, etc

- Spouse → Adult child → Parents → Siblings → Nearest living relative

Dementia verses Delirium

Dementia	**Delirium**
Setting: usually home/office	Setting: **Inpatient/Medical**: hospital, nursing home
Onset: **Gradual**	Onset: **Acute**
SX: Memory deficits, personality changes, Impaired judgment,	SX: Hallucinations, "wax and wane" level of consciousness, agitation, aggressive, disorganized thinking
Causes: Irreversible. Alzheimer's, Huntington's, Lewy Body Dementia, Creutzfeldt-Jakob Dz, Pick Dz, cerebral infarcts. Causes: Reversible. B12 Deficiency, hypothyroidism, Neurosyphilis, HIV	Causes: Reversible. Medications, illnesses, infections, electrolyte disturbances, trauma, substance withdrawal/abuse.
TX: Check labs: **TSH and B12**	TX: Treat underlying cause, provide: hydration, Oxygen. Labs: electrolytes (BMP). If aggressive: **Haloperidol**

Amnesia

- Anterograde Amnesia: Unable to remember anything **AFTER** a CNS injury. Difficulty in forming new memories.
- Retrograde Amnesia: Unable to remember anything **BEFORE** a CNS injury.
- Dissociative Amnesia: Causes by serious trauma or stress. Unable to remember who they are.
  Associated with **dissociative fugue**: wandering, travel or establishment of new identity due to inability to remember any identity, memories or personal information. Usually reversible.
- **Korsakoff Syndrome**: MC in alcoholics. Amnesia due to **deficiency of vitamin B1**. Destruction of the **mammillary bodies.** Individual will **confabulate** stories to fill in the blanks they do not remember.

Orientation

- Individual's ability to know who they are, where they are and in what time frame they are in.
- Order loss: 1st lost: time, 2nd: place, last lost: person.

Dissociative Disorders

Dissociative Disorder	Description
Dissociative Fugue	Wandering, travel or establishment of new identity due to inability to remember any identity, memories, or personal information. Individuals may actually set up another life in another location. Usually reversible.
Dissociative Identity Disorder	AKA: Multiple personalities. Individual presents with 2 or more separate personalities. Associated with abuse (sexual or substance), borderline personality, PTSD, severe depression, somatoform disorder.
Depersonalization Disorder	AKA: De-realization. Individuals feel estranged from their own body, thoughts or actions.

SLEEP DISORDERS

Stages of Sleep

	Stage 1	Stage 2	Stage 3	Stage 4	Stage 5
Amount of Time	5% of sleep (5 -10 minutes)	45 - 55% of sleep	5% of sleep	12 – 15% of sleep	20- 25% of sleep
Brain Waves	Alpha	Theta: **Spindles, K-complexes**	Delta	Delta	Beta **REM Sleep**
Characteristics	Beginning of sleep. Light sleep. Easily woken. Occasional twitching, muscle activity slows. Sense of falling can occur. No rapid eye movement.	Body temp decreases. ↓ heart rate. Light sleep. Sleep spindles (sudden bursts of brain activity). K-complexes (high brain wave peaks followed by low brain wave peaks – follows spindles. No rapid eye movement. **Bruxism** (grinding the teeth).	Transitioning from light sleep to deep sleep. Delta brain waves. Slow brain waves. No rapid eye movement. Difficult to wake, if awakened, individual could be agitated, groggy or disoriented. Growth hormone is released during this period. Restorative sleep. **Night terrors.** **Sleepwalking.**	Deepest sleep. Delta sleep. Essential for proper sleep. Easily woken up. No rapid eye movement.	Occurs from 70 – 90 minutes after falling asleep. Rapid eye movement. REM sleep. Beta waves. Low voltage, high frequency waves. REM stimulated by release of **acetylcholine**. REM is inhibited by secretion of serotonin. Parasympathetic activity is ↑ during REM. Memory is formed and revitalized. Arms and leg muscles paralyzed because **GABA and glycine** are inhibited. ↑ in heart rate and blood pressure. Breathing is rapid and shallow. Brain is very active: dreams, penis or clitoral erections.

Bedwetting (AKA: Enuresis)

- Occurs in deep non-REM sleep, **Delta** waveform
- Best TX: Reward, alarm setting
- Note: It is not considered abnormal if a child is still wetting the bed by the age of 7.
- Associated with family history of enuresis.
- TX: 1st: **Desmopressin** (ADH analog), DDAVP
  2nd: **Imipramine**

Night Terrors

- Occurs in deep non-REM sleep, **Delta** waveform
- No memory of occurrence

TX: **Benzodiazepines**

Sleepwalking	Bruxism
• Occurs in deep non-REM sleep, **Delta** waveform	• Teeth grinding • Occurs in non-REM sleep • Wave forms show: **Sleep Spindles, K-complexes**
Narcolepsy • Loss of the brain's ability to regulate sleep-wake cycles. • SX: **Excessive daytime sleepiness**, REM immediately after falling asleep, cataplexy, hypnogogic or hypnopompic hallucinations, sleep paralysis (individual is away but unable to move). • TX: **Amphetamines** and scheduled daytime naps. **Modafinil.**	**Insomnia** • Inability to go to sleep or stay asleep • Causes: depression, anxiety • TX: **Good sleep hygiene**: no caffeinated beverages, avoiding day time naps, do not do work/watch TV/read/eat in bed before going to sleep, not exercising just before going to sleep, going to bed at same time and getting up at the same time. • Medical TX: **Zolpidem, Zaleplon, Eszopiclone** **Primary Insomnia**: Difficulty falling asleep or staying asleep > 1 month.
Normal Aging • Nap during the day • Sleeplessness • Awakens more during all stages of sleep	**Poor Sleep Hygiene** • SX: Insomnia, poor sleep scheduling, variable sleep and awakening times, frequent daytime naps. • Causes: ↑ use of caffeine, alcohol or nicotine prior to sleep, engaging in mental and/or physical activities before sleep, eating late dinners, use of the bed for activities other than sleep or intimacy: ie: work, computer, television
Delayed Sleep Phase Syndrome • MC with jobs that work nights and changes to day • Circadian rhythm disorder. • Unable to fall asleep at the normal bedtime • Insomnia, ↑ daytime sleepiness • Is still able to sleep well during the sleep time used in the other schedule.	**Advanced Sleep Phase Syndrome** • Is unable to stay awake in the evenings (after 7 pm) so there is a ↓ in social function • Early morning insomnia because of early bedtime

EATING DISORDERS

Disorder	Description
Anorexia Nervosa	Fear of gaining weight. MC teenage girls. SX: **BMI ≤ 17**, **amenorrhea, electrolyte disturbances**, excessive exercise, purging/vomiting (will see eroded teeth, calluses on hands and inflamed parotid glands as in Bulimia), diarrhea (use of laxatives), lanugo (hair loss, fine hair), **cardiac atrophy**, cardiomyopathy, arrhythmia (due to electrolyte imbalances). Complications: Electrolyte imbalance (in particularly K = leads to arrhythmia), amenorrhea (due to no estrogen), **osteoporosis** (due to no estrogen). Treatment: Hospitalization: requires stabilizing the electrolytes to stop arrhythmias, requires nutrition specialist for nutrition rehabilitation and psychotherapy. TX: **Olanzapine** to ↑ weight.
Bulimia Nervosa	Binge eating (eating large amount of food in a short time) followed by guilt and purging. SX: **BMI normal to increased BMI (usually > 30)**, vomiting, diarrhea (due to laxatives), eroded teeth, calluses on hands, parotitis (inflamed parotid glands), anxiety, electrolyte imbalances, laxative, diuretics or enema use. TX: **SSRI**
NOTE: BOTH anorexia and bulimia can show **teeth erosion, calluses** on the hands and **inflamed parotid glands**. You **MUST** look at the weight **(BMI)** to determine the difference. Anorexia is severely underweight and bulimia is overweight.	

HUMAN SEXUALTIY DEFINITIONS

Sexuality	Description
Gender Role	Behaviors that identify with the inner gender identity of the individual
Gender Dysphoria (AKA: Gender Identity)	Person identifies themselves as a male or female. Established by 3 years old. Person persistently feels uncomfortable with the sex they were born. Presents by identifying with the opposite sex by wearing their clothes, playing with toys designed for the opposite sex, roll playing as the opposite sex. As the individual matures they may take hormones to alter their voice and appearance. They may also hide the physical features that identify them as the sex they do not want to be. TX: Individual therapy or consideration for surgery to change their sex.
Sexual Identity	Individuals secondary sexual characteristics
Sexual Orientation	Individuals choice: Heterosexual, homosexual, bisexual, asexual
Masturbation	Normal sexual behavior. Becomes a problem if it interferes with daily functions.
Homosexuality	Not considered a mental illness. May be normal experimentation in teenagers.

SEXUAL DYSFUNCTION

Erectile Dysfunction (Impotence)
- Inability to attain or maintain an erection until ejaculation
- Identify if cause is psychological or neurological.
  If the patient is still experiencing nighttime or early morning erections, problem is psychological.
- TX if psychological: **cGMP** phosphodiesterase inhibitors. **Sildenafil** *(Viagra)*, **Tadalafil** *(Cialis)*, **Vardenafil** *(Levitra)*.
- **CAUTION: Phosphodiesterase inhibitors cannot be taken together with Nitrates (angina) = severe hypotension and potentially death. They must be taken at least 4 hours apart.**

Premature Ejaculation
- Ejaculation before or just after penetration.
- MCC: anxiety.
- TX: Squeeze technique, start: stop when excitement builds till it subsides and start again.
- Medical TX: **SSRI**

Penetration Disorder (AKA: Vaginismus)
- Constriction of the vaginal opening preventing penetration
- TX: Psychotherapy, vaginal dilators

Dyspareunia
- Pain during sexual intercourse
- TX: Psychotherapy if no underlying medical causes
- Underlying medical causes: Endometriosis

Persistent Sexual Arousal Syndrome (PSAS)
- Spontaneous persistent genital arousal, with or without orgasm, not related to sexual desire.
- Failure to relieve the symptoms causes waves of spontaneous orgasms.
- Can be aggravated/stimulated by daily activities: vibrations from riding in automobiles, trains, and mobile phones, sitting on someone's lap.
- Believed to be due to an irregularity in sensory nerves or pudendal nerve entrapment.
- MC in post-menopausal women
- TX: Antidepressants, anesthesia gels, psychotherapy, nerve blocks.

Priapism
- Painful, sustained erection without the presence of physical or psychological stimulation. Blood stays to long in the penis causing ischemia to the penis.
- If it is not restored timely, disfigurement of the penis, erectile dysfunction or penile gangrene can occur.
- TX: Initial: Ice packs and **α-agonist (epinephrine or phenylephrine)**
- Erection should not go **beyond 4 hours**. Medical emergency.

Peyronie's Disease • Connective tissue disorder in which scar tissue forms in the tunica albuginea (thick sheath of tissue surrounding the corpora cavernosa). "Broken penis". • SX: pain, abnormal curvature, erectile dysfunction. • Cause: Trauma/injury to the penis usually through sexual activity. In particularly when positions are used cause the penis to hit in a straighter path (ie: woman on top).	**Anorgasmia** Individual can't achieve orgasm despite adequate stimulation. Causes: SSRI's, neuropathy (diabetics), pelvic trauma (straddle injury), childbirth, opiate (heroin) addiction. Alcoholism, prostatectomy, psychological problems (past abuse).
Genito-Pelvic Penetration/Pain Disorder (AKA: Dyspareunia) • No vaginal penetration due to vaginal or pelvic pain from tense pelvic muscles with intercourse or attempted intercourse > 6 months. • Due to fear or anxiety with no other underlying issues such as: relationship problems, drugs, and medical problems.	**Hypoactive Sexual Desire Disorder** Lack or absence of sexual fantasies and desire for sexual activity for a period of time. There is no response to their partner's desire for sexual activity. It causes distress or interpersonal difficulties not connected with any other mental disorder, drugs (illegal or legal) or any other medical condition.

PARAPHILIAS

Recurrent, sexually arousing disorders.
MC: men

Exhibitionism • Exposing one's self to strangers	**Fetishism** • Use of non-living objects for sexual pleasure
Frotteurism • Rubbing the pelvis/penis against another person (unknown to the person). MC: crowded buses/trains.	**Masochism** (Self-defeating personality disorder) • Behavior involving humiliation, feminine submissiveness
Sadism • Behavior involving inflicting pain (psychological or physically) on another for sexual excitement	**Transvestic Fetishism** • Cross dressing for sexual gratification. MC in heterosexual males. (**tip**: trans**VEST**tic = **VEST** is clothing)

CHILDHOOD and DEVELOPMENTAL DISORDERS

Note: The most important determining factor of compliance of an adolescent/teenager is if their peers are doing it.

Conduct Disorder • <18 years old • Child is destructive, breaks laws, sets fires, hurts animals, steals, **breaks rules** **After 18 years** old this same disorder is called **Anti-social.** (Criminals)	**Oppositional Defiant Disorder** • Defiant, hostile behavior toward any **authority figure** (teachers, parents, adults) lasting at least 6 months • This person is **NOT a rule breaker** (like Conduct disorder) • (**tip**: the exam will always put Oppositional Defiant up against Conduct Disorder: just look to see if the child is breaking the rules/laws. If so, it is conduct disorder. If all the child is doing is being hateful to people in positions of authority, it is Oppositional Defiant)

ADHD (Attention-deficit hyperactivity disorder)

- Onset after 6 months and before 12 years old
- Hyperactivity, impulsivity, inattention in **multiple settings.** (Multiple settings: MC: home and school),
  ↓ self-esteem.
- Normal intelligence
- Rate: 9% of the population. 9:1 of males over females.
- TX: Special classes in school.
- TX: **Amphetamines. Methylphenidate** *(Ritalin)*, **Atomoxetine** *(Strattera)*, **Adderall, Dextroamphetamine.**
- **↑ Dopamine and Epinephrine levels**
  <3 yrs: Dextroamphetamine, Modafinil (non-addicting), Atomoxetine *(Strattera)*, **(non-addicting and less side effects: can be used as DOC).**
  >6 yrs: Methylphenidate.
  Take kids off the medications during summer when school is out.
  Side effects: insomnia, anxiety, decreased appetite, GI disturbances.

Autism

- **Impaired verbal skills, ↓ communication** and social interaction skills, cognitive impairment (mental retardation in 75% of the cases). 25% will have seizures.
- Most signs appear **before the age of 3**, MC in boys
- SX: Repetitive actions (head banging to calm down), ritualized behavior (want things the same way all the time), preoccupation with a single subject, prefer to play alone, become upset if their routine is changed, unable to relate with others (in their own world), will not go to parent when upset, will choose to sit in the corner and rock, bizarre use of speech: will reverse pronouns (Will say "I" instead of "you"), avoids others, no eye contact, does not cry when parents leave, no separation anxiety, can be aggressive towards others, avoids pleasure and could injure himself in order to calm himself.
- Associated with Fragile X
- Prognosis: based on how well speech is developed.
- TX: Behavior management, family counseling, increase the use of language.
- TX: If child is aggressive: **Risperidone, Olanzapine**

Asperger's

- Impaired social interaction. There is **no impairment in speech/verbal communication** and normal cognitive development.

SX: Intense preoccupation with a single subject, clumsiness,

Tourette Syndrome

- Motor and/or vocal **tics** lasting > 1 year
  Tics: rapid, recurrent, sudden movements and utterances. (Ex: constant blinking of eyes, coughing, odd mouth movements, tapping or bouncing of foot/leg, grunting, throat clearing)
- Onset in childhood, usually by 7 years old. MC in boys.
- Due to ↓ dopamine in the caudate nucleus
- Includes: Coprolalia (spontaneous utterance of obscene words) Echolalia (repeating the words of others), Palilalia (repeating one's own words).
- Associated with OCD and ADHD.
- TX: Behavioral therapy, SSRI, antipsychotics

Disruptive Mood Dysregulation Disorder (DMDD)

- Mood disorder in children. MC in boys between ages 6 and 18. (Can't diagnose until the age of 6).
- First signs appear in the preschool years.
- Persistent irritable or angry moods with severe temper outburst (verbal or behavioral) that are disproportional to the situation in terns of intensity or duration.
- Children may throw objects, hit or bite others. Have rages or fits. They can scream, yell, cry, kick for long periods without provocation. These can occur daily and are noticed by others.
- Sad moods between the outbursts. (Higher likelihood of developing depression and anxiety as an adult).
- TX: Individualized therapy

Separation Anxiety	Selective Mutism
• 7 – 9 **years old** • Fear of separation. Example: Kids create excuses to not go to school. • TX: SSRI, cognitive behavior therapy **Stranger Anxiety** • 7 – 9 **months old.** Baby hangs onto mom and is afraid of others. Normal behavior.	• Child **speaks well at home** but speaks **little or not a all in public**. Generally happens at school: teacher will call parent and express concern about the child's verbal skills because they never speak in class only to find out the child speaks non-stop at home. This is usually due to the child's anxiety or shyness of public speaking.
Regression of Milestones	**Rett Syndrome**
• Rett Syndrome • Subacute Sclerosing Panencephalitis • Tay Sachs	• **X Linked, MC girls** • **Regression of milestones by the age of 4.** Loss of verbal skills, loss of development, loss of intellectual abilities, ataxia, **hand wringing** (repetitive stereotyped hand movements).

PSYCHOTIC DISORDERS

Disorder	Time Frame of Symptoms	Symptoms/Treatments
Brief Psychotic Disorder	**> 1 day to < 1 month**	Psychotic behavior: hallucinations, delusions, disorganized speech (aka: loose associations) and behavior, catatonic behavior. TX: **Antipsychotic medication**
Schizophreniform Disorder	**> 1 month to < 6 months**	Psychotic behavior: hallucinations, disorganized speech (aka: loose associations) and behavior, negative symptoms (flat effect), disheveled appearance (poor grooming), catatonic behavior. TX: **Antipsychotic medication** (**tip**: schizophreni**FORM** = **FORM**ing Schizophrenia)
Schizophrenia	**> 6 months**	Psychotic behavior: hallucinations, disorganized speech (aka: loose associations) and behavior, social withdrawal, negative symptoms (flat effect), disheveled appearance. Impaired daily functioning impaired Judgement and behavior, difficulty interpreting reality. TX: **Antipsychotic medication**
Schizotypal		Schizophrenia plus odd/eccentric behavior. Bizarre fantasy's/magical thinking. Believes in telepathy, clairvoyance, 6th sense, ↓ range of emotional expression, ↓ friends and relationships.

SCHIZOPHRENIA

- Disorder that impairs reality, judgment and behavior
- SX: hallucinations (MC: auditory: hears voices), ↓ IQ, ↓ functioning
- ↑ Dopamine and serotonin
- Psychotic behavior lasting > 6 months
- Associated with increased dopaminergic activity and decreased dendritic branching
- **Lifetime prevalence**: 1.5% Males = Females.
- MC onset in Men: ages 15 to 25. MC onset in women 25 – 35
- **Inheritance: Passing to monozygotic twins (identical twins, 1 egg splits): 47%**
  Both parents are schizophrenic: 47% inheritance rate.
  Passing to dizygotic twins (fraternal twins, 2 eggs): 12%
- Marijuana use is associated with schizophrenia development in teens
- Positive Symptoms: Hallucinations, Delusions, Disorganized Speech (loose associations), Disorganized or catatonic behavior
- Negative Symptoms: Flat affect, lack of motivation/energy, lack of speech, social withdrawal, lack of thought
- Diagnosis of Schizophrenia: Requires 2 more of any of the positive and/or negative symptoms
- Schizophrenia has a high attempted suicide rate. Be sure to hospitalize any patient that is a risk to themselves or others
- **Diagnosis: Must do a urinalysis (drug screen) to rule out amphetamine or cocaine use (these can mimic psychosis because they ↑ the level of dopamine).**

- **Other Differentials to rule out that can be confused with psychosis: Alcohol hallucinations, epilepsy, steroids, HIV or other DZ of the brain, personality disorders, hypo/hyperthyroidism (check TSH), syphilis (check VDRL), temporal lobe disorders, electrolytes (check BMP), calcium.**
- **Poor prognosis** and high rates of relapse is indicated in patients that present with: negative symptoms, early age at onset, family history of schizophrenia, higher in families with high emotion, poor premorbid functioning, and disorganized type.
- TX: Antipsychotic Medications: Long Term Treatments: **Haloperidol, Risperidone**
  The best atypical anti-psych med will ↓ dopamine and adjust levels of serotonin.
  Antipsychotic medicines can also sedate (Haloperidol) and suppress movement in disorders such as Tourette syndrome, tics and Huntington's DZ (CAG trinucleotide repeat).

Schizophrenia Type	**Description**
Catatonic	**Motor immobility** and abnormal behavior: Mutism, stupor. Holds rigid poses for long periods. They may not eat or drink so be aware of malnutrition or dehydration.
Disorganized	**Disheveled** appearances, disorganized speech and behavior, no contact with reality, child-like, flat affect, loose associations. Poor prognosis if develops at a younger age.
Paranoid	**Most common type. Delusions and/or hallucinations.** (MC: Auditory hallucinations). Individual is paranoid that everyone (government, banks, etc) are monitoring them, trying to take their thoughts, or persecuting them. **Delusions of Grandeur: false belief** that one is superior: a genius, wealthy, are famous, or in a relationship with a famous person.
Residual	No acute symptoms. Presence of negative symptoms (disheveled appearance, poor grooming, anhedonia, flat affect, social withdrawal) and an absence of positive symptoms (no hallucinations or delusion).
Undifferentiated	Behaviors not falling under any other criteria.

Schizophrenic Brain Traits

- **CT or MRI shows: Enlarged ventricles**
- Pet scan shows Hypodensity in frontal lobes
- Prominent sulci
- ↓ Hippocampus
- ↓ Temporal mass
- ↓ Cerebral mass

MOOD/AFFECTIVE DISORDERS
DEPRESSION

- Moods (emotional states) that cause an underlying disorder.
- **Symptoms of Depression** (tip: SIG E CAPS)
  - **S**leep disturbance: hypersomnia or insomnia
  - **I**nterest loss (**anhedonia**)
  - **G**uilt/worthlessness feelings
  - **E**nergy loss (fatigue) every day
  - **C**oncentration difficulty, decreased inability to think
  - **A**ppetite (weight changes)
  - **P**sychomotor difficulty/agitation most days
  - **S**uicidal thoughts
  - **D**epressed mood most of the day
- Sleep Changes
  - ↑ total REM sleep (with early REM cycle)
  - **Early morning awakening**
- Antidepressant Therapy
  - Prior to prescribing an antidepressant therapy: assess for suicidal ideation.
    During the first 2 weeks of therapy for depression, some patients become more prone to suicide ideas. If there is any concern for acute suicide ideas: hospitalize patient and evaluate for ECT therapy.

Mood Disorder	Time Frame	Description
Normal Depression		It is normal for everyone to become depressed at different points in time due to different stressors. The key is that their function at work or home is not affected.
Dysthymic Disorder	**> 2 years**	Less severe form of depression. It is a chronic, long-lasting depressed mood for most of the day on most days with at least 2 dysthymic symptoms: Feelings of hopelessness/helplessness, trouble sleeping, daytime sleepiness, poor appetite, eating too much, fatigue, low self-esteem, trouble concentrating, trouble making decisions.
Cyclothymic Disorder	> 2 years	Mild mood disorder. Recurrent depression and hypomania. Moods swings/fluctuations between short periods of mild depression and hypomania (elevated mood).
Seasonal Affective Disorder		Depressive symptoms associated with winter. Common in Alaska and other areas where it is dark throughout the day for days. TX: Phototherapy (Bright light exposure) and **Bupropion**.
Major Depressive Disorder	**≥ 2 weeks**	Individual must experience 5 of the 9 symptoms of depression listed above. TX: anti-depressants, ECT. **REMINDER**: Anti-depressants take up to 6 weeks to work. After 6 weeks if the medicine is not working then switch to another medication in the **SAME class** (ie: Start on SSRI, then switch to another SSRI). If the 2nd medication does not work, THEN it is ok to switch classes. REMINDER: Add a benzodiazepine if needed to help with depression while waiting for the anti-depressant to take affect. Major depressive disorder has been associated with fibromyalgia.
Atypical Depression		Depression presenting with opposite symptoms as seen in typical depression. SX: Increased: weight, sleep, and appetite. TX: MAOI's
Bipolar Disorder	**≥ 1 week**	Bipolar I: Minimum of 1 manic episode with/without depressive episode or hypomania episode. Bipolar II: Presence of both: depressive and hypomanic episode. Must have episodes of depression, mania (or mixed mania/depression) for ≥ 1 week, with impaired functioning. Bipolar Genetics: General public: 1% Individual with first Degree Relative with bipolar dz (parent/sibling/di-zygotic twin): 5 – 10% Individual with both parents with bipolar DZ: 60% Monozygotic twin with both parents with bipolar DZ: 70% TX: **Lithium, Valproic Acid, Carbamazepine, atypical antipsychotics**. CAUTION: Use of antidepressants can lead to ↑ risk for suicide or manic episode. The antidepressant will raise their mood enough to give them the energy to carry out these plans. CAUTION: Be sure to check urinalysis for amphetamine use causing the mania. CAUTION: If HTN is a symptom be sure to check TSH for hyperthyroidism and urine for VMA or metanephrine for Pheochromocytoma.
Hypomania	≥ 4 days	Less severe mood disturbance than a manic episode. No psychotic features and is not severe enough to cause impairment or require hospitalization.
Mania	≥ 1 week	Persistent **elevated** or irritable mood with **increase energy/activity** lasting ≥ 1 week. Symptoms: Distractibility, Irresponsibility, Grandiosity (inflated self esteem), Flight of ideas, Increase in agitation, **decreased need for sleep** (be up all nights for many nights in a row), pressured/fast speech, **spending sprees** that can deplete their savings, distractibility, racing thoughts. Examples: Will spend a lot of money, may even drain their savings. TX: Must hospitalize the patient to protect them from themselves (may spend all their money). TX with mood stabilizers for remission (**Lithium** is DOC) and antipsychotics to control mania (**Risperidone** is DOC). Caution: Before DX a bipolar disease or mania: Do a urinalysis to rule out use of amphetamine or cocaine.
Bipolar in Pregnancy		Discontinue Lithium. **ECT** (Electroconvulsive therapy) for the first trimester for manic episodes. For the 2nd and 3rd trimesters use **Lamotrigine**. (Lithium: birth defects: **Ebstein anomaly** (congenital cardiac defect that displaces leaflets of the tricuspid valve).

POST PARTUM DEPRESSION

Postpartum Blues	Postpartum Depression
• 50 – 80% incidence • Starts **birth to 2 weeks**. • SX: **Tearfulness (weeping), sadness, fatigue**, mild depression, difficulty sleeping. • **No negative feelings toward baby – cares about the baby** • TX: Supportive, no treatment. Self-limiting.	• 10- 15% incidence • Starts within **1 to 3 months** and can last **up to 1 year.** • Possible negative feelings toward the baby. • Most important: Be sure baby is safe. • Usually underlying psychiatric issues. • SX: **Anxiety**, poor concentration, severe depression. • TX: **Antidepressants (SSRI)**, psychotherapy
Postpartum Psychosis • 0.1 – 0.2 % Incidence • Starts 2 – 3 months after delivery • SX: **Delusions, hallucinations**, confusion, possible **homicidal thoughts (toward the baby)** or suicidal ideas. • Usually underlying psych issues. • Most important: Be sure baby is safe. • TX: Inpatient hospitalization, antipsychotics or mood stabilizers. ECT if patient is breastfeeding, antidepressants. • **Assess child safety.**	

Electroconvulsive Therapy (ECT)

- ECT is the most effective treatment for depression
- TX for Major Depressive
- TX for depression in **pregnancy**
- TX for immediate danger of suicide risk
- TX if there are contraindications for using antidepressants
- Side Effects: temporary memory loss, headaches
- ECT causes transient increases in intracranial pressure so do not use it in patients with brain metastasis (space-occupying lesions).

BEREAVEMENT (Grief)

Normal grief	• Normal grief: Begins after the death of a loved one and normally last ≤ 6 months, but can last up to a year or more. • Symptoms will alternate. • SX: Sadness, tearfulness, decreased appetite, decreased sleep, **can hallucinate and believe they see and/or hear their loved one**, can "bargain" in the hopes that their loved one will be returned, can feel guilt, can feel anger. (Statistic: when the loss involves the loss of a child when with one parent (typically in an automobile accident) the other parent usually places blame on the partner, ultimately ending in divorce). • SX are considered pathologic grief if they **impair daily functions after a 2 month time period after the death of the loved one**, or if more serious symptoms present • TX: Supportive
Pathologic Grief	• Serious side effects: Psychosis, thoughts of death/suicide, preoccupation with worthlessness, psychomotor impairment (slowing of thought and of physical movements). • TX: **SSRI**

BEREAVEMENT	DEPRESSION
• Tearfulness, sadness, decreased appetite • Supportive therapy • Symptoms < 1 year • Returns to normal daily functioning (base line) after 2 months • Guilt, shame, and suicidal thought's are rare • Symptoms alternate (wax and wane): Good days-bad days. • TX: Supportive psychotherapy	• Tearfulness, sadness, decreased appetite • Antidepressant therapy • Symptoms > 1 year • Does not return to normal daily functioning (base line) • Guilt, shame, and suicidal thoughts can be common • Symptoms are constant and continual (AKA: pervasive and unremitting) • TX: Anti-depressants

Stages of Bereavement

Bereavement can be in OTHER FORMS, not just death. It can occur with divorces, loss of job or a serious health diagnosis.
Stages do NOT have any specific order. (Note: If the vignette asks "what do you see first", the answer is "any of the above")

- Denial (shock)
- Anger (why did this happen?)
- Bargaining
- Depression
- Acceptance

Persistent Complex Bereavement Disorder (PCBD)

- MC with close relative's death. Significant impairment and reaction out of proportion to the normal
- Symptoms > 12 months
- DX if ≥ 1 of these symptoms last > 12 months: Persistent longing, ↑ sorrow/emotions, pre-occupation with the deceased or pre-occupation with the circumstance of the death.
- DX if ≥ 6 of these symptoms lasting > 12 months: Is unable to accept the loss, numbness and/or disbelief, bitterness or anger, self blame, avoids reminders of the person, desires to die in order to be with the deceased, unable to trust others, feels alone, ↓ sense of identity, stops pursuing plans or interest

DELUSIONAL DISORDER

- Presence of non-bizarre delusions (false beliefs) **> 1 month.**
- **No impairment in daily functioning**. Holds down a job, obeys laws, pays their bills.
- No hallucinations.
- TX: Atypical antipsychotics, psychotherapy

DEFENSE MECHANISMS (EGO)

Immature and Mature Defenses

Defense	Description	Example
Immature Defenses		
Acting Out	An anti-social form of expressing unacceptable feelings/thoughts through actions.	**Temper tantrums**
Blocking	Temporarily block of a thought for a moment.	"I can't remember his name"
Borderline AKA Splitting	Individual believes people or all good or all bad. Everything is either black or white – there is no gray. Associated with: **Suicide attempts and sexual abuse**. Is common to see scars on the wrist due to suicide attempts. MC: women.	Today the individual states that her doctor in the best doctor in the world, next week he is the worst.
Compensation	Individual over emphasizes their achievements in order to make up for another area they feel is a failure.	Unattractive individual focuses on scholastic success.
Displacement	When an individual **takes their anger**/feelings/emotions /words/actions **out on a neutral person or object**. (Verses Projection)	Man has a bad day at work and comes home and yells at wife.
Dissociation	Change in personality, memories, and behaviors in reaction to or to avoid stress.	Dissociative identity.
Denial	**Refusing to realize reality**. Usually seen with news of a terminal illness.	Individual is told they have terminal caner and they decides to start eating right and exercising.
Fantasy	Substitution of less disturbing view of the world in place of reality as a way to resolve conflict.	Mom dreams her son will live a long time (even though he as a serious disease). This fantasy offers a way for her to escape from anxiety about the son's illness.
Fixation	Individual **remains at earlier levels** of development. (**verses** regression)	Men fixated on video games.
Identification	Individual identifies and models their behavior after another person that is more powerful.	A mother dreams her son will liver a long time even though he has a terminal illness.
Intellectualization AKA: Isolation of Affect	Individual **separates their true feelings from the actual situation.** They try to understand what is wrong in order to decrease fear and anxiety.	Individual is told they have a terminal disease and they show no emotion and will then research/educate themselves on all aspects of that disease. They will also talk about it in an unemotional way.
Introjection	Individual interjects traits, thoughts or actions **into themselves.**	"What you think, I think. How you dress, I dress".

Defense Mechanisms cont'd

Projection	Individual with an unacceptable action/thought **projects this on to another person** (that is not doing it). This makes the individual feel that if "this other individual is doing it" then it justifies their actions. (**verses**: Displacement)	A husband that is cheating now believes his wife is cheating (and she is not) so that it makes him feel his actions are justified.
Rationalization	Individual **applies logical reasons** to why they did/or should do in order to avoid blame	An individual is fired from their job and tells himself/others that it really wasn't the job he had wanted anyway.
Reaction Formation	An individual has a social unacceptable habit/thoughts and goes out to do the **opposite so they can "undo" the feeling – BUT the underlying bad habit is not corrected.** (**Reaction Formation verses sublimation**) (**tip**: "R"eaction formation = behavior "R"emains the same)	An alcoholic goes to local schools to speak to children about not drinking. Yet he continues to drink. Person is angry for immigrants taking jobs but volunteers to help immigrants find jobs.
Regression	Individual **returns back** to an earlier (childhood) period in life to avoid dealing with issues. (**verses**: fixation)	**MC in children** when a new sibling enters their life. They may start wetting the bed again. **In adults**: when an adult may be going through something difficult and they want someone to stay with them, they do not want to be alone.
Repression	**Subconscious**/involuntary not remembering an event/person. (**Repression verses Suppression**)	An individual that has experienced a traumatic situation (accident, rape) will never remember it happened.
Mature Defenses		
Altruism	Principal or practice of the selfless concern for others. This can be at the cost or risk to ones own good. Giving of ones self not for recognition or out of obligation, but because it does good. Opposite of selfishness.	The widow of a serviceman gives his estate settlement to the VA hospital.
Humor	Using light hearted **humor** in order to make a difficult situation easier.	Individual makes jokes about hearts just before his heart surgery.
Sublimation	Individual replaces a socially unacceptable action/thought with the opposite so that it becomes socially acceptable. This **resolves the underlying bad habit**. (**Sublimation verses Reaction formation**) (**tip**: "S"ublimation = "S" for "S"witches behavior)	An individual enjoys cutting things so becomes a surgeon.
Suppression	Individual **consciously or semiconsciously chooses** not to think about an unpleasant situation/memory. This minimizes the discomfort/memory but does not take it away. (**Suppression verses Repression**)	Doctor's father was an alcoholic and he became angry when dealing with alcoholic patients. He chose to suppress the thought so he could take good care of his patients.

PERSONALITY DISORDERS

Disorder	Description
Cluster A (eccentric)	
Paranoid Disorder	**Suspiciousness and mistrust** of others. Their main defense mechanism is **projection**. Emotionally cold and often take legal action against others. Refusal to forgive, preoccupied with conspiracy ideas, excessive sensitivity to setbacks or criticism. (Do not confuse this with Paranoid Schizophrenia – there is no psychosis in paranoid disorder). EX: A 48-year-old male accuses his co-workers of conspiring against him to get him fired. He knows they have tapped his phone, open his mail and follow him when he goes on break or to lunch.
Schizoid Disorder	Individual has **no interest** in social relationships, including indifference toward sexual relationships. Usually solitary lifestyle, emotionless and apathy. This person does not want any kind of relationship. Their main defense mechanism is projection. (**tip**: schizoi**D**, **D** = Distant). (**verses Avoidant**). EX: The wife of a 58 year old male complains because her husband never wants to go anywhere with her, doesn't want any friends or people to come visit, and is upset because he seems to have no interest in any intimacy with her.
Schizotypal Disorder	Individual will avoid relationships and present with **odd behavior** (eccentric) and thinking. Superstitious, paranormal, clairvoyant, magical beliefs and peculiar speech mannerisms are normal for them. EX: A 32-year-old male makes a special breakfast drink everyday. He claims the ingredients have magical powers that guide him through his day.
Cluster B (dramatic and emotional)	
Conduct Disorder	Individuals are < 18. They **violate rules and are aggressive toward the rights of others, hurt animals,** destroy property, steal, lie, bully, pick fights, shoplift, **break laws,** do drugs and alcohol. Once the child becomes 18 the disorder is then called an **antisocial disorder** (AKA: psychopath). Rate: 9:1 of males over females. High in families with personality disorders. (**Conduct verses Oppositional defiant disorder**)

PERSONALITY DISORDERS cont'd

Antisocial Disorder AKA Psychopath or Sociopath	Individuals **over 18** years old that **violate rules and rights** of others. **Break laws**. Many criminals fall under this category. Individuals are manipulative, hostile, irresponsible and have a history of legal problems. They lack remorse, have no respect for the rights of others and are deceitful. (**Same as conduct disorder in children < 18.** At 18 years old it is called Antisocial) EX: A 26-year-old male is arrested for shooting out store windows. He is hateful to the police and brags to the others in jail that this was nothing new, he was always being arrested, even as a kid. Psychopaths tend to be due more to genetics. Sociopaths tend to be made by their environment.
Oppositional Defiant Disorder	Child is defiant against any figure of authority (parents, teachers, police). Seen in 10% of children: teens and pre-teens. Rate is equal between males and females. MCC: Inconsistent and poor parenting. Daily conflict escalates the disorder. TX: Work with the parents. Teach how to be good parents, consistency and how to reinforce good behavior. Behavior modification with the child: mentor program (Big Brothers/Sisters), boot camps. TX: Anti-psych meds if there is aggression. (Note: The vignette can make this disorder and conduct disorder the same, but child will break laws if it is conduct disorders. One a child with oppositional defiant disorder breaks the law, it is then considered conduct disorder).
Borderline/Splitting Disorder	Individual believes people or all good or all bad and are impulsive. They have mood swings, show inappropriate anger. They fear abandonment and are unable to have stable relationships. They frequently engage in dangerous behaviors and will harm themselves. They alternate between positive and negative feelings. Associated with: **Suicide attempts and sexual abuse.** Is common to see scars on the wrist due to suicide attempts. MC: women. The main defense mechanism used is **splitting**. (See also under defense mechanisms). EX: A 36-year-old female has been seeing a doctor for her cancer treatments. She tells everyone what a wonderful doctor he is. On one of her visits her doctor had asked a colleague to speak with her about an additional treatment. The treatment was not what she wanted and stormed out of the room stating that these doctors were the worst doctors she's ever had.
Histrionic Disorder	Individuals that present with **excessive attention** seeking **emotions**. They are very **dramatic**, enthusiastic and flirtatious. They need a lot of attention (they want to be the center of attention), exaggerate their emotions/behavior, **sexually provocative** behavior or appearance, manipulative behavior to achieve their needs, self-indulgence and impulsive. They will act inappropriately to get attention. They get upset if others do not praise them. (**Histrionic verses Narcissist**). EX: A 28-year-old woman dresses provocatively to go to her office party. Most everyone at the party spent their time talking to one of her co-workers that just announced she got engaged instead of showering her with praise and attention. She became very angry and left.
Narcissistic Disorder	Individual believes they are superior, arrogant and entitled, a **blown up perception of themselves**. They have an excessive desire for attention and admiration. Take advantage of others. They have no empathy for others and have little respect for other's feelings. They believe others envy them. Fantasize about power and success. Exaggerates their achievements or talents. Expect VIP treatment. They are unable to accept criticism and will usually respond in anger and seek vindication. They blame others for their failure. (BD, LG) (**Narcissist verses Histrionic**) EX: A 36-year-old female reports to the reception desk to check into a hotel. She is told that there will be a short wait. She immediately demands to see manger, stating that she is the president of a big company and should not be kept waiting. She wants their best room, concierge service and access to their executive lounge.

Cluster C (anxious or fearful)	
Avoidant Disorder	Individual is sensitive to rejection and feels inadequate, inferior or unattractive. Generally avoids social situation **but does want** relationships. Fears disapproval, embarrassment or ridicule so they stay away from social gatherings. They are hypersensitive to criticism (verses schizoid). (**Caution**: questions will make avoidant and schizoid sound exactly the same. But in avoidance look carefully something that indicates that the person "thought" about others – always very subtle. In schizoid, the person wants nothing to do with anyone else, even a spouse – it is never "thought" about.) (**Avoidant verses Schizoid**). EX: A 32-year-old female never goes anywhere, she stays at home alone. When her co-workers ask her to go out with them for dinner she considers and then declines the offer. She would rather just stay home. (Notice: it **did** cross her mind because she considered it).
Dependent Disorder	Individual has a **low self esteem and low self-confidence**. They need to be taken care of to the point they are **submissive and clingy**. They continually need to be reassured and complimented or they feel they failed or are not wanted. Tolerates poor or abusive treatment even if other options are available and will avoid disagreements with others. EX: A 40-year-old woman presents to her doctor for advice. She is distraught because another relationship has failed. She does not understand what went wrong. She states she did everything for him. She never did anything or went anywhere without checking with him first. She has become more concerned because he will not answer when she calls, yet she tries multiple times throughout the day.

PERSONALITY DISORDERS cont'd

Obsessive-Compulsive Disorder (OCD)	**Obsessive:** Are the continual **repetitive, intrusive thoughts**. (Example: constant thought to wash their hands). Many thoughts are due to fear of contamination. **Compulsive:** The **actions/rituals** taken to relieve the anxiety caused by the obsessions. (Example: constant washing of their hands). Individual is obsessed with repetitive thoughts or the need to perform repetitive actions. These individuals **recognize that they need help** and seek help. The obsessive/compulsiveness **interferes with their normal daily functions**. Example: continual washing of hands until they are raw or peel. The continual need to recheck to be sure a door is locked until they are always late for work. TX: **1st line: SSRI. 2nd line: TCA's: Clomipramine.**
Obsessive-Compulsive Personality Disorder (OCPD)	The individual is concerned with **orderliness and perfectionism**. They want to control their environment. Characteristics of these individuals include workaholics, miserliness and inflexible. They want things in exact order (example: grouping same colors together, lining up cans/boxes in the pantry by height). This person **doesn't recognize they have this issue** but everyone else around them does. EX: A 32-year-old woman confides in her friend that she is considering separating from her husband of 10 years. She claims that life is impossible it him. He demands the house is in perfect order and that they keep a regimented schedule each and every day, even down to the time meals are to be ready.
Misc. Disorders	
Passive Aggressive Behavior	Individual expresses his aggression (hostility) towards another person, **indirectly,** with repeated deliberate **failures to meet the other person's needs**. (Example: a doctor unable to get a patient in when the patient wanted so the patient intentionally reports late to future appointments). Passive Aggressive disorders are usually seen with self-mutilation or self-aggressive issues.
Self-Defeating Disorder	Individuals **avoid pleasurable experiences**; even to the extent they may undermine pleasurable experiences. Reject help and choose people or situations that lead to disappointment or failure.
Hoarding Disorder "Compulsive hoarding"	Individual that is unable or unwilling to discard their possessions, which leads to the accumulation of things that fill the living areas of their home. It is associated with increased health problems, economic loss, unsafe living conditions, dysfunctional relationships and impaired daily functioning. TX: **SSRI's**, Cognitive behavioral therapy and behavior modification techniques.

ANXIETY, PHOBIA, FEAR DISORDERS

Disorder	Time Line	Description
Normal Anxiety		Everyone experiences anxiety at points in their life. Example: a person gets a new promotion at work so is now very worried that they are doing a good job. In normal anxiety function at work and home are not affected.
General Anxiety Disorder	≥ 6 months	Excessive worry and anxiety over **various/multiple areas** of ones life, which can interfere with daily functioning. The anxiety is exaggerated as compared to the situation. SX: Fatigue, sleep problems, restlessness, and difficulties in concentration. Concerned about the job, about the bills, family, friends about the car, about a repair, etc. There is not one specific identifiable stressor. TX: **Cognitive behavior therapy, SSRI, SNRI's, Buspirone, Benzodiazepines, Venlafaxine.**
Adjustment Disorder AKA: Situational Depression	< 6 months (starts within 3 months)	Individual is unable to deal with a particular stress/change in their life. It can be anxiety, depression and irritability symptoms. There is always an **identifiable stressor** (divorce, move). Shows mild depressive symptoms and anxiety. (They need to adjust to a new situation). TX: Counseling to help patient adjust to the stressor. If needed can add SSRI.
Panic Disorder and Panic Attacks		**Panic Attack**: Recurrent periods of intense fear attacks with "**feelings of impending doom**". Presents to the ER afraid they are having a heart attack. SX: Sudden onset, palpitations, chest pain, sweating, chills, nausea, shortness of breath. MC in women 20 – 40 years old. DX: Must check drug screen and EKG to rule out other issues. TX: Panic Attack: **Alprazolam**. Cognitive behavior therapy, relaxation training, desensitization, Note: Alprazolam (Benzodiazepine): Can sedate: so advise patient to not drive, use machinery, or make any important decisions/contracts. Use the lowest dose in the elderly. Titrate doses. **Panic Disorder:** If the patient is not presenting to the ER and is just at the doctor's office telling the doctor about the panic attack, it is considered a **Panic Disorder**. TX: **SSRI** and Cognitive behavior therapy, relaxation training, desensitization,
Post-Traumatic Stress Disorder **(PTSD)**	> 1 month	Individual **repeatedly** relives a previous traumatic event. (Veterans from war, rape, robbery, automobile accident). SX: Intense fear, **flashbacks,** horror. Symptoms can begin anytime after the traumatic event. Avoidance of anything associated with the stressor, anxiety, sleep disturbances, emotional, impulsiveness. NOTE: The most important therapy TX: 1st line: **SSRI's** (ie: **Sertraline or Paroxetine**). Cognitive therapy and relaxation therapy. **Benzodiazepines can be added for acute needs.**

Acute Stress Disorder	3 days to 1 month	Re-living the stressor, avoidance of anything associated with the stressor, anxiety, sleep disturbances, emotional, impulsiveness. TX: **Benzodiazepines for acute need and SSRI for long term**
Performance Anxiety (Test anxiety)		Fear of performing or speaking in public. Stage fright, test anxiety. TX: **Propanolol or Atenolol.** (given 30 – 60 minutes prior to performance).
Specific Phobia		• Fear of heights, animals, objects • Arachnophobia: fear of spiders • Acrophobia: fear of heights • Aviophobia: fear of flying • TX: Behavioral therapy to desensitize. Exposure to item of fear a little at a time.
Social Phobia AKA: **Agoraphobia.** Social anxiety disorder		• **Fear of public places** due to fear that something embarrassing may happen and individual will be laughed at. Extreme fear and avoidance of settings requiring socialization. Impairs daily functions. • SX: Excess sweating, palpitations, nausea, rapid speech • Can cause **panic attacks**: intense fear, feeling of **"impending doom"** TX: **SSRI, SNRI's, MAOI's,** **Assertiveness training**
Trichotillomania		• Triggered by a stressful event. Can be associated with: OCD, Tourette's, eating disorders, anxiety disorders. • Repeatedly pulling out ones hair (hair, eyelashes, eyebrows, arm pits, pubic). • Anxiety present before pulling hair out and relief after it has been pulled out. • Not connected with other medical or dermatology issues. • Behavior causes distress SX: broken hair. It does not leave a bald spot such as in alopecia.
Excoriation Disorder		Repetitive, compulsive picking of the skin to the point it causes sores/damage. Can be brought on by stress or anxiety. Associated with OCD. TX: SSRI, cognitive behavior therapy

SOMATIC DISORDERS

Individuals present with physical symptoms that are unconscious and not intentional. Symptoms have no identifiable causes and all diagnostic test are negative.

Management of Somatic Disorders

- Establish a primary care physician that sees the patient once each month. Do not hospitalize the patient.
- The primary physician should avoid diagnostic test and/or therapies.
- Establish psychotherapy for the patient.

Disorder	Description
Somatoform Disorder	Multiple complaints of physical injury or illness in **multiple organ systems**. Symptoms usually appear in adolescence and the disorder is diagnosed before 30 years old. **Diagnostic test are negative** and patient will show numerous past medical visits and negative diagnostic test. (**Somatoform verses Hypochondriasis**). (**tip**: "S"omatoform = "S" for "S"everal problems)
Conversion Disorder	Individual that presents with a **sudden loss of sensory or motor function** (examples: blindness, numbness, paralysis, incontinence, seizures, pseudoseizure, diplopia, anesthesia, gait disturbance, aphonia). Neuro or medical disorders that can't be explained. All diagnostic tests will be negative. This is in **response to a major stressor** (such as a breakup with their partner). Most common in females. Patient is generally not concerned. **Self-limiting**. Recovery is spontaneous. TX: Supportive, psychotherapy. (Conversion verses Adjustment disorder).
Hypochondriasis	Persistent fear and preoccupation of having a serious illness (**one, not multiple problems**) despite medical diagnosis being negative. (Varies from munchausen: which is a focus on multiple problems). Individual is sure they have brain cancer and even after multiple test that show he does not, he still continues to worry about brain cancer and seeks more test. Hypochondriasis is most commonly seen in: histrionic, borderline or dependent personality disorders. (**Hypochondriasis verses Somatoform Disorder**)
Body Dysmorphic Disorder	Individuals' obsessive preoccupation that their **appearance** is flawed and is willing to do what is necessary to fix or hide it. It causes them to have difficulty functioning in most all aspects of their lives. Patient history may show **multiple plastic surgeries**. (If the focus is specifically only on their weight and body shape, it is considered to be an anorexia problem). TX: **SSRI**
Gender Identity Disorder	When the individuals concern about their body (as in body dysmorphic) is solely focused on sex characteristics.

FACTITIOUS DISORDERS

Individual's intentionally (consciously) fabricates/exaggerates medical symptoms for personal gain or attention.

Disorder	Description
Malingering	Individual intentionally fakes an illness or injury for **secondary gain**, usually financial. Secondary gains: getting out of work, insurance payoff. They have poor compliance in follow up and diagnostic procedures. Once the goal is achieved the injury/illness ceases. They will also decline invasive or painful procedures.
Munchausen Syndrome	Individuals continually and intentionally present with multiple symptoms of illness/injury for the purpose of gaining attention for themselves. There is no secondary gain being sought. They will have a history of multiple hospitalizations, doctors and negative diagnosis. They may demand treatment and are willing to undergo invasive and painful procedures. Many times this tends to be an individual with a medical background so they have a lot of medical knowledge. Example: individual exogenously injects insulin or takes sulfonylurea's to create hypoglycemia. (Varies from hypochondriasis: which is a focus on one major symptom)
Munchausen Syndrome by Proxy	Form of child or elderly abuse. Behavior in which the **caregiver fabricates or induces health problems in those they care for so that it brings attention to themselves**. Often times these individuals were admired as "mother of the year" type because their child was always sick and they were constantly there caring for them so everyone could see.

IMPULSE CONTROL DISORDERS

Individuals experience anxiety prior to the impulse. Once the person acts on the impulse the anxiety is relieved. They do not believe their actions are out of the ordinary or that they have any problem (just as in OCD).

Disorder	Description
Kleptomania	Individual that repeatedly steals items. They do not steal because they need too; it is to relieve the anxiety.
Pyromania	Individual that repeatedly starts fires. (If this individual is starting fires because they are angry or for secondary gain (insurance) it is considered a conduct disorder (if < 18) and anti-social (if > 18).
Pathologic Gambling	Individual is obsessed with gambling despite the consequences. TX: Psychotherapy: Gambling Anonymous
Explosive Disorder	Individual's anger explodes out of proportion to the inciting event. This explosion is not due to drugs. TX: SSRI, mood stabilizers

PSYCHIATRY PHARMACOLOGY

Antipsychotic, Typical (Neuroleptics)

High Potency

- Haloperidol
- Fluphenazine
- Trifluoperazine

Low Potency

- Highest risk of urinary retention, orthostatic hypotension (alpha blockade), dry mouth, vision disorder, delirium, impotence, weight gain. Switch to an atypical antipsychotic if needed.
- Chlorpromazine
- Thioridazine

DRUG **GENERIC name** **Trade name**	**Clinical Use**	**Mechanism of Action**	**Toxicity**
HALOPERIDOL *Haldol*	Schizophrenia Psychotic SX Agitation Acute Mania Tourette's	Dopamine receptor antagonist (D2) in the Mesolimbic and Mesocortical areas. Injectable if patient won't take it orally. Best for noncompliant patients (Haloperidol decanoate).	**Dystonia**, **tardive dyskinesia**, Parkinsonism, **Torsades de pointes**, Dyskinesia, hyperprolactinemia, Neuroleptic malignant syndrome. TX: **Tardive dyskinesia with Benztropine**
FLUPHENAZINE *Prolixin*	Schizophrenia Psychotic SX Agitation Acute Mania Tourette's	Dopamine receptor antagonist (D2) in the Mesolimbic and Mesocortical areas. Injectable if patient won't take it orally.	**Dystonia, tardive dyskinesia**, Parkinsonism, Dyskinesia, hyperprolactinemia, neuroleptic malignant syndrome. TX: **Tardive dyskinesia with Benztropine**
TRIFLUOPERAZINE *Stelazine*	Schizophrenia Psychotic SX Agitation Acute Mania Tourette's	Dopamine receptor antagonist (D2) in the Mesolimbic and Mesocortical areas	**Dystonia, tardive dyskinesia,** Parkinsonism, Dyskinesia, hyperprolactinemia, Neuroleptic malignant syndrome. TX: **Tardive dyskinesia with Benztropine**
CHLORPROMAZINE *Thorazine*	**Low potency** TX for Schizophrenia Psychotic SX	α-1 Antagonist, D2 Dopamine antagonist	Corneal deposits, anticholinergic and antihistamine effects, sedating, orthostatic hypotension (alpha blockade)
THIORIDAZINE	**Low potency** TX for Schizophrenia Psychotic SX	α-1 Antagonist, D2 Dopamine antagonist	Prolonged QT, arrhythmias (monitor EKG's), chest pain, palpitations, retinal deposits/pigmentations, anticholinergic and antihistamine effects, sedating, orthostatic hypotension (alpha blockade)

Antipsychotic Toxicities

Extrapyramidal Side Effects (EPS)

- **Dystonia:** within a few hours to days. Sustained or repetitive muscle contractions/spasms (torticollis) causing abnormal postures, difficulty swallowing. TX: Anticholinergics: Benztropine, **Diphenhydramine, Trihexyphenidyl.**
- **Akathisia**: within weeks and can be chronic. Restlessness causing one to be in constant motion (tapping legs/feet, rocking). TX: Add: **Beta Blockers or Benzodiazepines**.
- Bradykinesia (hypokinesia): Decreased body movements, tremors, muscle rigidity (Parkinsonism). Occurs within weeks. TX: Anticholinergics: Benztropine, **Diphenhydramine, Trihexyphenidyl**
- **Tardive Dyskinesia**: Develops in months to years. Choreoathetosis (twisting and writhing movements), usually irreversible, involuntary, repetitive movements (tongue movements, lip smacking). Switch to newer antipsychotics (ie: **Clozapine**).
  TX: **Benztropine**
  NOTE: Chronic use of any dopamine antagonists (it does not have to be an antipsychotic medication), can cause tardive dyskinesia. This includes: Melatonin, antiemetics: Metoclopramide and Prochlorperazine, Choline, tricyclic antidepressants: Clomipramine, Trimipramine, Amoxapine.
  Always stop the offending medication.

Neuroleptic Malignant Syndrome (NMS)

- MCC Antipsychotic medicines. NOTE: NMS can occur with Parkinson's patients that have recently discontinued Levodopa
- Similar to malignant hyperthermia in ETC uncoupling
- Muscle rigidity, fever, delirium, tachycardia, hyperthermia, autonomic dysfunction, altered mental status, loss of consciousness.
- Labs: ↑ Creatine Kinase and ↑ WBC
- TX: **Dantrolene** (D2 agonist. Blocks ryanodine receptors to stop Ca release from sarcoplasmic reticulum (↓ free intracellular calcium) which decreases muscle rigidity and administer **Bromocriptine** (Dopamine D2 receptor agonist) to overcome the dopamine receptor blockade.
  Stop the antipsychotic.

Atypical Antipsychotic's

Aripiprazole, Clozapine, Lurasidone, Olanzapine, Quetiapine, Risperidone, Ziprasidone

DRUG GENERIC name Trade name	**Clinical Use**	**Mechanism of Action**	**Toxicity**
ARIPIPRAZOLE *Abilify*	Schizophrenia (Positive and negative). OCD, Anxiety, Irritability in autism, Mania, Tourette's, Bipolar, Mania, Tic disorders. Insomnia. Used as adjunct in TX of major depressive disorders.	Neuroleptic agent with high affinity for $5HT_2$ and Dopamine (D4) receptors. (Partial dopamine agonist)	Anxiety, insomnia, GI effects, weight gain
CLOZAPINE	Schizophrenia (Positive and negative) Bipolar, Borderline personality disorder. TX: psychosis in Parkinson's Dz.	Neuroleptic agent with high affinity for $5HT_2$ and Dopamine (D4) receptors	**Agranulocytosis (requires weekly CBC labs), weight gain, seizures**, myocarditis, GI SX, megacolon, CNS SX. Least risk of tardive dyskinesia. Never used as a first line treatment. Only use if patient does not response to an appropriate trial of antipsychotic's first (typical or atypical).
OLANZAPINE *Zyprexa*	Schizophrenia (positive and negative). Bipolar. Insomnia.	Neuroleptic agent with high affinity for $5HT_2$ and Dopamine (D4) receptors	**Weight gain, Diabetes,** paradoxical effects on personality/behaviors. **Avoid in diabetic, obese patients.**
QUETIAPINE *Seroquel*	Schizophrenia (Positive and negative) Bipolar, antidepressant, Major depressive disorder. Insomnia. **TX: psychosis in Parkinson's Dz.**	Neuroleptic agent with high affinity for $5HT_2$ and Dopamine (D4) receptors	Dry mouth, somnolence, HTN, orthostatic HTN. Do not use in elderly with dementia. Has less incidence of movement disorders.
Lurasidone *Latuda*	Safe for use in pregnancy (Category B)	Partial agonist for $5\text{-}HT_{1A}$ receptor	
RISPERIDONE *Risperdal*	Schizophrenia (Positive and negative) Bipolar, irritability in autism	Neuroleptic agent with high affinity for $5HT_2$ and Dopamine (D4) receptors. Anti-serotonergic, anti-adrenergic, anti-histaminergic. Acts on receptors: 5HT, $\alpha1$, $\alpha2$, H1, D1, D2. Injectable if patient won't take orally.	**Galactorrhea, hyperprolactinemia** to cause lactation and gynecomastia, weight gain, pancreatitis Do not use in elderly with dementia. Greater incidence of **movement disorders**.

ZIPRASIDONE *Geodon,* *Zeldox*	Schizophrenia (Positive and negative). Bipolar, acute mania. Insomnia.	Neuroleptic agent with high affinity for $5HT_2$ and Dopamine (D4) receptors	**Prolong QT interval, torsades de pointes,** somnolence, Do not use in elderly with dementia. Do not use in patients with cardiac conduction defects.

(**Tip:** Atypical Side Effects:
"pines" (Asenapine, Clozapine, Olanzapine, Quetiapine): ↑ risk of diabetes, weight gain (metabolic syndrome.
"dones" (Iloperidone, Lurasidone, Risperidone, Ziprasidone): ↑ risk of cardiac and movement problems).

Injectable Psych Meds
Haloperidol decanoate, Risperidone, Fluphenazine

Psych Meds for Non-Compliant Patients to Prevent Relapses
Injectable
- Haloperidol: Give every 2 weeks to 1 months
- Fluphenazine: Give 2 times/month
- Risperidone: Give 2 times/month
- Paliperidone: Give 1 time/month

Antidepressants

- ↓ in serotonin, Norepinephrine, Dopamine = depression
- **Takes 4 – 6 weeks for antidepressants to take effect**
  - If patient comes in before this time, reassure them and recheck at 4 – 6 weeks.
  - **If it has been 6 weeks and the drug is not working, switch to another antidepressant in the SAME CATEGORY, do not change categories.**
  - If the same category of antidepressants has **failed twice, THEN** the patient can be **switched** to a different category (family/class) of antidepressant.
  - **Benzodiazepines (ie: Alprazolam) can provide immediate help for the patient while waiting for the effects of the SSRI to take affect.**

SSRI's (Selective Serotonin Reuptake Inhibitor)

1st Line drug choice for depression
Citalopram, Fluoxetine, Paroxetine (not safe in pregnancy), Sertraline

SSRI's are the drug of choice for: Depression, Post-partum depression, Bulimia nervosa, anxiety, PTSD, OCD, Panic Disorder, Social Phobia, Premature ejaculation.

DRUG GENERIC name Trade name	**Clinical Use**	**Mechanism of Action**	**Toxicity**
CITALOPRAM *Celexa* **FLUOXETINE** *Prozac* **PAROXETINE*** *Paxil* **SERTRALINE** *Zoloft*	**Depression, post-partum depression, panic disorder, OCD, eating disorders (bulimia), anxiety disorders, social phobia, PTSD.** **TX: Premature ejaculations**	5-HT (Serotonin) reuptake inhibitors	**Sexual dysfunction:** ↓ libido, anorgasmia, GI SX, Prolonged QT. **Serotonin Syndrome*** Avoid use with: SNRI, MOA's, TCA's, St John's Wart, Meperidine, Dextromethorphan, Triptans (Migraines). *Paroxetine **is NOT safe in pregnancy**. All other SSRI's are safe in pregnancy.

SNRI's (Serotonin-Norepinephrine Reuptake Inhibitor)

DRUG GENERIC name Trade name	Clinical Use	Mechanism of Action	Toxicity
DULOXETINE *Cymbalta*	Depression, Diabetic peripheral, Major depressive disorder, **neuropathy**, fibromyalgia, PTSD, panic disorder, OCD, social anxiety. Best for: patients with depression and neuropathic pain.	5-HT (Serotonin) and Norepinephrine reuptake inhibitors	**Sexual dysfunction**: ↓ libido, anorgasmia, GI sx, HTN Serotonin Syndrome* Avoid use with: SSRI, MOA's, TCA's, St John's Wart, Meperidine, Dextromethorphan.
VENLAFAXINE *Effexor*	Major depressive disorder, generalized anxiety disorder, panic disorder, social phobia	5-HT (Serotonin) and Norepinephrine reuptake inhibitors	↑ risk of suicide, ↑ eye pressure (glaucoma), lower seizure threshold, drug-drug interaction with St. John's Wart. Sexual dysfunction. Serotonin Syndrome*
Levomilnacipran Milnacipran Desvenlafaxine	Major depressive disorder, generalized anxiety disorder, panic disorder, social phobia	5-HT (Serotonin) and Norepinephrine reuptake inhibitors	↑ risk of suicide, ↑ eye pressure (glaucoma), lower seizure threshold, drug-drug interaction with St. John's Wart. Sexual dysfunction. Serotonin Syndrome*

Tricyclic Antidepressants (TCA's)

Amitriptyline, Nortriptyline, Doxepin, Amoxapine, Clomipramine, Desipramine, Imipramine

DRUG GENERIC name Trade name	Clinical Use	Mechanism of Action	Toxicity
AMITRIPTYLINE NORTRIPTYLINE DOXEPIN AMOXAPINE	Major depression, **Fibromyalgia** **TCA's are safe for use in pregnancy.**	Block reuptake of 5-HT and Norepinephrine TCA's have an anticholinergic effects (alpha blocker). They cause peripheral vasodilation leading to hypotension.	**Anticholinergic/Antimuscarinic effects** (**dry mouth**, urinary retention, tachycardia, **confusion**, **mydriasis**, hallucinations, constipation, sexual dysfunction, orthostatic hypotension, Parkinsonism. When a patient experiences anticholinergic affects on TCA's, switch them to an SSRI. (**tip:** ANTI depressants cause ANTIcholinergic effects). Amitriptyline is sedating and has anticholinergic effects: not good to use in the elderly. **Cardiotoxicity/arrhythmias** TCA's affect the sodium channels in the heart which can lead to arrhythmias, prolonged QT, QRS and PR intervals, V-tach and F-fib. It also causes: Seizures, Coma TX for OD: Cardiotoxicity: **NaHCO3 (Sodium Bicarb)** (stops fast Na channels) alkalinizes the blood which increases the extracellular sodium by releasing TCA from the hearts sodium channels. **NOTE: First step in TCA overdose is to check an EKG for potentially fatal arrhythmias.** **Serotonin Syndrome*** Avoid use with: SSRI, SNRI, MOA's, St John's Wart, Meperidine, Triptans, Dextromethorphan

Tricyclic Antidepressants (TCA's) cont'd

CLOMIPRAMINE	OCD (**SSRI are 1st line**), major depression	Block reuptake of 5-HT and Norepinephrine	**Same for all TCA's**
DESIPRAMINE	**Less sedating** for major depression	Block reuptake of 5-HT and Norepinephrine	**Same for all TCA's**
IMIPRAMINE	**Enuresis (bed-wetting)**	Block reuptake of 5-HT and Norepinephrine	**Same for all TCA's**

Monoamine Oxidase Inhibitors (MAOI)

MAOI's are the DOC for treating atypical depression.
Isocarboxazid, Phenelzine, Selegiline, Tranylcypromine

DRUG GENERIC name Trade name	**Clinical Use**	**Mechanism of Action**	**Toxicity**
ISOCARBOXAZID PHENELZINE SELEGILINE TRANYLCYPROMINE	Atypical depression, hypochondriasis, anxiety	Inhibits breakdown of Norepinephrine, Serotonin, and Dopamine. After discontinuation of MAO, it takes **4 weeks for the MAO enzyme to be replaced by the body.** MAOI's inhibit the breakdown of dietary amines, which allows the levels of **tyramine** to rise. The higher levels of tyramine displace norepinephrine causing the hypertensive crisis.	**MAOI Hypertensive Crisis (AKA: Tyramine crisis)** MAO interaction with **tyramine (from tyrosine)** rich foods/drinks: Foods/drinks that are **aged/fermented/dried**: pepperoni (pepperoni and cheese on pizza), wine, cheese, pickles, olives, salami, fava/broad beans, sauerkraut, all nuts, alcohol/fermented beverages. Can also occur when using an MAO with antihistamines and nasal decongestants. Hyperplasia, weight gain. Serotonin Syndrome* Avoid use with: SSRI, SNRI, TCA's, St John's Wart, Meperidine, Triptans, Dextromethorphan.

*Serotonin Syndrome (AKA: Serotonin toxicity)

- Drug-drug interaction. When an SSRI is mixed with any drug that ↑ levels of 5-HT (Serotonin) = excess serotonin in the CNS and/or PNS.
- Other drug that cause interaction: **MAO inhibitors, TCA's, SNRI's, Triptans** (Migraine TX)
- SX: **Rapid onset**. ↑ heart rate (tachycardia), dilated pupils, twitching (myoclonus), hyperactive reflexes, diaphoresis, confusion, agitation, nausea, diarrhea, flushing, high fever (hyperthermia), hallucinations, HTN, metabolic acidosis, shivering, rhabdomyolysis, renal failure, DIC
- TX: Discontinue medications.
- TX: Cyproheptadine (5-HT receptor antagonist. A 1st generation anti-histamine) that decreases serotonin production and give a Benzodiazepine to decrease muscle rigidity.

Atypical Antidepressants

Atypical depression: When the individual is depressed but is able to get into a better mood when good news is given.

DRUG GENERIC name Trade name	Clinical Use	Mechanism of Action	Toxicity
BUPROPION **Varenicline** *Wellbutrin*	Smoking cessation, Depression Best for patients with depression who are concerned about weight gain or sexual side effects. Also best for a smoker trying to quit.	Increases Norepinephrine, and Dopamine.	**NO sexual side effects.** **Seizures**, tachycardia, insomnia
MIRTAZAPINE	Depression and difficulty sleeping (**insomnia**) TX: for patients that need to gain weight: anorexia, elderly, chemotherapy.	**α-2 antagonist.** ↑ Norepinephrine and 5-HT. 5-HT receptor antagonist.	**Weight gain,** sedation, ↑ appetite
MAPROTILINE	Depression	Blocks Norepinephrine reuptake	Sedation, hypotension
TRAZODONE	Insomnia in depressed patients.	Blocks 5-HT and α-1 adrenergic receptors	**Priapism**, sedation, postural HTN. (**tip**: for side effect: trazo**BONE**)

Mood Disorders

Lithium, Carbamazepine, Valproic Acid, Lamotrigine

DRUG GENERIC name Trade name	Clinical Use	Mechanism of Action	Toxicity
LITHIUM	DOC for Bipolar. Acute mania, SIADH (Atypical antipsychotics: ie: Olanzapine, are better for acute mania due to a faster onset).	Unknown Lithium is reabsorbed in the PCT.	**NARROW THERAPUTIC WINDOW.** ↑Lithium toxicity if combined with: **Ace inhibitors, Thiazides, or NSAIDS**. **Nephrogenic Diabetes Insipidus** (causes resistance to ADH in collecting ducts by ↑ urinary prostaglandins which causes lysosomal degradation of the aquaporin water channels), **Hypothyroidism**, **Ebstein anomaly** (congenital cardiac defect that displaces leaflets of the tricuspid valve), Acne, weight gain, headaches, GI symptoms
CARBAMEZAPINE	**DOC: Trigeminal Neuralgia**, Bipolar, mania 3rd line for Bipolar disorder (Lithium is DOC and Valproic #2)	Inhibits voltage gated Na channels	**Agranulocytosis** (must follow weekly CBC labs), **aplastic anemia**, sedation, liver toxicity, Stevens-Johnson Syndrome, teratogen, **Inducer of Cytochrome P-450**
VALPROIC ACID **(AKA: Divalproex)** *(Depakote)*	**2nd line for Absence Seizures, myoclonic seizures, 2nd line for bipolar disorder** if Lithium is ineffective or contraindicated. First line for rapid-cycling bipolar disorders. Migraine headaches.	Inhibits Na channels, Inhibits GABA transaminase so ↑ GABA	**Severe Teratogen** (neural tube defects), **fatal hepatotoxicity** (must follow LFT's), weight gain. Do not use in pregnancy or with hepatitis. Dizziness, drowsiness, hair loss, blurred vision, tinnitus, diarrhea, tremor.

LAMOTRIGINE	**Mood disorders in pregnancy**, 2nd line drug for myoclonic seizures	Blocks voltage gated Na channels	Stevens-Johnson Syndrome

Anxiolytic Drugs

- Benzodiazepines
- Buspirone

DRUG GENERIC name Trade name	Clinical Use	Mechanism of Action	Toxicity
BENZODIAZEPINES **Short Acting:** ALPRAZOLAM TRIAZOLAM OXAZEPAM MIDAZOLAM **(tip: ATOM is very small)** **Long Acting:** CHLORDIAZEPOXIDE CLONAZEPAM DIAZAPAM FLURAZEPAM Intermediate Acting: LORAZAPAM TEMAZEPAM	**Anxiety – 1st line** Alprazolam: panic attacks and disorders. Clonazepam: used if there is concern for addiction (long half life). Lorazepam: Used in emergencies, given IM. Chlordiazepoxide, Oxazepam, Lorazepam: Used in alcohol withdrawal. Oxazepam and Lorazepam are used in patients with liver dz. Flurazepam, Triazolam, Temazepam: hypnotics	↑ **Frequency** of the opening of **Chloride channels** so that neuron firing is decreased and GABA ↑. (AKA: Allosterically binds GABA = ↑ GABA)	Sedation, confusion, potential for addiction, memory problems, respiratory depression. OD TX: **Flumazenil*** (GABA receptor antagonist) (***must not be used** in patients that are benzodiazepine dependent. It also stops the action of benzodiazepine that the patient is on, causing withdrawal and seizures).
BUSPIRONE *Buspar*	Generalize anxiety disorder. **(NOT FIRST LINE)** **1st line: SSRI unless** patient is worried about weight gain or sexual side effects.	Serotonin (5-HT) partial Agonist. Takes 2 weeks to take affect. During these first 2 weeks the patient can take benzodiazepines until Buspirone starts to work.	**NO sexual side effects.** No sedation, no addition, no tolerance. No interaction with alcohol. Headaches, dizziness, nausea.

MORTALITY and INCIDENCE RATES: DEATH and CANCER

MCC Death: Heart Disease

MCC Death in a smoker: Lung cancer
MCC Death in a non-smoker: Colon cancer
Mammograms lower the mortality more than any other cancer-screening test.

Cancer Mortality

MC in MEN	MC in Women
Lung Prostate Colon	Lung Breast Colon

Cancer Incidence

MC in MEN	MC in Women
Prostate	Breast

GYN Cancers

MC GYN Mortality	MC GYN Incidence
Ovarian Endometrial Cervical	Endometrial Ovarian Cervical

BIAS

- **Susceptibility Bias**: TX plan is selected for patient based on severity of their condition without taking into effect other possible confounding factors. Experimental and control group differ from prognostic standpoint b/c confounding variables. PREVENTION: Randomization
- **Verification Bias**: (work up or measurement bias). Insures that both sides (control and experimental group are handled the same) in measurements and selection. Measurement bias that selectively verifies results.
  Ex: BOTH women with positive and negative HPV test did colposcopy and biopsy.
- **Contamination Bias**: Control group accidently received the treatment.
- **Recall Bias**: Seen in CASE CONTROL (AKA: Odds Ratio) cases. When someone "Looks Back" to remember. Misclassification of exposure. People say what they think is true from the past even though it is incorrect = distorted information OR patient feels obligated to give info so they create info and believe it as a fact even though it is wrong. SOLUTION: Confirmation of the recall or triangulation: check with other sources to see if info is correct.
- **Confounding Bias**: A variable related to both groups and the response variable of interest. Confounding variables have a significant effect on response variable that confounds the explanatory variable. A confounding bias has a middle factor that is related to both exposure and outcome (EX: Smoking would be a confounder with: Alcohol (exposure) and Oral Cancer (outcome).
  EX 1: study showed heart problems with patients who owned a dog healed faster – So does a dog help a heart heal faster? CONFOUNDING FACTOR: Dog owners get more exercise because they walk their dog and this exercise helps heal hearts faster. Confounding Variable: Exercise. You must have this additional variable at work in order to achieve the result of a faster healing heart.
  EX 2: Study for 2 groups to study alcohol on heart dz. Group 1 also smokes and Group 2 drinks many varieties of alcoholic drinks. Results of test: Group 1 has higher rate of heart DZ than Group 2. **CONFOUNDER**: Smoking. Don't know if the higher rate is due to alcohol or smoking. (it is a known fact that smoking also leads to higher heart DZ).
  Confounding: "Found Within". Things are wrapped together therefore can't tell them apart. The factor being examined is related to other factors. There should be ONE and ONLY 1 difference b/t the treatment group and comparison group.
  EX: Treatment vs Non-Treatment: ALL ELSE must be the same in the beginning. ANY difference seen as an outcome at the end MUST be due to the 1 difference you started with. But if **MORE THAN 1 DIFFERENCE** is present at beginning then the outcome could be due to 1 or both of the factors. Confounding is NOT about what results you get (these are clear) it is about WHY you got the result (cause or interpretation of what happened). **PREVENTION: Matching,** Adjustments do multiple studies, Meta analysis (combine solutions to get one main one).
  NOTE: See "Effect Modification" below. Confounding bias is often confused with Effect Modification.

- **Effect Modification**: When the effect that occurs actually influences the results of the study.
  Many times an effect modification is confused with a confounding bias. Confounding is a bias (error), effect modification is not a bias. **Confounders affect BOTH the exposure and outcome**. Confounding is a bias for the ENTIRE population in the study and effect modification is stratified. Stratification is the process of dividing members of the population into a particular subgroups (or age group) in the population before sampling.
  The effect modification factor is ONLY related to the outcome, it has nothing to do with the exposure.
  (tip: "O"nly related to "O"utcome).
  EX 1: OCP's (exposure) and breast cancer (outcome). Family history is an effect modification because family history will modify the effect and will fasten the process of breast cancer. OCP (exposure) has nothing to do with family history.
  EX 2: Asbestos (exposure) and Lung cancer (outcome). Smoking is an effect modification. It is not related to asbestos (exposure) but smoking is a risk factor for lung cancer (outcome).
  EX 3: Estrogen (exposure) and DVT (outcome). Smoking is an effect modification because it has nothing to do with estrogen (exposure) but it is a risk for DVT's (outcome).
  EX: 4: Drug A worked on children but not on adults. This would be an effect modification because the drug worked ONLY on a specific age group (or subgroup) and not the entire population. This example can be modified into a confounding example by asking why the results of the drug test were not significant when the entire population (everyone: children and adults). Then the confounder would be age.
- **Lead Time Bias**: False estimate of survival time. This confuses early detection with that of added survival time. Patient still dies at the same time (no additional survival time), but is just aware of the dz earlier, so they know about it longer. Screening test for diseases with poor prognosis (ie: cancer) lead to a Lead Time Bias. SOLUTION: Never use how long a patient lives after diagnosis, only use life expectancy.
- **Late Look Bias**: Seen when studying a severe/fatal DZ (ie: cancer) because patients die before end of study so no way to get results. SOLUTION: Stratify by severity. Represent each level of sickness and severity. (tip: once a person has died, they are called "the **LATE** ....)
- **Design Bias**: Pieces of study are not done to allow the right comparisons to answer what is being asked/studied. Groups do not match/non-comparable control group. SOLUTION: Random Assignment (People already in the study after random selection, it is done to divide these groups).
- **Measurement Bias**: Poor data collection = inaccurate results. Gathering of info distorts information. Ex: "LEADING QUESTIONS: (word choice or tone) in how questions are done.
- **Hawthorn Effect**: Person changes or gives response based on the fact the person knows they are being measured/watched. SOLUTION: Control Group = Measurement Constant.
- **Pygmalion Bias**: Researchers belief in the studies efficacy.
- **Observer Bias**: Observer/Researcher prior knowledge of what is needed to sway study one way or the other to "see" the result of interest.
- **Experiment Expectancy Effect:** What the researcher THINKS they will find is WHAT they find. SOLUTION: Double Blind Design. This insures that neither the researchers nor the patients know what they are receiving.
- **Publication Bias** shown by a funnel plot
- **Interviewer Bias:** Solution: Use standardized questionnaire.
- **Selection Bias (Sampling Bias):** Manner in which people are chosen for the study. People in the study are NOT good representatives of those outside the population not in the study. "**LOST TO FOLLOW UP**".
  To PREVENT: Randomization in clinical trial.

  1. **Convenience Sample**: Selected because of convenient access and proximity to researcher. (EX: Study to determine cardio health of Springfield so researcher studies those that attend fitness club – this does NOT represent the general public)
  2. **Berkson's Bias**: Using **hospital** patients for your study – this does NOT represent the general public.
  3. **Non-Respondent Bias/ Volunteer Effect**: Study does not represent population, as a whole b/c volunteers are not the same as the general public. This only looks at one group of the population. SOLUTION: Random, independent sample: 1) Random Process: Those in the study match those outside the study and 2) Weigh the Data: Balance the % results so that they match the public.

DEFINITIONS

- **Generalizability**: Can the result of the study focused on one section (ie: such as one age group of women) be valid for all (generalized) ages of women?
- **Factorial Designs**: Factors in different goals. Randomization to different treatments with an additional goal/study of these into 2 additional variables. (ie: Group is divided into 3 separate drugs to use, then all groups are then given separate goals to meet with their own meds.)
- **Intension to Treat**: Preserves randomization
- **Internal Validity**: Are we observing/measuring what we think we are? (Threat of this is confounding bias). Are the results of the study valid (AKA: accurate) for the population of patients who were actually studied?
- **External Validity**: Dependent upon sample size (ie: large sample size is gives more generalized results/validity). Are the results of the study valid (AKA: accurate) for the other patients (not studied)?
- **Randomization:** Decreases confounding variables, selection bias, and design bias. Randomized control trials = least possibility of bias, therefore is ok with small numbers or decreased risk.

- **Community Trial:** test intervention in a non-medical setting. How does the treatment/test work in the "real world".
- **Time to Advent = Survival Analysis**
- **FDA Post Market Survey**: Monitors safety of drugs and treatments after they are approved for public use. Failure to find negative events in pre-testing is due to inadequate power (ie: lower number of people/low power).
- **Cross-Over:** Balances research b/c everyone in the project receives the experimental medicine/treatment at some point during the study.
- **Cross Sectional:** Assessed general prevalence of disease and factors in the general population. Sample of people at one certain point time and checks prevalence. How widespread is the disease? Uses Chi Square (categories).
  CROSS SECTIONAL = checks PREVELENCE = CHI SQUARE
- **Case Report:** Uses only a single patient (N=1).
- **Case Series/Study:** Study collects cases and looks at/for common elements. This is used with limited numbers of patients (more than 1 patient N>1), unknown diseases and is done quickly. This is for ONLY patients WITH disease of interest. Looks for all common elements in patients in the group and uses a list of criteria to describe the dz. Limitation: no control group.
- **Case Control (Odds Ratio):** Looks backwards in time - retrospective. Compares patients with the condition/disease to people without the condition/disease and looks for risk factors (exposure vs non-). It answers/informs: patient is more likely to have had the risk in their history AND determines the #1 risk factor of the disease. (Disease vs non-disease) Most common study to investigate acute outbreaks. HIGH: Recall Bias. Case Control is more prone to bias than cohort studies. **Case Control = Observational study = Selective Survival**
- **Cohort (Relative Risk):** Can go backward or forward in time. Identifies people WITH risk factors and then follows them forward looking for the development of the disease. Best study for causality. More prone to bias than randomized control trials. (Risk factor vs no risk factor). **COHERT (Relative Risk) = Differ in INCIDENCE (checks/compares incidence) = Confirmatory study**
- **SeNsitivity (AKA: Screening test): ability of a test is its ability to detect people who DO HAVE the disease. The best sensitivity test is a test with 100% sensitivity.**
  A Negative test rules OUT disease (tip: I hate to be withOUT my senses), a positive test = have disease.
  The sensitivity of a diagnostic test measures how effective it is in regards to detecting a disease in a patient that HAS the disease.
- **SPecificity (AKA: Confirmatory test) ability of a test to detect people that do NOT HAVE the disease.**
  A Positive test rules IN disease. (tip: SPIN), a negative test = no disease.
  The specificity of a diagnostic test measures how effective it is in regards to detecting a patient that does NOT have the disease.
- **Positive Predictive Value: the probability that if a patient is given a positive test result, that they actually have the disease.**
- **Negative Predictive Value: the probability that if a patient is given a negative test result, that they actually do NOT have the disease.**
- **PPV = indicate the prevalence of disease (Low disease = decreased PPV and High disease = high PPV)**
- **NPV is inversely proportional to prevalence.**
- **Prevalence is the number of total cases in the population at a specific time.**
  Prevalence and PPV always GO TOGETHER! If PPV decreases, Prevalence decreases, etc. NPV is inversely proportional to prevalence. If PPV is increased, NPV is decreased.
  Prevalence is greater than incidence for chronic disease.
  Prevalence is all current cases of the disease.
- **Prevalence and Incidence relationship (You will be tested on your understanding of what happens to prevalence and incidence when diseases increase or decrease.**
  Examples:
  1) **If a new treatment is given that decreases the duration of the illness, but does not alter the number of new cases or people dying = Prevalence decreases.**
  2) **If a new vaccine (or treatment) is found to improve the prevention of a on-fatal disease = BOTH the incidence and prevalence of the disease decreases.**
  3) **If a disease is stopped (cured) or if the disease process is shortened = the prevalence will decrease (less people will have it as long).**
  4) **Increase in deaths = decrease in prevalence.**
  5) **Increased long term survival = Increased prevalence.**
  6) **Acute disease = Increased incidence**
  7) **Chronic disease = Decreased incidence**
- **Incidence: All new cases that develop in a population.**
  Acute disease = Increased incidence.
  Chronic disease = Decreased incidence, but increased prevalence.

PRECISION (RELIABILITY)

- **Precision (AKA: Reliability):** Measures random error**. The width of the confidence interval reflects precision.** The tighter (closer) the Confidence Interval (CI) = more precise (AKA: highly precise). High precision = high sample size (AKA: higher power).
- **Precision:** A reliable (AKA: reliability) test is consistent, stable and dependable.
- **Precision:** A state of strict exactness – how often something is strictly exact.
- **Reliability (AKA: reproducibility, precision)** is the measure of random error.
- **Precision (random error) Random** variations are reliable and reproducible. Is affected by sample size.
- **Precision and the scatterplot:** The closer the scatter is to "1" the higher the precision.
- **Precision:** Means the measurements are ALL close to each other, but they may or my not be close to the target.
- **Precision =** Reliable = Reproducible = Range = In the Ballpark
- **Precision Examples:**
  1) If you obtain a weight of 2 lbs for a given object but the actual known weight is 8 lbs, then your measurement is not accurate (AKA: valid), it is not close to the known value.
  2) A golfer putting the ball: If the player putts with accuracy (AKA: validity) his aim will always take the ball close to or in the hole. If the player putts with precision, his aim will always take the ball to the same location which may or may be close to the hole. A good player will be both accurate and precise by putting the ball the same way each time and each time making it into the hole.

ACCURACY (VALIDITY)

- **Accuracy (AKA: Validity) =** Gold Standard = Valid = Will ALWAYS Be = Measure of truth = Specific = It measures exactly what it is supposed to.
- **Accuracy:** The degree to which an estimate is immune from error or bias.
- **Accuracy:** The measurements are very close to the true or absolute value. The measurements are very near the target.
- **Accuracy:** Scatterplots have no significant role in accuracy.
- **Accuracy (AKA: Validity (systematic error)** Flaws in study design. It is not affected by sample size.
- **Accuracy Examples:**
  1) If you obtain a weight of an object five times and get a 2 lb weight each time, then your measurements are very precise. Precision is independent of accuracy. You can be very precise but inaccurate. You can also be accurate but imprecise.
  2) In target shooting a high score indicates nearness to the bulls eye and is a measurement of the shooters accuracy.

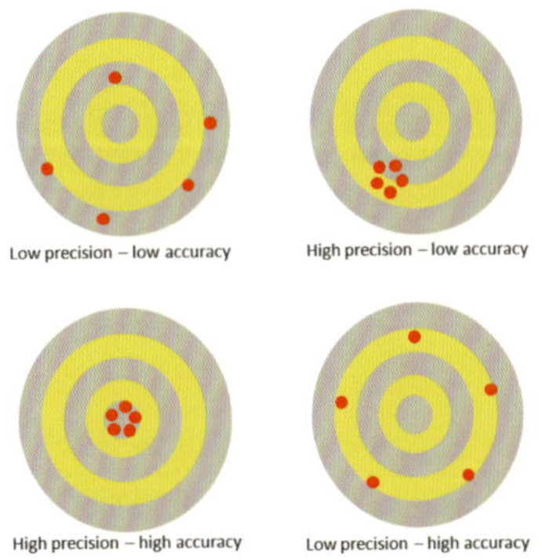

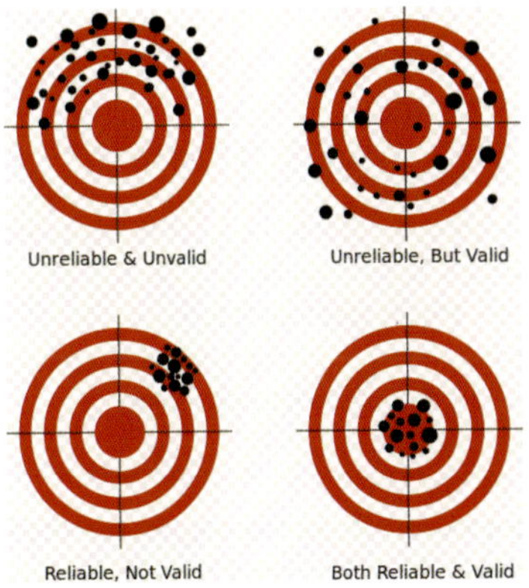

- Biased = Inaccurate, Imprecise = Random, Unbiased = Accurate, Precise = Not Random
- **Clinical Trial = Therapeutic comparisons.** It allows one to build the trail like they want (like putting Legos together to make a puzzle). **Control Group uses either: PLACEBOS**: Group gets all the treatments but does NOT get the drug, they get a "false" drug **OR "STANDARD of CARE**" group gets current best care verses new drug (ie: used in cancer). This answers: Does new drug work better than old drug?" **CONCLUSIONS**: Placebo determines does the treatment work better than no drug? And Standard of Care determines if the new drug works better than the old drug.

Clinical Trial Phases:

1. **Phase 1**: Safety. Drug given to small number of **healthy** volunteers and is the first time its given to people.
2. **Phase 2**: Drug is now given to a small number of **affected** volunteers. Drug is not given to patients to check on dose levels, protocol, processes and how best to administer and use drug for 100's of patients.
3. Phase 3: Key info to FDA for approval. Drug given to 1000's of patients/**large groups/public**. Checks on efficacy and side effects. If good efficacy and low side effects = FDA Approves.
4. Phase 4: Post marketing survey. Finding the side effects once it is released to the public. Physicians and patients report these side effects after the drug is out on the market.

- **Significance of Studies:** Randomized Controlled Trial best, then cohort (relative risk RR) and then case controlled (odds ratio OR). If an adjustment was made to a study with at least one known confounder to adjust it out: Results: If adjustment produces large decreases in the OR or RR, then the results are suspicious. If the adjustment produces increases in the OR or RR or they stay the same then the results are probably valid.
- **Double Blind:** Both researchers and subjects are "blind". Neither knows which is the treatment neither group nor control group. It is the LEAST SUBJECT TO BIAS.
- **Experimental Study = Clinical study trials = intervention study trials** (drugs/procedures/education)
- **Ecological Studies (ie: Correlation).** Only gives **population** information NOT individual patient results. (Ecologic fallacy)
- **Root Cause Analysis:** Identifies steps leading to preventable adverse outcomes in the health care system. (Ex: Over prescribing drugs between different physicians or when a physician makes an error (ie: surgery) and catches it **before** it affects patient).
- **Hazard Ratio = Relative Risk = Likelihood Ratio**
  Event rate in the treatment group (-) event rate in the non- TX group. The higher the ration the more likely the factor is associated with the incidence.
  Hazard Ratio: **<1 is a good prognosis (AKA: PROTECTIVE),** >1 = poor prognosis. 1= more test
  (tip: When you see this configuration in the vignette: 1.7 (1.2 – 3.3), the (1.2 – 3.3 is the confidence interval) and the 1.7 is the Relative Risk figure (AKA: hazard ration figure, likelihood ratio figure). Look at THIS number. Is it OVER 1 or LESS than 1. If it is over 1, then there is a high likelihood (AKA: hazard or relative risk) that the person has the disease. If this number is LESS than 1, there is a low risk (AKA: hazard or relative risk) that the person has the disease, **meaning this is PROTECTIVE.**
- **Likelihood Ratio:** Used when disease rate varies in different locations or groups but does not change with prevalence. What are the odds the patient has the disease.
  >1 = High odds of having the disease (poor prognosis)
  <1 = Low odds of having the disease (good prognosis = protective)

BIOSTAT EQUATIONS

These are the standard format for the biostat equations. For those that don't like math and prefer a more visual approach, look under the "Most Common Equations" under my illustrations following this section. It will simplify this process!

- **Incidence**
  Number of new cases / number of total people in given population at risk at that time period
  (Remember: do not count people in the population that were ALREADY sick with the disease before the time period specified. These people are NOT at risk, they have the disease and would not be NEW cases. New cases are considered people that develop the disease AFTER the start of the specified time period).
- **Prevalence (AKA: Point prevalence)**
  Number of existing cases / total population at risk
  Incidence rate X average disease duration
- **Positive Predictive Value (PPV)**
  TP / (TP + FP) or a / a + b
  Remember: read carefully in the vignette: the patient will have gotten a test and will ask the doctor: "Are you sure I HAVE this?" OR "What are the chances I HAVE the disease?" (these are both positive, "HAVE" comments)
- **Negative Predictive Value**
  TN / (FN + TN) or d / c + d
  Probability of NPV = 1 - NPV
  Remember: read carefully in the vignette: the patient have gotten a test back and will ask the doctor: "are sure I DON'T HAVE the disease" OR will say "What are the chances I DON'T HAVE the disease" (these are both negative, "NOT HAVE" comments).
- **Sensitivity**
  TP / (TP + FN) OR a / a + c
- **Specificity**
  TN / (TN + FP) OR d / b + d
- **Cohort (Prospective or Retrospective): (AKA: Relative Risk, RR, Hazard Ratio, likelihood ratio)**
  TP/(TP + FP) / FN/(FN + TN) OR a/(a+b) / c/(c +d)
- **Case Control (Observational and retrospective): (AKA: Odds Ratio, OR)**
  TP/FN divided FP/TN = TP x TN divided FP x FN OR a/c divided b/d = ad/bc

- **NNT (Number needed to treat)**
  NNT = 1 / ARR
  Means the number of people that would need to be treated before 1 would be helped. The ideal percent would be 100%. Meaning that everyone treated was helped.
- **NNH (Number needed to harm)**
  NNH = 1 / AR
  Means the number of people that would be exposed to a risk before 1 is harmed. The ideal percent is 0. Meaning that out of everyone that was exposed to the risk = none were harmed.
- **Relative Risk Reduction (RRR)**
  1 – RR (relative risk)
  The proportion of risk reduction attributable to the intervention verses the controls.
  This is the drug (experimental) group over the placebo (control) group
  EXAMPLE: There are 100 people in control group and 100 people in the experimental (drug) group.
  If 2% of the drug group get sick and 10% of the control group get sick then RRR = 2/10 = 0.20, so
  RRR = 1 – RR (0.20) = 0.80
- **Absolute Risk Reduction (ARR)***he % of event in control group minus the % of event in experimental (drug) group.*
  The difference (not proportion) in risk attributable to the intervention verses the controls.
  Event rate of the placebo (control) group minus even rate in the drug (experimental) group.
  EXAMPLE: There are 100 people in control group and 100 people in drug group. 10% of the people in the control group got sick and 4% of the people in the drug group got sick. 10% - 4% = 6% (ARR)
- **Population Attributable Risk (PARP)**
  Risk in population (-) Risk in exposed/Risk in Total Population
- Estimate of proportion of disease in a population that is attributable to exposure.
  The % calculated is the % of disease in the population that is attributable to the risk factor.
- **Correlation (Scatterplots)**
  No correlation between 2 factors = 0
  Positive correlation between 2 factors = 1
    (meaning that BOTH factors follow each other. If one of the factors increases the second factor increases.
    Example: Smoking and lung cancer have a positive correlation: meaning smoking is increased (UP) then lung cancer increases (UP)
  Negative correlation between 2 factors = negative 1
    (meaning that both factors go opposite directions. If the one of the factors increases then the second factor decreases.
    Example: Vegetables and stomach cancer have positive correlations. If the intake of vegetables increases (UP) then the risk of stomach cancer decreases (DOWN).
- **Proportion or Specific Mortality:**
  # of deaths from specific cause/# ALL deaths
- **Attack Rate:** % of people that get disease from all population at risk (who gets disease)
  # of deaths from specific cause/# total population
- **CASE RATE FATALITY**
  Those who died with the same condition
  # of deaths from specific DZ/total # of people with that DZ
- **Birth Rate:**
  # live births/# total population
- **Neonatal Mortality Rate**
  # deaths babies <28 days for year/# live births for year
- **Death Rate:**
  # of deaths/# total population
- **Maternal Death Rate**
  # maternal deaths/# live births
- **Standardized Mortality Ratio:** if # death in a group exceeds what is expected in a similar group
- **Median Survival Time:** Measure of prognosis when studying a disease. Length of time it takes for ½ of the population with the disease to die.

MEANINGS of the NUMBERS

- Odds Ratio: ad/bc = % (ex: 8100/100 = 81% If you have lung CA, you are 81 times more apt to have CA if you smoked)
- NPV (means a negative test means you do NOT have disease): (ex: if 96%, means: 96% of people do NOT have disease, leaving 4% that have the disease.
  Probability of NPV: Calculation: 1 – NPV
- Relative Risk: p= .01, means 1% chance/probability that the result observed was by chance.
- **NNT** – Number of people needed to treat before 1 gets better. Inverse of absolute risk reduction. The ideal NNT is 1, it means that everyone treated improves. The higher the NNT number is the less effective the treatment is.
- **NNH** – Number of people to be exposed to a risk factor before 1 is harmed. Inverse of attributable risk. The worst NNH is 1, meaning every person would be harmed.
- Probability: Ex: Probability of having CF: American mom has 1 in 30 and Asian dad is 1 in 100. What is probability of child having CF?
  Mom: (1/30 x ½) (1/100 x ½) = 1/60 x 1/200 = 1/12,000
  Ratio of Disease x Carrier Ratio
  *1/2 is b/c there is a 50/50 chance of a boy or a girl 50% = ½
- Hardy Weinberg (use if no family history)
  p2 x 2 pq x q2 = 1
  AA AaAa aa (A = Normal gene a = abnormal gene)
- **P Value** Ex: p = .01 Means: 1% possibility that there is NO association between factors. If P = .05 Means that there is a 5% probability that the null value is rejected and the alternative hypothesis is accepted. The P value is the probably that the null hypothesis is true.
- **Power: The greater the desired power then the greater the sample size must be.**
  High power = high sample size.
  Large differences between groups in studies means low power = low sample size. Smaller differences between groups means high power = high sample.
- If Sample Size Increases, then **Confidence Interval** (range) decreases (narrows – meaning the upper limit either decreases or the lower limit increases or both), ie: (.7 – 2.9) CI decreases to (.9 – 1.4).
  The distance between the 2 numbers decreases/narrows.
- If the Mean decreases then the Confidence Interval narrows (decreases)
- **Confidence Interval**: If the range contains the value "1" it is NOT a significant findings, **if the range does NOT contain the value "1" it IS significant.** (Ex: Not Significant = (.7 – 2.3).
  Significant = (1.2 – 2.3).
- **Null Hypothesis:** This is the "default" before any study. The null hypothesis is always pessimistic; it always expects that the study is **NOT** going to work. That there will be NO association between the disease and the risk. (Null = 0 It is N = Negative). So if you **"Accept"** the null hypothesis, you are accepting that the experiment/drug is NOT going to work. If you **"Reject"** the null hypothesis, you are saying that your experiment/drug IS going to work.
- **Type 1 Error (alpha).** It is a study (experiment) that says that your study DID find a different (example: your study showed that a drug did work), however, when in fact it did NOT work. So you **rejected the null hypothesis** by saying that the drug really did work. (tip: a (alpha) = to anxious. So **A**nxious the drug will work that you say it does work, when it really did not).
  Type 1 Error = Power (aka: Sample Size). Standard P (Type 1) is .05. < .05 is SIGNIFICANT. This means there is less than a 5% chance that the results from the study were due to chance. **The lower the number is (ex: .01 instead of .05) means that the results of the test are even stronger, there is a greater confidence**. To increase the power of this finding even more, you must increase the sample size (increase the number of participants).
  (**tip**: **A** for alpha) = **A** for **A**nxious. To Anxious that your drug works, so you say it does and it doesn't)
- **Type 1 Error (alpha) = A positive test is obtained in a person who does NOT the disease = False Positive.**
- **Type II Error (Beta).** It is a study (experiment) that says the experiment (drug) didn't work. So you accept the null hypothesis. (Example your study concluded that the drug did work, when in reality it actually did work.
  To calculate: 1 – B (1 is same as 100%), so 100% (-) error given is the %.
- **Type II Error = A negative test is obtained in a person who does have the disease = False Negative.**
- A True Negative test = A negative test obtained in a person who does NOT have the disease.
- A True Positive test = A positive test obtained in a person who DOES have the disease.
- Mental Retardation: If IQ is 70, this means it is 2 Standard Deviations (SD) below median = 2.5%.
  If IQ is 130 = 97.5%, If IQ is 70 = 2.5 %, if IQ is 115 = 84%

TEST

1. ANOVA (**Analysis of Variance**) Difference (variation) b/t the means of 3 or more **GROUPS** (ex: Diff in BP in 3 populations, based on exercise status).
2. META Analysis: Pools data from **several smaller studies** in order to make one larger study with more statistical power.
3. CHI SQUARE: 2 x 2 table that is used for results between 2 **CATEGORIES** in order to compare.
4. T TEST: **2 SAMPLES**: Compares 2 groups **MEANS** (Must show as numbers NOT words)
5. Z TEST: Measures of **populations** NOT individuals or subjects.
   Z Score is 1.96 SD if there is a 95% Confidence Interval
   Z Score is 2.58 SD if there is a 99% Confidence Interval

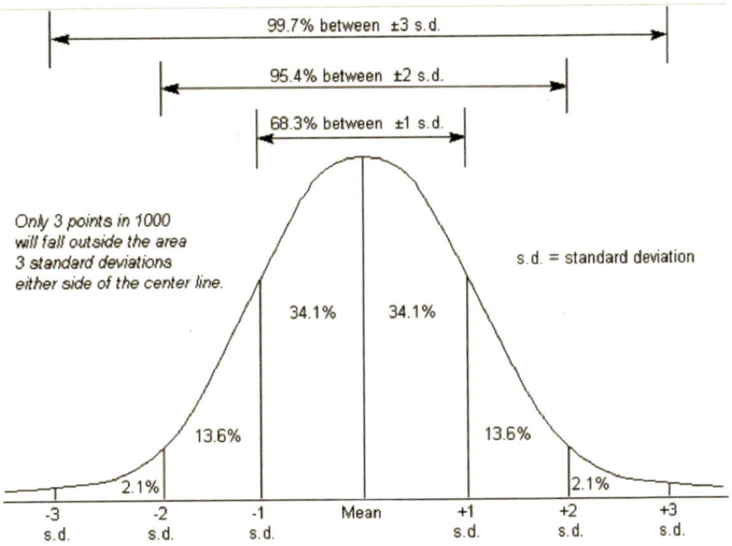

99.7% between ±3 s.d.
95.4% between ±2 s.d.
68.3% between ±1 s.d.
Only 3 points in 1000 will fall outside the area 3 standard deviations either side of the center line.
s.d. = standard deviation
34.1%
34.1%
13.6%
13.6%
2.1%
2.1%
-3 s.d.
-2 s.d.
-1 s.d.
Mean
+1 s.d.
+2 s.d.
+3 s.d.

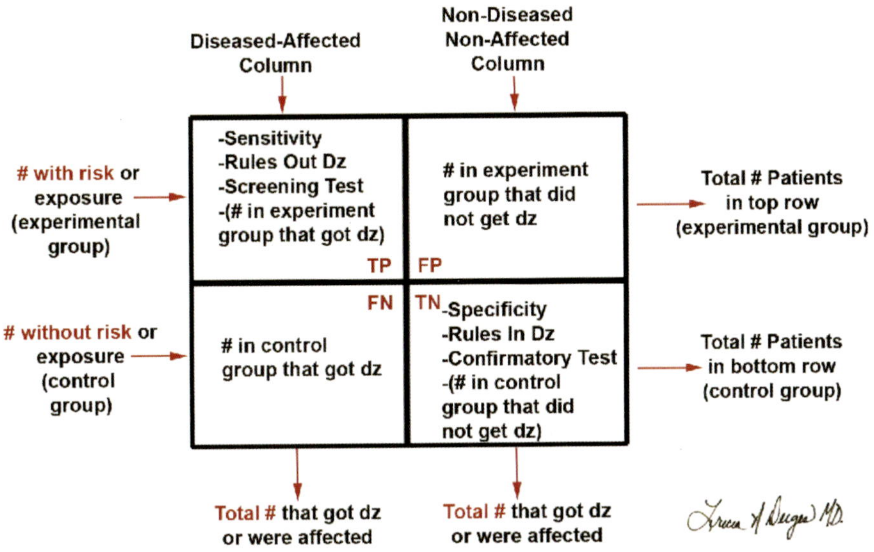

Diseased-Affected Column
Non-Diseased Non-Affected Column
with risk or exposure (experimental group)
-Sensitivity
-Rules Out Dz
-Screening Test
-(# in experiment group that got dz)
TP
in experiment group that did not get dz
FP
Total # Patients in top row (experimental group)
without risk or exposure (control group)
FN
in control group that got dz
TN
-Specificity
-Rules In Dz
-Confirmatory Test
-(# in control group that did not get dz)
Total # Patients in bottom row (control group)
Total # that got dz or were affected
Total # that got dz or were affected

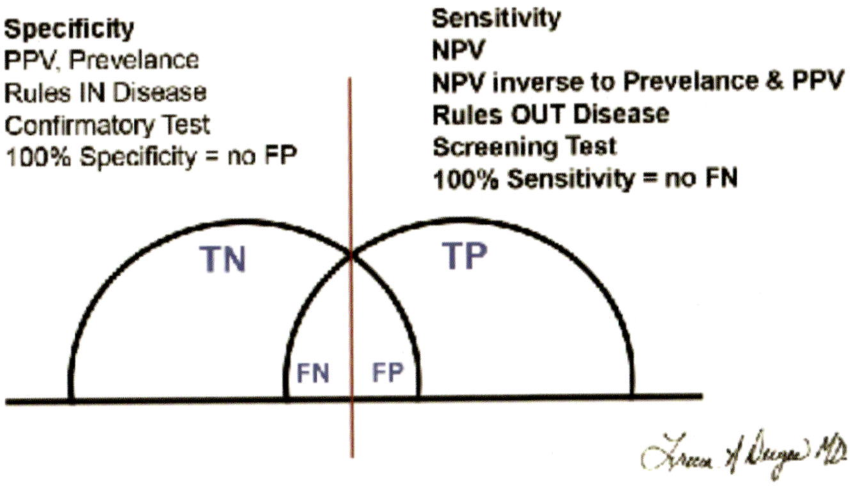

Specificity
PPV, Prevelance
Rules IN Disease
Confirmatory Test
100% Specificity = no FP
Sensitivity
NPV
NPV inverse to Prevelance & PPV
Rules OUT Disease
Screening Test
100% Sensitivity = no FN
TN
TP
FN
FP

Mean – Median – Mode

- Mean: The average of all numbers. Ex: 2, 4, 8, 12, 22.
  The average is 24.
  The Mean is the most sensitive to change – the most sensitive to an outlier.
- Median: The middle number (this includes ALL numbers (including repeated numbers). Ex: 18, 20, 21, 22, 22, 22, 30, 37, 41, 42, 42, 45, 58, 60. The middle number is 37).
- Mode: The number used most often. Ex: 1, 3, 3, 4, 6, 9, 14.
  The mode is 3. (the most common value).
  The mode is the least affected by outliers.
- In a normal (equal) bell distribution the mean, median and mode are all equal. AKA: Gaussian Curve.
- In a positively skewed distribution the Mean > Median > Mode.
- In a negatively skewed distribution the Mode > Median > Mean.

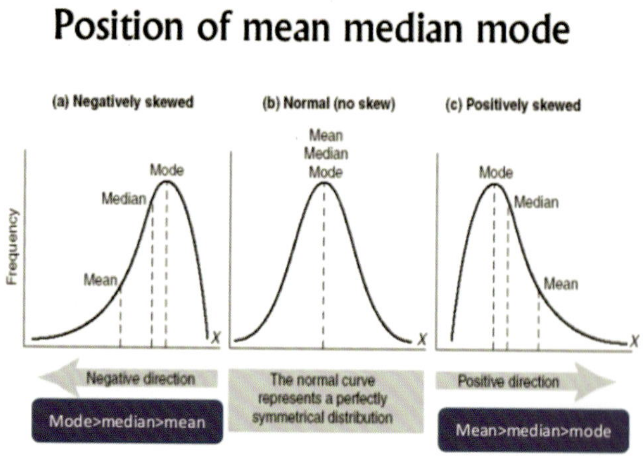

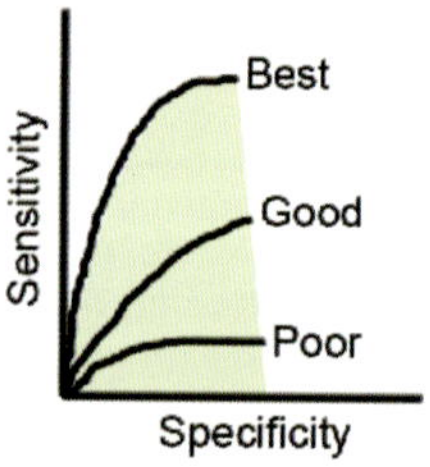

Area under the curve represents accuracy. More accuracy is the best.
The higher the sensitivity curve, the better.

Most Common Equations

Sensitivity Screening

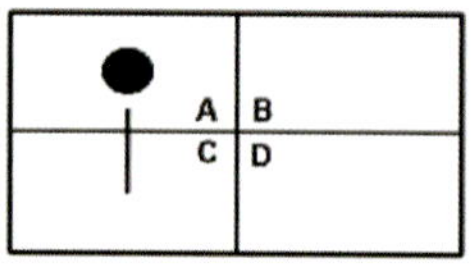

High Accuracy = High Sensitivity

$$\frac{A}{A + C}$$

Sensitivity Confirmatory

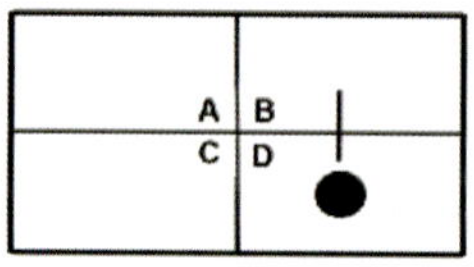

$$\frac{D}{B + D}$$

Case Control (Odds Ratio)

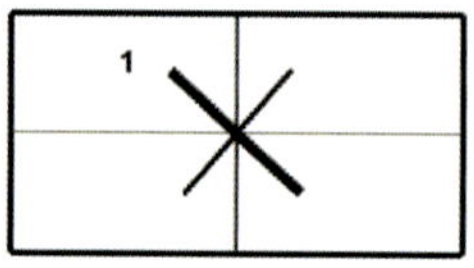

1 = No difference between groups
>1 = High risk of disease if exposed to risk
<1 = Protective, Low risk of disease

$$\frac{A \times D}{B \times C}$$

Cohert (Relative Risk)

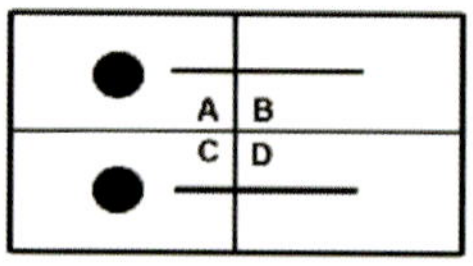

$$\frac{A}{A + B} \Big/ \frac{C}{C + D}$$

Positive Predictive Value (PPV)

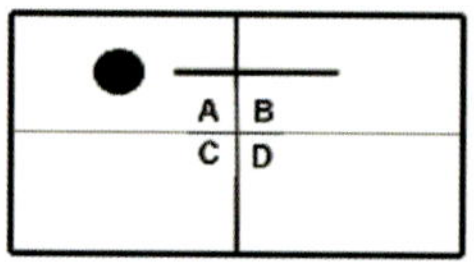

$$\frac{A}{A + B}$$

Negative Predictive Value (NPV)

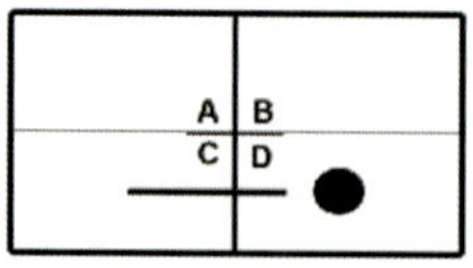

$$\frac{D}{C + D}$$

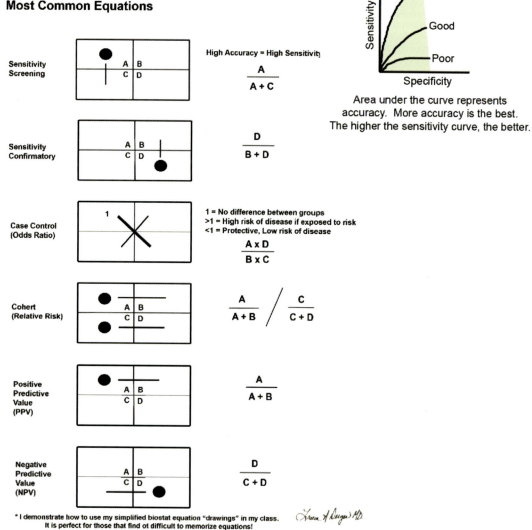

* I demonstrate how to use my simplified biostat equation "drawings" in my class. It is perfect for those that find ot difficult to memorize equations!

Meanings

- RR = .71 (p- .01)   Means there is a 1% chance that the result was observed by chance.
- P= <.01 = 1%   Means that there is no association between factors.

Linear Relationships (Scatter Plots)

- 0 = No relationship
- Negative relationship: -1 = Negative. The closer to -1, the stronger the correlation is.
  Negative correlation means that as the value of one of the variables increases, the values of the second variable decrease.
  They are inversely proportional: go in opposite directions.
  (X increases so Y decreases. X decreases so Y increases)
  Ex: Students that spend more time playing video games tend to have lower grades.

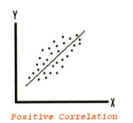

Positive Correlation

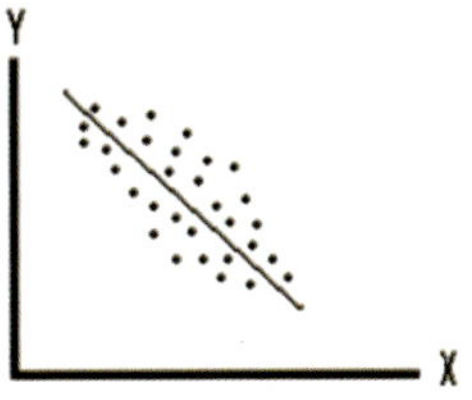

Negative Correlation

- Positive relationship: 1 = Positive. The closer to 1, the stronger the correlation is.
  Positive correlation means that as the value of one of the variables increases, the values of the second variable increases.
  (X increases so Y increases. X decreases so Y decreases)
  They go the same direction. (If one decreases, the other will decrease).
  EX: This past year the crime rate increased and during this period the number of gun sales increased.

Prevalence and Incidence

- Prevalence and Positive Predictive Value (PPV) always go in the same direction. Ex: If PPV goes up, Prevalence goes up.
- Prevalence and PPV are inversely proportional to Negative Predictive Value. If Prevalence or PPV goes up, then NPV goes down.
- High incidence = high prevalence.
- Prevalence = Incidence x duration (time)
- Incidence is NEW cases only. These are not cases that previously existed.
  Ex: If you are asked what the incidence is of a disease in 2010 – do **NOT** include ANY cases of the disease that were present in 2009. Incidence would be ONLY what NEW cases developed in 2010.
- **Incidence calculation**:   New Cases Only / All the population at risk (those that do NOT have the disease) x 100
- Prevalence: Is ALL cases of the disease. New cases and old cases. So in the example above, to calculate prevalence you would include all cases from 2009 and 2010.
- **Prevalence calculation**: All existing cases (new and old) / Total population x 100

	Incidence	**Prevalence**
New Treatment (treating something that is already occurring)	No change	Decrease in Prevalence
New Vaccine	Decrease in Incidence	Decrease in Prevalence
Increase in Deaths	No change	Decrease in Prevalence
Increase Long Term Survival (managing chronic issues, good medical practices)	No change	Increase in prevalence

Error Types

The NULL hypothesis (H0). The NULL (means NO, nothing, negative) always says to every study: "You **WILL NOT** be successful". It does not believe that any study will be successful. Therefore if you reject the "Null", then you are saying it is wrong and that you ARE successful. If you accept the "Null", then you are saying that you agree and were not successful.

Type I Error (aka: Alpha Error)

- Alpha is related to the level of significance.
- Type I is associated with the "P" value.
- If the "P" value is < .05 then this is significant. It means there is less than a 5% chance that the result of the study was due to chance.
- If the "P" value is > .05 then this means the study was not significant. The results may be due to chance.
- A Type I error means that you say your study WAS successful, but it really was not. Therefore you rejected the "Null".
  Ex: A scientist was sure his drug cured a disease because of his findings and told everyone. He was so excited, only to find out that his drug really did not cure the disease. Therefore, the "Null" was true all along, but the scientist rejected it – he did not believe it. (He believed a falsehood).
- False positive error.

Type II Error (aka: Beta Error)

- Beta error: 1 – B
- Beta error is related to statistical POWER.
- False negative error.
- A Type II error means that you say your study was NOT successful, but it really was. Therefore you accept the "Null".
  Ex: A scientist was sure his drug cured a disease but after his findings concluded that it did not. But later found that his drug really did cure the disease. Therefore, the "Null" was incorrect all along, but the scientist believed it.
- Type II errors are common when there is low power (small sample size). Therefore if you increase the sample size, you increase the power. (**tip**: There is always POWER in numbers).
- Many times studies will combine smaller studies so that they have many more involved which will then raise the power. This is called "Meta Analysis".
- The Power can be raised by: Increasing the sample size, increasing the precision of measurement or increasing the expected effect size.

Confidence Interval (CI)

- If CI is = 1 then there is no conclusion. More study is needed.
- If CI includes the number "1" in its range, then the study is insignificant. It is not effective. The "P" value > .05.
  Ex: (-5 – 45). When you go from – 5 up to 45, you must cross the number "1", therefore it is insignificant.
- If CI does NOT include the number "1" in its range, then the study is significant. It is effective, it is working.
  This means that the "P" value is < .05 (less than 5% chance the results are due to chance), therefore the "Null" is rejected.
  Ex: (1.05 – 12). When you go from 1.05 up to 12, you never cross the number "1", as you are already past it, therefore the study is significant.
- When the range of the CI becomes closer, then the findings of the study are more accurate (margin of error becomes smaller).
  Ex: CI #1: (2 – 12) CI #2: (2 – 5) CI #2 range is much closer, therefore much more accurate.
- A smaller sample size (smaller power) shows a wider CI (2 – 12)
- A larger sample (larger power) shows a more narrow CI (2 -5)
- CI and Z Score
  90% = 1.65
  95% = 1.96
  98% = 2.33
  99% = 2.58

Relative Risk (RR) (aka: Hazards Ratio)

- The risk (or event) of getting a disease
- RR – 1/RR
- If RR or Hazards Ratio is <1, this means that you are protective, low risk of getting the disease.
- If RR or Hazards Ratio is >1, this means that you are at a higher risk of getting the disease.
- Ex: .07 (1.2 – 4.3)
  In this example, the .07 is the RR (or Hazards Ratio). This number is <1, therefore the group is protected, they have a low risk of getting the disease. (the 1.2 – 4.3 represents the confidence interval).
- Ex: 1.70 (1.2 – 4.3)
  In this example, the 1.70 is the RR (or Hazards Ratio). This number is >1, therefore the group is at a high risk of getting the disease. (the 1.2 – 4.3 represents the confidence interval).

Central Tendency

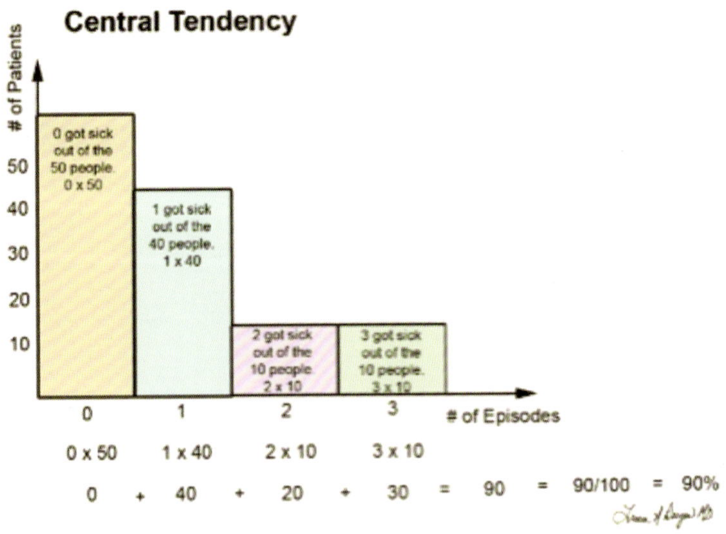

Range in Standard Deviation

- Generally always uses 2 Standard Deviations
- The Standard Deviation and the mode will be given.
- Ex: If the mode is 50 and the Standard Deviation is 5. Calculate the range.
  If it ask for the range within 2 Standard Deviations, then 5 will represent each Standard Deviation. There are 2 SD above the mode (50) and 2 SD below the mode (50). Each represents the value of 5.
  So 2 SD above would be: 2 x 5 = 10. So 10 added on to the mode (10 + 50) to account for the number above is 60.
  2 SD below would be: 2 x 5 = 10. So 10 subtracted from the mode (50 – 10) to account for then umber below is 40.
  Therefore the entire range of this SD would be 20. (It would range from 40 on the low end to 60 on the high end).

Number Needed to Treat (NNT)

- This is the number of people that you would need to treat before ONE person benefited.
  You would want this number to be as close to 1 as possible. Meaning: If it was "1", then every person treated would become better.
- 1/ARR

Number Needed to Harm (NNH)

- This is the number of people that you would need to treat before hurting one person.
  You would want this number to be as high as possible. Meaning, you do not want to hurt anyone.
- 1/AR

tip: A quick, good "estimate" of the NNT or NNH is to quickly look at the events between the 2 groups (control and experimental). Event means the number of people that were affected (or hurt) from the risk or drug. There will be people affected from both groups. Quickly subtract these 2 numbers (it doesn't matter what group you subtract from what: just subtract the small number from the large). Now, look at the answers and see what tense they want the answer to be in: % or decimal, etc). Then take the number you got from the subtraction and divide it into "1". Then take this answer and convert it into the final tense they want the answer to be in.
Ex: Group 1 had 10 people affected, Group 2 had 2 people affected. 10 – 2 = 8. Then take the 8 and divide into 1. This gives you .125 if they want a decimal or 12.5% if they want a %. So your NNT or NNH is 1 person (rounded down from 1.25) or 12.5%.

Funnel Plot

- Shows a bias or power of study
- If 95% of the dots are within the triangle, then there is no bias.
- The higher the power, the dots will all be inside the triangle and close to the top point.
- The lower the power, the dots will closer to the bottom of the triangle.

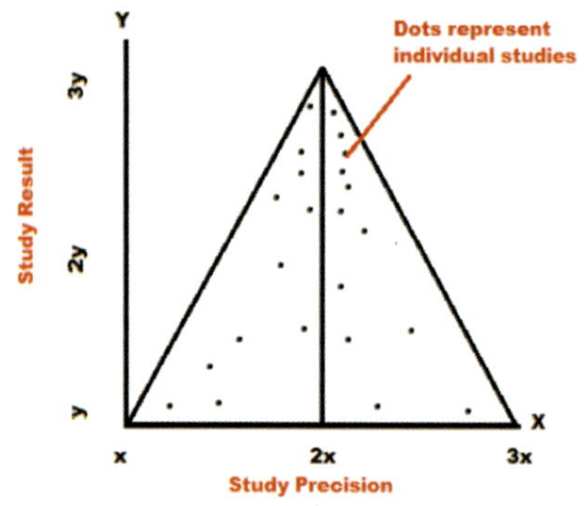

BIOSTAT PRACTICE QUESTIONS

Relative Risk (Cohort) AKA: Risk of RATIOS

How many times exposure to the risk increases the risk of disease between the exposed group and unexposed group.

Table: Risk	Lung CA	No Lung CA	Total
Exposed (smokers)	283	725	1008
Nonexposed (no smoker)	64	1010	1074
TOTAL	347	1735	2082

EX:

Test results from a cohort study of lung CA in which 1008 smokers and 1074 non smokers were followed. The **incidence** of lung CA over the time period of the study among those that were exposed to the risk (cigarettes) is 283/1008 (.28 or 28%) and the **incidence** among those not exposed (control group) was 64/1074 (.06 or 6%).

.28/.06 = 4.67 **(# affected in risk group / # affected in control group)**

Means: People that smoked were 4.67 times more likely to develop lung CA than nonsmokers

Attributable Risk
(aka: Risk Difference)
The difference in risk or incidence of the disease between two groups of people. (control vs experimental)

Incidence of disease in exposed (experimental) minus the incidence of disease in non-exposed (control)

Example (using the study in the previous slide, lung CA in smokers verses non-smokers) The attributable risk is .28 - .06 = .22 (or 22%)

Meaning of the 28% incidence of lung cancer among the smokers, 22% is attributable to smoking.

Relative Risk Reduction
1 – relative risk

EX: A double blind randomized clinical trial in which 6595 men with high cholesterol levels were randomly assigned to groups taking either a placebo or a cholesterol lowering drug for an average of 4.9 years. There were 73 death from cardiovascular disease in the placebo group (CONTROL) (mortality rate = 73/3293 = .022 or 2.2%) in the cholesterol drug group (EXPERIMENTAL GROUP) there was 50 deaths. (mortality rate = 50/3302 = .015 = 1.5%).

(Event rate in experimental group divided by event rate of control group)

Relative Risk: 1.5/2.2 = 0.68 1 - .068 = 0.32 or 32%

Meaning 32% of cardio deaths were prevented by the drug

Absolute Risk Reduction

SEE SLIDE ABOVE FOR STATS

(event rate of control group minus event rate in experimental group)

2.2% minus 1.5% = 0.7%

Which means that in the total time of the study, 4.9 years, that only 0.7% of the men were saved from a cardiovascular death.

NNT
of people needed to be treated before ONE person is helped

1/absolute risk reduction

AKA: Take the above slide: Event rate in control group minus event rate in experimental group and then put this figure under 1 and divide.

1 / 0.7% = 143

Need to treat 143 people in order to help 1 person

NNH
of people that are exposed to a risk factor before 1 is harmed

The SAME concept as in the above slide.

Event rate (percent) in experimental group minus event rate (percent) In control group = total

This answer is then put under the number 1 and then divide.

1 / answer = NNH

(Tip: Don't stress over what number needs to be subtracted from the other, Just always put the LARGER number on top. You can't subtract a larger Number from a smaller number! Don't worry about catagories: Control group (the one not receiving treatment) and the experimental group (the one receiving the treatment) **Watch for the PATTERN!!**

Example 1
Use the study below for the next ??'s

STUDY:

TREATMENT	DISEASE OUTCOME	
	Breast CA	No Breast CA
Placebo (control)	40	960
Drug (experimental)	10	990

1) What is the absolute risk (AKA: Incidence) of getting breast cancer for patients in the placebo group?
   a) 4%
   b) 1.6
   c) 24
   d) 67.5%
   e) 0.4

Answer #1 is A

Remember: **Absolute Risk is AKA: Incidence**
You are simply being asked what is the incidence of cancer in the control (placebo) group.

Overall incidence is the number of new cases divided by the number of total people.

For this question (they want to know the incidence for the control (placebo) group:

40/960 = .0416 round off to .04 = 4%

Example 2

What is the absolute risk of getting breast cancer for patients in the drug (experimental) group?

a) 30
b) 25%
c) 1%
d) 4
e) 0.5

Answer #2 is C

Same calculation as in example #1, except this is asking the incidence in the the drug (experimental) group.

10/990 = (always **ROUND OFF** to make it easy to calculate in your head so that it saves time on your exam!
10/1000 = .01 or 1%

Example 3

What is the relative risk reduction of breast cancer attributable to the drug?

a) 25%
b) 50%
c) 75%
d) 100%
e) 150%

Answer #3 is C

Remember the relative risk reduction is the drug (experimental) group OVER the placebo (control) group.
Equation = 1 – RR gives you what is attributable to the drug
**Be SURE to pay attention if they are wanting % or decimals in the answers.

Event rate in drug group: 10/990 = .01% = 1
Event rate in placebo group: 40/960 = .04% = 4

1 over 4 is ¼ or 25% = Relative Risk (meaning that patients exposed to the drug had 25% of the risk of cancer than those who took the placebo)

1 – 25% (.25) = 75% = Relative Risk Reduction (meaning 75% of the cancer was prevented by the drug)

Example #4

What is the absolute risk reduction in breast cancer attributable to the drug?

a) 1
b) 2
c) 3
d) 4
e) 5

Answer #4 is C

Remember Absolute risk reduction is the event rate of the placebo (control) group minus the event rate in the drug (experimental) group.

Event rate in placebo group = 4%
Event rate in the drug group = 1%

4% minus 1% = 3%

Example 5

What is the number needed to treat to prevent one case of breast cancer?

a) 2
b) 3
c) 4
d) 33.3
e) Cannot be calculated from the information given

Answer #5 is D

Remember NNT = 1 divided by absolute risk reduction

The absolute risk reduction (previous question) was 3%
This means that out of 100 women treated 3 fewer would get cancer.

100 / 3 = 33.3

OR ("pattern" method)
Event rate of group one = 40
Minus event of group two = 10
40 – 10 = 30 Therefore, 30 women would need to receive treatment before helping one

Example #6

If the drug cost $100 per month, what would be the cost of preventing 1 case of breast cancer in this 5 year study?

a) $1200
b) $6000
c) $20,000
d) $200,000
e) $330,000

Answer # 6 is D

$100 per month
$100 x 12 months per year = $1200
$1200 x 5 years = $6000
33 patients (NNT) to prevent 1 case = $6000 x 33 = $198,000
(or "pattern" 30 patients x $6000 = $180,000 (round off)

Prevalence and Incidence

New treatment decreases duration of illness, but does not alter the number of new cases or people dying = Decrease prevalence of disease.

A new vaccine (or treatment) is found to improve the prevention of a non-fatal disease = Decreases BOTH the incidence and prevalence of the disease.

If a disease is stopped (cured) or the disease process is shortened, the prevalence will decrease. (Less people will have it as long)

Question #1

Due to an effective prevention program, the prevalence of an infectious disease in a community has been reduced by 90%. A physician continues to use the same diagnostic test for the disease that she has always used. How have the test's characteristics changed?

a) Its sensitivity has increased
b) Its specificity has decreased
c) Its positive predictive value has increased
d) Its negative predictive value has increased
e) The test's characteristics have not changed

Answer #1 is D

Remember: P follows P Prevalence follows PPV
If one goes up, the other goes up.

NPV is opposite!

In this question, it states that the prevalence of the disease is reduced. Therefore, go look in the answer for either: PPV does down (decreased) or that NPV goes up (Increased). Answer D

Example #1

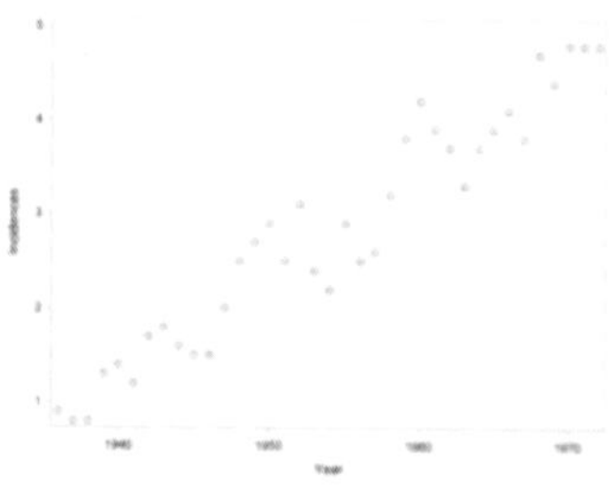

The best number representation on the graph above would be?
a) .8
b) -.3
c) .3
d) -.8

Answer #1 is A

The line is going upwards, there for there is a positive correlation.
A perfect positive correlation (an exact straight line) is "1".

The points on the graph are fairly close to each other therefore there is a strong correlation.

The closest number to "1" would indicate the strongest correlation.
The closest positive number to "1" is .8

Scattergraph/Scatterplot

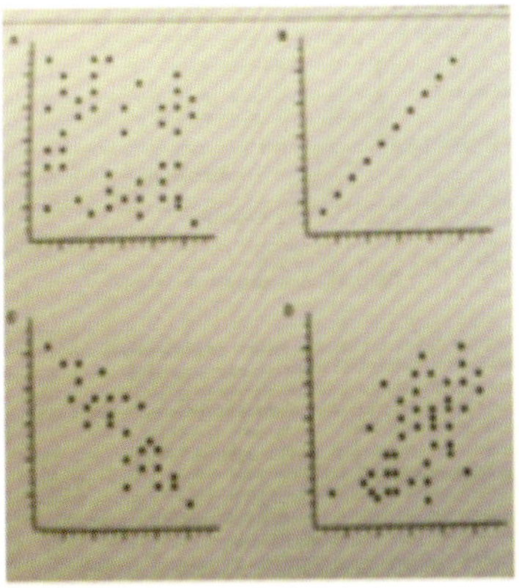

1) If no line can be drawn to fit the plotted points, there is **no correlation, value is 0**
   (Example A)
2) If an exact straight line can be drawn to plot all the points, the **correlation value is 1 (or -1)**
   (Example B)
3) If the points are fairly close together in a "line" format, there is a strong correlation.
   The closer the plots are located together, the stronger the correlation = meaning **closer to 1 or -1**
   (Example C)
4) If the points are further apart in a "line" format, then there is a weak correlation. The further the plots are apart, the weaker the correlation. = meaning **further away from 1 (or -1)**
   (Example D)

If the "line" is going upward from the Y axis, it is a positive correlation. The closer the number given is to +1, the stronger the correlation is. Example: .8 is a stronger correlation than .3 Examples: B and D
If the "line" is going downward from the Y axis, it is a negative correlation. The closer the number given is to -1, the stronger The correlation is. Example: C

Correlation / Scattergrams

Positive Correlation: high values of one variable are associated with high values of the other variable.
 Ie: high salt intact are associated with high blood pressure

Negative Correlation: high values of one variable are associated with low values of the other variable.
 Ie: high cigarette smoking are associated with low life expectancy

Sensitivity vs Specificity

SeNsitivity = sensitivity of a test is its ability to detect people who DO HAVE the disease.
 ie: Screening Test Best screening test: 100% sensitivity
 Negative Test RULES OUT DISEASE (tip: hate to be with**OUT** my senses)

sPecificity = specificity of a test is its ability to detect people that do NOT HAVE the disease
 ie: Confirmatory Test
 A POSITIVE TEST RULES IN DISEASE

BEWARE: Pay CLOSE attention to see if they are asking for sensitivity or specificity!!

FP: Type II error. A positive test is obtained in a person who does NOT have the disease

FN: Type I error. A negative test is obtained in a person who HAS the disease

TN: A negative test obtained in a person who does NOT have the disease

TP: A positive test obtained in a person who DOES have the disease

Precision vs Accuracy

Precision (AKA: Reliability) : The degree to which a figure (such as an estimate of a population) is immune from random variation.

A reliable (precise) test is consistent, stable and dependable.

The width of the confidence interval reflects precision. The wider the CI, the less precise.

Bias's cause precision to decrease.

A state of strict exactness – how often something is strictly exact.

Uses multiple measurements or factors. It is the degree to which several measurements provide answers very close to each other. It is an indicator of the scatter (scatterplot) in the data. The lesser the scatter (closer to 1), the higher the precision.

It means the measurements are ALL close to each other, but they may/may not be close to the target.

Ex: If you obtain a weight of 3.2 kg for a given substance but the actual known weight is 10kg, then your measurement is not accurate – it is not close to the known value.

Ex: A basketball player shoots baskets. If the player shoots with accuracy, his aim will always take the ball close to or in the basket. If the player shoots with precision, his aim will always take the ball to the same Location which may or may not be close to the basket. A good play will be both accurate and precise by Shooting the ball the same way each time and each time making it into the basket.

A measurement is VALID if it is both accurate and precise.

It is not necessary for precise measurements to be accurate or accurate measurements to be precise.

Accuracy vs Precision

Accuracy (AKA: Validity): The degree to which an estimate is immune from systematic error or bias.

The measurements are very close to the true or absolute value. The measurements are very near the target.

Scatter of the measurements does not have any significant role in accuracy.

Uses a single measurement or single factor.

It tests what it claims to test = the "Gold Standard"

The nearness of a measurement to the standard or true value. A highly accurate measuring device will provide measurements very close to the standard.

Internal validity: are the results of the study valid for the population of patients who were actually studied?

External validity: are the results of the study valid for other patients? (not studied)

Ex: If you obtain a weight of a given substance five times and get 3.2 kg each time, then your measurement is very precise. Precision is independent of accuracy. You can be very precise but inaccurate. You can also be accurate but imprecise.

Ex: In target shooting a high score indicates nearness to the bullseye and is a measure of the shooters accuracy.

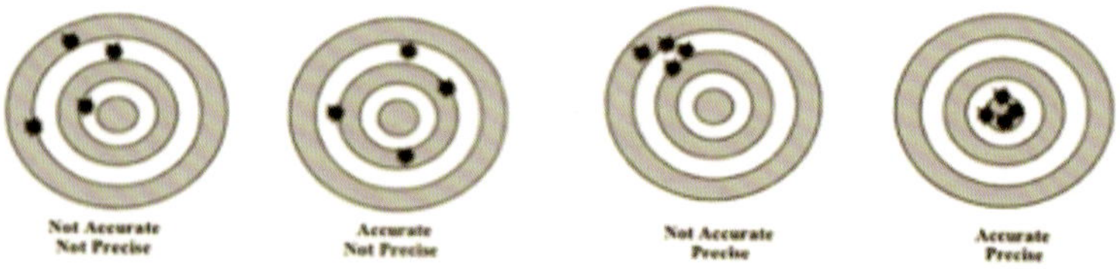

Question #1

A test for Hep C is performed for 200 patients with biopsy proven disease And 200 patients known to free from the disease. The test shows postive Results in 180 patients with the disease and negative results in 150 Patients without the disease. Among those tested, this test therefore.....

a) Has a positive predictive value of 90%
b) Has a negative predictive value of 75%
c) Has a sensitivity of 90%
d) Has a specificity of 82.5%
e) The information given is insufficient

ANSWER # 1 is C

The key to questions like this is that you must know:

1) How to set up your chart correctly
2) Correct equations

In this question:

1) There are 180 WITH a positive test for the Dz (goes in A)
2) There are 150 negative for the DZ (goes in D)
3) There are 200 patients in each group, so the total overall patients goes in the TOTAL column, vertically
4) Fill in the vertical blank spaces (B and C). Vertically under A, you would have to have 20 in C to equal 200 patients. Vertically under D you would have to have 50 in B to equal 200 patients.
5) Then add A and B columns horizontally to get the total of test that showed positive results
6) Then add C and D columns horizontally to get the total of test that showed negative results
7) Now, the answer is simply a matter of trying the different equations (sensitivity, specificity, PPV and NPV) and see which one is in the answer

Standard Deviation

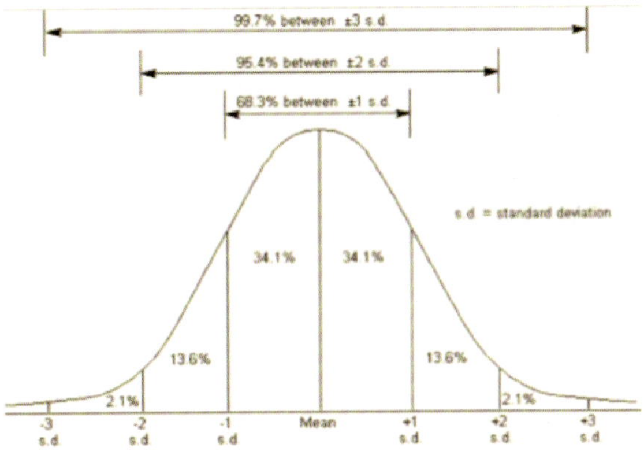

Standard Deviation Rules

Range:

1) They will give you the mean (average)
2) They will then give you what the standard deviation number is
3) They will give you how many standard deviations they want in the range
   ie: 1 or 2 (normally 2 is always used)
4) If they want 2 standard deviations, that the standard deviation number that was given and double that number (if they want 2 standard deviations)
5) Add that doubled number to the mean number you were given and this gives you the number of the upper range
6) Then subtract that doubled number from the mean given and this will give you the bottom number of that range
7) The bottom number to the top number you calculated is the range

Tip: Be careful to note if the question requires using the entire standard deviation Curve (meaning: 1 SD = 68%, 2 SD = 95% and 3 SD = 99%). If they are only using Half of the curve, use only that half, do not calculate in the other half. Esp. on The 2 SD which is 95%, which leaves 5% (meaning 2.5% on each end – not 5%)

ETHICS

Ethics can be one of the trickiest areas of the USMLE exam. Most people go into the exam expecting this area to be a "walk in the park" because most of ethics tends to be either obvious concepts or knowledge of the law. However, the test writers are amazingly gifted at wording ethics questions in such a way that you may find yourself stumped between two answer choices the majority of the time.

What you need to know

- The laws
- The exceptions to the laws
- General ethical decisions
- Do not "add" to an ethics question. When you read the question, consider yourself in that position at that EXACT minute. Don't think about what you would do a little later. This is critical in situations where you have a difficult job to carry out: Such KEY examples of this concept are:

  1) You have a signed advance directive from your patient, signed, stating that he does not want to be kept on life support. The patient is now unconscious and in a situation where he must go on life support. However, at this time family members are arguing or trying to convince you to put him on life support. There is NO doubt that you must honor your patients signed directive, you are going to "pull the plug", but NOT at this exact time. The USMLE (and in real practice) you are going to sit down and try to work with the family to help them understand what is happening. Remember, this is a hard thing for family members. You always do what you can as a physician to help people understand, to comfort and promote cooperation and accomodation.

  2) You have a male patient that has tested positive for HIV. He is married and contracted the disease when he was away on a business trip. He pleads with you to not tell his wife, that it will destroy his marriage. There is NO doubt that you have a legal obligation to report this to the CDC and you know that the man's wife WILL be informed, one way or the other. However, at this exact time, your job is to try and convince the man to inform his wife himself. This type of news would be much better coming from the husband rather than a stranger knocking on her door. So always choose the answer that promotes cooperation.

THE LAWS and EXCEPTIONS

- LIFESAVING PROCEDURES FOR CHILDREN (<18): When it comes to providing LIFE SAVING treatment to a minor, you do it. Regardless of what the parents wishes are or if you are unable to contact the parents.
  The typical case: A Jehovah's Witness adult and child will be brought into the ED after a major auto accident (MVA) with serious bleeding, both requiring a blood transfusion. The adult will tell you he/she does not want a transfusion and that they do not want the child to have a transfusion. In this case you will simply provide the adult with heavy fluids and Pressors in hopes their life may be spared, but you will immediately give the child a blood transfusion.
  You ALWAYS have the right and duty to save a minor's life.
- TREATING MINORS (<18): You can provide services, treatments and prescriptions to minors, without the parent's knowledge or approval for any issues regarding sex and drugs.
- TREATING MINORS (<18): You can provide treatment for minors without parental consent in these situations: The minor is married, in the military, is totally self-supportive (living on their own and paying their own bills), if it is an emergency and the parents are not reachable for consent.
- INFORMING CHILDREN ABOUT THEIR HEALTH CONDITION: Parents of the child are able to decide what information can be given to the child.
- MINOR THAT IS PREGNANT or HAS GIVEN BIRTH (<18): This patient has the right to make all decisions regarding her child (care, adoption, etc) despite what the parents of the minor want.
- CHILD ABUSE: Anytime, for any reason, you suspect child abuse, it MUST be reported to Child Services immediately. A physician is totally protected by law in this case. No actions may ever be brought against a physician for reporting a suspected child abuse.
- ELDERLY ABUSE: The same rules apply for elderly abuse as with child abuse. It is against the law. Suspected elderly abuse must be reported. (Be concerned about abuse when the elderly patient will not look at you when you ask them questions and/or the person that brought them in (usually one of their children) is domineering and answers all the questions for the parent. In this case, ask the accompanying person to leave the room so that you can speak to the elderly patient alone).
  Elderly abuse must be reported even if it is against the will of the patient.
- SPOUSE/SIGNIFICANT OTHER ABUSE: You cannot report abuse to a patient that has experienced/is experiencing spouse/significant other abuse. You CAN provide information on places to go for safety, etc. Never advise your patient to "leave" the person!
- CONFIDENTIALITY: Strict confidentiality is required of all doctors and their patients. A doctor may not discuss a patient with anyone (using the patients name or any other identifying information that would lead anyone to figure out the identity of the individual). This also includes any other doctor that is not involved with the case and patient. This also includes **ALL FAMILY MEMBERS** (including a spouse), the patient MUST give consent before any aspect of their health care can be discussed.
- CONFIDENTIALITY EXCEPTIONS: Anytime there are concerns for these issues a physician can break the rules of confidentiality: The patient threatens harm to themselves or others, reportable diseases, child or elderly abuse, impaired drivers (epileptics).
- CONFIDENTIALITY: Anytime any other individual informs you about issues regarding your patient, you should not discuss anything with the individual but should contact the patient to discuss.

- GIFTS: You cannot accept substantial gifts or money from patients. As long as the gift is small, thoughtful type gift, it is ok to accept this as you run the risk of hurting the feelings of a well meaning, appreciative patient.
  GIFTS: You can't accept any gifts from patients when the intention is to gain prescriptions.
- GIFTS FROM THE INDUSTRY: It is unacceptable to accept any gift, regardless of how small (pens, cups, t-shirts), from anyone from the medical industry (ie: drug companies/representatives). This does not pertain to accepting meals when the meals are in direct connection with educational programs.
- GUEST SPEAKERS FOR A DRUG COMPANY: If asked by a drug company to do a presentation for their drug, you are allowed to accept travel and accommodations. You cannot accept any type of a prepared presentation made by the company for that drug.
- TAKING PART IN A DRUG TRIAL: Before a physician can participate in any type of drug study, they must get consent from the National Institute of Health. (NIH)
- REFERRAL FEES FROM DRUG COMPANIES: If a physician is participating in a study and the drug company pays a referral fee, the physician is required to inform the patient about the referral fee.
- PREGNANCY: A pregnant woman has the right to make all decisions regarding herself, even at the risk of the fetus' life. She can refuse any treatment or procedure up until the time the baby is born. Once the baby is born and they are two separate people, the physician can intervene to care for the baby in life-threatening situations without the mother's consent
- ABORTION: These laws differ by state. Never advise a patient to get an abortion for any reason, including the fact there may be a medical condition with the fetus.
- ABORTION: A physician can refuse to do an abortion, but they must help refer the patient to a physician that will.
- ABORTION: You do not need the consent of the father for an abortion. Laws are dependent upon the states. Some states require the patient to consult with the parents.
- FIRING A PATIENT: A physician can "fire" a patient. However, before the patient can be fired, the physician MUST provide a referral to another physician that will take their case first. You can not abandon a patient.
- ACCEPTING A PATIENT: Physicians do not have any obligation to take a patient. But once you see or speak to (in person or on the phone) to a patient and give any advice/information, this patient is considered your patient.
- OBTAINING CONSENT: The physician that is performing the procedure/surgery must obtain the consent. They cannot ask another doctor to do it for them. This is to insure that the patient is properly informed about all aspects of the procedure/surgery.
- DATING A PATIENT: NO, NO, NO. Never even imply this is a possibility at a later date should they no longer be a patient. This also includes medical students and any patient they have ever treated.
- MISTAKE: If a physician (or staff) makes a medical mistake with a patient, no matter how minor, the physician MUST inform the patient of the error.
- "ALMOST A MISTAKE": In the event that a mistake is almost made but is caught, the patient does not need to be informed, however, the mistake must be reported to the hospital so that a "**Root Cause Analysis**" can be preformed. This is a study that determines the cause of the mistake so procedures can be put into place so that it does not happen again.
- ENDING A PATIENTS LIFE (AKA: euthanasia): These laws differ by state. Physicians should refuse any assisted suicide. However, physicians can prescribe medical analgesics or withhold medical treatment or care that "happen" to shorten the patient's life.
  Any adult patient may refuse nutrition. A physician cannot force a patient to have nutrition or fluids.
  Euthanasia: Physician directly administers the means of ending a life. This is NOT ethical and is wrong.
  Physician-assisted suicide: The physician provides the means for a patient to end their own life. This is NOT ethical and is wrong.
- EXECUTION of PRISONERS: Physicians are never to participate in an execution even if execution is legal in that state. This includes formulating the lethal injection or pronouncing death.
- TORTURE: Physicians are never to participate in the torture of anyone (prisoner), even if the physician is in the military and is commanded to participate by a superior. This also includes insuring that any torture administered by someone else will not be fatal or cause permanent harm.
- INSURANCE: When treating a patient a physician should never limit or deny any type of care or treatment to any patient, despite what is or is not covered by their insurance. All patients are entitled to all treatment options.
- REPORTING IMPAIRED COLLEAGUES: It is a physician's responsibility to report any behavior, by another physician that is ON DUTY, that is against hospital rules or that could **endanger a patient's care**. If the physician in question is ON DUTY: this includes: alcohol or drug use, sexual offense, any condition that would make the physician unfit to practice or potentially put a patient in harms way. NOTE: if the physician is off duty and their actions in no way affect a patient's care (ie: he is brought into the ED because he was involved in an accident and alcohol is smelled on his breath, he is caught stealing money – this is NOT reportable).
  Reporting chain of command: If the offending physician is a Resident, it is reported to the Program Director, if the offending physician is an employee of the hospital, it is reported to the hospital administration, if it is a physician at an independent clinic, it is reported to the states medical board and if it is a faculty member of a medical school, it is reported to the Dean or Department chair.
- HIV POSITIVE HEALTHCARE WORKERS: These individuals are not required to inform their patients or other hospital staff of their condition.
- HIV CONFIDENTIALITY: HIV patients have the right to confidentiality of their status. This confidentiality can be broken in order to protect those that are uninfected sexual partners or those sharing needles with the patient.
- TREATMENT of HIV PATIENTS: It is legal for a physician to refuse to treat a patient with HIV. (Unethical, but legal).
- EXTRAMARITAL AFFAIRS: The patient's confidentiality must be maintained at all times unless the situation involves a communicable/reportable disease or risk of safety (suicide/homicide).
- TB PROPHYLAXIS: If a healthcare employee or healthcare job applicant has a positive PPD test and a negative chest x-ray, they can refuse the INH/B6 prophylaxis and it not affect their job or ability to be hired.

- WITHHOLDING PATIENT INFORMATION: Every patient has the right to know everything about their condition as long as they are able mentally able to make their own decisions. If the family request that you not tell the patient because they feel the information would be detrimental, find out why the family believes this.
- PERFORMING SURGERY and FINDING ADDITIONAL PATHOLOGIES THAT COULD BE CORRECTED DURING THAT SURGERY: You must wake the patient to obtain consent to do the additional procedure.
- ORGAN DONOR: Even if the patient has signed the consent on the back of their drivers license giving permission for organ donor ship, the family can override this consent.
- ORGAN DONOR: The physician should never ask for consent for the donation of an organ. It is an ethical conflict. This request must only be done by the organ donor committee of the hospital.
- ORGAN DONOR: No one can be paid for organ donations.
- DONATIONS of SPERM and EGG: Anyone can donate sperms or eggs and they can receive pay for the donation.
- IMPAIRED DRIVERS: Physicians cannot take a patient's driver's license away (such as in the case of a seizure disorder). This must be done by the Dept. of Motor Vehicles.
- IMPAIRED DRIVERS REGARDING SEIZURES: This can differ from state to state. Physicians can't stop someone from driving, admit them to the hospital, take their keys or report them to the police. They can suggest the patient call someone for a ride or consider a different method of transportation.
- IMPAIRED DRIVERS REGARDING INTOXICATION: An intoxicated patient cannot be allowed to leave the hospital/ER as long as their alcohol level is above the legal limit. Once the level drops below the legal limit they are permitted to leave.
- DNR (Do not resuscitate. AKA: No code): Means that if a patient stops breathing or their heart stops beating that CPR (cardiopulmonary resuscitation or ACLS (advanced cardiac life support) is not given. They are not to be intubated or given CPR in order to keep them alive. This does NOT mean that other forms of treatment are not given. This includes: surgery, medicines, chemotherapy, procedures, etc.
- FUTILE CARE: A physician is not required (can refuse) to provide care or treatments that will not work or provide no benefit. This includes providing care to a patient that has been declared brain dead.
- MALPRACTICE: The factor that decreases the potential of a malpractice suit the most is that the patient feels that the physician truly cares and has compassion.

GENERAL ETHICAL SITUATIONS

- ALWAYS try and ask open-ended questions in order to encourage discussion. To try and find out what or why the person is doing/not doing what they should.
- ALWAYS try and promote cooperation and understanding.
- ALWAYS try and accommodate the patient.
- Always try and find out why the patient feels the way they do. Never say the "typical" feel good comments to a patient in order to make them feel better.
- Angry patients. This usually happens when a physician is late to the appointment. Always apologize for the inconvenience but do not explain the delay.
- Patients unhappy with another doctor: Recommend the patient to speak directly to the other physician, you do not speak to the other physician for them.
- Unnecessary procedures: As always, try to understand why the patient wants the procedure and discuss their concerns with them. Do not perform unnecessary procedures. You may help refer them to another physician.
- Even if something is legal a physician must never do anything unethical.

ETHICAL PRINCIPLES

- **Autonomy**: Respect each patient as an individual and their right to decide for themselves what they want regarding their medical care. Ex: A patient can refuse a life saving procedure or medicines.
- **Beneficence** (fiduciary duty): Act in the best interest of the patient.
- **Nonmaleficence**: To Do No Harm
- **Justice**: Treat patients fairly and equitably (this does not mean equally: in cases of triage, the most critical patients will be seen first).

INFORMED CONSENT: Must include: information, competence and voluntariness.

- Disclosure: Full disclosure about every part of the patient's care and treatment options. Discussing all positive benefits and risk of the procedure or treatment.
- Alternatives to the procedure/treatment are given.
- Understanding: The patient must understand/comprehend everything about the treatment/procedure. This includes that the information is provided/presented in a language that the patient can understand.
  If a patient speaks a different language you must wait until the translator for the hospital can be involved.
- Mental Capacity: Mentally able to make a decision.
- **Voluntariness**: The patient is no coerced or manipulated.
- The informed consent is required for each separate treatment/procedure that is being done/considered.

Exceptions to informed consent

- Patient is incompetent and can't make decisions
- Therapeutic privilege: withholding information that would severely harm the patient
- Patient waves the right of informed consent
- Implied consent in cases of emergencies

ADVANCE DIRECTIVES

- Medical Power of Attorney: (AKA: Health care proxy). Patient designates a person to make medical decisions on their behalf in the event they lose decision-making capabilities.
- Living Will (written advance directive): Patient writes the treatments that they wish to accept or decline in the event they lose decision-making capabilities.
- Oral Advance Directive: Patients oral statements that express their wishes prior to becoming incapacitated.
- Surrogate Decision Maker: In the case the patient has not provided an advance directive this individual would speak for the patient. **ORDER OF SURROGATES: Spouse, adult children, parents, adult siblings, other relatives**.
- DNR (Do Not Resuscitate): This order refusal for endotracheal intubation and cardiopulmonary resuscitation (CPR) (loss of ability to breath or if the heart stops). DNR does not mean the refusal of treatments, therapy, testing, etc.

ETHICS COMMITTEE

This committee is for purposes of making decisions in these situations:

- No clearly stated wishes/decisions on the part of the patient
- When the family/caregivers are in disagreement about the care of the patients
- The patient is a minor (not an adult) with capacity

COURT ORDER

- This is only used if all other attempts at agreement have been exhausted (including the ethics committee)
- No court order is necessary if the proxy makes the decision

PATIENT ABILITY

- Competent: Legal definition determined by courts
- Capacity: Used in medical situation to determine if someone has the ability to understand the informed consent as to make a decision in regards to receiving or refusing treatment/therapy.

PSYCHIATRIC EVALUTION

- If it is uncertain if a patient has the capacity to understand, a psychiatric evaluation may be needed.
- When it is clear the patient does not have the capacity (psychotic, delirious), no psychiatric evaluation is needed.

Payment Options to Doctors

1. **Capitation**: Paid fixed amount per patient, NOT service incentive to control cost b/c fixed budget given. **MOTIVATES to provide more PREVENTIVE CARE.** (Bigger tx or diseased tx = higher cost to provide and doctors are not paid for a lot of this.) Get more money for less expensive test (ie: screening) so catches DZ earlier and decreases the cost.
2. **Fee for Services**: Doctors are paid a fixed amount for each service or test. Face little financial risk so more apt to **increase # of services and increase # visits** per patient. No incentive to avoid costly test and procedures.
3. Discounted Fee For Service: Like "Fee for Service", but Doctor is reimbursed at a discounted amount. Causes doctors to be **more conservative and selective** if certain test or services are greatly discounted.
4. Salary: Paid fixed amount. Not tied to # patient or services. They face no risk (unless contracts have bonus's or withholdings). No financial incentive to change treatment patterns, services or # follow-ups.

MedicarE: Patients 65 and older or less than 65 with disabilities. (**tip**: MedicarE **E** = **E**lderly)
MedicaiD: Assistance for people with low income. (**tip**: Medicai**D** **D** = **D**estitute)

SCREENING – VACCINES – DIAGNOSTIC TEST - LABS

SCREENING SCHEDULES

Stages of Prevention

- Primary Prevention: Before patient develops disease
- Secondary Prevention: Action taken halts or delays the disease progress at the initial stage and stops complications
- Tertiary Stage: When disease progress is past the early stage and may disable or impair patient
- Quaternary Stage: Health activities that stop or limit unnecessary intervention or excessive intervention by health system

Screening Test	Age - Time of Screening	Notes
Cervical Cancer **PAP**	From 21 – 65 years of age: every 3 years. From 30 – 65: Can do PAP every 3 years or do PAP (cytology) and HPV every 5 years. If immunocompromised: first screen at the time of 1st sexual activity. Screen twice the first year and then yearly after this. (SLE, HIV, transplant, etc.) Can discontinue PAP's > 65 if there have been 3 consecutive negative test. No need to screen is there are no risk AND no DES exposure or hysterectomy with cervix Removed.	
Breast Cancer **Mammogram**	40 – 50 years of age: every 1 – 2 years 50 – 75 years of age: every 2 years > 75 years: no screening If there is a family history of breast cancer, begin mammograms 5 years before the age the family member was first diagnosed. Self-breast exams, MRI, CT, Ultrasound are not used for breast screening.	**NOTE: Mammograms lower the mortality more than any other cancer-screening test.**
Breast Cancer **BRCA Screen**	Test: If a family member has breast or ovarian cancer. ↑ Risk of the BRCA mutation if ≥ 2 or more close relatives had breast cancer before age 50, a male relative has breast cancer, a female relative has both breast and ovarian cancer, 2 relatives have ovarian cancer or you are of Ashkenazi Jewish ancestry and a close relative has breast or ovarian cancer. Low risk of having a BRCA mutation if: No relatives had breast cancer before age 50, no relatives with ovarian cancer and no male relatives that had breast cancer. BRCA mutation has an increased risk for breast and ovarian cancer. Note: Patients positive BRCA1 and BRCA2 test also have risk of developing: Pancreatic, colon, stomach, gallbladder, uterine or melanoma cancers. Men who test positive for BRCA run a risk for breast, pancreatic, testicular and prostate cancer.	
Bone Density **DEXA** (Dual Energy X-ray Absorptiometry)	≥ 65 years or under 65 and risk factors for osteoporosis: every 2 years. Hip fractures are more dangerous than myocardial infarctions in women. Bisphosphonates ("Dronates") are used to increase bone density. (Side effect: sit upright, drink lots of water to ↓ risk of pill esophagitis).	DEXA results: T-score -1.5 to – 2.5 = osteopenia T-score ≥ - 2.5 = osteoporosis
Lipid Screen	Cholesterol and LDL levels: Men > 35, Women > 45. Start screens at 20 years old if patient has: diabetes, family history, coronary artery DZ, aortic DZ, hyperlipidemia, CHD, peripheral vascular DZ (PAD).	

Screening Test cont'd

Diabetes Mellitus **HbA1c**	Normal HbA1c: 4 – 5.6% Pre-diabetic HbA1c 5.7 – 6.4% Diabetes: 2 separate measurements of an HbA1c ≥ 6.5% or fasting glucose > 126 or random glucose > 200 Screen if patient has hyperlipidemia and/or hypertension. Screening for the general public as long as there are no symptoms is not standard.	
Hypertension	Is standardly checked on all adults' ≥ 18 at all annual physicals.	
Lung Cancer Screen	Ages 55 – 80, yearly chest X-ray for those that are current smoker or persons that stopped smoking within the last 15 years. A one time CT scan in all long-term smokers with a 30 pack per year history at age 55. **Smoking cessation:** Oral meds: Varenicline, Bupropion. Non-oral: Nicotine gum and patches. Vapor cigarettes: fruit juice infused with nicotine that gradually decreases over time allowing the body to rid itself of nicotine.	Note: Most beneficial prevention: **stop smoking.**
Colon Cancer **Colonoscopy**	**Screening for Colon Cancer** • Normal patient: Begins screening by **colonoscopy at age 50**. Normal test results: **repeat every 10 years.** • Adenomatous polyps: Repeat colonoscopy every 3 to 5 years. • **CEA** (Carcinoembryonic antigen) marker is used to monitor therapeutic response. It is not used for screening. **Sigmoidoscopy** (similar to a colonoscopy): Exams only up to the sigmoid (most distal part of colon). Colonoscopy exams the entire large bowel. Positive test: If polyps or abnormal tissue is found the test will be followed up by a colonoscopy. Negative test (no cancer risk found): repeat sigmoidoscopy **every five years**. Sigmoidoscopy misses a large percent of cancers occurring proximal to the sigmoid colon. **Patient with family history of one member of the family:** Colonoscopy starting at age 40 or 10 years before the age of the family member that had cancer. (Which ever comes first) **Patient with family history of either 3 family members, 1 member with cancer < 50 or family history involving 2 generations:** (AKA: Lynch syndrome, Hereditary nonpolyposis colon cancer) Colonoscopy every 1 – 2 years starting at the age of 25. **Patient with ulcerative colitis**: start screening within 8 years of diagnosis of ulcerative colitis, then screen every 1 – 2 years later. **Patient with FAP** (Familial Adenomatous Polyposis) Autosomal Dominant. Must start colonoscopies at 12 years old and then every 1 – 2 years. **If a dysplastic polyp is found:** Repeat colonoscopy 3 – 5 years after the polyp was found.	Note: Colonoscopy is the best screening test for colon cancer.
Abdominal Aortic Aneurysm **AAA Screen**	Any men >65 that have EVER smoked, or are current smokers, receive one screening for AAA. Screen those from 65 – 75 with a family history of AAA.	If aneurysm is < 5mmrescreen in 6 months. If > 5 mm or has grown = surgical repair.
Chlamydia	<25 in all sexually active female 15 – 25 years old and in all prenatal test	
HIV, HBV	Prenatal testing	
Childrens: Hearing and Vision	Before the age of 5.	

Screening Test cont'd

Prostate Cancer	Not a standard screening test. PSA can be checked case by case **or if patient request**. From 40 – 70 prostate (PSA) is checked digitally. PSA screening does not provide any mortality benefit. It is used to monitor treatment and for reoccurrence.	
No Screening	Pancreatic Cancer Bladder Cancer	

VACCINE SCHEDULES/RECOMMENDATIONS

- **Immunocompromised defined as**: IC defined: **Steroid users**, COPD, asthma, emphysema, cardiovascular DZ, **diabetics**, chronic liver DZ, alcoholism, CSF leaks, chronic renal failure/dialysis, cochlear implants, **asplenic**, sickle cell, heme pathologies, **HIV**, chronic bronchitis and asthma, CSF leaks, SLE, transplants, **cancer**/chemotherapy, heart disease, autoimmune diseases and **chronic** diseases, alcoholics, smokers, IV drug users, anyone over 65.
- **Immunocompromised must have**:
    - Pneumococcal
    - Meningococcal
    - Influenza (annually to everyone, healthcare workers, pregnant women)
    - HEP A, HEP B
    - Tetanus every 10 years
- Pneumococcal, influenza and tetanus are the most beneficial vaccines for adults.

Childrens Vaccine Schedule

- If baby is preterm, vaccine schedule proceeds on chronologic age (day of birth being day 1)
- Do not adjust the dose on premature babies
- Do not give live vaccines to immunocompromised babies
- If children are mildly sick it is ok to get their vaccinations
- If children are sick (fever) it is best to wait. Antibodies are fighting off other antigens so they would not mount a response to the vaccine, therefore the vaccine would not work.
- It is ok to get all vaccinations at one time, there is no harm
- Egg Allergies:
  Contradictions: Do not give: Yellow fever vaccine
  No contraindications: It is ok to give vaccines if there are egg allergies with: MMR, Influenza (must use trivalent inactivated influenza vaccine and monitored for 30 minutes).

Vaccine	Age - Time – Situation for Vaccine	Notes
Pneumococcal (S. pneumonia)	Given to normal patient at 65 years. If vaccine is given prior to 65 years old, must give a booster in 5 years. Pneumococcal, influenza and tetanus are the most beneficial vaccines for adults. Immunocompromised from 2 – 64 years old: give at the time disease is diagnosed: COPD, asthma, emphysema, cardiovascular DZ, diabetics, chronic liver DZ, alcoholism, CSF leaks, renal failure, cochlear implants, asplenic, sickle cell, heme pathologies, chronic bronchitis, HIV, SLE, transplants	One vaccine, plus booster if given prior to 65 years. Vaccine is against the polysaccharide capsule. It can't present to T cells so it gives T cell independent with B cell response.
Meningococcal	Children at age 11. For anyone that is: collage age, lives in barracks, dorms, prisons, travel exposure, terminal complement deficiency, immunocompromised, asplenic.	One vaccine. The patient that benefits the most is the asplenic patient.
Shingles (Varicella zoster)	At 60 year old, even if the patient has had shingles. Prevents shingles.	1 vaccine
HPV	Non-pregnant females: 9 – 26 years old. Males: 9 – 21 years old. Do not give the vaccine to pregnant women. For the Gardasil vaccine do not give to those with yeast. For the Cervarix vaccine do not give to those with latex allergies.	2 vaccines

Tetanus	Td (toxoid) Everyone every 10 years. One Tdap (tetanus with pertussis) should be one of the boosters. Tetanus IG for those never vaccinated (used in post exposure prophylaxis). Prophylaxis: Clean wound: Booster at 10 years. Dirty wound: Booster if it has been more than 5 years since last tetanus shot. Never vaccinated or can't remember: Booster and IG. Pneumococcal, influenza and tetanus are the most beneficial vaccines for adults. **Babies/Children: Dtap: 5 doses before start of school (ages 4 – 6). Pertussis and Td given in the early teenage years.**	
Influenza (live or inactivated)	Everyone- **annually**. Immunocompromised must use injectable form, do not give nasal influenza vaccine (live). Pneumococcal, influenza and tetanus are the most beneficial vaccines for adults.	Egg allergy is NOT a contradiction. If there is an allergy to eggs: give only the inactivated form.
HEP A	Anyone that **travels out of the country**, immunocompromised, health care workers, HEP C, HIV, homosexual males, close contacts with HEP A, IV drug users.	2 vaccines
HEP B	Immunocompromised and healthcare workers, HEP C, HIV, homosexual males, close contacts with HEP B, IV drug users, dialysis, and diabetics. **Babies: If mother is HBsAg negative: Baby receives 1st dose at birth with 2 more doses before 18 months.** **If mother is HBsAg positive: Baby receives 1st dose and HEP B Ig at 2 different sites by 12 hours of birth with a total of 3 doses by 6 months.**	3 vaccines. Infants must be 2 Kg before getting their 1st HEP B vaccine. **HEP B vaccination ↓ lifetime chance of hepatic cancer.**
HiB (conjugated)	For influenza type B. Given before 5 years old.	
Pregnancy	Influenza is ok. If she has HEP C, ok to give HEP A and HEP B NO VACCINES in PREGNANCY FOR: MMR, Pneumococcal, HPV (If she received an MMR during pregnancy: it is OK, reassure the patient)	
Live Vaccines For immunocompromised	OK if CD counts > 200 to give MMR, Varicella Do not give BCG, Anthrax, oral typhoid, nasal influenza, oral polio, and yellow fever to immunocompromised.	
Neonatal vaccines	Vaccine schedule proceeds on chronologic age. Baby must be 2 Kg for 1st HEP B shot.	

Vaccines Required For Health Problems

Illness	**Vaccines Recommended**
Liver Disease	HEP A (series of 2) and B (series of 3), Tdap/Td (every 10 years, must have received one previous Tdap and then Td can be given thereafter), Influenza (annually – NOT nasal), Pneumococcal (with 5 year booster if original vaccine was given before age 65)
Asplenic	Td (every 10 years, must have received one previous Tdap), Influenza (annually – NOT nasal), Pneumococcal (with 5 year booster if original vaccine was given before age 65)
Immunocompromised	IC defined: COPD, asthma, emphysema, cardiovascular DZ, diabetics, chronic liver DZ, alcoholism, CSF leaks, renal failure, cochlear implants, asplenic, sickle cell, heme pathologies, HIV, chronic bronchitis, SLE, transplants. Pneumococcal (with 5 year booster), Influenza (annually), Td (every 10 years), meningococcal, HEP A and B.
HIV	Do not give these live vaccines (no BCG, anthrax, oral typhoid, nasal influenza, oral polio, yellow fever). Do give these live vaccines MMR, Varicella Zoster (if > 60 years old) if CD4 count > 200, Td/Tdap, Pneumococcus, influenza, HEP A, HEP B, meningococcal, HPV, HBV
Pregnancy	Do not give live vaccines (MMR), no pneumococcal. Do give influenza vaccine. (Note: If the vignette describes a pregnant woman concerned because she received an MMR vaccine while she was pregnant, the answer is to reassure her that it is ok). If pregnant woman has a HEP C infection it is ok to get both HEP A and HEP B vaccines.

Prophylaxis Post Exposure

Exposure	Treatment
Tetanus	Booster and IM immune globulin
Rabies	Booster and IVIG
Meningitis	Rifampin to close contacts
TB	INH and B6 for 9 months
Epiglottitis	Rifampin to household contacts
Hepatitis	HEP B series and immune globulin, HEP A Immune globulin
Varicella	Varicella zoster immune globulin
Measles	Rubeola IM immune globulin, Rubella IV immune globulin
Mumps	None
Rubella	None
Negative Rh	Rho-D Immune Globulin
Smallpox	Vaccinia Smallpox immune globulin
Infantile Botulism	Human-derived botulinum immune globulin
CMV	CytoGam, CMV immune globulin
RSV	RSV Immune globulin or Palivizumab

Birth	1 month	2 months	4 months	6 months	12 months	15 months	18 months	19-23 months	2-3 years	4-6 years
HepB	HepB			HepB						
		RV	RV	RV						
		DTaP	DTaP	DTaP		DTaP				DTaP
		Hib	Hib	Hib	Hib					
		PCV	PCV	PCV	PCV					
		IPV	IPV	IPV						IPV
				Influenza(Yearly)*						
					MMR					MMR
					Varicella					Varicella
					HepA§					

Shaded boxes indicate the vaccine can be given during shown age range.

Key:

HepB: HepB vaccine protects against hepatitis B.

RV: RV vaccine protects against rotavirus.

DTaP: DTaP vaccine protects against diphtheria, tetanus and pertussis (whooping cough).

Hib: Hib protects against *Haemophilus influenzae* type b.

PCV: PCV vaccine protects against pneumococcus.

IPV: IPV protects against polio.

Influenza: Influenza protects against flu.

MMR: MMR protects against measles, mumps and rubella.

Varicella: Varicella protects against chickenpox.

HepA: HepA vaccine protects against hepatitis A.

Footnotes:

*Two doses given at least four weeks apart are recommended for children aged 6 months through 8 years of age who are getting an influenza (flu) vaccine for the first time and for some other children in this age group.

§Two doses of HepA vaccine are needed for lasting protection. The first dose of HepA vaccine should be given between 12 months and 23 months of age. The second dose should be given 6 to 18 months later. HepA vaccination may be given to any child 12 months and older to protect against HepA. Children and adolescents who did not receive the HepA vaccine and are at high-risk, should be vaccinated against HepA.

If your child has any medical condition that put him at risk for infection or is travelling outside the United States, talk to your child's doctor about additional vaccines that he may need.

Note: If your child misses a shot, you don't need to start over, just go back to your child's doctor for the next shot. Talk with your child's doctor if you have any questions about vaccines.

7-10 years	11-12 years		13-18 years	
Tdap[1]	Tetanus,Diphtheria,Pertussis (Tdap) Vaccine		Tdap	
	Human Papillomavirus (HPV) Vaccine (3 Doses)[2]		HPV	
MCV4	Meningococcal Conjugate (MCV4) Vaccine Dose 1[3]		MCV4 Dose 1[3]	Booster at age 16 years
Influenza (Yearly)[4]				
Pneumococcal Vaccine				
Hepatitis A (HepA) Vaccine Series				
Hepatitis B (HepB) Vaccine Series				
Inactivated Polio Vaccine (IPV) Series				
Measles, Mumps, Rubella (MMR) Vaccine Series				
Varicella Vaccine Series				

These shaded boxes indicate when the vaccine is recommended for all children unless your doctor tells you that your child cannot safely receive the vaccine.

These shaded boxes indicate the vaccine should be given if a child is catching-up on missed vaccines.

These shaded boxes indicate the vaccine is recommended for children with certain health conditions that put them at high risk for serious diseases. Note that healthy children **can** get the HepA series[6]. See vaccine-specific recommendations at www.cdc.gov/vaccines/pubs/ACIP-list.htm

If you are this age ↓	talk to your healthcare professional about these vaccines ➡													
	Flu[1] *Influenza*	Td/Tdap[2] *Tetanus Diphtheria, pertussis*	Shingles[3] *Zoster*	Pneumococcal[4]		Meningococcal[5]	MMR[6], † *Measles, mumps, rubella*	HPV[7], † *Human papillomavirus*		Chickenpox† *Varicella*	Hepatitis A†	Hepatitis B†	Hib[8] *Haemophilus influenzae type b*
				PCV13	PPSV23			for women	for men				
19-21 years								3 doses	3 doses				
22-26 years		1 dose of Tdap[2]					1 or 2 doses		3 doses				
27-49 years	Flu vaccine every year			1 dose	1 or 2 doses	1 or more doses				2 doses			
50-59 years		Td booster every 10 years									2 doses	3 doses	1 or 3 doses
60-64 years			1 dose										
65+ year				1 dose	1 dose								

Recommended For You: This vaccine is recommended for you ***unless*** your healthcare professional tells you that you cannot safely receive it or that you do not need it.

May Be Recommended For You: This vaccine is recommended for you if you have certain risk factors due to your health, job or lifestyle that are not listed here. Talk to your healthcare professional to see if you need this vaccine.

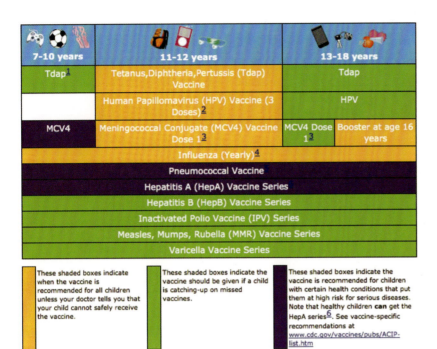

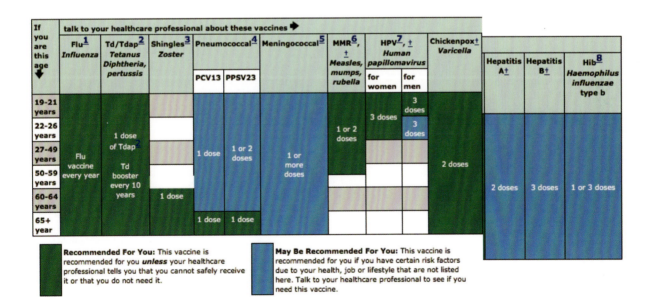

Pathologies required to be reported to the State Department of Health (DPH) for 2016.

Reports must contain: Full name and address of person reporting and attending physician, name of disease, illness or condition. Full name, address, date of birth, race/ethnicity, gender and occupation of the person affected. All mailed envelopes must be marked "CONFIDENTIAL".

Category 1:

Required to be reported by phone on the day of recognition or strong suspicion of the disease and to be mailed in within 12 hours:

- Anthrax, botulism, brucellosis, cholera, diphtheria, measles, melioidosis, meningococcal disease, foodborne illness involving ≥ persons/institutions, plague, poliomyelitis, Q Fever, rabies, ricin poisoning, SARS, Smallpox, Staph enterotoxin B pulmonary poisoning,, MRSA, tuberculosis, tularemia, Venezuelan equine encephalitis, viral hemorrhagic fever, yellow fever, Zika Virus, Ebola Virus.

Category 2:

Required to be reported by mail within 12 hours of recognition or strong suspicion of the disease.

- AIDS, acute flaccid myelitis, babesiosis, arbovirus, campylobacteriosis, carbon monoxide poisoning, chancroid, chickenpox, chickenpox-related death, chikungunya, chlamydia, cryptosporidiosis, cyclosporiasis, dengue, eastern equine encephalitis, Ehrlichia chaffeensis, E. coli O157:H7, gonorrhea, Group A Strep invasive, Group B Strep invasive, HUS, HEP A, HEP B, HEP C, HIV, HPV (CIN2, CIN3, AIS), Influenza associated death, influenza associated hospitalization, lead toxicity ≥ 15 μg/dL, legionellosis, listeriosis, lyme disease, malaria, mercury poisoning, mumps, neonatal bacterial sepsis, neonatal herpes ≤ 60 days of age, occupational asthma, pertussis, pneumococcal disease: invasive, rocky mountain spotted fever, rotavirus, rubella, congenital rubella, salmonellosis, Shiga toxin related disease (gastroenteritis) shigellosis, silicosis, St Louis encephalitis, syphilis, tetanus, trichinosis, typhoid fever, vaccinia disease, vibrio infection, West Nile virus.

DIAGNOSTIC TEST

Ultrasound Pathology DX	**Notes** **Best for:** Prostate, scrotum, uterus, ovaries, gallbladder, some kidney/gallbladder stones, kidneys, children, pregnant women, fetus, DVT, carotid.
Ovaries, Uterus, Adnexa	Monitoring fetus, Not for use in cervical carcinoma.
Testes, Prostate	Torsion,
DVT	
Gallbladder	Stones
Children, Infants	Appendix, hip alignment, Pyloric stenosis
Abdominal Aortic Aneurysm	
Pregnancy	Pathology or fetal check
Polycystic Kidney DZ	

CT Pathology DX Do not do CT's with contrast on patients with renal DZ (creatinine ≥ 1.5). Discontinue Metformin before a CT with contrast, resume at 48 hrs. Do not give IV contrast with renal failure or Multiple Myeloma. Insure all patients are well hydrated when using contrast dye.	**Notes** **Head CT's:** Non-Contrast CT's for: head trauma, stroke, intracranial bleeding. Contrast CT's for: Infection and Cancer. **Chest CT's:** Hilar nodes, tumors/cancer, Pulmonary emboli, interstitial lung disease, TB cavities. **Abdomen CT's:** Intraabdominal infections, appendicitis, pancreas, tumors/masses within abdominal organs, retroperitoneal structures. Diverticulitis
Cancers in the abdomen	
Pulmonary embolism	Preferred test for PE.
Diverticulitis	
Hemorrhage in the head	Noncontrast
Abdominal Cancers	Pancreas, gallbladder
Abdominal Metastasis	From prostate, colon, renal testicular cancers
Lung Cancers, Chest pathologies	Thymoma
Rule out ↑ ICP before doing a lumbar puncture	
Kidney Stones (uric acid)	Radiolucent
Abdominal Pathologies	Abdominal abscesses, spleen
Blood vessels	
Brain	Calcifications, abscesses, epidural or subdural hematomas
Skull	
Esophagus	Ruptured esophagus
Effusion	
Spleen	

MRI Pathology DX Do not do MRI's on patients with implanted metal. Do not do MRI's on patients with renal DZ (creatinine ≥ 1.5)	**Notes** **Best for** cerebellum, brainstem, demyelinating diseases, Pituitary, spinal cord, spinal column, vertebral lesions, Necrosis of the femoral head.
Multiple Sclerosis, Demyelinating DZ	
Tumors in the brain	Pituitary, acoustic neuromas
Spinal Cord, Spinal Column	
Osteonecrosis, Osteomyelitis	
Knee, hip, shoulder injuries	Joint spaces
Strokes, Cerebrovascular DZ	
Epilepsy, Infectious DZ in the brain,	
Joint DZ	

Nuclear Scan Pathology DX	Notes
V/Q Scan	BIT for Pulmonary Embolism. (CT is the preferred test for PE)
Bone Scan	Osteomyelitis, Avascular necrosis of femoral head. Metastatic bone lesions due to breast, kidney, prostate, lung, thyroid cancers. (Not as specific as an MRI)
HIDA Scan	Evaluate function of gallbladder, biliary obstruction, gallbladder evaluations, biliary tract evaluations
Adrenal Scan	Pheochromocytoma
Gallium Scan	Staging melanomas, Lymphomas, locating abscesses, adrenal glands. Gallium follows iron, which allows scan to identify areas of infection or cancer (cancers that increase iron deposits).
Indium Scan	Fever of unknown origin. White blood cells are tagged with indium to localize infection.
Multiple-gated Acquisition Scan (MUGA)	Most accurate measure of ejection fraction.

Endoscopy Pathology DX	Notes **Best for:** Pancreas, stomach (gastrinoma, ulcer), biliary disease)
Stomach	Upper GI
Intestines	Upper GI

Cystoscope Pathology DX	Notes
Bladder, Urethra	Bladder cancer, incontinence, cause of blood in urine
TURP	Prostate

Barium Pathology DX	Notes
Esophagus	Upper GI
Small Intestine	Upper GI: Intussusception, blockage, ulcers, tumors
Pharynx, Larynx	Upper GI
Colon, Rectum	Lower GI:
Hiatus Hernia	

Colposcopy Pathology DX	Notes
Cervix, Vagina	HPV, biopsies

Flat Film X-ray Pathology DX	Notes
Back	
Bones	Best imaging for osteomyelitis
Chest (initial)	Pneumonia and other pulmonary problems, Heart Size. Best: PA film (Posterior/anterior) if patient can stand. Best to detect a widened mediastinum. AP film (Anterior/posterior) if patient can't stand. Portable x-rays are usually used. Decubitus x-ray: Pleural effusion. Best to differentiate between effusions from an infiltrate in pneumonia. Lateral chest x-ray: Best to detect effusion.
Abdomen	Best for small bowel obstruction (gas/fluid levels). Be sure to get an upright chest (thorax) with abdomen view to identify air under the diaphragm.

TEE Pathology DX	Notes
Aortic Dissection	

ECRP Pathology DX	Notes
Pancreatic Duct, Head	
Common Bile Duct	

ECHO Pathology DX	Notes
Heart Function	EF, Valves, etc.

FAST Ultrasound (Focused Assessment with Sonography for Trauma)	Used with there has been traumatic injury. It identifies the presence of free intraperitoneal or pericardial fluid (in cardiac tamponade). MC due to hemorrhage. In the abdomen examines: perihepatic & hepato-renal space, perisplenic space and the pelvis. In the chest examines the pericardium.

Boards Ready LABS	NORMAL RANGES
Body Mass Index (BMI)	10 – 25 kg/m2 Adults
*Sodium	124 - 135 mEq/L
*Potassium	3.5 - 5.5 mEq/L
*Chloride	95 - 105 mEq/L
*Bicarbonate	22 - 26 mEq/L
Magnesium	1.5 - 2.0 mEq/L
*Calcium (serum)	8.0 - 10.4 mg/dL
Calcium ionized	4.24 - 5.25 mg/dL
Phosphorus	2.6 - 4.6 mg/dL
*Glucose (serum)	70 – 110 mg/dL Fasting <120 mg/dl 2 hr postprandial
*Anion Gap	8 – 12 mEq/L
Uric Acid	2.4 – 7.5 mg/dL
Albumin	3.4 – 8.4 g/dL
Total Bilirubin	0.2 – 1.5 mg/dL
Direct Bilirubin	0.0 – 0.3 mg/dL
Creatine Kinase (serum)	25 – 90 U/L Male 10 – 70 U/L Female
Creatinine (serum)	0.6 – 1.3 mg/dL
LDH	50 – 240 U/L
BUN	8 – 25 m/EqL
Alkaline Phos	25 – 115 U/L
CPK, CK	5 – 200 U/L
CPK, MB	<3.5 – 5.5%
Myoglobin	10 – 75 ng/mL
Troponin	0 – 0.5 ng/mL
*Total Cholesterol	<200 mg/dL
*LDL Cholesterol	30 – 135 mg/dL
*Triglycerides	30 – 135 mg/dL
*HDL Cholesterol	>40
Amylase	25 - 125 U/L
Lipase	4 – 25 U/L
Lactate Dehydrogenase	45 – 90 U/L
*ALT (Alanine)	10 - 30 U/L
*AST	8 - 46
*pH	7.35 – 7.45
*PCO2	33 – 4 mm Hg
*PO2	75 – 105 mm HG
*HCO2	22 – 28 mEq/L
*O2 Sat (artery)	97%
O2 Sat (vein)	60% - 85%
A-a Gradient	10 mm Hg
*RBC	3.2 – 5.2
*WBC (Leukocytes)	5000 – 10,000
*Neutrophils - Segmented	40 - 60
Bands	3% - 5%
*Eosinophils	1% - 3%
Basophils	0% - .75%
Lymphocytes	25% - 33%
Monocytes	3% - 7%
Plasma Volume	25 – 36 mL/kg Males 28 – 45 mL/kg Female
*OSM (serum)	275 – 295 mosmol/kg H20
Ethanol	0.1 – 0.4% Intoxicated 0.25% Toxic >0.5% Coma
Lead	0 – 4 ug/dL
Lab Chart© by Dr. Tricia Derges, MD	* Know These Labs

Boards Ready LABS	NORMAL RANGES
*Hemoglobin A1c	<5.7 (Pre-diabetic: 5.7 – 6.4; Diabetic: > 6.4
*Hematocrit	41% - 53% Male 35% - 46% Female
*Hemoglobin	13.5 – 17.5 g/dL Male 12.0 – 16.0 g/dL Female
Erythrocyte Count (ESR)	0 – 15 mm/h Male 0 – 20 mm/h Female
RDW	0 – 14.5
MCH (Mean Corpuscular Hb)	25.4 – 34.6 pg/cell
MCMC (Mean Corpuscular Hb Conc)	315 – 36% Hb/cell
*MCV (Mean Corpuscular Volume)	81 - 99 um3
Erythrocyte Count	4.3 – 5.9 million/mm3 Male 3.5 – 5.5 million/mm3 Female
*PTT (Partial Thromboplastin Time)	25 – 40 seconds
*PT (Prothrombin Time) PT/INR	11 – 15 seconds
Thrombin Time	<2 seconds deviation from control
*Reticulocyte Count	0.5% - 1.5%
*Platelet Count	150,000 – 400,000 mm3
Fibrinogen	152 – 376 mg/dL
FSH	4 – 30 mlU/mL Premenopause 40 – 250 mlU/mL Postmenopause
LH	5 – 30 mlU/mL Follicular Phase 30 – 200 mIU/mL Postmenopause
Testosterone	270 – 1070 Adult Males 15 – 70 Adult Female
Estrogen (Estradiol)	30 – 120 Follicular Phase 130 – 370 Ovulatory Peak 70 – 250 Luteal Phase 15 – 60 Postmenopause
PSA	<4.0 ng/mL
*TSH (serum)	0.5 – 5.0 uU/mL
T4 (Thyroxine) (serum)	5.0 – 12.0 ug/dL
T3	75 – 200 ng/dL
T3 Uptake	22% - 36%
Calcitonin	<75 pg/mL
Cortisol AM	6 – 24 ug/dL
Cortisol PM	2 – 10 ug/dL
Prolactin (serum)	<20 ng/mL
PTH (Parathyroid Hormone)	230 – 630 pg/mL
Iron	60 – 170 ug/dL
Ferritin	30 – 233 ng/mL
TIBC	240 – 450 mcg/dL
Transferrin Saturation	20% - 50%
Folate	>2.5 ng/mL
B12	>200 pg/mL
Growth Hormone	1 – 10 pg/mL
Calcium (urine)	100 – 300 mg/24 hrs
*Osmolality (urine)	50 – 1400 mosmol/kg H20
*Glucose (urine)	<300 mg/24 hrs
Oxalate (urine)	8 – 40 ug/mL
Proteins (urine)	<150 mg/24 hrs
Specific Gravity (urine)	1002 - 1030
Albumin (urine)	20 – 100 mg/24 hrs
Creatinine (urine)	0.75 – 1.5 g/24 hrs
Sodium (urine)	50 – 250 mEq/24 hrs
Uric Acid (urine)	50 – 700 mg/24 hrs
Potassium (urine)	25 – 115 mEq/24 hrs
Urea Nitrogen (Urine)	10 – 20 g/24 hrs
IgA	76 – 390 mg/dL
IgE	0 – 380 IU/mL
IgG	650 – 1500 mg/dL
IgM	40 – 345 mg/dL

The Boards Ready Study Clock© is a critical tool that I implement daily in my Boards Ready© course. This insures that you will be prepared for any possible way a question could be presented on the exam. This clock has been invaluable to students. My class is very focused on the 90% that can be expected on the exam. This clock has made tremendous differences in my students exam scores. To use the clock: Each category that is tested on the exam is noted on the clock. Start at the top category on the clock (Cell Biology), moving clockwise, take any given subject and ask yourself how a test question could be asked in each category. Understand that not every category will permit a question for any specific subject.
Example: *Subject: Cystic Fibrosis.* Start at the Cell Biology and Histology slot and ask: What question (s) can the exam make using Cell Biology and Histology for Cystic Fibrosis? Once you know these answers, move to the next category: Genetics and Biochemistry. Ask the same question: What question (s) can the exam make using Genetics and Biochemistry for Cystic Fibrosis. Continue this process for Cystic Fibrosis around the entire clock. Be sure you know the answers to each question before you move to the next category. Once you get to the end of the clock categories you will have covered any question that the exam could possibly ask you about Cystic Fibrosis (the subject). So when the question about Cystic Fibrosis comes up on your exam, you will be totally prepared for whatever direction they choose to go with their question.
This clock provides the most thorough study you can possibly do for your exam.

USMLE® Boards Ready Study Clock©

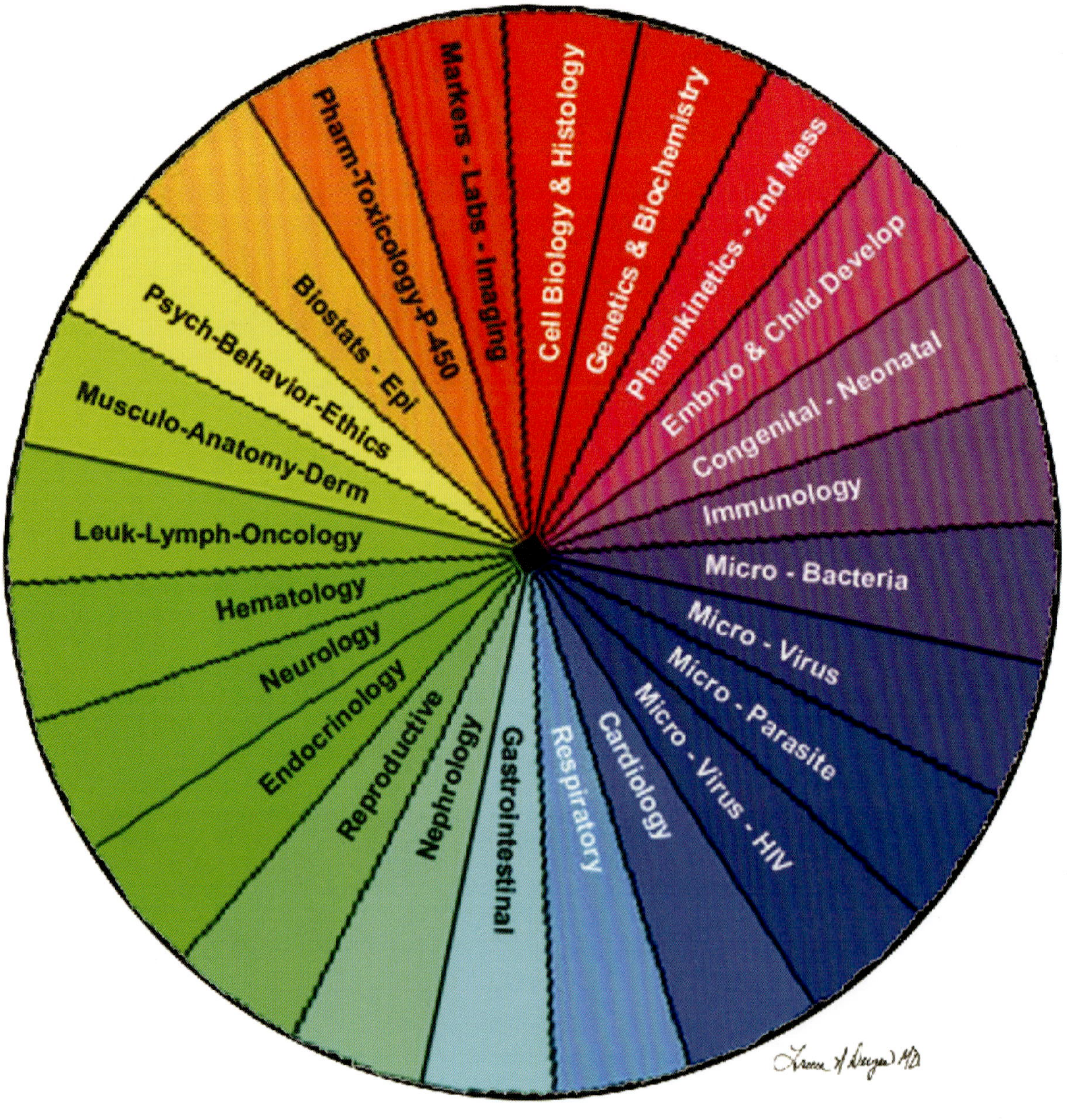

STEP 3 CS

Several bits of advice for Step 3 CS:

- Put yourself in the situation in **"real time"** thinking. **Do exactly what you would do in real life**. If you have to follow up with a patient in your office (waiting on lab results), schedule an appointment (during an actual week day and during real office hours 8 – 5). For the ER, never just let a patient sit in there forever, send them home or admit them to the hospital. It's no different on this test. But you do need to do this.
- **Practice heavily** on the USMLE Step 3 CS **software**. This is 90% of your battle! Get comfortable with it! Then simply do what you would do if you were at the clinic or hospital.
- Be aware, it is very common for your block to end early, before you are done with the treatments or management of the case. The computer is simply looking to see if you have gotten the key elements. Once the computer sees the proper management (test ordered, medicines ordered, etc.) and it matches with what you should actually be doing, then it will stop the block and move on. And likewise, if the computer detects that the management (test ordered, medicines ordered) is incorrect, or even worse, could hurt/kill the patient, it will also shut down early. The computer can tell very quickly if you have hit the diagnosis and treatment or missed it. Very few cases actually go to the end. So this part of the exam usually finishes early.
- If you get a 10-minute case, it WILL be a simple one. Do NOT overcomplicate it! If it is a 20-minute case, it will be a more involved one that will require much more work.
- Don't go to the trouble of learning a bunch of drugs for each problem. In most all cases you just need one. So keep this simple!
- For drugs: Be sure on Step 3 you give the route of administration of the drug as well as what drug you specifically want to give. You can't use "family" names (ie: you can't say give a beta blocker, you must order atenolol). You DO NOT need to know dosages for Step 3.
- You can always ask for a consult, but the consult will never give you any advice or information. It will simply tell you to continue treating the case, as you feel necessary.
- If you have a patient that comes in as a true emergency, automatically order a set group of stat tests before you even see them.
- Get RIGHT to the problem. Do a very focused exam. You do not need all of the typical H&P questions. You need to figure out the problem, diagnose it with the correct test, and then treat it.
- Step 3 CS drug names: You can use the chemical name or you can use the brand name.
- Never be afraid to order extra tests. It doesn't count against you and in many cases you may find a result that is extremely helpful that you may not have thought about otherwise.
- Order a lot of things at one time. There is no requirement when you order a group of tests as to which ones you must order first. Just get them all in. It's always a good idea to put certain tests on every single order, regardless: TSH, B12, **B-hCG** if it's a woman (**NEVER** FORGET THIS ONE-regardless of age!), finger stick glucose, EKG, CBC, BMP, UA, ESR.
- When you order several tests at once, this moves the clock forward nice chunks at a time. This way you will get more results back at one time versus moving the clock ahead every 15 minutes – you could do this all day.
- It is also VERY important to remember to order all "accessories" needed to do your treatment: If you are going to intubate someone, be sure to order the mechanical ventilator to go with it. If you order a drug that is IV, you need to order IV access.
- Other obvious things that are easy to forget: On D/C be sure to discontinue any IV meds and change them to PO meds to go home. Anytime anyone is in pain, be SURE to give a pain medication. Don't forget to order the appropriate diets for a patient you admit to the hospital so they don't starve! Just put yourself in the case – real time.
- Do not forget to take any samples, labs and cultures BEFORE you give any treatments!
- Don't forget to give nausea meds when giving pain meds.
- Don't forget to give a laxative when giving opiod pain meds.
- Don't forget to order IV antibiotics before surgery.
- I have bolded the test and treatments that are the most important. If you don't do or order anything else, don't miss these! These are the key to being sure you get what is needed. The non-bolded ones will give you a few extra points, but nothing major.
- Drugs: Do not memorize a bunch of drugs! Pick one drug in a category and just use this each time when needed. Ex: You know you will probably need a beta-blocker for a case. Just pick one beta-blocker and use it in every case. I've given these to you below.
- Mostly, enjoy this part of the exam, it is actually rather fun! Just make each case a "video" in your mind and play it through on test day – just as though you were on the floor in person. Do exactly what you would have done there!

The following are what I feel are the most likely cases that would be tested. Under each subject, I have kept the organization very simple. Under each case I have developed a simple format that contains the KEY things to do. Some books list dozens of things to do. I am sure if you were to list out the dozens of extra things for a treatment, it would be worth a couple of extra points, but that's probably all. The main points come from hitting the **KEY** treatments and drugs. Once you list those, the test will probably shut down. They know you are on target and so there is no reason to drag the case on.

I have created "KITS", your **Doctor's Bag,** to cover everything needed for each category of problems. Simply identify the category (breathing problem, bleeding, cancer, chest pain, etc.) and "grab" the appropriate "KIT" and treat. It's much easier to remember a "KIT" rather than dozens of individual items and cases. It is just like "real life" medicine, many things tend to get the majority of the same imaging, labs and treatments.

STANDARD DRUG KIT
Keep it simple: just get one main drug treatment down and use that for anything in that category.

Abdominal Surgery (ruptured organ) IV Piperacillin + Tazobactam	**Gut Surgery** IV Metronidazole + IV Cipro	**Diverticulitis** IV Ampicillin + Sulbactrum (Upon discharge: send PO drugs home: Metronidazole, Cipro, Percocet).
General Surgery IV Cefoxitin	**Post Partum Endometriosis** IV Gentamycin + IV Metronidazole	**PID** IV Cefoxitin + IV Doxycycline (admit) IM Ceftriaxone + PO Azithromycin (clinic)
Hypertensive Emergency Nitroprusside	**Endocarditis** IV Vanc + IV Gentamycin	**Sepsis** IV Vanc + IV Clindamycin
Allergies to Penicillin TMP/SMX Erythromycin Cephalosporins Cipro	**Cellulitis** TMP/SMX	**Septic Arthritis** IV Vanc IV Ceftriaxone
Croup Epinephrine nebulizer + PO Dexamethasone +humidified air	**Panic** IV Alprazolam	**DKA** IV Gentamycin + IV Cefotaxime
Bacterial Meningitis IV Vanc + IV Ceftriaxone IV Dexamethasone	**Any General Head Infection** (Strep, Ears, Bite) PO Amoxicillin	**Breathing Exacerbation** **COPD**: Albuterol Nebulizer + Ipratropium Nebulizer + IV Methylprednisone + IV Ceftriaxone. **Asthma:** Albuterol Nebulizer + IV Methylprednisone.
Drug OD **Heroin** (Opioids): IV Naloxone **Acetaminophen**: N-Acetylcysteine **Cocaine**: **TCA:** Sodium Bicarb + activated charcoal	**MI:** PO Aspirin, SL Nitroglycerin, IV Heparin, PO Clopidogrel, PO Lisinopril, IV Abciximab	**CHF** **IV Furosemide, Lisinopril**
A-Fib PO Warfarin + Metoprolol	**Eclampsia** IV Mg Sulfate + Hydralazine	**Acute Pancreatitis and Gallbladder** IV Phenergan + Piperacillin + Tazobactam
Gout Acute: Indomethacin Chronic: Allopurinol	**Sickle Cell** IV Morphine + Phenergan + PO Hydroxyurea. If chest infection: add IV Azithromycin	**Anaphylaxis** IM Epinephrine
Fungus Vaginal Candidiasis: Miconazole Tinea (feet, skin): Ketoconazole Tinea (hair, nails): Terbinafine Esophagitis: Fluconazole	**UTI and Pyelonephritis** UTI: TMP/SMX (Bactrim) UTI in Pregnancy: Nitrofurantoin Pyelonephritis: Inpatient: IV Ampicillin + IV Gentamycin. Outpatient: Ciprofloxacin	**TB** Prophylaxis: INH + B6 TB: INH, B6, Rifampin, Pyroxamide, Ethambutol
Pneumonias PCP: TMP/SMX + Prednisone + prophylaxis with Azithromycin. Community: Ceftriaxone or Fluoroquinolone Nosocomial: Pseudomonas: Piperacillin + Tazobactam	**STD and Sexual Associations** PID: PO Azithromycin + IM Ceftriaxone Trichomonas: Metronidazole BV: Metronidazole	**Pregnancy** Prenatal vitamins Folic acid (Folate) Iron Sulfate
Diverticulitis IV Ampicillin + Sulbactam + IV Phenergan	**DKA** **IV Regular Insulin,**	

KITS (DOCTOR'S BAG)

Think of these "Kits" as a doctor's bag. A "bag" that you open up and use when you identify the main problem you will be treating. Simply open your "kit" and place the orders for what is in the "kit". This keeps you from guessing or missing any test, imaging or treatment. Remember, it's okay to have extra tests. It is better to have too many tests than not enough and miss the diagnosis. Memorize the same order of items for each "kit", it will make it so much easier to remember.
Example: 1) H & P, 2) All labs, 3) All diagnostic/imaging test, 4) Treatments, 5) Counsel and Follow Up.
Treatments, management, and drugs will ultimately depend upon what you confirm as the diagnosis once all labs and test are back. The cases below list the standard treatments, management, and drugs for most cases.

STANDARD "KITS" (Standard Doctor's Bag)

In EVERY case you are given, regardless, you MUST DO the steps listed below. So I did NOT list them in the KIT descriptions.

- **H & P. For emergency cases, just do an H & P Limited. If a specific H & P is listed next to this, be SURE to do these**
- **Basic labs. Best to always do these. If there are labs listed beside "basic labs" this means BE SURE to do these**
- **Reassure and counsel patient/parents**
- **Control any pain (pain kit)**
- **For all admissions be sure to always monitor for: cardiac, blood pressure, pulse ox and urine output**
- **For all women in their reproductive years: always do a β-hCG.**
- **Always recommend to stop smoking and drinking and exercise appropriate to their ability**
- **ALWAYS add an ALLERGY BRACLET to anyone with ANY ALLERGIES BEFORE YOU ADMIT THEM**
- **ALWAYS add a Medical Alert Bracelet to anyone with a condition requiring this**

H&P: Vital Signs, Complete History and Physical Exam ***SHOULD DO FOR EVERYTHING***
H&P Limited: Vital Signs and Focused H & P ***SHOULD DO FOR ALL EMERGENCIES***
Basic Labs: CBC w/diff, BMP, TSH/Free T4, UA, B12, ESR, β-hCG (if woman) SHOULD ***DO FOR EVERYTHING***
B-hCG SHOULD DO FOR ALL WOMEN IN THEIR REPRODUCTIVE YEARS
Liver Panel: ALT, AST, TBG, PT/INR, PTT, D-Dimer, Albumin, Bilirubin, and Haptoglobin
Lipid and Diabetic Panel: HbA1c, Cholesterol, LDL, Triglycerides, HDL
Iron Panel: Ferritin, Iron, TIBC, and MCV
IV Kit: IV access, 9% normal saline, D/C upon discharge
Cardiac Kit: H & P Limited, MONA therapy, IV access, EKG, Monitor cardiac, CXR, ECHO, Cardiac Enzymes to repeat x 6 hrs, BNP, PT/PTT, CPK, LDH, UA drug screen, D-Dimer, monitor VS
SOB KIT: H & P Limited, Head of bed up, Oxygen, Pulse Ox and monitor hourly, Cardiac monitor, PEFR and monitor hourly, CXR, CT, ABG and monitor, PEFR and monitor, EKG, incentive spirometer, cardiac enzymes, D-dimer lab, monitor for need of intubation (add mechanical ventilation if intubated), monitor VS
PE-DVT Kit: Doppler US, Spiral CT, D-Dimer, LMWH, Warfarin, Monitor, PT/INR and Platelets
DVT Kit: Doppler US, liver panel, IV, LMWH and Warfarin plus standard labs. Consider IVC filter if contradictions to anticoagulation
Emergency Full Kit: EKG, CXR, Oxygen, IV Access, IV Naloxone, IV Thiamine, finger stick glucose, UA Drug screen, Ketones, ABG and monitor, urine output and monitor, CXR
Emergency Quick Kit: EKG, Oxygen, Pulse Oximeter monitor, BP Monitor, Cardiac Monitor, VS monitor, IV Access and Normal Saline
Pneumonia Kit: Pulse oximeter and monitor, oxygen, EKG, CXR, ABG and monitor
Surgery Kit: NPO, EKG, Liver panel, IV Cefazolin, Compression socks, consent, type and cross
Drug OD: Activated charcoal and NG tube, UA drug screen and report/consult: substance abuse, poison control, suicide support, psychiatric services, be prepared to intubate with mechanical ventilation, monitor VS
Pain Kit IV: IV access, IV morphine with Phenergan ***CONTROL PAIN APPROPRIATELY (oral or IV) for EVERYONE***
Pain Kit Oral: PO Acetominophen, Percocet, Ibuprofen ***CONTROL PAIN APPROPRIATELY (oral or IV) for EVERYONE***
Head Panel (ANY altered mental status or unconscious): H & P limited, Liver panel, lipid panel, EKG, EEG, Head CT, ECHO, UA Drug/Toxicology Screen, Finger Stick Glucose, Ammonia, B12
Infection Panel (Serum): ESR, CRP, Blood cultures
Infection *Panel* (**GI**): Infection labs plus urine culture, Stool O & P, Stool Gram Stains, KOH, D. Difficile toxin
Infection Panel (GU or STD): UA, Urine culture, Urine gram stain, blood culture
Bleeding Panel: Liver panel, Iron panel, FOBT, CEA, LDH, Haptoglobin, Reticulocyte count, Bilirubin, PT/PTT, Bleeding time, VWF, Factor VIII and IX, Coombs, Osmotic fragility, G6PD, HAM test, discontinue aspirin and anticoagulants
Bone and Joint Panel: PTH, Mg, Phosphate, CPK, ESR, X-Ray, serum uric acid, blood culture, viscosity, culture and sensitivity, Synovial Fluid Studied: synovial fluid glucose, synovial fluid cell count, Joint synovial fluid for gram stain and crystals, blood cultures
Joint-Tissue Autoantibody panel: RF, ANA, Anti-Citrullinated Protein, Parvo B-19, HLA, Anti-Jo, Anti-Mi-2, Anticentromere, Anti-Scl-70, Anti-cardiolipin, Anti-Ro, Anti-La
Thyroid Autoantibody panel: Antimicrosomal, Antithyroglobulin, Anti-TSH receptor
GI Autoantibody panel: IgA antiendomysial, Anti-smooth muscle antibody, p-ANCA, ASCA, Anti-flagellin antibody, CPR serum
Renal Autoantibody panel: c-ANCA, p-ANCA, Anti-basement membrane, Anti phospholipase A2
Renal Panel: BUN/Creatinine, Ca, Cl, Glucose, Filtration, Albumin, K, Sodium, microalbumin, urine output and monitor
GI Panel: NPO, Amylase, Lipase, Ultrasound, CT, Abdominal X-Ray, Liver panel, ESR, Stool 72 hour fat, Stool O & P, Stool culture and gram stain
Diarrhea Kit: Stool O & P, Stool Giardia antigen, Stool for C. difficile toxin, FBOT (if positive: do colonoscopy), P-ANCA, Sweat Test, Stool 72 hour fat
HIV Kit: ELISA, Western Blot, Viral Load, CD4 count, VDRL-RPR, HBV, HCV, TOXO, PPD, Prophylaxis with Azithromycin, vaccinations (influenza, pneumococcal), HAART Therapy, Report to Health Dept
Diabetic Kit: In Office: Diabetic panel, diabetic diet, Diabetic Meds (DMI or DMII), Lifestyle changes, Annual feet and eyes exam If hospital: Do all "Office" procedures and add: accucheck every 6 hours, serum Ketone bodies, Beta-hydroxybutyrate, Osmolality, ABG and monitor, BMP and monitor.
Cancer Panel: Check for metastasis in all other areas: CT abdomen, head, CXR, Bone scan, Tumor markers
GYN Panel: β-hCG, PAP, HPV DNA, Vaginal pH, gram stain, KOH, G & C culture and counsel about safe sex
Depression Panel: TSH, B12, UA, Depression Index, suicide contract, psychotherapy, mini mental status exam

Management

RS = Reschedule another appointment for lab or test results
C & R = Counsel about disease/problem, discuss medicines and side effects, compliance and reassure patient, advise no smoking, no alcohol and no drugs and exercise within capabilities
FU = Follow up and monitor treatment and progress over time
Inform Kit: Inform patient of their condition (cancer, etc.), management, prognosis, advance directives, support
Admit Kit: (this is in addition to your treatments for the condition): Cancel all outside drugs, Ambulation orders, diet orders, urine output and monitor
Admit ICU: NPO, IV, VS monitor, Foley, Urine output and monitor, bedrest, LMWH, IV Ranitidine, pulse ox and monitor, compression socks, EKG and monitor
Discharge Kit: Counsel about condition, discuss medicine compliance and side effects, discontinue all IV meds and change to PO, diet and FU

CASES – OFFICE

THYROID H & P Basic Labs – **TSH, Free T4** B-hCG **EKG** Liver Panel RS **RAI uptake** (not in pregnant patients) Thyroid autoantibodies Thyroid US RS If Hyperthyroid: Methimazole (PTU if pregnant) Or Propylthiouracil (PTU) If Hypothyroid Levothyroxine FU in 4 weeks Recheck TSH, Free T4 C & R FU ***If Thyroid Storm transfer to ER***	**MULTIPLE SCLEROSIS** H & P, **Neuro** Basic Labs B-hCG **Brain MRI** LP for **CSF for Myelin Basic Protein** RS **INF-β** C & R FU
CYSTIC FIBROSIS H&P Basic Labs **Sweat test** **CF DNA** 72 Hr Fat Stool **Pancreatic enzymes** CSR Sinus X-ray RS Consult genetic, dietary, endocrine. Enzyme replacement **Multivitamins** C & R FU If admitted: Admit Albuterol Amoxicillin + Clavulanic (Augmentin)	**ESSENTIAL HTN** H&P Basic Labs **EKG** **Lipid panel** **Fasting blood glucose** Counsel Lifestyle Changes (6 months): Decrease: Na, salt, fat, calorie intake. Exercise. Monitor BP and keep BP log Consult: Ophthalmology (eye exam) and Cardiac (ECHO) Repeat BP at appointments C & R **(lifestyle changes: weight loss/diet, low sodium diet, no smoking, no drinking)** RS: 3 months if BP < 140 – 160/90 - 100 RS: 3 months to check BP. If patient is 160-180/100-110 start on meds with lifestyle changes. C & R at every visit PO with appropriate Medicine: Lisinopril (if cough/angioedema use ARB's) African American: Amlodipine Diabetic: Lisinopril BPH: Terazosin

SLE - LUPUS H&P **Basic Labs** **Joint-Tissue-antibody panel – ds DNA** **Compliment level** ECHO CXR RS PO Hydroxychloroquine and PO Prednisone Consult: Rheumatology C & R FU	**TURNERS** H & P **FSH, LH** **Karyotype** **ECHO** Basic Labs, Lipid panel, renal panel, **fasting finger stick glucose** RS **Imaging:** Renal and Pelvic US, Skeletal survey, hearing test RS **SQ Growth hormone** **PO Estrogen-Progesterone TX** **PO: Vit D** **PO Calcium** **Consult: Dietary, Psychiatry, Genetics, Pediatric Endocrine** C & R RS 2 weeks FU
SHINGLES (HERPES ZOSTER) H & P limited Clinical Diagnosis Ibuprofen Cold compress **Valacyclovir** Varicella vaccine C & R RS 2 weeks	**ACUTE BACTERIAL SINUSITIS** H & P (Clinical Diagnosis) **PO Amoxicillin** PO Acetominophen PO Pseudoephedrine C & R RS 2 Weeks
POLYMYALGIA RHEUMATICA or TEMPORAL ARTERITIS H & P Basic Labs – **CBC, ESR** **Temporal artery biopsy** Inflammation labs Autoantibody panel RS FU H&P **PO Prednisone** **Calcium carbonate** C & R (**exercise**, eat healthy, reduce sugar/salt) RS in 2 weeks for recheck: ESR, CRP, Basic labs FU: monitor	**VAGINAL/CERVICAL** **CANDIDIASIS, BV, TRICHOMONAS, G & C** H & P limited **GYN panel** **C & R (safe sex)** FU Clinically Treat (don't wait for culture results) Note: If woman is vomiting: you MUST admit her for treatment. Candidiasis: Miconazole (cream or suppository) Trichomonas: **PO Metronidazole** BV: PO Metronidazole G & C: PO **Azithromycin plus IM Ceftriaxone**
OTITIS MEDIA H & P **PO Amoxicillin** C & R (counsel parent) FU	**SWIMMER'S EAR (ACUTE OTITIS EXTERNA)** H & P **Neomycin/polymyxin B/hydrocortisone otic ear drops** FU
CHRONIC CONSTIPATION H & P **Basic Labs** **FOBT** HbA1c, Mg, Phosphate RS If FOBT positive: Consult surgery: Polyethylene glycol prep and colonoscopy If FOBT negative: Metamucil C & R (increase: fiber in diet, exercise, hydration) FU	**IRRITABLE BOWEL SYNDROME** H & P Basic Labs **FOBT** **Diarrhea Kit** **Infection Panel GI** RS If FOBT positive: Consult surgery: Polyethylene glycol prep and colonoscopy If FOBT negative: **PO Dicyclomine** PO Loperamide C & R (limit: caffeine and alcohol, increase exercise and fiber) FU

ULCERATIVE COLITIS or CROHN'S

H & P
Basic labs
FOBT
Infection Panel GI
GI Autoantibody Panel – p-ANCA, ASCA
Liver panel
Folic
RS
Consult surgery: Polyethylene glycol prep and **colonoscopy** with biopsy
Consult dietary
PO Sulfasalazine or Mesalamine
PO Prednisone
PO Ferrous Sulfate
PO B12
C & R
FU to monitor ESR

GIARDIA and other INTESTINAL PARASITES GASTROENTERITIS

H & P
Basic Labs
Infection Panel GI
RS

Appropriate treatment based on lab results
Giardia: PO Metronidazole
Flukes: PO Praziquantel
Worms: PO Albendazole
C & R
FU

ALZHEIMERS

H & P - **Neuro**
Basic Labs
Liver Panel
Head CT, no contract (or MRI)
Depression Panel
UA Toxicology
RPR Serum
RS
Donepezil
(If depressed: add Fluoxetine
If delusions add Olanzapine)
C & R (advance directive, support groups, no driving, medical bracelet)
FU

MAJOR DEPRESSION

H & P
Basic Labs
Liver Panel
Depression Panel
RS
Fluoxetine
With anxiety/insomnia: add Lorazepam
If severe: ECT
C & R (exercise)
FU in 2 weeks

CYSTITIS

H & P limited
B-hCG
Infection panel: GU
If not pregnant: PO TMP/SMX
If sulfa allergies: PO Cipro
If pregnant: PO Nitrofurantoin
*If throwing up: must admit to treat IV
C & R
FU in 2 weeks

PYELONEPHRITIS

H & P
B-hCG
Infection panel: GU
Renal US
Outpatient: **Cipro**
Inpatient: Ampicillin + Gentamycin
C & R
FU in 3 days

OBSTRUCTIVE SLEEP APNEA

H & P
Basic Labs
Liver panel
ECHO
EKG
CXR
Pulse Ox
Polysomnography
RS
CPAP
C & R (weight loss)
FU in 4 weeks

PROSTATITIS

H & P limited
Basic Labs
Rectal exam
Infection panel: GU
PO **TMP/SMX**, Cipro
C & R
FU

EPIDIDYMITIS H & P limited Basic Labs **Infection Panel: GU** **Transilluminate (rule out malignancy)** US of testes **PO Azithromycin and IM Ceftriaxone** C & R (Scrotal elevation, ice packs, analgesics) FU	**HEPATITIS** H & P Basic Labs **Liver panel** **Antibodies HAV, HBV, HCV** RS Vaccines If Hepatitis A: Notify public health dept C & R FU to monitor Liver panel **Treatment based on DX: HEP C: Ribavarin, INFα** **HEP B: INFα, NRTI's**
DYSFUNCTIONAL UTERINE BLEEDING H & P Basic Labs – **TSH, CBC** **PT/PTT** **B hCG** PAP Prolactin (serum) OCP's to decrease estrogen and progesterone: **Medroxyprogesterone and Premarin if severe bleeding** **Ferrous sulfate** C & R FU in 3 months	**GESTATIONAL DIABETES** H & P Basic Labs HbA1c **UA** **3 hour glucose tolerance test** Lipid panel Diabetic panel RS **Diabetic diet** **Glucose control and monitor** C & R (weight loss and exercise) RS in 4 weeks Fetal US at 36 – 38 weeks FU
MENOPAUSE H & P Basic Labs **TSH, FSH** Prolactin RS Counsel: exercise, increase calcium and vitamin D, schedule screenings: PAP, colonoscopy, mammograms C & R FU	**PREGNANCY** H & P **B-hCG** **Basic Labs** **HEP B surface antigen, VDRL, HIV Elisa, Chlamydia, Rubella antibodies, Atypical antibodies, RPR,** **Urine culture** **PAP** **Blood type and RH** **Prenatal vitamins, folic acid, ferrous sulfate** **Counsel: Listeria, Toxo, Parvo B-19** High calorie diet Breastfeeding and childbirth classes 28 weeks: 1 hour glucose RS Ultrasound 2nd visit FU appointments
RENAL CELL CANCER H & P Basic Labs UA Urine cytology **Liver panel** **Iron panel** **Renal panel** RS Inform Kit **Abdominal CT** Admit to ward (NPO) **Cancer Kit** **Consult surgery and oncology** for **Nephrectomy** IV Kit Surgery Kit Pain Kit IV Discharge Kit C & R FU 1 week	**PROSTATE CANCER** H & P Basic Labs **Serum PSA** **US prostate – rectal exam** **X-Ray lumbosacral spine** **Prostate ultrasound** **Bone scan** RS Inform Kit **Cancer Kit** **FNB prostate** PSA Pain Kit PO RS **Consult urology, oncology, radiation for Prostatectomy** Counsel (advance directive, support groups)

CERVICAL CANCER	ENDOMETRIAL CANCER
H & P Basic Labs **GYN Panel** RS Inform Kit **Colposcopy** **Cervical biopsy** **Endocervical curettage** RS Consult oncology **LEEP** C & R (no smoking) FU PAP in 4 months	H & P Basic Labs **GYN Panel** **Endometrial biopsy** RS Inform Kit **Consult oncology and surgery for hysterectomy** Admit to ward (NPO) **Cancer Panel** CA-125 marker IV Kit Surgery Kit Pain Kit Discharge Kit C & R FU 1 week
OVARIAN CANCER H & P Basic Labs Pelvic US **GYN Panel - PAP smear** **HPV DNA probe** RS **Cervical biopsy** **Endocervical curettage** Inform Kit Cancer panel **LEEP** FOBT (if positive: colonoscopy) Mammogram Liver panel RS **Consult oncology and surgery for TAH-BSO** Admit to ward (NPO) IV Kit Surgery Kit Pain Kit Discharge Kit C & R FU 1 week	**COLON CANCER** H & P Basic Labs CEA FOBT Liver panel **Iron panel** PSA RS Polyethylene Glycol and **colonoscopy** RS Inform Kit Consult oncology and surgery for hemicolectomy Admit to ward (NPO) **Cancer Kit** **CEA marker** IV Kit Surgery Kit plus IV Metronidazole and IV Cipro **Oral Iron sulfate** Pain Kit – IV Discharge Kit C & R FU in 1 week and ongoing FU: Follow CEA every 3 months for 3 years. Repeat colonoscopy at 1, 3 and 5 years. Abdomen and Chest CT every year for 3 years.
LUNG CANCER H & P **CXR** Admit to ward Basic Labs **Chest CT with contrast** Liver panel **Sputum gram stain** **Sputum culture** **Sputum cytology** **Bronchoscopy** Consult thoracic surgery **Consult hematology/oncology** Consult radiation **Cancer Kit** (If lung cancer is due to small cell or squamous: must also treat other complications from ADH (SIADH), ACTH or PTH) **If SIADH: restrict water and Demeclocycline** C & R	**BLADDER CANCER** H & P **UA** Basic Labs RS **Urine cytology** **Cystoscopy** RS **Consult urology for TURP (Transurethral resection)** **Cancer Kit** C & R (no smoking)

HODGKIN LYMPHOMA H & P **CXR** RS **Chest CT with contrast** **Lymph node biopsy** RS Admit to ward **Consult with hematology/oncology** **Consult thoracic surgery** Consult radiation Cancer Kit C & R	**BREAST CANCER** H & P Basic Labs **B-hCG** Mammography **Breast ultrasound** **Breast FNB** RS **Consult general surgery, hematology/oncology, radiation** **Cancer Kit** C & R FU
PCOS POLYCYSTIC OVARIAN SYNDROME H & P Basic Labs **B-hCG** **Transvaginal ultrasound** Labs: **FSH, LH, Prolactin, Testosterone,** lipid panel, TSH, DHEA-S, Cortisol 24 hour urine, **fasting plasma glucose**, estrogen totals, RS PO Clomiphene (or **OCP high in estrogen and progestin**) **PO Metformin** C & R (lose weight, exercise) FU	**VON WILLEBRAND DISEASE** H & P Basic Labs **PT/PTT, Bleeding time** **Factor VIII** Iron Panel **VWF antigen** **Ristocetin cofactor** RX **DDAVP** **Iron sulfate** C & R (no NSAIDS, No aspirin, diet high in iron, ferrous sulfate) FU Admit to ward if transfusion is needed
RHEUMATOID ARTHRITIS H & P Basic Labs - **ESR** **Joint-Tissue Autoantibody Panel** **Bone and Joint Panel** Ibuprofen RS **Oral Methotrexate** Consult rheumatology C & R (exercise) FU	**OSTEOARTHRITIS** H & P **X-Ray of joints involved** X-Ray of spine: lumbosacral Rheumatoid factor **Pain Kit oral: PO Naproxen** C & R (lose weight, **exercise**, physical therapy) FU
OSTEOPOROSIS H & P Basic Labs **DEXA Scan** Lumbosacral XR **Calcium carbonate** **Vitamin D** **Alendronate** C & R – **high calcium diet, exercise** FU In case of compression fracture: Back brace Pain Kit - Oral	**GASTRITIS - GERD – PEPTIC ULCER DISEASE** H & P If < 45 and no alarm signs: PO Omeprazole If > 45 or has any alarm signs Basic Labs **Urea breath test** Liver panel **Iron panel if patient is anemic** H. pylori stool antigen **Endoscopy of upper GI** RS **PO Omeprazole plus Amoxicillin and Metronidazole** C & R **(no smoking, no alcohol, no NSAIDS)** FU in 4 weeks for H. pylori stool antigen

EMERGENCY ROOM

CELLULITIS	TB (with positive PPD)
H & P Admit to ward (normal diet, bedrest with BRP) Basic Labs Bone and Joint Kit **Infection Panel (serum)** IV Kit **IV Bactrim** Pain Kit PO FU on imaging and labs C & R Discharge Kit FU 2 weeks	H & P **CXR (if positive – admit) (If negative – TB prophylaxis: INH and B6 for 9 months)** Admit (normal diet, reverse isolation) Basic Labs **PPD** **HIV Elisa and Western Blot** **Sputum for AFB, Mycobacterium, PCR mycobacterium RNA** Check sputum daily. **PO INH plus B6** **PO Rifampin** **PO Pyrazinamide** **PO Ethambutol** **Notify public health** C & R Discharge Kit FU
DKA	**G6PD**
Emergency Full Kit H & P Limited Basic Labs IV Kit **UA** **Serum OSM** **Urine culture** **Urine Gram stain** **Blood Culture** IV Potassium **IV Regular Insulin** **9% Normal saline** If infection present: IV Gentamycin and IV Cefotaxime Admit to ICU **Glucose finger stick check every hour** **ABG every hour** **BMP every hour** C & R Discharge Kit FU	H & P Basic Labs **Hemolysis Kit** **G6PD serum** Admit to ward (dietary, bedrest with BRP) IV Kit Transfuse RBC Monitor Hb and Hct C & R Discharge Kit FU
ALCOHOL WITHDRAWL	**BENZODIAZEPINE OVERDOSE**
H & P Limited Basic Labs **UA Drug Screen** Liver panel Blood alcohol level Head CT IV Kit **IV Thiamine** **IV Naloxone** **IV 5% Dextrose** **IV Lorazepam** Admit to Withdrawal Ward Monitor K, Mg and Phosphorus labs Consult social worker C & R (AAA, support groups, no smoking) Discharge Kit FU 1 month	**Emergency Full Kit** H & P Limited **ABG monitor** Monitor need for intubation and mechanical ventilation Basic Labs **Drug OD Kit** (activated charcoal) IV Kit Admit to ICU **Consult psych, poison control, substance abuse** C & R Discharge Kit FU

TCA OVERDOSE **Emergency Full Kit** H & P Limited **ABG monitor** Monitor need for intubation and mechanical ventilation Basic Labs IV Kit **IV Sodium Bicarb** **Drug OD Kit** (activated charcoal) Admit to ICU **Consult psych, poison control, substance abuse** C & R Discharge Kit FU	**ACETOMENOPHEN OVERDOSE** **Emergency Full Kit** H & P Limited Monitor need for intubation and mechanical ventilation Basic Labs **ABG monitor** **BMP monitor** **Liver panel** **Acetominophen Toxicity – serum** IV Kit **Drug OD Kit** (activated charcoal) **IV N-Acetylcysteine** Admit to ICU **Consult psych, poison control, substance abuse** C & R Discharge Kit FU
HEROIN/OPIOD OVERDOSE **Emergency Full Kit** H & P Limited Monitor need for intubation and mechanical ventilation Basic Labs **Drug OD Kit** (activated charcoal) Acetominophen screen Blood alcohol screen IV Kit **IV Naloxone** IV Thiamine Admit to ICU **Consult psych, poison control, substance abuse** C & R Discharge Kit FU	**ANAPHYLAXIS** **Emergency Full Kit** **IM Epinephrine** H & P Limited Albuterol nebulizer IV Kit **IV Hydrocortisone** **IV Diphenhydramine** IV Ranitidine IV Dopamine if hypotensive Monitor Pulse and VS Consult immunology C & R Discharge Kit (PO steroids and PO diphenhydramine) FU
SICKLE CELL CRISIS **Emergency Quick Kit** H & P Limited Basic Labs **IV Pain Kit** **Reticulocyte count** **Blood culture** **Urine culture** **CXR** Type and Cross Admit to ward (NPO, Bedrest) Incentive spirometry PO Hydroxyurea If severe: transfusion RBC If infection: IV Azithromycin C & R Discharge Kit FU	**HEMOPHILIA** H & P Basic Labs **Liver panel** **Bleeding Kit** Admit to ward IV Kit **Test for Factor VIII, IX, XI** **Factor VIII therapy** Monitor until normal PTT and Factor VIII Consult genetics **Medic alert bracelet** C & R (no aspirin) Discharge Kit FU 1 week
DVT DEEP VEIN THROMBOSIS H & P Basic Labs IV Kit Pain Kit IV **PE-DVT Kit – Doppler of leg** C & R (diet, med side effects) Discharge Kit FU in 3 days to check platelet count FU to follow PT/INR	**PE PULMONARY EMBOLISM** **Emergency Quick Kit** H & P Limited Basic Labs IV Kit SOB Kit **PE-DVT Kit – Spiral CT, Doppler of leg** Admit to ward (regular diet, PT/INR and CBC daily) C & R (diet, med side effects) Discharge Kit FU to follow PT/INR and platelets

FOREIGN BODY ASPIRATION

Emergency Quick Kit
H & P Limited
Basic Labs – stat
Neck and CXR – stat
Consult pulmonary for **rigid bronchoscopy**
C & R
Discharge Kit
FU 2 weeks

PCP PNEUMOCYSTIS JIROVECI

H & P
Basic Labs
IV Kit
Pneumonia Kit
Admit to ward (ambulate, normal diet)
IV TMP/SMX
PO Prednisone
HIV Kit
Sputum pneumocystis stain
C & R (HIV support, med compliance and side effects)
Notify public health
Discharge Kit
FU with CD4 counts

COPD EXACERBATION

Emergency Quick Kit
H & P Limited
Basic Labs
SOB Kit
Sputum and blood cultures
Albuterol Nebulizer
Ipratropium Nebulizer
IV Methylprednisone
IV Ceftriaxone
Admit to ward (normal diet, bedrest with BRP)
Monitor pulse ox
Influenza and pneumococcal vaccine
C & R – no smoking, home oxygen
Discharge Kit
FU

ASTHMA EXACERBATION

Emergency Quick Kit
H & P Limited
Basic Labs
SOB Kit
Sputum and blood cultures
Monitor pulse ox
Albuterol Nebulizer
Oral prednisone
IV Methylprednisone
Ipratropium Nebulizer (if needed)
If better:
C & R (Beclomethasone and albuterol PRN)
FU

If not better:
Admit to ward (normal diet, bedrest with BRP)
PEFR every 2 hours
C & R (Beclomethasone and albuterol PRN)
Discharge Kit
FU

RSV – BRONCHIOLITIS

H & P
Pulse oximeter and monitor
Oxygen
CXR
RSV antigen
Albuterol Nebulizer
Epinephrine Nebulizer (if needed)
Recheck
Ribavirin Nebulizer (if needed)

If better
C & R
Discharge Kit
FU

If not better
Admit to ward

VIRAL CROUP

Pulse Ox monitor
Oxygen
H & P Limited
CBC
BMP
RSV antigen
Influenza swab
Neck X-ray
Humidified air
PO Dexamethasone if needed
Epinephrine Nebulizer if needed
If infection: PO 2nd generation Cephalosporin
Recheck every hour
Observe 3 hours

If better
C & R
Discharge Kit
FU
If not better admit to ward

TENSION PNEUMOTHORAX

Emergency Quick Kit
H & P limited
Needle thoracostomy
CXR
Pain Kit IV
Basic Labs
Cardiac Enzymes
Admit to ICU
Monitor cardiac, pulse ox, blood pressure
C & R

PNEUMONIA

H & P
Monitor pulse ox
Oxygen if needed
Basic Labs
Blood cultures
CXR

If pulse ox stays low or patient is unstable: **admit** to ward (ambulate, regular diet)
IV Levofloxacin

If pulse ox improves: will **discharge**
PO Azithromycin or
PO Ciprofloxacin if patient has additional complications

C & R (no smoking)
Discharge Kit
FU

PANIC ATTACK

H & P Limited
Basic Labs
D-dimer
CXR
EKG
Cardiac Enzymes
UA drug screen
Oral Alprazolam
Consult psych
C & R
Discharge Kit
FU

A-FIB

Emergency Quick Kit
H & P Limited
Basic Labs
Cardiac Kit
Consult cardio
IV Metoprolol
PO Warfarin
C & R (medicine compliance)
Discharge Kit
FU with EKG and PT/INR

ENDOCARDITIS

H & P
Basic Labs
Urine culture
Infection Panel - Blood culture
EKG
CXR
ECHO
IV Kit
IV Gentamycin and IV Vancomycin
Admit to ward
Consult Infectious Dz
Monitor blood cultures till negative
C & R
Discharge
FU

CHF EXACERBATION

H & P Limited
Emergency Quick Kit
SOB Kit
Basic Labs
Cardiac Kit
IV Furosemide
PO Lisinopril
PO Metoprolol
Admit to ward (ambulate, low sodium diet)
Monitor pulse ox, cardiac, blood pressure
C & R (meds, exercise, no alcohol)
Discharge
FU

HEART BLOCK
H & P Limited
Basic Labs
Cardiac Kit
IV Kit
Temporary pacemaker
Consult cardiac
Admit to ICU
Permanent pacemaker
C & R
Discharge Kit
FU

TAMPONADE
Emergency Quick Kit
H & P Limited
Consult thoracic surgery
Pericardiocentesis
Pain Kit IV
Cardiac Kit
FAST US
Admit to ICU
C & R
Discharge Kit
FU

<table>
<tr>
<td>UNSTABLE ANGINA

Emergency Quick Kit
H & P Limited
Cardiac Kit
IV Heparin
Monitor Cardiac enzymes every 8 hours
Monitor PTT every 6 hours
Admit to ICU
Consult cardiac
PO Metoprolol
PO Simvastatin
PO Clopidogrel
IV Abciximab
Lipid panel
Liver panel
Cardiac Catheterization - STAT
(if required: Cardiac angioplasty)
C & R (no alcohol, no smoking, exercise, decrease sodium and cholesterol from diet, meds: aspirin, metoprolol, statin, nitroglycerin, clopidogrel)
Discharge Kit
FU at 2 and 6 weeks</td>
<td>HTN EMERGENCY

H & P Limited
Emergency Quick Kit
Monitor BP and pulse oximeter and cardiac
Basic Labs
UA
Troponin serum
Head CT without contrast
Lipid panel
IV Nitroprusside or IV Labetalol
Admit to ICU
ECHO
C & R (no smoking, no alcohol, decrease salt. Meds: PO Labetalol, PO Lisinopril, PO Hydrochlorothiazide
Discharge Kit
FU</td>
</tr>
<tr>
<td>MYOCARDIAL INFARCTION

Cardiac Kit – Emergency Kit
H & P Limited
PO Metoprolol
IV Abciximab
IV Heparin
Coronary angiography
Consult cardiology for PCI (stent/angioplasty)
IV Furosemide (if CHF)
PO Clopidogrel
PO Lisinopril
Admit to ICU
C & R (no smoking)</td>
<td>MYOCARDIAL INFARCTION - COCAINE

Cardiac Kit – Emergency Kit
H & P Limited
IV Alprazolam
IV Diltiazem
IV Heparin
Coronary angiography
Consult cardiology for PCI (stent/angioplasty)
Admit to ICU
C & R (no smoking, no illicit drugs, no alcohol)</td>
</tr>
<tr>
<td>THYROID STORM

H & P
Emergency Quick Kit
Basic Labs - TSH
Liver Panel
Cardiac Kit
RAI uptake (not in pregnant patients)
Thyroid autoantibodies
Thyroid US
Methimazole (PTU if pregnant)
Propanolol
FU in 4 weeks
Recheck TSH, Free T4
C & R
FU</td>
<td>RUPTURE AAA

Emergency Quick Kit
IV Morphine and Phenergan
Basic Labs
Abdominal CT with contrast
Consult Vascular Surgery for laparotomy to repair AAA
Surgery Kit – type and cross
Admit to ICU
FU
Admit to ward
C & R (no smoking, no alcohol)
Discharge Kit
FU</td>
</tr>
</table>

TTP H & P Basic Labs **Bleeding panel** **Consult hematology** **Plasma Exchange (Plasmapheresis)** Transfer to ICU or ward **Monitor pulse ox and CBC** Check CBC daily C & R Discharge Kit FU	**TEMPORAL ARTERITIS** H & P Basic Labs – **ESR, monitor ESR** **Head CT without contrast** **PO Prednisone** Infection Panel – Serum Autoantibody panel Consult rheumatology **Temporal artery biopsy** C & R (**Increase calcium**, vitamin D, **calcium carbonate**, exercise) Discharge Kit FU with labs and biopsy
TIA **Emergency Quick Kit** H & P – **Neuro and Psych** Basic Labs Lipid panel **Head CT without contrast** Consult neurology **Carotid Doppler** **Carotid angiography** **Cardiac panel** Admit to ward (regular diet, ambulate) **PO Aspirin** **PO Dipyridamole** If > 70% stenosis: Consult vascular surgery for carotid endarterectomy C & R	**SEIZURE** **Emergency Kit** H & P Basic Labs **UA Drug screen** **Head CT without contrast** **MRI brain** Admit to ward **Consult neurology** C & R (no driving) Discharge Kit FU in 3 weeks
SUB ARACHNOIC HEMORRHAGE **Emergency Quick Kit** H & P Limited (be aware of breathing in case need for intubation and mechanical ventilation) **Head CT without contrast** **Cerebral angiography** **IV Labetalol** Monitor BP Monitor Cardiac Basic Labs Cardiac enzymes Pain Kit IV Admit to ICU **Monitor cardiac, pulse ox, blood pressure** **Contact neurosurgery** C & R	**STROKE** **Emergency Quick Kit** H & P – **Neuro and Psych** Basic Labs Lipid panel **Head CT without contrast** **IV Streptokinase (if no contradictions and <4 hours of SX)** Consult neurology **Carotid Doppler** **Carotid angiography** **Cardiac panel** Admit to ward (regular diet, ambulate) **PO Aspirin** **PO Dipyridamole** If > 70% stenosis: Consult vascular surgery for carotid endarterectomy C & R
SIGMOID VOLVULUS - OBSTRUCTION H & P Basic Labs IV Kit **NPO** **Abdominal X-Ray** Pain Kit IV NG Tube **Consult GI for surgery/sigmoidoscopy** Surgery Kit Admit to ward after surgery (bedrest, NPO) FU in 8 hours C & R Discharge Kit FU	**INTUSSUCEPTION** H & P Basic Labs IV Kit **NPO** **Abdominal X-Ray or US** Pain Kit IV NG Tube **Barium enema – STAT** Admit to ward (NPO, bedrest) Monitor urine output FU every 4 hours C & R Discharge Kit FU

DIVERTICULITIS H & P Basic Labs IV access **Pain Kit IV** **NPO** **Abdominal CT** **Blood cultures** **IV Ampicillin and Sulbactam** Admit to ward (NPO, bedrest with BRP) FU 12 and 24 hours C & R (oral meds: PO Percocet, PO Metronidazole, PO Ciprofloxacin, soft diet, increase dietary fiber, exercise) Discharge Kit FU	**PEPTIC ULCER RUPTURE** H & P Limited **Emergency Quick Kit** NPO Basic Labs **Pain Kit IV** Lipase Amylase **Liver panel - PT/PTT** **Abdominal X-Ray** **Abdominal CT** **Consult general surgery for laparotomy** IV Piperacillin and Tazobactam **IV Gentamicin** **IV Metronidazole** **IV Omeprazole** **Surgery Kit** NG tube Admit to ward or ICU after surgery (NPO, bedrest) **Monitor urine output, blood pressure, pulse ox, cardiac** C & R (no smoking, no alcohol)
ACUTE PANCREATITIS **Emergency Quick Kit** **NPO** H & P Basic Labs **Pain Kit IV with Meperidine or Dilaudid** **Amylase serum** **Lipase serum** **Liver panel** **Abdominal/Pelvis CT without contrast** Abdominal US IV Piperacillin and Tazobactam Admit to ICU **Monitor cardiac, blood pressure, pulse ox** Consult general surgery if gallstones C & R (no alcohol, no smoking) Discharge Kit FU	**ACUTE CHOLECYSTITIS** H & P Limited IV Kit Pain Kit IV **NPO** Basic Labs **Liver panel** **Amylase serum** **Lipase serum** Blood Cultures Abdominal X-Ray **Abdominal US** IV Piperacillin and Tazobactam IM Ketorolac Admit to ward **Consult with General Surgery for Laparoscope Cholecystectomy** Surgery Kit FU 8 hours C & R Discharge Kit FU
SPLEEN INJURY **Emergency Quick Kit** Cervical spine immobilization H & P NPO **Monitor cardiac, pulse ox, blood pressure** **Pain Kit IV** Basic Labs UA drug screen Blood alcohol level CXR **FAST Ultrasound** Spine X-RAY **Abdominal CT** **Consult general surgery** **Surgery Kit** Admit to ICU after surgery (NPO, bedrest) D/C Cervical spine brace FU 4 hours C & R Discharge Kit FU	**ACUTE APPENDICITIS** H & P NPO Basic Labs **B-hCG** Liver panel **Abdominal US or X-Ray** Pain Kit IV **Consult general surgery for laparotomy appendectomy** Surgery Kit Admit to ward after surgery (NPO, bedrest with BRP) C & R (counsel parent) Discharge Kit FU

PID H & P Basic Labs – **β-hCG** IV Kit **Transvaginal ultrasound** **GYN Panel** IV Kit **IV Cefoxitin** **Oral Doxycycline** Admit to ward (NPO, Bedrest with BRP) FU C & R (safe sex, PO Doxycycline) Discharge Kit FU	**OVARIAN TORSION – TESTICULAR TORSION** H & P Basic Labs – **β-hCG** NPO IV Kit **Pain Kit IV** **Pelvic US – STAT (ovarian torsion)** **US of testicles (testicular torsion)** **Consult GYN for Laparotomy STAT (ovarian torsion)** **Consult Urology for testicular torsion)** Surgery Kit Admit to ward after surgery (regular diet, bedrest with BRP) FU in 12 hours C & R Discharge Kit FU
ECTOPIC PREGNANCY H & P Basic Labs **Transvaginal US** **β-hCG qualitative** Admit to ward (**NPO**, bedrest) If β-hCG qualitative levels <5000 consult OBGYN for Methotrexate If β-hCG qualitative levels >5000 **consult OBGYN for laparoscope**. **Surgery Kit** **Pain Kit IV** FU C & R Discharge Kit FU in 4 days	**ECLAMPSIA, FETAL DISTRESS** **Emergency Quick Kit** Fetal monitor H & P NPO Basic Labs **UA** **Liver panel** Foley Monitor urine output Type and Cross **IV Magnesium Sulfate** **IV Hydralazine** **Consult OBGYN for C-section** Surgery Kit Admit to ward after surgery **Monitor cardiac, pulse ox, blood pressure, urine output** FU C & R
GOUT H & P Basic Labs **Uric acid- serum** **Bone and Joint panel** Liver panel **PO Indomethacin (Colchicine if allergies to NSAIDS)** C & R (decrease protein in diet, no alcohol, no smoking) Discharge Kit FU	**SEPTIC ARTHRITIS** H & P Basic Labs Pain Kit IV **Bone and Joint panel** Consult orthopedics for Arthrocentesis Admit to unit (NPO, bedrest) Aspirate joint fluid daily **Immobilize joint** **IV Ceftriaxone** C & R Discharge Kit FU

TOXIC SHOCK

Emergency Quick Kit
H & P
(Remove tampon or other blood filled item: nose pack)
IV Dopamine if hypotensive
ABG and monitor
Basic Labs
PT/INR
PTT
Vaginal gram stain (if female due to tampon)
Vaginal culture (if female due to tampon)
Serum Infection Panel - Blood cultures
IV Vancomycin
IV Clindamycin
Admit to ICU
Monitor cardiac, pulse ox, blood pressure, urine output
Consult Infectious Disease
FU
C & R
Discharge Kit
FU

Cryptococcus Meningitis: HIV

H & P
Basic Labs
IV Kit
Pain Kit IV
Serum Infection Panel - Blood cultures
Head CT
Cryptococcal Serum antigen
Lumbar Puncture for CSF – STAT
(CSF: glucose, protein, gram stain, Cryptococcus antigen, fungal cultures, bacterial antigen AFB stain, India Ink stain)
IV Amp B
PO Flucytosine
Transfer to ward (ambulate, regular diet)
HIV Kit
C & R (med compliance, no smoking, no alcohol, HIV support)
Discharge Kit
FU 2 weeks

BACTERIAL MENENGITIS

H & P
Basic Labs
IV Kit
Pain Kit IV
Serum Infection Panel - Blood cultures
Lumbar Puncture for CSF – STAT
(CSF: glucose, protein, gram stain, fungal cultures, bacterial antigen AFB stain)
Head CT
CXR
Elevate head
Monitor urine output
Pain Kit IV
IV Vancomycin and Ceftriaxone
IV Dexamethasone
Transfer to ward (NPO, Bedrest)
FU 8 hours
C & R (low salt diet)
Discharge Kit
FU

HERPES SIMPLEX ENCEPHALITIS

H & P
Basic Labs
UA Drug screen
IV Kit
Pain Kit IV
Blood cultures
PT/INR
PTT
Head CT
CXR
Elevate head
Monitor urine output
Pain Kit IV
IV Acyclovir
Lumbar Puncture for CSF – STAT
(CSF: PCR HSV, glucose, protein, gram stain, fungal cultures, bacterial antigen AFB stain)
Transfer to ward (NPO, Bedrest)
FU 8 hours
C & R (low salt diet)
Discharge Kit
FU

Hepatic Encephalopathy
H & P
IV Kit
Basic Labs
Ammonia serum
Liver panel
ABG and Monitor
UA Drug screen
Urine Culture
Blood Culture
Head CT
Oral Lactulose
Thiamine
Oral Neomycin
Admit to ICU
Monitor cardiac, pulse ox, blood pressure, urine output, ABG
FU
C & R

ANOREXIA
H & P
Basic Labs
Admit to ward (ambulate)
Consult with dietary specialist
Consult with psychiatry
BMP daily
EKG daily
Liver panel FSH,
Prolactin levels
FSH levels
PO Potassium chloride if hypokalemic
IV Calcium gluconate if hyperkalemic
PO Magnesium
PO Phosphate
Depression index: If depressed give SSRI
FU
C & R

MANIA	CHILD ABUSE or ELDER ABUSE
H & P Basic Labs **UA Drug screen** **PO Lithium** IM Olanzapine Admit to ward (ambulate, regular diet) **Consult with psychiatry** **Psychotherapy** Suicide contract C & R (medicine compliance, exercise)	H & P Basic Labs UA Drug screen **XR of any breaks and repair/cast breaks** **Head CT if head trauma or altered mental status** **Liver panel, Amylase, Lipase if abdominal indications** **GYN specimen if sexual abuse suspected** **Skeletal survey** **PT/ PTT, Bleed Time if bruising** **PO Acetaminophen** **Consult Child Protective Services** Consult Psych Admit to ward (regular diet, ambulate) – do NOT send home

INDEX

A

B

E

F

J

K

M

S

T

STEP 3 CS CASES

Illustration Credits

I have tried to give credit to the authors of each and every image or illustration in this medical textbook. Many hours were put into reaching out to all authors/sources. In the event that I was unable to find an author, I used images that were found in various places throughout the Internet and believe these to be within public domain. Public domain images used are believed to be within the US Copyright Fair Use Act (title 17, US Code). If you are the owner of any of these images and feel that it infringes your copyright please let me know, and I will be very happy to credit your work or remove the image on the next edition of this book. This book is solely used for the education of medical students and residents; therefore I greatly appreciate all of the authors and sources that have allowed us to use their work in order to provide excellent medical education to our future and current doctors.

Pg 27 Cell anatomy. Blausen.com staff. "Blausen gallery 2014". Wikiversity Journal of Medicine. DOI:10.15347/wjm/2014.010. ISSN 20018762. - Own work. Licensed under CC BY 3.0 via Wikimedia Commons.
Pg 29 Ribosomes. Illustration by Tricia Derges, MD.
Pg 30 Cilia. "Eukaryotic flagellum" by en:User:Smartse - File:Axoneme.JPG and Figure 19.28 on page 819 of "Molecular Cell Biology, 4th edition, Lodish and Berk" ISBN 0-7167-3706-X. Licensed under CC BY-SA 3.0 via Wikimedia Commons.
Pg 30 Dextrocardia. "Situs inversus chest Nevit" by Nevit - Own work. Licensed under CC BY-SA 3.0 via Wikimedia Commons.
Pg 30 mitochondria. https://commons.wikimedia.org/wiki/File%3AMitochondria%2C_mammalian_lung_-_TEM.jpg.
Pg 31 Cell histology. Illustration by Tricia Derges, MD.
Pg 33 Cellular junctions. Illustrations by Tricia Derges, MD.
Pg 34 Skin histology. http://commons.wikimedia.org/wiki/Image:Skin.jpg original license tag is "Public domain - Work of US fed. gov."
Pg 34 Langerhans cells: By Yale Rosen from USA. creativecommons.org/licenses/by-sa/2.0)], via Wikimedia Commons.
Pg 36 Pancreas cell. Illustration by Tricia Derges, MD.
Pg 38 Adrenal histology. By Jpogi [CC0], via Wikimedia Commons.
Pg 39 Neuron. Licensed under CC BY-SA 3.0 via Wikimedia Commons.
Pg 41 Mitosis and Meiosis. Illustrations by Tricia Derges MD.
Pg 42 Cell cycle. Illustrations by Tricia Derges, MD.
Pg 43 Cell cycle. Modification of work by Mariana Ruiz Villareal; credit "mitosis micrographs": modification of work by Roy van Heesbeen; credit "cytokinesis micrograph": modification of work by the Wadsworth Center, NY State Department of Health; donated to the Wikimedia foundation; scale-bar data from Matt Russell)
Pg 46 Apoptosis. Illustrations by Tricia Derges, MD.
Pg 46 Chromatin. By Sha, K. and Boyer, L. A. The chromatin signature of pluripotent cells (May 31, 2009), StemBook, ed. The Stem Cell Research Community, StemBook. creativecommons.org via Wikimedia Commons. Adapted by Dr. Tricia Derges, MD.
Pg 48 DNA Replication. By Bstlee (Own work) [Public domain], via Wikimedia Commons. Adapted by Dr. Tricia Derges, MD.
Pg 50 tRNA. Adapted by Dr. Tricia Derges, MD
Pg 50 Ribosome. Illustrations by Dr. Tricia Derges, MD.
Pg 51 mRNA. Illustrations by Dr. Tricia Derges, MD.
Pg 51 Poly Snake. Illustrations by Dr. Tricia Derges, MD.
Pg 56 Nondisjunction. By Tweety207 - Own work, CC BY-SA 3.0,
Pg 59 Brushfield spots. By Szymon Tomczak was the original author of this photo. [CC0], via Wikimedia Commons
Pg 59 Nuchal rigidity. [[File:Nuchal edema in Down Syndrome Dr. W. Moroder.jpg|Nuchal edema in Down Syndrome Dr. W. Moroder]]
Pg 59 Simean crease. סימיאני קו
Pg 59 Epicanthal folds. By Centers for Disease Control and Prevention, National Center on Birth Defects and Developmental Disabilities [Public domain], via Wikimedia Commons
Pg 62 "Lisch nodules" by National Eye Institute - National Eye Institute. Licensed under Public Domain via Commons.
Pg 62 Bilateral Schwannomas. Radipedia/WikiMedia. Hanleym.
Pg 66 Amino acid side chains. Illustrations by Dr. Tricia Derges, MD.
Pg 74 Glycolysis and Associated Cycles. Illustrations by Dr. Tricia Derges MD
Pg 75 Cori Cycle. Illustrations by Tricia Derges MD
Pg 75 TCA Cycle. By Narayanese, WikiUserPedia, YassineMrabet, TotoBaggins (uploaded to Commons by wadester16), CC BY-SA 3.0, https://commons.wikimedia.org
Pg 77 Electron Transport Chain. Illustrations by Dr. Tricia Derges, MD.
Pg 79 Gluconeogenesis. By Dwong527 - Own work, CC BY-SA 3.0, https://commons.wikimedia.org/w/index.php?curid=24993082
Pg 80 Galactose Pathway. Illustrations by Dr. Tricia Derges MD.
Pg 81 Fructose Pathway. Illustrations by Dr. Tricia Derges MD.
Pg 81 HMP Shunt (PPP): Illustrations by Dr. Tricia Derges MD
Pg 82 NADPH Pathway: Illustrations by Dr. Tricia Derges MD
Pg 83 Pyrimidine/Purine Synthesis. Illustrations by Dr. Tricia Derges MD
Pg 84 Purine Salvage Pathway. By Torres RJ, Puig JG - Torres RJ, Puig JG. Hypoxanthine-guanine phosphoribosyltransferase (HPRT) deficiency: Lesch-Nyhan Syndrome. Wikipedia Commons.
Pg 85 Urea Pathway. Illustrations by Dr. Tricia Derges, MD.
Pg 86 Phenylalanine and Catecholamine Pathway. Illustrations by Dr. Tricia Derges, MD.
Pg 88 Tryptophan Pathway. Illustrations by Dr. Tricia Derges, MD.
Pg 88 Homocysteine Pathway. Illustrations by Dr. Tricia Derges, MD.
Pg 91 Glycogen structure. Häggström, Mikael. "Medical gallery of Mikael Häggström 2014". Wikiversity Journal of Medicine 1 (2). [Public domain], via Wikimedia Commons
Pg 91 Glycogen structure and degradation. Illustrations by Dr. Tricia Derges, MD.
Pg 93 Fatty Acids, Cholesterol, Ketones. Illustrations by Dr. Tricia Derges, MD.
Pg 96 Lipid Transport. Illustrations by Dr. Tricia Derges MD.
Pg 96 Marasmus. "Starved child" by Photo Credit:Content Providers(s): CDC/ Don Eddins - This media comes from the Centers for Disease Control and Prevention's Public Health Image Library (PHIL), with identification number #1702.Note: Public Domain via Commons.
Pg 96 Kwashiorkor. "Starved girl" by Dr. Lyle Conrad - Centers for Disease Control and Prevention, Atlanta, Georgia, USAPublic Health Image Library (PHIL); via Wikimedia Commons, Flickr
Pg 97 Methanol, Ethanol Metabolism. Illustrations by Dr. Tricia Derges, MD.
Pg 98 Collagen Synthesis. Illustrations by Dr. Tricia Derges, MD.
Pg 100 Heme Synthesis. Illustrations by Dr. Tricia Derges, MD.
Pg 108 Action potential. By OpenStax College [CC BY 3.0) via Wikimedia Commons
Pg 108 Axon-Dendrite. By M.aljar3i - Own work, CC BY-SA 3.0, https://commons.wikimedia.org/w/index.php?curid=22116795
Pg 108 Action Potential. *Blausen.com staff. "Blausen gallery 2014". Wikiversity Journal of Medicine.*
Pg 110 CNS. By The original uploader was Fuzzform at अंग्रेज़ी Wikipedia - Transferred from en.wikipedia to Commons by Fredlyfish4 using Commons Helper., CC BY-SA 3.0, https://commons.wikimedia.org/w/index.php?curid=20086386
Pg 111 Spinal Nerves. By OpenStax College - Anatomy & Physiology, Connexions Web site. http://cnx.org/content/col11496/1.6/, Jun 19, 2013., CC BY 3.0, https://commons.wikimedia.org/w/index.php?curid=30148017
Pg 111 Parsympathetic vs Sympathetic. By Geo-Science-International (Own work) [CC0], via Wikimedia Commons
Pg 111 Vetebrae. By OpenStax College [CC BY 3.0 (http://creativecommons.org/licenses/by/3.0)], via Wikimedia Commons
Pg 111 Vertebrae. By user:debivort (Own work) [GFDL (http://www.gnu.org/copyleft/fdl.html) or CC-BY-SA-3.0 (http://creativecommons.org/licenses/by-sa/3.0/)], via Wikimedia Commons
Pg 114 Gs Pathways. Illustrations by Dr. Tricia Derges, MD.
Pg 115 Gi Pathway. Illustrations by Dr. Tricia Derges, MD.

Pg 115 *Gq Pathway. By Yikrazuul [CC BY-SA 3.0 (http://creativecommons.org/licenses/by-sa/3.0)], via Wikimedia Commons and adaptation by Dr. Tricia Derges, MD.*
Pg 118 *Cholinergic and Adrenergic NT Release. Illustrations by Dr. Tricia Derges, MD.*
Pg 126 *Vmax and Km. Illustration by Dr. Tricia Derges, MD.*
Pg 126 *Lineweaver-Burk plot. Bizz1111, own work, August 2016. Wikimedia Commons.*
Pg 128 *First Order-Zero Order. Wikispaces.com licensed under a Creative Commons Attribution Share-Alike 3.0 license.*
Pg 128 *First Order Metabolism. Illustration by Dr. Tricia Derges, MD.*
Pg 132 *Sympathomimetic Reactions. Illustrations by Dr. Tricia Derges MD.*
Pg 133 *Bioavailability. Illustration by Dr. Tricia Derges, MD.*
Pg 135 *Umbilical Cord. By pixgood.com*
Pg 135 *Twins. By Kevin Dufendach - Own work, CC BY 3.0, Creative Commons via Wikimedia Commons*
Pg 136 *Neural Crest Queen. Illustration by Dr. Tricia Derges MD.*
Pg 136 *Tongue Development. Illustration by Dr. Tricia Derges, MD.*
Pg 144 *Thyroglossal cyst. By Gzzz (Own work) [CC BY-SA 4.0 (http://creativecommons.org/licenses/by-sa/4.0)], via Wikimedia Commons*
Pg 144 *Brachial Cleft Cyst. Geneva Foundation for Medical Education and Research. Switzerland*
Pg 145 *Esophageal atresia. By see above - Lewis Spitz. Oesophageal atresia. Orphanet Journal of Rare Diseases. 2, 24. 2007. PMID 17498283., CC BY 2.0,* https://commons.wikimedia.org/w/index.php?curid=2576642
Pg 145 *Annular Pancreas. Illustration by Dr. Tricia Derges, MD.*
Pg 146 *Congenital diaphragmatic hernia.* https://radiopaedia.org/cases/congenital-diaphragmatic-hernia
Pg 146 *Intussusception. By Olek Remesz (wiki-pl: Orem, commons: Orem) (Own work) [CC BY-SA 3.0 Creative Commons via Wikimedia Commons*
Pg 148 *Duodenal Atresia.* "Radiograph with Double Bubble Sign" by Jason Robert Young MD - Own work. Licensed under CC BY-SA 4.0 via Wikimedia Commons
Pg 148 Apple Peel Atresia. Pixgood.com
Pg 149 Gastroschisis and Omphalocele. By Centers for Disease Control and Prevention, National Center on Birth Defects and Developmental Disabilities - Centers for Disease Control and Prevention, National Center on Birth Defects and Developmental Disabilities, CC BY-SA Wikipedia Commons.
Pg 151 Bicornuate Uterus, Hypospadias. Unable to locate author. Please contact us and we will credit in the next edition.
Pg 152 Caudal regression. *Geneva Foundation for Medical Education and Research. Switzerland*
Milium. By Serephine - Own work, CC0, commons.wikimedia.org
Pg 159 Microcephaly. By Sumaia Villela/Agência Brasil - http://agenciabrasil.ebc.com.br/geral/foto/2016-04/exercicios-simples-estimulam-bebes-com-microcefalia, CC BY 3.0 br, https://commons.wikimedia.org/w/index.php?curid=48094981
Pg 159 Macrocephaly. By See Source - The Cell Nucleus and Aging: Tantalizing Clues and Hopeful Promises. Scaffidi P, Gordon L, Misteli T. PLoS Biology Vol. 3/11/2005, e395 doi:10.1371/journal.pbio.0030395, CC BY 2.5, https://commons.wikimedia.org/w/index.php?curid=1432055
Pg 160 Syphilis. CDC/ Dr. Norman Cole - This media comes from the Centers for Disease Control and Prevention's Public Health Image Library (PHIL)
Pg 161 Congenital Rubella. By CDC - PHIL, Center for Disease Control (CDC) -- ID# 713, Public Domain, https://commons.wikimedia.org/w/index.php?curid=12841764
Pg 161 Congenital CMV. - This media comes from the Centers for Disease Control and Prevention's Public Health Image Library (PHIL)
Pg 161 Neonatal Chlamydia. By CDC/ J. Pledger - This media comes from the Centers for Disease Control and Prevention's Public Health Image Library (PHIL), with identification number #3766.
Pg 162 "Toxoplasma Gondii." J.P. Dubey 1996 http://gsbs.utmb.edu/microbook/ch084.htm 03/01/2009
Pg 162 Neonatal herpes. http://jillsafricamission.blogspot.com/2010/04/nalerigu-day-10-and-11-pics.html
Pg 163 Varicella-zoster. Imgarcade.com
Pg 164 Fetal Alcohol Syndrome. By Teresa Kellerman - http://www.come-over.to/FAS/fasbabyface.jpg, CC BY-SA 3.0, https://commons.wikimedia.org/w/index.php?curid=4847497
Pg 164 Premature. By Brian Hall (Own work) [Public domain], via Wikimedia Commons
Pg 171 Child abuse cigarette burns. By National Institute of Health - National Institute of Health, Public Domain, https://commons.wikimedia.org/w/index.php?curid=7848505
Pg 171 Child Abuse hot water burns. http://news.bbc.co.uk/2/hi/health/1879513.stm
Pg 171 Child abuse spiral fracture. By RSJThompson - Own work by uploader. Consent granted from patient., CC BY-SA 3.0, https://commons.wikimedia.org/w/index.php?curid=7752788
Pg 171 Mongolian spots. Imgarcade.com
Pg 171 Osteogenesis Fx. By Th. Zimmermann THWZ) - Own work, CC BY-SA 3.0 de, https://commons.wikimedia.org/w/index.php?curid=20683510
Pg 171 Spiral Fx. By RSJ Thompson - Own work by uploader. Consent granted from patient., CC BY-SA 3.0, https://commons.wikimedia.org/w/index.php?curid=7752788
Pg 180 Immune system pathway. . *Illustration by Dr. Tricia Derges, MD.*
Pg 187 *Antibody structure. Illustration by Dr. Tricia Derges, MD.*
Pg 188 *Complement pathway. By English text of 'Image:Complement pathway.png' by DO11.10 German translation of 'Image:Complement pathway.png' by Hduman Galician translation Miguelferig Catalan translation Leptictidium SVG by Perhelion [Public domain or Public domain], via Wikimedia Commons.*
Pg 190 *Margination: Leukocyte Extravasation. By Kuebi = Armin Kübelbeck (own work, made with InkScape) [CC BY 3.0 (http://creativecommons.org/licenses/by/3.0)], via Wikimedia Commons. Adapted by Dr. Tricia Derges, MD.*
Pg 191 *Arachidonic Acid Pathway. Illustration by Dr. Tricia Derges, MD.*
Pg 203 *Bacteria shapes. Illustration by Dr. Tricia Derges, MD*
Pg 203 *Gram Negative vs Gram Positive Bacteria. Illustration by Dr. Tricia Derges, MD*
Pg 211 *Splinter hemorrhages. By Splarka (Own work) [Public domain], via Wikimedia Commons.*
Pg 211 *Janeway lesions. By Wikinut.*
Pg 218 *Gram Positive Algorithm. By Huckfinne (Own work) [Public domain], via Wikimedia Commons.*
Pg 219 Cellulitis by RafaelLopez at the English language Wikipedia. Licensed under CC BY-SA 3.0 via Wikimedia Commons –
Pg 219 Septic arthritis. "Kneeffusion" by James Heilman, MD - Own work. Licensed under CC BY-SA 3.0 via Commons -
Pg 219 Impetigo-infected by Åsa Thörn - Own work. Licensed under CC BY-SA 3.0 via Commons -
Pg 221 Orbital cellulitis by Jonathan Trobe, M.D. - University of Michigan Kellogg Eye Center - The Eyes Have It. Licensed under CC BY 3.0 via Commons – Wikipedia.
Pg 224 Bacillus anthracis Gram by Photo Credit:Content Providers(s): CDC - This media comes from the Centers for Disease Control and Prevention's Public Health Image Library #2226. Licensed under Public Domain via Wikimedia Commons –
Pg 224 Neonatal tetanus 6374 by Photo Credit:Content Providers(s): CDC - This media comes from the Centers for Disease Control and Prevention's Public Health Image Library #6374.Note: Licensed under Public Domain via Commons.
Pg 225 Megacolon option. Ischemic bowel by haitham alfalah - Halfalah (talk) 14:34, 24 July 2008 (UTC). Licensed under CC BY-SA 3.0 via Commons - https://commons.wikimedia.org/wiki/File:Ischemic_bowel.JPG#/media/File:Ischemic_bowel.JPG
Pg 226 Pseudomembrane. Dirty white pseudomembrane classically seen in diphtheria 2013-07-06 11-07" by User:Dileepunnikri - Own work. Licensed under CC BY-SA 3.0 via wikimedia Commons –

Pg 226 Black colonies on tellurite agar option "Coli levine" by Witmadrid – Own work. Licensed under Public Domain via Commons

Pg 228 "Leprosy" by Pierre Arents - Pierre Arents printed the photographs for Leloir's monograph on leprosy titled, Traité pratique et théorique de la lèpre, published in 1886. This image is Plate VIII from that atlas. Vide: http://www.artandmedicine.com/biblio/authors/french/Leloir.html. Licensed under Public Domain via Commons –

Pg 228 miliary tuberculosis option. https://www.flickr.com/photos/pulmonary_pathology/7471756830

Pg 229 "Actinomycosis PHIL 2856 lores" by CDC/Dr. Thomas F. Sellers/Emory University - http://phil.cdc.gov/phil_images/20030110/21/PHIL_2856_lores.jpg. Licensed under Public Domain via Commons –

Pg 230 Septic arthritis. "Kneeffusion" by James Heilman, MD - Own work. Licensed under CC BY-SA 3.0 via Commons –

Pg 231 Pelvic inflammatory disease. "Perihepatic adhesions 2" by Hic et nunc - Own work. Licensed under Public Domain via Commons –

Pg 231 Gonorrhea male and gonorrhea female. Std-gov.org

Pg 237 Helicobacter pylori/AJC1/Flickr, Creative Commons.

Pg 238 Staghorn calculi. Kidney stones abdominal X-ray" by Bill Rhodes from Asheville - numerous stones kubU uploaded by Stevenfruitsmaak. Licensed under CC BY 2.0 via Commons –

Pg 242 SOA-Chlamydia-trachomatis-female". Licensed under CC BY-SA 3.0 via Commons –

Pg 242 Pap smear showing clamydia in the vacuoles 500x H&E" by http://visualsonline.cancer.gov/details.cfm?imageid=2331. Licensed under Public Domain via Commons –

Pg 242 Gonococcal ophthalmia neonatorum" by CDC/ J. Pledger - This media comes from the Centers for Disease Control and Prevention's Public Health Image Library #3766.Note: Licensed under Public Domain via Commons –

Pg 243 Pelvic inflammatory disease. "Perihepatic adhesions 2" by Hic et nunc - Own work. Licensed under Public Domain via Commons –

Pg 244 Leptospira interrogans strain RGA 01" by Obtained from the CDC Public Health Image Library. Image credit: CDC/NCID/HIP/Janice Carr (PHIL #1220). - http://en.wikipedia.org/wiki/Image:Leptospira_interrogans_strain_RGA_01.png CDC US Health. Licensed under Public Domain via Commons –

Pg 245 Syphilis lesions on back" es vum Office of Medical History, US Surgeon General - Adapted from http://history.amedd.army.mil/booksdocs/wwii/internalmedicinevolIII/chapter20figure64.jpg onger de Lezänz Allmende (jemeinfrei, public domain) jeschtallt woode, op udder övver <i lang="en">Wikimedia Commons</i> -

Pg 245 Ulcus-durum-am-Penis-01" by The original uploader was Pygmalion at German Wikipedia - Eigenes Archiv. Licensed under CC BY-SA 3.0 via Commons –

Pg 245 By Nephron (Own work) [CC BY-SA 3.0 (http://creativecommons.org/licenses/by-sa/3.0) or GFDL (http://www.gnu.org/copyleft/fdl.html)], via Wikimedia Commons

Pg 249 Bullseye Lyme Disease Rash" by Hannah Garrison Original uploader was Jongarrison at en.wikipedia - Transferred from en.wikipedia; transfer was stated to be made by User:Optigan13.(Original text : en:User:Jongarrison). Licensed under CC BY-SA 2.5 via Commons –

Pg 249 Maltese cross. "Babiesa spp" by Photo Credit:Content Providers(s): CDC/ Steven Glenn; Laboratory & Consultation Division – This media comes from the Centers for Disease Control and Prevention's Public Health Image Library #5943.Note: Licensed under Public Domain via Commons –

Pg 249 Rocky Mountain spotted fever PHIL 1962 lores" by Public Health Image Library Licensed under Public Domain via Wikimedia Commons –

Pg 249 Adult deer tick by Photo by Scott Bauer. - This image was released by the Agricultural Research Service, the research agency of the United States Department of Agriculture, with the ID k8002-3. Licensed under Public Domain via Commons –

Pg 249 Dermacentor andersoni by Centers for Desease and Prevention, part of Department of Health and Human Services - Licensed under Public Domain via Wikimedia Commons –

Pg 250 Xenopsylla cheopis flea PHIL 2069 lores" by CDC/Dr. Pratt - This media comes from the Centers for Disease Control and Prevention's Public Health Image Library #2069.Note: +/–. Licensed under Public Domain via Commons –

Pg 250 Louse nits. Licensed under CC BY-SA 3.0 via Wikipedia –

Pg 250 Male of head louse" by Kosta Mumcuoglu at the English language Wikipedia. Licensed under CC BY-SA 3.0 via Commons –

Pg 250 Body lice. public-domain-image.com/free-images/science/microscopy-images/lice-infestation/body-lice

Pg 250 Pubic louse. Pthirus pubis - crab louse. Commons. Wikimedia.

Pg 251 ScabiesD06. Licensed under Public Domain via Wikimedia Commons –

Pg 251 Bed bug, Cimex lectularius" by Content Providers(s): CDC/ Harvard University, Dr. Gary Alpert; Dr. Harold Harlan; Richard Pollack. Photo Credit: Piotr Naskrecki - http://phil.cdc.gov/phil. Licensed under Public Domain via Commons –

Pg 251 Bedbug bites by Original uploader was Andybrookestar at en.wikipedia - Transferred from en.wikipedia; transferred to Commons by User:Liftarn using CommonsHelper.. Licensed under Public Domain via Commons –

Pg 251 Bedbugb2 by James Heilman, MD - Own work. Licensed under CC BY-SA 3.0 via Commons

Pg 252 Antibiotic Mechanism of Action. *Illustration by Dr. Tricia Derges, MD.*

Pg 258 Antibiotics Chart. Illustration by Dr. Tricia Derges, MD, Concept by Dr. Hiram Isaac, MD.

Pg 262 PABA Path. Illustration by Dr. Tricia Derges, MD.

Pg 266 "Blastomyces dermatitidis GMS" by Medmyco (talk) (Uploads) - Own work. Licensed under CC0 via Wikipedia - https://en.wikipedia.org/wiki/File:Blastomyces_dermatitidis_GMS.jpeg#/media/File:Blastomyces_dermatitidis_GMS.jpeg

Pg 266 "Blastomycosis of skin" by Transferred from en.wikipedia to Commons. This media comes from the Centers for Disease Control and Prevention's Public Health Image Library #492. Licensed under Public Domain via Wikimedia Commons –

Pg 266 Endospores. "Coccidioidomycosis Spherule" by UNK - http://phil.cdc.gov/phil/. Licensed under Public Domain via Wikimedia Commons -

Pg 266 Coccidioidomycosis lesions. By CDC/ Dr. Lucille K. Georg [Public domain], via Wikimedia Commons

Pg 267 "Histoplasmosis capsulatum" by Photo Credit:Content Providers(s): CDC/Dr. Libero Ajello - This media comes from the Centers for Disease Control and Prevention's Public Health Image Library #4223.Note. Licensed under Public Domain via Commons –

Pg 267 "Paracoccidioides brasiliensis 01" by Photo Credit:Content Providers(s): CDC/ Dr. Lucille K. Georg - This media comes from the Centers for Disease Control and Prevention's Public Health Image Library #527. Licensed under Public Domain via Commons –

Pg 267 "Tinea versicolor1" by Sarahrosenau on Flickr.com - Flickr.com. Licensed under CC BY-SA 2.0 via Commons - https://commons.wikimedia.org/wiki/File:Tinea_versicolor1.jpg#/media/File:Tinea_versicolor1.jpg

Pg 269 Tinea pedis. Athletes" von User Falloonb on en.wikipedia - Eigenes Werk. Lizenziert unter Gemeinfrei über Wikimedia Commons –

Pg 269 Tinea capitis. Tinea capitis" by Teigne - Own work. Licensed under GFDL via Commons –

Pg 269 "Tinea corporis" by Corina G. - Corina G. (author wishes to remain partly anonymous). Licensed under Public Domain via Wikimedia Commons –

Pg 269 "Oncymycosis" by James Heilman, MD - Own work. Licensed under CC BY-SA 3.0 via Commons –

Pg 269 "Aspergillus fumigatus (257 15)" by Doc. RNDr. Josef Reischig, CSc. - Author's archive. Licensed under CC BY-SA 3.0 via Wikimedia Commons –

Pg 270 "Candida albicans 2" by GrahamColm - Own work. Licensed under CC BY-SA 3.0 via Wikimedia Commons –

Pg 270 "Candidal Vulvovaginitis" by Mikael Häggström - Own work. Licensed under CC0 via Commons –

Pg 271 "Cryptococcus neoformans" by see Source - Iron Regulation and an Opportunistic AIDS-Related Fungal Infection. Gross L, PLoS Biology Vol. 4/12/2006, e427. http://dx.doi.org/10.1371/journal.pbio.0040427. Licensed under CC BY 2.5 via Wikimedia Commons

Pg 271 Mucor sp. fungus" by Photo Credit:Content Providers: CDC/Dr. Lucille K. Georg - This media comes from the Centers for Disease Control #3960. Licensed under Public Domain via Wikimedia Commons –

Pg 271 Pneumocystis jirovecii. "PCPxray" by User InvictaHOG on en.wikipedia - Originally from en.wikipedia. Licensed under Public Domain via Commons –

Pg 272 Sporothrix **schenckii.** "Conidiophores and conidia of the fungus Sporothrix schenckii PHIL 4208 lores" by http://phil.cdc.gov/phil_images/20030721/16/PHIL_4208_lores.jpg. Licensed under Public Domain via Commons –

Pg 272 Rose gardener, "Sporotrichosis by the fungus Sporothrix schenckii PHIL 3940 lores" by Content Providers(s). CDC/Dr. Lucille K. Georg - http://phil.cdc.gov/phil_images/20030610/25/PHIL_3940_lores.jpg. Licensed under Public Domain via Wikimedia Commons –
Pg 272 Naegleria fowleri. Public domain. Wikimedia Commons.
Pg 273 African sleeping sickness. "Trypanosoma sp. PHIL 613 lores" by Photo Credit:Content Providers: CDC/Dr. Myron G. Schultz – This media comes from the Centers for Disease Control and Prevention's Public Health Image Library #613. Licensed under Public Domain via Wikimedia Commons –
Pg 273 Babesiosis. http://www.public-domain-image.com/free-images/science/microscopy-
Pg 274 Trophozoites, Merozoites. http://www.public-domain-image.com/free-images/science/microscopy-
Pg 274 Malaria life cycle. By Hill A [CC BY 3.0 (http://creativecommons.org/licenses/by/3.0)], via Wikimedia Commons
Pg 275 Cryptosporidium, Amebiasis, Giardiasis. http://www.public-domain-image.com/free-images/science/microscopy-
Pg 276 "Leishmania" by CDC/ Dr. Francis W. Chandler - This media comes from the Centers for Disease Control and Prevention's Public Health Image Library #30.Note: Licensed under Public Domain via Wikimedia Commons –
Pg 276 "Trichomoniasi02" di .cecco (msg) 12:57, 2 lug 2008 (CEST) - Esame clinico. Con licenza Pubblico dominio tramite Wikipedia –
Pg 277 "Trypanosoma cruzi crithidia" by Photo Credit:Content Providers(s): CDC/Dr. Myron G. Schultz - This media comes from the Centers for Disease Control and Prevention's Public Health Image Library #613. Licensed under Public Domain via Commons –
Pg 277 "Diphyllobothrium latum scolex x40" by - Own work. Licensed under CC BY-SA 3.0 via Commons –
Pg 277 "Echinococcus multilocularis" by http://www.cdc.gov/NCIDOD/EID/vol9no3/02-0320-G1.htm. Licensed under Public Domain via Commons –
Pg 278 "Taenia solium" by Unknown - Memorie sulla storia e notomia degli animali senza vertebre del regno di Napoli Chiaje, Stefano delle. Licensed under Public Domain via Commons –
Pg 278 "Neurocysticercosis". Licensed under Public Domain via Commons –
Pg 278 "Hookworm filariform A" by Fernandolive - Own work. Licensed under Public Domain via Wikimedia Commons –
Pg 278 "Ascaris lumbricoides adult worms" by SuSanA Secretariat - https://www.flickr.com/photos/gtzecosan/15701719491/in/set-72157648708895830. Licensed under CC BY 2.0 via Commons –
Pg 279 "Threadworm" (Pinworm). Licensed under Public Domain via Commons –
Pg 279 "Adult female Loa loa filarial worm - Extracted from a patient's conjunctiva in the left eye" by Nathan Reading from Halesowen, UK - Loa Loa. Licensed under CC BY 2.0 via Wikimedia Commons –
Pg 279 Onchocerca volvulus. bdracunculose" by Otis Historical Archives of "National Museum of Health & Medicine" (OTIS Archive 1) - http://www.flickr.com/photos/medicalmuseum/4951113771/in/photostream. Licensed under CC BY 2.0 via Commons –
Pg 279 "Strongyloides stercoralis larva". Licensed under Public Domain via Commons –
Pg 280 Toxocara canis . "T. canis adult worms wiki" by Flukeman - Own work. Licensed under CC BY-SA 3.0 via Commons –
Pg 280 Trichinellosis. Clinical appearance of eyes in trichinosis by trichinella 3MG0027 lores" de http://phil.cdc.gov/PHIL_Images/09041998/00033/3MG0027_lores.jpg. Sub licență Domeniu public via Wikimedia Commons –
Pg 280 Wuchereria bancrofti. "Elephanti" by O. G. Mason - Fox, George Henry. Photographic illustrations of skin diseases. E. B. Treat, New York, 1880. Licensed under Public Domain via Commons –
Pg 281 "Clonorchis sinensis 2" by Banchob Sripa, Sasithorn Kaewkes, Paiboon Sithithaworn, Eimorn Mairiang, Thewarach Laha, Michael Smout, Chawalit Pairojkul, Vajaraphongsa Bhudhisawasdi, Smarn Tesana, Bandit Thinkamrop, Jeffrey M. Bethony, Alex Loukas & Paul J. Brindley - Sripa B., Kaewkes S., Sithithaworn P., Mairiang E., Laha T., et al. (2007Licensed under CC BY 2.5 via Common
Pg 281 "Paragonimus westermani 01". Licensed under Public Domain via Commons
Pg 281 "Schistosome Parasite SEM" por Bruce Wetzel (photographer). Harry Schaefer =1762. Baixo a licenza Dominio público a través de Wikimedia Commons –
Pg 281 "Schistosoma 20041-300" by David Williams, Illinois State University - Transferred from en.wikipedia to Commons by User: Magnus Manske using CommonsHelper. Licensed under Public Domain via Commons
Pg 282 "Schistosoma mansoni2" by The original uploader was Waisberg at English Wikipedia - Transferred from en.wikipedia to Commons by Gliu.Davies Laboratory Uniformed Services University Bethesda, MD. Licensed under Public Domain via Commons –
Pg 283 Antifungal Pharmacology. Illustraion by Dr. Tricia Derges., MD.
Pg 287 Bacteriophage T4, Adenovirus, HIV retrovirus. By CNX OpenStax [CC BY 4.0 (http://creativecommons.org/licenses/by/4.0)], via Wikimedia Commons
Pg 287 Virus Structure. Work created by author, Graham Colm, Wikipedia Commons.
Pg 287 Viral Tegument. Work created by author, Ben Taylor. Wikipedia Commons.
Pg 289 DNA Virus. Nature Reviews/Microbiology.
Pg 290 DNA Virus Chart. Illustration by Dr. Tricia Derges, MD.
Pg 291 Herpes 1, Herpes labialis - opryszczka wargowa». Lisensiert under Offentlig eiendom via Wikimedia Commons.
Pg 291 Herpes 2. "SOA-Herpes-genitalis" by SOA-AIDS Amsterdam - SOA-AIDS Amsterdam. Licensed under CC BY-SA 3.0 via Commons.
Pg 292 "Child with chickenpox". Licensed under CC BY-SA 3.0 via Wikimedia Commons.
Pg 293 "Roseola" by Andrew Kerr - Own work. Licensed under Public Domain via Commons.
Pg 293 "Kaposi's Sarcoma" by Unknown - National Cancer Institute, AV-8500-3620. Licensed under Public Domain via Wikimedia Commons.
Pg 294 "HBV serum markers". Licensed under CC BY 3.0 via Wikipedia.
Pg 295 " Mulluscum contagiosum " by Evanherk from nl. Licensed under CC BY-SA 3.0 via Commons.
Pg 295 "Pink eye" by P33tr at English Wikipedia - Licensed under Public Domain via Wikimedia Commons.
Pg 296 „Conjuntivitis (RPS 03-06-2015)" von Raimundo Pastor - Eigenes Werk. Lizenziert unter CC-BY-SA 4.0 über Wikimedia Commons.
Pg 296 "Swollen eye with conjunctivitis" by Tanalai at English Wikipedia. Licensed under CC BY 3.0 via Commons.
Pg 296 "Allergicconjunctivitis" by James Heilman, MD - Own work. Licensed under CC BY-SA 4.0 via Commons.
Pg 296 " Fifth Disease" by Sandyjameslord - Own work. Licensed under CC BY-SA 4.0 via Commons.
Pg 299 RNA Virus Chart. Illustration by Dr. Tricia Derges, MD.
Pg 301 "Hand foot and mouth disease on child feet" by Ngufra at English Wikipedia. Licensed under CC BY-SA 3.0 via Commons.
Pg 301 "Hand Foot Mouth Disease" by MidgleyDJ at en.wikipedia. Licensed under CC BY-SA 3.0 via Commons.
Pg 301 "Trendelenburg" by User:Mikael Häggström. Licensed under Public Domain via Wikimedia Commons.
Pg 304 "Croup steeple sign" by Frank Gaillard - Own work. Licensed under CC BY-SA 3.0 via Commons.
Pg 305 "Morbillivirus measles infection" by Photo Credit:Content Providers(s): CDC/Dr. Heinz F. Eichenwald - This media comes from the Centers for Disease Control and Prevention's #3168.Note: Licensed under Public Domain via Commons.
Pg 305 "Mumps PHIL 130 lores" by Photo Credit:Content Providers: CDC/NIP/Barbara Rice - This media comes from the Centers for Disease Control and Prevention's Public Health Image #130.Note: Licensed under Public Domain via Commons.
Pg 306 "Rabies Virus Spikes" Licensed under Public Domain via Commons.
Pg 308 HIV Virus. By National Institutes of Health (NIH) - National Institutes of Health (NIH), Public Domain, Commons Wikipedia.
Pg 310 "Leukoplakiaaitor" by Aitor III - Own work. Licensed under Public Domain via Commons.
Pg 310 "Kaposis Sarcoma Lesions" by OpenStax College - Anatomy & Physiology, Connexions Web site. Licensed under CC BY 3.0 via Commons.
Pg 314 Antiviral Pharmacology. Illustrations by Dr. Tricia Derges, MD.
Pg 314 HIV Pharmacology. Illustrations by Dr. Tricia Derges, MD.
Pg 318 *Margination: Leukocyte Extravasation. By Kuebi = Armin Kübelbeck (own work, made with InkScape) [CC BY 3.0 (http://creativecommons.org/licenses/by/3.0)], via Wikimedia Commons. Adapted by Dr. Tricia Derges, MD.*
Pg 319 "Complications of Hypertrophic Scarring" by Aarabi S, Longaker MT, Gurtner GC (2007). Licensed under CC BY 3.0 via Commons.

Pg 319 "Keloid" by Michael Rodger - Own work. Licensed under CC BY 3.0 via Commons.
Pg 321 Lipofuscin. By Nephron (Own work) via Wikimedia Commons.
Pg 322 Apoptosis. Illustrations by Dr. Tricia Derges, MD.
Pg 322 Extrinsic Apoptosis. By B1357M (Own work) via Wikimedia Commons.
Pg 331 "Cardiac muscle". By Dr. S. Girod, Anton Becker (Own work) via Wikimedia Commons.
Pg 335 Normal chest X-ray. Image from Radiology Assistant, Robin Smithuis, Otto van Delden. The Netherlands.
Pg 335 Normal chest CT's. Images from "About Cancer".
Pg 336 Aortic arch branches. Images from "In Colors Club".
Pg 336 Profile of the aortic branches into the head. Unable to locate author. Please contact us and we will credit in the next edition.
Pg 336 Aortic arch distribution. Illustration by Dr. Tricia Derges, MD.
Pg 337 Physio affects of low BP, Additional physio affects on the heart. Illustrations by Dr. Tricia Derges, MD.
Pg 337 Physio affects of high BP. Illustration by Dr. Tricia Derges, MD.
Pg 340 Cardiac function curve. By Huckfinne - Own work, Public Domain, commons.wikimedia.org
Pg 342 Conducting system of the heart. By Madhero88 (original files); Angelito7 (this SVG version); creativecommons.org/licenses via Wikimedia Commons
Pg 342 Pacemaker action potential. By Pacemaker_potential.svg: Diberri derivative work: Silvia3 (Pacemaker_potential.svg) by creativecommons.org/licenses/by-sa/3.0/) via Wikimedia Commons
Pg 343 Ventricular Cardiac Action Potential. : User:Quasar derivative work: Mnokel (talk) derivative work: Silvia3 (Action_potential2.svg) creativecommons.org/licenses/by-sa/3.0/) or GFDL via Wikimedia Commons.
Pg 343 Cardiac Action Potential. Anatomy & Physiology, Connexions Web site. Wikipedia Commons.
Pg 343 Sympathetic, Parasympathetic Effects on Heart. Illustration by Dr. Tricia Derges, MD.
Pg 344 Cardiac Pressure. Unable to locate author. Please contact us and we will credit in the next edition.
Pg 344 Cardiac Pressure-Volume Loop. Illustration by Dr. Tricia Derges, MD.
Pg 345 Cardiac Curve. By Daniel Chang MD revised original work of Destiny Qx [CC BY-SA 2.5, creativecommons.org/licenses via Wikimedia Commons
Pg 346 Cardiac Pressure-Volume examples. Illustration by Dr. Tricia Derges, MD.
Pg 347 JVP Waveforms. Illustration by Dr. Tricia Derges, MD.
Pg 348 Murmurs. By Madhero88 (Own work Reference netter image) [CC BY-SA 3.0. creativecommons.org/licenses via Wikimedia Commons.
Pg 353 Lines of Zahn. By Nephron (Own work) [CC BY-SA 3.0. creativecommons.org/licenses/by-sa/3.0) or GFDL via Wikimedia Commons
Pg 356 Fibromuscular dysplasia. See page for author [CC BY 2.0 (http://creativecommons.org/licenses/by/2.0)], via Wikimedia Commons
Pg 359 "Papilledema" by Jonathan Trobe, M.D. - University of Michigan Kellogg Eye Center - The Eyes Have It. Licensed under CC BY 3.0 via Commons.
Pg 359 Blood vessel "Onion skinning". By Nephron (Own work) [CC BY-SA 3.0 (http://creativecommons.org/licenses/by-sa/3.0) or GFDL via Wikimedia Commons.
Pg 361 Coronary Artery Disease..com staff (2014). "Medical gallery of Blausen Medical 2014". Wiki Journal of Medicine. commons.wikimedia.
Pg 361 Atherosclerosis timeline. See page for author [GFDL or CC-BY-SA-3.0 (http://creativecommons.org/licenses/by-sa/3.0/)], via Wikimedia Commons.
Pg 361 Carotid Artery Disease. By Bruce Blaus. Blausen.com staff (2014). "Medical gallery of Blausen Medical 2014". Wiki Journal of Medicine 1 via Wikimedia Commons.
Pg 361 Xanthelasma. By Klaus D. Peter, Gummersbach, Germany (Own work) [CC BY 3.0 de (http://creativecommons.org/licenses/by/3.0/de/deed.en)], via Wikimedia Commons
Pg 361 Xanthoma. Unable to locate author. Please contact us and we will credit in the next edition.
Pg 362 Aortic dissection. By en:National Institutes of Health [Public domain], via Wikimedia Commons.
Pg 362 Aortic aneurysms. By James Heilman, MD (Own work) [CC BY-SA 3.0 (http://creativecommons.org/licenses/by-sa/3.0) or GFDL (http://www.gnu.org/copyleft/fdl.html)], via Wikimedia Commons.
Pg 362 Aortic dissection types. EmergencyPedia.
Pg 362 Aortic dissection CT. By James Heilman, MD (Own work) [CC BY-SA 3.0 (http://creativecommons.org/licenses/by-sa/3.0)], via Wikimedia Commons.
Pg 364 STEMI vs NSTEMI. Multiple sources for EKG slide and ACS slide. Could not locate original artist.
Pg 367 V Lead EKG Placement. First Aid For Free.
Pg 368 Coronary blood supply. By Coronary.pdf: Patrick J. Lynch, medical illustrator derivative work [1]: Fred the Oyster (talk) adaption and further labeling: Mikael Häggström (Coronary.pdf). creativecommons.org/licenses/by-sa/3.0)], via Wikimedia Commons.
Pg 368 Coronary Sinus. By Chris Talbot (Own work) [CC BY-SA 3.0 (http://creativecommons.org/licenses/by-sa/3.0)], via Wikimedia Commons.
Pg 372 Left Ventricular Hypertrophy CXR. Professor Peter Anderson DVM PhD, University of Alabama at Birmingham, WikiDoc.
Pg 372 Siderophages, heart failure cells. Unable to locate author. Please contact us and we will credit in the next edition.
Pg 374 Pitting edema. By James Heilman, MD - Own work, CC BY-SA 3.0. Commons.wikimedia.org/w/index.php?curid=11787530.
Pg 374 Kearley B Lines. By James Heilman, MD - Own work, CC BY-SA 3.0, Commons.wikimedia.org/w/index.php?curid=11787530.
Pg 375 Dilated cardiomyopathy illustration. By Blausen.com staff (2014). "Medical gallery of Blausen Medical 2014". WikiJournal of Medicine. Creativecommons.org/licenses/by/3.0)], via Wikimedia Commons.
Pg 375 Hypertrophic cardiomyopathy: Unable to locate authors. Please contact us and we will credit in the next edition.
Pg 376 Nutmeg liver. Unable to locate author. Please contact us and we will credit in the next edition.
Pg 377 Cardiac disease comparisons illustration. N patchett at English Wikipedia. creativecommons.org/licenses/by-sa/3.0)], via Wikimedia Commons.
Pg 378 Constrictive pericarditis. Radiopaedia, case by Dr. Julian L. Wichmann.
Pg 380 Splinter hemorrhages. By Splarka (Own work) [Public domain], via Wikimedia Commons.
Pg 380 Janeway lesions. By Wikinut.
Pg 381 Pericardiocentesis. By Npatchett (Own work). creativecommons.org/licenses/by-sa/4.0)], via Wikimedia Commons.
Pg 381 Cardiac Tamponade. By Npatchett (Own work). creativecommons.org/licenses/by-sa/4.0)], via Wikimedia Commons.
Pg 382 Cardiac Myxoma. By G.steph.rocket (Own work). creativecommons.org/licenses/by-sa/3.0) via Wikimedia Commons.
Pg 394 Takayasu Arteritis. Unable to locate authors. Please contact us and we will credit in the next edition.
Pg 394 Buerger Disease. Unable to locate author. Please contact us and we will credit in the next edition.
Pg 395 Kawasaki Disease. Kawasaki_symptoms.jpg: Dong Soo Kimderivative work: Natr (talk) - Kawasaki_symptoms. commons.wikimedia.org =12776137.
Pg 395 Livedo reticularis. By Nantsupawat T et al. creativecommons.org/licenses/by-sa/3.0)], via Wikimedia Commons.
Pg 396 Henoch-schonlein-purpura. By Madhero88. creativecommons.org/licenses/by-sa/3.0)], via Wikimedia Commons.
Pg 397 Wegners Granulomatosis CXR. By Tom Buur (Own work). creativecommons.org/licenses/by-sa/4.0)], via Wikimedia Commons.
Pg 397 Tracheal stenosis. By Rn cantab (Own work). creativecommons.org/licenses/by-sa/3.0) via Wikimedia Commons.
Pg 397 C-ANCA. By Malittle at English Wikipedia (Transferred from en.wikipedia to Commons.) [Public domain], via Wikimedia Commons.
Pg 397 P-ANCA. By Malittle at English Wikipedia (Transferred from en.wikipedia to Commons.) [Public domain], via Wikimedia Commons.
Pg 398 Cellulitis. Wikimedia Commons. Photograph by Colm Anderson. Wikipedia.org.
Pg 398 Varicose Veins. By Open Stax College [CC BY 3.0 (http://creativecommons.org/licenses/by/3.0)], via Wikimedia Commons.
Pg 398 Carotid Artery Stenosis. By Blausen.com staff (2014). "Medical gallery of Blausen Medical 2014". WikiJournal of Medicine 1. Via Wikimedia Commons.

Pg 399 Peripheral Artery Disease. Photograph by Wfnicdao for public use with Wikimedia commons.
Pg 399 Reynauds. By Niklas D (Own work). creativecommons.org/licenses/by-sa/3.0)], via Wikimedia Commons.
Pg 400 Osler – Weber – Rendu. By Herbert L. Fred, MD and Hendrik A. van Dijk - Images of Memorable Cases: Cases 115 & 116, commons.wikimedia.org =11084865.
Pg 400 Angiosarcoma. Unable to locate author. Please contact us and we will credit in the next edition.
Pg 400 Cystic Hygroma. By Timothyjosephwood (Own work). creativecommons.org/licenses/by-sa/4.0)], via Wikimedia Commons.
Pg 401 Glomus Tumor. By Skoch3 (Own work). creativecommons.org/licenses/by-sa/3.0)], via Wikimedia Commons.
Pg 401 Kaposi's Sarcoma. Author unknown. Public domain: Wikimedia commons.
Pg 401 Lymphangiosarcoma. Unable to locate author. Please contact us and we will credit in the next edition.
Pg 401 Pyogenic Granuloma. By Angus Johnson - Own work, CC BY 3.0, wikipedia.org =39262356.
Pg 402 Cardiac Action Potential (drug affects) By Architha Srinivasan (Own work). creativecommons.orgvia Wikimedia Commons.
Pg 411 Lipid Pharmacology. Illustration by Dr. Tricia Derges, MD.
Pg 412 Respiratory Illustration. By UNSHAW (Own work) [CC BY-SA 4.0 via Wikimedia Commons.
Pg 412 Respiratory zone. By OpenStax College. creativecommons.org/licenses/by/3.0)], via Wikimedia Commons.
Pg 413 Aspiration of foreign object (coin). By Samir (talk) (Uploads) - Own work, CC BY 3.0, wikipedia.org. 5445137.
Pg 414 Lung Volumes. Public domain, Wikimedia.org.
Pg 416 Lung Zones. Redrawn with modification from West JB: *Ventilation/Blood flow and gas exchange,* ed 4, Oxford, 1970, Blackwell Scientific, 1970.
Pg 417 Breathing patterns. Unable to locate author. Please contact us and we will credit in the next edition.
Pg 418 Oxygen exchange illustration. Illustration by Dr. Tricia Derges, MD.
Pg 419 Oxyhemoglobin Dissociation Curve. Illustration by Dr. Tricia Derges, MD.
Pg 422 Flow – Volume Loop. Public domain by Creative Commons.
Pg 424 Ferruginous Bodies. Yale Rosen microphotography via Creative Commons.
Pg 428 Pleural Effusion. By James Heilman, MD (Own work). http://creativecommons.org via Wikimedia Commons.
Pg 428 Bronchopneumonia. Yale Rosen photography via Creative Commons.
Pg 428 Lobar Pneumonia. By James Heilman, MD - Own work, commons.wikimedia.org.
Pg 428 Emphysema. Yale Rosen photography via Creative Commons.
Pg 435 Bronchiectasis. By Laura Fregonese, Jan Stolk. creativecommons.org/licenses via Wikimedia Commons.
Pg 436 Charcot-Leyden crystal. By Patho (Own work). creativecommons.org/licenses/by-sa/3.0)], via Wikimedia Commons.
Pg 440 Pulmonary embolism. By Walter Serra, Giuseppe De Iaco, Claudio Reverberi and Tiziano Gherli. creativecommons.org/licenses/by/2.0)], via Wikimedia Commons.
Pg 442 Pneumothorax. By Hellerhoff (Own work) creativecommons.org/licenses/by-sa/3.0)], via Wikimedia Commons.
Pg 442 Tension pneumothorax. By James Heilman, MD (Own work). creativecommons.org/licenses/by-sa/3.0)], via Wikimedia Commons.
Pg 444 Invasive Aspergillosis. Unable to locate author. Please contact us and we will credit in the next edition.
Pg 447 Chest anatomy. By Mikael Häggström [Public domain], via Wikimedia Commons.
Pg 449 Keratin Pearls in Squamous Cell Carincoma. Yale Rosen photography via Creative Commons.
Pg 450 Ferruginous Bodies. Yale Rosen microphotography via Creative Commons.
Pg 457 Alimentary Canal. Illustration by OpenStax College via Wikimedia Commons.
Pg 460 Secretory cells of the GI. CC BY-SA, commons.wikimedia.org. Adapted by Dr. Tricia Derges, MD.
Pg 461 Portal System. By OpenStax College [CC BY 3.0 (http://creativecommons.org/licenses/by/3.0)], via Wikimedia Commons.
Pg 461 Celiac Trunk. By Dr. Muhammad Osama (Own work) [CC BY-SA 3.0 (http://creativecommons.org via Wikimedia Commons.
Pg 462 IVC and Portal Blood Supply. Illustration by Dr. Tricia Derges, MD.
Pg 464 Pancreas. By OpenStax College [CC BY 3.0 (http://creativecommons.org/licenses/by/3.0)], via Wikimedia Commons.
Pg 464 Pancreatic cells. Illustrations by Dr. Tricia Derges, MD.
Pg 465 Liver histology. By OpenStax College - Anatomy & Physiology, Connexions Web site. commons.wikimedia.org.
Pg 465 Hepatic zones. Illustrations by Dr. Tricia Derges, MD.
Pg 466 Gall bladder. Henry Vandyke Carter [Public domain], via Wikimedia Commons.
Pg 467 Gall Bladder and liver. By OpenStax College [CC BY 3.0 (http://creativecommons.org/licenses/by/3.0)], via Wikimedia Commons.
Pg 467 Stomach anatomy. By OpenStax College [CC BY 3.0 (http://creativecommons.org/licenses/by/3.0)], via Wikimedia Commons.
Pg 470 Salivary gland. By OpenStax College [CC BY 3.0 (http://creativecommons.org/licenses/by/3.0)], via Wikimedia Commons.
Pg 471 Sinuses. By OpenStax College [CC BY 3.0 (http://creativecommons.org/licenses/by/3.0)], via Wikimedia Commons.
Pg 472 Achalasia. By Farnoosh Farrokhi, Michael F. Vaezi. [CC BY 2.0 Creative Commons via Wikimedia Commons.
Pg 473 Esophageal stricture. Unable to locate author. Please contact us and we will credit in the next edition.
Pg 475 Retropharyngeal abscess. By James Heilman, MD (Own work) [CC BY-SA 3.0 Creative commons via Wikimedia Commons.
Pg 475 Glossitis. Schariach via Wikipedia Commons.
Pg 475 Esophageal manometry. Unable to locate author. Please contact us and we will credit in the next edition.
Pg 481 Stomach cancer. Unable to locate author. Please contact us and we will credit in the next edition.
Pg 481 Krukenberg Tumor. By Department of Pathology, Calicut Medical. Creativecommons.org via Wikimedia Commons.
Pg 481 Sister Mary Joseph Nodule and Virchow Node. Unable to locate author. Please contact us and we will credit in the next edition.
Pg 486 Dermatitis Herpetiformis. Unable to locate author. Please contact us and we will credit in the next edition.
Pg 488 Diverticulitis. By Haymanj, a retired pathologist from Melbourne, Australia. - Self-photographed, Public Domain, Commons.wikimedia.
Pg 488 Small bowel obstruction. собственная работа. Creative Commons via Wikimedia Commons.
Pg 490 Mega Colon. Unable to locate author. Please contact us and we will credit in the next edition.
Pg 495 Heterotopic Gastric Mucosa. Dr. Jean-Christophe Fournet, Paris, France.
Pg 496. Tubular Adenoma of the colon. Image by Ed Uthman, Creative Commons via Wikimedia Commons.
Pg 496 Tubular Adenoma. By The original uploader was J. Guntau at German Wikipedia [Public domain], via Wikimedia Commons.
Pg 496 Tubulovillous Polyp of the colon. Image by Ed Uthman, Creative Commons via Wikimedia Commons.
Pg 496 Blood supply to the colon: By OpenStax. creativecommons.org/licenses/by/3.0)], via Wikimedia Commons.
Pg 497 Colon cancer "Apple Peel". Unable to locate author. Please contact us and we will credit in the next edition.
Pg 497 Familial Adenomatous Polyposis (FAP). By Department of Pathology, Calicut Medical creativecommons.org via Wikimedia Commons
Pg 497 Peutz-Jeghers Syndrome. By Abdullah Sarhan (Own work) [CC BY-SA 4.0 Creativecommons.orgvia Wikimedia Commons.
Pg 498 Adenoma to Carcinoma. Illustration by Dr. Tricia Derges, MD.
Pg 499 Portal anastomosis. Unable to locate author. Please contact us and we will credit in the next edition.
Pg 502 Kayser Fleischer Rings. By Herbert L. Fred, MD, Hendrik A. van Dijk [CC BY 3.0 Creative Commons via Wikimedia Commons.
Pg 504 Nutmeg liver. Unable to locate author. Please contact us and we will credit in the next edition.
Pg 507 Cavernous Liver Hemangioma. By Nephron. Own work. CC BY-SA 3.0. Creative Commons via Wikimedia Commons.
Pg 507 Ethanol Pathway. Illustration by Dr. Tricia Derges, MD.
Pg 509 Cirrhosis of the liver and liver disease comparisons. Images from cirrhosis of the liver.org.
Pg 510 Wernicke's and Broca's area. By Peter Hagoort [CC BY 3.0 (http://creativecommons.org/licenses/by/3.0)], via Wikimedia Commons.
Pg 510 Mammillary bodies. By Yukaizou2016 ([1]) [CC BY-SA 4.0 Creative Commons via Wikimedia Commons.
Pg 511 Biliary System. By Drriad (Own work) [Public domain], via Wikimedia Commons.
Pg 512 Hepatocytes. By Boumphreyfr (Own work) [CC BY-SA 3.0 Creative Commons via Wikimedia Commons.
Pg 512 Architecture of the liver. By Zorn, A.M., Liver development (October 31, 2008), StemBook, ed. The Stem Cell Research Community, StemBook, Creative Commons via Wikimedia Commons.
Pg 512 Primary Sclerosing Cholangitis. Unable to locate author. Please contact us and we will credit in the next edition.

Pg 514 Porcelain gallbladder. Unable to locate author. Please contact us and we will credit in the next edition.

Pg 515 Gallstones. By Tomáš Vendiš (http://radiologieplzen.eu) CC BY-SA 3. Creative Commons via Wikimedia Commons.

Pg 516 Gallstones. Unable to locate author. Please contact us and we will credit in the next edition.

Pg 520 Indirect and direct hernia. Unable to locate author. Please contact us and we will credit in the next edition.

Pg 520 Sliding and Diaphragmatic Hiatal Hernia. By Mysid, adapted by Dr. Tricia Derges, MD. Creative Commons, Wikimedia Commons.

Pg 521 Umbilical hernia. By Rocco_Cusari [CC BY-SA 2.5 (http://creativecommons.org/licenses/by-sa/2.5)], via Wikimedia Commons.

Pg 521 Incisional and Femoral hernias. Unable to locate author. Please contact us and we will credit in the next edition.

Pg 527 Kidney structure. By OpenStax College [CC BY 3.0 (http://creativecommons.org/licenses/by/3.0)], via Wikimedia Commons.

Pg 527 Glomerulus. By OpenStax College [CC BY 3.0 (http://creativecommons.org/licenses/by/3.0)], via Wikimedia Commons.

Pg 527 Nephron. By Artwork by Holly Fischer. Urinary Tract Slide 20, 26, CC BY 3.0, Commons Wikimedia.

Pg 527 Renal blood supply. By OpenStax College [CC BY 3.0 (http://creativecommons.org/licenses/by/3.0)], via Wikimedia Commons.

Pg 527 Nephron. By Davidson, A.J., Mouse kidney development (January 15, 2009), StemBook, ed. The Stem Cell Research Community, creativecommons.org via Wikimedia Commons

Pg 528 Fluid Balance. Illustration by Dr. Tricia Derges, MD.

Pg 528 Osm flow. Unable to locate author. Please contact us and we will credit in the next edition.

Pg 529 Osm and fluid movement. Illustrations by Dr. Tricia Derges, MD.

Pg 530 Diffusion. Public domain, Wikimedia.

Pg 532 Collecting tubule. By OpenStax College [CC BY 3.0 (http://creativecommons.org/licenses/by/3.0)], via Wikimedia Commons

Pg 532 Aquaporin Channels. By Lennert B creativecommons.org via Wikimedia Commons, adapted by Dr. Tricia Derges, MD.

Pg 532 Nephron. By Nephron-urine.svg: M•Komorniczak, polish wikipedist. Kidney. Derivative work: Juvo415, derivative work: Mcstrother, Creative Commons.org via Wikimedia Commons.

Pg 538 Compensation response for acid base. By Huckfinne (Own work) [Public domain], via Wikimedia Commons.

Pg 541 Solute reabsorption. Adaptation by Dr. Tricia Derges, MD.

Pg 542 Renal physiology. Haisook at English Wikipedia. Creative Commons.org via Wikimedia Commons.

Pg 543 Renin-Aldosterone System. By A. Rad (me) (Own work) CC-BY-SA-3.0 . Creative Commons via Wikimedia Commons.

Pg 545 Chloride Shift. Unable to locate author. Please contact us and we will credit in the next edition.

Pg 553 Henoch-Schonlein Purpura. Henoch-schonlein-purpura. By Madhero88. Creative Commons via Wikimedia Commons.

Pg 560 Fibromuscular dysplasia. See page for author [CC BY 2.0. Creative Commons via Wikimedia Commons.

Pg 561 Polycystic Kidney Disease gross speciman. Public domain. Creative Commons via Wikimedia Commons.

Pg 561 Polycystic Kidney Disease CT. By Sb2207 (Own work by CC BY-SA 3.0 Creative Commons via Wikimedia Commons.

Pg 562 Aniridia. By The original uploader was Gardar Rurak at English Wikipedia. Creative Commons via Wikimedia Commons.

Pg 563 Calcium oxalate stones. By NASA/JSC [Public domain], via Wikimedia Commons.

Pg 564 Struvite Stones. Creative Commons Αναφορά προέλευσης-Παρόμοια διανομή 3.0 Μη εισαγόμενη.

Pg 566 Renal physiology. Haisook at English Wikipedia. Creative Commons.org via Wikimedia Commons.

Pg 571 Female anatomy. By OpenStax College [CC BY 3.0 (http://creativecommons.org/licenses/by/3.0)], via Wikimedia Commons.

Pg 574 Male anatomy. By OpenStax College [CC BY 3.0 (http://creativecommons.org/licenses/by/3.0)], via Wikimedia Commons.

Pg 574 Testicle anatomy. By OpenStax College [CC BY 3.0 (http://creativecommons.org/licenses/by/3.0)], via Wikimedia Commons.

Pg 574 Penis anatomy. By OpenStax College [CC BY 3.0 (http://creativecommons.org/licenses/by/3.0)], via Wikimedia Commons.

Pg 577 Female and Male lymph system. Unable to locate author. Please contact us and we will credit in the next edition.

Pg 579 Follicular phase. By Procedureready (Own work) [CC BY 3.0. Creative Commons via Wikimedia Commons.

Pg 580 Menstrual cycle. By Lyrl [GFDL CC-BY-SA-3.0. Creative Commons via Wikimedia Commons.

Pg 582 Oogenesis. By OpenStax College [CC BY 3.0 (http://creativecommons.org/licenses/by/3.0)], via Wikimedia Commons.

Pg 582 Spermatogenesis. By OpenStax College [CC BY 3.0 (http://creativecommons.org/licenses/by/3.0)], via Wikimedia Commons.

Pg 582 Sperm anatomy. By Mariana Ruiz Villarreal spermatozoa [Public domain], via Wikimedia Commons.

Pg 583 Male feedback. Illustrations by Dr. Tricia Derges, MD.

Pg 585 Egg fertilization. By OpenStax College [CC BY 3.0 (http://creativecommons.org/licenses/by/3.0)], via Wikimedia Commons.

Pg 594 Molar pregnancy. By Mikael Häggström. (2014) used with permission. (Own work) [CC0], via Wikimedia Commons.

Pg 595 IURG. Mt Sinai Hospital, Fetal medicine.

Pg 597 Caudal regression. By Stanislav Kozlovskiy (Own work (Own photo)) Creative Commons via Wikimedia Commons.

Pg 599 Positive Ferning Test. By Paul_012 Creative Commons via Wikimedia Commons.

Pg 599 Rh Factor. Unable to locate author. Please contact us and we will credit in the next edition.

Pg 599 Cervical cerclage. By BruceBlaus (Own work) CC BY-SA 4.0. Creative Commons via Wikimedia Commons.

Pg 601 Placenta previa. By OpenStax College [CC BY 3.0 (http://creativecommons.org/licenses/by/3.0)], via Wikimedia Commons.

Pg 601 Abrupto placenta. Blausen.com staff (2014). "Medical gallery of Blausen Medical 2014". WikiJournal of Medicine 1, creativecommons via Wikimedia Commons.

Pg 602 Placenta percreta. The New Messiah at English Wikipedia [Public domain], via Wikimedia Commons.

Pg 609 Fetal monitoring.

Pg 610 Fetal stations. Abnormal birth presentations. Unable to locate authors. Please contact us and we will credit in the next edition.

Pg 610 Breech presentations. Unable to locate author. Please contact us and we will credit in the next edition.

Pg 611 Cesarean delivery. Unable to locate author. Please contact us and we will credit in the next edition.

Pg 612 McRoberts maneuver. (Modified from Gabbe, S., Niebyl, J., & Simpson, J. [2002]. Obstetrics: Normal and problem pregnancies [4th ed.]. New York: Churchill Livingstone.

Pg 615 Fitz Hugh-Curtis Syndrome. By Hic et nunc (Own work) [Public domain], via Wikimedia Commons.

Pg 615 Gonorrhea mucopurulent discharge. Unable to locate author. Please contact us and we will credit in the next edition.

Pg 616 Lichen Sclerosus. By Mikael Häggström (Own work) [CC0], via Wikimedia Commons.

Pg 620 Condylomata acuminate. Unable to locate author. Please contact us and we will credit in the next edition.

Pg 622 Paget's disease of the vulva. Unable to locate author. Please contact us and we will credit in the next edition.

Pg 622 Leiomyoma. By Hic et nunc, CC BY-SA 3.0 (http://creativecommons.org/licenses/by-sa/3.0)], via Wikimedia Commons.

Pg 623 Dermoid (Teratoma) Cyst. By The Armed Forces Institute of Pathology (AFIP) [Public domain], via Wikimedia Commons.

Pg 624 Krukenberg Tumor. By Department of Pathology, Calicut Medical. Creativecommons.org via Wikimedia Commons.

Pg 625 Sarcoma Botryoides. Unable to locate author. Please contact us and we will credit in the next edition.

Pg 626 Luteoma of Pregnancy. By Ed Uthman from Houston, TX, USA [CC BY 2.0 creativecommons.org via Wikimedia Commons.

Pg 627 Ductal and Lobular Carcinoma: In situ and Invasive. By Cancer Research UK (Original email from CRUK) creativecommons.org via Wikimedia Commons

Pg 627 Breast anatomy illustration. Patrick J. Lynch. Use via Creative Commons via Wikimedia Commons.

Pg 627 Ductal Carcinoma: In situ and Invasive. By Don Bliss (artist) [Public domain], via Wikimedia Commons.

Pg 630 Gynecomastia. By JMZ1122 Dr. Mordcai Blau (Own work) Creativecommons.org via Wikimedia Commons.

Pg 631 Intraductal Papilloma. ADAM Medical Encyclopedia.

Pg 631 Comedocarcinoma. By Difu Wu (Own work) Creativecommons.org via Wikimedia Commons.

Pg 632 Paget's Disease of the Breast. Radiopaedia.org.

Pg 632 Cribriform Breast Cancer. By Difu Wu (Own work) Creativecommons.org via Wikimedia Commons.

Pg 632 Lobular Carcinoma: Invasive. By Cancer Research UK (Original email from CRUK) creativecommons.org via Wikimedia Commons.

Pg 632 Ductal Carcinoma: Invasive. By Don Bliss (artist) [Public domain], via Wikimedia Commons.

Pg 633 Peau d'orange. Unable to locate author. Please contact us and we will credit in the next edition.

Pg 635 Benign Prostatic Hyperplasia. By ناطق1 (Own work) [CC BY-SA 3.0 creativecommons.org via Wikimedia Commons.

Pg 636 Varicocele. Unable to locate author. Please contact us and we will credit in the next edition.
Pg 636 Hydrocele. Transillumination. Unable to locate author. Please contact us and we will credit in the next edition.
Pg 637 Hypospadias. CCO 1.0 Universal Public Domain Dedication under Creative Commons.
Pg 637 Testicular torsion. Unable to locate author. Please contact us and we will credit in the next edition.
Pg 639 Indirect and Direct inguinal hernia. Unable to locate author. Please contact us and we will credit in the next edition.
Pg 639 Direct inguinal hernia. Photograph by Dr. Tricia Derges, MD.
Pg 640 Anal cancer. Unable to locate author. Please contact us and we will credit in the next edition.
Pg 640 Penile Squamous Cell Carcinoma. Unable to locate author. Please contact us and we will credit in the next edition.
Pg 651 Adrenal gland. By OpenStax College [CC BY 3.0 (http://creativecommons.org/licenses/by/3.0)], via Wikimedia Commons.
Pg 651 Adrenal gland histology. By Jpogi [CC0], via Wikimedia Commons.
Pg 656 Cortisol negative feedback. Illustration by Dr. Tricia Derges, MD.
Pg 657 Metabolic Syndrome. Photograph by Dr. Tricia Derges, MD.
Pg 657 Cushing's Syndrome. By Mikael Häggström (Own work) [CC0], via Wikimedia Commons.
Pg 660 Adrenal gland layers. By Copyright © 2014 Matthew Colo, CC BY-SA 3.0, commons.wikimedia.org.
Pg 663 McCune Albright Syndrome. Creativecommons.org/licenses/by/2.0)], via Wikimedia Commons.
Pg 664 Waterhouse-Friderichsen Syndrome. Unable to locate author. Please contact us and we will credit in the next edition.
Pg 667 Pituitary. By OpenStax College [CC BY 3.0 (http://creativecommons.org/licenses/by/3.0)], via Wikimedia Commons.
Pg 669 Pituitary adenoma. Unable to locate author. Please contact us and we will credit in the next edition.
Pg 670 Gigantism. By Wouter W. de Herder [CC BY 2.0 (http://creativecommons.org/licenses/by/2.0)], via Wikimedia Commons.
Pg 670 Dwarfism. Mathew Brady [Public domain], via Wikimedia Commons.
Pg 670 Acromegaly sequence. Unable to locate author. Please contact us and we will credit in the next edition.
Pg 671 Pancreas cell. Illustration by Tricia Derges, MD.
Pg 673 Insulin Release. By Attribution details, CC BY-SA 3.0, https://en.wikipedia.org.
Pg 673 Insulin Receptor. By Attribution details, CC BY-SA 3.0, https://en.wikipedia.org.
Pg 680 Parathyroid Glands. By OpenStax College [CC BY 3.0 (http://creativecommons.org/licenses/by/3.0)], via Wikimedia Commons.
Pg 681 Parathyroid Action. . Unable to locate author. Please contact us and we will credit in the next edition.
Pg 682 Metabolism of Vitamin D. Michael Holick: Journal Clinical Investigation 2006.
Pg 682 Rachitic Rosary in Rickets. Unable to locate author. Please contact us and we will credit in the next edition.
Pg 683 Pseudohypoparathyroidism. Unable to locate author. Please contact us and we will credit in the next edition.
Pg 684 PTH and Calcium pathologies. Illustration by Dr. Tricia Derges, MD.
Pg 685 Thyroid Hormone Synthesis. Illustration by Dr. Tricia Derges, MD.
Pg 687 Goiter. By Drahreg01 (Own work) creativecommons.org via Wikimedia Commons.
Pg 687 Pretibial Myxedema. By Herbert L. Fred, MD and Hendrik A. van Dijk. Creativecommons.org via Wikimedia Commons.
Pg 687 Exophthalmos. Unable to locate author. Please contact us and we will credit in the next edition.
Pg 690 Congenital Hypothyroidism. Unable to locate author. Please contact us and we will credit in the next edition.
Pg 694 MEN differential chart. Illustration by Dr. Tricia Derges, MD.
Pg 699 Neuro Crest Queen. Illustration by Dr. Tricia Derges, MD.
Pg 700 Tongue Development. Illustration by Dr. Tricia Derges, MD.
Pg 702 Brain Summary. Illustration by Dr. Tricia Derges, MD.
Pg 703 Brain Sagittal Plane. Unable to locate author. Please contact us and we will credit in the next edition.
Pg 703 Brain Coronal Plane. Unable to locate author. Please contact us and we will credit in the next edition.
Pg 703 Cranial nerves. By Brain_human_normal_inferior_view.svg: Patrick J. Lynch, medical illustrator derivative work: Creativecommons.org via Wikimedia Commons
Pg 704 Cranial Nerves. Encyclopedia Britannica.
Pg 704 Cranial Nerves Chart. Dr. Tricia Derges, MD.
Pg 707 Neuron cell. By LadyofHats [Public domain], via Wikimedia Commons.
Pg 707 Nodes of Ranvier. By OpenStax [CC BY 4.0 (http://creativecommons.org/licenses/by/4.0)], via Wikimedia Commons.
Pg 708 Skin anatomy. By Madhero88 and M.Komorniczak. Creativecommons.org via Wikimedia Commons.
Pg 709 Dermatones. By Grant, John Charles Boileau (An atlas of anatomy, / by regions 1962) [Public domain], via Wikimedia Commons.
Pg 709 Vertebra anatomy. By OpenStax College [CC BY 3.0 (http://creativecommons.org/licenses/by/3.0)], via Wikimedia Commons.
Pg 710 Dopamine pathways. Illustration by Dr. Tricia Derges, MD.
Pg 711 Cerebral Cortex (Broca's and Wernicke's area). By BruceBlaus. "Medical gallery of Blausen Medical 2014". WikiJournal of Medicine 1. (Own work). Creativecommons.org via Wikimedia Commons.
Pg 713 Thalamus. By Madhero88 [CC BY-SA 3.0 (http://creativecommons.org/licenses/by-sa/3.0)], via Wikimedia Commons.
Pg 714 Brain gyrus. By John A Beal, PhD. Dep't. of Cellular Biology & Anatomy, Louisiana State University Health Sciences Center Shreveport. Creativecommons.org via Wikimedia Commons.
Pg 714 Brain sulcus. By Allan Ajifo. creativecommons.org/licenses/by/2.0)], via Wikimedia Commons.
Pg 714 Brain sinus. By OpenStax - [CC BY 4.0 (http://creativecommons.org/licenses/by/4.0)], via Wikimedia Commons.
Pg 715 Brain ventricles. By OpenStax [CC BY 4.0 (http://creativecommons.org/licenses/by/4.0)], via Wikimedia Commons.
Pg 716 Normal Pressure Hydrocephalus. By Nevit Dilmen (Own work). Creativecommons.orgvia Wikimedia Commons.
Pg 718 Caudate Nucleus. By OpenStax [CC BY 4.0 (http://creativecommons.org/licenses/by/4.0)], via Wikimedia Commons.
Pg 718 Substantia Nigra. Blausen.com staff (2014). "Medical gallery of Blausen Medical 2014". WikiJournal of Medicine 1 (Own work) [CC BY 30. Creative Commons via Wikimedia Commons.
Pg 720 Vertebrae. By OpenStax College [CC BY 3.0 (http://creativecommons.org/licenses/by/3.0)], via Wikimedia Commons.
Pg 729 Strokes. Illustration by Dr. Tricia Derges, MD.
Pg 730 Epidural hematoma. By Hellerhoff (Own work) CC BY-SA 3.0. Creativecommons.org via Wikimedia Commons.
Pg 730 Subdural hematoma. By James Heilman, MD (Own work). CC BY-SA 3.0. creativecommons.org via Wikimedia Commons.
Pg 730 Subarachnoid hemorage. By James Heilman, MD (Own work). CC BY-SA 3.0. creativecommons.org via Wikimedia Commons.
Pg 730 Cerebral Contusion. By Lucien Monfils (Own work) CC BY-SA 3.0. Creativecommons.org via Wikimedia Commons.
Pg 732 Spinal Nerves. By Mysid (original by Tristanb) CC-BY-SA-3. Creativecommons.org via Wikimedia Commons.
Pg 734 Spinal Tracts. Illustration by Dr. Tricia Derges, MD.
Pg 734 Location of spinal tracts. By Polarlys and Mikael Häggström. CC BY-SA 3.0. creativecommons.org via Wikimedia Commons.
Pg 735 Doral Column and Spinothalamic Tracts. By OpenStax College. Creativecommons.org via Wikimedia Commons.
Pg 735 Corticospinal Tract. By OpenStax College [CC BY 3.0 (http://creativecommons.org/licenses/by/3.0)], via Wikimedia Commons.
Pg 736 Golgi and Spindle Organ Feedback. Unable to locate author. Please contact us and we will credit in the next edition.
Pg 737 Homunculus. Unable to locate author. Please contact us and we will credit in the next edition.
Pg 737 Levels of spinal cord. Adapted by Dr. Tricia Derges, MD.
Pg 738 Bells Palsy. Center for Disease Control and Prevention. Creativecommons.org via Wikimedia Commons. Adapted by Dr. Tricia Derges. MD.
Pg 738 Central nerve lesion. Unable to locate author. Please contact us and we will credit in the next edition.
Pg 739 Metastasis to the brain. By Jmarchn (Own work). CC BY-SA 3.0. Creativecommons.org via Wikimedia Commons.
Pg 739 Metastasis to the brain. By Hellerhoff (Own work). CC BY-SA 3.0. Creativecommons.org via Wikimedia Commons.
Pg 740 Meningioma and Schwannoma. Unable to locate author. Please contact us and we will credit in the next edition.
Pg 740 Glioblastoma. By Christaras A (Created myself from anonymized patient MR) Creativecommons.orgvia Wikimedia Commons.
Pg 741 Pituitary Adenoma. By Hellerhoff - Own work, CC BY-SA 3.0, Commons.wikimedia.org/w/index.php?curid=10860698.
Pg 742 Medulloblastoma. By Hellerhoff (Own work) [CC BY-SA 3.0, Commons.wikimedia.org via Wikimedia Commons.

Pg 742 Ependymoma. By The Armed Forces Institute of Pathology [Public domain], via Wikimedia Commons.
Pg 742 Craniopharyngioma. By Hellerhoff (Own work) CC BY 3.0, Creativecommons.org via Wikimedia Commons.
Pg 743 Multiple Sclerosis MRI. Unable to locate author. Please contact us and we will credit in the next edition.
Pg 744 MS Nerve cell. Creative Commons via Wikimedia Commons. Adapted by Dr. Tricia Derges, MD.
Pg 744 Charcot-Marie-Tooth Disease. Unable to locate author. Please contact us and we will credit in the next edition.
Pg 750 "Lisch nodules" by National Eye Institute - National Eye Institute. Licensed under Public Domain via Commons.
Pg 750 Bilateral Schwannomas. Radipedia/WikiMedia. Hanleym.
Pg 751 Sturge-Weber Syndrome CT. Radiop.paedia.org.
Pg 751 Sturge-Weber Trigeminal Regions. Unable to locate author. Please contact us and we will credit in the next edition.
Pg 751 Tuberous sclerosis angiofibromas. By Herbert L. Fred, MD and Hendrik A. van Dijk. Creativecommons.org via Wikimedia Commons.
Pg 751 Koenen's tumors and Coloboma of the Iris. Unable to locate author. Please contact us and we will credit in the next edition.
Pg 756 Eye anatomy. By Rhcastilhos. Public Domain. Commons.wikimedia.org via Wikimedia Commons.
Pg 756 Blood supply of the eye. Dr. Amer A. Shamsulddin.
Pg 757 Pupillary controls. By Open Stax College [CC BY 3.0 (http://creativecommons.org/licenses/by/3.0)], via Wikimedia Commons.
Pg 757 Pupillary sympathetic and parasympathetic control. Unable to locate author. Please contact us and we will credit in the next edition.
Pg 758 Myopia and Hyperopia. By National Eye Institute [Public domain], via Wikimedia Commons.
Pg 758 Cranial nerves and the eye. Unable to locate author. Please contact us and we will credit in the next edition.
Pg 759 MLF Syndrome. Author: Suraj Rajan. ml.wikipedia.org. Creative Commons via Wikimedia Commons.
Pg 760 Pg. 760 – 767. Images used are found in various places throughout the internet and are believed to be within public domain. We have searched to identify and credit all images. Images used are believed to be within our rights as stated within the US Copyright Fair use Act (title 17, US Code). If you are the owner of any of these images and feel that it infringes your copyright please let us know, and we will credit your work or remove the image on the next edition of this book.
Pg 762 Macular degeneration example. Photograph by Dr. Tricia Derges, MD.
Pg 768 Eye Tract Lesions. Illustration by Dr. Tricia Derges, MD.
Pg 770 Anatomy of the ear. Blausen.com staff (2014). "Medical gallery of Blausen Medical 2014". WikiJournal of Medicine 1. creativecommons.org via Wikimedia Commons.
Pg 770 Sound waves. By OpenStax [CC BY 4.0 (http://creativecommons.org/licenses/by/4.0)], via Wikimedia Commons.
Pg 772 Bilateral Schwannomas. Radipedia/WikiMedia. Hanleym.
Pg 774 Anatomy of the larynx. Public domain in Creative Commons via Wikimedia Commons.
Pg 774 Vocal cords and polyp. Unable to locate author. Please contact us and we will credit in the next edition.
Pg 784 Structure of Hemoglobin. Encyclopaedia Britannica.
Pg 784 Adult and fetal hemoglobin. Wikipendia, Wikibooks.
Pg 785 Hematopoiesis in humans. By A. Rad (Own work). CC-BY-SA-3.0. Creativecommons.org via Wikimedia Commons.
Pg 786 Anemia: sizes and color chart. McGill physiology, McGill University.
Pg 786 Pg. 786-788. Images used are found in various places throughout the internet and are believed to be within public domain. We have searched to identify and credit all images. Images used are believed to be within our rights as stated within the US Copyright Fair use Act (title 17, US Code). If you are the owner of any of these images and feel that it infringes your copyright please let us know, and we will credit your work or remove the image on the next edition of this book.
Pg 791 Lead lines: Unable to locate author. Please contact us and we will credit in the next edition.
Pg 792 MCV levels. David Wickes, D.C. Sizing Up Anemias.
Pg 794 Iron deficiency anemia signs: nails and tongue. Unable to locate author. Please contact us and we will credit in the next edition.
Pg 794 B-thalassemia chipmunk face and crew cut skull. Public domain.
Pg 799 Dactylitis. Wikispaces. Public domain.
Pg 799 Sickle Cell Anemia. By Diana grib (Own work). Creativecommons.org via Wikimedia Commons.
Pg 804 Diamond-Blackfan Anemia. Unable to locate author. Please contact us and we will credit in the next edition.
Pg 804 Fanconi Anemia. Imgarcade.
Pg 806 Clotting pathway. By Dr Graham Beards (Own work). Creativecommons.org via Wikimedia Commons.
Pg 810 Vitamin K Pathway. Illustration by Dr. Tricia Derges, MD.
Pg 815 Platelet plug formation. Illustration by Dr. Tricia Derges, MD.
Pg 817 HIT. Unable to locate author. Please contact us and we will credit in the next edition.
Pg 824 Pg. 824 – 831. Images used are found in various places throughout the internet and are believed to be within public domain. We have searched to identify and credit all images. Images used are believed to be within our rights as stated within the US Copyright Fair use Act (title 17, US Code). If you are the owner of any of these images and feel that it infringes your copyright please let us know, and we will credit your work or remove the image on the next edition of this book.
Pg 828 Burkitt's Lymphoma. Public domain, Wikipedia.
Pg 832 Polycythemia Vera. By by Herbert L. Fred, MD and Hendrik A. van Dijk. CC BY 2.0 Creativecommons.orgvia Wikimedia Commons.
Pg 843 Cancer drugs. Cancer drug illustration by Dr. Tricia Derges, MD. Cell cycle illustration by By Brat Ural (Own work. Creativecommons.org via Wikimedia Commons.
Pg 844 dUMP to dTMP. Illustration by Dr. Tricia Derges, MD.
Pg 850 Paranasal sinuses. By OpenStax College [CC BY 3.0 (http://creativecommons.org/licenses/by/3.0)], via Wikimedia Commons.
Pg 851 Tongue development. Illustration by Dr. Tricia Derges, MD.
Pg 851 Facial Nerve. Public domain.
Pg 852 Arteries supplying the head and neck by von Phil Schatz Lizenz. CC by 4.0.
Pg 853 Bones of the upper extremities. Wikipedia, author: Lady of Hats Mariana Ruiz Villarreal.
Pg 853 Muscles of the upper extremities. By CFCF (Own work) CC BY-SA 4.0, Creativecommons.org via Wikimedia Commons.
Pg 854 Dermatones of the arms. Henry Vandyke Carter [Public domain], via Wikimedia Commons.
Pg 854 Muscles of the upper back, shoulder. By OpenStax, CC BY 4.0 Creativecommons.org via Wikimedia Commons.
Pg 854 Muscles of the neck. By OpenStax [CC BY 4.0 (http://creativecommons.org/licenses/by/4.0)], via Wikimedia Commons.
Pg 854 Blood supply of the arms. By OpenStax College [CC BY 3.0 (http://creativecommons.org/licenses/by/3.0)], via Wikimedia Commons
Pg 854 Nerves of the arm. Slideshare.
Pg 855 Brachial plexus. By Patrick John Duggan (Own original computer diagram.) [Public domain], via Wikimedia Commons.
Pg 855 Erb Palsy. Unable to locate author. Please contact us and we will credit in the next edition.
Pg 856 Klumpkey's Palsy. Unable to locate author. Please contact us and we will credit in the next edition.
Pg 857 Annular ligament and median nerve damage. Unable to locate author. Please contact us and we will credit in the next edition.
Pg 858 Ulnar injury and biceps rupture. Unable to locate author. Please contact us and we will credit in the next edition.
Pg 859 Tennis elbow. By BruceBlaus (Own work) [CC BY-SA 4.0. Creativecommons.org via Wikimedia Commons.
Pg 859 Golfers elbow. By www.scientificanimations.com [CC BY-SA 4.0, creativecommons.org via Wikimedia Commons.
Pg 859 Olecranon bursitis and Cubital fossa. Unable to locate author. Please contact us and we will credit in the next edition.
Pg 860 Muscle of the hand. By OpenStax [CC BY 4.0 (http://creativecommons.org/licenses/by/4.0)], via Wikimedia Commons.
Pg 860 Nerve supply of the hand. Unable to locate author. Please contact us and we will credit in the next edition.
Pg 860 Blood supply of the hand. By Rhcastilhos (Gray1237.png) [Public domain], via Wikimedia Commons.
Pg 860 Joints of the hand. By Original by LadyofHats. Translated by Rodrigo.dst. (Derivative of Image:Scheme human hand bones-en.svg) [Public domain], via Wikimedia Commons
Pg 861 Wrist bones. By OpenStax College [CC BY 3.0 (http://creativecommons.org/licenses/by/3.0)], via Wikimedia Commons.
Pg 862 Rotator cuff muscles. Imgarcade.
Pg 862 Shoulder anatomy. Paul B. Roache, MD.
Pg 863 Muscles of the leg. By OpenStax [CC BY 4.0 (http://creativecommons.org/licenses/by/4.0)], via Wikimedia Commons.
Pg 863 Nerves of the leg. Unable to locate author. Please contact us and we will credit in the next edition.
Pg 863 Veins of the leg. Blausen.com staff (2014). "Medical gallery of Blausen Medical 2014". WikiJournal of Medicine 1 (2). (Own work) [CC BY 3.0. Creativecommons.org via Wikimedia Commons.
Pg 863 Arteries of the leg. By OpenStax College [CC BY 3.0 (http://creativecommons.org/licenses/by/3.0)], via Wikimedia Commons.

Pg 863 Knee blood supply. Henry Vandyke Carter [Public domain], via Wikimedia Commons.
Pg 865 Ankle ligaments. Creative commons via Wikimedia Commons.
Pg 869 Knee x-ray. © Nevit Dilmen [CC BY-SA 3.0. creativecommons.org/licenses/by-sa/3.0) via Wikimedia Commons.
Pg 869 Posterior knee x-ray. Radiopaedia.
Pg 870 Hip injections. Unable to locate author. Please contact us and we will credit in the next edition.
Pg 871 Chest anatomy. By Mikael Häggström (All used images are in public domain.) [Public domain], via Wikimedia Commons.
Pg 871 Heart location. Blausen.com staff (2014). "Medical gallery of Blausen Medical 2014". WikiJournal of Medicine 1 (2). (Own work) [CC BY 3.0. Creativecommons.org via Wikimedia Commons.
Pg 871 Thoracic blood supply. By OpenStax College [CC BY 3.0 (http://creativecommons.org/licenses/by/3.0)], via Wikimedia Commons.
Pg 871 Kidney location. By OpenStax College [CC BY 3.0 (http://creativecommons.org/licenses/by/3.0)], via Wikimedia Commons.
Pg 873 Thoracic wall. Slideshare.
Pg 873 Abdominal wall. Unable to locate author. Please contact us and we will credit in the next edition.
Pg 874 Skull layers. Author: Mysid, original by SEER development team. Creative commons via Wikimedia Commons.
Pg 876 Portal Anastomosis. Unable to locate author. Please contact us and we will credit in the next edition.
Pg 877 Knee Anastomosis. Henry Vandyke Carter [Public domain], via Wikimedia Commons.
Pg 877 Shoulder Anastomosis. Unable to locate author. Please contact us and we will credit in the next edition.
Pg 879 Anterior, Posterior Triangles of Neck. By Olek Remesz (wiki-pl: Orem, commons: Orem) Modified by user:madhero88 – original image File:Musculi coli base.svg, CC BY 3.0, commons.wikimedia.org.
Pg 879 Carotid Triangle. By Olek Remesz (wiki-pl: Orem, commons: Orem) Modified by user:madhero88 – original image File:Musculi coli base.svg, CC BY 3.0, commons.wikimedia.org.
Pg 879 Carotid Sheath. Unable to locate author. Please contact us and we will credit in the next edition.
Pg 880 Hesselbach's Triangle. Unable to locate author. Please contact us and we will credit in the next edition.
Pg 880 Femoral Triangle. Slideshare.
Pg 880 Babinski reflex. Creative commons via Wikimedia commons.
Pg 882 Skeletal muscle contraction. Unable to locate author. Please contact us and we will credit in the next edition.
Pg 882 Skeletal muscle. By Open Stax [CC BY 4.0 (http://creativecommons.org/licenses/by/4.0)], via Wikimedia Commons.
Pg 882 Electron microscope: skeletal muscle. Unable to locate author. Please contact us and we will credit in the next edition.
Pg 884 Smooth muscle relaxation and contraction. Illustration by Dr. Tricia Derges, MD.
Pg 886 Bone anatomy. By SEER - U.S. National Cancer Institute's Surveillance, Epidemiology and End Results (SEER) Program. Public Domain. commons.wikimedia.org
Pg 886 Anatomy of long bone. By Open Stax College [CC BY 3.0 (http://creativecommons.org/licenses/by/3.0)], via Wikimedia Commons.
Pg 886 Spongy bone. By Open Stax College [CC BY 3.0 (http://creativecommons.org/licenses/by/3.0)], via Wikimedia Commons.
Pg 887 Osteoporosis. By Aisha Huseynova (Own work) [CC BY-SA 4.0. creative commons via Wikimedia Commons.
Pg 888 Pagets dz of the bone. By dr Laughlin Dawes (radpod.org) CC BY 3.0 creativecommons.org via Wikimedia Commons.
Pg 888 Adult achondroplasia. By User:Sonia Sevilla (Own work) [CC0 or Public domain], via Wikimedia Commons.
Pg 888 Achondroplasia x-ray. 1994, George Tiller.
Pg 888 Achondroplasia twins. Unable to locate author. Please contact us and we will credit in the next edition.
Pg 889 Pectus carinatum. By Tolson411 (Own work) [CC BY-SA 3.0. creativecommons.org via Wikimedia Commons.
Pg 889 Rickets and osteopetrosis. Unable to locate author. Please contact us and we will credit in the next edition.
Pg 890 Charcot-Marie-Tooth Disease. Unable to locate author. Please contact us and we will credit in the next edition.
Pg 892 Osteoarthritis. By James Heilman, MD (Own work) [CC BY-SA 3.0.creativecommons.org via Wikimedia Commons.
Pg 893 Rheumatoid Arthritis. By James Heilman, MD (Own work) [CC BY-SA 3.0.creativecommons.org via Wikimedia Commons.
Pg 893 Arthritis comparisons. Arthritis foundation.
Pg 894 Pg 894 – 897. Images used are found in various places throughout the internet and are believed to be within public domain. We have searched to identify and credit all images. Images used are believed to be within our rights as stated within the US Copyright Fair use Act (title 17, US Code). If you are the owner of any of these images and feel that it infringes your copyright please let us know, and we will credit your work or remove the image on the next edition of this book.
Pg 902 Osteochondroma. Radiopaedia.
Pg 902 Liposarcoma. Unklekrappy - Personal digital camera, CC0, Wikimedia Commons.
Pg 903 Lipoma. Photography by Dr. Tricia Derges, MD.
Pg 904 Gottron's papules. By Elizabeth M. Dugan, Adam M. Huber, Frederick W. Miller, Lisa G. Rider [CC BY-SA 3.0 creativecommons.org via Wikimedia Commons.
Pg 905 Muscle fiber. Public domain. Creative Commons via Wikimedia Commons.
Pg 915 Pg. 915 – 947. Images used are found in various places throughout the internet and are believed to be within public domain. We have searched to identify and credit all images. Images used are believed to be within our rights as stated within the US Copyright Fair use Act (title 17, US Code). If you are the owner of any of these images and feel that it infringes your copyright please let us know, and we will credit your work or remove the image on the next edition of this book.
Pg 1005 Reliability vs validity. © Nevit Dilmen [CC BY-SA 3.0. creativecommons.org via Wikimedia Commons.
Pg 1009 1009 – 1014. Biostatistics Charts and Drawings. Illustrations by Dr. Tricia Derges, MD.
Pg 1027 Pg 1027 - 1028: Vaccination schedules. Public domain. Health Dept.
Pg 1037 Boards Ready Study Clock©. Illustration by Dr. Tricia Derges, MD.

NOTES

NOTES

NOTES

NOTES

NOTES

NOTES

NOTES

NOTES